Section Editors	Section
Douglas H. Slatter	*Development of Veterinary Surgery*
Alan J. Lipowitz	*Surgical Biology*
Andreas Von Recum	*Surgical Methods*
Michael M. Pavletic	*Skin and Adnexa*
Melvin Helphrey	*Body Cavities*
Eberhard Rosin / Colin E. Harvey	*Alimentary System*
C. R. Bellenger	*Hernias*
A. Wendell Nelson	*Respiratory System*
George Eyster	*Cardiovascular System*
Anthony Schwartz	*Hemolymphatic System*
Stephen T. Simpson	*Nervous System*
Douglas H. Slatter	*Eye and Adnexa*
Dudley E. Johnston	*Male Reproductive System*
Dudley E. Johnston	*Female Reproductive System*
Bruce A. Christie	*Urinary System*
Anthony Schwartz	*Endocrine System*
Colin E. Harvey	*The Ear*
Stephen P. Arnoczky	*Musculoskeletal System*
Dennis D. Caywood	*Oncology*
Donald C. Sawyer	*Anesthetic Considerations*

TEXTBOOK OF
SMALL
ANIMAL SURGERY

Volume I

Edited by

Douglas H. Slatter,
B.V.Sc., M.S., Ph.D., F.R.C.V.S.

Diplomate, American College of Veterinary Surgeons
Diplomate, American College of Veterinary Ophthalmologists

Animal Eye and Surgical Associates
San Diego, California

1985
W.B. SAUNDERS COMPANY
Philadelphia   London   Toronto   Mexico City   Rio de Janeiro   Sydney   Tokyo

W. B. Saunders Company: West Washington Square
Philadelphia, PA   19105

1 St. Anne's Road
Eastbourne, East Sussex BN21 3UN, England

1 Goldthorne Avenue
Toronto, Ontario M8Z 5T9, Canada

Apartado 26370—Cedro 512
Mexico 4, D.F., Mexico

Rua Coronel Cabrita, 8
Sao Cristovao Caixa Postal 21176
Rio de Janeiro, Brazil

9 Waltham Street
Artarmon, N.S.W. 2064, Australia

Ichibancho, Central Bldg., 22-1 Ichibancho
Chiyoda-Ku, Tokyo 102, Japan

Library of Congress Cataloging in Publication Data

Main entry under title:

Textbook of small animal surgery.

1. Veterinary surgery—Collected works.   I. Slatter, Douglas H.
II. Title: Small animal surgery.   [DNLM: 1. Surgery, Operative—Veterinary. SF 911 T355]

SF911.T49   1985   636.089'7   83–14294

ISBN 0–7216–8348–7

Complete Set   ISBN   0–7216–8348–7
Volume I   ISBN   0–7216–8349–5
Volume II   ISBN   0–7216–8350–9

Textbook of Small Animal Surgery

Last digit is the print number: 9   8   7   6   5   4   3   2   1

To Our Patients

Contributors

Shehu U. Abdullahi, D.V.M., Ph.D.
Lecturer, Department of Surgery and Medicine, Faculty of Veterinary Medicine, and Director, Small Animal Medicine Section, Veterinary Teaching Hospital, Amadu Bello University, Zaria, Nigeria.

J. W. Alexander, D.V.M., M.S.
Diplomate, American College of Veterinary Surgeons. Professor and Chairman, Division of Agricultural and Urban Practice, and Director, Veterinary Medical Teaching Hospital, Virginia–Maryland Regional College of Veterinary Medicine, Blacksburg, Virginia.

Lorel K. Anderson, D.V.M.
Assistant Professor, Department of Small Animal Clinical Sciences, College of Veterinary Medicine, and Staff Veterinarian, Veterinary Clinical Center, Michigan State University, East Lansing, Michigan.

Steven Paul Arnoczky, D.V.M.
Diplomate, American College of Veterinary Surgeons. Associate Professor of Surgery, Cornell University Medical College; Associate Research Scientist, Division of Research, Director, Division of Laboratory Animal Care, and Director, Laboratory of Comparative Orthopaedics, The Hospital for Special Surgery, New York, New York.

Michael Aronsohn, V.M.D.
Clinical Assistant Professor of Surgery, School of Veterinary Medicine, Tufts University; Staff Surgeon, Angell Memorial Animal Hospital, Boston, Massachusetts.

John D. Bacher, D.V.M., M.S.
Chief, Surgery Unit, National Institutes of Health, Bethesda, Maryland.

J. E. Bartels, B.S., D.V.M., M.S.
Diplomate, American College of Veterinary Radiology. Professor of Radiology and Head, Department of Radiology, College of Veterinary Medicine, Auburn University, Auburn, Alabama.

Christopher R. Bellenger, B.V.Sc., Ph.D.
Associate Professor of Veterinary Surgery, Faculty of Veterinary Science, University of Sydney, New South Wales, Australia.

R. John Berg, D.V.M.
Resident in Surgery, Veterinary Teaching Hospital, Colorado State University, Fort Collins, Colorado.

Jeffrey L. Berzon, D.V.M.
Diplomate, American College of Veterinary Surgeons. Veterinary Specialists of Connecticut, P. C., West Hartford, Connecticut.

C. W. Betts, D.V.M.
Diplomate, American College of Veterinary Surgeons. Professor of Surgery, School of Veterinary Medicine, and Staff Surgeon, Veterinary Teaching Hospital, North Carolina State University, Raleigh, North Carolina.

A. G. Binnington, D.V.M., M.S.
Diplomate, American College of Veterinary Surgeons. Associate Professor, Department of Clinical Studies, Ontario Veterinary College, University of Guelph, Ontario, Canada.

Stephen I. Bistner, D.V.M.
Diplomate, American College of Veterinary Surgeons. Associate Professor of Comparative Ophthalmology, College of Veterinary Medicine, University of Minnesota, St. Paul, Minnesota.

Dale E. Bjorling, D.V.M., M.S.
Assistant Professor, Department of Small Animal Medicine and Surgery, College of Veterinary Medicine, University of Georgia, Athens, Georgia.

Charles E. Blass, D.V.M., M.S.
Assistant Professor of Veterinary Surgery, Department of Veterinary Clinical Sciences, College of Veterinary Medicine, Louisiana State University, Baton Rouge, Louisiana.

Mark S. Bloomberg, D.V.M., M.S.
Diplomate, American College of Veterinary Surgeons. Associate Professor and Chairman, Department of Surgical Sciences, College of Veterinary Medicine, and Associate Professor of Orthopaedic Surgery, Veterinary Medical Teaching Hospital, University of Florida, Gainesville, Florida.

Julia T. Blue, D.V.M., Ph.D.
Assistant Professor, Clinical Pathology, New York State College of Veterinary Medicine, Cornell University, Ithaca, New York.

David L. Bone, D.V.M.
Assistant Professor of Surgery, Department of Small Animal Clinics, College of Veterinary Medicine, Purdue University, West Lafayette, Indiana.

Harry W. Boothe, D.V.M., M.S.
Diplomate, American College of Veterinary Surgeons. Associate Professor, Department of Small Animal Medicine and Surgery, College of Veterinary Medicine, and Veterinary Teaching Hospital, Texas A&M University, College Station, Texas.

Adele L. Boskey, Ph.D.
Associate Professor, Biochemistry, Cornell University Medical College; Senior Scientist and Director, Laboratory of Ultrastructural Biochemistry, The Hospital For Special Surgery, New York, New York.

K. C. Bovée, D.V.M., M.Med.Sc.
Professor of Medicine, School of Veterinary Medicine, University of Pennsylvania, Philadelphia, Pennsylvania.

Gale Gilbert Bowman, D.V.M.
Practitioner, Raleigh, North Carolina.

Kyle G. Braund, D.V.M., M.S., Ph.D., F.R.C.V.S.
Diplomate, American College of Veterinary Internal Medicine. Associate Professor, School of Veterinary Medicine, and Staff Neurologist, Department of Small Animal Surgery and Medicine, School of Veterinary Medicine, Auburn University, Auburn, Alabama.

William R. Brawner, Jr., D.V.M., Ph.D.
Diplomate, American College of Veterinary Radiology. Assistant Professor, Department of Radiology, School of Veterinary Medicine, Auburn University, Auburn, Alabama.

Eugene M. Breznock, D.V.M., M.S., Ph.D.
Diplomate, American College of Veterinary Surgeons. Associate Professor, Department of Veterinary Surgery, School of Veterinary Medicine, and Chief, Small Animal Surgery Service, Veterinary Medical Teaching Hospital, University of California, Davis, California.

Ronald M. Bright, D.V.M., M.S.
Diplomate, American College of Veterinary Sur-
geons. Department of Urban Practice, College of Veterinary Medicine, University of Tennessee, Knoxville, Tennessee.

Alan H. Brightman II, D.V.M., M.S.
Diplomate, American College of Veterinary Ophthalmologists. Associate Professor, Department of Veterinary Clinical Medicine, College of Veterinary Medicine, and Ophthalmologist, Veterinary Medicine Teaching Hospital, University of Illinois, Urbana, Illinois.

Nancy O. Brown, V.M.D.
Diplomate, American College of Veterinary Surgeons. Practitioner, Hickory Veterinary Hospital, Plymouth Meeting, Pennsylvania; Consultant in Surgery, The Animal Medical Center, New York, New York.

Philip A. Bushby, B.S., D.V.M., M.S.
Diplomate, American College of Veterinary Surgeons. Associate Professor, College of Veterinary Medicine, Mississippi State University, Mississippi State, Mississippi.

Rhondda B. Canfield, B.V.Sc.
Tutor in Veterinary Anatomy, Department of Veterinary Anatomy, Faculty of Veterinary Science, The University of Sydney, New South Wales, Australia.

Joseph M. Carillo, D.V.M.
Diplomate, American College of Veterinary Internal Medicine. Staff, Internal Medicine—Neurology, The Animal Medical Center, New York, New York.

Dennis D. Caywood, D.V.M., M.S.
Diplomate, American College of Veterinary Surgeons. Associate Professor of Small Animal Surgery, Department of Small Animal Sciences, College of Veterinary Medicine, University of Minnesota, St. Paul, Minnesota.

Elizabeth D. Chambers, D.V.M., M.S.
Veterinary Ophthalmologist, Animal Eye & Surgical Associates, San Diego, California.

Bruce A. Christie, M.V.Sc.
Diplomate, American College of Veterinary Surgeons. Senior Lecturer in Veterinary Anatomy, Veterinary Preclinical Sciences, University of Melbourne, Parkville; Consultant in Soft Tissue Surgery, Veterinary Clinical Sciences, University of Melbourne, Werribee, Victoria, Australia.

William G. Connor, Ph.D.
Associate Professor, Division of Radiation Oncology,

Department of Radiology, University of Arizona Medical Center, Tucson, Arizona.

Cynthia S. Cook, D.V.M.
Resident, Ophthalmology, School of Veterinary Medicine, North Carolina State University, Raleigh, North Carolina.

Daniel M. Core, D.V.M.
Staff Surgeon, Martin Animal Hospital, Shreveport, Louisiana.

Susan M. Cotter, D.V.M.
Diplomate, American College of Veterinary Internal Medicine. Associate Professor of Medicine, School of Veterinary Medicine, Tufts University; Angell Memorial Animal Hospital; Lecturer in Cancer Biology, Harvard School of Public Health, Boston, Massachusetts.

Stephen W. Crane, D.V.M.
Diplomate, American College of Veterinary Surgeons. Professor of Surgery, School of Veterinary Medicine, North Carolina State University, Raleigh, North Carolina.

Dennis T. Crowe, Jr., D.V.M.
Diplomate, American College of Veterinary Surgeons. Assistant Professor of Surgery, Department of Small Animal Medicine, College of Veterinary Medicine, and Staff Surgeon, Small Animal Teaching Hospital, University of Georgia, Athens, Georgia.

William R. Daly, D.V.M.
Diplomate, American College of Veterinary Surgeons. Houston Veterinary Referral Surgery Service, Houston, Texas.

A. P. Davies, D.V.M., M.S.
Diplomate, American College of Veterinary Internal Medicine. Clinical Associate Professor, Department of Small Animal Clinical Sciences, College of Veterinary Medicine, and Lewis Hospital for Companion Animals, University of Minnesota, St. Paul, Minnesota.

Mark W. Dewhirst, D.V.M., Ph.D.
Assistant Professor, Division of Radiation Oncology, Duke University Medical Center, Durham, North Carolina.

Bonnie DeYoung
Surgery Research Technician, School of Veterinary Medicine, North Carolina State University, Raleigh, North Carolina.

David J. DeYoung, D.V.M.
Diplomate, American College of Veterinary Surgeons. Associate Professor of Surgery, Department of Companion Animal and Special Species Medicine, School of Veterinary Medicine, North Carolina State University, Raleigh, North Carolina.

W. Jean Dodds, D.V.M.
Chief, Laboratory of Hematology, Center for Laboratories and Research, New York State Health Department, Albany, New York.

Mary L. Dulisch, D.V.M., M.S.
Diplomate, American College of Veterinary Surgeons. Staff Surgeon, Angell Memorial Animal Hospital, Boston, Massachusetts.

Erick L. Egger, D.V.M.
Diplomate, American College of Veterinary Surgeons. Assistant Professor of Small Animal Surgery, College of Veterinary Medicine and Biomedical Sciences, and Orthopedic Surgeon, Veterinary Teaching Hospital, Colorado State University, Fort Collins, Colorado.

J. E. Eigenmann, D.V.M., Dr.Med.Vet., Ph.D.
Assistant Professor of Medicine, Department of Clinical Studies, School of Veterinary Medicine, University of Pennsylvania, Philadelphia, Pennsylvania.

Glenn S. Elliott, D.V.M.
Resident, Internal Medicine/Clinical Oncology, Purdue University, West Lafayette, Indiana.

Gary W. Ellison, D.V.M., M.S.
Diplomate, American College of Veterinary Surgeons. Assistant Professor, College of Veterinary Medicine, University of Florida, Gainesville, Florida.

T. Evans, D.V.M., M.S.
Diplomate, American College of Veterinary Anesthesiologists. Associate Professor, College of Veterinary Medicine, and Section Chief, Anesthesia, Veterinary Clinical Center, Michigan State University, East Lansing, Michigan.

George E. Eyster, V.M.D., M.S.
Diplomate, American College of Veterinary Surgeons. Professor of Thoracic and Cardiovascular Surgery, College of Veterinary Medicine, and Veterinary Clinical Center, Michigan State University, East Lansing, Michigan.

Roy T. Faulkner, D.V.M., M.S.
Staff Surgeon, Skyway Animal Hospital, St. Petersburg, Florida.

Daniel A. Feeney, D.V.M., M.S.
Diplomate, American College of Veterinary Radiology. Associate Professor of Radiology, College of Veterinary Medicine, University of Minnesota, St. Paul, Minnesota.

Beverly Ann Gilroy, D.V.M.
Diplomate, American College of Veterinary Anesthesiologists. Associate Professor of Anesthesiology, Department of Anatomy, Physiological Sciences and Radiology, School of Veterinary Medicine, and Head, Anesthesia Section, Veterinary Teaching Hospital, North Carolina State University, Raleigh, North Carolina.

Norman Gofton, B.V.Sc.
Assistant Professor, Ontario Veterinary College, University of Guelph, Ontario, Canada.

John Grandage, B.Vet.Med.
Associate Professor of Anatomy, School of Veterinary Studies, Murdoch University, Perth, Western Australia.

Jacqueline L. Grandy, D.V.M.
Diplomate, American College of Veterinary Anesthesiologists. Assistant Professor, College of Veterinary Medicine and Biomedical Sciences, and Veterinary Teaching Hospital, Colorado State University, Fort Collins, Colorado.

Kenneth M. Greenwood, D.V.M.
Private referral surgery practice, Ellenwood, Georgia.

C. R. Gregory, D.V.M.
Assistant Professor of Surgery, School of Veterinary Medicine, University of California, Davis, California.

Ronald L. Grier, D.V.M., Ph.D.
Diplomate, American College of Veterinary Surgeons. Professor, Department of Veterinary Clinical Sciences, College of Veterinary Medicine, Iowa State University, Ames, Iowa.

C. B. Grindem, D.V.M., Ph.D.
Diplomate, American College of Veterinary Pathologists. Assistant Professor, School of Veterinary Medicine, North Carolina State University, Raleigh, North Carolina.

L. R. Grono, B.V.Sc., M.Sc., Ph.D.
Associate Professor and Head, Department of Veterinary Surgery, and Surgeon, Veterinary Clinic, University of Queensland, St. Lucia, Queensland, Australia.

Nancy L. Hampel, D.V.M., M.S.
Staff Surgeon, Broadway Animal Hospital, El Cajon, California.

H. W. Hannah, B.S., J.D.
Professor of Agricultural and Veterinary Medical Law, emeritus, University of Illinois, Urbana; Adjunct Professor of Law, Southern Illinois University, Springfield, Illinois.

Reinier P. Happé, D.V.M., Ph.D.
Lecturer in Small Animal Gastroenterology, Faculty of Veterinary Medicine, State University of Utrecht, The Netherlands.

R. M. Hardy, D.V.M., M.S.
Diplomate, American College of Veterinary Internal Medicine. Associate Professor, College of Veterinary Medicine, University of Minnesota, St. Paul, Minnesota.

David E. Harling, D.V.M.
Visiting Instructor in Ophthalmology, Department of Companion Animals and Special Species, School of Veterinary Medicine, North Carolina State University, Raleigh; Director and Clinician, Battleground Veterinary Hospital, Greensboro, North Carolina.

Benjamin L. Hart, D.V.M., Ph.D.
Professor of Neurobiology and Behavior, Department of Physiological Sciences, School of Veterinary Medicine, and Director, Behavioral Service, Veterinary Medical Teaching Hospital, University of California, Davis, California.

Sandee M. Hartsfield, D.V.M., M.S.
Diplomate, American College of Veterinary Anesthesiologists. Professor, Department of Small Animal Medicine and Surgery, College of Veterinary Medicine, and Veterinary Anesthesiologist, Veterinary Teaching Hospital, Texas A&M University, College Station, Texas.

Colin E. Harvey, B.V.Sc.
Diplomate, American College of Veterinary Surgeons. Professor of Surgery, School of Veterinary Medicine, University of Pennsylvania, Philadelphia, Pennsylvania.

Steve C. Haskins, D.V.M., M.S.
Diplomate, American College of Veterinary Anesthesiologists. Associate Professor, Department of Veterinary Surgery, School of Veterinary Medicine, and Section of Anesthesiology and Intensive Care, Veterinary Medical Teaching Hospital, University of California, Davis, California.

Joe Hauptman, D.V.M., M.S.
Diplomate, American College of Veterinary Surgeons. Assistant Professor of Surgery, Department of Small Animal Clinical Sciences and Veterinary Clinical Center, College of Veterinary Medicine, Michigan State University, East Lansing, Michigan.

Melvin L. Helphrey, D.V.M.
Diplomate, American College of Veterinary Surgeons. Private practice, Seminole, Florida.

Ralph A. Henderson, D.V.M., M.S.
Diplomate, American College of Veterinary Surgeons. Associate Professor, Department of Small Animal Surgery and Medicine, and Chief, Small Animal Surgery, School of Veterinary Medicine, Auburn University, Auburn, Alabama.

H. Philip Hobson, B.S., D.V.M., M.S.
Diplomate, American College of Veterinary Surgeons. Professor and Chief, Department of Small Animal Surgery, College of Veterinary Medicine, Texas A&M University, College Station, Texas.

Richard E. Hoffer, D.V.M., M.S.
Diplomate, American College of Veterinary Surgeons. Professor of Surgical Sciences, School of Veterinary Medicine, University of Wisconsin, Madison, Wisconsin.

David L. Holmberg, D.V.M., M.V.Sc.
Diplomate, American College of Veterinary Surgeons. Associate Professor of Surgery, Department of Veterinary Anesthesiology, Radiology and Surgery, Western College of Veterinary Medicine, University of Saskatchewan, Saskatoon, Saskatchewan, Canada.

R. D. Horne, D.V.M., M.S.
Diplomate, American College of Veterinary Surgeons. Professor of Surgery, School of Veterinary Medicine, Auburn University, Auburn, Alabama.

Don A. Hulse, B.S., D.V.M.
Diplomate, American College of Veterinary Surgeons. Professor of Surgery, College of Veterinary Medicine, Texas A&M University, College Station, Texas.

Richard J. Indrieri, M.S., D.V.M.
Diplomate, American College of Veterinary Internal Medicine (Neurology). Assistant Professor, Neurology and Neurosurgery, Department of Small Animal Clinical Sciences, College of Veterinary Medicine, Michigan State University, East Lansing, Michigan.

Wolfgang Janas
Veterinary Research Assistant, Biomedical Engineer-

ing Center, Purdue University, West Lafayette, Indiana.

K. Ann Jeglum, V.M.D.
Assistant Professor of Medical Oncology, School of Veterinary Medicine, and Head of Clinical Oncology Service, Veterinary Hospital, University of Pennsylvania, Philadelphia, Pennsylvania.

Richard G. Johnson, D.V.M.
Director of Surgery, Broadway Animal Hospital, El Cajon, California.

Dudley E. Johnston, M.V.Sc.
Professor of Surgery, School of Veterinary Medicine, University of Pennsylvania, Philadelphia, Pennsylvania.

Gary R. Johnston, D.V.M., M.S.
Diplomate, American College of Veterinary Radiology. Associate Professor of Comparative Radiology, College of Veterinary Medicine, University of Minnesota, St. Paul, Minnesota.

Shirley D. Johnston, D.V.M., Ph.D.
Diplomate, American College of Theriogenologists. Assistant Professor, Small Animal Medicine, College of Veterinary Medicine, University of Minnesota, St. Paul, Minnesota.

R. L. Jones, D.V.M., Ph.D.
Assistant Professor, Department of Microbiology and Environmental Health, and Head, Bacteriology Section, Diagnostic Laboratories, College of Veterinary Medicine and Biomedical Sciences, Colorado State University, Fort Collins, Colorado.

J. Michael Kehoe, D.V.M., Ph.D.
Professor and Chairman, Department of Microbiology/Immunology, Northeastern Ohio Universities College of Medicine, Rootstown, Ohio.

Mark D. Kittleson, D.V.M., Ph.D.
Diplomate, American College of Veterinary Internal Medicine. Assistant Professor, Department of Small Animal Clinical Sciences, College of Veterinary Medicine, and Cardiologist, Veterinary Clinical Center, Michigan State University, East Lansing, Michigan.

J. S. Klausner, D.V.M., M.S.
Diplomate, American College of Veterinary Internal Medicine. Associate Professor, Veterinary Internal Medicine, College of Veterinary Medicine, University of Minnesota, St. Paul, Minnesota.

L. Klein, V.M.D.
Diplomate, American College of Veterinary Anesthesiologists. Associate Professor of Anesthesia, School

of Veterinary Medicine, University of Pennsylvania, New Bolton Center, Kennett Square, Pennsylvania.

Alan Klide, V.M.D.
Diplomate, American College of Veterinary Anesthesiologists. Associate Professor of Anesthesia, School of Veterinary Medicine, University of Pennsylvania, Philadelphia, Pennsylvania.

Charles D. Knecht, V.M.D., M.S.
Diplomate, American College of Veterinary Surgeons and *American College of Veterinary Internal Medicine (Neurology).* Professor and Head, Department of Small Animal Surgery and Medicine, School of Veterinary Medicine, Auburn University, Auburn, Alabama.

Ronald J. Kolata, D.V.M., M.S.
Diplomate, American College of Veterinary Surgeons. Research Associate Professor, Departments of Surgery and Comparative Medicine, School of Medicine, St. Louis University, St. Louis, Missouri.

Joe N. Kornegay, D.V.M., Ph.D.
Diplomate, American College of Veterinary Internal Medicine. Associate Professor, Department of Companion Animal and Special Species Medicine, School of Veterinary Medicine, and Veterinary Teaching Hospital, North Carolina State University, Raleigh, North Carolina.

D. J. Krahwinkel, D.V.M., M.S.
Diplomate, American College of Veterinary Surgeons and *American College of Veterinary Anesthesiologists.* Head, Department of Urban Practice, College of Veterinary Medicine, and Professor of Surgery, Veterinary Teaching Hospital, University of Tennessee, Knoxville, Tennessee.

Gary C. Lantz, D.V.M.
Diplomate, American College of Veterinary Surgeons. Assistant Professor of Surgery, Department of Small Animal Clinics, College of Veterinary Medicine, Purdue University, West Lafayette, Indiana.

J. D. Lavach, D.V.M., M.S.
Diplomate, American College of Veterinary Ophthalmologists. Associate Professor of Ophthalmology, College of Veterinary Medicine and Biomedical Sciences, Colorado State University, Fort Collins, Colorado.

M. P. Lavery, R.N., B.S.N.
Surgical Nurse, Veterinary Medical Teaching Hospital, Virginia-Maryland Regional College of Veterinary Medicine, Blacksburg, Virginia.

George E. Lees, D.V.M., M.S.
Diplomate, American College of Veterinary Internal Medicine. Associate Professor, Department of Small Animal Medicine and Surgery, College of Veterinary Medicine, and Veterinary Teaching Hospital, Texas A&M University, College Station, Texas.

Arnold S. Lesser, V.M.D.
Diplomate, American College of Veterinary Surgeons. Director, Flushing Veterinary Hospital, Flushing; Staff Surgeon, Surgical Referral Service, Huntington, New York.

Stephen H. Levine, D.V.M., M.S.
Veterinary Medical Associate, Department of Small Animal Clinical Sciences, College of Veterinary Medicine, University of Minnesota, St. Paul; Director of Surgery, Minneapolis Veterinary Referral Services, Minneapolis, Minnesota.

Alan J. Lipowitz, D.V.M., M.S.
Diplomate, American College of Veterinary Surgeons. Associate Professor of Surgery and Chairman, Department of Small Animal Clinical Sciences, College of Veterinary Medicine, University of Minnesota, St. Paul, Minnesota.

William D. Liska, D.V.M.
Diplomate, American College of Veterinary Surgeons. Research Instructor in Orthopedics, Baylor College of Medicine; Staff Surgeon, Westbury Animal Hospital, Inc., Houston, Texas.

Philip Litwak, D.V.M., Ph.D.
Diplomate, American College of Veterinary Surgeons. Thoratec Laboratories Corporation, Berkeley, California.

A. A. M. E. Lubberink, D.V.M., Ph.D.
Lecturer in Soft Tissue Surgery, Small Animal Clinic, Faculty of Veterinary Medicine, State University of Utrecht, The Netherlands.

Charles L. Martin, D.V.M., M.S.
Diplomate, American College of Veterinary Ophthalmologists. Professor, Department of Small Animal Medicine, College of Veterinary Medicine, and Chief, Small Animal Medicine Service, Veterinary Teaching Hospital, University of Georgia, Athens, Georgia.

Louis McCoy
Senior Surgical Technician, Henry Bergh Memorial Animal Hospital, A.S.P.C.A., New York, New York.

D. M. McCurnin, D.V.M.
Diplomate, American College of Veterinary Surgeons. Professor of Surgery, Department of Clinical

Sciences, College of Veterinary Medicine and Biomedical Sciences, and Hospital Director, Veterinary Teaching Hospital, Colorado State University, Fort Collins, Colorado.

Wayne N. McDonell, D.V.M., Ph.D.
Diplomate, American College of Veterinary Anesthesiologists. Professor of Anesthesiology, Ontario Veterinary College, and Veterinary Medical Director, Veterinary Teaching Hospital, University of Guelph, Ontario, Canada.

H. Vince Mendenhall, D.V.M., Ph.D.
Senior Surgical Research Specialist, 3M Center, and Chief Surgeon, Veterinary Surgical Specialists, St. Paul, Minnesota.

David F. Merkley, D.V.M., M.S.
Diplomate, American College of Veterinary Surgeons. Associate Professor, Department of Veterinary Clinical Sciences, College of Veterinary Medicine, Iowa State University, Ames, Iowa.

Jennifer N. Mills, B.V.Sc., M.Sc.
Lecturer in Clinical Pathology, School of Veterinary Studies, Murdoch University, Murdoch, Western Australia.

J. L. Milton, D.V.M., M.S.
Diplomate, American College of Veterinary Surgeons. Associate Professor, School of Veterinary Medicine, Auburn University, Auburn, Alabama.

Robert W. Moore, D.V.M., M.S.
Staff Surgeon, South Shores Pet Clinic, San Pedro, California.

Robert J. Munger, D.V.M.
Diplomate, American College of Veterinary Ophthalmologists. Staff Veterinarian, Alcon Laboratories, and Veterinary Ophthalmologist, Animal Ophthalmology Clinic, Dallas, Texas.

A. Wendell Nelson, D.V.M., M.S., Ph.D.
Diplomate, American College of Veterinary Surgeons. Professor of Clinical Sciences, College of Veterinary Medicine and Biomedical Sciences, and Small Animal Surgeon, Veterinary Teaching Hospital, Colorado State University, Fort Collins, Colorado.

Teresa Nesbitt, D.V.M.
Research Associate, Duke University Medical Center, Durham, North Carolina.

M. E. Newman, D.V.M.
Resident in Surgery, Small Animal Clinic, School of Veterinary Medicine, Auburn University, Auburn, Alabama.

Alan M. Norris, D.V.M.
Diplomate, American College of Veterinary Internal Medicine. Assistant Professor, Department of Small Animal Medicine, Ontario Veterinary College, University of Guelph; Staff Internist, Veterinary Referral Clinic of Toronto, Toronto, Ontario, Canada.

Phillip N. Ogburn, D.V.M., Ph.D.
Associate Professor of Cardiology, Department of Small Animal Clinical Science, College of Veterinary Medicine, University of Minnesota, St. Paul, Minnesota.

N. Bari Olivier, D.V.M.
Instructor and Resident, Internal Medicine and Cardiology, Veterinary Clinical Center, College of Veterinary Medicine, Michigan State University, East Lansing, Michigan.

Marvin L. Olmstead, D.V.M., M.S.
Diplomate, American College of Veterinary Surgeons. Associate Professor, College of Veterinary Medicine, Ohio State University, Columbus, Ohio.

Don B. Olsen, D.V.M., Ph.D.
Research Professor of Surgery, School of Medicine, College of Medicine, University of Utah, Salt Lake City, Utah.

Patricia N. Olson, D.V.M., Ph.D.
Diplomate, American College of Theriogenologists. Assistant Professor, College of Veterinary Medicine and Biomedical Sciences, Colorado State University, Fort Collins, Colorado.

E. Christopher Orton, D.V.M., M.S.
Assistant Professor, Department of Clinical Sciences, College of Veterinary Medicine and Biomedical Sciences, and Veterinary Teaching Hospital, Colorado State University, Fort Collins, Colorado.

Carl A. Osborne, D.V.M., Ph.D.
Diplomate, American College of Veterinary Internal Medicine. Professor, Department of Small Animal Clinical Sciences, College of Veterinary Medicine, University of Minnesota, St. Paul, Minnesota.

Richard D. Park, D.V.M., Ph.D.
Diplomate, American College of Veterinary Radiology. Professor of Radiology, Department of Radiology and Radiation Biology, College of Veterinary Medicine and Biomedical Sciences, and Radiologist, Veterinary Teaching Hospital, Colorado State University, Fort Collins, Colorado.

Robert B. Parker, D.V.M.
Diplomate, American College of Veterinary Sur-

geons. Associate Professor and Chief, Small Animal Surgery, College of Veterinary Medicine, University of Florida, Gainesville, Florida.

Michael A. Pass, B.V.Sc., M.Sc., Ph.D.
Senior Lecturer in Physiology and Pharmacology, University of Queensland, St. Lucia, Queensland, Australia.

Clark S. Patton, D.V.M., M.S.
Diplomate, American College of Veterinary Pathologists. Associate Professor, Department of Pathobiology, College of Veterinary Medicine, University of Tennessee, Knoxville, Tennessee.

Michael M. Pavletic, D.V.M.
Diplomate, American College of Veterinary Surgeons. Assistant Professor of Surgery, School of Veterinary Medicine, Tufts University; Member, Surgical Staff, Angell Memorial Animal Hospital, Boston, Massachusetts.

Robert D. Pechman, Jr., D.V.M.
Diplomate, American College of Veterinary Radiology. Associate Professor, Department of Veterinary Clinical Sciences, School of Veterinary Medicine, Louisiana State University, Baton Rouge, Louisiana.

Robert L. Peiffer, Jr., D.V.M., Ph.D.
Diplomate, American College of Veterinary Ophthalmologists. Associate Professor, Departments of Ophthalmology and Pathology, School of Medicine, University of North Carolina, Chapel Hill, North Carolina.

Roger C. Penwick, V.M.D.
Assistant Professor of Small Animal Surgery, Department of Medicine and Surgery, College of Veterinary Medicine, and Clinician, Small Animal Surgery, Boren Veterinary Medical Teaching Hospital, Oklahoma State University, Stillwater, Oklahoma.

Victor Perman, D.V.M., Ph.D.
Diplomate, American College of Veterinary Pathologists. Professor and Chairman, Department of Veterinary Pathobiology, College of Veterinary Medicine, and Clinical Pathologist, Veterinary Teaching Hospital, University of Minnesota, St. Paul, Minnesota.

David J. Polzin, D.V.M., Ph.D.
Diplomate, American College of Veterinary Pathologists. Assistant Professor, Department of Small Animal Clinical Sciences, College of Veterinary Medicine, and Staff Internist, Lewis Hospital for Companion Animals, University of Minnesota, St. Paul, Minnesota.

Dennis L. Powers, D.V.M.
Assistant Professor of Bioengineering, Clemson University, Clemson, South Carolina.

Raymond G. Prata, D.V.M.
Diplomate, American College of Veterinary Surgeons. Surgeon, Neurosurgery and Orthopedics, Oradell Animal Hospital, Inc., Oradell, New Jersey.

Kenneth R. Presnell, D.V.M., M.Sc.
Diplomate, American College of Veterinary Surgeons. Professor of Small Animal Surgery, Head, Department of Veterinary Anesthesiology, Radiology and Surgery, Western College of Veterinary Medicine, University of Saskatchewan, Saskatoon, Saskatchewan, Canada.

Curtis W. Probst, D.V.M.
Assistant Professor, Small Animal Surgery, Department of Small Animal Clinical Sciences, Veterinary Clinical Center, Michigan State University, East Lansing, Michigan.

Maralyn R. Probst
Cardiology Research Technician, Department of Small Animal Clinical Sciences, Veterinary Clinical Center, Michigan State University, East Lansing, Michigan.

Peter I. Punch, B.Sc., B.V.M.S.
Practitioner, Perth, Western Australia.

Marc R. Raffe, D.V.M., M.S.
Assistant Professor of Comparative Anesthesiology, College of Veterinary Medicine, University of Minnesota, St. Paul, Minnesota.

Richard Read, B.V.Sc.
Postgraduate student, School of Veterinary Medicine, Murdoch University, Murdoch, Western Australia.

R. W. Redding, D.V.M., M.Sc., Ph.D.
Diplomate, American College of Veterinary Internal Medicine (Neurology). Professor, Departments of Veterinary Physiology and Pharmacology and Small Animal Surgery and Medicine, School of Veterinary Medicine, Auburn University Auburn, Alabama.

Daniel C. Richardson, D.V.M.
Diplomate, American College of Veterinary Surgeons. Assistant Professor of Surgery, School of Veterinary Medicine, North Carolina State University Raleigh, North Carolina.

Ken Richardson, B.Sc., B.V.Sc., Ph.D.
Lecturer, Veterinary Anatomy, School of Veterinary Studies, Murdoch University, Perth, Western Australia.

Ralph C. Richardson, D.V.M.
Diplomate, American College of Veterinary Internal Medicine. Associate Professor of Medicine, and Chief, Clinical Oncology, College of Veterinary Medicine, Purdue University, West Lafayette, Indiana.

Robert C. Rosenthal, D.V.M., M.S.
Diplomate, American College of Veterinary Internal Medicine. Assistant Professor, Department of Medical Sciences, School of Veterinary Medicine, University of Wisconsin, Madison, Wisconsin.

Anne E. Rosin, D.V.M.
Instructor, Clinical Pathology, Department of Pathobiological Sciences, School of Veterinary Medicine, University of Wisconsin, Madison, Wisconsin.

Eberhard Rosin, D.V.M., Ph.D.
Diplomate, American College of Veterinary Surgeons. Associate Professor, School of Veterinary Medicine, University of Wisconsin, Madison, Wisconsin.

Donald C. Sawyer, D.V.M., Ph.D.
Diplomate, American College of Veterinary Anesthesiologists. Professor of Anesthesia, Department of Small Animal Clinical Sciences, College of Veterinary Medicine, and Veterinary Clinical Center, Michigan State University, East Lansing, Michigan.

Anthony Schwartz, D.V.M., Ph.D.
Diplomate, American College of Veterinary Surgeons. Professor and Chairman, Department of Surgery, School of Veterinary Medicine, Tufts University; Member, Surgical Staff, Angell Memorial Animal Hospital, Boston, Massachusetts.

Peter D. Schwarz, D.V.M.
Assistant Professor, Department of Clinical Sciences, College of Veterinary Medicine and Biomedical Sciences, Colorado State University, Fort Collins, Colorado.

Kay L. Schwink, D.V.M.
Resident in Ophthalmology, College of Veterinary Medicine, Iowa State University, Ames, Iowa.

Peter K. Shires, B.V.Sc., M.S.
Diplomate, American College of Veterinary Surgeons. Associate Professor, School of Veterinary Medicine, and Surgeon, Veterinary Teaching Hospital, Louisiana State University, Baton Rouge, Louisiana.

Andy Shores, D.V.M., M.S.
Neurology/Neurosurgery Resident, Department of Small Animal Surgery and Medicine, School of Veterinary Medicine, Auburn University, Auburn, Alabama.

Stephen T. Simpson, D.V.M., M.S.
Diplomate, American College of Veterinary Internal Medicine (Neurology). Associate Professor, School of Veterinary Medicine, and Staff Neurologist, Small Animal Clinic, Auburn University, Auburn, Alabama.

Douglas H. Slatter, B.V.Sc., M.S., Ph.D., F.R.C.V.S.
Diplomate, American College of Veterinary Surgeons and *American College of Veterinary Ophthalmologists.* Veterinary Ophthalmologist and Surgeon, Animal Eye and Surgical Associates, San Diego, California.

D. D. Smeak, B.S., D.V.M.
Assistant Professor of Surgery, College of Veterinary Medicine, and Surgeon, Ohio State University, Columbus, Ohio.

C. W. Smith, D.V.M., M.S.
Diplomate, American College of Veterinary Surgeons. Professor, Department of Veterinary Clinical Medicine, College of Veterinary Medicine, and Chief, Small Animal Surgery, Veterinary Medical Teaching Hospital, Urbana, Illinois.

Donald C. Sorjonen, D.V.M.
Assistant Professor, School of Veterinary Medicine, and Staff Neurologist, Small Animal Clinic, Auburn University, Auburn, Alabama.

Eugene P. Steffey, V.M.D., Ph.D.
Diplomate, American College of Veterinary Anesthesiologists. Professor and Chairman, Department of Surgery, School of Veterinary Medicine, and Chief of Anesthesia/Critical Patient Care, Veterinary Medical Teaching Hospital, University of California, Davis, California.

Sharon Stevenson, D.V.M., M.S.
Diplomate, American College of Veterinary Surgeons. Postgraduate Research Pathologist, Department of Pathology, School of Veterinary Medicine, University of California, Davis, California.

Steven L. Stockham, B.V.M., M.S.
Diplomate, American College of Veterinary Pathologists. Assistant Professor of Veterinary Clinical Pathology, College of Veterinary Medicine, University of Missouri, Columbia, Missouri.

Elizabeth A. Stone, D.V.M., M.S.
Diplomate, American College of Veterinary Surgeons. Assistant Professor of Surgery, Department of Clinical Studies, School of Veterinary Medicine, University of Pennsylvania, Philadelphia, Pennsylvania.

Steven J. Susaneck, D.V.M., M.S.
Diplomate, American College of Veterinary Internal Medicine. Staff Oncologist, Westbury Animal Hospital, Inc., Houston, Texas.

Steven F. Swaim, D.V.M., M.S.
Professor of Surgery, Department of Small Animal Surgery and Medicine, School of Veterinary Medicine, Auburn University, Auburn, Alabama.

James Tomlinson, B.S., D.V.M., M.V.Sc.
Assistant Professor of Surgery, College of Veterinary Medicine, and Head of Orthopedic Surgery, University of Missouri, Columbia, Missouri.

James P. Toombs, D.V.M., M.S.
Assistant Professor of Surgery, Department of Small Animal Medicine, College of Veterinary Medicine, and Staff Surgeon, Small Animal Orthopedics, Veterinary Teaching Hospital, University of Georgia, Athens, Georgia.

Cynthia M. Trim, B.V.Sc.
Associate Professor and Anesthesiologist, College of Veterinary Medicine, University of Georgia, Athens, Georgia.

Alan Tucker, Ph.D.
Associate Professor, Department of Physiology and Biophysics, College of Veterinary Medicine and Biomedical Sciences, Colorado State University, Fort Collins, Colorado.

David C. Twedt, D.V.M.
Diplomate, American College of Veterinary Internal Medicine. Associate Professor, Department of Clinical Sciences, College of Veterinary Medicine and Biomedical Sciences, and Staff Gastroenterologist, Veterinary Teaching Hospital, Colorado State University, Fort Collins, Colorado.

Frederik J. Van Sluys, D.V.M.
Lecturer in Small Animal Surgery, Faculty of Veterinary Medicine, State University of Utrecht, The Netherlands.

P. B. Vasseur, D.V.M.
Diplomate, American College of Veterinary Surgeons. Assistant Professor, Department of Surgery, School of Veterinary Medicine, University of California, Davis, California.

William Ardene Vestre, D.V.M., M.S.
Diplomate, American College of Veterinary Ophthalmologists. Assistant Professor, School of Veterinary

Medicine, Purdue University, West Lafayette, Indiana.

Andreas F. von Recum, D.V.M., Dr. med.vet., Ph.D.
Professor and Head, Department of Bioengineering, College of Engineering, Clemson University, Clemson, South Carolina.

Stanley D. Wagner, D.V.M.
Instructor, College of Veterinary Medicine, Kansas State University, Manhattan, Kansas.

Tom L. Walker, B.S., D.V.M., M. S.
Diplomate, American College of Veterinary Surgeons. Associate Professor of Surgery, Department of Urban Practice, College of Veterinary Medicine, University of Tennessee, Knoxville, Tennessee.

Richard Walshaw, B.V.M.S.
Diplomate, American College of Veterinary Surgeons. Associate Professor, Department of Small Animal Clinical Sciences, College of Veterinary Medicine, and Surgeon, Veterinary Clinical Center, Michigan State University, East Lansing, Michigan.

Andy Wasilewski, M.S.
Director of Data Processing, School of Veterinary Medicine, North Carolina State University, Raleigh, North Carolina.

Joseph P. Weigel, B.S., D.V.M.
Diplomate, American College of Veterinary Surgeons. Associate Professor of Surgery, Department of Urban Practice, College of Veterinary Medicine, University of Tennessee, Knoxville, Tennessee.

Walter E. Weirich, D.V.M., Ph.D.
Diplomate, American College of Veterinary Surgeons. Professor and Head, Department of Small Animal Clinics, School of Veterinary Medicine, Purdue University, West Lafayette, Indiana.

Pamela G. Whiting, D.V.M.
Fellow, Liver Disease Research, National Institute of Arthritis, Diabetes, Digestive and Kidney Diseases, National Institutes of Health; Veterinary Medical Teaching Hospital, School of Veterinary Medicine, University of California, Davis, California.

James W. Wilson, B.S., D.V.M., M.S.
Diplomate, American College of Veterinary Surgeons. Department of Surgical Sciences, School of Veterinary Medicine, University of Wisconsin, Madison, Wisconsin.

Stephen J. Withrow, D.V.M.
Diplomate, American College of Veterinary Surgeons. Professor of Surgery, College of Veterinary Medicine and Biomedical Sciences, and Chief, Clinical Oncology Service, Veterinary Teaching Hospital, Colorado State University, Fort Collins, Colorado.

Peggy M. Wykes, D.V.M., M.S.
Private practice (surgical specialty), Reference Surgical Veterinary Practice, Englewood, Colorado.

Preface

Surgery is that fascinating and stimulating branch of therapeutic science that deals with the treatment of disease and injury by manipulative or operative methods. It requires of its practitioners not only a knowledge of diseases and their diagnosis, but also specific technical skills necessary for the operative treatment of disease. Although it is often fashionable to decry the importance of one or the other of these aspects of surgery, a surgeon's clinical results nevertheless reflect his expertise in both areas. This requirement places an additional burden on the aspiring surgeon, who must acquire both the knowledge and skills through arduous training, either by means of graduate institutional training programs or in veterinary practice.

Textbook of Small Animal Surgery is directed to the student as a text and to the veterinary practitioner and surgeon-in-training as a reference, in the hope that the rigors of training will not relegate him to the "surgical technician" category—the present-day equivalent of the barber-surgeon of previous centuries—but rather to development as a complete surgeon, whose diagnostic and treatment methods are firmly based in modern surgical science and compare favorably in results and methods with those of his colleagues. The book is also directed to the busy clinician as a source of information in routine clinical situations, when the unusual, stimulating, and challenging may become submerged in a sea of necessary but mundane procedures.

As in other specialties, the volume of new information in surgery is awesome, and the authors have attempted to distill the clinically and scientifically relevant material in one place. It is often difficult to differentiate material that will be necessary to an understanding of treatment methods currently under development from that of lesser importance. Where more than one method of treatment exists, authors have been encouraged to compare them, where possible, and the reasons for their apparent success or lack of it. The information presented is keyed to the vast literature of surgical science and published knowledge. I hope that the contents will stimulate users to read further in the literature of the subject and will assist them in the daily and effective treatment of our trusting patients.

Constructive suggestions by veterinarians, students, and other users of the text are welcome for the continued development of *Textbook of Small Animal Surgery*.

DOUGLAS H. SLATTER

Acknowledgments

I am endebted to the Section Editors, who have labored with skill and diligence in planning their sections and coordinating their respective contributing authors, and with patience when confronted with constant reminders of the task at hand. The efforts of each author are appreciated—the fruits of their intense labors are very evident. To the many veterinary and medical colleagues and farsighted teaching institutions who have allowed publication of illustrations previously published or otherwise, without charge, I extend my sincere thanks, for it is only by contributions such as this that illustration of a surgery text of this type is possible. Ray Kersey as well as the staff of the W. B. Saunders Company, especially Sandy Reinhardt, Virginia Ingaran, Amy Grodnick, and Janet Macnamara-Barnett, have been outstanding in the assistance, forbearance, and encouragement they have offered in the many phases of production of the book.

Contents

Volume I

Volume II

Contents

Contents

Section

Development of Veterinary Surgery

Douglas H. Slatter
Section Editor

1 Development of Veterinary Surgery

History of Small Animal Surgery

Colin E. Harvey and Douglas H. Slatter

Dogs and cats have been man's companions since before recorded time. As with other animal species, the diagnosis and management of the diseases of dogs and cats have had a checkered history. The available historical accounts of veterinary medicine, which largely consist of descriptions of practices current at the time of writing, are heavily weighted with diseases of horses until the middle of the 19th century. The companionship of a dog or cat was valued, but the animal was easily and cheaply replaced, and, since professions develop in response to a market for their services, companion animal medicine did not flourish until the 20th century.

Veterinary hospitals functioned in India from at least 1800 B.C., although their patients consisted mainly of horses, cattle, and elephants. Dogs were treated with respect in ancient Egypt; fractures were splinted, hemorrhage was controlled with cautery, and castration was practiced. Phlebotomy was a common treatment for many conditions until this century.

The classical Greek period is considered an important era in the development of human medicine. There are many veterinary parallels, with detailed accounts of the management of diseases of domestic animals that remained in use for several hundred years. These include a treatise on dogs written in 284 B.C. One common medical fallacy first recorded in Greek manuscripts is the surgical prevention or treatment of rabies by resection of the "lyssa," the sublingual fold believed to be the "worm" that caused rabies—this remedy was still in use through the 19th century.

The Romans added little to advance the understanding of diseases of dogs and cats. Tail docking joined resection of the "lyssa" as a specific prophylactic against rabies.

Little progress was made for hundreds of years until men of vision were willing to observe and then seek explanations for their observations. Meanwhile, most animals suffered in silence or in noisy misery while subjected to the cruel and ineffective manipulations and nostrums used by untrained animal doctors. Until the 19th century, there were no training requirements or practice standards for veterinarians. Most practitioners learned their trade by apprenticeship, a system that perpetuated such nonsense as removal of the frog of the equine foot.

Progress came slowly. Access to books was limited, particularly among the uneducated providers of "veterinary" services. Those who did manage to rise above their colleagues because of force of personality were often men of immense ego as well as incredible ignorance.

The spaying of bitches was described at least as early as 1576, the procedure being performed through the flank in pregnant bitches. The use of ligatures (first described in detail by Paré 20 years earlier) was not mentioned.

The situation did not begin to improve until the training of veterinarians was put on a scientific basis with the establishment of veterinary schools, starting with the school at Lyon in 1762. A major advance was the required training in anatomy and pathology. As more graduates became available, the animal-owning public became more aware of the differences between veterinarians and untrained practitioners. This trend culminated with legislation in the 19th century limiting the practice of veterinary medicine and surgery to licensed individuals.

The first comprehensive account of diseases of the dog appeared in 1817.[1] The author, Blaine, relied more on medications (of great variety) than on surgery but described drainage of aural hematoma, aspiration of ascites and pleural effusions, external reduction of joint luxations and external fixation of fractures, open resection of callus followed by external fixation for fracture nonunions, castration and spaying, urethrotomy for calculus, and excision of superficial growths or bite wounds caused by rabid animals. The beneficial effects of canine saliva on open wounds are acknowledged, although this had been described at least 250 years earlier. Cats received very little attention.

Major advances in the surgery of dogs and cats could not occur until reliable anesthetics became available. Narcotic analgesia and sedation were investigated in the 17th century, and the effects of inhaling nitrous oxide were reported in 1779, but these observations were not followed up for many years. The anesthetic effect of ether and chloroform was discovered in the first half of the 19th century, but this mode of anesthesia was only slowly adopted for veterinary practice. A second major advance was the understanding of the cause and detrimental effect of infection. The era of "laudable pus" is not as well-described for veterinary surgeons as it is for human counterparts, but the same deplorable surgical conditions prevailed. Following the observation, by Semmelweiss and others, of the connection between contamination and subsequent infection, the use of antiseptic techniques considerably improved results in human surgery. These techniques were slowly, and often half-heartedly, accepted in veterinary practice. Aseptic technique, the logical extension of antiseptic technique, was not fully adopted in some veterinary schools until the middle of this century. Coincident with the major advances in anesthesia and aseptic technique were advances in the design and manufacture of surgical instruments, although here again veterinary surgery lagged behind human surgery because of financial realities and the range in size of animal species.

Surgical textbooks appearing before 1900 contained little detailed information on anesthesia and rarely contained much systematic information on the dog. The English veterinary literature owes much to the translation of standard German veterinary surgical texts written in the late 1800s, although these did not include a comprehensive review of the surgical diseases of dogs and cats.

Early specialists in companion animal surgery, such as F. T. G. Hobday, who wrote the first comprehensive text on surgical diseases of the dog and cat,[3] were master clinicians and surgeons but were limited because of a lack of understanding of pathophysiology. Hobday's book includes details of intricate surgical procedures, such as corneal dermoid and cataract removal and entropion and ectropion repair, and sections on dentistry, intestinal surgery, cystotomy, and even nephrolithotomy. The section on orthopedic procedures is very limited, and the discussion of thoracic disease is limited to thoracocentesis.

The tradition of technical excellence and innovation was continued by J. G. Wright and later several others in British veterinary schools. General practice conditions in the early part of the 20th century remained rather primitive, surgery being relegated to procedures performed in a back room in poor light and with rather minimal instrumentation. Surgical specialists established themselves by reputation. These days are retold with rare literary style by James Herriot in his descriptions of practice in Darrowby[2] and the miracles wrought by Granville Bennett in his specialist practice.

In the United States, energetic private practitioners such as Ehmer, Hoskins, and LaCroix were pioneers in disseminating information to the practicing veterinarian. The founding of the American Animal Hospital Association in 1933 expedited the advance of practice standards and continuing education. The first edition of *Canine Surgery*, published in 1939, was a compilation of articles from The North American Veterinarian and mentioned shock and the importance of fluid therapy; a comprehensive section on orthopedic procedures included chapters by some still familiar names such as Ehmer, Schroeder, Stader, and Morris. Advances made by veterinarians during this period that were to have effects beyond small animal surgery included the Ehmer and Stader orthopedic devices.

The pathophysiological effects of thoracotomy on the dog were observed as early as 1733; however, reliable techniques for thoracic surgery did not appear until the principles of positive pressure ventilation were understood, almost 200 years later. Descriptions of lung surgery are included in Markowitz's book, *Experimental Surgery*,[7] along with other information recorded in human or experimental surgery journals on topics previously closed to veterinary surgeons.

The lack of innovation in small animal surgery in the veterinary schools in the United States in the first 40 years of this century is notable compared with the period since then.

FROM 1945 ONWARD

In the last 40 years, many major influences have affected the current state of veterinary surgery, primarily by initially affecting the North American veterinary profession. In some cases these influences have been felt in other parts of the world.

It was not until the 1940s that aseptic surgical principles were widely applied in veterinary surgery; until that time lack of asepsis and consequent infection had been major inhibiting factors in surgical interventions. In the 1900 edition of Hobday's *Canine and Feline Surgery*,[3] the discussion of asepsis is limited to washing of the operator's hands with soap and the application of alcohol or ether "in serious operations" to remove grease from the fingers prior to surgery. Even after significant progress in the application of asepsis had been made in small animal surgery, resistance was often seen among large animal surgeons.

Major contributions were made in applying the principles of asepsis and modern physiology to veterinary surgery by the staffs of the Angell Memorial Animal Hospital in Boston (Schroeder, Schnelle, and Blakely), Colorado State University (Farquharson), Cornell University (Leonard), and the Ontario Veterinary College (Archibald) in association with physicians such as Markowitz during the late 1940s and early 1950s. Markowitz's writings stand as a monument to the surgical application of physiological principles and philosophies. As with many outstanding veterinary surgeons over the next several decades, Markowitz, a physician, received postgraduate training in a human surgical research laboratory, in his case at the Mayo Foundation, where he worked with C. F. Schlotthauer.

The influence of persons trained in these schools was widespread; e.g., Larsen, after a period at Colorado State University, greatly advanced veterinary surgery at the University of Sydney, Australia. The Angell Memorial Animal Hospital and its association with Harvard Medical School greatly influenced the standards of veterinary surgery and medicine in general, especially by its internship programs and its prominent and influential staff veterinarians. Many of the recipients of such training, including Jenny and Lumb, subsequently taught in veterinary schools and further disseminated the application of modern surgical techniques. Schnelle also aided the development of surgery with his improvements and wide usage of radiology for diagnosis and a teaching file of radiographs, previously rare practices. The more consistent performance of necropsies on clinical patients and the introduction of the clinical laboratory into diagnosis were also notable at this institution.

The association between veterinarians and physicians was especially fruitful during the postwar period at the University of Pennsylvania and resulted in considerable stimulus for the development of specialties in veterinary medicine including surgery. This influence has endured to the present day. Jacque Jenny and Robert Brodey were notable for their contributions to orthopedics and oncology, respectively.

The widespread introduction of gaseous anesthesia during the 1960s, largely replacing the intravenous use of long-acting barbiturates for major surgery, greatly facilitated the development of more sophisticated surgical techniques, especially when the patient was at risk or when better muscle relaxation was needed. Although cyclopropane had been used to some extent in the United Kingdom during the 1950s, it was never widely used in North America because of its explosive properties. By the middle 1950s, the use of halothane and methoxyflurane in anesthetic machines had become more common.

The availability of antibiotics and the more widespread use of aseptic procedures stimulated the development of many orthopedic procedures, including open reduction of fractures, that had not been commonly practiced before. In addition, the anatomical approach to surgery as exemplified in Piermattei and Greeley's *Surgical Approaches to the Bones of the Dog and Cat* significantly influenced the development of veterinary orthopedics.

ASSOCIATIONS

The establishment of the American College of Veterinary Surgeons in 1965 was a major factor in the development of veterinary surgery. A forum for the presentation of surgical material became available, and, more importantly, the training of future surgeons was given major emphasis. An internship followed by a two-year surgical residency and an additional two years of training supervised by a Diplomate of the College are required prior to theoretical, practical, and oral examinations. A number of surgical societies have been formed in other countries, but none emphasizes formal training and examination. The distinction between graduate training and clinical training in surgery emerged as the di-

ploma of the A.C.V.S. was accepted as the standard of specialist clinical training in both institutions and private practice. A number of combined programs exist, offering both residency training and a higher degree, usually at the Master's level. From 1964 to 1977, the Surgical Laboratory at Colorado State University offered a wide range of training programs in comparative surgical research at the graduate level.

The dissemination of surgical knowledge by the American Animal Hospital Association, its journal, and its major annual conference has continued. The first Archibald edition of *Canine Surgery* in 1965 marked a step forward in the application of anatomy and pathology to small animal surgery in a form readily available to practicing veterinarians. The Archives of the A.C.V.S. eventually evolved into the *Journal of Veterinary Surgery* in 1970, the first English journal devoted entirely to the subject. In addition, a number of societies have been established, the members of which have special interests in different fields of veterinary surgery and associated disciplines, including oncology, cryosurgery, and orthopedics.

In 1974, the A.C.V.S. began conducting the annual Surgical Forum, devoted to the presentation of current clinical material on a systems basis for practicing veterinarians. The American Colleges of Veterinary Ophthalmologists and Veterinary Anesthesiologists later joined The Surgical Forum, which has become the largest meeting of its kind devoted primarily to small animal surgery. At the current stage of scientific and technical development in veterinary surgery, there are few procedures available for humans that cannot be performed on animals by trained veterinary surgeons, the major barrier, however, being cost. In most major cities appropriately trained surgeons are available in either institutions or private practice to offer services of a high standard to dog and cat owners.

1. Blaine, D.: *Canine Pathology: A Description of the Diseases of Dogs.* Boosey and Sons, London, 1817.
2. Herriot, J.: *All Creatures Great and Small.* St. Martins Press, New York, 1971.
3. Hobday, F. T. G.: *Canine and Feline Surgery.* W. and A. K. Johnston, London, 1900.
4. Lacroix, J. V., and Hoskins, H. P. (eds.): *Canine Surgery,* 1st ed. The North American Veterinarian, Evanston, IL, 1939.
5. Leonard, E.: *Orthopedic Surgery of the Dog and Cat.* W. B. Saunders, Philadelphia, 1961.
6. Lumb, W. V.: Personal communication, 1983.
7. Markowitz, J.: *Experimental Surgery,* 1st and 2nd eds. Williams & Wilkins, Baltimore, 1937 and 1949.
8. Ormrod, A. N.: *Surgery of the Dog and Cat.* Baillière, Tindall and Cassell, London, 1966.
9. Pettit, G. D.: Personal communication, 1983.
10. Smithcors, J. F.: *The Evolution of the Veterinary Art.* Veterinary Medical Publishing Co., Kansas City, 1957.

Legal Aspects of Veterinary Surgery*

H. W. Hannah

INTRODUCTION†

The American Veterinary Medical Association Code of Ethics states in succinct language that veterinarians shall comply with all laws affecting them and that they shall not engage in illegal practices.

What kinds of laws affect the veterinarian? A legislative act prescribes the conditions under which he can be licensed and can practice and whether or not he can incorporate; administrative regulations determine when and how he shall fill out a health certificate; both statutes and common-law principles determine when he has failed to "measure up" in his treatment of animals; the civil law (as distinguished from the criminal law) determines his contractual rights and obligations; the criminal law can come into play if he uses narcotics illegally or issues a false certificate; and even local ordinances play an important role, for example, a zoning classification that precludes him from establishing a practice except in certain areas or an air pollution ordinance that forces him to buy a new incinerator.

Constitutional law, both federal and state, is of special importance to a veterinarian because the interstate commerce clause in the former is the basis upon which Congress has provided for an extensive animal disease control authority; and limitations on the authority of state legislatures contained in state constitutions protect the veterinarian from arbitrary and discriminatory use of police power.

Although the litigation experience of veterinary practitioners does not match that of their human medicine counterparts, it has nevertheless been significant, and for those practitioners involved sometimes costly and traumatic. In the preface to *Veterinarian in Litigation*,[1] the author states that in writing the book "Literally hundreds of cases have been read and digested . . . ." In *Law for the Veterinarian and Livestock Owner*,[2] the author footnoted 375 legal references, most of which were citations of appeals court cases.

Who can practice veterinary medicine and surgery? Those who meet the requirements expressed in governmental practice acts. In the United States these acts are the product of state legislatures, legalized by the right of these legislatures to pass laws for the protection of the health, safety, and welfare of the citizens of the state—a right referred to as the "police power." Although these practice acts vary from state to state, there are some common features. Most significant are provisions regarding minimal educational requirements; examinations for licensure; what constitutes the practice of veterinary medicine and surgery; exemptions from the act; continuing veterinary medical education; license renewal; administration of the act; reciprocity; causes for revocation or suspension of license and the hearing procedure to be followed when complaints are lodged; animal technicians, veterinary assistants, or other lay help; and unlicensed practice.

What do such acts mean to the practitioner? They mean, on the one hand, that he is protected from unlicensed competition (providing there is enforcement) and, on the other, that the continuation of his practice depends on his remaining within the law. Although this is not particularly difficult for most practitioners, there are requirements or prohibitions in these acts that could "trap" the unknowing, including:

1. Using technicians or lay help beyond the guidelines established by law and regulation (e.g., not providing "direction and control" or letting them in fact substitute for the veterinarian in making judgments and performing surgery).

2. Not meeting continuing veterinary medical education requirements established by law and regulation.

3. Being too casual about preparing and signing health certificates or reporting on tests required by law.

4. Loose practice in storing, safeguarding, and dispensing controlled substances.

5. Failure to maintain adequate sanitary standards.

There are many causes for revocation or suspension of license other than those mentioned. But most of these involve an intent to circumvent or flout the law. "Gross malpractice," included in some acts as cause for revocation of license, is not likely to "trap the unknowing," since it is difficult to imagine that a practitioner whose activities would support such a charge would not know about his own shortcomings.

Concern is often expressed by veterinarians about the competition they receive from unlicensed persons. Typical complaints name the salesman who makes an off-the-cuff diagnosis and sells a remedy, or a person (sometimes quite able) who diagnoses, treats, performs surgery, and assumes the role of a licensed veterinarian. What can be done? Practice acts generally contain two provisions that are pertinent to this point. One directs the state or district attorney, upon filing of the proper complaint, to prosecute. If there is a conviction, a fine and possibly a jail sentence can be imposed. Another, more effective remedy provides that any person who has reason to believe a practitioner is unlicensed may seek an injunction. If the action is successful the practitioner will then be enjoined from further practice. Violation of this court order amounts to contempt, for which

---

*Certain sections of this chapter contain excerpts from legal briefs prepared by the author that appeared in the *Journal of the American Veterinary Medical Association*.

†Excerpted from What should a veterinarian know about the law? J. Am. Vet. Med. Assoc. *161*:1074, 1972.

proper penalties are provided. Before proceeding under either of these laws the informer should first ascertain that the acts complained of are in fact within the practice of veterinary medicine and surgery.

A prime source of client discontent and one leading, in some cases, to a malpractice action is failure of the veterinarian to establish a friendly and considerate relationship with a client. Clients who are treated well, who are informed about the veterinarian's findings and future plans, and who are given an opportunity to ask questions are likely to forgive mistakes that could otherwise lead to a malpractice claim or at least to a complaint to the state veterinary medical association. There are economic as well as legal overtones to communication. A veterinarian who is always too busy to talk to his clients, who "talks down" to them, or who tries to brush off a bad result will assuredly drive some of his clientele to veterinarians who treat them differently. There is a further consideration, that having to do with "informed consent." This is discussed in a subsequent section of this chapter.

Scope of Chapter

As far as possible, the sections that follow concentrate on subjects that, although not in every instance peculiar to veterinary surgeons, are nevertheless of concern to them.

WHAT CONSTITUTES VETERINARY SURGERY WITHIN THE DEFINITIONS PROVIDED BY LAW?*

Despite efforts made by legislators to adequately define "practice," gray areas exist to perplex those responsible for applying the law. The gray areas seem to grow larger with the advent of procedures not contemplated when the definitions were coined.

Courts have distinguished between "medicine" and "surgery"; the former " . . . denotes the treatment of disease by the administration of drugs or other sanitave substances," whereas the latter is " . . . that branch of medical science which treats of mechanical or operative measures for healing diseases, deformities or injuries."[3] Practice acts employ both terms, recognizing that it is not possible for one to be qualified to render either kind of treatment without being grounded in the other.

Without exploring the specific language in state veterinary acts, it is safe to assume that in all of them anything that can be defined as "surgery" constitutes the practice of veterinary medicine. Difficulties arise in determining if a particular procedure, especially a new or different one, is surgery. Acupuncture, arti-

ficial insemination, and embryo transplantation are cases in point. Some state practice acts resolved the artificial insemination problem by exempting such from the definition of "practice." Acupuncture has been defined as the practice of medicine by the Supreme Court of Ohio[4] and thus by inference would also constitute the practice of veterinary medicine. The court was not impressed by the argument that acupuncture is only "minor surgery" and thus permissible to chiropractors. It was impressed by the fact that needles had to be inserted beneath the skin. An Oregon appeals court reached the same conclusion,[5] and a note on this case discloses that several other jurisdictions are in accord.[6]

Court decisions strongly intimate that if the skin is punctured or bodily tissues are disrupted in some way this amounts to surgery and hence the practice of veterinary medicine.

Pressure groups have been able to have certain activities excluded from the definition of practice. These exclusions vary by state, and some acts may contain none. The most common ones are castration, spaying, docking, and dehorning. But some inroad has been made on these exclusions. In Illinois, for example, where castration has from the first passage of the practice act been excluded, the exclusion is now limited to farm animals; neutering of dogs, cats, and other pet, exotic, or companion animals is the practice of veterinary medicine.

Certain categories of persons are also exempt from the application of state veterinary practice acts. Because of their official duties many persons perform acts that could otherwise be defined as the practice of veterinary medicine. These exemptions generally apply to Federal or state veterinarians actually engaged or employed in their official capacity, to out-of-state veterinarians called in for consultation, to students and staff of veterinary colleges pursuing their educational duties, and to employees of other colleges and research institutions engaged in their research activities. Without exception, also, state practice acts exempt individuals who treat their own animals. However, some state laws have qualified this right by saying such treatment must be "in a humane manner."

Practice acts are worded so that medical doctors and dentists do not have a right to treat animals; similarly, a veterinarian does not have a right to treat human patients.

With respect to gratuitous treatment, practice acts vary. Some permit treatment by neighbors as long as it is in exchange for work and not for any other kind of remuneration. This again is a concession to previous practices, e.g., when neighbors helped each other with vaccination or other activities that now constitute the practice of veterinary medicine unless performed by the owner himself. The tendency to disallow exemption to those who render gratuitous services stems from an interest in the humane treatment of animals and the control of transmissible diseases.

---

*Excerpted from Your practice act—Do you know how it affects you? J. Am. Vet. Med. Assoc. *162*:600, 1973.

The Standard of Skill and Care for Veterinary Surgeons

The standards of professional performance exhibited by a veterinarian in treating animals and in dealing with his clients are the key issues in malpractice actions. Malpractice has been defined as

. . . bad, wrong, or injudicious treatment of a patient, professionally and in respect to the particular disease or injury, resulting in injury, unnecessary suffering, or death to the patient, and proceeding from ignorance, carelessness, want of proper professional skill, disregard of established rules or principles, neglect or a malicious or criminal intent.[7]

It is obvious, therefore, that some appraisal or measurement must be made of a veterinary surgeon's performance to determine if it was "bad, wrong, or injudicious." This determination is made by the court after evidence has been presented by a plaintiff attempting to show that the defendant's treatment fell below the standard of his fellow practitioners. This raises another question. Against the standards of which practitioners will his standards in this particular case be measured?

At one time a "locality rule" was generally applicable. Under this rule a veterinarian's performance would be compared with that of practitioners in his area or locality. With improved communications, better travel facilities, greater availability of professional journals and literature, and the growth of continuing veterinary medical education courses, seminars, and conferences, an increasing number of courts are abandoning the locality rule in favor of a more comprehensive rule that allows the admission of evidence on standards and procedures used throughout the profession.[8]

Veterinary surgeons are not held to a "standard of perfection." One work of law states that "a veterinary surgeon is bound to use, in performing the duties of his employment, such reasonable skill, diligence, and attention as may ordinarily be expected of careful, skillful and trustworthy persons in his profession, and if he does not possess and exercise these qualities he is answerable for the result of his want of skill or care."[9] He is not required to exercise an extraordinary amount of care or to have an extraordinary amount of knowledge and skill.

In an action against the United States for alleged erroneous certification of tick-infested cattle for interstate shipment, the court said:

The nearest analogy that occurs to us is the duty of one who undertakes a matter requiring expertness to bring reasonable skill and knowledge to his task according to the then state of the art, and to execute it with ordinary care, but involves no guaranty of the results. Such is the duty of a medical practitioner on man or beast.[10]

Although veterinary surgeons are not held to a standard of perfection, they are expected to keep up with discoveries and new methods. This means that the move toward requiring completion of a specified amount of continuing veterinary medical education as a prerequisite to relicensure has important legal overtones. For example, the Supreme Court of South Dakota upheld the revocation of an optometrist's license for failure to submit satisfactory evidence of having met the continuing professional educational requirements imposed by law and regulation.[11] In a malpractice action, failure to possess knowledge imparted in such programs could mean that the practitioner has not met the required standard. Significant also is the trend toward adding lay members to veterinary medical examining boards and changing the names of such boards to reflect the public interest in the competent delivery of veterinary services. For example, a California law changed the name of the "Board of Medical Examiners" to "Board of Medical Quality Assurance."

What is the standard for the specialist? Although there appear to be no cases directly involving veterinary surgeons, at least two courts have stated that, with respect to human medicine, the standard is that of other specialists in the particular field.[12] Furthermore, it has been indicated by the courts that if one in fact considers himself as a specialist, although not board certified, he will be held to the standard of a specialist. A zoo veterinarian may, for example, be regarded by the law as a specialist even though there is no formal recognition of that fact.

The standard of skill and care involves more than the veterinarian's performance; it also involves the equipment he maintains and has available for diagnosis and treatment. If he is not equipped to meet the standard of other veterinarians in this regard he has but three alternatives: refer the animal to another veterinarian; arrange for access to equipment he does not have; or refuse to treat the animal.

Standards of practice as viewed by the law may be affected by the formal adoption of practice standards. Such standards may emanate from the legislature as part of the practice act; they may be established as regulations of the veterinary examining board; or they may be adopted as bylaws or as part of the code of ethics of a state veterinary medical association. Thus, in a malpractice action there could be presented to the court not only evidence of the standards of the profession generally but the specific standards applicable to the defendant veterinarian.

Veterinarians frequently ask if it is possible to excuse themselves from or at least decrease the likelihood of liability by including in their admission forms statements that they will not be liable for their negligence in treating or caring for animals. Such provisions are termed *exculpatory clauses*, and they do not have a very good record in court. Unless the clause is specific with regard to the action to be excused and unless it can be shown that the client understood its intent and extent, a court is not likely to uphold it. Although a veterinarian was held not liable for the death of an elephant in his care, where the contract for care stated that he would be held harmless ". . . from any liability in the event of the death of the elephant,"[13] this case hardly sets a precedent. The trial court had ruled for the plaintiff elephant owner, and one of the appellate court judges wrote a strong dissent to that court's reversal of the trial court.

INFORMED CONSENT*

The principle of informed consent holds that if surgery is performed or a substantial change in treatment is made without adequately informing the client of the risk and cost involved and without procuring the client's consent, such surgery or treatment is unauthorized and the veterinarian can be held liable in a malpractice action. In such an instance the client's case is not based on an alleged lack of skill or care but rather on a change in the original conditions and understanding that constituted the client-veterinarian contract. The courts have said that the consent must be "informed." If a veterinarian makes a hasty explanation to the client and the change in treatment does not achieve a good result, the client may say, "Yes, I agreed to have you go ahead, but I didn't understand what might happen."

There may be circumstances under which it is impossible to communicate with the client or get his consent about a treatment that the veterinarian regards as essential. In such a circumstance the veterinarian must use his own judgment about what to do and hope that the client agrees. If the client disagrees about what was done and attempts to collect damages, the veterinarian's defense would be that under similar circumstances other veterinarians would have pursued a like course.

It is apparent that failure to establish good communications with clients and particularly to get an informed consent when circumstances indicate has several legal overtones. Among the possibilities are the following:

1. The client may institute a malpractice action claiming that he was not properly informed.

2. The client may refuse to pay the veterinarian's fee.

3. If sued for the fee the client may defend, claiming that there was a lack of informed consent.

4. If the client can show that the veterinarian is of an uncommunicative nature and that other clients have suffered as he claims he did, a request that the veterinarian's license be revoked or suspended might be filed with the state licensing agency.

In human medical cases the physician is frequently confronted with the question of what to do when the patient is unconscious. This has given rise to theories regarding the right of a spouse to make a decision and the authority of other members of the family

when there is no spouse capable of making a decision. Although veterinarians are not confronted with this problem, they may nevertheless be unable to contact a client at a critical time and thus may have to decide for themselves whether additional surgery or additional procedures are so important that they should be implemented without waiting for a client's consent. There may, however, be a question of agency. If a household pet is involved and either the husband or wife can be contacted, the court may find that the veterinarian had a duty to attempt such a contact although he may have dealt with only one of the parties when the animal was received. When animals are in the custody of someone other than the owner (a boarding stable or a kennel, for example), the veterinarian should inquire about the authority of the custodian to procure veterinary services.

In human medicine a physician may attempt to defend his failure to obtain informed consent by saying that full disclosure would, in his opinion, have so upset the patient that more harm than good would have been done or that the patient might then decide against an essential procedure. Although an exact parallel does not exist in veterinary medicine, there are nevertheless owners so attached to a pet that the same argument might be made. The courts have not viewed this as an adequate defense, and a study conducted by the medical profession itself concluded that most patients not only have a right to know but want to know the possible complications regardless of how they may feel. Since risk disclosure is likely to be more traumatic for a human patient than for an animal owner, this defense seems even less plausible for a veterinarian.

A natural result of an increase in malpractice cases based on failure to obtain informed consent is the attempt of hospitals and physicians to obtain consent in advance through their admission forms or through separate consent forms. The legal effect of such waivers is minimal. If they can be made sufficiently specific—after a consultation with the client has indicated the probable course of treatment—they may have some value. But a form that lists in general terms all the things a veterinarian might determine the animal needs, although read and signed by the client, will not excuse liability when the client is in fact not informed about a treatment he had no reason to believe would be necessary.

SOME CAUSES OF MALPRACTICE ACTIONS

Some cases alleging a cause of action against a veterinarian that have reached the appeals court level are listed here for their informative value. In subsequent sections of this chapter reference will be made to additional cases.

1. Suit based on allegation that veterinarian's method of handling a valuable thoroughbred resulted in an undesirable temperament.[14] The court ruled for the veterinarian.

2. Plaintiff alleged that veterinarian gave his horse

---

*Excerpted from Informed consent and consent forms. J. Am. Vet. Med. Assoc. *180*:720, 1982.

an intramuscular injection in the wrong place, resulting in abscess and loss of the horse. The appeals court remanded for further hearing, saying that the trial judge should have admitted expert testimony regarding the proper place to give the injection.[15]

3. Claim of negligence in examining the uterus of a mare.[16] A directed verdict for the defendant veterinarian was affirmed.

4. Action against veterinarian alleging negligent vaccination of pregnant gilts. Jury verdict for the plaintiff was reversed.[17]

5. Action for negligent treatment of Norwegian elkhound puppies. Negligence was not proved.[18]

6. Alleged improper treatment of a dog that had been bitten by a rabid dog. Plaintiff failed to show that veterinarian had not exercised required degree of care and skill.[19]

7. Alleged negligence in the storage and use of hog cholera vaccine and virus. A directed verdict for the defendant veterinarian was reversed.[20]

8. Alleged negligence in handling cattle during vaccination. Judgment for the defendant veterinarian was reversed.[21]

9. Owner of dog counterclaimed for alleged improper treatment of dog in suit by veterinarian for his fee. The court ruled for the veterinarian and disallowed the counterclaim.[22]

10. Alleged failure to properly diagnose and treat hogs for cholera. The plaintiff made his case.[23]

11. Claim for death of sheep caused by improper administration of remedy for intestinal worms. Held for the plaintiff sheep owner.[24]

12. Owner of mule claimed that veterinarian's negligence in confining mule prior to an operation resulted in paralysis and the necessity to destroy. Held for the mule owner.[25]

13. Horse owner sued veterinarian for damages claiming that the latter's advice that horses with nasal gleet should be destroyed was erroneous. The court held for the veterinarian.[26]

14. Alleged erroneous diagnosis and vaccination of hogs for cholera. Held for the defendant veterinarian.[27]

15. Hogs died owing to alleged negligent treatment by veterinarian. Held for the plaintiff.[28]

16. Suit for death of dogs alleged to be caused by improperly prepared mange dip. Held for the dog owner.[29]

STATUTES OF LIMITATION*

State legislatures have determined as a matter of policy that if a law suit is to be commenced it should be within a reasonable period of time after an injury occurs or a cause of action arises. Otherwise memory fades, witnesses die or move away, exhibits disappear, and proof is more difficult to obtain. Accordingly, in every state there are "statutes of limitation" specifying the time period within which particular kinds of actions can be commenced. A customary period for such involving rights in real estate is 20 years; for suits on written contracts, ten years; oral contracts, five years; and torts (civil wrongs involving damage to persons or property), generally three or two years. Some states specify an even shorter period for particular kinds of torts, slander and libel, for example.

When a client sues a veterinarian he must commence his action within the applicable statutory period. To determine what this period is, the law of the particular state must be consulted. But this may not produce a definite answer for three reasons.

Courts from state to state have reached varying conclusions about the nature of a malpractice action— is it based on contract or tort? If based on the former, the longer period for contracts applies.

Some states, to resolve the contract-tort argument, have established a specific limitation period for "malpractice" actions. This is generally a short period, either one or two years. This should benefit veterinarians, but in a recent Ohio Court of Appeals decision the Court held that the Ohio law requiring malpractice actions to be commenced within one year did not apply to veterinarians.[30] The Appeals Court said the law applied only to the professional misconduct of members of the medical profession and attorneys. Although the law was no doubt passed because of the increasing number of human medical malpractice suits, there is no reason why such laws could not also apply to veterinarians.

Probably the most important question regarding the statute of limitations in veterinary medical malpractice cases is *when* the statute commences to run. The Federal Circuit Court of Appeals in deciding a case in Colorado said that the claim commences to run "when the claimant discovers or, in the exercise of reasonable diligence, should have discovered the alleged malpractice."[31] Recovery was denied because the plaintiff knew of his injury in December, 1969, but did not file his claim until July, 1972. Veterinarians and their attorneys should be aware that the statute of limitations may commence to run on a date later than the surgery or treatment giving rise to the injury. This would be true when the plaintiff is not remiss in discovering the cause of the injury at an earlier date.

COUNTERSUITS BY VETERINARIANS*

Lawyers who have successfully defended a malpractice action sometimes institute a countersuit against the losing plaintiff claiming that the suit was brought maliciously and without probable cause.

*Excerpted from Veterinarians and statutes of limitation. J. Am. Vet. Med. Assoc. *162*:267, 1973.

*Excerpted from Malicious prosecution. J. Am. Vet. Med. Assoc. *171*:625, 1977.

Such countersuits are called actions for "malicious prosecution" or "malicious use of process."

The odds in favor of a suit of this kind are not good. It is not a favored action, and in a few states the courts will not entertain it unless there has been an arrest, a property seizure, or some special injury to the defendant. However, in most jurisdictions such a suit can succeed if the facts support it.

The difficulties besetting a plaintiff (the winning defendant in the original suit) are illustrated by a Louisiana Court of Appeals case.[32] A physician sought damages against plaintiff's attorney for embarrassment, discomfort, and lost time. In her petition the physician alleged that she won the case, that the defendant called only two witnesses and they both testified in her favor, that the hospital records showed that four doctors had examined the child and found no damage, that witnesses were not consulted prior to trial, that the attorney could have determined the condition of the patient prior to trial following which there would have been no suit, and finally that it was the duty of the attorney " . . . to refrain from frivolously filing a suit which had no basis in law or in fact."

The Court ruled against the plaintiff because she did not allege and prove malice. Although courts will sometimes imply malice from the evidence brought forth, the court in this case found that such was not implied, saying "At worst the allegation is that defendant went to trial with a poor case and got his just desserts, to wit, he lost. If that constitutes malice, the courtrooms are full of malicious attorneys."

This decision was rendered by a court composed of three judges, one of whom registered a vigorous dissent. Apparently the basis for his dissent was that Louisiana is different from the common-law states in that malice is unimportant and negligence only need be proved, along with proof of lack of probable cause. The dissenting judge said that while the lawyer may be justified in filing the case to escape a statute of limitations, he was not for that reason compelled to go forward with it upon discovering that there was lack of probable cause.

The rule generally throughout the United States is that to maintain an action for malicious prosecution there must be proof of both malice and a lack of probable cause.[33] One without the other is not sufficient. How far a particular court will go in implying malice is uncertain. At least malice should be alleged in the petition. Another point made in this case was that malice should be proved against the plaintiff, not against the plaintiff's attorney.

THE STANDARD OF DIAGNOSIS*

Veterinarians are not held to a standard of perfection in determining what ails an animal. The standard

---

*Excerpted from Diagnosis—What is the standard of care? J. Am. Vet. Med. Assoc. *181*:664, 1982.

of skill and care against which they will be measured in making a diagnosis is the same as that used by the courts to determine if they were negligent in the treatment of an animal. In either case the standard followed by veterinarians generally is the yardstick. And in either case, expert testimony is usually required to determine what this yardstick is.

In an Iowa Supreme Court case,[34] a veterinarian was sued for the loss of 93 hogs out of a total of 137 treated by him. He diagnosed their disease as cholera and vaccinated them. The plaintiff alleged that the veterinarian made an erroneous diagnosis. The Court denied recovery, holding that the alleged improper diagnosis " . . . was at most an error of judgment at a point where there is no guide." However, in a Minnesota case[35] in which the veterinarian failed to diagnose cholera he was held liable in damages to the owner. The facts in that case indicated that the veterinarian may have suspected cholera but did not inform the owner, one of his defenses being that he had been told by the livestock sanitary board that he could not administer serum. The Court stated that inability to administer a particular kind of treatment was no excuse for an inaccurate diagnosis.

A Georgia Appellate Court held a veterinarian not liable for failing to properly diagnose the disease of a dog when he did not see the dog but relied on the owner's description of its condition.[36] However, this case suggests that if the veterinarian has inadequate information it would be legally hazardous to prescribe treatment.

In an early New York State case,[37] a veterinarian failed to recover his fees because the client was able to show that his diagnosis was negligent. The Appeals Court concluded that the trial court, based on the evidence before it, " . . . could properly determine that defendant's horse was suffering from an impaction of the colon instead of inflammation of the bowels and that therefore the plaintiff who prescribed for the latter disease did not exercise a reasonable degree of skill . . . ."

A physician or a veterinarian must at some risk decide how much testing to do and what test to make in arriving at a proper diagnosis. In a Louisiana Court of Appeals case,[38] a physician was held not liable for failure to make a Pap test on a patient who, during his course of treatment, presented no symptoms relating to her female organs. Expert witnesses testified that the physician's treatment did not fall below the requisite standard. This case suggests, however, that if a course of treatment does not help a patient, further exploration is indicated to determine the cause of the patient's illness.

In a Georgia Court of Appeals case,[39] suit was based not on failure to make a proper diagnosis but on an alleged wasting of valuable time performing a diagnosis when the physician and his assistant should have been performing resuscitative procedures to ensure the flow of oxygen and nutrients to the brain of a five-month-old infant who had lapsed into coma and shock. The Court held that there was no liability, thus reaffirming the principle that a doctor will be protected in his judgment about the nature and extent of a diagnosis so long as he does not depart from the standard of his fellow practitioners.

Although it is clear that a veterinarian is not liable for a misdiagnosis unless he is negligent, there are an increasing number of factors to be considered, among them the patient's reaction to drugs or procedures that might be used in making a diagnosis. Failure of a veterinarian to "keep up," to have the equipment regarded as essential to make a proper diagnosis, to refer cases when he is not adequately experienced or equipped to make such a diagnosis, and to acquire as much pertinent patient history as possible could mean liability to an otherwise skillful practitioner.

USING TECHNICIANS AND LAY HELP*

Veterinary practice acts are in agreement on one point: the only persons who can legally practice veterinary medicine in the state are those who hold a "valid and existing license." If the state legislature provides for the certification of "animal technicians," how will it define their "practice" so that it does not violate this prohibition?

Regardless of certification, the courts have held that medical or veterinary medical lay personnel may assist in many ways, providing certain tests are met: that the activity be under the supervision of a licensed professional, that the assistants be skilled and competent to do what they undertake, that they make no decisions that require professional judgment, and that they not hold themselves as licensed veterinarians.

The laws providing for technicians in human and animal medicine require that an agency of the state adopt suitable standards and administer an examination. An educational requirement of some duration, such as two years of college-level work designed for such technologists, is required. Also, the law may attempt to define a "veterinary technician" in terms of what he can legally do. This is likely to mean that the veterinary practice act is amended to state that certain procedures (inoculation and implantations, for example) shall not constitute the practice of veterinary medicine when done by a licensed technician under the supervision of a veterinarian.

Does this narrow the rule that already seems to have been established by common law for lay help? It is not certain. When the law "particularizes," there is always a danger that other reasonable activities may be excluded and the licensed technician thus restricted from carrying out procedures that by common law and without licensing would have been upheld by the courts as not violating the practice act.

Instead of trying to define the particular acts that shall "not be deemed the practice of veterinary medicine," it would be better to use the tests that the courts have developed. This would prevent the assistant from "practicing" by any fair definition of the term but would not prevent the assistant or technician from performing many acts for which he has the competence but that may not have been specifically exempted.

The amount of necessary supervision or control required is a question of fact. The veterinarian does not have to "stand over" an assistant skilled in making injections. On the other hand, it would clearly be a violation of the practice act to send an assistant out on a call or put him in any position in which there is a need to decide what treatment the animal needs. A provision in the regulations developed under the Illinois Veterinary Medical Practice Act states that "Animal health technician means a person . . . qualified . . . to provide veterinary service under the control and direction of a licensed veterinarian. . . . Such veterinarian shall be continuously available to observe and monitor the activities and performance of each technician . . . and for such purpose shall be in sufficiently close proximity to such technician to permit such personal observance and monitoring by such veterinarian." As a practical matter, technicians should be trusted to perform many services without the direct supervision of the veterinarian. Unless this is true the advantage in hiring technicians will be impaired. However, there are and will continue to be activities "on the fringe"; opinions on these activities will differ, and moving too far in the direction of either tighter or looser control will produce undesirable results.

If a technician is permitted to overstep the bounds, the license of his professional employer may be in jeopardy "for having professional connection with . . . any illegal practitioner of veterinary medicine . . . ." This quote is from the section of the Illinois Veterinary Medical Practice Act that specifies causes for revocation or suspension of license. Other states have similar provisions. In a Minnesota Supreme Court case,[40] revocation of a veterinarian's license was upheld when it was proved that he permitted an unlicensed assistant to diagnose and treat a sick mare and divided the fee with him.

It should be noted that the question of illegal practice is an issue distinct from the possible right of a client to recover from the veterinarian because of the negligence of the technician or veterinary assistant. With respect to a veterinarian's civil liability, it does not matter whether the assistant's negligence occurred in the performance of acts that he was legally permitted to perform or whether such negligence occurred with respect to acts that by law, regulation, or court interpretation he was not permitted to perform.

The doctrine of *respondeat superior*, i.e., an employer is liable for damages caused by the negligent

---

*Excerpted from Veterinarians and their employees. J. Am. Vet. Med. Assoc. *164*:682, 1974; and Using animal technicians—Some legal considerations. J. Am. Vet. Med. Assoc. *177*:218, 1980.

acts of his employee while on the job, applies to veterinarians who employ kennel men, laboratory technicians, or other personnel.

This liability exists regardless of the kind of work the assistant performs provided it occurred in the course of duty. If an employee negligently injures someone while driving a car or truck on business; leaves a cage door open and a dog escapes; carelessly mixes feed that proves to be harmful; or injures an animal while making an injection, the veterinarian can be held liable. In a Supreme Court of Wisconsin case, for example, a veterinarian was held liable for the loss of a client's hogs when his son, a veterinary student helping his father during vacation, gave the client a can of creosote instead of a can of mange oil for treatment of the latter's hogs.[41] However, contributory negligence and other common-law defenses would be available to the veterinarian. For example, a plaintiff has the burden of proving not only that his animal was injured but that the employee was negligent and that his negligence was the proximate cause of the injury.

The fact that an employer is liable for the negligent acts of his employee does not bar a suit against the employee. Although the "deep pocket" theory may mean that the professional is the only one sued, anyone else negligently involved may also be sued.

In human medicine, lawsuits against doctors and hospitals are frequently predicated on the alleged negligence of hospital employees. Under what circumstances may a veterinarian be held liable for the negligent acts of assistants who are not employees? There are a number of variables in determining if the veterinarian should be held liable: What was the nature of the act? Was it a procedure for which the assistant was trained and which he would be expected to perform without direct supervision? What degree of skill did the assistant in fact possess, and how much knowledge did the doctor have about his degree of skill? Was there direct supervision and control (as during surgery, for example)?

From medical malpractice cases the courts have constructed a theory of liability based on the idea that surgery is a team or "crew" effort and that the surgeon is the "captain." Hence, any mistakes that occur during this closely controlled procedure are imputed to the doctor in charge—he is the "captain of the ship."

The "captain of the ship" theory, or "concert of action" theory, as it is sometimes called, does not apply during the presurgery and postoperative care periods. Nurses and others must be relied upon to perform certain tasks for which they are skilled with no immediate supervision. The patient's doctor is not liable for the negligence of hospital employees under these circumstances. He may, of course, be liable for their acts if he is personally at fault, e.g., if he fails to give proper instructions or prescribes harmful medications or aftercare procedures. Sometimes the courts use the "borrowed servant" concept. This is simply another way of raising the question of supervision and control.

Although the probability of legal action against a veterinarian for the alleged negligence of nonemployees may not be great, the principles established in human medicine would apply. With an increase in the number, size, and complexity of animal hospitals, similar cases may arise.

Liability to others for the actions of his employees is only one aspect of a veterinarian's legal vulnerability. Another has to do with liability to his employees when they are injured in the course of their employment. If he is subject to the Workmen's Compensation Act of his state, his employees can ordinarily recover for any injury received during the course of their employment. However, the compensation allowable is fixed by law, with limitations on the amount that can be recovered for particular kinds of injuries. Insurance under such a program is mandatory and must be written by companies that qualify under state law.

Whether or not an employer is automatically covered by the Workmen's Compensation Act depends on the particular state law. Agricultural and some other pursuits may be exempt. But even exempt pursuits may be included if the employer elects to come under the Compensation Act. Veterinarians should determine first if they are automatically covered; if not, then they should consider whether or not to elect. If they do not elect, common-law rules of liability apply. This means that an employee is less likely to recover for his injury because certain defenses eliminated by worker's compensation laws may still be made by the employer, the principle ones being that there was contributory negligence or an assumption of risk by the employee and that the injury was caused by a fellow workman. Employees are frequently able to overcome all these hurdles and secure a judgment against their employer. There is no limitation on the amount of damages that can be claimed. Hence, liability insurance is a must.

Under what circumstances are employees likely to seek damages from a veterinarian employer? There is no limit to the factual situations that may lead to a suit. Generally, however, they can be categorized as follows:

1. Failure to repair equipment and keep it safe,
2. Failure to give adequate instructions to employees,
3. Asking or knowingly permitting employees to engage in activities for which there is reason to believe they are lacking in ability and skill, and
4. Asking employees to handle or work with dangerous products or dangerous animals without taking extra care to inform them. (In a Florida Appellate Court case a veterinarian's helper was bitten by a German shepherd dog while assisting him in taking a blood sample from the dog's leg.[42] Although the helper sued the owner of the dog, she could have sued the veterinarian for negligence in relying on the

owner's word that the dog would not bite and thus failing to use a muzzle.)

How can a veterinarian minimize the risk of liability to his employees? Some suggestions follow.

No matter how small the operation or how few employees may be hired, have a safety program and keep it current and viable.

Follow high standards of equipment care and maintenance.

Know your employees, their limitations, and their skills. A physical handicap may indicate that a particular employee should not be asked to do a certain job.

Take extra care to have the employees learn about the products and animals they handle, especially about the possibility of injury to themselves or others.

CONTINUING SURVEILLANCE AND POSTOPERATIVE CARE*

Once a veterinarian has accepted a call a contract arises, and he is then under obligation to give the animal reasonable attention, the amount and kind of attention resting largely with the judgment of the veterinarian. In a New York case a veterinarian was denied compensation for his treatment of a client's horse. In affirming the judgment the higher court said, "The evidence produced by defendant, which the trial judge had the right to believe, showed that plaintiff, being called to treat the animal, and having undertaken its cure, on the day of his last visit—the horse at that time being very ill—agreed to call the next morning early but neglected to ever call again. I think the action of the plaintiff in leaving the animal he had assumed to take charge of in such a dangerous condition and failing again to call according to his promise was such clear negligence as justified the judgment rendered by the trial court."[43] In an action against a veterinarian for negligence in gelding a colt, the Supreme Court of Maine held that, in the absence of special agreement or reasonable notice to the contrary, it was the duty of the defendant to give the colt such continued further attention, after the operation, as the necessity of the case required.[44] The prevailing rule is well stated in the *Cyclopedia of Law and Procedure*: "A physician, responding to the call of a patient, thereby becomes engaged, in the absence of a special agreement, to attend to the case so long as it requires attention . . . and he is bound to use ordinary care and skill . . . in determining when it may be safely and properly discontinued."[45] But if a patient is treated at the office of the practitioner and fails to return for further treatments, he cannot hold the practitioner liable for the consequences.[46] Likewise, if a veterinarian were to treat an animal and prescribe certain things for the owner to do, the veterinarian could not be held liable for any damage resulting from a failure of the owner to follow instructions. On the other hand, a veterinarian may be held responsible, even when animals are brought to him for treatment, if their condition clearly indicates further care and treatment and he fails to instruct the client to leave the animal or return with the animal or does not himself call at the client's premises.

What is the duty of a veterinarian and others who may be assisting him in the treatment of an animal, particularly during surgery, to maintain close observation of the animal so a proper response can be made to changes that occur? Cases arising in human medicine indicate that this duty is considerable. In a United States Circuit Court of Appeals case arising in the District of Columbia, the Court said, "The theory of abandonment presupposes the duty on the part of the physician to remain with his patient until he can properly withdraw. . . . The doctor should not be heard to say, 'Even if I abandoned the patient, how do I know I could have helped if I had stayed?' "[47]

One of the problems in both human and veterinary medicine is the proper monitoring of objects inserted into a patient's body during surgery or, for that matter, during other types of treatment. Sponges and surgical instruments are the usual culprits.

Can a veterinarian be held liable for failure to have the necessary equipment to handle situations that may arise during surgery? Assuming that there is a causal connection between such failure and the damage alleged to have occurred, the answer would depend on what is usual and customary for veterinarians performing surgery to have in the way of facilities and equipment. Such failure could amount to negligence.

With respect to the performance of surgery or other treatment by a veterinarian, the following generalizations seem in point:

Once the patient enters surgery, it should not be left without professional observation until its condition is judged stable.

Since surgery is closely controlled by the veterinarian performing the operation, he may be held liable for the negligence or failure to observe of those assisting him.

To avoid a claim of malpractice or negligence, the veterinary surgeon should have on hand such equipment and materials as might be needed to care for foreseeable events that could arise during surgery. Before commencing surgery, the veterinarian should make a reasonable effort to discover any allergies or reactions that could condition his response to situations arising during surgery.

Many of the complaints against veterinarians arise not from their lack of skill or knowledge in treatment but rather from alleged negligence in caring for an animal while it is in the custody of the veterinarian. Following are some of the complaints that have been registered.

Animals escaping from the veterinarian's clinic.

---

*Excerpted from Monitoring patients during treatment. J. Am. Vet. Med. Assoc. *171*:244, 1977; and Animals in custody—The degree of care required. J. Am. Vet. Med. Assoc. *170*:1286, 1977.

No matter how careful the veterinarian and his employees are, it is possible for an animal to escape. Although there is no absolute liability for an escaped animal, it might be difficult for the veterinarian to refute an allegation of negligence. At any rate, he should have insurance to cover this contingency either as a rider on his malpractice policy or as a separate policy.

Animals injured in cages. From time to time a client complains about loss or injury resulting from his animal's being caught in a cage. Here again, although there is no absolute liability there would be a strong presumption of negligence.

Injuries occurring during handling or restraint. The best assurance that this kind of complaint will not arise is to have well-trained assistants and proper facilities.

Animals injured by other animals. This is always a possibility, even though the veterinarian may use every precaution to keep animals segregated and prevent such an occurrence.

Animals contracting disease. If precautions are not taken to prevent animals with a contagious disease from infecting other animals, liability on the part of the veterinarian could be established.

Unsanitary condition of the premises. Failure to maintain sanitary standards, besides being a possible cause for revocation of the veterinarian's license, may give rise to a claim for damages by a client alleging that failure to maintain such standards resulted in loss or deterioration in the condition of his animal.

Other elements of care, such as those listed in animal welfare acts and having to do with adequate and wholesome feed, clean water, exercise, ventilation, proper temperature, and sufficient space, could very well be the basis for a claim by a client who is able to prove that his animal was injured as a result of failure to meet acceptable standards in these regards.

The amount of aftercare and surveillance necessary in animal hospitals is a matter of professional judgment, and the veterinarian's lapse in this regard could make him liable for malpractice.

ASSISTANCE FROM CLIENTS*

What are the legal implications when a client assists the veterinarian or when he simply observes the veterinarian treat or perform surgery on an animal?

Although there appear to be no American Appellate Court cases involving suit by a client against a veterinarian for damages under these circumstances, there have been suits and threats of suits at the trial court level.

A circuit court in Wisconsin sitting with a jury absolved two veterinarians from any negligence in connection with injury to a client by her cat while the client was holding the cat during administration of a worm pill by the veterinarian.

A local court in Adelaide, Australia, held a veterinarian liable to a client who was holding his cat during an examination. The judge said that permitting the client to expose himself to the risk of injury *without warning* was a breach of duty on the part of the veterinarian.

In her book, *Clinical Aspects of Some Diseases of Cats*, J. O. Joshua states with regard to the danger from cat bites " . . . but a warning must also be given as to the dangers from a bite and the method of holding advisable . . . the veterinarian has an equal public health duty to himself, his clients, and his staff in this respect." In addition to the physical injury that may result, the writer also points out that infection might occur following a cat bite.

In another instance suit was filed by a client who fainted after smelling the ether being used to anesthetize his cat. Apparently this was settled out of court.

What should be the veterinarian's attitude about permitting the client or even asking the client to help? As in all situations involving negligence, the answer must be it depends on the circumstances. To my knowledge there is no law or provision in any practice act that states that a veterinarian should not use the client's assistance. But there are some important considerations. A veterinarian's defense will be strengthened if it can be shown that he warned the client about the possibility of bites, scratches, or other kinds of injury. But a good defense can be built, even if there were no warnings, if it can be shown that:

1. The client is experienced with the kind of animal involved,

2. The veterinarian had no previous knowledge of the animal's temperament,

3. The animal had no defects or diseased or tender spots that would have made it unusually sensitive when held and that the veterinarian knew about or should have discovered,

4. It is accepted custom among veterinarians in the locality (the larger the locality the better, in view of the trend toward exclusion of the "locality rule" by courts in human medicine) for clients to hold their own pets while the veterinarian examines them or administers medication, and

5. The client has held the animal on other occasions while it was being examined or treated.

These principles are applicable whether the animal involved is large or small. Traditionally, large animal owners have been knowledgeable and competent in handling animals and have been expected to assist as a matter of course. But even in these situations, if the veterinarian knows that an animal is particularly dangerous or that the client is likely to faint when he sees blood, he has an additional duty either to warn the client or to dispense with the client's assistance.

A young person with a recently acquired pony or horse and no experience around livestock presents a

---

*Excerpted from Assistance from clients. J. Am. Vet. Med. Assoc. *164*:882, 1974.

different problem from an experienced Four-H member with a club calf. The veterinarian's best defense in these situations must come before the fact, in the veterinarian's consideration of the client's ability and experience, the kind of animal being handled, the nature of the treatment being administered, and other factors that the veterinarian is in a position to appraise and that might indicate that it is either reasonable or unreasonable to use the client's assistance.

Permitting clients, or for that matter other individuals, to witness the treatment of an animal, particularly surgery, also carries some legal hazards. Fainting, nausea, or even "shocking the sensibilities" could lead to the threat of legal action. If the veterinarian pays no heed to those who watch him perform, is unmindful of the effect it might have on observers, or in fact invites such observation, he is legally vulnerable.

Although veterinarians should not "run scared" about using clients to assist—because there are many situations in which this is a reasonable and nonnegligent thing to do—they should keep in mind that any negligence or lack of foresight on their part that might lead to a client's injury can also lead to a damage suit. As the number of a veterinarian's clients increases and relationships become less personal, this danger increases and may lead a veterinarian to decide that as a matter of policy clients should not be permitted to assist in the treatment of their animals.

Although out of considerations of good will a veterinarian is not likely to consider legal action against a client whose negligence in assisting or restraining an animal results in injury to the veterinarian, such an action is possible. In a Missouri Appellate Court case a veterinarian recovered for injuries inflicted on him by a large Airedale when the owner negligently dropped the leash.[48]

EUTHANIZING—THE DEAD ANIMAL*

Does a veterinarian have a right to euthanize a client's animal without the client's consent or to euthanize a badly injured and crippled animal at the scene of an accident as an act of mercy? The answer is no, based on cases that have arisen and on the common law's jealous protection of one's property rights. There undoubtedly are situations in which killing as an act of mercy is justified, but in such circumstances veterinarians have no greater right than lay persons. Any person, including veterinarians, may kill an animal in self-defense or to abate a dangerous threat or nuisance.

This suggests, therefore, that before euthanizing an animal the consent of the rightful owner or authorized agent should be given, preferably in writing on a consent form. When children or several members of a family are involved it is doubly important to determine who has the right to give consent. The question of who has authority may be complicated by livestock-share leases, partnerships, or other forms of cooperative or group ownership.

What discretion does a veterinarian have in disposing of the body of an animal that he has euthanized or that dies on his premises? He has none, unless moving the body from his premises would violate state law or regulations on the movement of an animal that has died of a contagious disease, in which case he could refuse the owner's demand for the body. An owner has a property right to the body and may either remove it or ask the veterinarian to dispose of it.

Whether or not a lien that a veterinarian might have on the animal for board and services persists against the body of a dead animal has apparently not been litigated. The better view would be that it does not persist since the animal has lost its economic value and disposition by incineration, burial, or some other method must be made within a short time. Hence, refusal to yield the body to a client might be regarded as a punitive act rather than a sound collection procedure.

The veterinarian should properly identify the animal to be euthanized. Destroying the wrong one could result in two malpractice suits. This is not a fanciful or impossible occurrence, just as performing an operation on the wrong patient has not been wholly precluded in human hospitals.

The death of an animal under treatment or following surgery creates no presumption that the veterinarian was at fault, and he is entitled to recover in full for his services.

Public veterinarians have the authority to destroy or order the destruction of diseased animals when they proceed in accordance with valid laws or regulations.

What is the veterinarian's right to perform a necropsy? Although the reasons for obtaining consent before doing a necropsy on an animal may not be as compelling as when a human body is involved, such consent should nevertheless be obtained. The body belongs to the client, and the veterinarian should at least assure himself that the client does not object. There may be circumstances in which a necropsy is necessary: to perfect a claim under an insurance policy or to determine the presence of a communicable animal disease, for example. In the latter case the law may require a necropsy.

What is the legal position of a veterinarian who, after being requested to euthanize a dog or other animal, keeps the animal and disposes of it in some other way? This is a violation of the owner's contractual rights. Furthermore, it could possibly give rise to other legal complaints, fraud and a suit for punitive damages, for example.

Communication with a client becomes especially

*Excerpted from Property rights in animals—Postmortems. J. Am. Vet. Med. Assoc. *163*:1352, 1973; and Euthanasia—Some legal aspects. J. Am. Vet. Med. Assoc. *168*:32, 1976.

important when euthanasia is contemplated. The client may be in an emotional condition that makes it more difficult to explain clearly the veterinarian's assessment of an animal's condition. "Informed consent" takes on additional meaning, and failure to show that it was given leaves the veterinarian vulnerable even though he may have performed without fault.

Before destroying an animal, the veterinarian should ask the client about livestock insurance. If an animal is insured, the policy will contain provisions regarding destruction. If these provisions are not followed the insurance may be voided. Issues regarding coverage when an animal is destroyed have arisen on several occasions when horses have been insured. But other valuable animals, including small animals, may be insured, so the question becomes important. Although the veterinarian would not be liable to a client for euthanizing an animal under circumstances that voided the insurance, he would be rendering a service to the client by raising the question before the animal is destroyed.

CORPORATE INSULATION—HOW REAL?*

Until state legislatures adopted laws permitting the incorporation of doctors, lawyers, veterinarians, and other professionals, American courts held that since it is impossible for a corporation, being an artificial person, to take an examination and qualify as a professional, these professionals could not incorporate. Among the arguments made by the courts in support of this view was one that held that the professional-client relationship can exist only between natural persons and that nothing should be permitted to interfere with any rights of the client that might grow out of such a relationship. Hence, incorporation acts for professionals, when finally adopted by state legislatures, contained language making it clear that the professional-client relationship was not to be disturbed by the presence of a corporation. For example, the Illinois Act provides:

It is the legislative intent to provide for the incorporation of an individual or group of individuals to render the same professional service or related professional services to the public for which such individuals are required by law to be licensed or to obtain other legal authorization while preserving the established professional aspects of the personal relationship between the professional person and those he serves professionally.[49]

When a member of a professional corporation has been negligent and a malpractice action is commenced, who can be sued? Obviously the individual himself may be sued, even in the absence of a provision such as that contained in the Illinois legislation, which states as a matter of law that a professional relationship exists between the treating professional and the client. But can other members of the

corporation be sued and can the corporation be sued? Two cases, one arising in Indiana and one in Illinois, speak definitively on this point. Fortunately, the cases are in accord.

In the Indiana case a malpractice action was brought against the treating physician who was a member of a medical corporation and also against other physician members of the corporation. The Court had no difficulty finding that an action would lie against the treating physician, saying:

It is thus apparent that our legislature intended that the IMPCA (Indiana Medical Professional Corporation Act) should not destroy the traditional relationship between a professional and his patient through the creation of a corporate shield . . . the malpracticing physician is liable to the extent of his personal assets and such malpractice insurance as he or the corporation may possess. In addition it is beyond question that the corporate entity is liable for malpractice committed by one of its members.[50]

Thus we have a statement of what appears to be sound law, namely, that a corporation itself is liable for the act of its members or agents and that the negligent member or agent may also be liable, but the corporation does shield other members who were not involved in the alleged negligent act. The Illinois Court reached the same conclusion, saying:

Under both acts (the Medical Corporation Act and the Professional Corporation Act), a physician-shareholder has the same privileges and liabilities as a shareholder of any other Illinois corporation. In this state a shareholder, officer, director, agent, or employee of a corporation is insulated from personal liability for the tortious acts of the corporation and its officers, agents, employees and shareholders in which he does not participate and resultant injuries to which he does not contribute.[51]

In view of these court decisions, of the language in the professional corporation acts, and of the traditional theory that the corporation insulates innocent members from acts of negligent members, the position of members of a professional veterinary corporation or veterinary professional association would be precisely the same as that of the physicians involved in these two cases.

A harder question has to do with the liability status of a professional member who may have assisted or been involved with the member against whom a claim of negligence is made. Does it matter if the one who assisted was himself negligent in any way or can he be held liable simply because he participated? It is likely that, by an extension of the "captain of the ship" doctrine or "concert of action" theory, he could also be held liable regardless of personal negligence. It should be noted that although other professionals not involved cannot be sued for the malpractice of one, the corporate assets can be reached. This means, therefore, that the corporation itself as well as its individual members should be insured.

An additional observation is in order. It is well

---

*Excerpted from Malpractice and the professional corporation. J. Am. Vet. Med. Assoc. *175*:888, 1979.

known that in professional partnerships all of the partners may be held liable for the malpractice of any one, the theory being that each is an agent for the other. Attorneys for the losing parties in the previously mentioned two cases made similar arguments with respect to the members of a professional corporation, saying that there is just as much reason for vicarious liability among members of a professional corporation as there is among members of a partnership. It is just possible that another court in another case may agree with this point of view.

PUNITIVE DAMAGES*

Pet owners have been allowed to recover more than compensatory damages for the loss of or injury to a pet alleged to have resulted from the negligent treatment of a veterinarian. Such additional damages are referred to as "punitive." The objective in awarding them, so the courts say, is to discourage the reckless, malicious, or grossly negligent conduct of the defendant. In a sense the awarding of such damages amounts to civil "punishment." Compensatory damages, on the other hand, are simply to make the injured party whole by paying for the value of the loss and any additional expenses incurred because of the loss.

In addition to compensatory or punitive damages, a court may also award a client damages for "pain and suffering" or "mental anguish." A classic example of an award for mental anguish is *La Porte v. Associated Independents Inc.*[52] decided by a Florida Appeals Court. In that case a garbage collector, without any reason, threw a garbage pail at a miniature dachshund, causing it to expire. The owner, who was in her kitchen when the event occurred, rushed out in time to hear the collector laugh and depart. In overturning a lower court decision denying punitive damages, the Florida Court of Appeals upheld a $1,000 verdict. The Court, among other things, said:

The restriction of the loss of a pet to its intrinsic value in circumstances such as the one before us is a principle we cannot accept. Without indulging in a discussion of the affinity between "sentimental value" and "mental suffering," we feel that the affection of a master for his dog is a very real thing and that the malicious destruction of the pet provides an element of damage for which the owner should recover irrespective of the value of the animal.

How does a holding such as that in the *La Porte* case affect veterinarians? If the courts in a particular state are willing to award punitive damages or damages for mental anguish, a veterinarian guilty of the required degree of culpability could be required to pay such damages. There is early precedent for such a holding. In an 1855 Alabama Supreme Court case, *Parker v. Mise*, the Court said:

In addition to actual damages the owner of a dog may be entitled to recover punitive damages if the defendant's actions contain some element of wantonness or maliciousness.

Volume 1, *American Law Reports Third* (page 997), summarizes cases involving this question. According to this summary, courts in Iowa, Kentucky, Michigan, New York, Texas, and Vermont have said that punitive damages are allowable for damage to or loss of a pet. However, courts in Alabama (apparently the 1855 decision has been overruled), New York, Louisiana, Missouri, New Mexico, and Texas have said that sentiment is not recognized as an element of damage.

In *Levine v. Knowles*,[53] a case that was in and out of the courts over a period of years, a Florida Appellate Court finally ruled that a summary judgment for the veterinarian must be reversed. It ordered a retrial on the plaintiff's claims for both compensatory and punitive damages. In that case a toy Chihuahua died while undergoing apparently routine treatment for a skin condition. The owner instructed the veterinarian to retain the body. However, employees of the veterinarian cremated the body before it could be reclaimed. The defendant veterinarian admitted receiving the owner's instructions but said that the body had been cremated by "unknown employees." In its opinion the Court said: "The change of form does not deprive the owner of title to or right of possession of property."

The Court further said that if compensatory damages " . . . are too lenient for admonitory purposes or if the payment of compensatory damages only would not handicap the defendant sufficiently to discourage such conduct in the future . . . " then punitive damages should be awarded. In discussing the conduct that gives rise to an award of punitive damages the Court said it must be " . . . willful, wanton, reckless, malicious, or oppressive. . . . "

In a more recent Florida case decided in 1978, *Knowles Animal Hospital v. Wills*,[54] a dog was placed on a heating pad in its cage following an operation. It was given no care or attention for more than a day. As a result it was severely burned, complications developed, and it had to be destroyed. Suit was brought against the animal hospital and the veterinarian, the plaintiff alleging gross negligence. He asked for compensatory damages and damages for physical and mental pain and suffering. The trial court ruled in favor of the veterinarian but against his hospital with a judgment of $1,000 compensatory and $12,000 punitive damages. This was upheld on appeal. The Court cited the *La Porte* and *Levine* cases and said: " . . . on the evidence the jury could and no doubt did view the neglectful conduct which resulted in the burn injury to the dog to have been of a character amounting to great indifference to the property of the plaintiff such as to justify the jury award."

In summary, it can be said that if treatment by a veterinarian is sufficiently reprehensible the courts

*Excerpted from Pet owners and punitive damages. J. Am. Vet. Med. Assoc. *179*:224, 1981.

in many states will allow punitive damages. However, some courts that allow punitive damages will not allow damages for mental anguish. Whether or not there can be such a recovery in a particular jurisdiction depends on the courts and not on statutory law. To my knowledge there are no state statutes defining situations in which punitive damages or damages for mental anguish should or should not be allowed.

There are a limited number of American jurisdictions that allow recovery by third parties who suffer emotional distress when under the circumstances the defendant could have foreseen this result. Thus, if a veterinarian were to handle or treat an animal in what the law would describe as an "outrageous manner" in the presence of bystanders, especially children or persons who the veterinarian should realize are particularly sensitive or emotionally disturbed, a cause of action would exist in some jurisdictions. The law, however, has been slow to accept an interest in peace of mind as entitlement to independent legal protection, even as against intentional invasions. Various reasons have been advanced for this reluctance to redress purely mental injuries. One such reason is the difficulty of proof or measurement of the damages. Another objection to protecting such an interest lies in the difficulty of containing or restricting such actions to bona fide claims when emotional distress has been truly severe. One court said, "Once the tort of outrage is recognized, the doors of the courts are opened wide, not only to fictitious claims but to litigation in the field of trivialities and mere bad manners."

There are two threshold requirements for recovery: the defendant's conduct must in fact be extreme and outrageous, and the emotional distress suffered by the plaintiff must be extreme and real. At least one court has said that an action for emotional distress will not be sustained when it arises from witnessing injury to property. In that case the plaintiff witnessed an attack on her poodle by a St. Bernard, as a result of which the poodle died.[55] The court did not mention distinctions that could be made between animate and inanimate property, a distinction that has been recognized by many courts in phrases such as "the affection of an owner for his pet is very real."

Any veterinarian who views good client relations as an important aspect of his practice and who does not make public displays of his own temper or emotions should not find himself a defendant in an emotional distress case.

THE VETERINARY SURGEON AS AN EXPERT WITNESS*

Expert testimony is that which is needed to inform the jury and the court about things they would not otherwise be able to fully understand. It is testimony concerning some principle or procedure in a specialized area of learning such as medicine, veterinary medicine, engineering, or any one of a number of scientific disciplines.

Expert testimony is not needed if the point in question is one on which a layman is able to pass judgment. Many things "speak for themselves," and the law has coined a Latin phrase, *res ipsa loquitor*, to characterize these kinds of things. Typical are sponges or surgical instruments left in an incision, removal of the wrong organ, or physical damage resulting from the way in which a patient is handled. Some of the circumstances in which expert testimony from a veterinarian is likely to be required follow:

1. To determine the cause of death of an animal,
2. To determine the cause and exact nature of injury to an animal,
3. To determine if there is "incurable suffering" justifying destruction of an animal under an insurance policy that will pay for voluntary destruction only if there is such suffering,
4. To determine whether a veterinarian has made an illegal use of lay help, or
5. To testify regarding the standard of skill and care required by a fellow veterinarian in a malpractice case.

A veterinary surgeon cannot be compelled to testify as an expert, but if he was involved in a case he can be compelled to testify as a witness of fact.

The party calling the veterinarian must qualify him as an expert by examination in open court. The opposing party has a right to cross-examine. An expert witness may charge for his services as much as the party calling him is willing to pay. It is implied that he will study the case and prepare himself with guidance and information from the attorney for the party calling him. His demeanor on the witness stand should be firm but respectful. Only the questions asked should be answered. The cross-examining attorney may try to "needle" him. This will be evident, and the witness should respond by controlling his feelings, asking for a clarification of questions if required, and by all means not trying to respond in kind to an approach that is obviously meant to irritate him.

In a case that involves explanation of an injury, charts and visual aids may be used to help the jury and judge understand the nature and cause. During preparation for trial the attorney should describe to the expert witness the "courtroom scene" and should supply him with all the information that is available. If asked to give a deposition the expert should be informed and prepared and should conduct himself in the same manner as for an appearance in court.

GOOD SAMARITAN LAWS*

American courts have said that one who volunteers to help in an emergency or at the scene of an accident

*Excerpted from The veterinarian as an expert witness. J. Am. Vet. Med. Assoc. *181*:444, 1982.

*Excerpted from Veterinarians as Good Samaritans. J. Am. Vet. Med. Assoc. *169*:198, 1976.

is at most required to exercise the skill and care usually bestowed by like persons under like circumstances; that to hold otherwise would discourage the "kindly offices" that should be rendered to those in need. Nevertheless, many state legislatures have passed statutes that provide that one who renders such kind offices shall not be liable for ordinary negligence. These are known as Good Samaritan laws.

Some Good Samaritan laws are for the benefit of anyone who stops to help; others apply only to specified professionals in the health field. The Illinois law, for example, is a limited one applying only to physicians, dentists, and nurses "who in good faith provide emergency care without fee to a victim of an accident at the scene of an accident or in case of nuclear attack . . . ." Policemen and firemen are accorded similar protection. There is no reason why veterinarians should not be included in such limited laws.

The counterpart of such a law of special significance to veterinarians is an "animal Good Samaritan law," which states that if a veterinarian renders emergency aid to an animal without expectation of a fee and other than at the request of the owner he will be liable only for gross negligence. Illinois has such a law.

VETERINARY MEDICAL RECORDS*

In view of the increase in litigation in veterinary medicine, the importance of records kept by the veterinarian is evident. That they should be made promptly and should be complete and accurate perhaps sounds "old hat" and to a busy veterinarian may seem like a useless waste of energy. However, winning one law suit because good records were kept could more than justify the extra expense of having them well done on a daily basis.

By definition, the medical record includes all information that a veterinarian might compile about a client's animal. Laboratory reports and x-rays are a part of this record, along with any notes made by attendants, professional or otherwise, who under the direction of the veterinarian have any connection with the animal. The value of such records as evidence is increased by the ability of the veterinarian to show that they are regularly made, that they were done promptly in the course of his professional business, and that a standard form is used to make sure that different kinds of basic information are recorded. It is also helpful to show that there is a systematic method of filing and maintaining files and of determining retention periods. Particularly important are records of consent to change in treatment or to surgery when such was not contemplated at the beginning of treatment.

Are veterinarian-client communications privileged? According to the Iowa Supreme Court they are not. In *Hendershot v. Western Union Telegraph Co.*,[56] a veterinarian was not required to answer certain questions because the lower court held that his communications with his client were privileged. The Supreme Court of Iowa reversed this finding, saying that a veterinarian is not in the same position as a physician regarding privileged communications. Although there may be rare exceptions to this holding, it probably represents the law generally and would be followed in other states.

Although veterinary medical records may not enjoy the privileged status of human medical records, they are nevertheless the property of the veterinarian. They should be carefully and promptly made for the protection of both the veterinarian and his client and should not be disclosed to anyone but the client except with the client's consent or a court order. If suit is threatened, the records should be retained until the threat is resolved by a law suit (plus the appeals period) or by the statute of limitations. If there is a possibility that the records might be used for research or historical purposes, they should be retained and catalogued in such a way as to make them useful.

MALPRACTICE INSURANCE*

Assuming that all practicing veterinary surgeons carry professional liability insurance, questions arise about the coverage of such insurance and about the veterinarian's role when a malpractice suit is threatened.

Unless a malpractice policy has a rider or language in the policy specifically covering nonprofessional negligence, it does not protect the veterinarian against such negligent acts as permitting an animal to escape or damaging a client's property while on the client's premises. Also, policies should be checked to make certain that they cover the liability that may derive from the acts of the veterinarian's employees and agents. There are special requirements when one is a partner, generally that all partners and the partnership itself be insured.

When sued, how does the veterinarian decide whether to settle or defend? Ordinarily he will be guided by the advice of his insurer. There are pros and cons on both sides. Any settlement, however small, even though there is clearly no malpractice, creates the impression that the veterinarian did something wrong. On the other hand, defending a claim, no matter how strong the case for the veterinarian, involves time and expense and, even more important, the risk that the judgment will go against the veterinarian even if the claimant's case is a poor one. Settling regardless of the fault of the veterinarian

---

*Excerpted from Veterinary medical records. J. Am. Vet. Med. Assoc. *166*:137, 1975.

*Excerpted from Malpractice—Settle or defend? J. Am. Vet. Med. Assoc. *165*:36, 1974.

could lead to a belief on the part of the public that the standards of the veterinary profession are lower than they really are and also to more claims, since fault on the part of the veterinarian would appear to be unimportant. Despite cost, loss of time, and risk involved, cases should be defended when there is clearly no negligence on the part of the veterinarian.

The courts in American jurisdictions have varied in their opinions regarding the liability of a malpractice insurer to pay punitive damages. Although the language in an insurance policy may in some instances be decisive, there are courts—including the Federal Courts—that hold that it is against public policy for an insurer to come to the rescue of a professional who has conducted himself in such a manner as to cause a court to award punitive damages.

1. Morris, W. O.: *Veterinarian in Litigation.* Veterinary Medical Publishing Co., Inc., Bonner Springs, KS, 1976.
2. Hannah, H. W., and Storm, D. F.: *Law for The Veterinarian and Livestock Owner,* 3rd ed. Interstate Printers & Publishers, Inc., Danville, IL, 1974.
3. *Black's Law Dictionary,* 4th ed. West Publishing Co., St. Paul, 1968.
4. *State v. Rich,* 339 N.E.2d 630 (S.C. of Ohio 1975).
5. *State of Oregon v. Sam Won,* 528 P.2d 594 (1974).
6. 72 A.L.R. 3d 1253.
7. *Black's Law Dictionary.*
8. In *Ruden v. Hansen,* 206 N.W.2d 713 (1973), the Supreme Court of Iowa said: "we have omitted reference to the veterinarian's duty 'in the neighborhood or vicinity' . . . because we no longer approve that limitation. The standard of care practiced in the particular community or like communities may be one of the elements to be considered but it is not conclusive. We are convinced the correct standard of the veterinarian's care should be held to that exercised generally under similar circumstances."
9. 21 Ruling Case Law 657.
10. *United States v. Russell and Tucker,* 95 F.2d 684 (1938).
11. *Brown v. State Board of Examiners in Optometry,* 263 N.W.2d 490 (S.C. of S.D., 1978).
12. *Helling v. Carey,* 519 P.2d 981 (S.C. of Wash. 1974); *Robbins v. Footer,* 553 F.2d 123 (D.C. Cir. Ct. of Appeals 1977).
13. *Elephant, Inc. v. Hartford Accident & Indemnity Co.* 216 So.2d 837 (La. App. 1968); *Elephant, Inc. v. Hartford Accident & Indemnity Co.,* 239 So.2d 692 (La. App. 1970).
14. *Southall v. Gabel,* 293 N.E.2d 891 (Ohio 1972).
15. *Spilotro v. Hugi,* 417 N.E.2d 1066 (Ill. App. Ct. 1981).
16. *Posnien v. Rogers* 533 P.2d 120 (S.C. of Utah 1975).
17. *Supra,* note 8.
18. *Dyess v. Caraway,* 190 So.2d 666 (La. Ct. of App. 1966).
19. *McNew v. Decatur Veterinary Hospital,* 68 S.E.2d 221 (1951).
20. *Kinney v. Cady,* 4 N.W.2d 225 (S.C. of Iowa 1942).
21. *Breece v. Ragan,* 138 S.W.2d 758 (K.C. Ct. of App., Mo. 1940).
22. *Smith v. Quayle,* 14 N.Y.S.2d 741 (S.C., App. Div., N.Y. 1939).
23. *Bekkemo v. Erickson,* 242 N.W.617 (S.C. of Minn. 1932).
24. *Erickson v. Webber,* 237 N.W.558 (S.C. of S.D. 1931).
25. *Beck v. Henkle-Craig Livestock Co.,* 88 S.E.865 (S.C. of N.C. 1916).
26. *Carroll v. Bell,* 15 West. Law Rept. 327 (Canada 1910).
27. *Phillips v. Leuth* 204 N.W.301 (S.C. of Iowa 1925).
28. *Hohenstein v. Dodds,* 16 N.W.2d 236 (S.C. of Minn. 1943).
29. *Kerbow v. Bell,* 259 P.2d 317 (S.C. of Okla. 1953).
30. *Supra,* note 14.
31. *Casias v. U.S.,* 532 F.2d 1339 (C.A. 10, Colo. 1976).
32. *Spencer v. Burglass,* 337 So.2d 596 (1976).
33. *Supra,* note 32.
34. *Supra,* note 27.
35. *Supra,* note 23.
36. *Supra,* note 19.
37. *Boom v. Read,* 23 N.Y.S. 421 (1893).
38. *Lambert v. Michel,* 364 So.2d 248 (La. Ct. of App. 1978).
39. *Moore v. Carrington et al.,* 270 S.E.2d 222 (Ga. Ct. of App. 1980).
40. *In Re Walker's License,* 300 N.W.800 (S.C. of Minn. 1941).
41. *Acherman v. Robertson,* 3 N.W.2d 723 (1942).
42. *Wendlund v. Akers,* 356 So.2d 368 (1978).
43. *Supra,* note 37.
44. *William v. Gilman,* 72 Me. 21 (1880).
45. 30 C.Y.C. 1573.
46. *Dashiell v. Griffith,* 35 A. 1094 (S.C. of Md.).
47. *Ascher v. Gutierrez,* 533 F.2d 1235 (U.S. Ct. of App., D.C. 1976).
48. *Brune v. Debenedetty,* 261 S.W. 930 (Mo. App.).
49. Ill. Rev. Stat. ch. 32, §415–2 (1981).
50. *Birt v. St. Mary Mercy Hospital of Gary, Inc.,* 370 N.E.2d 379 (Ind. Ct. of App. 1977).
51. *Fure v. Sherman Hospital,* 371 N.E.2d 143 (Ill. App. Ct. 1977).
52. *LaPorte v. Associated Independents, Inc.,* 163 So.2d 267 (Dist. Ct. of App., Fla. 1964).
53. *Levine v. Knowles,* 197 So.2d 329 (Fla. App. 1967).
54. *Knowles Animal Hospital v. Wills,* 360 So.2d 37 (Fla. App. 1978).
55. *Roman v. Carroll,* 621 P.2d 307 (Ct. of App., Ariz. 1980).
56. *Hendershot v. Western Union Telegraph Co.,* 79 N.W.2d 828 (S.C. of Iowa).

Section **II**

Surgical Biology

Alan J. Lipowitz
Section Editor

Chapter 2 Tissue Regeneration

Alan J. Lipowitz

Tissue repair is the formation of nonfunctional scar tissue preceded by an inflammatory reaction in which all mediators of inflammation participate. In contrast, tissue regeneration is influenced by growth-regulating factors that foster the replacement of lost tissue with normal, functioning cells.[24] Obviously, regeneration is the ideal method for healing a tissue gap; repair is the second best method.

Certain tissues have the capacity to regenerate, some do not; those that can may not always do so. Whether regeneration or repair occurs depends primarily on the type of tissue and the extent of the defect, the duration and repetition of the trauma causing the defect, and the tissue's ability to overcome the acute irritation so that chronic inflammation and granuloma formation do not occur.

The relationship between the degree of differentiation and the regenerative capacity of tissues is well known; neurons, well-differentiated cells, never divide, central nervous system defects being replaced by glial scar; so-called less-differentiated cells, such as the basal cells of the epidermis, actively divide and reproduce themselves.[24]

Tissues may be categorized according to their mitotic capacity as renewing, expanding, and static.[6] Renewing tissues have a continuously active subpopulation of dividing cells from which functioning cells are recruited. These functional end cells have a limited life span. Hematopoietic cells and epithelial cells, such as those lining the small intestine and those of the epidermis, belong to this category.

In expanding tissue, cell division is more limited; cells still retain their mitotic ability, but a subpopulation of continually active mitotic cells is absent. Mitosis occurs during normal growth and development; in mature tissue the original volume of tissue mass is maintained by the replacement of dead cells. Liver and bone belong in this category.

Cells of static tissue do not have the ability to divide; once lost, these cells cannot be replenished. Neurons are composed of cells of static tissue.

Tissue regeneration, a form of growth, is distinct from hypertrophy and hyperplasia. Hypertrophy is an increase in organ volume, the result of an increase in the volume of individual cells; theoretically the number of cells remains constant as the size of the organ increases. In hyperplasia an increase in organ volume results from an increase in cell numbers. Hypertrophy is frequently an adaptive phenomenon, the stimulus being mechanical in nature, such as cardiac ventricular hypertrophy as seen with the increased pulmonary resistance of patent ductus arteriosus. Hyperplasia is frequently seen in renewing tissues and, in particular, in those tissues under the direct influence of hormones such as the prostate, endometrium, thyroid, and pancreatic islet cells. Hyperplasia, by definition, is only possible in renewing or expanding tissues; it is frequently combined with hypertrophy.[24]

Regeneration and hyperplasia are both associated with active mitosis and therefore have similar mechanisms for the production of new cells; however, the stimulus for each may be different. Regeneration begins with tissue loss or damage and is preceded by the classical inflammatory reaction associated with tissue trauma. Hyperplasia does not occur in response to trauma and is not usually preceded by inflammation. It is a normal phenomenon, e.g., endometrial hyperplasia occurring with estrus or the pathological changes such as thyroid hyperplasia seen in response to excess thyroid-stimulating hormone.

The well-being of individual cells and their ability to divide depend to a great extent on the influence and activities of various chemical mediators. The function of some, such as thyroid-stimulating hormone, are reasonably well understood. Other "growth-stimulating factors" have been identified; in some cases their role or importance is not yet appreciated. Chalones are tissue-specific mitotic inhibitors.[3, 19, 24] At proper concentrations they prevent continuous or excessive cell division. A decrease in the local concentration of chalone occurs in wounded tissues; therefore there is less inhibitory effect on cells. Cell mitotic rate then increases. Although much investigation and evidence support the existence of chalones, their chemical structure is not known. The nature and precise mechanisms of chalone production, release, transport, and action on target cells also are yet to be determined.

Steroid and polypeptide hormones, poietins, and many other factors with potential influence on tissue regeneration and repair are continually being recognized, including vitamins. Autocoid mediators are formed within the tissues they influence and have a limited radius of action; important variations in tissue concentrations may not be accurately reflected in the plasma. They are secreted by platelets, monocytes, fibroblasts, polymorphonuclear leukocytes, and other cells of the healing wound.[3] Many of the substances have been identified only in laboratory animals, or their influence has been shown *in vitro*. Nonetheless, their actions are real. Whether these substances have clinical relevance remains to be determined. Table 2–1 lists several mediators that stimulate connective tissue growth.[3]

Although renewing and expanding tissues have the capacity to heal by regeneration, this does not occur unless conditions are favorable. Assuming that the intrinsic controlling mechanisms of cell replication are intact, the choice between healing by repair and regeneration is primarily influenced by extrinsic factors. The type of initiating agent and the chronicity of its effects affect tissue healing. An irritant (etiological agent) that is easily neutralized during the

TABLE 2–1. Factors Stimulating Growth or DNA Synthesis in Connective Tissue*

Substance	Source	Target Cells
Connective tissue–activating peptide III (CTap)	Platelets (human)	Synovium, cartilage, dermal fibroblasts (human)
Primate factor	Platelets (primate)	Arterial smooth muscle, dermal fibroblasts (primate)
Ctap-PMN	Polymorphonuclear leukocytes (human)	Synovial fibroblasts (human)
Somatomedin B and C	Plasma (human)	Human glial cells, embryonic lung cells; cartilage (rat)
Tumor angiogenesis factor	Tumor cells	Host capillaries
Nerve growth factor	Submaxillary gland (mouse)	Sympathetic nerve ganglia

*Modified from Castor, C. W.: Autocoid regulation of wound healing. *In* Glynn, L. E. (eds.): *Tissue Repair and Regeneration*. Elsevier-North Holland, Amsterdam, 1981.

very early inflammatory stages of healing will have no adverse effect on the progression of healing by regeneration. For instance, lesions such as bacterial infection of bone cause cell death and, therefore, loss of bone substance. If the host defense mechanisms can overcome the infection in a relatively short period of time, the events of normal bone healing (i.e., regeneration) are not disturbed. However, if the irritant cannot be overcome a chronic inflammatory reaction occurs and some lost tissue is replaced by fibrous scar, as seen with a sequestrum involucrum.

The environment of the damaged tissue can influence the path between regeneration and repair. Motion at a fracture site prevents or delays healing by regeneration; indeed, a fibrous nonunion may result. The nonunion may be perceived as a failure to heal; however, at the cellular level a "healing process" has occurred even though the organ's function was not restored.

Other environmental influences include the immunological status of the host and the chemical and hormonal factors that stimulate cell activity. Cells with the intrinsic capacity for regeneration may be prevented from carrying out this healing process unless the proper biochemical and immunological milieu is established.

All adult tissues are derived from the embryologically distinct ectoderm, mesoderm, or endoderm.[18] Some organs, such as the intestine, are compound, being derived from endoderm and mesoderm. The embryological origin of tissues offers little information regarding the derivation of renewing, expanding, or static tissues of the adult. Neurons, derived from ectoderm, are static; dermal epithelium, which is renewing, is also of ectodermal origin; the liver, which has miraculous regenerative properties, is of endodermal origin. Bone is classified as an expanding tissue with the ability to regenerate under the appropriate conditions; fascia, which, like bone, is of mesodermal origin, does not regenerate but heals by fibrosis and scar formation instead.

Continued differentiation of embryologically similar tissues eventually produces tissues that have lost their capacity for replication, but their ability to heal has not been lost. How, why, and at what point during embryological maturation and tissue differentiation certain tissues lose their capacity to regenerate are not known. It is well known that not all animals lose tissue regenerative capacity; this depends on the stage of organ development and the level of phylogenetic sophistication. Recently, it has been learned that even genetically elevated mammals, including humans, may have the intrinsic capacity for regeneration; the expression of this regenerative capacity is related to the local environment of the area of tissue loss.[2]

REGENERATION OF SELECTED TISSUES

Skeletal Muscle

Cellular mechanisms of skeletal muscle regeneration are still not entirely understood. Currently two theories are in favor.[17, 28] The first suggests that new muscle fibers develop from myotubes that have budded from injured muscle fibers, their new nuclei being formed by mitosis. Myotubes are smaller than muscle cells; the muscle myofibrillar system is synthesized within these multinucleated cells. The second and more recent theory suggests that when mononuclear muscle precursor cells are formed, the cells multiply by mitosis and subsequently fuse, forming myotubes from which muscle fibers develop. The growing evidence suggests that these precursor cells are probably derived from satellite cells.[17, 29] Satellite cells are structurally undifferentiated cells that lie between the basement and plasma membranes of skeletal muscle.[15] The term *myoblast* is used for those cells that can be shown by immunofluorescence and electron microscopy to contain skeletal muscle myofibular protein such as myosin and organizing myofibers.[28] The sequence of cellular events in muscle fiber regeneration, incorporating both theories, is depicted in Figure 2–1.[28]

Skeletal muscle does have the capacity to regenerate in the sense that transected fibers heal together, reconstituting the normal histological appearance of the muscle. It is uncertain whether regeneration occurs when there is a loss of significant muscle fiber

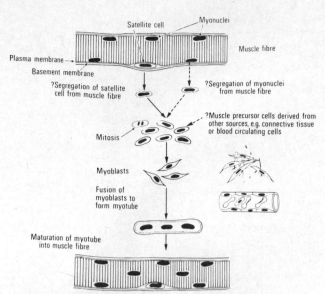

Figure 2–1. Theories of skeletal muscle regeneration involving muscle cell precursors (myoblasts). Myoblasts are supposedly derived from satellite cells, segregated myonuclei, connective tissue cells, or circulating cells. Muscle precursor cells multiply, fuse, and form multinuclear myotubes that mature into muscle fibers. (Reprinted with permission from Sloper, J. C., and Partidge, T. A.: Skeletal muscle: regeneration and transplantation. Br. Med. Bull. 36:153, 1980.)

mass. The regenerative healing of transected muscle fibers, like the healing of long bone fractures, can be delayed or even prevented if substances are interposed between the transected ends or if the distance between the transected ends is too great. Skeletal muscle regeneration studies have been conducted on muscles that have been burned or frozen in a relatively narrow band perpendicular to the long axis of the muscle and on muscle that has been incompletely transected perpendicular to its long axis.[17] Although such studies reveal a great deal about muscle fiber regeneration and reconstitution of muscle mass, they do not mimic the clinical situation seen when muscle mass transection produces large gaps between the transected ends or the loss of large amounts of muscle mass seen with shearing injuries of limbs. Such injuries may result in a fibrous union between the transected ends of muscle rather than muscle fiber regeneration.[11]

Muscle regeneration is affected by denervation. Recent denervation (one to two weeks) has little effect on regenerative healing capacity, although all muscle fibers become thinner owing to denervation atrophy. If denervation atrophy precedes muscle fiber injury, the regenerative response is significantly decreased. Muscle that has been denervated for long periods of time loses its regenerative capacities, healing by fibrosis instead.[17]

Smooth Muscle

In studies using visceral and vascular smooth muscle, cells grown in culture pass through stages of dedifferentiation and then redifferentiation into spontaneously active cells. Initially, there is a period of contractile activity immediately after plating; this is followed by a period of cell division or proliferation during which the cells no longer contract or have the appearance of smooth muscle cells. Finally, the cells redifferentiate into well-defined smooth muscle cells that contract spontaneously.[5]

Regeneration of functionally normal visceral smooth muscle has been studied for some time. In several studies, re-formed urinary bladder wall, following partial and total cystectomy in rabbits and dogs, contained smooth muscle fibers.[10, 12, 26] The source of regrowth of the bladder wall components was believed to be either the small portion of remaining bladder following resection or undifferentiated cells that produce muscle tissue by induction or budding. In more recent studies in the dog involving healing of cystotomy incisions and alloplastic replacement of partially resected urinary bladder, no smooth muscle fiber regeneration was found.[8, 9]

Regeneration of the urinary bladder has been regarded by some as the exception to the general principle that only tissues, and not compound organs, can regenerate. Uroepithelium has great regenerative properties. If a mold stent is placed in the proper position and intermittent storage and expulsion of urine continued, a fibrous storage sac lined by uroepithelium forms. Regeneration and cell-for-cell reconstitution of the bladder following subtotal cystectomy do not occur. The sac, which may indeed act as an effective bladder, results from a combination of epithelial regeneration, synthesis and remodelling of fibrous scar, hypertrophy and some proliferation of smooth muscle, and stretching of the bladder remnant. Regeneration of urinary bladder smooth muscle probably does not occur.[19]

Gastrointestinal tract wounds heal in a manner similar to that seen with urinary system wounds. The epithelium of the stomach, duodenum, small intestine, and colon regenerates rapidly, covering defects or incisions. The underlying muscular layers to not regenerate but heal by fibrous protein reconstitution.[1, 19]

Liver

Regeneration of the liver and reconstitution of liver mass following partial hepatectomy are well known. Histological and biochemical studies of liver resection in dogs have shown that repair and regeneration begin within 12 hours following resection, reaching peak activity by three days.[4] Six weeks following removal of 70 per cent of the liver, the regenerated and reconstituted liver attains 83 per cent of its estimated preoperative weight.[13] A startling feature of liver regeneration following partial resection is that the entire remnant participates in the regenerative process, unlike other tissues in which the repair and regenerative processes are confined to the margin from which the transected portion was removed.[17] As the original volume is reached, the regenerative processes cease. This suggests that liver regeneration is under the control of chalones; regeneration occurs as a result of the abolition of normal inhibition of cellular activity rather than a stimulation of these cells.[24] In addition, the influence of portal blood flow and, in particular, the pancreatic contribution to portal blood are critical in the maintenance of normal liver size in the dog and the regenerative capacity of the liver. In a portal blood flow diversion model it was found that lobes of normal liver receiving portal blood from the pancreas maintained their size and weight, whereas lobes of the same liver not receiving pancreatic portal blood but an equal quantity of portal blood atrophied.[14]

The histological appearance of the regenerated liver varies, assuming the characteristics of fetal liver in some areas and those of normal adult liver in others.[13, 19] Liver function tests, including serum bilirubin, alkaline phosphatase, SGPT, SGOT, total protein, albumin, and bromsulphthalein (BSP) retention, are, as expected, significantly altered by 70 per cent liver resection. Each parameter returns to near normal levels, although with varying speed.[13] During active liver regeneration the intrahepatic biliary ducts also proliferate. The epithelial lining of the biliary tree can readily migrate and undergo mitosis. New intrahepatic ducts are formed by budding and penetration between parenchymal cells.[17]

Epithelium and Endothelium

The lining cells of hollow viscera and the superficial cells of exposed surfaces are in a continual renewal process. Although the normal rate of replacement varies with location, these cells are replaced with ones identical to those lost. This is continuous regeneration.

Epithelial replacement is well understood. The processes of mobilization, migration, and mitosis of cells at the periphery of a lesion are the same, regardless of whether the lesion is of the cornea or the gallbladder. However, full thickness lesions of compound organs heal according to the characteristics of intrinsic regenerative capacities of each tissue layer. Consider the small intestine following an end-to-end anastomosis. The epithelial lining of the mucosa covers the anastomotic site in a very short period of time, mainly by the regeneration of new epithelial cells and the migration of those at the periphery of the incision.[1, 19] The serosal surface, the visceral peritoneum, also reconstitutes itself to cover the anastomotic site. The new mesothelial covering is derived mainly from subperitoneal fibroblasts.[23] Only the muscular layers fail to regenerate. However, the muscular layers heal by fibrous union rather than by replacement of lost tissue.[1, 19]

Peripheral Nerves

In most body systems regeneration involves the replacement of lost cells and the restoration of bulk or continuity. A different situation exists in the nervous system. During fetal development nervous tissue develops from the mitotic proliferation of neuronal precursors; once neuronal differentiation is achieved, mitotic activity ceases. Once the adult nervous system is fully developed, the capacity for mitosis is lost forever.[25] New nerve cells cannot be formed, unlike cells in other systems. Repair and regeneration can only be accomplished by the regrowth and re-organization of damaged neuronal processes. Should the cell body be injured, all is lost.

Injuries to peripheral nerves are classified according to their severity.[22] Neuropraxia is the mildest form of injury. It is a reversible acute disruption of impulse transmission most likely due to transient microvascular ischemia associated with mild but reversible morphological changes. Physical disruption of one or more axons without injury to the stromal tissue is axonotmesis. In this injury the axoplasm and cell membrane of the axon are damaged but the Schwann cells and supporting connective tissues remain intact. Neurotmesis is complete severance of all elements of a peripheral nerve trunk; physical continuity is lost and proximal and distal nerve trunk segments are created. The regenerative activities of the proximal and distal segments are very different.

As with other tissues, the regenerative capabilities of peripheral nerves vary with the type and extent of injury and the local tissue environment. The ability of an injured nerve to regenerate following injury depends on the degree of continuity remaining in the nerve trunk. Neuropraxic lesions have a greater chance of regeneration than axonotmesic or neurotmesic lesions because the supporting structures and Schwann cells remain intact, maintaining continuity of the trunk structure.

The healing or continuity restoration of a severed peripheral nerve relies on the normal slow flow of axoplasm from the cell body along the axon.[17, 22] Cutting an axon leads to a spilling out of axoplasm. Following peripheral nerve transection, the cell body undergoes several visible as well as chemical changes. The nucleus moves to an eccentric position, the cell body swells, and intracytoplasmic organelles change in their staining characteristics. The last-mentioned change is called chromatolysis and is due to the transformation of RNA into a more active molecular complex needed for nerve regeneration.[19] Retraction of both the proximal and distal nerve stumps occurs owing to the action of elastic fibers within their supporting structures. Degeneration of the proximal stump occurs for a distance of two to three nodes of Ranvier from the site of injury. Schwann cells assume a phagocytic role, aiding in the removal of degenerating axon, myelin fragments, and other cellular debris.[17, 19]

The distal stump undergoes wallerian degeneration.[17, 19] Distal stump degeneration proceeds most rapidly in unmyelinated fibers and least rapidly in those with thick myelin sheaths. Separated from the nurturing flow of axoplasm, the distal segment of a transected nerve quickly loses its histological conformation. Within four to five days axoplasm and myelin have degenerated. The injury site is invaded by inflammatory cells, and the accumulation of degenerating myelin in phagocytes gives rise to "foam cells," which are a histological feature of wallerian degeneration.

Successful regeneration of a transected peripheral nerve is measured by the return of neurological function distal to the point of transection. Two features, among many, that deserve mention because of their importance in nerve continuity restoration are neuromas and axial re-alignment of individual axons and axon bundles.

Neuromas at the distal end of the proximal segment may be an impediment to restoration of continuity. They are composed of a microscopic mesh work of fibers upon which migrating axoplasm travels distally.[19] Migrating axons follow regenerating Schwann tubules; the orientation of the Schwann tubules is dictated to a significant degree by the alignment of the fibrin mesh work. If the Schwann tubules cannot align themselves with the proximal end of the distal segment, axonal migration across the gap is inhibited. In addition, extraneural connective tissue proliferation at the site of transection may also inhibit axonal migration by altering the fiber orientation of the scaffold for Schwann tubule alignment.

The first sign of regeneration after transection is an outflow of axoplasm from the cut end of the proximal nerve fiber. New axoplasm is transported by migration from its site of synthesis in the cell body to the area of injury. Outflow may begin as early as several hours following injury. Sprouting or branching axoplasmic outgrowths may also appear from the proximal cut end. These misguided axons and axonal branches caught in a labyrinth of connective tissue proliferation form a neuroma. Extension of the Schwann cell tubules and other connective tissue elements provides the initial reconnection between the proximal and distal stumps of a transected peripheral nerve.[22] As mentioned, the migrating axoplasm follows the lead of the Schwann cells.

Axonal migration across the site of transection and down the distal segment occurs, assuming there is no impediment to axonal flow. The connective tissue union between proximal and distal stumps should assure restoration of continuity. The key to a clinically successful outcome is the return of as many axons as possible to their original position within the distal segment. In crush injuries endoneural sheaths are intact and axons grow down their own sheaths and eventually regain their original peripheral connections. In a transected nerve united by scar or sutures, axons grow randomly down the endoneural sheaths. The chances of a motor fiber reaching its original

end-plate are remote.[17] The probability of original fiber–original end-plate reunion is reduced to some degree by axonal sprouting.

The growth rate of the regenerating axon varies according to the species studied, the time of study following injury, the type of injury to the axon, and the location within the axon where regeneration rate is being measured. The growth rate curve of animals appears to be linear (i.e., the velocity is constant), whereas that of humans is curvilinear with a gradual deceleration. Growth rate in animals ranges between 1 and 3 mm per day.[17, 22]

Motor end-plates and sensory endings undergo degeneration following axonal transection. Neurogenic muscle atrophy also occurs if reinnervation is not established in a short period of time. After cutting motor nerves, the nerve endings degenerate and are phagocytized by Schwann cells. Axon growth proceeds along the re-established pathways in the distal segment of a transected nerve to make contact with former synaptic junctions. Studies have shown that re-innervation occurs at previous myoneural junctions. That is, under ideal conditions topographically precise muscle re-innervation occurs, with over 90 per cent of the original synaptic sites once again activated. Although the re-activation of original end-plates may be high, their connection rate to original axons is low.[16]

Appendages

The ultimate achievement of tissue regeneration may be the nearly complete replacement of amputated appendages by certain amphibians. First recorded in 1768 by Spallanzani,[7, 27] many questions still remain regarding this seemingly miraculous biological feat.

Regeneration of amputated appendages in amphibians is dependent on many factors: ambient temperature, season of the year, size of the appendage, and age and species of the animal.[27] Repeated studies have shown the following: (1) the resulting regenerated parts never achieve the full size of the portion removed, even after one year; (2) repeated regeneration follows repeated amputation; (3) appendages regenerate independently of other amputated appendages in the same animal; (4) restricted diet affects regeneration rate but not the capacity to regenerate; (5) regenerating tissue is continuous with that of the amputation stump; and (6) the level of amputation is critical to the development of regeneration; high amputations produce little or no regeneration.[27]

It is important to note that not all amphibians have the capacity for limb regeneration. Certain types of adult frogs have varying capacities for limb regeneration. In addition, some animals may be able to regenerate one appendage and not another. For example, tail regeneration occurs following amputation in certain lizards, but forelimb regeneration does not; limbs of tadpoles regenerate faster and more anatomically correctly than do the limbs of the adult frogs they are destined to become.[20, 21, 27]

It is not the intent of this chapter to review in detail the intimate cellular, biochemical, and other physiological events of amphibian appendage regeneration. Suffice it to say that, following amputation, the regenerating limb passes through three recognizable but overlapping phases.[27] Each is grossly distinct and reminiscent of embryogenesis. The preblastemic phase begins immediately following amputation. Within 24 hours the wound is covered by migrating epithelium, beneath which a substantial inflammatory response is occurring. This phase of acute inflammation lasts for approximately 15 days, to be followed by the blastemic phase, which is recognizable by its smooth conical outgrowth of the already growing limb bud. This conical protuberance may be the most critical stage in amphibian limb regeneration, for it is the advanced blastema that serves as the basis for subsequent new limb morphogenesis. On about the twenty-sixth day the broad-based conical or oval pointed blastema begins to flatten dorsoventrally, evolving into the so-called paddleform regenerate. Thus begins the phase of morphogenesis and differentiation. In the adult newt the paddleform stage rarely lasts more than two days, at which time a groove becomes visible, signaling the formation of digits. All four digits do not form simultaneously; the fourth appears much later than the first and requires more time to develop to a useful size. The final result approaches, but seldom equals, the original lost limb. This may be a function of time, however, as observations of limb regeneration have rarely exceeded one year after the original amputation. Nevertheless, the regenerate is unequivocally a new limb, in every way as functional as the original.[27]

After more than two centuries of study, the exact cellular mechanisms of appendage regeneration are still not known. Among the still unanswered questions is whether each individual tissue type transected at amputation produces cells responsible for its own regeneration or whether one precursor cell arises from which all tissues are derived. There is little doubt, however, that a dedifferentiation of cells occurs at the site of amputation. It is believed that one of the differences in cellular response following appendage amputation in mammals and amphibians is the loss of tissue or cellular ability for dedifferentiation at the site of transection in mammals.[6, 7, 20, 21, 27] Another difference is the rapid development of cicatrix formation over the amputation stump in mammals.[2, 27] This does not occur in animals that have appendage regeneration capabilities. Following amputation in mammals and amphibians, there is surface epithelial migration across the amputation site. In the mammal, collagen deposition, scar tissue formation, and epidermal migration (wound contraction) begin to cover and close the open wound. In the amphibian neither epidermal migration nor scar tissue formation occurs. Rather, beneath the conical cap of the blastema, cellular dedifferentiation and tissue restoration occur.

It is not accurate to describe mammals as being entirely devoid of appendage regenerative capacity. Neonatal mice and opossums do have the capacity for digit regeneration, if experiments are conducted within several days after birth, and if the level of amputation is not very high. Indeed, it was recently shown that adult mice replace amputated tips of their foretoes when the amputation is distal to the last interphalangeal joint.[2] Also, regrowth of the very tips of human fingers has been reported, but only when the amputation stump was treated by debridement and dressings without surgical intervention. If the amputation surface is closed, a stump results.[2]

Regeneration of tissue is an obviously complicated and astounding physiological process. The nearly accurate replacement of structures that are no longer present brings forth a great many questions and an equal amount of wonder. Healing (i.e., replacement) of bone or liver is more easily understood. One type of tissue is involved and an orderly progression of events is known, beginning with identifiable precursor cells and ending with a reconstitution of lost mass identical or nearly so to that which was lost. Appendage and, in particular, limb regrowth, with the many different tissues involved; and the regrowth of bones and joint surfaces, muscles and nerves, and lymphatics and blood vessels rival a biological event that is even more amazing, i.e., embryogenesis following ovum fertilization.

 1. Bellenger, C. R.: Comparison of inverting and appositional methods for anastomosis of the small intestine in cats. Vet. Rec. 110:265, 1982.
 2. Borgens, R. B.: Mice regrow the tips of their foretoes. Science 217:747, 1982.
 3. Castor, C. W.: Autocoid regulation of wound healing. In Glynn, L. E. (ed.): Tissue Repair and Regeneration. Elsevier-North Holland, Amsterdam, 1981.
 4. Francavilla, A., Porter, K. A., Benichou, J., Jones, A. F., and Starzl, T. E.: Liver regeneration in dogs: morphologic and chemical changes. J. Surg. Res. 25:409, 1978.
 5. Garfield, R. E.: Regeneration of smooth muscle: ultrastructure and multipotential properties of smooth muscle. In Mauro, A. (ed.): Muscle Regeneration. Raven Press, New York, 1979.
 6. Gross, R. J.: The strategy of growth. In Teir, H., and Rytomaa, T. (eds.): Control of Cellular Growth in Adult Organisms. Academic Press, New York, 1967, pp. 3–27.
 7. Gross, R. J.: Principles of Regeneration. Academic Press, New York, 1969.
 8. Hansen, O. H., Rasmussen, F., and Hansen, J. P. H.: Alloplastic replacement of the partially resected urinary bladder in dogs. Scand. J. Nephrol. 8:7, 1974.
 9. Hastings, J. C., Van Winkle, W., Jr., Barker, E., Hines, D., and Nichols, W.: The effect of suture materials on healing wounds of the bladder. Surg. Gynecol. Obstet. 140:933, 1975.
10. Hinman, F., Jr., Cox, C. E., and Ayres, R. D.: Smooth muscle regrowth in experimental defects in bladder tubes. Invest. Urol. 1:45, 1963.
11. Jones, D. S.: Effects of various incisions on the rectum abdominis muscle (abstract). Anat. Rec. 103:473, 1949.
12. Kretschmer, H. L., and Barber, K. E.: Regeneration of

bladder following resection: preliminary report on an experimental study. JAMA 90:355, 1928.

13. Mackenzie, R. J., Furnival, C. M., O'Keane, M. A., and Blumgart, L. H.: The effect of hepatic ischemia on liver function and the restoration of liver mass after 70% partial hepatectomy in the dog. Br. J. Surg. 62:431, 1975.

14. Mathie, R. T., Leiberman, D. P., Harper, A. M., and Blumgart, L. H.: The role of blood flow in the control of liver size. J. Surg. Res. 27:139, 1979.

15. Mauro, A.: Satellite cells of skeletal muscle fibers. J. Biophys. Biochem. Cytol. 9:493, 1961.

16. McMahan, V. J., Edgington, D. R., and Kuffler, D. P.: Factors that influence regeneration of the neuromuscular junction. J. Exp. Biol. 89:31, 1980.

17. McMinn, R. M. H.: Tissue Repair. Academic Press, New York, 1969.

18. Patten, B. M., and Carlson, B. M.: Foundations of Embryology, 3rd ed. McGraw-Hill, New York, 1974, pp. 132–143.

19. Peacock, E. E., Jr., and Van Winkle, W., Jr.: Wound Repair, 2nd ed. W. B. Saunders, Philadelphia, 1976.

20. Polezhaev, L. V.: Loss and Restoration of Regenerative Capacity in Tissues and Organs of Animals. Harvard University Press, Cambridge, 1972.

21. Polezhaev, L. V.: Organ Regeneration in Animals: Recovery of Organ Regeneration Ability in Animals. Charles C Thomas, Springfield, 1972.

22. Raffe, M. R.: Principles of peripheral nerve repair and regeneration. In Newton, C. D., Nunamaker, D. (eds.): Textbook of Small Animal Orthopedics. J. B. Lippincott, Philadelphia, 1984.

23. Raftery, A. T.: Regeneration of parietal and visceral peritoneum: a light microscopic study. Br. J. Surg. 60:293, 1973.

24. Roels, H.: Hyperplasia versus atrophy—regeneration versus repair. In Glynn, L. E. (ed.): Tissue Repair and Regeneration, Vol. 3. Elsevier-North Holland, Amsterdam, 1981.

25. Scaravilli, F., and Duchen, L. W.: Regeneration in the central nervous system. In Glynn, L. E. (ed.): Tissue Repair and Regeneration, Vol. 3. Elsevier-North Holland, Amsterdam, 1981.

26. Schiller, H.: Regeneration of resected urinary bladders in rabbits. Surg. Gynecol. Obstet. 36:24, 1923.

27. Schmidt, A. J.: Cellular Biology of Vertebrate Regeneration and Repair. University of Chicago Press, Chicago, 1968.

28. Sloper, J. C., and Partridge, T. A.: Skeletal muscle: regeneration and transplantation studies. Br. Med. Bull. 36:153, 1980.

Chapter **3**

Wound Healing

Curtis W. Probst and Ronald M. Bright

INTRODUCTION

A wound is a bodily injury caused by physical means resulting in disruption of the normal continuity of structures. Wound healing is the restoration of continuity. The biological processes of wound healing include cell regeneration, cell proliferation, and collagen production. Higher animals possess limited regenerative capabilities; therefore, epithelial, endothelial, and fibroblastic proliferation with collagen production replaces regeneration. These events occur in an orderly fashion, beginning with wounding, and continue for several months (Fig. 3–1).

The response of tissue to injury forms the foundation of all surgical practice. Unfortunately, because wound healing represents such a basic response of living tissue to injury, the biology of repair is taken for granted. An understanding of the biology of wound healing is essential to the surgeon so that he can minimize any adverse consequences and use these processes for the patient's benefit.

STAGES OF WOUND REPAIR

The Inflammatory Stage

Regardless of the nature of the injury, the body's response is basically the same. The immediate response to injury is vasoconstriction of the small vessels in the area of the wound. Actual vascular occlusion occurs at the point of trauma, tending to control hemorrhage. This response lasts five to ten minutes and is followed by active vasodilation. This vasodilation involves all elements of the local vasculature.[19–22, 25, 34, 35, 43–45]

As vasodilation occurs, fluid having the same composition as plasma and containing enzymes, proteins, antibodies, and complement begins to leak from the venules. This fluid leakage occurs before any cells leave the affected vasculature and in the absence of obvious gaps in the vessel walls. Increased vascular permeability, which is actually confined to small venules, soon occurs and is the key to all subsequent inflammatory events. This increased vascular permeability may be caused by histamine; however, serotonin and kinins are also involved. The major source of histamine is the mast cell; however, histamine is also found in platelets. Serotonin is also released from mast cells, and kinins are released from α_2-globulin of plasma. The action of these amines results in swelling or "rounding" of vascular endothelial cells, creating gaps between these cells. The basement membrane is not visibly affected. This effect is short-lived. Prolongation of the inflammatory reaction occurs owing to prostaglandins in the presence of complement.[19–21, 34, 43, 45]

Fragile lymphatics are usually more severely damaged than the vasculature. Fluid leaking from the venules provides fibrinogen and other clotting elements, which form fibrin clots. These fibrin clots quickly plug the damaged lymphatics, preventing drainage from the injured area. Thus, the inflammatory reaction is localized to an area immediately

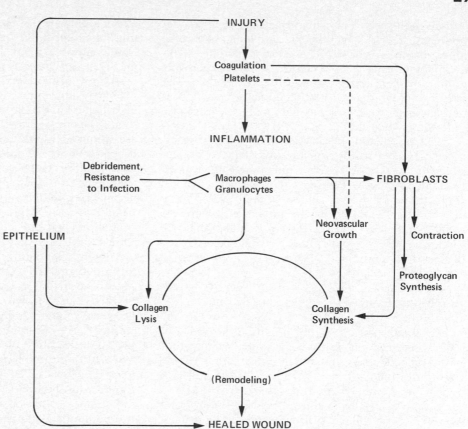

Figure 3–1. Schematic diagram of wound healing. (Reprinted with permission from Hunt, T. K., and Van Winkle, W., Jr.: *Fundamentals of Wound Management.* Appleton-Century-Crofts, 1979.)

surrounding the injury. Eventually, activation of fibrinolysin relieves the obstruction and lymphatic drainage resumes.[19–21, 34, 45]

Soon after injury, leukocytes in the local vasculature become "sticky" and adhere to the endothelium. Within 30 to 60 minutes, the entire endothelium of local venules may be covered with adherent leukocytes, which begin to move through the gaps in the vessel walls and eventually concentrate at the site of injury. Initially, the predominate cell is the polymorphonuclear leukocyte (PMN), whose primary role is the destruction of bacteria. As the PMNs degenerate and die, their outer membranes rupture and release enzyme-containing granules. These enzymes are released and attack extracellular debris. In clean wounds, PMNs are soon superseded by monocytes. At one time, it was thought that the PMNs migrated first and were followed later by the monocytes. However, careful studies have shown that the migration of these cells is in the same proportion as that which occurs in the peripheral blood. The PMN is short-lived compared with the monocyte; therefore, the monocyte predominates in older wounds.[19–21, 25, 34, 43–45]

Monocytes are essential for wound healing. Circulating monocytes originate from precursor cells found in the bone marrow. Upon entrance into the wound, they become macrophages, which phagocytize necrotic tissue and debris. Monocytes may coalesce to form multinucleated giant cells, which are also phagocytic. Monocytes may also evolve into epithelioid cells and histiocytes. The persistence of mononuclear cells at the site of injury indicates the presence of foreign material that granulocytes have been unable to dispose of. Once the acute inflammatory reaction subsides, local vascular permeability is restored and blood cells cease to pass into the extravascular space. If an inciting agent is still present in the wound, mononuclear cells undergo local proliferation, characteristic of chronic inflammation, and respond to the continued presence of foreign material, including bacteria.[19–21, 34, 35, 45]

Macrophages precede the onset of fibroplasia during wound healing and might even regulate the process. Macrophages can be activated by products of activated lymphocytes (lymphokines), immune complexes, and a complement cleavage product. This activation results in several specialized responses, including enhanced lysosomal enzyme activity, increased secretion of proteases, released complement components, production of interferon, secretion of endogenous pyrogen, formation of tissue thromboplastin, and synthesis of prostaglandins. These cellular responses are important because several of these enzymes, such as proteases, help remove foreign material from the wound, while complement aids in combating infection and tissue thromboplastin facilitates hemostasis. There is good evidence that macrophages release a chemotactic substance that not only attracts mesenchymal cells to the area but also influences their differentiation into fibroblasts.[10, 19–21, 34–36, 45]

Lymphocytes are also found at sites of inflammation. Both T- and B-lymphocytes are found in chronic inflammatory reactions. These are important in inflammation caused by bacteria but are relatively unimportant in inflammation caused by trauma. The presence of lymphocytes in inflammatory reactions is perhaps indicative of some immunological response to foreign material.[34, 45]

Local vasodilation, leakage of fluid into the extravascular space, and lymphatic occlusion are responsible for the classic signs of inflammation: redness, swelling, and heat. Pressure, and perhaps chemical stimulation, produces the fourth sign—pain.[34] The duration and intensity of the inflammatory process are dependent on the severity of trauma;[19–21, 24, 34, 45] therefore, the surgeon must strive to keep tissue damage to a minimum.

The Repair Stage

The repair processes begin almost immediately after wounding and continue as rapidly as necrotic tissue, blood clots, and other debris are removed from the wound.[19–21, 34, 45] PMNs are the first cells to appear in numbers in the wound. The PMN is important to wound healing if sepsis is present, as wound healing will not proceed until the infection is under control. In the absence of infection, however, wound repair proceeds normally in the complete absence of granulocytes. Macrophages normally appear in the wound, phagocytize dead cells and debris, and perform normally in all respects. Fibroblasts also migrate into the wound and deposit collagen normally.[34, 35]

Macrophages, however, are essential for normal wound repair. If monocytes are prevented from migrating into the wound, the appearance of fibroblasts is delayed, and those that are eventually seen are immature. The amount of collagen laid down is reduced. The primary functions of active macrophages are disposal of necrotic tissue, removal of foreign material, and, although the exact mechanism is not understood, attraction of fibroblasts and perhaps influencing them to undergo maturation and collagen synthesis.[10, 19–21, 34, 35, 44]

Experiments with antilymphocyte serum indicate that lymphocytes, like granulocytes, are not essential for wound healing. Wounds in humans receiving large doses of antilymphocyte serum following organ transplantation heal normally.[34]

Fibroblastic Phase

The term *fibroblast* is used to describe the cell actively engaged in the production of connective tissue matrix, in contrast to its dormant phase as a fibrocyte. The origin of wound fibroblasts is controversial. It was initially thought that white blood cells served as progenitors for fibroblasts in healing wounds; however, it has not been possible to verify this hypothesis. Present evidence indicates that wound fibroblasts are derived from local mesenchymal cells, particularly those associated with blood vessel adventitia.[19–21, 25, 34, 35, 44]

Shortly after injury, undifferentiated mesenchymal cells begin to change into migratory fibroblasts. As soon as necrotic tissue, blood clots, and other debris are removed by granulocytes and macrophages, fibroblasts move into the injured area. In the initial inflammatory response, the inflammatory exudate contains a considerable amount of fibrinogen, which is converted to fibrin by the release of enzymes from blood and tissue cells. This fibrin is laid down in the wound and acts as a hemostatic barrier and a framework for other elements of repair.[19–21, 25, 34, 35, 44]

Although migrating fibroblasts seem to use the fibrin network as a scaffold, whether or not the fibrin strands provide orientation or contact guidance is still debated. However, there is a close association between migrating fibroblasts and the fibrin network.[19–21, 34, 44] Fibroblasts move by forming a cytoplasmic extension called a ruffled membrane, which extends from the cell and adheres to a solid substrate (e.g., fiber or capillary). The cell then moves in the direction of the ruffled membrane. When the ruffled membranes of two like cells meet, the cells adhere to one another and movement ceases. This process is called contact inhibition. Cell edges free of cellular contact continue to form ruffled membranes, and the cells move in the direction of ruffling.[25, 34, 45]

Although fibrin appears to provide a scaffold for fibroblast migration, large amounts of fibrin may interfere with cell migration of not only fibroblasts but epithelial cells as well. Fibroblasts do not contain fibrinolytic enzymes but, when migrating into a wound, are closely followed by new capillaries. New capillaries are formed by endothelial budding and are a prominent feature of new granulation tissue. The endothelial cells of these new capillaries contain a plasminogen activator. Thus, as new capillaries grow into a wound immediately behind the fibroblasts, fibrinolysis occurs and the fibrin network is broken down and removed. If large hematomas, necrotic tissue, or bacteria are present in a wound, the migration of fibroblasts and the formation of new capillaries are blocked. In uncomplicated wounds, debris is usually removed by the third to the fifth day, and fibroblasts and new capillaries invade the entire wound.[19–21, 25, 34, 45]

After the fibroblasts have entered the wound, they secrete protein polysaccharides and various glycoproteins that make up the ground substance. Mucopolysaccharides of the ground substance surround the fibroblast and influence the aggregation and orientation of collagen.[19–21, 34, 35, 45] Collagen is synthesized by the fibroblasts from hydroxyproline and hydroxylysine beginning on about the fourth or fifth day. The polypeptide chains of these proteins, in the form of three separate alpha helices, are joined together by disulfide bonds. These are passed into the Golgi vesicles before being secreted into the extracellular environment as procollagen molecules. Two endopeptidase enzymes are required for the complete conversion of procollagen to collagen fibrils. As young collagen fibrils bond together, collagen fibers are formed and the collagen becomes less soluble. The collagen bundles are small but gradually enlarge to form dense collagen that binds the edges of the wound. [15, 19–21, 25, 34, 35, 45]

Several factors control and finally lead to the cessation of collagen production. Native collagen is remarkably resistant to the action of most proteolytic enzymes; however, denatured collagen is completely digested by such enzymes. [13] There are specific collagenases that can cleave native collagen into fragments that are denatured at body temperature. The denatured fragments can be completely digested by proteases. [16] Collagenases are produced by epithelial cells proliferating at the wound edge and by fibroblasts coming in contact with new epithelial cells. [15, 19–21, 34, 35, 45]

The fibroblastic phase of wound healing lasts two to four weeks, depending on the wound. As the collagen content of a wound increases, the glycoprotein and mucopolysaccharide content and synthesizing fibroblast numbers decrease. Capillaries begin to regress, and the rate of total collagen synthesis decreases and eventually balances the rate of collagen destruction. [19–21, 34, 35, 45]

Epithelialization Phase

Epithelialization, proliferation, and migration are the first signs of repair and occur before any new connective tissue has been formed in the wound. The initial response of cells immediately adjacent to a wound is mobilization. These cells must detach from their substrate and prepare for migration. Normally, epidermal basal cells adhere to each other and to the underlying layers of the dermis. The exact nature of these adhesive forces is not known. It is thought that some readily hydrolyzable protein is involved in all adhesions because cell attachment can be severed by treating living tissue with trypsin. It is possible that such a proteolytic enzyme is released from damaged cells or leukocytes and is involved in cell mobilization. [19–21, 30, 34]

Following mobilization, epithelial cells enlarge and begin to migrate down and across the wound. The main regenerative activity occurs in the marginal basal cell layer. Transected hair follicles also contribute to the number of migrating epithelial cells. Migrating epidermal cells appear to move by rolling or sliding over one another. Isolated cells move randomly if the substrate on which they are placed is not oriented. Epithelial cells migrating across a wound usually move across the rest of the basal lamina or along fibrin deposits. This phenomenon is called contact guidance and is an important factor in epithelial migration. As with fibroblasts, the migrating epithelial cells stop moving when they come in contact with a like cell ("contact inhibi-

tion"). [19–21, 25, 30, 34, 45] Cell migration plays an important role in epithelial repair, as increased mitosis of epidermal cells is not usually observed until one to two days after restoration of epidermal continuity when the migrating cells have reached their final positions and ceased to move. [5]

The stimulus for increased mitotic activity has not yet been defined. Normally, mitosis in epidermal epithelium has a diurnal rhythm, being most active during sleep and least active during wakefulness. Wounding abolishes the diurnal mitotic rhythm in cells immediately adjacent to the wound and results in an absolute increase in mitotic activity. This increased mitosis led investigators to postulate the release of a wound hormone that directly stimulates cells to divide. Attempts to isolate such a substance have been unsuccessful. Recent evidence suggests that a water-soluble, heat-labile substance known as "chalone" controls mitosis. This substance seems to require epinephrine to be effective and may exist as an epinephrine-chalone complex. It is normally present in the epidermis and seems to inhibit mitosis. When tissue is damaged, the concentration and production of "chalone" fall and a decreasing concentration gradient exists from normal tissue to the edge of the wound, where it is presumed to be near zero. This could explain why increased mitotic activity is confined to a narrow (1 to 2 mm) zone around the edge of the wound. "Chalone" has been shown to be tissue-specific but not species-specific. [5, 6, 19–21, 30, 34, 45]

In a sutured wound, even though the surgeon takes care to evert the skin edges while suturing, the epidermal edges invert into the dermal portion of the incision. If hemostasis is perfect, the dermal and subcutaneous parts of the incision are held together by an acellular fibrin clot. Within 24 hours, the inverted epidermis thickens and marginal basal cells become mobile, enlarge, and begin to migrate across the wound (Fig. 3–2). The epithelial cells have bridged the gap within 48 hours. It is important to remember that no new connective tissue has been formed during this time and that the epidermis is largely responsible for wound strength up to five days post incision. As the epithelium thickens, the cells become more columnar and mitotic activity increases. Keratinization occurs in the uppermost epithelial cells of a wound, and the overlying scab is loosened and dislodged. [19–21, 25, 30, 34, 37, 45]

Downward invasion of the epidermis occurs not only at the incision but also in the suture tracts. Keratinization of epithelial cells in the suture tracts occurs when these cells come in contact with connective tissue. This incites an inflammatory reaction, which is often mistaken for an infected suture abscess. Early suture removal can minimize this problem. [19–21, 25, 30, 34, 45]

In open wounds, epithelial regeneration begins by cell mobilization and migration at the wound edges, just as it does in the sutured wound. If the full thickness of dermis has not been removed, as with split thickness skin grafts, mobilization and migration

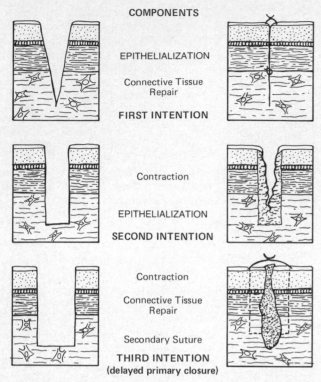

COMPONENTS

EPITHELIALIZATION

Connective Tissue
Repair

FIRST INTENTION

Contraction

EPITHELIALIZATION

SECOND INTENTION

Contraction

Connective Tissue
Repair

Secondary Suture

THIRD INTENTION
(delayed primary closure)

Figure 3–2. First, second, and third intention healing. (Reprinted with permission from Hunt, T. K.: Wound healing. *In* Dunphy, J. E., and Way, L. W. (eds.): *Current Surgical Diagnosis and Treatment*, 2nd ed. Lange Medical Publishers, Los Altos, 1975.)

of epithelial cells from skin appendages (primarily hair follicles) also occur. Almost always, an open wound is initially covered by a blood clot and then by granulation tissue. The migrating epithelium moves under the clot (not through it) and over or into the granulation tissue. The epithelial cells secrete a proteolytic enzyme that dissolves the base of the clot and permits unhindered cell migration. The undermining of the clot, and later the scab, by migrating epithelium is seen grossly as separation of the scab as epithelialization progresses. Epithelial cells migrate over a wound as a sheet. The cells at the leading edge do not drag the other cells with them, but all the cells in the sheet contribute to the movement.[19–21, 25, 30, 34, 45]

In large open wounds, all stages of epithelial repair occur simultaneously. Epithelial migration is rapid initially, but as the migrating cells move further from the wound's edge the epithelium becomes a monolayer and progresses more slowly. Days or even weeks may be required for epithelialization to become complete. In some large wounds, epithelialization may never be complete, or the epithelium in the wound's center may be so delicate that it is continually traumatized, leaving exposed granulation tissue.[19–21, 34, 45]

Contraction Phase

Contraction, as defined by Peacock and Van Winkle, is "the process by which the size of a full-thickness open wound is diminished, and is charac-

terized by the centripetal movement of the whole thickness of surrounding skin."[34] Contraction involves the movement of existing tissue at the wound edge, not the formation of new skin. Most animals possess a well-developed layer of cutaneous muscle called the panniculus carnosus. This muscle and the lack of substantial attachment of the skin to the underlying structures allow contraction to occur to its fullest extent and with little functional interference by underlying structures. Because of this, relatively large wounds on the trunk of animals can be completely closed by contraction, leaving minimal scar tissue.[19–21, 25, 30, 45]

The basic morphological and chemical processes involved in the healing of sutured wounds are also involved in the healing of open wounds. In healing open wounds, contraction becomes an important feature and epithelialization assumes a more prominent role; however, the two processes are independent of one another[25, 30, 45] (Fig. 3–2B).

When a full thickness portion of skin is lost, the wound edges initially retract, enlarging the wound. A fibrin clot is formed over the wound by the immediate exudation of blood and tissue fluids. The clot dehydrates, forming a scab. Leukocytes and macrophages move into the wound to remove debris. Epithelial cells become detached and begin migrating down the wound edge and beneath the scab. Fibroblasts invade the wound, followed by new capillaries. The fibroblasts begin secreting collagen, and granulation tissue is formed. It is over this granulation tissue base that the skin moves. In the dog, there is a lag period of five to nine days before significant contraction is seen. This lag phase is the time necessary for significant fibroblastic invasion of the wound to occur.[19–21, 25, 30, 34, 35]

The mechanism of wound contraction has been the subject of extensive investigation. It was once thought that contraction occurred by shortening of the collagen fibers that are laid down in the granulation tissue. It is now known that collagen fibers are not contractile. Also, contraction proceeds at the same rate and to the same extent in scorbutic guinea pigs as in normal guinea pigs, although the scorbutic wounds contained only 15 per cent as much collagen as normal wounds. This evidence eliminates collagen as a factor in contraction.[25, 34, 35]

There are five theories of contraction of open wounds. These are (1) the push theory, in which the wound edges are pushed inward by extension of surrounding skin; (2) the growth and push theory, in which the wound edges grow; (3) the sphincter theory, in which contractile material at the wound margin acts as a constricting sphincter; (4) the picture frame theory, in which active cells within the wound margin migrate inward, pulling the edges of the defect; and (5) the pull theory, in which material within the defect exerts tension. The first three theories are unlikely to be correct, because the surrounding skin stretches as the wound contracts and the contracting wound takes on a stellate shape.[19–21, 25, 30, 34, 38]

The picture frame and pull theories are the two most plausible current theories used to explain the mechanism of wound contraction. The picture frame theory states that active cells, presumably fibroblasts, within the wound margin migrate toward the center of the wound, pulling the skin edge with them. This theory was based on experiments in which wound edge retraction did not occur following excision of the central portion of the wound unless 0.5 mm of the skin margin was included. Wound edge retraction also occurred when just the wound margin (the "picture frame" area) was excised and the central granulation tissue was left intact. In contrast, the pull theory suggests that the mechanism of pull is distributed equally throughout the granulation tissue of a contracting wound. This theory is based on experiments in which wound edge retraction did occur following excision of the central granulation tissue of contracting wounds.[1, 8, 14, 38, 47]

All evidence points to contraction as a cell-mediated phenomenon. Electron microscopic studies have shown that some of the fibroblasts in contracting wounds have the appearance of smooth muscle cells. These fibroblasts are called myofibroblasts. They share features of both fibroblasts and smooth muscle cells (i.e., they have potentially contractile myofilaments in their cytoplasm, and cell membrane modifications capable of interconnecting and transmitting contraction other cells). Immunofluorescent studies show that myofibroblasts bind antibody against smooth muscle. In vitro pharmacological studies demonstrated that strips of granulation tissue contract and relax, as do strips of smooth muscle. In vivo studies showed that wound contraction can be inhibited by topical application of smooth muscle relaxants. Wound contraction was inhibited as long as the chemical was applied, but contraction resumed when the chemical was discontinued.[2, 12, 17, 19–21, 26–29, 30, 34, 38, 41]

The life cycle of myofibroblasts parallels the behavior of the contracting wound. There is an initial rapid rise in myofibroblast numbers, with a large percentage of fibroblasts having a myofibroblastic appearance during active wound contraction. As the rate of wound contraction decreases, there is a decrease in myofibroblast numbers. When wound contraction ceases, no myofibroblasts are found. Full thickness skin grafts speed up the life cycle of myofibroblasts, as there is a faster decline in myofibroblast numbers in grafted wounds than in open wounds. This parallels the clinical observation that wounds covered with full thickness grafts contract less than open wounds or wounds covered with split thickness grafts.[39, 40] Once contraction begins, skin grafts are less effective in limiting contraction unless the entire granulation bed is excised.[2, 34, 45]

It is not known whether myofibroblasts are derived from normal fibroblasts, multipotential stem cells, or perivascular cells. Although differentiation of the hybrid myofibroblast occurs in an inflammatory environment and prostaglandins play a role in inducing inflammation, prostaglandin inhibitors do not affect the production or activity of myofibroblasts.[28, 40]

Clearly, myofibroblasts play a key role in wound contraction. No matter how these cells contract or what the stimulus for contraction is, there must be some sort of attachment of these cells to the wound edge. Observations of the myofibroblasts reveal that they have cell-to-cell attachments and adherent processes that attach them to the wound bed, the panniculus, and the dermis at the wound edge. Thus, there is a mechanical apparatus for the exertion and transmission of the contractile force. Although the stimulus that causes contraction remains unknown,[19–21, 25, 34, 44, 45] nerve growth factor, which is secreted by fibroblasts, is thought to be involved.[24]

Once contraction begins, it continues until the wound edges meet and contact inhibition halts the process or until the tension in the surrounding skin equals or exceeds the force of contraction. In the latter circumstance, epithelial migration may cover the wound unless it is large, in which case the wound becomes a chronic open ulcer.[19–21, 25, 34, 45] In some wounds, contraction may stop before the wound edges meet, although there is still some laxity in the surrounding skin. In these wounds, the granulation tissue is pale and probably composed primarily of collagen and ground substance, thus lacking contractile myofibroblasts.[19–21, 45]

During contraction, the skin surrounding the wound is stretched, thinned, and under tension; however, this state does not persist. Gradually, new collagen is laid down in the dermis and new epithelial cells are formed. This process continues until the full thickness of the stretched skin is restored. This process is called intussusceptive growth.[19–21, 34, 45]

Wound contraction is an extremely valuable process in the healing of open wounds, but it is not without some disadvantages. Contraction of wounds near joints may result in the formation of a tight band of scar tissue limiting flexion or extension of the joint. Also, contraction of wounds near body openings, such as the anus, may result in stenosis. Deformity and loss of function resulting from wound contraction are less of a problem in animals than in humans but must still be considered when one manages open wounds.[19–21, 45]

Remodeling Phase

Early Wound Strength. Although there is not an appreciable gain in wound strength during the first four to six days following injury (the lag phase, or, more properly termed, the proliferative phase), a properly coapted wound has effective strength even during the first 24 hours. This strength is the result of the formation of a fibrin clot within the wound. Epithelialization across the wound also contributes to early wound strength, as does ingrowth of new capillaries into the wound's ground substance. There is no evidence that glycoproteins, mucopolysaccharides, or other elements of ground substance contribute to wound strength at this stage.[3, 18–21, 34, 45]

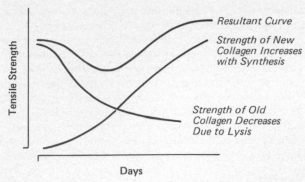

Figure 3–3. Tensile strength is ultimately determined by the strength of old collagen undergoing lysis and new collagen laid down by synthesis due to lysis. (Reprinted with permission from Hunt, T. K.: Wound healing. *In* Dunphy, J. E., and Way, L. W. (eds.): *Current Surgical Diagnosis and Treatment,* 2nd ed. Lange Medical Publishers, Los Altos, 1975.)

After the initial proliferative phase, wound strength increases significantly to reach an early maximum at 14 to 16 days. This increase in wound strength is during the period of rapid fibroplasia and parallels the rise of collagen content in the wound. Hydroxyproline, a measure of collagen concentration, increases rapidly on the fourth day, with the highest rate seen between days 5 and 12, a lesser rate of increase between days 12 and 21, and a markedly lower rate from days 21 to 60.[19–21, 34]

Late Wound Strength. The collagen content of a wound begins to stabilize after the first three weeks. As new collagen fibers are laid down, others are digested and removed by various tissue collagenases. Generally, the collagen fibers that are oriented along the lines of tension remain in the scar.

Wounds continue to increase in strength even after the wound collagen content stabilizes. This increase in wound strength may continue over a period of years, but the rate of gain in strength becomes gradually less with time. The increased strength results from intramolecular and intermolecular crosslinking of collagen fibers that renders the collagen less accessible to tissue collagenases. Although the arrangement of collagen fibers within the scar also has an effect on tensile strength, a scar is never as strong as the tissue it replaces[19–21, 34, 45] (Fig. 3–3).

SYSTEMIC AND ENVIRONMENTAL FACTORS AFFECTING WOUNDS

Secondary Wound Healing

Many surgeons have made the observation that a wound created within a week or so after an initial injury seemed to heal faster. Early investigations showed that secondary skin wounds in rabbits healed more rapidly than primary ones. Because the wounds were on opposite sides of the body, many investigators postulated the existence of a wound hormone that was responsible for accelerating the healing of the secondary wounds. Further investigation showed that the secondary wounds did not heal faster but that the primary wounds healed more slowly owing to the effect of cold vasoconstriction.[34]

Primary wounds allowed to heal undisturbed for short periods and then dehisced and resutured immediately show a significantly greater strength on the third day after resuturing than primary wounds after the same time. This seems to be due to the immediate onset of fibroplasia in the resutured wounds without the usual lag phase. The reason for this is that dehiscence of the original wound did not destroy the macrophages and fibroblasts that were present, and, after resuturing the wound, the healing process already under way in the original wound continued unaltered. No time was necessary to activate and mobilize cells.[25, 34, 42, 45]

Biochemical studies showed that the total collagen content in secondary wounds is less than that in primary wounds, although the rate of collagen synthesis is significantly higher. This suggests that there is more degradation of collagen in the secondary wounds. The rapid gain in tensile strength of secondary wounds may be due more to organization and crosslinking of existing collagen than to its amount.[9, 34, 45]

These observations on secondary wounds do not show that the rate of wound healing is increased. The rate of gain in breaking strength is the same in primary as in secondary wounds, and the ultimate strength attained in each wound is also the same. It has also been shown that the secondary healing phenomenon can be abolished by excising a 1-cm strip from around the primary wound, thus demonstrating that the secondary wound effect is purely local.[25, 34, 42, 45]

Hypoproteinemia

Although the rate of wound healing is not well correlated with plasma protein levels,[25, 34, 45] if serum protein concentration is below 2 gm/100 ml, wound healing is inhibited. It seems that decreased plasma protein levels decrease fibroplasia rather than prolong the lag phase.[21, 34, 45]

Incised wounds in animals fed a protein-free diet for prolonged periods gain strength slowly. Feeding DL-methionine or cystine alone prevents delayed healing. Methionine is converted to cystine, which is the critical amino acid needed in wound healing in protein-deficient animals. Cystine may be needed as a component of one of the cellular enzymes in collagen synthesis.[21, 25, 34, 45]

Anemia and Blood Loss

Anemia per se does not delay wound healing providing the blood volume is normal. The healing wound depends on the local microcirculation to furnish necessary oxygen and other nutrients; therefore, anything that interferes with the microcirculation inhibits wound healing. In anemia, particularly that due to blood loss, there may be varying degrees of hypovolemia. It is well documented that hypovolemia is the major deterrent to wound healing in anemia, hemorrhage, and shock. In severe trauma, microvascular coagulation or sludging may interfere with wound oxygenation and nutrition. Thus, even though blood volume is restored, healing may be delayed.[21, 25, 34, 45]

Oxygen

Oxygen is required for normal wound healing. However, the wound environment is characterized by low levels of pO_2. An oxygen gradient exists between the nearest functioning capillary and the wound edge. The oxygen tension near a wound capillary is between 60 and 90 mm Hg; however, near the advancing edge of the granulation tissue, about 150 microns away, the oxygen tension approaches zero. This decrease is due to the diffisuion gradient and the oxygen consumption of cells in the wound margin.[21, 25, 32, 34]

Measurements of oxygen tension near the leading fibroblasts suggest that oxygen supply is at the lower limit for migration and too low for replication or protein synthesis. Therefore, the activities of fibroblasts depend on the rate at which new capillaries are formed. Anything that interereferes with this process interferes with wound healing.[32,,34, 45]

Animals kept in 10 per cent oxygen have a small but significant decrease in wound strength compared with controls, and animals kept in 40 per cent oxygen have a small but significant increase in wound strength compared with controls. These differences, although statistically significant, were of no clinical significance. Thus, it seems unlikely that, in the absence of factors interfering with tissue oxygenation, administering high oxygen concentrations to patients will significantly affect wound healing.[21, 34, 45]

Temperature

Wounds have been reported to heal faster at an environmental temperature of 30°C than at normal room temperature (18 to 20°C). Decreasing room temperature from 20 to 12°C decreases wound tensile strength by 20 per cent. It is thought that reflex vasoconstriction is responsible for the decreased healing, as denervation of the skin before the temperature is decreased abolishes the inhibition of healing.[25, 34, 45]

Uremia

Uremia decreases wound healing by altering enzyme systems, biochemical pathways, and cellular metabolism. Wound strength is decreased in acute uremia, although the total hydroxyproline content of wounds is not decreased. The total hydroxyproline content of healing wounds does not differentiate between collagen synthesis and collagen degradation; therefore, the decreased wound strength could be explained by synthesis of poor-quality collagen or increased collagen degradation.[7, 21]

Anti-Inflammatory Drugs

Phenylbutazone, Aspirin, and Indomethacin

Experimentally, large doses of aspirin decreased wound tensile strength in rats. However, these commonly used anti-inflammatory agents have no effect on the course or quality of wound healing providing they are administered in pharmacological doses.[13, 21, 23, 25, 34, 45]

Steroids

Cortisone and its derivatives decrease the rate of protein synthesis, stabilize lysosomal membranes, and inhibit the normal inflammatory reaction. High doses of corticoids limit capillary budding, inhibit fibroblast proliferation, and decrease the rate of epithelialization. There is good evidence to suggest that chronic stress or repeated administration of very large doses of corticosteroids, particularly if given before or at the time of wounding, inhibits wound healing. The effects of cortisone are greatly enhanced in the presence of mild starvation and protein depletion, such that relatively low doses markedly inhibit fibroplasia. Acute stress or single doses of cortisone have no effect on healing. Generally, even with high doses of steroids, wound healing proceeds to completion but at a slower rate.[11, 21, 25, 33, 34, 45]

Vitamins and Minerals

Vitamin A

Excessive doses of vitamin A have been reported to increase inflammatory reactions. One of the effects of vitamin A is the labeling of lysosomes through an action on lysosomal membranes. The inhibition of wound healing caused by high doses of cortisone can be completely reversed with high doses of vitamin A. This suggests that the effect of cortisone is, in part, mediated through the lysosome. Vitamin A has been found to stimulate fibroblasts and the accumulation of collagen; however, there is no evidence that the administration of vitamin A alters the wound healing rate in animals not under the influence of steroids or vitamin E.[11, 34, 45]

Vitamin E

Vitamin E, like cortisone, stabilizes membranes. High doses of vitamin E significantly retard wound healing and collagen production.[34, 45]

Vitamin C

A deficiency of vitamin C delays wound healing. Vitamin C is necessary for hydroxylation of proline and lysine for the synthesis of collagen. Without vitamin C, the collagen molecules remain incomplete and may not be secreted by the fibroblast. Dogs and cats do not require exogenous sources of vitamin C.[21]

Zinc

Normal epithelial and fibroblastic proliferation requires the zinc-dependent enzymes DNA-polymerase and reverse transcriptase. Without adequate zinc levels, epithelial cells and fibroblasts may migrate normally, but they cannot multiply. Thus, epithelialization cannot occur and collagen synthesis is inadequate to hold the wound together.[21, 34, 45, 46]

Zinc can also be detrimental to healing. Zinc stabilizes lysosomal and cell membranes and at high levels can inhibit macrophages and thus decrease phagocytosis. High zinc levels may also interfere with collagen crosslinking.[34, 45]

The administration of zinc to patients with low blood and tissue zinc levels can restore normal wound healing, but zinc administration to patients with normal zinc levels will not accelerate wound healing.[34, 45, 46]

Radiation and Cytotoxic Drugs

Any agent that inhibits the division of local fibroblasts or epithelial cells could delay or prevent wound healing. Acute radiation and other cytotoxic agents influence the rate of wound healing. Most cytotoxic agents have their greatest effect on dividing cells. The systemic administration of nitrogen mustard (mechlorethamine chloride), 5-fluorouracil, and other antimetabolites rarely reaches high enough wound concentrations to influence cell division. However, chronic, local application of these agents can prevent wound healing. High doses of radiation, especially during the first three days following wounding significantly delays gains in wound strength.[21, 25, 34, 45]

Dehydration and Edema

Dehydration delays wound healing, but moderate edema has little or no effect on gain in wound tensile strength. Marked edema has a slight and temporary inhibiting effect on healing. The edema per se does not seem to inhibit wound healing, but the factors that initiate edema do.[45]

Infection

Infection has been shown to delay healing. Infected wounds in rats were found to be weaker but had a higher hydroxyproline content than noninfected controls. Bacteria produce collagenases, which degrade collagen, and this, in combination with granulocyte and macrophage collagenases, may account for the decreased wound strength in spite of the high hydroxyproline content. The infected wounds also had decreased fibroblastic activity. Bacteria change wound pH, which may also affect local mediators of healing.[4]

Antiseptics

Antiseptics destroy bacteria, but they also injure body cells. Any solution that is not isotonic can injure cells. Only isotonic solutions should be directly applied to wounds.[21, 45]

1. Abercrombie, M., et al.: Wound contraction in rabbit skin. J. Anat. 94:170, 1960.
2. Ariyan, S., et al.: Wound contraction and fibrocontractive disorders. Arch. Surg. 113:1034, 1978.
3. Botsford, T. W.: The tensile strength of sutured skin wounds during healing. Surg. Gynecol. Obstet. 72:690, 1941.
4. Bucknall, T. E.: The effect of local wound infection upon wound healing: An experimental study. Br. J. Surg. 68:851, 1980.
5. Bullough, W. S., and Laurence, E. B.: The control of epidermal mitotic activity in the mouse. Proc. Roy. Soc. Bull. 151:517, 1960.
6. Bullough, W. S., and Laurence, E. B.: Mitotic control by internal secretion: The role of the chalone-adrenaline complex. Exp. Cell Res. 36:192, 1964.
7. Colin, J. F., et al.: The effect of uremia upon wound healing: An experimental study. Br. J. Surg. 66:793, 1979.
8. Cuthbertson, A. M.: Contraction of full thickness skin wounds in the rat. Surg. Gynecol. Obstet. 108:421, 1959.
9. Danielsen, C. C., and Fogdestam, I.: Delayed primary closure: collagen synthesis and content in healing rat skin incisions. J. Surg. Res. 31:210, 1981.
10. Diegelmann, R. F., et al.: The role of macrophages in wound repair: A review. Plast. Reconstr. Surg. 68:107, 1981.
11. Ehrlich, P., and Hunt, T. K.: Effects of cortisone and vitamin A on wound healing. Ann. Surg. 167:324, 1968.
12. Gabbiani, G., et al.: Granulation tissue as a contractile organ: A study of structure and function. J. Exper. Med. 135:719, 1972.
13. Gorman, H. A., et al.: Effect of oxyphenylbutazone on surgical wounds in horses. J. Am. Vet. Med. Assoc. 152:487, 1968.
14. Grillo, H. C., et al.: Studies in wound healing—I. Ann. Surg. 148:145, 1958.
15. Gunson, D. E.: Collagen in normal and abnormal tissue. Equine Vet. J. 11:97, 1979.
16. Harris, E. D., and Krane, S. M.: Collagenases. N. Engl. J. Med. 291:557, 1974.
17. Hirschel, B. J., et al.: Fibroblasts of granulation tissue: Immunofluorescent staining which antismooth muscle serum. Proc. Soc. Exp. Biol. Med. 138:466, 1971.
18. Howes, E. L., et al.: Rate of fibroplasia and differentiation in the healing of cutaneous wounds in different species of animals. Arch. Surg. 38:934, 1939.
19. Johnston, D. E.: The processes in wound healing. J. Am. Anim. Hosp. Assoc. 13:186, 1977.
20. Johnston, D. E.: The healing process in open skin wounds. Comp. Cont. Ed. 1:789, 1979.
21. Johnston, D. E.: Skin and subcutaneous tissue. In Bojrab, M. J. (ed.): Pathophysiology in Small Animal Surgery. Lea & Febiger, Philadelphia, 1981, p. 405.
22. Kolata, R. J.: The body's response to trauma. In Archibald, J. (ed.): Management of Trauma in Dogs and Cats. American Veterinary Publications, Inc., Santa Barbara, CA, 1981, p. 21.

23. Lee, K.: Studies on the mechanism of action of salicylate II. Retardation of wound healing by aspirin. J. Pharm. Sci. 57:1042, 1968.

24. Li, A. K. C., and Koroly, M. J.: Mechanical and humoral factors in wound healing. Br. J. Surg. 68:738, 1981.

25. Madden, J. W.: Wound healing: biologic and clinical features. *In* Sabiston, D. C. (ed.): *Davis-Christopher Textbook of Surgery*, 10th ed. W. B. Saunders, Philadelphia, 1972, p. 249.

26. Madden, J. W., et al.: Contraction of experimental wounds: I. Inhibiting wound contraction by using a topical smooth muscle antagonist. Surgery 76:8, 1974.

27. Majno, G., et al.: Contraction of granulation tissue in vitro: Similarity to smooth muscle. Science 173:548, 1971.

28. McGrath, M. H.: The effect of prostaglandin inhibitors on wound contraction and the myofibroblast. Plast. Reconstr. Surg. 69:74, 1982.

29. Montandon, D., et al.: The contractile fibroblast: Its relevance in plastic surgery. Plast. Reconstr. Surg. 52:286, 1973.

30. Montandon, D., et al.: The mechanism of wound contraction and epithelization. Clin. Plast. Surg. 4:325, 1977.

31. Morton, D., Jr., et al.: Effect of a local smooth muscle antagonist on wound contraction. Surg. Forum 23:511, 1972.

32. Niinikoski, J.: Oxygen and wound healing. Clin. Plast. Surg. 4:361, 1977.

33. Oxlund, H., et al.: The influence of cortisol on wound healing of the skin and dstant connective tissue response. Surg. Gynecol. Obstet. 148:876, 1979.

34. Peacock, E. E., and Van Winkel, W.: *Wound Repair*, 2nd ed. W. B. Saunders, Philadelphia, 1976.

35. Ross, R.: The fibroblast and wound repair. Biol. Rev. 43:51, 1968.

36. Ross, R., and Benditt, E. P.: Wound healing and collagen formation: I. Sequential changes in components of guinea pig skin wounds observed in the electron microscope. J. Biophys. Biochem. Cytol. 11:677, 1961.

37. Rovee, D. T., and Miller, C. H.: Epidermal role in the breaking strength of wounds. Arch. Surg. 96:43, 1968.

38. Rudolph, R.: Location of the force of wound contraction. Surg. Gynecol. Obstet. 148:547, 1979.

39. Rudolph, R.: Inhibition of myofibroblasts by skin grafts. Plast. Reconstr. Surg. 63:473, 1979.

40. Rudolph, R., et al.: The life cycle of the myofibroblast. Surg. Gynecol. Obstet. 145:389, 1977.

41. Rudolph, R., et al.: Ultrastructure of active versus passive contracture of wounds. Surg. Gynecol. Obstet. 151:396, 1980.

42. Savlov, E. D., and Dunphy, J. E.: The healing of the disrupted and resutured wound. Surgery 36:362, 1954.

43. Schilling, J. A.: Wound healing. Surg. Clin. North Am. 56:859, 1976.

44. Silver, I. A.: Basic physiology of wound healing in the horse. Equine Vet. J. 14:7, 1982.

45. Swaim, S. F.: Wound healing. *In* Swaim, S. F. (ed.): *Surgery of Traumatized Skin: Management and Reconstruction in the Dog and Cat*. W. B. Saunders, Philadelphia, 1980, p. 70.

46. Tengrup, I., et al.: Influence of zinc on synthesis and the accumulation of collagen in early granulation tissue. Surg. Gynecol. Obstet. 152:323, 1981.

47. Watts, G. T., et al.: Studies in wound healing—II. The role of granulation tissue in contraction. Ann. Surg. 148:153, 1958.

Wound Infections

Chapter **4**

William R. Daly

Infection has been associated with wounding, both accidental and intentional, since the beginning of recorded history.[37] Sepsis has been associated with hospitals for centuries, especially with the practice of surgery, and was so common that surgeons regarded it as a normal part of healing. The doctrine that suppuration was a normal and necessary part of wound healing grew out of the teachings of Galen, a surgeon to gladiators and Roman emperors in the 2nd century A.D. Galen's teachings persisted for centuries, and until the surgical renaissance in the 13th and 14th centuries, disagreement with Galenical thought was heresy. In the 13th century Theodoric wrote:

For it is not necessary, as Roger and Roland have written, and as many of their disciples teach, and as all modern surgeons profess, that pus should be generated in wounds. No error can be greater than this. Such a practice is indeed to hinder nature, to prolong the disease, and to prevent the conglutination and consolidation of the wound.

The reversal of the concept of "laudable pus" came with the introduction of antisepsis by Joseph Lister in 1865. Prior to that time, infection was the common sequela to surgery. Amputations were associated with a mortality of 25 to 60 per cent in hospitalized patients and 75 to 90 per cent in military practice. Most of these deaths were from overwhelming sepsis. Lister's application of carbolic acid to surgical wounds and dressings led to a dramatic reduction in wound sepsis and enabled Lister and his contemporaries to undertake operations that previously would have failed owing to sepsis.

The understanding of the growth of bacteria and their mode of spread led to the development of aseptic techniques, which eventually supplemented antisepsis. Asepsis differs from antisepsis in its emphasis on prevention of wound contamination by bacteria rather than on killing of bacteria after they have entered the wound.

The use of sulfas and antibiotics to prevent and treat wound infection has created another significant reduction in infection rates. The administration of these agents at the proper time, by the proper route, and in the proper dosage to be effective should, theoretically, prevent or treat all wound infections caused by organisms susceptible to the agents. The proliferating use of antibiotics, however, has not eliminated infection. Surgeons have tended to concern themselves more with the nature and control of the bacteria than with the management and control of the tissues into which the organisms have been introduced. The result has been the production of antibiotic-resistant organisms. Reducing the chance of infection to its minimum requires an understanding of the factors that determine whether an infection will occur in a wound.

THE DETERMINANTS OF WOUND INFECTION

Homeostasis is a word coined by Cannon to indicate the totality of physiological responses that return the internal environment to a normal steady state after an acute challenge such as injury.[42] Every infectious process, regardless of its location, involves an upset of the normal homeostatic mechanisms that tend to keep the body free from infection. In its simplest form this homeostatic mechanism can be described as a delicate balance between (1) the microorganism causing the infection, (2) the environment in which the infection takes place, and (3) the host defense mechanisms that control the invasion of bacteria into any environment.[38] Each of these factors is intimately involved with the development of, or protection against, any infectious process.

THE ROLE OF BACTERIA IN WOUND INFECTIONS

One of the major advances in the understanding of wound infection is the recognition that the mere presence of bacteria in a wound is far less important than the numbers of bacteria. It has been estimated that 35,000 to 60,000 bacteria drop into the average surgical field each hour.[45] Despite this apparently large number of bacteria, relatively few wounds become infected. In addition, despite a significant reduction in the number of airborne bacteria entering a wound, the overall wound infection rate does not appear to be affected.[45]

Numerous clinical and experimental studies have revealed that a critical level of bacterial contamination is required before a wound infection results. In nearly all studies it has been found that the critical level of contamination for most bacteria is 10^5 to 10^6 organisms/gm of tissue or ml of biological fluid. Remarkable correlation exists between these studies, which have included pustule production in human skin,[21] bacteriuria in pyelonephritis,[30] skin grafts in rabbits and humans,[33] *Clostridium* in wounds of goats,[35] healing of decubital ulcers,[6] and delayed closure of wounds.[48, 49] These studies show that as long as environmental (wound) factors and host defense mechanisms are relatively normal, a bacterial load of 10^6 organisms/gm of tissue is required before the equilibrium is upset enough for a wound to become infected.

This number varies suprisingly little despite the multitude of organisms that have been studied. Only the beta-hemolytic *Streptococcus* appears capable of routinely causing infection at lower levels.[44] In managing infection in his patients, the surgeon should first evaluate whether the patient's balance is in equilibrium or is upset in favor of the bacteria. If equilibrium exists, efforts are directed toward maintaining it to prevent infection. If the balance is upset, efforts are directed toward re-establishment of normal equilibrium.

Time is an important factor in the diagnosis of equilibrium imbalance. In a series of 80 wounds seen in a human hospital emergency department, the mean time following injury of patients who had fewer than 10^2 bacteria/gm of tissue in their wounds was 2.2 hours; the mean time of patients with 10^2 to 10^5 organisms/gm of tissue was 3 hours; and in those with more than 10^5 organisms/gm of tissue, the mean time following wounding was 5.17 hours.[19] It appears that, for the average wound, a "golden period" of around five hours exists in which the bacterial inoculum is at low enough levels that primary closure of the wound can be safely undertaken.

Other factors that must be considered in evaluating the bacteria-host equilibrium are age of the patient, metabolic diseases such as diabetes mellitus and Cushing's disease, presence of existing infections at other sites, neoplasia, malnutrition, drug therapy, and necrotic tissue or ischemia in the wound. All of these factors may affect the defense mechanisms or the local wound environment to such a degree that relatively few bacteria are required to produce clinical infection.

SOURCES OF BACTERIA

All wounds are contaminated to some degree. Antisepsis and asepsis have markedly reduced the degree of contamination of surgical wounds. The fact remains, however, that despite extraordinary success at reducing the numbers of exogenous airborne bacteria entering the surgical wound, clean wound infection rates do not show a significant decrease. In a study conducted by the National Research Council,[1] a reduction of airborne bacteria of up to 74 per cent was possible using ultraviolet light in the operating room. Despite this, the overall postoperative infection rate remained relatively unchanged.

Laminar airflow systems with high-efficiency particle-absorbing (HEPA) filters which remove all particles larger than 0.3 μ with a 99.97 per cent efficiency, have successfully reduced the number of colony-forming units to nearly 0; however, wound infections are still a major problem. Charnley's work with total hip replacement in humans demonstrated that, despite a 25-fold improvement in air cleanliness, the infection rate was only cut in half when compared with procedures done in modern operating rooms without laminar airflow and HEPA filters.[5, 20]

Studies of operating rooms during periods of inactivity indicate that although the walls and floors contain considerable numbers of bacteria, these organisms do not enter the room air. Movement in the operating room is responsible for the air currents that disperse the bacteria.[5, 23, 53]

Numerous studies have shown little correlation between bacteria isolated from the operating room air, from the wound at the time of operation, and from resultant postoperative wound infections.[44] There is considerable evidence to support the theory that endogenous sources of bacteria account for the majority of wound infections.

Several mechanisms exist whereby bacteria from endogenous sources may colonize a wound.[44, 45] The first, called *primary lodgement,* results from direct contact of bacteria within the body with the wound edges. Clinical examples of this type of mechanism are operations requiring invasion of the bowel and biliary and urinary tracts. An increased wound infection rate is found in these clean-contaminated wounds, and the majority of organisms cultured from the infected wound are the same as those cultured at the time of surgery from the hollow organ entered.[46, 47]

The second mechanism of endogenous wound infection is seen in patients that have an established infection at a distant site from the new wound. The bacteria periodically invade the blood and lymphatic systems and ultimately invade and colonize the second wound. Increased venular permeability and capillary endothelial adhesiveness during the inflammatory process may promote collection of these bacteria in the area of the new wound.

The lymphatic system may be responsible for the transport of bacteria to the wound site in some instances. It was found that 37 of 38 dogs undergoing gastrointestinal surgery had enteric organisms in lymph taken from the thoracic duct. Of these dogs, only 12 of the 38 had positive blood cultures.[12]

Remote infections in humans have been associated with a threefold increase in wound infection rates compared with patients in whom no remote infection exists.[1]

QUANTITATIVE MEASUREMENT OF BACTERIAL CONTAMINATION

Many techniques have been described that quantitate the number of bacteria in a wound. From a clinical standpoint the major drawback of these techniques has been that, since they require serial dilutions of tissue biopsies and subsequent colony counts of growth on nutrient agar, they offer no immediate information to aid in the decision of whether a wound is safe to close primarily. To avoid this delay, a rapid slide technique was devised to obtain immediate quantitative information on the level of bacterial contamination.[26] This technique has been used on thousands of wounds and has a greater than 95 per cent correlation with standard colony count methods.[26] The technique is as follows:

1. The open wound surface is cleaned with isopropyl alcohol.
2. A tissue biopsy sample is obtained.
3. The specimen is aseptically weighed.
4. It is dipped in alcohol, air dried, and flamed to remove surface contamination.
5. The specimen is diluted 1:10 w/v in thioglycollate broth and homogenized.
6. Using a 20-λ Sahli pipette, exactly 0.02 ml of the suspension is spread evenly on a glass slide, confining the area to 15 mm in diameter.
7. The slide is oven dried at 75° C.
8. The slide is stained with either the Gram stain or the Brown and Brenn modification to highlight the gram-negative bacteria.
9. The smear is read under the $97\times$ objective, and all fields are examined for the presence of bacteria.
10. The presence of a single bacterium indicates that the original tissue specimen contains a level of bacterial growth greater than 10^5 bacteria/gm of tissue.

THE ROLE OF HOST DEFENSE MECHANISMS IN WOUND INFECTION

The host defense mechanisms are the local and systemic factors involved in the containment and resolution of infection once an organism has penetrated. Typically, these mechanisms are described as (1) the inflammatory response, (2) the humoral component (immunoglobulins), (3) the phagocytic system (neutrophils and macrophages), (4) cell-mediated immunity (lymphocytes), and (5) the complement system.[38]

The first component, the inflammatory response, is a complex series of vascular changes coordinated to allow the delivery of the other components (immunoglobulins, neutrophils, macrophages, lymphocytes, and complement) to the site of the impending or existing infection.

The Inflammatory Response[29, 39, 40, 41, 43, 50]

Inflammation occurs at the site of any injury, and, within limits, the magnitude of the inflammatory response is proportional to the degree of injury. Initially, broken small vessels allow loss of blood into the tissue spaces. The immediate response to injury is a temporary (five to ten minutes) vasoconstriction of the small vessels. An active vasodilation follows that appears to involve all elements of the circulation.

The initial vasodilation is caused by the degranulation of mast cells and the subsequent release of histamine. Serotonin from platelets also plays a part in active vasodilation. Concurrent with vasodilation is an increase in vascular permeability and a tendency for leukocytes, red cells, and platelets to begin to adhere to the vascular endothelium in the area of the injury. The vascular permeability increases as a result of separation of the endothelial cells, particularly in the small venules, leading to transudation of plasma proteins, antibodies, complement, water, electrolytes, and all circulating humoral substances into the wound, including biologically active polypeptides, which may play a role in chemotaxis and the emigration of white blood cells into the wound. Vasodilation caused by histamine and serotonin is enhanced by the production of the kinins bradykinin and kallidin. The activation of Hageman factor, clotting factor XII, by the exposed endothelial collagen in the wound allows activation of the plasma enzyme kallikrein, which in turn splits these vasoactive kinins from circulating alpha-2 globulins.

Following the margination of leukocytes on the vascular endothelial walls, these cells begin to move into the inflammatory site by a process known as diapedesis. The cells pass through capillaries and small venules in the areas of separated endothelium in approximately the same concentration as in the blood stream.

The inflammatory response is localized owing to fibrin clots, which form in broken lymphatics, preventing drainage from the site. The fibrin also provides a matrix against which polymorphonuclear leukocytes can phagocytize bacteria. The inflammatory response is important in controlling wound infection because it localizes the injured areas and provides a mechanism for the transport of the components of the defense mechanism to the injury site. Both the resistance of an animal to the development of bacterial infection and the ability of the animal to overcome an existing infection depend primarily on the animal's ability to deliver phagocytic cells to the area of bacterial invasion and the effectiveness of intracellular digestion of the bacteria by the cells.

Humoral Immunity and Complement[2, 3, 25, 27, 39, 41, 50]

For phagocytosis to occur, there first must be recognition of the bacteria as foreign to the host. The animal's immune system, particularly the humoral component, is directed primarily toward the recognition of foreign molecules (antigens). Immunoglobulins (antibodies) are specific serum proteins synthesized by cells in the lymphoid system (B-lymphocytes and plasma cells) in response to a specific antigenic stimulus.

During the phase of increased vascular permeability in the inflammatory response, serum proteins, including the immunoglobulins and complement, ooze into the tissues at the injury site. If bacteria are present, immunoglobulins, the most important of which are IgG and IgM, react with specific antigenic sites of the bacterial cell wall. The union of the antibody with a specific antigenic site causes a phys-

ical change in the antibody that reveals or produces a site on one of the heavy protein chains that attracts and activates another protein, C_1, thereby triggering the enzymatic cascade of the complement system. The term *complement* refers to a complex system of distinct serum proteins that react with one another in an orderly sequence. As in the blood clotting cascade, there is a progressive increase in the number of molecules involved at each step, thus amplifying the effects of interaction between a specific antigen and its antibody.

A detailed description of complement activation is beyond the scope of this discussion. The effects of complement activation, however, are critical in the success of the host defense mechanism in overcoming bacterial invasion. As the complement cascade proceeds, biologically active particles are produced in the medium that help to increase vascular permeability, cause chemotactic attraction of leukocytes, neutralize viruses, cause lysis of some bacterial membranes, promote immune adherence, and, most importantly, complete the process called *opsonization*. Opsonization, the deposition of antibody, usually IgG, and the complement breakdown product C_3b on the bacterial surface, is important because the deposited proteins serve as a means of recognition by phagocytic cells (neutrophils and macrophages) that chemically attach to the deposited complement and antibody by specific receptor sites on their surfaces. Binding of an opsonized microbe to a leukocyte is followed by engulfment, or phagocytosis.

The Phagocytic System[3, 38, 50]

Phagocytosis of microbes in an inflammatory site depends first on the infiltration of active phagocytic cells, primarily neutrophils and monocytes, to the infection site. This process begins with the attachment of the leukocytes to the venular endothelium in the inflammatory site. The mechanism for this apparent leukocyte "stickiness" is not well known; however, it does not appear to be related to the increased vascular permeability. Relatively few leukocytes adhere to the venules following a histamine injection; however, massive sticking is noted in the presence of a bacterial infection. Presumably leukocytes adhere in these circumstances because of alteration of the venular endothelium by bacteria-produced mediators.

Leukocyte migration across the venular wall occurs at the junction of the endothelial cells, which appear to separate to allow diapedesis. Again, the stimulus for leukocyte emigration is not known; however, it appears that chemotactic substances are released during interaction of the microbe with antibody and complement that initiate the process. These substances provide directional motility for the leukocytes, which would otherwise exhibit random motion. Once binding of an active leukocyte with an opsonized bacterium occurs, phagocytosis follows.

Pseudopods extend to totally surround and engulf the bacteria. Once surrounded, the cell membranes fuse, and the organism becomes trapped inside a "bubble" of cell membrane, now called a *phagosome*. Cytoplasmic granules called *lysosomes* converge on the membrane-bound bacteria and discharge their contents into the vacuole, causing bacterial death and digestion.

In the normal patient the neutrophil provides most of the phagocytic function and is the most predominant cell in the initial cellular response. Neutrophils are the initial bactericidal cell and are essential to the maintenance of an intact host defense. Although the initial inflammatory response results in large numbers of neutrophils accumulating at the injury site, these cells are relatively short-lived and must be constantly replaced in the circulation and at the inflammatory site. Neutrophils die at the inflammatory site and are phagocytized and removed by macrophages.

The second line of phagocytic response is the monocyte. Once a monocyte enters an inflammatory site, it is activated to become a macrophage with phagocytic and bactericidal properties and a long half-life. The macrophage, like the neutrophil, requires antibody and complement for effective phagocytosis. It also contains lysosomal structures with hydrolytic enzymes but, unlike the neutrophil, relatively small amounts of the enzymes lysozyme and phagocytin and a group of basic proteins with antibacterial properties. Following phagocytosis and digestion by a macrophage, microbial antigens are transported either locally or regionally to lymphocytes for specific antibody production.

In addition to the monocyte or "wandering macrophage," numerous tissue macrophages are essential to host defense. These cells, which comprise the mononuclear-phagocytic system or reticuloendothelial system (RES), are the Kupffer cells of the liver, littoral cells of the spleen, microglial cells of the brain, and pulmonary alveolar macrophages. Macrophages are also found in other tissues but in lesser numbers and are greatly supplemented by circulating monocytes when required.

Cell-Mediated Immunity[3, 25, 27, 28, 38, 39, 41]

The term *cell-mediated immunity* generally refers to immune reactions that require the presence of living lymphocytes. These reactions have profound importance in antimicrobial defense, autoimmune disease, allergy, cancer, and transplantation reactions and are further discussed in Chapter 15.

Acquired Defects in the Host Defense Mechanism[3, 28, 39]

Defects in the host defense mechanism may be primary (congenital) or secondary (acquired). Primary

TABLE 4–1. Factors Known to Have Deleterious Effects on Host Defense Mechanisms

Malnutrition	Diabetes mellitus
Sepsis	Shock
Chronic fistulae	Burns
Trauma	Cancer
Major surgery	Uremia
Advanced age	Pancreatitis

immunological deficiency was discovered in man in 1952 with the recognition of agammaglobulinemia. At least 11 clinical entities have been recognized in man in which there is a primary failure of lymphoid function.[3] It is likely that some or all of these clinical entities exist in animals as well. The vast majority of defects in the host defense mechanism are acquired secondary to a disease process, traumatic event, or drug treatment.[28] Events that cause defects in host defense generally produce a variety of abnormalities in the mechanisms that regulate host defense rather than affecting only one component.[39]

The list of factors that affect host defense mechanisms is long. A partial list is presented in Table 4–1. For convenience it is helpful to classify these abnormalities as those involving the inflammatory response, those involving the opsonic substances, and those involving the phagocytic cells. Any factor that alters the inflammatory response by the relative impairment of delivery of phagocytic cells to the microenvironment where bacterial contamination has occurred will encourage the development of infection. Conditions in which this is likely include inhibition of the mediators of inflammation, insufficient blood flow to the affected area (such as in shock, vascular injury, or the application of constricting dressings), the presence of devitalized tissue, the presence of foreign bodies, and collections of blood or other fluids in the tissues.

Abnormalities of the phagocytic cells are regularly seen in association with the development of sepsis. When there is an impairment of the ability of phagocytic cells to ingest and kill bacteria, the critical number of bacteria required for the development of infection decreases considerably. Abnormalities that develop in the phagocytic cell may involve chemotaxis, phagocytic ability, or bactericidal ability once the bacteria have been phagocytized.

Many tests have been developed to quantitatively evaluate the immune system in an attempt to predict which patients are at an unusually high risk for the development of infection. Random evaluations of the host defense mechanisms measuring the numbers of circulating immunoglobulins (IgA, IgM, IgG) and complement, neutrophil phagocytic and bactericidal function, and lymphocyte reactivity have proved to be expensive and of no significant value in the prediction of sepsis. One test that has shown promise in humans is the cutaneous reactivity to recall antigens.[36]

In this test the patients are injected intradermally

with five separate recall antigens (PPD, mumps, *Trichophyton*, Varidase, and *Candida*) and evaluated for skin reaction. Those patients that demonstrated anergy, i.e., no response to any antigen, showed a highly significant predisposition to sepsis. One-third, in fact, died of a septic episode. It appears that skin test responses, a classic reflection of cell-mediated immunity, have predictive value in terms of patient sepsis and mortality. No test has been described to test animals in a similar manner; however, it is likely that a method can be developed that can serve as a nonspecific indicator of altered antibacterial host defense.

THE ROLE OF LOCAL ENVIRONMENT ON WOUND INFECTION

Nonspecific Factors Influencing Local Environment[25, 41]

In addition to the components of the inflammatory response that function to resist the development of infection, many nonspecific defense mechanisms function to prevent the lodgement of microbes in the body. The skin and mucous membranes provide the first line of defense against a microbial invasion.

The skin provides a tough flexible covering for the entire body. In addition to the physical barrier provided by the dry keratin layer, the skin secretions themselves are bacteriostatic or bactericidal. The normal dryness of the skin's keratin layer protects against staphylococci. The products of cornification, such as sterols, amino acids, pentoses, phospholipids, and complex polysaccharides, are antimicrobial, as are the lactic acid, uric acid, ammonia, fatty acids, triglycerides, and waxy alcohols present in sweat and sebaceous gland secretions.

The respiratory tract is protected by tracheobronchial secretions, which contain IgA, lysozyme, lactoferrin, and alpha$_1$-antitrypsin. In addition, the cilia of the respiratory tract provide a mucociliary transport mechanism that moves particulate matter from the recesses of the bronchial tree.

Several mechanisms function to protect the gastrointestinal tract from microbial invasion. The acidity of the stomach reduces bacterial levels to maintain an effective balance between the host and the bacteria. As ingesta proceed distally down the GI tract, bacterial levels increase. Peristaltic motion is essential to eliminate waste, which prevents overpopulation of the resident flora. Ileus or obstructive lesions that prevent motility compromise the host by allowing microbial overgrowth.

The normal bacterial flora of a tissue may prevent the establishment of pathogenic bacteria. The presence of bacteria on the skin and mucous membranes and in the gut is protective in the sense that these bacteria are not pathogenic to the animal as long as the normal homeostatic mechanisms are active and

TABLE 4–2. Halsted's Principles of Surgery

Gentle tissue handling
Accurate hemostasis
Preservation of adequate blood supply
Strict asepsis
No tension on tissues
Careful approximation of tissues
Obliteration of dead space

they successfully compete with the possibly pathogenic organisms for nutrients, space, and moisture.

The Influence of Surgical Technique on Wound Environment[7, 10, 11, 31, 43–45, 52]

Once wounding has occurred, the principle responsibility of the tissues and their defenses is to prevent bacteria from establishing themselves as pathogens. To be successful, the tissues must be able to function in as normal a manner as possible. Of all of the factors that contribute to the development of wound infection or its prevention, the surgeon probably has the most control over the wound environment. Meticulous surgical technique is essential to prevent postoperative wound infection. Just as the number of bacteria entering a wound is a major factor in the development of sepsis, tissue trauma also plays a critically important role. The number of bacteria needed to create an infection varies with the physiological state of the tissues. Surgical technique that adheres to Halsted's principles (Table 4–2) results in significantly lower infection rates.

Accurate and complete hemostasis reduces retention of blood clots and development of hematomas, which provide a coagulum for bacterial growth. Avoidance of necrotic or severely traumatized tissue is essential. Particularly important in this regard are the judicious use of electrocautery; the avoidance of ligatures, which strangulate large amounts of tissue; and the gentle use of tissue retractors. The presence of ischemic tissue or significant amounts of foreign material, including suture, can convert a wound that would ordinarily resist millions of bacteria into one that is susceptible to hundreds.

The suture should be carefully selected, choosing the smallest size and least number of sutures required to do the job. Accurate anatomical apposition of tissue is required for successful primary closure. This is important for all tissues, as it restores proper anatomical alignment, which minimizes the number of spaces for the collection of blood or serum and allows the healing process to occur at an optimal rate with a minimal risk of infection.

DIAGNOSIS OF WOUND INFECTION

A complete definition of wound infection is difficult to provide; however, for our purposes we can define it as a pathological process caused by the growth of microorganisms in the tissues. In an effort to aid early diagnosis of a wound infection, the National Research Council has adopted the classification of wounds as infected, possibly infected, or noninfected.[1] From a clinical standpoint we must consider a wound to be infected when it discharges pus or accumulates pus in an abscess cavity. Many wounds do not fall neatly into the infected and noninfected categories. These wounds are classified as possibly infected and are evaluated frequently until they either become obviously infected or resolve and heal.

Generally the first sign of a wound infection is pyrexia. Fever is not clearly understood; however, it has been postulated that an elevation in temperature is beneficial because it produces an environment detrimental to the invading microbe. All wounded patients should have their body temperature monitored frequently. Fever must be evaluated in relation to both the magnitude of stress and trauma incurred and the time since the wounding occurred.

It is not uncommon for a febrile response to develop in the first 24 to 48 hours following a major traumatic event, particularly anesthesia and surgery. Infection is not likely to be manifest in a clean wound for three to four days. An elevation of temperature of one or two degrees on the day following a major orthopedic surgical procedure is expected and does not indicate a developing infection. This fever should subside without medication within two days. A febrile response starting three to five days following surgery should alert the surgeon to the possibility of an infectious process. As the febrile response is a very early sign of infection and can be easily measured, it is recommended that all patients that appear to be at an increased risk of infection because of compromised host defenses have their temperature taken three or four times daily. In addition, body temperature is a valuable aid in the evaluation of a treatment regimen once an infection is diagnosed.

Measurement of total leukocyte numbers in the peripheral blood and differential counts of stained smears provide other means of diagnosing and monitoring wound infections. Total white blood cell counts provide a measurement of the inflammatory response. Serial white cell counts may provide some evidence of the clinical progression of the problem.

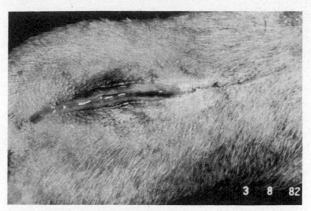

Figure 4–1. Early wound infection in an incision of the distal forelimb. Skin edges have separated and are edematous and erythematous. A thin watery exudate is present in the wound.

White cell counts must always be evaluated in relation to the relative numbers and maturity of the white cell types in the peripheral blood. For this reason, white cell counts without a differential count of the cell types lose a great deal of their value.

The surgeon should examine all wounded patients regularly until it is clear that no infection exists. Examination consists of temperature measurement and careful assessment with gentle palpation of the wound itself. The signs of infection are the signs of inflammation, i.e., pain, heat, redness, swelling, and loss of function. It may be difficult to differentiate a normal inflammatory response from an early wound infection. The signs of early infection are fever, slight edema of the skin edges, tight sutures, erythema, and occasionally a drop or two of serous fluid exuding from the suture line (Fig. 4–1). Palpation of a pocket of fluid beneath the skin or the induration of large muscle masses may suggest the presence of infection not yet draining to the outside. An occasional infection may appear as a cellulitis, particularly those caused by *Streptococcus* sp. In this case the aspiration of significant amounts of fluid from the wound is generally unsuccessful.

Drainage material should be collected from a wound that is infected or possibly infected for Gram staining and culture. The Gram stain of a wound exudate or aspirate offers immediate, valuable information on the character of the exudate. In addition

---

TABLE 4–3. Wound Classification*

Clean Wound   No infection encountered, no break in aseptic technique, and no hollow muscular organ opened. Hysterectomy for sterilization should be included in this category if no acute inflammation is present

Clean-Contaminated Wound   A hollow muscular organ is opened but minimal spillage of contents occurred, the oropharynx or vagina is entered, or a minor break in technique occurs.

Contaminated   A hollow muscular organ is opened with gross spillage of contents, or acute inflammation without pus is encountered. A traumatic wound less than four hours old falls in this group, as do operations associated with a major break in technique.

Dirty Wound   Pus is encountered at operation or a perforated hollow organ is found. A traumatic wound of more than four hours duration is included in this category.

*Based on the recommendations of the Committee on Control of Surgical Infections of the Committee on Pre- and Postoperative Care of the American College of Surgeons.

TABLE 4–4. Analysis of Wound Infection Rates Related to Wound Classification*

Classification	Total Number	Number Infected	Percentage
Clean	47,054	732	1.5
Clean- contaminated	9,370	720	7.7
Contaminated	442	676	15.2
Dirty	2,093	832	40.0
Overall	62,939	2,960	4.7

*Reprinted with permission from Cruse, P.J.E., and Foord, R.: The epidemiology of wound infection: a 10-year prospective study of 62,939 wounds. Surg. Clin. North Am. *60*:27, 1980.

TABLE 4–6. Orthopedic Procedures— Nonfracture*

Classification	No. Cases	No. Infected (%)	No. Positive Cultures (%)
Clean	74	2 (2.7)	1 (1.3)
Clean- contaminated	0	0 (0)	0 (0)
Contaminated	0	0 (0)	0 (0)
Dirty	4	0 (0)	0 (0)
Overall	78	2 (2.5)	1 (1.2)

*Cases include ruptured ligaments, patellar luxations, coxofemoral luxations, total hip prostheses, femoral head ostectomies, and tendon surgeries.

to guiding the choice of antibiotic if an infection is present, it can help differentiate a seroma from a leukocytic inflammatory response. Samples from any significant discharge from a wound should be submitted for microbial culture. It should be realized that diagnosis of wound infection is made on physical examination. Laboratory cultures should not be expected to provide a diagnosis of infection; they merely guide the treatment of an infected patient, revealing the presence of organisms resistant to a particular antibiotic.

CLASSIFICATION OF SURGICAL WOUNDS

To focus attention on those wounds that have a higher risk of infection, it is convenient to classify wounds based on an estimate of contamination. Four categories are generally described (Table 4–3).

In a published prospective study performed at human teaching hospitals, 62,939 surgical wounds were observed.[15] Infections occurred in 2,960, yielding an overall infection rate of 4.7 per cent. An analysis of wound infection rates in this study related to wound classification appears in Table 4–4. In a similar unpublished prospective study comparable data have been collected.[16] This study was performed in a private veterinary referral surgical facility over a period of 17 months. In an effort to determine the

actual risk of wound infection, no animal was given antibiotics, regardless of the wound classification, until either a Gram stain showed evidence of bacteria in a wound exudate or a positive microbial culture was reported by the laboratory. The results of this study are presented in Tables 4–5 through 4–12.

Several comments should be made concerning the population of animals in this study. As noted in Table 4–5, the greatest number of cases that became infected were in the clean fracture category. A review of these cases revealed three situations in which infections were most likely to occur. Severely traumatized patients with severe or multiple fractures appeared to become infected most easily. This is to be expected, as host defenses are most likely to be depressed in these patients. Traumatic surgical procedures such as carpal arthrodesis appeared to increase infection rates. This most likely reflects surgical technique. A third situation in which infections appear more commonly is clean fractures of the distal radius or tibia in which a plate is used for fixation. In these cases very little soft tissue is available to cover the plate, and in this series several animals developed low-grade infections, necessitating removal of the plate after the fracture had healed.

The purpose of classification of surgical wounds is to determine the risk of infection and decide which patients require prophylactic antibiotics. Both the human and veterinary series lead to the same conclusion. Antibiotics are probably indicated in cases in the contaminated and dirty categories owing to the exceptional risk of postoperative infection. Clean and

TABLE 4–5. Orthopedic Procedures—Fractures of the Pelvis and Long Bones

Classification	No. Cases	No. Infected (%)	No. Positive Cultures (%)
Clean	165	12 (7.2)	9 (5.4)
Clean- contaminated	2	0 (0)	0 (0)
Contaminated	8	1 (12.5)	0 (0)
Dirty	7	0 (0)	0 (0)
Overall	182	13 (7.1)	9 (4.9)

TABLE 4–7. Orthopedic Procedures—Fractures of the Mandible/Maxilla

Classification	No. Cases	No. Infected (%)	No. Positive Cultures (%)
Clean	2	0 (0)	0 (0)
Clean-contam- inated	0	0 (0)	0 (0)
Contaminated	4	1 (25.0)	1 (25.0)
Dirty	7	2 (28.6)	2 (28.6)
Overall	13	3 (23.1)	3 (23.1)

TABLE 4–8. Urogenital Procedures*

Classification	No. Cases	No. Infected (%)	No. Positive Cultures (%)
Clean	2	0 (0)	0 (0)
Clean-contaminated	28	1 (3.5)	1 (3.5)
Contaminated	0	0 (0)	0 (0)
Dirty	3	0 (0)	0 (0)
Overall	33	1 (3.0)	1 (3.0)

*Cases include urethrostomies, cystotomies, cesarean sections, nephrotomies, and ruptured bladders.

clean-contaminated cases do not require prophylactic antibiotics unless some other condition exists that is likely to reduce host defense mechanisms to such a degree that infection is probable. Examples of such conditions are noted in Table 4–13.

Some surgeons depend on antibiotics to prevent infection and neglect proper wound management. Antimicrobials are not substitutes for careful surgical technique, the principle elements of which are gentleness, preservation of vascularity, accurate hemostasis, removal of devascularized tissue and foreign particles, and accurate anatomical closure without tension or dead space.

PREVENTION OF WOUND INFECTION

Prevention of wound infection requires conscientious and strict attention to a great number of details, including design of the operating room; conduct of the surgical team; pre-, intra-, and postoperative patient management; and observation of wounds to determine infection rates.

The Operating Room

The design of the operating room and its airflow system has a great effect on the number of airborne organisms. Elaborate operating theaters with laminar airflow and highly efficient air filtration systems are very effective at reducing the number of airborne particles.[53] These systems are probably not economically feasible for the veterinary surgical facility.[5]

TABLE 4–9. Neurosurgical Procedures*

Classification	No. Cases	No. Infected (%)	No. Positive Cultures (%)
Clean	40	3 (7.5)	2 (5)
Clean-contaminated	0	0 (0)	0 (0)
Contaminated	1	0 (0)	0 (0)
Dirty	0	0 (0)	0 (0)
Overall	41	3 (7.3)	2 (4.8)

*Cases include hemilaminectomies, laminectomies, spinal fractures, and disc fenestrations.

TABLE 4–10. Gastrointestinal Procedures*

Classification	No. Cases	No. Infected (%)	No. Positive Cultures (%)
Clean	0	0 (0)	0 (0)
Clean-contaminated	4	0 (0)	0 (0)
Contaminated	1	0 (0)	0 (0)
Dirty	1	0 (0)	0 (0)
Overall	6	0 (0)	0 (0)

*Cases include esophageal, gastric, and intestinal biopsies; foreign bodies; tumors; and gastric torsions.

Studies have shown that the operating team significantly affects air contamination. An increase in airborne particles of nearly 100 times occurs when the surgical team enters the room.[5, 23] Obviously, the size and movement of the operating team should be kept to a minimum. Procedures that carry a higher risk of infection, such as vascular grafts or total joint replacement, warrant the absolute exclusion of any nonessential personnel from the operating room. Talking in the operating room should be discouraged except for profession and educational necessities. Talking significantly increases the number of bacteria in the environment, even with proper masking.[17]

Preoperative Preparation

Preoperative preparation of the patient's skin is aimed at reduction of the numbers of bacteria in the surgical field (see Chapter 22). The patient's hair should be shaved immediately prior to surgery. Small nicks in the skin provide a perfect coagulum for the proliferation of surface bacteria. Shaving the day before surgery, as is done in many human hospitals, has been shown to increase infection rates.[15]

The use of impermeable plastic drapes has been advocated to prevent skin contamination of the surgical wound. In practice, these drapes prove costly and have been associated with an increase in infection rates in clean wounds from 1.5 per cent when cotton drapes are used to 2.3 per cent when plastic drapes are used.[15]

Preoperative hospitalization and age of the patient have been shown to affect wound infection rates.

TABLE 4–11. Miscellaneous Procedures*

Classification	No. Cases	No. Infected (%)	No. Positive Cultures (%)
Clean	32	1 (3.1)	1 (3.1)
Clean-contaminated	6	0 (0)	0 (0)
Contaminated	5	2 (40.0)	2 (40.0)
Dirty	10	6 (60.0)	6 (60.0)
Overall	53	9 (17.0)	9 (17.0)

*Cases include tumors, mucoceles, hernias, ear drainages, fistulas, biopsies, abscesses, and thoracic surgeries.

TABLE 4–12. Overall Results

Classification	No. Cases (%)	No. Infected (%)	No. Positive Cultures (%)
Clean	315 (77.5)	18 (5.7)	13 (4.1)
Clean-contaminated	40 (9.8)	1 (2.5)	1 (2.5)
Contaminated	19 (4.7)	4 (21.0)	3 (15.7)
Dirty	32 (7.9)	8 (25.0)	8 (25.0)
Overall	406 (100.0)	31 (7.6)	25 (6.1)

One study in humans showed an infection rate of 1.2 per cent with one-day preoperative stays, 2.1 per cent with seven-day preoperative stays, and 3.4 per cent with two-week preoperative stays.[15] It is likely that the patient's skin becomes colonized with bacteria to which he is not resistant. This same study also showed that elderly patients (over 66 years of age) were six times more likely to develop infections than patients under 14 years of age. It is likely that these principles hold true for veterinary patients as well.

A significant difference in infection rates has not been shown for five-minute scrubs of the surgeon's hands as opposed to ten-minute scrubs. *In vitro* tests suggest that a one-minute surgical scrub might be adequate.[17] Holes in surgical gloves might be expected to have an effect on infection rates. One study showed an overall incidence of glove punctures in 11.6 per cent of all cases.[15] Not a single infection occurred in 141 cases with glove punctures.

The duration of the surgical procedure has an effect on postoperative sepsis. The infection rate in clean wounds roughly doubles with every hour of surgical time.[15] Explanations proposed for this are (1) increased bacterial contamination with increased surgical time, (2) more wound trauma due to air drying of tissues and damage by retractors, (3) increased

TABLE 4–13. Conditions That May be Indications for Antibiotic Prophylaxis in Clean Surgical Wounds

Shock
Multiple severe trauma
Lengthy surgical procedures
Traumatic surgical procedures
Poor blood supply or tissue oxygenation
Foreign bodies (organic and inorganic)
Seromas and hematomas
Malnutrition
Obesity
Any other inherent or iatrogenic factor that alters host immune mechanisms

amounts of suture and electrocoagulation in more difficult, lengthy cases, and (4) more blood loss and shock and longer anesthesia associated with longer procedures, thereby reducing the overall host resistance to infection.

Drainage Systems

The use of drains has been studied in association with infection rates. The presence of fluid or hematoma clearly inhibits the ability of normal host defenses to neutralize contaminating bacteria in a wound. If large collections of fluid occur, neutrophils necessary for phagocytosis of microbes are less able to penetrate in sufficient numbers to kill bacteria. Studies show that fluids collecting in wounds progressively lose their ability to support opsonization of bacteria for phagocytosis and killing by neutrophils.[4] It seems desirable to improve tissue apposition by preventing the accumulation of fluids as much as possible and removing the collections as they occur. The removal of stagnant wound fluid allows fresh fluid with opsonic proteins to enter the wound. It is toward this end that the use of drains is directed.

Open drains, such as the Penrose or sump drain, have been shown to allow bacteria from the skin and air to gain entrance to the wound bed. If the site is perfectly drained, this may be of little consequence. However, if a fluid cavity remains despite the drain, an abscess is likely to result. Penrose drains, when used, should always leave a site away from the main wound. In a study of gall bladder surgeries, infection rates were 4.5 per cent when no drain was used compared with 7.8 per cent when a Penrose drain was brought out the main incision.[15] Closed suction drainage has been advocated to avoid the problems of contamination with open drain systems, and studies have shown lower infection rates.[4] The major problem with any drainage system for small animals is the lack of a cooperative patient. Experience has shown that many animals remove their drain, or worse, part of the drain.

Observation

Observation of wounds and determination of infection rates are important in the prevention of infections. A clean wound infection rate of less than 1 per cent is exemplary, 1 to 2 per cent is acceptable, and over 2 per cent is cause for concern (see Table 4–2).

Host Defense Mechanisms

Whether or not an infection develops in a clean wound is probably to the greatest extent a measurement of the effectiveness of the host defense mechanisms. Although there is still a great deal to be learned about the intricacies of the immune response to microbial contamination, experience has shown that the manner in which the surgeon deals with the wounded tissues greatly influences how the wounded tissues deal with microbial contamination. The principles of gentle tissue handling, accurate hemostasis, and closure without excessive foreign material or potential dead space are effective because they preserve the host defense mechanisms to the greatest degree.

Debridement

Prevention of infection in open traumatic wounds requires application of the principles of wound debridement and proper timing of wound closure. Wound debridement is basically the removal of all foreign material and devitalized or badly compromised tissue from the wound.[24] Debridement is an exacting technique that requires experience, judgment, patience, and the proper facilities. Compromise of the debridement technique will definitely compromise results.

Debridement of an open wound should be done as soon as possible in the course of treatment. At times this may require the use of spinal or local anesthesia in patients judged to be poor risks for general anesthesia. The initial step in debridement is adequate clipping of hair from the periphery of the wound and a thorough soap and water wash (Figs. 4–2 and 4–3). While clipping, it is important to prevent clipped hairs from falling into the wound. This can be accomplished by either packing the wound with gauze or filling the wound with a water-soluble lubricant such as K-Y jelly.* Occasionally a razor blade is used to trim hair from wound edges or from areas difficult to reach with the electric clippers. Strong soaps and detergents are best used only on the skin surrounding the wound and not in the wound itself. The wound is gently washed with sterile saline or a very mild soap solution.

---

*Johnson & Johnson, New Brunswick, NJ.

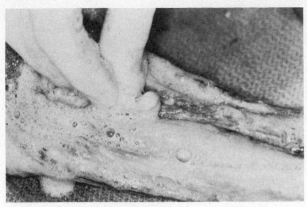

Figure 4–3. The wound is thoroughly cleaned with soap and water following clipping of hair surrounding the wound.

Once the general area around the wound is cleaned, attention is turned to the wound itself. Initially, a thorough examination is made of the wounded tissues. This may require extension of the margins of the wounded skin, particularly in the case of destructive injuries, e.g., those produced by high-velocity bullets (Fig. 4–4). Areas of the skin that are badly damaged or that have no capillary oozing from the margins are excised. Any fascia in the wound should be excised, as it is normally relatively avascular and particularly susceptible to colonization by bacteria. Areas of muscle that are avascular, pale, friable, badly damaged, or heavily contaminated should be excised. In most areas the loss of muscle is well-tolerated, and it is far better to excise it with a scalpel than have it undergo liquefactive necrosis four to five days later.[7]

Some of the principles of debridement must be compromised when dealing with bone, nerve, major vessels, and tendons.[7] In general, bony fragments should be removed only if they are totally avascular and small enough that they are not essential to stabilization of the fracture. Large fragments, regardless of their vascular state, should be left in place.

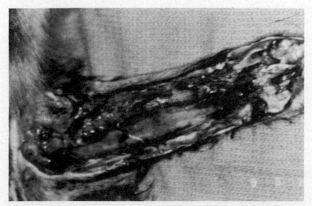

Figure 4–2. A contaminated traumatic wound on the medial aspect of the forelimb of a dog. Debridement and healing of this wound are presented in Figures 4–3 through 4–6 and 4–8 through 4–13.

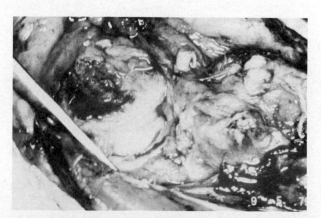

Figure 4–4. Wound exploration: extension of skin margins and incision of fascia revealed an open injury and subluxation of the elbow joint. The medial collateral ligament and a portion of the medial humoral condyle have been ground off.

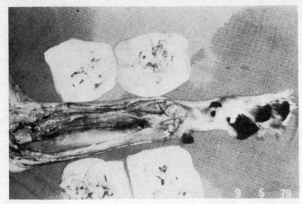

Figure 4–5. Wound exploration: removal of foreign material and obvious necrotic tissue.

Pik.* The Water-Pik unit is relatively inexpensive and quite effective. Its major disadvantage is the difficulty of providing a sterile fluid pathway. This requires ethylene oxide sterilization of a completely dry unit. If care is taken to thoroughly clean the unit before and after each use, its advantages in cleaning a contaminated wound probably outweight the risk of introducing new pathogens with an unsterilized unit.

The fluid used for lavage is ideally sterile, isotonic, and isosmotic. Saline, Ringer's, and lactated Ringer's solutions work well. The addition of antiseptics and antibiotics to this fluid is not essential and is possibly detrimental. Some advocate the addition of povidone-iodine solutions to the fluid (1 part povidone-iodine solution to 9 parts of electrolyte solution), and this can be done without apparently harmful effects on the tissues. Chemicals act indiscriminately on microbial and tissue cells, and the major benefit of the lavage is the physical removal of debris.

Nerves, major vessels, and tendons should be cleaned as well as possible and preserved unless they are obviously avascular or avulsed. Foreign bodies such as hair, organic material, skin, and dirt should be removed as they are encountered (Fig. 4–5). No attempt is made to remove fragments of lead bullets, as they rarely cause problems unless in a joint. The use of steel shot is becoming more common in shotgun shells, and injuries involving this type of shot may require some reconsideration of this principle.

The removal of damaged or avascular tissues and all foreign bodies also removes a great number of contaminating bacteria. Further removal of bacteria, tissue fragments, and foreign bodies is accomplished by thorough lavage of the wound. Merely flooding the wound with fluid is not effective. The wound should be thoroughly explored and flushed with a thin stream of fluid under pressure (Fig. 4–6). This can be accomplished with a bulb syringe or by gravity flow from a bottle of fluid held high over the wound and delivered through a large-bore hypodermic needle. The thin stream of fluid helps to flush out small debris and microbes.

A more effective method is the use of a pulsating jet lavage, such as that provided by a dental Water-

Wound Closure

Once the wound is made as clean as possible, the surgeon must make a decision regarding closure of the wound. Unfortunately, some surgeons have an irresistible urge to close a wound. They interpret an open wound as an incomplete treatment or a challenge not met.[7] Unfortunately, some wounds are closed to the detriment of the wound and the patient (Fig. 4–7). The best defense of a contaminated tissue against infection is good circulation; conversely, anything that compromises circulation encourages bacterial infection. Wounds closed under tension, with dead or potentially dead tissue spaces, fluid accumulation, lack of fluid egress, or foreign materials in tissues with compromised vascularity, are at exceptional risk for the development of infection.

The surgeon must consider the condition and location of the wound, the health of the tissues and

---

*Teledyne Aquatec, Fort Collins, CO.

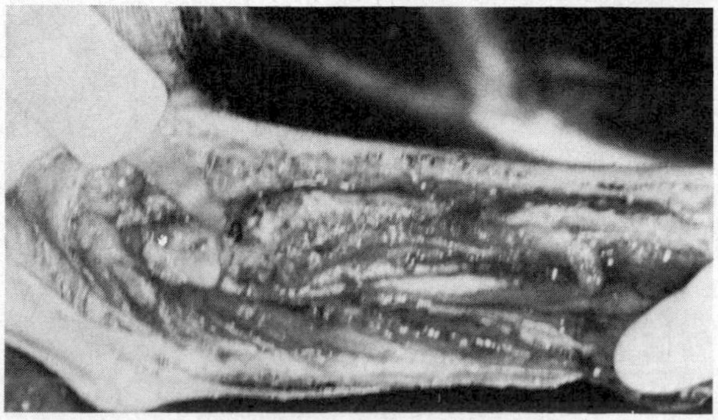

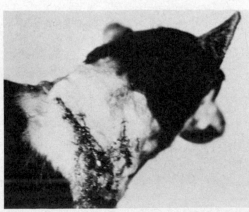

Figure 4–6. Wound lavage: extensive and copious lavage with isotonic fluid at body temperature delivered under pressure further aids in removal of debris and bacteria.

Figure 4–7. Infection and partial dehiscence five days following debridement and primary closure of a bite wound.

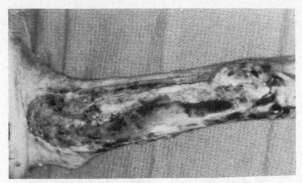

Figure 4–8. Five days following initial injury and debridement: early granulation tissue formation in the wound bed. Wound has been protected with bandages that were changed daily.

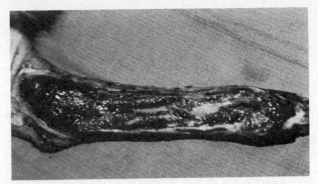

Figure 4–10. Twenty days following injury and debridement: wound bed contains proliferation of granulation tissue. Wound contraction has begun with skin edge migration toward the center of the wound. Sutures have not been used to close this wound.

adequacy of debridement, the forces involved in wounding, the degree of contamination, the treatment given, the overall health of the patient, and how long the wound has been open. Only when all factors are favorable and the surgeon is firmly convinced with no reservations that the wound will heal without complications should the wound be closed primarily.

When there is some question as to the adequacy of debridement, degree of contamination, or health of the tissues, the options of delayed primary closure, secondary closure, and nonclosure must be considered. The formation of granulation tissue in an open wound starts on about the fifth day (Figs. 4–8 through 4–10). Until this time a wound may be closed and healing will occur by primary intention. When there is some question about the ability of a wound to heal by primary closure without infection, it should be left open and the bandages changed frequently. Gauze sponges can be placed in the wound bed and moistened with saline or a dilute antiseptic solution such as povidone-iodine. The wound is gently and effectively debrided each time the gauze sponges are changed. Small bits of dead tissue cling to the gauze and are removed with it. If examination of the wound shows all tissues to be healthy with no evidence of

infection, the wound can be closed. The advantage of this process (delayed primary closure) is that the wound is examined daily and can undergo secondary debridement of devitalized tissues missed initially.

Once granulation tissue has formed over the wound, generally in five to seven days, healing can usually be expected without complication and the wound can be closed. By this time the skin edges are often adherent to the granulation tissue and must be dissected free. Secondary closure, that is, closure of the wound after the formation of granulation tissue, is generally not required in animals. Most wounds on dogs and cats have a tremendous potential for wound contraction and close spontaneously by contraction and epithelialization with minimal scarring and loss of function (Figs. 4–11 through 4–13).

Full circumference skin loss of the distal portion of the limb is one of the few cases in the dog and cat in which wound contraction creates a significant problem. In most cases if a wound cannot be closed primarily or as a delayed primary closure, nonclosure is the procedure of choice. If disfiguring scars occur, they can be revised after healing is completed and the danger of infection is passed.

The principle behind wound closure is to close the wound at a time when all tissues of that wound are

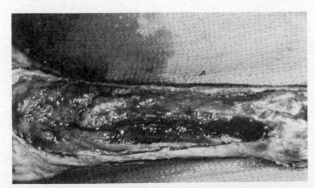

Figure 4–9. Nine days following injury and debridement: wound bed is completely covered by granulation tissue. Wound infection is not present; systemic or topical antibiotics were not used in the treatment of this wound.

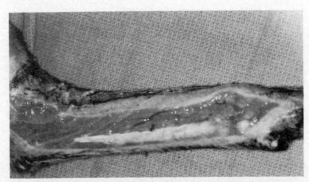

Figure 4–11. Twenty-seven days following injury and debridement: skin edge migration continues. Granulation tissue is covered by a thin fragile layer of epithelium.

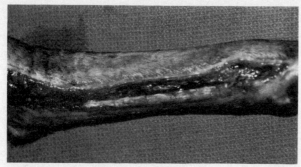

Figure 4–12. Thirty days following injury and debridement: further reduction in size of open wound by continuing skin edge migration. Wound has been protected by bandages.

ready to accept closure. Any attempt before this time represents premature closure and is an invitation to wound infection, dehiscence, and all of the resultant consequences.[7] If the principles of wound management are applied well, the use of antibiotics becomes quite secondary. The importance of prophylactic antibiotics has become overemphasized, and when reliance is placed on them to the neglect of proper tissue management, the incidence of wound breakdown and infection increases.[7]

MANAGEMENT OF WOUND INFECTION

Once a wound infection becomes apparent, treatment is directed toward restoring the tissues to a normal homeostatic state. When wounds accumulate a pocket of exudate, i.e., abscess, the initial immediate treatment is to remove the sutures and open the wound completely. Those wounds in which infection is present as a cellulitis probably do not require disruption, as an abscess cavity does not exist.

The purpose of intentional dehiscence is to provide drainage of the abscess. Once drained, the wound is thoroughly debrided as discussed for the prevention of wound infection in open wounds. Closure of the wound can be done only if debridement has been

adequate and perfect drainage has been provided. Generally this is not the case and the wound should be either closed at a later time or allowed to close by contraction and epithelialization.

At the time of drainage and debridement of the wound, samples should be taken for Gram staining and culture. The Gram stain can provide a great deal of early information about the microbe causing the infection and frequently allows the choice of an antibiotic to which the organism is susceptible. Knowledge of which organisms are most common in each situation and the typical antibiogram for the organisms allows a potential 48-hour head start on effective antimicrobial therapy. Cultures and antimicrobial susceptibility patterns of the organisms are used to confirm the information gained by Gram staining and to reveal the presence of resistant organisms.

If possible, infected wounds should remain bandaged. Bandages protect the wound from additional heavy contamination and licking and chewing by the animal. They also provide gentle debridement as the bandage is changed and an assessment of the volume and character of wound exudate. It is particularly important for infected wounds with Penrose drains to be bandaged whenever possible. The bandages help prevent ascending infections from the drain exit site and prevent the drain from being removed prematurely by the animal. More importantly, they give some assessment of the volume and character of the drainage, which in turn dictates the time for removal of the drain.

1. Ad Hoc Committee of the Committee on Trauma, Division of Medical Sciences, National Research Council Report: Postoperative wound infections: the influence of ultraviolet irradiation of the operating room and the influence of various other factors. Ann. Surg. *160*(Suppl. 1):1, 1964.
2. Alexander, J. W.: The role of host defense mechanisms in surgical infections. Surg. Clin. North Am. *60*:107, 1980.
3. Alexander, J. W., and Good, R. A.: *Immunobiology for Surgeons.* Philadelphia, W. B. Saunders, 1970.
4. Alexander, J. W., Korelitz, J., and Alexander, N. S.: Prevention of wound infections. A case for closed suction drainage to remove wound fluids deficient in opsonic proteins. Am. J. Surg. *132*:59, 1976.
5. Amstutz, H. C.: Prevention of operative infections. Cleve. Clin. Q. *40*:125, 1973.
6. Bendy, R. H., Nuccio, P. A., Wolfe, E., et al.: Relationship of quantitative wound bacterial counts to healing of decubitus: Effect of topical gentamicin. Antimicrob. Agents Chemother. 4:147, 1964.
7. Brown, P. W.: The prevention of infection in open wounds. Clin. Orthop. Rel. Res. *96*:42, 1973.
8. Burke, J. F.: Identification of the sources of staphylococci contaminating the surgical wound during operation. Ann. Surg. *158*:898, 1963.
9. Burke, J. F.: Infection. *In* Hunt, T. K., and Dunphy, J. E. (eds.): *Fundamentals of Wound Management.* Appleton-Century-Crofts, New York, 1980.
10. Burke, J. F.: The physiology of wound infection. *In* Hunt, T. K. (ed.): *Wound Healing and Wound Infection—Theory and Surgical Practice.* Appleton-Century-Crofts, New York, 1980.
11. Burke, J. F.: Risk factors predisposing to wound infection and means of their prevention. *In* Dineen, P. (ed.): *The Surgical Wound.* Lea & Febiger, Philadelphia, 1981.

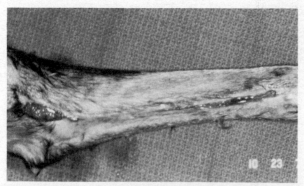

Figure 4–13. Forty-eight days following injury and debridement: wound contraction is almost complete and has nearly closed the entire wound.

12. Cole, W. R., Petit, R., Brown, A., et al.: Lymphatic transport of bacteria in surgical infection. Lymphology 1:52, 1968.

13. Committee on Control of Surgical Infections of the Committee on Pre- and Postoperative Care of the American College of Surgeons: *Manual on Control of Infection in Surgical Patients.* J. B. Lippincott Co., Philadelphia, 1976.

14. Cruse, P. J. E.: Incidence of wound infection on the surgical services. Surg. Clin. North Am. 55:1269, 1975.

15. Cruse, P. J. E., and Foord, R.: The epidemiology of wound infection: A 10-year prospective study of 62,939 wounds. Surg. Clin. North Am. 60:27, 1980.

16. Daly, W. R.: Unpublished data, 1983.

17. Dineen, P.: Influence of operating room conduct on wound infections. Surg. Clin. North Am. 55:1283, 1975.

18. Duboc, F., Guimont, A., Roy, L., and Ferland, J. J.: A study of some factors which contribute to surgical wound contamination. Clin. Orthop. Rel. Res. 96:176, 1973.

19. Duke, W. F., Robson, M. C., and Krizek, T. J.: Civilian wounds, their bacterial flora, and rate of infection. Surg. Forum 23:518, 1972.

20. Eftekhar, N. S.: The surgeon and clean air in the operating room. Clin. Orthop. Rel. Res. 96:188, 1973.

21. Elek, S. D.: Experimental staphylococcal infections in the skin of man. Ann. N.Y. Acad. Sci. 65:85, 1956.

22. Fry, D. E.: Wound infection. *In* Flint, L. M., and Fry, D. E. (eds.): *Surgical Infections.* Medical Examination Publishing Co., Garden City, NY, 1982.

23. Goodrich, E. O., and Whitfield, W. W.: Air environment in the operating room. Bull. Am. Coll. Surg. 55:7, 1970.

24. Haury, B., et al.: Debridement: An essential component of traumatic wound care. *In* Hunt, T. K. (ed.): *Wound Healing and Wound Infection—Theory and Surgical Practice.* Appleton-Century-Crofts, New York, 1980.

25. Heggers, J. P.: Natural host defense mechanisms. Clin. Plast. Surg. 6:505, 1979.

26. Heggers, J. P., Robson, M. C., and Doran, E. T.: The quantitative assessment of bacterial contamination of open wounds by a slide technique. Trans. Roy. Soc. Trop. Med. Hyg. 63:532, 1969.

27. Herbert, W. J.: Reviews in immunology. The immune responses. J. Small Anim. Pract. 17:9, 1976.

28. Howard, R. J., and Simmons, R. L.: Acquired immunologic deficiencies after trauma and surgical procedures. Surg. Gynecol. Obstet. 139:771, 1974.

29. Jones, E. W.: Inflammation, pain, pyrexia, prostaglandins, and antiprostaglandins. Equine Med. Surg. 1:364, 1977.

30. Kass, E. H.: Bacteriuria and the diagnosis of infections of the urinary tract. Arch. Intern. Med. 100:709, 1957.

31. Keighley, M. R. B., and Burdon, D. W.: Aetiology of surgical infection. *In Antimicrobial Prophylaxis in Surgery.* Pitman Medical Publishing Ltd., Kent, England, 1979.

32. Frizek, T. J., and Robson, M. C.: Biology of surgical infection. Surg. Clin. North Am. 55:1261, 1975.

33. Krizek, T. J., Robson, M. C., and Kho, E.: Bacterial growth and skin graft survival. Surg. Forum 18:518, 1967.

34. Ledger, W. J.: Prevention, diagnosis, and treatment of postoperative infections. Obstet. Gynecol. 55:203s, 1980.

35. Lindsey, D., Wise, H. M., Knocht, M. S., et al.: The role of Clostridia in mortality following an experimental wound in the goat. I. Quantitative bacteriology. Surgery 45:602, 1959.

36. Maclean, L. D., Meakins, J. L., Taguchi, K., et al.: Host resistance in sepsis and trauma. Ann. Surg. 182:207, 1975.

37. Majno, G.: *The Healing Hand—Man and Wound in the Ancient World.* Harvard University Press, Cambridge, 1975.

38. Meakins, J. L.: Pathophysiologic determinants and prediction of sepsis. Surg. Clin. North Am. 56:847, 1976.

39. Meakins, J. L.: Host defense mechanisms. wound healing, and infection. *In* Hunt, T. K., and Dunphy, J. E. (eds.): *Fundamentals of Wound Management.* Appleton-Century-Crofts, New York, 1979.

40. Miles, A. A.: The inflammatory response in relation to local infections. Surg. Clin. North Am. 60:93, 1980.

41. Miller, C., and Trunkey, D. D.: Immunobiology of sepsis. *In* Flint, L. M., and Fry, D. E. (eds.): *Surgical Infections.* Medical Examination Publishing Co., Garden City, NY, 1982.

42. Moore, F. D.: Homeostasis: Bodily changes in trauma and surgery. *In* Sabiston, D. C. (eds.): *Davis-Christopher Textbook of Surgery.* W. B. Saunders, Philadelphia, 1972.

43. Polk, H. C., Fry, D. E., and Flint, L. M.: Dissemination and causes of infection. Surg. Clin. North Am. 56:817, 1976.

44. Robson, M. C.: Infection in the surgical patient: An imbalance in the normal equilibrium. Clin. Plast. Surg. 6:493, 1979.

45. Robson, M. C.: Biology of Infection. *In* Kerstein, M. D. (ed.): *Management of Surgical Infections.* Futura Publishing Co., Mt. Kisco, NY, 1980.

46. Robson, M. C., Bogart, J. N., and Heggers, J. P.: An endogenous source for wound infections based on quantitative bacteriology of the biliary tract. Surgery 86:471, 1975.

47. Robson, M. C., Funderburk, M. S., Heggers, J. P., and Dalton, J. B.: Bacterial quantification of peritoneal exudates. Surg. Gynecol. Obstet. 130:267, 1970.

48. Robson, M. C., and Heggers, J. P.: Bacterial quantification in open wounds. Mil. Med. 134:19, 1969.

49. Robson, M. C., Krizek, T. J., and Heggers, J. P.: Biology of surgical infection. *In: Current Problems in Surgery.* Year Book Medical Publishers, Chicago, 1973.

50. Ryan, G. B.: Inflammation and localization of infection. Surg. Clin. North Am. 56:831, 1976.

51. Sandusky, W. R.: Use of prophylactic antibiotics in surgical patients. Surg. Clin. North Am. 60:83, 1980.

52. Schilling, J. A.: Wound healing. Surg. Clin. North Am. 56:859, 1976.

53. Schonholtz, G. J.: Maintenance of aseptic barriers in the conventional operating room. J. Bone Joint Surg. 58A:439, 1976.

54. Wiley, A. M., and Barnett, M.: Clean surgeons and clean air. Clin. Orthop. Rel. Res. 96:168, 1973.

Chapter 5

Use of Antimicrobial Drugs in Surgery

Roger C. Penwick

Chemotherapy and antibiotic therapy have had a tremendous impact upon the practice of surgery.[7] Despite irrefutable evidence of the benefits of antimicrobial therapy and 40 years of antibiotic use, clinical and laboratory studies indicate that such use has failed to reduce the overall incidence of infection in surgical patients.[4, 7, 47]

Surgical infections may be divided into two categories. Many infections among surgical patients develop spontaneously and are considered *community-acquired infections*—the infectious process constitutes, at least in part, the reason for operative intervention. Infected bite wounds, perforation of the gastrointestinal tract with secondary bacterial peritonitis, and pyometritis are among such instances. The majority of infections occur in incisions and are operating-room–based, postoperative nosocomial infections.[6] Thus, antibiotic use in surgery has been for chemoprophylactic purposes.[34, 45, 53] There is continued debate as to the appropriate use of antimicrobial agents in preventing surgical infection.[2, 47]

Antimicrobial agents have been used to prevent postoperative infection on the assumption that if a drug is effective in eradicating bacteria that have already become established, it should easily discourage their implantation.[13] Such extrapolation seems so logical and the specter of surgical infection is so dreaded that it has become dogma to administer antibiotics to "high-risk" patients even in instances in which studies are not available to support their use.[47]

Consequently, the indiscriminate use of antibiotics has become widespread. In several studies conducted in human hospitals more than 50 per cent of the total antimicrobial use was for prophylaxis.[13, 28, 39, 45] If antibiotics were innocuous, with beneficial potential only, the single objection to their irrational use would be cost. However, cost is not the only, nor the most significant, objection to the improper use of antibiotics.[39] There are many avenues by which the unnecessary or inappropriate use of these agents may be harmful to the individual patient or to the population in general.

ADVERSE EFFECTS OF ANTIBIOTIC ADMINISTRATION

The adverse reactions produced by the antimicrobial drugs are of three general types: (1) toxic effects, (2) hypersensitivity reactions, and (3) biological alterations affecting the microbial ecosystem. No antibiotic presently available is entirely free of side effects; any of these reactions may be induced in varying degrees by their administration.[5, 55]

Toxic Effects

Because drugs are concentrated and metabolized by the liver and kidney, damage to these organs by a direct toxic effect is not uncommon.[55] Intrarenal precipitation of the less soluble sulfonamides is a major cause of nephrotoxicity. Ototoxicity and nephrotoxicity of certain aminoglycosides is also well known.[55] Certain other antibiotics, such as chloramphenicol, may inhibit protein metabolism and cell growth and thus may potentially interfere with host antibacterial responses and wound healing.[12, 24] The short duration of administration consistent with properly applied chemoprophylaxis should minimize these problems.

Acute adverse effects may occur independent of the duration of drug administration. Under certain circumstances commonly used antibiotics may induce cardiovascular or respiratory depression through direct effects upon specific physiologic functions. These acute pharmacologic effects have no relationship to immune system phenomena or to cytotoxicity.[1]

In most instances, other contributing factors such as pre-existing pathological conditions, cardiac or renal dysfunction, systemic illness, and the simultaneous administration of other drugs (e.g., general anesthetics, neuromuscular blocking drugs, other antibiotics) have been present. The potential for such adverse reactions dictates that the use of some antibiotics should be approached with caution under certain clinical conditions.[1]

Hypersensitivity Reactions

Drug allergy may take many forms, including the full spectrum of immediate and delayed types of allergic phenomena produced by foreign macromolecules.[55] These immunologic reactions vary from rapidly fatal anaphylactic shock to mild allergic dermatitis requiring no specific therapy.[24] The full importance of drug sensitivity in veterinary medicine has yet to be defined.[1] Table 5–1 lists some of the adverse effects of antibiotics.

Biological Alterations

Biological alterations that occur in the host owing to antibiotic administration may produce many serious problems.[24] These include alterations in the normal microbial flora of the host, superinfection, and emergence of antibiotic-resistant strains of microorganisms.[55]

Practically all individuals receiving therapeutic doses of antimicrobial agents undergo alterations in the normal microbial population of the intestinal, upper respiratory, and genitourinary tracts[20] secondary to antibiotic therapy.[40] These changes commonly include a significant increase in the total number of strains of gram-negative organisms in the enteric flora. Presumably, the administered antibiotics alter the normal flora, permiting drug-resistant gram-negative bacilli to persist in the intestinal tract.[40] Thus, the gastrointestinal tracts of treated patients may become important reservoirs of pathogenic gram-negative bacilli.

Development of superinfection in certain patients may also be related to changes in the endogenous microbial flora.[55] Superinfection, the appearance of a new infection during the chemotherapy of a primary one, is a relatively common and potentially dangerous complication because the new microorganisms are often Proteus strains, drug-resistant staphylococci, Pseudomonas, Klebsiella, Candida, and fungi that may be difficult to eradicate with anti-infective drugs.[55] The range or spectrum of antibacterial activity of single or combined drugs is a factor in the pathogenesis of superinfection. The more "broad" the effect of an antibiotic, the greater the possibility that a single component of the normal or acquired microflora will predominate, invade, and produce infection.[55]

In addition to the adverse effects on the individual patient, the injudicious use of antimicrobials may pose severe hazards to the general population. Paramount among these is the emergence of resistant bacterial strains.

The development of resistance to an antibiotic involves a stable genetic change heritable from generation to generation, and thus any of the mechanisms that can result in the alteration of bacterial genetic composition can operate. Bacteria may become resistant to antimicrobial agents by mutation, transduction, transformation, or conjugation. The first three mechanisms are particularly involved in the development of drug resistance in gram-positive cocci, and all four may be responsible for the acquisition of resistance by gram-negative bacilli.[55]

Regardless of the genetic mechanism involved, the basic alterations in susceptibility are related to (1) elaboration of drug-metabolizing enzymes such as penicillinase, cephalosporinase, and adenylating, phosphorylating, and acetylating enzymes; (2) alteration of the permeability of the bacterial cell to the drug; (3) increased amount of an endogenous antagonist of drug action; or (4) alteration of the amount of drug receptor or the binding characteristics of the compound to its critical target.[55]

There is no evidence that mutations resulting in microbial resistance to an antibiotic are caused by exposure to the drug. On the contrary, mutations are random events, and the appearance of microbial resistance during therapy merely represents selective multiplication of the mutants that have been present

from the beginning of the infection or of a resistant strain introduced from the environment. Selection also accounts for an increase in the number of resistant strains present in a community or hospital. Widespread and prolonged use of a particular antibiotic agent, by eliminating the bulk of sensitive microorganisms, selects for the resistant ones, which then become the predominant forms.[55]

Conjugation, essentially asexual mating incorporating transfer of resistance factors (R factors) among bacterial organisms, is important in acquisition of drug resistance.[50] Because the R factors may contain genetic information coding for resistance to multiple drugs, all of this information may be acquired by a sensitive bacterium as a single event.[55] Within a given nosocomial setting, a prevalent R factor may be sustained by the use of any drug that is encompassed in its resistance package.[20]

The use of antimicrobial drugs may have undesirable side effects because organisms with multiple drug resistance are given a selective advantage.[50] However, the accumulated evidence also suggests that drug-resistant bacteria that are selected by the pressure of antibacterial drugs are at a disadvantage, however slight, in the absence of the selection pressure.[20]

Many of these concepts are illustrated in striking form in a 1970 report from Glasgow, Scotland, concerning the natural history of epidemic Klebsiella infection in a neurosurgical intensive care ward.[37] In 1966, postoperative infections due to coagulase-positive staphylococci and antibiotic-sensitive coliforms had become "troublesome," resulting in the institution of antimicrobial prophylaxis with ampicillin and cloxacillin in patients at special risk. During the winter of 1967–1968, antibiotic-resistant Klebsiella was cultured from sputum and urine of patients in the ward. By July of 1968, this organism was recovered from the sputum of 25 per cent of the patients. After the death of a 12-year-old boy from Klebsiella meningitis, bacterial cultures performed on specimens from the environment and personnel demonstrated that Klebsiella species were widespread in the unit.

By chance, the ward was due for renovation, and all of the infected patients were transferred to other wards or hospitals. The ward was modernized, all equipment was sterilized, and nursing techniques were reviewed. Despite these measures, infections due to Klebsiella reappeared within four weeks of the ward's reopening in October, 1968.

From October, 1968, to May, 1969, of 228 patients admitted to the ward, 28 per cent developed respiratory tract infection and 20 per cent urinary tract infection due to Klebsiella. Seven more patients contracted Klebsiella meningitis and died. Eighty per cent of the patients with these infections had had previous chemotherapy—generally with ampicillin, to which all the Klebsiella strains were resistant.

Despite efforts to eradicate the epidemic through varying antibiotic protocols and isolation procedures,

TABLE 5–l. Adverse Effects of Some Common Antimicrobial Compounds

Antimicrobial Drug	Adverse Effects
Aminoglycosides	Nephrotoxicity Ototoxicity—vestibular and auditory—cats are especially sensitive to vestibular abnormalities Cardiotoxicity Neuromuscular blockage Malabsorption (neomycin)
Carbenicillin, ticarcillin	Inhibition of platelet aggregation Hypokalemia due to renal distal tubular overload with nonreabsorbable anions with massive drug doses
Cephalosporins	Hypersensitivity reactions (rare); there is cross allergenicity with the penicillins Nephrotoxicity with large doses of cephaloridine or cephalothin Nausea, vomiting, minor GI disturbances In cats, chronic use of cephaloridine results in anemia
Chloramphenicol	Reversible dose-dependent bone marrow depression with aplastic anemia and other dyscrasias—cats are especially sensitive Vomiting and diarrhea Anorexia and depression in cats—possibly severe reactions in kittens Inhibition of the anamnestic immune response
Clindamycin	GI disturbances, enterocolotoxicity Neuromuscular blockade
Colistin	Nephrotoxicity and neurotoxicity (by parenteral administration)
Lincomycin	GI disturbances are common—including diarrhea and vomiting in cats Neuromuscular blockage and skeletal muscle paralysis at high concentrations
Macrolides (erythromycin, tylosin)	GI disturbances
Metronidazole	Enterocolotoxicity Neuropathy
Nitrofurantoin	Polyneuritis GI disturbances Pulmonary infiltrates Hemolytic anemia

Table continued on opposite page

control of the infection was not achieved, and by September, 1969, the staff was faced with closure of the unit. They therefore reluctantly adopted the drastic measure that both prophylactic and therapeutic antibiotics be entirely discontinued, on the hypothesis that the Klebsiella organisms were opportunists ready to colonize the respiratory tract of patients whose normal flora had been suppressed by broad-spectrum antibiotics. This course of action was ruthlessly adhered to for four months. Institution of the program was followed by an immediate decrease in the incidence of Klebsiella chest and urinary tract infections. Within four weeks, the Klebsiella chest infection rate fell to 2 per cent. In the subsequent year, no patient developed Klebsiella meningitis.

It had been feared that the rate of infections due to more antibiotic-sensitive organisms might increase, but in fact the total infection rate in the ward fell—respiratory tract infections from 45 to 15 per cent and urinary tract infections from 21 to 8 per cent within weeks of instituting the "no antibiotic" regimen.[37]

Finally, there are more subtle adverse sequelae pursuant to injudicious operative antimicrobial use. These problems may be collectively referred to as deterioration of the "surgical conscience." Surgical infection has been de-emphasized in the education of students and physicians. Many surgeons have developed a blind reliance on antibiotic agents for prophylaxis. Relaxation of the strict disciplines of established aseptic and antiseptic techniques has occurred, tending to remove some of the safety factors of surgical practice.[6, 7] Such attitudinal alterations within the surgical community may be among the most significant hazards associated with the indiscriminate administration of antibiotics in surgery.

The major factor that leads to wound sepsis is bacterial contamination during operation.[15, 42] A system of classification of surgical procedures has been developed to predict the amount of bacterial contamination likely to occur and by extension, the possibility of infection and the relative merits of chemoprophylaxis (Table 5–2). This classification can guide the use of antibiotics. It is also clear that bacterial contamination at operation does not have a linear relationship to postoperative infection. Many heavily

TABLE 5–1. Adverse Effects of Some Common Antimicrobial Compounds (*Continued*)

Antimicrobial Drug	Adverse Effects
Penicillins	Hypersensitivity, with skin reactions, angioedema, fever, serum sickness, eosinophilia, and anaphylaxis being most common
Ampicillin	GI disturbances
Oxycillin	Hepatotoxicity
Methacillin	Interstitial nephritis
Polymixin B	Nephrotoxicity Neuromuscular blockade
Sulfonamides	Adverse reactions may be allergic or toxic—fever, skin rashes, photosensitization, nausea, vomiting and/or diarrhea, stomatitis, conjunctivitis and keratitis sicca, arthritis, hepatitis Crystal formation in urine may lead to hematuria and obstruction; crystal formation in the glomeruli and pelvis of the kidney can be fatal Hemolytic or aplastic anemia, thrombocytopenia, granulocytopenia (esp. with sulfadiazine) Acute toxicity may result from overdosage by IV or oral routes or excessively rapid IV administration (blindness, tremors, dilated pupils, and collapse)
Tetracyclines	GI disturbances due to suprainfection may occur (can be serious in cats) Staining of erupting teeth IV injection can cause cardiac arrhythmias and hemolysis resulting in hemoglobinuria if the preparation is not diluted sufficiently Antianabolic effect—may inhibit weight gain and produce an elevated BUN Phototoxicosis
Trimethoprim-sulfadiazine	Side effects are rare Slight to moderate decrease in hematopoietic activity after high and prolonged doses
Vancomycin	Hypersensitivity—skin reactions Chills, fever, shocklike state may develop with IV infusion Ototoxicity Nephrotoxicity

(Reprinted with permission from Jenkins, W. L., and Riviere, J. E., *in* Johnston, D. E. (ed.): *The Bristol Veterinary Handbook of Antimicrobial Therapy*, Veterinary Learning Systems Co., Inc., Syracuse, NY, 1982; and from Goodman, L. S., and Gilman, A. (eds.): *The Pharmacological Basis of Therapeutics*, 5th ed. New York, Macmillan Pub. Co., Inc., 1975.)

TABLE 5–2. National Research Council Classification of Operative Wounds in Relation to Contamination and Increasing Risk of Infection*

Clean	Nontraumatic No inflammation encountered No break in technique Respiratory, alimentary, genitourinary tracts not entered
Clean-contaminated	Gastrointestinal or respiratory tracts entered without significant spillage Oropharynx entered Vagina entered Genitourinary tract entered in absence of infected urine Biliary tract entered in absence of infected bile Minor break in technique
Contaminated	Major break in technique Gross spillage from gastrointestinal tract Traumatic wound, fresh Entrance of genitourinary tract or biliary tract in presence of infected urine or bile
Dirty and infected	Acute bacterial inflammation encountered, without pus Transection of "clean" tissues for the purpose of surgical access to a collection of pus Traumatic wound with retained devitalized tissue, foreign bodies, fecal contamination and/or delayed treatment, or from dirty source

*Adapted from Altemeier, W. A., Burke, J. F., Pruitt, B. A., Jr., and Sandusky, W. R. (eds.): Definitions and classifications of surgical infections. *In: Manual on Control of Infection in Surgical Patients*. Philadelphia, J. B. Lippincott, 1976; reprinted with permission from Cruse, T. J. E.: Wound infections: Epidemiology and clinical characteristics. *In* Simmons, R. L., and Howard, R. J. (eds.): *Surgical Infectious Diseases*. New York, Appleton-Century-Crofts, 1982.

contaminated wounds heal without complication, whereas others become infected, implying that infection will occur only when host defenses are insufficient to keep bacterial proliferation under control.[18] Factors such as advanced age, concurrent infection, hepatic or renal dysfunction, and extreme obesity increase postoperative infection. Additionally, host resistance is abnormal in disorders such as leukemia, diabetes mellitus, pneumonia, burns, severe pancreatitis, and malnutrition, and following trauma.[5] Anesthesia, ischemia, shock, and depletion of complement also enhance the size of a standard infective lesion.[11, 38] Under such conditions, microbes that normally have low virulence may be able to escape local and systemic host defenses, invade tissue, and cause disease.[23]

The importance of endogenous host factors in wound infection is now being given much consideration. To be effective, host defense requires the integrated and efficient function of the component parts.[27, 31] The interplay of phagocytic cells, lymphocytes, and mediators of both cell-mediated and humoral immunity, opsonins, and the complement system is complex and can be impaired by a variety of congenital and acquired abnormalities.[31] Disorders of neutrophil production, leukocyte migration or degranulation, opsonization, monocyte or macrophage dysfunction, T- or B-cell immunodeficiencies, and defects of the complement system may be caused by a variety of physiologic derangements. Not all patients exhibiting such physiologic alterations have detectable abnormalities in host defense.[31] Because of the significance of these host defenses and their variability from patient to patient, the decision to employ chemoprophylaxis cannot be based solely upon the type of operation to be performed. The important factor is the ability of the patient to withstand the operation without developing infection.[24]

Although such systemic host defenses are of unquestionable importance in the pathogenesis of postoperative infection, the local resistance of the wound is much more important than the general resistance of the patient.[18] Local factors that influence postoperative infection encompass endogenous host variables as well as technical and environmental concerns. Surgical technique is one of the most significant of these variables. Kocher and Von Bergman first demonstrated that meticulous hemostasis and gentle tissue handling were associated with lower wound sepsis rates.[18] Halstead adopted their views and stressed finite attention to operative detail with his principles of complete hemostasis, adequate blood supply, removal of devitalized tissue, obliteration of dead space, use of fine nonabsorbable suture material, and wound closure without tension.[18] Since their time, many investigators have demonstrated the basis for these concepts and reinforced their validity.

Infection is closely and inversely related to blood flow through injured and contaminated tissue.[31] Unnecessary trauma to tissue, dead space, hematoma formation, foreign body implantation, duration of operation, and other factors have effects upon local vascular dynamics. Additionally, there are normal differences in capillary density in various areas of the body. Therefore, the space of unperfused tissue associated with wounding is larger in the extremities than in the face, and larger in connective tissue than in parenchymatous organs.[31] The increased susceptibility to infection in the hypovascular and therefore hypoxic wound space may be related to impaired function of the wound leukocyte. Leukocytes in a hypoxic environment are less capable of killing bacteria than those kept in an arterial or even venous pO_2 owing to failure of the oxidative bactericidal pathway.[31]

Observations that wounds made with an electric scalpel or laser are roughly twice as susceptible to infection as those made with a cold knife, and that avulsed wounds are more prone to infection than cleanly cut ones may be explained on the basis of alterations in local blood flow.[31] Also, hypovolemia or the use of vasoconstrictive drugs enhances wound infection when present in the first few hours after wounding. Shock and ischemia in this early determinative period are particularly detrimental. Because of local blood flow effects, the induction of shock to the point of impairment of skin perfusion reduces the minimal dose of bacteria necessary to initiate infection 10,000-fold.[18]

In addition to the impairment of phagocyte function that occurs in hypoxic tissue, embarrassment of local blood flow also results in decreased delivery of these cells to the involved area. Many other conditions also contribute to decreased influx of wound leukocytes and any such situation promotes infection.[5]

PRINCIPLES OF ANTIMICROBIAL CHEMOPROPHYLAXIS IN SURGERY

When a single effective drug is used to avoid implantation of a specific microorganism or to eradicate it immediately or shortly after it has become established, but not yet clinically evident, chemoprophylaxis is, with uncommon exception, highly successful. However, if the aim of prophylaxis is to prevent colonization and/or infection by any and all microorganisms that may be present in the patient's internal or external environment, failure is the rule.

Weinstein—1954[54]

The basic tenets of safe and rational chemoprophylaxis are few and straightforward. The antibiotic must be selected and administered in such a fashion that there is a therapeutically effective concentration of an appropriate antibiotic in the interstitial fluid space during the time of risk of primary bacterial lodgement. The drug chosen should possess as narrow an antimicrobial spectrum as possible consistent with providing adequate protection against the most likely offending microorganisms. Finally, the duration of administration should be kept to a minimum to decrease the risks associated with protracted courses of antibiotic therapy.[6, 28, 49]

These principles have been condensed from a large body of clinical and experimental data. Experimental work has clearly demonstrated that there is a short period during which developing primary bacterial lesions are susceptible to treatment.[13] This susceptibility is maximal if the antibiotic is in the tissue when the bacteria arrive. As the interval between the introduction of the bacteria and the administration of the antibiotic increases, the antibiotic effect decreases. The major antibiotic effect is over in approximately one hour, and the systemic antibiotics have no effect on primary bacterial infection if the bacteria creating the infection have been in the tissue longer than three hours before the antibiotic is given.[13]

The basis for these observations lies in the mode of genesis of the primary bacterial lesion. It had usually been assumed that for the experimental primary staphylococcal lesion, the period of development covered approximately 24 hours.[13] Although the physical events necessary to produce a mature primary lesion require 24 hours, there is evidence that the biochemical interactions between tissues and bacteria that control the size of the lesion occur in a much shorter time.[13, 32] The extensive physical changes such as induration and necrosis, looked upon as the direct action of the bacteria on tissue, are only the slowly evolving indirect results of bacterial action. If this is true, a developing primary bacterial lesion could be modified during the early short period of decisive biochemical action but not during the period of slowly evolving induration and necrosis.[13] Considering these findings, there is not a six- to eight-hour "golden period" when tissue is free of infection after contamination.[13] Nontraumatic surgical wounds, however, are usually seeded during operation, and thus the time of primary bacterial lodgement is easily predicted.

This evidence suggests that the antibacterial agent must be present in an effective concentration at the time of primary bacterial lodgement for maximal effect to be obtained. The evidence also indicates that it is unnecessary to begin administration of antibiotics as early as 24 hours before operation. Such practice unnecessarily prolongs the duration of drug administration, increasing the hazards of selection of resistant strains.[3, 6, 24, 49] Instead, the length of time that a prophylactic antimicrobial should be given preoperatively should be dictated by the rate at which that compound reaches an effective concentration in the interstitial fluid by the route of administration to be employed.[24]

In any experimental or clinical treatment in which drugs are tested, it is essential that time/dose relationships to drug concentration at the site of action be determined for proper evaluation of the effect of the agents. Many studies have measured serum concentrations of the drugs or concentrations in tissue homogenates.[14, 51] The interstitial fluid concentration is more representative of the required concentration, since intracellular infections by the bacteria commonly implicated in postoperative infection do not occur except in cells of lymphatic and hematopoietic origin.[51] Also, because infections caused by these bacteria are not intravascular except in septicemia,

TABLE 5–3. Time Required to Attain Peak Concentrations in Wound Fluid for Selected Antibiotics*

Penicillin-G, ampicillin, and nafcillin	Concentrations in wound fluid exceed serum concentrations by one hour.
	Serum concentrations of nafcillin fall rapidly—wound fluid concentrations always low in comparison to those of the other agents.
Oxacillin and carbenicillin	At one hour, the ratios of wound fluid concentration to serum concentration are much less than for the other penicillins.
	Highest concentrations in the wound fluid are seen at 30 minutes; then they gradually decrease to approximately equal serum concentrations by two hours.
Cephalosporins (cefazolin, cephalothin, cephaloridine)	All reached significant wound fluid levels with a peak between one and two hours.
	Highest concentrations were found with cefazolin, followed by cephaloridine and finally cephalothin. The degree of protein binding has little influence upon the kinetics of transfer (serum to wound fluid).
Gentamicin	Peak wound fluid levels at two hours. Relatively low concentrations of drug present in wound fluid.
Erythromycin	Relatively low concentrations produced in wound.
	Peak at one hour—at that time wound fluid level is approximately half the serum level.
	Wound fluid concentrations do not exceed serum concentrations until five hours after administration.
Polymyxin-B and tetracycline	Peak concentrations in wound at one hour.
	Wound fluid concentrations never reach serum concentrations.

*A single dose of drug administered intravenously. (Reprinted with permission from Alexander, J. W., Sykes, N. S., Mitchell, M. M., and Fisher, M. W.: Concentration of selected intravenously administered antibiotics in experimental surgical wounds. J. Trauma 13:423, 1973.)

the concentration of the antibiotics in the interstitial fluid that bathes the wound is of greater significance than serum concentrations.[51]

There are considerable differences among various antibiotics in the rate at which they reach the operative wound, with peak levels reached in less than one hour by some and more than five hours by others (Table 5–3).[24] Some experimental results indicate that tissues may never be exposed to an adequate concentration of some antibacterial agents administered in clinically acceptable fashion (Table 5–4).[14]

The reasons for the marked differences in the distribution of antibacterial agents are complex. The capillary endothelium does not restrict the distribution of drugs (except in the brain), and most drugs, whether ionized or un-ionized, diffuse into the interstitial fluid.[21] The overall disposition within the body is limited by such factors as plasma protein binding, the drug's rate of absorption, distribution, and elimination, the dose of the drug, the plasma peak, the volume of distribution, ability to penetrate tissue barriers, the dissociation constant of the drug, the extent of hepatic biotransformation, reabsorption through enterohepatic circulation, renal excretion and secretion, and specific interactions with coadministered therapeutic agents.[14, 24, 27, 38]

The interchange between plasma and wound or interstitial fluid is a passive process regulated by simple diffusion. Curves generated by plotting the respective concentrations of antibiotic in wound fluid and blood as a function of time exhibit the phenomenon of diffusion along a concentration gradient across a semipermeable barrier.[2, 10] This distribution can be described in terms of transfer between a well-perfused central compartment and a tissue compartment composed of less-perfused areas, including the interstitial fluid.[38] There is a phase of initial distribution, during which the drug introduced to the body is distributed from the central to the tissue compartment. When this has occurred, a second or elimination phase begins. Peak tissue concentrations of antibiotic are not realized until the early distribution phase is complete (Fig. 5–1).[38]

It is important that the peak levels achieved are sufficient to establish the desired antibacterial effect and that these levels persist as long as necessary to protect against primary bacterial lodgement.

For any antibiotic, the concentration necessary to inhibit a particular strain of bacterium *in vitro* is referred to as the *minimal inhibitory concentration* (MIC). A bacterium is "sensitive" to the antibiotic if it is inhibited by the concentration of antibiotic attained in the tissues by the recommended clinical dosage.[25] For a wide range of antibiotics, the peak non–protein-bound concentration achieved in plasma is approximately twice the *in vitro* MIC for bacteria sensitive to that antibiotic.[25] Accordingly, the principle has been advanced in the veterinary literature that the goal should be to maintain free plasma levels "well in excess" of the MIC for the bacteria concerned.[25] Considering the intricacies of equilibration

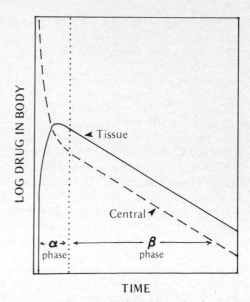

Figure 5–1. Plot of the amount of intravenously administered drug in the central and tissue compartments as a function of time. α, distribution; β, elimination. (Reprinted with permission from Riviere, J. E., Kaufman, G. M., and Bright, R. M.: Prophylactic use of systemic antimicrobial drugs in surgery. Comp. Cont. Ed. 3:345, 1981.)

of antibiotics between plasma and interstitial fluid, this principle is a gross oversimplification. Another commonly accepted guideline is to attempt to achieve a blood level that exceeds the MIC for a given organism by two- to eight-fold. This is an arbitrary concentration of drug and obviously does not take into account all the variations in penetration into different tissues or the role of host defense mechanisms.[26]

The concentration of antibiotic in wound fluid reflects but does not parallel serum concentrations.[2, 3] The tissue fluid concentration is always lower than the peak concentration in serum, and the concentration of antibiotic in interstitial fluid is not necessarily similar to that in serum.[14] For those drugs that are slowly excreted (e.g., trimethoprim, sulfamethoxazole, chloramphenicol, metronidazole, tetracycline) the tissue fluid concentration is similar to the serum concentration after approximately six hours. With more rapidly excreted compounds (e.g., carbenicillin, cephalothin, ampicillin, gentamicin, cloxacillin, erythromycin) the concentration in tissue fluid is unpredictable—being either negligible and of no benefit, or maintained at levels significantly better than those in serum.[14] Such facts further demonstrate the potential hazards of inferring wound fluid activity by extrapolation from serum concentrations. In the study of distribution of drugs in body fluids there is no substitute for direct measurement.[14]

Prophylactic antibiotics should be given shortly prior to surgery in quantities and via a route that results in therapeutic interstitial fluid concentrations at the appropriate time.[51] The surgical incision should be made during the early elimination phase.[38]

Considering that the fundamental basis for distri-

TABLE 5–4. Tissue Distribution of Several Antimicrobial Drugs*†

	Penicillins	Streptomycin	Tetracyclines	Sulfonamides	Erythromycin	Chloramphenicol	Novobiocin	Lincomycin
Tissue concentration								
Prostate	Low	Negligible	++++	++	++++	++	—	+++
Synovial fluid	Low	++	Low	++	+++	+++	+++	+++
Peritoneal fluid	Low	++++	Low	++++	+++	+++++	+++	++++
Pleural fluid	Low	+++++	Low	+++++	+++	+++++	+++	++++
Bile	+++	+++++	++	+++++	++++	+++++	+++++	+++
Urine	++++	+++++	+++	+++++	Low	Low	Negligible	+++
Brain	Negligible	Negligible	Negligible	Some compounds	++	+++	Negligible	Negligible
Eye (aqueous)	Negligible	+++	Low	Some compounds	Negligible	++	Negligible	Negligible
Lung	++	+++	+++	++++	+++	+++	+++	+++
Kidneys	++++	+++	+++	+++	+++	+++	Low	++++
Liver	++++	+++	+++	+++	+++	+++	++++	++++
Skin	+++	+++	++	+++	+++	+++	++	++
Intestine	++	++	+++	++	—	++	—	+
Milk	Low	—	+++	Low	Low	—	—	++
Bone	Low	++	+++	+++	++	+++	+++	+++
Muscle	+++	++	+++	+++	+++	+++	—	++
Fetus	Low	++	++	+++	+	+++	—	+++
Intracellular	No	No	Yes	Yes	No	Yes	—	Yes
Elimination								
Renal	++++	++++	++++	+++	Low	Low	Low	+++
Biliary	Low	Low	++	++	++++	++	+++	+++
Biotransformation	+	No	+	+	—	+++++	++	—

*Concentrations of antimicrobial drugs found in various tissues and the principal route of elimination are indicated in relative terms. Negligible = nil; ++++ = concentrations higher than those found in other tissues or principal route of elimination. Modified from Davis, L. E.: Syllabus on Clinical Pharmacology and Therapeutics. Fort Collins, Colorado State University, 1976.

bution of antibiotic to the wound fluid is simple passive diffusion, it is clear that the magnitude of the initial serum peak exerts a profound influence upon the concentration gradient realized. It is important that initial plasma peaks be high in order to obtain high concentrations in the wound.

The clinician has greatest control over the two factors that determine the peak serum concentration, which are dose of the drug and the route of administration. As dosage is increased, the peak concentration is increased without change in the time at which the peak effect occurs.[21, 51] The implication is that doubling, tripling, or quadrupling the dose usually administered to raise the concentration quickly in the interstitial fluid would be required or beneficial. However, increasing the dose of the drug also increases the risks of toxic reactions, the amount of drug released into the environment, and the cost—a significant factor with some of the drugs.[51]

A more practical method of assuring therapeutic interstitial fluid levels is to administer the drug by a route that guarantees high plasma peaks.

The problem of assessing the influence of route of administration on the wound fluid concentration of prophylactic antibiotics has been addressed.[3] Major inconsistencies in the manner in which antibiotics were first administered to trauma patients in human hospitals had been observed. Patients occasionally received antibiotics for prophylaxis of infection after trauma by continuous intravenous infusion rather than by bolus. Therefore, attempts were made to establish what differences actually existed. The result was an experimental study carried out using the dog in which 13 antibiotics were used to assess the distribution in serum and wound fluid after different modes of administration.

Each antibiotic had different patterns of distribution in serum and wound fluid compartments, but in general, intravenous bolus administration showed comparable levels in the wound four to 12 times faster than continuous intravenous infusion. After 12 hours, the highest sustained antibiotic concentration in wound fluid was usually obtained via intramuscular administration.

The intravenous bolus yields high peak plasma levels instantaneously.[21, 25] Therefore, owing to markedly higher initial serum concentration, the antibiotics appeared more promptly in the tissue fluid when first administered by this route. Because of more rapid excretion, administration by intravenous bolus generally resulted in less sustained serum levels than when the agent was first given by the intramuscular route. Accordingly, antibiotics administered intramuscularly generally demonstrated higher peak levels in the interstitial fluid, since a concentration gradient forcing antibiotic into the tissue compartment persisted longer.[3] When a similar total dose of antimicrobial was given by continuous intravenous infusion, peak levels were often not achieved in wound fluid until after 18 hours, and the appearance of effective antibiotic concentrations in the wound

fluid was usually longer than the three-hour period considered to be maximum if drug administration is to be effective in preventing wound infection after contamination.[3] Therefore, for chemoprophylaxis, simultaneous administration of both intravenous boluses and intramuscular doses is recommended, followed by intermittent intramuscular injections if necessary.

Oral administration for prophylaxis is not suitable for a number of reasons. Low plasma levels are consistently produced by oral administration. The same dose of ampicillin given orally results in only 20 per cent of the peak plasma levels achieved when it is given intramuscularly in the dog.[17] Additionally, absorption from the gastrointestinal tract may be varied, unpredictable, and influenced by other enteric factors.[15, 21, 22]

For chemoprophylaxis to be beneficial, therapeutic concentrations of the antibiotic agent must be present in the interstitial spaces throughout the duration of risk of bacterial lodgement. If the surgical procedure is exceedingly long (i.e., longer than three to four hours) or if the antibacterial agent chosen is excreted rapidly, tissue levels of antibiotic may not persist as long as the risk of contamination exists.[38] Therefore it is necessary to give some consideration to maintenance of therapy.

In the simple kinetic model upon which fundamental pharmacodynamic principles are based, the body is a single compartment within which distribution of a drug is relatively uniform.[21] Absorption and elimination of the drugs in general follow exponential or first-order kinetics; that is, a constant fraction of the drug present is eliminated per unit time.[21] The rate of such an exponential process can be expressed in terms of its "half-life"—the time required for completion of 50 per cent of the process. The half-life is independent of drug dose and of concentration of the drug preparation.[21]

The process of elimination of the antibiotic from the body is 93.75 per cent complete after four half-lives. Because first-order kinetics dictate that a constant fraction of drug is lost per unit time, a graph of the logarithm of drug concentration *versus* time is linear during the elimination phase (see Fig. 5–1).[21]

Since more than four half-lives are required for complete elimination, repeated administration of a drug at intervals shorter than this may result in drug accumulation.[21] Accumulation continues to occur until the amount of drug eliminated per dosage interval equals the amount administered per dose.[21] As long as first-order kinetics apply, elimination of drug also increases as accumulation occurs. If a drug is administered intermittently at intervals shorter than that necessary to achieve complete elimination (or by continuous intravenous infusion), it accumulates exponentially to a plateau with a half-life equal to the elimination half-life.[21] Ninety-four per cent of this plateau is attained after four half-lives. The drug concentration maintained during the plateau state is directly proportional to the total dose of drug given per unit time and to the elimination half-life of the drug.[21] When a drug is administered at intervals equal to its elimination half-life, the average concentration during the plateau state is about 1.5 times the peak concentration after the initial dose.[21] Half doses at half intervals maintain the same average concentration with smaller fluctuations.[21] Table 5–5 lists pertinent pharmacokinetic data for some common antimicrobial drugs.

Fluctuations in drug concentration that can be tolerated without loss of efficacy or excess toxicity are important in selecting a maintenance schedule. For most drugs, a dosage interval less than or equal to the elimination half-life is recommended.[21] Proper intervals for multiple-dose administration of various antimicrobial drugs are listed in Table 5–6. If such a schedule is followed from the inception of therapy, partial effect is achieved promptly, but the full therapeutic effect is not achieved for four elimination half-lives.[21] In chemoprophylaxis, the desired effect must be realized more promptly; thus the recommendation for the initial "loading" regimen described earlier.

This "loading" regimen was devised for use in trauma patients with contaminated wounds in whom considerable time may have elapsed before institution of therapy. The antibiotic must then be chosen on the basis not only of the most likely contaminating organisms but also of the rapidity of penetration and ultimate concentration in wound fluids. The experiment investigating these effects measured the antibiotic concentration in interstitial fluid in tissues that had not undergone recent dissection or wounding. The results are therefore more applicable to the circumstances of surgical chemoprophylaxis, in which the time of bacterial contamination can be predicted and tissue levels of antibiotic can be reached prior to operation.

Diffusion of antibiotics into dissected tissues does occur but is delayed in comparison with that in uninjured tissue.[2, 16, 51] This emphasizes the importance of achieving a therapeutic concentration in the interstitial space prior to the beginning of surgery.

As noted earlier, the duration of administration of chemoprophylactic agents should be minimized to avoid undesirable sequelae. Thus, a maintenance regimen as discussed previously needs to be implemented only when a source of contamination persists for a protracted period. Indwelling venous catheters, drains, and so on, afford continuing opportunity for

TABLE 5–5. Pharmacokinetic Data for Selected Antimicrobial Drugs in Dogs*

Drug	Route	Percentage Absorbed	Absorption Half-Life (hr)	Volume of Distribution (% of body weight)	Elimination Half-Life (hr)	Rate Constant of Elimination (hr^{-1})
Amoxicillin	PO	80	0.5	20	1.5	0.462
Ampicillin	IM	100	0.3	40	1.5	0.462
	PO	50	0.5	40	1.5	0.462
Carbenicillin	IM	—	—	20	1.5	0.462
Cephalothin	IM	100	0.3	30	0.5	1.386
Chloramphenicol succinate	IM	70	0.3	177	4.2	0.165
Chloramphenicol	PO	100	1.0	177	4.2	0.165
Cloxacillin	IM	—	—	20	0.5	1.386
Erythromycin	PO	60	1.5	70	1.5	0.462
Gentamicin	IM	100	0.2	20	1.5	0.462
Kanamycin	IM	100	0.2	20	2.0	0.347
Methicillin	IV	—	—	20	0.5	1.386
Metronidazole	PO	100	0.5	90	4.4	0.158
Oxacillin	IM	100	0.3	30	0.5	1.386
	PO	50	0.5	30	0.5	1.386
Oxytetracycline	PO	—	—	90	5.0	0.139
Potassium penicillin G	IM	100	0.2	30	0.5	1.386
	PO	25	0.5	30	0.5	1.386
Procaine penicillin G	IM	100	4.0	30	0.5	1.386
Steptomycin	IM	100	0.3	20	2.5	0.277
Sulfadimethoxine		30	1.5	40	13.2	0.053
Sulfamethazine	PO	100	0.5	70	6.0	0.116
Sulfisoxazole	PO	—	—	30	4.5	0.154
Tetracycline	PO	70	0.5	120	7.0	0.099
Trimethoprim		—	—	400	3.9	0.178
Tylosin	IM	100	0.25	170	0.9	0.770

*Modified from Davis, L. E.: Antimicrobial therapy. *In* Kirk, R. W. (ed.): *Current Veterinary Therapy: Small Animal Practice.* Philadelphia, W. B. Saunders, 1980; and from a personal communication to Dr. Davis from Dr. G. C. Conzelman, Jr., School of Veterinary Medicine, University of California, Davis.

TABLE 5–6. Conventional Regimens for Some Antimicrobial Drugs in Dogs and Cats

Drug	Dosage	Route	Repeat Dose
Amphotericin B	0.5 to 1.0 mg./kg.	IV	See below*
Ampicillin	10 to 20 mg./kg.	PO	6 hours
	5 to 10 mg./kg.	IV,IM,SC	6 hours
Amoxicillin	11 mg./kg.	PO,IM	12 hrs
Carbencillin	15 mg./kg.	IV	8 hours
Cephalexin	30 mg./kg.	PO	12 hours
Cephaloridine	10 mg./kg.	IM,SC	8 to 12 hours
Cephalothin	35 mg./kg.	IM,SC	8 hours
Chloramphenicol	50 mg./kg.	PO,IV,IM,SC	8 hours (dog), 12 hours (cat)
Chlortetracycline	20 mg./kg.	PO	8 hours
Cloxacillin	10 mg./kg.	PO,IV,IM	6 hours
Colistin	1 mg./kg.	IM	6 hours
Dihydrostreptomycin	20 mg./kg.	PO	6 hours (not absorbed)
	10 mg./kg.	IM,SC	8 hours
Erythromycin	10 mg./kg.	PO	8 hours
Framycetin	20 mg./kg.	PO	6 hours (not absorbed)
Gentamicin	4 mg./kg.	IM,SC	12 hours first day, then 24 hours
Griseofulvin	20 mg./kg.	PO	24 hours, with fat
	140 mg./kg.	PO	1 week, with fat
Hetacillin	10 to 20 mg./kg.	PO	8 hours
Kanamycin	10 mg./kg.	PO	6 hours (not absorbed)
	7 mg./kg.	IM,SC	6 hours
Lincomycin	15 mg./kg.	PO	8 hours
	10 mg./kg.	IV,IM	12 hours
Methicillin	20 mg./kg.	IV,IM	6 hours
Metronidazole	60 mg./kg.	PO	24 hours
Nafcillin	10 mg./kg.	PO,IM	6 hours
Neomycin	20 mg./kg.	PO	6 hours (not absorbed)
	10 mg./kg.	IM,SC	12 hours
Nitrofurantoin	4 mg./kg.	PO	8 hours
	3 mg./kg.	IM	12 hours
Nystatin	100,000 U	PO	6 hours (not absorbed)
Oxacillin	10 mg./kg.	PO,IV,IM	6 hours
Oxytetracycline	20 mg./kg.	PO	8 hours
	7 mg./kg.	IV,IM	12 hours
Penicillin G, Na or K	40,000 U/kg.	PO	6 hours (not with food)
	20,000 U/kg.	IV,IM,SC	4 hours
Penicillin G, benethamine	40,000 U/kg.	IM	5 days
Penicillin G, procaine	20,000 U/kg.	IM,SC	12 to 24 hours
Penicillin V	10 mg./kg.	PO	8 hours
Phenethicillin	10 mg./kg.	PO	8 hours
Phthalylsulfathiazole	50 mg./kg.	PO	6 hours (not absorbed)
Polymyxin B	2 mg (20,000 U)/kg.	IM	12 hours
Pyrimethamine	1 mg./kg.	PO	24 hours for 3 days, then
	0.5 mg./kg.	PO	24 hours
Streptomycin	20 mg./kg.	PO	6 hours (not absorbed)
	10 mg./kg.	IM,SC	8 hours
Sulfadiazine, sulfamerazine, sulfamethazine	50 mg./kg.	PO,IV	12 hours
Sulfadimethoxine	25 mg./kg.	PO,IV,IM	24 hours
Sulfamethizole, sulfisoxazole	50 mg./kg.	PO	8 hours
Sulfasalazine	15 mg./kg.	PO	6 hours (Dog only)
Tetracycline	20 mg./kg.	PO	8 hours
	7 mg./kg.	IV,IM	12 hours
Trimethoprim plus sulfadiazine	30 mg./kg.	PO	12 hours
Trimethoprim plus sulfadoxine	15 mg.(combined)/kg.	IV,IM	24 hours
Tylosin	10 mg./kg.	PO	8 hours
	5 mg./kg.	IV,IM	12 hours

*Amphotericin B must be diluted with 5 per cent dextrose and water. It can be given IV two to three times weekly. It is very toxic; treatment should be stopped if vomiting, proteinuria, or an increase in BUN develops. Toxicity may preclude its use in cats. (Reprinted with permission from Davis, L. E.: Antimicrobial therapy. In Kirk, R. W. (ed.): *Current Veterinary Therapy VII: Small Animal Practice.* Philadelphia, W.B. Saunders, 1980.)

metastatic bacterial lodgment in surgically disrupted tissues.[24] However, the thesis that antibiotic administration must continue for the period of maintenance of such devices is not widely accepted, and one or two doses of drug during the perioperative period are sufficient for prophylactic purposes.[6, 20, 48] There is no conclusive evidence to support the use of prophylactic antibiotic agents beyond three to six hours postoperatively.[48]

Antibiotic prophylaxis should be limited to patients with a significant risk of postoperative infection. The clinical merit of this concept presupposes a sufficient frequency of infection to warrant the use of agents that may be both directly and indirectly hazardous.[33]

Uncontaminated Surgery

Although there are instances in which the usual low risk of infection following a clean, elective surgical procedure is changed to a substantial risk of infection owing to the patient's compromised defense mechanisms, prophylactic antibiotics should not be administered to patients undergoing clean surgery.[2, 5, 6, 15, 20, 24, 28, 35, 47] Antibiotics are also less likely to be beneficial when host resistance is diminished, whereas strict asepsis prevents contamination and reduces the risk of infection.[28, 29] In clean surgery, meticulous technique must take preference over chemoprophylaxis to avoid infection.

Regardless of other qualifying factors, the postoperative infection rate for clean procedures should remain at less than 5 per cent.[2, 18, 24, 47] If such a rate is exceeded in a given hospital, regardless of the patient population, an investigation of surgical technique, ventilation, or other variables known to contribute to postoperative infection is more appropriate than the institution of chemoprophylaxis.[2, 24]

Contaminated Surgery

Clean-contaminated procedures present the greatest quandary in consideration of chemoprophylaxis, because operations in this category vary considerably in degree of contamination. In contaminated and "dirty" or infected surgery, antibiotic administration by some route is usually appropriate. Whether such drug use is more properly termed *prophylactic* or *therapeutic* is often debated.

PRINCIPLES OF SURGICAL ANTIMICROBIAL THERAPY

Rational implementation of chemotherapy in surgery may be less controversial than that of chemoprophylaxis. Careful consideration is necessary to most effectively employ antimicrobial agents. The basic tenets of antimicrobial therapy are: (1) the organism must be sensitive to the drug; (2) the drug must be distributed to the site of infection; and (3) conditions at the site of infection must be favorable for the drug to exert its action.[8]

Chemotherapy is used in community-acquired infections, in heavily contaminated traumatic wounds, for elective surgical procedures in which significant spillage occurs (e.g., "dirty" wounds), and in postoperative infections that may relate to failure of chemoprophylaxis.

Antibiotic use is indicated in those community-acquired infections in which surgery is an important facet of management. As with chemoprophylaxis, the selection of antibiotic is based on the most likely offending organisms and the pharmacokinetic characteristics of the drugs. Prior to treatment, it is important to document that an infectious process necessitating chemotherapy actually exists. The mere presence of leukocyte changes is not adequate evidence. Samples of exudates, discharges, urine, cerebrospinal fluid, transtracheal aspirates, synovial fluid, and so on, should be examined microscopically and bacteriologically to assess microorganisms in the disease.[19]

In serious infectious processes, antimicrobial use may consist of *initial therapy*, in which the emphasis is on broad antibiotic coverage, and *definitive therapy*, in which the choice of specific drugs depends on bacterial isolation and *in vitro* sensitivity testing.[22]

In the initial 24 to 48 hours, when microbiological information is not available, treatment is based upon clinical information and results of simple laboratory tests.[22] From the history and physical examination, knowledge may be gained regarding the major site of involvement (e.g., pneumonia, pyometritis, pyelonephritis), and possible complications (e.g., bactermia, renal damage, metastatic infection). On the basis of the primary site of infection, hospital antibiograms (if available), and previous experience, treatment may be initiated with agents likely to be effective against probable pathogens (Table 5–7).[19]

For example, when there is suspicion of intra-abdominal infection with possible bacteremia, *Escherichia coli*, Klebsiella, Proteus, Group-D streptococci (enterococci), and various anaerobes are likely to be involved. Treatment is directed against all potential pathogens capable of causing infection in pure culture. The assumption that one strain is more important than another should not be made.[20] Therefore, such potentially overwhelming infections may merit "shotgun" use of drug combinations in the initial phase. Penicillin G, ampicillin, or trimethoprim-sulfadiazine is effective against enterococci; clindamycin, chloramphenicol, carbenicillin, or cefoxitin against *Bacteroides fragilis*; and gentamicin or trimethoprim-sulfadiazine against the Enterobacteriaceae. Combinations of these drugs may be employed in this situation; different combinations may also be useful in the initial aggressive treatment of other processes in which mixed infections are likely. Mixtures of drugs that are known or suspected to be

TABLE 5–7. Possible Etiologic Agents in Typical Clinical Infections

Diagnosis	Commonly Isolated Organisms
Stomatitis	Streptococcus,* Staphylococcus,* Proteus, Pseudomonas, *Escherichia coli, Fusobacterium fusiforme, Candida albicans*
Tonsillitis, pharyngitis	Streptococcus,* Staphylococcus
Bronchitis, pneumonia	*Bordetella bronchiseptica,* Pseudomonas aeruginosa,* Klebsiella, *Staphylococcccus aureus, Streptococcus pyogenes,* viruses
Pyothorax	*Pasteurella multocida,* Escherichia coli,* Streptococcus, Staphylococcus, Nocardia, viruses
Pyodermas	*Staphylococcus aureus,* Streptococcus,* Proteus,* Pseudomonas, Corynebacterium, *Escherichia coli,* Enterobacter aerogenes*
Vulvitis, vaginitis	*Proteus mirabilis,* Escherichia coli,* Streptococcus

Metritis
  Chronic
  Acute
	
	Streptococcus,* *Brucella canis, Escherichia coli,* Hemophilus
	Streptococcus,* *Proteus mirabilis,* Escherichia coli

Pyometra	*Escherichia coli,* Streptococcus
Balanoposthitis	Escherichia coli,* Klebsiella, Enterobacter, Proteus, Pseudomonas, Staphylococcus
Cystitis	*Escherichia coli,* Proteus mirabilis,* Pseudomonas,* Streptococcus, Staphylococcus
Prostatitis	*Escherichia coli,* Proteus, Pseudomonas, Streptococcus, Staphyloccus
Infectious enteritis	Salmonella,* *Escherichia coli,* Pseudomonas (?Steptococcus, Proteus), Giardia, coccidia, distemper virus
Superficial ocular infections	Staphylococcus, Streptococcus
Osteomyelitis	*Staphylococcus aureus,* Escherichia coli,* Streptococcus, Proteus
Wound infections	Staphylococcus,* coliforms,* Clostridium
Bacterial endocarditis	Streptococcus,* *Escherichia coli,* Pseudomonas, Staphylococcus
Puppy septicemias	Streptococcus,* *Escherichia coli,* Proteus mirabilis, Pseudomonas aeruginosa,* Staphylococcus, viruses
Otitis media	Staphylococcus,* Streptococcus,* Pityrosporum, Pseudomonas, *Escherichia coli, Proteus mirabilis*
Otitis externa	*Staphylococcus aureus,* Streptococcus,* Pityrosporum* Secondary: *Proteus mirabilis,* Pseudomonas,* Corynebacterium, *Bacillus subtilis, Candida albicans*
Burns	Pseudomonas,* Proteus, *Escherichia coli,* Staphylococcus

*Most commonly isolated. (Reprinted with permission from Davis, L. E.: Antimicrobial therapy. *In* Kirk, R. W. (ed.): *Current Veterinary Therapy VII: Small Animal Practice.* Philadelphia, W. B. Saunders Co., 1980; modified from Aronson, A. L., and Kirk, R. W.: Antimicrobial drugs. *In* Ettinger, S. J. (ed.): *Textbook of Veterinary Internal Medicine.* Philadelphia, W. B. Saunders, 1975.)

antagonistic must be avoided (Table 5–8). One should also bear in mind that in such polymicrobial infections as peritonitis, otitis media, and urinary tract infections, a single drug is as effective as a combination and that cure is achieved by the single most effective agent within a combination.[8]

The choice of appropriate drugs may be aided by rapid laboratory procedures such as smear and Gram stain of exudates, aspirates, tissue biopsy specimens, or discharges and examination of urine sediment. Interpretation of Gram stain results may be altered if: (1) the preparation is carelessly obtained from superficial exudate or from contaminated mucosal surfaces; or (2) fewer than 10^5 organisms per ml of exudates are present, because Gram stains may not reveal bacteria; during a clinically obvious or highly suspicious infection, negative Gram stain results should be ignored until both the aerobic and anaerobic cultures are sterile.[43]

On the other hand, the need to start antibiotic therapy prior to drainage or surgical exploration and the procurement of appropriate specimens for micro-

TABLE 5–8. Antibiotic Combinations Claimed to Be Antagonistic

Antibiotic Combination	Antagonism
Aminoglycoside plus tetracycline or chloramphenicol	Antagonism of the aminoglycoside against gram-negative bacilli. Most pronounced in neutropenia. Mechanism: inhibition of cellular penetration by aminoglycoside.
Erythromycin plus chloramphenicol	Antagonism of activity against staphylococci and streptococci.
Penicillin plus tetracycline	Antagonism of penicillin in streptococcal and pneumococcal infections.
Penicillin plus chloramphenicol	Antagonism of penicillin effect on pneumococcus, streptococcus, Klebsiella. No antagonism occurs when penicillin concentrations are high. No antagonism when ampicillin and chloramphenicol are combined to treat Hemophilus and pneumococcal meningitis or brain abscesses.

(Modified from Sabath, L. D., Simmons, R. L., Howard, R. J., and Canafax, D. M.: Antimicrobial agents. *In* Simmons, R. L., and Howard, R. J. (eds.): *Surgical Infectious Diseases.* New York, Appleton-Century-Crofts, 1982.)

biological study can render the cultures sterile. The Gram-stained smear is therefore sometimes a better guide to therapy than the results of bacterial culture.[43] Every effort is made to collect all pertinent samples for microbiological study prior to chemotherapy.

With severe infections, antibiotics must be administered parenterally, at least initially. Intravenous bolus administration is preferable, as this route guarantees therapeutic blood levels and consequently higher tissue levels.[3, 22] Depending upon the site of infection and the microorganisms involved, intravenous administration may be changed to oral therapy after the patient has responded satisfactorily or after five to seven days. In some situations, notably osteomyelitis, endocarditis, and severe infections caused by Gram-negative bacilli, therapy should be continued by the intravenous route throughout the full course of treatment.[22]

Intramuscular administration is also suitable, but after a few days animals become refractory to multiple daily intramuscular injections. Therefore, if parenteral administration several times daily is required, the intravenous route is preferable for both patient comfort and cooperation.[22] Subcutaneous administration is also a viable route of parenteral drug use but can be used only with compounds that are not irritating to tissue. Gentamicin, chloramphenicol, and ampicillin are commonly administered subcuta-

neously, whereas the parenteral form of trimethoprim-sulfadiazine is available only for subcutaneous use. The injection of this latter preparation often produces pain. Irritating substances that cannot be administered subcutaneously can often be given intramuscularly.[21]

In the initial treatment of fulminating infections, it is also important that optimal doses of the antibiotics be used. This is particularly pertinent with the aminoglycosides, because there may be a tendency to use inadequate doses owing to concerns about toxic effects.[22]

It is advisable that the initial therapy be with bactericidal rather than bacteriostatic antibiotics. Such a practice appears to improve results in treatment of serious infections (Table 5–9).[20]

The phase of definitive therapy begins when microbiological information becomes available; the species of the organism(s) involved may be sufficient. In some instances, further laboratory testing is unnecessary, as many bacteria have stable and predictable sensitivities—e.g., *Streptococcus pyogenes* and *Streptococcus pneumoniae* are extremely sensitive to penicillin G, and *Pseudomonas aerguinosa* is often sensitive only to carbenicillin, gentamicin, and polymyxin B.

Other organisms have unpredictable sensitivity patterns requiring sensitivity profiles or specific information regarding the MIC of the offending bacteria for formulation of definitive therapy. For example, once *Staphylococcus aureus* is identified as a pathogen, initial treatment should always be with penicillinase-resistant penicillins (PRP). If sensitivity testing demonstrates that the strain is sensitive to penicillin G, the drug should be used for definitive therapy, because it is more effective weight for weight than the semisynthetic penicillinase-resistant penicillins.

When infection is by gram-negative bacilli and

TABLE 5–9. Bacteriostatic *versus* Bactericidal Antibiotics*

Bactericidal	Penicillins
	Cephalosporins
	Polymyxins
	Aminoglycosides
	Vancomycin
	Trimethoprim-sulfadiazine
Bacteriostatic	Tetracyclines
	Chloramphenicol
	Erythromycin
	Lincomycin
	Sulfonamides

*Antibacterial and antifungal drugs are generally considered to be either bactericidal—if they are capable of killing susceptible organisms at concentrations close to those required to inhibit the organism and readily achievable clinically—or bacteriostatic—if the action of the drugs at clinically achievable concentrations is primarily to inhibit growth rather than to kill the organism.

therapy has been initiated with an aminoglycoside, a less toxic agent such as ampicillin or a cephalosporin should be substituted if *in vitro* testing indicates that the organisms are sensitive to these drugs. This practice is suggested even if the infection is responding satisfactorily to the aminoglycoside.[22]

In extraurinary infections, all *Enterobacteriaceae* require determination of their sensitivity to the aminoglycosides, cephalosporins, and ampicillin. Strains have been reported as variously resistant or sensitive to these compounds.[22]

In vitro testing is only one method of assessing the appropriateness of antibiotic choice. Careful consideration is also necessary in using these studies. Selecting therapy simply by matching the microorganism to an antimicrobial agent to which it is susceptible is a superficial approach to chemotherapy that is likely to have unsatisfactory results.[41] Some common errors in the interpretation of *in vitro* sensitivity studies are listed in Table 5–10.

Combination chemotherapy is sometimes indicated in the definitive treatment of severe infections, especially those caused by *Pseudomonas aeruginosa* (gentamicin + carbenicillin), Group D streptococci (penicillin or ampicillin + aminoglycoside), *Klebsiella pneumoniae* (cephalosporin + aminoglycoside), and *Cryotococcus neoformans* (amphotericin B + flucytosine). However, multiple-antibiotic use should be implemented only when specifically justified, since superinfection is more common and the risk of other adverse effects is increased.[22]

The appropriate duration of therapy for infectious processes may be difficult to define precisely and is unknown for many infections. There is considerable variation in the length of time antimicrobial drugs are administered from one center to another.[26] Effective therapy should not be stopped arbitrarily after a predetermined period unless the infection is well controlled.[43] The animal's response may be assessed both clinically and via laboratory study. Clinical response may be contingent upon the age of the animal; the presence of immunosuppressive disease or drug therapy; the extent and location of infection; the necessity for surgical drainage of infectious foci; the adequacy of dosage of the antimicrobial drugs; the ability of the drugs to reach the site of infection in effective concentration; and the susceptibility of the infecting microbes to the drugs used.[41]

As a general rule, antibiotic treatment should be carried out for a minimum of three days and continued for two to three days after body temperature returns to normal and other signs of infection have subsided.[52] Undue emphasis must not be placed on the febrile response of the patient. In addition to infectious processes, pyrexia may be related to immune-mediated disease, neoplasia, drug reactions, and dehydration. Even when related to infection, fever can continue. For example, pyrexia can continue for several weeks after successful chemotherapy owing to sterile effusions complicating pneumonias. Conversely, persistence of fever may represent superinfection or failure to diagnose and drain abscesses or may be related to clinical or microbiological errors.[22]

Laboratory information can also lead to inappropriate duration of therapy. Cerebrospinal fluid abnormalities can persist for a considerable period after bacterial meningitis, leading to continuation of chemotherapy for longer than necessary.[26] The opposite situation may pertain in chronic osteomyelitis, in which culture of fine needle aspirates or other specimens of the infectious site may yield no microbial growth even though viable colonies of bacteria persist within microsequestra of avascular bone. Such information may lead to premature cessation of drug therapy.

In surgical practice, the guidelines for duration of treatment must be sufficiently flexible to accommodate the animal being treated. Three to five days of therapy should be adequate to indicate whether resolution of infection is occurring. If at the end of such a period the animal's condition has not improved, several possibilities should be considered.[46, 51] The reason for a poor response can almost always be identified in the answers to the following questions:

TABLE 5–10. Common Errors in the Interpretation of *in vitro* Sensitivity Tests

1. Using drugs mainly intended for treatment of urinary tract infections for systemic infections instead (e.g., nitrofurantoin, methenamine mandelate, nalidixic acid) because the laboratory indicated the pathogenic organism was sensitive.

2. Failing to use some nontoxic antibiotics for urinary tract infections (e.g., ampicillin, cephalothin) because the laboratory reported the organism as resistant when in fact the high urinary concentration of these antibiotics would make them suitable (some knowledge of the degree of "resistance" should be available before using the antibiotic to which the organism is resistant).

3. In endocarditis, using an antibiotic which the organism is sensitive to by disc test but which is bacteriostatic and therefore unsuitable for this infection (e.g., tetracycline, chloramphenicol).

4. Using drugs for the treatment of central nervous system infections which do not penetrate the blood-brain barrier (e.g., aminoglycosides).

(Reprinted with permission from Sabath, L. D., Simmons, R. L., Howard, R. J., and Canafax, D. M.: Antimicrobial agents. *In* Simmons, R. L., and Howard, R. J. (eds.): *Surgical Infectious Diseases.* Appleton-Century-Crofts, 1982.)

TABLE 5–11. Possible Causes of Antibiotic Treatment Failure

Inappropriate antibiotic	Organism not susceptible to antibiotic at concentrations achievable at focus of infection
	Suprainfection (or erroneous initial diagnosis)
	New, unrelated infection elsewhere in body
	Failure of drug to reach site of infection (because of shock or poor penetration of drug into appropriate body compartment, as in failure of gentamicin and polymycin to pass into central nervous system and CSF)
	Bacteria in a dormant state or present as wall-deficient form when growth of cell wall must be present for antibiotic action
Appropriate antibiotic but insufficient treatment	Too small a dose of drug or dose given too infrequently
	Course of therapy too short
	Drug administered by inappropriate route (e.g., orally rather than intravenously)
	Wrong preparation of appropriate drug (e.g., procain penicillin, which yields very low blood levels, rather than aqueous crystalline penicillin, which yields very high serum levels, when high levels are required)
Appropriate antibiotic but other therapy required	Failure to institute appropriate measures in addition to prescribing antibiotics (e.g., surgical drainage, debridement, replacement of blood volume, correction of metabolic disorders)
	Failure to prescribe necessary adjuvant medication (e.g., acidify or alkalize urine when appropriate)
	Presence of substances (indigenous or prescribed) that antagonize the antibacterial activity of the drug being used
	Impaired host defenses (cellular, humoral, or nutritional; naturally occurring or secondary to physical or chemical injury)
	Treatment started too late, i.e., after changes were initiated that cannot be stopped or reversed by effective chemotherapy

(Modified from Sabath, L. D., Simmons, R. L., Howard, R. J., and Canafax, D. M.: Antimicrobial agents. *In* Simmons, R. H., and Howard, R. J. (eds.): *Surgical Infectious Diseases*. New York, Appleton-Century-Crofts, 1982.)

1. Was the original clinical and bacteriological diagnosis correct?

2. Is the pathogen being treated susceptible to the drug being given?

3. Is the drug being given by a route and in a dosage appropriate to the clinical situation?

4. Is there an unidentified or undrained focus of infection?

5. Is a new infection superimposed on the original one?

6. Are host defense mechanisms relatively intact or severely compromised?[20]

Potential reasons for antibiotic treatment failure are given in Table 5–11.

In many perioperative infections, a cure is not achieved with antibiotic therapy alone. In such situations the antibiotic administration is a valuable adjunct to surgical therapy. This situation pertains when large amounts of pus, exudate, necrotic or avascular infected tissue, or foreign bodies are present. Some examples are empyema (pyothorax), abscesses, urinary tract infections in which vesicular or renal calculi or hydronephrosis is present, pyometritis, chronic osteomyelitis in which necrotic bone must be removed, and suppurative arthritis.

These local factors may profoundly influence the animal's response. Other local factors may also directly impair the efficacy of the antimicrobial drugs. The aminoglycosides are inactivated by purulent material as are the polymyxins.[43] Aminoglycoside activity also decreases with decreasing pH.[41] An anaerobic environment, as occurs in abscesses, also has deleterious effects upon aminoglycoside activity because oxygen is required for transport of these drugs into bacterial cells. In this same situation of low redox potential, leukocyte phagocytosis and bacterial killing are less effective than normal, and bacteriostatic agents lose their efficacy. Because the penicillins and tetracyclines are bound by hemoglobin, they may be less effective when hematomas are present.[43]

Renal Insufficiency

Many antibiotics are excreted via the urinary system. In patients with renal failure or insufficiency, the delayed excretion of the drugs may result in accumulation to potentially toxic levels. One approach to this problem is to employ antibiotics of low toxicity that spare the kidneys from metabolic or excretory functions, such as chloramphenicol, clindamycin, erythromycin, lincomycin, and doxycycline.[9] When this approach is not practicable and the clinician must employ drugs such as the penicillins, cephalosporins, or aminoglycosides, the regular initial dose should be given followed either by reduced dosage or by increased dosage intervals.[9, 43] One suggestion for the use of gentamicin is to divide the regular dose by the patient's serum creatinine level to arrive at a reduced-dose regimen.[9] Other protocols have also been suggested. However, all such schedules are not totally reliable, and toxicity may still occur.[43]

A useful monitoring technique is frequent examination of the urine. Changes indicative of drug-related nephrosis are often demonstrated earlier by urinalysis than by evaluation of serum creatinine or blood urea nitrogen.[44] The sudden appearance of proteinuria, tubular casts, or red or white blood cells in the urine mandates further reduction in drug dosage or discontinuation of therapy.

With gentamicin the nephrotoxic effects continue to increase in severity for five to 30 days after cessation of administration. The changes that occur are generally reversible, but as long as five months may be required for complete resolution. Table 5–12 lists dosages and potential side effects regarding antibiotic use in animals with renal insufficiency.

Hepatic Disease

With liver disease most antibiotics, such as the penicillins, cephalosporins, and aminoglycosides, require no modification in dosage owing to the preponderance of renal excretion. Other antibiotics, such as the tetracyclines, chloramphenicol, and sulfonamides, are primarily metabolized by the liver. Little data exist about how these drugs should be used in patients with abnormalities of the hepatobiliary system,[43] and it is probably reasonable to avoid their use. Lincomycin, clindamycin, chloramphenicol, and erythromycin should probably be administered in reduced dosage if therapy is necessary for more than three days. One-half of the normal dose after two to three days may be appropriate and has been suggested in humans.[43] However, evidence for drug accumulation in patients with obstructive or hepatocellular disease is lacking, at least with lincomycin, chloramphenicol, clindamycin, and erythromycin. Normal doses may be used at least initially. The ideal regimen requires monitoring of serum concentrations of the drugs every three to seven days, but this is rarely feasible in small animal patients.

Pregnancy

Tetracyclines should be avoided in pregnant animals owing to adverse effects on fetal dentition and to hepatotoxic effects in the pregnant female.[43] All suspected teratogenic drugs must also be avoided. Metronidazole and ticarcillin are teratogenic in rodents. The teratogenic potential of many other antibiotics is unresolved.[43] Drug clearance of ampicillin is accelerated during pregnancy, and doses must be revised upward. Similar data for other antibiotics are not available.[43]

The Neonate

The neonatal liver is underdeveloped. Drugs such as chloramphenicol that are metabolized by hepatic conjugation must therefore be administered only in reduced dosage or, preferably, should be avoided entirely. Sulfonamides and novobiocin should be avoided in the neonate because they interfere with bilirubin metabolism.[43] Tetracyclines should also be avoided in young animals with deciduous dentition,

TABLE 5–12. Suggested Dosage and Potential Side Effects of Drugs in Dogs and Cats with Renal Insufficiency

Drugs	Route of Excretion	Nephrotoxic	Extrarenal Toxicity	Dosage
Amphotericin B	Unknown	Yes	Hepatic, renal	Normal
Ampicillin	Hepatic and renal	No	Gastrointestinal	Reduce
Cephaloridine	Renal	No	?	Reduce(?)
Chloramphenicol	Hepatic and renal	No	Anorexia, diarrhea, bone marrow depression (esp. cats)	Normal
Doxycycline	Gastrointestinal (dog), ?(cat)	?	?	Normal
Erythromycin	Hepatic and renal	No	Gastrointestinal, hepatic	Normal
Gentamicin	Renal	Yes	Ototoxic, gastrointestinal	Reduce
Kanamycin	Renal	Yes	Ototoxic	Reduce
Lincomycin	Hepatic	No	Gastrointestinal	Normal
Neomycin	Renal	Yes	Ototoxic	Reduce
Nitrofurans	Renal	No	Gastrointestinal, CNS	Avoid
Penicillin G	Renal and hepatic	No	Encephalopathy	Normal
Polymyxin B	Renal	Yes	CNS(?)	Avoid
Streptomycin	Renal	Yes	Ototoxic	Reduce
Sulfonamides	Renal	Yes	Gastrointestinal, CNS	Reduce
Tetracycline	Renal and Hepatic	Yes	Hepatotoxic	Avoid
Tylosin	Hepatic and renal	?	?	Normal (?)
Vancomycin	Renal	Yes	Ototoxic	Reduce

(Reprinted with permission from Osborne, C. A., and Klausner, J. S.: Adverse drug reactions in the uremic patient. *In* Kirk, R. W. (ed.): *Current Veterinary Therapy VI: Small Animal Practice.* Philadelphia, W. B. Saunders Co., 1977.)

because they bind to developing teeth, resulting in a characteristic yellow staining. The drug combinations containing corticosteroids and tetracyclines that are often administered to young dogs with infectious tracheobronchitis are notorious in this regard.

Fixed-Dose Combinations

Until recently, more than 100 fixed-dose combinations were commercially available in the United States for oral or parenteral use. Virtually all have been ordered off the market by the Food and Drug Administration, since controlled studies could not show that both agents contributed to the claimed therapeutic effects. Also, the concentrations of each agent present were often not appropriate, and patients were exposed to the potential hazards of two drugs when only one was needed.[26]

In veterinary medicine, the best-known fixed-dose combinations are penicillin G/streptomycin and antibiotic/corticosteroid mixtures. Pharmacological studies have adequately demonstrated the irrationality of the combination of penicillin and streptomycin. Effective concentrations of penicillin G persist in the body for 24 hours after administration. However, for streptomycin the duration is only eight to 12 hours. If such a preparation is administered every 24 hours, the dosage of streptomycin is inadequate. Induced bacterial resistance to streptomycin can occur more readily than to any other antimicrobial agent. One of the best ways to induce resistance is to employ an inadequate dosage regimen.[9]

It is irrational to mix drugs of different durations of effect and degrees of toxicity in fixed-dose ratios that cannot be adapted to the needs of a specific patient. Combinations of penicillin G/streptomycin can be used correctly by administering the drugs as individual preparations with consideration of the appropriate dosage and dosage interval for each drug.[9]

In the treatment of infections, corticosteroid therapy is rarely indicated and may cause harm by suppressing the host defense mechanisms or masking signs of infection. Drug preparations containing mixtures of antibiotics and corticosteroids are particularly irrational and should rarely, if ever, be used.[52]

Recommendations have been made for combining an aminoglycoside such as gentamicin with a cephalosporin. There is controversy regarding the interaction of these combinations, specifically with reference to potential nephrotoxicity. Some studies in people have demonstrated a marked increase in nephrotoxicity of aminoglycosides when cephalothin was administered concurrently. Another study has failed to confirm this effect.[36]

In animal studies, coadministration of cephalosporins failed to augment the nephrotoxicity of gentamicin. On the contrary, concurrent administration of the cephalosporins with the aminoglycosides exerted a protective effect against aminoglycoside nephrotoxicity.[36] The question is still unresolved. In the clinical experience of the author, frequent use of this combination has been associated with no nephrotoxic complications of clinical significance.

New Agents

Finally a comment is in order with regard to the continued proliferation of new antimicrobial agents. It is important to develop a sound skepticism with reference to the many claims testifying to alleged superiority of newer antimicrobial drugs.[22] Several years of careful clinical assessment are required to document such claims. In general, it is better to be thoroughly familiar with a number of well-established antibiotics with which many infections can be treated than to use every new agent that reaches the marketplace.[22]

1. Adams, R. H.: Acute adverse effects of antibiotics. JAVMA, 66:983, 1975.
2. Alexander, J. W., Sykes, N. S., Mitchell, M. M. and Fisher, M. W.: Concentration of selected intravenously administered antibiotics in experimental surgical wounds. J. Trauma 13:423, 1973.
3. Alexander, J. W., and Alexander, N. S.: The influence of route of administration on wound fluid concentration of prophylactic antibiotics. J. Trauma, 16:488, 1976.
4. Altemeier, W. A., Hummel, R. P., Hill, E. O., and Lewis, S.: Changing patterns in surgical infections. Ann. Surg., 178:436, 1973.
5. Altemeier, W. A., and Alexander, J. W.: Surgical infection and choice of antibiotics. In Sabiston D. C., Jr. (ed.): Christopher's Textbook of Surgery: The Biological Basis of Modern Surgical Practice, 11th ed. Philadelphia, W. B. Saunders, 1977.
6. Altemeir, W. A.: Surgical infections: Incisional Wounds. In Bennett, J. V., and Brachman, P. S. (eds.): Hospital Infections. Boston, Little, Brown, 1979.
7. Altemeier, W. A.: Sepsis in surgery. Presidential Address of 1st Annual Meeting of Surgical Infection Society. Arch. Surg. 117:107, 1982.
8. Aronson, A. L., and Kirk, R. W.: Antimicrobial drugs. In Ettinger, S. J. (ed.): Textbook of Veterinary Internal Medicine. Philadelphia, W. B. Saunders, 1975.
9. Aronson, A. L., and Kirk, R. W.: Antimicrobial Drugs. In Ettinger, S. J. (ed.): Textbook of Veterinary Internal Medicine, 2nd ed., Vol. I., Philadelphia, W. B. Saunders, 1983.
10. Baker, G., and Hunt, T. K.: Penicillin concentrations in experimental wounds. Am. J. Surg., 115:531, 1968.
11. Bowers, W. H., Wilson, F. C., and Greene, W. B.: Antibiotic prophylaxis in experimental bone infections. J. Bone Joint Surg., 55A:795, 1973.
12. Brock, T. D.: Chloramphenicol. Bact. Rev., 25:32, 1961.
13. Burke, J. F.: The effective period of preventive antibiotic action in experimental incisions and dermal lesions. Surgery 50:161, 1961.
14. Chisholm, G. D., Waterworth, P. M., Calnan, J. S., and Garrod, L. P.: Concentration of antibacterial agents in interstitial tissue fluid. Brit. Med. J., 1:569, 1973.
15. Chodak, G., and Plant, M.: Use of systemic antibiotics for prophylaxis in surgery: a critical review. Arch. Surg. 112:346, 1977.
16. Clark, C. H.: Prophylactic use of antibiotics in surgery, Part I. Mod. Vet. Prac., Jan. 1980, p. 30.
17. Clark, C. H.: Use of antibiotics in wounds. Mod. Vet. Prac., April 1980, p. 307.
18. Cruse, P. J. E.: Wound infections: epidemiology and clinical characteristics. In Simmons, R. L., and Howard, R. J.

(eds.): *Surgical Infectious Diseases*. New York, Appleton-Century-Crofts, 1982.

19. Davis, L. E.: Antimicrobial therapy. *In* Kirk, R. W. (ed.): *Current Veterinary Therapy VII: Small Animal Practice*. Philadelphia, W. B. Saunders, 1980.

20. Eickhoft, T. C.: Antibiotics and nosocomial infections. *In* Bennett, J. V., and Brachman, P. S. (eds.): *Hospital Infections*. Boston, Little, Brown, 1979.

21. Fingl, E., and Woodbury, D. M.: General principles. *In* Goodman, L. S., and Gilman, A. (eds.): *The Pharmacological Basis of Therapeutics*, 5th ed. New York, MacMillan, 1975.

22. Hermans, P. E.: General principles of antimicrobial therapy. Mayo Clin. Proc. *52*:603, 1977.

23. Howard, R. J.: Microbes and their pathogenicity. *In* Simmons, R. L., and Howard, R. J. (eds.): *Surgical Infectious Diseases*. New York, Appleton-Century-Crofts, 1982.

24. Hunt, T. K., Alexander, J. W., Burke, J. F., and MacLean, L. D.: Antibiotics in surgery. Arch. Surg. *110*:148, 1975.

25. Keen, P.: Some aspects of the pharmacology of antibiotics in the cat and dog. J. Small Animal Prac. *16*:767, 1975.

26. Kirby, W. M. M., and Petersdorf, R. G.: Chemotherapy of infection. *In* Wintrobe, M. M., Thorn, G. W., Adams, R. D., et al. (eds.): *Harrison's Principles of Internal Medicine*, 7th ed. New York, McGraw-Hill, 1974.

27. Klausner, J. S., and Osborne, C. A.: Management of canine bacterial prostatitis. JAVMA *182*:292, 1983.

28. Lewis, R. T.: Advances in antibiotic prophylaxis in gastrointestinal surgery. Can. Med. Assoc. *121*:265, 1979.

29. Lewis, R. T., Allan, C. M., Goodell, R. G., et al.: The discriminate usage of antibiotic prophylaxis in gastroduodenal surgery. Am. J. Surg. *138*:640, 1979.

30. Ling, G. V., and Hirsh, D. C.: Principles of antimicrobial therapy. *In* Kirk, R. W. (ed.): *Current Veterinary Therapy VIII: Small Animal Practice*. Philadelphia, W. B. Saunders, 1983.

31. Meakins, J. L., Hohn, D. C., Hunt, T. K., and Simmons, R. L.: Host defenses. *In* Simmons, R. L., and Howard, R. J. (eds.): *Surgical Infectious Diseases*. New York, Appleton-Century-Crofts, 1982.

32. Miles, A. A., Miles, E. M., and Burke, J.: The value and duration of defense reactions of the skin to the primary lodgement of bacteria. Br. J. Exp. Pathol. *38*:79, 1957.

33. Polk, H. C., Lopez-Mayor, J. F.: Postoperative wound infection: a prospective study of determinant factors and prevention. Surgery *66*:97, 1969.

34. Polk, H. C., Trachtenberg, L., and Finn, M. P.: Antibiotic activity in surgical incisions—the basis for prophylaxis in selected operations. JAMA *244*:1353, 1980.

35. Polk, H. C., and Finn, M. P.: Chemoprophylaxis of wound infections. *In* Simmons, R. L., and Howard, R. J. (eds.): *Surgical Infectious Diseases*. New York, Appleton-Century-Crofts, 1982.

36. Powers, T. E., and Garg, R. C.: Pharmacotherapeutics of newer penicillins and cephalosporins. JAVMA, Colloq. on Clin. Pharm. *176*:1054, 1980.

37. Price, D. J. E., and Sleigh, J. D.: Control of infections due to *Klebsilla aerogenes* in a neurosurgical unit by withdrawal of all antibiotics. *Lancet* *2*:1213, 1970.

38. Riviere, J. E., Kaufman, G. M., and Bright, R. M.: Prophylactic use of systemic antimicrobial drugs in surgery. Compend. Cont. Educ. *3*:345, 1981.

39. Roberts, A. W., and Visconti, J. A.: The rational and irrational use of systemic antimicrobial drugs. Am. J. Hosp. Pharm. *29*:828, 1972.

40. Rose, H. D., and Schreier, J.: The effect of hospitalization and antibiotic therapy on the gram-negative fecal flora. Am. J. Med. Sci. *225*:228, 1968.

41. Rosenblatt, J. E.: Laboratory tests used to guide antimicrobial therapy. Mayo Clin. Proc. *52*:611, 1977.

42. Rowlands, B. J., Clark, R. G., and Richards, D. G.: Single-dose intraoperative antibiotic prophylaxis in emergency abdominal surgery. Arch. Surg. *117*:195, 1982.

43. Sabath, L. D., Simmons, R. L., Howard, R. J., and Carefax, D. M.: Antimicrobial agents. *In* Simmons, R. L., and Howard, R. J. (eds.): *Surgical Infectious Diseases*. New York, Appleton-Century-Crofts, 1982.

44. Senior, D.: Drug use in renal failure. Lecture Notes, Medicine Course #7501, University of Pennsylvania, 1978.

45. Shapiro, M., and Townsend, T. R., Rosner, B., and Kass, E. H.: Use of antimicrobial drugs in general hospitals. N. Engl. J. Med. *301*:351, 1979.

46. Smith, H.: *Antibiotics in Clinical Practice*, 3rd ed. Baltimore, University Park Press, 1977.

47. Spievack, A. R.: The prophylactic antibiotic puzzle. Surg. Gynecol. Obstet. *147*:80, 1978.

48. VanScoy, R. E.: Prophylactic use of antimicrobial agents. Mayo Clin. Prac. *52*:701, 1977.

49. Veterans Administration Ad Hoc Interdisciplinary Advisory Committee of Antimicrobial Drug Use: (1) Prophylaxis in surgery. JAMA *237*:1003, 1977.

50. Waterman, N. G.: The transfer of gram-negative bacterial resistance. Surg. Gynecol. Obstet. *134*:656, 1972.

51. Waterman, N. G., and Kastan, L. B.: Interstitial fluid and serum antibiotic concentrations. Arch. Surg. *105*:192, 1972.

52. Watson, A. D. J.: Antimicrobial therapy. *In* Kirk, R. W. (ed.): *Current Veterinary Therapy VI: Small Animal Practice*. Philadelphia, W. B. Saunders, 1977.

53. Weiner, J. P., Gibson, G., and Munster, A. M.: Use of prophylactic antibiotics in surgical procedures: peer review guidelines as a method for quality assurance. Am. J. Surg. *139*:348, 1980.

54. Weinstein, L.: The complications of antibiotic therapy. Bull. N.Y. Acad. Med. *31*:500, 1954.

55. Weinstein, L.: Antibiotics agents: general considerations. *In* Goodman, L. S., and Gilman, A. (eds.): *The Pharmacological Basis of Therapeutics*, 5th ed. New York, MacMillan, 1975.

Chapter 6

Physiology of Hemostasis

W. Jean Dodds

Hemostasis involves three major components and physiological events that follow blood vessel injury: (1) reflex vasoconstriction of the blood vessel wall, (2) participation of blood platelets, and (3) blood coagulation.[3–6] Once a stable hemostatic plug has formed, the process of fibrinolysis dissolves the newly developed thrombus to re-establish patency of the vessel. Each of these events will be briefly described. More detailed accounts can be found in the references listed at the end of this chapter.

BLOOD VESSEL WALL

Following blood vessel injury or severance, a brief, local, reflex vasoconstriction reduces blood flow at the site. Release of vasoactive components from adjacent platelets and surrounding tissues maintains vascular contraction. Concomitantly, platelets in the vicinity of the injury adhere to the exposed collagen fibers of the subendothelium. The role of platelets in this process is discussed hereafter.

Other important functions of the vessel wall include the role of vessel constituents, especially the endothelial cells lining the intima, in the formation and dissolution of hemostatic plugs, thrombi, and atherosclerotic lesions. Thorgeirsson and Robertson[7] and Wight[8] have reviewed this complex subject.

An important basic function of intact, healthy vascular endothelium is to present a surface resistant to thrombosis to the flowing blood.[7] Such intact vessel linings are passive to leukocytes, platelets, and coagulation. Apparently both active and passive mechanisms are involved in maintaining resistance to thrombosis. Endothelial cells, particularly in the pulmonary microcirculation, contribute actively to this resistance by removing from the circulating blood compounds that promote platelet aggregation (prostaglandin $F_1\alpha$, serotonin, adenine nucleotides, bradykinin, and angiotensin I). In addition, all blood vessel layers synthesize and release prostacyclin (prostaglandin I_2, or PGI_2), a potent inhibitor of platelet aggregation and thus a promoter of resistance to thrombosis.

Proteoglycans comprising the matrix of the blood vessel wall also directly influence thrombogenicity.[8] Three of these compounds—heparin, heparan sulfate, and dermatan sulfate—possess anticoagulant activity; other glycosaminoglycans and hyaluronic acid do not. Vascular tissues, such as veins, that have the highest concentrations of these compounds are the most resistant to thrombosis. The antithrombotic proteoglycans differ in their potency and mechanism of action. They act against coagulation factors (thrombin, antithrombin III, factor X, and fibrinogen) and affect platelet functions (inhibit thrombin- and collagen-induced aggregation and bind to platelet factor 4 and growth factor derived from platelets).

Passive mechanisms of resistance to thrombosis are less important. These include the glycocalyx or carbohydrate-rich coat, which protects the cell surface; the negative surface charge of the vessel lumen, which repels similarly charged cells such as platelets; the continuous renewal of cell membranes; and the presence at the cell surface of α_2-macroglobulin, a protease inhibitor.

Endothelial cells also have important synthetic, metabolic, and pathological functions.[7] They synthesize von Willebrand factor protein, plasminogen activator, fibronectin, types III and IV basement-membrane collagens, elastin, many enzymes, and prostacyclin. The pathological processes to which the endothelium contributes are atherosclerosis; thrombosis; disseminated intravascular coagulation; defective hemostasis; inflammation, especially from viral, rickettsial, or gram-negative bacterial injury; immune disorders; vascular neoplasia; metastasis; prolonged hypotension, acidosis, or hypoxia; and dysproteinemias. Depending on the nature of the incitant to vascular injury, these conditions predispose to thrombosis, increased vascular permeability, purpura, or hemorrhage.[3, 7]

PLATELETS

Blood platelets are 1- to 4-μm particles that are extruded as buds from the extremities of megakaryocytes in the bone marrow, lung, and spleen. Circulating platelets are disc-shaped but appear in Wright's-stained blood films as pale-blue cells—spherical, oval, or rod-shaped—containing reddish granules. The numerous functions of platelets are listed in Table 6–1.

Platelets promote hemostasis by adhesion, aggregation, and secretion (release) reactions, among other ways, and are an essential component of the initial hemostatic plug. Recent reviews on the subject include those of Sixma and Wester,[6] DeGaetano and Garattini,[1] and Zucker.[9]

Platelets accumulate rapidly at the site of vessel injury. They adhere to the vessel wall and then to each other, after which they become involved in the intrinsic coagulation pathway (Fig. 6–1). Contact be-

Supported, in part, by research grants HL09902 and HL07173, awarded by the National Heart, Lung, and Blood Institute, PHS/DHHS.

TABLE 6–1. Functions of Blood Platelets

Hemostasis and thrombosis (endothelial cells, coagulation, von Willebrand factor,
    collagen, adenosine diphosphate, adrenalin, thrombin)
Atherogenesis (platelet-derived growth factor, mitogens, cell-proliferating activity)
Specialized smooth muscle cell role (clot retraction)
Inflammation (specialized type of intravascular leukocyte; chemotaxis and
    phagocytosis)
Prostaglandin metabolism
Immunologic reactions (immune-complex disease)
Endotoxin reactivity (Shwartzman reaction)
Monoamines and serotoninergic synaptosomes (epinephrine, serotonin)
Interactions with tumor cells (adhesion, aggregation, cell transformation,
    metastases)
Synthesis of proteins, lipids, carbohydrates, and nucleotides

tween platelets and collagen fibers in the subendothelium in the presence of von Willebrand factor
causes a release of arachidonic acid from platelet
membrane phospholipids, which initiates the prostaglandin pathway and generates thromboxane A_2
(TXA$_2$), a potent platelet aggregator. This in turn
stimulates the secretion of adenosine diphosphate
(ADP) from platelet-dense granules. The collagen-
adhering platelets change shape, spread out along
the collagen fibers, and degranulate. Degranulation
also provides ADP as well as other platelet constituents, such as serotonin, histamines, and platelet
factor 4. At the same time, thrombin is being formed
by coagulation; it stimulates platelet secretion and
"viscous metamorphosis" as well as converts fibrinogen to fibrin. Platelets thus become aggregated in
response to collagen, ADP, and thrombin. Strands of
fibrin reinforce this hemostatic plug.

In addition to the initiating agonist, platelet aggregation sufficient to seal the vessel requires calcium
ions, fibrinogen, and metabolic energy. An active
function of platelets is to generate metabolic energy
in the form of adenosine triphosphate (ATP) from
platelet glycolysis, glycogenolysis, citric- and fatty-
acid oxidation, and oxidative phosphorylation. Platelet factor 3, a platelet surface phospholipoprotein
with thromboplastic activity, is made available to
accelerate blood coagulation during the initial platelet
activation steps.

The final and extremely important function of
platelets is their regulatory role, in conjunction with
the vessel wall, in maintaining endothelial resistance
to thrombosis via the prostaglandin pathways.[1, 7] The
arachidonic acid released from membrane phospholipids is acted upon by cyclooxygenase to produce
cyclic endoperoxides. These, in turn, form either the
potent platelet aggregator and vasoconstrictor TXA$_2$
(by the action of thromboxane synthetase) or the
potent platelet inhibitor and smooth muscle relaxant
prostacyclin, or PGI$_2$ (by the action of prostacyclin

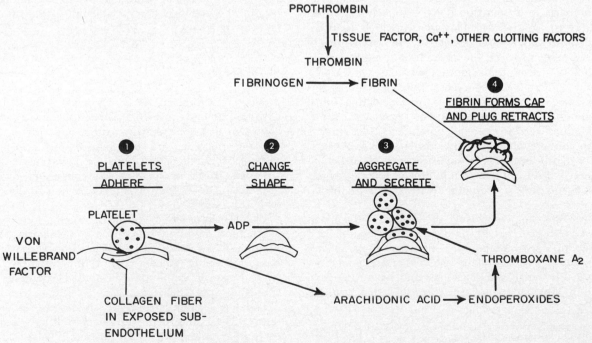

Figure 6–1. Interactions of blood vessel, blood platelets, and coagulation in hemostasis.

synthetase). Thus, platelets produce TXA_2, a stimulator of aggregation, whereas blood vessels produce PGI_2 to inhibit aggregation and maintain homeostatic balance. Platelet and vessel phospholipid and lipid metabolism plays a crucial role in providing the necessary substrates and metabolites for these reactions.

The use of aspirin as a pharmacological inhibitor of platelet aggregation is based on its ability to acetylate cyclooxygenase and thus block the production of TXA_2. A four- to fivefold higher dose of aspirin is inhibitory to PGI_2 production, so the inhibitory effect of low-dosage aspirin on TXA_2 production can be reversed by higher doses. Indomethacin, another antiplatelet drug, also blocks platelet prostaglandin metabolism. Dipyridamole achieves its antiplatelet effect by blocking platelet phosphodiesterase, thus causing cyclic AMP, an endogenous inhibitor of aggregation, to accumulate.

A last point to emphasize about platelets is the marked species differences encountered in their morphological and functional expression.[2, 3]

COAGULATION

The process of blood coagulation, a complex series of reactions of inactive precursor proteins and active enzymes (Fig. 6–2), becomes involved in hemostasis after the initial interactions of platelets with the vessel wall and each other.[3–5] The exposed foreign surfaces of an injured vessel activate the contact phase of intrinsic pathway coagulation via the Hageman factor (factor XII), and the injured cells release tissue thromboplastin, which activates the extrinsic pathway via factor VII. Thus, coagulation proceeds by an intrinsic (intravascular) pathway and an extrinsic (tissue juice) pathway to convert prothrombin to thrombin, the potent coagulant enzyme.

In the intrinsic pathway, factors XII, XI, IX, and VIII become activated sequentially to produce plasma thromboplastin. This thromboplastin, together with phospholipid—from platelets (platelet factor 3), tissues, and red cells—and calcium ions, activates factor X, the final common pathway to prothrombin conversion. Similarly, in the extrinsic pathway, tissue

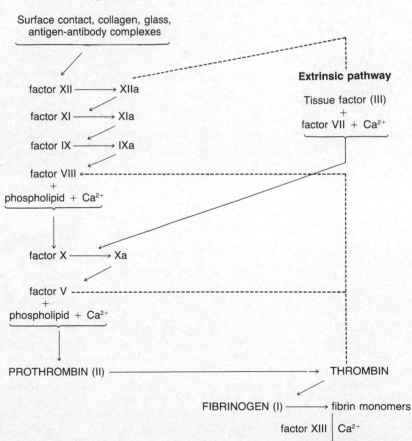

Figure 6–2. Intrinsic and extrinsic pathways of blood coagulation. (Adapted with permission from Dodds, W. J. *In* Kaneko, J. J. (ed.): *Clinical Biochemistry of Domestic Animals*, 3rd ed. Academic Press, New York, 1980, p. 677.)

factor and calcium ions activate factor VII, forming prothrombinase, which also activates factor X conversion. Factor VII also activates factor XII, albeit slowly, which provides another route of intrinsic coagulation.

In the final common pathway, activated factor X activates factor V; and in the presence of phospholipid and calcium ions, factor V converts prothrombin to thrombin. Thrombin acts on fibrinogen and converts it to fibrin in the presence of factor XIII (fibrin-stabilizing factor) and calcium ions. The clotting mechanism of "cascade" can best be described, therefore, as a series of sequential activating steps that results in conversion of prothrombin to thrombin and then fibrinogen to fibrin in the presence of calcium ions.

Several new clotting factors have been described that participate in the contact phase (factors XII and XI) of the intrinsic system.[3] These factors are components of the plasma kallikrein-kinin system, which is responsible for capillary permeability and smooth muscle contraction; they include Fletcher factor (prekallikrein) and Fitzgerald, Williams, and Flaujeac factors (high-molecular-weight kininogens). Deficiencies of these factors, such as factor XII deficiency, are not associated with a bleeding tendency but produce very long clotting times in screening tests of intrinsic clotting (APTT). Of the contact-phase clotting factors, only factor XI deficiency produces a bleeding diathesis.

The thrombin generated during coagulation also plays a key role in the growth and stabilization of the initial platelet plug. Even at concentrations much too low to produce visible fibrin formation, thrombin causes platelet aggregation, induces viscous metamorphosis and the release reaction, and makes platelet factor 3 available on the platelet surface for coagulation. Thus, platelet functions are directly enhanced by products evolved by activation of coagulation. As with platelets, there are many differences in the activities of coagulation factors in man and other animals.[3]

FIBRINOLYSIS

Fibrinolysis involves a series of events that produce plasmin, the enzyme that digests fibrin and initiates dissolution of hemostatic plugs to support vessel healing and repair. The process parallels that of coagulation, as either direct or indirect activation of the fibrinolytic pathway converts plasminogen (zymogen precursor) to its active enzyme (plasmin). Plasmin also digests fibrinogen and factors V and VIII.

Physiologic control of this process is maintained by natural fibrinolytic inhibitors (antiplasmins). Fibrinolysis is thereby usually restricted to the area in and around a fibrin deposit.

1. DeGaetano, G., and Garattini, S. (eds.): *Platelets: A Multidisciplinary Approach.* Raven Press, New York, 1978.
2. Dodds, W. J.: Platelet function in animals: species specificities. *In* DeGaetano, G., and Garattini, S. (eds.): *Platelets: A Multidisciplinary Approach.* Raven Press, New York, 1978, pp. 45–59.
3. Doods, W. J.: Hemostasis and coagulation. *In* Kaneko, J. J. (ed.): *Clinical Biochemistry of Domestic Animals*, 3rd ed. Academic Press, New York, 1980, pp. 671–718.
4. Dodds, W. J.: The normal hemostatic mechanism. *In* Bojrab, M J. (ed.): *Pathophysiology in Small Animal Surgery.* Lea & Febiger, Philadelphia, 1981, pp. 460–462.
5. Owen, C. A., Jr., Bowie, E. J. W., Didisheim, P., and Thompson, J. H.: *The Diagnosis of Bleeding Disorders.* Little, Brown and Co., Boston, 1975.
6. Sixma, J. J., and Wester, J.: The hemostatic plug. Sem. Hematol. *14*:265, 1977.
7. Thorgeirsson, G., and Robertson, A. L., Jr.: The vascular endothelium: pathobiologic significance. Am. J. Pathol. *93*:803, 1978.
8. Wight, T. N.: Vessel proteoglycans and thrombogenesis. *In* Spaet, T. H. (ed.): *Progress in Hemostasis and Thrombosis*, Vol. 5. Grune and Stratton, New York, 1980, pp. 1–39.
9. Zucker, M. B.: The functioning of blood platelets. Sci. Am. *242*:86, 1980.

Chapter **7**

Blood Transfusion

George E. Lees

Administration of blood or blood components is generally intended to relieve a critical shortage of blood cells, proteins, or volume in the recipient. To optimize the therapeutic benefits of transfusion, care must be taken during collection, processing, storage, and administration of the blood. The goal is to harvest, preserve, and deliver the needed blood components so that they are functional and sufficiently abundant. Economic and practical considerations require that this goal be attained efficiently.

Standards of good medical practice require that the blood be of excellent quality and that it be used appropriately. Additionally, precautions must be taken to prevent any avoidable complication or adverse outcome.

Recommended methods for accomplishing these objectives are described in this chapter, as well as indications, contraindications, and precautions for administration of blood products to animals with specific conditions.

SELECTION AND USE OF BLOOD DONORS

Healthy young adult animals that have never had a transfusion are generally the best individuals to use as blood donors.[9] Females should not have been pregnant and should be spayed. To facilitate blood collection, donor animals should possess a cooperative temperament, have a short haircoat, and not be obese. Dogs should weigh at least 20 kg.

Prospective blood donors must be free of infections and infestations that might be transferred by blood transfusion.[9] In dogs, brucellosis, ehrlichiosis, and microfilaremia must be excluded. Similarly, cats must be free of feline leukemia virus and feline infectious peritonitis infections. Infestations by blood parasites such as *Haemobartonella*, *Babesia*, and so on should be excluded in dogs and cats. Because these blood parasites may otherwise be difficult to detect, examination of appropriately stained blood smears obtained following splenectomy is recommended. Blood donors should be vaccinated and kept free of ticks, fleas, and intestinal parasites, particularly hookworms.

Eight blood groups determined by specific dog erythrocyte antigens (DEAs) have been identified in dogs.[4, 9, 20] Among these antigens, DEA 1.1, DEA 1.2, and DEA 7 have the potential to induce clinically important isoantibody production in recipient dogs whose own erythrocytes lack these antigens. Use of blood typing to select donors that are negative for DEAs 1.1, 1.2, and 7 is recommended and is especially important when recipient animals may require sequential transfusions.[4, 15, 20] Feline blood groups and their clinical importance are less well studied than those of dogs.[4, 9, 20] Two erythrocyte antigen groups, designated A and B, have been identified in cats.[2] Although adverse reactions attributed to transfusions of mismatched blood have been reported in cats,[2] use of blood typing to select feline blood donors is not a common practice, and reactions are rarely observed.[4, 5, 9, 10] Further considerations regarding compatibility of blood administered to dogs and cats are discussed subsequently in the section on complications of transfusions.

With adequate husbandry and nutritional support, donors can routinely provide as much as 20 to 25 ml of blood per kg body weight every 14 to 21 days.[9] Intervals between withdrawals of whole blood should always be at least seven days for dogs and ten days for cats. Maintenance of hematopoiesis in blood donors that are used regularly requires adequate dietary intake of vitamins, minerals, and protein. Dietary supplementation with vitamin B_{12}, folic acid, pyridoxine, and iron intake is advisable. To sustain optimum bone marrow productivity, proteins of meat rather than plant origin are required. Hematological findings should be monitored to detect evidence of deficiencies.

Scheduled periodic collection of blood is suggested to maximize the availability of erythrocytes and plasma from the donors in use.[4, 9] If stored whole blood is not used before its shelf life expires, its plasma can be separated, frozen, and stored up to two years for later use. Fresh blood must be used if functional thrombocytes are required. Therefore, it is advisable to keep at least one blood donor available for immediate use. When only thrombocytes are needed by the recipient, an individual donor can be used as often as two or three times a week. This is accomplished by separating the platelet-rich plasma from the erythrocytes, which are returned to the donor.

BLOOD COLLECTION

Blood for transfusion may be collected in glass containers, such as vacuum bottles, plastic bags, or syringes.[4, 9, 15, 20] Each method has advantages and limitations that vary in their importance depending on the clinical situation. The chief advantage of vacuum bottles is the simplicity of their use. Large volumes of blood can be obtained easily and rapidly from the jugular veins of conscious dogs.[9] To minimize hemolysis, however, it is important to tilt the collection bottle sideways so that the entering stream of blood flows down the side of the container rather than jetting to the bottom. Blood collection bottles have the disadvantage of allowing bacterial contamination of their contents as air is admitted if the vacuum is broken during blood collection or when the bottle is vented during blood administration.[9] Separation of blood components is most difficult if glass bottles are used and at best involves additional risks of contamination. Additionally, glass surfaces have a tendency to cause contact activation of coagulation factors and to activite platelets.[9] Adhesion of platelets to glass bottles may decrease delivery of platelets to recipient animals.

The major disadvantages associated with vacuum bottles are overcome by the use of plastic bags for blood collection.[9] The sterilized container remains closed throughout blood collection and administration, and contamination of the contents is not a problem when bags are used properly. Especially when interconnected plastic bags (so-called double or triple packs) are used, separation of blood components is easily accomplished, again without risk of contamination. Surfaces of plastic blood collection bags activate coagulation factors and platelets less than do the glass surfaces of vacuum bottles. The principal shortcoming of the use of plastic bags is that blood collection is less easily accomplished. To collect blood in plastic bags efficiently, it is necessary to obtain the blood from the arterial circulation (e.g., from a femoral artery) or to use a vacuum-assist device if a venipuncture is performed. Blood can be collected by gravity flow into bags from the jugular veins of dogs, but with this method blood flow is slow, and clot formation in the tubing leading to the bag is often a problem. Further, blood collection should be completed within eight minutes using standard (400 to 500 ml) blood packs if ultimate delivery of platelets or coagulation factors to the recipient is to be optimized.[12] A rate of blood flow sufficient to meet this criterion is difficult to accomplish using gravity flow from a venipuncture in dogs.

To collect blood from the arterial circulation into a bag, the donor dog is lightly anesthetized with a short-acting barbiturate. I prefer to use the femoral artery of the top leg (i.e., right leg with the dog in left lateral recumbency, or vice versa), which is exposed by abducting and extending the leg until the medial aspect of the thigh is facing upward. A large-bore needle attached to the collection apparatus is used to perform a percutaneous puncture of the femoral artery, and blood collection is usually completed in five to seven minutes. Hemorrhage from the artery following blood collection is successfully controlled by applying broad, firm pressure over the vessel for five to ten minutes. The need to repeatedly anesthetize a valuable donor animal and the development of vessel scarring are potential disadvantages of arterial collection.

A vacuum-assist device can be purchased or constructed to facilitate blood collection into bags from large veins. In this situation, rapid blood flow is accomplished by creating negative pressure around the bag rather than by blood pressure. The vacuum chamber is a rigid-walled container large enough to accommodate a filled blood collection bag. It must have an orifice that can be connected to suction and must have a tight-fitting lid. Tubing leading from the donor to the bag passes through a notch in the rim of the container. Sources of suction that can be connected to the chamber after venipuncture include surgical suction machines and Venturi devices attached to water faucets.

Blood for transfusion may also be collected into syringes. This technique is most suitable when the blood is to be given to a cat, puppy, or other small dog. Anticoagulant is placed in a large (e.g., 60 ml) plastic syringe, and an appropriate quantity of blood, usually 50 ml, is drawn from the donor animal's jugular vein. Cardiac puncture can be performed to obtain the blood and has been recommended,[4] particularly for cats, but it is more hazardous to the donor animal than is venipuncture. Good blood donors are valuable animals, and it is prudent to avoid unnecessary risks to their welfare.

Regardless of the technique used for blood collection, the site should be surgically prepared and aseptic procedures should be employed. A single, "clean" puncture of the blood vessel followed by continuous flow of blood until the collection is completed is important. Blood and anticoagulant in the collection vessel should be gently mixed during the collection process, and the container should be immediately and appropriately labeled when the collection is completed.[12]

ANTICOAGULANTS

Acid, citrate, dextrose (ACD); citrate, phosphate, dextrose (CPD); and heparin solutions have been used as anticoagulants for blood intended for transfusion. Of these, heparin is not recommended because it activates platelets, resulting in presentation of clumped, nonfunctional thrombocytes to the recipient's microcirculation. Additionally, the coagulation systems of the recipient may be impaired by heparin's antithrombotic effect. Furthermore, blood containing heparin has accelerated glycolysis and deteriorates rapidly; therefore it is not safe for use after 48 hours.[17]

For routine use, and especially when storage of blood products is intended, ACD or CPD anticoagulant solutions are recommended.[9, 20] Erythrocyte preservation is generally considered to be better in CPD than in ACD solutions for reasons that will be discussed subsequently, but it has been suggested that microaggregate formation during refrigerated storage is greater in CPD.[9] It is important to use the proper amount of anticoagulant solution for the volume of blood collected.[12] This is generally accomplished by filling commercially prepared blood collection containers with the volume of blood for which they were intended; when collection of a lesser volume of blood is planned, the amount of anticoagulant solution used should be reduced proportionately (i.e., use approximately 14 ml of ACD or CPD solution per 100 ml of blood).

STORAGE

Blood products are stored under refrigeration or are frozen. Platelets cannot be stored without special additives and preparation, so blood must be freshly drawn and administered promptly (i.e., within a few hours) when transfusion of functional platelets is desired. Blood coagulation factors are also labile but can be preserved if they are frozen shortly after collection. Fresh plasma and plasma components or concentrates should be stored in plastic containers at $-20°C$ or less, preferably -40 to $-70°C$, if they are to be used to correct deficiencies of clotting factors.[6, 13]

Although erythrocytes can be frozen for long-term storage, the necessary technology is generally not available to veterinarians, so that animal red blood cells are usually stored under refrigeration. Two factors affect the ultimate function and survival of erythrocytes that are transfused following storage. The first are the metabolic changes that alter erythrocyte oxygen affinity in refrigerated blood during storage.[11, 13, 19] Erythrocyte adenosine triphosphate (ATP) and 2,3-diphosphoglycerate (DPG) concentrations and the pH of the storage medium all decline during storage.[8, 19] These changes cause the oxygen dissociation curve to shift to the left, producing decreased oxygen delivery to tissues.[14] Compared with ACD solution, CPD solution maintains higher values for these variables, particularly pH, during storage. For this reason, CPD is generally preferred to ACD for blood storage.[7, 13] Satisfactory oxygen dissociation curves are maintained by canine erythrocytes for four weeks in CPD solutions but only for two weeks in ACD solutions.[14] However, this is of particular importance only when the transfused red cells are required to have optimum functional capacity immediately. The metabolic changes in stored erythrocytes are largely reversible and are corrected *in vivo* during the first 24 hours following transfusion.[19] For this reason, stored erythrocytes should be administered to anemic patients 12 to 24 hours before predictable blood loss (e.g., during surgery) occurs.

In addition to changes in their oxygen-carrying capacity, stored erythrocytes undergo changes in their shape and cell membrane characteristics.[11, 20] Because erythrocytes must remain deformable to survive in the circulation, these changes can lead to accelerated destruction of transfused cells. During storage, erythrocytes gradually become rigid spherocytes. Their volume is reduced by the hypertonicity of the anticoagulant solution, the fluidity of cell contents (primarily hemoglobin) decreases, and intrinsic membrane deformability is impaired. Metabolic changes in the erythrocytes during storage, including the changes in ATP and pH mentioned previously, are responsible for these alterations. These metabolic changes are reversible, at least initially, and some of the abnormalities of transfused erythrocytes can be repaired *in vivo*. The accepted standard for satisfactory survival (viability) of transfused red cells following storage is greater than 70 per cent.[12, 13] This standard is met by erythrocytes stored in ACP solution for up to three weeks and by erythrocytes stored in CPD solution for up to four weeks (some studies suggest up to six weeks).[17]

Gentle mixing of refrigerated blood periodically (e.g., weekly) during storage helps to minimize erythrocyte deterioration.[20] Sedimentation of erythrocytes to the bottom of the container, where there is less plasma, causes the cells to deteriorate more rapidly. Erythrocytes should be stored at 4 to 6°C, and the temperature should be kept uniform. Once stored blood has been warmed to 10°C or more (i.e., out of refrigeration for 30 minutes) or the container has been opened, it should be used within 24 hours. Studies of storage methods for canine blood have shown that plastic bags containing CPD solution are superior to bags or bottles containing ACD solution.[7] It is recommended that erythrocytes not be used after storage in ACD for three weeks or in CPD for four weeks. An anticoagulant solution that was satisfactory for storage of canine blood in bags for up to six weeks has been described, but it is not readily available.[18]

Once separated from blood cell components, plasma can be frozen and stored for extended periods. Although fresh or fresh-frozen plasma must be used if coagulation factors are needed, plasma harvested from outdated, stored whole blood is satisfactory when other plasma components (e.g., albumin) are needed.

PREPARATION AND USE OF BLOOD COMPONENTS

Blood component therapy is the practice of administering specific constituents of blood to recipients based on their individual requirements.[11, 13] This allows more efficient use of blood from available donors and produces greater therapeutic benefits. Needed blood components are delivered in a more concentrated product, reducing expansion of circulatory volume and infusion of superfluous or potentially detrimental components. For example, a patient's posttransfusion hematocrit will be greater if the available erythrocytes are given as packed cells rather than as whole blood. Coincidentally, risks of circulatory overload (an important consideration in patients with severe chronic anemia) and adverse reactions to plasma constituents are reduced. Similarly, administration of platelet-rich plasma or platelet concentrates can be used to control hemorrhage due to thrombocytopenia when clinically significant anemia is not also a problem. Serial fresh whole blood transfusions for thrombocytopenia might ultimately produce an excessive hematocrit in the recipient if the effort to prevent hemorrhage is successful.

Blood components can be separated by gravity (sedimentation) or by centrifugation.[13, 15] Sedimentation is adequate only for preparation of units of concentrated erythrocytes and old (i.e., not fresh) plasma, because platelets and coagulation factors deteriorate in the time required for separation. Units of sedimented red cells, however, have hematocrits of 60 to 75%, and the plasma can be used for volume expansion or treatment of hypoproteinemia.

Preassembled plastic bags with multiple compartments are safely and conveniently used to prepare blood components.[13, 17] Blood is collected into the primary pouch, which contains anticoagulant, and separation is accomplished by sedimentation or centrifugation. Transfer of blood components is then accomplished by placing the primary pouch in a press that propels the supernatant through connecting tubing to a separate compartment. Presses manufactured specifically for this purpose are available, but a large book will also suffice.

Availability of a large centrifuge with a rotor head equipped with buckets that can accommodate filled blood bags allows production of packed red cells (hematocrit 80 to 90%), platelet-rich plasma, platelet concentrates, and plasma. Centrifugation at $375 \times g$ for 15 to 20 minutes separates packed red cells from platelet-rich plasma.[4] Subsequent centrifugation of platelet-rich plasma at $2,000 \times g$ for 30 minutes produces a platelet concentrate and platelet-poor plasma. If platelet separation is not desired, initial centrifugation at the higher speed increases the yield of plasma. Placing water around the bags in the centrifuge buckets prevents bursting of the bags by the forces that are generated to separate the blood components. Other sources should be consulted regarding methods for preparing concentrates of coagulation factors (e.g., cryoprecipitate) from fresh plasma.[6, 13]

Blood collected in bottles or syringes can be separated into component products. Usually, sedimentation is allowed to occur under refrigeration with the container in an upright position.[4] Plasma is then withdrawn, frozen, and stored separately. Great care must be taken to avoid contamination of blood products that are prepared in this way.

ADMINISTRATION

Inexpensive, sterilized, disposable blood administration sets are commercially available, and their use is recommended.[4, 9] Standard (170 micron pore size) filter screens that are incorporated in these units restrain blood clots and other large particles, but microaggregates are allowed to pass. Microaggregates are particulate debris composed of red cells, platelets, leukocytes, and fibrin that form primarily during the first seven days of storage.[19] Because their diameters are usually less than 164 microns, filters with pore sizes of 20 to 40 microns (i.e., micropore filters) must be used if this debris is to be removed. Routine use of such filters, however, is not necessary. If properly obtained, freshly collected blood does not contain microaggregates. Clinically evident complications are rarely observed when massive transfusions of stored blood are given through standard filters.[19]

Blood collected in syringes (as for cats, pups, and small dogs) is frequently administered without filtration.[4, 9, 20] This procedure is acceptable provided that the blood is free of large particles such as clots. Indeed, given the mechanical problems of working with such small patients and the severe degree of physiological distress that often accompanies the need for transfusion, injection of blood directly from the syringe into the recipient can be the optimum alternative. Blood in syringes may also be given through standard blood administration sets. A long needle (e.g., a 3.5-inch spinal needle) attached to the syringe is passed through the input portal of the drip chamber so that air is not trapped in the chamber when it is filled with blood from the syringe. As blood flows to the recipient the drip chamber is refilled from the syringe as needed to prevent air from entering the administration line. At the end of the transfusion, most of the blood remaining in the administration tubing can also be delivered to the patient by filling the drip chamber with saline. Although this system is not closed, risks of contamination are minimal if aseptic technique is used.

Blood should be warmed to room temperature or preferably to 37°C before its administration.[4, 9] Blood warming should not be accelerated by the use of excessive heat.[9] Fibrinogen precipitates at 56°C, and autoagglutination occurs when temperatures exceed 45°C. Water baths for warming blood products should not exceed 40°C. Blood can be warmed en route to the patient by placing part of the administration tubing in a warm water bath. Devices designed for this purpose are available.

Blood is best administered intravenously. When venous administration is impossible, however, blood can be given by intramedullary or intraperitoneal injection.[9] Absorption from the peritoneal cavity is delayed, and some of the erythocytes given by either of these alternative routes will never reach the circulation. Blood can be mixed with normal saline for administration or can be administered through tubing or catheters that are also carrying this fluid, but other commonly used intravenous fluids cannot be given with blood.[9] Dextrose solutions may cause autoagglutination, hemolysis, or both, and the calcium in fluids such as Ringer's solution may cause coagulation.

Appropriate dosage and rate of administration for blood or blood products are highly variable, depending on the clinical circumstance, the disease or condition being treated, and the physiological status of the patient. Specific recommendations for transfusion therapy will be found in discussions of treatment of those conditions in other chapters. However, several principles of transfusion therapy are worthy of mention. First, laboratory test results (e.g., hematocrit, platelet count, and so on) alone are poor guides for the use of transfusion therapy. Clinical signs, physiological status, and the direction and rate of anticipated changes (whether spontaneous or induced by other therapeutic efforts) must be considered as well. Second, the amount of blood or blood product required to produce a desired effect can be estimated by computations based on the size of the animal, approximate blood volume per unit weight (i.e., 88 ml/kg for dogs and 66 ml/kg for cats), composition of the blood or blood product, and desired composition of the recipient's blood following transfusion. For example, if a 20-kg dog's blood volume is about 1,760 ml and the hematocrit is 11%, the circulation contains about 200 ml of erythocytes. To have a posttransfusion hematocrit of 25%, the dog would need 440 ml of erythocytes; 240 ml of erythocytes need to be administered. The amount of blood required to deliver 240 ml of erythocytes depends on the hematocrit of the product administered; i.e., 400 ml if it is 60% (e.g., sedimented red cells), 600 ml if it is 40% and so on. The actual posttransfusion hematocrit will usually be somewhat less than that predicted because of volume expansion caused by fluid infusion. Third, blood products should be infused slowly unless the animal is hypovolemic.[9, 20] Because the administered cells and proteins tend to remain within the circulation, infusions of blood products produce greater volume expansion than do infusions of crystalloid solutions. Circulatory overload and cardiac insufficiency are more easily produced, particularly in chronically anemic animals.

AUTOTRANSFUSION

Autotransfusion is the practice of administering autologous blood or blood products to a patient. The patient's own blood is obtained and is subsequently returned. Compared with the use of homologous donor blood, autotransfusion has several advantages.[3] The potential problems of disease transmission; isoimmunization to erythrocyte, leukocyte, platelet, or protein antigens; and hemolytic, febrile, allergic, or graft versus host reactions are avoided. Blood typing and crossmatching are unnecessary, and availability of blood for the patient can sometimes be assured when it would otherwise be insufficient. Lastly, blood that is collected for autologous use but is not needed can be used for homologous transfusion. Because of its numerous advantages in various clinical circumstances, the increased use of autotransfusion has been advocated.[3, 21]

Three types of autotransfusion strategies have been described:[3] (1) storage of blood obtained periodically for several weeks prior to an anticipated episode of blood loss; (2) immediate preoperative phlebotomy and hemodilution to produce a state of normovolemic anemia; and (3) salvage of blood hemorrhaged during surgery or as a result of trauma. In each instance, blood is administered to the patient when needed, and the requirements for homologous blood are reduced or eliminated. Although autotransfusion techniques are more widely used in human than in veterinary medicine, many of the procedures were originally evaluated in canine models.[3] The successful clinical use of autotransfusion in animals has been reported.[21]

Provided that the patient's bone marrow and erythropoietin system are intact, one or more phlebotomies performed over a three-week period prior to a surgical procedure known to produce substantial blood loss can be beneficial and safe.[3] Obviously, the blood can be refrigerated, stored, and then given during or following surgery. It must be remembered that this blood is depleted of functional platelets and coagulation factors. In addition, the hematopoietic response by the bone marrow to phlebotomy can be maximized by oral iron administration. Thus, the animal is subjected to surgery with a state of maximal hematopoiesis already developed. Because bone marrow response to blood loss requires several days to develop fully, optimum hematopoiesis is delayed following surgical blood loss when preoperative phlebotomy is not performed. Following phlebotomy, plasma volume is rapidly replenished. Provided that the interval between phlebotomy and surgery is at least three days and that the patient's hematocrit is not below 30% immediately prior to surgery, the animal's tolerance of anesthesia and surgery will not be altered.

The rationale for acute production of normovolemic anemia by hemodilution and phlebotomy just prior to surgery is that fewer erythrocytes are lost during intraoperative hemorrhage.[3] Diminished red cell loss reduces the requirement for homologous blood. Blood removed from the patient at the outset of the procedure is not only available for use during or following surgery but is fresh and contains more platelets and coagulation factors that stored blood. Compensatory responses to acute normovolemic anemia maintain a satisfactory physiological state if the hematocrit is reduced by less than half. In people, this type of autotransfusion is particularly useful for patients undergoing extracorporeal circulation; in this setting, a 10% hematocrit is sufficient.

Re-infusion of blood salvaged from patients suffering massive intraoperative or posttraumatic hemorrhage has proven to be life-saving in human and veterinary medicine.[3, 21] In certain circumstances, the quantity and immediate availability of compatible blood make this type of autotransfusion far superior to homologous donor blood. The technique is most often used in human trauma centers. Systems varying in complexity from simple to elaborate have been designed to collect, filter, and, in some instances, wash and re-infuse hemorrhaged blood.

The basic principles of autotransfusion of salvaged blood include minimizing problems associated with trauma to blood components (e.g., hemolysis); coagulation; and dissemination of microorganisms, neoplastic cells, or particulate debris prior to re-infusion.[3, 21] In traumatized dogs with hemothorax, this has been accomplished by aspirating blood through chest drains into vacuum blood collection bottles containing ACD solution, followed by infusion through standard blood administration sets.[21] To minimize hemolysis, blood aspiration should be gentle and should not occur at a blood-air interface. Administration of large quantities of hemolyzed blood can cause disseminated intravascular coagulation (DIC) or hemoglobin nephropathy, but these complications usually do not occur if hypotension and hypovolemia are prevented. Contact of blood with air or tissue surfaces causes platelet aggregation and activation of coagulation. Thrombocytopenia consistently develops with the use of extracorporeal bypass, including autotransfusion, but it is usually not a problem unless platelet counts fall below 50,000/mm[3] Although infusion of activated coagulation factors may initiate DIC, the greater risk is usually exacerbation of a preexisting coagulopathy. Microaggregates, particularly composed of platelets, will be infused with salvaged blood unless a micropore filter is used; however, the clinical importance of microaggregate infusion is controversial.[11, 19] Malignancy and infection are contraindications to autotransfusion.

COMPLICATIONS OF BLOOD TRANSFUSIONS

Therapeutic administration of blood or blood components can cause numerous complications or adverse reactions.[4, 9] Hemolytic reactions are of obvious concern; however, they are certainly not the only type of potential complication. Indeed, they may not even be the most frequently occurring.[9, 11] Nonhemolytic reactions, microcirculatory blockade, cardiovascular overload, and disease transmission are other potential complications of transfusions. Additionally, there is an increase in the metabolic workload of the recipient of transfused blood. This extra metabolic effort may be difficult for a debilitated patient to meet.

Accelerated destruction of circulating erythrocytes may occur following transfusion in several ways.[4, 9, 16] Hemolysis can be immediate, because of pre-existing isoantibodies, or delayed until the recipient mounts an immune response to the infused incompatible cells. Hemolysis can occur intravascularly, producing hemoglobinemia and hemoglobinuria, or extravascularly (in the reticuloendothelial system), producing only hyperbilirubinemia and bilirubinuria. Usually the donated red cells are destroyed, but the recipient's own erythrocytes can also be hemolyzed by antibodies in the donor plasma. Immunological mechanisms are generally involved in hemolytic reactions, but transfused red cells can be destroyed at an accelerated rate because of mechanical factors such as decreased deformability or increased fragility.

Blood typing and crossmatching procedures are used to minimize the risks of hemolytic reactions, but random blood transfusions (i.e., those performed without benefit of such tests) are relatively safe in dogs provided the patient does not have immune-mediated hemolytic anemia and does not require sequential transfusions.[4, 15, 20] There are several reasons for this. Only DEA 1.1, 1.2, and possibly 7 are sufficiently immunogenic to pose clinically important red cell incompatibility problems. Approximately 60 per cent of dogs are DEA 1.1 and 1.2 positive (i.e., are universal recipients), and 40 per cent are DEA 1.1 and 1.2 negative (i.e., are universal donors). The random chance of transfusing a DEA 1.1 and 1.2 negative dog with blood from a DEA 1.1 or 1.2 positive dog is about one in four. Even in that instance, however, an immediate hemolytic reaction is unlikely following the first transfusion because DEA 1.1 and 1.2 negative dogs rarely develop significant anti-DEA 1.1 or 1.2 antibody titers spontaneously. However, approximately 50 per cent of the random dog population is DEA 7 negative and has naturally occurring anti-DEA 7 antibody that may cause destruction of transfused cells *in vivo*. Nonetheless, transfusion of incompatible cells would stimulate an immune response, and destruction of the cells would occur when antibody production commenced (i.e., delayed hemolysis). Additionally, the animal would be sensitized and immediate hemolytic reactions would be expected to occur if subsequent transfusions of DEA 1.1 or 1.2 positive blood were performed. If such a sensitized animal was a female and was mated to a DEA 1.1 or 1.2 positive male, DEA 1.1 or 1.2 positive offspring might suffer neonatal isoerythrolysis caused by anti-DEA 1.1 and 1.2 isoantibodies received from the dam's colostrum.[4] Thus, transfusions from randomly selected donors usually produce clinically acceptable results provided

that sequential transfusions are not required and the recipient is not a female to be used for breeding.

Crossmatching detects antibodies that produce red cell agglutination or lysis. The procedure is simple and can be performed in the office.[4, 15] A major crossmatch is the most important and checks for antibodies in the recipient's serum that will interact with the donor's cells. A minor crossmatch detects antibodies in the donor's serum that will react with the recipient's cells. Crossmatching detects the presence of pre-existing antibodies that produce an immediate hemolytic reaction, but a compatible crossmatch does not preclude sensitization to a subsequent transfusion. Thus, the random odds of sensitizing the recipient by transfusing DEA 1.1 and 1.2 positive blood (i.e., one in four) are not altered by crossmatch testing. Therefore, once a random transfusion has been given, crossmatching before a subsequent transfusion is essential.[15]

To prevent sensitization of recipient animals to erythrocyte antigens, it is necessary to determine the blood type of potential donors and select for use only those that are DEA 1.1, 1.2, and 7 negative.[9, 15, 20] Canine blood typing, however, is a specialized procedure that is not widely available. Because of this and because the use of randomly selected blood donors is safe in many instances, failure to utilize blood typing may not be detrimental, provided the previously mentioned precautions are taken.

Signs of an immediate hemolytic reaction develop within an hour following blood administration and may include fever, nausea, vomiting, urticaria, tachycardia, dyspnea, hypotension, and hemoglobinuria.[4, 9, 20] Laboratory evaluations should demonstrate evidence of red cell destruction and may reveal leukopenia and thrombocytopenia as well. Therapy consists of cessation of blood administration and institution of supportive measures. Disseminated intravascular coagulation, acute renal failure, or both may ensue, particularly if shock and hypotension are not adequately combated.[16] Signs of delayed hemolytic reactions are more subtle and may be limited to fever, anorexia, jaundice, and increased urinary bilirubin. These signs coincide with laboratory findings indicative of hemolysis.

In contrast to dogs, cats have been reported to spontaneously develop antierythrocyte isoantibodies that produce potentially lethal reactions following initial transfusions.[2] Approximately 75 per cent of cats in Brisbane, Australia, were found to be group A positive; the remaining 25 per cent were group B positive. High titers of anti-A isoantibody, a potent agglutinin and hemolysin, were prevalent in group B cats. Administration of A positive erythrocytes to group B cats frequently produced adverse reactions characterized by profound hypotension, tachycardia, transient apnea, tachypnea, and sometimes atrioventricular blockade. Group A cats generally had low titers of anti-B isoantibody, and administration of B positive blood to these cats did not produce adverse reactions. Use of crossmatching, even for initial transfusions, was advocated to prevent the administration of incompatible blood to cats.[2]

Although these studies of transfusion reactions in cats are noteworthy, their implications remain uncertain. The reactions were produced by intravenous injection of 1.0 ml of a 50% suspension of red cells in saline, which supports the premise that erythrocyte antigen-isoantibody interactions were responsible for the reactions. It is remarkable that hemolysis of so few red cells would have such profound effects. Furthermore, the random chances of such reactions are 3 in 16 (using the population distribution of feline blood groups in Australia); the general experience of clinicians in the United States is that transfusion reactions rarely occur in cats.[4, 5, 9, 10]

A variety of nonhemolytic reactions can occur following administration of blood or blood components.[17] Immunological mechanisms involving antigens associated with thrombocytes, leukocytes, or plasma proteins may produce hypersensitivity reactions. Additionally, vasoactive amines emanating from activation of the kallikrein-kinin system by contact coagulation factors (e.g., factor XII) have been implicated in the genesis of "plasma reactions."[1, 9] Fever, chills, restlessness, nausea, vomiting, and urticaria can be produced by nonhemolytic reactions. Signs typically develop rapidly but are usually mild and transient. Depending on the severity of the reaction, it may be necessary to slow or stop the infusion or to administer antipyretics (e.g., dipyrone, salicylates), antihistamines, or glucocorticoids. Urticarial reactions (e.g., facial swelling, hives) are fairly common during transfusion of dogs, but discontinuation of transfusion for this reason is rarely necessary.[9]

Administration of blood containing bacteria or bacterial endotoxins may cause fever, chills, hypotension, and shock.[9, 17] Infusion must be stopped, blood cultures should be obtained, and administration of antibiotics, corticosteroids, and replacement fluids may be required. Practices such as warming and rechilling stored blood and failing to administer warmed blood promptly should be avoided.[17] Dark discoloration (i.e., black or dark brown) of the plasma in a unit of blood indicates bacterial digestion of hemoglobin, and such blood must not be used.[9]

Microcirculatory blockade, particularly in the lungs, may be of concern when large volumes of stored blood are administered.[9] Microaggregates that form in stored blood have been implicated in the genesis of adult respiratory distress syndrome in severely injured people receiving massive transfusions during resuscitation. In a large human trauma center, however, the incidence of adult respiratory distress syndrome was reported to be extremely low even though micropore filters were not routinely used during massive transfusions of stored blood.[19]

Blood transfusion can produce circulatory overload, cardiac insufficiency, and pulmonary edema, particularly in normovolemic animals.[9, 20] The existence of functionally important cardiac disease also greatly increases the risk of these complications. Signs of circulatory overload include vomiting, urticaria, tachycardia, coughing, dyspnea, and cyanosis. Fulminant pulmonary edema and death may occur. Treatment includes slowing or stopping the infusion and administering diuretics (e.g., furosemide). Slower infusion rates and the use of packed red cells instead of whole blood for anemia help to prevent volume overload.[9, 20]

A variety of infectious diseases can be transmitted from an affected donor animal to a susceptible recipient by blood transfusion. Adequate investigation of the background and current health status of prospective blood donors is the only way to prevent this complication. The fact that apparently healthy animals may be carriers of important infectious agents bears emphasis. Procedures discussed in the section on selection of blood donors should be followed.

Administration of stored blood, especially a large volume, imposes a substantial metabolic burden on the recipient.[19] *In vivo* restoration of normal erythrocytic composition and metabolism or excretion of by-products and debris that have accumulated during storage requires expenditure of energy. In people, the metabolic "cost" for the regeneration of intracellular ATP and DPG has been estimated to exceed 13,000 micromoles of ATP per unit of stored blood.[19] Phagocytosis of cellular debris increases oxygen consumption and lactate production. The metabolic demands imposed by transfusion of stored blood often must be met in a setting of poor tissue perfusion and impaired oxygen availability, the latter condition being created, at least in part, by the increase in hemoglobin oxygen affinity exhibited by stored erythrocytes that are depleted of DPG.

Significant quantities of ammonia accumulate in blood during storage.[17, 19] Adverse metabolic effects of ammonia include increased hepatic energy requirements for urea production and stimulation of glycolysis and tricarboxylic acid cycle activity in muscle.[19] The latter effect is counterproductive to a general effort to reduce metabolic rate in nonessential peripheral tissues while perfusion and oxygen availability are impaired. Additionally, ammonia toxicity (which is potentiated by hypoxia) can be a problem, particularly if hepatic function is reduced.

1. Alving, B. M., Hojima, Y., Pisano, J. J., Mason, B. L., Buckingham, R. E., Mosen, M. M., and Finlayson, J. S.: Hypotension associated with prekallikrein activator (Hageman-factor fragments) in plasma protein fraction. N. Engl. J. Med. 299:66, 1978.
2. Auer, L., Bell, K., and Coatcs, S.: Blood transfusion reactions in the cat. J. Am. Vet. Med. Assoc. 180:799, 1982.
3. Brzica, S. M., Jr., Pineda, A. A., and Taswell, H. F.: Autologous blood transfusion. Mayo Clin. Proc. 51:723, 1976.
4. Buening, G. M.: Transfusions. In Bojrab, M. J. (ed.): *Pathophysiology in Small Animal Surgery*. Lea & Febiger, Philadelphia, 1981, pp. 478–501.
5. Cotter, S. M.: Blood transfusion reactions in cats. J. Am. Vet. Med. Assoc. 181:5, 1982.

6. Dodds, W. J.: Management and treatment of hemostatic defects. In Bojrab, M. J. (ed.): *Pathophysiology in Small Animal Surgery.* Lea & Febiger, Philadelphia, 1981, pp. 475–477.
7. Eisenbrandt, D. L., and Smith J. E.: Evaluation of preservatives and containers for storage of canine blood. J. Am. Vet. Med. Assoc. *163*:988, 1973.
8. Eisenbrandt, D. L., and Smith, J. E.: Use of biochemical measures to estimate viability of red blood cells in canine blood stored in acid citrate dextrose solution, with and without added ascorbic acid. J. Am. Vet. Med. Assoc. *163*:984, 1973.
9. Greene, C. E.: Blood transfusion therapy: An updated overview. Proc. 49th Ann. Mtg. Am. Anim. Hosp. Assoc. 1982, pp. 187–189.
10. Hayes, A., Mastrota, F., Mooney, S., and Hurvitz, A.: Safety of transfusing blood in cats (letter). J. Am. Vet. Med. Assoc. *181*:4, 1982.
11. Isbister, J. P., and Scurr, R. D.: Blood transfusion therapy: Components, indications, complications, and controversies. Anaesth. Intensive Care 6:297, 1978.
12. Miller, W. V. (ed.): *Technical Manual of the American Association of Blood Banks.* J. B. Lippincott, Philadelphia, 1977.
13. Myhre, B. A., and Harris, G. E.: Blood components for hemotherapy. Clin. Lab. Med. 2:3, 1982.
14. Ou, D., Mahaffey, E., and Smith, J. E.: Effect of storage on oxygen dissociation of canine blood. J. Am. Vet. Med. Assoc. *167*:56, 1975.
15. Owen, R. R., and Glen, J. B.: Factors to be considered when making canine blood and blood products available for transfusions. Vet. Rec. *91*:406, 1972.
16. Pineda, A. A., Brzica, S. M., and Taswell, H. F.: Hemolytic transfusion reaction. Recent experience in a large blood bank. Mayo. Clin. Proc. 53:378, 1978.
17. Silver, D.: Blood transfusions and disorders of surgical bleeding. In Sabiston, D. C. (ed.): *Textbook of Surgery*, 11th ed. W. B. Saunders, Philadelphia, 1977, pp. 131–138.
18. Smith, J. E., Mahaffey, E., and Board, P.: A new storage medium for canine blood. J. Am. Vet. Med. Assoc. *172*:701, 1978.
19. Sohmer, P. R., and Scott, R. L.: Massive transfusion. Clin. Lab. Med. 2:21, 1982.
20. Tangner, C. H.: Transfusion therapy for the dog and cat. Comp. Cont. Ed. Pract. Vet. *4*:521, 1982.
21. Zenoble, R. D., and Stone, E. A.: Autotransfusion in the dog. J. Am. Vet. Med. Assoc. *172*:1411, 1978.

Chapter **8** # Metabolism of the Surgical Patient

Ronald M. Bright and Gary C. Lantz

An animal reacts to a stressful stimulus with a variety of metabolic and endocrine responses, depending on the severity of the insult. These responses are minimal when a simple skin incision is made and more complex in shock or following major surgery. An insufficient response may result when the stimuli affecting the equilibrium of the patient are so severe that homeostatic mechanisms are overwhelmed (Fig. 8–1). Hypovolemia, general anesthesia, major surgery, nonsurgical trauma, psychic stresses, and sepsis are the stimuli of most concern in surgical patients.

The normal reaction to stressful stimuli is a certain degree of resistance to the effects of trauma. The response is basically the same but varies in magnitude with the severity of the insult. The response may continue until the pretrauma status has returned.

HYPOTHALAMIC-PITUITARY SYSTEM

Adrenocorticotropic Hormone (ACTH)

Endocrine responses following injury depend on an intact nerve supply. Experiments in dogs have demonstrated a lack of endocrine response to injury when the part of the body traumatized has suffered prior denervation. Sensory input into the hypothalamic-pituitary system comes from the brain stem, reticular formation system, limbic system, and sub-cortex.[15] Endotoxins may stimulate the hypothalamus directly, the hormone released varying with the stimulus.

ACTH is released from the anterior pituitary as a result of stimulation by corticotropin-releasing factor (CRF) from the hypothalamus. This in turn causes the zona fasciculata of the adrenal cortex to produce higher levels of glucocorticoids. In acute and severe trauma, higher ACTH levels may also release aldosterone from the zona glomerulosa. The primary result is the mobilization of free fatty acids (lipolysis), which can act as an energy source, and the impairment of hepatic enzymes that normally inactivate cortisol. This allows larger amounts of unconjugated (active) corticosteroids to become available even though the rate of secretion may remain constant.[11]

Cortisol affects the metabolism of carbohydrates by stimulating gluconeogenesis by the liver and decreasing the rate of glucose utilization by the body cells.[25]

During stress, amino acids are released from the extrahepatic tissues, mainly muscle, and converted into glucose. This metabolism is stimulated by the increased cortisol levels and accounts for the muscle wasting often seen in patients suffering chronic stress.[22]

The presence of cortisol in adequate amounts is extremely important if the animal is to withstand the stress of surgical trauma. Patients with unrecognized adrenal insufficiency or those who become that way

Figure 8–1. Threshold stimuli (group I) produce minor changes in the organism. Should any of these stimuli be prolonged or of extreme severity, they may be fatal. Generally they are of short duration and low magnitude and constitute little trauma to the animal. Group II evokes a strong homeostatic response. The longer the challenges remain unopposed or uncorrected (e.g., bleeding, anoxia), the more severe the injury. These are correctable by the body as long as necessary steps are taken to enhance homeostasis (e.g., blood replacement, tracheostomy). Group III (tissue-killing injury) produces dead tissues that release products of tissue necrosis into the circulation as well as deprive the organism of the function of the organ undergoing ischemic necrosis. (Reprinted with permission from Moore, F.D.: *Metabolic Care of The Surgical Patient.* W. B. Saunders, Philadelphia, 1959.)

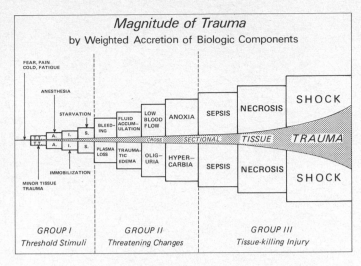

as a result of their condition will not tolerate stress well unless supplemented with an exogenous corticosteroid. Adrenal insufficiency is rarely the cause of death after surgical trauma in adrenally compromised patients if corticosteroids are given. The need to recognize adrenal insufficiency is obvious. Anorexia, muscle weakness, and ECG changes consistent with hyperkalemia, plus dehydration, collapse, and coma are a few of the clinical findings associated with hypoadrenocorticism.[25]

Cortisol decreases inflammatory and immune responses. Sodium and water retention also occur in varying degrees, with potassium being excreted by the renal tubules. It is possible that cortisol binds with specific complexes of protein in all cytoplasm and nuclei, causing the RNA molecule to help the cell adapt to its altered environment.

Antidiuretic Hormone (ADH)

The release of ADH is controlled by carotid and atrial volume receptors and central nervous system (CNS) osmoreceptors. The production and release of ADH is increased following stimuli such as hyperosmolarity and hypovolemia owing to dehydration and hemorrhage, respectively. Additional stimuli resulting in ADH release include trauma, pain, and some anesthetic agents. Any water solute distortion or blood volume reduction stimulates ADH and, in turn, exerts its effect on the renal tubules. ADH (vasopressin) affects the renal tubules by increasing renal tubule permeability and resorption of water (Fig. 8–2). The result is reduced urine volume and increased urine osmolality. Sodium is retained and extracellular water volume restored by transcapillary refill within hours after hemorrhage.[27]

The antidiuresis that follows surgery is inappropriate since it is activated by tissue trauma and isotonic volume reduction. The administration of hypotonic solutions or water may, therefore, produce hyponatremia and hypotonicity rather than merely shut off ADH production.[22]

Renin-Angiotensin-Aldosterone Response

This response aids in the preservation of circulatory volume and, therefore, cell metabolism. This system is activated by any condition that results in an ineffective circulatory volume. In man, an increased urinary potassium excretion and a decreased sodium excretion were noted in the first four days following a moderate form of surgical insult.[10, 20] Hyperaldosteronism in the postoperative patient is caused by an increased production of aldosterone by the adrenal cortex and an impaired rate of destruction by the liver.[10, 17, 24]

Aldosterone secretion results primarily from the renin-angiotensin stimulus (Fig. 8–3). ACTH further

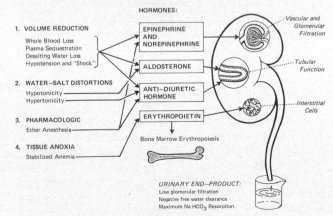

Figure 8–2. Mechanisms activated to conserve effective volume of body water, plasma, and interstitial fluid. The pituitary can be considered the "master gland" of the endocrine system, whereas the catecholamines are the primary hormones in the response to injury. Besides local effects on the kidney, their widespread effects on the circulatory system conserve blood flow to critical areas. Significant effects of catecholamines on the intermediary metabolism of fat, nitrogen, and carbohydrate are also important. (Reprinted with permission from Moore, F. D.: Homeostasis: Bodily changes in trauma and surgery. *In* Sabiston, D. C., Jr.: *Textbook of Surgery,* 12th ed. W. B. Saunders, Philadelphia, 1981, p. 36.)

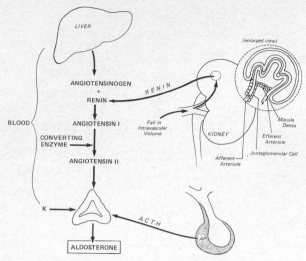

Figure 8–3. Stimuli of aldosterone secretion. The primary stimulus is a decrease in intravascular volume. (Reprinted with permission from Schwartz, S. I. et al.: *Principles of Surgery*, 2nd ed. McGraw-Hill Book Co., New York, 1969.)

enhances its secretion. Renin is secreted from the renal juxtaglomerular cells and results in the transformation of hepatically derived angiotensinogen into angiotensin I in the plasma. This substance is enzymatically converted into angiotensin II, which stimulates the adrenal cortex to secrete aldosterone while acting as a potent vasopressor. Both eventually act to maintain blood pressure, angiotensin II by its vasoconstrictive properties and aldosterone by causing the kidney to conserve sodium, thereby supporting the plasma volume. Besides the renin source of stimulation, an increased output of aldosterone results from high ACTH levels, hyperkalemia, surgical and nonsurgical trauma, and hemorrhage (hypovolemia). Following the acute loss of blood, aldosterone secretion may increase thirtyfold, with an increased urinary excretion of aldosterone as well.[22]

Sympathetic Adrenal Medulla System

A number of events related to surgical trauma stimulate the sympathetic system and the subsequent output of catecholamines. Stimuli such as pain, fear, hypercarbia, hypoxia, hypovolemia, and trauma trigger the release of epinephrine and norepinephrine from the adrenal medulla. Norepinephrine is released from other sites as well. Moderate surgical trauma causes a transient rise of catecholamines in the blood, which is sustained for 24 to 48 hours.[10] Epinephrine has several functions, including vasoconstriction of vessels of the skin, adipose tissue, kidneys, and splanchnic bed, thereby preserving blood flow to more vital structures, including the heart and brain. It also increases heart rate and myocardial contractility. The principal action of norepinephrine is its vasomotor effect on blood vessels, causing a vasocon-

striction throughout the body except for the myocardium.[22]

Catecholamine may be considered the primary endocrine response to injury.[22] It has widespread effects and is a stimulator of the pituitary, producing ACTH and, therefore, glucocorticoids and aldosterone. Gluconeogenesis results as well as a shift of potassium from the intracellular to the extracellular space.[10]

The short-lived catecholamine response is beneficial to the animal.[22] If catecholamine levels remain elevated for a prolonged period of time, deleterious effects, such as exhaustion of energy stores and ischemia of cellular tissues, may occur (Fig. 8–4).

Some studies have suggested a benefit from inhibition of the beta-adrenergic response in stress conditions. It is known that beta-adrenergic activity plays an important role in certain metabolic responses, primarily by inducing muscular glycogenolysis, lactate formation, and lipolysis. Alpha receptor stimulation results in hepatic glycogenolysis.[31] In experimental shock produced by hemorrhage or endotoxin injection, the administration of a beta blocker, propanolol, resulted in fewer deaths.[28, 31] In the operative management of human diabetics, the inhibitory effects of epidural analgesia on beta-adrenergic activity and, subsequently, on metabolic responses have been beneficial.[12] Although propanolol inhibits lactate, nonesterified fatty acid, and glucose levels in humans

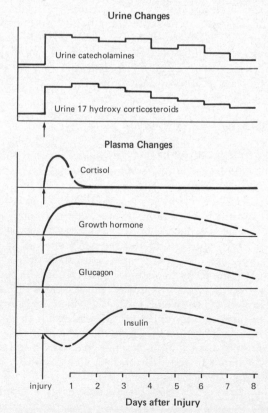

Figure 8–4. Hormonal changes after injury, including both urine and plasma changes. (Reprinted with permission from Ledingham I. McA., and Mackay, C. (eds.): *Jamieson and Kay's Textbook of Surgical Physiology*, 3rd ed. Churchill Livingstone, Edinburgh, 1977.)

following gastrectomies, it does not have any deleterious effects.[6, 31]

CARBOHYDRATE METABOLISM

Carbohydrate is needed as an energy source for DNA and RNA synthesis, the formation of cellular components, and the transfer of nutrients and electrolytes. The stress of surgery and anesthesia results in hyperglycemia and glucosuria. The inhibition of the pancreatic production of insulin and its peripheral activity, probably via catecholamine production, is in part the cause of the hyperglycemia.[22] Other factors contributing to increased blood glucose include peripheral carbohydrate breakdown by cortisol, the mobilization of carbohydrate by growth hormone and its antagonistic effect on insulin in the periphery, and gluconeogenesis due to the release of glucagon.[11] Carbohydrate metabolism is most important to the animal during the initial phases of trauma.[11] Later, when the glucose demand exceeds mobilization and gluconeogenesis, the breakdown of fat and protein to produce energy occurs.[30]

PROTEIN METABOLISM

Surgical trauma results in tissue wasting and weight loss (Fig. 8–5). Although this is minimal in elective surgery, it takes on added importance when a catabolic state exists owing to the nature of the illness. In one study in humans, preoperative weight loss was the only factor that correlated with operative mortality rates.[13]

The extent of weight loss in man has been shown to be influenced by the patient's sex, body build,

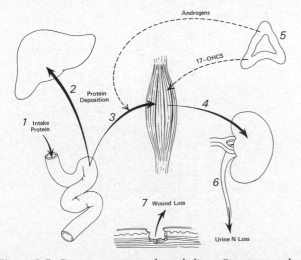

Figure 8–5. Protein storage and catabolism. Protein may be preferentially stored in the liver while being catabolized from muscle stores. Its catabolism is increased by glucocorticoids and decreased by adrenal androgens. (Reprinted with permission from Schwartz, S. I., et al.: *Principles of Surgery*, 2nd ed. McGraw-Hill Book Co., New York, 1969.)

Resting Energy Expenditure

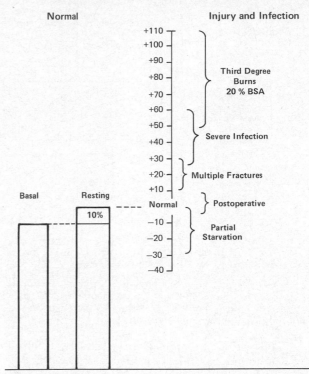

Figure 8–6. The effect of injury, sepsis, and nutritional depletion on resting energy expenditure. The extent to which expenditure of energy increases varies markedly with the nature and degree of injury. (Reprinted with permission from Kinney, J. M. (ed.): *Assessment of Energy Metabolism in Health and Disease, Report of the First Ross Conference on Medical Research*. Columbus, Ohio, Ross Laboratories, 1980, p. 48.)

preoperative nutritional status, degree of injury associated with the procedure, and the presence of any complicating factors such as infection[13] (Fig. 8–6). Tissue loss is the result of both nutritional deficit and neuroendocrine mechanisms activated by injury.

Following surgery, normal caloric intake is usually decreased, whereas catabolism is increased.[9] The intensity and duration of the postoperative catabolic period depend on the nature of the injury and whether sepsis or another major complication is present. An elective procedure has little effect on the expenditure of energy. However, severe fractures or major abdominal surgery may cause a 10 to 30 per cent increase in energy expenditure, whereas sepsis and severe burns can increase energy expenditure by 60 and 200 per cent, respectively.

Plasma protein levels decline after injury, and this is primarily reflected in the albumin fraction[11] (Fig. 8–7). This fraction decreases in man by 25 to 30 per cent on the fourth or fifth day following moderate injury and gradually returns to normal thereafter.[16] The return to normal depends on the extent and duration of the injury.[16] Burns depress albumin for a prolonged period of time, sometimes requiring months to return to normal.[16]

Urinary nitrogen excretion increases after injury and is primarily in the form of urea nitrogen[11] (Fig.

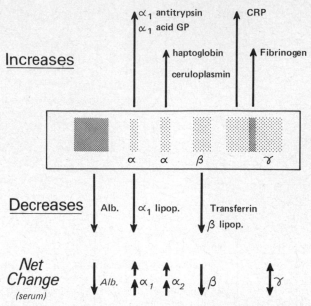

Figure 8–7. Changes in plasma proteins after injury. (Reprinted with permission from Ledingham, I. McA., and Mackay, C. (eds.): *Jamieson and Kay's Textbook of Surgical Physiology*, 3rd ed. Churchill Livingstone, Edinburgh, 1977.)

Since carbohydrates serve as the main source of energy following surgical trauma, protein stores are spared but eventually are converted to carbohydrates for energy through gluconeogenesis.[27] During this period of stress, exogenous protein does not contribute to tissue repair but serves as an energy source. Only when large amounts of readily utilized calories and protein are provided during the catabolic period can the net nitrogen loss be halted.[27] This means that the metabolic effects of trauma on protein nutrition are mainly attributable to factors other than starvation. The severe stimulus for protein catabolism during the early posttrauma period is, as mentioned before, quite difficult to overcome by providing exogenous nutrients.[27] The main hormonal trigger for the catabolism of trauma is probably due to the release of catecholamines from the adrenal medulla.[27]

Following most uncomplicated surgeries, the patient enters the catabolic phase of surgical convalescence on the third or fourth postoperative day. The action of anabolic steroids on protein is the opposite of that of glucocorticoids. Anabolic steroids cause protein to re-enter the skeletal muscles and form

8–8). This excretion begins soon after surgical insult and sometimes continues for weeks (Fig. 8–9). Urinary loss is not only from simple catabolism of body protein but also from protein synthesis. The catabolic source of protein is primarily skeletal muscle, with the liver and other active organs being spared.[11] More athletic muscular animals presumably have a higher urinary protein loss, since the major source of protein is protein stores in the muscle.[11] Multiple surgeries done over a short period of time usually result in less protein loss, probably owing to storage protein being lost by previous surgery.[11]

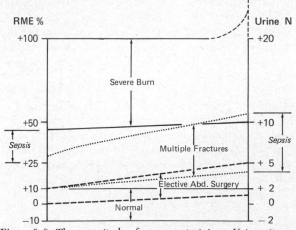

Figure 8–8. The magnitude of response to injury. Urine nitrogen is expressed as gm/day. Even minor surgical procedures lead to a transient negative nitrogen balance and slight weight loss. The alteration in resting metabolic expenditure (RME) is usually not detectable. In more serious injuries the loss of body nitrogen corresponds approximately to the increase in RME, as illustrated. Severe burns result in the greatest losses in body weight. (Reprinted with permission from Ledingham, I. McA., and Mackay, C. (eds.): *Jamieson and Kay's Textbook of Surgical Physiology*, 3rd ed. Churchill Livingstone, Edinburgh, 1977.)

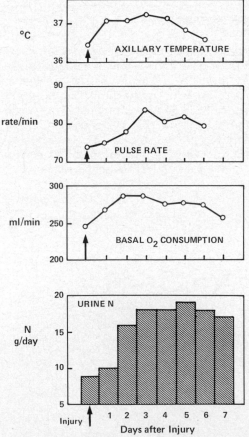

Figure 8–9. Response to bone injury. The predominant effect of injury is a net increase in catabolism, which leads to a generalized loss of body protein. An increase in oxygen consumption as well as temperature and pulse rate was observed. Urinary loss of protein was also observed after injury. (Reprinted with permission from Ledingham, I. McA., and Mackay, C. (eds.): *Jamieson and Kay's Textbook of Surgical Physiology*, 3rd ed. Churchill Livingstone, Edinburgh, 1977.)

connective tissue.[10] Ingested protein is retained, and a positive nitrogen balance is finally achieved. Urinary nitrogen losses decrease later to further enhance the positive nitrogen balance.

FAT METABOLISM

The importance of endogenous fat stores as sources of energy is often unappreciated. Although tissues such as the brain, erythrocytes, and peripheral nerves utilize glucose as their sole energy source, other tissues can catabolize fatty acids and their metabolic products (ketones) for energy.[27] This occurs as carbohydrate availability diminishes.

During starvation, increasing amounts of fatty acids derived from body fat can provide an energy source by converting into acetylcoenzyme A and participating in the tricarboxylic acid cycle. By-products of this shift in metabolic pathways are excreted in the urine, and ketoacidosis may exist when these substances are produced in excess.[10]

The increase in plasma unesterified fatty acids normally seen soon after surgery can be counteracted by the injection of glucose.[10, 31] Fat metabolism can also be markedly decreased by early food intake after surgery. When fats again start to be stored, the patient enters the fat gain phase of convalescence. Fat is stored in adipose tissue, mostly as triglycerides, to be readily available again as an energy source.[10] The fat gain phase lasts for several weeks after a moderately severe surgical procedure or longer following more severe surgical trauma.[10]

FLUID AND ELECTROLYTE SHIFTS

In the injured animal several mechanisms conserve extracellular fluid and maintain blood volume.[37] The volume of extracellular fluid has a higher biological priority than the maintenance of its precise chemical composition.[21] Sodium conservation is the key, and renal retention of water is important as well. The fluid-conserving mechanism (ADH) causes a sharp restriction in excretion of free water. Urine osmolality rises owing to distal tubular resorption.[21] Combined with fluid therapy during and after surgery, dilutional hyponatremia often results despite sodium retention caused by the release of aldosterone in response to a surgical-anesthetic episode.[19] The angiotensin secreted during this response causes some degree of vasoconstriction and subsequently decreases the glomerular filtration rate (GFR). These effects last only a few days, especially if the condition is not complicated by major and severe surgery, prolonged anesthesia, infections, and severe hemorrhage.

ADH secretion can be suppressed to varying degrees by maintaining good hydration preoperatively and during anesthesia. However, these measures have little effect on ADH secretion during a major operation or in the postoperative period. Water re-

tention, oliguria, and hyponatremia are compounded by giving solute-free fluids and, to a minor degree, by water released during the oxidation of fat.[11]

Potassium is lost via renal excretion in relatively large quantities after injury. This loss is promoted by aldosterone and cortisol. The potassium stored with glycogen is released during glycogenolysis and from severely damaged tissues. Acidosis drives potassium from the cell, whereas alkalosis drives it into the cell.

The phosphate anion rises immediately after a prolonged operation and reflects a decrease in GFR. It is also released from muscle and liver.

The hydrogen ion (HI) usually increases in concentration (acidosis) with the magnitude of the injury. Shock and renal failure contribute greatly to acidosis. An elevated HI concentration is also associated with a release of organic and inorganic acids. Acids contributing to a lower pH include lactate, fatty acids, ketones, phosphate, and sulfate. The lactate ion increases greatly when tissues are poorly perfused with blood.

RENAL RESPONSE TO INJURY

The risk of irreversible renal damage following surgery is greatest if there is any degree of renal disease prior to surgery and anesthesia. The kidney is easily insulted because it is the target organ for a wide variety of influences following trauma. The mechanism that triggers water or sodium retention may, at the same time, have a deleterious effect on the kidney. Differential renal vasoconstriction is a response to any blood volume or flow challenge.[22]

Extrinsic causes of oliguria include external fluid loss, hemorrhage, dehydration, gastrointestinal fluid loss, or internal "third space" accumulation of fluid as seen with bowel obstruction, gastric dilation-volvulus complex, pancreatitis, peritonitis, or limb trauma.[22]

Intrinsic renal damage causing oliguria is due to acute tubular necrosis.[2] This results from renal vasoconstriction coupled with shunting of blood away from the renal cortex, decreased filtration fraction of renal blood flow, and a maximal resorptive stimulus by aldosterone and ADH.[22] Adequate hydration and solute loading help protect the kidney from these normal responses to surgical trauma.

RESPIRATORY DISEASE AND ITS EFFECT ON THE SURGICAL PATIENT

Because of the increased morbidity and mortality of surgical patients with lung disease, it is mandatory that the risks of surgery be given prime consideration. The risks depend on the clinical status of the animal and the type of surgery to be performed. One can anticipate a more unfavorable outcome in pulmonary cripples if thoracic surgery is done compared with a minor nonthoracic procedure.

Alterations of pulmonary function after all kinds of surgical trauma are common and can develop into postoperative pulmonary complications in previously normal patients. Prophylactic measures taken in higher risk patients ensure a better outcome.[32]

Pulmonary abnormalities following surgery are due to stimuli to which patients are exposed during the operative period, including the surgical procedure itself, anesthesia, restrictive bandages, sensorium changes, postoperative medications (specifically analgesics), and lateral recumbency on one side for a prolonged period.[30] There are four areas in which these events can exert an influence: (1) lung volumes, (2) pattern of ventilation, (3) gas exchange, and (4) defense mechanisms.[30]

Total lung capacity and its subdivisions are often affected, especially if abdominal or thoracic surgery is performed.[30] In one human study nonabdominal, nonthoracic surgery did not affect vital capacity, whereas abdominal surgery decreased the vital capacity by 25 to 50 per cent.[1, 3-5, 7] Decreased functional residual capacity is an added problem in animal patients if the thorax has been surgically invaded and a pleural filling defect (pneumo- or hemothorax) remains postoperatively.

Surgery often affects the pattern of ventilation as well as the work of breathing, the degree of which depends on the nature of the surgical injury. Tidal volume is severely affected in thoracic surgical procedures in which pain and discomfort play an important role in preventing good chest excursion. The fall in tidal volume may be due to a decrease in lung compliance. The elastic work required to inflate the lung increases with the square of the increase in tidal volume.[23] Tachypnea combined with shallow breathing can severely decrease tidal volume to the point of hypoxia and hypercarbia in the postoperative period.

The importance of good ventilation under anesthesia is indicated by several studies in dogs demonstrating a clear-cut decrease in compliance if periodic hyperinflation was not performed.[18, 30] Functional residual capacity was also decreased in these dogs.[8, 18] This decrease in compliance was noted during postmortem examination to be due, at least in part, to airway closure.[8] This appeared to be most severe in the dependent portions of the lungs.

A gas exchange problem is often seen postoperatively in animals. The decrease in $P_{A_{O_2}}$ is thought to be directly related to positioning, lack of turning, and the type of surgery on the ventilation-perfusion (V/Q) ratio. Studies in rabbits undergoing thoracotomies revealed an increase in venous admixture, thought to be produced by perfusion of collapsed alveoli.[26] More severe lung disease in thoracic surgery patients could result in retention of carbon dioxide as well as a more severe gas exchange problem.

The cough mechanism is an important defense against the accumulation of secretions and particulate matter, both of which tend to deposit in the upper airways during surgery and anesthesia. Clearance from lower airways depends on maintaining the integrity of the mucociliary system, the alveoli, the cellular components, and lymphatic drainage.[30] Tracheobronchial secretions and their evacuation are of prime importance if the normal pulmonary defense mechanisms are to be preserved.

A variety of posttrauma factors can threaten the integrity of the lungs.[22] Airway compromise may result from aspiration of gastric contents or prolonged immobilization.[22] Other factors include fluid overload with oncotic dilution and pulmonary edema and underlying heart failure. Vasoactive substances affecting pulmonary perfusion can contribute to poor pulmonary function, especially serotonin from platelets, catecholamines, and the kinins.[22] Chest wall mechanisms threaten lung integrity and can be due to an unstable rib cage or sternum following closure of the chest wound. If open chest surgery is prolonged, collapsed or underperfused lungs can also contribute to pulmonary dysfunction.

Prophylactic measures recommended to decrease postoperative complications include operative considerations such as decreased length of anesthesia, evacuation of secretions, prevention of aspiration, and intermittent hyperinflation. Postoperative measures include the continuation of hyperinflation, good tracheobronchial toiletry, early ambulation, no antitussive medication, and analgesics to control pain with special emphasis on monitoring the effects of the analgesic on the pattern of breathing.[30]

CARDIAC FUNCTION OF THE PATIENT UNDERGOING SURGICAL TRAUMA

Surgical metabolism and the ability of the patient to withstand surgical trauma depend greatly on good cardiovascular function. The heart is a "flow-sensitive organ," as are the brain and kidneys.[22] It is one of the organs that should be closely evaluated when subjecting the patient to any form of surgical trauma.

Many factors during surgery and anesthesia are potentially deleterious to good cardiac function, including acidosis, hypoxemia, hypercapnia, decreased systemic vascular resistance, decreased myocardial contractility, and hypotension due to hypovolemia or other non–volume-related factors. Dysrhythmias due to catecholamine release, bradycardia associated with some muscle relaxants (e.g., succinylcholine), and decreased coronary flow due to a diminished systemic flow are additional cardiac hazards.

Although cardiac output decreases intraoperatively owing to a decrease in stroke volume,[11] an elevated postoperative cardiac output is the normal response in man.[22] This is due to catecholamine influence and a left shift of the hemoglobin dissociation curve in those patients hyperventilated during surgery or those that have hypocarbia due to hyperventilation secondary to pain, stress, and anxiety.[22] Massive blood transfusions can cause a deficiency in 2,3 DPG and can complement the effect of respiratory acidosis on the oxyhemoglobin dissociation curve. Because of decreased oxygen extraction by the tissues, cardiac output is increased by a compensatory mechanism working to correct an oxygen transport disorder. Some patients with other underlying pathology such as lactic acidosis, congestive heart failure, cardiac dysrhythmias, or renal failure may not accept this challenge of increased cardiac output and must be cautiously monitored postoperatively. The heart is also affected by the nutritional status of the patient, as proposed by investigators who have shown adverse effects on the hearts of rats maintained in a protein-deficient state.[14]

THE GASTROINTESTINAL SYSTEM AND THE SURGICAL PATIENT

Following surgical trauma, the stomach shows decreased motility and delayed emptying. Increased sympathetic influence is responsible for most of this effect. With severe trauma, achlorhydria may be present.[15]

Intestinal secretions are usually unaffected by surgery, but motility and absorption of fluids are decreased, sometimes to the point of gastrointestinal "pooling" of fluid. During recovery, motility usually returns before absorption, and, as a result, the initial stools may be watery.

SURGICAL CONVALESCENCE

Barring unforeseen complications, there is usually a shorter catabolic phase and a longer anabolic phase following a surgical procedure. The four phases associated with the postoperative recovery are (1) injury (catabolic) phase, (2) turning point (equilibrium), (3) anabolic phase, and (4) fat gain.[22]

The catabolic phase can be influenced by the knowledge and skill of the surgeon, as the extent and duration of the injury during the surgical procedure can be diminished in many cases. Minimal trauma to tissues, accurate restoration of fluid volumes, careful placement of sutures, and adequate immobilization of bone injuries minimize pain, the degree of endocrine response, and the total stimulus of injury.[22]

The turning point phase is the most dramatic period. The animal returns to normal eating, ambulation, and elimination habits and displays behavior seen in a better state of health (e.g., grooming in cats).

The anabolic phase is characterized by an increase in strength, a further increase in appetite and ambulation, and the maintenance of a positive nitrogen balance until pre-injury levels have been restored.[22]

The fat gain phase follows the return of nitrogen metabolism to 0 balance.[22] Any caloric intake that exceeds the 0 balance now results in the deposition of body fat and further weight gain. This weight gain

may be a problem in some animals, especially those that are immobilized and have a decrease in activity due to their surgical illness, must notably neurosurgical and orthopedic patients. Some degree of dietary restraint may be necessary if normal activity and exercise cannot be regained after postinjury anabolism is complete.[22]

1. Anscombe, A. R., and Buxton, R. S.: Effect of abdominal operations on total lung capacity and its subdivisions. Br. Med. J. 2:84, 1958.
2. Arieff, A. I.: In Dunphy, J. E., and Way, L. W. (eds.): *Current Surgical Diagnosis and Treatment*, 3rd ed. Lange Medical Publications, Los Altos, CA, 1977, p. 54.
3. Beecher, H. K.: The measured effect of laparotomy on the respiration. J. Clin. Invest. 12:639, 1933.
4. Beecher, H. K.: Effect of laparotomy on lung volume: demonstration of a new type of pulmonary collapse. J. Clin. Invest. 12:651, 1933.
5. Churchill, E. D., and McNeil, D.: The reduction in vital capacity following operation. Surg. Gynecol. Obstet. 44:483, 1927.
6. Cooper, G. M., Paterson, J. L., Mashiter, K., et al.: Beta-adrenergic blockade and the metabolic response to surgery. Br. J. Anaesth. 52:1231, 1980.
7. Diament, M. L., and Palmer, K. N. V.: Postoperative changes in gas tensions of arterial blood and in ventilatory function. Lancet 2:180, 1966.
8. Dubois, A. B., Botelho, S. Y., Bedell, G. N., et al.: A rapid plethysmographic method for measuring thoracic gas volume: Comparison with a nitrogen washout method for measuring functional residual capacity in normals. J. Clin. Invest. 35:322, 1956.
9. Elwyn, D. H., Kinney, J. M., and Askanazi, J.: Energy expenditure in surgical patients. Surg. Clin. North Am. 61:545, 1981.
10. Henegar, G. C.: Metabolic and endocrine effects of injury and surgery. In Preston, F. W., and Beal, J. M. (eds.): *Basic Surgical Physiology*. Year Book Medical Publishers, Chicago, 1969, p. 65.
11. Hume, D. M.: Endocrine and metabolic responses to injury. In Schwartz, S. (ed.): *Principles of Surgery*, 2nd ed. McGraw-Hill Book Co., New York, 1974, p. 3.
12. Kehlet, H., Brandt, M. R., Hansen, A. P., et al.: Effect of epidural anesthesia on metabolic profiles during and after surgery. Br. J. Surg. 66:543, 1979.
13. Kinney, J. M., Long, C. L., Gump, F. E., et al.: Tissue composition of weight loss in surgical patients I. Elective operation. Ann. Surg. 168:459, 1968.
14. Kyger, E. R., Block, W. J., Roach, G., et al.: Adverse effects of protein malnutrition on myocardial function. Surgery 84:147, 1978.
15. Lantz, G.: *Small Animal Surgery Course Outline*. Purdue University, West Lafayette, IN, 1981.
16. Ledingham, I. McA., Mackay, C., Jamieson, R. A., and Kay, A. W.: Metabolic response to injury. In Ledingham, I. McA., and Mackay, C. (eds.): *Jamieson and Kay's Textbook of Surgical Physiology*, 3rd ed. Churchill-Livingstone, New York, 1978, p. 42.
17. Llaurado, J. G., and Woodruff, M. F. A.: Postoperative transient aldosteronism. Surgery 42:313, 1957.
18. Mead, J., and Collier, C.: Relation of volume history of lungs to respiratory mechanics in dogs. J. Appl. Physiol. 14:669, 1959.
19. Michell, A. R.: The metabolic consequences of trauma. J. Small Anim. Pract. 15:279, 1974.
20. Moore, F. D.: Bodily changes in surgical convalescence. I. Normal sequence—observations and interpretations. Ann. Surg. 137:289, 1953.
21. Moore, F. D.: *Metabolic Care of The Surgical Patient*. W. B. Saunders, Philadelphia, 1959. pp. 20–24, 28–48, 109–114, 197.

22. Moore, F. D.: Homeostasis: Bodily changes in trauma and surgery. *In* Sabiston, D. C., Jr. (ed.): *Textbook of Surgery*, 10th ed. W. B. Saunders, Philadelphia, 1972, p. 26.
23. Peters, R. M., Wellons, H. A., Jr., and Htwe, T. M.: Total compliance and work of breathing after thoracotomy. J. Thorac. Cardiovasc. Surg. 57:348, 1969.
24. Riveron, E., Kukral, J. C., and Henegar, G. C.: Blood volume, water, and electrolyte spaces in human beings with cirrhosis and in dogs with Eck's fistula. Surg. Forum 17:365, 1966.
25. Rosin, E.: The systemic response to injury. *In* Bojrab, M. J. (ed.): *Pathophysiology in Small Animal Surgery*. Lea & Febiger, Philadelphia, 1981, p. 3.
26. Sackur: Zur lehre vom pneumothorax. Zentralbl. Khnical Med. 29:25, 1896.
27. Sheldon, G. F., Harper, H. A., and Way, L. W.: *In* Dunphy, J. E., and Way, L. W. (eds.): *Current Surgical Diagnosis*

and Treatment, 3rd ed. Lange Medical Publications, Los Altos, CA, 1977, p. 160.
28. Snow, P. J. D.: Treatment of acute myocardial injection with propanolol. Am. J. Cardiol. 18:458, 1966.
29. Sokolow, M.: *In* Dunphy, J. E., and Way, L. W. (eds.): *Current Surgical Diagnosis and Treatment*, 3rd ed. Lange Medical Publications, Los Altos, CA, 1977, p. 50.
30. Tisi, G. M.: State of the art preoperative evaluation of pulmonary function. Am. Rev. Resp. Dis. 119:293, 1979.
31. Tsuji, H., Asoh, T., Shirasaica, C., et al.: Inhibition of metabolic response to surgery with beta adrenergic blockage. Br. J. Surg. 67:503, 1980.
32. Wilson, J. L.: Respiratory disease in the surgical patient. *In* Dunphy, J. E., and Way, L. W. (eds.): *Current Surgical Diagnosis and Treatment*, 3rd ed. Lange Medical Publications, Los Altos, CA, 1977, p. 54.

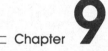

Chapter **9**

Fluid Therapy in the Surgical Patient

Marc R. Raffe

Parenteral fluid administration has been used for decades in small animal practice. However, in many cases fluid is administered empirically. Balanced polyionic solutions are administered to maintain physiological support during the operative period. The administration of solutions similar in composition to extracellular fluid is generally prudent. However, in surgical candidates with specific requirements or pre-existing electrolyte imbalance, fluid administration assumes increased importance. Fluid therapy should be formulated and administered on a therapeutic rather than an empirical basis. This chapter reviews the principles of fluid therapy and electrolyte balance, provides a review for rational, therapeutic decisions relevant to fluid administration, and establishes guidelines for the selection of appropriate fluid and electrolyte therapy in the surgical patient.

NORMAL BODY FLUID BALANCE

Intravascular compartment measurements are used as an indication of the dimensions of the extracellular and intracellular spaces. The validity of this concept is based on the relationship between total body water and various subcompartments: the two major subcompartments—intracellular (ICF) and extracellular (ECF)—and the subdivisions of the latter, the intravascular and interstitial compartments. Approximately 60 to 70 per cent of the functional adult mammalian mass is water. The distribution of total body water varies among species, from an ICF:ECF ratio of 1 in the horse to 2:1 in small animals and humans. Therefore, the ECF represents only a frac-

tion of total body water, and the vascular compartment is approximately one-fourth of this value.[13, 24]

Water equilibrium between intravascular and extracellular spaces is maintained by oncotic pressure of plasma protein, lipids, and erythrocytes. Distribution of body water depends on the osmolality of a fluid compartment. Protein segregated in the plasma compartment exerts an oncotic pressure that attracts free water from surrounding tissue spaces. This activity is opposed by intravascular hydrostatic pressure generated by the heart. These two forces balance under normal conditions in accordance with Starling's law of the capillary to distribute free water between the intravascular and interstitial spaces. Several homeostatic mechanisms maintain appropriate balance between the size of the intravascular space and the intravascular volume. Lymph mobilization and hepatic protein release may increase intravascular protein concentration, allowing for free water transfer into the intravascular space. Vasoconstriction of the capacitance vessels diminishes the intravascular volume required for maintenance. Hypothalamic release of antidiuretic hormone and aldosterone also contributes to stabilization of vascular water volume. Distribution of water in the intracellular compartment is governed by factors similar to those found in the extracellular compartment. If interstitial and intracellular pressure become imbalanced, free water transfer occurs in the direction of higher oncotic pressure.[5, 13, 19, 24]

Extracellular and intracellular compartments have approximately equal tissue pressure; however, the constituents of these compartments are markedly different. Each tissue compartment has electrolytes that contribute to the total osmotic pressure of the fluid space. The cell membrane separating fluid spaces is semipermeable and partitions ions between compartments. This partition establishes intercompartmental pressure gradients. The composition of electrolytes in the intracellular and extracellular compartments differs. This has important implications for diagnosis and therapy of specific electrolyte deficiencies, because measurement of extracellular electrolyte levels may not accurately reflect intracellular composition. The predominant extracellular electrolytes are sodium and chloride, whereas potassium, magnesium, and phosphates are the dominant intracellular ions. The partition across cell membrane surfaces is maintained by active energy-consuming pump mechanisms that maintain the segregation of electrolytes. This stabilizes osmotic pressure between the intracellular and interstitial compartments.[19]

Regulation of extracellular water balance and osmotic pressure is controlled by the kidney and may be influenced by a neuroendocrine response. Renal water balance is controlled by antidiuretic hormone (ADH). Appropriate stimulation triggers the release of ADH from the neurohypophyseal region. ADH is carried by the vasculature to the distal nephrotubules and interacts to increase the size of aqueous channels in this area, promoting enhanced water resorption. Numerous factors, both osmotic and nonosmotic, may initiate ADH release. An increase in plasma osmolarity as small as 2 per cent can initiate ADH release. Decreased cardiac output and increased baroreceptor response, diminished circulating blood volume, emotional stress, hyperthermia, pharmacological agents including anesthetic drugs, and mechanical ventilatory support may increase ADH release. Pharmacological agents that suppress ADH activity include alcohol, phenytoin, epinephrine, and atropine.[20]

Sodium, the principal extracellular ion, contributes to tonicity and has specific regulatory mechanisms to maintain extracellular levels. The juxtaglomerular apparatus of the kidney is sensitive to changes in extracellular fluid volume. A decreased ECF volume stimulates the renin-angiotensin response, which in turn initiates aldosterone release. Alteration in extracellular fluid volume may also initiate sodium conservation mediated by direct sympathetic influence on renal tubules to modulate sodium excretion. Sodium conservation is associated with water balance modulated by ADH release. Increased extracellular volume prompts an increased glomerular filtration rate. Sodium excretion concurrently increases because of an increased filtered sodium load; however, the primary mechanism for fine regulation of sodium balance involves glomerulotubular balance. Redistribution of intrarenal blood flow between cortical and juxtamedullary nephrons may also influence fine control of sodium excretion. Peritubular hydrostatic and oncotic pressure also interact in sodium balance. The composition of extracellular and intracellular fluid, as well as tonicity, is listed in Table 9–1.[7, 36, 42]

Potassium regulation is also a function of the renal

TABLE 9–1. Osmolar Substances in ECF and ICF*†

Component	Plasma	Interstitium	Intracellular Fluid
Na$^+$	144.0	133.0	10.0
K$^+$	5.0	4.7	141.0
Ca^{++}	2.5	2.4	0
Mg^{++}	1.5	1.4	31.0
Cl$^-$	107.0	113.0	4.0
HCO$_3$$^-$	27.0	28.3	10.0
HPO$_4$$^{--}$, H$_2PO_4$$^-$	2.0	2.0	11.0
SO$_4$$^{--}$	0.5	0.5	1.0
Glucose	5.6	5.6	—
Protein	1.2	0.2	4.0
Urea	4.0	4.0	4.0
Other	3.4	3.4	84.2
Total mOsm	303.7	302.2	302.2
Corrected osmolar activity (mOsm)	282.6	281.3	281.3
Total osmotic pressure (37°C)	5454.0	5430.0	5430.0

*in mOsm/L H$_2$O.
†Adapted from Guyton, A. C.: *Textbook of Medical Physiology,* 4th ed. W. B. Saunders, Philadelphia, 1971.

tubules. Most filtered potassium is actively resorbed in the proximal tubule. In the distal tubule, passive secretion of potassium in exchange for sodium maintains transcellular electroneutrality. Alkalosis and increased concentrations of sodium and potassium facilitate potassium secretion. An obligatory renal potassium loss of 20 milliequivalents (mEq) per day has been documented in man.[34]

On a daily basis, water and electrolyte balance is maintained through the regulation of gain and loss. Water is gained in healthy animals by the ingestion of free water or water in foodstuffs, and the synthesis of water as a byproduct of metabolism. Routes of water loss are varied and include sensible (quantitative) and insensible (qualitative) components. Routes of sensible loss are renal and gastrointestinal; pulmonary and cutaneous routes constitute insensible loss. Electrolyte supplementation is provided by oral foodstuffs containing electrolytes. The gastrointestinal tract and kidney regulate absorption and conservation of electrolytes. Cutaneous electrolyte loss is minimal in small domestic animals owing to the poor development of eccrine sweat glands. Significant pulmonary electrolyte loss has not been documented.[14, 30]

DIAGNOSIS OF FLUID AND ELECTROLYTE ABNORMALITIES

Quantitative and qualitative assessments aid in the clinical determination of fluid balance in the surgical patient. History prior to surgery may provide qualitative indications of alterations in water balance. Observation of diarrhea, emesis, fistulous drainage, cutaneous denudation, polyuria, and overt hemorrhage may provide an estimation of water and electrolyte balance. Clinical evaluation of the patient provides an assessment of dehydration. At approximately 5 per cent dehydration, increased skin turgor with doughy, inelastic consistency is noted. Dry, tacky, oral mucous membranes may also be seen. With 7 per cent dehydration, definite changes in skin consistency are noted. Ten to twelve per cent dehydration may be assessed by the presence of the previously mentioned signs and the presence of hypovolemic shock in debilitated animals. Involuntary muscular clonus may also be present. Twelve to fifteen per cent dehydration is accompanied by severe shock and death. Sequential monitoring of total body weight may aid in evaluating total body water. If caloric intake is adequate, alteration in body weight reflects total water balance. With inadequate caloric intake, a weight loss of 0.1 to 0.3 kg/day/1000 calories can be attributed to tissue catabolism. Weight loss in excess of calculated values can be attributed to water loss. Estimation of peripheral pulse quality may provide valuable information in conjunction with clinical evaluation to aid in estimation of vascular volume. Blood pressure measurements may provide information regarding vascular status. Evaluation of fluid balance during therapy may be provided by measurement of water balance. Records of fluid volume administered and sensible loss measurements may provide valuable data regarding initial patient status.[14]

Clinicopathological data may also quantitate fluid balance. Packed red blood cell volume (PCV) using the microhematocrit technique is useful in estimating intravascular fluid balance. The noncellular fraction of the sample may be measured by an optical refractometer to determine the concentration of total plasma solids (TS). Simultaneous assessment is needed to interpret these values. Since the values for PCV and TS depend on the ratio of erythrocytes and protein to free water, the values may reflect variations in either component. Deviations from normal for either value should cause the surgeon to investigate the etiology of the imbalance. If both values are abnormally elevated, hemoconcentration should be included in a differential diagnosis. Conversely, diminution of both values during fluid administration may indicate overhydration. Baseline values prior to fluid administration should be obtained, as all patients may not have normal values prior to surgery. Absolute percentage dehydration cannot be calculated from these values, as all fluid compartments may not be equilibrated. Values can be used to confirm or adjust clinical impressions of dehydration as well as for monitoring hydration status during fluid administration.[14]

Definitive assessment of vascular water status may be obtained by measurement of osmolality. Freezing point depression techniques may be used to quantitate plasma osmolality. This information may be useful, along with clinical assessment, PCV, and TS, in making an overall patient evaluation. Osmolality may also be estimated by knowing serum sodium, glucose, and BUN values. These may be applied to the formula

$$mOsm/kg = 1.86\,Na + \frac{Glucose}{18} + \frac{BUN}{28}$$

to calculate serum osmolality. An elevated value may be correlated with a number of clinical syndromes; water loss is indicated by elevated levels.[14, 18]

Alterations in water balance may be accompanied by changes in electrolyte levels. Altered sodium, potassium, chloride, and phosphorus levels can be appreciated on biochemical analysis and may be clinically evident in some cases. In the surgical patient, sodium balance may be altered by administration of large volumes of sodium free or hypoosmotic fluids, pain, anesthetic agents, and positive pressure ventilation. If functional sodium loss occurs, redistribution of free water occurs owing to osmolality gradients. In man, serum sodium levels of less than 125 mEq/L may be accompanied by clinical signs of altered mental status, muscle clonus, hyperreflexia, and hypotension from intercompartmental water shifts. Tachycardia, weak pulse pressure, and decreased skin compliance as assessed by the skin fold test may also be apparent. In acute cases, circulatory shock may be a complicating factor. Serum sodium levels of less than 120 mEq/L have resulted in convulsions, stupor, coma, and death in man. Laboratory data used to confirm clinical impressions includes PCV and TS to measure hemoconcentration, serum sodium levels, and plasma osmolality. Hyponatremia may also be noted when ADH is inappropriately released during free water administration. This complication may be noted in the surgical patient in which ADH release from pain and anesthetic drugs is seen in conjunction with free water administration from sodium free fluid sources. Diuretics and chemotherapeutic agents may also augment vasopressin release by direct or indirect pathways.[12, 18, 36, 40, 42]

Hypernatremia is a less frequent, but potentially life-threatening, complication of excess free water loss. Hypernatremia may be noted in diabetes insipidus, high output renal failure, the diuretic phase of oliguric renal failure, and any condition resulting in increased evaporative water loss. Clinical signs include alteration of mental status and reflexes, hypotension, and dry oral membranes. Diagnosis is confirmed by the clinicopathological tests previously described.

Disturbances in potassium balance are more common in surgical patients than sodium imbalances. Hypokalemia (< 3.5 mEq/L) can result from a variety of pre-existing medical or surgical conditions represented by alterations in acid-base status, emesis, diarrhea, gastrointestinal volvulus, renal disease, administration of diuretics or insulin, and the presence of potassium free replacement fluids. Potassium is the predominant intracellular electrolyte; diminished serum levels may reflect either redistribution to the ICF or total body depletion of the ion. Complications related to hypokalemia may be metabolic, neuromuscular, renal, or cardiovascular. Insulin release from pancreatic beta cells may be impaired with hypokalemia, resulting in glucose intolerance. Skeletal muscle weakness, paralytic ileus, gastric atony, and altered response to pharmacological agents affecting neuromuscular function may be clinically apparent. Decreased urine concentrating capacity and ADH resistance may be present and clinically noted as polyuria, polydipsia, and nocturia. Cardiovascular changes reflect altered electrical conduction of excitable membranes. The changes noted on electrocardiography (ECG) reflect alterations in repolarization and re-establishment of transmembrane potential. Reported ECG alterations of hypokalemia include S-T segment depression, changes in T wave configuration, presence of a U wave, and prolongation of the QT interval. These findings are less consistent in small animals than in other species. In man, changes in P wave amplitude are noted. A variety of atrial, atrioventricular, nodal, and ventricular arrhythmias have been documented. Potentiation of digitalis-class agents may produce signs of drug intoxication. Diagnosis is confirmed by determination of serum potassium levels.[2, 34, 42]

Hyperkalemia (> 5.5 mEq/L) is a potentially life-threatening electrolyte disturbance. Acute renal failure, urinary tract obstruction, adrenocortical insufficiency, respiratory or metabolic acidosis, musculoskeletal injury, excessive potassium administration, and administration of potassium-sparing diuretics and banked blood have all been associated with hyperkalemia. Alteration in transmembrane resting potential of excitable tissue causes muscle weakness and disturbance in propagation of cardiac action potential. Potentiation of the physiological effects of hyperkalemia may occur in the presence of hyponatremia, hypocalcemia, or acidosis or during the administration of succinylcholine. Alterations in myocardial excitation and conduction velocity may contribute to the development of arrhythmias in these patients. Changes in T wave configuration, P wave flattening and disappearance, PR interval prolongation, QRS complex widening, irregular RR intervals, atrioventricular block, and electrical arrest have been described in conjunction with hyperkalemia. The serum potassium levels attendant with these changes vary with the underlying etiology and the presence of the interactive factors previously listed. In general, a progression of ECG-related changes occurs with increased serum potassium levels. T wave amplitude and base width changes and loss of P waves are noted at a potassium level of approximately 6 mEq/L. Levels in excess of 8 mEq/L may be accompanied by widened QRS complexes; bradycardia related to con-

duction delays in atrioventricular node, His-Purkinje system, and ventricular myocardium; idioventricular rhythm; and escape beats. Serum levels in excess of 10 mEq/L are manifested by idioventricular rhythm and ventricular fibrillation or arrest. Diagnosis is confirmed by evaluation of serum potassium levels.[2, 34]

Alterations in calcium and phosphorus levels are not frequently noted in the surgical patient. The majority of patients with abnormal serum levels of one of these electrolytes do not exhibit simultaneous alteration in the corollary value, although both should be quantitated owing to interrelated regulation and control. Hypercalcemia can be found in a variety of conditions including normal growth, neoplasia, hypoadrenocorticism, renal failure, hyperparathyroidism, hypervitaminosis D, and bone lesions. Many of these conditions are potentially reversible or ameliorated by surgery, and therefore the surgeon should be aware of the potential for hypercalcemia in the preoperative period. Clinical signs of hypercalcemia may include renal, gastrointestinal, nervous, and cardiovascular system involvement as well as secondary signs from coexisting electrolyte disturbance or acid-base alteration. Emesis, anorexia, stupor, myoclonus, polyuria, polydipsia, and azotemia have been reported. Electrocardiographic alterations include PR interval prolongation and shortening of the QT interval. Ventricular fibrillation can occur in severe cases. Hypocalcemia can be associated with a variety of medical or surgical diseases. Gastrointestinal or renal disease, pancreatitis, hypoalbuminemia, hypoparathyroidism, intoxication, postparturient eclampsia, and iatrogenic causes (blood transfusion, phosphate enemas, EDTA administration) may be contributory. Clinical signs of increased neuromuscular excitability (tremor, twitching, cramps, muscle spasms), seizures, hyperthermia, and altered QT interval on electrocardiography may be noted. Acid-base alterations may shift ionized calcium levels to protein-bound fractions; therefore, total serum calcium values may remain within normal limits with altered active fraction levels until acid-base values are corrected.[2, 6]

Alterations in phosphorus levels are not common. Hyperphosphatemia is most frequently noted as a component of renal or gastrointestinal disease. Orthopedic injury, trauma, peritonitis, inflammation, and iatrogenic causes may also be correlated with increased phosphorus levels. Transient elevations of phosphate produce no signs or require therapy other than correction of the primary disorder. Chronic elevation may risk soft tissue mineralization or contribute to hypocalcemia. Hypophosphatemia may be noted in patients experiencing neoplasia, orthopedic surgery, or trauma. Usually, clinical signs are vague or absent and do not appear until serum levels reach less than 1.0 mg/dl. Neuromuscular weakness, alteration in 2,3 diphosphoglycerate function, and leukocyte impairment have been described with chronic phosphorus deficiency.[6]

THERAPY OF FLUID IMBALANCE

The quantity and composition of fluids administered should be determined prior to surgical intervention. Patient evaluation, clinicopathological data, pharmacological agents administered, the proposed surgical technique, and attendant complications must be considered when selecting an appropriate fluid for administration. Quantitation of fluid requirements has been calculated based on (1) recognition of preoperative deficits of water and electrolytes; (2) maintenance water and electrolyte requirements during the period; and (3) estimation of losses during the operative and postoperative periods. Caloric requirements should also be considered and energy substrates provided as a component of the fluid therapy. However, complete nutritional requirements are not met by this approach.[18, 31]

Patients at risk for significant deficits in water and electrolytes include those with gastrointestinal disease, peritonitis, renal failure, thermal injury, pyrexia, diuretic therapy, hemorrhage, deprivation of water and foodstuffs, and radiographic contrast media administration. The degree of deficit is evaluated using criteria previously described. Stabilization of the cardiovascular system is essential prior to induction of anesthesia, because further decompensation may result from administration of many anesthetic drugs.[42] Acute resuscitation in the immediate preoperative period is beneficial; however, equilibration across fluid compartments may not occur. Ideally, replacement therapy over a longer period (24 to 48 hours) allows for intercompartmental equilibration of both free water and electrolyte components and minimizes complications during the operative period. Caution should be exercised in animals with chronic water and electrolyte deficits (depletion syndrome), because re-establishing water and salt balance may require more time. Significant disturbances of amino acids, glycogen, fats, and caloric reserves as well as deficits in total body water, electrolytes, and serum proteins make these individuals poor candidates for anesthesia and surgery. These cases are stable until acutely decompensated during exposure to anesthesia and surgery. Poor response to resuscitative measures usually occurs.[13]

Deficit replacement and maintenance fluids can be administered by several routes. Preoperatively, oral administration is preferred unless underlying disease precludes this route. Physiological absorption of water and electrolytes occurs and allows for autoregulation relative to requirements. If an oral route cannot be used, parenteral administration of fluids and electrolytes must be considered. Routes of parenteral fluid administration include intravenous, subcutaneous, and intraperitoneal. Intravenous administration is the most direct route, and its advantages include (1) direct introduction into the intravascular space; (2) fluids with tonicity other than isotonic may be administered; (3) fluids with alkaline or acid pH may be administered without tissue injury; (4) col-

loids and blood may be directly replaced; and (5) supplemental drugs may be rapidly introduced. Disadvantages of intravenous infusion include (1) thrombophlebitis and endocarditis; (2) perivascular "leakage" of administration fluid; (3) pyrogenic reactions; (4) air embolism; (5) hemorrhage; (6) volume overload; and (7) reactions to excessive administration rate. Despite the potential drawbacks, venous cannulation is a relatively safe therapeutic procedure if precautions related to aseptic technique and catheter placement are followed.[8, 35]

Subcutaneous fluid administration may be used for preoperative rehydration of active or uncooperative patients. Advantages of this technique include (1) ease of administration; (2) longer period of fluid uptake; and (3) circumvention of drawbacks of intravenous infusion. Disadvantages of the technique include (1) discomfort from large volumes or irritating fluids; (2) gravitation of fluid to ventral sites; (3) dermal necrosis; and (4) limitations in tonicity of solutions administered by this route.[8]

Intraperitoneal fluid administration can be used in chronic stabilization. A needle is introduced into the abdomen midway between the umbilicus and pubis, and the calculated volume of fluid is administered until abdominal distension is apparent. Advantages include (1) ease of administration; (2) large reservoir for fluid introduction; and (3) slower absorption than direct intravascular access. Disadvantages include (1) uncontrolled fluid uptake; (2) potential for peritoneal sepsis; (3) chemical peritonitis from alkaline, acidic, or other irritant fluid components; (4) emesis or shock from cold solutions; and (5) interference with surgical procedures. This route is probably the least controlled and should be reserved for cases in which other routes cannot be used.[23]

Estimation of water deficit is based on clinical evaluation of dehydration and clinicopathological data. Microhematocrit (PCV) values may be used to estimate water loss by the following formula

$$\text{Plasma deficit} = \text{Normal blood volume} - \frac{\text{Normal blood volume} \times \text{Normal PCV}}{\text{Measured PCV}}$$

Crystalloid solutions should be administered for replacement therapy so that 75 per cent of the total estimated correction occurs in the first 24 hours, with complete correction by 48 hours after initiation of therapy.[18]

Therapy should be monitored to evaluate cardiovascular response, minimize hemodilution, and prevent significant alterations in plasma oncotic pressure. In the patient with severe dehydration, depletion syndrome, or "third space" sequestration of fluid, monitoring of changes in central venous pressure is an indirect method of measuring left atrial pressure and preload volume. Patients with impairment of myocardial function or severe pulmonary disease benefit from pulmonary artery pressure measurement if rapid volume replacement is indicated.

Assessment of blood pressure and pulse quality may provide information regarding the patient's response to therapy by evaluating changes in intravascular volume. Monitoring total solids with packed cell volume alerts the clinician to significant hemodilution or diminished plasma protein concentration. Administration of colloids such as separated plasma or albumin may be indicated if total solid and albumin levels fall below 4.0 and 1.5 gm/dl, respectively.[18, 42]

Electrolyte deficits may be corrected by administration of polyionic fluids with supplemental electrolyte salts as necessary. Fluid composition should be checked prior to administration to determine if adequate replacement salts are incorporated. Most commercial preparations of polyionic fluids are deficient in potassium, calcium, and magnesium salts. Buffer base precursors may also be incorporated. Therapy of specific electrolyte deficits is described elsewhere.[6, 11, 18, 34, 36]

After correction and stabilization of preoperative fluid deficits, maintenance and contemporary fluid requirements should be determined for the operative period. Maintenance fluid requirements should include both sensible and insensible water requirements. Maintenance fluid requirements must take into account normal water requirements during the anticipated operative period, evaporative water loss from respiratory tract and surgical site, vascular effects of anesthetic agents, and sequestration of interstitial fluids from surgical trauma. Fever, trauma, infection, and immobilization may increase endogenous water production as a consequence of increased fat oxidation and body mass catabolism. Careful evaluation of hydration status and operative fluid restriction may be indicated in affected patients.[28, 31]

Unless specific conditions dictate alternate fluid regimens, polyionic isotonic maintenance fluids are used in most surgical patients. A polyionic fluid retards the formation of excess free water that occurs with dextrose base fluids or hypotonic preparations. Initiation of fluid therapy in the preoperative period decreases alterations in water balance from preoperative fasting. Inhibition of antidiuretic hormone levels and induction of mild diuresis counterbalances anesthetic drug-related oliguria and maintains urinary output during the operative period. Most references suggest an infusion rate of 10 ml/kg/hr for maintenance requirements. Hemodynamic alterations occur during the surgical period, and long-term procedures may benefit from tapered administration.[15, 16, 29, 30, 33, 38, 41]

Losses during the operative period should be replaced with a similar fluid. Tissue desiccation, evaporative losses from pulmonary tissue and surgical site, redistribution of extracellular fluid from surgical injury (third space loss), and continuing fluid deficits from the preoperative period are iso-osmotic and can be replaced by iso-osmotic solutions. Losses due to protein-rich exudation should be replenished with albumin or plasma substitutes to maintain oncotic

pressure. Blood loss during the operative period may be replaced with crystalloid solutions as long as significant diminution in packed cell volume or plasma proteins does not occur. If packed cell volume decreases to values less than 25 per cent and plasma proteins are less than 4.0 gm/dl, whole blood transfusion is indicated to restore red cell mass and protein content. In man, insensible water loss is calculated at 1.5 ml/kg/hr during the operative period. This factor may also be used to estimate normal water deficits expected during the preoperative fast period. Isotonic solutions are recommended for replacement therapy except under patient conditions described previously.[17, 37, 42]

Therapy in the postoperative period should be considered for patients who cannot tolerate oral fluid administration within 12 hours postoperatively. Metabolic response to surgical trauma includes increased plasma levels of cortisol, catecholamines, glucagon, aldosterone, and antidiuretic hormone. The net effects of alterations in these hormones include increased metabolizable energy requirements (discussed in Chapter 17) and oliguria with sodium retention. This "injury" phase may persist as long as 48 to 72 hours postoperatively and may predispose the surgical patient to further renal and metabolic impairment. Attenuation of the antidiuresis can be achieved by replacement fluid therapy during surgery and continuing into the early postoperative phase. Fluid composition for support during this period is controversial; however, balanced polyionic solutions containing sodium enhance free water clearance and urine output better than free water infusion as a 5% dextrose solution. Water and sodium retention does not occur to significant degrees when polyionic fluids are administered in the postoperative period.[5, 21, 23]

Postoperative disorders related to fluid therapy include volume, electrolyte, and acid-base alterations. Overhydration may occur if aggressive infusion of isotonic solutions has occurred. Retention of free water from elevated levels of antidiuretic hormone may result in decreased serum osmolality, hypertonic urine with increased sodium levels, dehydration, and hypotension. This syndrome is common in elderly patients during the postoperative period owing to decreased tolerance of vascular overexpansion. Predisposing factors include preoperative desiccation, narcotic and barbiturate premedication, apprehension, surgical stimulation, hemorrhage, positive pressure ventilation, and general anesthetic administration. All factors contribute to sustained ADH release in the postoperative period. Water restriction is used until extracellular balance is re-established. Clinical signs of overhydration include weight gain, edema, elevated central venous pressure, increased pulse pressure, moist rales, dyspnea, and cyanosis. Restriction of fluid intake or use of loop diuretics, such as furosemide or ethacrynic acid, is adequate unless respiratory signs occur. Supplemental oxygenation may be required in such cases.[12, 22, 40, 42]

Continued losses from the gastrointestinal tract, surgical site, or traumatized tissue or due to renal disease should be replaced to avoid volume deficit in the postoperative period. Redistribution of extracellular water to other compartments occurs in volume depletion, resulting in decreased ECF. Signs of volume deficit include weight loss, tachycardia, hypotension, and oliguria. Packed cell volume, total solids, azotemia of prerenal origin, and concentrated urine levels may be elevated. Replacement therapy is with fluid of appropriate composition. Balanced salt solutions are satisfactory in the majority of cases; losses of enteral origin may be replaced with normal saline and potassium supplementation as necessary. Response to therapy may be assessed by the previously mentioned parameters and re-establishment of adequate urine output.[42]

Disorders related to sodium, potassium, and acid-base balance may also be noted in the postoperative period. Previous discussions of sodium and potassium imbalance apply during this phase. Therapy of acid-base imbalance is discussed elsewhere in this text.

COMMERCIALLY AVAILABLE SOLUTIONS FOR FLUID THERAPY

Selection of appropriate fluid should be based on the criteria established in the previous discussion. In most cases, a commercially available solution is appropriate. In certain cases, a base fluid is selected and specific electrolyte or component supplementation is added. Specific additive incompatibilities should be noted in preparation of these solutions. Available fluids can be classified as follows.[1, 18, 27]

Carbohydrate Solutions

Dextrose is available in 2, 5, 10, 20, 25, and 50% solutions, and fructose is available in 5 and 10% solutions. These solutions are beneficial for (1) supplying free water, (2) providing calories, and (3) inhibiting glycogen depletion and protein catabolism. Pure water is supplied as an isotonic solution in 5% dextrose. Free water remains after metabolism of the carbohydrate substrate. When free water supplementation is appropriate, this solution is preferred. Oxidation of the carbohydrate contributes to caloric requirements. A gram of dextrose provides 4.1 calories. Hypertonic solutions or large volume infusion is required for significant calorie contribution. However, administration of carbohydrates reduces use of alternate energy substrates such as glycogen and protein and prevents endogenous catabolism. Fructose has several theoretical advantages: (1) its metabolism is independent of insulin levels, and (2) a higher concentration may be administered without glucosuria induction. However, glucose still maintains popularity as the primary carbohydrate source.[29]

Sodium Chloride Solutions

Solutions are available in various concentrations and may be combined with other solution classes. Examples of available solutions include the following:

1. 5% sodium chloride
2. 3% sodium coloride
3. 0.9% sodium chloride: plain
   with 2.5, 5, or 10% dextrose
   with 10% fructose
4. 0.45% sodium chloride: plain
   with 2.5, 5, or 10% dextrose
5. 0.33% sodium chloride   with 5% dextrose
6. 0.3% sodium chloride   with 3.3 or 5% dextrose
7. 0.225% sodium chloride   with 5% dextrose
8. 0.2% sodium chloride   with 5% dextrose

Physiological saline (0.9%) has excess chloride concentration relative to blood values; a severe hyperchloremic metabolic acidosis can occur if administered aggressively in patients with poor renal function. However, it is an isotonic solution and does not cause intravascular hemolysis when infused alone or in combination with dextrose, fructose, electrolytes, and dextrans. Indications for saline administration are those syndromes involving sodium loss, such as diabetic ketoacidosis, gastrointestinal disease, adrenocortical insufficiency, and burns. Saline alone at 0.45 or 0.9% may be given intravenously. Hypertonic solutions are indicated in syndromes associated with severe sodium loss or primary water excess. Pulmonary edema may occur with rapid administration of hypertonic saline solutions.

Multiple Electrolyte Solutions

A variety of maintenance and replacement solutions are commercially available with and without carbohydrates (Table 9–2). Two types of solutions are available: maintenance solutions, which are hypotonic in composition, and replacement solutions of isotonic composition. The development of multiple electrolyte solutions was originally based on the premise of eliminating unnecessary constitutents by renal mechanisms. This premise has been successfully used in patients with (1) water and electrolyte maintenance requirements met by parenteral routes; (2) replacement for fluid lost by emesis, diarrhea, or fistulae; (3) moderate sodium or potassium loss; and (4) metabolic alkalosis or acidosis. Balanced solutions may not be appropriate in patients with (1) severe hyponatremia; (2) significant thermal injury; (3) adrenocortical insufficiency; (4) diabetes insipidus; (5) water intoxication; (6) renal disease; (7) hypoparathyroidism; and (8) hypocalcemia. Regulatory mechanisms may be altered during the operative period, altering nor-

Text continued on page 100

TABLE 9–2. Commercially Available Multiple Electrolyte Solutions

Solution	Tonicity*	Manufacturer	Carbohydrate	Na^+	K^+	Ca^{+2}	Mg^{+2}	Cl^-	HCO_3^-	HPO_4^{--}
Ionosol MB	H	Abbott	5% dextrose	25	20	5	3	22	23 (as lactate)	3
Isolyte R	H	McGaw	5% dextrose	40	16	5	3	40	24 (acetate)	—
Normosol M	H	Abbott	plain 5% dextrose	40	13	—	3	40	16 (acetate)	—
Polysal M	H	Cutter	2.5, 5, 10% dextrose	40	16	5	3	40	24 (lactate 12) (acetate 12)	—
Plasmalyte 56	H	Travenol	plain 5% dextrose	40	13	—	3	140	16 (acetate)	—
Ringer's	I	several	plain 2.5, 5% dextrose	147	4	5	—	156	—	—
Lactated Ringer's	I	several	plain 2.5, 5% dextrose	130	4	3	—	109	28 (as lactate)	—
Hartmann's	I	several	plain 5% dextrose	131	4	4	—	111	27 (as lactate or acetate)	—
Normosol R	I	Abbott	plain 5% dextrose	140	5	—	3	98	50 (acetate 27) (gluconate 23)	—
Plasmalyte 148	I	Travenol	plain 5% dextrose 10% invert sugar	140	10	5	3	103	55 (acetate 47) (lactate 8)	—
Polysal	I	Cutter	plain 5% dextrose	140	10	5	3	103	55 (acetate 47) (lactate 8)	—
Isolyte E	I	McGaw	plain 5% dextrose	140	10	5	3	103	55 (acetate 47) (acetate 8)	—

*H = hypotonic, I = isotonic.

TABLE 9–3. Physical Compatibility of Parenteral Admixtures*

Agent	5% Dextrose in Lactated Ringer's Solution	5% Dextrose in Water	Ionosol MB with 5% Dextrose	Lactated Ringer's Solution	Normosol-R	Normosol-R in D5W	Ringer's Solution	0.9% Sodium Chloride	Dextrose 2.5% in Half-Strength Ringer's Solution
Antimicrobial Agents									
Ampicillin	—	C	—	—	—	—	—	—	—
Chloramphenicol	C	C	C	C	C	C	C	C	C
Penicillin Na/K 1,000,000 U	C	C	C	C	C	C	C	C	C
Oxytetracycline	C	C	—	—	—	—	—	—	—
Tetracycline	C	C	Z	C	Z	C	C	C	C
Anesthetic Agents									
Diazepam	—	—	—	I	—	—	—	—	—
Doxopram	—	—	—	—	—	—	—	—	—
Edrophonium	—	—	—	—	—	—	—	—	—
Fentanyl (Innovar)	—	C	—	—	—	—	—	—	—
Meperidine (100 mg)	C	C	C	C	C	C	C	C	C
Morphine (16.2 mg)	C	C	C	C	C	C	C	C	C
Oxymorphone	—	—	—	—	—	—	—	—	—
Pentobarbital sodium	C	C	C	C	C	C	C	C	C
Phenobarbital	C	C	C	C	C	C	C	C	C
Phenothiazines	C	C	C	C	C	C	C	C	C
Procaine	C	C	C	C	C	C	C	C	C
Thiopental	I	C	I	I	I	I	I	C	I
Intravenous Solutions and Ions									
Calcium chloride/ glucoheptonate	C	C	C	C	C	C	C	C	C
Insulin	—	C	—	C	C	C	C	C	—

Mannitol			C	C	C			
Potassium chloride	C	C	C	C	C	C	C
Sodium bicarbonate	X	C	C	C	C	X	X
Cardiovascular Drugs							
Ammophylline	C	C	C	C	C	C	C
Antihistamines	C	C	C	C	C	C	C
Digitalis class	I	I	—	—	I	I	I
Dopamine/dobutamine			I	I	I			
Dexamethasone	C	C	C	C	C	C	C
Epinephrine	C	C	C	C	C	C	Z
Ephedrine (50 mg)	C	C	C	C	C	C	C
Hydrocortisone sodium succinate	C	C	C	C	C	C	C
Isoproterenol			C	C	C		C
Lidocaine (2 gm)	C	C	C	C	C	C	C
Phenylephrine (10 mg)	C	C	C	C	C	C	C
Procainamide								

*Adapted from Abbott Laboratories: *Physical Compatibility of Parenteral Admixtures.* Abbott Laboratories, North Chicago, 1973; and McGrath, C. J., and McGrath, D. H.: Pharmacology. *In* Sattler, F. P., Knowles, R. P., and Whittick, W. G. (eds.): *Veterinary Critical Care.* Lea & Febiger, Philadelphia, 1981.

Notes: C = compatible. No haze or precipitation within 24 hours.
I = incompatible. Haze or precipitation in one hour or less.
X = haze or precipitation in less than six hours but more than 1 hour.
Z = color change.
— = data are currently unavailable.

mal conservation and excretion of water and electrolytes. Balanced solutions should be administered intravenously, although subcutaneous administration may also be used.

Acidifying Solutions

Ammonium chloride may be considered for metabolic alkalosis. Ammonium chloride undergoes hepatic metabolism to urea and chloride. The chloride combines with hydrogen in the ECF, forming hydrochloric acid. Animals with hepatic disease, hyperammonemia, or azotemia should not be treated by this approach. Ammonium chloride is available as an isotonic (0.9%) or hypertonic (2.14%) solution. It may be administered by oral or intravenous routes. Replacement therapy calculation is based on restoration of serum chloride levels to normal. Calculation of ECF chloride deficit and knowledge of chloride concentration in the solution allow calculation of the dose required.

Alkalinizing Solutions

Commercially available alkalinizing solutions include sodium bicarbonate, sodium lactate, sodium acetate, and THAM (tromethamine). Sodium bicarbonate is most commonly used. Commercially available sodium bicarbonate is hypertonic and should be diluted to a 1.5% solution prior to administration. If alkalinization is required urgently or the patient is hyponatremic with metabolic acidosis (renal failure), hypertonic solutions may be used. Lactate requires hepatic metabolism to glycogen, allowing Na^+ to combine with carbonic acid to form sodium bicarbonate. THAM can also promote osmotic diuresis during renal excretion, increasing glomerular filtration and excretion of fixed acids and electrolytes.

Electrolyte Supplement

The availability of potassium and calcium salts for replacement therapy allows for correction of deficits encountered in the surgical patient. Generally, these preparations are available as potassium chloride and calcium chloride or calcium gluconate. These salts are added to intravenous solutions to supplement levels present in the base solution. Mixture incompatibilities of calcium and phosphorus should be recognized during preparation.

COMPLICATIONS OF FLUID THERAPY

Despite widespread use of fluid therapy, complications can occur and must be anticipated. Some complications are minimal in their influence, whereas others may be life-threatening. General complications involving venous cannulation and routes of administration are described earlier in this chapter and in Chapter 17. The reader is referred to these sections for further discussion.[26] Complications pertinent to fluid selection and administration include the following.

Volume Overload

Acute overhydration may be encountered with aggressive fluid therapy. Small animals may have a greater predisposition because the margin of error in fluid administration is less. Studies in normal dogs and cats suggest that administration rates of 90 ml/kg/hr may be tolerated for one hour without adverse reactions. Animals with significant cardiovascular disease, renal disease, Cushing's disease, pulmonary disease, or chronic depletion of fluid and electrolytes are intolerant of high administration rates. Use of isotonic fluids represented by 0.9% NaCl or lactated Ringer's solution may induce overhydration by retention of administered fluids within the intravascular space. Selection of fluid composition and administration rates should be made accordingly.[2, 8, 10]

The fluid administration rate must be monitored in high-risk patients. Measurement of central venous pressure provides information regarding response to fluid administration. Central venous pressure (CVP) measurement has limitations in isolated left heart or biventricular failure. Placement of a catheter into the pulmonary artery and use of pulmonary capillary wedge pressure is valuable in these cases. The normal value range for CVP is 0 to 5 cm H_2O, with values up to 10 to 15 cm H_2O noted in high administration rate therapy. In general, it is best not to exceed CVP values of 10 to 12 cm H_2O except in emergency replacement. Pulmonary capillary wedge pressures range from 2 to 20 mm Hg, and measurements can be used to estimate the tendency to form pulmonary edema by subcategorizing low (< 7 mm Hg), optimal (10 to 14 mm Hg), or elevated (> 20 mm Hg) venous pressures and adjusting administration rates appropriately.[4]

Clinical signs of overhydration may include cough, moist rales on pulmonary field auscultation, tissue chemosis, hypothermia, and alteration in mental status (water intoxication). Reassessment of the goals of fluid therapy, calculated administration rate, and current patient status is imperative to prevent further complications. Therapy would include discontinuation of fluid administration, treatment for pulmonary edema (oxygen, bronchodilators, diuretics), thermal support, and assessment of serum electrolyte values if altered mentation is noted.[4, 23]

Particulate Contamination

Particulate contamination occurs in commercially prepared solutions. The presence of rubber, metal fragments, fibers, mold, and plastics has been reported. Glass fragments from ampules opened to mix in the administered fluids and coring of rubber injection ports from large bore needles have also been described. Improved manufacturing techniques have diminished production-related contamination. Particles of less than 50 microns diameter are invisible, although particles as small as 12 microns may become trapped in the pulmonary vascular bed. Particulate-related injury has occurred subclinically in many animals receiving fluid therapy.[25]

Little data regarding the implications of particulate matter infusion have been reported. Most likely, pulmonary entrapment of particles occurs in most cases. Reports have appeared regarding pulmonary hypertension and respiratory failure related to parenteral fluid administration.

Mixture Incompatibility

Numerous studies of component incompatibility with pharmacological, electrolyte, acidifying, or alkalinizing agents and antimicrobials have been reported. Various charts and tables have been prepared by fluid manufacturers and others detailing incompatibility. As a general rule, dextrose preparations are safe in most instances, whereas electrolyte-containing solutions are less compatible (Table 9–3).[1, 25, 27]

Inappropriate Fluid Selection

Disturbances in electrolyte, acid-base status, osmolality, and metabolic response to surgery and anesthesia should be considered in the selection of an appropriate fluid and its administration rate. Discussions concerning osmolality, electrolyte balance, and metabolic response to surgical injury may be reviewed for further information.[12, 13, 32, 40]

1. Abbott Laboratories: *Physical Compatibility of Parenteral Admixtures*. Abbot Laboratories, North Chicago, 1973.
2. Bellet, S.: *Essentials of Cardiac Arrhythmias*. W. B. Saunders, Philadelphia, 1972, p. 312.
3. Bjorling, D. E., and Rawlings, C. A.: Relationship of intravenous administration of Ringer's lactate solution to pulmonary edema in halothane-anesthetized cats. Am. J. Vet. Res. *44*:1000, 1983.
4. Bonagura, J. D.: Fluid and electrolyte management of the cardiac patient. Vet. Clin. North Am. *12*:501, 1982.
5. Breivick, H.: Preoperative hydration with lactated Ringer's solution versus a salt free restrictive fluid regimen. Acta Anesth. Scand. *13*:113, 1969.
6. Chew, D. J., and Meuten, D. J.: Disorders of calcium and phosphorous metabolism. Vet. Clin. North Am. *12*:411, 1982.
7. Clark, C. H.: Fluid therapy. *In* Sattler, F. P., Knowles, R. P., and Whittick, W. G. (eds.): *Veterinary Critical Care*. Lea & Febiger, Philadelphia, 1981, p. 415.
8. Cohen, J. S.: A summary of complications of fluid therapy. Vet. Clin. North Am. *12*:545, 1982.
9. Cornelius, L. M.: Fluid therapy in small animal practice. J. Am. Vet. Med. Assoc. *176*:110, 1980.
10. Cornelius, L. M., Finco, D. R., and Culver, D. H.: Physiologic effects of rapid infusion of Ringer's lactate solution into dogs. Am. J. Vet. Res. *39*:1185, 1978.
11. Dent, D. M.: Immediate preoperative correction of electrolyte balance. S. Afr. Med. J. *50*:1656, 1976.
12. Deutsch, S., Goldberg, M., and Drupps, R. D.: Postoperative hyponatremia with the inappropriate release of antidiuretic hormone. Anesthesiology *27*:250, 1966.
13. Dripps, R. D., Eckenhoff, J. E., and Vandam, L. D.: *Introduction to Anesthesia: The Principles of Safe Practice*, 6th ed. W. B. Saunders, Philadelphia, 1982, p. 253.
14. Finco, D. R.: Fluid therapy. *In* Kirk, R. W. (ed.): *Current Veterinary Therapy*, 6th ed., W. B. Saunders, Philadelphia, 1977, p. 3.
15. Finlayson, D. C.: Fluid and electrolyte requirements during anesthesia and surgery. Anesth. Analg. *51*:69, 1972.
16. Foster, P. A.: Intravenous fluid therapy during prolonged surgery. S. Afr. Med. J. *50*:1659, 1976.
17. Gieseke, A. H.: Intraoperative fluid therapy. Refresher Courses, Am. Soc. Anes. 1980, No. 110.
18. Goldberger, E.: *A Primer of Water, Electrolytes, and Acid-base Syndromes*, 5th ed. Lea & Febiger, Philadelphia, 1975.
19. Guyton, A. C.: The body fluids: osmotic equilibria between extracellular and intracellular fluids. *In* Guyton, A. C. (ed.): *Textbook of Medical Physiology*, 4th ed. W. B. Saunders, Philadelphia, 1971, p. 380.
20. Hardy, R. M.: Disorders of water metabolism. Vet. Clin. North Am. *12*:353, 1982.
21. Immelman, E. J.: Routine, early postoperative fluid therapy. S. Afr. Med. J. *50*:1663, 1976.
22. Jenkins, M. T., Gieseke, A. H., and Johnson, E. R.: The postoperative patient and his fluid and electrolyte requirements. Br. J. Anes. *47*:143, 1975.
23. Kirk, R. H., and Bistner, S. I.: *Handbook of Veterinary Procedures and Emergency Treatment*, 3rd ed. W. B. Saunders, Philadelphia, 1981, p. 573.
24. Kohn, C. W.: Preoperative management of the equine patient with an abdominal crisis. Vet. Clin. North Am. *2*:289, 1979.
25. Lawson, D. H., and Henry, D. A.: Intravenous fluid therapy. J. Maine Med. Assoc. *68*:432, 1977.
26. Maki, D. G.: Preventing infection in intravenous therapy. Anesth. Analg. *56*:141, 1977.
27. McGrath, C. J., and McGrath, D. H.: Pharmacology. *In* Sattler, F. P., Knowles, R. P., and Whittick, W. G. (eds.): *Veterinary Critical Care*. Lea & Febiger, Philadelphia, 1981, p. 298.
28. Miller, T. A., and Duke, J. H., Jr.: Fluid and electrolyte management. *In* American College of Surgeons (eds.): *Manual of Preoperative and Postoperative Care*. W. B. Saunders, Philadelphia, 1983, p. 38.
29. Moffitt, E. A., Schnelle, N., Rodriquez, R., et al.: Effects of intravenously administered solutions on electrolytes and energy substrates during surgery. Can. Anes. Soc. J. *21*:285, 1974.
30. Polzin, D. J.: Fluid, acid-base, and electrolyte therapy in small animals. Course Notes, University of Minnesota, 1981.
31. Randall, H. T.: Fluid and electrolyte therapy. *In* American College of Surgeons (eds.): *Manual of Preoperative and Postoperative Care*. W. B. Saunders, Philadelphia, 1967, p. 15.
32. Rose, R. J.: Some physiological and biochemical effects of the intravenous administration of five different electrolyte solutions in the dog. J. Vet. Pharmacol. Therapy *2*:279, 1979.
33. Roth, E., Lax, L. C., and Maloney, J. V.: Ringer's lactate solution and extracellular fluid volume in the surgical patient. Ann. Surg. *169*:149, 1969.
34. Schaer, M.: Disorders of potassium metabolism. Vet. Clin. North Am. *12*:399, 1982.
35. Schall, W. D.: General principles of fluid therapy. Vet. Clin. North Am. *12*:453, 1982.
36. Scott, R. C.: Disorders of sodium metabolism. Vet. Clin. North Am. *12*:375, 1982.
37. Shires, T., Williams, J., and Brown, F.: Acute changes in

extracellular fluid associated with major surgical procedures. Ann. Surg. *154*:803, 1961.

38. Steffey, E. P.: Circulatory effects of inhalation anaesthetics in dogs and horses. Proc. Assoc. Vet. Anes. G. Brit. and Ireland (Suppl. 10):82, 1982.

39. Stephen, M., Loewenthal, J., Wong, J., et al.: Complications of intravenous therapy. Med. J. Aust. 2:557, 1976.

40. Thomas, T. H., and Morgan, D. B.: Post-surgical hyponatre-

mia: the role of intravenous fluids and arginine vasopressin. Br. J. Surg. *66*:540, 1979.

41. Virtue, R. W., LeVine, D. S., and Aikawa, J. K.: Fluids shifts during the surgical period. Ann. Surg. *163*:523, 1966.

42. Wharton, R. S., and Mazze, R. I.: Fluid and electrolyte problems. In Orkin, F. K., and Cooperman, L. H. (eds.): *Complications in Anesthesiology*. J. B. Lippincott, Philadelphia, 1983, p. 381.

Acid-Base Balance

Chapter **10**

Marc R. Raffe

Disorders of acid-base balance transcend individual disciplines. The interaction of pulmonary, renal, gastrointestinal, and hematologic factors in regulation and response to acid-base disturbance demonstrate an integrated response. This presentation reviews principles of acid-base function, current methods for assessment of acid-base balance, and the contribution of all factors to acid-base regulation. The organization reflects factors and techniques that have been applied to clinical medicine in the past decade for assessment of acid-base profiles.

THE OXYGEN SYSTEM[7, 13, 16, 18, 25, 29]

The lungs assist gas transfer from the environment to the vascular compartment and, ultimately, to the body tissues. The process of gas exchange–oxygen transfer at the lung-blood interface is commonly referred to as *arterialization*. The oxygen transferred in this process is secondarily distributed to metabolically active tissues. Although this basic concept is a simple one, it is often disregarded during evaluation of laboratory data. Oxygen transport is not as uncomplicated as described. Factors related to (1) pulmonary function, (2) gas tension and laws of gas behavior, (3) hemodynamic competency, (4) available sites of oxygen transport, and (5) balance between gas transfer and blood exchange all affect oxygenation. The three steps in oxygenation are: oxygen uptake, oxygen transport, and oxygen delivery and utilization.

Oxygen Uptake

Oxygen uptake is the process by which lungs extract oxygen from the atmosphere and deliver it to blood through a series of diffusion gradients (see also Chapter 62). The gas laws of Boyle, Charles, and Guy-Lussac govern this process. Net transfer of oxygen occurs only across a gradient of gas pressure. The process is a passive one, requiring no energy consumption, and occurs until an equilibrium is

reached. Dry gas (oxygen) is inspired and humidified by the respiratory epithelium and upper airways. Addition of moisture (water vapor) decreases the concentration of oxygen by principles stated in the gas laws. Oxygen concentration (partial pressure of oxygen or P_{O_2}) is further diminished by mixture with dead space and exhaled gases in the alveolus. A continuously diminished oxygen gradient occurs during this phase of gas transfer.

A further concentration gradient exists between alveolar P_{O_2} and the gas pressure in venous blood presented to the alveolus. Venous blood, previously undergoing oxygen extraction at the tissue level, has a lower P_{O_2} than alveolar gas, thus allowing transfer across the gas-permeable tissue membrane (capillary-alveolar membrane) into the plasma compartment. Concurrently, carbon dioxide transfer occurs into the alveolar space as described by similar application of gas laws. The only energy consumption required for gas exchange is in conjunction with transfer of gas from the environment to conducting pathways and alveoli. This is supplied by respiratory muscles and involves mechanical expansion and contraction of pulmonary tissue to generate gas exchange. Although gas transfer exists by this mechanism, pressure gradients are important in gas transfer across the membrane surface and in portions of lower conducting airways.

Once the alveolar gas tension has been equilibrated among water vapor pressure, dead space gas, and gas diffusion from the adjacent capillary to the alveolus, consideration must be given to factors that affect the relationship to gas exchange between the alveolar and capillary compartments. The relationship between alveolar and capillary function is the ventilation:perfusion ratio (V/Q). The ratio is not uniform in all areas of the lung, with the net result being decreased efficiency in gas exchange where V/Q balance does not exist (see Chapter 62). Four separate circumstances may co-exist in pulmonary parenchyma to impede gas exchange:

1. Venous blood may travel through pulmonary zones that are nonfunctional owing to alveolar col-

lapse or are occupied by transudate or exudate (atelectasis, pulmonary edema, pneumonia, or contusion).

2. Blood may pass areas that are not exposed to functional alveoli (bronchial veins, thebesian veins, congenital vascular anomalies).

3. Alveoli may have adequate gas exchange without adequate capillary circulation (hypotension, vascular blockage).

4. A relative imbalance may exist between alveolar gas exchange and pulmonary circulation.

The first two examples represent instances in which $V < Q$ (V may be zero) and are called venous admixtures, or *shunt*. Alveolar gas exchange in the absence of perfusion is referred to as *dead space ventilation* ($V > Q$, Q approaches zero). Imbalance in V and Q is referred to as *V/Q mismatch;* it occurs in dependent pulmonary areas and may by accentuated by shallow ventilation and increased resistance to gas flow. These alterations may occur in normal or diseased lung tissue; altering any component may retard gas exchange and inhibit oxygen uptake by the lung. Another factor in gas exchange is the capillary-alveolar membrane integrity. Thickening of the membrane due to inflammatory, transudative, or structural disease results in retarded gas diffusion. Attenuation of oxygen diffusion usually precedes carbon dioxide interruption.

The net effect of reduced oxygen levels is development of *hypoxemia,* which is defined as a relative deficiency of oxygen in the blood. Because clinical evaluation utilizes measurement of oxygen tension in plasma, hypoxemia is defined on the basis of this measurement. In general, hypoxemia occurs when oxygen tension in arterial blood is less than 60 to 70 torr. Physiologic causes of hypoxemia include changes of inspired gas concentration, alterations in gas exchange, alterations in ventilation or perfusion factors, and cardiovascular changes. As a result of these factors, blood returning to the left atrium may not be adequately arterialized. The fraction of total blood perfusion that does not arterialize ultimately mixes with adequately arterialized blood, decreasing the final plasma concentration of oxygen. Increased ventilation may not fully compensate for diminished oxygen concentration. Increased ventilation may attenuate or reverse carbon dioxide retention. Hemoglobin saturation of the blood fraction ideally exposed to arterialization is little changed by increased ventilation. The major factor governing change in the oxygen tension of blood is the concentration of inspired oxygen. Most circumstances, except absolute shunts, respond to increased oxygen concentrations, which will be reflected in increased plasma values after administration of enriched gas mixtures.

When oxygen tensions fall below 60 to 70 torr, rapid oxygen desaturation from hemoglobin occurs, diminishing oxygen availability to tissues. As oxygen tension diminishes, so does preferential oxidative metabolism, with resulting anaerobic glycolysis. Accumulation of lactic acid and development of lactic

acidemia progressively increase, causing intracellular injury and death. Tissue hypoxia cannot be directly evaluated but is inferred from measuring arterial and mixed venous oxygen tensions. Mixed venous oxygen values less than 30 torr along with arterial oxygen values less than 60 torr indicate tissue hypoxemia. Clinical signs related to acute hypoxemia include restlessness, tachycardia, hypotension, increased ventilatory depth and rate, tremors, and unconsciousness. If chronic hypoxemia related to lung disease exists, compensatory mechanisms for physiologic adaptation occur. Increased cardiac output, erythropoietin-mediated polycythemia, and alteration in 2, 3-diphosphoglycerate (2,3-DPG) activity compensate for altered oxygen uptake to minimize hypoxemia in the affected animal.

Differences exist in oxygen tension measured at various levels in the respiratory tract and systemic circulation. Usually, evaluations of arterialized samples reflect changes that occur during gas transfer and uptake. Normal Pa_{O_2} at sea level is 89 to 104 torr in dogs and 102 to 112 torr in cats with no evidence of preexisting pulmonary disease. Normal values diminish with altitude elevations because inspired oxygen concentrations decrease.

Oxygen Transport

Once alveolar levels of oxygen increase and oxygen diffuses across the capillary-alveolar membrane, transport of oxygen occurs. Oxygen is transported by one of two mechanisms: free or dissolved oxygen in plasma and reversible binding to respiratory pigments, primarily hemoglobin (Hb). A relatively small, but important quantity of oxygen is dissolved in plasma. Oxygen is relatively insoluble in plasma, thereby limiting the quantity that can be carried by this means. Plasma exposure to oxygen diffused across the capillary-alveolar membrane establishes the partial gas pressure of oxygen in arterialized blood. This gas pressure secondarily effects transfer of oxygen onto respiratory pigments (Hb), the predominant method of oxygen transport to tissue sites. The amount of oxygen physically dissolved in blood is directly and linearly proportional to the blood oxygen tension. If an inspired gas tension of 100 torr exists at the alveolar level, only 0.3 ml/dl of oxygen is *dissolved* in plasma. Measured oxygen tension is 100 torr. This point is important to discriminate between gas partial pressure and *quantity* carried by plasma. Arterial gas tension (Pa_{O_2}) reflects efficiency of gas transfer through the pulmonary parenchyma. However, abnormal oxygen delivery, tissue hypoxia, and low blood oxygen content (discussed later) are not reflected by this evaluation.

The gas tension in plasma facilitates oxygen transfer to hemoglobin. The hemoglobin molecule in the erythrocyte is synthesized during the development of the erythrocyte in bone marrow. This development continues for several days after the cell leaves the marrow. The globin molecule consists of four amino acid chains, each of which carries a heme group. The nucleus of the heme group is a ferrous (Fe^{+2}) ion that has the capacity to reversibly combine with an oxygen molecule. This iron-containing subunit is a ferrous-protoporphyrin complex, ferroheme. Oxygen combines with ferrohemoglobin in the ratio of one gas molecule per ferroheme. Hemoglobin release is regulated principally by changes in erythropoietin production by the kidney. The release stimulates bone marrow production of additional erythrocytes.

Exposure of hemoglobin to oxygen results in attachment of oxygen to the ferroheme subunits. This process may be analogously viewed as a "magnetic" interaction between the two and continues until available binding sites are filled or "saturated." The saturation process is governed by a variety of factors, but under ideal circumstances full saturation occurs under normal conditions of oxygen tension. Each gram of hemoglobin combines with approximately 1.34 ml of oxygen. The amount of oxygen carried by hemoglobin can be measured by oxygen saturation. This value is a ratio of concentrations, and can be described as shown at the bottom of the page.

Clinical instrumentation and methodology exist to measure this value. Calculated oxygen-hemoglobin saturation values can be obtained from the oxyhemoglobin dissociation curve and are expressed as the percentage of actually measured Pa_{O_2}.

Evaluation of total oxygen concentration in blood is measured by oxygen content. This value is equal to the oxygen capacity of hemoglobin (total saturation) plus the free oxygen in plasma. The quantity of dissolved oxygen in plasma is relatively small at normal oxygen tension. If 100 per cent saturation of hemoglobin is present, with a theoretical hemoglobin concentration of 15 gm/dl, then oxygen content is:

$$O_2 \text{ content} = O_2 \text{ capacity} + \text{free } O_2$$

O_2 content = (1.34 ml O_2/gm Hb) × (15 gm Hb) + 0.003 ml O_2/ml plasma; or O_2 content = 20.1 ml/dl + 0.3 ml/dl = 20.4 ml/dl. Oxygen content depends on the degree of hemoglobin saturation. Hemoglobin concentration, inspired oxygen tension, and factors affecting the interactions between hemoglobin and oxygen may all influence oxygen content. Adequate hemoglobin concentration and appropriate oxygen tension do not guarantee appropriate oxygen kinetics. This subject is further elaborated in relation to the oxygen dissociation curve.

Oxyhemoglobin Dissociation Curve

Oxygen transfer from alveolus to hemoglobin occurs until a gas pressure gradient no longer exists. According to Henry's law, when alveolar and plasma driving pressures are equal, the hemoglobin is "saturated" for that oxygen tension. Graphic representation comparing hemoglobin saturation and oxygen tension shows that the relationship is not linear but curvilinear or sigmoid in character and describes the loading and unloading of hemoglobin at various oxygen tensions. The affinity of hemoglobin for oxygen increases progressively as more oxygen molecules combine with the heme pigment. The flat upper portion of the curve relates this fact to the ease of oxygen loading in the lung over a broad range of alveolar oxygen tensions. The oxygen content remains high and generally constant despite momentary fluctuations in alveolar and plasma oxygen tension. Thus, a "buffer" opposing variations in delivered oxygen concentration is present. Additionally, a steep slope, facilitating oxygen desaturation, occurs in the oxygen tension range associated with tissue oxygen tension. This "reverse" gradient favors greater delivery for relatively small changes in oxygen tension. Reversibility of the ferrous-oxygen bond within hemoglobin is described by the zone of curve that correlates with the surrounding oxygen tension.

Under normal conditions, arterialization of blood results in 97 per cent hemoglobin saturation with oxygen. Little additional benefit is gained by increasing ventilation rate. The flat portion of the curve precludes further large gains in saturation with increased oxygen delivery. Additional gains may be realized by increasing the oxygen tension through addition of enriched oxygen mixtures, but large changes in saturation do not occur in healthy animals. If pulmonary disease results in altered V/Q relationship, increased dead space, or large differences in $(A\text{-}a)d_{O_2}$, enriched gas mixtures are beneficial. The steep middle portion of the curve allows release of large quantities of oxygen at lower oxygen tensions that exist at tissue levels. Normally, hemoglobin is still over 75 per cent saturated even when oxygen delivery to tissues has been completed.

The oxygen tension (P_{O_2}) at which 50 per cent of the hemoglobin is saturated under ideal conditions of gas pressure and pH has been used extensively as a hallmark of the position of the oxyhemoglobin dissociation curve. This value is denoted by the symbol P_{50}. A P_{50} value greater than normal suggests a low affinity of hemoglobin for oxygen; a P_{50} value less than normal signifies an increased affinity of hemoglobin for oxygen.

A change in affinity of hemoglobin for oxygen changes the position of the oxyhemoglobin dissociation curve (a left or right "shift"). Shifts in the oxyhemoglobin dissociation curve produce minimal effects on the loading of oxygen from the normal lung because of the convergence of the flat portions of the curve in the plateau area associated with relatively

$$S_{O_2} = \frac{\text{Actual quantity of } O_2 \text{ bound to hemoglobin}}{\text{Potential quantity of } O_2 \text{ that can be bound to Hb}} \times 100$$

high oxygen tension. Alteration in delivery of oxygen at tissue levels occurs because the steep slope of the curve is moved, producing differences in relative ability to release oxygen from ferroheme at the appropriate gas tension.

Increased affinity of hemoglobin for oxygen results in a shift of the oxyhemoglobin dissociation curve to the left. Hemoglobin saturation at a given oxygen tension is increased, thereby diminishing the capacity for oxygen movement from blood to tissue, because the ability to release oxygen is impeded. Through a shift of the curve in this direction, a small increase in oxygen loading at the pulmonary level results; however, this small benefit is of no physiologic significance because tissue oxygen delivery is impeded.

Decreases in hydrogen ion concentration, body temperature, carbon dioxide gas tensions, and enzyme activity in 2,3-DPG all influence a left shift. The role of 2,3-DPG in the process of oxygen-hemoglobin activity merits further consideration. 2,3-DPG, which directly affects hemoglobin-oxygen interaction, is a product of glucose metabolism by glycolytic pathways via the Rapoport-Luebering shunt. The role of 2,3-DPG is two-fold in influencing oxyhemoglobin affinity. First, 2,3-DPG preferentially binds to deoxyhemoglobin, causing a displacement of oxygen from oxyhemoglobin. Second, 2,3-DPG locally affects erythrocyte pH. The resultant diminished pH reduces oxygen affinity by the Bohr effect. The importance of 2,3-DPG is increased in relation to blood storage. Anticoagulant composition may contribute to left shifts in the oxyhemoglobin curve with a reduction in P_{50} values. Maintenance of 2,3-DPG concentration has improved with the use of citrate-phosphate-dextrose (CPD) anticoagulant. Increased 2,3-DPG levels have been noted in alkalosis, chronic hypoxemia, anemia, and diminished cardiovascular function. Decreased levels accompany acidosis. Studies suggest that acid-base balance influences 2,3-DPG levels, and restoration of normal levels may require 24 to 48 hours after the insult. Thus, acute acid-base disturbances produce acute oxyhemoglobin dissociation curve shifts that can be attenuated or reversed as 2,3-DPG accommodates to the imposed changes.

Decreased oxygen affinity for hemoglobin results in a shift of the oxyhemoglobin dissociation curve to the right. A shift in this direction is physiologically advantageous because at a given oxygen tension, a greater net movement of oxygen from blood to tissue occurs. A right shift usually occurs to prevent development of tissue hypoxia. Although a right shift may slightly reduce the capacity of blood to bind oxygen and, ultimately, the total amount of oxygen delivered to the tissues, this effect is minimized by convergence of the plateau portion of the curve at high oxygen tension. Thus, the ability to deliver oxygen at tissue level is significantly increased with minimal effects on oxygen loading. Increases in hydrogen ion concentration, carbon dioxide levels, body temperature, and 2,3-DPG concentration all favor right shifts. A

measured P_{50} is increased, representing a right curve shift.

Alteration in hemoglobin configuration or affinity also occurs during physiologic events. The cycle between oxyhemoglobin and deoxyhemoglobin and accompanying changes in oxygen affinity are governed by three factors: (1) carbon dioxide, which forms specific interactions with carbamino groups, (2) hydrogen ion, which strengthens salt bridges, and (3) 2,3-DPG concentration. Another factor important in this cycle is the Bohr effect. The Bohr effect is physiologically advantageous because it enhances oxygen uptake in the lungs and oxygen release in tissues. The affinity of hemoglobin for oxygen is increased in the blood of pulmonary capillaries as carbon dioxide is eliminated and hydrogen ion is decreased. In the peripheral tissues, the opposite process occurs. As oxygen is released from hemoglobin, a hydrogen ion enters the erythrocyte as a result of carbon dioxide buffering, reducing the affinity of hemoglobin for oxygen (right shift) and favoring increased oxygen availability in the tissues.

The last factor in oxygen delivery is systemic circulation. Perfusion of appropriate tissues is regulated by an active balance between central and regional circulation. Under normal conditions, oxygen transport and delivery to tissues exceed requirements. Deficits in oxygenation that may occur are tolerated or overcome by increased cardiac output. However, increasing cardiac output is an expensive mechanism of compensation as total oxygen requirements increase. Additionally, cardiac output is the limiting factor in oxygen delivery. Minute ventilation of the lungs can be increased to provide 15 to 20 times baseline values in oxygen delivery. However, cardiac output can only increase four- to five-fold, limiting oxygen transport. In addition, cardiac output is not affected unless changes in oxygen tension are large. Local and neurohumoral reflexes relative to regional tissue oxygenation also contribute to deliver oxygen to appropriate tissue sites. Vascular tissue regulates regional blood flow by autonomous regulation of perfusing vessels. Sympathetic nerve fibers and receptor sites coordinate regional flow with local modulation to protect the brain, heart, and other vital organs. Autoregulation of capillary beds controls oxygen delivery at the local tissue level. Combined, adjustments in peripheral or regional perfusion can compensate for about one-third of the cardiac output or one-half of the basal body oxygen requirements.

Oxygen Utilization

Internal respiration, exchange of gases between blood and tissues, is a function of metabolic rate, vascular perfusion, local microcirculation, and oxygen demands of tissue cells. Oxygen delivery requires maintenance of tissue tension of at least 3.5 to 10 torr and an intramitochondrial tissue tension of more

TABLE 10–1. Causes of Inadequate Ventilation, Hypercapnia, or Hypoxemia

Cause	Treatment
I. *Neuromuscular complication (bradypnea/apnea)*	
Temporary absence of chemical stimuli (hypocapnia) associated with hyperventilation or anesthetic induction agent.	
Inactivity of the central control unit due to organic lesions, cerebral edema, anesthetic depression, severe metabolic disturbances, hypothermia (mid-80s°F; 29 to 30°C), trauma, and hemorrhage.	Hypoventilate 1/30 sec until spontaneous ventilation begins. Weaning procedure should be limited to 10 to 15 minutes.
Interference with motor efferents: (a) spinal cord edema due to trauma of surgery, vertebral fractures, or disc prolapse; (b) neuromuscular blocking agents.	Treat the primary disorder. Support ventilation.
II. *Loss of integrity of the bellows*	
Open pneumothorax, flail chest.	
III. *Upper airway obstruction*	Remove or bypass obstruction.
Laryngeal edema, foreign body.	
Collapsing cervical trachea, laryngeal collapse.	
Recurrent laryngeal nerve injury.	
Brachycephalic syndrome.	
Occluded endotracheal tube (endobronchial or esophageal intubation; dried lubricant occluding the lumen; occlusion of the end of the tube by the wall of the trachea at the carina; evagination of the inflated cuff over the end of the tube; accumulation of mucus, blood, and debris in the lumen; collapse of the tube by excessive cuff inflation or by tying the gauze roll too tightly; kinking of the tube; excessively small hole in the tracheal tube adaptor).	
IV. *Pleural filling defect*	
Hydrothorax, chylothorax, hemothorax.	No treatment in absence of dyspnea. Thoracentesis. If fluid returns rapidly, consider insertion of a chest drain.
Pneumothorax.	Avoid IPPV until after chest drain placement.
Diaphragmatic hernia.	Surgical repair; caution during anesthetic induction.

Table continued on opposite page

than 1 torr. Unfortunately, cellular oxygen tensions cannot be directly measured but must be inferred from comparison of arterial and mixed venous samples. Mixed venous samples are usually collected from the right ventricle or pulmonary artery. The mixed venous sample represents the ratio of:

$$P\overline{v}_{O_2} = \frac{O_2 \text{ consumption}}{O_2 \text{ delivery}}$$

In ideal cases, this value is usually 40 to 46 torr or higher and represents residual hemoglobin saturation, under ideal circumstances, of approximately 75 per cent. Oxygen consumption reflects normal metabolic requirements and any alteration in oxygen demand related to exercise, fever, or hypermetabolic states. In humans, the usual value attributed to oxygen consumption at rest is 250 ml/min. Fever increases this value by 7 per cent per 1°F.

Mixed venous oxygen partial pressure can be used to estimate capillary oxygen tension (Pc_{O_2}) by the following relationship:

$$Pc_{O_2} = P\overline{v}_{O_2} + 1/3 \, (Pa_{O_2} - P\overline{v}_{O_2})$$

When $P\overline{v}_{O_2}$ is less than 30 torr, tissue hypoxia is generally present. Adaptation to this hypoxia can occur with time. Augmentation of oxygen release from hemoglobin at lower oxygen tensions may provide a partial explanation for this adaptive process.

Significance of Abnormalities in Oxygen Utilization

Arterial oxygen tension of less than 60 torr evokes a biologic response mediated by the carotid and aortic bodies. In stimulus-mediated respiratory responses, oxygen chemoceptor function is relatively insensitive. Chemoceptor stimulation evokes an integrated response consisting of alterations in: (1) respiratory rate and depth, (2) vascular tone, (3) heart rate, (4) myocardial contractility and blood pressure, (5) functional reserve capacity of the lung, and (6) increased secretory activity of the adrenal cortex and medulla plus posterior pituitary function. These changes are designed to increase oxygen delivery at tissue level. Because other variables attempt to minimize the

TABLE 10–1. Causes of Inadequate Ventilation, Hypercapnia, or Hypoxemia (*Continued*)

Cause	Treatment

V. *Parenchymal disease*
    Atelectasis, hypostatic congestion.
    Pulmonary edema.
    Pneumonia, aspiration, inhalation injury.
    Neoplasia.
    Trauma and hemorrhage.
    Embolic phenomena.
    Secondary to shock, intravascular coagulation,
        pancreatitis, uremia.
	Symptomatic treatment depends on the underlying disease mechanism, e.g., oxygen for V/Q mismatching, impaired diffusion, and small shunts, or IPPV for physiologic shunting due to atelectasis from any cause.

VI. *Apparatus-related problems*
    Excessive circuit resistance.
    Exhausted soda lime or "channeling" of gas flow
        through the path of least resistance.
    Excessive dead space (e.g., improperly functioning
        unidirectional valves, insufficient flows with the
        nonrebreathing system or face masks, small
        patient/large machine).	

VII. *Apparent or associated problems to consider*
    Hypermetabolic states such as hyperthermia or
        hyperthyroidism cause hyperventilation.
    A false hypercapnia may result if blood sample is
        taken immediately following a large dose of
        bicarbonate, especially with a marginal ventilatory
        capacity.
    Failure to correct the measured value for
        hypothermia will cause an apparent increase in
        P_{CO_2}; for hyperthermia it will cause an apparent
        decrease in P_{O_2}.
    Drug-induced methoglobinemia causes cyanosis and a
        decrease in blood oxygen content without a
        decrease in Pa_{O_2}.	

(Reprinted with permission from Haskins, S. C.: Blood gases and acid-base balance: Clinical interpretation and therapeutic implications. *In* Kirk, R. W. (ed.): *Current Veterinary Therapy VIII.* W. B. Saunders Co., Philadelphia, 1983.)

detrimental effects of oxygen starvation (hypoxemia), the danger level of Pa_{O_2} is difficult to predict, although unconsciousness occurs at 36 torr in the absence of other abnormalities. For this reason, maintenance of Pa_{O_2} in excess of 60 torr is desirable to minimize evoked physiologic response and to maintain adequate hemoglobin saturation for tissue delivery, in order to minimize stress-mediated responses that increase oxygen consumption from ventilatory efforts.

Delivery of high inspired oxygen tensions may not be required because little additional oxygen-carrying capacity is mediated by hemoglobin in excess of 200 torr, and 97 per cent saturation occurs at 100 torr. High concentrations of oxygen may create pulmonary epithelial injury if prolonged (greater than 24 hours) exposure occurs. If extended oxygen therapy is anticipated, inspired oxygen concentrations of 40 to 50 per cent (with Pa_{O_2} greater than 60 torr) are appropriate. Obviously, higher concentrations may be temporarily required until the underlying cause and corrective procedures are initiated.

The effect of hemoglobin concentration on oxygen-carrying capacity should be considered. As noted earlier, oxygen content reflects the contribution of both oxygen in plasma and hemoglobin-associated oxygen. Partial oxygen pressure (Pa_{O_2}) is not adequate evidence of oxygen-carrying capacity. In the anemic animal, Pa_{O_2} is adequate but *total* capacity is diminished. Therefore, elevating Pa_{O_2} does not produce a linear response in oxygen-carrying capacity. Augmenting hemoglobin-carrying capacity by administering whole blood or synthetic fluorocarbon products capable of reversible oxygen transport is indicated to increase oxygen delivery.

A variety of insults may result in hypoventilation, hypoxemia, or hypercapnia (Table 10–1). Irrespective of cause, initial therapy should be directed at reversing hypoxemia and should consist of: (1) ensuring of airway patency, (2) adequate ventilation by spontaneous or artificial support, and (3) delivery of enriched oxygen to inspired gas. Many preexisting conditions alter the V/Q ratio. Enriched oxygen will improve alveolar oxygenation to underventilated alveoli. If no improvement is noted with enriched oxygen administration, reevaluation and application of supplemental therapy may be indicated. Use of manual or mechanical ventilatory assistance to improve alveolar gas exchange and evaluation of hemodynamic perfusion to pulmonary tissue is warranted. Alveolar collapse related to accumulation of fluids or exudates may be reversed by application of positive-pressure airway support. Reinflation of these alveoli improves pulmonary volumes and facilitates oxygen exchange. In some cases, cardiovascular support may be indicated to improve perfusion to alveoli and facilitate arterialization. Maintenance of a slight positive airway pressure at all times may be required to pneumatically "splint" the alveoli and prevent atelectasis from redeveloping.

Effectiveness of therapy is evaluated on the basis of repetitive sampling of Pa_{O_2}, physical appearance of the animal, auscultation of pulmonary fields to monitor gas exchange, and radiography. Diminished restlessness, respiratory rate and effort, heart rate, and blood pressure are all signs of therapeutic response to oxygen therapy. If no response to oxygen therapy, ventilatory support, and positive airway pressure occurs, a shunt may exist. Shunts are usually related to congenital cardiovascular anomalies and should be differentiated from primary pulmonary lesions.

Normal Pa_{O_2} is 90 to 100 torr. Variations in alveolar ventilation and minute volume affect alveolar and arterial P_{O_2} in pulmonary tissue. Pa_{O_2} alone may reflect efficiency in gas exchange. Because Pa_{O_2} and Pa_{CO_2} are interrelated parameters, combining them provides a "standardized" guideline beneficial if hyperventilation or hypoventilation is evident. A calculation referred to as the alveolar-arterial difference in oxygen tension—$(A-a)d_{O_2}$—may be used, which is reached using the equation:

$$(A-a)d_{O_2} = PA_{O_2} - Pa_{O_2}$$

The arterial component comes directly from measurement of arterial oxygen tension. The alveolar component must be derived by subtracting interrelated gas partial pressures that exist at the alveolar level, requiring interpolation of barometric pressure, water vapor saturation, and carbon dioxide values as follows:

$$PA_{O_2} = PI_{O_2} - Pa_{CO_2} (1.1)$$

where PI_{O_2} (inspired oxygen tension) = 20.93% × barometric press −50 torr (water vapor pressure). The factor of 1.1 corrects the respiratory quotient. This factor may be ignored if inspired oxygen tension exceeds 90 per cent. If barometric pressure is at STP (765 torr) and Pa_{CO_2} is 40 torr, then:

$$PA_{O_2} = [(20.93\% \times 765 \text{ torr}) - 50 \text{ torr}]$$
$$- 40 \text{ torr} (1.1)$$
$$= 110 \text{ torr} - 4.4 \text{ torr}$$
$$= 105.6 \text{ torr}$$

This value can be used to calculate $(A-a)d_{O_2}$ difference if the PA_{O_2} is 95 torr:

$$(A-a)d_{O_2} = 105.6 \text{ torr} - 95 \text{ torr}$$
$$= 10 \text{ torr}$$

A value of 10 torr is normal, because V/Q varies even under ideal circumstances. A value in excess of 15 torr indicates increased venous admixture and a diminished oxygenating efficiency.

If high inspired oxygen tensions are administered, a similar calculation is used, neglecting the correction factor of respiratory quotient (1.1). If pure oxygen (100 per cent) is administered, acceptable $(A-a)d_{O_2}$ is 100 torr; values in excess of 150 torr indicate increased venous admixture. A crude approximation of $(A-a)d_{O_2}$ can be calculated by multiplying the inspired oxygen concentration by a factor of 5. An animal ventilating on 20 per cent oxygen should have a Pa_{O_2} of 100 torr, and one ventilating on 50 per cent oxygen should have a Pa_{O_2} of 250 torr and so forth.

THE CARBON DIOXIDE SYSTEM[1, 16, 18, 25, 29]

The quantity of carbon dioxide (CO_2) present in the blood reflects a balance between generation of CO_2 and elimination from pulmonary tissue during gas exchange. Although elimination of CO_2 depends on pulmonary blood flow and alveolar ventilation, its production depends on the metabolic state of the animal. CO_2 diffuses from venous blood into the alveolus as a result of a partial pressure gradient. A direct relationship can be established between quantity of gas exchange from the alveolus and the blood level of carbon dioxide. More efficient removal of CO_2 improves the capillary-alveolar gradient and enhances further clearance of CO_2.

Carbon dioxide is generated by mitochondrial utilization of glucose under aerobic conditions, and its production is a function of oxygen consumption and utilization of energy sources. Under basal metabolic conditions, a relationship referred to as the respiratory quotient (R) can be described by the equation:

$$R = \frac{\text{Rate of } CO_2 \text{ output}}{\text{Rate of } O_2 \text{ uptake}}$$

With mixed substrates, R is 0.8; that is, only 80 per cent as much CO_2 is produced as O_2 is consumed. This value is based on a normal dietary intake. Increased carbohydrate substrate produces a greater amount of CO_2 and raises the R value to 1.0. Lipid metabolism, conversely, utilizes oxygen for water formation and diminishes the R value to 0.7.

Carbon dioxide is approximately 20 times more soluble than oxygen in biologic tissues and is easily absorbed or transferred across tissue spaces. For this reason, an efficient mechanism has developed to handle this potentially toxic waste product. This mechanism is enhanced by the high volatility, solubility, and diffusibility of CO_2. Carbon dioxide may be transported in several ways: (1) by physical dissolution in blood, (2) as carbonic acid, (3) as bicarbonate ion, (4) as carbamino hemoglobin plus other carbamino compounds, and (5) as small quantities of carbonate ion.

Carbon Dioxide Transport in Plasma

When carbon dioxide is produced as an end-product of metabolism, the local tissue carbon dioxide partial pressure (P_{CO_2}) rises above arterial levels. Carbon dioxide molecules diffuse from the tissue into the plasma of capillary blood. A variable percentage of CO_2 remains physically dissolved in plasma as transit occurs to the pulmonary alveoli for elimination. The gas pressure exerted by the dissolved carbon dioxide is the partial pressure (P_{CO_2}) that is sampled in clinical evaluation of samples for blood gas parameters. A small quantity of CO_2 is actually dissolved in plasma in addition to the free CO_2. The quantity of dissolved CO_2 is expressed as:

$$\text{Physically dissolved } CO_2 = \alpha(P_{CO_2})$$

where α is the solubility coefficient of carbon dioxide in plasma (0.03 mmol/liter/mm Hg at 37°C.). Therefore, in each liter of blood, 1.2 mmol of CO_2 is dissolved in plasma.

Carbon dioxide may also be transported in plasma by two other routes. It may reversibly interact with free amino groups of plasma proteins to form plasma carbamino groups. As there are relatively few protein sites that can combine with carbon dioxide, only about 0.5 moles of CO_2 can be carried per liter of plasma. Oxygenation does not appear to influence this process, because similar values have been measured in both arterial and venous samples. Hydrogen ions released by carbamino reactions are sequestered by plasma buffers. A small quantity may also interact with water to form bicarbonate and hydrogen ions. This reaction is relatively slow and takes several minutes to equilibrate. The limitation of this route is the slow formation of the intermediate product, carbonic acid, owing to absence of the enzyme carbonic anhydrase. The concentration of carbonic acid in plasma is 0.0017 mmol/l. Any hydrogen ion formed in this process is readily buffered by plasma buffering systems.

Hemoglobin-Related Carbon Dioxide Transport

After being transferred across the erythrocyte membrane, carbon dioxide may (1) remain dissolved in erythrocytes, (2) undergo transformation to bicarbonate ion, or (3) combine directly with hemoglobin. Small quantities of carbon dioxide may remain dissolved in erythrocytes. The contribution of this factor is relatively small, 0.34 mmol/l in arterial blood and 0.39 mmol/l in venous blood.

Most carbon dioxide undergoes reversible reactions within the erythrocyte. Approximately two-thirds of generated carbon dioxide is transported in this manner, the remaining one-third being transported in the plasma by methods described previously. The plasma component is important in determining directional "drive pressure" for all associated reactions. On entry into the erythrocyte, approximately 15 to 30 per cent of CO_2 is transferred directly to the hemoglobin molecule, exchanging on a 1:1 basis with molecular oxygen and forming carbamino hemoglobin. Carbon dioxide combines with hemoglobin at free amino sites of the globin moiety. Presence of oxygen on the heme pigment inhibits carbon dioxide combination with amino sites. A decreased P_{O_2} aids in the association of CO_2 with hemoglobin, and an increased P_{CO_2} aids in the unloading of oxygen at tissue levels. The dissociation curve for carbon dioxide is linear over the physiologic range, as opposed to the sigmoid shape of the oxyhemoglobin curve. Deoxyhemoglobin exerts a greater affinity for carbon dioxide.

In the erythrocyte, most carbon dioxide combines with tissue water in the presence of the enzyme *carbonic anhydrase* (C.A.) to form hydrogen ion and bicarbonate ion. This reaction may be expressed as:

$$H_2O + CO_2 \underset{}{\overset{C.A.}{\rightleftharpoons}} H_2CO_3 \rightleftharpoons H^+ + HCO_3^-$$

Carbonic anhydrase facilitates the speed of reaction and is found in erythrocytes and renal tubular cells, as well as the choroid of the eye. This zinc-containing enzyme facilitates the reaction at a rate 1000 times faster than in plasma. Further, 99.9 per cent of carbonic acid dissociates to bicarbonate and hydrogen ions. The bicarbonate ion combines mainly with intracellular potassium and effluxes into plasma to perform a buffering role. This diffusion process disturbs electroneutrality between the plasma and erythrocyte compartments. To compensate for this disturbance, an ionic exchange with chloride ion, known as *chloride shift*, occurs. This process increases plasma bicarbonate levels, enhances carbon dioxide transfer by plasma, and preserves electroneutrality. The hydrogen ion formed in this process is buffered by hemoglobin, as discussed in the section on buffer base. The reaction indirectly facilitates CO_2 transport by the Haldane effect.

The Haldane effect describes the relationship of carbon dioxide to hemoglobin in the presence of oxygen. As oxygen is released from tissue, an enhancement of carbon dioxide affinity by hemoglobin occurs because deoxyhemoglobin becomes a weaker acid (increased H^+ ion binding capability), allowing an increase in hemoglobin's ability to transport carbon dioxide that is entering the blood. At the alveolus, increased oxygen pressures aid in the displacement of carbon dioxide from hemoglobin. This reaction is the opposite of the one occurring at the tissue level. The displacement of carbamino hemoglobin dissociation curve by alteration in oxygen tension is defined as the *Haldane effect*. Thus, a constant "oscillatory" cycle exists within the erythrocyte. The *Bohr effect* occurs at tissue level and reflects the addition of CO_2 to the hemoglobin molecule. The addition creates a right shift in the oxyhemoglobin dissociation curve that favors further release of oxygen. The Haldane effect describes the corollary relationship, whereby addition of oxygen to the blood facilitates release of carbon dioxide from carbamino hemoglobin. Hemoglobin activity is favorably altered in both the lungs and tissues to facilitate delivery and exchange of oxygen and carbon dioxide at the appropriate moment.

Clinical Evaluation of Carbon Dioxide Pressure

The partial pressure of carbon dioxide can be readily measured with the Severinghaus electrode. The P_{CO_2} is the driving pressure necessary for gas to go into solution; when CO_2 leaves the blood in the lungs, this value is called the escape pressure. The pooled venous P_{CO_2} ($P\bar{v}_{CO_2}$), which represents pooled carbon dioxide output from all tissues, varies by species but is approximately 45 ± 4 torr. This gas pressure gradient is exposed at the pulmonary level to lower gas pressures within the alveolus, and re-equilibration occurs across the capillary-alveolar membrane. The re-equilibration sets the arterial gas tension, which in dogs is 36.8 ± 3.0 torr and in cats is 31.0 ± 2.9 torr. Ventilation has a direct influence upon P_{CO_2}.

Total carbon dioxide content in blood reflects the sum of various transport methods in the plasma and erythrocytes. Plasma carbon dioxide content is the sum of dissolved CO_2, bicarbonate, and plasma protein–bound CO_2 concentrations:

$$\begin{aligned} \text{Plasma } CO_2 &= \text{dissolved } CO_2 + HCO_3^- + \text{plasma-} \\ &\quad \text{bound } CO_2 \\ &= 1.2 \text{ mmol/l} + 25.4 \text{ mmol/l} \\ &= 26.6 \text{ mmol/l in arterial blood} \end{aligned}$$

Erythrocyte (RBC) carbon dioxide content is, similarly, a sum of all components described above:

$$\begin{aligned} \text{RBC } CO_2 &= \text{dissolved } CO_2 + \text{carbamino } CO_2 + \\ &\quad HCO_3^- \\ &= 0.85 \text{ mmol/l} + 2.43 \text{ mmol/l} + 10.7 \\ \text{mmol/l} \\ &= 13.98 \text{ mmol/l in arterial blood} \end{aligned}$$

Combined contents for whole blood require knowledge of the proportion of erythrocyte mass determined by packed cell volume (PCV). Assuming a PCV of 40 per cent:

$$\begin{aligned} \text{Whole blood } CO_2 &= 26.6 \, (0.6 \text{ plasma factor}) + \\ &\quad 13.98 \, (0.4 \text{ erythrocyte factor}) \\ &= 15.96 + 5.59 \\ &= 21.5 \text{ mmol/l} \end{aligned}$$

Components of Acid-Base Regulation[4, 11, 13, 18, 20, 21, 31]

Maintenance of cellular function requires an exacting environment. Temperature, osmolarity, and concentrations of electrolytes, nutrients, and oxygen must remain within narrow limits to maintain normal metabolic function. One of the most important factors is the hydrogen ion concentration (H^+), a by-product of normal metabolism. Substances that can donate hydrogen ion are called *acids*, and substances that can receive hydrogen ion are called *bases*. A constant interaction between acids and bases occurs *in vivo* to maintain systemic homeostasis. A substance that prevents extreme changes in free hydrogen ion concentration within a solution is called a *buffer*. Buffers allow normal cell function to continue unimpeded when cells are subjected to significant changes in hydrogen ion concentration. Four major buffer systems exist: hemoglobin, bicarbonate, phosphate, and serum proteins.

Quantification of hydrogen ion is important. The most widely accepted method of assessing H^+ concentration is the use of pH units, first described by Sorenson. Water can be dissociated into hydrogen and hydoxy ions. This fractionation is referred to as the ionization constant of water and is quantified as the dissociation constant (Kw):

$$\begin{aligned} H_2O &= H^+ + OH^- \\ Kw &= 1 \times 10^{-14} \\ Kw &= [1 \times 10^{-7}] [1 \times 10^{-7}] \end{aligned}$$

In this form, equal numbers of H^+ and OH^- ions occur, and the solution is therefore *neutral*. Sorenson first proposed the use of an exponent on a base 10 logarithmic scale to simplify interpretation. This concept was refined by Karl Hasselbalch to arrive at the term pH, by which:

$$pH = - \log [H^+]$$

The use of a negative log term allows for all values to be expressed as positive numbers. In clinical medicine, blood levels of hydrogen ion fall between 6.3×10^{-6} (pH = 6.8) and 6.3×10^{-7} (pH = 7.8). The average value for hydrogen ion concentration is 0.4×10^{-8} mole/l (pH = 7.4). Measurement of pH reflects the net result of all acidotic and alkalotic processes in the body.

A pH value reflects one moment in time; it does not contribute to an understanding of the dynamics of acid-base balance. This balance is best described by the Henderson-Hasselbalch equation, which expresses the relationship between acids and conjugate base substances:

$$K = \frac{[H^+] [A^-]}{[HA]}$$

describing the relationship between dissociated and undissociated components of a chemical buffer system. K is the ionization constant of that system. Transformation of this equation can be performed to yield:

$$[H^+] = \frac{K [HA]}{[A^-]}$$

which in turn can be expressed in log form as:

$$- \log [H^+] = - \log K + \log \frac{[A^-]}{[HA]}$$

or

$$pH = pK = \log \frac{[Base]}{[Acid]}$$

This last form, the Henderson-Hasselbalch equation, is the foundation for discussion of acid-base physiology. Alteration in the relationship of acid and conjugate base will result in changes in net hydrogen ion (pH) activity. The equation may be further combined, enabling it to be easily used in the clinical evaluation of acid-base status. A pH value of 7.4 has been determined as the mean value in most biologic systems. In addition, the ionization constant (pK) is 6.1 for most acid-base calculations. By using these values in the equation:

$$7.4 = 6.1 + \log \frac{[Base]}{[Acid]}$$
$$1.3 = \log \frac{[Base]}{[Acid]}$$
$$\text{antilog } 1.3 = \frac{[Base]}{[Acid]}$$
$$\frac{20}{1} = \frac{[Base]}{[Acid]}$$

a constant ratio of 20:1 is derived during homeostasis. We can now use this value to create a "formula":

$$pH \sim \frac{Base}{Acid} = \frac{20}{1}$$

to predict the effects of fluxes in acid and base components on the net effect on pH. Systemic disturbances in equilibrium evoke a response to minimize net changes or reestablish equilibrium by mechanisms described in succeeding sections.

Most domestic species have a blood pH near 7.4. A fall in pH (hydrogen ion increases) is *acidemia*. Conversely, an elevation in blood pH (hydrogen ion decreases) is *alkalemia*. The terms acidosis and alkalosis are commonly interchanged with acidemia and alkalemia to describe biochemical alteration. *Acidosis* refers to a medically significant gain of acid or loss of base by the body. *Alkalosis* means a medically significant loss of acid or gain of base by the body. Gains and losses are not necessarily paralleled by blood pH, which only measures *net* effect. It is possible for alkalemia to exist in an animal with a generalized intracellular acidosis.

Metabolism produces a continuous source of acidic by-products that challenge the buffering capacity of any species. The predominant product generated is hydrogen ion; short-chain organic acids also contribute to the acidity. To maintain homeostasis, the acid produced is constantly neutralized by a series of buffer systems. The buffers involved in the response to acid production include bicarbonate, hemoglobin, plasma protein, and phosphate.

Bicarbonate

The bicarbonate system is the predominant and most rapidly responding of the major buffering mechanisms. In addition, it is the most complex and integrated system for buffering volatile and fixed acid components. The bicarbonate system is the only "open" buffer system. Buffered acids may be subsequently excreted by lungs or kidneys. Appreciation of this system is fundamental to an overall comprehension of acid-base balance. The bicarbonate system is:

$$CO_2 + H_2O \rightleftharpoons H_2CO_3 \rightleftharpoons H^+ + HCO_3^-$$

This equation is referred to as the *hydration equation*. The relationship between metabolic acid (H^+ ion) and carbon dioxide allows for chemical transformation of a metabolic product (fixed acid) into a volatile product (carbon dioxide). In addition, carbon dioxide (volatile acid) can be transformed to a fixed product for more efficient systemic transport to the organs of excretion. Owing to physical laws governing gas solubility in fluids, much less carbon dioxide–carrying capacity can occur from solubility than can occur by transformation into a chemical by-product. Thus, CO_2 can be transformed into bicarbonate at the cellular level for transportation to sites of elimination. When the sites of elimination are reached, reconversion to volatile acid can occur for ultimate excretion by ventilation. Virtually all produced acid is handled in this manner. Various ratios of excretion by pulmonary and metabolic routes have been reported; however, the lung is at least 1000 times more active in acid excretion than other routes in a homeostatic situation. Free bicarbonate is re-formed upon elimination of carbon dioxide.

The bicarbonate system can be represented by the generalized Henderson-Hasselbalch equation. The relationship of carbon dioxide value (P_{CO_2}) and H_2CO_3 in body fluids is such that H_2CO_3 is proportional to αP_{CO_2} (in torr). The factor of 0.03 is the constant of carbon dioxide (H_2CO_3) that relates CO_2 and carbonic acid. Relatively little CO_2 can be carried by physical solution. Thus the equation becomes:

$$pH = 6.1 + \log \frac{[HCO_3]}{[H_2CO_3] + [CO_2]}$$
$$= \frac{[HCO_3]}{0.03 \times P_{CO_2}}$$

Assuming a normal P_{CO_2} value of 40 torr:

$$pH = 6.1 + \log \frac{[HCO_3]}{40 \times 0.03}$$
$$= 1.2$$

Observed values of bicarbonate are approximately 24 mEq/l at pH of 7.4. Thus, a constant relationship

$$7.4 = 6.1 + \log \frac{24}{1.2}$$
$$1.3 = \log 20$$

is established for the bicarbonate system. Stated alternatively:

$$pH = \frac{HCO_3}{\alpha CO_2}$$

This ratio is useful in interpretation of blood gas data and is referred to later.

Hemoglobin

The bicarbonate–carbonic acid system is important in regulation of acid-base balance and is easily sampled for *in vitro* analysis. However, early investigations determined that separated plasma was not as efficient in buffering acid as whole blood and that some metabolic acids could not be volatilized. Therefore, alternate systems must exist to deal with these acids. The other buffer systems in blood include phosphate, plasma protein, and hemoglobin.

Systems in erythrocytes include both bicarbonate and hemoglobin buffers. Hemoglobin is a complex molecule with 540 amino acid residues in its structure, 36 of which are histidine. The imidazole subunit of histidine possesses chemical properties that allow for combination of hydrogen ion on an amine group. This combination is a reversible process and has pK values in the physiologic range. In addition, *N*-terminal valine groups have a pK of 7.8 and can serve as buffer sites. When fixed acids are buffered, approximately 60 per cent of the buffering capacity resides in the hemoglobin buffer system, with 30 per cent in the bicarbonate buffer system. The remaining 10 per cent is provided by organic phosphate buffers that are present intracellularly. The hemoglobin buffer system is integral in buffering carbonic acid, as described later.

Addition of oxygen onto the hemoglobin molecule alters the pK of the hemoglobin buffer system. The alteration is a reflection of changes in stereochemical configuration of the hemoglobin molecule and a result of relative interactions between oxygen, carbon dioxide, and hemoglobin. This effect, central to smooth uptake and delivery of oxygen and carbon dioxide, is referred to as the Bohr-Haldane effect, which is discussed further in the section on oxygen and carbon dioxide transport systems because of its importance to gas transit and buffering capacity.

The erythrocyte also contains carbonic anhydrase that facilitates the conversion of bicarbonate to carbonic acid. Because CO_2 is freely diffusible through cell membrane surfaces, diffusion into the erythrocyte initiates the mass action relationship with formation of new bicarbonate ion. This ion migrates to the extracellular space in exchange for chloride ion (chloride shift), representing new bicarbonate formation.

Protein

Plasma proteins provide a broad spectrum of histidine residue buffer pairs with a pK range of 5.5 to 8.5. Their function is similar to that of the hemoglobin system. Plasma proteins are a heterogenous group of buffers usually thought of as a single entity. The contribution of this system to total buffering capacity is relatively small; however, proteins can buffer acids of respiratory and nonrespiratory origin, making them valuable in counteracting the effects of carbonic acid in plasma spaces.

Phosphate

The phosphate buffer system is similar to the bicarbonate buffer system and is capable of buffering both strong and weak alkali components. However, its contribution is limited by the relatively low concentration of phosphate in plasma. Its main importance is acid-base balance in renal tubules. Phosphate is also an important buffer system in intracellular fluids.

Distribution of Buffers

Buffering systems are not equally distributed in body spaces. Extracellular fluid has bicarbonate, protein, and phsophate systems. Intracellular fluid (including erythrocytes) has hemoglobin, phosphate, and protein buffering systems. Bicarbonate buffering does not occur in significant amounts except in cells where carbonic anhydrase activity is present (erythrocytes, renal tubular cells, choroid plexus). Interstitial fluid (lymph) has a high concentration of bicarbonate buffer. In bone, the calcium hydroxyapatite matrix can participate in buffering of hydrogen ion in acute or chronic acidosis, perhaps at the expense of solubilizing bone minerals and conversion of one insoluble salt form to another.

Principles of Buffer Function

The different buffer systems have the same goal, to buffer hydrogen ion. When a change in hydrogen ion concentration occurs, the responses of the various buffer systems are qualitatively similar, but of dissimilar magnitude. Change in balance in one system can also change the balance of all coexisting systems, demonstrating that buffer systems interact to prevent large changes in proton concentration.

Buffering in Extracellular Fluids

Addition of hydrogen ion to extracellular fluid alters the ratio of $H_2PO_4^-$ and HPO_4^{-2} as well as forming carbonic acid from bicarbonate. The process could terminate at this point with buffering completed. The volatile component then comes into play. A rise in carbonic acid occurs owing to equilibrium with carbon dioxide and water. The increased amounts of carbon dioxide are eliminated by increased pulmonary ventilation. The result is a concurrent decline in bicarbonate and gas pressure of carbon dioxide (P_{CO_2}). The directions of change for the components are similar, and the ratio of the pair is decreased, extending the effectiveness of the buffer. Carbonic acid and carbon dioxide are both membrane permeable; thus, changes in extracellular buffer capacity may be further distributed to the larger intracellular space.

As hydrogen ion conversion and excretion occurs through the carbonic acid system, a redistribution of ion occurs. The phosphate buffer system has a pK value that favors release of hydrogen ion at normal pH levels. The release of hydrogen ion and transfer to the carbonic acid system for ultimate disposition can occur as volatilization of acid progresses.

Buffering by Ionic Shifts

In addition to extracellular buffering systems as represented by carbonic acid—bicarbonate, phosphate, and protein—intracellular and extracellular compartments are linked by a system of proton-cation exchange. This exchange is frequently encountered in clinical medicine as a shift in sodium and potassium concentration between intracellular and extracellular spaces. Giebisch investigated the importance of this exchange relative to total buffering capacity. Experimentally produced respiratory acidosis and alkalosis was created, and changes in proton-anion balance were measured. Respiratory acidosis was buffered approximately 37 per cent by sodium-proton exchange, 14 per cent by potassium-proton shifts, and 29 per cent by chloride-bicarbonate exchange. Respiratory alkalosis was buffered 16 per cent by sodium-proton shifts, 4 per cent by potassium-proton movement, and 37 per cent by chloride-bicarbonate handling. In addition, buffering was partially provided from lactic acid accumulation as a result of metabolic pathway stimulation.

A corollary experiment using nephrectomized dogs administered acid or alkali was reported by Swann and Pitts. Similar patterns of transcellular distribution of infused acid/alkali by shifts in sodium, potassium, and chloride concentrations were demonstrated, although significant contribution of extracellular buffer systems (bicarbonate and protein) were also demonstrated. Respiratory-related alteration in acid-base balance can be effectively buffered in the intracellular fluid compartment, because diffusion of carbon dioxide occurs equally throughout the body water. Metabolic origin disturbance requires a greater contribution of extracellular buffer systems for compensation. However, direct infusion of acid or alkali into extracellular space can still effectively be distributed to intracellular fluid space by buffer reactions, thereby allowing increased buffering to occur.

Buffering by Bone

Although not normally considered a buffering reservoir, bone is an available storage site of bicarbonate and phosphate. Acute buffering may occur from a small, readily accessible pool and a much larger, inaccessible pool. Bone requires several days to exhibit maximum buffering capacity. Parathyroid hormone plays a role in the ability of bone to play an active role in buffering. The mechanism for this activation has not been fully elucidated; however, bone buffering does not occur without parathyroid hormone. Paradoxically, parathyroid hormone also promotes excretion of bicarbonate ion by renal tubules. The net effect of these factors may be highly significant with regard to bone structure, tissue mass, and acid-base balance.

Evaluation of Buffer Function

Clinical measurement of acid-base balance utilizes arterial or venous blood samples. Evaluation of blood as a reflection of acid-base status has become standard in human and veterinary medicine. Several laboratory techniques have been described to evaluate the role of bicarbonate either singularly or in combination with other buffer systems. Although bicarbonate is measured as the primary *in vitro* buffer base, all other systems should be in equilibrium.

Use of Nomograms

In vitro sample analysis includes the actual measurement of pH, P_{CO_2}, and P_{O_2} by direct methods. The other components of a blood gas analysis are not measured but are derived from the relationships between these values. Previously, presentation and manipulation of the Henderson-Hasselbalch equation resulted in the relationship:

$$pH \sim \frac{[HCO_3]}{[CO_2]}$$

If pH and CO_2 values are known, bicarbonate value can be derived. This relationship has been graphically represented in the Davenport diagram. If the pH and CO_2 values determined by tonometry are plotted, the bicarbonate value is extrapolated. An essential feature of this diagram is the multiple "isobars" of carbon dioxide. This feature is essential to encompass the range of carbon dioxide levels encountered in clinical and laboratory medicine. By *in vitro* manipulation of a collected blood sample, equilibration with one or more additional known concentrations of carbon dioxide gas allows plotting of a buffer line with a "slope" that reflects the buffering capacity and bicarbonate values under these different conditions. This line allows one to predict the behavior of blood or blood components under these various values of carbon dioxide tension. This function has been called a "buffer titration curve."

In vivo blood analysis incorporating both bicarbonate and hemoglobin buffer systems differs in line slope from separated plasma, thus confirming the contribution of hemoglobin to buffer capacity. The slope of this line is referred to in Slyke units. Whole blood slope is 28 to 30 Slyke units; this value represents the change in bicarbonate value across the physiologic range (pH 6.8–7.8). Therefore, 28 to 30 mmol/l bicarbonate change can be expected across this range. Change in slope, and therefore buffer capacity, reflects hemoglobin concentration. An anemic animal exhibits reduced buffering capacity.

An alternative, multifunction nomogram has been described by Siggaard-Andersen (Fig. 10–1). The nomogram is a result of *in vitro* addition of known amounts of acid or base to human blood samples with different hemoglobin concentrations. It allows for linear alignment of pH and P_{CO_2} values, with extrapolation of bicarbonate, base excess, and total CO_2 values (discussed later). *In vitro* analysis differs from *in vivo* dynamics. To minimize these variations, incorporation of isobars representing hemoglobin contribution to base buffer is included. The intersection of the two lines representing pH-P_{CO_2} relationship

and hemoglobin concentration allows for extrapolation of buffer base data.

Errors are inherent in construction and use of all nomograms, and assumptions must be made. Components of the Henderson-Hasselbalch equation (pK of H_2CO_3 and CO_2 solubility) have been shown to be variable. Variations in blood/extracellular fluid volume ratio and H^+ or HCO_3^- distributions affect *in vivo* buffer slope. Species variation in buffer capacity and normal values also influence the results obtained. Correction of the hemoglobin contribution to extracellular water must be performed to reflect accurately the base alteration in a replacement formula. All body cells can generate bicarbonate, which is equally distributed through all tissue spaces. *In vitro* analysis requires equilibration of blood with gas in a closed system (tonometry). This artificial manipulation differs from *in vivo* systems, where a continuous pulmonary "escape" route exists (open system). In addition, complex regulatory mechanisms are not

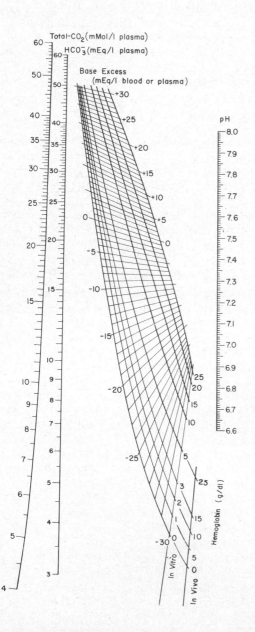

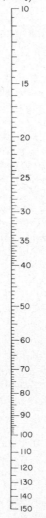

Figure 10–1. The Siggaard-Andersen blood acid-base alignment nomogram. The base deficit/excess and bicarbonate and total CO_2 concentrations can be estimated by aligning the measured values of pH and P_{CO_2} with a straight edge and reading the respective values (any two values would permit the calculation of the other three). The base excess/deficits should be read from the isopleth of the effective, in vivo hemoglobin concentration. (Reprinted with permission from Siggaard-Andersen, O.: Blood acid-base alignment nomogram. Scales for pH, P_{CO_2}, base excess of whole blood of different hemoglobin concentrations, plasma, bicarbonate, and plasma total CO_2. Scand. J. Clin. Lab. Invest. *15*:211, 1963.)

present *in vitro*. Because of these factors, *in vivo* response can differ from *in vitro* analysis. Despite these limitations, bicarbonate changes are a good "indicator" and reflect acid-base balance.

The interrelationship of bicarbonate to carbon dioxide should also be remembered. Independent evaluation of one parameter does little to indicate the source of change. For example, a low bicarbonate value may indicate bicarbonate consumption from a metabolic acid challenge or simply may reflect shifts as a result of CO_2 elimination that is greater than normal. The differentiation of these two possibilities occurs during *in vitro* analysis by re-equilibrating the blood sample to a standardized pH or P_{CO_2} tension and analyzing a single factor. Through maintenance of constant (normal) values, a correction for one of the two factors influencing measurement occurs, establishing an independent analysis.

Base Measurements

Base Excess Concept. Several different systems of base measurement have been described and used in clinical medicine. Currently, the concepts of *base excess* and *total carbon dioxide* are used frequently. Base excess specifies the number of milliequivalents of acid or base needed to titrate one liter of blood to pH 7.40 at 37°C while the P_{CO_2} is held constant at 40 torr. This concept is a derived binding index, developed for its potential practical application, and consists of the bicarbonate concentration corrected for alterations in P_{CO_2} (respiratory component) plus the buffering capacity or contribution of hemoglobin, phosphates, and protein. The concept depends upon a relationship between pH and HCO_3^- and does not include any respiratory component. Measurement of bicarbonate does not reflect total base excess values if pH and buffering capacity are unknown, because the contribution of hemoglobin and other nonbicarbonate buffers would not be evaluated. To correct for these factors, the base excess equation becomes:

$$\text{Base Excess/l} = [HCO_3^-] \text{ measured} \\ - [(\text{pH normal} - \text{pH measured}) \\ 28 \text{ Slykes}] + [HCO_3^-] \text{ normal}$$

which mathematically states:

$$\text{Base Excess/l} = \Delta[HCO_3^-] + \Delta[\text{nonbicarbonate buffer}]$$

This concept is expressed in mEq/l above or below the normal buffer-base range and has a normal value of 0 ± 2 mEq/l. In any patient, the base excess may be higher (more positive) or lower (more negative) than the bicarbonate value, reflecting alteration in corollary buffer systems.

Expression of base excess allows assessment of the metabolic contribution to acid-base balance. The terminology can be confusing, because "negative" and "positive" are used in conjunction with the concept. A negative base excess implies a true base deficit; a positive base excess signifies a true base excess. Once the base excess value is known, calculation of replacement base therapy (if required) can be performed. Several formulas have been published for correction calculation. The most frequently used is:

$$\text{Base needed (mEq)} = 0.3 \times [\text{body weight (kg)}] \\ \times \text{base excess}$$

The factor 0.3 represents the extracellular fluid (in liters) to which bicarbonate is administered. This formula predicts the *total* base requirement for correction. Administration of buffer base replacement therapy should be performed judiciously, because most ions do not immediately equilibrate across membrane partitions. To compensate for this factor, and to prevent broad variations in acid-base balance, one-quarter to one-half the calculated amount is administered for acute replacement purposes, with the remaining base infused over a period of 12 to 24 hours. When one provides bicarbonate replacement on the basis of base-excess calculations, the blood base excess, not the total body base excess, is "treated."

Total Carbon Dioxide

Total carbon dioxide, the amount of carbon dioxide that can be recovered from a plasma sample that has been collected and processed under anaerobic conditions, represents the sum of carbon dioxide dissolved in plasma as carbonic acid and bicarbonate. Since the ratio of these two components is approximately 20:1, total CO_2 is a relatively good index of bicarbonate activity.

The procedure is relatively inexpensive and rapid. Reagents can be commercially purchased and come in prepackaged vials. A blood sample (serum or plasma) is introduced into the vial along with a dilute acid. The liberation of carbon dioxide gas that occurs can be quantitated by syringe plunger displacement. A standard is concurrently evaluated, and the two values are incorporated into a formula to calculate total CO_2. The limitations of this test are: (1) constant specific temperature is needed for testing; (2) it evaluates *only* metabolic acid-base profile; (3) absence of blood pH data requires the clinician to appreciate the effects of underlying disease contributing to the acid-base disturbance; and (4) pulmonary disease that causes carbon dioxide retention interferes with its accuracy. Despite these drawbacks, total CO_2 measurement is relatively inexpensive, technically uncomplicated, and relatively accurate. This evaluation can easily be incorporated into veterinary practice.

Normal values for total carbon dioxide approximate those for bicarbonate measurement. Owing to the incorporation of the carbonic acid component, mean values reported for normal are 24 mEq/l (HCO_3^-) + 1.2 mEq/l (H_2CO_3) = 25.2 mEq/l. The range of normal overlaps the range of bicarbonate ion and, therefore, bicarbonate values may be practically used in most cases.

RESPIRATORY ACID-BASE BALANCE

Arterial Carbon Dioxide Tension

Arterial carbon dioxide tension is the direct and immediate reflection of adequacy of alveolar ventilation in relation to metabolic rate. Elevated carbon dioxide tension can usually be attributed to increased metabolic rate or diminished effective ventilation. Alternatively, carbon dioxide partial pressure is inversely proportional to effective minute ventilation. If blood carbon dioxide level is higher than normal, decreased elimination due to hypoventilation is assumed to be the cause. Conversely, increased elimination (hyperventilation) is assumed if the measured blood carbon dioxide is low.

In contrast to the oxygen dissociation curve, the shape of the carbon dioxide dissociation curve is relatively linear over the physiologic range. This permits a greater compensatory capacity of the lung to balance P_{CO_2} values between areas of high and low ventilation-perfusion ratios. Thus, Pa_{CO_2} values may be relatively normal in the presence of even moderately severe hypoxemia due to ventilation-perfusion abnormalities.

Normal values for arterial carbon dioxide in the awake animal are 36.8 ± 3.0 in the dog and 31.0 ± 2.9 in the cat.

Pulmonary elimination of carbon dioxide (volatile acids) is a major component in acid-base balance. Physiologically, pulmonary excretion of volatile acid is the predominant mechanism. The excretion of volatile acid (CO_2) is mediated through the mass action equation:

$$CO_2 + H_2O \rightleftharpoons H_2CO_3 \rightleftharpoons H^+ + HCO_3^-$$

Carbon dioxide is carried as bicarbonate, carbamino hemoglobin, carbonic acid, and physically dissolved gas in both arterial and venous blood. An increase in one component of the equation causes a proportional elevation in all other component concentrations. Ineffective alveolar ventilation creates retention of carbon dioxide and effectively induces retention of hydrogen ion (acidosis). Conversely, increased alveolar ventilation enhances removal of carbon dioxide and effectively reduces hydrogen ion concentration (alkalosis). Thus, the lungs are indispensable in regulation of acid-base balance. This can be appreciated by comparing the effects of respiratory and metabolic lesions. Apnea (ventilatory failure) is accompanied by a rapid deterioration in acid-base balance; renal failure requires several hours to days to achieve similar effects. Thus, respiratory acid-base balance is integrally linked to *effective alveolar ventilation*. Disruption of this balance is described in subsequent sections.

Regulation of Ventilation

Maintenance of P_{CO_2} under physiologic conditions requires a feedback control mechanism to regulate carbon dioxide levels, and indirectly, acid-base balance. This regulation necessitates an integrated neurologic response of both central and peripheral chemoceptor components sensitive to carbon dioxide. Extreme sensitivity to changes in CO_2 is apparent in the immediate response in effective ventilation to fluctuations in blood carbon dioxide levels. The control mechanism comprises peripheral (carotid and aortic body) and central components; the relative contribution of each is still not well defined. Central chemoceptors located on the ventral surface of the medulla are sensitive to alterations in cerebrospinal fluid pH mediated by elevated carbon dioxide tension. This mechanism may be the predominant stimulus for ventilation. Peripheral chemoceptor response to CO_2 elevations is mediated through cranial nerve reflexes that augment the ventilatory response. Thus, an integrated response is initiated when arterial CO_2 levels increase.

METABOLIC ACID-BASE BALANCE[2, 10, 16, 17, 18, 23, 27, 31]

Renal Regulation of Acid-Base Balance

Acute alterations in P_{CO_2} are pulmonary in origin, whereas changes in bicarbonate ion concentration, and indirectly in buffer base, reflect renal regulation and excretion of fixed (noncarbonic) acids. The processes are interrelated through the Henderson-Hasselbalch equation, with pulmonary regulation controlling the denominator and metabolic regulation controlling the numerator. The net result of extracellular fluid bicarbonate buffering is the formation of acid anions. The anion generated in this process ultimately undergoes renal elimination. The overall process would deplete whole body buffer base unless regeneration or conservation of bicarbonate occurred. The pathways associated with this process interact by eliminating intact fixed acids and conserving bicarbonate buffer.

Acid Excretion

There is continuous production of hydrogen ion by normal metabolism. Hydrogen ion initially interacts with plasma buffer base resulting in consumption of bicarbonate and other buffers. The kidneys are principally responsible for excretion of the hydrogen ion resulting from endogenous metabolism. As hydrogen ion is eliminated, bicarbonate is conserved on a 1:1 basis. The kidney thus regenerates the bicarbonate used in neutralization of endogenous acid. This process occurs in a balanced manner, providing that the animal is normal in acid-base balance initially and has a constant diet.

The quantity of hydrogen ion excreted can be measured by titrating the urine to neutral pH (7.4) and adding the amount of ammonium ion present in the urine. The amount of alkali required to titrate hydrogen ion carriers is the *titratable acidity* (TA) of the urine. The sum of TA and ammonium ion excreted is the total urinary acid excretion. This amount is also equivalent to the quantity of bicarbonate ion lost in this process. In humans, a value of 50 mEq/day of hydrogen ion is removed by this process, representing approximately 0.2 per cent of total hydrogen ion loss per day. Hydrogen ion eliminated by this route, as reflected in urine pH, is approximately 400 to 800 times more acidic than plasma, signifying a steep concentration gradient. The quantity of hydrogen ion lost in the urine is a function of the quantity of urinary buffers available to bind protons.

In addition to excretion of hydrogen ion, the kidney generates approximately 5000 mEq of bicarbonate per day by reabsorbing filtered bicarbonate load. The kidney excretes hydrogen ion through (1) resorption of bicarbonate, (2) excretion of titratable acidity, and (3) excretion of ammonium ion. Although it is technically inaccurate to suggest that metabolically derived bicarbonate is the same molecule that was lost by glomerular filtration, this concept is a "working" definition and is used in further discussion.

Bicarbonate Reabsorption

Bicarbonate undergoes dynamic, interrelated regulations in the nephron unit. Reabsorption takes place through hydrogen ion secretion and selective recirculation of bicarbonate ion. Bicarbonate is delivered, primarily as the sodium salt, to the renal tubular lumen by glomerular filtration. Hydrogen ion in the lumen interacts with bicarbonate to form water and carbon dioxide. These products are membrane-permeable and diffuse into the proximal tubular epithelium and eventually the venous blood. In the proximal tubular cell, bicarbonate and hydrogen ions are re-formed by the corollary reaction, and differential transfer of bicarbonate to plasma occurs. As hydrogen ion is excreted, disturbance in electroneutrality occurs, which is rectified by resorption of sodium ion from the tubular lumen. The exact mechanism of this sodium-hydrogen exchange is not fully understood. Sodium may play a role in initiating an exchange with hydrogen ion, thus providing a driving pressure for the reaction. This reaction is rate-limited, as plasma bicarbonate values in excess of 27 to 28 mEq/l are accompanied by increased excretion of bicarbonate.

Bicarbonate resorption is related to a variety of regulatory factors. Extracellular volume (ECV) is a major controlling factor. Expansion of ECV inhibits sodium and, secondarily, bicarbonate resorption. Potassium is related to bicarbonate levels and appears to intrinsically control bicarbonate resorption, independent of ECV. Plasma P_{CO_2} affects bicarbonate resorption by changes in intracellular hydrogen ion concentration. Glucose levels affect bicarbonate resorption by unknown mechanisms. Elevations in glucose enhance bicarbonate resorption in normal dogs. Parathyroid hormone (PTH), calcium, and phosphorus also influence bicarbonate resorption. Elevation in PTH levels depress, and increased calcium levels enhance, the resorption by altering hydrogen ion secretion. Phosphorus responds in similar fashion. Aldosterone enhances acid excretion and indirectly enhances bicarbonate resorption.

Ammonium Ion

Bicarbonate conservation may also occur in distal renal tubules, where intraluminal volumes are diminished and the previous interaction is exhausted. To further conserve bicarbonate, ammonia (NH_3) formed from amino acid deamination diffuses into the tubular cells and combines with hydrogen ion to form ammonium ion (NH_4^+). By this process, ammonia is acting as a urine buffer. Once NH_4^+ is formed, it penetrates cell membranes poorly and remains in the tubular lumen. Thus, a unidirectional flow is established. Excretion of NH_4^+ preserves a bicarbonate ion, thus maintaining the alkali reserve.

Ammonium excretion is influenced by urine pH and metabolic acidosis. Lower urine pH values favor ammonium ion formation. Infusion of sodium bicarbonate or acetazolamide diminishes NH_4^+ formation. Chronic metabolic acidosis favors greater deamination of glutamine, furthering NH_3 production, enhancing the contribution of ammonia to acid excretion, and lessening further bicarbonate loss.

Titratable Acidity

Weak anions of monobasic and dibasic phosphate interact with hydrogen ions to further preserve bicarbonate ion. The interaction of this group is commonly considered *titratable acidity*. In general, a majority of phosphates in the tubular lumen are of the dibasic variety that become monobasic by the acceptance of hydrogen ion. Titratable acidity can be influenced by buffer system pK, buffer quantity, and urine pH. Buffer system pK and pH interact in a manner whereby the system is most efficient at urine pH in the range of 6.8 to 7.4. As urine pH diminishes, a lower proportion of dibasic phosphate is present, diminishing buffering capacity of this component.

Potassium Ion

Potassium ion is also regulated by renal tubular cells and has an important role in acid-base physiology. Potassium is inversely exchanged with hydrogen ion on a one-to-one basis. Potassium is resorbed in proximal renal tubular cells in a passive process and is reabsorbed in the loop of Henle as an active process. When plasma potassium concentration is elevated because of hydrogen ion entry into the intracellular space with liberation of sodium and potassium, acid secretion in the kidney is depressed, resulting in moderate bicarbonate retention and development of *hypokalemic alkalosis*.

Extracellular Fluid Volume

The kidneys can regulate the bicarbonate concentration in plasma indirectly by altering extracellular fluid volume. This effect occurs in extreme cases because other nonbicarbonate buffers attenuate buffer base disturbance. Rapid volume expansion with sodium-containing fluids may create a *dilutional acidosis* and serve as a stimulus for bicarbonate conservation by the kidney. Conversely, and more clinically significant, loss of extracellular fluid volume may induce *contraction alkalosis* with elevation in bicarbonate buffer base.

Measurement of Acid-Base Balance

A variety of measurement techniques are used to evaluate the metabolic contribution to acid-base balance. Currently, the indirect evaluations of bicarbonate concentration and base excess are the most common. Indirect analysis with confirmation by anion gap measurement is also useful.

Base Excess

Base excess specifies the number of milliequivalents of acid or base required to titrate one liter of blood to pH 7.40 at 37°C with constant P_{CO_2} of 40 torr. The concept includes the buffering contribution of bicarbonate corrected for P_{CO_2} plus the buffering capacity of hemoglobin, phosphates, and other blood proteins. Base excess may be determined by actual titration or can be derived from nomogram calculations following measurement of pH, P_{CO_2}, and hematocrit values. An index of deviation from the normal base concentration, the base excess is expressed in mEq/l above or below the normal buffer-base range. Thus, a "normal" value has been assigned. It varies with species. In the dog, $-1.5 + 1.1$ mEq/l and in the cat, -5.9 ± 3.9 mEq/l are accepted normals. Base excess is altered only by nonvolatile acids and measures the true nonrespiratory acid-base status.

The value of the base excess concept is in formulating therapeutic guidelines. A negative base excess (base deficit) suggests a metabolic disturbance that may require base replacement. Conversely, a positive base excess indicates a metabolic alkalosis. The numerical values provide a guideline for calculation of base replacement (sodium bicarbonate is routinely selected) according to standard formulas discussed in the therapy section.

The *in vitro* analysis of blood differs from *in vivo* dynamics of the extracellular fluid compartment. To minimize this difference, the Siggaard-Anderson nomogram has been modified to include effective hemoglobin concentrations. The *effective hemoglobin concentration* is the contribution of hemoglobin to the buffer base capacity of the extracellular compartment. This amounts to about 20 per cent of the actual hemoglobin concentration. Accurate measurement of *in vivo* base excess or deficit may be obtained by using the modified isobars on the nomogram representing "effective" hemoglobin concentration.

Carbon Dioxide Content (Total CO₂)

Carbon dioxide content represents the total amount of CO_2 that can be recovered from a plasma sample collected under anaerobic conditions. It is equal to the bicarbonate plus carbonic acid concentrations. Because the bicarbonate to carbonic acid ratio is 20:1, the carbon dioxide content is also a relatively good index of total bicarbonate activity. Measurement of carbon dioxide content is an estimate of the *metabolic* component of acid-base balance.

Several techniques may be used to measure total CO_2. A kit for individual tests is commercially available. Alternatively, the direct titration technique may be used (Oxford titrator). Either method produces satisfactory results under appropriate conditions.

Anion Gap

The anion gap accounts for the difference between measured cations and anions. Clinically measured ions are sodium (Na^+), potassium (K^+), chloride (Cl^-), and bicarbonate (HCO_3^-). Unmeasured cations include calcium, magnesium, and gamma globulins. Unmeasured anions include phosphate, sulfate, lactate, pyruvate, alpha and beta globulins, and albumin. Generally, changes in unmeasured anion concentration are principal determinants of changes in anion gap.

The anion gap is derived from a concentration equation, which by mathematical rearrangement results in:

$$\text{Anion gap (mEq/l)} = (Na^+ + K^+) - (Cl^- + HCO_3^-)$$

The normal value for anion gap in domestic species has been debated. Values range from 12 to 24 mEq/l, with 10 mEq/l frequently accepted as normal. An elevation in anion gap represents metabolic acidosis, and a decline represents metabolic alkalosis. The value of an anion gap measurement is to alert the clinician to alterations in a metabolic acid-base profile that are not detectable by standard measurement techniques. An additional benefit is confirmatory data supporting the presence of acid-base disturbances. For example, metabolic acidosis consumes bicarbonate ion, creating an imbalance in the anion gap classified as a high anion gap metabloic acidosis. Examples of high anion gap acidosis include uremia, ketoacidosis, lactic acidosis, and intoxication with ethylene glycol, salicylate, methanol, and paraldehyde. Independently, acidosis unassociated with an increased anion gap is usually associated with a hyperchloremia relative to serum sodium concentration. Hyperchloremia can result from hemoconcentration, hyperchloremic metabolic acidosis, or chronic respiratory alkalosis.

The anion gap should be calculated whenever it is

necessary to define precisely the existence of an acidosis independent of base excess. It may also be used to define the major source of the acidosis, to serve as an index of the severity of the disease process, and to evaluate the effectiveness of therapy.

ABNORMALITIES OF ACID-BASE BALANCE[2, 4–7, 9, 18, 19, 22, 23, 25–30]

Table 10–2 summarizes the types of acid-base disturbances.

Simple Acid-Base Disturbances

The Henderson-Hasselbalch equation illustrates that pH is a result of the base/acid ratio or pH:HCO_3^-/CO_2. This may also be thought of as a renal function/respiratory function ratio. The standard "ratio" of the equation is:

$$pH \sim \frac{[HCO_3]}{[CO_2]}$$

during normal balance in most mammalian species. Disturbances can be categorized by alterations in [HCO_3^-] (metabolic component) or P_{CO_2} (respiratory component). Use of the equations aids the clinician in determining the component of primary imbalance and whether compensatory change is present. Acid-

TABLE 10–2. Types of Acid-Base Disturbances

Simple acid-base disorders	Respiratory
	  Acidosis (acute or chronic)
	  Alkalosis (acute or chronic)

	Metabolic
	  Acidosis
	  Alkalosis

Mixed acid-base disorders	Mixed metabolic disorders
	  Metabolic acidosis + metabolic alkalosis
	  Anion gap acidosis + hyperchloremic acidosis
	  Mixed anion gap or hyperchloremic acidosis

	Mixed respiratory-metabolic disorders
	  Respiratory acidosis + metabolic acidosis
	  Respiratory acidosis + metabolic alkalosis
	  Respiratory alkalosis + metabolic acidosis
	  Respiratory alkalosis + metabolic alkalosis
	"Triple" disorders
	  Metabolic acidosis + metabolic alkalosis + respiratory acidosis
	  Metabolic acidosis + metabolic alkalosis + respiratory alkalosis

base disturbances are categorized as four primary disturbances: primary CO_2 retention (respiratory acidosis), primary CO_2 depletion (respiratory alkalosis), primary HCO_3^- depletion (metabolic acidosis), and primary HCO_3^- retention (metabolic alkalosis). Two or more primary problems may coexist in the same animal.

Respiratory Acidosis

Under normal circumstances production, transport, and elimination of CO_2 exist in balance as defined by the respiratory quotient. The rate of excretion is balanced primarily against the production rate and is modulated by a neurogenic control mechanism. If an imbalance occurs at any step in the process, compensatory mechanisms are initiated. Compensation consists of increased alveolar ventilation in the initial period. This response, in general, is adequate; however, in circumstances such as CNS disease, thoracic lesions, pulmonary parenchymal disease, and related problems, inadequate elimination occurs. Production of CO_2 then exceeds elimination, resulting in elevated levels of carbonic acid (H^+ ion) and diminished pH values (respiratory acidosis).

In the initial period, CO_2 is generated more rapidly than bicarbonate, and pH falls immediately along the blood buffer isobar and in all body fluids. The initiation of higher respiratory rate increases the metabolic component of ventilation (work of breathing), imposing another site of CO_2 generation. Augmented ventilatory work increases CO_2 production and may further exacerbate the underlying problem. For any given increase in effective alveolar ventilation, the Pa_{CO_2} rises further with progressive metabolic cost. Therefore, the respiratory system cannot correct or adapt itself effectively for primary pathologic conditions involving ventilation. During the acute phase, acidosis is buffered by titration of non-bicarbonate tissue buffers. Carbonic acid protons are taken up by buffers such as hemoglobin, allowing HCO_3^- to be spared. Although HCO_3^- is produced through mass action, the quantity produced is limited, and little renal compensation exists. Clear and predictable changes have been demonstrated regarding changes in CO_2 and pH during this period. Experimental evidence suggests that HCO_3^- does not exceed 31 to 32 mEq/l when P_{CO_2} is 80 to 90 torr. A relationship between these two factors may be expressed as: [HCO_3^-] increases 1 mEq/l for each 10-torr P_{CO_2} elevation in acute phase. A similar relationship between pH and P_{CO_2} is that anticipated pH changes are 0.8 of P_{CO_2} alterations; this may be expressed as: 0.01 pH unit change accompanies each 1-torr change in P_{CO_2} (Table 10–3).

If carbon dioxide retention persists, within 12 to 24 hours the plasma bicarbonate concentration increases beyond the initial mass action response. This elevation is a result of renal conservation and synthesis of bicarbonate. Carbonic acid loading stimulates renal ammonia production, causing increased excre-

TABLE 10–3. Summary of Responses to Simple Acid-Base Disorders

Primary Disturbance	Acid-Base Abnormality	Compensatory Response	Predicted Compensation Range of Values
Respiratory Acidosis	Hypoventilation ($\uparrow P_{CO_2}$)	Production of HCO_3^- (cell buffering)	Acute: HCO_3^- increases 1 mEq/l for 10-torr increase in P_{CO_2} Chronic: HCO_3^- increases 3.5 mEq/l for every 10-torr increase in P_{CO_2}
Alkalosis	Hyperventilation ($\downarrow P_{CO_2}$)	Consumption of HCO_3^- (cell buffering and renal)	Acute: HCO_3^- falls 2 mEq/l for each 10-torr decrease in P_{CO_2} Chronic: HCO_3^- falls 5 mEq/l for each 10-torr decrease in P_{CO_2}
Metabolic Acidosis	Loss of HCO_3^- or gain of hydrogen ion	Increase in ventilation (chemical buffering)	$Pa_{CO_2} = (1.5 \times [HCO_3^-]) + 8$
Alkalosis	Gain of HCO_3^- or loss of hydrogen ion	Decrease in ventilation	$Pa_{CO_2} = (0.9 \times [HCO_3^-]) + 9$

tion of titrated buffer (NH_4Cl) with net gain of bicarbonate ion. Addition of bicarbonate in exchange for chloride ion in the distal tubules results in hypochloremia. This response maintains overall electroneutrality. With the change in pH, transcellular shifts of potassium ion may also occur with liberation into the extracellular fluid and plasma. Because renal conservation is poor, potassium loss may be present in chronic cases. The integration of bicarbonate resorption and synthesis stabilizes serum pH by permitting a sustained increase in serum bicarbonate concentration. The compensation normalizes overall balance, but pH values do not return to normal, as confirmed in experimental studies in dogs and humans. Relevant factors in this finding are the continued metabolic cost of breathing, and the readjustment of neurogenic control to "accept" less than optimal parameters. Compensatory adaptation balances oxygen and carbon dioxide levels to maximize alveolar ventilation in the presence of less than optimal circumstances. If successful adaptation occurs, *respiratory insufficiency* is present. Tolerance of less than optimal P_{O_2} and P_{CO_2} levels is a result of the predisposing circumstances, but the capability for eliminating CO_2 is present. If inability to eliminate CO_2 and O_2 exists, then *ventilatory failure* is present. The animal is intolerant of the circumstances that are present and cannot compensate despite maximal efforts. With the introduction of metabolic compensation, the relationship of P_{CO_2} and bicarbonate is altered. Bicarbonate values increase 3 to 4 mEq/l for every 10-torr elevation in P_{CO_2}, reflecting the additional metabolic compensation present in the chronic period (see Table 10–3).

Systemic effects of respiratory acidosis are reflected in the cardiovascular and neuromuscular systems. Hypercapnia causes increases in cardiac output and vasodilation. Blood pressure is usually maintained near normal values. The overall hemodynamic status usually reflects mixed influences of hypoxemia, hypercapnia, and acidosis. Ventricular dysrhythmias may be noted, but the frequency is variable and may be a reflection of multiple disturbances. During anesthesia, the interaction of acidemia and anesthetic agents renders the animal more susceptible to development of this complication. Respiratory acidosis also increases susceptibility to digitalis intoxication.

Acute hypercapnia has been associated with neuromuscular dysfunction, altered mental status, delirium, seizures, papillary edema, stupor, and coma. Tremors, myoclonus, and alteration in deep tendon reflexes also occur. Many of these signs are attributed to elevation in cerebral blood flow caused by the vasodilating properties of carbon dioxide. Not all, or even a majority of, animals exhibit these signs, because chronic elevations of 90 to 100 torr can be tolerated if oxygenation is adequate. Signs are more frequently noted in cases of chronic hypercapnia, especially if concomitant hypoxemia is treated with supplemental oxygen. The depression of hypoxemic ventilatory stimulus in these cases diminishes minute volume, further decompensating carbon dioxide elimination.

Causes of hypercapnia reflect conditions that reduce effective alveolar ventilation. Specific causes are listed in Table 10–4. In a general sense, any underlying disease related to carbon dioxide elimination may predispose to hypercapnia and resultant acidosis. Alterations in pulmonary perfusion, parenchymal ventilation, or thoracic integrity, muscle lesions, central and peripheral nerve lesions, and improper ventilatory support all result in respiratory acidosis. In

TABLE 10–4. Etiology of Simple Acid-Base Disturbances

Origin and Type	Etiology	Origin and Type	Etiology
Metabolic acidosis	Increased anion gap 　Generalized renal failure 　Diabetic ketoacidosis 　Lactic acidosis 　Toxicity 　　Methanol 　　Ethylene glycol 　　Paraldehyde 　　Salicylate Normal anion gap (hyperchloremic acidosis) 　Gastrointestinal lesion 　　Diarrhea, emesis 　　Pancreatic lesion 　Ingestion of acid or potential acid 　Parenteral nutrition 　NH_4Cl, $CaCl_2$, HCl 　Dilutional acidosis (rapid saline infusion) 　Carbonic anhydrase inhibitor (acetazolamide) 　Renal tubular acidosis 　Secondary to prolonged respiratory alkalosis 　Hypoaldosteronism	Respiratory acidosis *continued*	Hemothorax Hydrothorax Abdominal distension 　Muscular defects 　Hypokalemia 　Myasthenia gravis Control-mediated 　Central nervous system 　　Anesthesia 　　Analgesics, sedatives 　　Trauma, tumor 　Spinal cord and peripheral nerves 　　Cervical injury 　　Guillain-Barré syndrome 　　Neurotoxins (e.g., tetanus) 　　Drugs (succinylcholine, pancuronium) 　　Diaphragmatic paralysis Failure of mechanical ventilation
Metabolic alkalosis	Gastric loss 　Emesis Renal origin 　Mineralocorticoid excess 　Hypercapnia compensation 　Hypokalemia, hypochloremia 　Diuretics 　Hypoparathyroidism Bicarbonate retention 　Base infusion Volume depletion 　Secondary to respiratory acidosis Contraction alkalosis	Respiratory alkalosis	Cortical influences 　Anxiety 　Pain 　Fever 　Primary CNS disease Hypoxemia 　Altitude 　Pulmonary shunts 　Pulmonary V/Q imbalance 　Diffusion disease 　Hypotension 　Pulmonary edema Physical stimuli 　Decreased chest wall or diaphragm movement 　Interstitial fibrosis 　Inflammatory lesions Drugs or hormones
Respiratory acidosis	Pulmonary-mediated 　Perfusion 　　Pulmonary embolism 　　Cardiac arrest 　Ventilation 　　Pulmonary edema 　　Pneumonia 　　Airway obstruction 　　Interstitial fibrosis 　Thorax, lung restriction 　　Flail chest 　　Pneumothorax		Salicylates 　Thyroid hormone 　Progesterone 　Catecholamines 　Xanthines Primary disease 　Septicemia 　Pregnancy 　Hyponatremia 　Heat exposure 　Compensation for metabolic acidosis 　Mechanical ventilation

many cases, hypoxemia may also be present (hypoventilation) and may pose additional threats to homeostasis.

Diagnosis of respiratory acidosis is made on the basis of the clinical signs described and results of arterial blood gas analysis. Typically, a pH value in the acidotic range is present as well as an elevation in P_{CO_2} level. Alterations in bicarbonate and base excess values vary with time. In the acute phase,

limited response will be noted, as suggested by experimental data. Later on, renal compensatory mechanisms operate and may involve a greater change in bicarbonate values.

Respiratory Alkalosis

Arterial P_{CO_2} falls whenever pulmonary CO_2 excretion exceeds CO_2 production. The enhanced rate of

CO_2 excretion is self-limited, however, since a falling P_{CO_2} acts to offset increased ventilation, and in the steady state, the rate of CO_2 production once again equals that of excretion, at a lower arterial P_{CO_2}.

Hypocapnia and a corresponding decline in carbonic acid concentration characterize respiratory alkalosis. Nonbicarbonate cellular and extracellular buffers respond to elevated HCO_3^--CO_2 ratio by consuming HCO_3^- in order to attenuate pH changes. Respiratory alkalosis is initiated by a fall in P_{CO_2}, which in turn stimulates processes to lower the HCO_3^-. Laboratory data demonstrate hypocapnia ($P_{CO_2} < 35$ torr), causing an alkalemia (pH > 7.45) and low bicarbonate values (< 20 mEq/l). Mild hypokalemia may also occur, reflecting renal wasting of potassium and translocation of extracellular cation into the cellular space. Chloride is retained to offset bicarbonate loss and maintain electroneutrality. Mild hypokalemia and hyperchloremia are characteristic electrolyte changes associated with respiratory alkalosis. It is unusual to note serum HCO_3^- values less than 15 mEq/l in respiratory alkalosis; lower values may reflect concurrent acidosis of metabolic origin. In severe cases, hyperventilation also results in tissue release of lactic acid and pyruvic acid, producing a base deficit that contributes to compensatory mechanisms.

The acute period is characterized by bicarbonate alterations that are independent of renal function. An adaptive fall in bicarbonate values occurs within minutes and is unassociated with any significant renal bicarbonate loss. Within hours, a diminution in renal acid excretion occurs, resulting in retention of endogenous acid and consumption of reserve bicarbonate. Changes in respiratory alkalosis mirror those in acute respiratory acidosis. Guidelines relating alterations in bicarbonate and P_{CO_2} have been established. Bicarbonate (HCO_3^-) increases 3 to 4 mEq/l for every 10 torr increase in P_{CO_2} (see Table 10–3).

Hypocapnia for more than six hours results in renal adjustment to increase bicarbonate excretion and reduces loss of ammonium and titratable acid. A new "steady state" is reached within 1½ to three days. This response is directly related to P_{CO_2} and is independent of the preexisting metabolic state. The magnitude of change in chronic respiratory alkalosis is greater than in the acute period. A change in bicarbonate values of up to 5 mEq/l occurs for every 10-torr change in P_{CO_2}. Of the simple acid-base disturbances respiratory alkalosis is unique in its ability to return pH to normal. The return occurs in humans over seven to nine days. The underlying mechanism of the complete compensation has not been determined.

Systemic effects of respiratory alkalosis mirror those of respiratory acidosis. Acute hypocapnia produces cerebral vasoconstriction with consequent fall in cerebral blood flow. Alterations in mental status, syncope, and seizures have been reported in humans. Paresthesia, muscle clonus, tetany, and exaggerated deep tendon reflexes may also be present. Tachycardia, S-T segment depression on electrocardiography, and arrythmias have also been demonstrated. Nausea and vomiting have been reported in extreme cases. Many of these signs disappear with persistence of low Pa_{CO_2}.

Causes of respiratory alkalosis are diverse (see Table 10–4). Central nervous system factors, hypoxemia, physical stimuli, pharmacologic agents or intoxication, and specific physiologic insults may all be involved.

Diagnosis is made on the basis of history and physical evaluation and is confirmed by results of blood gas analysis. Typically, elevated pH and diminished P_{CO_2} and bicarbonate values are noted in the acute period. Chronic respiratory alkalosis may not affect pH values as compensation occurs. Diminished P_{CO_2} and bicarbonate values persist until the disturbance is corrected.

Metabolic Acidosis

Nonrespiratory acidosis is referred to as metabolic acidosis, although primary metabolic changes often have little influence on its development. In acidosis of this origin, plasma bicarbonate values diminish significantly with development of an acidic pH. The diminished bicarbonate level may be caused by secretory loss (diarrhea, certain renal diseases) or by consumption of bicarbonate in response to the production of fixed nonvolatile acid (ketoacidosis, lactic acidosis). Buffering of the nonvolatile acid results in transformation of hydrogen ion to carbon dioxide and permits elimination by ventilation. Nonbicarbonate buffers can sequester some of the exogenous acid but may not contribute to ultimate excretion. If the fixed acid is not fully buffered by bicarbonate, pH initially falls without respiratory response. It may take 12 to 24 hours for full ventilatory response to develop, reflecting the delayed passage of hydrogen ion across the blood-brain barrier to stimulate central ventilatory control mechanisms. Despite the delay, CSF pH reflects blood pH values and ventilatory drive is initiated, causing pulmonary acid excretion as carbon dioxide. The degree of ventilatory response is proportional to the underlying metabolic component, but the compensatory process stops short of normalizing pH; this may be a reflection of the interrelated aspects of hydrogen ion and carbon dioxide on control of respiration.

With low plasma bicarbonate concentration, less bicarbonate is filtered through the glomeruli. Increased bicarbonate absorption occurs in the proximal tubule to maintain a higher blood level of HCO_3^-. The additional hydrogen ion appears in the urine as titratable acid. The lower the plasma bicarbonate levels, the more acid the urine. The acid loss adds buffer to the blood, and pH rises in the presence of normal renal function. Increased excretion of ammonium ion also occurs. This process is more active as acidosis persists. In many cases, potassium ion moves into the extracellular space and may be lost through renal elimination.

Metabolic acidosis may be a component of a variety of medical and surgical disorders. The gastrointestinal tract and the kidney can excrete bicarbonate. Excessive loss of bicarbonate from either source can contribute to metabolic acidosis. Diminished microcirculation from hypoperfusion allows accumulation of metabolic acids. Factors contributing to development of metabolic acidosis may be divided into those occurring with normal renal function and those occurring with abnormal renal function.

With normal renal function, bicarbonate losses are confined to gastrointestinal losses. Copious quantities of bicarbonate are secreted daily by the pancreas and small intestine. Diarrhea, emesis, or fistula drainage can lead to acid-base disturbance. The kidney attempts to secrete excess acid to compensate for the bicarbonate loss but is not successful in all cases, especially if the loss is large and rapid. Dehydration may further contribute to the severity of acidosis. Exogenous or endogenous accumulation of metabolic acid is also important. Administration of ammonium chloride, salicylates, paraldehyde, or ethylene glycol may result in metabolic acidosis. Disturbances in normal metabolism may result in production of acidic compounds in excess of renal excretory capacity. Altered substrate metabolism (diabetes) or the inability to utilize oxygen for metabolism (exercise, shock, cyanide intoxication, lactic acidosis) are factors in acid production during abnormal metabolic states.

Functional disturbance in renal hydrogen ion secretion and bicarbonate conservation produces or exacerbates metabolic acidosis. Functional disturbance may be broadly subcategorized into disturbances in renal tubular balance and reductions in parenchymal mass. Disturbances in renal tubular balance may occur in either the proximal or the distal tubule, with renal tubular acidosis (RTA) the result. Proximal RTA is characterized by bicarbonate loss, and distal RTA results from hydrogen ion secretion failure. Proximal RTA is associated with loss of sodium bicarbonate due to absence of hydrogen ion secretion. Distal RTA reflects one of several factors: carbonic anhydrase inhibiting agents, failure of ammonium production, hypoaldosteronism, and hyperchloremia of the distal tubules. Reduction in nephron mass to 25 per cent of normal invariably results in metabolic acidosis because of the reduction in ammonium ion excretion. Individual nephrons may excrete ammonium ion in higher quantities, but total ammonium elimination is reduced. Bicarbonate resorption remains unchanged or is mildly increased when there is a loss of functional nephrons.

In the acute phase, signs of metabolic acidosis reflect cardiovascular and central nervous system changes. Severe acidosis (pH < 7.1) predisposes the myocardium to arrhythmias. Diminished myocardial contractility (ionotrophy) and alterations in vascular tone also occur. Signs of altered mental status have been documented, but the incidence appears lower than in respiratory-mediated disturbances. Ventilatory response occurs shortly after initiation of the disturbance. In chronic acidemia, decalcification of bone salts to buffer hydrogen ion has been noted. Growth retardation occurs in the young patient with marked metabolic acidosis; serum HCO_3^- levels decrease approximately 1 mEq/l for every 1-mEq/l increase in the anion gap (elevated anion gap acidosis); P_{CO_2} decreases 1.2 torr for every 1-mEq/l reduction in HCO_3^- (see Table 10–3).

Two groups of metabolic acidosis can be identified on the basis of the anion gap equation. A normal "gap" of measured cations and anions exists, reflecting the presence of unmeasured ions. Using this principle, two classes of acidemia have been identified: elevated anion gap and normal anion gap, or hyperchloremic acidosis (see Table 10–4). Acidosis of elevated anion gap origin may be due to uremia, ketoacidosis, lactic acidosis, or intoxication with ethylene glycol and salicylates. Hyperchloremic acidosis results from diarrhea, renal tubular acidosis, carbonic anhydrase agents, or rapid intravenous therapy. Elevated anion gap usually reflects direct or indirect losses of bicarbonate ion. Hyperchloremic acidosis generally reflects accumulation of hydrogen ion by incomplete elimination of bicarbonate loss with chloride retention.

Metabolic Alkalosis

Metabolic alkalosis is a common acid-base disorder characterized by primary elevation of plasma bicarbonate concentration with a reciprocal reduction in plasma chloride concentration. Development of metabolic alkalosis generally reflects increased activity of buffer base or buffer base precursors as well as loss of nonvolatile acid. Contributory factors in the development of metabolic alkalosis include administration of exogenous base substances, gastrointestinal loss or sequestration of nonvolatile acid, and increased loss of urinary hydrogen ion from many causes. Regardless of the underlying disturbance, most compensatory mechanisms of metabolic alkalosis are renally mediated. Renal integrity, electrolyte values, and therapeutic course must be evaluated to prevent further metabolic disturbances.

With excess bicarbonate load, the normal kidney excretes bicarbonate in order to eliminate excess base buffer. The renal response to elevations in blood bicarbonate is rapid under these circumstances. However, certain factors can cause the kidney to maintain bicarbonate. These factors, including chloride and potassium deficiencies and hypermineralocorticoidism, cause excess renal resorption of bicarbonate and prevent bicarbonate loss; metabolic alkalosis is thus sustained. Three mechanisms participate in the retention of bicarbonate: (1) Glomerular filtration rate (GFR) may fall reciprocally as arterial bicarbonate concentration rises; if GFR remains constant, then (2) enhanced proximal tubular resorption of bicarbonate or (3) distal nephron conservation must occur. One or more of these factors can be activated by potassium and chloride deficiencies or hypermineralocorticoidism. The relationship between these factors has not fully been defined. The role of potassium in maintenance of alkalosis is unclear, but the interaction of hypokalemia and hyperchloremia to sustain metabolic alkalosis is well established. Mineralocorticoids promote distal tubular acidification. Activation of mineralocorticoids may be related to enhanced sodium delivery, nonresorbable anions, and potassium deficiency. Whether hyperadrenocorticoidism is a primary or secondary event, the net result is development of sustained alkalosis.

Clinical examples of metabolic alkalosis include overalkalinization in acidosis therapy, gastric alkalosis from emesis, overadministration of thiazide or potent loop diuretics (furosemide), and secondary response to chronic respiratory retention of carbon dioxide. Primary hyperadrenocorticism (aldosteronism) also induces metabolic alkalosis (see Table 10–4). Signs are uncommon in metabolic alkalosis, but they may mimic those of hypocalcemia. They include: alteration in mental status, seizures, paresthesia, and tetany. Dysrhythmias may be seen. Signs attributable to coexistent electrolyte abnormalities, such as hypokalemia and hypophosphatemia, may also occur. Slight respiratory depression may occur in severe cases.

Diagnosis is made on the basis of blood gas parameters and coexisting electrolyte changes. Measuring urine pH may be beneficial in discriminating the disorder. P_{CO_2} increases 0.5 to 1.0 torr for every 1-mEq/l increase in HCO_3^- (see Table 10–3).

Mixed Acid-Base Disturbances

The previous discussion defined the four primary alterations in acid-base disturbance and indicated the expected response. Changes in individual parameters induced by the initial disturbance provide two distinct, but important conclusions: *Overcompensation* of the primary disorder is rare, and deviation from the guidelines may suggest coexistence of more than one primary disturbance.

Multiple disturbances are not usually encountered but should be considered in interpretation of values (see Table 10–2). It is not possible for primary respiratory acidosis and alkalosis to coexist in the same animal. Under rare circumstances, triple acid-base disorders have been documented. The key to recognition is an underlying comprehension of the pathophysiologic effects of simple disorders. Each disorder, individually, alters acid-base and electrolyte parameters in a predictable manner.

Compensation

The two major acid-base regulatory components, metabolic and respiratory, are complementary in their effects. Maintenance of normal acid-base equilibrium frequently results in a mixed response for compensation. Respiratory compensation is rapidly responsive to alterations in metabolic acid-base equilibrium. An adjustment in alveolar ventilation either reduces or accentuates elimination of carbon dioxide. The adjustment to alveolar ventilation is controlled by pH-sensitive receptors in the carotid bodies and by respiratory centers on the ventrolateral surface of the brain. These "sensitive" areas mediate the degree of response to the metabolic abnormality. Because hydrogen ion does not rapidly traverse the blood-brain barrier, a slow equilibration of bicarbonate levels occurs between the circulation and the cerebrospinal fluid. The normal pH of cerebrospinal fluid is between 7.30 and 7.36. These factors cause an opposite change in CSF pH with metabolic disorders and a negative influence by the medullary centers on the carotid bodies' attempt to compensate. An additional factor is the effect of P_{O_2} on the carotid body. Pa_{O_2} values less than 70 torr stimulate the carotid bodies more than pH. This fact partially explains the inability of the lungs to compensate effectively for metabolic alkalosis by marked hypoventilation. Although chemoreceptors respond to pH, pH is determined by the $HCO_3^- = CO_2$ ratio, thus influencing ventilatory response. Transport of HCO_3^- is slow, and CSF pH requires up to 48 hours to readjust following a disturbance in Pa_{CO_2}. This temporal disparity reduces the maximum compensatory response initiated by the carotid body.

Metabolic compensation is mediated by the kidneys but requires activation and may not be fully functional for 10 to 48 hours after initial disturbance, suggesting that metabolic compensation cannot be relied upon in many cases of acute disturbance.

Respiratory compensation is seldom complete, whereas metabolic mechanisms can restore normal pH values. Overcompensation probably does not exist as a primary process but may reflect additional factors. The duration of acid-base disturbance is useful in evaluating the patient's response. Metabolic compensation is deferred as long as three to five days after initial disturbance. Respiratory compensation for nonrespiratory disorders is maximal within eight to 12 hours.

COLLECTION OF BLOOD GAS SAMPLES

Accurate blood gas analysis or titration technique depends upon adherence to appropriate collection technique. Arterial sites are preferred. Central venous samples provide data with respect to acid-base status, but no conclusions regarding respiratory function can be inferred from their analysis. Peripheral capillary samples for microassay may be accurate if free-flowing capillary blood is collected by appropriate methods. Use of tourniquets or flow impedance from vasoconstriction produces inaccuracies.

Arterial blood collection sites include the femoral

and dorsal metatarsal arteries in the awake animal; the brachial, lingual, and radial arteries may be used in the anesthetized animal. Restraint-induced excitement should be minimized to prevent inaccuracies. The hair and skin over the sample site should be appropriately prepared prior to sample collection. Indwelling catheters may be used for repetitive sampling.

Glass syringes are preferred for blood collection for gas analysis. Oxygen tension in excess of 120 torr may fall in plastic syringes, but blood P_{CO_2}, pH, and bicarbonate values are not affected. Although syringe material was reported to affect measurement, early reports of oxygen absorption by plastic syringes have been subsequently refuted. Most authors still suggest that glass syringes are preferred for several reasons: (1) minimal friction between the glass barrel and plunger allows confirmation of arterial puncture and filling pressure; (2) minimal plunger withdrawal decreases the risk of air bubble introduction; and (3) small air bubbles are dislodged more easily from a glass syringe barrel. Despite these theoretical advantages, most clinicians routinely use plastic syringes with acceptable results. New designs allow for collection without air bubble introduction and circumvent some of the previously cited disadvantages. Needle size varies with personal preference but a 25-gauge, ⅝-inch needle is useful in all but large dogs. In large dogs, a 22- or 23-gauge, 1-inch needle is preferred. If arterial catheterization is desired, a variety of indwelling catheters are available. Polyethylene or Teflon catheter materials are preferred, as silicone catheters are gas-permeable and may affect values obtained from the sample.

Prior to collection, an anticoagulant is introduced into the syringe-needle unit. Heparin is preferred because other anticoagulants (EDTA, CPD, ACD, sodium fluoride, concentrated heparin) may induce changes in acid-base status. Sodium heparin (1000 U/ml) is introduced into the syringe and expelled until residual heparin remains only in the syringe hub (dead space). A consistent volume of blood (i.e., 2 ml) is collected, because dilution of the blood sample by heparin induces changes in measured pH values. Consistency in technique produces repeatable results. Newer prepackaged collection units contain a lyophilized heparin pellet.

Sample collection should be performed anaerobically, so that room air cannot influence results. Slow aspiration of the sample is preferred to minimize air entrapment. Excessive negative pressure on the syringe may cause separation of gases from the collection sample. Room air has a P_{O_2} of approximately 150 torr and a P_{CO_2} of essentially zero. Mixture with the collected sample results in gas equilibration between the air and the blood. Significant lowering of P_{CO_2} and resulting alteration in pH may occur. Also, P_{O_2} will approach the room air value of 150 torr. The greater air volume mixed in, the greater the chance of error. Therefore, collected samples with more than minor gas bubbles should be discarded. Numerous small bubbles with a "foamy" appearance to the blood indicate poor sampling technique, and collection should be repeated. After the needle is withdrawn, rotation of the syringe barrel with the needle pointed up enhances dispersion of heparin and allows air to collect at the liquid surface, thereby facilitating gas expulsion. Blood is introduced to the needle tip and a rubber or cork stopper is placed over the needle tip to maintain an anaerobic environment. Needle crimping is not satisfactory. Newer prepackaged collection units (Auto Stik, Marquest) incorporate a plunger vent to expel gas bubbles automatically during collection.

After collection, immediate analysis is preferred to provide accurate measurements. Delay in evaluation (longer than 15 minutes) permits continued oxygen consumption by the citric acid and cytochrome systems in leukocytes and reticulocytes as well as glycolysis in erythrocytes. Alterations in oxygen, carbon dioxide, and pH values result. If a delay longer than 10 minutes between collection and analysis is expected, the sample should be placed in an ice bath. Failure to cool samples can result in significant alteration in P_{O_2}, P_{CO_2}, and pH.

INTERPRETATION OF BLOOD GAS VALUES [1, 3, 13, 16, 25, 28, 29]

The goal of interpetation of acid-base disorders is to establish a diagnosis on which rational treatment can be based. Prior to interpretation of laboratory "values," a clinical impression should be established by reviewing the patient's history and the clinical findings. Information about preexisting drug therapy, disease, and current therapy and support techniques should also be considered. Results of urinalysis and plasma electrolyte determinations are also useful.

Blood is the most accessible medium for evaluation. Although bicarbonate/carbonic acid is not the only acid-base system present in the blood, it is extensively evaluated because: (1) the variables of pH, P_{CO_2}, and bicarbonate ion are easily measured or derived; (2) a direct relationship exists between P_{CO_2} and pulmonary ventilation; (3) quantification of changes in metabolic acid-base balance can be expressed by bicarbonate ion change; (4) quantitatively, the bicarbonate/carbon dioxide system accounts for 50 per cent of the body's buffering capacity; and (5) evaluation of oxygen dynamics in the vascular compartment can be appreciated. The most important factors in interpretation of acid-base disturbances are: to determine the involvement of respiratory/metabolic components, to ascertain the cause(s) of the disturbance, and to devise therapeutic regimens appropriate for the underlying disorder. As previously discussed, the four primary alterations in acid-base balance form the basis for data interpretation. In addition, the Henderson-Hasselbalch equation is useful in determining the primary disturbance and direction, or trend, of response.

Analysis of obtained data should be performed in a logical, consistent manner. The interrelationship of pH, P_{O_2}, and P_{CO_2} can be appreciated for evaluation of the respiratory component. Similarly, pH, HCO_3^-, and base excess values represent measured metabolic parameters. Once the primary disturbances are established, one must determine whether compensation is present and evaluate the magnitude of the response (compensated, partially compensated, uncompensated); this evaluation is the most interpretative and prone to discussion. Analytical breakdown of blood gas data follows.

The first consideration is evaluation of pH. Subsequent evaluation of the metabolic and respiratory components determines the contribution to this value as described by the Henderson-Hasselbalch equation. Multiple studies have shown a general range of pH in normal dogs and cats to be 7.35 to 7.45. Values of pH less than 7.35 represent an increase in hydrogen ion concentration (acidosis), and values greater than 7.45 represent a decrease in hydrogen ion concentration (alkalosis).

Similar normal values have been noted for P_{O_2}, P_{CO_2}, and bicarbonate levels in arterial blood. Only pH, P_{O_2}, and P_{CO_2} are directly measured; bicarbonate, base excess, and total CO_2 are derived from nomograms. The normal ranges of P_{O_2} in dogs and cats are 86 to 97 torr and 101 to 112 torr, respectively. The normal ranges of P_{CO_2} in dogs is 34 to 40 torr and in cats 28 to 34 torr. Normal bicarbonate levels are 20 to 24 mEq/l in dogs and 16 to 19 mEq/l in cats. Using these values for normal, one can note differences and infer underlying disorders.

Quantitation of Respiratory Disturbances

Evaluation of pH, P_{O_2}, and P_{CO_2} values aid assessment of respiratory status. Arterial P_{CO_2} values reflect effective minute ventilation of the lungs. Oxygen values may also reflect change if inspired oxygen concentration is not enriched. If hypoventilation occurs with retention of carbon dioxide ($Pa_{CO_2} > 45$ torr), elevation in carbonic acid concentration occurs with development of respiratory acidosis. Conversely, augmentation of minute ventilation with elevated carbon dioxide elimination ($Pa_{CO_2} < 35$ torr) diminishes carbonic acid levels and results in respiratory alkalosis. The relationship of pH to P_{CO_2} is fairly predictable over a wide spectrum. Starting at a Pa_{CO_2} of 40 torr, for every 20-torr increase in Pa_{CO_2}, the pH decreases by 0.1 unit, and for every 10-torr decrease in Pa_{CO_2}, the pH increases by 0.1 unit. Change in Pa_{CO_2} is slower (about 3 to 4 torr/minute in apnea), the rate being limited by CO_2 production. Additional information gained from the pH and bicarbonate values indicates chronicity of the disturbance and the primary or compensatory nature of the respiratory change.

The time course of the disturbance may be reflected in the compensation in the metabolic com-

ponent. If compensation is present, changes in metabolic parameters (HCO_3^-, base excess) may be noted. Bicarbonate concentration varies with ventilation, because of the interrelationship noted in the mass action equation. Retention of CO_2 elevates bicarbonate concentration, and lowering CO_2 lowers bicarbonate values. The alterations in bicarbonate levels are reasonably linear and may be summarized as follows:

1. Acute changes in P_{CO_2} above 40 torr change bicarbonate concentration by 1 mEq/l for each 10-torr change in P_{CO_2}.

2. The change in bicarbonate concentration with an acute change in P_{CO_2} below 40 torr is 2 mEq/l for each 10-torr change in P_{CO_2}.

3. The change in bicarbonate concentration with a chronic change in P_{CO_2} greater than 40 torr is 4 mEq/l for each 10-torr change in P_{CO_2}.

4. The change in bicarbonate with a chronic change in P_{CO_2} of less than 40 torr is 5 to 6 mEq/l for each 10-torr change in P_{CO_2}.

Changes in metabolic indices in excess of these values suggest a primary metabolic component in addition to respiratory-induced changes.

Arterial oxygenation should be evaluated for the presence of hypoxemia ($Pa_{O_2} < 70$ torr). This is the only direct information that can be obtained about ventilatory status. Hypoxemia can be diagnosed only if the patient is breathing room air; however, indications may be obtained with the patient breathing air enriched with oxygen. Significance of the disturbance in oxygenation may be derived by analysis of alveolar-arterial difference in oxygen values or calculation of $\dot{Q}s/\dot{Q}t$ (shunt). If either of these parameters is increased, hypoventilation or elevation of intrapulmonary vascular shunting should be considered.

Quantitation of Metabolic Disturbances

Evaluation of metabolic disturbance relies on analysis of pH and parameters reflecting nonvolatile (metabolic) components. These components usually consist of bicarbonate and base excess values. Analysis of anion gap is also meaningful in aiding evaluation. Decreased bicarbonate levels with lowered pH values suggest metabolic acidosis. Elevated pH values with increased bicarbonate levels suggest metabolic alkalosis. Base excess values are also useful in measurement of metabolic contribution, although respiratory-mediated influences may also be operating.

Analysis of pH is the cornerstone of interpretation. Interaction of pH and bicarbonate during interpretation suggests the contribution of changes in metabolic parameters. A decrease in pH (acidosis) with simultaneous decrease in bicarbonate values suggests metabolic acidosis. A pH-HCO_3^- interrelationship can indicate the severity of the disturbance. Conversely, elevation in pH values concurrent with an

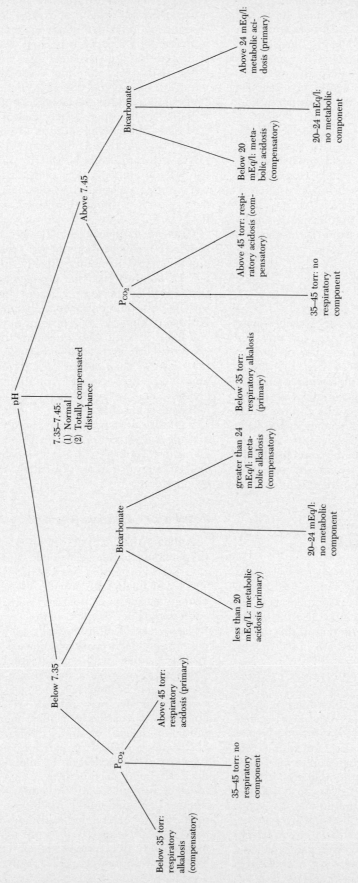

Figure 10–2. Interpretation of acid-base balance in an arterial sample.

increase in bicarbonate level may reflect metabolic alkalosis. Interactive changes in ventilation, as reflected by P_{CO_2} values, also indicates magnitude and duration of disturbance as well as of compensation. The parameter that has changed in the direction of the pH is the primary disturbance, with compensation occurring through the alternate pathway.

From Figure 10–2, the interaction of metabolic and respiratory components can be appreciated. Disturbance in one component usually elicits a compensatory response in the opposite component. If both are altered in the same direction, the presence of two primary problems must be considered. pH values in the normal range may signify a totally compensated disturbance in acid-base balance. Primary respiratory disorders are seldom fully compensated; metabolic disorders may chronically result in full compensation. This aspect may be appreciated from the history and underlying pathophysiologic processes.

THERAPY [5, 6, 9, 12, 16, 26, 28, 29]

Once an acid-base disturbance or oxygen-related disease is identified, appropriate therapy must be instituted. The progression and severity of the underlying lesion is determined so that therapy is appropriate. As a general principle, acute lesions are treated quickly and chronic lesions are treated slowly. Rapid intervention and correction of a chronic lesion may unbalance compensatory mechanisms that have begun to operate. Likewise, conservative management of an acute lesion may not be appropriate. In certain cases, such as diabetic ketoacidosis, correction of the underlying metabolic lesion results in restoration of acid-base balance.

Respiratory-Related Disturbances

Primary respiratory-related disturbances are usually associated with an inadequate delivery of oxygen or retention of carbon dioxide. Compensation for primary metabolic disturbances may also be noted. Therapy is directed toward correction of the underlying lesion.

Oxygen Disturbances

If hypoxemia is confirmed by blood gas analysis, oxygen therapy is indicated. The only direct effects of supplemental oxygenation are improved alveolar oxygen tensions, decreased work of breathing, and decreased myocardial work to maintain oxygenation. Clinical response to oxygen supplementation may be dramatic. Usually, concentrations less than 100 per cent effect clinical response. Diminution of respiratory rate and effort and of apprehension are noted.

Oxygen may be delivered by artificial airway (tracheostomy, endotracheal catheter), face mask, or nasal catheter. Commercially available oxygen enclosures (cages) may also improve inspired oxygen tension. Therapy may be titrated by use of an air-oxygen mixer or by adjustment of oxygen flow rates. Clinical response is indicative of adequate support as well as improvement of oxygen tension ($Pa_{O_2} > 60$ torr) as indicated by arterial blood gas analysis. Diseases other than true shunting respond rapidly (15–20 minutes) to oxygen therapy. Failure of response suggests that additional factors should be considered. If there is no response, mechanical ventilatory support and further identification of underlying disease should be considered. Refractory hypoxemia usually exists with cardiovascular shunts, pulmonary vascular fistulas (i.e., neoplastic metastasis), alveolar atelectasis, surfactant-related diseases, and acute pulmonary injury (respiratory distress syndrome, shock lung).

High levels of oxygen (70–100 per cent) may be required during cardiopulmonary resuscitation or cardiopulmonary instability. Ideally, high levels should not be administered for prolonged periods (longer than 24–48 hours) to prevent development of oxygen toxicity with pulmonary epithelial injury and fibrosis. However, high oxygen concentrations should not be withheld if they are indicated. In general, little additional benefit is achieved from oxygen concentrations greater than 50 per cent. True shunting is not improved, hemoglobin saturation cannot be increased, and tissue tensions are not improved by higher concentrations.

If coexistent hypercapnia is noted with diminished oxygen concentration, ventilatory failure is present. Clinical response will not be achieved solely by oxygen administration; ventilatory support must also be provided.

Respiratory Acidosis (Ventilatory Failure)

Animals that exhibit retention of carbon dioxide (hypercapnia) with or without diminished oxygenation have respiratory acidosis or ventilatory failure. They are unable to provide muscular work to exchange an adequate volume of air for elimination of carbon dioxide. Hypercapnia may be accompanied by a variety of clinical signs, e.g., the animal may have rapid, labored respiration or apnea. Little response is noted with supplemental oxygen. Accompanying tachycardia, hypertension, and altered mental state may be noted.

Many insults may produce respiratory acidosis; alteration in ventilatory control mechanisms, neuromuscular disease or injury, thoracic injury, airway obstruction, pleural or parenchymal disease, anesthesia, and compensation for metabolic disturbances have all been documented. Support of ventilation must be provided until the underlying factor can be reversed or ameliorated. Application of supplemental techniques, positive end expiratory pressure, or continuous positive airway pressure may also be considered. These techniques are described elsewhere. Ventilatory support is palliative until therapy of the underlying disorder is instituted and response is noted.

Respiratory Alkalosis

Respiratory alkalosis may be secondary to pulmonary disease. There are three primary causes of respiratory alkalosis: chemoceptor response to hypoxemia, ventilatory response to metabolic acidosis, and central nervous system stimulation (e.g., pain, excitement, disease-mediated response). If hypoxemia is present, primary cardiopulmonary lesions should be considered. Alveolar disease, myocardial lesions, pulmonary edema, postoperative compromise, pregnancy, and musculoskeletal disease affecting ventilation represent possible causes in which carbon dioxide exchange is adequate but oxygen demands are not met. In these cases, hyperventilation reflects oxygen deficiency and may be corrected by the administration of oxygen. Respiratory alkalosis without hypoxemia is usually secondary to CNS-mediated events represented by pain and excitement. Anemia or carbon monoxide poisoning may also be reflected in respiratory alkalosis. In these cases, correction of the underlying disturbance eliminates the alkalosis.

Metabolic Disturbances

Metabolic Acidosis

With the exception of lactic acidosis, metabolic acidosis is rarely due to primary pulmonary disease. The underlying cause of the metabolic acidosis should be treated. If pH is 7.20 or greater, metabolic therapy is the only intervention necessary. However, if the pH is 7.20 or less, or if the underlying cause cannot be corrected in a reasonable time, administration of alkalizing salts is indicated.

Sodium bicarbonate is the preferred alkalizing agent. Sodium lactate and sodium acetate have also been used for this purpose, but they offer no advantage over administration of sodium bicarbonate. The deficit of bicarbonate is usually derived from the formula:

$$0.3 \times \text{body weight (kg)} \times \text{base deficit} = \text{net bicarbonate requirement}$$

Base deficit is derived from the base excess equation or by subtracting actual bicarbonate values from desired bicarbonate values. The factor of 0.3 is a value for interstitial fluid volume. In severe acidosis, a factor of 0.6 (total body water) may be substituted. If total correction is not desired, an alternative formula may be used:

$$\text{Bicarbonate dose} = (\tfrac{1}{2} P_{CO_2} - [HCO_3^-] \times 0.5 \text{ body wt (kg)}$$

Alternatively, one may infuse a portion ($\tfrac{1}{4}$ to $\tfrac{1}{2}$) of the total calculated deficit and remeasure parameters in 30 to 60 minutes. In this time, distribution in the interstitial space is almost complete (98 per cent). The distribution of bicarbonate into the intracellular space is slow, requiring up to 18 hours. Acid-base measurements of extracellular fluid may not reflect intracellular pH. Therefore, conservative replacement and measurement are recommended. A dynamic state exists during therapy. Therefore, the calculated requirement may require modification. Origin of acidosis, distribution of bicarbonate, and correction of the underlying disorder affect therapy. Continuous bicarbonate loss, production of metabolic acids, and depletion of bicarbonate and other buffer systems in chronic, severe metabolic acidosis may require therapy in excess of calculated values.

Potential hazards of bicarbonate infusion exist. Hyperosmolality in a range detrimental to cerebral function has been observed to occur with rapid infusion of bicarbonate. An increase in CO_2 production as hydrogen ion is buffered may exacerbate preexisting pulmonary disease and cause respiratory acidosis. Alkalization of blood is not immediately accompanied by pH equilibrium in cerebrospinal fluid. This paradoxic shift in CSF pH is attributed to an increase in P_{CO_2} and an absence of change in bicarbonate concentration. A decrease in minute volume due to extracellular pH change mediates retention of P_{CO_2} centrally with development of acidosis in CSF. Hypokalemia may result from transcellular shift in hydrogen ion in exchange for potassium. Hypocalcemia has also been noted. Hypernatremia can occur from administration of sodium salts of bicarbonate and intravascular volume expansion may be noted.

Metabolic Alkalosis

Metabolic alkalosis may be pure or mixed. It is compensated by depression of ventilation with development of respiratory acidosis, but the compensatory mechanism is limited by activation of oxygen receptors from decreased Pa_{O_2}. Compensation may also be impaired by chronic respiratory disease, cardiac failure, and hepatic coma. Adverse effects of chronic alkalemia include: (1) left shift of the oxyhemoglobin dissociation curve, inhibiting release of oxygen, (2) muscle irritability, (3) decrease in hypoxic respiratory drive, and (4) cardiac dysrhythmias. Mortality rate increases with pH values consistently in excess of pH 7.54 and reaches 80 per cent when pH exceeds 7.65.

Therapy of metabolic alkalosis involves correction of underlying disturbances. Administration of normal saline (0.9 per cent NaCl) corrects volume depletion associated with alkalosis as well as replaces chloride ions. It also attentuates alkalosis associated with elevated aldosterone levels. Administration of supplemental potassium salts is beneficial. Efficacy of potassium administration without chloride ion is controversial, as most studies suggest that chloride is the therapeutic ion. Saline-resistant metabolic alkalosis has also been documented and is associated with elevated mineralocorticoid production, e.g., due to

Cushing's syndrome, corticosteroid therapy, magnesium deficiency, and diuretic-induced potassium loss. Treatment consists of removal of the cause, correction of electrolyte balance, and blockage of mineralocorticoid activity.

Immediate therapy may be provided by giving acetazolamide or dilute hydrochloric acid, if the underlying etiology cannot be corrected.

1. Adams, A. P., and Hahn, C. E. W.: Principles and Practice of Blood-Gas Analysis. W. S. Cowell Ltd., Butler Market, Ipswich, 1979.
2. Arruda, J. A. L., and Kurtzman, N. H.: Metabolic acidosis and alkalosis. Clin. Nephrol. 7:201, 1977.
3. Bright, R. M., and McIntosh, J. J.: Clinical application of arterial blood gases in companion animals. Calif. Vet. 7:20, 1981.
4. Brobst, D.: Evaluation of clinical disorders of acid-base balance. J. Am. Vet. Med. Assoc. 166:359, 1975.
5. Brobst, D.: Pathophysiologic and adaptive changes in acid-base disorders. J. Am. Vet. Med. Assoc. 183:773, 1983.
6. Cogan, M. G., Liu, F., Berger, B. E., et al.: Metabolic alkalosis. Med. Clin. North Am. 67:903, 1983.
7. Comroe, J. H.: Physiology of Respiration. 2nd ed. Year Book Medical Publishers, Chicago, 1974.
8. Dohoo, S. E., McDonell, W. N., and Dohoo, I. R.: A comparison of fresh gas flows during anesthesia with nitrous oxide in the dog. J. Am. Anim. Hosp. Assoc. 18:900, 1982.
9. DuBose, T. D.: Clinical approach to patients with acid-base disorders. Med. Clin. North Am. 67:799, 1983.
10. Garella, S., Chang, B. S., and Kahn, S. I.: Dilutional acidosis and contraction alkalosis. Kidney Int. 8:279, 1975.
11. Guyton, A. C.: Textbook of Physiology. 4th ed. W. B. Saunders, Philadelphia, 1971.
12. Hartsfield, S. M., Thurmon, J. C., and Benson, G. J.: Sodium bicarbonate and bicarbonate precursors for treatment of metabolic acidosis. J. Am. Vet. Med. Assoc. 179:914, 1981.
13. Haskins, S. C.: An overview of acid-base physiology. J. Am. Vet. Med. Assoc. 170:423, 1977.
14. Haskins, S. C.: Sampling and storage of blood for pH and blood gas analysis. J. Am. Vet. Med. Assoc. 170:429, 1977.
15. Haskins, S. C., and Knapp, R. G.: Effect of low carrier gas flows on inspired oxygen tension in anesthetized dogs. J. Am. Vet. Med. Assoc. 180:735, 1982.
16. Haskins, S. C.: Blood gases and acid-base balance: Clinical interpretation and therapeutic implications. In Kirk, R. W. (ed.): Current Veterinary Therapy VIII. W. B. Saunders, Philadelphia, 1983.
17. Holt, J. C.: Blood pH and plasma bicarbonate determination: A practitioner's viewpoint. J. Am. Anim. Hosp. Assoc. 8:448, 1972.
18. Huber, G. L.: Aarterial blood gas and acid-base physiology. Upjohn Company, Kalamazoo, 1978.
19. Kaehny, W. D.: Respiratory acid-base disorders. Med. Clin. North Am. 67:915, 1983.
20. Laski, M. E.: Normal regulation of acid-base balance: Renal and pulmonary response and other extrarenal buffering mechanisms. Med. Clin. North Am. 67:771, 1983.
21. Masoro, E. J., and Siegel, P. D.: Acid-Base Regulation: Its Physiology, Pathophysiology and the Interpretation of Blood-Gas Analysis. 2nd ed. W. B. Saunders, Philadelphia, 1977.
22. Nauns, R. G., and Emmett, M.: Simple and mixed acid-base disorders: A practical approach. Medicine 59:161, 1980.
23. Polzin, D. J., Stevens, J. B., and Osborne, C. A.: Clinical application of the anion gap in evaluation of acid-base disorders in dogs. Comp. Cont. Ed. Pract. Vet. 4:102, 1982.
24. Rodkey, W. G., Hannon, J. P., Dramise, J. G., et al.: Arterialized capillary blood used to determine the acid-base and blood gas status of dogs. Am. J. Vet. Res. 39:459, 1978.
25. Rosenthal, M. H.: Acid-base equilibrium and blood-gas measurement. In Miller, R. D. (ed.): Anesthesia. Churchill Livingstone, New York, 1981.
26. Sabatini, S., Arruda, J. A. L., and Kurtzman, N. A.: Disorders of acid-base balance. Med. Clin. North Am. 62:1223, 1978.
27. Sabatini, S.: The acidosis of chronic renal failure. Med. Clin. North Am. 67:845, 1983.
28. Schaer, M.: A practical review of simple acid-base disorders. Vet. Clin. North Am. 12:439, 1982.
29. Shapiro, B. A., Harrison, R. A., and Walton, J. R.: Clinical Application of Blood Gases. 3rd ed. Year Book Medical Publishers, Chicago, 1982.
30. Shoemaker, W. C.: Fluids and electrolytes in the acutely ill adult. In Shoemaker, W. C., Thompson, W. L., and Holbrook, P. R. (eds.): Textbook of Critical Care. W. B. Saunders, Philadelphia, 1984.
31. Stevens, J. B.: Teaching Monograph of Acid-Base Physiology. University of Minnesota, 1982.

Chapter **11**

Shock: Pathophysiology and Management

Sandee M. Hartsfield

INTRODUCTION

The term *shock* has been used medically for more than 200 years.[119] One definition, "inadequate blood flow to vital organs or the inability of the body cell mass to metabolize nutrients normally,"[84] indicates that the pathophysiology of shock includes primary cellular alterations as well as secondary cellular derangement. Therefore, shock is a severe pathophysiological abnormality due to or associated with abnormal cellular metabolism, which is usually due to poor tissue perfusion.[124]

Shock initially described clinical injury, that is, the typical appearance of a hypovolemic patient and the lack of explanation for death. With increased monitoring, shock was equated with hypotension. In World War II, studies of battle casualties led to the conclusion that the major cause of shock was hemorrhage and fluid loss, which resulted in metabolic acidosis.[84] Blalock stated that "shock is a peripheral circulatory failure, resulting from a discrepancy in the size of the vascular bed and the volume of intravascular fluid."[109] In the 1960s, cardiac output measurements influenced the definition; shock was described as "decreased blood flow to vital organs."[84] Thus, blood pressure might be low, but cardiac output could vary; some patients could survive with low blood pressure if cardiac output and tissue perfusion remained adequate.

Recent studies of septic shock indicate that some patients have sufficient blood flow to vital tissues but develop characteristic signs of shock (elevated arterial blood lactate level, hypotension, and oliguria). Therefore, shock includes those situations in which utilization of nutrients is impaired, even with apparently normal nutrient availability.[84, 85] Shock as a medical term has progressed from a clinical description of typical signs and responses following severe injury to implications regarding abnormalities of metabolism at the cellular and subcellular levels related to decreased total blood flow, maldistribution of blood flow, or a primary cellular defect.[67, 84, 111]

Various kinds of shock have been studied extensively in various animal species using experimental methods, but there are inherent problems in the transfer of information from species to species. Also, erroneous assumptions can result from the application of information from "pure" shock models to clinical shock, in which multiple forms may coexist.

TYPES OF CIRCULATORY SHOCK

Shock has been classified according to the factors producing the characteristic circulatory changes. The broad categories of circulatory insults include decreased effective circulating blood volume and inadequate cardiac function. Circulating blood volume may be impaired by extracellular fluid loss or by increased vascular capacitance.[30] Recent outlines[77, 84] expand shock to include another major etiological division, maldistribution of blood flow. Thus, the classification of shock includes hypovolemic, vasculogenic, cardiogenic, and maldistributive categories (Table 11–1).

Hypovolemic Shock

Hypovolemic shock is characterized by low blood pressure, cardiac output, and central venous pressure (CVP); increased peripheral vascular resistance; and increased arteriovenous O_2 difference.[77, 84, 111] It may result from acute hemorrhage, plasma loss, or generalized depletion of extracellular fluid, but it is a real loss of fluid volume compared with vasculogenic shock, in which volume depletion is relative.[30]

Trauma and hemorrhage are considered one entity in the production of shock and often occur together.[111]

TABLE 11–1. Classification of Shock with Some Inciting Factors

I. *Hypovolemic Shock* (reduced blood volume)
   A. Blood loss (external, internal, "third space")
   B. Plasma loss (burns, gastrointestinal obstruction, pancreatitis)
   C. Loss of water and electrolytes (vomiting, diarrhea)
II. *Vasculogenic Shock* (peripheral pooling)
   A. Loss of tone in resistance and capacitance vessels
      1. Spinal or epidural anesthesia
      2. Central nervous system lesions causing vasomotor paralysis
      3. Anaphylaxis
   B. Trapping in capacitance vessels—endotoxin infusion in dogs
   C. Prolonged, severe increase in peripheral resistance
III. *Cardiogenic Shock* (decreased ability of the heart as a pump)
   A. Interference with effective cardiac filling
      1. Cardiac tamponade
      2. Positive pressure ventilation
      3. Hemopneumothorax
   B. Improper ventricular emptying
      1. Acute cor pulmonale
      2. Abrupt increase in systemic vascular resistance
      3. Ruptured chordae tendineae
      4. Deep anesthesia or other toxic causes of myocardial depression
      5. Cardiac dysrhythmias
      6. Late hypovolemia
      7. Cardiac infarction
      8. Hemopneumothorax
IV. *Maldistributive Shock* (failure of normal cellular metabolic function related to blood flow maldistribution and oxygen utilization)
   A. Sepsis
   B. Trauma

If trauma is complicated by blood loss greater than 20 per cent of the blood volume, the early cardiorespiratory pattern of traumatic shock is similar to that of hemorrhagic shock.[77] Either can cause "third space" loss of extracellular fluid, probably into ischemic cells and injured tissues.[102] Surgical suction may remove a large quantity of blood and fluid from a surgical site, the total volume of which can be easily underestimated without regular, accurate measurements. Plasma loss occurs with chemical or physical burns and in acute intestinal obstruction by transudation. Loss of water and electrolytes is associated with vomiting, diarrhea, diuresis, and natriuresis of adrenocortical failure.[30] Such fluid loss becomes more significant if fluid and electrolyte replacement is restricted. With reduction of actual fluid volume comes an increase in blood viscosity, causing sluggish blood flow.[100]

Vasculogenic Shock

Vasculogenic shock has been termed *neurogenic shock* because of the associated loss of vasomotor tone.[58] Venous capacitance vessels contain about 80 per cent of the regional blood volume, and changes in smooth muscle tone can shift blood volume and alter venous return.[21]

Shock due to increased venous capacitance is associated with direct infusion of endotoxin in dogs.[84] The syndrome is characterized by failure of venous return, low cardiac index, low blood pressure, rapid pulse, low CVP, and low Pa_{O_2} with increased arteriovenous oxygen difference. Much of the increased vascular capacity in the dog is in the liver and splanchnic vascular beds.[30, 84] Endotoxins from gram-negative bacteria such as *Escherichia coli* or various *Proteus* species may act to release vasoactive substances (e.g., serotonin, histamine, kinins) to produce a rapid decrease in circulating fluid volume. Increased capillary permeability, venoconstriction (in the area of the postcapillary sphincter), and increased capillary pressure promote plasma loss from the vascular system, which compounds the effects of increased vascular capacitance.[30]

Spinal or epidural anesthesia, central nervous system (CNS) depression due to lesions or drugs, and anaphylaxis induce vasculogenic shock by decreasing tone in arteriolar resistance and venous capacitance vessels, thereby increasing vascular capacity. The term *shock* may be misleading in these instances because of differences in syndromes and treatments compared with other types of shock.[83]

Anaphylactic shock is associated with sequestration of as much as 60 per cent of the blood volume in portal vascular beds of dogs.[100] Although clinical responses vary among species,[44, 103] anaphylaxis is caused by a specific antigen-antibody reaction involving previously sensitized cells. Cellular damage releases vasoactive substances, resulting in increased vascular capacity and increased capillary permeability, which promotes extravasation of fluid. Cardiac output is reduced.[100]

Subarachnoid or epidural injections of local analgesics increase vascular capacitance by interfering with sympathetic vasoconstriction.[58] The propensity to develop circulatory shock is determined by the segmental extent of the blockage. There are four potential influences of epidural analgesia on cardiovascular dynamics.[21]

1. Segmental sympathetic efferent blockade with dilation of resistance and capacitance vessels.

2. Paralysis of cardiac sympathetic fibers from the cranial four or five thoracic segments, decreasing chronotropic and inotropic drive, heart rate, and ejection force.

3. Vascular absorption of anesthetic leading to depression of smooth muscle function and cardiac output by beta-receptor blockade, the depressant effects being seen most likely with concurrent acidosis.

4. Vascular absorption of epinephrine, which may be mixed with the local anesthetic, resulting in beta-receptor stimulation leading to an increase in cardiac output but a fall in peripheral vascular resistance.

Spinal or epidural analgesia produces more profound blood pressure changes if a low level of general anesthesia or alpha-blocking drugs (e.g., phenoxybenzamine or acetylpromazine) have been administered previously. Otherwise, unblocked sympathetic activity may maintain a relatively normal cardiovascular status.[21] Subarachnoid and epidural analgesia produce similar neural effects, but less vascular absorption of local anesthetic occurs with the former.[34] Typically, shock due to sympathetic block produces low blood pressure, variable cardiac output, relatively normal pulse rate, and decreased peripheral vascular resistance.[124]

Central nervous system abnormalities due to trauma, disease, or pharmacological depression may promote vasomotor paralysis and increase vascular capacitance. The medullary area of the brain and the thoracolumbar region of the spinal cord are particularly important.[30] However, neurogenic shock from acute head injury in man is rare,[87] and shock is infrequently encountered in uncomplicated head or spinal cord trauma in veterinary patients.[42, 106] In humans and other primates, a sudden, complete, transverse spinal cord injury in which the cord ceases to function below the level of the injury induces a state of "spinal shock."[41, 87] A lesion that affects most of the thoracolumbar area can have significant effects on blood pressure owing to impaired tonic vasoconstrictor impulses from the medullary vasomotor centers. In most instances, perfusion is well maintained, but postural compensation does not occur. The neurological effects of spinal shock are less significant in domestic animals.[41]

The vasomotor centers may be depressed by general anesthetic agents and anesthetic adjuncts, impairing effective vasomotor outflow,[30] vasoconstrictor activity, and cardiac function. Also, prolonged medullary ischemia may induce neurogenic shock by inactivation of vasomotor neurons.[58]

Other initiating causes of vasculogenic shock include acute, severe pain (may be associated with trauma)[58] and other psychological stimuli.[92, 109] In addition, rapid reduction in abdominal pressure by removal of ascitic fluid, an abdominal tumor, or a gravid uterus increases the capacity of abdominal blood vessels and blood reservoirs (e.g., liver and spleen).[58, 100] Finally, a prolonged, severe increase in peripheral vascular resistance has been implicated in the production of vasculogenic shock as a part of the terminal phase of hypovolemic shock;[92] paradoxically, prolonged infusions of potent vasoconstrictors (e.g., norepinephrine) may induce shock.[30]

Cardiogenic Shock

Cardiogenic shock results from a decreased ability of the heart to function as a pump. Cardiac insufficiency develops if the heart does not fill or empty effectively.[30] Classically, cardiogenic shock is associated with human myocardial infarction. Usually, shock occurs after damage to 40 to 70 per cent of the left ventricular myocardium.[124] Unusual in the dog and cat, myocardial infarcts are rarely involved in promoting cardiogenic shock.[47, 100] The patient with cardiogenic shock usually has lowered arterial blood pressure, elevated CVP, decreased cardiac index, lowered arterial O_2 tension, and increased arteriovenous O_2 difference.[30, 84]

Inadequate ejection of blood from the heart that has filled properly can be due to myocardial depression (e.g., deep anesthesia, high epidural or spinal anesthesia with bradycardia),[21] dysrhythmias, or structural alterations such as ruptured chordae tendineae.[30] Also, increased systemic or pulmonary vascular resistance may decrease emptying.

The heart may fail to function effectively if ventricular filling is impaired. Cardiac tamponade (e.g., pericardial effusion), hemo- or pneumothorax, inappropriately applied positive pressure ventilation, and cardiac dysrhythmias can contribute to poor ventricular filling. Pulmonary emboli have been related to cardiogenic shock in man.[84] Some authors have used a classification of obstruction for shock induced by pulmonary embolism or tamponade.[102]

Maldistributive Shock

Maldistribution of blood flow to tissues or a primary impairment in cellular and subcellular utilization of nutrients may cause shock. Septic shock is common in man and is recognized in animals,[62, 77, 123] but the pathophysiology has not been elucidated. Although septic shock is related to endotoxin, the human response is different from that produced by direct infusion of endotoxin in the dog.[84] There are hyperdynamic (warm) and hypodynamic (cold) phases of septic shock. The principal abnormality leading to septic shock may be a cellular defect impairing oxygen and nutrient utilization before any hemodynamic changes are present. However, maldistribution of blood flow has been implicated as well.[84, 124]

In man, fungi, viruses, rickettsiae, gram-positive aerobic bacteria, and gram-negative anaerobic bacteria have been associated with circulatory collapse.[45] In most instances, gram-negative aerobic rods capable of producing endotoxins produce septic shock. *Escherichia coli*, *Klebsiella pneumoniae*, *Proteus* spp., and *Pseudomonas aeruginosa* are the most common pathogens.[11] Human septic shock occurs primarily in hospitalized patients, and a number of predisposing factors have been identified.[45, 84]

1. Neoplastic disease
2. Diabetes mellitus
3. Old age
4. Hypovolemia
5. Steroid therapy
6. Other immunosuppressive therapy
7. Indwelling urinary or intravenous catheters
8. Indiscriminate use of prophylactic antibiotics
9. Cancer chemotherapy
10. Cirrhosis of the liver
11. Tracheostomy
12. Radiation therapy

Such conditions and treatments are common in veterinary patients and may contribute to shock. Common causes of septic shock in veterinary patients have been listed as peritonitis, pyometra, gastroenteritis, and intestinal strangulation.[89] Mastitis, bowel infarction or strangulation, penetrating abdominal wounds, prostatic infections, and contaminated skin wounds can be sources of infection leading to sepsis.[62]

Hyperdynamic shock is the early phase of septic shock. It is characterized by high CVP, increased cardiac output, hyperventilation and respiratory alkalosis, profound hypotension, low peripheral resistance, oliguria, and warm, dry extremities.[84] A hyperdynamic state with nearly twice the normal cardiac output has been demonstrated in canine cecal ligation models of sepsis.[3] Impaired cellular metabolism prevents the proper utilization of oxygen and energy substrates and, therefore, the formation of ATP.[124] This hyperdynamic state may be the result of immunological reactions to various toxins including endotoxin.[104]

Hypodynamic shock appears if sepsis persists and therapy is not aggressive. Endotoxin and lysosomal enzymes contribute to capillary fluid leakage. With fluid loss, cardiac output and CVP are reduced. Cardiac dysfunction promotes the development of hypodynamic shock.[62] At this point, septic shock is similar to vasculogenic or hypovolemic shock.[30, 84]

Traumatic shock, without hypovolemia, produces hemodynamic changes similar to those seen in septic shock.[77] Increased cardiac output, heart rate, stroke volume, and O_2 delivery and decreased arterial pressure, systemic vascular resistance, oxygen extraction, arteriovenous oxygen difference, and O_2 consumption are typical responses. Minute ventilation increases to produce respiratory alkalosis, even without metabolic acidosis.[111] As in septic shock, traumatic shock may progress to a hypodynamic state.

PATHOPHYSIOLOGY OF SHOCK

Basic Changes and Reflex Mechanisms

Although shock may be due to different causes, a common feature is decreased or ineffective blood flow through the microcirculation. When the circulation fails, several mechanisms attempt maintenance of homeostasis,[30] including autoregulation, sympathoadrenal discharge, transmural capillary effects, and conservation and expansion of plasma volume.[26]

Autoregulation maintains renal, coronary, and cerebral blood flow until perfusion pressure is significantly reduced. Because of passive pressure-flow relationships, other tissues are inadequately perfused before the brain, heart, and kidney. Blood flow is maintained in the renal circulation until arterial blood pressure is less than approximately 70 to 80 mm Hg, in the coronary circulation until 60 to 70 mm Hg, and in the cerebral circulation until 50 to 60 mm Hg.[26, 78, 97]

Sympathoadrenal discharge, mediated through baroreceptors, causes arteriolar constriction and increased cardiac rate and contractility, leading to increased perfusion pressure. Sympathoadrenal-induced venoconstriction reduces venous capacitance, leading to improved venous return.[26, 30] This response inhibits circulation to the skin, kidneys, gastrointestinal tract, and muscle mass. Cerebral and coronary circulations are preferentially perfused, both areas showing minimal response to even very intense sympathetic stimulation.[23, 84]

Transmural capillary changes initially favor fluid movement to increase plasma volume. Decreased capillary hydrostatic pressure occurs owing to arteriolar constriction. Thus, oncotic pressure favors interstitial fluid movement into the capillary to restore plasma volume.[26, 30, 84]

Further conservation and expansion of plasma volume are achieved through other mechanisms. Antidiuretic hormone (ADH) and aldosterone promote sodium and water retention. Decreased renal blood flow (pressure) stimulates renin secretion and the subsequent formation of angiotensin, leading to arteriolar constriction and adrenal production of aldosterone. Sodium and water resorption and potassium excretion are enhanced.[26, 30, 84]

If these mechanisms do not restore circulating blood volume adequately, cellular damage occurs owing to ischemia. If tissue ischemia is present long enough prior to the initiation of therapy, shock becomes irreversible and even intense treatment is unsuccessful. Because of these reflex mechanisms, some patients are able to recover from mild or only moderately severe shock.[30]

The Cell in Shock

A recent hypothesis explains progressive cell injury with ischemia.[26, 27] Initially, changes occur when cell membrane potential decreases, possibly owing to circulating catecholamines or other substances. Because of alterations in ion transport systems, sodium moves into the cell, and increased ion transport requires greater utilization of adenosine triphosphate (ATP). Mitochondria are stimulated to produce more energy, decreasing cyclic adenosine monophosphate (AMP) levels and altering the adenyl cyclase system responsiveness. The response to various hormones (e.g., insulin and glucagon) may be impaired. As ATP continues to decrease, more sodium enters the cell, impairing volume regulation of the cell, the mitochondria, and the endoplasmic reticulum. All of these organelles swell. Ultimately, there is decreased metabolic capability (loss and use of ATP substrates),

lysosomal leak, and cellular destruction. Adjoining cells can be damaged, and a cycle of deterioration occurs.

Because of altered cellular function, metabolic substrates that could favorably influence the outcome of shock have been studied. Such compounds were usually administered along with fluids in amounts needed to provide adequate vascular volume. Energy compounds and substrates including glucose, Krebs cycle intermediates, and ATP have been used.[26] Some beneficial effects occur following fumarate or oxaloacetate plus alpha-ketoglutarate infusion.[29] However, other studies suggest both beneficial and nonbeneficial effects of glucose or Krebs cycle intermediates in the treatment of shock.[26] The use of ATP infusion as a direct energy source (along with $MgCl_2$ to improve the availability of ATP)[26, 28] has been successful in improving patient survival following shock. Although the use of ATP in shock remains controversial, a number of studies strongly suggest it is useful. Such evidence seems logical, since ATP is vital to membrane function, carbohydrate metabolism, tissue respiration, and intracellular reactions.[26] Depletion of ATP occurs in shock, and restoration of ATP or prevention of its depletion could minimize cellular dysfunction. Prostacyclin (PGI_2) and fructose-1, 6-diphosphate are beneficial in the survival of experimentally shocked dogs. Both increase levels of ATP.[18]

Organs and Organ Systems in Shock

Once shock begins, ischemia can lead to cell, tissue, and organ failure and, finally, death. All organ systems can become involved, depending on the duration of ischemia and treatment. Some tissues, such as skeletal muscle, appear resistant to anoxia,[36] whereas others are susceptible. The brain is the organ most vulnerable to shock.[102]

The liver is at risk because of the large amount of blood with a low O_2 tension that enters through the portal system. Hepatic dysfunction is more likely following severe rather than minor hemorrhage, which may be related to the tendency to maintain hepatic arterial flow in shock.[78] Impairment of cellular integrity in isolated perfused cat livers occurred after 60 to 90 minutes of simulated shock.[25] The perfused liver is sensitive to local stimuli, particularly hypoxia, and releases lysosomal and cytoplasmic enzymes. Centrilobular necrosis is typical in animals following shock, and generalized intracellular edema is present.[35] Manipulation of the traumatized, hypoxic liver during surgical operations results in the release of emboli of liver tissue, bile salts, and toxic or vasoactive substances, promoting pulmonary insufficiency in trauma patients.[78] Hepatic and splenic capillary blood flow is reduced in shock owing to vasoconstriction, and the resulting reduction in reticuloendothelial function renders hepatic cells incapable of detoxifying bacterial cytotoxins. Thus, in any form of shock, a depressed hepatic reticuloendothelial system may allow a build-up of endotoxins.[100] In general, changes in hepatic structure and function during shock can contribute to increased gluconeogenesis, increased protein degradation with alteration of serum levels, and altered blood coagulation.[36]

Ischemia and shock affect the gastrointestinal tract. Erosions of the mucosa of the small intestine occur in carnivorous animals. Intestinal lesions promote loss of water, electrolytes, and protein into the intestinal lumen. As the barrier function of the gut becomes impaired, gram-negative bacteria and endotoxins enter the systemic circulation.[88] Splanchnic vasoconstriction is typical for dogs in shock. In early shock, the gastrointestinal tract is reduced in volume, the vascular system contains no red blood cells, and intestinal villi slough at the tips. After treatment to enhance blood volume, the gastrointestinal tract becomes congested, with fluid loss into the lumen, and microthrombi are present in villous capillaries.[78]

Reduced blood flow to the pancreas and the resulting ischemia may influence the severity of shock. The pancreas may affect hepatic energy metabolism and may help to regulate splanchnic and celiac blood flow during shock. Autophagic vacuoles in pancreatic tissue may continue self-destruction with the release of enzymes and myocardial depressant factor.[73] Digestive enzymes may increase intestinal damage, since hemorrhagic enteritis following shock can be eliminated by pancreatectomy, pancreatic duct ligation, or the use of trypsin inhibitors prior to shock.[78]

Myocardial depressant factor (MDF) has been found in plasma from several animal species following different types of shock.[80] It accumulates in plasma and reaches toxic levels two to seven hours after the onset of shock, the critical factor in its formation being splanchnic hypoperfusion, particularly to the pancreas. Pancreatic acidosis, hypoxia, and ischemia occur during hypoperfusion. Hypoxia and ischemia are potent stimuli for lysosomal damage and activation of zymogenic enzyme (e.g., conversion of trypsinogen to trypsin). Release of these enzymes into acinar cells with enhanced activity due to acidosis results in proteolysis and stimulation of MDF production.[80] Experimental evidence for the pancreas as a major source of MDF is convincing.[55, 80] MDF is released through acinar cell membranes, taken up by capillaries or lymphatics, and delivered to the systemic circulation. In intact animals and isolated tissue preparations, MDF produces negative inotropic effects, splanchnic vasoconstrictor effects, and depression of phagocytosis by the reticuloendothelial system. Thus, shock is promoted by direct myocardial depression and further impairment of tissue perfusion. MDF may also increase vascular permeability.[51, 80] Apparently, glucocorticoids prevent formation of MDF by stabilization of lysosomal membranes if given early in shock.[56, 81]

Pulmonary function in dogs following trauma and shock has been described.[78] Clinical syndromes have been categorized into three groups, although clear distinctions are not always possible. The first is progressive pulmonary insufficiency, which has increased in incidence owing to improved management of patients in shock after survival of the initial insult. Pulmonary failure occurs from a few hours to several days after injury. The syndrome in man is characterized by four phases.

Phase I includes the period of shock, its treatment, and a favorable response with adequate arterial O_2 tension.

Phase II is a period of cardiovascular stability but deteriorating respiration including hyperventilation and borderline arterial O_2 tensions.

Phase III includes increased respiratory difficulty characterized by increased tidal volume, hypocarbia, and hypoxemia. Oxygen therapy becomes less effective.

Phase IV is the terminal phase with hypoxia and hypercarbia leading to pulmonary and cardiac arrest.

Microemboli, sepsis, and overhydration were identified as likely causes of progressive pulmonary failure.[78]

The second pulmonary syndrome is induced by nonpenetrating blunt trauma.[78] This may cause pneumothorax, hemothorax, or diaphragmatic herniation leading to lung collapse. This injury may include pulmonary contusion. Interstitial and alveolar hemorrhage may occur. The prognosis varies depending on the extent of injury. If the injury involves hepatic damage, respiratory failure may follow (1) thoracic and abdominal trauma, (2) hepatic damage, (3) general anesthesia and surgical manipulation of the liver, and (4) respiratory failure and death. Respiratory failure occurs after hepatic manipulations cause liver emboli, bile salts, and toxic or vasoactive substances to pass into the lung.[78]

The third pulmonary failure syndrome is related to irreversible shock induced by various causes.[78] The pathology is dictated by the severity and duration of shock. The release and absorption of toxins, vasoactive substances, and metabolites from areas of tissue ischemia plus the infusion of particulate matter from stored blood may contribute to the pathology.[13, 78, 113, 115]

Finally, pulmonary edema can be related to CNS damage due to trauma or shock. The mechanism for neurogenic pulmonary edema is unclear.[102]

In sepsis, animal studies have shown a primary change in the permeability of pulmonary exchanging vessels as a likely cause of increased lung water. Specifically, endotoxin can increase alveolar-capillary permeability in dogs.[113] Increased permeability in the dog lung following hemorrhage is associated with increased lymph flow (which reflects transvascular fluid filtration rate).[43] Pulmonary hypertension occurs in shock. Thus, increased capillary hydrostatic pressure and alveolar-capillary permeability may cause fluid leakage.[43] However, dogs may be more resistant to the acute pulmonary changes induced by sepsis in other species.[62]

Lysosomal enzymes, histamine, serotonin, bradykinin, and prostaglandin are associated with and may mediate pulmonary injury. Lysosomal enzymes indicate cell injury and are likely to produce further damage because of their autolytic properties. They may be released from leukocytes sequestered in the pulmonary circulation during shock and sepsis. The elevation of lysosomal enzymes seems to correlate with the magnitude of lung injury in animal studies. Endotoxin and sepsis drastically elevate pulmonary lymph flow, and lysosomal enzyme activity is a possible cause of permeability changes in the lung associated with shock. Histamine is present in large amounts in various body tissues, particularly white blood cells, platelets, and lung mast cells. Histamine increases pulmonary vascular tone (including pulmonary venules) and vascular permeability, probably through H_1 receptors. Histamine may also affect platelet aggregation in lung tissue. Serotonin is found in high concentrations in circulating platelets, and it increases pulmonary vascular resistance in sheep and dogs. Bradykinin is particularly notable after endotoxemia, possibly being increased by the effects of endotoxin on granulocytes. It decreases peripheral vascular resistance. Since the lung is responsible for metabolism of bradykinin, pulmonary injury may decrease metabolism and prolong or exaggerate systemic effects. Systemic levels of prostaglandins are increased after hemorrhagic, endotoxic, anaphylactic, and burn-induced shock. These agents can be synthesized and metabolized by the lung, and prostaglandins are potent with regard to pulmonary hemodynamic, barrier, and respiratory functions. However, their exact roles in shock have yet to be elucidated. They may cause injury, modulate the effects of injury, or have no significant role.[43]

The kidney receives decreased blood flow during hypotension. Acute renal failure may occur from ischemia following shock or cardiac arrest. In septic shock, there may be both ischemic and toxic components in renal pathology.[10] Tubular dysfunction can begin within seconds to minutes following ischemic injury and, probably, toxic damage as well. However, it is uncommon for hypotensive renal failure to occur if fluid volume is restored rapidly.[78]

Acute renal failure following shock has not been a significant complication in dogs and cats. Organ systems more sensitive to hypotension may fail prior to the onset of renal failure.[118] However, with low blood flow and pressure, the superficial cortical nephrons are underperfused with redistribution of flow to medullary and juxtamedullary nephrons. This is consistent with the patchy pattern of tubular necrosis that may occur following ischemia. Prolonged renal ischemia (complete occlusion of the renal pedicle) produces acute tubular necrosis in two hours, resulting in detectable but reversible changes, and in four hours causes irreversible changes.[118] Renal vasoconstriction has been related to catecholamines[30] and to the renin-angiotensin system. Prolonged vasoconstriction and hypotension lead to oliguria, isosthenuria, glycosuria, and tubular cells in the urine sediment. Renal vasoconstriction lasting for more than 12 to 24 hours has been associated with renal tubular damage.[78]

During hypotension, blood flow is maintained preferentially to the coronary, cerebral, diaphragmatic, and hypophyseal-thyroid-adrenal areas.[23] Coronary blood flow is adequate with mean arterial blood pressures greater than 70 mm Hg.[78] With further hypotension, especially during diastole, coronary perfusion decreases. Also, elevation of the heart rate as a response to hypotension results in a shorter cardiac filling time. Thus, there is less opportunity for adequate cardiac perfusion during a period of greater myocardial work.[93] In experimental shock, a 50 per cent decrease in cardiac output results in a 40 per cent decrease in coronary blood flow.[78] Myocardial dysfunction in experimental septic shock has been postulated to be caused by coronary hypoperfusion and depressed responses to beta adrenergic stimuli. Acidosis may impair cardiac responsiveness to catecholamines, and it may depress the heart directly.[100] Intracardiac disturbances, including myocardial edema, ionic imbalances (K^+ and probably Ca^{++}), elevated ventricular end-diastolic pressure and depression of the rate of change of intraventricular pressure to its maximum (dP/dt_{max}), decreased cardiac power, and reduced cardiac efficiency also play important roles.[67] The effects of MDF have been discussed.

Cerebral circulation is adequately maintained with arterial pressure greater than 50 mm Hg,[78] but it begins to decrease with a mean arterial pressure of 60 mm Hg.[65, 79] Further blood pressure reduction, depending on duration, results in ischemia and possibly irreversible effects. The brain is absolutely dependent on the supply of glucose, which becomes limited following ischemia, the CNS requiring oxidative glucose metabolism. Thus, reduced oxygenation limits mitochondrial ATP synthesis, and hypoxia results in unconsciousness fairly rapidly. Cellular swelling is probably a major factor in CNS damage owing to ischemia or anoxia, possibly because of de-energization of the sodium-potassium ATPase system and the Gibbs-Donnan effect. Cellular swelling becomes significant because of the CNS confinement in a rather nonexpandable compartment leading to further reduction in cerebral blood flow.[38]

In shock, the endocrine response includes increased concentrations of adrenocorticotropic hormone (ACTH), cortisol, ADH, prolactin, and aldosterone, all of which come from areas of the CNS or are stimulated by hormones from the CNS. The adrenal glands have preferential perfusion. With depletion of 40 per cent of the blood volume, adrenal perfusion increases up to 108 per cent. The adrenal cortex is quite resistant to hypoxia, but it requires an adequate perfusion volume. The adrenals play important roles in shock when levels of glucocorticoids (cortisol) and mineralocorticoids (aldosterone) are generally elevated. The benefits of cortisol include the following:[23]

1. Acceleration of ATP formation from inorganic phosphate
2. Gluconeogenesis from amino acids
3. Decreasing lactic acidosis to oppose glycolytic and lipolytic effects of epinephrine
4. Shifting of the oxyhemoglobin dissociation curve to the right
5. Stabilization of capillary membranes and intracellular membrane systems that contain enzymes.

Disseminated Intravascular Coagulation

Disseminated intravascular coagulation (DIC) can occur in and be a complication of shock, and it may involve numerous organ systems. It is "an acute, transient coagulation occurring in the flowing blood throughout the vascular tree and which may obstruct the microcirculation."[60] Numerous factors are involved in DIC, but DIC is difficult to produce without deficient capillary blood flow. Decreased capillary flow can be caused by decreased cardiac output, systemic arteriolar constriction, opening of arteriovenous shunts, low arterial blood pressure, opening of all capillaries at once, and increased viscosity of blood. Coagulation may be initiated by red blood cell hemolysis, bacterial toxins, amniotic fluid with cellular debris, tissue fluids such as those from injury, malignant cells gaining access to the circulation, antigen-antibody complexes, ischemic tissue, anaphylaxis, absorption of trypsin, pit viper venoms, thermal burns, heat stroke, contact of blood with foreign substances (e.g., glass), damage to the reticuloendothelial system, and damage to vascular walls (e.g., by infectious agents). Certain conditions may increase blood coagulability including acidosis, high levels of clotting factors (pregnancy), increased platelet adhesiveness, catecholamines and sympathetic stimulation, and fibrinolysin inhibition.[60]

There are significant aspects of DIC related to shock.[61, 118] First, the consumption of various components of the clotting mechanism can promote bleeding and further fluid loss. The bleeding tendency is associated with excessive activation of profibrinolysin to fibrinolysin, with dissolution of any fibrin formed.[60] Second, focal tissue infarction caused by microthrombi in capillary beds of important organs, including lung, liver, kidney, and heart, may impair perfusion and lead to ischemia. If these clots are not resolved, cellular damage can occur, and organ failure may result.[60, 61, 118] For irreversible shock related to DIC to occur, slow capillary blood flow and the presence of thromboplastic material in the blood are required.[61]

Oxygen Consumption and Arterial Venous Oxygen Difference

In early hemorrhagic shock, total oxygen consumption is decreased (reflecting decreased tissue perfusion), but arteriovenous (A-V) oxygen difference and oxygen extraction are increased (reflecting increased removal of oxygen from blood that does perfuse tissues). With treatment, O_2 consumption begins to exceed normal values, suggesting repayment of the oxygen debt that developed during hypovolemia. In late stages of irreversible shock, the A-V oxygen difference and O_2 extraction are small. This may indicate impaired utilization or uptake by the cell.[77] Cardiogenic shock and vasculogenic shock follow similar patterns of oxygen consumption, A-V O_2 difference, and O_2 extraction. In maldistributive forms of shock (early septic or traumatic shock), O_2 consumption, A-V O_2 difference, and O_2 extraction are all decreased.[77] In terminal stages, all are depleted, further reflecting deficient capillary blood flow or nutritional uptake of O_2 by the cell. Based on studies in the dog,[126] animals with hyperdynamic sepsis have no significant degree of capillary arteriovenous shunting, but decreased oxygen uptake occurs probably because of a primary cellular defect. The hyperdynamic state of the circulation is possibly a compensatory mechanism to supply blood flow and oxygen to deficient cells.[84]

MANAGEMENT OF SHOCK

Recognition of Shock and Initial Evaluation

The recognition and diagnosis of shock is based on historical data, physical examination, and laboratory evaluation. Typical signs of shock include the following:[30, 78, 100]

1. Tachycardia
2. Diminished heart sounds
3. Hypotension
   a. Lower pulse pressure (weak or absent in peripheral vessels)
   b. Slow capillary refill time (greater than two seconds)
   c. Muscle weakness
   d. Cold extremities
4. Depressed mental state (indifference to stimuli)
5. Hyperventilation (tachypnea)
6. Decreased urine output (oliguria and anuria)
7. Pale or slightly cyanotic mucous membranes

There may be some variations in the signs, particularly in hyperdynamic septic shock and certain types of vasculogenic shock, in which skin and mucous membranes may be warm and hyperemic.[45, 100, 124] Also, in cardiogenic shock, peripheral veins may be distended rather than collapsed.[30] Table 11–2 lists several variables and their usual alterations in the

TABLE 11–2. Clinical Indications of Shock

	Hypovolemic Shock	Vasculogenic Shock	Cardiogenic Shock	Hyperdynamic Maldistributive Shock	Hypodynamic Maldistributive Shock
Blood pressure	↓	↓	↓		↓
Heart rate or pulse rate	↑	↑	↓ or ↑	↑	↑
Central venous pressure	↓	↓	↑	↑	↑
Cardiac output/index	↓	↓	↑	↑	↓
Urine flow	↓	↓	↓	↓	↓
Pa_{O_2}	↓	↓	↓	↓	↓
Arteriovenous O_2 difference	↑	↑	↑	↓	↑
Blood lactate	↑	↑	↑	↑	↑
Peripheral vascular resistance	↑	↓	→ or ↑	↓	↑
Skin	Cold	Cold	Cold	Warm	Cold

various forms of shock. After rapid patient evaluation, treatment should begin immediately.

Treatment of Shock and Monitoring to Assess Patient Response

The aims of treatment include (1) restoration of an adequate, properly distributed circulating blood volume to prevent tissue ischemia, (2), management of inciting causes of shock such as sepsis, hemorrhage, or cardiac failure, and (3) reversal of the consequences of ischemia. A patent airway and control of hemorrhage are assumed for initial management.

Blood Volume Expanders and Diuretics

Blood volume expansion has priority. Various fluids can be used including crystalloids, colloids, plasma, and whole blood. Immediate volume expansion is usually accomplished by crystalloids because of ready availability. In most cases, electrolyte solutions are the only fluids necessary.[77] Saline, lactated Ringer's, Ringer's, or other balanced electrolyte solutions are adequate. Ideally, crystalloids should be isotonic, nearly isoionic for major ions, easily adjusted to normal pH, nontoxic, nonallergenic, safe to give rapidly in large volumes, readily available, and inexpensive.[20] The resuscitative value of electrolyte solutions involves movement of these fluids into interstitial fluid as well as expansion of vascular volume. During shock, interstitial fluid moves intercellularly, is bound to collagen, and must be replaced during the resuscitation period.[77, 110] The rate, type, and amount of fluid are based on patient response and various monitored variables. The importance of avoiding electrolyte solutions containing benzyl alcohol as a preservative in cats has been emphasized. Cats have a decreased capacity for metabolism of the compound.[40]

The principal factors affecting oxygen delivery to tissue are blood flow, hemoglobin level, and oxyhemoglobin dissociation.[115] Restoration of fluid volume alone will increase blood flow, improve O_2 delivery, and increase O_2 consumption.[112, 115] Hemodilution with fluids increases total oxygen transport capacity even in a clinically normal animal. Optimal O_2 transport capacity occurs at a hematocrit of 25 to 30 per cent. Although hemodilution may decrease total plasma protein, protein levels return toward normal as lymph flow increases following re-absorption of interstitial fluid.[20] Hemodilution also decreases viscosity of blood and helps to prevent cellular aggregation[77] and DIC.[61] Blood flow through the microcirculation is enhanced both by decreasing viscosity and increasing the pressure head for fluid movement.[54] Therefore, temporary hemodilution is not considered dangerous and is associated with excellent survival in shock patients.[20]

When re-establishing oxygen delivery to tissues, hemoglobin levels should be evaluated after blood flow is increased.[115] In hemorrhaged patients, hematocrits below 25 to 30 per cent are less than optimal for O_2 delivery.[20, 54] Thus, red blood cell (RBC) and hemoglobin replacement becomes necessary with severe blood loss. Recently, autotransfusions have been used in traumatized animals,[39] particularly when fresh or stored donor blood is not readily available. When donor blood is used, typed and crossmatched compatible blood is desirable. Fresh blood is most desirable. However, stored blood is acceptable and is normally filtered (microfilter, 10 to 40 microns) to avoid microembolization. The significance of microemboli in posttransfusion pulmonary disease has been recently questioned.[22] Stored blood should be warmed on delivery to the patient to prevent cardiac arrest from cardiac hypothermia. Coil-type, water bath blood warmers avoid high temperatures that may denature protein.[102] For resuscitation of the hemorrhaged patient, whole blood is more effective if accompanied by one or two equal volumes of balanced electrolyte solution.[77, 120] Although blood has certain potential disadvantages, it is necessary when O_2 carrying capacity has been diminished significantly by blood loss.

Along with adequate blood volume and RBCs, the hemoglobin of the RBCs must be in a correct amount and biochemical state to assure proper O_2 exchange at the tissue level. Fresh blood from healthy, nonanemic donors usually has appropriate levels and states of hemoglobin. However, stored blood may be less effective, depending on duration of storage and the storage medium. Because of its better maintenance of RBC function, citrate phosphate dextrose (CPD) is a more desirable preservative than acid citrate dextrose (ACD).[115, 120] It maintains 2,3-DPG and hemoglobin function better.[46, 115] Stored blood has hemoglobin with a greater O_2 affinity (left shift in the oxyhemoglobin dissociation curve), which may reduce the volume of oxygen delivered to tissues at a given oxygen tension. The significance of this is related to the duration of storage, the amount of blood transfused, and the pretransfusion condition of the patient. Regeneration of 2,3-DPG begins shortly after transfusion and is normal within 24 hours. Abnormal 2,3-DPG seems to be of most clinical significance in animals with substantially reduced total red cell mass prior to transfusion.[115]

In blood volume expansion, the ability of the vascular system to retain fluids should be considered. This is especially important, since it may be necessary to elevate the circulating volume to 10 per cent above normal to assure filling of all dilated vessels and adequate tissue perfusion.[77] The total amount of fluid required for survival, when bleeding has reached 75 per cent of normal blood volume, must equal two or three times the patient's normal blood volume.[20]

Colloid osmotic pressure (COP) is vital for fluid retention and depends on the size and shape of various macromolecules. In plasma, COP is produced primarily by albumin. Plasma albumin is reduced by increased venular permeability following hemorrhage, major surgery, burns, and sepsis. Reduction in plasma albumin leads to fluid movement away from the vascular system and into interstitial spaces.[54] Colloids may be needed if total plasma protein is less than 4 gm/dl.[120] In comparison to resuscitation with Ringer's acetate, colloids produce more durable elevations in plasma volume and less extravascular water gain.[54] Blood, plasma, and dextran are most likely to be used for increasing COP. Blood or plasma provides the obvious advantage of protein replacement. Plasma can be frozen and stored for long periods, and plasma infusion does not produce immune problems.

Dextrans, with molecular weights of 40,000 (dextran 40) and 70,000 (dextran 70), are available colloids, and dextran molecules with an average molecular weight of 70,000 create a higher COP than equal concentrations of plasma proteins.[54] Dextran 40 is initially more effective than dextran 70 in expanding plasma volume, but the effect of dextran 40 is shorter owing to urinary excretion.[102] The plasma half-life of dextran 40 is two to three hours, whereas that of dextran 70 is six hours.[120] Molecules smaller than 50,000 readily pass through the glomerular membrane. Dextran 40 has the potential to produce renal failure if administered during hypotension and should be used only after urine flow is started with other fluids. Both dextrans increase bleeding times.[102] Clotting abnormalities may be associated with dextran 40, particularly if it exceeds 20 per cent of the blood volume. Therefore, the dose should not exceed 15 ml/kg/24 hr of the usual 6 or 10 per cent solutions.[120] Dextran 70 increases RBC aggregation.[54] Dextran 40 decreases blood viscosity, opens the microcirculation, and reduces platelet aggregation.[57] It is more commonly used in veterinary patients.

Plasma expanders, other than whole blood, cause hemodilution. Their benefits include expansion of vascular volume to increase perfusion; decreased blood viscosity, which improves venous return; and dispersion of aggregated blood cells to improve oxygen availability and decrease venous stasis. In a comparison of various expanders, colloids provide more prolonged maintenance of blood volume expansion than crystalloids, and albumin and dextran 40 are more effective than gelatin, plasma, or dextran 70 based on rheological properties and ability to restore oxygen consumption and base excess in shocked animals. Maintenance of water balance remains important with the use of colloids.[54] Logically, both colloids and crystalloids have value in resuscitating animals in shock. Crystalloids are indicated for rapid, economical volume expansion, and colloids are useful for elevation of COP.

When fluids for volume expansion have been chosen, the total amount and rate of administration must be determined. Most clinical estimates of fluid needs are inaccurate and low.[78] One blood volume (90 ml/ kg, dog) is an initial loading dose.[20] Cats have a total blood volume of about 70 ml/kg.[116] Recently, healthy cats have been shown to safely tolerate Ringer's lactate administered at 90 ml/kg/hr.[17] Although the initial physical examination gives much information about the need for fluid, the amount of fluid required is best judged by the response of the patient.

Monitoring of central venous pressure (CVP) provides substantial information for assessing the effects of rapid fluid infusion.[71] The CVP is a function of blood volume in the central veins, the distensibility and contractility of the right heart, the venomotor activity in the central veins, and intrathoracic pressure. Excluding abnormal causes for increased CVP such as pneumothorax, the CVP is related to the volume of venous return and to right and left cardiac contractility.[84] Low CVP suggests inadequate blood volume, and high CVP implies excessive volume or a failing heart. Serial CVP measurements are most helpful in assessing fluid needs.[78, 84]

CVP is measured by a jugular catheter placed aseptically with the distal tip in the anterior vena cava near the right atrium. A saline manometer is attached to the catheter, and the zero is adjusted to the level of the right atrium, which is usually aligned with the sternum in patients in lateral recumbency. Normal CVP values vary between 0 and 5 cm H_2O in the dog and cat.[78] Generally, CVP values within or below the normal range during blood volume expansion of a shocked patient indicate that more fluid should be given. Rising values imply a need for reducing the rate of infusion, and a CVP of 10 cm

H_2O is consistent with blood volume expansion.[78] However, such a value does not necessarily mean that fluid administration should be stopped. In evaluation of CVP in man, rapid test infusions are used. A physician may administer 200 ml of fluid per 70 kg over ten minutes, and if the CVP rises more than 2 cm H_2O and the elevation persists for ten minutes, fluid administration is slowed or stopped temporarily.[102] A similar fluid challenge has been described for veterinary patients using ten-minute infusion rates of 1 to 4 ml/kg/min.[120] An elevated or rising CVP indicates that the fluid volume is approaching the heart's capacity to pump the fluid effectively. Values above 15 cm of H_2O indicate right heart failure.[78] Certainly, as CVP rises toward this value, caution is indicated, and such elevations are cause to consider withdrawal of blood, improvement of cardiac contractility (inotropic drug), or diuresis.[102]

In recent years, measurement of *pulmonary artery wedge pressure* (PAWP) has been used in patients with significant cardiopulmonary disease because it coincides closely with left atrial pressure, giving a better indicator of the effectiveness of cardiac function with fluid loading.[84] Swan-Ganz flow-directed catheters have been used for this purpose in humans and animals. However, such measurements in small animals are not practical in most clinical situations.[120] When it is possible to obtain both CVP and PAWP values, assessment of fluid needs and evaluation of cardiac function are more reliable. Collection of valuable information concerning cardiac output and arteriovenous oxygen content differences can be facilitated by pulmonary artery and systemic arterial catheters.[84]

Although not as useful as CVP values, *arterial blood pressure* measurements are helpful.[82, 120] Internal (direct) or external (indirect) methods may be used. Pulse pressure is indicative of blood flow, larger values implying better tissue perfusion.[84] Systolic, diastolic, mean, and pulse pressures measured serially reflect the patient's response to therapy, but CVP responds more rapidly to changes in fluid volume.

Blood pressure can be estimated by palpation of peripheral arteries (dorsal pedal or lingual) if monitoring equipment is unavailable.[78] Although these are gross approximations, femoral blood pressure is not palpable at pressures less than 50 mm Hg, is detectable but weak between 50 and 70 mm Hg, and is usually full at pressures greater than 80 mm Hg. Detection of a peripheral pulse in a small artery can be equated (very roughly) with improvement of tissue perfusion if the peripheral pulse was absent prior to the onset of treatment.

Urine output is a relatively good indicator of tissue perfusion, since renal blood flow is reduced during hypovolemia and hypotension.[82] Glomerular filtration ceases when arterial blood pressure falls below 60 mm Hg.[78, 100] Return to normal urine output after an episode of hypotension is indicative of improved organ perfusion and the value of therapy. The normal cat or dog should produce 0.5 to 1.0 ml/kg hr of urine.[78]

If volume expansion does not restore urine output, *diuretics* may be indicated. Furosemide (0.5 to 1.0 mg/kg) and mannitol (0.15 to 0.3 gm/kg) intravenously have been recommended.[120] The use of mannitol must be carefully monitored in patients in shock[96] or with borderline cardiac function.[120] Rebound oliguria is a potential risk with furosemide and other loop diuretics.[120] Administration of any diuretic concurrently with volume depletion may aggravate renal insufficiency.[53] Therefore, diuretics should be used only after restoration of an adequate circulating blood volume.[100]

Mannitol has been advocated in acute renal failure in man to promote urine production in patients with altered renal function without histological damage. Since the onset of histological damage is unpredictable, early use of the drug is suggested. Diuresis with mannitol may remove toxic substances from the kidney through improved glomerular filtration. The mechanism may include arteriolar dilation, decreased plasma COP and improved effective filtration pressure, and reduced interstitial edema within the renal parenchyma that could compress renal tubules and impair glomerular filtration. The benefits of furosemide in acute renal failure are controversial, but human patients in nonoliguric renal failure showed decreased mortality when compared with those in oliguric renal failure.[7, 53] When either of these drugs alone fails to produce adequate diuresis, combination therapy may be used to promote additional diuresis.[8, 53] Although diuretics are not definitive in resuscitation following shock, evidence suggests that maintenance of urine production is associated with a better clinical outcome than allowing oliguria or anuria.[53]

Ventilation and Oxygenation

Inadequate ventilation and oxygenation complicate shock, particularly in traumatized patients. Prior to or concurrent with blood volume expansion, a patient in shock should receive emergency attention to assure an adequate patent airway. Endotracheal intubation, aspiration of foreign material from the airways, or tracheostomy may be necessary. Protection of the respiratory tract from foreign material may necessitate the use of cuffed tubes or properly sized Cole tubes for intubation. Removal of inhibitions to ventilation, such as aspiration of pleural air or fluid, may be necessary to assure respiratory function.

Depending on the condition and temperament of the patient, ventilation should be controlled if hypoventilation is apparent or is reflected in arterial CO_2 tensions. Carbon dioxide retention contributes to acidemia, and it should not be allowed to complicate the acid-base status of the patient in shock. Since alkalosis increases hemoglobin affinity for oxygen,[12, 107] artificial hyperventilation should be avoided.

If Pa_{O_2} values are less than 70 torr, oxygen administration can be of particular benefit.[120] By maintaining the Pa_{O_2} at values greater than 70 torr, hemoglobin loading with oxygen approaches maximum levels. Oxygen therapy improves O_2 tensions in alveolar-capillary diffusion impairment (e.g., pulmonary edema), hypoventilation, and alveolar ventilation-perfusion mismatching,[70] all of which may be present in some forms of shock. Elevated tensions of inspired oxygen (FI_{O_2} greater than 30 per cent) can be delivered using endotracheal or tracheostomy tubes, percutaneous intratracheal catheters, masks, nasal catheters, or oxygen cages, depending on the temperament and condition of the patient. The inspired fraction of O_2 necessary depends on the condition of the patient, and humidification and temperature control of gases may be required if O_2 use is prolonged.

Ventricular arrhythmias, tachypnea, restlessness, and cyanosis may be induced by hypoxemia.[78] Continued hypoxemia impairs other forms of treatment in the shock patient, and prolonged tissue ischemia is likely to produce irreversible shock. The importance of O_2 therapy in shock seems obvious. The oxygen saturation of portal venous blood can be increased to approximately 95 per cent by the administration of oxygen. Hyperbaric oxygen improves survival in several animal models of shock.[35] In addition to these benefits, elevating Pa_{O_2} to 600 torr by raising FI_{O_2} to 1 can add 1.5 ml of O_2 per 100 ml of blood, which can be a significant portion of the total arterial O_2 content in severe anemia following hemorrhage.[102]

Corticosteroids

Glucocorticoids are adjunctive in the treatment of shock. In septic shock their use is almost mandatory.[19] Administration of glucocorticoids in pharmacological doses during the period from one hour prior to the onset of hemorrhage to approximately one hour after the onset of hemorrhage will, in association with adequate volume replacement, significantly improve survival of animals in experimental hemorrhagic shock. In similar situations, administration of corticosteroids late in severe hemorrhagic shock does not improve survival or produce consistent hemodynamic or metabolic improvement. From experimental studies, it appears the bolus administration of appropriate doses of steroids is more effective than frequent, smaller-than-optimal doses.[108] In animal models, early steroid therapy combined with antibiotic therapy for gram-negative bacteremia was more beneficial than antibiotic therapy alone.[68] Most animal studies of gram-negative shock confirm that large doses of steroids increase survival if the steroids are given early. However, large doses of steroids are greater than amounts equivalent to 30 mg/kg/day of methylprednisolone.[69, 108]

Glucocorticoids may be beneficial in shock because of inotropic cardiac effects, stabilization of lysosomal and endothelial membranes, augmentation of microcirculatory function leading to decreased peripheral resistance (small vasodilating effect) and increased perfusion of vital organs, an anticoagulant effect, and detoxification of endotoxin. Corticosteroids inhibit the interaction of endotoxin with complement,[77] preventing the release of autocoids (e.g., histamine) that cause vasodilation, increase membrane permeability, and release lysosomal enzymes.[19, 69] Given early in shock, glucocorticoids prevent MDF formation.[108] They prevent leakage of acid hydrolases into the circulation from ischemic liver and pancreas and prevent swelling and vacuolization of lysosomes in liver, pancreas, and heart during ischemia,[80] direct evidence of lysosomal stabilizing effects. Prevention of the release of lysosomal enzymes may protect mitochondria and help to maintain cellular oxygen utilization.[84] Even given later in the course of hemorrhagic shock in dogs, corticosteroids restored adenyl cyclase activity, demonstrating a direct cellular effect.[108]

Thus, corticosteroids are useful in the treatment of shock. To be most effective, they should be used as early as possible and in appropriate doses. The importance of using water-soluble steroids for the treatment of canine septic shock has been emphasized recently.[121] Current veterinary recommendations include dexamethasone at 5 to 15 mg/kg (others[77] recommend 4 to 8 mg/kg), methylprednisolone at 15 to 30 mg/kg, and prednisolone sodium succinate at 5 to 10 mg/kg (others[19] recommend 35 to 40 mg/kg).[120] Dosing should be repeated at four- to six-hour intervals until the patient is stabilized.[19, 77] Corticosteroids should not be used alone as treatment for shock.[19]

Cardiac, Vasoactive, and Antiarrhythmic Drugs

Based on animal experiments, vasodilators such as phenoxybenzamine or phenothiazine derivatives (alpha-adrenergic blockers) have been recommended to counter pre- and postcapillary vasoconstriction.[102] They improve regional blood flow and reverse ischemia.[1] However, venodilation in acute hemorrhage can lead to a reduction in venous return, cardiac output, coronary perfusion, and finally, cardiac arrest. Also, in shock, reducing mean arterial blood pressure can result in cerebral ischemia. However, clinical improvement has been reported in patients given vasodilators after volume replacement was ineffective.[102] If vasodilators are to be used in shock, appropriate blood volume expansion must precede their administration.[77] If a vasodilator can be given without inducing severe diastolic pressure reduction and tachycardia, the reduced peripheral resistance and decrease in cardiac wall tension might benefit the heart by reducing myocardial oxygen consumption.[102] This justifies the use of afterload-reducing agents in ischemic heart disease or congestive heart failure. Assuming that preload (left ventricular end-diastolic pressure) and cardiac contractility remain unchanged, an afterload-reducing agent (vasodilator such as sodium nitroprusside) may increase cardiac output. However, coronary perfusion depends on diastolic blood pressure. Below the range of 60 to 120 mm Hg, coronary flow becomes pressure dependent. Therefore, afterload reducers must be used carefully to avoid a reduction in coronary perfusion.[84]

Adrenergic drugs have variable effects depending on the particular agent. Their use in shock is adjunctive to blood volume expansion, particularly if the response to volume replacement is not adequate.[77] Alpha-adrenergic stimulating drugs (norepinephrine, phenylephrine, methoxamine, metaraminol, and dopamine in large doses) are not indicated as prolonged infusions.[102] A vasoconstrictor, given to act nonselectively on various vascular beds, causes peripheral vascular shutdown.[1] Used to produce rapid vasoconstriction in acute, severe hemorrhage, a vasoconstrictor could restore cerebral and coronary circulation briefly while blood volume is being expanded.[102] Even epinephrine with its beta dilating effects is contraindicated as an infusion to restore blood pressure except in neurogenic shock. Most of its vasodilating effect occurs in skeletal muscle, and its alpha-adrenergic vasoconstrictor effects predominate in splanchnic and renal areas, resulting in greater impairment of blood flow to these vital areas.[1] The use of a vasoconstrictor as a primary agent in shock is limited to vasculogenic shock.

Inotropic drugs to increase cardiac output and tissue perfusion without causing peripheral vasoconstriction can be beneficial in shock. Isoproterenol, dopamine, and dobutamine have been used. Isoproterenol is a beta$_1$ and a beta$_2$ agonist. It increases heart rate, myocardial contractility, and peripheral vasodilation.[1] Isoproterenol causes dilation of arterioles of mesenteric vascular beds, reduces the volume of capacitance vessels, and thus improves cardiac output and peripheral blood flow. Vasodilation also occurs in skin and muscles.[77, 84] However, the drug is arrhythmogenic and may elevate the heart rate excessively if given too rapidly. With vasodilation accompanying tachycardia, coronary blood flow and delivery of oxygen to the myocardium may be decreased.[1] Consequently, isoproterenol may be less desirable for augmenting cardiovascular function in the shock patient than drugs that promote myocardial contractility with less influence on heart rate, myocardial oxygen consumption, and myocardial blood flow. However, dilute isoproterenol infusions at slow rates with concurrent volume expansion are useful clinically. Although a dosage range of 0.2 to 0.8 µg/kg/min has been recommended,[77] a dilute infusion given to effect a heart rate of 120 to 150 per minute in dogs is clinically valuable.

Dopamine has alpha, beta, and dopaminergic effects. It may be used at various dosages to achieve the desired effect. Dopamine is likely to cause alpha-induced blood pressure elevation if given in high doses. In lower doses, it is a dopaminergic agonist and causes vasodilation in splanchnic and renal vascular beds, leading to increased perfusion of the microcirculation. By its beta agonist activity, the drug increases myocardial contractility and improves cardiac output.[1] The dose rate for dopamine is 1 to 10 µg/kg/min,[77, 120] the lower end of the range being less likely to induce vasoconstriction and dysrhythmias. The rate of administration should be slow enough to avoid inducing tachycardia.

Dobutamine[75] is a synthetic beta agonist, producing most of its effect on beta$_1$ receptors that produce inotropic effects.[1] There are fewer chronotropic and vasodilatory effects in the suggested dosage range of 2 to 10 µg/kg/min.[120] Thus, the ability of the drug to increase cardiac output without significantly promoting dysrhythmias or impairing perfusion pressure seems advantageous. However, too rapid infusions can be associated with arrhythmias in clinical patients.

The chronotropic effects of adrenergic drugs can reverse bradyarrhythmias. Heart rates of less than 60 per minute dramatically decrease cardiac output and arterial blood pressure.[90] If slow heart rates are associated with shock, dilute isoproterenol can be infused to produce a heart rate of approximately 130 per minute, which is optimal in the average dog. The rate of infusion should be assessed with electrocardiographic monitoring for detection of ventricular arrhythmias. Use of a continuous oscilloscopic trace is most practical for long-term evaluation.

Anticholinergic drugs such as atropine or glycopyrrolate also reverse bradyarrhythmias. Atropine should be used cautiously because of its tendency to produce tachycardia,[120] increasing cardiac oxygen demands without increasing coronary perfusion in proportion to those demands. Although it may provide some protection to the gastrointestinal tract,[1] atropine's disadvantages have been enumerated,[90] and its use in shock must be carefully weighed against potential complications. Glycopyrrolate produces an elevation in heart rate when given intravenously at recommended dosages (0.011 mg/kg), but the heart rate is usually lower than that produced by atropine, an observation consistent with the effects of the drug in man.[98] It usually elevates the heart rate of the dog to about 160 per minute with a return toward 120 to 140 per minute within 15 to 30 minutes. Such rates are more consistent with optimal cardiac output in the dog.

Ventricular dysrhythmias may develop during shock or the resuscitation period. The ventricular arrhythmias are potentially serious because they may impair cardiac output and may lead to more serious arrhythmias. Ventricular extrasystoles, although not highly significant as occasional occurrences, may precede ventricular tachycardia or ventricular fibrillation. Therefore, extrasystoles should be treated with lidocaine (1 to 2 mg/kg intravenously) if they occur in large numbers or are multifocal.[91] The drug acts for about 20 minutes, since it is readily metabolized by the liver.[15] For recurrent extrasystoles, repeated boluses of lidocaine may be given or a lidocaine infusion (30 to 60 μg/kg/min) may be used. With continued arrhythmias, other antiarrhythmic agents can be considered including procainamide, quinidine, phenytoin, and propranolol.[1]

Antibiotics

Antibiotics are used in septic shock and are probably indicated after two hours or more of hypotension (50 mm Hg).[92] Identification of the etiological agent is important in the selection of antibiotics for treatment of septic shock, since various organisms can be involved.[69] However, antibiotic therapy is usually started before culture results can be obtained in suspected septic shock. Broad spectrum antibiotic therapy is indicated, and it should be continued until definitive culture and sensitivity results are available or for a minimum of four days.[100] The effects of antibiotic administration should be taken into account, realizing the possible complications. For example, muscle relaxing and respiratory depressant effects of the aminoglycoside antibiotics may complicate their use and require control of ventilation.

In septic or endotoxic shock, antibiotics are indicated to stop endotoxin production. However, the use of bactericidal antibiotics increases endotoxin in the blood as bacteria die. Therefore, the concurrent use of corticosteroids to prevent detrimental effects of endotoxin is essential and is associated with improved patient survival.[19, 121]

Alkalinizing Agents

Metabolic acidosis develops in shock when tissue perfusion is inadequate. The decrease in pH depends on the degree of hypoperfusion and its duration.[100] As the degree and duration of hypoperfusion increase, a metabolic acid load accumulates due to anaerobic glycolysis. If blood pH falls below 7.2, myocardial depression and vasodilation may occur.[77, 117] Acidosis also inhibits the effectiveness of catecholamines.[117] If pH is low, alkalinizers are indicated.

Sodium bicarbonate and metabolizable anion alkalinizers can be used.[63, 64] Various guidelines may be followed, but repeated evaluation of arterial blood gases and acid-base values are most reliable. A formula using base deficit for calculation of sodium bicarbonate need is 0.3 × body weight (kg) × base deficit = milliequivalents of bicarbonate. This amount can be given over a period of approximately two hours, the first half being given within the first 30 minutes. Since the factor of 0.3 estimates the acute distribution volume of bicarbonate[66] and does not estimate total body water, complete correction of acidosis cannot be expected. Follow-up blood gas and acid-base measurements should guide further administration of alkalinizers. Excessively rapid infusion should be avoided to prevent CO_2 build-up at a faster rate than it can be eliminated by the respiratory system. Carbon dioxide accumulation may contribute to a further decrease in pH,[95] and patients receiving alkalinizers should have adequate ventilation to prevent excessive CO_2 build-up.[63, 64] Carbon dioxide production from rapid infusion of alkalinizers can cause cerebrospinal fluid acidosis owing to the ease with which CO_2 diffuses into cerebrospinal fluid.[14, 16] In addition, hyperosmolality of extracellular fluid due to hypernatremia and intracranial hemorrhages have been reported as complications of excessive or rapid bicarbonate infusions.[114]

Anion alkalinizers such as lactate, acetate, and gluconate can be substituted for bicarbonate with some limitations.[63, 64] Adequate tissue perfusion is required for lactate metabolism, and lactate is not useful as an alkalinizer if the pH is very low.[105] Therefore, another alkalinizer (e.g., bicarbonate, acetate) must be used to elevate pH before the lactate can be adequately utilized. Usefulness of acetate depends on the adequacy of tissue perfusion, since it must be metabolized in muscle or other tissues to be effective as an alkalinizer.

Excessive alkalinization has several potential detrimental effects. Alkalosis is associated with a shift in the oxyhemoglobin dissociation curve, and rapid alkalinization may produce increased hemoglobin-oxygen affinity, leading to a decrease in cellular oxygen availability.[12, 107] Such a change has been associated with arrhythmias following rapidly induced alkalosis.[9] In addition, arrhythmias can be due to pH-related variations in serum levels of calcium, potassium, and sodium.[52, 77] Increased O_2 consumption occurs with induced metabolic or respiratory alkalosis.[24, 74] Therefore, alkalosis may inhibit O_2 delivery and increase consumption concurrently.[32] Because extracellular alkalosis has a more profound effect on the intracellular environment than extracellular acidosis[4, 5] and because of the effects of alkalosis, conservative use of alkalinizers with maintenance of normal to slight acid pH is recommended.

Body Temperature in Shock

Patients in shock have cool extremities, and body temperatures can be variable[78] but are usually low.[100] Patients should be insulated from cold tables by blankets or pads, and if core temperature is below 38°C, the patient should be further insulated from cooler ambient air. Active warming with warm water circulating blankets may be needed if temperature is low or continues to drop. Fluids used for volume replacement should be warmed. The potential benefits of hypothermia to shock patients have been explained,[100] but the effects of hypothermia can be difficult to manage.

Measurements of peripheral temperatures in shock patients have been suggested for evaluation of peripheral blood flow. The temperature of the toe web of the rear paw of the dog is usually 1 to 5°C less than rectal temperature. In shock, the difference increases, correlating well with changes in cardiac index and peripheral blood flow.[76–78] With treatment, a favorable response is a decrease in the difference.

Lactic Acid and Lactate Measurements

Since lactic acid accumulates when oxygen is not available to accept hydrogen ions in anaerobic metabolism, lactate concentration rises and is an indication of the general state of tissue oxygenation.[117] There is an inverse correlation between oxygen consumption and total lactate in the blood.[94, 117] Some workers[94] have calculated excess lactate (the disproportionate elevation of lactate in relation to pyruvate) instead of total lactate because only lactate rises in response to cellular oxygen deprivation, whereas both pyruvate and lactate are elevated under other circumstances, for example, following glucose administration.[117] However, total blood lactate is a useful prognostic tool.[72, 122] In man, arterial blood lactate levels, when a shock patient is first seen, are well correlated with final mortality. In addition, serially measured lactate levels are helpful in the evaluation of therapy.[84] Elevation of lactate in shock is usually associated with decreased tissue perfusion or decreased oxygen availability. However, in maldistributive shock, such as septic shock, lactate elevation may be due to failure of oxygen utilization.[84, 117]

The cause-and-effect relationship between lactate elevation and tissue hypoxia has been questioned.[84] Other factors elevate blood lactate, e.g., nonhypoxic hyperventilation.[127] One study of canine shock induced by hemorrhage, cardiac tamponade, or endotoxin showed that elevation of lactate did not correlate with oxygen lack or decreased CO_2 production. The conclusions were that lactate utilization and production are increased in shock even if O_2 uptake and CO_2 production are normal, that metabolic clearance of lactate is decreased, and that abnormal substrates (decreased use of fatty acids and increased metabolism of liver glycogen and amino acids) are involved in energy production. Thus, lactate in the dog may relate more to abnormal substrate utilization than to oxygen debt, and nutritional support may be one of the prime concerns in the management of shock patients.[84]

Lactate values may be useful in assessing therapy. Appropriate treatment of shock in a patient able to respond should reverse a rising trend in lactate levels. Lactate levels may rise initially as increased perfusion causes tissue washout of lactate, but such an increase should be temporary. As tissue oxygenation improves, production of lactate should decrease, and hepatic and muscle metabolism should reduce lactic acid levels. Continued elevation of lactate levels or stable levels indicate inadequate therapy or inability of the patient to respond. A normal, well-perfused liver should metabolize lactate faster than it can be produced in tissues.[117] In severe acidosis, the liver may not efficiently metabolize lactate, and alkalinization with sodium bicarbonate may be required to initiate normal lactate metabolism. However, infusion of sodium lactate in shock does not contribute to the state of acidemia, but it may not function as an alkalinizer until perfusion and acid-base balance are partially restored.[33]

Lactate concentrations in the normal, resting dog range between 5 and 20 mg/dl in venous blood and 12.6 and 36 mg/dl in plasma, with slightly lower concentrations in arterial blood samples.[117] Serial lactate values exceeding 35 mg/dl (two to three times normal) suggest a guarded prognosis.[59]

Disseminated Intravascular Coagulation

Diagnosis of DIC is usually by association with various disease processes. These may contribute to DIC and development of shock, or shock may initiate DIC. The clinical signs of DIC are often related to hemorrhage or a tendency to bleed. Various sites bleed, including skin, mucous membranes, and various organ systems (e.g., urinary, gastrointestinal, respiratory),[50] particularly at locations of trauma or surgical incisions. In some cases, formation of thrombin leads to deposition of microthrombi and other debris, causing occlusion of small vessels within the microcirculation. In these patients, thrombosis can lead to infarction and tissue necrosis.[84] When DIC is diagnosed, treatment should be instituted and the cause corrected.[101, 118]

Analgesics and Anesthetics in Shock

Because of pain or the need for surgical intervention, the patient that is or has recently been in shock may require analgesics or anesthetics. The use of such drugs should be delayed until volume expansion can be initiated. Most of the drugs available for analgesia or anesthesia have some deleterious cardiopulmonary effects that are pronounced in the shock patient.

In shock, three major factors affect the response of the patient to anesthetics and analgesics: CNS depression, decreased blood volume with preferential perfusion of vital organs, and acidemia. All produce a more pronounced effect from a given amount of anesthetic or analgesic.

SUMMARY OF MANAGEMENT

Management of Hypovolemic Shock

"Prompt treatment with adequate volume replacement based on hemodynamic and metabolic monitoring is the keystone to uncomplicated survival from hypovolemic shock."[84] As much as possible, the causes of hypovolemic shock must be managed along with corrective treatment. For example, external hemorrhage should be controlled by pressure or ligation, and internal hemorrhage must be assessed to determine the need for immediate surgery. Fluid replacement with crystalloids should be started immediately. Based on assessment of CVP, arterial blood pressure, heart rate, urine production, response of the patient, and other variables, the rate of fluid administration and the total needed volume can be adjusted. Selection of fluids to accompany the crystalloids should be based on serial hematocrit and total protein values; blood or colloids may be necessary to maintain a reasonable packed cell volume and total serum protein. Other monitoring, such as electrocardiogram and arterial acid-base and blood gas analyses, should direct the use of antiarrhythmic and alkalinizing drugs. Monitoring of urine output should control the use of diuretics. Vasoactive drugs may be necessary to support cardiac function and maintain tissue perfusion. Corticosteroids, although controversial, should be administered as early as possible.

Management of Vasculogenic Shock

Management of vasculogenic shock is variable, depending on the initiating factors. In most instances, fluid infusion corrects the perfusion deficit by increasing venous return. However, use of vasoactive drugs is often beneficial. With anaphylaxis, vasoconstrictors, corticosteroids, and antihistamines have proved useful, and epinephrine is still the mainstay of therapy. In overdosage of spinal or epidural analgesics, volume expansion concurrently with ephedrine, phenylephrine, or desoxyephedrine administration has been recommended (along with ventilation). Treatment of shock related to head trauma and brain lesions should include therapy to decrease brain edema and prevent the consequences of ischemia (e.g., corticosteroids and mannitol) as well as support of cardiac output. Shock related to pain and psychological stimuli may require judicious use of sedatives and analgesics, along with attention to the cardiovascular system.

Management of Cardiogenic Shock

Cardiogenic shock, as a single entity, is rare in the dog and cat but may complicate later stages of other types of shock. When inadequate cardiac function occurs, the factors contributing to the process should be eliminated, e.g., anesthesia can be discontinued, application of positive pressure ventilation can be altered, fluid surrounding the heart in cardiac tamponade can be aspirated, and hemo- or pneumothorax can be controlled. If the cause of cardiogenic shock is direct generalized myocardial depression, drugs may be indicated to improve cardiac function, that is, to increase cardiac contractility or control the rate. Dopamine has been useful, but all adrenergic drugs should be used carefully, as some may increase cardiac contractility while increasing peripheral resistance and cardiac oxygen consumption. Recent advances in improving myocardial performance have relied on afterload reduction and decreasing aortic diastolic pressure. Ideally, vasodilators that affect arteriolar resistance vessels without dilating venous capacitance vessels are used because they do not reduce venous return. Even these drugs carry the potential of significantly reducing coronary perfusion. The management of cardiogenic shock should be based on good monitoring including CVP, ECG, acid-base balance, arterial blood pressure, and other procedures to direct the use of fluids, diuretics, corticosteroids, antiarrhythmics, and other drugs. Use of pulmonary artery wedge pressure has been very helpful for treatment of human cardiogenic shock, but practicability of the technique inhibits its use in small animal patients.

Management of Maldistributive Shock

Management of septic shock must be based on prevention when possible. Potentially contaminated wounds or surgical sites must be properly cared for. Vascular and urinary catheters are placed and managed to prevent infection. Use of appropriate antibiotics, based on culture and sensitivity, should be a part of the preventive regimen.

Early detection of the development of sepsis is important. If the source of infection can be reached surgically, drainage is beneficial. Early use of fluids to maintain an elevated cardiac output and normal hematocrit is helpful, and vasoactive drugs may be needed to maintain cardiac output. Finally, the use of corticosteroids is important. Although there is no clinical proof that steroids change mortality in clinical septic shock, the literature generally supports their use. Aggressive fluid therapy is of great importance in preventing cardiorespiratory progression of hyperdynamic to hypodynamic shock.

RECENT DEVELOPMENTS IN THE TREATMENT OF SHOCK

Based on economics and practical usage (partially owing to patient size), newer developments are more likely to be applied to humans before they are used on veterinary patients. Fluids superior to blood, e.g., fluorocarbon emulsions,[31, 37] may increase oxygen carrying capacity and flow to tissues in hypovolemic states. Gelatin polymers may prove beneficial as colloids for volume expansion.[1] Hyperbaric oxygen may also be useful.[37] Nutritional support and methods of altering cellular function may become important in therapy of hyperdynamic septic or traumatic shock.[84] Already, studies with glucose infusions in humans; glucose, insulin, and potassium infusions in dogs; Krebs cycle intermediates in rabbits; adenosine or creatine phosphate in animals; ATP, ATP-$MgCl_2$, and agents promoting ATP formation have shown beneficial effects on survival and improvements in certain cardiovascular and biochemical measurements in various experimental models of shock.[18, 26, 28, 29]

The study of prostaglandins has revealed more information about control of blood vessel function that could be of importance in ischemia and shock. Knowledge of the prostacyclin-thromboxane system will be helpful in the study of shock. Thromboxane A_2 promotes vasoconstriction and platelet aggregation, whereas prostacyclin (PGI_2) protects vessels from the effects of thromboxanes.[80] Thromboxane inhibition and infusion of PGI_2 appear helpful in various states of ischemia and shock.

Naloxone, a narcotic antagonist, is being investigated in shock. With the discovery of endorphins and their profound cardiovascular effects, endorphins and narcotic antagonists have been studied. Naloxone increases survival time in animals subjected to shock[48, 99] and has improved blood pressure in hypotensive animals due to endotoxic, neurogenic, and hypovolemic shock; several species have been studied, including rats, cats, dogs, and pigs.[2, 48, 49] The mechanism of action of naloxone in shock is unknown, but it may protect the sodium-potassium pump mechanism from the effects of endorphins.

Flow-directed pulmonary artery catheters presently provide much useful hemodynamic data in human shock patients regarding pulmonary artery wedge pressure;[125] such measurements could be used in small animals, particularly larger dogs. The use of transcutaneous measurements of O_2 tension may also help in evaluation of the shock patient.[31] Transcutaneous oxygen tensions in hypovolemic dogs follow oxygen delivery rather than arterial oxygen tensions. Thus, transcutaneous oxygen tensions may prove valuable in alerting the clinician monitoring the potential shock patient.[31, 86]

1. Adams, H. R.: Cardiovascular emergencies—drugs and resuscitative principles. Vet. Clin. North Am. *11*:77, 1981.
2. Albert, S. A., Shires, G. T. III, Illner, H., et al.: Effects of naloxone in hemorrhagic shock. Surg. Gynecol. Obstet. *155*:326, 1982.
3. Albrecht, M., and Clowes, G. H. A., Jr.: The increase of circulatory requirements in the presence of inflammation. Surgery 56:158, 1964.
4. Alder, S., Roy, A., and Relman, A. S.: Intracellular acid-base regulation. 1. The response of muscle cells to changes in CO_2 tension or extracellular bicarbonate concentration. J. Clin. Invest. *44*:8, 1965.
5. Alder, S., Roy, A., and Relman, A. S.: Intracellular acid-base regulation. 1. The interaction between CO_2 tension and extracellular bicarbonate in the determination of muscle cell pH. J. Clin. Invest. *44*:21, 1965.
6. Altemeier, W. A., Todd, J. C., and Wellford, W. I.: Gram-negative septicemia: a growing threat. Ann. Surg. *166*:530, 1967.
7. Anderson, R. J., Linas, S. L., Berns, A. S., et al.: Nonoliguric acute renal failure. N. Engl. J. Med. *296*:1134, 1977.
8. Auger, G., Dayton, A., Harrison, C. E., et al.: Use of ethacrynic acid in mannitol resistant oliguric renal failure. J. Am. Vet. Med. Assoc. *206*:891, 1968.
9. Ayres, S. M., and Grace, W. J.: Inappropriate ventilation and hypoxemia as a cause of cardiac arrhythmias. Am. J. Med. *46*:495, 1969.
10. Barnes, J. L., and McDowell, E. M.: Pathology and pathophysiology of acute renal failure—a review. *In* Cowley, R.

A., and Trump, B. F. (eds.): *Pathophysiology of Shock, Anoxia and Ischemia*. Williams & Wilkins, Baltimore, 1982, pp. 324–339.
11. Barnett, J. A., and Sandford, J. P.: Bacterial shock. JAMA *209*:1514, 1969.
12. Bellingham, A. J., Detter, J. C., and Lenfant, C.: Regulatory mechanisms of hemoglobin-oxygen affinity in acidosis and alkalosis. J. Clin. Invest. *50*:700, 1971.
13. Bennett, S. H., Geelhoed, G. W., Aaron, R. K., et al.: Pulmonary injury resulting from perfusion with stored bank blood in the baboon and dog. J. Surg. Res. *13*:295, 1972.
14. Berenji, K. J., Wolk, M., and Killip, T.: Cerebrospinal fluid acidosis complicating therapy of experimental cardiac arrest. Circulation 52:319, 1975.
15. Bigger, J. T., Jr., and Hoffman, B. F.: Antiarrhythmic drugs. *In* Gilman, A. G., Goodman, L. S., and Gilman, A. (eds.): *The Pharmacological Basis of Therapeutics*, 6th ed. MacMillan Publishing Co., New York, 1980, pp. 761–792.
16. Bishop, R. L., and Weisfeldt, M. L.: Sodium bicarbonate administration during cardiac arrest. J.A.M.A. *235*:506, 1976.
17. Bjorling, D. E., and Rawlings, C. A.: Relationship of intravenous administration of Ringer's lactate solution to pulmonary edema in halothane anesthetized cats. Am. J. Vet. Res. *44*:1000, 1983.
18. Bland, P.: Investigations into the hemodynamic and metabolic effects of fructose 1, 6 diphosphate and prostacyclin in hypovolemic shock. Dissertation, Texas A & M University, 1982.
19. Bowen, J. M.: Are corticosteroids useful in shock therapy? J. Am. Vet. Med. Assoc. *177*:453, 1980.
20. Brasmer, T. H.: Fluid therapy in shock. J. Am. Vet. Med. Assoc. *174*:475, 1979.
21. Bromage, P. R.: *Epidural Analgesia*. W. B. Saunders, Philadelphia, 1978, pp. 348–351.
22. Brzica, S. M.: Practical aspects of transfusion therapy. Proc. 33rd Ann Refresher Course Lecture Program of the American Society of Anesthesiologists. 1982, Course 125, pp. 1–7.
23. Bucur, A. I., and Cafrita, A.: The neuronal and endocrine system. *In* Suteu, I., Bandila, T., Cafrita, A., Bucur, A. I. and Candea, V.: *Shock*. Abacus Press, Kent, England, 1977, p. 129.
24. Cain, S. M.: Increased oxygen uptake with passive hyperventilation of dogs. J. Appl. Physiol. 28:4, 1970.
25. Carlson, R. P., and Lefer, A. M.: Hepatic cell integrity in hypodynamic states. Am. J. Physiol. *231*:1408, 1976.
26. Chaudry, I. H., and Baue, A. E.: Overview of hemorrhagic shock. *In* Cowley, R. A., and Trump, B. F. (eds.): *Pathophysiology of Shock, Anoxia and Ischemia*. Williams & Wilkins, Baltimore, 1982, pp. 203–219.
27. Chaudry, I. H., Clemens, M. G., and Baue, A. E.: Alterations in cell function with ischemia and shock and their correction. Arch. Surg. *116*: 1309, 1981.
28. Chaudry, I. H., Sayeed, M. M., and Baue, A. E.: Effects of adenosine triphosphate-magnesium chloride administration in shock. Surgery 75:220, 1974.
29. Chick, W. L., Weiner, R., Cascarano, J., et al.: Influence of Krebs cycle intermediates on survival in hemorrhagic shock. Am. J. Physiol. *215*:1107, 1968.
30. Clark, D. R.: Circulatory shock: etiology and pathophysiology. J. Am. Vet. Med. Assoc. *175*:78, 1979.
31. Clark, L. C., Jr.: Theoretical and practical considerations of fluorocarbon emulsions in the treatment of shock. *In* Cowley, R. A., and Trump, B. F. (eds.): *Pathophysiology of Shock, Anoxia and Ischemia*. Williams & Wilkins, Baltimore, 1982, p. 507.
32. Cohen, P. J.: More on lactate. Anesthesiology 43:614, 1975.
33. Cohen, R. D., and Simpson, R.: Lactate metabolism. Anesthesiology 43:661, 1975.
34. Cousins, M. J.: Epidural neural blockade. *In* Cousins, M. J., and Bridenbraugh, P. O. (eds.): *Neural Blockade in Clinical Anesthesia and Management of Pain*. J. B. Lippincott, Philadelphia, 1980, pp. 176–274.
35. Cowley, R. A., Hankins, J. R., Jones, R. T., et al.: Pathology

and pathophysiology of the liver. *In* Cowley, R. A., and Trump, B. F. (eds.): *Pathophysiology of Shock, Anoxia and Ischemia*. Williams & Wilkins, Baltimore, 1982, pp. 285–301.

36. Cowley, R. A., and Trump, B. F.: Organ dysfunctions in shock (editor's summary). *In* Cowley, R. A., and Trump, B. F. (eds.): *Pathophysiology of Shock, Anoxia and Ischemia*. Williams & Wilkins, Baltimore, 1982, pp. 281–284.

37. Cowley, R. A., and Trump, B. F.: Strategies for future diagnosis and therapy (editor's summary). *In* Cowley, R. A., and Trump, B. F. (eds.): *Pathophysiology of Shock, Anoxia and Ischemia*. Williams & Wilkins, Baltimore, 1982, p. 499.

38. Cowley, R. A., and Trump, B. F.: Injury of the central nervous system (editor's summary). *In* Cowley, R. A., and Trump, B. F. (eds.): *Pathophysiology of Shock, Anoxia and Ischemia*. Williams & Wilkins, Baltimore, 1982, pp. 555–557.

39. Crowe, D. T.: Autotransfusion in the trauma patient. Vet. Clin. North Am. *10*:581, 1980.

40. Cullison, R. F., Menard, P. D., and Buck, W. B.: Toxicosis in cats from use of benzyl alcohol in lactated Ringer's solution. J. Am. Vet. Med. Assoc. *182*:61, 1983.

41. de Lahunta, A.: Spinal cord disease. *In Veterinary Neuroanatomy and Clinical Neurology*. W. B. Saunders, Philadelphia, 1977, pp. 169–220.

42. de Lahunta, A.: Diagnosis and evaluation of traumatic lesions of the nervous system. *In Veterinary Neuroanatomy and Clinical Neurology*. W. B. Saunders, Philadelphia, 1977, pp. 333–343.

43. Demling, R. H., and Flynn, J. T.: Humoral factors and lung injury during shock, trauma and sepsis. *In* Cowley, R. A., and Trump, B. F. (eds.): *Pathophysiology of Shock, Anoxia and Ischemia*. Williams & Wilkins, Baltimore, 1982, pp. 395–407.

44. Douglas, W. W.: Histamine and 5-hydroxytryptamine (serotonin) and their antagonists. *In* Gilman, A. G., Goodman, L. S., and Gilman, A. (eds.): *The Pharmacological Basis of Therapeutics*, 6th ed. MacMillan Publishing Company, New York, 1980, pp. 609–646.

45. Duff, P.: Pathophysiology and management of septic shock: J. Reprod. Med. *24*:109, 1980.

46. Eisenbrandt, D. L., and Smith, J. E.: Evaluation of preservatives and containers for storage of canine blood. J. Am. Vet. Med. Assoc. *163*:988, 1973.

47. Ettinger, S. J., and Suter, P. F.: *Canine Cardiology*. W. B. Saunders, Philadelphia, 1970, p. 400.

48. Faden, A., and Holaday, J.: Opiate antagonists. Science *205*:317, 1979.

49. Faden, A., and Holaday, J.: Naloxone treatment of endotoxin shock. J. Pharmacol. Exp. Therap. *212*:441, 1980.

50. Feldman, B. F.: Disseminated intravascular coagulation. Comp. Cont. Ed. *3*:46, 1981.

51. Ferguson, W. W., Glenn, T. M., and Lefer, A. M.: Mechanisms of production of circulatory shock factors in the isolated perfused pancreas. Am. J. Physiol. *222*:450, 1972.

52. Garilla, S., Dava, C. L., and Chazan, J. A.: Severity of metabolic acidosis as a determinant of bicarbonate requirements. N. Engl. J. Med. *289*:121, 1973.

53. Gehr, M., Gross, M., Schmitt, G., et al.: Treatment of acute renal failure. *In* Cowley, R. A., and Trump, B. F. (eds.): *Pathophysiology of Shock, Anoxia, and Ischemia*. Williams & Wilkins, Baltimore, 1982, pp. 341–357.

54. Gelin, L., and Dawidson, I.: Plasma expanders and hemodilution in treatment of hypovolemic shock. *In* Cowley, R. A., and Trump, B. F. (eds.): *Pathophysiology of Shock, Anoxia and Ischemia*. Williams & Wilkins, Baltimore, 1982, pp. 454–463.

55. Glenn, T. M., and Lefer, A. M.: Significance of splanchnic proteases in the production of a toxic factor in hemorrhagic shock. Circ. Res. *29*:338, 1971.

56. Glenn, T. M., and Lefer, A. M.: Antitoxic action of methylprednisolone in hemorrhagic shock. Eur. J. Pharmacol. *13*:230, 1971.

57. Greene, C. E.: Disseminated intravascular coagulation in the dog: a review. J. Am. Anim. Hosp. Assoc. *11*:674, 1975.

58. Guyton, A. C.: Circulatory shock and physiology of its treatment. *In Textbook of Medical Physiology*, 4th ed. W. B. Saunders, Philadelphia, 1971, pp. 325–336.

59. Hankes, G. H., and Dillion, A. R.: Parameters and measurements of evaluation. *In* Sattler, F. P., Knowles, R. P., and Whittick, W. G. (eds.): *Veterinary Critical Care*. Lea & Febiger, Philadelphia, 1981, p. 111.

60. Hardaway, R. M.: Pathology and pathophysiology of disseminated intravascular coagulation. *In* Cowley, R. A., and Trump, B. F. (eds.): *Pathophysiology of Shock, Anoxia, and Ischemia*. Williams & Wilkins, Baltimore, 1982, pp. 186–197.

61. Hardaway, R. M. III: Cellular and metabolic effects of shock. J. Am. Vet. Med. Assoc. *175*:81, 1979.

62. Hardie, E. M., and Rawlings, C. A.: Septic shock, Part I. Pathophysiology. Comp. Cont. Ed. *5*:365, 1983.

63. Hartsfield, S. M., Thurmon, J. C., and Benson, G. J.: Sodium bicarbonate and bicarbonate precursors for treatment of metabolic acidosis. J. Am. Vet. Med. Assoc. *179*:914, 1981.

64. Hartsfield, S. M., Thurmon, J. C., Corbin, J. E., et al.: Effects of sodium acetate, bicarbonate and lactate on acid-base status in anesthetized dogs. J. Vet. Pharmacol. Therap. *4*:51, 1981.

65. Haskins, S. C.: Prevention of inadequate intraoperative tissue oxygenation. Vet. Clin. North Am. *6*:257, 1976.

66. Haskins, S. C.: An overview of acid-base physiology. J. Am. Vet. Med. Assoc. *170*:423, 1977.

67. Hinshaw, L. B.: Overview of endotoxin shock. *In* Cowley, R. A., and Trump, B. F. (eds.): *Pathophysiology of Shock, Anoxia and Ischemia*. Williams & Wilkins, Baltimore, 1982, pp. 219–235.

68. Hinshaw, L. B., Beller, B. K., Archer, L. T., et al.: Recovery from lethal *Escherichia coli* shock in dogs. Surg. Gynecol. Obstet. *149*:545, 1979.

69. Hruska, J. F., and Hornick, R. B.: Treatment of infection in septic shock. *In* Cowley, R. A., and Trump, B. F. (eds.): *Pathophysiology of Shock, Anoxia and Ischemia*. Williams & Wilkins, Baltimore, 1982, pp. 482–497.

70. Hyde, R. W.: Clinical interpretation of arterial oxygen measurements. Med. Clin. North Am. *54*:617, 1970.

71. Jennings, P. B., Anderson, R. W., and Martin, A. M., Jr.: Central venous pressure monitoring: a guide to blood volume replacement in the dog. J. Am. Vet. Med. Assoc. *151*:1283, 1967.

72. Jennings, P. B., Whitten, N. J., and Sleeman, H. K.: The diagnosis and treatment of shock in the critical care patient. *In* Sattler, F. P., Knowles, R. P., and Whittick, W. G. (eds.): *Veterinary Critical Care*. Lea & Febiger, Philadelphia, 1981, pp. 486–523.

73. Jones, R. T., and Linhardt, G. E., Jr.: Pathology and pathophysiology of the exocrine pancreas in shock. *In* Cowley, R. A., and Trump, B. F. (eds.): *Pathophysiology of Shock, Anoxia and Ischemia*. Williams & Wilkins, Baltimore, 1982, pp. 309–324.

74. Karetsky, M. S., and Cain, S. M.: Oxygen uptake stimulation following Na-L-lactate infusion in anesthetized dogs. Am. J. Physiol. *216*:1486, 1969.

75. Kittleson, M. D.: Dobutamine. J. Am. Vet. Med. Assoc. *177*:642, 1980.

76. Kolata, R. J.: The significance of changes in toe web temperature in dogs in circulatory shock. Proc. 28th Gaines Vet. Symp. 1979, pp. 21–26.

77. Kolata, R. J.: The clinical management of circulatory shock based on pathophysiological patterns. Comp. Cont. Ed. *2*:314, 1980.

78. Kolata, R. J., Burrows, C. F., and Soma, L. R.: Shock: pathophysiology and management. *In* Kirk, R. W. (ed.): *Current Veterinary Therapy VII*. W. B. Saunders, Philadelphia, 1980, pp. 32–48.

79. Lassen, N. A.: Control of cerebral circulation in health and disease. Circ. Res. *34*:749, 1974.

80. Lefer, A. M.: Vascular mediators in ischemia and shock. *In*

Cowley, R. A., and Trump, B. F. (eds.): *Pathophysiology of Shock, Anoxia and Ischemia*. Williams & Wilkins, Baltimore, 1982, pp. 165–181.

81. Lefer, A. M., and Glenn, T. M.: Corticosteroids and the lysosomal protease-MDF system. *In* Glenn, T. M. (ed.): *Corticosteroids in the Therapy of Shock*. University Park Press, Baltimore, 1974, pp. 233–251.

82. Longnecker, D. E.: The patient in shock: Perioperative and anesthetic care. *In* Hershey, S. G. (ed.): *ASA Refresher Courses in Anesthesiology*. J. B. Lippincott, Philadelphia, 1981, pp. 85–96.

83. Lumb, W. V., and Jones, E. W.: *Veterinary Anesthesia*. Lea & Febiger, Philadelphia, 1973, p. 580.

84. MacLean, L. D.: Shock: Causes and management of circulatory collapse. *In* Sabiston, D. C. (ed.): *Textbook of Surgery*, 11th ed. W. B. Saunders, Philadelphia, 1977, pp. 65–94.

85. MacLean, L. D., Mulligan, W. G., McLean, A. P. H., et al.: Patterns of septic shock in man—a detailed study of 56 patients. Ann. Surg. *166*:543, 1967.

86. Matsen, F. A. III, Wyss, C. R., King, R. V., et al.: Effect of acute hemorrhage on transcutaneous, subcutaneous, intramuscular and arterial oxygen tensions. Pediatrics *65*:881, 1980.

87. McComish, P. B., and Bodley, P. O.: Anesthesia for surgery of the spine. *In Anaesthesia for Neurological Surgery*. Year Book Medical Publishers, Chicago, 1971, pp. 264–280.

88. Mittermayer, C., and Riede, U. N.: Human pathology of the gastrointestinal tract in shock, ischemia and hypoxemia. *In* Cowley, R. A., and Trump, B. F. (eds.): *Pathophysiology of Shock, Anoxia and Ischemia*. Williams & Wilkins, Baltimore, 1982, pp. 301–308.

89. Morgan, R. V.: Shock. Comp. Cont. Ed. *3*:533, 1981.

90. Muir, W. W.: Electrocardiographic interpretation of thiobarbiturate-induced dysrhythmias in dogs. J. Am. Vet. Med. Assoc. *170*:1419, 1977.

91. Muir, W. W.: Effects of atropine on cardiac rate and rhythm in dogs. J. Am. Vet. Med. Assoc. *172*:917, 1978.

92. Nelson, A. W.: The unified concept of shock. Vet. Clin. North Am. *6*:173, 1976.

93. Nelson, A. W.: Hypovolemic shock. Vet. Clin. North Am. *6*:187, 1976.

94. Oliva, P. B.: Lactic acidosis. Am. J. Med. *48*:209, 1975.

95. Ostea, E. M., and Odell, G. B.: The influence of bicarbonate administration on blood pH in a "closed system": clinical implications. J. Pediatr. *80*:671, 1972.

96. Parker, A. J.: Blood pressure changes and lethality of mannitol infusions in dogs. Am. J. Vet. Res. *34*:1523, 1973.

97. Prys-Roberts, C.: *The Circulation in Anesthesia*. Blackwell Scientific Publications, London, 1980, pp. 150, 213, 231.

98. Ramamurthy, S., Ylagan, L. B., and Winnie, A. P.: Glycopyrrolate as a substitute for atropine: a preliminary report. Anesth. Analg. *50*:732, 1971.

99. Raymond, R., Harkema, J., Stoffs, W., et al.: Effects of naloxone therapy on hemodynamics and metabolism following a superlethal dosage of Escherichia coli endotoxin in dogs. Surg. Gynecol. Obstet. *152*:159, 1981.

100. Ross, J. N., Jr.: Heart failure and shock. *In* Ettinger, S. J. (ed.): *Textbook of Veterinary Internal Medicine*. W. B. Saunders, Philadelphia, 1975, pp. 825–864.

101. Ruehl, W., Mills, C., and Feldman, B. F.: Rational therapy in disseminated intravascular coagulation. J. Am. Vet. Med. Assoc. *181*:76, 1982.

102. Safar, P.: Resuscitation in hemorrhagic shock, coma and cardiac arrest. *In* Cowley, R. A., and Trump, B. F. (eds.): *Pathophysiology of Shock, Anoxia and Ischemia*. Williams & Wilkins, Baltimore, 1982, pp. 411–438.

103. Scherago, M.: Bacterial allergy. Vet. Clin. North Am. *4*:91, 1974.

104. Schumer, W.: General treatment of septic shock. *In* Cowley, R. A., and Trump, B. F. (eds.): *Pathophysiology of Shock, Anoxia and Ischemia*. Williams & Wilkins, Baltimore, 1982, pp. 479–482.

105. Schwartz, W. B., and Waters, W. C.: Lactate versus bicarbonate (editorial). Am. J. Med. *32*:831, 1962.

106. Selcer, R. R.: Trauma to the central nervous system. Vet. Clin. North Am. *10*:619, 1980.

107. Shappell, S. D., and Lenfant, C. J. M.: Adaptic, genetic and iatrogenic alterations of the oxyhemoglobin dissociation curve. Anesthesiology *37*:127, 1972.

108. Shatney, C. H.: The use of corticosteroids in the therapy of hemorrhagic shock. *In* Cowley, R. A., and Trump, B. F. (eds.): *Pathophysiology of Shock, Anoxia and Ischemia*. Williams & Wilkins, Baltimore, 1982, pp. 465–478.

109. Shires, G. T.: Principles and management of hemorrhagic shock. *In Care of the Trauma Patient*, 2nd ed. McGraw-Hill, New York, 1979, pp. 3–51.

110. Shires, G. T., and Canizaro, P. C.: Fluid resuscitation in the severely injured. Surg. Clin. North Am. *53*:1341, 1973.

111. Shoemaker, W. C.: Pathophysiology and therapy of hemorrhage and trauma states. *In* Cowley, R. A., and Trump, B. F. (eds.): *Pathophysiology of Shock, Anoxia and Ischemia*. Williams & Wilkins, Baltimore, 1982, pp. 439–446.

112. Shoemaker, W. C., and Bryan-Brown, C. W.: Resuscitation and the immediate care of the critically ill and injured patient. Semin. Drug. Treat. *3*:249, 1973.

113. Sibbald, W. J., and Driedger, A. A.: Pulmonary alveolarcapillary permeability in human septic respiratory distress syndrome. *In* Cowley, R. A., and Trump, B. F. (eds.): *Pathophysiology of Shock, Anoxia and Ischemia*. Williams & Wilkins, Baltimore, 1982, pp. 372–387.

114. Simmons, M. A., Adcock, E. W., Bard, H., et al.: Hypernatremia and intracranial hemorrhage in neonates. N. Engl. J. Med. *291*:6, 1974.

115. Sohmer, P. R., and Dawson, R. B.: Transfusion therapy in hemorrhagic shock. *In* Cowley, R. A., and Trump, B. F. (eds.): *Pathophysiology of Shock, Anoxia and Ischemia*. Williams & Wilkins, Baltimore, 1982, pp. 447–454.

116. Sprink, D. R., Malvin, R. L., and Cohen, B. J.: Determination of erythrocyte half life and blood volume in cats. Am. J. Vet. Res. *27*:1041, 1966.

117. Stevens, J. B.: Laboratory procedures in shock diagnosis and prognosis. Vet. Clin. North Am. *6*:203, 1976.

118. Stevens, J. B.: Post-shock complications. Vet. Clin. North Am. *6*:297, 1976.

119. Suteu, I.: General introduction. *In* Suteu, I., Bandila, T., Cafrita, A., Bucur, A. I., and Candea, V.: *Shock*. Abacus Press, Kent, England, 1977, pp. 1–50.

120. Webb, A. I.: Fluid therapy in hypotensive shock. Vet. Clin. North Am. *12*:515, 1982.

121. White, G. L., White, G. S., Kosanke, S. D., et al.: Therapeutic effects of prednisolone sodium succinate vs dexamethosone in dogs subjected to E. coli septic shock. J. Am. Anim. Hosp. Assoc. *18*:639, 1982.

122. Whittick, W. G.: Clinical evaluation of shock in small animals. Vet. Clin. North Am. *6*:227, 1976.

123. Wichterman, K. A., Baue, A. E., and Chaudry, I. H.: Sepsis and septic shock—a review of laboratory models and a proposal. J. Surg. Res. *29*:189, 1980.

124. Wilson, R. F.: The pathophysiology of shock. Intensive Care Med. *6*:89, 1980.

125. Wilson, R. F.: Future treatment of shock. *In* Cowley, R. A., and Trump, B. F. (eds.): *Pathophysiology of Shock, Anoxia and Ischemia*. Williams & Wilkins, Baltimore, 1982, p. 500.

126. Wright, C. J.: The effects of severe progressive hemodilution on regional blood flow and oxygen consumption. Surgery *79*:299, 1976.

127. Zborowska-Sluis, D. T., and Dossetor, J. B.: Hyperlactatemia of hyperventilation. J. Appl. Physiol. *22*:746, 1967.

12 Cardiopulmonary Arrest and Resuscitation

Sandee M. Hartsfield

Cardiopulmonary arrest (CPA) is a medical emergency that requires prompt attention and effective management to prevent irreversible deterioration of vital body tissues, particularly the brain. CPA can be defined as cessation of effective external respiration and cardiac function. Cardiopulmonary resuscitation (CPR) must begin in the absence of detectable arterial pulses and heart sounds. In the arrested patient, apneustic gasps may mimic effective breaths but produce inadequate alveolar ventilation. Cardiac electrical activity may be present, even in an apparently normal configuration, while mechanical myocardial movements produce no systolic arterial blood pressure elevation, resulting in inadequately perfused tissues. Similarly, direct inspection of the heart may reveal muscular contractions of the atria or fibrillatory motions by the ventricles with no cardiac output. One should not be deceived by such dissembled signs. The attending veterinarian must recognize the urgency of CPA, and all CPR plans must include the rapid institution of oxygen delivery to tissues.

CAUSES AND PREVENTION OF CPA

Numerous causes for CPA exist, and certain ominous indications of impending CPA have been determined. Knowledge of a patient's medical history, physical condition, and changes in physical status is the basis for prevention of CPA in critical or anesthetized patients. Pre-existing diseases, biochemical or physiological abnormalities, and anesthesia and surgical manipulations may contribute to the development of CPA.

Inadequate ventilation may be the most likely cause of CPA encountered by veterinarians.[89] Causes for insufficient ventilation include administration of general anesthetics and other pharmacological respiratory depressants (e.g., narcotics); airway obstruction due to acquired or congenital oropharyngeal, nasal, or respiratory abnormalities; and thoracic trauma and other abnormalities (e.g., pneumothorax, diaphragmatic hernia, obesity) that hinder diaphragmatic, lung, or thoracic wall movements. Ventilatory embarrassment may result in hypercapnia and hypoxemia, both of which contribute to a higher probability of CPA.[89, 105]

Hypoxemia can be caused by alveolar-to-capillary diffusion abnormalities (e.g., pulmonary edema), pulmonary ventilation-perfusion imbalances (e.g, pneumonia, collapsed lung), cardiac or pulmonary shunts (e.g., right to left intracardiac or intrapulmonary flow of unoxygenated blood), hypoventilation, or decreased inspired fractions of oxygen (e.g., abnormal anesthetic machine function).[60] In mild hypoxemia, tachycardia is consistent. However, prolonged or severe hypoxemia results in decreasing heart rate and can lead to circulatory failure.[100] In anesthetized patients, severe hypoxia may produce bradycardia that progresses to asystole (Fig. 12–1). Similarly, ventricular fibrillation has been related to arterial hypoxemia.[25]

Hypercarbia may contribute to CPA by predisposing to arrhythmias.[105] Unanesthetized patients may tolerate elevated CO_2 levels without arrhythmias, but arrhythmias related to hypercarbia are more prevalent in the presence of halogenated hydrocarbon anesthetics[100] and hypoxia.[25]

Acidemia, either metabolic or respiratory in origin, may contribute to CPA.[89] Acidosis increases catecholamine output in dogs,[53] which may play a role in the development of arrhythmias in patients with sensitized, hypoxic, diseased hearts.[25] Acidemia also enhances the depressant effects of some anesthetics (e.g., thiobarbiturates)[82] and may be partially responsible for relative overdosage of these drugs in certain critical patients.

Moderate to severe changes in body temperature are associated with CPA. Hypothermia produces an anesthetic effect, reducing apneic and anesthetizing alveolar concentrations of inhalation anesthetics in a rectilinear fashion below 37°C in dogs.[83] With halothane or methoxyflurane, the requirement for anesthesia drops by 5 per cent for each degree centigrade below 37°C.[39] Consequently, as the duration of anesthesia increases and hypothermia becomes more pronounced, patients tend to become too deeply anesthetized unless the inspired anesthetic concentration is reduced.[49] Concurrently, the cardiovascular system is affected by low body temperature. Cardiac dysrhythmias, decreased circulating blood volume, hemoconcentration, bradycardia, and depressed cardiac output are possible complications.[49] Clinically significant cardiovascular abnormalities are most likely if body temperature falls below 32°C for an extended period.[19] With further cooling, there is increased myocardial irritability and increased probability of cardiac arrest.[113] Following hypothermia, rewarming is associated with shivering and increased metabolic rate. Oxygen consumption may increase from 80 to 400 per cent, and hypoxemia may develop.[71, 113]

Hyperthermia from various causes is associated with respiratory arrest and cardiovascular abnormalities in later stages. Dysrhythmias and acid-base and

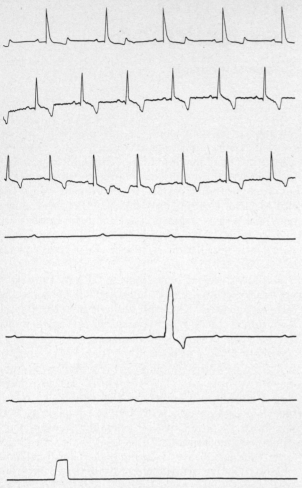

Figure 12–1. Progressive bradycardia leading to asystole due to hypoxia.

blood gas changes may be marked.[50, 96] In malignant hyperthermia, cardiac arrhythmias are common, are often associated with hyperkalemia, and may progress to asystole or ventricular fibrillation.[63]

Electrolyte imbalances, particularly changes in potassium or calcium, have been related to CPA.[25, 89, 105] Hyperkalemia, with potassium values of 5 to 7 mEq/L, may produce "tented" T waves and a minor acceleration of cardiac electrical conduction. With increasing potassium levels, the P-R interval of the electrocardiogram lengthens and the P wave ultimately disappears. Impulse generation and conduction are depressed in all cardiac tissues with QRS widening, eventually leading to asystole. Ventricular tachycardia or fibrillation may precede asystole in some instances.[73] Potassium elevation results in lower resting membrane potentials, weakened action potentials, and decreased strength of contractions.[79] Causes of potassium elevation include renal failure or urinary obstruction, adrenal cortical failure, acidosis, tissue trauma, use of succinylcholine, and inappropriate administration of potassium-containing solutions (e.g, potassium penicillin).[25] Depolarizing muscle relaxants such as succinylcholine must be given carefully, if at all, in traumatized patients (e.g., those with muscle damage and burns) to avoid elevation of serum potassium levels leading to severe dysrhythmias or cardiac arrest.[93]

Hypokalemia may induce abnormal cardiac rhythm and has been reported as a complicating factor in veterinary anesthesia leading to complete atrioventricular heart block.[76] Various cardiac arrhythmias including ventricular fibrillation have been reported in humans.[95, 103] Patients with low serum potassium levels are also subject to increased sensitivity to vagal stimulation.[31, 103] Hypokalemia augments the resting membrane potential of cardiac cells, and the difference between resting and threshold potential is increased, making the cell more difficult to depolarize. Repolarization of cell membranes is prolonged.[66, 95] It decreases conduction and enhances the automaticity of ventricular pacemaker cells.[38] Hypokalemia should be regarded as a possible complication in patients with diarrhea, vomiting, gastrointestinal obstruction and fluid accumulation, prolonged anorexia, long-term diuretic therapy, long-term steroid therapy, and certain renal disturbances. Treatment with alkalinizing agents (e.g., bicarbonate, lactate, and acetate) and hyperventilation may exacerbate the degree of hypokalemia in patients with marginal serum potassium levels and induce dysrhythmias, which may be of most significance in patients with pre-existing cardiovascular disease.[38]

Along with potassium changes, calcium may also influence arrhythmias in critical patients and may predispose to CPA. Increased serum calcium can cause a prolonged P-R interval, shortened Q-T interval,[24] myocardial excitability, and diminished ventricular systole. Ventricular premature contractions and ventricular tachycardia have been reported.[36] Ventricular fibrillation may occur with extreme hypercalcemia or can be related to cardiac mineralization.[24] Potential causes for hypercalcemia are numerous,[24] but increased calcium is commonly associated with malignant neoplasms.

Hypocalcemia may also produce certain electrocardiographic changes and hypotension. Ventricular extrasystoles may be associated with hypocalcemia of pregnancy, and hypotension has been successfully managed in man with calcium infusions.[108] Atrioventricular dissociation has been related to hypocalcemia in the dog.[70] Electrocardiographic signs include tachycardia and a prolonged Q-T interval.[25] Neuromuscular effects of hypocalcemia can include status epilepticus and muscular paralysis leading to respiratory arrest.[24]

Cardiovascular abnormalities place animals at risk for the development of CPA.[89] Hypovolemia and hypotension contribute to cardiovascular insufficiency owing to poor venous return, reducing tissue perfusion and possibly promoting acidosis. Therefore, maintenance and restoration of blood volume are important in the prevention of CPA.[89] Preanesthetic loading of fluids in cardiovascularly debilitated patients has been recommended.[55]

In providing tissue oxygenation, the amount of hemoglobin is critical. Anemia may impair oxygenation of vital tissues and predispose a patient to CPA,[105] although the significance of a reduction in hematocrit varies with the rapidity of its onset. In contrast, hemoconcentration may lead to increased blood viscosity, impaired blood flow in the microcirculation, and poor oxygenation of vital tissue.

In addition to these predisposing factors, significant arrhythmias and cardiac arrest may follow intense vagal stimulation. The effects of vagal stimulation are likely to be more pronounced in conjunction with hypoxia, hypercarbia, or electrolyte imbalance (e.g., hypokalemia).[65] Common stimuli for vagus-induced arrhythmias include endotracheal intubation, carotid sinus pressure, extraocular muscle manipulation, exteriorization or retraction of abdominal or thoracic viscera, diffuse or discrete stimulation of the central nervous system,[65] and direct stimulation of the vagus nerve.[105]

Surgical manipulations may contribute to the possibility of CPA if they create physiological embarrassment that produces one of the major abnormalities already mentioned—hypoxemia, acidemia, hypotension, electrolyte imbalance, or body temperature changes. Surgical packing may interfere with venous return by compressing the vena cava. Patient positioning presumably has the potential to create physiological abnormalities (e.g., large rolls positioned under the abdomen for spinal surgery) of both respiratory and cardiovascular function. Tilting of the surgical table to create head-down positioning may alter lung volume, blood pressure, and cerebral perfusion.[81] Exteriorization of an abdominal mass (e.g., a gravid uterus or a large abdominal tumor) may lead to hypotension by creating vasculogenic shock[46] or by interfering with venous return. Blood loss during surgery with inadequate hemostasis may contribute to hypotension and resultant hypoxemia and acidemia if tissue perfusion is impaired. Prolonged exposure and manipulation of the gastrointestinal tract may promote decreased blood pressure and plasma volume loss.[32, 33] In traumatized patients, the surgical manipulation of the liver can result in release of vasoactive substances and emboli that can contribute to an abnormal patient status.[69] Surgical manipulations of the stomach in canine gastric dilation-torsion can result in dysrhythmias,[75] probably related to changes in the autonomic nervous system. Finally, my clinical impression is that surgical handling of infected, necrotic tissues may promote hypotension. Examples include radical mastectomy, pyometra, and exploration of large areas of fistulous tracts. Nearly all surgical procedures produce increased tissue exposure that will potentiate anesthetic-induced hypothermia, but those that create the most tissue exposure are most significant (e.g., radical mastectomy, abdominal exploration with exteriorization of viscera, and thoracic surgery).[49] Obviously, direct interference with the heart, great vessels, or lungs may create physiological abnormalities, and surgery that impairs perfusion of the heart or central nervous

system, particularly the brain, must be considered hazardous with regard to the potential development of CPA. Such interference can be related to direct organ manipulation or interference with the major blood vessels related to those organs.

Venous air embolism is another cause of acute CPA. It has been reported in association with cryotherapy[52] as well as other surgical procedures.[106] If the operative site is elevated above the level of the right heart, there may be increased risk.[113] Air may be drawn into exposed vessels, leading to cardiovascular collapse. The cause may be an air lock in the heart with failure of cardiac output (rapid air uptake) or a sympatholytic reflex initiated by receptors in the pulmonary vasculature leading to decreased peripheral resistance and shock (slow uptake of air).[1]

Although the specific patient that responds unfavorably to surgery or general anesthesia cannot be predicted with accuracy,[55] certain types of surgeries and anesthetics are associated with greater mortality in human patients.[37, 72, 107] Emergency surgery results in the most instances of CPA. In elective procedures, mortality is highest in neurosurgery and cardiovascular surgery, followed by intra-abdominal surgery; mortality is lowest in other types of surgery.[72]

The best determinant of the likelihood of CPA may be assessment of the preanesthetic physical status of the patient. Assignment of patients to classes I, II, III, IV, and V[71] prior to anesthesia and surgery is of value in this regard. As the physical status deteriorates, the patient is classed in a higher numbered category, and the occurrence of CPA is greater.[37, 107] The age of the patient does influence mortality, but only in that more aged patients tend to fall into higher physical status categories.[72] In veterinary patients, one report indicates that a substantial number of malpractice claims involved cosmetic surgical procedures of the ears and tail in small and giant breeds of dogs.[34] Although this does not reflect the incidence of CPA in such elective procedures compared with nonelective and emergency surgeries, it does indicate the need for careful monitoring and evaluation of all patients during all surgeries despite the apparent simplicity or low risk involved.

In anesthetizing patients for diagnostic, surgical, and therapeutic manipulations, the fact that anesthetics and anesthetic adjunctive agents may induce CPA in themselves or may contribute to physiological derangement that can lead to CPA should be foremost in the mind of the veterinarian. General anesthesia is definitely associated with CPA. A British high court judge once gave the following opinion: "It is a fact that to anesthetize a human being, to deprive him of consciousness outright, is to take a considerable step along the road to killing him."[56, 107] Although CPA may occur during anesthesia owing to unusual patient responses to particular drugs, the true relationship between anesthesia and CPA probably involves errors in anesthetic administration, patient monitoring, and clinical judgment rather than the specific drug chosen or the anesthetic state itself. However, it is unlikely that gross overdosage of anesthetics plays a significant role in CPA in clinical practice.[47] Relative overdosage probably remains an important factor in the development of CPA. There are numerous examples of patients that can be easily given a relative excess of anesthetic drug: (1) hypovolemic patients that have reduced circulating blood volumes, allowing greater than normal percentages of an injectable drug to reach vital organs (e.g., brain and heart),[82] (2) acidotic patients that respond more dramatically to thiobarbiturates because acidemia results in more of the undissociated, active drug,[82] and (3) patients with pre-existing cardiopulmonary abnormalities that respond more profoundly than normal to a given dose of drug owing to decreased volume of drug distribution, physiological abnormalities induced by the disease state (e.g., acidemia), or pre-existing cardiac depression that appears synergistic with the effect of the drug.

In addition to gross or relative overdosages, there are other obvious errors in anesthetic protocol that should be avoided. These include use of epinephrine in the face of halogenated hydrocarbon anesthesia (particularly halothane) in unprotected patients; failure to use anticholinergic premedication prior to the use of narcotics, xylazine, or antiacetylcholinesterase drugs (reversal agents for nondepolarizing muscle relaxants); failure to use anticholinergic premedication when profound vagal stimulation is likely; failure to intubate the anesthetized patient or assure a patent airway in any patient; failure to support breathing when hypoventilation develops; failure to attend to fluid volume and acid-base abnormalities; use of certain antibiotics concurrently with or shortly after administration of muscle relaxants (without prolonged attention to ventilation), allowing extreme hypothermia to develop; failure to evacuate the pleural space adequately post thoracotomy; use of succinylcholine as a muscle relaxant for recently traumatized patients; and failure to regularly monitor heart rate, pulse quality, and respiration in any anesthetized or heavily sedated patient. In contrast, the ability to control the airway and the immediate availability of a means of assuring a patent airway are given as reasons for the low incidence of malpractice claims against veterinarians using inhalation anesthesia.[34]

Knowledge of each patient's medical history and physical status will help the veterinarian to recognize a group of animals that should be monitored carefully, possibly requiring intensive observation in a critical care unit or extremely close management during anesthesia and surgery. By monitoring, one can prevent the onset of CPA through early recognition and treatment of inadequate or abnormal cardiopulmonary function.[55] Monitoring and observation are keys to the prevention of CPA.[89] Regular or continuous evaluation of respiratory, cardiovascular, renal, and central nervous system function should be performed.

Sophisticated mechanical and electronic monitors can be utilized with profit, but adequate monitoring can be done for many patients without such devices. Palpation, thermometry, and stethoscopy are basic for an evaluation of heart and respiration rate and sounds, body temperature, and pulse rate and quality. Some arrhythmias may be noted by detection of pulse deficits. Fluid administration for critical patients should include records of fluid input, urine production and other fluid losses, and central venous pressure. An electrocardiographic tracing gives valuable information about electrical activity of the heart and the numerous influences on it. Measurements of acid-base balance and blood gases can also prove helpful. Various blood and urine tests can be done serially to evaluate the status of a critical patient (hematocrit, serum protein, electrolytes, urine specific gravity, and pH). Other variables can be monitored and other equipment used. All monitoring should be done to allow early detection of conditions that predispose to CPA, allowing prevention if possible. If CPA occurs despite all efforts, continuous monitoring will allow early recognition so that resuscitation procedures can begin before extensive organ system damage has occurred due to ischemia, anoxia, and shock.

RECOGNITION OF CPA

It is imperative that impending or existing CPA be recognized immediately, because hypoxic damage to central nervous tissue occurs after approximately three minutes in animals with normal body temperature.[55] Usually, patients will not survive cardiac arrest that exceeds four minutes,[25, 89] although patients that are hypothermic at the time of circulatory arrest may be revived after slightly longer periods.[13]

Diminished respiration, decreasing amplitude of heart sounds, cyanosis, failing pulse quality, rapid or pronounced reduction in heart rate, and prolonged capillary refill time may be indicative of impending cardiac arrest.[25] Some electrocardiographic changes are warnings of the potential development of cardiac arrest. These include ventricular tachycardia, multifocal ventricular extrasystoles, diminishing amplitude of QRS, and T wave or ST segment changes.

Signs of existing cardiac arrest are fairly consistent.[25, 55] The presence of cardiac arrest is indicated by lack of a palpable pulse, apex heart beat, and heart sounds as well as an absence of effective ventilation. Cyanosis or pallor of mucous membranes may be present along with pupillary dilation. Unconsciousness also accompanies the onset of cardiac arrest.

If electronic or mechanical monitoring is being used prior to the onset of CPA, these devices are valuable in determining CPA. Electrocardiographic monitoring has become common in intensive care facilities, and the characteristic appearance of the oscilloscopic trace in asystole or ventricular fibrillation confirms a diagnosis of CPA. If central venous pressure (CVP) is being monitored, it increases rapidly following cardiac arrest and reaches values between 20 and 25 cm H_2O within seconds.[25] The use of external blood pressure monitoring can be helpful in the early detection of CPA. Reduction of arterial blood pressure to 0 is indicative of CPA. Although each mechanical device offers advantages, nothing has replaced observation of the surgical, anesthetized, or critical patient by veterinarians or technicians trained in intensive monitoring techniques. Therefore, stethoscopy and evaluation of the patient by palpation are invaluable. In all instances, cardiopulmonary resuscitation (CPR) techniques should be begun if heart sounds and a palpable pulse are not present.

INITIAL MANAGEMENT OF CPA—CPR

The initial goal of CPR is effective cardiopulmonary support[55] to prevent deterioration of vital organs, particularly the brain, until appropriate cardiopulmonary function can be re-instituted. In nearly all CPA patients, the basic steps of CPR are necessary to allow time for definitive therapy. The steps in CPR have been given as ABCs[55, 89]: Airway, Breathing, Circulation, Drugs, Electrocardiographic monitoring.

The first three steps must be immediate, almost simultaneous, and continuous for CPR to be effective. Some patients respond to the initial establishment of artificial ventilation and circulation by resumption of spontaneous, effective cardiopulmonary function.[89]

Artificial Ventilation

Airway

In small domestic animals, a patent airway is established with an endotracheal tube, but occasionally a tracheostomy tube is used. Appropriate devices for intubation should be available in any veterinary facility, and all anesthetized patients should have protected airways following induction. When an endotracheal tube is placed, it should be secured adequately. Failure to secure a patent airway may be a factor in unsuccessful resuscitation. The endotracheal tube may be placed correctly initially, but it can be dislocated owing to failure to tie it in place. Although the endotracheal tube for CPR does not have to be perfectly sized, tubes that are too long can be easily introduced into one bronchus, creating an unventilated lung and a pulmonary vascular shunt, which will promote hypoxemia. Extremely short tubes may be displaced during external cardiac massage or cuff inflation. A tube with a diameter near that of the tracheal lumen is desirable to reduce resistance to breathing, particularly when the patient begins to ventilate spontaneously after resuscitation.

Breathing—Intermittent Positive Pressure Ventilation

After endotracheal intubation has been effected, intermittent positive pressure ventilation (IPPV) should be applied to the patient's respiratory system to assure adequate alveolar ventilation.[55] In itself, external cardiac compression does not provide adequate ventilation.[25] The importance of properly applied artificial respiration cannot be overemphasized. Adequate ventilation is necessary to alleviate hypercapnia, and the CO_2 produced by a combination of sodium bicarbonate and metabolic acids during pharmacological correction of metabolic acidosis must be eliminated through the respiratory system.[25] Without an open end to the bicarbonate buffer system, CO_2 accumulates, thus contributing to acidosis rather than eliminating it.[77] During application of positive pressure ventilation, one can assess the need for internal cardiac massage. In patients with significant quantities of pleural air or fluid, the lungs appear rather poorly compliant and resist inflation, indicating that CPR can probably be better applied with internal cardiac compression.[25] Such decreased respiratory compliance may be discovered early in certain patients (e.g., traumatic emergencies), or compliance may be reduced later and recognized as a complication of the CPR procedure, particularly when CPR is inappropriately applied (e.g., development of pneumothorax due to alveolar rupture). To provide adequate tidal volume for elimination of CO_2 and to prevent alveolar damage leading to pneumothorax, ventilation should be coordinated with external massage. That is, the thorax should not be compressed at the same time that the lungs are being inflated.[55] Coordination of massage and ventilation is obviously unimportant during open chest cardiac compression, and artificial ventilation can be applied in the same manner as that for intrathoracic surgery.

During external massage, the patient should be ventilated regularly. Massage rhythm should not be interrupted for breathing, but breathing should be strategically interspersed between two compressions of the thorax. The rate of ventilation should be approximately 12 respirations per minute.[89] One breath for each five to seven external compressions has been recommended.[25, 55, 89, 97] This rate is usually appropriate for internal cardiac massage also. The use of large tidal volumes in resuscitation has been suggested.[55] The proper application of artificial ventilation is necessary for it to be most effective and cause the least cardiovascular interference. In normal or anesthetized patients, positive pressure ventilation impairs thoracic blood flow by decreasing venous return to both sides of the heart, by increasing pulmonary vascular resistance, and by interfering with ventricular diastolic filling.[54] These effects are pronounced by a long duration of inspiration (greater than 1.0 to 1.5 seconds), by high intrathoracic pressures (greater than 20 cm H_2O), and by excessive respiratory rate (greater than 8 to 15 respirations per minute). Pressures greater than 40 cm H_2O applied to the respiratory system may cause physical damage,[54] and continuous pressure on the respiratory system may decrease venous return significantly.[55, 58]

The device chosen to facilitate artificial ventilation is based on the preference of the veterinarian and the available equipment. An anesthetic machine with either an adult circle system or a pediatric system is most likely to be used. However, a self-inflating resuscitation bag is useful, and mouth-to-tube ventilation can be substituted.[55] Automatic, pressure-limited, or pressure-cycled mechanical ventilators are not desirable for artificial ventilation during external cardiac massage.[89] The inflation cycle will be prematurely terminated by each compression of the thorax.[45] With other types of ventilators, it is difficult to coordinate the inspiratory cycle of the ventilator with external compression of the chest unless manual cycling is employed.[45, 55]

Oxygen

During positive pressure ventilation, the make-up of gases supplied to the patient must be considered. In CPR, oxygen is an essential drug.[45] Since reduced tissue blood flow, hypoxia, and acidosis develop during CPA, adequate tissue oxygenation is vital during CPR. External cardiac compression contributes to pulmonary arteriovenous shunting, which increases arterial CO_2 and decreases arterial O_2 tensions.[25] Hypoxemia is common after shock or cardiac arrest.[92, 99]

Basic causes of hypoxemia include low inspired fraction of oxygen (FI_{O_2}), hypoventilation, diffusion impairment, pulmonary ventilation, perfusion mismatching, and right-to-left shunting of blood. All are potential problems in CPA. A low FI_{O_2} is unlikely unless room air is used for resuscitation or gas flowmeters are improperly adjusted (e.g., inadvertent increase in N_2O). Certainly, once CPA is recognized, all anesthetic gases must be eliminated, and 100 per cent O_2 should be used. Adjustments of all flowmeters and vaporizers should be double-checked early in resuscitation. Hypoventilation is usually eliminated as a cause of hypoxemia during CPR by IPPV, assuming proper application. Pulmonary edema may interfere with gas diffusion across the alveolar-capillary membrane and promote hypoxemia. External massage reduces functional residual capacity and promotes small airway closure. Ventilation and perfusion mismatching can occur owing to an imbalance of perfusion and gas flow into various areas of the lungs.[25] Portions of the lung that are completely unventilated but are still perfused are extremes of V/Q mismatching called *pulmonary arteriovenous shunts*. Hypoxemia can be at least partially corrected by allowing the patient to breathe high levels of oxygen.[60] For shock or CPR in man it is recommended that FI_{O_2} be maintained at a minimum of 60 torr in conscious patients and at a minimum of 100 torr in unconscious patients.[92] These minimums may

not be met in patients ventilated with room air if significant shunts or other abnormalities leading to hypoxemia exist.

In the CPA patient, the factors leading to hypoxemia should be reversed as quickly as possible. Increasing cardiac output, providing artificial ventilation, and elevating the inspired concentration of oxygen are used together to improve tissue perfusion, restore aerobic metabolism, and inhibit further development of acidosis.

Analeptics

In CPA, veterinarians may be tempted to use analeptics to restore spontaneous respiration. These drugs cannot be recommended for routine use. Probably the greatest disadvantage to their use is the delay in initiation of more appropriate therapy.

Artificial Circulation

Blood flow to vital organ systems during CPA can be partially restored by either internal cardiac compression (ICC) or external chest compression (ECC). Immediately upon recognition of CPA, ECC should begin. Since the amount of ventilation produced by ECC is inadequate, endotracheal intubation and artificial respiration must also be used. However, ECC should not be delayed even for the few seconds required to obtain an endotracheal tube and establish IPPV. When appropriate equipment is available, ECC can be interrupted for 15 seconds for intubation.[89] Assessment of the patient after the initial application of ECC and IPPV should indicate whether to continue ECC or begin ICC.

Precordial Thump

The value of precordial thump in dogs and cats has yet to be determined, but one study in dogs showed no particular benefit and even some detrimental effects.[89, 114] Institution of ECC and IPPV should not be delayed by this procedure.[89]

External Chest Compression

Regardless of the situation, external chest compression (ECC) should be instituted as the initial step in CPR (except when the thorax has been incised prior to CPA). This method can be continued if patient evaluation shows it to be effective, usually indicated by a palpable pulse in the area of the large femoral vessels, improved mucous membrane color, and pupillary response to light.[45, 55, 57]

Generally, the patient is placed in right lateral recumbency for ECC.[57] Some authors recommend dorsal recumbency for barrel-chested dogs.[25] Patient size determines the technique and force of compression, and the resuscitator's preference may alter positioning of the hands.[55] The following techniques are useful:

1. **Very small patients (<3 kg):** The dorsum (vertebrae) is stabilized with one hand. The other hand is placed so that the thumb is on one side of the thorax and the fingers are on the other side. Palpation of the heart through the thorax allows appropriate placement of the thumb and fingers.

2. **Small patients (approximately 3 to 5 kg):** One hand is placed on the sternum and one on the dorsum. The thumbs are used to compress the thorax over the heart.

3. **Medium patients (5 to 10 kg):** With one hand stabilizing the dorsum, the heart can be compressed between the heel of the hand on one side of the thorax and the fingers on the other.

4. **Medium to large patients (10 to 25 kg):** The heel and palm of one hand are used to compress the thorax. The dorsum of the patient is stabilized with the other hand if the resuscitator is standing on the sternal side of the patient. If the resuscitator prefers to stand on the dorsal side, the free hand is used to stabilize the sternum.

5. **Large patients (>25 kg):** The resuscitator stands on the sternal side of the patient and compresses the thorax over the heart using both hands (interlocking fingers as in human CPR). The dorsum of the patient is stabilized by a second person or by moving the dorsum of the patient next to a solid surface such as a wall.

General recommendations for ECC are 60 to 80 compressions per minute, although higher rates have been suggested for smaller dogs.[25, 55, 57, 89] The force should vary with the size of the patient, but compression should be directly over the heart. In ECC in humans sufficient pressure is required to depress an adult's lower sternum a minimum of 4 to 5 cm, young children 2 to 4 cm, and infants 1 to 2 cm.[45] This may give some rough guidelines for veterinary use.

Positioning of the patient is important in ECC. Horizontal positioning, without any elevation of the head, is expected to produce more cerebral blood flow.[101] Smooth, regular, and uninterrupted compressions, with complete release between compressions, should be applied. A time cycle requiring equal time for compression and release has been recommended in man.[101] Others have recommended cycles of one-third compression and two-thirds release.[55] The release time is important to allow adequate blood flow (venous return) to the heart and thorax.[101] The hand used in ECC should maintain contact with the thoracic wall during the release time, but there should be a period during which no pressure is applied to the chest.[101]

The main advantages of ECC are its ease of application, lack of necessity for surgical intervention, and proven effectiveness. It appears that properly performed ECC provides 25 to 50 per cent of normal basal cardiac output.[25] In humans, ECC is expected to produce peak systolic blood pressures of approximately 100 mm Hg. However, the diastolic pressure is low and mean blood pressure in the carotid arteries usually does not exceed 40 mm Hg, producing only about one-third or less of normal carotid blood flow.[101] In dogs, a diastolic blood pressure of 40 mm Hg has been shown necessary for successful resuscitation.[115]

Venous return to the heart must be adequate for ECC to be effective. Measures for improving venous return during ECC include abdominal binding.[55] However, abdominal binding is not recommended in human CPR because of the danger of hepatic entrapment and rupture during ECC.[48, 101, 112] Other techniques for maximizing venous return include fluid loading and administration of certain pharmacological vasoconstrictors.[55]

Various complications may arise owing to ECC. Proper performance of the technique prevents some problems, but rib fractures, costochondral separations, pneumothorax, hemothorax, lung contusions, liver damage, and fat emboli are possible.[5, 57 101] Because of the potential for trauma with ECC, internal massage should be considered after 10 to 20 minutes,[55] even if the technique is effective.

Internal Cardiac Compression

Internal cardiac compression (ICC) is indicated when ECC is ineffective (determined within one to two minutes after initiating ECC) or when a thoracic surgical procedure is already in progress. In patients with suspected intrathoracic pathology[92] (pneumothorax, pericardial effusion or pleural fluid) and in barrel-chested patients (e.g., English bulldogs), ICC may be indicated almost immediately to assure adequate circulation.[55, 101] Penetrating chest wounds and extensive thoracic wall injury with rib fractures are also indications for ICC.[55, 92]

There are several advantages of ICC over ECC.[55, 92] (1) ICC allows direct visualization of the heart, necessary to determine adequacy of venous return. (2) ICC permits examination and correction of intrathoracic pathology that may interfere with CPR (e.g., hemorrhage). (3) It affords direct detection of ventricular fibrillation. (4) It allows aortic compression to enhance coronary and cerebral blood flow. (5) It allows direct intracardiac injections without the potential for laceration of a coronary vessel.

ICC usually involves thoracotomy at the fourth or fifth intercostal space of the left thoracic wall. The ribs should be separated with surgical retractors (basic CPR emergency equipment [Table 12–1]). Upon entry into the chest, the pericardial sac is incised longitudinally below the phrenic nerve.[55] Following resuscitation, closure of the pericardium may constrict the heart, which usually becomes dilated during massage. Also, transudate from the traumatized epicardium may collect in a closed pericardial sac.[55] Therefore, the pericardium is closed loosely or left open in a manner that will not allow the heart to become entrapped in the opening of the sac.

TABLE 12–1. Drugs, Equipment, and Supplies for Use in Cardiopulmonary Resuscitation

Surgical Pack (for venous cut-down and thoracotomy)
Scalpel handle
Scalpel blade
Scissors
Several hemostats
2-0 silk suture
Rib retractors

Needles
18, 20, and 23 gauges

Syringes
1, 3, 5, 10, 20, 60 ml

Catheters
Around-the-needle type (4 to 7 cm)—18 and 20 gauge
Inside-the-needle type (25 to 28 cm)—18 and 20 gauge
Butterfly type (2.5 cm)—19 and 23 gauge

Supplies
Tape—1 and 2 cm
Gauze (roll type)—4 to 6 cm
Gauze sponges—8 × 8 cm or 10 × 10 cm
Electrode paste
Tourniquet
Three-way stopcock
Thoracic drain tubes
Heimlich valves
Assorted endotracheal tubes—2.5 to 12 mm inside diameter
Elastic bandage—5 to 7 cm
Tongue depressors
Ophthalmic ointment
Laryngoscope and blade

Equipment
Electrocardiograph with appropriate leads
Direct current defibrillator with appropriate internal and external paddles
Complete anesthetic machine and system

Drugs
Sodium bicarbonate
Prednisolone sodium succinate
Dexamethasone
Atropine
Glycopyrrolate
Lidocaine
Epinephrine
Isoproterenol
Dopamine
Calcium chloride
Heparin
Procainamide
Oxygen

Fluids—250, 500, and 1000 ml
5% dextrose
Balanced electrolyte solution

Since emergency thoracotomy does not allow time for aseptic surgical technique, appropriate steps must be taken as for a contaminated surgical site. Flushing, thoracic drainage, and operative and postoperative antibiotic therapy are usually indicated.

Massage is begun at a rate of 60 to 80 compressions per minute using the palmar surfaces of the hand (not the finger tips, which could create enough pressure to "dig into" and damage the myocardium).[57] The heart should be compressed from apex to base, similar to the normal contraction mechanism. Small hearts can be compressed effectively between the palmar surfaces of the thumb and one or two fingers, medium-sized hearts can be massaged between the palmar surfaces of the fingers and the palm of the hand, and large hearts can be compressed between the palm of one hand and the opposite thoracic wall.[55] In some medium to large patients, both hands may be used to compress the ventricles and generate effective ejection of blood from the heart.[57] Large hearts can be compressed with one hand behind and one hand in front of the heart.[92] Since filling of the ventricles is necessary for adequate stroke volume with ICC, adequate time for venous return must be allowed after each compression.

Effective ICC may supply 50 to 60 per cent of the normal cardiac output. This greater output compared with that of ECC is due to selective ventricular compression without compression of the atria or vena cava.[25] To be effective, venous return must be adequate. This may be improved by fluid loading, vasoconstrictor administration, or abdominal binding.[7, 55] When holding the heart, the resuscitator must be careful to avoid occlusion of the great vessels that supply venous return by twisting or excessively elevating the heart,[55] especially in small patients. To improve cerebral and coronary blood flow during ICC, the resuscitator may compress the descending aorta with the fingers of the free hand.[55] After effective mechanical cardiac function begins, ICC should be continued for five to ten minutes to augment cardiac output.[57]

Physiology of ECC and ICC

Two mechanisms of blood flow during CPR using external compression of the chest—the cardiac pump and the thoracic pump—have been suggested.[7] Both may be effective in certain cases. In ECC, equally high pressures may be generated simultaneously in all four cardiac chambers.[25] In studies using large dogs (20 to 40 kg), there was essentially an equal rise in central venous, right atrial, pulmonary artery, and aortic blood pressures.[91] The pressure in the intrathoracic vasculature was nearly equal to the general intrathoracic (esophageal) pressure. Since forward carotid blood flow occurred only during chest compression, a pressure gradient must have existed to create flow. Since all pressures were equal in the heart during ECC, the heart did not create a pressure gradient between the aorta and the central veins, as it does during normal function. Thus, an extrathoracic peripheral arterial-venous pressure gradient was confirmed by measuring extrathoracic pressures in the carotid artery and the jugular vein. Thoracic pressures generated during ECC were transmitted to the carotid artery but not to the jugular vein. Three mechanisms may contribute to this pressure differential, including venous valves, greater venous than arterial capacitance, and greater arterial resistance to collapse. During ECC, extrathoracic venous pressure rises[91] (although not as high as extrathoracic arterial pressure). Between compressions, intrathoracic pressure falls, and blood flows from the periphery to the central veins. Compression of the right heart *per se* may be involved in pulmonary blood flow.[109] However, during release of chest compression,[26, 109] pulmonary blood flow occurs because an extrathoracic venous-to-intrapulmonary pressure gradient exists.[109] Even if the heart is compressed appreciably during ECC, cardiac compression is not likely to be responsible for generating peripheral or systemic blood flow.[109] However, significant compression of the heart during ECC may promote a higher arterial pressure and, more importantly, a higher diastolic pressure. This could, if present, improve coronary perfusion.[109] Therefore, ECC should be applied directly over the heart during CPR.

Direct cardiac compression during ECC may be the more significant mechanism in smaller dogs (less than 10 kg), since positive systolic arteriovenous pressure differences in the thorax have been recorded during CPR.[7] When such a difference exists, the heart functions as a pump. In either mechanism, the determinants of venous return are very similar. Fluid loading, venoconstrictor administration, and abdominal binding are effective in promoting venous return.[7]

Abdominal binding has been shown to augment carotid blood flow in the dog,[109] and the procedure has been recommended for veterinary use.[55] The mechanisms have been postulated to be increased intrathoracic pressure during ECC, direction of blood flow away from the abdominal viscera, and increased effective circulating blood volume.[109] Whereas some workers have shown significant cardiovascular benefits and lowered mortality from abdominal binding,[84, 109] others have suggested a higher incidence of hepatic rupture.[48] In one canine study, evidence of hepatic damage was not found.[91]

Recent studies indicate that synchronous use of ECC and high-airway pressure ventilation approximately doubles carotid blood flow.[20] However, in some dogs, carotid flow may be less than with conventional CPR.[109] At present, the procedure is still experimental, and the use of asynchronous ECC and ventilation appears most appropriate in the uncontrolled clinical setting.

In comparison with ECC, ICC produces significantly better blood pressures and flows.[25, 92] The increased cardiac output with ICC results from selective ventricular compression without greatly affecting the atria or the vena cavae.[25, 44] If CPR is prolonged, ICC provides a better chance for restarting the heart and brain recovery.[4, 92]

Initial Pharmacological Management of Cardiopulmonary Arrest (CPA)

Following establishment of an airway, artificial ventilation, and artificial circulation, the type of pharmacological or mechanical intervention used varies with each patient. In acute ventricular fibrillation in a monitored patient, electrical defibrillation can be done immediately without drug therapy. In acute asystole, epinephrine may be used for initial management. However, patients that undergo cardiac arrest may need, in addition to tissue oxygenation, alkalinization to improve the effectiveness of cardiac arrest therapy.

During CPA, numerous factors contribute to decreased tissue perfusion, hypoxemia, and inadequate tissue oxygenation.[101] With inadequate oxygenation of tissues, anaerobic metabolism leads to metabolic acidosis. Acidosis may impair the beneficial effects of pharmacological and electrical therapies.[101] Shock, ischemia, and hypoxemia are associated with cellular damage in various organ systems. Cellular and subcellular membrane dysfunction probably leads to decreased metabolic capability, lysosomal leakage, and cellular destruction.[21, 22] In CPA that is recognized and reversed very quickly, such considerations are not extremely significant. However, if CPA has existed for several minutes, if CPA occurs in a patient with pre-existing abnormalities, or if CPR is prolonged, tissue hypoperfusion and its effects must be countered. Blood volume expansion, correction of acidemia, and prevention of cellular deterioration are important factors.

Creation of a more effective circulating blood volume can be accomplished in several ways. Recent considerations include abdominal binding, medical antishock garments, and vasoconstrictors.[55, 101, 109] The most common procedure for increasing venous return in veterinary CPR is probably fluid loading. The purpose of increasing venous return is to assure adequate central blood volume between thoracic or cardiac compressions. Procedures that promote elevation of arterial blood pressure, specifically diastolic pressure, are likely to increase survival.[55, 86-88, 114] If diastolic blood pressure can be increased, coronary blood flow is improved, increasing the chances of resumption of spontaneous cardiac function. Indeed, it has been concluded that the main benefit of epinephrine in resuscitation is alpha-adrenergic stimulation, causing increased peripheral vasoconstriction, diastolic blood pressure, and coronary blood flow.[78, 88]

Since fluid loading should be accomplished early in CPR to supplement venous return,[55] an appropriate intravenous catheter must be inserted. A short, large-bore catheter should be placed and secured to assure rapid fluid delivery. A venous cut-down should be performed if percutaneous catheter insertion is difficult and causes delay. A peripheral vein (cephalic or saphenous) is a good location for insertion, since the catheter can be secured easily. It is usually more difficult to manage placement and stabilization of a jugular catheter during CPR.

The fluid chosen for initial volume expansion during CPR is not critical, since increasing venous return is its main purpose. However, 5% dextrose in water has been suggested[101] because of the absence of both sodium and calcium. Since sodium bicarbonate is often a part of CPR therapy, hyperosmolar effects are possible, and 5% dextrose can help to counteract them. In addition, some drugs may precipitate if administered in calcium-containing fluids.

Establishment of a reliable intravenous route is essential in advanced human CPR.[101] It is not only useful for fluid administration but also for other medications. Unnecessary cardiac punctures can be avoided. Even though repeated cardiac punctures appear to be relatively safe,[17, 30] the potential exists for complications following intracardiac puncture. Pneumothorax caused by intracardiac needle placement during positive pressure breathing, hemopericardium, cardiac tamponade, and coronary artery puncture or laceration are possible. However, the main disadvantage of the intracardiac route is the need to stop ECC.[101] Although some clinical reports indicate that intracardiac epinephrine may be more effective than intravenous epinephrine,[101] the advantages of the intracardiac route remain to be proved.[30] For cardiac effects, intracardiac punctures have been recommended for such drugs as epinephrine and calcium.[55] For peripheral effects, intravenous administration is effective,[55] and drugs such as sodium bicarbonate and glucocorticoids are usually administered intravenously. Many clinicians use the intravenous route almost exclusively for CPR drugs if possible.

In CPR, adequate ventilation is used to combat respiratory acidosis (CO_2 retention) due to respiratory arrest, and sodium bicarbonate is used to counter metabolic acidosis (increased hydrogen ion) due to inadequate tissue oxygenation, anaerobic metabolism, and lactic acid build-up. As acidosis increases, several detrimental effects are possible. The myocardium is less responsive to electrical defibrillation in the presence of acidosis,[25, 101] and acidosis enhances myocardial irritability, making ventricular fibrillation more likely. In addition, the acidotic heart does not respond as well as the normal heart to catecholamines,[92] and severe acidosis impairs myocardial contractility.[89]

A number of factors influence the need for bicarbonate during CPR. These include the duration of CPA prior to institution of CPR, the degree of prearrest hypoperfusion and acidosis, the effectiveness of ECC or ICC during CPR, and the duration of CPR before establishment of a normal beat. Therefore, the decision to administer bicarbonate must be based on good clinical judgment, and the administration must be accompanied by repeated measurements of arterial acid-base and blood gas values.[89]

In human CPR, an amount of bicarbonate equal to 1 mEq/kg is recommended as an initial dose, to be followed by no more than one-half that amount at ten-minute intervals during CPA.[101] Greater doses (0.5 to 1.0 mEq/kg/5 min) have been recommended in the veterinary literature,[55] although bicarbonate may not be needed if the heart is restarted within five minutes (if acidosis did not precede CPA).[55]

If acid-base and blood gas values can be determined, more accurate evaluation of bicarbonate needs can be made. During resuscitation, the calculated bicarbonate needs can be based on the volume of the vascular fluid compartment (8 per cent of body weight) to avoid excessive alkalinization.[55] Following shock or resuscitation, the increased perfusion of various organ systems may result in removal of lactic acid and reduced pH.[92, 101] Therefore, it is appropriate to re-evaluate acid-base balance following CPR. In many cases of mild acidosis, hepatic metabolism of lactate can effectively raise pH without the use of alkalinizers. However, if pH is very low, alkalinizers are indicated, and administration should be based initially on the following formula: 0.3 × body weight (kg) × base deficit = bicarbonate (mEq) to be given over approximately two hours. Acid-base and blood gas values should be measured again after this period.[51]

When alkalinizers are used, CO_2 forms as a product of bicarbonate and hydrogen ion, leading to carbonic acid and, ultimately, CO_2 and H_2O. Without adequate ventilation, CO_2 accumulates and may contribute to acidemia.[77] Owing to the ease of CO_2 diffusion into cerebrospinal fluid (CSF), CSF acidosis is a potential complication.[10, 12] Other possible side effects of sodium bicarbonate administration include excessive alkalinization, sodium overload, and dysrhythmias.[51] Rapid alkalinization may produce increased hemoglobin-oxygen affinity, leading to decreased cellular oxygen availability.[9, 35, 98] Following rapid alkalosis, arrhythmias may develop, possibly related to variations in serum levels of calcium, potassium, and sodium or due to hypoxemia.[6, 40, 68] Since increased oxygen consumption is associated with alkalosis,[18, 64] alkalosis may both inhibit O_2 delivery and increase consumption.[27] Also, extracellular alkalosis has a more profound effect on the intracellular environment than does extracellular acidosis.[2, 3] Severe hyperventilation, causing CO_2 elimination and respiratory alkalosis, has been associated with increased cerebral ischemia in shock.[92] Therefore, the use of alkalinizers and IPPV demands care, and excessive alkalinization should be avoided.

In situations of poor tissue perfusion, ischemia, or anoxia, the use of glucocorticoids remains controversial. However, the literature suggests numerous beneficial effects. Corticosteroids are obviously not an immediate need compared with other treatments already discussed. However, based on the results of glucocorticoid administration in various shock studies, early use of these agents gives the most beneficial effects. The use of large bolus dosages seems most appropriate. Steroids may be helpful if they prevent production of the myocardial depressant factor, sta-

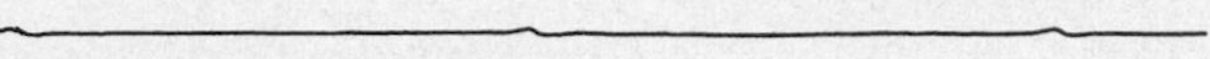

Figure 12–2. Electrocardiographic tracing in a patient in cardiac arrest due to asystole.

bilize cellular and subcellular membranes, produce inotropic cardiac effects, and improve perfusion of the microcirculation. Also, steroids may help to counter cerebral edema. Therefore, when volume replacement has been started, glucocorticoids may be given, but their administration should not interrupt the orderly progression of CPR (see Chapter 11).

Electrocardiographic Monitoring

The next step in the initial management of CPA is evaluation of an electrocardiographic tracing to determine the type of cardiac arrest present so that definitive therapy can be instituted. There are three kinds of cardiac arrest: ventricular asystole, ventricular fibrillation, and electromechanical dissociation. Since each requires different management procedures, diagnosis of the type of arrest is essential.

Ventricular Asystole

In ventricular asystole,[101] there is an absence of electrical (Fig. 12–2) and mechanical cardiac activity. The electrocardiographic tracing is generally a flat line, and direct observation of the heart reveals no contractile activity in the ventricles. In asystole, pacemaker tissue fails to initiate propagated electrical impulses. The SA node, AV node, bundle of His, bundle branches, and Purkinje fibers usually generate cardiac electrical activity.[25] If the more automatic tissue fails to depolarize spontaneously, other automatic tissues generally depolarize, providing an escape mechanism to sustain electrical activity. However, spontaneous depolarization may be suppressed by vagal activity,[16, 101] hyperkalemia, acidemia, hypoxemia, or anesthesia.[25] Ventricular asystole generally is associated with a severe metabolic defect or extensive myocardial damage. Asystole may be the end result of ventricular fibrillation or electromechanical dissociation.[101]

Electromechanical Dissociation

Electromechanical dissociation is characterized by normal electrocardiographic tracings (Fig. 12–3) in the absence of mechanical cardiac contractions. The mechanism is not completely understood but is sus-

pected to involve calcium transport at the level of the sarcoplasmic reticulum.[62, 101] Calcium is an essential ion involved in excitation-contraction coupling, the process that results in mechanical activity after depolarization in cardiac muscle cells.[101] Hypoxia, acidemia, anesthetics, certain cardiac drugs (e.g., propranolol), and hyperkalemia have been identified as factors that may cause profound myocardial depression (absence of mechanical contraction) while electrocardiographic activity remains essentially normal.[25]

Ventricular Fibrillation

Ventricular fibrillation[28] is characterized by the presence of disorganized electrical activity (Fig. 12–4) on the electrocardiogram (fibrillation waves) and the lack of effective mechanical activity. Fine to coarse movements over the ventricular mass may be observed. Abnormal impulse formation (automaticity) and abnormal impulse conduction (re-entry) can precipitate fibrillation and probably are important in its development and perpetuation.[28, 101] In the ventricles, without orderly electrical activation, there is no net contraction, rise in intraventricular pressure, pumping of blood, or tissue perfusion. This loss of tissue blood flow results in organ failure, including eventual myocardial irreversibility. However, if perfusion of the heart is maintained artificially, it can be defibrillated after long periods of fibrillation,[25, 28] a fact that has long been useful in human intracardiac surgery. Countershock with a sufficiently strong electrical stimulus to the entire ventricular mass is the only effective treatment for ventricular fibrillation. Arterial hypoxemia, certain anesthetics and anesthetic adjuncts, endogenous or exogenous catecholamines, digitalis preparations, electrolyte imbalance (especially acute changes in potassium or calcium), and electric shock have been identified as promoting or causing ventricular fibrillation, especially if multiple factors are present in the same patient.[25] Ischemia, hypoxia, hypothermia, acidosis, and electrolyte imbalance can lower the ventricular fibrillation threshold.[101]

Cardiovascular Collapse

Cardiovascular collapse is the inability of the vascular system to return adequate blood volume to the heart[55] to achieve significant cardiac output. Since both electrical activity and mechanical contractions are normal and coordinated,[55] cardiovascular collapse is basically circulatory shock that may be initiated by different types of insults. If untreated, the heart may be adversely affected, and any of the three forms of cardiac arrest may develop, or cardiovascular collapse

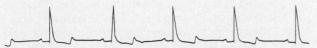

Figure 12–3. Electrocardiographic tracing in a patient in cardiac arrest due to electromechanical dissociation.

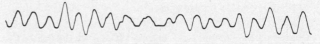

Figure 12–4. Electrocardiographic tracing in a patient in cardiac arrest due to ventricular fibrillation.

may occur as a sequela to any of the forms of cardiac arrest. Cardiovascular collapse is normally managed effectively by fluid loading and possibly, in acute situations, by vasoconstrictor administration.[55] Rapid exsanguination results in cardiac arrest, which, if treated rapidly, responds to blood volume expansion and CPR. If not, epinephrine is effective in restarting spontaneous activity in most cases. In some instances, ventricular fibrillation occurs, and defibrillation is required.[92]

SUBSEQUENT MANAGEMENT OF CPA

Management of CPA requires appropriate pharmacological and electrical intervention. After initial management has been accomplished (airway, breathing, circulation, volume expansion, bicarbonate, and ECG diagnosis), specific therapy must be directed toward the type of cardiac arrest present. The aim of therapy is to restore spontaneous, effective electrical activity that will support spontaneous, normal mechanical activity. Although there is evidence supporting the immediate use of certain drugs (epinephrine) and techniques (defibrillation) in cardiac arrest, effective massage and ventilation supported by increased venous return and normalization of pH may improve the response of the patient to specific therapy.

Management of Asystole

Epinephrine is probably the drug most commonly used to treat asystole. Its benefit has been related to beta stimulation (chronotropic effect) eliciting pacemaker activity.[44] However, recent studies have suggested that alpha-adrenergic stimulation is the primary mechanism for beneficial effects of epinephrine in asystole.[59, 78] The increase in peripheral vasoconstriction may augment venous return or improve diastolic blood pressure and, thus, restore coronary perfusion, allowing resumption of spontaneous cardiac function.[78] Beta-adrenergic receptor activity is not necessary for successful resuscitation[78, 115] and is unimportant for initial CPR.[80, 92] However, the beta effects of epinephrine may be advantageous because, in a comparison of various therapeutic agents, epinephrine produced the greatest increase in coronary blood flow. This was presumed to be related to generalized vasoconstriction (alpha) and coronary vasodilation (beta).[59]

In veterinary practice, the use of epinephrine in patients in asystole may be questioned because of its ability to induce ventricular fibrillation. Since most veterinary practitioners do not have access to a defibrillator, conversion of asystole to fibrillation can be devastating. However, the tendency of epinephrine to induce fibrillation can be reduced by using low

dosages and increasing the amount administered with each succeeding injection until the desired effect is achieved.[55]

Epinephrine is supplied as a 1:1000 solution, but some recommendations suggest use of a 1:10,000 solution in CPR at a dosage rate of 0.05 to 0.5 mg for an average dog (15 kg).[55] Therefore, dilution is necessary (1 ml of a 1:1000 solution diluted with 9 ml of saline). Others recommend a 1:20,000 solution dosed at 2 to 5 μg/kg by intracardiac injection or 5 to 15 μg/kg intravenously to be repeated as needed.[67] If effective, intravenous administration is preferred over intracardiac injection for reasons previously stated. When injecting epinephrine intravenously, it should not be given concomitantly with sodium bicarbonate, which would inactivate its effects.[89, 90]

Isoproterenol was a favorite drug in the late 1960s and early 1970s for the treatment of asystole. Even today when beta effects have been shown to be of lesser significance in initial resuscitation,[59] isoproterenol is useful in patients with extremely slow heart rates. However, even with such historical perspective, the use of isoproterenol as a treatment for asystole must be condemned based on its peripheral vasodilating effect, which decreases diastolic blood pressure and coronary blood flow.[59] It should be reserved for bradyarrhythmias following initial resuscitation and restoration of blood volume.

Since vagal influences are believed to cause cardiac arrest in some instances, anticholinergic drugs must be included in the treatment of asystole. Atropine may be helpful in the treatment of asystole.[16, 55, 101] It increases sinus node discharge and improves atrioventricular conduction.[29, 101] The dose rate is recommended at 0.05 to 0.2 mg/kg intravenously, intramuscularly, or subcutaneously.[67] Although atropine is capable of inducing an increase in heart rate, even to the point of tachycardia, small doses may slow heart rate by peripheral parasympathomimetic or central vagal stimulating action.[101] Therefore, it is important to use a dose that causes an anticholinergic action. For asystole, 0.05 mg/kg intravenously, repeated at five-minute intervals, appears appropriate. Unnecessary dosing of atropine should be avoided owing to the potential detrimental effects of the drug. In particular, large intravenous dosages may alter cardiac rhythm. Atropine increases airway dead space; impairs tracheal mucous flow; produces tachycardia, which may interfere with cardiac output by decreasing diastolic filling time; and elevates heart rate, which may make monitoring more difficult in the post-CPR period.

Calcium administration has classically been a part of CPR. Calcium is an antagonist of potassium. If hyperkalemia is the cause of cardiac arrest, calcium is indicated for immediate administration.[55] Also, it has been reported that calcium may enhance ventricular automaticity.[101] Calcium is used at a dose of 0.05 to 0.2 ml/kg when using a 10% solution of calcium chloride (5 to 20 mg/kg) intravenously. When using calcium gluconate, the dosage can be at least doubled.[101, 111]

Calcium should be used carefully in digitalized patients.[55] When infused in the same intravenous line with sodium bicarbonate, insoluble complexes may form. Generally, it is best to administer calcium solutions in 5% dextrose rather than in fluids containing other ions. Recently, the use of calcium has been questioned because of simultaneously increased myocardial oxygen consumption and decreased myocardial blood flow.[97] Indeed, calcium chloride was ineffectual at restarting the arrested heart in some studies.[87, 116]

Direct current countershock is unproved as a treatment for asystole, but it has been used in apparent asystole. Since it may be difficult to differentiate true asystole from very fine (low-voltage) ventricular fibrillation, this may explain the success of the technique in patients that appear to be asystolic.

Management of Electromechanical Dissociation

Since excitation-contraction coupling is a calcium-dependent process occurring at the level of the sarcoplasmic reticulum, the treatment for this form of cardiac arrest attempts to assure adequate plasma calcium concentration, which may help to ensure an adequate calcium level in the cellular organelles of the heart. Epinephrine is also commonly used in electromechanical dissociation.[101] Theoretically, it may redistribute calcium within cardiac tissue and improve excitation-contraction coupling. The prognosis is grave.[101]

Management of Ventricular Fibrillation

The definitive treatment for ventricular fibrillation is electrical defibrillation. In man, witnessed ventricular fibrillation or ventricular fibrillation diagnosed in a patient arrested for less than two minutes is treated with direct current (DC) defibrillation as soon as possible. With longer periods of arrest, basic massage and ventilation are recommended prior to defibrillation.[101] In man, it is clear that a shorter time between CPA and defibrillation gives better results.[97]

To terminate fibrillation, a large enough mass of myocardial tissue must be defibrillated to allow organized electrical impulse formation and transmission.[97] Factors involved in correctly delivering enough energy to successfully defibrillate the heart include body weight, paddle position, electrical wave form, and resistance to electrical current flow. To assure lack of resistance to current flow, electrode paste on external paddles and saline pads on internal paddles are useful. Larger paddles have lower resistance. Applying firm pressure and forcing the paddles closer to each other (which removes air from the lungs, since air is a poor conductor) also reduces resistance to electrical current flow.[97]

Available defibrillators commonly supply direct current and half-sinusoidal wave forms.[97] Low-energy DC defibrillators deliver a maximum of 360 joules,[101] which is usually adequate for small animal patients.

For best results, the paddles should be positioned so that most of the current passes through the ventricular mass.[97] Care should be taken not to position both external paddles too close to the sternum. One external electrode should be centered over the left sixth intercostal space near the sternum and the other electrode more dorsal at the right third or fourth space.[25] Paddles should not contact each other during the defibrillation process, either directly or through electrode paste bridging.[55]

Based on experimental reports,[41, 42] the following values have been recommended for DC defibrillation[55]:

1. Internal defibrillation: 0.2 to 0.4 joule or watt-second per kg of body weight
2. External defibrillation:
   Patients less than 7 kg: 2 joules/kg
   Patients 8 to 40 kg: 5 joules/kg
   Patients over 40 kg: 5–10 joules/kg

Others have recommended the following[57]:

1. Large patients: 200 to 400 joules external
   100 to 200 joules internal
2. Medium patients: 100 to 200 joules external
   50 to 100 joules internal
3. Small patients: 50 to 100 joules external
   25 to 50 joules internal

Defibrillation safety is important to prevent injury to the operator and others involved in CPR. Combustible materials such as alcohol should not be used to improve ECG electrode contact, because fires can occur during defibrillation. When defibrillation is in progress, all bystanders should be clear of the patient and table. The operator's hands should not be contaminated with electrode paste. With older defibrillators, an electrical charge often builds up immediately after discharge without requiring action by the operator. Therefore, paddles should be assumed to be capable of discharge at all times and handled with care. Newer machines tend to have better safety features and generally do not charge without action by the operator.

When ventricular fibrillation is prolonged, defibrillation may become more difficult. Correction of acidosis[25] with bicarbonate, appropriate ventilation with oxygen, and cardiac massage may make defibrillation easier. In addition, epinephrine may be used to lengthen fibrillation waves to facilitate defibrillation.[85, 92, 101] In some patients, defibrillation may result in a period of asystole or normal cardiac activity that quickly reverts to ventricular fibrillation. In some instances, this may be managed by defibrillating twice in succession to assure defibrillation of as much of the ventricular mass as possible. Lidocaine has been reported to make defibrillation more difficult[8, 55]; however, it has been useful clinically to administer lidocaine to patients that tend to refibrillate.[101] Bretylium tosylate lowers the defibrillation threshold in dogs,[104] allowing some refractory dysrhythmias to be converted.[97] However, the drug also has certain effects that may inhibit complete resuscitation.[104] Although electrical dosage for defibrillation is controversial, the least number of conversion attempts with the smallest electrical dosage appears to produce the least electrical injury to the myocardium. Generally, start in the low range for a particular sized patient and increase the amount of energy as needed.[55]

Chemical defibrillation is often discussed in veterinary CPR because of the lack of defibrillators in many practices. It has been well-stated that "attempts to induce reversion by drug or electrolyte therapy alone are ill-advised and impractical."[25] However, administration of potassium chloride followed by calcium chloride has been reported for this purpose.[55] Also, an ionic-choline cocktail using potassium chloride (1 mEq/kg) and acetylcholine (6 mg/kg) has been suggested.[14, 15, 55, 67]

In definitive treatment, attempts at therapy must be continued based on the cardiac rhythm present. Although each treatment is designed to establish a relatively normal spontaneous rhythm, various abnormal electrical configurations may persist or change from one form to another. When spontaneous electrical and mechanical activity is restored, the patient must be supported to avoid regression or permanent organ system damage due to ischemia or anoxia.

MORTALITY AND SUCCESS OF CPR

The success of CPR depends on the preanesthetic condition of the patient, the reason for CPA, the duration of CPA prior to the onset of CPR, and whether or not an intravenous catheter was in place prior to arrest.[94] A success rate, defined as the percentage of patients returned to relatively normal condition following CPR, is excellent if it exceeds 25 per cent; a more realistic figure of 10 per cent has been suggested.[94] In clinical patients, successful CPR is more likely if patients are healthy prior to the onset of CPA, if CPR is started immediately after the onset of CPA, and if volume expansion and supportive therapy can be instituted promptly.

Termination of CPR is a necessary decision in each patient that does not respond to resuscitation. Resuscitation in man can be discontinued if evidence of brain or cardiac death exists for one hour of adequate CPR or if CPA was known to be present for greater than six minutes before institution of CPR.[89] However, CPR may be successful after periods approaching one hour.[94]

CONCLUSIONS

Cardiopulmonary arrest is an emergency that must be managed without delay. The CPA patient must receive artificial ventilation and circulatory support immediately to sustain vital organs, and definitive therapy for CPA must be instituted as soon as possible. Appropriate treatment is based on electrocardiographic evaluation and includes pharmacological therapy and various monitoring techniques. Following successful CPR, monitoring and support of all body systems are needed to prevent organ deterioration from sequelae to CPA.

1. Adornato, D. C., Gildenberg, P. L., Ferrario, C. M., et al.: Pathophysiology of intravenous air embolism in dogs. Anesthesiology 49:120, 1978.
2. Alder, S., Roy, A., and Relman, A. S.: Intracellular acid-base regulation. 1. The response of muscle cells to changes in CO_2 tension or extracellular bicarbonate concentration. J. Clin. Invest. 44:8, 1965.
3. Alder, S., Roy, A., and Relman, A. S.: Intracellular acid-base regulation. 2. The interaction between CO_2 tension and extracellular bicarbonate in the determination of muscle cell pH. J. Clin. Invest. 44:21, 1965.
4. Alifimoff, J. K., Safar, P., Bircher, N., et al.: Cardiac resuscitability after closed chest, MAST-augmented and open-chest cardiopulmonary resuscitation (CPR); Cerebral recovery after prolonged closed chest, MAST-augmented and open-chest cardiopulmonary resuscitation (CPR). Anesthesiology 53:S147, S151, 1980.
5. Atcheson, S. G., and Fred, H. L.: Complications of cardiac resuscitation. Am. Heart J. 89:263, 1975.
6. Ayres, S. M., and Grace, W. J.: Inappropriate ventilation and hypoxemia as a cause of cardiac arrhythmias. Am. J. Med. 46:495, 1969.
7. Babbs, C. F.: New versus old theories of blood flow during CPR. Crit. Care Med. 8:191, 1980.
8. Babbs, C. F., Yim, G. K. W., Whistler, S. J., et al.: Elevation of ventricular defibrillation threshold in dogs by antiarrhythmic drugs. Am. Heart J. 98:345, 1979.
9. Bellingham, A. J., Detter, J. C., and Lenfant, C.: Regulatory mechanisms of hemoglobin-oxygen affinity in acidosis and alkalosis. J. Clin. Invest. 50:700, 1971.
10. Berenji, K. J., Wolk, M., and Killip, T.: Cerebrospinal fluid acidosis complicating therapy of experimental cardiac arrest. Circulation 52:319, 1975.
11. Bircher, N., and Safar, P.: Comparison of standard and new closed-chest CPR and open-chest CPR in dogs. Crit. Care Med. 9:384, 1981.
12. Bishop, R. L., and Weisfeldt, M. L.: Sodium bicarbonate administration during cardiac arrest. J.A.M.A. 235:506, 1976.
13. Blair, E.: Hypothermia. In Soma, L. R. (ed.): Textbook of Veterinary Anesthesia. Williams & Wilkins, Baltimore, 1971, p. 555.
14. Breznock, E. M., Kagan, K. G., and Attix, E. S.: Chemical cardioversion of electrically induced ventricular fibrillation in dogs. Am. J. Vet. Res. 39:971, 1978.
15. Breznock, E. M., Kagan, K. G., and Attix, E. S.: Effects of ionic salts or acetylcholine, or both on electrically induced ventricular fibrillation in dogs. Am. J. Vet. Res. 39:977, 1978.
16. Brown, D. C., Lewis, A. J., and Criley, J. M.: Asystole and its treatment: The possible role of the parasympathetic nervous system in cardiac arrest. J. Am. Coll. Emerg. Phys. 8:448, 1979.
17. Buchanan, J. W., and Botts, R. P.: Clinical effects of repeated cardiac punctures in dogs. J. Am. Vet. Med. Assoc. 161:814, 1972.
18. Cain, S. M.: Increased oxygen uptake with passive hyperventilation of dogs. J. Appl. Physiol. 28:4, 1970.
19. Calvert, D. G.: Inadvertent hypothermia in pediatric surgery and a method for its prevention. Anesthesia 17:29, 1962.
20. Chandra, N., Rudikoff, M., Tsitlik, J., et al.: Augmentation of carotid blood flow during cardiopulmonary resuscitation

(CPR) in the dog by simultaneous compression and ventilation with high airway pressure. Am. J. Cardiol. *43*:422, 1979.

21. Chaudry, I. H., and Baue, A. E.: Overview of hemorrhagic shock. *In* Cowley, R. A., and Trump, B. F. (eds.): *Pathophysiology of Shock, Anoxia and Ischemia*. Williams & Wilkins, Baltimore, 1982, p. 203.
22. Chaudry, I. H., Clemens, M. G., and Baue, A. E.: Alterations in cell function with ischemia and shock and their correction. Arch. Surg. *116*:1309, 1981.
23. Chazan, J. A., Stenson, R., and Kurland, G. S.: The acidosis of cardiac arrest. N. Engl. J. Med. *278*:360, 1968.
24. Chew, D. J., and Meuten, D. J.: Disorders of calcium and phosphorous metabolism. Vet. Clin. North Am. *12*:411, 1982.
25. Clark, D. R.: Recognition and treatment of cardiac emergencies. J. Am. Vet. Med. Assoc. *171*:98, 1977.
26. Cohen, J. M., Alderson, P. O., Van Aswegen, A., et al.: Timing of intrathoracic blood flow during resuscitation with high intrathoracic pressure. Circulation 59 and 60:II, 1979.
27. Cohen, P. J.: More on lactate. Anesthesiology *43*:614, 1975.
28. Cranfield, P. F.: Ventricular fibrillation. N. Engl. J. Med. *289*:732, 1973.
29. Dauchot, P., and Gravenstein, J. S.: Bradycardia after myocardial ischemia and its treatment with atropine. Anesthesiology *44*:501, 1976.
30. Davidson, R., Barresi, V., Parker, M., et al.: Intracardiac injections during cardiopulmonary resuscitation, a low risk procedure. J.A.M.A.*244*:1110, 1980.
31. Davidson, S., and Surawicz, B.: Ectopic beats and atrioventricular conduction disturbances. Arch. Intern. Med. *120*:280, 1967.
32. Dawidson, I., Appelgren, L., Gelin, L. E., et al.: Skeletal muscle microcirculation and oxygenation in experimental intestinal shock: a study on the efficacy of different plasma substitutes. Circ. Shock 7:435, 1980.
33. Dawidson, I., Gelin, L. E., and Haglind, E.: Plasma volume, intravascular protein content, hemodynamic and oxygen transport changes during intestinal shock in dogs. Crit. Care Med. 8:73, 1980.
34. Dinsmore, J. R.: Malpractice claims in small animal practice. J. Am. Vet. Med. Assoc. *168*:944, 1976.
35. Douglas, M. E., Downs, J. B., Mantini, E. L., et al.: Alterations of oxygen tension and oxyhemoglobin saturation: a hazard of sodium bicarbonate administration. Arch. Surg. *114*:326, 1979.
36. Drazner, F. H.: Hypercalcemia in the dog and cat. J. Am. Vet. Med. Assoc. *178*:1252, 1981.
37. Dripps, R. D., Lamont, A., and Eckenhoff, J. E.: The role of anesthesia in surgical mortality. J.A.M.A. *178*:261, 1961.
38. Edwards, R., Winnie, A. P., and Ramamurthy, S.: Acute hypocapneic hypokalemia: an iatrogenic anesthetic complication. Anesth. Analg. *56*:786, 1977.
39. Eger, E. I. (ed.): Changes in solubility. *In Anesthetic Uptake and Action*. Williams & Wilkins, Baltimore, 1974.
40. Garilla, S., Dava, C. L., and Chazan, J. A.: Severity of metabolic acidosis as a determinant of bicarbonate requirements. N. Engl. J. Med. *289*:121, 1973.
41. Geddes, L. A., Tacker, W. A., Rosborough, J. P., et al.: Electrical dose for ventricular defibrillation of large and small animals using precordial electrodes. J. Clin. Invest. *53*:310, 1974.
42. Geddes, L. A., Tacker, W. A., Rosborough, J. P., et al.: The electrical dose for ventricular defibrillation with electrodes applied directly to the heart. J. Thorac. Cardiovasc. Surg. *68*:593, 1974.
43. Gilroy, B. A., Rockoff, M. A., Dunlop, B. J., et al.: Cardiopulmonary resuscitation in the nonhuman primate. J. Am. Vet. Med. Assoc. *177*:867, 1980.
44. Goldberg, A. H.: Cardiopulmonary arrest. N. Engl. J. Med. *290*:381, 1974.
45. Gordon, A. S.: Standards for cardiopulmonary resuscitation (CPR) and cardiac care (ECC). J.A.M.A. 277(Suppl.):833, 1974.
46. Guyton, A. C. (ed.): Circulatory shock and physiology of its treatment. *In Textbook of Medical Physiology*, 4th ed. W. B. Saunders, Philadelphia, 1971.
47. Hall, L. W.: Anesthetic accidents and emergencies. Vet. Rec. 76:713, 1964.
48. Harris, L. C., Kirmili, B., and Safar, P.: Augmentation of artificial circulation during cardiopulmonary resuscitation. Anesthesiology *28*:730, 1967.
49. Hartsfield, S. M.: Body temperature variations associated with general anesthesia: A review. Part I: Hypothermia. Southwest. Vet. *32*:95, 1979.
50. Hartsfield, S. M.: Body temperature variations associated with general anesthesia: A review. Part II: Hyperthermia. Southwest. Vet. *32*:179, 1979.
51. Hartsfield, S. M., Thurmon, J. C., and Benson, G. J.: Sodium bicarbonate and bicarbonate precursors for treatment of metabolic acidosis. J. Am. Vet. Med. Assoc. *179*:914, 1981.
52. Harvey, H. J.: Fatal air embolization associated with cryosurgery in two dogs. J. Am. Vet. Med. Assoc. *173*:175, 1978.
53. Haskins, S. C.: An overview of acid-base physiology. J. Am. Vet. Med. Assoc., *170*:423, 1977.
54. Haskins, S. C.: Standards and techniques of equipment utilization. *In* Sattler, F. P., Knowles, R. P., and Wittick, W. G. (eds.): *Veterinary Critical Care*. Lea & Febiger, Philadelphia, 1981. p. 60.
55. Haskins, S. C.: Cardiopulmonary resuscitation. Comp. Cont. Ed. *4*:170, 1982.
56. Hawkins, W. G.: Medicolegal hazards of anesthesia. J.A.M.A. *163*:746, 1957.
57. Heavner, J. E.: Cardiac arrest and cardiopulmonary resuscitation. Vet. Clin. North Am. 3:33, 1973.
58. Hodgkin, B. C., Lambrew, C. T., Lawrence, F. H., et al.: Effect of PEEP and of increased frequency of ventilation during CPR. Crit. Care Med., 8:123, 1980.
59. Holmes, H. R., Babbs, C. F., and Voorhees, W. D.: Influence of adrenergic drugs upon vital organ perfusion during CPR. Crit. Care Med. 8:137, 1980.
60. Hyde, R. W.: Clinical interpretation of arterial oxygen measurements. Med. Clin. North Am. *54*:617, 1970.
61. Iseri, L. T., Humphrey, S. B., and Siner, E. J.: Prehospital brady-asystolic cardiac arrest. Ann. Intern. Med., *88*:741, 1978.
62. James, T. N.: The coronary circulation and conduction system in acute myocardial infarction. Prog. Cardiovasc. Dis. *10*:410, 1968.
63. Jones, E. W., Nelson, T. E., Anderson, I. L., et al.: Malignant hyperthermia of swine. Anesthesiology *36*:42, 1972.
64. Karetsky, M. S., and Cain, S. M.: Oxygen uptake stimulation following Na-L-lactate infusion in anesthetized dogs. Am. J. Physiol. *16*:1486, 1969.
65. Katz, R. L., and Bigger, J. T.: Cardiac arrhythmias during anesthesia and operation. Anesthesiology *33*:193, 1970.
66. Kleeman, K., and Singh, B. N.: Serum electrolytes and the heart. *In* Maxwell, M. H., and Kleeman, C. R. (eds.): *Clinical Disorders of Fluid and Electrolyte Metabolism*, 3rd ed. McGraw-Hill Book Co., New York, 1980.
67. Knauer, K. W.: *American Animal Hospital Association Cardiopulmonary Arrest Emergency Procedures*. American Animal Hospital Association, South Bend, IN, 1981.
68. Kolata, R. J.: The clinical management of circulatory shock based on pathophysiological patterns. Comp. Cont. Ed. 2:314, 1980.
69. Kolata, R. J., Burrows, C. F., and Soma, L. R.: Shock: Pathophysiology and management. *In* Kirk, R. W. (ed.): *Veterinary Therapy VII*. W. B. Saunders, Philadelphia, 1980, p. 32.
70. Kunze, R., Wingfield, W. E.: ECG of the month. J. Am. Vet. Med. Assoc. *174*:1080, 1979.
71. Lumb, W. V., and Jones, E. W. (eds.): Anesthetic emergencies. *In Veterinary Anesthesia*. Lea & Febiger, Philadelphia, 1973, p. 21.
72. Marx, G. F., Mateo, C. V., and Orkin, L. R.: Computer

analysis of postanesthetic deaths. Anesthesiology *39*:54, 1973.

73. Mudge, G. H.: Agents affecting volume and composition of body fluids. *In* Gilman, A. G., Goodman, L. S., and Gilman, A. (eds.): *The Pharmacological Basis of Therapeutics*, 6th ed. Macmillan Publishing Co., New York, 1980, p. 848.

74. Muir, W. W.: Electrocardiographic interpretation of thiobarbiturate-induced dysrhythmias in dogs. J. Am. Vet. Med. Assoc., *170*:1419, 1977.

75. Muir, W. W.: Gastric dilation-volvulus in the dog, with emphasis on cardiac arrhythmias. J. Am. Vet. Med. Assoc. *180*:739, 1982.

76. Musselman, E. E., and Hartsfield, S. M.: Complete atrioventricular heart block due to hypokalemia following ovariohysterectomy. Vet. Med./Sm. Anim. Clin. *71*:155, 1976.

77. Ostea, E. M., and Odell, G. B.: The influence of bicarbonate administration of blood pH in a "closed system": clinical implications. J. Pediatr. *80*:671, 1972.

78. Otto, C. W., Yakaitis, R. W., and Blitt, C. D.: Mechanism of action of epinephrine during resuscitation. Anesthesiology *51*:S152, 1979.

79. Parks, J.: Electrocardiographic abnormalities from serum electrolyte imbalance due to feline urethral obstruction. J. Am. Anim. Hosp. Assoc., *11*:102, 1975.

80. Pearson, J. W., and Redding, J. S.: Influence of peripheral vascular tone on cardiac resuscitation. Anesth. Analg. *44*:746, 1965.

81. Prentice, J. A.: The Trendelenburg position, anesthesiologic considerations. *In* Martin, J. T. (ed.): *Positioning in Anesthesia and Surgery*. W. B. Saunders, Philadelphia, 1978, p. 98.

82. Price, H. L.: The pharmacodynamics of thiobarbiturates. *In* Soma, L. R. (ed.): *Textbook of Veterinary Anesthesia*. Williams & Wilkins, Baltimore, 1971, p. 105.

83. Reagan, M. J., and Eger, E., III: Effect of hypothermia in dogs on anesthetizing and apneic doses of inhalation agents. Anesthesiology *28*:689, 1967.

84. Redding, J. S.: Abdominal compression in cardiopulmonary circulation. Anesth. Analg. *50*:668, 1971.

85. Redding, J. S.: Drug therapy during cardiac arrest. *In* Safar, P. (ed.): *Advances in Cardiopulmonary Resuscitation*. Springer-Verlag, New York, 1977, p. 113.

86. Redding, J. S.: Cardiopulmonary resuscitation: an algorithm and some common pitfalls. Am. Heart J. *98*:788, 1979.

87. Redding, J. S., and Pearson, J. W.: Evaluation of drugs for cardiac resuscitation. Anesthesiology *24*:203, 1963.

88. Redding, J. S., and Pearson, J. W.: Resuscitation from ventricular fibrillation. J.A.M.A. *203*:255, 1968.

89. Ross, J. N., Jr., and Breznock, E. M.: Resuscitation. *In* Sattler, F. P., Knowles, R. P., and Whittick, W. G. (eds.): *Veterinary Critical Care*. Lea & Febiger, Philadelphia, 1981, pp. 435–466.

90. Rothwell-Jackson, R. L.: The adjuvant use of pressor amines during cardiac massage. Br. J. Surg. *55*:545, 1968.

91. Rudikoff, M. T., Maughan, W. L., Effron, M., et al.: Mechanisms of blood flow during cardiopulmonary resuscitation. Circulation *61*:345, 1980.

92. Safar, P.: Resuscitation in hemorrhagic shock, coma and cardiac arrest. *In* Cowley, R. A., and Trump, B. F. (eds.): *Pathophysiology of Shock, Anoxia and Ischemia*. Williams & Wilkins, Baltimore, 1982, p. 411.

93. Sawyer, D. C. (ed.): The anesthetic period. *In The Practice of Small Animal Anesthesia*. W. B. Saunders, Philadelphia, 1982, p. 45.

94. Sawyer, D. C. (ed.): The nobody wins period: cardiac arrest and resuscitation. *In The Practice of Small Animal Anesthesia*. W. B. Saunders, Philadelphia, 1982, p. 213.

95. Schaer, M.: Disorders of potassium metabolism. Vet. Clin. North Am. *12*:399, 1982.

96. Schall, W. D.: Heat stroke (heat stress, hyperpyrexia). *In* Kirk, R. W. (ed.): *Current Veterinary Therapy VI*. W. B. Saunders, Philadelphia, 1977.

97. Schwartz, A. J.: Current concepts in cardiopulmonary resuscitation. American Society of Anesthesiologists Annual Refresher Course Lectures. Las Vegas, Nevada, 1982, Number 140, p. 1.

98. Shappell, S. D., and Lenfant, C. J. M.: Adaptic genetic and iatrogenic alterations of the oxyhemoglobin dissociation curve. Anesthesiology *37*:127, 1972.

99. Smith, J., Penninckx, J. J., Kampschulte, S., et al.: Need for oxygen enrichment in myocardial infarction, shock and following cardiac arrest. Acta Anaesthesiol. Scand. *29*(suppl.):127, 1968.

100. Smith, T. C., Cooperman, L. H., and Wollman, H.: The therapeutic gases. *In* Gilman, A. G., Goodman, L. S., and Gilman, A. (eds.): *The Pharmacological Basis of Therapeutics*, 6th ed. Macmillan Publishing Co., New York, 1980, p. 321.

101. Standards and guidelines for cardiopulmonary resuscitation (CPR) and emergency cardiac care. J.A.M.A. *244*:453, 1980.

102. Stevens, J. B.: Laboratory procedures in shock diagnosis and prognosis. Vet. Clin. North Am. *6*:203, 1976.

103. Surawicz, B.: Electrolytes and the electrocardiogram. Postgrad. Med. *55*:123, 1974.

104. Tacker, W. A., Niebauer, M. J., Babbs, C. F., et al.: The effect of newer antiarrhythmic drugs on defibrillation threshold. Crit. Care Med. *8*:177, 1980.

105. Tavernor, W. D.: Cardiac resuscitation. *In* Soma, L. R. (ed.): *Textbook of Veterinary Anesthesia*. Williams & Wilkins, Baltimore, 1971, pp. 500–509.

106. Thayer, G. W., Carrig, C. B., and Evans, A. T.: Fatal venous air embolism associated with pneumocystography in a cat. J. Am. Vet. Med. Assoc. *176*:643, 1980.

107. Vacanti, C. J., VanHouten, R. J., and Hall, R. C.: A statistical analysis of the relationship of physical status to postoperative mortality in 68,388 cases. Anesth. Analg. *49*:564, 1970.

108. VanLeenwen, A. M., St. Van Eps, L. W., Boen, S. T., et al.: Hypotension accompanying ECG changes in two uremic patients with severe hypocalcemia. Am. Heart J. *61*:264, 1961.

109. Weisfeldt, M. L., and Chandra, N.: Physiology of cardiopulmonary resuscitation. Ann. Rev. Med. *32*:435, 1981.

110. White, B. C.: Pulseless idioventricular rhythm during CPR: an indication for massive intravenous bolus glucocorticoids. J. Am. Coll. Emerg. Phys. *5*:449, 1976.

111. White, R. D., Goldsmith, R. S., Rodriguez, R., et al.: Plasma ionic calcium levels following injection of chloride, gluconate and gluceptate salts of calcium. J. Thorac. Cardiovas. Surg. *72*:609, 1976.

112. Wilder, R. J., Weir, D., Rusch, B. F., et al.: Methods of coordinating ventilation and closed-chest cardiac massage in the dog. Surgery *53*:186, 1963.

113. Wylie, W. D., and Churchill-Davidson, H. C. (eds.): Hibernation and hypothermia. *In A Practice of Anesthesia*, 3rd ed. Year Book Medical Publishers, Chicago, 1972.

114. Yakaitis, R. W., Ewy, G. A., Otto, C. W., et al.: Influence of time and therapy on ventricular defibrillation in dogs. Crit. Care Med. *8*:157, 1980.

115. Yakaitis, R. W., Otto, C. W., and Blitt, C. D.: Relative importance of alpha and beta adrenergic receptors during resuscitation. Crit. Care Med. *7*:293, 1979.

116. Yakaitis, R. W., and Redding, J. S.: Precordial thumping during cardiac resuscitation. Crit. Care Med. *1*:22, 1973.

Most operations proceed without unplanned complications that detrimentally affect the patient. The incidence and severity of problems that do arise are influenced by many factors. Certain complications, such as wound infection, may follow any major operation. In addition, each type of operation has its own special problems. Complications may be minor and easily treated without delay in patient recovery, or they may be major, resulting in lengthened hospitalization, prolonged patient discomfort, and even death.[8] Some complications are preventable, others are not; there are some for which we are not directly responsible but must still assume responsibility. The latter category is a result of the unpredictable tendencies of small animal patients. Complications of veterinary surgery, although similar to complications of human surgery, involve one factor that is not faced by the surgeon who operates on people: whereas human patients may not follow instructions, they can understand the consequences of not doing so.

Surgical principles are not static, and some of our closest held standards change, but there remain rules of general surgical patient management that must be followed. Frequently, it is the pressure of time or expense that causes rules to be broken. Simple steps, such as thorough preoperative patient evaluation, good aseptic technique, fluid therapy, gentle tissue handling, and adequate postoperative nursing, may be overlooked. Often these short cuts do not lead to problems, but eventually the price is paid, and a patient may suffer because of our conscious disregard of surgical principles. There are times when the emergent nature of the problem forces short cuts. But these emergencies are few and the risks usually cannot be justified in daily surgical practice.

Postoperative complications may occur immediately following surgery, while the patient is still hospitalized, or following discharge from the hospital. It is easy to be cynical when a noncooperative owner neglects the simplest postoperative instructions. On the other hand, instructions must be understood and should not present difficulties for the owner. What we might interpret as total disregard for our instructions may in reality be total confusion on the part of the owner.[2] Written instructions help lessen the problem.

Each major surgical procedure usually has its own specific set of potential complications. Complications common to many surgical procedures are summarized here.

HYPOVOLEMIA, HEMORRHAGE, AND SHOCK
(See also Chapter 11)

Shock may be categorized in several different ways. Shock as a complication of surgery is frequently seen as hypovolemia. Inadequate circulating blood volume may be due to a preoperative volume deficit, unreplaced blood loss during surgery, or continuing hemorrhage in the postoperative period.[8] Postoperative hemorrhage may not be readily apparent but should be suspected in those patients who appear to be recovering from anesthesia more slowly than expected, especially when exhibiting prolonged hypotension. Other signs of hypovolemic shock include diminished capillary filling, weak pulse, rapid heart rate, and reduced or absent urine output.

Hypovolemia in the preoperative or operative period is usually easily recognized. Not only must postoperative hypovolemic shock be recognized during anesthetic recovery, but the cause of the hypovolemia must also be identified. Central venous pressure, urine output, and heart rate and rhythm should be monitored immediately if hypovolemic shock is suspected. Central venous pressure may be monitored either by direct or indirect means; a sterile catheter should be placed in the urinary bladder and the rate and volume of urine production measured; heart rate and rhythm may be assessed frequently by auscultation or constant electronic monitoring.

Postoperative Hemorrhage

Postoperative hemorrhage sufficient to cause hypovolemic shock is a rare occurrence following orthopedic procedures in small animals. This may be due to the compression placed on a hemorrhaging vessel by a hematoma forming within a closed space between muscle bundles. Serious postoperative hemorrhage is more usually associated with thoracic or abdominal procedures. Once the signs are recognized and the appropriate monitoring begun, little doubt should remain as to whether hypovolemia is present. The dilemma then arises as to whether the blood loss and hypovolemia should be treated solely by infusion or whether the abdomen or thorax should be reinvaded and the offending vessel ligated. Prior to this critical decision, it is imperative that coagulation defects be ruled out. Disseminated intravascular coagulation (DIC) may also produce intra-abdominal or intrathoracic hemorrhage and, therefore, hypovolemic shock. Appropriate laboratory assessment of blood-clotting efficacy should be undertaken, and two simple tests may add valuable information and save precious time: if a smear of peripheral blood shows an adequate number of platelets, and if the peripheral blood clots promptly upon standing in a test tube, the odds favor unligated vessels rather than a clotting defect as the cause of hemorrhage.[8]

Suspected thoracic or abdominal hemorrhage may be further assessed by radiographs and paracentesis. The surgeon should have some idea of the likelihood of hemorrhage occurring at the operative site and its severity. If the operative field was free of blood at the time of closure, and if all vessels were adequately managed, the chances of reoperation are decreased and hypovolemia can be treated by volume replacement and continued monitoring.

Based on the patient's hemoglobin and packed cell volume and the severity of the signs of shock, appropriate amounts of whole blood or crystalloid fluids are given intravenously. A rise in central venous pressure, an increase in urine output, and a slowing heart rate are favorable responses to fluid replacement. The amount of fluid given is calculated based on the body weight of the patient and the estimated amount of blood loss. Intravenous fluid replacement must continue until the previously mentioned parameters have been stabilized.

Reoperation may be necessary, particularly if the response to therapy is less than satisfactory. In some situations, more blood may be needed than is available. The decision to reoperate is always difficult. The surgeon faced with a postoperative patient suffering from hypovolemic shock due to hemorrhage must learn to take immediate inventory of all available resources and establish a point at which the risk of reoperation is no greater than that of continued supportive therapy. If that point is reached despite vigorous therapy, there should be no hesitation in the decision—reoperate.

A certain margin of safety should be maintained when the decision to operate has been reached. One should not wait until the patient is near death.

DISSEMINATED INTRAVASCULAR COAGULATION

Disseminated intravascular coagulation (DIC) occurs secondary to many disease processes, surgery, and trauma. It is the most common coagulopathy encountered in veterinary medicine.[6] Every surgical procedure stimulates the blood coagulation system. Only when disease or trauma induces an exuberant response by the blood clotting system does DIC occur. The essential features of DIC are a generalized stimulation of the normal blood clotting mechanisms with a simultaneous overstimulation of clot lysis. This leads to rapid depletion of blood clotting factors and platelets.

DIC may occur following trauma, exposure to endotoxin, prolonged hypotension, vascular stasis, and damage to vascular endothelium and in association with neoplasia. Clinically, it may be associated with heartworm disease, prolonged abdominal surgical procedures, gastric dilation-volvulus, severe trauma, and shock.

Because DIC occurs subsequent to other conditions, its presence is frequently overlooked or not recognized initially. As the clotting elements are consumed and bleeding time is increased, spontaneous hemorrhage occurs. Most often, the first recognizable signs of DIC are petechial hemorrhages and prolonged venipuncture bleeding. In addition, bleeding from incision sites may occur. In the immediately postoperative patient, these signs are usually sufficient to establish a tentative diagnosis of DIC.

Laboratory confirmation should be obtained when possible. An elevation of fibrin degradation products (FDP), prolongation of activated partial thromboplastin time (APTT) and activated clotting time (ACT), and the presence of thrombocytopenia and hypofibrinogenemia confirm the diagnosis.[6] Some practices are not equipped to perform these tests, and use of an outside laboratory may mean a delay in obtaining results. Confirmation of DIC is needed rapidly. Some of these tests can be performed by the average practitioner; they do not require expensive special equipment and greatly add to the diagnostic capabilities of the practice. Activated clotting time is a simple test that may be performed in minutes;[3] platelet counts can also be done easily and rapidly. Platelet numbers may also be estimated by examining peripheral blood smears. It is suggested that a diagnosis of DIC should not be based solely on the results of ACT tests and an estimation of platelet numbers taken from peripheral blood smear. However, in an emergency situation, and in conjunction with the appropriate clinical signs, the results of these tests more firmly establish the possible existence of DIC.

The usual therapy for DIC consists of removal of the cause, replacement of clotting factors, and heparinization.[6] Because DIC is a secondary condition, the primary focus of therapy must be on removal of the underlying cause. This includes supportive treatment for shock, acidosis, electrolyte imbalances, infection, or renal failure.[6]

Fresh blood is given to DIC patients that are actively hemorrhaging. Heparin should not be given to bleeding patients that have thrombocytopenia and severe factor depletion—fatal hemorrhage may result. Heparin is given only after fresh whole blood administration has produced a platelet count in excess of $30,000/\mu l$ and fibrinogen levels greater than 50 mg/dl.[6] Initial heparinization is begun by giving 50 units/kg/hr by continuous intravenous drip or subcutaneous administration of 500 units/kg t.i.d. The goal is to achieve a steady state of anticoagulation of an approximate 1.5- to 2.5-fold increase in normal APTT, or a 1.33 times normal increase in ACT (i.e.,

92 to 108 sec).[6] Favorable responses to therapy are cessation of hemorrhage, decreased levels of fibrinogen degradation products and ACT, and an increasing fibrinogen level. Platelet counts return to normal very slowly following successful treatment.[6]

COMPLICATIONS INVOLVING THE RESPIRATORY SYSTEM

Bacterial pneumonia is a rare surgical complication in dogs and cats. It most frequently occurs in those patients already compromised by disease that are further stressed by surgery. Immunosuppressed animals or those with chronic upper airway disease are especially at risk.[12] Bacterial pneumonia may also occur as a secondary complication of other pneumonias. In the postoperative patient, aspiration pneumonia may precede bacterial pneumonia.

Fever is a frequent prodromal sign of bacterial pneumonia in the postoperative patient. Typically, bacterial pneumonia manifests itself fully within four to five days after surgery. Signs include fever, anorexia, listlessness, depression, and restrictive breathing. A frequent postoperative cough has not been a common feature of postoperative bacterial pneumonia. Other clinical findings include auscultation of abnormal sounds, mainly in the ventral thorax. Fine to coarse crackles or rhonchi may be heard depending on the extent of lung involvement.[12] Similarly, the radiographic appearance of the lungs indicates the degree of involvement; mild cases may have a mixed pattern of alveolar-bronchial-interstitial involvement; more extensive cases show severe alveolar disease with air bronchograms.[12]

Leukocytosis with a left shift is a usual accompanying feature. White blood cell counts rarely exceed $30,000/\mu l$. It may be difficult initially to differentiate the leukocytosis of bacterial pneumonia from the usual stress of surgery.

Gram-negative bacteria are the most frequent infectious agents causing bacterial pneumonia. Among the most common are *Klebsiella* spp., *Escherichia coli*, *Pseudomonas*, *Pasteurella*, and *Bordetella*. Diagnosis is based on clinical signs, radiographic appearance of the lungs, bacterial cultures, and blood gas values. Treatment includes antibiotics dictated by the bacterial culture and sensitivity results, maintenance of hydration, supplemental feeding, expectorants if indicated, and aerosol therapy in severe cases.[12]

Arterial blood gases should be obtained if possible. They reflect the degree of lung involvement and can serve as an accurate indicator of treatment progress. A continued increase of Pa_{CO_2}, especially after vigorous therapy for several days, is an ominous sign.[12]

Aspiration Pneumonia

Aspiration pneumonia most commonly occurs in dogs and cats owing to chronic aspiration of saliva or small amounts of food, as seen in animals with incomplete hard palate, megaesophagus, or persistent right aortic arch.[12] In the surgical patient, it may occur as a result of aspiration of regurgitated gastric contents during anesthetic induction or while under anesthesia. In addition, aspiration of blood and debris can occur during oral or facial surgical procedures such as tonsillectomy, dentistry, repair of mandibular fractures, and nasal cavity or sinus exploration.

Signs depend on the degree of airway blockage and whether the material aspirated acts as a nidus for bacterial colonization and pneumonia. Dyspnea, tachypnea, coughing, tachycardia, and various degrees of cyanosis may be seen. If the aspirated material was infected or if infection occurs, signs and symptoms are similar to those of bacterial pneumonia.[12]

Prevention is the easiest and best therapy for aspiration pneumonia in the surgical patient. Withholding food for the prescribed length of time prior to surgery; careful observation of the patient from the time of preanesthetic medication to full recovery from anesthesia; careful attention to hemorrhage and irrigation solutions during head, neck, and oral surgical procedures; and the use of well-fitting, cuffed endotracheal tubes greatly reduce complications of aspiration pneumonia.

Prognosis depends on the degree of lung involvement, the type and quantity of material aspirated, and the initial physical findings. Lung and bronchial lavages are usually ineffective unless done immediately after aspiration.[12] Saline only should be used, and no attempt should be made to use pH-corrective materials to "neutralize" acidic gastric secretions. A bronchoscope may be used to remove particulate matter. Oxygen should be administered as needed. Corticosteroids given early after the aspiration incident may be beneficial. The use of antibiotics has been discouraged unless a specific bacterial component has been identified.[12] However, the immediate postoperative surgical patient is usually in a state of mild to moderate immunosuppression from the stress of surgery and anesthesia; for this reason, antibiotics are advocated following surgically related episodes of aspiration.

Pleural Space

In the normal animal, the pleural space is almost nonexistent, with the parietal and visceral pleura in immediate contact.[9] Separation of these surfaces may reduce alveolar inflation. The degree of ventilatory capacity and lung expandability is inversely related to any increase in the pleural space.

In dogs and cats, pneumothorax is the most common pleural space abnormality. All thoracic surgical procedures produce pneumothorax. In addition, iatrogenic pneumothorax may be caused by an unrecognized puncture of the pleura during nonthoracic surgical procedures. The pleural space may be inadvertently punctured during dissection for lateral intervertebral disc fenestration of the caudal thoracic vertebrae or during surgical procedures near the thoracic inlet. Pneumothorax may also result from alveolar rupture caused by lung overinflation during anesthesia. Surgical procedures of the lung, trachea, or bronchi can also lead to air leakage and pneumothorax.[1] A sometimes overlooked source of postoperative pneumothorax is the esophagus. Air can leak from the esophageal lumen into the thorax through an incision or tear in the esophagus. The entry of air into the thorax through an improperly sutured thoracotomy incision in quantities sufficient to cause respiratory distress is rare.

Pneumothorax is not difficult to manage if diagnosed and treated early. A high index of suspicion, plus radiographs of the thorax and needle aspiration, confirms the presence of air in the pleural space. Signs of pneumothorax vary from none in mild cases to severe dyspnea in others.[9] Accentuated respiratory movements, open-mouth breathing (rather than panting), tachypnea, and cyanosis, especially in severe cases, may be seen. In cases involving thoracic surgery initially, it may be difficult to differentiate postoperative patient discomfort from respiratory difficulty caused by pneumothorax.

Pneumothorax following surgery may be one of two types or a combination. Open pneumothorax refers to a direct communication between the pleural space and the outside atmosphere, usually through a traumatic tear in the thoracic wall. Air moves freely in and out of the chest and pleural space through this opening, and lung expansion is inhibited. Tension pneumothorax results when there is a valvelike defect at the source of air entrance.[9] Air is drawn into the pleural space during inspiration but cannot escape during expiration. The condition is progressive, with air rapidly accumulating in the pleural space, decreasing lung expansion, ventilation, and venous return to the heart. Of the two, tension pneumothorax more rapidly produces respiratory distress and death.

Most cases of postoperative pneumothorax can be managed conservatively. Chest drains are advocated following most intrathoracic surgical procedures.[1, 11] The drains are placed in the thorax just prior to incision closure and left in place for several hours to several days, depending on the condition of the patient and the procedure performed. In uncomplicated cases, they are removed after the patient has regained consciousness and is breathing spontaneously and the likelihood of significant amounts of air or fluid remaining in the chest is low.

In cases not involving a thoracotomy and, when there is little ventilatory distress, the only treatment required is cage rest and careful observation. Air in the pleural space is absorbed in several days. Animals with moderate signs of distress may be successfully treated by needle aspiration of the thorax. Those patients in severe distress and those originally treated by needle aspiration only to have pneumothorax recur are probably best managed by tube drainage.[1, 9, 11] If considerable amounts of air are still withdrawn from the chest 48 to 72 hours following tube placement, reassessment is indicated; surgical exploration and closure of the leak may be necessary.

Chest Wall

Poor postoperative ventilation may be the result of inadequate chest wall function. Without normal chest wall excursion and occasional respiratory sighing, pulmonary atelectasis gradually increases and tidal volume falls. The cause may be pain—from injury such as rib fractures, blunt trauma to the chest wall, and fractured sternum or after thoracotomy. Also, large, repeated doses of narcotics to reduce pain seriously depress ventilation. Restrictive bandages around the chest almost always result in decreased motion of the chest wall. Decreased chest wall movement following surgery may compound the problems of atelectasis and small airway obstruction that frequently occur in animals that have been anesthetized for any length of time. Body bandages following thoracotomy should be applied so that inhibition of chest wall movement is minimal.

In the immediate postoperative period, human patients are frequently encouraged to cough to reexpand collapsed alveoli and dislodge mucoid material from the smaller airways. Atelectasis and small airway obstruction probably occur in dogs following surgery. However, it is difficult to encourage dogs to cough. If properly stimulated by the veterinarian, the owner, another dog, or the hospital blood donor cat, most dogs will forget their chest discomfort and give a vigorous bark or two. Alveoli are inflated, mucus is expelled from small airways, and ventilation improves.

Probably the most serious complication involving the chest wall is respiratory paresis or paralysis. This is a neurological problem involving the muscles of respiration. Iatrogenic damage during surgery to the cervical spinal cord and ascending myelomalacia associated with thoracolumbar spinal disc disease or surgery are usually associated with this rare surgical complication. If a mechanical respirator is used during surgery, the paresis is not apparent until the patient is removed from the respirator. The usual delay or apnea is frequently the result of moderate hyperventilation or too deep anesthesia. Patients with respiratory paresis or paralysis do not begin spontaneous respiration, and mechanical respiratory assistance must be resumed.

COMPLICATIONS INVOLVING THE URINARY SYSTEM

Acute renal failure is a rapid decrease in renal function, recognized clinically by rapidly progressive azotemia. It may be associated with either oliguria or polyuria; oliguria is usually present in the initial phase and may remain or progress to polyuria. Acute renal failure is often precipitated by renal ischemia or nephrotoxic injury.[5] In the surgical patient, prolonged renal hypotension is a likely cause of acute renal failure. However, nephrotoxic injury from antibiotics, anesthetics, and iodinated radiocontrast materials should not be overlooked.

Glomerular filtration and urine production normally occur at a relatively constant rate regardless of changes in renal arterial blood pressure. Glomerular perfusion and urine production are maintained with varying renal arterial pressures by elaborate mechanisms that alter glomerular efferent or afferent blood flow and tubular absorption of solutes and solvents.

Reduced renal perfusion or reduced tension of afferent arterioles stimulates release of renin from the juxtaglomerular apparatus, leading to activation of angiotensin. Angiotensin I converted to angiotensin II affects renal function by its effect on vascular tone and stimulation of aldosterone release from the adrenal cortex.[15]

Aldosterone promotes tubular reabsorption of water and sodium and tubular secretion of potassium. Renal function and urine production are pressure-driven mechanisms; despite ongoing water reabsorption and secretion and ion exchange, without adequate pressure these processes cannot occur. The renin angiotensin system and the effects of aldosterone maintain intrinsic renal pressure in the face of falling systemic arterial pressure. The supposed minimal arterial pressure that supports adequate renal function is 60 mm Hg.[5] Prolonged pressures below this level lead to acute renal failure.

Acute renal failure has not been recognized as a frequent complication of surgery in dogs and cats. However, the potential for renal failure exists, especially in those patients entering surgery with pre-existing renal disease.

Acute renal failure is recognized clinically by rapidly progressive azotemia; the patient may be oliguric. Oliguria is the first and most obvious clinical sign. Without laboratory confirmation, azotemia may be clinically misinterpreted as a slow recovery from the effects of anesthesia. Lethargy, depression, and stupor may accompany azotemia.[5] Normal urine production in the dog and cat is 2 ml/kg/hr—oliguria in dogs is generally accepted as present when urine output is less than 0.6 to 1.0 ml/kg/hr. Azotemia is present with blood urea nitrogen and creatinine levels greater than 20 mg/dl and 4 mg/dl, respectively, in dogs and 30 mg/dl and 4 mg/dl, respectively, in cats.[5, 15]

Prerenal azotemia is defined as a decreased perfusion of normal kidneys with blood, most often due to hypovolemia or decreased cardiac output. Postrenal azotemia is due to urine retention within the body, caused by outflow obstruction or urinary tract rupture and leakage of urine into tissues. It is important to differentiate pre- and postrenal azotemia from acute parenchymal failure.[5, 15]

Prerenal azotemia is treated by restoration of circulating blood volume. Intravenous administration of crystalloid solutions is preferred; the amount of fluid given and the rate at which it is administered depend on the defects and the patient's condition. Prompt urine output is the usual response. Patients in acute renal failure are susceptible to infection. Urinary catheterization should be done as aseptically as possible, and catheters should be kept clean. Urine production can be measured and the rate of intravenous fluid administration altered, based on the hourly urine output.

Patients that remain oliguric may benefit from the administration of diuretics, such as furosemide (2 mg/kg IV). If within two hours the response is less than anticipated, the drug may be given again at a dose of 4 mg/kg intravenously. Furosemide may be given every eight hours for 24 to 36 hours to maintain diuresis.[5] Serum electrolyte levels must be closely monitored in patients receiving furosemide.

Postrenal azotemia, like prerenal azotemia, is unusual in small animal surgical patients. When it occurs, it is usually associated with surgery of the urinary tract and obstruction of urine outflow. Unilateral obstruction of a renal pelvis or ureter will not result in azotemia as long as the opposite kidney is functioning normally without impedance to urine outflow. Therefore, outflow obstruction sufficient to cause azotemia most likely occurs in the lower urinary tract, from the urinary bladder and the cystic-urethral junction through the entire length of the urethra. Exceptions are bilateral renal surgery or ureteral surgery or injury. It is rare for both kidneys or ureters to be operated on during the same surgical episode. Inadvertent incorporation of both ureters in a circumferential suture for ligation of the uterine body during an ovariohysterectomy has been reported.[18]

Blood clots, calculi, and iatrogenic stricture can prevent urine outflow. Hemorrhage sufficient to cause large blood clots may follow a nephrotomy or cystotomy. These clots could accumulate in the bladder lumen and cause obstruction at the cystic urethral junction. Partial prostatectomy may also cause hemorrhage and clots to form within the urethra.

Patients that have undergone surgery for calculi removal may have calculi that were not removed, causing urinary obstruction. In such situations the calculi are almost always lodged in the urethra. Careful preoperative evaluation of the urinary tract, careful manipulation of the calculi during surgery, and careful assessment of urinary tract patency during surgery prior to closure can prevent such occurrences. Treatment is dislodgment and removal of the calculi and restoration of urine outflow.

Postrenal azotemia may also occur when there is leakage of urine into body tissues. Although an unusual sequela to common surgical procedures of the urinary tract, this has been reported as a complication following total prostatectomy that requires urethral anastomosis.[7] Urine may leak either into the abdominal cavity or outside into the retroperitoneal space. Normal-appearing urine may be voided even while some urine is leaking into the surrounding tissue. Urine leakage has also been reported following perineal urethrostomy in the cat.[10, 19] Urine is very irritating to tissues, causing severe inflammation and even tissue necrosis. These problems must be dealt with promptly in addition to the resulting azotemia.

Urinary tract stricture severe enough to cause urine outflow obstruction resulting in postrenal azotemia is unusual postoperatively and is most commonly associated with urethral surgery. Anastomosis of a healthy pelvic urethra is usually a straightforward procedure; when done properly, there is little danger of stricture. A traumatically ruptured urethra is a far different matter. Trauma, urine leakage, and damage to blood supply contribute to fibrotic healing and eventual stricture. Urethral strictures that occur after perineal urethrostomy in cats are believed to be due to poor apposition of tissue, leaving a urethral orifice of insufficient size, and, in some cases, excessive fibrosis due to urine leakage and surgical trauma.[10, 19] Treatment involves relief of the obstruction, either by bougienage or surgery. In addition, intravenous crystalloid fluids are given to stimulate diuresis.

COMPLICATIONS INVOLVING THE GASTROINTESTINAL SYSTEM

Most patients exhibit some change in alimentary tract function following major surgery, regardless of what region of the body was operated on. This is usually manifested as a temporary loss of appetite and lack of defecation. In uncomplicated cases, appetite and bowel function usually return by the second or third postoperative day. Dogs and cats are not affected with significant postoperative gastrointestinal ileus. Prolonged lack of bowel motility and painful gaseous distension of the stomach and small bowel are not frequent problems of the postoperative period. Indeed, two studies, one involving parietal and visceral peritoneal irritation[13] and the other involving cholecystectomy and small bowel enterectomy and anastomosis,[4] have shown that the gastrointestinal tract of dogs is extremely resistant to paralytic ileus.

However, ileus not caused by foreign body obstruction does occur in small animals and is frequently associated with severe hypokalemia, intra-abdominal sepsis or irritation, and conditions that may alter the normal autonomic influence on the gastrointestinal tract, such as intervertebral disc disease. The role of autonomic imbalance in the production of gastrointestinal upset and even perforation in dogs with intervertebral disc disease has recently been described.[17] Spinal cord lesions, stress of surgery, corticosteroids, and bowel stasis or ileus all contribute to the pathogenesis, particularly in colonic perforation. Diarrhea, melena, depression, anorexia, and vomiting are common clinical features of gastrointestinal hemorrhage, necrosis, and pancreatitis in these patients.[14, 17]

Treatment of postoperative ileus requires identification and elimination of the primary problem. Hypokalemia is treated with intravenous fluids containing appropriate amounts of potassium. Septic peritonitis is dealt with by eliminating the primary etiology and cleansing the abdominal cavity. Ileus resolves as the peritoneal infection and irritation are controlled. If gastrointestinal disturbances occur in intervertebral disc cases, corticosteroid administration is stopped at once and the patient given antibiotics and oral gastrointestinal protectants and antacids.[14, 17]

OTHER POSTOPERATIVE PROBLEMS

Common problems affecting the surgical patient include peripheral vascular disorders resulting from irritation from intravenous catheters or perivascular infiltration of drugs, paresis or paralysis from improper pressure on nerves during prolonged surgery, foreign material such as surgical sponges or instruments left in wounds, skin burns from improper use of electrocautery, and infections from improperly placed urinary catheters. The complications of wound infection and dehiscence; nutritional defects; and fluid, electrolyte, and acid-base imbalances are described in detail elsewhere in this text. In addition, complications related to specific operations are also discussed elsewhere.

Two further problems of the postoperative period are worthy of mention. The first is the recognition and control of postoperative pain, and the second is the prevention and treatment of decubital ulcers.

An accurate method of assessing postoperative pain in animals does not exist.[20] Acute pain, such as that produced by a broken bone, can usually be identified by eliciting manifestations of discomfort on palpation of the affected bone. Sometimes pain produces clear clinical signs of discomfort, such as dyschezia, dysuria, or lameness. In some cases, animals may cry. In other cases, manifestations of pain are less apparent and are demonstrated by behavioral or attitude changes. Affected animals may be depressed or less lively.[20] The decision to administer analgesics is based solely on subjective criteria. Certain operations cause more postoperative discomfort than others; for example, most veterinary surgeons agree that median sternotomy produces more discomfort than ventral midline celiotomy. Careful observation and monitoring of the postoperative patient are required. When signs of pain are present, a careful search for their cause should be made. In some situations, patients are in pain because bandages, casts, or splints have been improperly applied. Removing and replacing these offending devices may be all that is necessary to restore patient comfort. Analgesics should be given whenever a patient is experiencing more than a justifiable amount of discomfort.

Decubital ulcers occur almost exclusively in patients that have been recumbent for long periods.

Animals suffering spinal cord lesions, such as trauma or intervertebral disc disease, and those recovering from repair of severely fractured long bones or multiple pelvic fractures are most frequently affected.[16]

The lesions are brought on by excessive pressure on soft tissue that overlies bony prominences of the greater trochanter, tuber ischii, tuber coxae, lateral condyles of the humerus and tibia, tuber calcis, olecranon, acromion of the scapula, and the fifth digits. Large dogs, especially those that are thin, may be more prone to develop the lesions. Attentive nursing care is the best prevention. Keeping the animal's skin free of soilage from urine and feces, frequent changes in patient body position, frequent whirlpool baths, use of foam or air-filled mattresses, and early restoration of normal ambulation and nutritional balance are all helpful.[16]

Once the lesions develop, they should be cared for daily and kept clean and protected from further pressure and self-injury by the patient. Severe lesions may require surgical treatment.

1. Archibald, J., and Harvey, C. E.: Thorax. *In* Archibald, J. (ed.): *Canine Surgery.* 2nd ed. American Veterinary Publications, Inc. Santa Barbara, 1974.
2. Bomzon, L.: Short-term antimicrobial therapy—A pilot compliance study using ampicillin in dogs. J. Small Anim. Pract. *19*:697, 1978.
3. Byars, T. D., Ling, G. V., Ferris, N. A., and Keeton, K. S.: Activated coagulation time (ACT) of whole blood in normal dogs. Am. J. Vet. Res. 37:1359, 1976.
4. Carmichael, M. J., Weisbrodt, N. W., and Copeland, E. M.: Effect of abdominal surgery on intestinal myoelectric activity in the dog. Am. J. Surg. *133*:34, 1977.
5. Cowgill, L. D.: Diseases of the kidney. *In* Ettinger, S. J. (ed.): *Textbook of Veterinary Internal Medicine*, 2nd ed. W. B. Saunders, Philadelphia, 1983.
6. Green, R. A.: Bleeding disorders. *In* Ettinger, S. J. (ed.): *Textbook of Veterinary Internal Medicine*, 2nd ed. W. B. Saunders, Philadelphia, 1983.
7. Greiner, T. P., and Johnson, R. G.: Diseases of the prostate gland. *In* Ettinger, S. J. (ed.): *Textbook of Veterinary Internal Medicine*. 2nd ed. W. B. Saunders, Philadelphia, 1983.
8. Hardy, J. D.: Surgical complications. *In* Sabiston, D. C., Jr. (ed.): *Textbook of Surgery*, 12th ed. W. B. Saunders, Philadelphia, 1981.
9. Krahwinkel, D. J., Jr.: Thoracic trauma. *In* Kirk, R. W. (ed.): *Current Veterinary Therapy VII.* W. B. Saunders, Philadelphia, 1980.
10. Kusba, J. K., and Lipowitz, A. J.: Repair of strictures following perineal urethrostomy in the cat. J. Am. Anim. Hosp. Assoc. *18*:308, 1982.
11. Lipowitz, A. J., and Schenk, M.: Surgical approaches to the abdominal and thoracic viscera of the dog and cat. Vet. Clin. North Am. 9:169, 1979.
12. McKiernan, B.: Canine and feline pneumonia. *In* Kirk, R. W. (ed.): *Current Veterinary Therapy VII.* W. B. Saunders, Philadelphia, 1980.
13. Mishra, N. K., Appert, H. E., and Howard, J. M.: Studies of paralytic ileus: Effects of intraperitoneal injury on motility of the canine small intestine. Am. J. Surg. *129*:559, 1975.
14. Moore, R. W., and Withrow, S. J.: Gastrointestinal hemorrhage and pancreatitis associated with intervertebral disc disease in the dog. J. Am. Vet. Med. Assoc. *180*:1443, 1982.
15. Osborne, C. A., Finco, D. R., and Low, D. G.: Pathophysiology of renal disease, renal failure, and uremia. *In* Ettinger, S. J. (ed.): *Textbook of Veterinary Internal Medicine*, 2nd ed. W. B. Saunders, Philadelphia, 1983.
16. Swaim, S. F.: *Surgery of Traumatized Skin: Management and Reconstruction in the Dog and Cat.* W. B. Saunders, Philadelphia, 1980, pp. 60–62, 199–201.
17. Toombs, J. P., Caywood, D. D., Lipowitz, A. J., and Stevens, J. B.: Colonic perforation following neurosurgical procedures and corticosteroid therapy in four dogs. J. Am. Vet. Med. Assoc. *177*:68, 1980.
18. Wilson, G. P., and Hayes, H. M.: Ovariohysterectomy in the dog and cat. *In* Bojrab, M. J. (ed.): *Current Techniques in Small Animal Surgery*, 2nd ed. Lea & Febiger, Philadelphia, 1983.
19. Wilson, G. P., and Kusba, J. K.: Perineal urethrostomy in the cat. *In* Bojrab, M. J. (ed.): *Current Techniques in Small Animal Surgery*, 2nd ed. Lea & Febiger, Philadelphia, 1983.
20. Yoxall, A. T.: Pain in small animals—Its recognition and control. J. Small Anim. Pract. *19*:423, 1978.

Biological Implants

Chapter **14**

Marvin L. Olmstead and H. Vince Mendenhall

Biological implants are foreign materials placed in the body to either temporarily or permanently assist or assume the function of a body part. They are made of substances that are relatively inert or that stimulate a biological response that enhances their intended function. The body's response to these implants is dependent on a number of factors including the material from which the implant is made and the microenvironment surrounding the implant.

SOFT TISSUE IMPLANTS

Modern materials and the knowledge of their fabrication represent the real keystones of the success and rapid growth in the use of surgical implants over the last two decades. Design engineers working closely with surgeons played the greatest part in this development. Until the emergence of materials in response to military needs, there was relatively little advance in the field of surgical implants.[20] The aerospace program finally made the commercial production of these unique materials practical.

Man-made materials cannot, given the current state of the art, duplicate the characteristics of the structures that make up the body. Very few synthetic materials exhibit physical properties comparable to those of living tissue or have the ability to withstand the hostile environment of the body for a prolonged period. The few materials that do must also be nontoxic and noncarcinogenic. The extensive testing currently required to prove an acceptable level of biocompatibility for a new material is so time-consuming and expensive that the number of implant materials increases very slowly.

Soft tissue implant materials in popular use are classified as polymers, including plastics, rubbers, gels, and fluids. Polymers are large, long-chain molecules synthesized from simple molecules called monomers. An example of a plastic polymer used as an implant material and also commonly used for milk containers is polyethylene. Polyethylene is made by the polymerization of the simple organic compound ethylene. Many thousands of ethylene molecules are joined together to form polyethylene. The polyethylene chain could typically contain 150,000 carbon atoms and be 18 microns long.

The criteria for selection of a synthetic material for an implantable device would include the following:[23]

1. It must be possible to reproduce the polymer.

2. Fabrication of the polymer must be possible without significant adverse changes in its properties.

3. The material should possess the necessary chemical, physical, and mechanical properties to permit indefinite tissue support, including adequate tensile strength, resistance to flex fracture, and lack of biodegradability.

4. The material should not provide a site for bacterial proliferation.

5. The polymer should not interfere with normal blood coagulation.

6. The substance should be inert so that it will not incite an inflammatory reaction. Connective tissue growth about the material should not be excessively stimulated.

7. The polymer should not be allergenic.

8. The polymer should not be carcinogenic.

Biocompatibility of implant materials has been evaluated most often by limited animal implantation followed by tentative clinical application. The criterion for rejection was usually gross tissue "reaction" adjacent to the implant.

Selection of a prosthetic implant material must also involve appraisal of *in vivo* chemical reactivity and functional stability. Although contiguous tissue may respond to the simple physical presence of an inert implant in ways that modulate function, chemical reactivity and functional stability are usually interrelated. This interaction exhibits a spectrum over which either criterion may cause implant failure.[11]

Nontoxic chemical interaction of an implant with the *in vivo* milieu may lead to changes in surface physical chemistry and related mechanical performance. This occurs in the adsorption of lipids by silicone rubber spheres in heart valve prostheses. The adsorption aggravates surface stress/crack tendencies, leading to sphere deformation and subsequent malfunction. Cracking of prosthetic hand joints made of silicone rubber may also be caused by this mechanism.[11]

Implantation of a prosthetic material involves surgical trauma at the implant site. Without implantation of a foreign material, a complex series of biochemical processes directed at healing of the incision site occurs. Briefly, there is acute cellular activity characterized by an influx of polymorphonuclear cells and edema, which is soon followed by the appearance of mononuclear cells, i.e., lymphocytes and macrophages, and fibroblasts, the latter producing collagenous tissue. This fibrous tissue provides a framework on which reconstruction of preoperative tissue structures proceeds. In time, a major part of this scar tissue is replaced by normal tissue.[30]

The presence of an implant may impede the normal healing sequence. If the implant surface is significantly extensive to present an impervious barrier to body fluids, the healing process previously described leads to a fibrocartilaginous membrane of low cellularity, isolating the implant from normal tissue. This capsule is the body's response to the presence of an inert foreign material impervious to body fluids.[30]

It has been demonstrated that perforated or porous structures with a pore size of 1 mm or less allow sufficient body fluid movement through and around the implant to lead to infiltration with tissue rather than sequestration.[7, 13, 24] The woven or knitted fiber vascular prosthesis was the first clinical device to demonstrate this phenomenon. Seamless knitted tubular grafts of polyethylene terephthalate, retrieved up to seven years after implantation, in most cases exhibit luminal surfaces of fibrin and outer surfaces of thicker fibrous connective tissue.[10]

Soft tissue implants are characterized by a so-called foreign body reaction:[1]

1. Shortly after implantation, the implant surface is modified by protein adsorption from the implant site exudate.

2. The implant site is infiltrated by various cell types whose functions include phagocytosis and connective tissue synthesis.

3. The implant is encapsulated by a thin wall of dense, nonadherent collagenous material whose individual fibers are aligned parallel to the implant surface.

There is great variation in the number and types of cells, the duration of cellular activity, the degree of tissue necrosis, the size of the tissue reaction zone, and the final capsule thickness between implants. These differences may be attributed to varying levels of additives or biodegradation products. Although implant chemistry does not appear to significantly affect this soft tissue response, there are a number of other variables that do, including the implant's porosity, rigidity, and shape and the presence of sharp or smooth surfaces.[1] A rigid implant or one with sharp surfaces tends to enhance capsule formation, whereas smooth surfaces tend to enhance giant cell formation.

Any attempt to correlate deliberate alterations in implant surface chemistry with subsequent tissue response must take into account not only the effect of inadvertent surface changes in addition to the chemical change but also the formidable array of other variables that are recognized qualitatively but have never been fully quantified.

Biocompatibility may also be related to the material's hydrophobic or hydrophilic nature. Hydrophilic polymers with a surface excess of anions are known to elicit minimal soft tissue response.[2] However, a certain critical hydrophobic character does exist that promotes irreversible plasma protein adsorption. All surfaces with this level of hydrophobicity are likely to elicit minimal soft tissue response similar to that seen with a hydrophilic surface.

The initially bound adsorbed layer of macromolecules reflects the implant surface chemistry in such a way that equilibrium occurs between the implant and the host tissue through the development of an interface of several adsorbed protein layers. The outermost layer has minimum interfacial free energy adsorption. All surfaces with this level of hydrophobicity are likely to elicit a similar response with the surrounding tissue fluid. This characteristic promotes the absence of a significant interface because of the adsorbed host macromolecules and correlates well with a significant lack of tissue response.[1] This is fortunate, since most polymeric plastics are hydrophobic.

Unfortunately, the number of biocompatible polymers that can be made into fibers is limited and none possess all the ideal characteristics. Materials presently available are polyethylene terephthalate (Dacron), polypropylene, and various forms of nylon. For all filaments, the polymerization process determines the molecular weight, density, and mechanical properties of the resulting fiber. Therefore, only generalities can be stated about any group of polymers.

Polyethylene

Polyethylene is a thermoplastic polymer that is so well tolerated when implanted *in vivo* that it is used as a standard of comparison in toxicity testing of biomaterials.[20] It is resistant to all acids, alkalis, and inorganic chemicals and is insoluble at room temperature. It has a very low coefficient of friction and outstanding wear resistance. Consequently, the ultra-high-molecular-weight (UHMW)* polyethylene, which is the strongest type, is used for articulation

surfaces in joints. Other applications include otological implants and mesh* used in repairs of the chest wall and diaphragm. Porous, high-density polyethylene readily accepts the ingrowth of bone and soft tissue and can be used as a bond coating for joint prostheses; it is also used in otological implants.

Polytetrafluoroethylene†

A direct reaction between polyethylene and fluorine converts the polyethylene to polytetrafluoroethylene (PTFE). It is probably the most inert of the plastic materials and has the lowest coefficient of friction.[20] Despite these attributes, its use in the body is quite limited because of poor physical properties, particularly its tendency to cold flow. In an expanded, reinforced form, ‖ it is used as a blood vessel replacement, and small quantities are used for otological prostheses.

Polyester

The polyester polyethylene terephthalate is produced as a fiber‡ to make a variety of fabrics used as implants. Its greatest use is probably in knit arterial prostheses. Felt and open-weave polyesters have been used as stroma on silicone and other implants to permit tissue fixation. Although polyester is quite stable as an implant material, it does cause more tissue reaction than other implant material, encouraging the growth of tissue into open-weave structures and promoting quick fixation.[20] Polyester mesh is used to re-inforce silicone rubber sheets used in a variety of surgical reconstructive procedures. The monofilament form is used in the manufacture of strong nonabsorbable sutures; the suture surface is usually treated with Teflon or silicone.

Silicone

Silicone is a popular term used to describe a whole family of organosilicon polymers based on a backbone or molecular chain of alternating silicon and oxygen atoms. Depending on the length of the chain and the organic groups attached to the silicon atoms, these compounds range from wafer-thin to heavy, oil-like fluids, to greases, gels, rubbers, and solid resins.

The silicones are exceptionally stable and highly biocompatible. The bioacceptability of the silicones is supported by a great volume of research.[8, 25, 26] Even the fluids are stable. They do not break down in the body, and it is a well-established fact that medical-grade silicones do no physiological harm.

Silicone rubber is the material of choice for soft

---

*The most serviceable combination of physical properties appears to accompany a molecular weight of 2×10^6.

*Marlex Phillips Chemical Co., Bartlesville, OK.
†Teflon, DuPont, Wilmington, DE.
‡Gore-Tex, W. L. Gore and Assoc., Elkton, M.D.
‖Dacron, DuPont; Terylene, Imperial Chemical Industries, Wilmington, DE.

tissue restoration in plastic surgery, and as such is the most versatile of all elastomers. It can be produced over a broad range of hardnesses and moduli without the addition of plasticizers; nor does it need antioxidants, ultraviolet absorbers, or the many additives that are regularly mixed with other elastomers and that reduce their biocompatibility.[20]

Silicone rubber can be easily fabricated into a variety of tubes and molded shapes that, because of high thermal stability, can be sterilized repeatedly by steam or even dry heat.[19]

The applications for implant grades of silicone rubber in human medicine include prostheses for ophthalmology, otology, neurology, laryngology, and esophagology; facial reconstruction; breast augmentation and reconstruction; augmentation and reconstruction of the genitalia; urinary conduit reconstruction; finger, toe, and wrist joint replacement; and tendon replacement. Also incorporating silicone rubber are implantable heart pacer leads and power source, neurostimulator leads and loop antennae, and drug release capsules.

Carbon

Carbon occurs in a number of forms displaying an extraordinarily wide range of properties, including a unique immunity to fatigue. Some forms of carbon exhibit outstanding biocompatibility and are being used increasingly as a tissue interface in a variety of implant applications.[5]

Carbon fibers are made by the pyrolization of polymer fibers such as polyacrylonitrile or rayon at very high temperatures in an inert atmosphere. They can be felted, woven into cloth, or used as monodirectional filaments when applied as composite reinforcements. Besides their use in composites, carbon fibers have been successfully used as tendon- and ligament-forming implants.[2]

Proplast* is an ultraporous (70 to 90 per cent by volume) implant material composed of Teflon and carbon fibers. It has the appearance and resiliency of a black felt sponge, is easily carved into shape with a scalpel, and can be safely sterilized by autoclaving. The carbon fibers present a highly wettable surface to body fluids; thus tissue growth, which serves to stabilize the implant, takes place rapidly. The wettable characteristic also allows Proplast to be bonded to metal or plastic prostheses to secure fixation to adjoining tissue.[12] Proplast has found applications in maxillofacial, otological, orthopedic, and plastic surgery.

Collagen

Collagen is a generic term for the main supportive material of skin, tendon, cartilage, and connective

*Vitek, Inc., Houston, TX.

tissue. It represents a group of fibrous proteins composed largely of three amino acids: glycine, proline, and hydroxyproline.[20] Collagen fibers are laid down by fibroblasts in the body in definite patterns according to the requirements of the particular tissue (e.g., parallel in tendons, woven pattern in skin, and so on).

Collagen may be chemically crosslinked to stabilize it, as when hides are tanned to become leather. The collagen fibers of porcine heart valves are stabilized by using glutaraldehyde as the crosslinking agent. These natural valves have become quite popular as replacements for diseased human heart valves.[28]

On the other hand, collagen may be made soluble by controlled proteolytic digestion. The resulting, almost clear, viscous solution of collagen spontaneously forms a firm, white, opaque gel within ten minutes upon warming to 37°C. It has been used for the repair of soft tissue contour defects in humans; upon injection into the site requiring augmentation, body heat quickly causes gelation, with resultant preservation of contour reconstruction.[16]

ORTHOPEDIC IMPLANTS

The earliest attempts at implanting orthopedic materials in the body were performed by physicians who used their patients for pseudoresearch efforts. In the 16th century, Petronius and Paré separately described the use of gold as a biological implant.[22, 27] Between 1875 and 1890, Thomas Gluck implanted prosthetic joints made of ivory cylinders and hinges, fixed in place with ivory nails.[27] Such clinical experimentation sometimes led to interesting results. One patient's hand contracted whenever the surgeon contacted an implanted aluminum plate with a brass screw.[22] Another surgeon discovered that when a magnesium plate and steel screws were used together, the implants completely dissolved.[22] Although the early results were sometimes disastrous for the individual, the cumulative data of these uncontrolled experiments have fostered a more scientific approach to the development of modern implants.

Metals, polymers, and ceramics are the materials currently used in orthopedic implants. Of these, metals are the most widely used in veterinary medicine. Polymers are being used with greater frequency in a number of different orthopedic treatments. Ceramics, on the other hand, have been used only sparingly in clinical cases.

Metallic Implants

For metal to be used as an orthopedic implant, it must be resistant to corrosion, have adequate mechanical strength to perform those functions for which it was designed, and be accepted by the body. Although platinum, gold, and tantalum are corrosion resistant and accepted biologically, their inadequate mechanical properties have caused them to be discarded.[27] Crystalline alloys, which have a stainless steel, cobalt chrome, or titanium base, have been developed that meet the criteria necessary to be acceptable implants. Pure titanium is also acceptable.[3]

All metals are subject to different types and varying degrees of corrosion, which may occur by one or more of three processes.[4] Ionization is the direct formation of metallic cations. When a metal reacts directly with oxygen, it is referred to as oxidation. Hydroxylation is the reaction of metal with water under alkaline conditions, such as the combination of the metal or metallic ions with other cations and anions. Local pH and electrical potential determine which process occurs. An acid pH favors corrosion, whereas an alkaline pH reduces the rate of corrosion. Thus, corrosion causes degradation of the metals through chemical changes, electrochemical changes, or physical dissolution. The rate of corrosion is controlled by the type of metal used and the environment surrounding the metal. The metals currently used for orthopedic implants are highly resistant to corrosion.

General corrosion of the exposed metal surface occurs when the ions of the metal are not in equilibrium with the bathing extracellular solutions. Galvanic corrosion occurs when two different metals are in physical contact and are surrounded by a conducting fluid medium. The metal with the most positive electrochemical potential releases its metallic ions into solution. The phenomenon of crevice corrosion occurs whenever there is a defect in the metal surface or a crevice in the plate–screw head interface. The crevice is oxygen depleted; thus corrosion occurs at its contact surfaces. The mouth of the crevice is protected from corrosion. Pitting corrosion is a special form of crevice corrosion that occurs when the metal is scratched or damaged in handling or has inclusion impurities. Stress corrosion occurs when a flexed metal plate is under tension on its convex side and under compression on its concave side. This produces a difference in the metal's electrochemical potential. Stress corrosion combined with crevice corrosion may lead to fatigue corrosion. In fatigue corrosion, the total amount of stress an implant can endure without failing decreases as the number of load cycles increases. Another type of corrosion seen at the plate–screw head interface is referred to as fretting corrosion. This occurs when motion between the plate and screw physically removes metal.

A number of advances have improved the corrosion resistance of metals.[22] The original stainless steel used for implantation was type 18–8. The inclusion of molybdenum in the manufacture of this alloy greatly improved its corrosion resistance. This substance became known as 18–8 SMo stainless steel. The lettering "SMo" symbolized surgical grade material. Today this stainless steel is known as 316 stainless steel. The problem of pitting corrosion was greatly

reduced when the carbon content of 316 stainless steel was reduced from 0.08 per cent to a maximum of 0.03 per cent.[20, 21] This gave rise to the currently used 316 L stainless steel. 316 LVM stainless steel, which is virtually free of all impurities, is made by the vacuum melting process. Metals used for orthopedics also resist corrosion by forming an oxide film on their surfaces. Titanium and its alloys are extremely resistant to corrosion because the dioxide coating formed is extremely insoluble. Should this oxide layer be disrupted, it re-forms by a process known as repassivation. Only during the repassivating interval does the exposed metal surface undergo corrosion. Thus, every time the oxide film is interrupted, a small amount of corrosion occurs at the metal surface.

All implants are subjected to various mechanical forces through weight bearing or the action of muscle groups. Therefore, an implant must have sufficient mechanical strength to perform its intended function. A standard stress/strain curve demonstrates the mechanical properties that are expected of implant materials (Fig. 14–1). Stress is defined as the load applied divided by the original area of the material. Strain is defined as the change in length divided by the original length of the material. Strain is proportional to stress until the elastic limit of the material has been reached. The slope of the linear aspect of the stress/strain curve, $\tan \theta$, establishes the modulus of elasticity (Young's modulus) for a given substance. This is a measure of the stiffness of that material. If the slope is very steep, the material is very stiff.

The transition phase between the elastic properties and the plastic behavior of a given material is often difficult to precisely identify. Thus, it is accepted that 0.2 per cent proof stress is the amount of stress that causes 0.2 per cent irrecoverable strain. The precise elastic limit lies within this part of the curve. Once the plastic phase has been reached, a relatively small amount of stress results in a marked increase in the

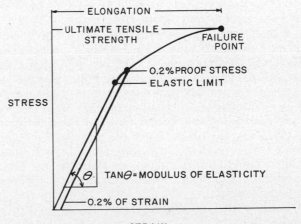

Figure 14–1. Stress-strain curve.

length of the substance, until the ultimate tensile strength has been achieved and the material fractures.

The elongation of a substance is a measure of the permanent changes in physical dimensions during mechanical testing. The amount of elongation is an indication of the brittleness or ductility of a given substance. A substance with a very small amount of elongation is very brittle, whereas one with a large amount of elongation is very ductile. The stress/strain curve can be applied not only to those materials that are used as orthopedic implants but also to hard tissues of the body.

Of the three metals used for orthopedic implants, stainless steel is the least resistant to corrosion and titanium the most resistant. Titanium has a lower ductility than either stainless steel or cobalt chromium; thus it is relatively more brittle than those two metals. On the other hand, its yield strength is greater than either stainless steel or cobalt chrome. Stainless steel has a lower yield and lower ultimate strength than cobalt chrome, but it has better ductility. When all of the properties of the metals used for orthopedic implants are compared and contrasted, no one metal is inherently superior to the other.

In 1892, Julius Wolf, a German anatomist, postulated that bone remodels in an attempt to maintain a constant pressure or stress.[6] This ultimately became known as Wolf's law. Through this law, we understand some of the effects of placing metallic implants on or within bone. It has been shown that there is a reduction of the load in a bone underneath a bone plate while the opposite cortex may be loaded at the normal rate.[17] This reduction in normal mechanical stimulus has been referred to as stress protection. A bone plate that is relatively stiff compared with bone causes osteoporosis to develop. The woven bone that is laid down underneath a plate is disorganized and incompletely mineralized. Axial alignment of the woven bone does not occur until after plate removal.[29] When the stiffness of the plate more closely matches that of bone, the osteoporosis is not as pronounced. Strain gauge studies have demonstrated that surface strain on the femur can be reduced up to 84 per cent by the use of a compression plate.[9]

Osteoporosis observed under a plate can be explained in part by the normal healing process. The Haversian system in the normal bone is widened by osteoclasts forming resorption cavities. Because of the widening of the Haversian system, the normally dense lamellar bone becomes temporarily more porous until new bone is laid down in the resorption cavities by osteoblasts. Since the plate has taken up some stress, there is no need for a large healing callus. Thus, until the new bone formation has been completed, the healed fracture underneath a plate is relatively weak.

Because the metallic implants are foreign to the body, they evoke some reaction. The degree of response is dependent upon the reactivity of a given implant. If there is corrosion of the metal, however limited, the particles released evoke a response.[4] For example, stainless steel corrosion products, if they are large, are surrounded by multinucleated giant cells or macrophages, and if small are found within macrophages and fibroblasts. The corrosion of stainless steel results in a mild leukocytic inflammatory response. Particles of titanium may be released even if there is no corrosion present on the implant surface.[21] These particles are found in the cytoplasm of fibrocytes and concentrated around small blood vessels. The corrosion particles of cobalt chromium alloys cause considerable local tissue reaction and granuloma formation when the products are present in large quantities. For this reason, cobalt chromium alloys are used primarily for prosthetic devices with metal-plastic contact surfaces. This eliminates the possibility of fretting or pitting corrosion on the cobalt chrome surface.

Whenever a tissue response occurs around an implant, causes other than those directly related to the implant's composition must be considered. As red blood cells within a hematoma break down, they release hemosiderin, which contains iron particles. These particles are engulfed by macrophages and histologically appear to be corrosion products. A loose implant may mechanically cause tissue damage and necrosis. Infection can also result in a reaction around an implant.

Although there may be a definite histological reaction to an implant, it may be insignificant in clinical terms. Whenever there is a clinical reaction, all causes of the reaction must be eliminated before the implant is implicated.

Any tissue insult results in an inflammatory response. In traumatized tissue where no implant is used, the response is usually completed in two to three weeks. In the presence of an implant the response does not completely subside but becomes chronic.[5] Mildly reactive implants reach a static reactive state within three to four weeks, whereas highly reactive implants take six to eight weeks to reach the same state (Fig. 14–2). A relatively acellular fibrous capsule covers the mildly reactive implants now in use by the fourth week. A few fibroblasts and small macrophages will be present, but the appearance of multinucleated giant cells suggests that small particles of corrosion have been produced.

Corrosion particles move about the body by two different methods. If the particle is large and asymmetrical, it will move through soft tissues by the massaging action of muscles. However, if these particles are spherical, they stay in position indefinitely. Particles that have been phagocytized can pass into the blood stream or the lymphatics with the engulfing cell. When the cell dies within the lymphatic system, the particles are released and accumulate in the lymph nodes.

Recent interest has centered on the advantages of tissues growing into implants. Biological ingrowth is

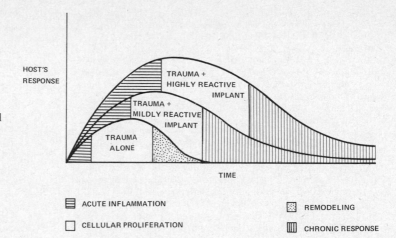

Figure 14–2. Host's response to trauma and biological implants.

entirely dependent on the pore size at the implant's surface.[6] The minimum optimum pore size for ingrowth of soft tissues is 1 to 5 μm; for mineralized tissues, 50–100 μm, and for organized osteomal bone, 250 μm. The rate of ingrowth increases with pore sizes above 50 μm and peaks at pore sizes of 400 to 500 μm. The ingrowth of tissue into an implant provides stability to that implant and to the tissue. It takes 8 to 16 weeks for the maximum holding strength to develop between the tissue and the implant.

Polymers in Orthopedics

Implants made of polymers are a more recent addition to orthopedics. High-density polyethylene is made of molecules that rarely branch and are tightly packed. This substance is highly resistant to wear and has good mechanical properties. It is used to make the acetabular cups for total hip replacement. Polymethylmethacrylate is made by mixing prepolymerized granules of methylmethacrylate with a liquid monomer that contains 1 to 2 per cent of dimethylparatoluidine. The substances react through polymerization to form a long-chain polymethylmethacrylate. This is an exothermic reaction. The substance initially forms as a liquid, which then hardens into a solid. Methacrylate is stiffer than cancellous bone but not as stiff as either compact bone or the alloys used to make the metallic portion of a prosthesis.

There are three phases of the bone's response to the implantation of polymethylmethacrylate for stabilization of a prosthesis.[18] In phase one, primary necrosis occurs at the bone-methacrylate interface owing to the bone-reaming process, which prepares the prosthetic beds, and not to either the leaching of methacrylate monomer or the exothermic reaction of polymerization. The necrosis generally is present for the first three weeks after implantation. In the second phase, the injured bone undergoes repair. This can last up to two years. A fibrous tissue bed forms around the methacrylate that may be up to 1.5 mm wide. This bed constitutes a satisfactory basis for function of the prosthesis. In the third phase of tissue response, there are remodeling of the bone and stabilization of the prosthesis. The fibrous tissue bed is replaced with fibrocartilage and new bone.

Ceramic Implants

Ceramics have found limited application as orthopedic implants. These substances mainly contain metallic elements of aluminum and calcium and nonmetallic elements of carbon and oxygen. Unlike industrial ceramics, medical-grade alumina ceramics contain no silica and are over 99.5 per cent aluminum oxide.[27] In this pure state the ceramics are very biocompatible and have high hydrophilic properties. When the ceramics are made with 100- to 150-μm surface pores, bone readily grows into the openings. Extremely smooth surface finishes can be applied to ceramics, giving them excellent durability.

Although ceramics have some very desirable characteristics, they also have some bad traits. They are very brittle and have poor tensile properties. Poor flexural strength makes this material unsuitable for intramedullary fixation. Owing to these limitations, they have not been used frequently in veterinary orthopedics.

1. Bagnall, R. B.: An approach to the soft tissue/synthetic material interface. J. Biomed. Mater. Res. *11*:939, 1977.
2. Barvic, M., Kliment, K., and Zavadie, M.: Biologic properties and possible uses of polymer-like sponges. J. Biomed. Mater. Res. *1*:313, 1967.
3. Black, J.: Biomaterial for internal fixation. *In* Heppenstall, R. B. (ed.): *Fracture Treatment and Healing.* W. B. Saunders, Philadelphia, 1980, pp. 113–123.
4. Black, J.: Corrosion and dissolution. *In: Biological Performance of Materials.* Marcel Dekker Inc., New York, 1981, pp. 27–45.
5. Black, J.: The inflammatory response. *In: Biological Performance of Materials.* Marcel Dekker Inc., New York, 1981, pp. 87–101.
6. Black, J.: Adaptation. *In: Biological Performance of Materials.* Marcel Dekker Inc., New York, 1981, pp. 116–127.
7. Calnan, J. S.: The use of inert plastic materials in reconstructive surgery. Br. J. Plast. Surg. *16*:1, 1963.

8. Child, G. P., Paquin, H. O., and Deichman, W. B.: Chronic toxicity of the methylpolysiloxane, DC antifoam A in dogs. Arch. Ind. Hyg. Occupational Med. *3*:479, 1951.
9. Cochran, G. V. B.: Effects of internal fixation plates on mechanical deformation of bone. Surg. Forum *20*:469, 1969.
10. DeBakey, M. E., Jordan, G. L., and Beall, A. C.: Basic biological reactions to vascular grafts and prostheses. Surg. Clin. North Am. *45*:477, 1965.
11. Homsy, C. A.: Biocompatibility and selection of materials for implantation. J. Biomed. Mater. Res. *4*:341, 1970.
12. Homsy, C. A., Cain, T. E., Kessler, F. B., Anderson, M. S., and King, J. W.: Porous implant systems for prosthesis stabilization. Clin. Orthop. *89*:220, 1972.
13. Hulbert, S. F., Young, F. A., Mathews, R. S., Klawitter, J. J., Talbert, C. D., and Stelling, F. H.: Potential of ceramic materials as permanently implanted skeletal prostheses. J. Biomed. Mater. Res. *4*:433, 1970.
14. Jenkins, D. H. R.: The repair of tendons with carbon fiber. International Biomaterials Symposium, 1976.
15. Jenkins, G. M., and Kawamura, K.: *Polymeric Carbons— Carbon Fibre, Glass and Char.* Cambridge University Press, Cambridge, 1976.
16. Knapp, T. R., Luck, E., and Daniels, J. R.: Behavior of solubolized collagen as a bioimplant. J. Surg. Res. *23*:96, 1977.
17. Lanyon, L. E.: Mechanical function and bone remodeling. *In* Sumner-Smith, G. (ed.): *Bone in Clinical Orthopaedics.* W. B. Saunders, Philadelphia, 1982, pp. 299–301.
18. Ling, R. S. M.: The bonding of internal implants of bone. *In* Owen, R., Goodfellow, J., and Bullough, P. (eds.): *Scientific Foundations of Orthopaedics and Traumatology.* W. B. Saunders, Philadelphia, 1980, pp. 474–478.
19. Lynch, W.: *Handbook of Silicone Rubber Fabrication.* Van Nostrand Reinhold Company, New York, 1978.
20. Lynch, W.: Materials. *In Implants: Reconstructing the Human Body.* Van Nostrand Reinhold Co., New York, 1982, p. 1.
21. Meachin, G.: Histological interpretation of tissue changes adjacent to orthopaedic implant. *In* Williams, D.: *Biocompatibility of Implant Materials.* Sector Publishing Limited, London, 1976, pp. 120–127.
22. *Medical Metals.* Richard Technical Publication No. 3922, Richards Manufacturing Company Inc., Memphis, TN, 1980, pp. 2–7.
23. Miller, J. M.: Evaluation of a new surgical suture (Prolene (tm)). Am. Surg. *39*:31, 1973.
24. Oppenheimer, E. T., Fishman, M. M., Stout, A. P., Wilhite, M., and Danishefsky, I.: Autoradiographic studies of the connective tissue pocket formed around imbedded plastics. Cancer Res. *20*:654, 1960.
25. Paul, J., and Pover, W. F. R.: The failure of absorption of DC silicone fluid 703 from the gastrointestinal tract of rats. Br. J. Ind. Med. *17*:149, 1960.
26. Rowe, V. K., Spencer, H. S., and Bass, S. L.: Toxicological studies on certain commercial silicones. II. Two year dietary feeding of DC antifoam A to rats. Arch. Ind. Hyg. Occupational Med. *1*:529, 1950.
27. Scales, J. T.: Implant materials. *In* Owen, R., Goodfellow, J., and Bullough, P. (eds.): *Scientific Foundations of Orthopaedics and Traumatology.* W. B. Saunders, Philadelphia, 1980, pp. 456–471.
28. Stenzel, K. H., Miyata, T., and Rubin, A. L.: Collagen as a biomaterial. Ann. Rev. Biophys. Bioeng. *3*:231, 1974.
28. Uhthoff, H. K., and Dubuc, F. L.: Bone structure changes in the dog under rigid internal fixation. Clin. Orthop. Rel. Res. *81*:165, 1971.
30. Williams, D. F.: The response of the body to implants. *In* Williams, D. F., and Roaf, R. (eds.): *Implants in Surgery.* W. B. Saunders, Philadelphia, 1973, pp. 203–297.

Chapter **15** # Surgical Immunology

Fundamentals of Immunology

Anthony Schwartz and J. Michael Kehoe

Modern immunology involves many fields, including basic chemistry (structure of humoral mediators of immune reactions), cell biology (origin and nature of cells active in immunity), genetics (transmission and activation of genetic information required in immunological responses), and clinical medicine and surgery (selective induction or suppression of immune reactivity). The application of these principles to clinical problems is illustrated in several chapters of this text. This chapter provides background information necessary to an understanding of the role of immunological processes in disease and in important biological phenomena such as allograft rejection.

THE LYMPHOID SYSTEM

Cellular Interactions in Antibody-Mediated (Humoral) Immunity

Although the ability to mount an immune response has been attributed to cells from lymphoid tissues for some time, it is only in the last 25 years that it has become recognized that a complex division of labor exists between different populations of lymphocytes as well as nonlymphoid cells. The thymus is involved in both graft rejection and antibody formation, whereas the bursa of Fabricius in chickens and its mammalian equivalent (which is still not definitely identified but may be the liver) is important only to antibody formation.[27] Thymus-derived cells (T cells) and bursa-derived cells (B cells) interact to result in an antibody response,[15] and, although T cells do not make antibody, they can proliferate in response to antigen[19, 47] and "help" the B cells produce antibody.

A third type of cell has been shown to be required for an effective immune response.[52] These are non-lymphoid, bone marrow–derived "accessory cells" that consist primarily of macrophagelike cells that are glass adherent. They include fixed cells in the spleen, lymph nodes, lung alveoli, liver (Kupffer's cells), and skin (Langerhans' cells) and free cells in the peritoneal cavity and circulation. Accessory cells are important for both the production of antibody and the expression of cell-mediated immune (CMI) responses.

Phagocytic cells function by trapping antigenic molecules, most of which are ingested and degraded. Some of this processed antigen is presented to T lymphocytes. Some, but not all, macrophages can function as accessory cells (bone marrow macrophages cannot), whereas some adherent cells are nonphagocytic (dendritic cells of the spleen and lymph nodes) but are excellent antigen presenters.[66] Macrophages can form soluble substances such as lymphocyte activating factor (LAF,[26] now termed *interleukin I*), which can activate certain T cells. In addition, macrophages comprise the main component of the inflammatory response in certain CMI reactions and may be the effector cells in such responses (described hereafter).

Central Lymphoid Organs: Lymphocyte Differentiation

Immunologically competent lymphoid cells originate from *pluripotent stem cells,*[74, 75] which reside first in the fetal yolk sac and then in the bone marrow. Through some unknown mechanism, stem cells appear to become either hematopoietic or lymphocyte *progenitor cells,* which are now precommitted to "education" in one of the inducing microenvironments, called primary or central lymphoid organs[70] (the thymus or bursal equivalent). In the bursa or its equivalent, cells mature to B cells, which leave the bursa and produce and secrete antibody.

The other primary lymphoid organ, the thymus, is the site where some precursors become T cells. This lymphoepithelial gland, the epithelial portion of which is derived from the third and fourth branchial pouches, is located in the anterior mediastinum. Immature thymocytes comprise over 90 per cent of thymic lymphoid cells. Under the influence of thymic hormones (such as thymopoietin; see Chapter 87, The Thymus Gland), they reproduce repeatedly and somehow become committed to differentiate into T cells that have antigen specificity and the added ability to recognize self components as self and non-self components as foreign. These cells leave the thymus and enter the peripheral functional T lymphocyte pool in the spleen and lymph nodes (secondary lymphoid organs).

Secondary Lymphoid Organs

Lymph Nodes

In the superficial cortex ("thymus-independent area") of lymph nodes, there are follicles that consist mainly of B lymphocytes. Less well-organized groups of lymphocytes are found between the follicles. During an immune response the follicles enlarge to become secondary follicles and develop a germinal center, which contains proliferating lymphocytes. The deep cortex ("thymus-dependent area") contains three T cells for each B cell. About 95 per cent of lymphocytes that leave an unstimulated lymph node are recirculating cells derived from the blood and not the node itself. Drainage of recirculating lymphocytes by exteriorizing the thoracic duct will primarily cause depletion of the thymus-dependent areas of the lymph nodes, demonstrating that most recirculating lymphocytes are T cells.

Antigen enters the lymph node via the afferent lymph and is trapped by accessory cells, partially digested, and presented to T cells to initiate the immune response. The trapping of antigen is facilitated if it is already antibody-coated. Within two to five days, lymphocytes specific for the antigen in question increase in number in the node and antibody formation is detected. After five days, these lymphocytes leave the node, thus disseminating the response. Plasma cells, the antibody-producing end state of the differentiation of B cells, become abundant in germinal centers after seven days.

The Spleen

The spleen is predominantly responsible for responses to blood-borne antigens. It is made up of the lymphoid cell–rich white pulp and blood-filled sinuses of the red pulp. The thymus-dependent area of the white pulp surrounds arterioles and is called the *periarteriolar lymphoid sheath*. The thymus-dependent area is made up of the follicular or nodular B cell regions surrounding the T cell areas.[70] See Chapter 84 for a further discussion of splenic anatomy and physiology.

TABLE 15–1. Distinguishing Characteristics of Mouse B and T Cells

Property	B Cell	T Cell
Antigen binding receptor	IgM (heavy concentration) IgD Single idiotype	Unclear and controversial. Idiotype and V_H segment present.
Surface antigens:		
Thy-1	−	+
TL	−	+
Ly	Lyb	Lyt
Pc	+	−
H-2	+	+
Inactivated by		
X-rays	Strongly	Slightly*
Corticosteroids	Moderately	Slightly*
Anti-lymphocyte serum	Slightly	Strongly
Functions:		
Memory	Yes	Yes
Ig secretion	Yes	No
Helper function	No	Yes (Ly 1)
Cell mediated immunity	No	Yes (Ly 23)
Suppression	Yes	Yes (Ly 23)
Tolerance	Late and transient	Early and long lasting
Differentiation	Bone marrow, then Bursa of Fabricius in birds (liver in mammals), then general circulation	Bone marrow, then thymus, then general circulation
Response to mitogens	Lipopolysaccharide (LPS)	Concanavalin A (Con A) Phytohemagglutinin (PHA)

*Ly 123 cells appear more sensitive.

Identification of Lymphoid Cell Sets

Table 15–1 presents the characteristics of T and B lymphocytes in the mouse, the most extensively studied species. There have been attempts to similarly identify sets of canine and feline lymphocytes. Canine B lymphocytes bear surface immunoglobulin and receptors for the third component of complement.[17, 46] Canine T lymphocytes are thought to react specifically with human or guinea pig erythrocytes to form "E-rosettes"; however, the specificity of this marker is in question.[46] Similarly, canine T lymphocytes respond to the plant lectins phytohemagglutinin (PHA) and concanavalin A (Con A). Although lipopolysaccharide (LPS) is a specific B cell mitogen for mouse cells, there are no known B cell–specific mitogens for canine cells. Anti–T cell sera have been developed for dog lymphocytes, but there are, as yet, no reagents available comparable to the anti-Lyt reagents of mice or similar antibodies of man that can functionally separate helper from killer and suppressor cells. It may only be through the development of monoclonal antibodies specific for such cells that we will have reagents suitable for the study and manipulation of canine and feline lymphocyte subsets for clinical and research purposes.

THE CONCEPT OF ANTIGENICITY AND THE NORMAL IMMUNE RESPONSE

The term *antigenicity* denotes the capacity of given substance (antigen) to induce a state of altered reactivity in an individual such that subsequent encounters with that specific antigen result in an augmented secondary, or anamnestic, response. This reaction, which can take many forms, is called an *immune response*. The ability to induce an immune response is a function of certain molecular characteristics of the antigen (molecular size, rigidity, net charge, stereospecificity) as well as certain biological characteristics of the host (genetic constitution, species, age). Normally, an antigenic substance differs from constituents of the responding host's own body. In other words, the immune response is capable of distinguishing "self" from "nonself." Loss of this discriminating capacity can lead to disease (autoimmunity).

Requirements for Antigenicity

A *complete* antigen can both induce an immune response and react with the humoral products of the response (antibodies). However, an incomplete antigen, or *hapten* (part of a complete antigen), is unable to induce an immune response but can be bound by specific antibodies previously generated in response to the complete antigen. Haptens (such as metals or small chemical moieties such as dinitrophenol) will lead to an immune response only if they are attached to a *carrier* molecule (e.g., a "self" protein). Such hapten-carrier relationships have clinical relevance in *contact hypersensitivity* to various chemicals, including drugs (see hereafter).

Larger antigens (bacteria, viruses, or mammalian cells) are actually mosaics of a number of individual antigens. Even in a single protein molecule, certain local regions, called *antigenic determinants*, stimulate the formation of antibodies whose specificity is directed against these local regions only.

Proteins are the most common antigens known. In addition, certain carbohydrates are very strongly antigenic, e.g., bacterial polysaccharides and blood group substances. Nucleic acids are weak antigens, but anti–nucleic acid antibodies can be induced by appropriate laboratory manipulations and are seen spontaneously in certain diseases, such as systemic lupus erythematosus. Lipids normally are not antigenic, but exceptions do occur.

Adjuvants

The immune response can be enhanced by combining antigens with adjuvants. These substances exert their enhancing effect on the host in several ways, some of which are still unknown. Some adjuvants, such as mineral oil or alum precipitates, retard the destruction of antigen (depot effect), whereas others, such as Freund's complete adjuvant (which combines a mineral oil depot with killed mycobacteria), cause inflammatory reactions that permit the recruitment and activation of larger numbers of immunocompetent cells.

The Normal Immune Response

The typical humoral immune response to an antigen such as an invading bacterium or virus is graphically illustrated in Figure 15–1. A "primary" response to antigenic stimulation in a previously unstimulated individual is followed by a lag phase and then an exponential increase in antibody titer to a steady state. The titer then rapidly falls off. Restimulation of a previously sensitized individual leads to a secondary (anamnestic) response. In this case, the lag phase is shorter, the rate of titer increase is greater, a higher final titer is reached at the steady state phase, and the falloff is less rapid than in a primary response. The expansion of antigen-specific clones of T and B cells occurs during the primary response. Secondary stimulation with the same antigen can lead to rapid triggering of these "memory" cells, resulting in an augmented secondary response.

Thymus-Dependent Antibody Responses

An obligatory synergism exists between T and B cells in the antibody response to most antigens. This is called a *thymus-dependent* response. T cells *can* respond to the same immunogenic components (determinants) of most antigens as do B cells. However, during a response to complex antigens (or to model

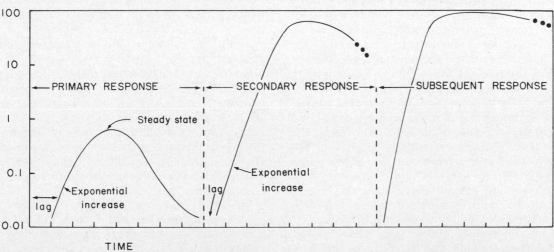

Figure 15–1. Graphic illustration of the normal humoral immune response. The secondary (anamnestic) response is characterized by a greater rate of antibody rise, a higher plateau region, and a more modest titer decrement after challenge. The difference is due primarily to the presence of memory T and B lymphocytes subsequent to an initial antigen sensitization. (Reprinted with permission from Schwartz, A., and Kehoe, J. M.: Fundamental principles of immunology. *In* Ettinger, S. J.: *Textbook of Veterinary Internal Medicine,* 2nd ed. W. B. Saunders, Philadelphia, 1983, pp. 2102–2139.)

antigens made up of hapten and carrier), T cells generally respond to a different determinant (the carrier) on the same molecule than the B cells, which respond to the hapten itself.

T Cell–Independent B Cell Responses

Optimal specific humoral immune responses to certain antigens can occur without T cell cooperation. Such antigens usually consist of repetitive sequences of identical subunits. Some thymus-independent antigens, such as polysaccharides, often behave as B cell mitogens (e.g., LPS). The response caused by these antigens is generally restricted to the IgM class, and little effective memory results (i.e., there is no augmented secondary response on re-exposure to the same antigen). The special structure of T cell–independent antigens somehow substitutes for the "second signal" given to B cells by T cells (antigen is signal 1 and the T cell signal to the B cell is signal 2) in T cell–dependent responses.[72] Such responses are of considerable practical significance, since a number of vaccines (e.g., killed bacterial products) contain antigens with repetitive determinants of the sort described previously.

Control Mechanisms in the Immune Response

As with other body systems, the immune apparatus is finely tuned. Thus, in addition to positive (helper), or "on," signals, negative (suppressor), or "off," signals exist as well. Therefore, the net observed level of the immune response is a balance between positive and negative regulatory interactions. Only by comprehending this concept can one understand why the response to a particular antigen does not continually progress to overwhelm the entire lymphoid system, why the fetus as an allotransplant is not rejected by a maternal immune response, and why immune responses to our own tissue antigens are the exception rather than the rule. In such a complex system there are multiple levels of control.

Antigen. Whether an immune response occurs following exposure to an antigen depends on the dose, timing, and nature of the antigen involved. For example, the lethal dose of tetanus toxin in mice is 20 pg (2×10^{-11} gm), whereas the dose required for immunization is 2 µg (2×10^{-6} gm). Therefore, even though it is a highly immunogenic molecule, tetanus toxin must be detoxified before it can be used. Certain antigens have, for unknown reasons, low intrinsic immunogenicity. In this case, adjuvants may be used. Other antigens that have proven immunogenicity do not provoke an immune response, possibly because they fail to reach lymphoid tissues. Thus, ocular lens protein is in a privileged site inaccessible to lymphocytes. Some antigens on tumor cells appar-

ently fail to elicit a response because they are covered with sialic acid, which somehow prevents the appropriate cell interaction required for immunity.

Antibody. The administration or production of antibody results in feedback inhibition of antibody production.[68] For example, although the exact mechanism is not known, the appearance of IgG results in a shut-off of IgM antibody production.

Immunological Tolerance—Central Effects Mediated by Antigen. Immunological tolerance is defined as the inability to respond to a specific antigenic determinant.[8, 49-51] It may be manifested by diminished or absent cell-mediated or humoral immunity or both. Specific tolerance is the reason that an animal exists without immunologically attacking its own tissues and cells while specifically and strongly rejecting everything else that is foreign (e.g., infectious agents, toxins, neoplastic cells, tissue grafts). When something occurs to interrupt this "self-tolerance," the consequences may be minimal or catastrophic, depending on the extent to which the tolerant state is lost. When disease occurs, autoimmunity is said to exist.

Fetuses and neonatal animals are more susceptible to tolerance induction than are adult animals. However, adult animals can be rendered essentially immunologically immature and more amenable to tolerance induction by whole-body irradiation with x-rays or the use of immunosuppressive drugs, such as cyclophosphamide. In addition, even normal adults can be made tolerant if the following conditions prevail:

1. The antigen is *poorly immunogenic* in its native state.

2. The antigen is *in the proper form.* That is, bovine gamma globulin, when in soluble form (monomeric), readily induces tolerance in adult animals, but if it is given with an adjuvant or if it is in aggregated form, it is immunogenic. This leads to the suggestion that molecules that are in a form not readily phagocytized by macrophages are shifted toward tolerogenicity.

3. Either *very high or very low doses* of antigen are used.

4. *The host is unable to catabolize the substance;* e.g., high doses of pneumococcal polysaccharides are tolerogenic. Such substances can be phagocytized but are resistant to digestion.

The work of Chiller and Weigle[14] demonstrated that both T and B cells can be rendered tolerant. However, the susceptibilities of these two lymphocyte classes differ considerably with respect to the required dose of tolerogen (lower for T than for B cells) and the time required after treatment for tolerance induction (less for T than for B cells). In addition, the duration of tolerance is significantly less in B cells than in T cells. Finally, the specific immune response of the whole animal reflects that of the T cell population in the case of a thymus-dependent response; i.e., the animal appears tolerant if its T cells are, even when its B cells are not tolerized.

The Mechanisms of Immunological Tolerance

Burnet[11] hypothesized that self-tolerance is due to clonal deletion (death of responsible clones following exposure to antigen). Tolerance to certain antigens induced early in life (especially self-antigens) may be the result of death of clones of B cells ("clonal abortion"[53]). Tolerance induced with high doses of antigen (high-zone tolerance) was hypothesized to be due to such clonal deletion. When Mitchison[48] found that tolerance could also be induced by extremely *low* doses of antigen, this explanation seemed untenable. In many cases, this low-zone tolerance has been found to be due to suppressor T cells. Suppressor T cells have been shown to play a critical role in both T and B cell tolerance by acting in a way to actively "turn off" T or B cell function.[22] These cells may be required for prevention of excessive or harmful (autoimmune) responses. To further complicate the situation, the recent work of Gershon and colleagues[25] has indicated that not only can T cell help for B cells be prevented by suppressor T cells, but the ability of suppressor cells to function also is regulated by other, "contrasuppressor," cells.

Mechanism of Cell Cooperation

Although the possibility that lymphoid cells may deliver their signals to one another by direct, intimate contact cannot be ruled out, there is mounting evidence that T cells generally exert their regulatory influence on other T cells and on B cells by release of biologically active soluble factors. Helper, suppressor, and contrasuppressor factors from T cells have been described[23] some of which are antigen-specific.

Recently it has been discovered that some populations of both helper and suppressor T cells and some of the factors derived from them have specificity not for antigen but for "idiotypes," which are antigenic determinants found on antibody molecules in their V_H region (Fig. 15–2). Such factors could regulate the function of cells bearing these determinants, as was first suggested by Jerne.[33] This mechanism and the other complex regulatory interactions previously described are believed to be operative, with some variations, in all mammalian species and to influence the nature and degree of immune responsiveness that such individuals show.

IMMUNOGLOBULIN STRUCTURE AND FUNCTION

Antibodies as Proteins

Antibody molecules are B cell products that are elicited in response to an antigen and react, specifically, with that antigen. In serum, most antibodies are found in a slowly migrating electrophoretic fraction termed *gamma globulin* and are thus termed *immunoglobulins* (Ig). Ig molecules are a heterogeneous family of complex, related proteins that differ in their functional properties according to differences in their chemical structure.

Ig molecules from a wide variety of mammalian species can be subcategorized into five distinct classes according to differences in the structure of one of the constituent polypeptide chains, termed the *heavy* chain (see Fig. 15–2). Structural studies of antibody molecules have been greatly aided by the availability of homogeneous, pure Ig proteins that are produced in large quantities by certain tumors of B lymphocytes called *myelomas* (see hereafter, Tumors of the Immune System). Recently, the technology for fusing normal B cells with malignant B cells (hybridomas)

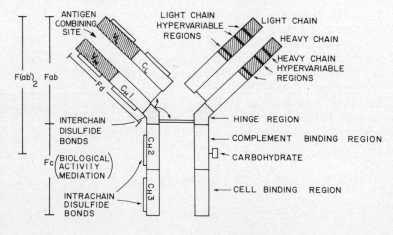

Figure 15–2. A prototype mammalian IgG molecule. The two constituent polypeptide chains—heavy and light—are indicated, as are three major proteolytic fragments that can be produced from this antibody protein [F(ab')₂, Fab, Fc]. The usual locations of the disulfide bonds and the hypervariable (complementarity-determining) regions of the variable regions of both the heavy (V_H) and light (V_L) chains are also shown. See text for additional details. (Reprinted with permission from Schwartz, A., and Kehoe, J. M.: Fundamental principles of immunology. *In* Ettinger, S. J.: *Textbook of Veterinary Internal Medicine*, 2nd ed. W. B. Saunders, Philadelphia, 1983, pp. 2102–2139.)

TABLE 15–2. Mammalian Immunoglobulin Classes

Characteristics and Functions	IgG	IgA	IgM	IgD	IgE
$S_{20,w}$	7.0	7,10,13,15,16	19	7	8
Molecular weight	150,000	180,000–500,000	850,000	160,000	196,000
Carbohydrate (%)	2.9	7.5	6–10	12	10.7
Approximate concentration in normal serum (mg/100 ml)	700–1500	140–420	50–190	3–40	0.01–0.14
Major biological functions	Principal serum antibody Complement activation, opsonization Passive transfer to fetus or newborn	Secretory antibody, active at mucosal surfaces Polymeric (dimer to higher order polymers)	Initial antibody produced Prominent serum antibody Polymeric (pentamer in serum) Complement activation B lymphocyte antigen receptor as monomer	Important cell surface antibody of developing B lymphocytes	Reagin-humoral mediator of immediate hypersensitivity reactions (e.g., anaphylaxis)

has allowed selective production of homogeneous antibodies of any desired specificity in essentially limitless quantities. Some general characteristics of the five classes of mammalian immunoglobulins (IgG, IgM, IgA, IgD, and IgE) are provided in Table 15–2.

Some further subdivision of certain of these classes, also attributable to differences in heavy chain structure, exists in numerous species. For example, the IgG class of the dog is known to comprise four distinct *subclasses* termed IgG1, IgG2a, IgG2b, and IgG2c.[17, 35]

IgG as an Immunoglobulin Prototype

The importance of IgG is illustrated by the finding that approximately 80 per cent of antibacterial, antiviral, and antitoxin antibodies belong to this class. A schematic representation of an intact IgG molecule is shown in Figure 15–2, since the structure of this protein has become the prototype for relating the structural features of antibodies to their functions. As illustrated, IgG proteins (and antibodies in general) are characterized by a remarkable degree of regional differentiation. At a first level, the IgG molecule can be split by proteolytic cleavage into two fragments termed *Fab* and *Fc*. The Fab region binds antigen, whereas the Fc region mediates the biological functions of the molecule (see hereafter).

Antigen Receptors on B Cells and T Cells

The immunoglobulins are either attached to the lymphocyte cell membrane or released into the serum to become serum antibody. The antigen receptor for such antibodies (and for a B cell carrying such an antibody) is the combined variable regions of the light and heavy chain (see Fig. 15–2) and is

formed specifically by the *hypervariable* segments situated within the variable regions as a whole.[13] Since T cell–mediated immunological responses are also highly antigen specific, T cells must also have surface receptors that render them able to recognize and bind specific antigenic determinants. However, whether conventional immunoglobulin is also the T cell receptor is open to controversy.[41] Conventional IgG, IgA, IgM, IgD, or IgE has not been detectable on T cells. As noted previously, serologically detectable *antigenic determinants* have been found in the variable region of Ig molecules. These markers, called *idiotypes*, are associated with the hypervariable regions that comprise an antibody combining site and, when found, are indicative of a characteristic antigenic specificity of the IgG. Anti-idiotypic antibodies have been used to show that some T cells and some B cells reactive for a given antigen *share* similar idiotypes.[9] Therefore, at least a portion of the T cell receptor is composed of the same variable region found in the Ig produced by B cells. The other portion of the T cell receptor may comprise a new Ig heavy chain type.[41]

Biological Properties (Effector Functions) of Antibodies

Immunoglobulin molecules are multifunctional. These functions can be divided into two main categories: antigen binding, mediated by the variable regions of heavy and light chains (part of the Fab fragment); and biological properties, or effector functions, mediated by the Fc region.[34, 36]

The effector functions are very important physiologically, since they often determine exactly what biological *consequences* follow the union of a given antigen with its antibody. Such effector activities include interaction with complement proteins, fixa-

TABLE 15–3. Effector Functions of Immunoglobulin Classes

Class	Classic Complement Fixation	Skin Attachment
IgG	+ (some subclasses)	+ (some subclasses)
IgM	+	−
IgA	−	−
IgD	−	−
IgE	−	+

tion to skin, reactivity with rheumatoid factors, fixation to macrophages and lymphocytes, membrane passage (placenta, intestine), augmented phagocytosis (opsonization), regulation of immunoglobulin catabolism, and interaction with staphylococcal "A" protein. Not all immunoglobulin molecules are capable of all these activities, and some correlations have been made between the class or subclass of given molecules and their capacity to mediate some of these functions. For example, certain classes lack certain effector function capabilities, as illustrated by Table 15–3. These various differences are thought to reflect differences in chemical structure among the Fc regions of the various immunoglobulins, but the exact nature of these differences is not yet known.

Some of these activities, such as complement fixation, are expressed by antibodies only after union with antigen has occurred, whereas others, such as skin fixation, do not require prior antigen union. In those cases in which antigen-antibody interaction is required for the expression of the biological activity, it has been presumed that some antigen-induced conformational alteration of the antibody molecule might occur, perhaps exposing a previously buried active site. Alternatively, much recent experimental evidence supports the view that antigen-induced aggregation may be adequate to initially activate the complement system.

The Antigen–Antibody Reaction

The antigen-antibody reaction itself may be separated into two stages. The first is concerned with the actual union (combination), which occurs very rapidly. The second stage (consequences of the antigen-antibody reaction) evolves more slowly. Antigen-antibody interactions are noncovalent and relatively weak and reversible. Second-stage events can include effects that depend only on the union itself (antitoxin activity, virus neutralization, bacterial agglutination) or those that involve the effector function capabilities of the antibody molecule (complement fixation, opsonic activity). Previously, these distinctions led to the designation of different "kinds" of antibodies (lysins, agglutinins, antitoxins, and so forth). Such categorizations have less meaning now that the struc-

tural and functional relationships of antibodies are understood in greater detail.

The Precipitin Reaction and Lattice Theory

An important consequence of the union of *soluble* antigens with their specific antibody is the precipitin reaction. This reaction is used in a variety of formats in clinical immunology, especially as a diagnostic tool. In addition, precipitin antibodies play a dominant role in *immune complex* diseases. The behavior of these antibodies in solution is explained by the lattice hypothesis, which assumes the interaction of multivalent antibody with multivalent antigen. The most common precipitin antibody, IgG, is divalent. Most antigens involved in the precipitin reaction are highly multivalent with many antigenic determinants that can interact with antibody. The characteristic precipitin curve can be demonstrated in the laboratory by adding increasing antigen to constant aliquots of antibody. A curve is formed by measuring the *total* amount of precipitate at various points as the ratio of antigen to antibody is increased (Fig. 15–3).

Precipitin antibodies are involved in immune complex diseases. In the zone of antigen excess in the precipitin curve, soluble complexes of antigen and antibody are formed that can lodge in tissues (kidney, joints) and be biologically active (by activating complement, for example). These reactivities are responsible for many aspects of the pathogenesis of immune complex diseases.

The maximum precipitation zone (zone of equivalency, see Fig. 15–3) is widely used in clinical im-

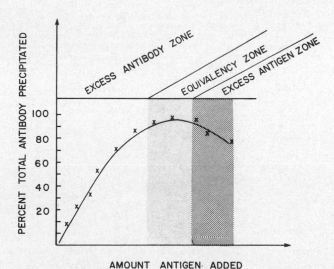

AMOUNT ANTIGEN ADDED

Figure 15–3. The quantitative precipitin reaction characteristic of the interaction of soluble, multivalent antigen with multivalent antibody. The three zones can be discerned when antigen is progressively added to a standard aliquot of antibody. (Reprinted with permission from Schwartz, A., and Kehoe, J. M.: Fundamental principles of immunology. *In* Ettinger, S. J.: *Textbook of Veterinary Internal Medicine,* 2nd ed. W. B. Saunders, Philadelphia, 1983, pp. 2102–2139.)

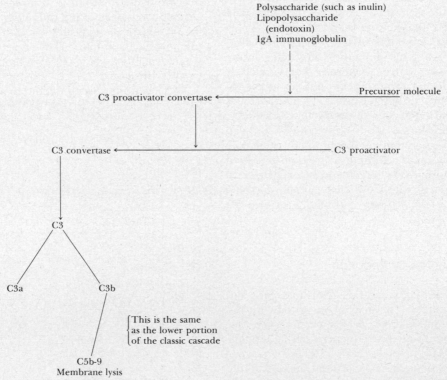

Figure 15–4. A, The classical complement cascade. *B,* The alternate complement cascade. See text for detailed discussion. (Reprinted with permission from Schwartz, A., and Kehoe, J. M.: Fundamental principles of immunology. *In* Ettinger, S. J.: *Textbook of Veterinary Internal Medicine,* 2nd ed. W. B. Saunders, Philadelphia, 1983, pp. 2102–2139.)

munology, especially when antigen-antibody precipitin reactions are allowed to occur in semisolid media such as gels (immunodiffusion).

THE COMPLEMENT SYSTEM

The complement system is an interrelated complex of serum proteins that is closely associated with the humoral antibody system. Although the system, with some variations, is present in all mammals, the most detailed information has been obtained for man and the guinea pig. The general principles are known to hold for other mammalian species, however.

It is now clear that there are two distinct activation schemes for the complement system—one initiated by appropriate antigen-antibody complexes leading to the *classical* cascade, and a second, the *alternate* or *properdin* pathway, that occurs because of initiation of the cascade at the C3 level. Both pathways have important *in vivo* implications for the prevention and production of disease.

The Classical Complement System

The classical complement system is composed of 12 serum proteins that interact in a closely ordered and integrated sequence termed the *complement cascade*. The complete cascade occurs as shown in Figure 15–4A. The reaction sequence is initiated by antibody, produces a series of soluble degradation products, some of which have important physiological properties, and terminates by generating the capacity to damage a cell membrane.

The classical cascade is initiated by certain Ig molecules that have bound their specific antigen. The IgM class and at least some of the IgG subclasses are active in starting the cascade, whereas the IgD, IgE, and IgA classes are not. The complement-fixing region of the IgM and IgG molecule resides in the Fc portion (see Fig. 15–2) and involves the C_H2 domain of IgG.[36] The cascade is activated by an initial interaction between Ig and C1q. Under usual circumstances, an antibody molecule alone will not initiate the cascade; it must be bound to its antigen before its latent potential for stimulating the entire cascade is revealed.

The complement proteins are able to associate with each other in a specific reaction sequence following the initial interaction of antibody with C1q. As indicated in Figure 15–4A, the complement components have been given numbers and in some instances additional letters. A bar over the symbol indicates that enzymatic activity has been induced during the cascade.

The reaction sequence continues until the C5b-9 complex is formed. A variety of studies have shown that the C5b-9 complex is the active moiety in producing damage to the membrane. Available evidence indicates that C8 is primarily responsible for the actual membrane damage, with C9 serving mainly a potentiating role. *In vivo*, bacterial cell membranes, red blood cell membranes, and, perhaps, tumor cell membranes are most commonly damaged.

The Alternate (Properdin) Pathway of Complement Activation

A summary of the general features of the alternate pathway is presented in Figure 15–4B. Certain substances—including such polysaccharides as inulin, bacterial endotoxins, and IgA—are capable of activating the precursor of a molecule called C3 proactivator convertase. This causes a sequence of events in which the terminal components of the complement cascade are activated.

Biological Importance of Complement Cascade Peptides

The fragments C3a and C5a interact with mast cells and basophils, leading to histamine release; cause contraction of smooth muscle; and are chemotactic for neutrophils, so they clearly participate in various inflammatory responses. Another component is formed when C5b binds to C6 and C7 to form a trimolecular complex, which, because it is highly chemotactic for neutrophils, is an important participant in inflammatory reactions. It is likely that additional important biological properties will ultimately be assigned to other soluble degradation products of the complement cascade.

There are important and necessary controls on the complement system. One is the short life of certain complexes, which decay to inactivity if the next component in the cascade is not contacted. Another is a series of specific inhibitor molecules in serum. Selected genetic deficiencies of either these inhibitor molecules or complement components themselves have been described in some species. These conditions may lead to serious disease, usually involving recurrent infections.

ANTIBODY-MEDIATED HYPERSENSITIVITY

From a clinical perspective, the most significant antibody-mediated hypersensitivity syndromes are acute anaphylaxis or atopy (immediate hypersensitivity), which is mediated by specific antibody of the IgE class that is bound to mast cells or basophils, and serum sickness, which is due to complement-fixing immune complexes that develop subsequent to the administration of a large protein dose to a previously sensitized individual (e.g., an animal that has previously received foreign serum in an attempt to provide passive immunity). Various antibody-me-

TABLE 15–4. Antibody-Mediated Hypersensitivity Reactions

Reaction	Characteristics	Immunoglobulin Involved	Special Features
Direct Arthus Reaction	Repeated local injection of antigen leads to local erythema, edema, and necrosis at that tissue site, principally as a result of blood vessel reaction. Antibodies are produced by the animal receiving the injections	IgG, IgM (complement fixing)	1. No tissue fixation of antibody 2. Complement participates 3. Polymorphonuclear leukocytes attracted by antigen-antibody-complement complexes leads to tissue injury 4. Antigen-antibody-C' precipitates in tissues 5. Antihistamines have no ameliorating effect
Direct Passive Arthus Reaction	Antigen injected locally, then antibodies injected intravenously	As above	As above
Reverse Passive Arthus Reaction	Antibodies injected into skin, then antigen injected intravenously	As above	As above
Systemic Arthus Reaction	Slow development over several hours of fatal reaction characterized by widespread circulatory changes and hemorrhages. Takes place when antigen exposure occurs in a protracted way (slow absorption from tissue sites) in individuals that already have high levels of circulating antibodies	As above	As above (details depend on where precipitates occur in tissues)
Prausnitz-Küstner (P-K) Reaction	Local injection into skin of antibody-containing serum followed by later (24-hr) injection of antigen (allergen) into same site leads to a reaction at that site (wheal and erythema)	IgE	Mediated solely by reaginic antibodies (IgE), which bind to mast cells in the skin
Systemic Anaphylaxis	Entry of antigen into the systemic circulation of a previously sensitized individual (i.e., one that has antibodies in serum and fixed to cells) leads to a severe general reaction that can be fatal. Details of the general reaction vary with species	IgE	Antigen interaction with specific IgE molecules that have been previously fixed to cells (mast cells) leads to release of pharmacologic mediators (histamine, serotonin), which then results in smooth muscle contraction and increased vascular permeability

Table continued on opposite page

diated hypersensitivity conditions have been described in several species and are presented in Table 15–4. Some of those listed are experimentally induced. Immune complex disorders are covered later in the chapter.

Although the existence of IgE has not yet been definitely established in all species, general indications and the existence of acute anaphylaxis in most species imply that this antibody occurs in most mammals. Thus, the *immunological* component of the IgE-mediated conditions described in Table 15–4 is thought to be comparable in the various species. That is, IgE bound to mast cells of a previously sensitized individual can rapidly trigger the degranulation of this cell when a subsequent encounter with that antigen occurs. This leads to release by the mast cell of pharmacological mediators (which vary from species to species) that cause subsequent clinical signs. If the antigen exposure is massive, mast cell degran-

ulation can be extensive, rather than just local, and can lead to death from acute anaphylaxis.

CELL-MEDIATED IMMUNE REACTIONS

Sensitized (antigen-specific) T cells either are the primary effectors of cell-mediated immunity (e.g., cytotoxic T cells) or induce other cells to be effectors. As in humoral immune responses, antigen must be trapped, digested, and presented to T cells by macrophagelike cells.

Delayed Hypersensitivity Reactions (Classical Type IV Hypersensitivity)

Delayed hypersensitivity (DH) reactions are the prototype of cell-mediated immunity (CMI). An ex-

TABLE 15–4. Antibody-Mediated Hypersensitivity Reactions (*Continued*)

Reaction	Characteristics	Immunoglobulin Involved	Special Features
Passive Cutaneous Anaphylaxis	Injection of antibody containing serum into skin of experimental animal of a different species; results in antibody fixation to cells, if they are so capable. After an appropriate waiting period, antigen is injected intravenously together with a marker dye. A circular colored spot develops in a positive reaction	IgG, IgE	Antibodies must fix to cells in skin (probably mast cells); then Ab-Ag reaction leads to release of pharmacologic mediators, circulatory changes, and dye deposition. This is a very sensitive test for antibodies. Antibodies involved are always heterocytotropic
Reverse Passive Cutaneous Anaphylaxis	A test immunoglobulin molecule is injected into the skin. If the molecule is capable of cell fixation, it will be fixed to certain cells (probably mast cells) near the injection site. After a waiting period, an antiserum containing anti-immunoglobulin antibodies is injected intravenously together with a marker dye. The anti-immunoglobulin antibodies will react with the immunoglobulin that has fixed to the cells, and cell degranulation will occur	IgG, IgE	The anti-immunoglobulin antibodies usually react with determinants in the Fc region of the immunoglobulin that is cell fixed. The RPCA reaction is used most to test for the skin fixing property of immunoglobulins
Serum Sickness	Administration of a single injection of antigen is followed by a slowly developing illness characterized by hives, edema, and fever. The reaction peaks 7 to 10 days following the antigen injection and is usually not fatal	IgG (with or without IgE?)	The antibody induced by the antigen(s) reacts with some remaining antigen, often on cell surfaces. The complement system is activated, leading to anaphylatoxin release, and histamine is released from cells. Serum sickness thus involves several different types of hypersensitivity responses

General comments on cell-fixing antibodies:
1. Cell-fixing antibodies are called "cytotropic" and have been found in both the IgG and IgE classes.
2. Homocytotropic antibodies will fix to cells of the *same* species that synthesized them.
3. Heterocytotropic antibodies will fix only to cells in species *different* from that in which the antibody has been produced.

cellent review of the current concepts of DH has been presented by Askenase.[4] DH exemplifies the ability of T cells to recruit effector leukocytes to a tissue site. The term *DH*, or, more precisely, *tuberculin-type hypersensitivity*, is now reserved for the classical T cell–dependent reaction associated with either immunization with antigens augmented by a water-in-oil, mycobacteria-containing adjuvant (complete Freund's adjuvant) or infection with mycobacteria. Therefore, these reactions may be elicited by intradermal challenge with either tuberculin or antigens administered with the mycobacteria. The development of DH reactions, in contrast to that of anaphylactic reactions, requires 24 to 48 hours, probably because it involves interaction of a number of different cell types, such as *recirculating cells*, antigen-specific immune T cells; *resident cells*, vascular endothelial cells, which must be traversed by both recirculating cells and recruited cells, tissue macrophagelike cells, and mast cells; and *recruited cells*, bone marrow–derived effector leukocytes, such as monocytes, basophils, and neutrophils, which comprise more than 95 per cent of the cellular infiltrate in a DH reaction.[39, 43]

The involvement of vasoamines in DH has been reviewed by Askenase.[2] T cells mediating DH (which are Lyt 1^+2^- in the mouse[28]) are recirculating cells. During normal rounds, they leave the circulation by passing directly through the cytoplasm of high endothelial cells of the postcapillary venules by a process called *emperipolesis*.[42] When a rare, passing, specifically immune T cell meets the antigen-presenting cell, it stops its migration and becomes activated. In the process of activation, it releases a number of soluble substances called *lymphokines* (Table 15–5). Some of these substances are chemotactic and may cause recruited cells to be attracted to and stick to the endothelial wall of blood vessels near the lesion. Recent data imply that T cells may also be responsible for inducing the release of vasoactive amines from local mast cells. These amines (serotonin or histamine, depending on the species) cause an increase

TABLE 15–5. Representative Lymphokines

Lymphokine	Activity
Affecting Lymphocytes	
Blastogenic or mitogenic factor (BF or MF)	Induces blast cell formation and thymidine incorporation in normal lymphocytes
Potentiating factor (PF)	Augments or enhances ongoing transformation in MLC or antigen-stimulated cultures
Cell cooperation or helper factor	Produced by T cells, increases the number or rate of formation of antibody-producing cells *in vitro*
Suppressor factors	Inhibits activation of and/or antibody production by B cells
Interleukin II (TCGF)	An Ly 1 cell factor that helps T cells, such as CTL precursors, to proliferate
Affecting Macrophages	
Migration-inhibitory factor (MIF)	Inhibits the migration of normal macrophages
Macrophage-aggregation factor (MAF)	Agglutinates macrophages in suspension
Macrophage-spreading inhibition factor (MSIF)	Prevents the flattening and spreading of primary macrophages in culture
Migration-enhancement factor (MEF)	Promotes the migration of macrophages in agarose (antagonistic with MIF)
Affecting Granulocytes	
Inhibitory factor	Inhibits the migration of buffy coat cells or peripheral blood leukocytes from capillary tubes or wells in agar plates
Chemotactic factor	Causes granulocytes to migrate through micropore filter against a gradient
Affecting Cultured Cells	
Lymphotoxin (LT)	Cytotoxic for certain cultured cells, e.g., mouse L cells or HeLa cells
Proliferation inhibitory factor (PIF)	Inhibits proliferation of cultured cells without lysing them
Interferon	Protects cells against virus infection

in the spaces between endothelial cells, which are apparently required for the migration (diapedesis) of recruited, bone marrow–derived cells into the tissues.[24, 61] Once these cells enter the tissues, their migration is halted by lymphokines such as macrophage inhibitory factor (MIF, which can be detected *in vitro* in the correlate of DH, the MIF assay). Some of these bone marrow–derived macrophages also become activated by lymphokines and can kill the invading pathogen. Although the elicitation of the response is specific at the level of the T cell, the effector arm is not antigenically specific. This is because an activated macrophage can ingest and destroy not only the eliciting antigen (e.g., mycobacteria) but other "intracellular" bacteria as well (such as *Listeria* spp.)

DH lesions require the presence of antigen, because once antigen is removed, the lesion subsides. In the case of a tuberculin skin test, this may take several days, whereas in chronic diseases in which the pathogen reproduces and cannot be eliminated, systemic or local lesions can last for long periods of time.

Contact sensitivity (CS) is another form of delayed onset reaction. In CS, the immunogen is an exogenous, simple haptenic reactive chemical (such as dinitrophenol [DNP] or a metal) or an environmental allergen (such as in poison ivy sensitivity) that be-

comes covalently linked with host skin components. This complex becomes the complete antigen, which is necessary for the induction of immune T cells and the elicitation of the response as previously described. These lesions are usually rich in basophils in man and guinea pigs and are considered to be a subset of the type of delayed reaction called *cutaneous basophil hypersensitivity* (CBH).[3, 65] Important differences between DH and CBH are that CBH reactions can be induced without mycobacterial adjuvants and that some of these reactions may be antibody mediated.

In delayed reactions, the identity of cells recruited into the tissues by T cells varies with (1) the *species*—monocytes are the principal cells recruited in human DH reactions, whereas neutrophils are common in the mouse and the dog; (2) the *mode of immunization*—basophils are preferentially recruited when the immunization does not involve mycobacteria; and (3) the type of *immunogen*—eosinophils are recruited for delayed responses to helminthic parasites and basophils for responses to ectoparasites such as ticks. The release of vasoactive mediators by basophils and mast cells may serve other functions. For example, vasoactive mediators may be protective at sites where reactions are expelling parasites. In addition, there is mounting evidence that at least one of the vasoactive amines, histamine, may have a regulatory role through its ability to interact with functional histamine$_2$ receptors on various leukocytes. These include cytotoxic T cell lymphocyte (CTL) precursors or effectors[56, 62] and suppressor T cell precursors and effectors.[5, 59, 63] Along with the effect on lymphocytes, the effect of histamine on other leukocytes leads to a net suppressive or anti-inflammatory effect and contributes to the diminution of these reactions.[2]

CMI and Resistance to Pathogens

The most convincing proof of the relative importance of cellular versus humoral immune mechanisms in protection against pathogens has come from studies of congenital "immunological cripples." Information derived from these human patients and, in selected instances, from other species, is presented in Table 15–6, which summarizes protective mechanisms in infectious diseases.

Bacterial Diseases. The involvement of cell-mediated immunity in resistance to bacterial infections has been the subject of an extensive review.[12] The primary immune defense against extracellular bacteria is antibody-mediated (see Table 15–6). This is often by complement-dependent lysis, especially in the case of IgM. The cellular components of these reactions include phagocytic cells, primarily macrophages and neutrophils. Specific antibody coats and thereby opsonizes bacteria, making them more susceptible to engulfment by phagocytic cells that bear Fc receptors on their surface. Engulfed organisms are subsequently destroyed in phagolysosomes. The antibodies involved in opsonic activity are usually IgG. Complement components, most notably C3b, may aid in this specific opsonization by virtue of C3b receptors on the surface of the phagocyte. Phagocytes can also be specifically *armed* by local antibody, making them more capable of specifically engulfing bacteria.

Intracellular Infections. DH-like CMI responses deal primarily or exclusively with intracellular infec-

tions. These include infections caused by bacteria (such as mycobacteria, salmonellae, *Listeria monocytogenes*, and *Brucella*); fungi (e.g., *Coccidioides immitis*[6] and *Candida*); viruses; and certain protozoal parasites (e.g., *Toxoplasma*, those causing malaria, *Leishmania*, and various trypanosomes) (see Table 15–6). When bacteria are able to invade and grow inside cells, they are safe from antibody-mediated attack. The primary defense against such agents is phagocytosis and killing by *activated* macrophages. It appears that less mature macrophages, with few hydrolytic granules, are susceptible to and can support the growth of intracellular bacteria. Once influenced by lymphokines in a DH-like response, the macrophage becomes activated, gains many motile cytoplasmic processes and well-developed intracellular lysosomal granules, and becomes able to kill engulfed bacteria.[40]

Viral Infections. CMI responses are important protection against viral diseases as well. Activated macrophages can kill their virus-infected targets by a mechanism that is not totally understood. It has been demonstrated that CTLs are also induced during virus infections and may be the primary mediators of protection.[76] These cells (as well as macrophages) are able to kill infected targets prior to assembly of infectious particles and can break the cycle of viral replication. As in the B cell response, helper T cells are needed to help CTL precursors become killers.[69] In order to kill a target cell, in all virus systems tested (i.e., in man, mice, rats, and chickens), the effectors must recognize not only the relevant virus-associated antigen but self, major histocompatibility complex (MHC)–coded antigens as well. There is evidence that pathological effects of the immune response may result in host cell destruction in some viral infections, as in lymphocytic choriomeningitis (LCM).[21]

Other mechanisms of immune protection against virus infections have been described, such as T cell–dependent antibody formation by B cells, which is critical to protection against re-infection with most viruses; IgA secretion at mucosal surfaces; macro-

TABLE 15–6. Defense Mechanisms*

	Bacteria		Viruses†	Fungi	Parasites‡
	Extracellular	*Intracellular*			
CMI	±	+++	+++	+++	+
Antibody	+++	±	++	±	++
Complement	+++	−	++	?	**
NK cells	−	−	++	−	+
Granulocytes	+++	−	+	+	+++§

*From Robert S. Schwartz, personal communication, 1980.

†Depends on nature of virus and stage of infection. Antibody most important for reinfection. Interferon may induce NK cells.

‡Mixed cell mediated response and eosinophils plus antibody.

**Complement may be important in protection against certain blood-borne metazoal parasites via the activation of the alternate pathway.

§Eosinophils, depending on type of parasites.

phage phagocytosis and killing of certain large viruses; and antibody-dependent, cell-mediated cytotoxicity by non-B, non-T (null) lymphoid cells.

Immunity to Parasitic Infections

Helminths. Peripheral blood and tissue eosinophilia are characteristic of helminth infestations. The eosinophil is a major effector cell in CMI to such parasites, probably by Fc receptor–bound IgG antibody–dependent destruction of the parasites and their eggs.[73] Eosinophils produce large quantities of superoxide, which may be a mechanism by which they damage nonphagocytosable parasites. It appears that one major mechanism of protection involves parasite antigen–induced release of eosinophil chemotactic factors both from specifically immune T cells and (by virtue of Fc receptor–bound cytophilic antibody) by degranulation of mast cells. Eosinophils invade the region and attack the parasite specifically by antibody-dependent cytotoxic mechanisms. It should be emphasized that other effector mechanisms may also be involved, including complement-dependent, antibody-mediated killing; macrophage or neutrophil antibody–dependent killing; and nonspecific inflammatory responses (see Table 15–6).

Parasitic disease can be chronic and granulomatous, in many cases associated with an inability of the host to reject the invading parasites. This is because the parasites have evolved a great variety of mechanisms to survive natural and acquired immune attack by the host.[10] For example, although some parasitic larvae are immunogenic and induce a high level of T cell and antibody responses, as they develop they are no longer recognized as foreign.

Protozoa. Most intracellular protozoal infections are dealt with in much the same way as intracellular bacteria, i.e., T cell–dependent killing by activated macrophages.[45] Immunity to the hemoprotozoa such as malaria organisms and *Babesia* is complex.[1] B cells, T cells, and macrophages are all involved in the recovery from these infections.

Protozoan parasites survive by their ability to escape the immune response of the host. Antigenic variation in trypanosomes is well known.[18] This is explained by the sequential expression of alternative cell surface glycoproteins by the parasite. In addition, suppressor T cells are activated in experimental trypanosomiasis.[32]

Ectoparasites. There is not a great deal known about immunity to ectoparasites. Askenase[3] has studied the CBH response to ticks. Basophils may play an effector role, since they comprise up to 90 per cent of the infiltrate, although eosinophils appear to be required as well. Nearly complete resistance can be achieved in guinea pigs (80 to 100 per cent rejection of ticks), which can be transferred to normal animals with sensitized cells or immune serum.

THE MAJOR HISTOCOMPATIBILITY COMPLEX (MHC)

The MHC is discussed in depth in the subsequent subchapter. How the MHC is involved in the normal immune response to other antigens will be described here.

Structure of the MHC

Table 15–7 summarizes the major traits attributed to specific regions of the H-2 complex of the mouse (Fig. 15–5). More limited, but comparable, information is accumulating for other species (e.g., the dog; see "Transplantation Immunology"), but the mouse is the best prototype.

K and D Regions

The K and D regions of the mouse and similar regions of all other mammals code for antigens on the surface of virtually all cells of adult animals with the exception of mature erythrocytes of some species. Such antigens readily stimulate the formation of antibodies and are, therefore, called *serologically defined* (SD) *antigens*. Products of the K and D loci are present separately on the surface of cells. There is structural homology between H-2K- and H-2D-coded antigens as well as between the SD antigens of man and mouse and probably other species as well.

TABLE 15–7. Partial List of Genes Localized to the Mouse MHC (H-2) Region

Biological Trait	Segment of Mouse H-2 Complex					
	K	*I-A*	*I-B*	*I-C*	*S*	*D*
H-2 (SD) antigens	+					+
Target antigens for CTL	+					+
Transplantation antigens	+	+				+
Immune response genes		+	+	+		
Ia (LD) antigens		+	+	+		
MLR, GVHR	+	+	+	+		+
Serum proteins					+	

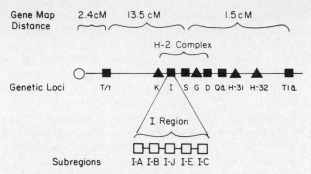

Figure 15–5. A map of the 17th chromosome of the mouse. The positions of the centromere (○) and identified genes (△) and complexes of two or more genes (□) are shown, which code for cell-surface alloantigens. T/t codes for short tail, and H-31 and H-32 are minor histocompatibility genes. See the text for descriptions of the other loci. One centimorgan (cM) represents a recombination frequency of 1.0 per cent; for example, there is approximately a 13.5 per cent recombination rate between T/t and H-2K, and a 1.5 per cent recombination rate between H-2D and T1a. (Reprinted with permission from Schwartz, A., and Kehoe, J. M.: Fundamental principles of immunology. *In* Ettinger, S. J.: *Textbook of Veterinary Internal Medicine*, 2nd ed. W. B. Saunders, Philadelphia, 1983, pp. 2102–2139.)

The I (Immune Response) Region

The I region of the murine MHC, and similar loci of other species, codes for certain I region–associated (Ia) cell-surface antigens. In the mouse it is composed of at least five genetic loci: I-A, I-B, I-J, I-E, and I-C. Ia antigens are a group of cell-surface glycoproteins against which antibodies are difficult to raise but which lymphocytes can recognize. Consequently, they have been called *lymphocyte-defined* (LD) *antigens*. Ia antigens are selectively expressed on B lymphocytes, some macrophages (I-A and I-E), and some T cell subsets (I-J and I-C). The Ia antigens are primary stimulators of mixed leukocyte responses (MLR) and graft-versus-host (GvH) responses.

The I region has been identified as the site where most immune-response (Ir) genes are found. These autosomal dominant genes are defined on the basis of the differences in the response levels of different inbred strains of mice and guinea pigs[7] to branched, relatively simple, synthetic polypeptide antigens. The I region also controls the cell's ability to make a vigorous cellular or humoral immune response to a variety of other thymus-dependent antigens in several species, such as rats, rhesus monkeys, and man. All species probably have such genes. The entire MHC is inherited as a package or "haplotype" and is codominantly expressed. That is, genes coding for histocompatibility antigens from one of the paired chromosomes of each parent are expressed in each offspring.

The Biological Role of the MHC

The MHC is important in graft rejection and graft-versus-host responses and probably has an important biological function. CTLs are induced by and are specific for SD (K or D) antigens on allogeneic cells. They are induced, as well, by syngeneic cells bearing tumor-specific antigens or cells that are virally or chemically (i.e., hapten) modified. Zinkernagel and Doherty[76] discovered that host CTL appear to "recognize" such antigens in association with the MHC K or D products (T helper cells and T cells reactive in DH also recognize antigen in association with MHC products but, generally, with Ia and not K or D antigens). Recognition is strong enough to lead to rejection of virus-infected cells, which might be recognized in a similar manner as for foreign MHC antigens. (This is also one explanation for autoimmune responses; see hereafter.) Certain murine regulatory T cells have been found to display one or another of the Ia antigens on their surface. For example, suppressor cells often bear I-J antigens. In addition, there is evidence that the presence of I-A and I-C antigens on macrophages and B cells allows certain T cells to interact preferentially with them. Thus, these antigens may act as specific interaction molecules.

In all species there are large numbers of alleles for different LD and SD antigens. One explanation for this diversity could be that MHC-coded antigens serve as the binding site for microorganisms, and different microorganisms may have different affinities for different MHC-coded antigens. This variation in affinity of viral binding site might render some members of a given animal species more resistant to infection than others, and the population might therefore be protected from annihilation by that infectious agent. However, in spite of numerous similar observations, the general biological role of the MHC is not yet totally clear.

Association of MHC and Disease

In man and in some animal species, an increased predilection for the occurrence of certain infectious, allergic, autoimmune, and other diseases has been associated with individuals bearing one or more specific MHC-coded antigenic specificities on their cell surface. The reason for these associations is not known, although the microorganism receptor theory in the preceding paragraph has been suggested. Other explanations might include the following: (1) Structural similarity of the MHC-coded antigen to the antigens of an infectious agent. The host thus recognizes the agent as self, leading to tolerance, which then increases susceptibility to the infection. Conversely, this could lead to the recognition of a self component as foreign and, therefore, autoimmunity. (2) "Defective" Ir genes (coding for incorrect responses) might be associated more frequently with one of the genes coding for Ia antigens. Ia antigens might even be directly involved in the pathogenesis of the disordered immune response, perhaps by affecting the events associated with antigen recognition. (3) The genes of the MHC might merely be tightly linked to other genes affecting the pathogenesis of a disease without being directly involved in immune reactivity (linkage disequilibrium).

IMMUNOLOGICAL REACTIONS AND DISEASE

This section deals with general characteristics of some disorders that relate to the fundamental immunological principles discussed previously.

Autoimmunity

Autoimmunity is defined as an immune response to self components and represents a breakdown of self-tolerance. Autoimmune reactions can involve T cell– or antibody-mediated processes. The mere presence of circulating antibody to a self component is not adequate evidence for the involvement of that antibody in the pathogenesis of an autoimmune disease state. For example, in systemic lupus erythematosus (SLE), there are circulating antibodies to DNA. Such antibodies to intracellular antigens are not known to *cause* cell damage but could have been the *result* of an immune response to DNA released following cell death from another cause. (However, this issue is complicated by recent findings that some putative anti-DNA antibodies can also react with the phosphate moiety of phospholipids, which are constituents of cell membranes.) Autoimmunity to circulating (serum) proteins present in large quantities is not found, possibly because the level of circulating protein maintains both B and T cell tolerance. On the other hand, autoimmunity to circulating proteins that are present in small amounts, such as thyroglobulin, does occur, perhaps relating to only T cell tolerance and not B cell tolerance. The state of tolerance to intracellular antigens is poor, and autoantibodies are often induced after trauma. Examples are the nonpathogenic antibodies to cytoplasmic antigens of the liver that are made after chemically induced hepatonecrosis and the autoantibodies to prostatic antigens that develop after cryotherapy.

It is possible to induce loss of self-tolerance by immunizing an animal to its own tissues in complete Freund's adjuvant (strong immunization) or with antigens cross-reactive with self components (e.g., immunization of rabbits with human thyroglobulin results in autoantibodies to rabbit thyroglobulin). This might stimulate T cell help for already existing nontolerant B cells. Therefore, it is possible to have no response but no tolerance (hidden antigens), only B cell tolerance, or both T and B cell tolerance to self antigens.

Spontaneous autoimmune diseases in both man and animals have been described. These include Goodpasture's syndrome, in which antibodies are deposited on the glomerular basement membrane (GBM) of the kidney. Such antibodies are occasionally also associated with pulmonary damage. Hashimoto's thyroiditis is a disease associated with the formation of antibodies to thyroglobulin resulting in cellular infiltrates of the thyroid. Other examples of clinically significant autoimmune disease are autoimmune hemolytic anemia in which autoantibodies to erythrocytes result in premature destruction of the cells, idiopathic thrombocytopenic purpura in which antibodies destroy circulating platelets, SLE, and rheumatoid arthritis in which immune complexes formed in response to altered host IgG are deposited in synovial tissue, leading to destruction of articular cartilage.

A number of factors have been postulated to lead to autoimmune disease. These include viruses, disordered immunoregulation, and genetic predisposition. The involvement of viral infection in autoimmunity is still unclear.[58, 64] For example, autoantibodies to T cells have been discovered in NZB mice, humans, and dogs with autoimmune disease.[31, 67] This could result in a lack of suppressor cells, which might lead to a breakdown of self-tolerance. There is also convincing evidence for *genetic* influences in human SLE, and some strains of mice routinely get autoimmune disorders. In addition, some dogs that had been bred for SLE developed not only SLE but rheumatoid arthritis, autoimmune hemolytic anemia, pernicious anemia, thrombocytopenic purpura hemorrhagica, celiac disease, autoimmune thyroiditis, Sjögren's-like syndrome, and a variety of autoantibodies as well.[57] Studies with autoimmune disease–prone mice and dogs have shown that many animals may have autoantibodies without autoimmune disease.

Immune Complex Diseases

In immune complex diseases, which include serum sickness, Arthus reactions, and certain autoimmune diseases, antigen-antibody complexes formed in antigen excess are deposited in tissues or blood vessels. The serum complement cascade is activated by the classical or alternative pathway, leading to formation of chemotactic factors. Neutrophils that are drawn in can cause severe tissue necrosis. They bind to the complexes via C3 receptors, phagocytose the complexes, and release lysosomal enzymes and vasoactive peptides. IgG is the usual antibody class involved in these reactions. IgM can fix complement also but is present in considerably smaller concentration in the serum.

The immune complex can be a combination of antibody with antigen circulating in the serum or soluble in the tissue fluid phase or unmodified or antigen-modified tissue antigens. The classic form of a systemic immune complex disease is serum sickness that occurs following deposition of circulating immune complexes that are developed by antibodies induced by administration of foreign serum proteins such as horse serum[20] (see Table 15–4). The kidney probably suffers most from immune complex accumulation, because complexes are readily trapped owing to the high blood flow and the fine fenestrated capillary network of this organ, which exposes the glomerular basement membrane.

Local Immune Complex Disease: Arthus Reactions and Related Maladies

The Arthus reaction is an acute immune complex vasculitis produced when antigen is injected intradermally into an animal that has preformed circulating antibodies to that antigen (see Table 15–4). The reaction is usually seen after an immediate response but before a typical DH response, i.e., at four to ten hours after administration of antigen. The pathogenesis of the reaction is essentially the same as that described for serum sickness except that the antigen is deposited extravascularly. Damage is restricted to where serum antibody and antigen come in contact. Thus, severe neutrophilic infiltrates are seen along regional vessel walls, occasionally in association with thrombosis and necrosis, and with leakage of proteins and erythrocytes into the extravascular space.

The chronic inflammatory disease of the joints known as *rheumatoid arthritis* also has immune complexes as part of its pathogenesis. Immune complexes are found in joint fluids, together with neutrophils and a low level of complement proteins. Antibodies called *rheumatoid factor* (which are IgM or, more rarely, other Ig classes) complex with IgG antibodies specific for bound microbial antigens. Another example of a local immune complex disease is *farmer's lung,* in which inhaled fungal antigens complex in the lung with circulating antibodies to that fungus. Other environmental antigens cause similar processes and undoubtedly produce disease that is not accurately diagnosed.

Examples of diseases in man and animals in which immune complexes have been implicated include the following, in addition to classic serum sickness: (1) *Poststreptococcal (or other bacterial) glomerulonephritis.* This is due to the acute release of a large amount or the continuous slow release of small amounts of bacterial antigens. (2) *Malaria.* Plasmodial antigens may result in glomerulonephritis. (3) *Viruses.* In such cases viruses often circulate for prolonged periods without disease. Animals infected with lymphocytic choriomeningitis (LCM) virus suffer from CTL-mediated damage of virus-modified nervous tissue cells. In addition, when neonatal mice are infected with LCM virus and thereby become partially tolerant to the virus, no acute disease develops.[54] Rather, a moderate antibody response gradually develops that results in antigen-excess, immune complex glomerulonephritis. Similar problems occur in Aleutian disease of mink and equine infectious anemia in horses and probably many other diseases. (4) *Autoantigens.* In a variety of species, antibodies to DNA are developed in association with SLE. Immune complex glomerulonephritis occurs. Complexes are also deposited in various other tissues.

(5) *Unknown antigen.* In many instances the identity of the antigen is not known; however, Ig with or without complement may be deposited along the glomerular basement membrane with typical pathological changes. Other diseases, such as polyarteritis nodosa, are likely to be immune complex–mediated as well.

Autoantibodies to erythrocytes, platelets, neutrophils, and other cells may bind to such cells and eliminate them from the circulation. In some cases a drug may bind to self components and the complex antigen may be recognized as foreign. These drug-induced autoimmune disorders have been induced by a variety of agents such as quinidine, aspirin, and sulfonamides. The disorder abates once the drug is removed from the system.

Tumors of the Immune System

In man and in many domestic species lymphoid tumors that are derived from B cell, T cell, and stem cell lineages have been discovered. The characterization of the tumor type often depends on using markers similar to those employed for classifying normal lymphoid cells. Such studies have shown, for example, that the majority of leukemias in cats are of the T cell lineage. Perhaps the most thoroughly studied of the lymphoid tumors, however, is the myeloma or malignant plasma cell tumor. Although most of the proteins that have been studied extensively are from the mouse and man, some myeloma proteins from dogs and cats have been isolated and characterized as well.[29, 36–38] These B cell tumors are generally the products of single clones of plasma cells that have escaped regulation. Each cell of the clone secretes an identical immunoglobulin. Therefore, the serum of affected animals often contains a large amount of homogeneous Ig.

Immunoglobulin light chains (see Fig. 15–2) appear in the urine of animals that suffer from myeloma, since light chains are often secreted in excess by malignant plasma cells. These proteins have been described in dogs.[30] Urinary light chains are called *Bence Jones proteins.* Heating the urine of individuals affected with myeloma to 56°C for 15 minutes results in the formation of a proteinaceous precipitate. Further heating at 100°C for three minutes results in its return to solution. Some tumors make only light chains (light-chain disease), whereas others make only heavy chains (heavy-chain disease). The heavy chains are often abnormal in such patients, with variable deletions of amino acids near the amino terminal end of the heavy chain.

Immunodeficiency States

Immunodeficiencies can be classified as congenital or acquired. The congenital immunodeficiency states are often genetic diseases and have been termed *experiments of nature.* This is because by studying each disease state, the lack of a given component of the immune apparatus may be associated with the absence of a given spectrum of normal functions (see Table 15–6). Although many of these disorders have not been described in domestic animals, many conditions comparable to those described in man have been studied.

Congenital Immunodeficiency Diseases

Refer to Figure 15–6, which indicates the cellular location of the defect keyed by the following numbers:

1. **Severe Total Deficiency of Stem Cells.** Even under the best conditions, animals affected live only a few days. These neonates lack granulocytes, megakaryocytes, erythrocytes, and lymphoid cells and therefore have no resistance to any microorganism.

2. **Severe Combined Immunodeficiency Disease (SCID) or Swiss-Type Agammaglobulinemia.** This X-linked recessive or autosomal recessive trait is due to absence of early committed lymphoid stem cells. There are few or no T or B cells. Combined immunodeficiency has been discovered in Arabian foals in association with lymphopenia, thymic aplasia, absent cell-mediated immunity, Ig deficiency, marked decreases in spleen and lymph node lymphocytes, and increased susceptibility to infection. The trait is inherited in an autosomal recessive manner.[44] Pneumonia is the most common secondary disease and is caused by viral, fungal, bacterial, or protozoal agents. Bone marrow grafts have been employed as a means of treatment of stem cell defects.

3. **DiGeorge's Syndrome.** This syndrome is due to congenital (not hereditary in man) lack of the third and fourth branchial pouches. Affected individuals lack both epithelial thymus and parathyroid glands. The disease varies from total absence to severe underdevelopment of the thymus with hypocalcemic tetany. Although the lymphoid cell precursor pool is normal, owing to lack of a thymic developmental microenvironment and thymic hormones affected individuals have few or no T cells and marked hypocellularity of T cell areas of lymphoid organs. Such individuals, in the partial forms, might be likened to neonatally thymectomized mice in that they have a relative lack of T cell function. Total lack of the thymus is hereditary in the nude mouse, which also lacks T cell function. Unless placed in a controlled environment, in complete thymic aplasia death occurs owing to overwhelming infection with viruses such as herpes viruses, fungi, or, often, normally nonpathogenic agents such as *Candida albicans* or protozoa such as *Pneumocystis carinii.* Fetal thymus transplants have been used for treatment of human patients and might be applicable to affected animals.

4. **Bruton's Agammaglobulinemia.** This condition is an X-linked complete B cell deficiency characterized by recurrent pyogenic bacterial infections; no circulating IgM, IgA, IgE, or IgD; and less than 10 per cent of the normal level of IgG. Affected individuals make no antibody responses, although they have normal T cell numbers and function (no increased susceptibility to fungi or most viruses). In man, this condition is usually treated with gamma globulin and the requisite supportive therapy. An exact equivalent has not been described in domestic animals.

5. **Common Variable Agammaglobulinemia.** This human condition is a late-onset disease, often not observed until adulthood in either sex. It is characterized by both hypogammaglobulinemia and a deficiency in cell-mediated immunity. Patients have B cells, but these cells fail to mature to Ig-secreting cells in response to antigens. T cell function decreases with time, especially in patients developing thymomas. The spectrum of disease susceptibility is similar to that in Bruton's disease. Certain forms of this condition are thought to be related to a severe derangement of regulation, particularly that by suppressor T cells, in that T cells from affected patients can suppress Ig production by normal B cells *in vitro.*[71] Such patients are very susceptible to autoimmune disease. This syndrome most likely exists in other mammalian species but is yet to be formally described.

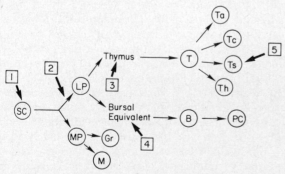

Figure 15–6. Points of defect in some congenital immunodeficiency diseases. *SC,* Stem cell; *LP,* lymphocyte precursor; *MP,* myeloid cell precursor; *T,* T cell; *B,* B cell; *Gr,* granulocyte; *M,* monocyte; *PC,* plasma cell; *Th,* T helper cell; *Tc,* cytotoxic T cell, *Ta,* amplifier T cell; *Ts,* suppressor T cell. Numbers 1 through 5 relate to text paragraph numbers for defects. (Reprinted with permission from Schwartz, A., and Kehoe, S. J.: Fundamental principles of immunology. *In* Ettinger, S. J.: *Textbook of Veterinary Internal Medicine,* 2nd ed. W. B. Saunders, Philadelphia, 1983, pp. 2102–2139.)

Acquired Immunodeficiencies

Naturally occurring acquired immunodeficiency diseases of the dog and cat have been reviewed by Cockerell.[16]

Viral Infections. In man, nonspecific immunodeficiency associated with measles infection has been detected by a transient lack of response (anergy) to tuberculin in otherwise sensitive individuals. A closely related paramyxovirus of dogs, canine distemper virus, also results in immunodeficiency. Lymphopenia is observed in the acute phase, and dogs with active distemper reject kidney grafts less well.

DH and T cell mitogen responses are also decreased. Immunosuppression is likely owing to virus replication in cells of the lymphoreticular system and their subsequent destruction or functional alteration.

Cats infected with feline leukemia virus (oncornavirus) may also become immunologically crippled and may show thymic atrophy and T cell depletion. Bone marrow cells are also infected and may be a target. T cell responses are decreased, including allograft rejection and lectin-induced DNA synthesis stimulation. There also appears to be a B cell functional deficiency. Many animals infected with feline leukemia virus that do not develop lympyhosarcoma succumb to secondary infection with other agents such as feline infectious peritonitis virus. A protein constituent of the virus is believed responsible.[55] Feline panleukopenia virus also causes a mild degree of T cell immunosuppression.

Parasitic Infestations, Chronic Bacterial Diseases, and Malignancy. All these can be nonspecifically immunosuppressive, in some cases involving nonspecific suppressor T cell activation.

Chemotherapy and Radiotherapy for Cancer. With the increasing use of antimetabolites, alkylating agents, and adrenal corticosteroids, the occurrence of secondary immunodeficiency states is increasing. In many instances there is an increase in susceptibility to herpes viruses, *Candida* spp., *Aspergillus* spp., *Nocardia* spp., gram-negative flora, *Pneumocystis* spp., and other organisms. The primary defect is usually in T cells. In very high doses, however, many of the agents are general bone marrow depressants and general immunosuppressants. The use of immunosuppressive agents in organ transplantation has been associated with a great increase in lymphoreticular neoplasia.

Other Factors. Malnutrition, aging, failure of colostrum transfer, and protein-depleting enteropathies and nephropathies have been associated with acquired immunodeficiencies.

LIST OF ABBREVIATIONS

B cell	Bursa (equivalent)-derived lymphocytes
CBH	Cutaneous basophil hypersensitivity
CMI	Cell-mediated immunity
Con A	Concanavalin A
CS	Contact sensitivity
CTL	Cytotoxic T lymphocyte
DNP	Dinitrophenol
DH	Delayed hypersensitivity
Fab fragment	Antigen-binding portion of Ig molecule
Fc fragment	Biological activity (effector function)–containing portion of Ig molecule
GBM	Glomerular basement membrane
GvH	Graft versus host
Ia antigen	I region–associated antigen
Ig	Immunoglobulin
I region	Genetic region of MHC containing Ir genes and coding for Ia antigens
Ir gene	Immune response gene
LAF	Lymphocyte activating factor (also called interleukin I)
LCM	Lymphocytic choriomeningitis
LD	Lymphocyte-defined MHC antigens (Ia in mouse)
LPS	Lipopolysaccharide
Lyt antigens	T lymphocyte differentiation antigens of mice
MHC	Major histocompatibility complex
MIF	Macrophage inhibitory factor
MLR	Allogeneic mixed leukocyte response
PHA	Phytohemagglutinin
SD	Serologically defined MHC antigens (K/D in mouse)
SLE	Systemic lupus erythematosus
T cell	Thymus-derived lymphocyte
TL antigen	Thymus leukemia antigen of mice

1. Allison, A. C., and Clark, I. A.: Specific and nonspecific immunity to haemoprotozoa. Am. J. Trop. Med. Hyg. 26:216, 1977.
2. Askenase, P. W.: Role of basophils, mast cells and vasoamines in hypersensitivity reactions with a delayed time course. Prog. Allergy 23:199, 1977.
3. Askenase, P. W.: Basophil arrival and function in tissue hypersensitivity reactions. J. Allergy Clin. Immunol. 64:79, 1979.
4. Askenase, P. W.: Effector cells in late and delayed hypersensitivity reactions that are dependent on antibodies or T cells. In Fougereau, M., and Dausset, J. (eds.): *Progress in Immunology IV.* Academic Press, London, 1980, p. 829.
5. Askenase, P. W., Schwartz, A., Siegel, J. N., and Gershon, R. K.: Role of histamine in the regulation of cell mediated immunity. Int. Arch. Allergy Appl. Immunol. 66(Suppl. 1):225, 1981.
6. Beaman, L., Pappagianis, D., and Benjamini, E.: Significance of T cells in resistance to experimental murine coccidioidomycosis. Inf. Immun. 17:580, 1977.
7. Benacerraf, B., and McDevitt, H. O.: Histocompatibility-linked immune response genes. Science 175:273, 1972.
8. Benacerraf, B., and Unanue, E. R.: *Textbook of Immunology.* Williams & Wilkins, Baltimore, 1979.
9. Binz, H., Frischknecht, H., Shen, F. W., and Wigzell, H.: Idiotypic determinants on T-cell subpopulations. J. Exp. Med. 149:910, 1979.
10. Bloom, B. R.: Games parasites play: How parasites evade immune surveillance. Nature 279:21, 1979.
11. Burnet, F. M.: *The Clonal Selection Theory of Acquired Immunity.* Cambridge University Press, Cambridge, 1959.
12. Campbell, P. A.: Immunocompetent cells in resistance to bacterial infections. Bact. Rev. 40:284, 1976.
13. Capra, J. D., and Kehoe, J. M.: Hypervariable regions, idiotypy, and the antibody combining site. Adv. Immunol. 20:1, 1975.
14. Chiller, J. M., and Weigle, W. O.: Cellular interactions during induction of immunological unresponsiveness in adult mice. J. Immunol. 106:1647, 1971.
15. Claman, H. N., Chaperon, E. A., and Triplett, R. F.: Thymus-marrow cell combinations. Synergism in antibody production. Proc. Soc. Exp. Biol. Med. 122:1167, 1966.
16. Cockerell, G. L.: Naturally acquired immunodeficiency diseases of the dog and cat. Vet. Clin. North Am. 8:613, 1978.
17. Colgrove, G. S., and Shifrine, M.: Canine immunology: Current status. In Shifrine, M., and Wilson, F. D. (eds.): *The Canine as a Biomedical Research Model: Immunologi-*

cal, Hematological and Oncological Aspects. U.S. Dept. of Energy, Washington, D.C., 1980, p. 43.

18. Cross, G. A. M.: Antigenic variation in trypanosomes. Am. J. Trop. Med. Hyg. 26:240, 1977.

19. Davies, A. J. S.: The failure of thymus derived cells to produce antibody. Transplantation 5:222, 1964.

20. Dixon, F. J.: The role of antigen-antibody complexes in disease. Harvey Lect. 58:21, 1963.

21. Doherty, P. C., and Zinkernagel, R. M.: T cell-mediated immunopathology in viral infection. Transplant. Rev. 19:89, 1974.

22. Gershon, R. K.: A disquisition on suppressor T cells. Transplant. Rev. 26:170, 1975.

23. Gershon, R. K.: Suppressor T cells: A miniposition paper celebrating a new decade. *In* Fougereau, M., and Dausset, J. (eds.): *Progress in Immunology IV*. Academic Press, London, 1980, p. 375.

24. Gershon, R. K., Askenase, P. W., and Gershon, M. D.: Requirement for vasoactive amines for production of delayed type hypersensitivity skin reactions. J. Exp. Med. 143:732, 1975.

25. Gershon, R. K., Eardley, D. D., Durum, S., Green, D. R., Shen, F. W., Yamauchi, K., Cantor, H., and Murphy, D. B.: Contrasuppression: A novel immunoregulatory activity. J. Exp. Med. 153:1533, 1981.

26. Gheri, I., Gershon, R. K., and Waksman, B. H.: Potentiation of the T-lymphocyte responses to mitogens. I. The responding cells. J. Exp. Med. 136:128, 1972.

27. Good, R. A., and Gabrielson, A. E. (eds.): *The Thymus in Immunobiology*. Harper and Row, New York, 1964.

28. Huber, B., Devinsky, O., Gershon, R. K., and Cantor, H.: Cell mediated immunity. Delayed type hypersensitivity and cytotoxic responses are mediated by different T cell subclasses. J. Exp. Med. 143:1534, 1976.

29. Hurvitz, A. I., Kehoe, J. M., and Capra, J. D.: Characterization of three homogeneous canine immunoglobulins. J. Immunol. 107:648, 1971.

30. Hurvitz, A. I., Kehoe, J. M., and Capra, J. D.: Bence-Jones proteinuria associated with canine plasma cell malignancy. J. Am. Vet. Med. Assoc. 159:1112, 1972.

31. Imai, Y., Nakano, T., Sawada, J. I., and Oswawa, T.: Specificity of natural thymocytotoxic autoantibody developed in New Zealand Black Mice. J. Immunol. 124:1556, 1980.

32. Jayawardena, A. N., Waksman, B. H., and Eardley, D. D.: Activation of distinct helper and suppressor T cells in experimental trypanosomiasis. J. Immunol. 121:622, 1978.

33. Jerne, N. K.: The somatic generation of immune recognition. Eur. J. Immunol. 1:1, 1971.

34. Kehoe, J. M.: The structural basis for the biological properties of immunoglobulins. *In* Good, R. A., and Day, S. B. (eds.): *Comprehensive Immunology*, Vol. 5, Immunoglobulins. Plenum Press, New York, 1978.

35. Kehoe, J. M.: Selected aspects of the canine immune response. *In* Hay, J. B. (ed.): *Animal Models of Immunological Processes*. Academic Press, London, 1982.

36. Kehoe, J. M., Bourgois, A., Capra, J. D., and Fougereau, M.: Amino acid sequence of a murine immunoglobulin fragment that possesses complement fixing activity. Biochemistry 13:2499, 1974.

37. Kehoe, J. M., Hurvitz, A. I., and Capra, J. D.: Characterization of three feline paraproteins. J. Immunol. 109:511, 1972.

38. Kehoe, J. M., Tomasi, T. B., Ellouz, F., and Capra, J. D.: Identification of "J" chain in a homogeneous canine IgA immunoglobulin. J. Immunol. 109:59, 1972.

39. Lubaroff, D. M., and Waksman, B. H.: Bone marrow as a source of cells in cellular hypersensitivity. I. Passive transfer of tuberculin sensitivity in syngeneic systems. J. Exp. Med. 128:1425, 1968.

40. Mackaness, G. B.: The mechanisms of macrophage activation. *In* Mudd, S. (ed.): *Infectious Agents and Host Reactions*. W. B. Saunders, Philadelphia, 1970.

41. Marchalonis, J. J., and Moseley, J. M.: The immunoglobulin-like T cell receptor problem. *In* Müeller-Ruchholtz, W.,

and Muller-Hermelink, H. K. (eds.): *Function and Structure of the Immune System*. Plenum Press, New York, 1979

42. Marchesi, V. T., and Gowans, J. L.: The migration of lymphocytes through the endothelium of venules in lymph nodes. Proc. R. Soc. Lond. (Biol.) 157:283, 1964.

43. McCluskey, R. T., Benacerraf, B., and McCluskey, J. W.: Studies on the specificity of the cellular infiltrate in delayed hypersensitivity reactions. J. Immunol. 58:466, 1976.

44. McGuire, T. C., Banks, K. L., and Davis, W. C.: Alterations of the thymus and other lymphoid tissues in young horses with combined immunodeficiency. Am. J. Pathol. 84:39, 1976.

45. McLeod, K., and Remington, J. S.: Influence of infection with *Toxoplasma* on macrophage function and the role of macrophages in resistance to *Toxoplasma*. Am. J. Trop. Med. Hyg. 26:170, 1977.

46. Miller, C. H., and Mackenzie, M. R.: Cell surface markers of canine lymphocytes. *In* Shifrine, M., and Wilson, F. D. (eds.): *The Canine Biomedical Research Model: Immunological, Hematological and Oncological Aspects*. U.S. Dept. of Energy, Washington, D.C., 1980, p. 67.

47. Miller, J. F. A. P., and Mitchell, G. F.: Immunological activity of thymus and thoracic duct lymphocytes. Proc. Natl. Acad. Sci. USA 59:296, 1968.

48. Mitchison, N. A.: Induction of immunological paralysis in two zones of dosage. Proc. R. Soc. Lond. (Biol.) 161:275, 1965.

49. Möller, G. (ed.): Mechanism of B cell tolerance. Immunol. Rev. 43:1, 1979.

50. Möller, G. (ed.): Transplantation tolerance. Immunol. Rev. 46:1, 1979.

51. Möller, G. (ed.): Unresponsiveness to haptenated self molecules. Immunol. Rev. 50:1, 1980.

52. Mosier, D. E.: A requirement for two cell types for antibody formation *in vitro*. Science 158:1573, 1967.

53. Nossal, G. J. V., Pike, B. L., Stocker, J. W., Layton, J. E., and Goding, J. W.: Hapten-specific B lymphocytes: enrichment, cloning, receptor analysis, and tolerance induction. Cold Spring Harbor Symp. Quant. Biol. 41:237, 1976.

54. Oldstone, M. B. A., and Dixon, F. J.: Immune complex disease in chronic viral infections. J. Exp. Med. 134:325, 1971.

55. Olsen, R. G., and Krakowka, S.: *Immunology and Immunopathology of Domestic Animals*. Charles C Thomas, Springfield, IL, 1979.

56. Plaut, M., Lichtenstein, L. M., and Henney, C. S.: Properties of a subpopulation of T cells bearing histamine receptors. J. Clin. Invest. 55:856, 1975.

57. Quimby, F. W., Jensen, C., Nawrocki, D., and Scollin, P.: Selected autoimmune diseases in the dog. Vet. Clin. North Am. 8:665, 1978.

58. Quimby, F. W., Lewis, R. M., and Datta, S.: Characterization of a retrovirus that cross reacts serologically with canine and human systemic lupus erythematosus. Clin. Exp. Immunol. 9:194, 1977.

59. Rocklin, R. E., Greineder, D., Littman, B. N., and Melman, K. L.: Modulation of cellular immune function *in vitro* by histamine receptor bearing lymphocytes: mechanism of action. Cell. Immunol. 37:162, 1978.

60. Schultz, R. D.: Practical immunology. Vet. Clin. North Am. 8:553, 1978.

61. Schwartz, A., Askenase, P. W., and Gershon, R. K.: The effect of locally injected vasoactive amines on the elicitation of delayed type hypersensitivity. J. Immunol. 118:159, 1977.

62. Schwartz, A., Askenase, P. W., and Gershon, R. K.: Histamine inhibition of the *in vitro* induction of cytotoxic T cell responses. Immunopharmacology 2:179, 1980.

63. Schwartz, A., Askenase, P. W., and Gershon, R. K.: Histamine inhibition of Concanavalin A-induced suppressor T cell activation. Cell Immunol. 60:426, 1981.

64. Schwartz, R. S.: Viruses and systemic lupus erythematosus. N. Engl. J. Med. 293:132, 1975.

65. Stadecker, M. J., and Leskowitz, S.: The cutaneous basophil response to particulate antigens. Proc. Soc. Exp. Biol. Med. 142:150, 1973.

66. Steinman, R. M., and Witmer, M. D.: Lymphoid dendritic cells are potent stimulators of the primary mixed leukocyte reaction in mice. Proc. Natl. Acad. Sci. USA 75:5132, 1978.

67. Strelkauskas, A. J., Schauf, V., Wilson, B. S., Chess, L., and Schlossman, S. F.: Isolation and characterization of naturally occurring subclasses of human peripheral blood T cells with regulatory functions. J. Immunol. 120:1278, 1978.

68. Uhr, J. W., and Möller, G.: Regulatory effect of antibody on the immune response. Adv. Immunol. 8:81, 1968.

69. Wagner, H., Rollinghoff, M., Pfizenmaier, K., Hardt, C., and Jonscher, G.: T-T interactions during in vitro cytotoxic T lymphocyte (CTL) responses. J. Immunol. 124:1058, 1980.

70. Waksman, B. H.: Atlas of Experimental Immunology and Immunopathology. Yale University Press, New Haven, 1970.

71. Waldmann, T. A., Blaeze, R. M., Broder, S., and Krakauer, R. S.: Disorders of suppressor immunoregulatory cells in the pathogenesis of immunodeficiency and autoimmunity. Ann. Intern. Med. 88:226, 1978.

72. Watson, J., Trenkner, E., and Cohn, M.: The use of bacterial lipopolysaccharides to show that two signals are required for the induction of antibody synthesis. J. Exp. Med. 138:699, 1973.

73. Weller, P. F., and Göetzl, E. J.: The regulatory and effector roles of eosinophils. Adv. Immunol. 27:339, 1979.

74. Wilson, F. D., and Shifrine, M.: The canine as a model for studies on stem and progenitor cells of lymphohematopoiesis. In Shifrine, M., and Wilson, F. D. (eds.): The Canine as a Biomedical Research Model: Immunological, Hematological and Oncological Aspects. U. S. Dept. of Energy, Washington, D.C., 1980, p. 3.

75. Wu, A. M., Till, J. E., Siminovitch, L., and McCulloch, E. A.: Cytological evidence for a relationship between normal colony-forming cells and cells of the lymphoid system. J. Exp. Med. 127:455, 1968.

76. Zinkernagel, R. M., and Doherty, P. C.: MHC-restricted cytotoxic T cells: studies on the biological role of polymorphic major transplantation antigens determining T-cell restriction, specificity, function and responsiveness. Adv. Immunol. 27:51, 1979.

Transplantation Immunology

Sharon Stevenson and Anthony Schwartz

The field of transplantation is an excellent example of a symbiotic relationship between two disciplines in which advances in one field allow and often stimulate advances in the other. The complicated surgical techniques of organ transplantation would be of little use without sophisticated immunological tests to identify appropriate organ donors and monitor the recipient's response to donor tissues. The word transplantation is derived from the Latin trans- (through, beyond, across) and plantare (to plant). Transplantation immunology is the study of the inherent capacity of an individual to distinguish self from nonself (foreign) antigens and of the immune response to those foreign antigens present on tissues or organs that have been surgically transplanted. This immune response is the major factor limiting organ transplantation. To understand and control this response, one must have an appreciation of the antigens involved, their mode of inheritance and relative importance, and tissue differences in antigenicity.

Because the dog has been used extensively as an experimental model for transplantation studies, much information has been gathered on canine immunogenetics, transplantation surgery, and immunosuppression.[57, 71] This subchapter summarizes the current knowledge of canine transplantation immunology. Extrapolations of general principles may be made to the cat, although few studies have been published using cats as the experimental model.[66]

Transplantation immunology has its own vocabulary. The most commonly used terms are

Graft   Any tissue or organ for transplantation (in its most exact usage the word graft implies living cells)

Implant A material that is inserted or transplanted into the body (includes metals, ceramics, fabrics, and dead tissue, e.g., autoclaved bone); implants are rarely immunogenic

Autograft A tissue or organ removed from and then transplanted into the same individual (adjective—autologous)

Isograft A tissue or organ transplanted between two members of the same species that have identical genomes, e.g., identical twins; called a syngraft or isograft (adjective—syngeneic) when the donor and recipient are members of an artificially inbred, virtually genetically identical strain of laboratory animal (adjective—isologous)

Allograft A tissue or organ transplanted between genetically nonidentical members of the same species; formerly called a homograft (adjective—allogeneic)

Xenograft A tissue or organ transplanted between two members of different species; formerly called a heterograft (adjective—xenogeneic)

Heterotopic Placement of a transplanted tissue or organ into an abnormal site, e.g., a kidney transplanted into a subcutaneous pocket and attached to the external iliac rather than renal vessels

Orthotopic Placement of a transplanted tissue or organ into the anatomically appropriate site, e.g., a kidney attached to host renal vessels in the site of the excised kidney

The authors wish to thank Dr. R. Scibienski, University of California, Davis, and Dr. Joe W. Templeton, Texas A&M University, for their critical review of this manuscript.

HISTOCOMPATIBILITY AND TRANSPLANTATION ANTIGENS

The response of the recipient to foreign donor tissues is immunological in nature; thus, the lymphoid system of the recipient recognizes foreign cell-surface antigens on donor tissues. These cell-surface antigens are termed *histocompatibility* (H) *antigens,* and the genes that code for these antigens are called *histocompatibility* (H) *genes.*[2] Only those H antigens shown to induce graft rejection are termed *transplantation antigens.* There are many loci (specific sites of genes on chromosomes) that code for histocompatibility antigens, but in all species studied there is only one cluster of loci on one autosomal chromosome that contains the genes that code for the "strong," or major, histocompatibility antigens.[40] This cluster is called the *major histocompatibility complex* (MHC). The MHC of dogs is named *DLA* (*dog leukocyte antigen*); in human beings, *HLA;* mice, H-2; swine, *SLA;* cattle, *BOLA;* and so on. An allele is one of two or more alternate forms of a gene that occupies the same locus on homologous (paired) chromosomes. Polymorphism, or the presence of many alleles at each locus, is a particular characteristic of the genes of the MHC. Each individual will, therefore, have two (one on each of the paired chromosomes) of many possible alleles in his genome. Because the loci of the MHC are closely linked, the group of alleles of the MHC genes contributed by each parent is inherited as a bloc. This group of alleles is called the *DLA haplotype;* an offspring obtains one haplotype from each parent. MHC genes are expressed codominantly,[76] so that gene products (cell-surface antigens) derived from each parent may be detected on the cells of the offspring.

MAJOR AND MINOR HISTOCOMPATIBILITY SYSTEMS

Without immunosuppression, allograft survival usually is short in unrelated donor-recipient pairs; prolonged survival is found only in those extremely rare cases in which the donor and recipient tissues are histocompatible. A summary of the results of a typical kidney allograft experiment in which no immunosuppressive drugs are given is presented in Figure 15–7.[6, 7] In completely mismatched littermate pairs (two haplotype difference), allograft survival is as short as that in unrelated donor combinations (8 to 12 days). In littermates mismatched by one haplotype, kidney allografts survive for a longer period (between 12 and 35 days). Finally, in totally matched littermate pairs, the kidneys survive the longest period after transplantation (150 days or more). These results can be explained by simple mendelian genetics for one system (i.e., MHC-*DLA*). As stated previously, each offspring inherits one haplotype from each parent (Fig. 15–8). Large population studies have shown that approximately 25 per cent of littermates are *DLA*-identical, 50 per cent share one

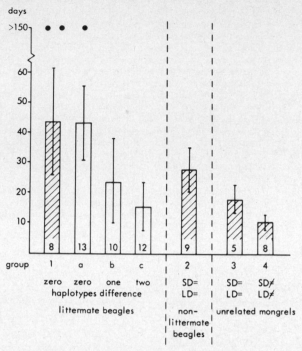

Figure 15–7. Survival of kidney allografts (mean ± standard deviation) exchanged between serologically typed littermate beagles, nonsibling beagles, and unrelated mongrels. The numbers at the bottom of the bars indicate the number of kidneys allografted in each group. ▨ MLR also performed (one way, with responder cells derived from the recipient and stimulator cells derived from the donor); ● long-term surviving kidneys that are not included for the calculation of the mean ± SD. Groups a, b, and c and 1, 2, 3, and 4 came from different experiments. In Groups 1, 2, and 3, the MLR were negative (LD =), whereas in Group 4 the MLR were positive (LD ≠). (Reprinted with permission from Bijnen, A. B., Westbroek, D. L., Obertop, H., et al.: Genetics of kidney allograft survival in dogs. Transplantation 28:191, 1979.)

haplotype, and 25 per cent share no haplotype. However, as shown in Figure 15–7, even when *DLA*-identical donors and recipients are used, indefinite survival of kidney allografts in littermate pairs does not occur. Therefore, although the MHC is obviously the most important determinant of transplant survival, other histocompatibility systems must exist. These minor H systems prevent a complete match between unrelated individuals or siblings, even if they are *DLA*-identical. It is of clinical importance that minor H antigen–induced responses, although difficult to identify prospectively, are relatively easy to suppress with drugs (Table 15–8). Therefore, the

	Male	Female
Parents	9,4/3,6	7,5/1,13

	W	X	Y	Z
Progeny	9,4/1,13	9,4/7,5	3,6/7,5	3,6/1,13

Figure 15–8. An example of en bloc inheritance of *DLA*-SD specificities in the dog. For the sake of simplicity, only alleles (specified by numbers) of loci A and B are shown. In this example, pairs WY and XZ share no haplotypes, and pairs WX, WZ, XY, and YZ share one haplotype. Should a fifth puppy be born, one of the sibling genomes would have to be repeated, resulting in a complete match with that sibling.

TABLE 15–8.   Differences Between Major and Minor Histocompatibility Systems

No. of Different Systems	Influence on Graft Survival	Inactivation by Immunosuppression	Prospective Identification of Antigens	Histology of Rejection
Major Histocompatibility System				
One	Pronounced	Difficult	Easy	Acute graft ischemia; severe cellular infiltrate
Minor Histocompatibility System				
Many	Weak; only demonstrated when identity present for the major histocompatibility complex; sometimes sensitization required	Easy	Difficult	Chronic graft ischemia due to endarteritis; mild, sometimes disappearing, cellular infiltrate

combination of matching the donor and recipient at the MHC and treating with immunosuppressive drugs to control the immune response to minor H differences should afford prolonged graft survival.[72]

The Major Histocompatibility Complex of Dogs

Figure 15–9 illustrates the genetic organization of the *DLA* complex, and Table 15–9 summarizes current nomenclature of the canine MHC.[73] The size of a genetic region, such as the MHC, may be inferred from the frequency of recombination between known H genes (as detected by H antigens). The greater the frequency of recombination, the larger the distance and the more genes that can be present between the

known loci. The recombination frequencies between various loci in the *DLA* area indicate that there are still many (more than 100) undefined loci within the *DLA* complex.[73, 80] It is likely that not all the unidentified loci are important in transplantation rejection. In an effort to summarize and unify the available knowledge of MHC in many species, the genes within the MHC have been divided into three classes based on genetic origin or function: class I corresponds to SD regions (K and D, mouse; *DLA*-A, -B, -C, dog; *HLA*-A and -B, human). There is similarity in the amino acid sequences of class I products in several species. Class II regions include the LD (LAD) regions and Ir and Ia loci, which may, in fact, be identical. Class III consists of genes that control the expression of certain components of the complement system, particularly those involved in the activation

TABLE 15–9.   Regions of *DLA* Complex

Class	Type*	Loci	Alleles	Method of Detection	References
I	SD	A	1–3, 7–10, Blk	Antisera in microcytotoxicity test	1, 68, 73, 80
		B	4–6, 13, Blk		
		C	11, 12, R15, Blk		
II	LD (LAD)	D + E	50–58, R1–R4, Blk	MLR and homologous typing	4, 64, 68
II	Ir	IrGA	IrGA	Antibody formation after low-dose antigen inoculation	76
		IrGL	IrGL		
		IrGY	IrGT		
II	Ia*	Unknown	Unknown	Antisera in microcytotoxicity test	76
Unknown	LD	PLT	Unknown	Secondary MLR	44
Unknown	R	R	Unknown	Hematopoietic regeneration after TLI and BM transplantation	79
Unknown	PGM-3	PGM-3	3.1, 3.2, 3.3	Electrophoresis of leukocyte lysate on cellulose acetate gel	46
III	Complement	Unknown	Unknown	Polymorphism of C_3	76

*The presence of these types is suggested but not proved in the dog. Ia and Ir loci may be identical with LD loci. See text for further information.

Notes: Blk = Blank; additional alleles remain to be defined.

MLR = Mixed lymphocyte response.

TLI = Total lymphoid irradiation.

BM = Bone marrow.

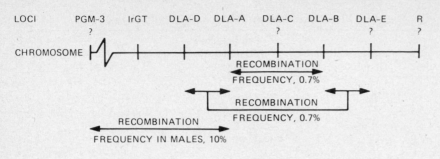

Figure 15–9. Current model of the genetic organization of the *DLA* complex. (Reprinted with permission from Vriesendorp, H. M.: Canine histocompatibility testing. *In* Shifrine, M., and Wilson, F. D. (eds.): *The Canine as a Biomedical Research Model: Immunological, Hematological, and Oncological Aspects.* Technical Information Center/U.S. Department of Energy, Oak Ridge, TN, 1980.)

of C_3. Currently recognized loci (Table 15–10) are as follows:

Serologically Defined (SD) Loci (Class I). The products (antigens) of these loci are found on the surface of virtually all cells with the exception of mature erythrocytes. These antigens induce the production of humoral antibodies, which are detectable by a variety of serological methods. In the dog there are three SD loci termed *DLA*-A, -B, and -C; alleles of these loci have been numbered sequentially in the order of discovery. Antisera are obtained from postpartum bitches or by immunization with lymphoid cells bearing the antigen in question. The antisera are rendered monospecific by absorption with lymphoid cells bearing other SD antigens to which antibodies are present. These reagents are used to identify SD antigens on peripheral lymphocytes in a complement-dependent microcytotoxicity test.[76] If the antigen for which the serum is specific is present on the lymphocytes, the cells are killed. When a large panel of sera is tested, most SD antigens can be identified and suitable donor-recipient pairs can be selected. Family studies (see Fig. 15–8) simplify the selection of sibling transplantation pairs. Both parents and all offspring are tested. Each of the four different haplotypes (two from each parent within a family) has an equal chance of being present in a given offspring. Some haplotypes are more common than others (i.e., certain MHC alleles of different loci are associated more often than expected based on the gene frequencies in the general population). This phenomenon is known as linkage disequilibrium and is discussed hereafter.

SD antigens are also the major stimulator and target antigens of cytotoxic T lymphocytes (CTLs), which are active in graft rejection. Lymphocyte-defined antigens on the graft induce another cell population (T helper), which enhances the maturation of CTL precursors into killer cells (see hereafter and previous subchapter).

Lymphocyte-Defined (LD) Loci and Immune-Response (Ir) Loci (Class II). The gene products (antigens) of the LD loci (also termed *LAD*, lymphocyte activating determinants) readily induce T cell activation, leading to blast transformation, but do not easily induce antibody formation. LD antigens are found primarily on B cells and on antigen-presenting cells such as dendritic cells and macrophages. The presence of LD antigens is most commonly detected *in vitro* by the mixed leukocyte response (MLR). In the MLR, leukocytes from the potential donor and recipient are cultured together. The cells of the potential donor are rendered incapable of dividing by irradiation (γ or x) or by treatment with mitomycin C. These cells are termed *stimulator cells*. If the lymphocytes of the potential recipient recognize foreign antigens on the donor cells and are capable of responding (responder cells), they synthesize DNA and divide. When H^3-thymidine is added to the culture medium while the cells are synthesizing DNA, the isotope is incorporated into responder cell DNA. Cell-bound radioactivity, which reflects LD antigen disparity, can then be determined. Homozygous typing cells may be used as stimulator cells in the MLC to identify specific antigens. For example, cells of dog A, which is homozygous for *DLA*-LD allele 50 (designated 50/50), are cultured with cells from dog B, which is heterozygous, i.e., 50/53. When dog A's cells are the stimulator cells, there is no response by dog B's cells, which look upon antigen 50 as self. However, if dog B's lymphocytes are the stimulator cells, dog A's lymphocytes respond to the foreign antigen 53. In the dog, two LD loci (*DLA*-D and -E) have been identified. Until international standards can be set, antigens produced by LD alleles provisionally have been numbered consecutively starting from 50. At the time of this writing, assignment of specific LD

TABLE 15–10. Influence of *DLA* Matching on Organ Survival in Littermate Donors*

Organ	Survival Time (days) DLA-*Different Donor*	DLA-*Identical Donor*	References for Techniques
Skin	12	18 to 24	26, 77
Kidney	20	27 to 43	6, 7, 26, 84
Small intestine	15	45	83
Pancreas	10	46	13, 28, 43, 45
Lung	13	43	10, 29
Heart	18	33 to 110	11, 19, 20, 25
Liver	8 to 11	76 to 210	21, 25, 50

*No immunosuppressive treatment was given.

alleles to the D or E locus has not been done. Linkage disequilibrium also occurs between SD and LD loci; for example, 47 per cent of MLC between unrelated mongrel dogs matched for *DLA*-A but mismatched for *DLA*-B are negative.[68] Generally, no significant MLR stimulation occurs between the cells of SD identical littermates.[68]

Ir loci are involved in the regulation of the immune response to a variety of thymus-dependent antigens. To detect gene products of these loci, dogs are immunized with L-glutamic acid copolymerized with another amino acid. The dogs are classified as responders or nonresponders based on the resultant humoral immune response. The loci are named after the synthetic polypeptide copolymerized with L-glutamic acid that induces the response—e.g., L-alanine, IrGA; L-lysine, IrGL; and L-tyrosine, IrGT. In several species immune-response genes are linked to genes controlling antigens present on antigen-presenting cells, B cells, and some populations of T cells. Such antigens are termed *Ia* (I-region associated) *antigens* and may be the primary stimulators in the MLC. To date, Ia antigens have not been detected by antisera in dogs. LD, Ia, and Ir loci are all class II loci and may be identical.

PGM-3 (Phosphoglucomutase-3) Locus. Phosphoglucomutase-3 is a polymorphic leukocyte enzyme in human beings as well as in dogs. Linkage has been demonstrated between PGM-3 and DLA, but the exact location of the PGM-3 locus is unknown.[76]

R (Resistance) Locus. The R locus codes for products that affect the survival of transplanted allogeneic bone marrow cells. There is currently no direct *in vitro* test to identify products of the R locus; its effects are only known retrospectively following *in vivo* bone marrow transplantation. After total-body irradiation, more allogeneic bone marrow cells must be injected to ensure survival of the recipient than when autologous or isologous bone marrow is injected.[79] Experimental data suggest that the R locus is separate from the *DLA* LD and SD loci but that marked linkage disequilibrium exists between these loci.[76] For example, in one study bone marrow transplants survived in 33 of 33 *DLA*-identical littermate pairs.[76] In another study, bone marrow transplants survived in 8 of 8 unrelated LD- and SD-identical pairs in contrast to 2 of 11 *DLA*-mismatched unrelated pairs. The number of bone marrow transplant "takes" in random, unrelated donor-recipient pairs indicates that there is at least one R locus with six alleles of equal strength and frequency.[79]

PLT (Primary Lymphocyte Test) Locus. In the PLT, lymphocytes (responder cells) that previously recognized and responded to foreign antigens present on stimulator cells in the MLC are challenged again in secondary cultures with fresh stimulator cells. Positive PLT results are strongly, but not absolutely, correlated with similar LD antigens on both the first cells to which the responder became "primed" and the second cells. However, about one-third of positive PLT results occur when the first and second stimulators have no *DLA*-LD antigens in common. Conversely, about 10 per cent of PLT results are negative when the original cells that clearly stimulated a response in the MLC are used for the secondary PLT. These data suggest not only a difference between genetic control of the MLC and PLT but that both are controlled from within the *DLA* complex.[44]

Other Markers

Complement Markers (Class III). The biosynthesis and activation of several complement components appear to be under the control of loci within MHC in some species (human beings, mice, guinea pigs, rhesus monkeys, and chickens). Recently, variations that may be genetically controlled have been found in a complement component (probably C_3) of dogs. No linkage was found between this marker and *DLA* in preliminary family studies.[76]

Linkage Disequilibrium and the DLA Complex

The high degree of linkage disequilibrium in the dog makes discrimination between alleles of different, linked loci more difficult than in other outbred species.[72] *Linkage equilibrium* describes the independent inheritance of alleles of linked loci (e.g., A and B) after they have reached an equilibrium state in a random population. For example, the presence of a certain allele *a* of locus A does not influence the chance that another allele *b* of locus B is present in that individual. On the other hand, if *linkage disequilibrium* exists, *a* and *b* are found more often in the same individual than would be predicted; consequently, the frequency of the phenotype *ab* is much higher than the product of the population frequencies (the expected frequency) of *a* and *b*. In unrelated individuals linkage disequilibrium leads to positive associations between antigens of different series. In dogs, a high degree of linkage disequilibrium exists between SD alleles of different loci as well as between SD and LD alleles and between LD alleles of different loci.[35, 70] The higher degree of linkage disequilibrium in the *DLA* region than in the *HLA* region may be explained by the "founder" effect[70]; i.e., by natural selection or extensive breeding of a few champion dogs within a breed, the genes, and thus the *DLA* haplotypes, of a few animals come to be over-represented in the population. The founder effect should not be equated with inbreeding, which would increase the frequency of homozygosity for polymorphic genetic systems. Canine genetic systems show Hardy-Weinberg equilibrium,[73, 80] which indicates that the observed frequency of homozygosity is not significantly different from the expected frequency from random mating.[18] Thus, the founder effect will lead to some loss of genetic variation through "gene drift," but the effect is not the same as that with inbreeding.

The inadvertent matching for several loci that occurs in unrelated donor-recipient pairs owing to linkage disequilibrium is different from the concurrent matching that occurs in sibling pairs. Since the loci of the *DLA* complex are closely linked and are therefore inherited *en bloc,* matching between siblings for several *DLA* antigens of a haplotype implies a match for the entire parental haplotype. Linkage disequilibrium between alleles *a* and *b,* on the other hand, simply increases the chances that allele *b* will be present (and therefore matched) when allele *a* is found in two unrelated dogs.

Minor Histocompatibility Systems

The sites of minor histocompatibility loci are unknown but are outside the MHC. The antigens coded for by these loci account for late rejection of transplanted tissues between *DLA*-identical donors and recipients. There are many minor H systems, the antigens of which, in contrast to SD and LD antigens, are difficult to identify prospectively because of the lack of appropriate tests. The effects of minor H differences, in contrast to MHC differences, are easy to suppress by drug therapy. As for the MHC, the function of minor histocompatibility loci probably is not related to the rejection of transplanted tissues (see following section). The minor H loci code for polymorphic enzymes, structural proteins, or hormones of a very diverse nature. The only feature the products of these loci have in common is their presence on the cell surface. Because of their expression on the cell membrane, they are recognized as nonself by the MHC-dependent recognition system, and an immune response is mounted against cells bearing them. Thus, their involvement in transplantation rejection simply is an artifact of their allelic nature and cell-surface location.

Currently there are four recognized minor histocompatibility systems in the dog, although others probably exist:

Blood Groups. Blood groups of the dog are considered minor histocompatibility systems because they influence the survival of allogeneic blood cells after transfusion. There are no preformed antibodies to dog erythrocyte antigens (DEA) as there are for the ABO system of human beings. However, DEA 1 and 5 donor-recipient differences have led to shortened red cell survival subsequent to repeated transfusions.[76]

Canine Secretory Alloantigen (CSA) System. The CSA has some similarities with the human ABO blood group; i.e., when a given CSA alloantigen is not present, an animal antibody to it may be and vice versa. In dogs, CSA incompatibility apparently offers some protection against graft-versus-host reactions following bone marrow allografts in DLA-identical donor-recipient pairs. The mechanism of the protective effect is unknown.[74, 87]

Phosphoglucomutase-2 (PGM-2). Phosphogluco-mutase-2 is a red cell enzyme that shows polymorphic electrophoretic variation in dogs. Disparities in PGM-2 have been associated with graft-versus-host (GvH) reactions following bone marrow transplantations, and both the PGM-2 and GvH loci may be on the same chromosome.[74, 81] Thus, two similar linkage groups are present in dogs: (1) PGM-2 and a minor GvH locus and (2) PGM-3 and DLA. Typing for the PGM-2–linked GvH locus by serological or other immunogenetic methods is not yet possible.

Sex Chromosomes. Suggestive evidence for both X- and Y-linked minor histocompatibility systems has been obtained in the dog as in other species.[3, 72] The H-Y antigen is presumed to be responsible for the rejection of male-to-female skin grafts in syngeneic mice.[59]

Biological Significance of the MHC Complex in Dogs

Both class I and class II gene products seem to serve as a means of recognition between cells. For example, the recognition of shared MHC specificities is necessary for certain T and B cell interactions. Thus, one of the functions of the MHC is *self-recognition.*[33]

Self-recognition or *altered* self-recognition may explain the association between certain *HLA* alleles and diseases, particularly autoimmune diseases. However, very little information is available in the dog regarding *DLA*-disease associations. Possible associations between *DLA* haplotypes and the clinical course of transmissible venereal tumor (TVT) and between *DLA* haplotypes and the occurrence of lymphoid neoplasia or atopy have been investigated. The demonstration of *DLA* antigens on TVT cells and the production of alloantigen-specific antibodies by regressor animals suggest that the MHC may influence the clinical course of the tumor.[31] The immune response to TVT may also be influenced by the *DLA* haplotype of the host. For example, in one study dogs of known *DLA* haplotypes were inoculated experimentally with TVT cells. Tumors inoculated into *DLA*-identical siblings either grew or were rejected similarly in both siblings, whereas tumors inoculated into *DLA*-different siblings behaved differently.[63] No association between certain *DLA* specificities and atopy or lymphoid neoplasia has been demonstrated[75, 78]; information on other diseases is not yet available.

Correlation of Histocompatibility Testing and Graft Survival—Related Donors

Matching of the donor and recipient for class I and class II histocompatibility antigens prolongs allograft survival in human beings, dogs, and other species.[6, 7, 55] In dogs the longest allograft survival has been achieved in littermate donor and recipient pairs matched for histocompatibility antigens. However, even when matched sibling donor-recipient pairs are used, allografts of some organs survive much longer than allografts of other organs (see Table 15–10).

Organ- or Tissue-Specific Differences

The data in Table 15–10 show that skin grafts benefit the least and liver grafts the most from donor selection. There are several possible explanations for the differences in effectiveness of MHC matching for different organs.

1. Different End Points. The subjective interpretation of when a 100 per cent rejection of a skin graft occurs is more difficult than the determination of azotemia or the death of an animal due to rejection of a kidney or heart transplant.

2. Difference in Susceptibility to Rejection. Some organs or tissues are more susceptible to immunological attack by the host than others. Allografts of cortical bone serve mostly as a scaffold for the ingrowth of host bone, so even if osteocytes bearing H antigens are killed, the ultimate function of the allograft is maintained. Additionally, nonvascularized grafts such as skin are more sensitive to rejection than vascularized organs such as kidneys, perhaps because of longer periods of hypoxia. Differences in susceptibility of the cells of different organs to antibodies, cytotoxic lymphocytes, and so on are important, as is the presence of a particularly crucial, immunologically vulnerable structure within an organ; e.g., rejection of the conduction system of the heart renders the entire organ useless.

3. Blood Transfusions. Either prior to or during long or complicated procedures such as heart or liver transplant operations, blood transfusions are given that may cause intentional or accidental immunosuppression in the recipient. This may be due to the induction of "blocking" antibodies or tolerance (see "Management of Rejection"). Prior transfusion of the recipient with donor blood depleted of Ia antigen–bearing cells prolonged the survival of pancreatic islet cell allografts in mice.[32]

4. Minor Tissue-Specific Histocompatibility Differences. The survival of each organ may be influenced by a different set of tissue-specific minor histocompatibility systems. For example, kidney and vascular endothelium–specific antigens have been demonstrated.[22, 36, 52, 69]

5. Differences in Immunization Procedures. Since it is membrane-bound, the amount of H antigen presented to the host varies with the cell type and cell number transplanted. For example, bone marrow is very cellular and has a high concentration of relevant antigens, cortical bone has few cells and therefore very little H antigen, and kidney has an intermediate amount. Furthermore, the route of antigen presentation may affect the immunogenicity of the transplanted organ. The intradermal route (e.g., sensitization via skin grafting) may be more immunogenic than the intravenous route (e.g., sensitization by "passenger leukocytes" in a kidney graft).

Histocompatibility Testing and Unrelated Donors

Although the survival of allografts from matched sibling donors has been encouraging, much shorter graft survival occurs in matched, *unrelated* pairs (see Fig. 15–7). The most likely explanations for this disparity are as follows:

1. Imperfect *DLA* SD and LD Matching. Perhaps owing to inadequate absorption of unwanted specificities, *DLA* SD antisera are not always totally specific and therefore may react with more than one antigen. Owing to haplotype inheritance patterns, imperfect *DLA* typing in littermates will not lead to erroneous matching if the inheritance patterns are properly interpreted; this is not true in unrelated pairs.

2. Minor Histocompatibility Differences. A pronounced influence of minor histocompatibility differences was found in studies of kidney allograft survival in beagles.[6] Through a comparison of groups of appropriately selected animals it was shown that cumulative minor histocompatibility differences had about the same effect on graft survival as a one *DLA* haplotype difference (when one haplotype is shared by donor and recipient and the other is not).

3. Other Regions Within the MHC That Have Not Been Identified. Because of haplotype inheritance patterns in dogs, matching for known regions in littermate pairs simultaneously may match for unknown, closely linked regions that may affect transplantation rejection. In unrelated pairs this concurrent matching does not occur.

Relative Importance to Transplant Survival of Matching for LD versus SD Antigens

Matching for the LD region appears to be more important than matching for the SD region, at least in kidney transplantation. In a kidney allograft study in unrelated mongrel dogs, kidneys functioned longest in donor-recipient pairs that were both SD- and LD- compatible or SD- incompatible and LD- compatible; kidneys functioned shortest in pairs that were SD- compatible and LD- incompatible or SD- and LD- incompatible.[85] In addition, a correlation has been found between mixed lymphocyte culture (MLC) stimulation and kidney allograft survival time; i.e., the kidney allografts of unrelated pairs with low stimulation indices (a measure of LD-antigen relatedness) functioned longer than those with high stimulation indices.[23]

ALLOGRAFT REJECTION

Immunological Aspects of Rejection

Transplant rejection is defined as the destruction or loss of function of all or part of an allograft by the immune system of the recipient. The end point depends on the cells, tissues, or organ transplanted and the anatomy, function, and vulnerability of the graft. Rejection is a very complex process in which both humoral and cellular responses to a variety of immunogens participate; the relative contribution of the two responses varies among grafts, and the degree of involvement of one mechanism or the other often is reflected in the histology of the rejected organ. For rejection to occur there must be both sensitization of the host (the afferent arc) and an immunological attack on the transplanted organ by the host (the efferent arc).[16]

The *afferent arc* of transplantation immunity includes the recognition of foreign cell-surface antigens and stimulation of an immune response to those immunogens. The immune response involves the cooperation of several cells (T and B lymphocytes and accessory cells, e.g., macrophages). The end products of the response are differentiated plasma cells capable of making antibody and T cells. T cells are involved in delayed hypersensitivity (DH)- like responses in which macrophages and other leukocytes are often the effector cells and in cytotoxic responses in which killer T cells are induced. Antibody and killer T cells are induced primarily against SD antigens, whereas DH T cells tend to respond to LD

antigens. The graft alloantigens that stimulate this response may travel to host lymphoid tissue via lymphatics (e.g., from a skin graft) or the vasculature (from a kidney or heart graft), or the host cells may travel to the graft and be sensitized there.[86] Other organ- or tissue-specific antigens besides *DLA* products (e.g., minor H antigens such as antigens specific to skin or kidney epithelium or vascular endothelium) also may elicit an immune response leading to rejection.

The *efferent arc* of the transplantation rejection reaction consists of two major phases: *recognition of the target antigen* and *recruitment of effector systems*. This results in removal of the antigen or destruction of the graft.[48] With the exception of cytotoxic responses, the reaction of an immune T cell or an antibody with an antigen will not by itself eliminate the antigen or destroy the graft. The recognition phase triggers the activation of several cascading enzyme systems that include the complement, clotting, and probably kinin pathways (Fig. 15–10). In addition, a number of effector cells (lymphocytes, macrophages, platelets, and neutrophils) are recruited both as a consequence of the specific immunological response and as a result of the subsequent

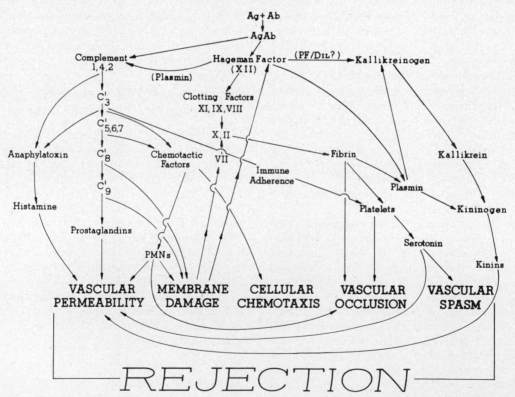

RECOGNITION

Figure 15–10. Integration of the humoral amplication system in graft rejection. This diagram suggests the complexity of allograft rejection. The three main cascade pathways—complement, clotting, and kinin—generate many active molecules, including the kinins, chemotactic factors, anaphylatoxins, histamine, and serotonin. These molecules, together with platelets and neutrophils, produce the destructive effects on the graft. The most prominent consequences include increased vascular permeability (edema), spasm, and occlusion as well as cell and basement membrane damage and cellular chemotaxis (infiltration).

These systems do not operate singly but tend to activate each other. Not shown are the many interlocking inhibitory factors that keep these systems in check once they are activated. (Reprinted with permission from Najarian, J. S., and Fokker, J. E.: The expression of immunity: The efferent arc. *In* Najarian, J. S., and Simmons, R. L. (eds.): *Transplantation.* Lea & Febiger, Philadelphia, 1972, p. 109.)

enzymatic events. Thus, the recognition phase of the efferent limb of the allograft reaction is immunologically specific, whereas the effector phase has both specific (e.g., cytotoxic T cells and antibody) and nonspecific components (macrophages, enzyme systems, and so on).

Cell-Mediated Immunity. An extensive cellular infiltrate (predominantly lymphocytes) within transplanted tissues has long been recognized as a hallmark of acute allograft rejection.[37] These lymphocytes are predominantly alloantigen-specific T cells that participate in rejection by at least two different mechanisms: (1) Sensitized killer T cells are generated that are specific primarily for SD antigen–bearing target cells. Such T cells kill target cells by direct cell-to-cell contact. (2) LD antigen-specific activated T cells also have an important DH-like function in allograft rejection. These cells release lymphokines that recruit other lymphocytes, promote chemotaxis of neutrophils, inhibit the migration of and activate macrophages, and increase vascular permeability. Thus, such T cells are not the true effectors of rejection but are necessary to recruit and activate the effectors.

Humoral Immunity. It should be emphasized that humoral (antibody-mediated) immunity is not necessary for graft rejection. Furthermore, antibody is not directly damaging to tissues, but provides instead the specific recognition portion of graft rejection. Antibody and antigen interactions activate nonspecific effector mechanisms such as the complement and coagulation cascades. Humoral antibody is important in at least two types of rejection: (1) Preformed circulating antibody may be present in the circulation of patients exposed to transplantation antigens via previous organ transplants that bear one or more antigens in common with the new donor, via pregnancy, blood transfusions, or infections with bacterial antigens that crossreact with transplantation antigens. This presensitization may result in hyperacute rejection (see hereafter). (2) After transplantation, the host may become sensitized to MHC antigens released into the circulation on passenger leukocytes or on vascular endothelium. The target of these antibodies is the graft vasculature, and the result of this antibody-dependent rejection is vasculitis. Antibodies may cause injury to the vascular endothelium by complement-dependent cytotoxicity, antibody-dependent cell-mediated cytotoxicity, deposition of antigen-antibody complexes, and the activation of other mediators of inflammation such as the complement, coagulation, and kinin systems.[15] Both IgG and IgM have been identified in organs undergoing rejection, and elevated levels of specific immunoglobulins have been measured *in vitro* after transplantation.[36, 52]

Soluble Mediators. Once an antibody-antigen complex is formed, whether fixed or circulating, the complement, coagulation, and kinin cascades are activated. This results in the production of factors that attract and hold active cells, increase vascular permeability, release enzymes capable of degrading proteins and cell membranes, cause smooth muscle contraction, and precipitate the formation of fibrin clots. Therefore, macrophages, neutrophils, and platelets are attracted to the site of rejection by both the specific immune response and the products of the cascade systems and participate actively in graft destruction[15] (see Fig. 15–10).

In summary, rejection is an extremely complicated reaction in which both specific humoral and cellular responses participate in addition to many nonspecific effector systems, leading to damage or death of a graft.

Kinetics of Rejection. When an allograft of skin, for example, is placed on a recipient animal, the graft first becomes vascularized and its cells proliferate; after about ten days it quite abruptly becomes the seat of inflammation, withers, and is sloughed (*first-set reaction*). If a second graft from the same donor is then made to the same recipient, it is rejected much more rapidly, perhaps in five to six days. This accelerated rejection is known as the *second-set reaction* and is specific for the transplantation antigens of the donor. The shorter survival time of the second graft results from persistence of the immunity acquired from the first graft or from an anamnestic response. Since potential recipients may be sensitized by pathways other than prior grafting (e.g., pregnancy, transfusions, and so on), these older terms have been replaced by descriptive morphological classifications of rejection.

Morphological Types of Rejection[42]

There are three morphological types of rejection, classified by the intensity and timing of the rejection phenomena. The morphological changes in these three types are described as they relate to renal transplants. Similar changes are seen in any vascularized organ transplant.

Hyperacute Rejection. Hyperacute rejection results from the presence of *preformed* circulating antibodies to donor-specific alloantigens. Rejection occurs within minutes to hours after transplantation and can be recognized by the lack of normal perfusion. Previously pink, blood-filled kidneys become soft, blue, and mottled, and urine output drops markedly. Histologically, hyperacute rejection resembles a classic Arthus reaction. Within hours, increased numbers of neutrophils are present on the endothelium of arterioles and capillaries, and the walls show characteristic fibrinoid necrosis. Immunoglobulin and complement are demonstrable in the vessel walls, and fibrin-platelet thrombi may be detectable. These changes point to an antigen-antibody reaction in the vascular endothelium. Thrombi eventually are formed, and the organ undergoes infarction and necrosis. Fortunately, this complication now is rare because pre-existing antibody can be identified prior to transplantation by testing leukocytes of the potential donor with serum of the recipient in the presence of complement.

Acute Rejection. Both cellular and humoral immunity are involved in acute rejection, which may occur within days after transplantation in untreated patients or may appear months to years later when immunosuppression has been used and then terminated. Either the cellular or humoral immune system may predominate in causing tissue damage. In acute cellular rejection, an extensive interstitial mononuclear cell infiltrate consisting of small and large lymphocytes, macrophages, and a few plasma cells is present in addition to edema and mild interstitial hemorrhage. These lesions usually respond to immunosuppressive therapy (see hereafter). Acute humoral rejection is manifested by vasculitis. Histological lesions consist of endothelial necrosis; neutrophilic infiltration; and deposition of immunoglobulins, complement, and fibrin. These lesions may result in thrombosis and infarction. This type of acute rejection does not respond well to immunosuppressive therapy. A milder form of humoral rejection, which is more common, is termed *subacute vasculitis*. The major lesions are in the arterial intima, which is markedly thickened by proliferating fibroblasts, myocytes, and macrophages leading to luminal narrowing or obliteration.[54] The walls of most of these arteries show deposits of immunoglobulin and complement.

Chronic Rejection. Chronic lesions are seen when acute rejection is more or less controlled with immunosuppression. Both humoral and cellular immunity are undoubtedly involved, but it is difficult to differentiate the lesions induced by the two mechanisms. Vascular changes consist of dense intimal fibrosis, probably the end stage of the proliferative arteritis of the acute and subacute stages. In the kidney these vascular lesions result in renal ischemia, interstitial fibrosis, tubular atrophy, and shrinkage of the parenchyma. Interstitial infiltrates containing large numbers of plasma cells and eosinophils are usually present.

These classifications are somewhat arbitrary, and lesions typical of acute and chronic rejection may exist concomitantly.

Special Types of Rejection

Graft versus Host and Host versus Graft

Bone marrow cells transplanted into an immunocompetent nonidentical recipient are rejected following recognition of MHC-coded alloantigens, as is the case for rejection of other kinds of grafts.[72] Allogeneic bone marrow transplants usually take if the donor and recipient are MHC-identical siblings but not if they are MHC-different siblings. However, this is not always the case. There are instances in which a recipient will reject an LD and SD antigen–identical bone marrow transplant even from a sibling. The implication of this finding is that rejection of a bone marrow graft, i.e., a host-versus-graft (HvG) response, is controlled by a locus or loci different from, but linked to, known LD and SD loci.

Acceptance of antigenically nonidentical bone marrow grafts occurs in severely immunodeficient recipients. Such recipients can be congenitally immunodeficient (see previous subchapter) or clinical patients treated so as to eliminate their immune responsiveness, e.g., with total-body irradiation. Unfortunately, immunodeficient recipients of antigenically different bone marrow grafts are at risk for a condition called *graft-versus-host* (GvH) *disease*, in which T cells of donor origin attack host tissues. There are three categories of GvH disease.[34, 79] One type, called *acute GvH disease*, is caused by infusion of thymus-derived cells along with bone marrow cells. In this instance, the mature T cells that are transferred attack host tissues and usually result in death of the recipient within four weeks after transplantation. The second type, *delayed GvH disease*, develops between 30 and 100 days after transplantation. This delay reflects the time required for hematopoietic stem cell precursors transferred in the graft to mature into immunocompetent T cells. The latter form of GvH disease has a lower degree of associated mortality and may resolve spontaneously. The third type of GvH disease has been observed in human beings and is called *chronic GvH disease*. This type occurs later and persists longer than either acute or delayed GvH disease. The classic targets of GvH disease include skin, lymph nodes, liver, and the gastrointestinal tract, although histological lesions have been observed in other organs and tissues such as the lung, trachea, neuroepithelium, prostate, salivary gland, and pancreatic duct. GvH disease is under the control of the MHC, athough there are data that indicate that the known LD and SD loci of the MHC *(DLA)* of dogs are not involved but are linked to the relevant loci. In addition, minor H loci are involved in GvH disease following transplant between MHC-identical donors and recipients. Evidence has been found indicating that elimination of thymus-derived cells from bone marrow grafts by *in vitro* treatment with antibodies specific for lymphocytes of T cell lineage can help prevent GvH disease.

Diagnosis of Rejection

The specific manifestations of rejection depend primarily on the function of the transplanted organ. ECG abnormalities and congestive heart failure are present when a transplanted heart is being rejected. Similarly, there are diminished urinary output and azotemia in association with failing kidney allografts.[84] These are somewhat late changes; biopsies have shown that rejection is well under way histologically by the time these clinical changes are discovered. Although biopsies are quite useful in diagnosing rejection, their use is limited by trauma to the biopsied organ and the necessity for multiple anesthetic periods.[9, 54] Elevations of organ-specific enzymes or isoenzymes (e.g., LDH) may also help in the diagnosis of rejection.[24]

Another approach to the diagnosis of rejection has been to monitor nonspecific activation of circulating lymphoid cells by measuring the uptake of H³-thymidine by unstimulated peripheral blood lymphocytes *in vitro*. Uptake (predominantly by LD antigen–responsive T cells) increases significantly during active rejection.[19, 51, 65] However, it also increases during systemic infections and hemolytic episodes, so care must be taken when interpreting the results of this test.[30] Antibodies and activated T cells specific for graft antigens may also be measured.[36, 52, 69] A significant correlation has been demonstrated between the presence of circulating antigraft antibodies and rejection.[52]

Treatment of Rejection

When faced not only with the near inevitability of a host immune response to foreign transplantation antigens but the remarkable efficiency of that response in destroying the graft, the clinician must disrupt or at least redirect the host defenses. The immune response can be reduced by radiation or drugs that nonspecifically reduce or destroy the host's ability to respond to immunogens. This is termed *immunosuppression*. Because this method of immunosuppression is nonspecific, the immune response to many antigens is decreased, leading to an increased risk of infection, particularly with intracellular pathogens, and an increased incidence of certain types of neoplasia. A better approach would be to specifically immunosuppress by manipulating the host response to graft antigens. For instance, the immune system of the host may be deceived into producing a response that is protective of the graft. Such protection would be nontoxic and specific for graft antigens and would leave general host protective mechanisms intact. One form of specific immunosuppression is immunological enhancement.

Immunological enhancement involves the use of protective antibodies specific for transplantation antigens. These antibodies may be passively administered or induced by immunization with antigens prior to transplantation. These protective antibodies may work by (1) blockade of lymphocyte sensitization by covering antigenic determinants on the graft, (2) blockade of the effector function of sensitized cells by a similar mechanism, or (3) central suppression of the immune response to the graft, perhaps by activating suppressor T lymphocytes.[12, 47] Attempts to induce enhancing or "blocking" antibodies have not

TABLE 15–11. Immunosuppressive Regimens in the Dog

Agent	Class	Drug Schedule	Toxicity	Tissues Tested	References
Cyclosporin-A	Antifungal	20 mg/kg/day PO	Nephrotoxicity, increased lymphomas, hepatotoxicity	Kidney, bone marrow	27, 38
Cyclophosphamide	Alkylating	1.0 to 2.0 mg/kg/day IV or PO	Leukopenia, sterile hemorrhagic cystitis, retardation of new hair growth	Heart, kidney	20
Azathioprine	Antimetabolite	1.2 to 2.0 mg/kg/day IV or PO	Bone marrow suppression, GI disturbances, retardation of new hair growth	Kidney, heart	8, 20
Prednisone	Hormone	1.0 to 3.0 mg/kg/day PO or IV	Corticosteroid side effects	Kidney, heart, bone marrow	8, 49, 53
Antilymphocyte	Biological	Variable	Sensitization to foreign animal protein, thrombocytopenia, anemia	Kidney, parathyroid gland	17, 39, 60, 82
Methotrexate	Antimetabolite	0.2 mg/kg once a week PO or IV	Bone marrow suppression, GI disturbances	Skin	53
Total lymphoid irradiation		1800 rads divided into 18 fractions	GI disturbances	Heart	41
With bone marrow graft from organ donor			GI disturbances, GvH disease	Kidney	56, 58
Blood transfusions with low-dose immunosuppression	Biological	Variable	None	Kidney	5, 14, 49

been successful in dogs.[62] Immunological tolerance is a state of antigen-specific nonreactivity induced by administration of an antigen. As yet, these two methods are research tools.

Another specific method of immunosuppression is removal of "passenger" leukocytes from grafts by *in vitro* culture techniques or graft pretreatment with cytotoxic drugs or LD-specific antibodies.[12, 62]

Prior to transplanting an organ, as good a donor-recipient histocompatibility antigen match as possible must be achieved. As mentioned, even the most stringent immunosuppression is unable to prevent rejection when major mismatches of the MHC exist in a donor-recipient pair. The rejection phenomenon resulting from minor histocompatibility mismatches is often manageable by either nonspecific immunosuppression or, experimentally, specific immunosuppression. At present, chemotherapeutic immunosuppression, usually involving combinations of drugs, remains the most effective method of reducing immune injury to a graft by the host. The most frequently used methods are summarized in Table 15–11.

SUMMARY

A large body of knowledge has accumulated over the last 15 years relating not only to the *DLA* complex but also the MHC of many species. The key role of the MHC is self-recognition, which allows cooperation among immunocompetent cells, has been elucidated and is the subject of active research. The incredible complexity of the MHC is now appreciated. Clinical manipulations of the host response to transplanted tissues are becoming more sophisticated. At present, human beings are the recipients of most of the benefits from canine transplantation research because of economic constraints on the application of this technology to individual dogs. However, the surgical technology currently exists for transplantation; batteries of *DLA*-specific antisera are available for tissue typing; and newer approaches to specific and nonspecific immunosuppression are being developed. It is quite possible that clinical transplantation may become a reality in institutional veterinary practice in the next decade.

1. Albert, E. D., Erickson, V. M., Graham, T. C., et al.: Serology and genetics of the DLA system. I. Establishment of specificities. Tissue Antigens 3:417, 1973.
2. Bach, F. H., and van Rood, J. J.: The major histocompatibility complex—genetics and biology. N. Engl. J. Med. 295:806, 872, 927, 1976.
3. Bailey, D. W.: Histocompatibility associated with the X-chromosome in mice. Transplantation 1:70, 1963.
4. Bijnen, A. B., Dekkers-Bijma, A. M., Vriesendorp, H. M., et al.: Value of the mixed lymphocyte reaction in dogs as a genetic assay. Immunogenetics 8:287, 1979.
5. Bijnen, A. B., Vriesendorp, H. M., de Gruyl, J., et al.: Host responses to blood transfusions after transplantation of a DLA identical kidney. Transplant. Proc. 7:431, 1975.
6. Bijnen, A. B., Westbroek, D. L., Obertop, H., et al.: Genetics of kidney allograft survival in dogs. I. Relevance of subregions of the major histocompatibility complex in recipients without immunosuppressive therapy. Transplantation 28:186, 1979.
7. Bijnen, A. B., Westbroek, D. L., Obertop, H., et al.: Genetics of kidney allograft survival in dogs. II. Relevance of minor histocompatibility systems in recipients without immunosuppressive therapy. Transplantation 28:191, 1979.
8. Benfield, J. R., Shors, E., and Schick, P.: Monitoring of immunosuppression in beagles. J. Surg. Res. 23:207, 1977.
9. Billingham, M. E., Caves, P. K., Dong, E., et al.: The diagnosis of canine orthotopic cardiac allograft rejection by transvenous endomyocardial biopsy. Transplant. Proc. 5:741, 1973.
10. Blumenstock, D. A., Cannon, F. D., Vlahovic, V. L., et al.: Transplantation of the lung from mongrel dogs into DLA-nonidentical beagles. Transplant. Proc. 13:863, 1981.
11. Bos, E., Meeter, K., and Stibbe, J.: Histocompatibility in orthotopic heart transplantation in dogs. Transplant. Proc. 3:155, 1971.
12. Brent, L., and Hutchinson, I. V.: Specific immunosuppression and graft survival. Transplant. Proc. 13:541, 1981.
13. Britt, L. D., Scharp, D. W., Lacy, P. E., et al.: Transplantation of islet cells across major histocompatibility barriers after total lymphoid irradiation and infusion of allogeneic bone marrow cells. Diabetes 31:63, 1982.
14. Bull, R. W., Vriesendorp, H. M., Obertop, H., et al.: Effect of prior third-party blood transfusions on canine renal allograft survival. Transplantation 26:249, 1978.
15. Burrows, L., Haimiov, M., Aledort, L., et al.: The platelet in the obliterative vascular rejection phenomenon. Transplant. Proc. 5:157, 1973.
16. Butcher, G. W., and Howard, J. C.: Genetic control of transplant rejection. Transplantation 34:161, 1982.
17. Caradis, D. T., Liegeois, A., Barrett, I., et al.: Enhanced survival of canine renal allografts of ALS-treated dogs given bone marrow. Transplant. Proc. 5:671, 1973.
18. Cavalli Storza, L. L., and Bodmer, W. F.: *The Genetics of Human Populations.* W. H. Freeman and Co., San Francisco, 1970.
19. Caves, P. K., Dong, E., Morris, R. E., et al.: The immunologic diagnosis of orthotopic cardiac allograft rejection in dogs. Transplant. Proc. 5:745, 1973.
20. Caves, P. K., Dong, E., and Shumway, N. E.: Immunosuppression with cyclophosphamide in dogs following cardiac transplantation. Transplant. Proc. 5:517, 1973.
21. Chandler, J. G., Villar, H., Lee, S., et al.: The influence of histocompatibility matching according to lymphocyte types on orthotopic liver. Surgery 71:807, 1972.
22. Claas, F. H. J., Paul, L. C., van Es, L. A., et al.: Antibodies against donor antigens on endothelial cells and monocytes in eluates of rejected kidney allografts. Tissue Antigens 15:19, 1980.
23. Cochrum, K. C., Perkins, H. A., and Payne, R. O.: The correlation of MLC with graft survival. Transplant. Proc. 5:391, 1973.
24. Codd, J. E., Garvin, P. J., Morgan, R., et al.: Allograft viability determined by enzyme analysis. Transplantation 28:477, 1979.
25. Dausset, J., and Contu, L.: MHC in general biologic recognition: Its theoretical implications in transplantation. Transplant. Proc. 13:895, 1981.
26. Dausset, J., Rapaport, F. T., Cannon, F. D., et al.: Histocompatibility in a closely bred colony of dogs. J. Exp. Med. 134:1222, 1971.
27. Deeg, H. J., Storb, R., Weiden, P. L., et al.: Cyclosporin-A: Effect on marrow engraftment and graft-versus-host disease in dogs. Transplant. Proc. 13:402, 1981.
28. de Gruyl, J., Westbroek, D. L., Dijkhuis, C. M., et al.: Influence of DL-A matching, ALS and 24 hour preservation on isolated pancreas allograft survival. Transplant. Proc. 3:755, 1973.
29. de Langen, Z. J., de Jong, B., Eysink Smeets, H., et al.: Unmodified lung allograft survival related to the major

histocompatibility complex in the dog. *In* Cochera, J. P. (ed.): *Abstracts of the 10th Congress of the European Society for Experimental Surgery*, 1975, p. 166.

30. Dent, P.: (Letter). *In* Harris, J. E. (ed.): *Proceedings of the Fifth Leukocyte Culture Conference*. Academic Press, New York, 1971, pp. 274–276.

31. Epstein, R. B., and Bennett, B. T.: Histocompatibility testing and the course of canine venereal tumors transplanted into unmodified random dogs. Cancer Res. *34*:788, 1974.

32. Faustman, D., Lacy, P., Davie, J., and Hauptfeld, V.: Prevention of allograft rejection by immunization with donor blood depleted of Ia-bearing cells. Science *217*:157, 1982.

33. Gotze, D.: The major histocompatibility system. *In* Gotze, D. (ed.): *The Major Histocompatibility System in Man and Animals*. Springer-Verlag, New York, 1977.

34. Graze, P. R., Ho, W., and Gale, R. P.: Chronic graft versus host disease in man. Exp. Hematol. *6*(Suppl. 3):44, 1978.

35. Grosse-Wilde, H., Vriesendorp, H. M., Netzel, B., et al.: Immunogenetics of seven LD alleles of the DL-A complex in mongrels, beagles and labradors. Transplant. Proc. *7*(Suppl. 1):159, 1975.

36. Hart, D. N. J., and Fabre, J. W.: Kidney-specific alloantigen system in the rat. J. Exp. Med. *151*:651, 1980.

37. Haskill, J. S., Hayry, P., and Radov, L. A.: Systemic and local immunity in allograft systemic and local immunity in allograft and cancer rejection. Contemp. Top. Immunobiol. *8*:107, 1978.

38. Homan, W. P., French, M. E., Millard, P. R., et al.: A study of eleven drug regimens using cyclosporin-A to suppress renal allograft rejection in the dog. Transplant. Proc. *13*:397, 1981.

39. Jeekel, J., Obertop, H., Vriesendorp, H. M., et al.: Effect of anti-donor serum and donor cells on renal allograft survival in DLA tissue-typed littermate beagles. Transplant. Proc. *7*:435, 1975.

40. Klein, J.: Evolution and function of the major histocompatibility system: Facts and speculations. *In* Gotze, D. (ed.): *The Major Histocompatibility System in Man and Animals*. Springer-Verlag, New York, 1977, pp. 339–378.

41. Koretz, S. H., Gottlieb, M. S., Strober, S., et al.: Organ transplantation in mongrel dogs using total lymphoid irradiation (TLI). Transplant. Proc. *13*:443, 1981.

42. Kumar, V.: Diseases of immunology. *In* Robbins, S., and Cotran, R. S. (eds.): *Pathologic Basis of Disease*. W. B. Saunders, Philadelphia, 1979, pp. 288–292.

43. Kyriakides, G. K., Nuttall, F. Q., and Miller, J.: Segmental pancreatic transplantation in pigs. Surgery *85*:154, 1979.

44. Landsdorp, P. M., Vriesendorp, H. M., Betton, G. R., et al.: Secondary responses of alloantigen-primed dog lymphocytes. Tissue Antigens *15*:40, 1980.

45. Martin, X., Faure, J., Amiel, J., et al.: Systemic versus portal vein drainage of segmental pancreatic transplants in dogs. Transplant. Proc. *12*:138, 1980.

46. Meera Khan, P., Vriesendorp, H., Saisson, R., et al.: Linkage between PGM3 and the genes determining the major histocompatibility complex (MHC) in *Canis familiaris* (the domestic dog). Cytogenet. Cell Genet. *22*:585, 1978.

47. Morris, P. J.: Suppression of rejection of organ allografts by alloantibody. Immunol. Rev. *49*:93, 1980.

48. Najarian, J. S., and Fokker, J. E.: The expression of immunity: The efferent arc. *In* Najarian, J. S., and Simmons, R. L. (eds.): *Transplantation*. Lea & Febiger, Philadelphia, 1972, pp. 94–122.

49. Obertop, H., Bijnin, A. B., Vriesendorp, H. M., et al.: Prolongation of renal allograft survival in DLA tissue-typed beagles after third-party blood transfusions and immunosuppressive treatment. Transplantation *26*:255, 1978.

50. Otte, J. B., Lambotte, L., Westbroek, D. L., et al.: Liver transplantation in DL-A identical beagles. Europ. Surg. Res. *8*(Suppl. 1):63, 1976.

51. Page, D., Posen, G., Stewart, T., et al.: Immunological detection of renal allograft rejection in man. Transplantation *12*:341, 1971.

52. Paul, L. C., van Es, L. A., van Rood, J., et al.: Antibodies directed against antigens on the endothelium of peritubular capillaries in patients with rejecting renal allografts. Transplantation *27*:175, 1979.

53. Pedersen, N. C.: Immunosuppressive drugs and their role in the treatment of immunologic diseases of the dog. Proceedings 28th Gaines Veterinary Symposium, Tuskegee, Alabama, 1978, pp. 13–20.

54. Penn, O. C., McDickin, I., Leicher, F., et al.: Histopathology of rejection in DLA-identical canine orthotopic cardiac allografts. Transplantation *22*:313, 1976.

55. Persijen, G. G., Cohen, B., Lansbergen, M. M., et al.: Effect of HLA-A and HLA-B matching on survival of grafts and recipients after renal transplantation. N. Engl. J. Med. *307*:905, 1982.

56. Raaf, J., Bryan, C., Monden, M., et al.: Bone marrow and renal transplantation in canine recipients prepared by total lymphoid irradiation. Transplant. Proc. *13*:429, 1981.

57. Rapaport, F. T., and Bachvaroff, R. J.: Experimental transplantation and histocompatibility systems in the canine species. Adv. Vet. Sci. Comp. Med. *22*:195, 1978.

58. Rapaport, F. T., Bachvaroff, R. J., Watanabe, K., et al.: Induction of tolerance to third-party donor organs in canine radiation chimeras. Transplant. Proc. *7*:471, 1975.

59. Selden, J. R., and Wachtel, S. S.: H-Y antigen in the dog. Transplantation *24*:298, 1977.

60. Shanfield, I., Wolf, J. S., Wren, S. F. G., et al.: Mechanism of permanent survival of canine renal allografts following a limited course of ALS treatment. Transplant. Proc. *5*:533, 1973.

61. Silvers, W. K., Fleming, H. L., Naji, A., et al.: The influence of removing passenger cells on the fate of skin and parathyroid allografts. Diabetes *31*(Suppl. 4):60, 1982.

62. Soulillou, J. P., Keribin, D., Lecoquie, G., et al.: Attempts to enhance kidney allografts in DLA-identical dogs with specific anti-Ia-like sera. Transplantation *29*:314, 1980.

63. Taylor Bennett, B., Taylor, Y., and Epstein, R.: Segregation of the clinical course of transmissible venereal tumor with DL-A haplotypes in canine families. Transplant. Proc. *7*:503, 1975.

64. Templeton, J. W., and Thomas, E. D.: Evidence for a major histocompatibility locus in the dog. Transplantation *11*:429, 1971.

65. Tennenbaum, J. I., St. Pierre, R. L., Vasko, J. S., et al.: Early detection of allograft rejection: In vitro lymphocyte transformation. *In* Harris, J. E. (ed.): *Proceeding of the Fifth Leukocyte Culture Conference*. Academic Press, New York, 1971, pp. 261–276.

66. Tomford, W. W., Schachar, N. S., Fuller, T. C., et al.: Immunogenicity of frozen osteoarticular allografts. Transplant. Proc. *13*:888, 1981.

67. Van der Feltz, M. J. M., Van der Korput, J. A. G. M., Giphart, M. J., et al.: The major histocompatibility complex of the dog. Isolation and partial characterization of the SD antigens. Transplantation *32*:253, 1981.

68. Van der Tweel, J. G., Vriesendorp, H. M., Termijtelen, A., et al.: Genetic aspects of canine mixed leukocyte cultures. J. Exp. Med. *140*:825, 1974.

69. Vegt, P. A., Burman, W. A., Van der Linden, C. J., et al.: Cell-mediated cytotoxicity toward canine kidney epithelial cells. Transplantation *33*:465, 1982.

70. Vriesendorp, H. M.: Major histocompatibility complex of the dog. Thesis, Erasmus University, Rotterdam, 1973.

71. Vriesendorp, H. M.: Applications of transplantation immunology in the dog. Adv. Vet. Sci. Comp. Med. *23*:229, 1979.

72. Vriesendorp, H. M.: Canine histocompatibility testing. *In* Shifrine, M., and Wilson, F. D. (eds.): *The Canine as a Biomedical Research Model: Immunological, Hematological, and Oncological Aspects*. Technical Information Center/ U.S. Department of Energy, Washington, D.C., 1980, pp. 134–153.

73. Vriesendorp, H. M., Albert, E. D., Templeton, J. W., et al.: Joint report of the second international workshop on canine immunogenetics. Transplant. Proc. *8*:289, 1976.

74. Vriesendorp, H. M., Bijnen, A. B., Zurcher, C., et al.: Donor selection and bone marrow transplantation in dogs. *In*

Kissmeyer-Nielsen, F. (ed.): *Histocompatibility Testing 1975.* Munksgaard, Copenhagen, 1975, p. 963.

75. Vriesendorp, H. M., D'Amaro, J., Van der Does, J. A., et al.: Analysis of the DL-A system in families and populations of healthy and diseased individuals. Transplant. Proc. 5:311, 1973.

76. Vriesendorf, H. M., Grosse-wilde, H., and Dorf, M. E.: The major histocompatibility system of the dog. *In* Gotze, D. (ed.): *The Major Histocompatibility System in Man and Animals.* Springer-Verlag, New York, 1977.

77. Vriesendorp, H. M., Rothengalter, C., Bos, E., et al.: The production and evaluation of dog allolymphotoxins for donor selection in transplantation experiments. Transplantation *11*:440, 1971.

78. Vriesendorp, H. M., Smid-Mercx, B. M. J., Visser, T. P., et al.: Serological DL-A typing of normal and atopic dogs. Transplant. Proc. 7:375, 1975.

79. Vriesendorp, H. M., and van Bekkum, D. W.: Bone-marrow transplantation in the canine. *In* Shifrine, M., and Wilson, F. D. (eds.): *The Canine as a Biomedical Research Model: Immunological, Hematological, and Oncological Aspects.* Technical Information Center/U.S. Department of Energy, Washington, D.C., 1980, pp. 153–202.

80. Vriesendorp, H. M., Westbroek, D. L., D'Amaro, J. D., et al.: Joint report of 1st international workshop on canine immunogenetics. Tissue Antigens 3:145, 1973.

81. Vriesendorp, H. M., Zurcher, C., Bull, R. W., et al.: Take and graft vs. host reactions of allogeneic bone marrow in tissue typed dogs. Transplant. Proc. 7(Suppl. 1): 849, 1975.

82. Wells, S. A., Burdick, J. F., Christiansen, C., et al.: Long-term survival of dogs transplanted with parathyroid glands as autografts and as allografts in immunosuppressed hosts. Transplant. Proc. 5:769, 1973.

83. Westbroek, D. L., Rothengatter, C., Vriesendorp, H. M., et al.: Histocompatibility and heterotopic segmental small bowel allograft survival in dogs. Europ. Surg. Res. 2:401, 1970.

84. Westbroek, D. L., Silberbusch, J., Vriesendorp, H. M., et al.: The influence of DLA histocompatibility on the function and pathohistological changes in unmodified canine renal allografts. Transplantation *14*:582, 1972.

85. Westbroek, D. L., Vriesendorp, H. M., Van den Tweel, J. G., et al.: Influence of SD and LD matching of kidney allograft survival in unrelated mongrel dogs. Transplant. Proc. 7:427, 1975.

86. Wolman, M., Bleiberg, I., and Leibovici, J.: Histological criteria for immunological rejection of mouse skin homografts. J. Pathol. *122*:1, 1977.

87. Zwiebaum, A., Oriol, R., Feingold, N., et al.: Studies on canine secretory alloantigens (CSA). Tissue Antigens 4:115, 1974.

Chapter **16**

Epidemiology and Mechanisms of Trauma in Companion Animals

Stephen W. Crane

DEFINITION OF TRAUMA

Trauma is defined as any force or exposure from the environment that causes undesirable changes, injury, or death in the affected animal. This encompassing definition includes exposure to indirect environmental factors that predispose to future disease, stress syndromes, or disability. Among these are exposure to acute or chronic psychological injury, carcinogens, and chemical or physical agents with cumulative deleterious effects. Trauma in companion animals is an extremely important facet of the typical veterinary practice. The purpose of this chapter is to describe certain epidemiological features of pet animal trauma and their general mechanisms of injury. Comments regarding specific organ system injuries and their treatment are found in appropriate sections elsewhere in this text.

PREVALENCE AND INCIDENCE OF TRAUMA

The epidemic of human trauma in the United States produces 75 million injuries each year of sufficient magnitude to require medical care or hospitalization. Trauma is the leading cause of death until the fourth decade of life and the fourth leading cause of death overall. Although the morbidity and mortality from many diseases are decreasing, traumatic diseases and their aftereffects are increasing.[2]

The major studies by Kolata and associates of trauma in dogs and cats have been valuable in establishing period prevalence rates and risk factors based on the emergency service records of two teaching hospitals.[13-16] The following descriptions refer to this information (Tables 16–1 through 16–6) as well as to my notes and case studies. These surveys have also been valuable in contrasting the location of injury for a variety of etiological agents and in differentiating risk factors between urban and rural environments.

Kolata's group noted that hospital admissions for trauma-related problems were about 12 per cent of the total admissions, with dogs being presented more frequently than cats.[16] The case fatality rate for trauma patients seen at these established emergency services was approximately 9 per cent, including the option of owner-elected euthanasia. Thirty-five per cent of the patients manifested severe injury (see

Text continued on page 215

TABLE 16–1. Causes of Trauma in Dogs Examined at the University of Pennsylvania Veterinary Hospital (UPVH) and the University of Georgia Small Animal Teaching Hospital (UGSATH)*

	UPVH (970 Dogs)		UGSATH (129 Dogs)	
	Number	*Per Cent*	*Number*	*Per Cent*
Motor vehicle accident	516	53.2	69	53.5
Unknown cause	118	12.2	22	17.0
Animal interaction	108	11.1	18	13.9
Sharp object	109	11.2	7	5.3
Fall from height	61	6.3	5	3.8
Crush	25	2.6	1	0.8
Weapon	21	2.2	7	5.3
Burn	12	1.4	0	0

*Reprinted with permission from Kolata, R. J.: Trauma in dogs and cats: An overview. Vet. Clin. North Am. *10*:515, 1980.

TABLE 16–2. Causes of Trauma in Cats Examined at the University of Pennsylvania Veterinary Hospital (UPVH) and the University of Georgia Small Animal Teaching Hospital (UGSATH)*

	UPVH (156 Cats)		UGSATH (35 Cats)	
	Number	*Per Cent*	*Number*	*Per Cent*
Unknown cause	57	36.5	9	25.7
Motor vehicle accident	28	17.9	10	28.6
Animal interaction	25	16.0	8	22.8
Fall from height	21	13.5	1	2.8
Crush	17	10.9	1	2.8
Sharp object	5	3.2	4	11.4
Burn	3	1.9	0	0
Weapon	0	0	2	5.7

*Reprinted with permission from Kolata, R. J.: Trauma in dogs and cats: An overview. Vet. Clin. North Am. *10*:515, 1980.

TABLE 16–3. Body Regions Injured by Specific Cause in 970 Dogs at University of Pennsylvania Veterinary Hospital (A) and 129 Dogs at University of Georgia Small Animal Teaching Hospital (B)*

	Motor Vehicle		Unknown		Animal Interaction		Sharp Object		Fall from Height		Crush		Weapon		Burn	
	A	B	A	B	A	B	A	B	A	B	A	B	A	B	A	B
Head	128	15	24	3	41	4	15	2	7	0	2	1	7	1	8	0
Neck	8	0	6	2	27	6	0	1	0	0	1	0	1	0	1	0
Thorax	84	13	5	3	15	7	2	1	5	0	2	0	5	2	1	0
Abdomen	73	10	6	3	12	4	2	0	2	0	1	0	6	0	6	0
Pelvis	105	20	7	2	3	2	1	0	6	0	1	0	2	2	4	0
Extremity	335	32	74	14	36	8	91	3	7	5	25	0	5	4	3	0
TOTAL	733	90	122	27	134	31	111	7	27	5	32	1	26	9	23	0

*Reprinted with permission from Kolata, R. J.: Trauma in dogs and cats: An overview. Vet. Clin. North Am. *10*:515, 1980.

TABLE 16–4. Body Regions Injured by Specific Cause in 156 Cats at University of Pennsylvania Veterinary Hospital (A) and 35 Cats at University of Georgia Small Animal Teaching Hospital (B)*

	Unknown		Motor Vehicle		Animal Interaction		Fall from Height		Crush		Sharp Object		Burn		Weapon	
	A	B	A	B	A	B	A	B	A	B	A	B	A	B	A	B
Head	19	3	12	6	8	2	5	0	5	0	3	2	0	0	0	0
Neck	2	1	1	0	2	1	0	0	1	0	0	1	1	0	0	1
Thorax	6	1	3	4	1	2	5	0	0	0	0	1	2	0	0	2
Abdomen	4	1	2	2	5	3	3	0	0	0	0	1	0	0	0	1
Pelvis	8	2	11	4	2	3	1	1	2	0	0	1	0	0	0	0
Extremity	25	2	7	3	13	6	9	0	8	0	3	2	1	0	0	0
Total	64	10	36	19	31	17	23	1	16	0	6	8	4	0	0	4

*Reprinted with permission from Kolata, R. J.: Trauma in dogs and cats: An overview. Vet. Clin. North Am. *10*:515, 1980.

TABLE 16–5. Index for Rating the Severity of Injury*

0	No definable injury	No physically or radiographically definable injury.
1	Minor	Small lacerations or abrasions, undisplaced pelvic fractures (animal can walk). Simple metacarpal or metacarpal metatarsal fractures.
2	Moderate	Large or deep lacerations; skull or spinal fractures without neurologic signs. Luxation; ligament ruptures. Simple fractures of long bones, rib, or pelvis.
3	Severe (not life-threatening)	Multiple deep extensive lacerations; skull or spinal fractures with minimal neurologic deficit. Pneumothorax, hemothorax, or large contusion with minimal respiratory embarrassment. Multiple fractures of pelvic or long bones.
4	Severe (life-threatening)	Multiple extensive lacerations with shock. Skull and spinal fractures with neurologic deficits. Thoracic trauma with respiratory embarrassment; abdominal trauma with signs of shock. Major disruption of pelvis and open multiple fractures of long bones with signs of shock.

*Reprinted with permission from Kolata, R. J.: Trauma in dogs and cats: An overview. Vet. Clin. North Am. *10*:515, 1980.

TABLE 16–6. Severity of Injuries (Per Cent) in Dogs and Cats Examined at the University of Pennsylvania Veterinary Hospital (UPVH) and the University of Georgia Small Animal Teaching Hospital (UGSATH)*

	UPVH		UGSATH	
	Dogs	*Cats*	*Dogs*	*Cats*
Minor to moderate	64.4	58.3	66.4	40.0
Severe to greater	35.6	41.7	33.6	60.0

*Reprinted with permission from Kolata, R. J.: Trauma in dogs and cats: An overview. Vet. Clin. North Am. *10*:515, 1980.

Table 16–6). Automobile-induced trauma accounted for a majority of deaths, but burns and firearm injuries were the most likely injuries to place the animal in a severely injured group or to express fatality on a percentage basis.[13, 18] Examination of these data clearly defines accidental injury and death as a major veterinary health problem.

From the practicing veterinarian's standpoint, lacerations and fight wounds often assume significance in the overall pattern of patient presentations. Management of major injury and resuscitation from extensive trauma are routinely accomplished in many hospitals and emergency facilities. Additionally, the development and proliferation of the specialized emergency facility in many areas has increased public awareness of and expectations for effective primary care of the animal accident victim. From the perspective of the emergency service practitioner there are few professional satisfactions greater than the successful resuscitation, initial care, and stabilization of the injured animal.

RANGE OF TRAUMATIC AGENTS

Direct trauma often causes injuries requiring surgical care. Such agents include physical impact, penetration and impalement, crushing, laceration, and burns. Kolata and coworkers catégorized nine major etiologies for trauma, including motor vehicle accidents, animal fights, injury from sharp objects, falls, crushing injuries, burns, injuries from firearms, animal abuse by humans, and unknown causes.[16]

Less frequent forms of direct physical injury in clinical practice include electrical burns, electrocution, friction with soft tissue and orthopedic avulsions, barotrauma due to explosions, drowning, frostbite, systemic hypothermia, systemic hyperthermia with or without "heatstroke," and ingestion of linear and nonlinear gastrointestinal foreign bodies.

Other important direct traumatic agents are agricultural, industrial, household, and garden chemicals with which the animal may accidentally come in contact (Fig. 16–1). Among the toxic preparations commonly available to pet or working companion

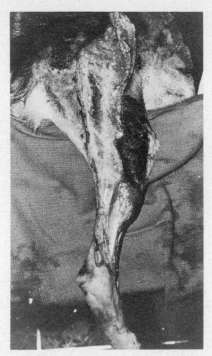

Figure 16–1. A chemical burn wound following a hydrochloric acid spill. Note the superficial necrosis into muscle bellies. Following debridement, porcine dermal xenografts were applied every other day for 12 days, and then delayed primary closure was performed with an excellent functional and cosmetic result.

animals are field and orchard sprays and powders for insect control, warfarin-based rodenticides, glycol-based antifreeze, methaldehyde snail baits, and lead. Accidental or mistaken drug overdosage, particularly with externally applied insecticides or aspirin and aspirin substitutes, is also encountered. Malicious poisoning of pet animals is occasionally seen, and most veterinarians have had some experience in the diagnosis and treatment of this form of trauma.

In addition to injury from fire, inhalation of toxic smoke and gases such as carbon monoxide, cyanide, and oxides of nitrogen and sulfur must be considered in those patients escaping from house fires.[19] In fact, pulmonary injury may be the predominant or exclusive feature of many patients trapped in burning buildings. Accidental contact with hot floor furnace

Figure 16–2. The groin of a dog that had been intentionally irrigated with kerosene and ignited. Full thickness burns covered over 70 per cent of the body surface, and a cellulitis was present under the desiccated burn eschars. Cultures of the burn fluid exudate revealed high numbers of gram-positive cocci.

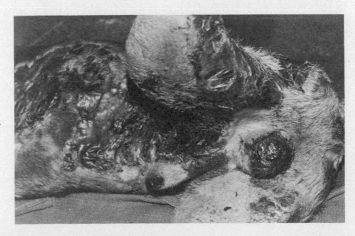

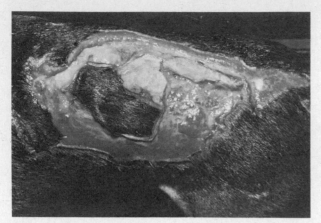

Figure 16–3. Full thickness burns in a patient allowed to recover from anesthesia on a household electrical heating pad.

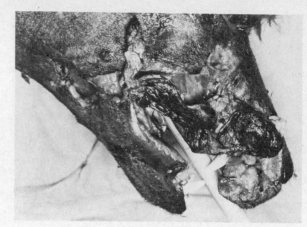

Figure 16–5. Full-thickness skin and subcutaneous facial necrosis in a Kerry blue terrier nine days following envenomation by an Eastern diamondback rattlesnake. Although many pit viper bites are innocuous, the bite of this snake is often fatal or produces exceptional morbidity.

registers can burn feet. Scalding from fluids such as spilled hot water or beverages or cooking oil spilled from stovetops and contact with steam constitute other forms of thermal injury. Malicious ignition of an animal is one pattern of abuse that is particularly tragic (Fig. 16–2). Unfortunately, thermal burns in anesthetized or immobile animals placed on electrical heating pads or "warmed" by heat lamps is also encountered (Figs. 16–3 and 16–4).

Exposure to cold is usually well tolerated in breeds of dogs and cats adapted to the outdoors and acclimatized to inclement conditions. However, systemic hypothermia and frostbite can occur in either the acclimatized or nonadapted animal that becomes immobilized or exposed in a cold environment.

Bites from venomous insects, arachnids, and reptiles may be occasionally encountered. Bees, wasps and hornets, scorpions, brown recluse and black widow spiders, and venomous snakes are all potentially dangerous, especially in the smaller animal in which high venom concentrations are easily reached. In my experience, the brown recluse spider (extensive local necrosis) and the Eastern diamondback

rattlesnake (neurolytic, hemolytic, and local necrosis) possess the most dangerous venoms (Fig. 16–5).

Iatrogenic trauma from internal diagnostic or therapeutic instrumentation or misapplied or mismanaged external orthopedic coaptation devices is another possible source of injury.

RISK FACTORS IN COMPANION ANIMAL TRAUMA

Supervision of the Animal by Humans

A consistent and major risk factor relates to the available level of responsible human supervision of the pet. In both urban and suburban emergency patient populations, 70 to 80 per cent of animals presented had suffered injuries caused by motor vehicle accidents, animal fights, or unknown factors.[16] This suggests that injury frequently occurs when the level of human supervision is low. Since reliable voice command control for dog obedience is infrequently seen, these injuries are much less likely to occur if the animal is confined to the home, yard, or leash. Adherence to municipal or self-imposed leash laws is excellent insurance against the animal's being hit by a car or becoming involved in an animal fight. Direct leash control also establishes the image of the "good neighbor." Such pets are less likely to be retaliated against with traps, poisons, beatings, or a firearm than one who roams at will, pillages in garbage, eliminates indiscriminately in the neighborhood, or disturbs others with barking.

Cats that are kept indoors, either primarily or exclusively, experience fewer environmental hazards than free-roaming outdoor animals.

Age

The median age for trauma presentation was 1.9 years among dogs and 1.3 years among cats in the

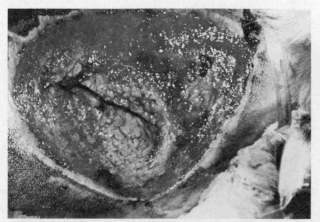

Figure 16–4. Full-thickness burn over the shoulder in an animal that had been placed under a heat lamp to combat postoperative hypothermia. Tissues are infected and wound healing is arrested.

study of urban trauma.[16] The median age at death was 3.7 years for another group of 28 canine trauma victims.[3] However, animals hit by cars were younger than those in a standardized hospital population.[15] Empirically, it is suspected that the frequency of trauma is somewhat higher in younger animals. Whether it be chewing on electrical cords, inexperience at the roadside, or exploring perceived openings in the "pecking order," puppies and kittens seem to make more misjudgments than older animals. The death rate from injury is probably higher in puppies and kittens and in geriatric patients, although substantial data have not been gathered in veterinary medicine. A higher case fatality rate in these age groups would presumably be due to the propensity for medical complications or the tendency of owners to elect euthanasia in older injured animals.

Sex

In the United States, the risk for fatal injury in human males is 2.5 times the rate for females. Additionally, males have 50 per cent more nonfatal injuries and a greater proportion of very severe injuries.[2] Gender as a risk factor in veterinary trauma seems important. Common observations in veterinary practice implicate males as more subject to trauma because they are more likely to roam, defend territory, and fight for females. In a general hospital population consisting of 55 per cent male dogs and 60 per cent male cats, 65 per cent of the male dogs and 69 per cent of the male cats were presented for trauma evaluation.[14] Thus, there were significantly more males seen in general, and significantly more males were evaluated for animal fight injuries. Female animals are more likely to be sexually neutered and remain in a more predictable and homeostatic environment. Falls, crush injuries, and burns occurred more frequently in the female.[16]

Species

Species-specific habit patterns, as well as age and sex, modulate the risk of injury. Of those animals presented for treatment, dogs were about 2.5 times more likely than cats to have been hit by a vehicle.[16] The risk for falls from high places is higher in cats than in dogs and probably reflects the tendency of cats to sit on open window sills, navigate over rooftops, and climb trees.

The frequency of animal fights was higher for dogs than for cats, at least in the group of animals presented for care. This finding may be open to question because of the large number of variables in detecting fights and fight wounds. The propensity of the cat to form visible subcutaneous abscesses following wounds inflicted by teeth or claws is a clinical feature that probably brings many cats to professional attention. Cats were about twice as likely as dogs to be

presented with trauma of unknown causes, which may reflect the nocturnal roaming habits of many unconfined cats.[16]

Position of the Pet in the Family Social Hierarchy

Veterinarians have long been aware of the tremendous spectrum of expression of the human–companion animal bond. Observations of extremes in the manner in which people relate to their pets is a continual source of fascination to most clinicians. It is accepted among experienced veterinarians that they may be psychologically "treating" the owner of the pet as well as the pet itself. The descriptions of his analysis and management of the bonding proclivities between the owner and the animal, as much as the veterinary ailments of his patients, create the compelling and entertaining substance of many of the James Herriot stories.

The qualitative aspect of this bond may be a risk factor in trauma. For example, some pets fill child surrogate roles and are consciously protected from exposure to injury. Other animals are, of course, not in such a protected position.

Since animals and humans may interact and relate in negative as well as positive ways, it is of concern when an animal becomes a patient through intentional trauma by humans. Although animal abuse and cruelty is a well-known clinical entity, there is scant social or clinical literature regarding its general nature or epidemiology. Abused animals, like abused children, may or may not be presented for professional evaluation. If the animal is presented for attention, the owner may or may not give a misleading history. In the survey of urban trauma, 12 out of 1000 patients presented with a voluntary owner history of willful abuse.[16] In my opinion, there is considerable underreporting of the abused animal syndrome. Substantiation for this position is extrapolated from recent experience regarding battered children.[11] In 1967 there were 7000 cases of battered children reported, escalating to over 200,000 cases in 1974 after education efforts were directed toward physicians and the public.

Some work has suggested that children who torture animals may be at significant risk for later life aggression and that the triad of bedwetting, firesetting, and animal torture may be linked signs or symptoms of an aggression dyscontrol syndrome.[8] In a recent study, two groups of psychiatric patients, one with a childhood history of general assault and one with a history of childhood animal cruelty, were compared for common and differentiating etiological features underlying their behavioral disorders. Those in the animal cruelty group, which was exclusively male, were about three times more likely to abuse cats than dogs. Methods of torture and resultant injury to the animals testified to incredible sadistic creativity, and multiple episodes of animal torture per patient were usually reported.[8] Both groups had a high incidence of general aggressive behavior in childhood. Such behavior probably results from generalized parental abuse or brutality. However, those in the assaultive group were specifically more likely to have suffered unjustified maternal punishment or brutality, whereas patients in the animal cruelty group were more likely to have had an alcoholic father figure, prolonged or permanent absence of the father, or other forms of paternal deprivation.[8]

Child and animal abuse by adults may be parallel elements in aggression dyscontrol behaviors. Females as well as males may be involved. The battered child, and presumably the abused animal as well, is in an especially dangerous situation because of the high repeatability of battering and abuse. As pointed out in the literature of human trauma, a battered child who is returned to its parents without professional counseling has a 5 per cent chance of being killed and a 35 per cent chance of suffering serious re-injury.[11] Morse has noted that injury from the battered child syndrome is more common than appendicitis and the mortality is many times higher.[18]

The veterinarian may occasionally be in a position to suspect possible sociopathic tendencies within the client family. The index of suspicion for animal abuse should be especially high if the animal seems "accident prone" for such major injuries as fractures, head and ocular injuries, extensive blunt contusions, or abdominal ecchymoses. A high "turnover" of young animals in the client household is another possible danger signal. The possibility of concomitant animal and child abuse calls for judgment and professionalism when it becomes apparent that the veterinarian may be in a primary position to identify battering and thus help protect the physical or psychological health of innocent parties. Questioning a regional or local human services agency or using a child abuse hotline service should provide enough information with which to make further decisions regarding a specific course of action.

Whereas the consumption of alcohol is a major and widely appreciated risk factor in human trauma (driving, fighting, or falling while under the influence), it is a minor factor in animal trauma. In my experience, the misjudgment and violence sometimes associated with overindulgence in alcoholic beverages does extend to abuse of animals within the household. However, it is nearly impossible to guess the threat potential posed by this risk factor prior to an actual injury and a determination of contributory events.

PATHOPHYSIOLOGY OF TRAUMA

General Considerations of Impact Trauma

The physical principles regarding force vectors and acceleration of mass pertain to the patient's body at the time of impact. Since kinetic energy equals the product of one-half the mass times the square of the velocity, it is clear that faster rather than heavier objects possess more potential for trauma. Upon impact at the body surface, "loading" of kinetic energy into the animal's body produces stress and strain within organs and tissues.

Stress is the internal force that develops within a certain plane in an object in response to an externally applied load. Stress resists forces tending to deform the object and is measured in force per unit area. Strain is defined as deformation or change in geometric configuration of the object from the resting shape in response to an externally applied load.[10]

For example, high-speed cinephotography combined with simultaneous strain gauge measurements in a long bone model reveal that initial loading of force does not cause deformation; rather, stress accumulates within the bone to prevent collapse of the structure. The stress is measured by force per unit area such as kilograms per square centimeter. As loading continues, the transferred energy is stored as potential energy, while compressional and torsional stresses accumulate further. With more loading, the elastic limit of the bone is reached (the yield point), and bending and torsional deformation begin to occur. Strain can then be measured as the new length or shape divided by the original length or shape. In objects with high elasticity, the object tends to return to its original shape; objects exhibiting high plasticity tend to stay deformed. In wet-bone preparations, it is surprising how much elasticity and plasticity are present before fracture occurs. When the compression, torsion, shear, or tension strain limits are finally exceeded, mechanical failure occurs. The principles relating load, stress-strain, elasticity and elastic limit, tensile and bursting strength, and mechanical failure apply to all biological tissues as well as to inert materials.[10]

Soft Tissue Injury

The type and amount of trauma suffered following direct impact are highly individualized and depend on several factors in addition to the total quantity of kinetic energy delivered. The angle of collision as well as the force can be represented by a force vectorgram of the actual physical impact. The elastic limits and the tensile and bursting strength of the specific tissues involved are important variables. For example, skin has high tensile strength, whereas that of liver or kidney is much lower. Another important factor modifying injury is the mass of the animal, because mass at rest represents inertia or the tendency to resist acceleration. Accordingly, larger animals resist displacement by a given force and have a larger volume into which impact forces may be dissipated. The surface area over which the force is distributed is a factor in predicting trauma production. Energy density per unit area and per unit time has obvious clinical implications; penetration may occur with a smaller sharp object that makes quick

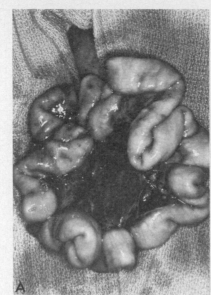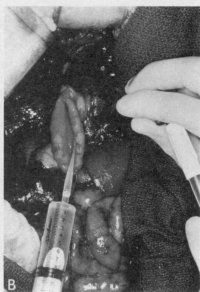

Figure 16–6. A, Appearance and surgical exploration of the biliary system for bile peritonitis in a dog that had been hit by a car two weeks previously. *B,* Surgical diagnosis was avulsion of the right hepatic duct from the common bile duct with extensive bile peritonitis and adhesions. (Reprinted with permission from Crane, S. W.: Evaluation and management of abdominal trauma in the dog and cat. Vet. Clin. North Am. *10*:655, 1980.)

contact but not with a blunt, flat, or slower-moving object.[14]

The quantity of tissue damage is further determined by the duration of the impact. In the transfer of the same total energy, the energy density per unit time is higher in a quicker impact. Therefore, trauma levels may be greater in the longer impact. During the initial phase of collision, compression waves travel outward from the impact point. The radial dispersion of compression waves functionally increases the surface area over which energy is able to dissipate, and the energy accumulations per unit of tissue volume are thereby reduced.[10, 14] The compression waves forming at initial impact result from the incompressibility of tissue water. As the transfer of kinetic energy into the impact zone extends into an event of longer duration, the compression waves are converted into shear waves, which generate tissue strain and distortion. Recoil and rebounding events from the travel of the shear waves add further trauma to that caused by the impact itself. The shear waves often produce cavitation and sonication effects, with extensive tissue destruction, at considerable distances from the impact point. This observation is especially apparent in the tissues surrounding a missile path when ultra-high-energy bullets penetrate the body.

The disruption of loose connective tissue, bursting of organ capsules, parenchymal shattering, vascular avulsion, and other damage to soft tissue are due to shear and compressional strain, shear wave formation, and recoil effects that exceed the tissue's tensile strength and elasticity limits.[10] Clinically, such tissue strain is frequently caused by sudden acceleration or deceleration. Shear strain development is due to the differences between density and inertia of structures and organs attached to one another. Density and inertia are due to the blood, water, and air content of the organ as well as its mass. The degree of support and anchoring by ligaments and mesenteries also influences the vector of interorgan displacement that

may occur. Anatomical examples include tearing and avulsions between the air-filled bronchus and the air- and blood-filled lung, the bile ducts and the liver lobes, the urinary bladder and the urethral neck, the fluid-filled intestine and its filmy supporting mesentery, and the heart and great vessels (Fig. 16–6).

Transient and direct compressive forces can cause organ contusion, organ capsule bursting, or organ shattering. Such injury can also be caused by organ acceleration and rebound from fixed skeletal elements such as ribs and the spinal column. Examples include liver injury from the rib cage during injury to the cranial abdomen (Fig. 16–7). Blunt cardiac contusions and rupture of the urinary bladder may also occur. I have observed vascular avulsion within the small intestinal mesentery or the splenic and renal pedicles on several occasions. Gastrointestinal tract rupture is infrequent.

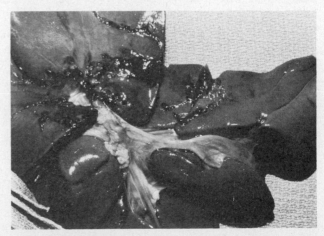

Figure 16–7. Abdominal aspect of traumatized liver. Note the "road map" mosaic of superficial capsule and parenchymal breakage as well as deep laceration into the hilus of the right lateral lobe. Injury resulted from a fall of 10 meters. (Reprinted with permission from Crane, S. W.: Evaluation and management of abdominal trauma in the dog and cat. Vet. Clin. North Am. *10*:655, 1980.)

Another important aspect of impact injury is the transient compression of air to high pressure within the conducting airways following impact. If the injury is anticipated by the animal and the glottis is reflexly closed to "brace" for collision, the kinetic energy of impact may be transferred through the body wall and diaphragm to mechanically compress the air in the closed spaces of the tracheobronchial tree. Such transient yet high-airway pressures may rupture the conducting airways or pulmonary parenchyma.[12] This is one proposed mechanism for the development of pneumothorax or tension pneumothorax, which is commonly associated with significant blunt trauma as well as penetrating wounds of the thorax.

If impact has not been anticipated by the animal there will be no opportunity for it to reflexly "brace" for impact by closing the glottis and applying abdominal pressure. The latter maneuver equalizes pressures between the abdomen and the thorax and results in a more limited excursion of the diaphragm and the abdominal wall. This may prevent the liver from moving cranially toward the thorax and tearing the diaphragm.[12]

Orthopedic Injury

In contrast to the dried preparation of the museum skeleton, living lamellar bone is a dynamic, diphasic material with distinct organic and inorganic components. The soft tissue—blood vessels, collagen fibers, and cells—is surrounded by mineral matrix. The trabecular support as well as vascular and mineral structure of the cortices gives maximal strength with minimal weight and volume of tissue. This exceptional volumetric efficiency is further enhanced because bone can be produced, thickened, remodeled, and removed along internal lines of stress according to need. Thus, static and dynamic loading patterns strongly influence the configuration of elastic fiber and mineral deposition. Because of its structure, bone has great tensile strength and surprising elasticity with considerable capacity to store potential energy prior to fracturing.

When a bone is abnormally loaded at the time of impact, compression, shearing, and torsional forces may be very high, and the bone passes through phases of elastic and plastic deformation. When mechanical strength limits are surpassed, the anatomical point at which stress forces and strain deformation meet may influence the region of the bone in which fracture first occurs. Since considerable potential energy can be stored within living bone before the deformation and mechanical failure points are reached, the reconversion of potential energy back into kinetic energy at the time of fracture can be of considerable magnitude. Such a "high-energy" fracture is typically multiple or comminuted with extensive secondary damage to muscle, nerves, lymphatics, and blood vessels.

Ligaments and tendons are longitudinally orga-nized bundles of collagen that assume the function of cables and straps in an inanimate mechanical system. Because of their fiber orientation they have a different modulus of strain and a much greater tensile strength in tension than in shear or torsion.[10] Therefore, the effect of lateral shear forces can be especially disruptive, particularly to a short collateral ligament. Both cruciate ligaments of the stifle might be considered anatomically and functionally "compound," since they possess distinct intraligamentous bands that stabilize the stifle during different phases of joint motion.[1] Additionally, there is complementary and functional interdependence between the cranial and caudal cruciate ligaments as they twist and untwist relative to one another as the stifle flexes and extends. The greatest potential for cranial cruciate ligament failure occurs with sudden internal rotation of the tibia on the femur with the stifle in 20 to 50° of flexion.[1] Cranial cruciate ligament rupture is readily produced from external trauma and can even occur from routine spontaneous activity in some patients. Unlike the stifle, other joints usually undergo ligamentous disruption or luxation only with considerable external violence.

EFFECTS OF SPECIFIC INJURIES

Burns and motor vehicle accidents are the most serious injuries in dogs, resulting in mortality rates of 36 and 12 per cent, respectively.[14] Crushing injuries and motor vehicle accidents cause the highest mortality among cats, at 30 and 24 per cent, respectively.[14] The effects and seriousness of other categories of injury are less predictable and depend on individual circumstances.

Falls

Owing to the relationship between mass and acceleration, larger animals absorb considerably more kinetic energy than smaller animals from falls of equal distance. Since the kinetic energies can be extremely high, death or multiple trauma is not unusual in animals falling from heights. Forelimb long bone fractures are common because many animals, especially cats, land on the head or forequarters. Fractures of the axial skeleton, including facial bones, skull, mandible, and teeth, and longitudinal splitting of the hard palate are often seen (Fig. 16–8). Broken or cracked ribs and compression fractures or fracture-luxations of the vertebrae and pelvic fractures occur as well.

Soft tissue injuries resulting from falls include lacerations, abrasions, avulsions, impalements, brain damage, ocular proptosis or internal injury to the globe, pneumothorax, diaphragmatic rupture, tearing of the muscular body wall, and visceral organ disruption. Each patient must be carefully and frequently monitored for delayed or occult vital organ or other soft tissue injury following resuscitation.

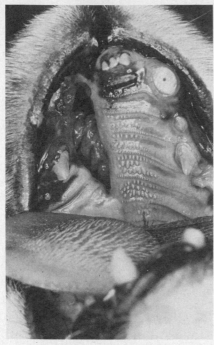

Figure 16–8. Extensive facial, palatine, and dental injuries resulting from a fall from a windowsill onto a sidewalk. Note the chronic rhinitis resulting from a long-standing oronasal fistula. A mucoperiosteal flap resulted in satisfactory closure.

Burns

Specific systemic changes and effects of burns, as documented in human patients, are summarized in Table 16–7. For further information regarding burn injuries, see Chapter 40.

Friction Injury

Friction injury results from sliding contact with highways and is a commonly encountered injury in companion animals (Fig. 16–9). Following acceleration along the pavement, avulsions of soft tissue often

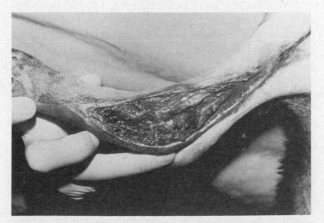

Figure 16–9. Avulsion of tissue secondary to friction injuries commonly associated with being dragged along the road after being hit by a car.

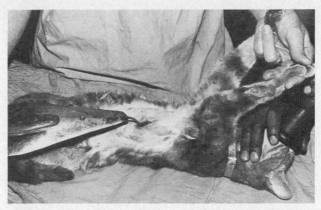

Figure 16–10. Penetrating wounds are usually low-energy wounds with tissue or organ damage, depending on the individual circumstances. Exploration is indicated for most deep wounds.

extend into the bones of the extremities. Such wounds are frequently challenging to treat owing to initial contamination and the necessity of reconstructing ligaments to maintain both range of motion and stability in the joint.[7]

Penetrating Wounds

Penetrating wounds are almost always low-energy penetrations unless the animal has fallen from some height onto a projection. However, a tremendous variety of objects can potentially enter the body to cause bizarre injuries (Fig. 16–10). Acute mortality from impalement usually relates to penetration of vital structures. Morbidity from impalement is influenced by concomitant injuries including the degree of contamination and the location and nature of established infections and occult foreign bodies. Infections of soft tissues and body cavities by wooden sticks or splinters can be difficult to diagnose and are usually impossible to treat without direct surgical removal of the entire foreign body. Migrating plant awns, such as the California foxtail, pose similar hazards.

Gunshot Wounds

As would be expected, rural animals are more likely to sustain injuries from firearms than urban animals. Although this has not been confirmed in specific studies, hunting dogs would presumably be at high risk for such injuries, especially superficial wounds from birdshot. Although the cause of some bullet wounds is obvious, the cause of others can be elusive. Therefore, all gunshot wounds should be considered serious until proved otherwise because of the tremendous kinetic energies and penetration effects potentially present. While taking the patient's history, performing a physical examination, and establishing resuscitation, certain general features regarding firearm injury should be kept in mind.

TABLE 16–7.   Changes in Selected Physiological and Metabolic Parameters Associated with Burns*

Parameter	Changes Following Burning
Free fatty acids	Elevated proportional to burn size for short time.
Triglycerides	Elevated proportional to burn size for short time.
Cholesterol	Depressed proportional to burn size.
Phospholipids	Depressed proportional to burn size.
Fibrinogen	Initial fall with prolonged rise following. Consumption great but production greater.
Renin	Increase proportional to burn size, especially children.
Angiotensin	Increase proportional to burn size, especially children.
ACTH	Increase proportional to burn size, especially children.
Protein	Rapid and persistent drop.
Albumin	Prompt and persistent drop persisting until wound closed. Production depressed and catabolism two to three times normal.
Globulin	Initial drop with rise to supranormal levels by five to seven days. Catabolism two to three times normal but production vastly increased.
IgG	Immediate depression followed by slow rise.
IgM	Altered little by burn in adults but in children follows pattern of IgG.
IgA	Altered little by burn in adults but in children follows pattern of IgG.
Red blood cells	Immediate loss proportional to burn size and depth. Life span 30 per cent of normal owing to plasma factor.
White blood cells	Initial and prolonged rise. May drop with sepsis.
Cardiac output	Precipitous drop to 20 to 40 per cent of normal with slow spontaneous recovery in 24 to 36 hours. Myocardial depressant factor demonstrated.
Blood viscosity	Sharp rise proportional to hematocrit.
Carboxyhemoglobin	Not significant after 72 hours (< 2 per cent). Most prominent with inhalation injury (80 per cent). Exists with or without surface burns.
BSP	Retention proportional to burn size with rapid rise and persistence for several weeks.
Cortisol	Prompt rise to two to four times normal.
Aldosterone	Usually returns to normal by end of first week but may remain elevated for long periods. Varied response to ACTH often nil in early period.

Table continued on opposite page

The primary determinant of kinetic energy is the muzzle velocity of the weapon. Doubling the mass of the projectile doubles the energy, but doubling the velocity quadruples the energy.[21] The amount of energy released into the tissue, however, may be modified by several factors. For example, nonjacketed projectiles that flatten, deform, or disintegrate upon impact give up more energy as they pass through tissue and can produce extensive secondary wound cavities and devitalized tissue. These effects are due to the cavitation and sonication effects associated with secondary shear wave formation.[21] The ultimate expression of this effect occurs in ultra-high-velocity military weapons; extensive tissue destruction occurs with small-caliber and small-weight bullets fired from such weapons. Debridement a considerable distance from the missile path is the only way of removing such shattered tissue.

Shotgun injuries are extremely variable and depend on the pattern, distance, shot size, and, perhaps, blast effects. Close-range injuries involving much of the shot pattern cause severe tissue damage. Long-range injuries, particularly with birdshot, are not usually fatal, since the pellets lodge in subcutaneous or muscular tissue.

Generally, all gunshot wounds of the thorax and abdomen should be surgically explored without delay.[5, 21] It is frequently noted that the predicted path of the projectile, based on the location of the wounds of entrance and exit, may not be followed. Rather, a zigzag course of the projectile may be noted at celiotomy.[5] Such deflections may be caused by areas of different density and specific gravity as the missile penetrates and then passes through and around a body cavity or extremity. Tumbling and deforming effects also may affect the route of passage of projectiles.[21] Thus, a dangerous clinical generalization can occur if one attempts to predict internal organ dam-

TABLE 16–7. Changes in Selected Physiological and Metabolic Parameters Associated with Burns* (Continued)

Parameter	Changes Following Burning
Peripheral resistance	Rises sharply; slow fall.
Pulmonary vascular resistance	Rises sharply; slow fall.
Pulmonary artery pressure	Prompt rise and slow return.
Left arterial pressure	Normal or low.
	High with failure.
P_{O_2}	Both low with delay or inadequate therapy.
PH	Prompt response to therapy.
p_{CO_2}	Initial alkalosis or hyperventilation promptly resolves.
Blood lactate	May rise to high levels with hyperventilation or poor perfusion.
Excess lactate	Mild elevations characteristic but may rise to high levels with inadequate or delayed resuscitation.
SGOT	Prompt rise with peak at two to three days and persistence
SGPT	for several weeks owing to liver damage; not release of
A-P	skin enzymes.
Renal function	Renal plasma flow depressed more than glomerular filtration rates.
	Free water clearances down.
	All values promptly return to normal with adequate resuscitation.
Evaporative water loss	Donor sites and partial-thickness burns have intermediate loss rates.
	Full-thickness burns lose at same rate as open pan of water.
	Estimate (25 + % burn) × m² body surface.
	15 to 20 times normal skin rates.
Pulmonary function	Proportional to magnitude of burn.
(in absence of pneumonia)	Independent of inhalation injury.
	Minute ventilation (V_e) increased up to 500 per cent. Peak at five days.
	Static compliance (C_{stat}) usually normal but may change with onset pneumonia.
	Lung clearance index (LCl) normal until terminal.
	Oxygen consumption greatly increased.
	Forced vital capacity (FVC) normal even with V_e increase.
	May drop with pneumonia.

*Reprinted with permission from Moncrief, J. A.: The body's response to heat. *In* Artz, C. P. (ed.): *Burns: A Team Approach*. W. B. Saunders, Philadelphia, 1979, pp. 41–42.
Note: Some changes are dependent upon burn size and severity.

age solely on the basis of entrance and exit wounds. If there are doubts, the clinician should establish a visual diagnosis or rule out organ injury with such reliable methods as diagnostic peritoneal lavage.

treatment includes mechanical and hydraulic debridement. Major surgical reconstructions, often under difficult circumstances, usually await the veterinarian caring for severe trauma from animal fights.

Animal Fights

Depending on the circumstances surrounding animal fighting, which can be highly mutable, the resulting injuries can range from trivial to fatal. Bite wounds to the neck, head, and extremities are most commonly encountered.[16] The devastating combination of crush and impalement wounds seen in small animals caught and shaken in the mouth of a larger animal is especially serious (Fig. 16–11). Such wounds are particularly insidious and dangerous because innocent-appearing external tooth marks may not indicate extensive damage (Fig. 16–12). Because of the bacterial flora of an oral puncture wound,

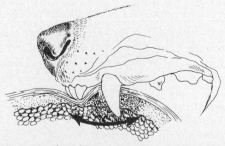

Figure 16–11. Combined penetrating and crushing wounds result from bite wounds and cause extensive damage to underlying tissues as the tooth moves through the tissue. At extreme risk for serious injury is the small animal bitten upon and shaken by a larger animal. (Reprinted with permission from Swaim, S. F.: *Surgery of Traumatized Skin: Management and Reconstruction in the Dog and Cat.* W. B. Saunders, Philadelphia, 1980, p. 43.)

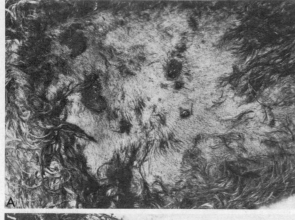

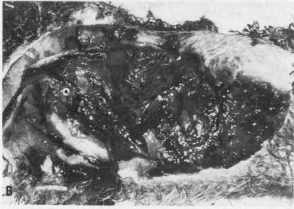

Figure 16–12. *A*, Superficial-appearing external fang marks in a small dog attacked by a larger dog. *B*, Following removal of the skin over a wide area, an extensive subcutaneous hematoma and macerated lateral thoracic wall are seen. Deeper examination revealed the entire intercostal musculature to be destroyed. Flail chest was present and multiple pulmonic puncture wounds of the lung hilus and heart base were found.

Motor Vehicle Accidents

Motor vehicle accidents are a major cause of morbidity and mortality in pets. Combinations of lacerations and crushing injuries are frequently found in animals sustaining roadside trauma. One study designed to quantitate the specific injury patterns in dogs found that about 30 per cent of the injuries were superficial, but nearly 60 per cent of the patients presented had major skeletal injury consisting of fractures or luxations. The pelvis was the most commonly fractured bony region.[15] Fractures of the femur, radius, lumbar vertebrae, and skull and coxofemoral luxations also accounted for a significant percentage of all skeletal injuries. The liver was the most frequently injured internal organ, and neurological damage was seen in half of the dogs, which were subsequently euthanized for failure to respond to treatment.

It should be noted that this study excluded animals dead on arrival. The patterns of multiple trauma present in nonsurvivors could be quite different in that more vital organ and major vessel injury would be expected. Generally speaking, major trauma to organs of the thorax, abdomen, and head is the most frequent cause of early mortality following motor vehicle trauma.[14, 15]

COMMENTS

The veterinarian's management of trauma cases must rapidly and comprehensively consider resuscitation from hypoventilation and hypoperfusion, the arrest of hemorrhage, prevention of additional iatrogenic injuries, the choice of anesthesia if needed, the establishment of priorities for treatment of obvious injuries, preplanning for postoperative nursing care, and adequate communication with the pet's owner. Detecting occult injury is an additional concern in later convalescence. The precise and definitive surgical treatment of specific injuries and concerned postoperative care are paramount to successful results and are considered elsewhere in this book.

Finally, the veterinarian and organized veterinary medicine should assume an active role in reducing the frequency of injury through client and public education programs.

 1. Arnoscky, S. P., and Marshall, J. L.: Pathomechanics of cruciate and meniscal injuries. *In* Bojrab, M. J. (ed.): *Pathophysiology of Small Animal Surgery.* Lea & Febiger, Philadelphia, 1981, pp. 590–660.
 2. Baker, S. P., and Dietz, P.: The epidemiology and prevention of injuries. *In* Zuidema, G. D., Rutherford, R. B., and Ballinger, W. F. (eds.): *The Management of Trauma.* W. B. Saunders, Philadelphia, 1979, pp. 794–821.
 3. Bronson, R. T.: Variation in age at death of dogs of different sexes and breeds. Am. J. Vet. Res. *43*:2057, 1982.
 4. Collins, J. A.: Post-traumatic pulmonary insufficiency. *In* Zuidema, G. D., Rutherford, R. B., and Ballinger, W. F. (eds.): *The Management of Trauma.* W. B. Saunders. Philadelphia, 1979, pp. 114–147.
 5. Crane, S. W.: Evaluation and management of abdominal trauma in the dog and cat. Vet. Clin. North Am. *10*:655, 1980.
 6. Davis, L. E.: Thermal burns. *In* Swaim, S. F. (ed.): *Surgery of Traumatized Skin: Management and Reconstruction in the Dog and Cat.* W. B. Saunders, Philadelphia, 1980, pp. 214–233.
 7. Earley, T. D., and Dee, J. F.: Trauma to the carpus, tarsus and phalanges of dogs and cats. Vet. Clin. North Am. *10*:717, 1980.
 8. Felthouse, A. R.: Aggression against cats, dogs, and people. Child Psychiatry Hum. Dev. *10*:169, 1980.
 9. Friedman, G. D.: *A Primer of Epidemiology.* McGraw-Hill, New York, 1979, p. 9.
10. Frost, H. M.: *An Introduction to Biomechanics.* Charles C Thomas, Springfield, IL, 1967, pp. 6–20.
11. Haller, J. A., Talbert, J. L., and Shermeta, D. W.: Trauma and the child. *In* Zuidema, G. D., Rutherford, R. B., and Ballinger, W. F. (eds.): *The Management of Trauma.* W. B. Saunders, Philadelphia, 1979, pp. 731–734.
12. Kagan, K. G.: Thoracic trauma. Vet. Clin. North Am. *10*:641, 1980.
13. Kolata, R. J.: Trauma in dogs and cats: an overview. Vet. Clin. North Am. *10*:515, 1980.
14. Kolata, R. J.: Patterns and incidence of trauma. *In* Archibald, J. (ed.): *Management of Trauma in Dogs and Cats.* American Veterinary Publications, Santa Barbara, 1981, pp. 2–8.
15. Kolata, R. J., and Johnston, D. E.: Motor vehicle accidents

in urban dogs: A study of 600 cases. J. Am. Vet. Med. Assoc. 167:938, 1975.

16. Kolata, R. J., Kraut, N. H., and Johnston, D. E.: Patterns of trauma in urban dogs and cats: A study of 1000 cases. J. Am. Vet. Med. Assoc. *164*:499, 1974.

17. Moncrief, J. A.: The body's response to heat. *In* Artz, C. P. (ed.): *Burns: A Team Approach*. W. B. Saunders, Philadelphia, 1979, pp. 23–44.

18. Morse, T. S.: Child abuse: A neglected form of trauma. J. Trauma *15*:620, 1975.

19. Robson, M. C., Krizek, T. J., and Wray, R. C.: Care of the thermally injured patient. *In* Zuidema, G. D., Rutherford,

R. B., and Ballinger, W. F. (eds.): *The Management of Trauma*. W. B. Saunders, Philadelphia, 1979, pp. 666–730.

20. Teplitz, C.: The pathology of burns and the fundamentals of burn wound sepsis. *In* Artz, C. P. (ed.): *Burns: A Team Approach*. W. B. Saunders, Philadelphia, 1979, pp. 45–94.

21. Swaim, S. F.: Etiology of skin trauma and defects. *In* Swaim, S. F. (ed.): *Surgery of Traumatized Skin: Management and Reconstruction in the Dog and Cat*. W. B. Saunders, Philadelphia, 1980, pp. 55–59.

22. Wilmore, D. W.: Nutrition. *In* Artz, C. P. (ed.): *Burns: A Team Approach*. W. B. Saunders, Philadelphia, 1979, pp. 120–131.

Chapter **17**

Total Parenteral Nutrition

Marc R. Raffe

Many surgical patients can tolerate acute withdrawal of nutritional support without complications. Preoperative fasting has little effect on the nutritionally sound patient.[76] Unfortunately, surgery must sometimes be performed on debilitated patients with poor nutritional status. In these cases, supplemental oral (enteral) caloric feeding is valuable to partially reverse a negative nutritional balance. Some patients will not tolerate this approach owing to conditions for which the surgery may be indicated, such as facial fractures; parenteral administration of nutrients has been advocated for these patients. Intravascular infusion of carbohydrate is one common approach. However, the nutritional needs of the patient are not met by the administration of carbohydrate alone. Calories, vitamins, minerals, and essential fatty acids are important components of a nutritionally balanced diet. These basic substances must be given in appropriate amounts to overcome a negative nutritional state.

There are two forms of parenteral nutrition: (1) total parenteral nutrition (TPN), which is the maintenance of body weight and normal metabolic function by parenteral methods, and (2) hyperalimentation, which is the administration of essential nutrients in excess of a patient's calculated normal requirements, providing a "positive" metabolic state for reversal of poor nutrition.[1]

Historically, a variety of domestic and laboratory animal species have been used in experimental trials of various nutrients.[18-21, 31] Difficulties in animal management, excessive cost, potential complications, and limitations in diseases amenable to nutritional support have impeded the development of this discipline in veterinary practice.[18-21] Despite these drawbacks, nutritional care can be a valuable therapeutic technique and may be lifesaving in the severely debilitated surgical or medical patient.

Patient Selection

Total parenteral nutrition should be considered in any patient that cannot be nutritionally maintained by conventional means. If oral diets can be modified to supply essential nutritional requirements, this approach should be used.[1] Patients with medical or surgical conditions that affect ingestion, transport, or digestion of nutrients may be considered for total parenteral support.

Parenteral nutrition can be used in surgical and medical patients as either support or primary therapy. Support therapy may be considered in cases of poor preoperative nutrition as well as in the management of a variety of disorders, including gastrointestinal disease, pancreatitis, trauma, burns, massive degloving injuries, and organ failure.[1, 37, 45, 55] These conditions create a nutritional imbalance by altering oral ingestion or basal metabolic requirements. Parenteral supplementation of conventional intake may prevent a negative nutritional balance in these patients.

Primary therapy is indicated when the only nutritional support is to be provided by parenteral means.[1, 37, 45, 55] Indications may overlap with those of support therapy and are differentiated by the severity of the inciting disease, the surgical procedure, and intensity of the postoperative rehabilitation program. Specific indications may include short bowel syndrome from massive gastrointestinal resection, acute pancreatitis, enterocutaneous fistula, inflammatory bowel disease, neoplasia, burns, trauma, acute renal or hepatic failure, and reversible medical disease that precludes ingestion.[1, 37, 45, 55]

The indications for parenteral nutrition may appear diverse, and undoubtedly other indications exist. The common feature is the inability to provide adequate nutritional support by conventional means. Any patient that can be so categorized should be considered for parenteral nutrition support.

NUTRITIONAL REQUIREMENTS

Complete nutrition by parenteral methods requires consideration of nutrient components that normally are provided by oral intake. The water, metabolizable energy, protein, essential fatty acids, vitamins, and mineral needs of the patient must be carefully calculated. These must then be accurately administered

to provide a "balanced" dietary intake.[31] In the following discussion, requirements are presented for domestic animals as reported. Many parameters have not been defined, and human values are listed for guideline information when values are unknown.

Metabolizable Energy

The caloric requirements of the human parenteral nutrition patient are calculated from a basal energy expenditure formula. Weight, height, and age are all

TABLE 17–1. Basal Nutrient Requirements in Dogs and Cats*

Component	Canine Oral	Canine Intravenous	Feline Oral†
Metabolizable energy (Kcal/kg$^{0.75}$/day)			
Growth	200	140–200	130–250
Adult	132	—	80
Protein (g/kg/day)			
Growth	9.6	4.0	10.5
Adult	4.8	4.0	6.0
Lipid (g/kg/day)			
Growth	2.2	2.2	3.4
Adult	1.1	1.1	1.91
Linoleic acid (g/kg/day)			
Growth	0.22	—	0.21
Adult	0.44	—	0.38
Minerals (mg/kg/day)			
Sodium	210	100	121
Potassium	140	115	66
Chloride	315	225	121
Calcium	242	72	242
Phosphorus	198	58	198
Magnesium	8.8	4	8.8
Iron	1.3	0.058	2.15
Copper	0.16	0.065	0.11
Cobalt	1.055	0.041	—
Manganese	0.11	0.04	0.22
Zinc	0.22	0.14	0.66
Iodine	0.034	0.046	0.02
Vitamins			
A (I.U./kg/day)	200	100	212
D (I.U./kg/day)	20	10	21
E (I.U./kg/day)	1.1	0.05	1.6
Thiamine (mg/kg/day)	0.03	0.5	0.1
Riboflavin (mg/kg/day)	0.09	0.1	0.1
Pyridoxine (mg/kg/day)	0.05	0.15	0.08
Niacin (mg/kg/day)	0.04	0.1	0.9
Pantothenic acid (mg/kg/day)	0.1	0.25	0.2
C (mg/kg/day)	—	—	—
K (mg/kg/day)	—	0.1	—
Folic acid (mg/kg/day)	0.01	0.01	0.02
Choline (mg/kg/day)	60	25	40
Biotin (mg/kg/day)	—	0.007	0.001

*Adapted from *Nutritional Requirements of Cats. Nutritional Requirements of Domestic Animals*, Vol. 13. National Academy of Sciences, Washington, D.C., 1978; *Nutritional Requirements of Dogs. Nutritional Requirements of Animals*, Vol. 8. National Academy of Sciences, Washington, D.C., 1974; Dudrick, S. J., et al.: Long-term total parenteral nutrition with growth, development, and positive nitrogen balance. Surgery *64*:134, 1968; and Carter, J. M., and Freedman, A. B.: Total intravenous feeding in the dog. Am. J. Vet. Res. *171*:71, 1977.

†Feline values are derived from NRC requirements by dividing dry basis formulation per kilogram (4.0 Kcal/gm) into metabolizable energy requirement for adult cat (85 Kcal/kg) and multiplying the product by unit percentage for daily recommendations.

considered to arrive at a basal energy expenditure value. This value is multiplied, if necessary, by a factor estimating the per cent increase in energy required in excess of basal expenditure to calculate kilocalorie requirements per day.[7, 31, 32] In veterinary practice, calculation of required metabolizable energy is the product of (body weight in kilograms)$^{0.75}$ and the basal energy expenditure factor determined by the National Research Council (NRC).[11] In the adult dog this value is 132 Kcal.[11, 50, 52] Table 17–1 lists values of other nutritional components. Similar values are available for the cat, and calculations are performed in a like manner. The factor in the adult cat is 85 Kcal multiplied by (body weight in kilograms$^{0.75}$).[53] Other components are listed in Table 17–1.

Additional energy requirements must be considered in patients with pyrexia, surgical or metabolic stress, and wound healing requirements.[2, 49, 64] The availability of additional metabolizable energy (calories) is critical to prevent body weight losses from increased energy demands. Estimation of this additional requirement is dependent upon the underlying physiological insult.[31] Experimental data on metabolic response to injury and illness in humans suggest a 24 per cent increase in energy requirements over baseline for elective surgery patients, a 32 per cent increase in skeletal trauma patients, a 61 per cent increase in trauma patients in whom corticosteroids have been administered, and an 80 per cent increase in septic patients.[49] Pyrexia requires an increase in energy expenditure of 12 per cent per degree centigrade in excess of basal body temperature per day.[31] These values are approximate requirements for metabolizable energy calculation based on clinical practice. Actual values may be derived from measurement of oxygen consumption, by either closed or open collection technique, and conversion to caloric expenditures.[5, 31] Appropriate calculation values are available in cited reference sources.

Nitrogen

The provision of an adequate nitrogen (protein) source is an important consideration. Nitrogen is utilized for integral support of high-density protein-base tissue as well as a secondary energy substrate in the absence of metabolizable energy (gluconeogenesis).[15, 26, 60, 68, 76] Muscle mass catabolism may occur with inadequate protein intake, as noted by diminished lean body mass, resulting in decreased weight.[15, 68] Inadequate protein administration may occur even in the presence of adequate energy substrate and is clinically noted by sodium retention, ascites, anasarca, and depletion of visceral protein storage.[31] Visceral protein depletion, indicated by decreased serum albumin levels, transferrin activity, and thyroxin-binding prealbumin levels, has also been described. Immune reactivity may also be diminished.[31]

Studies in adult and growing dogs using the NRC protein requirements of 4.0 to 4.8 gm/kg/day have not resulted in any signs referrable to protein malnutrition.[11, 18-21, 50] The suggested minimum carbohydrate:nitrogen ratio of 150:1 in humans has been shown to prevent the utilization of protein substrate as an energy source.[31] Highly stressed patients may require additional carbohydrate resources, and in these cases the carbohydrate:protein ratio may approach 100:1.

Ten amino acids have been identified as essential in the dog[54]: arginine, histidine, isoleucine, leucine, lysine, methionine, phenylalanine, threonine, tryptophan, and valine. These amino acids cannot be synthesized by the body or stored for a significant time period. Any consideration of dietary formulation should include these components in minimum daily values.

Similar essential amino acids have been identified in the cat.[53] An additional requirement for long-term parenteral nutrition is taurine. Unlike other domestic species, the cat does not have the biochemical capability to convert methionine to taurine.[53] Taurine is an essential component for retinal function; retinal degeneration occurs in its absence.[53] Dietary sources high in taurine include mammalian muscle, liver, and kidney. Parenteral dietary formulations should include taurine, especially in chronically ill cats.

Lipids

Lipid preparations provide essential fatty acids required for daily homeostasis. Acute effects do not result from lipid deprivation.[11] In dogs, changes in haircoat and skin texture are not demonstrable until three months after initiation of a lipid-free diet.[54] In cats, linoleic acid has been described as essential for homeostasis. Soybean and linseed oil are good sources of this lipid.[53] Like the dog, clinical signs referrable to fatty acid deprivation in the cat appear to be more chronic than acute.[53, 54] Lipids may also be used to provide metabolizable energy in parenteral nutrition. Current recommendations suggest that 4 to 10 per cent of daily caloric requirements should be present as essential fatty acids. Linoleic, linolenic, and arachidonic acids are essential nutritional components.[53, 54]

Minerals

Mineral requirements are empirical in formulation, as basic dietary requirements have not been determined in the dog and cat.[53, 54] Recommended levels for daily nutrition are listed in Table 17–1. These levels have been used in several experimental trials and have been adequate for long-term support of both adult and growing dogs.[11, 18-21] Essential minerals for acute parenteral support are sodium, potassium, chloride, and phosphorus. Calcium and magnesium should be included during chronic patient support. Caution should be exercised in selection and determination of salts used in parenteral solution. Excess chloride salts may result in clinical signs related to hyperchloremia.[31, 66] In general, the chloride concentration (in mEq/L) should not exceed values normally found in plasma. Alternate salt forms such as acetate, lactate, and gluconate should be used if possible. However, lactate and acetate may be contraindicated in patients with hepatic disease.[31]

Vitamins

Fat- and water-soluble vitamins must be administered during parenteral nutrition. Specific requirements are presented in Table 17–1. Commercially available multivitamin infusion preparations meet most requirements for the dog and cat, except for niacin (B_5), vitamin B_{12}, and biotin (B_7).[11] These may be added by supplementing the infusion preparations with injectable B vitamin or using complete commercial preparations, e.g., MVI-12.*

Fluids

Water balance must be considered in the parenteral nutrition patient. Fluid requirements are generally calculated based on body surface area (Table 17–2). Daily fluid balance matches intake with loss. Routes of loss normally include urinary excretion and insensible loss. Additional routes of loss experienced by the surgical patient include fever, third space fluid losses (surgical site, burns, open wounds, fistula), gastrointestinal losses, and drainage devices.[31] Normal body water gain is a combination of both metabolic water production (endogenous) and normal water ingestion (exogenous). Parenteral nutrition may

*Armour Pharmaceutical Co., Tarrytown, NY.

TABLE 17–2. Fluid Requirements*

Body Weight (kg)	Maintenance Water Requirement (cc/day)
1.4	80
2.7	160
4.0	240
5.5	320
7.0	400
9.0	475
13.0	625
17.5	875
22.0	1000
27.5	1130
32.5	1250
37.5	1400
42.0	1500

*Adapted from Harrison, J. B., Sussman, H. H., and Pickering, D. E.: Fluid and electrolyte therapy in small animals. J. Am. Vet. Med. Assoc. 37:637, 1960.

paradoxically increase exogenous water requirements. Conversion to a positive anabolic state diminishes proteolysis and fat oxidation, thereby diminishing endogenous water production. Additional fluid volume may be required to restore this loss.[31]

Metabolic Response to Starvation and Injury

In the healthy presurgical patient, brief fast periods of 12 to 24 hours may be accommodated without metabolic expense.[76] Normal caloric requirements are provided by the conversion of muscle and hepatic glycogen reserves to carbohydrate substrates. After 24 hours, however, glycogen reserves are depleted and alternate forms of energy substrates must be utilized. In the presence of decreased carbohydrate intake, protein catabolism with release of amino acids occurs.[32, 52, 55, 68] These amino acid substrates are converted to glucose by hepatic gluconeogenesis. In addition, mobilization of adipose tissue to free fatty acids and glycerol begins.[32] This metabolic pathway is not predominant for several days; therefore, protein catabolism provides the primary energy source during this time. After 72 hours, lipid catabolism for gluconeogenesis is the predominant metabolic pathway.[28, 32, 33] However, protein catabolism continues to provide some calories. The net result is loss in both lean and nonlean body mass, reflected as weight loss.[28, 32, 38] This system is not ideal from the body's standpoint, as lipid metabolism without protein catabolism is preferred. The use of amino acids for energy substrate defers their use for other physiological and reparative processes.[28, 30, 38] Deterioration in organ function, immune surveillance, wound healing, and poor early ambulation have all been described in calorie-deficient surgical patients.

This sequence of events is applicable to patients with normal basal metabolic requirements prior to withdrawal of nutritional support. Many surgical patients are presented after a traumatic incident and have additional metabolic burdens owing to trauma and shock. Increased levels or activity of catecholamines, ACTH, TSH, and glucagon can be demonstrated following insults. Increased levels of these substances result in increased steroid synthesis, glucose oxidation and gluconeogenesis, lipolysis, and glycogen mobilization.[2, 49, 64, 68] These activities result in increased calories available after an injury. Unfortunately, carbohydrate uptake by cells is impaired owing to diminished function of insulin. This has been described as the "diabetes of trauma."[64, 66] Because of this "diabetes," alternate energy sources, namely, protein and lipid, become predominant under these circumstances to respond to increased energy requirements.

A more favorable metabolic picture cannot occur simply by the addition of a carbohydrate source, as impairment of cellular uptake of carbohydrate is the underlying cause. Caloric sources may be altered by the use of other carbohydrates (xylitol, sorbitol) or the supplemental administration of crystalline insulin to enhance cellular uptake of available carbohydrate. Additional insulin administration may re-establish the balance of glucagon and insulin, enhancing cellular glucose uptake.[24, 31, 44, 64]

Patients presented for surgery with chronic illness may exhibit signs of long-term nutritional debilitation. These patients are best managed by re-establishment of a favorable metabolic and nutritional profile prior to the *stress* of anesthesia and surgery. Hyperalimentation to restore a positive metabolic state (anabolism) is preferred.[31, 64] Even with this approach, conversion to anabolism is not acute. Chronic deterioration of the patient has occurred, and hyperalimentation should be used for seven to 14 days prior to re-evaluation of the patient. Metabolic changes in chronic nutritional deterioration are similar to those seen in the acutely traumatized patient. The intensity and magnitude of change may differ from those seen in the acute state.[31]

COMPONENTS OF PARENTERAL NUTRITION

Nitrogen Sources (Protein)

Nitrogen requirements for nutritional support have been described previously and are based on oral maintenance requirements in the dog and cat.[53, 54] Currently, two forms of nitrogen source are commercially available in the United States—protein hydrolysates and crystalline amino acid compounds.[25] Neither is optimum in all respects, but both have been used in animal experiments with favorable results.

Protein hydrolysates are the products of acid or enzyme hydrolysis of casein, fibrin, or meat products[25, 31] and are a heterogeneous mixture of amino acids, di- and tripeptides, and large proteins. These products are assayed by the manufacturer and listed on each bottle.[31] Analyses of commercial preparations of 5% and 10% Amigen,* 5% Aminosol,† and 5% CPH,‡ indicate that they contain acceptable levels of essential amino acids for the adult dog. Hyprotigen 5%§ is deficient in histidine and arginine. All solutions exclude the amino acid taurine, which is essential in the cat. Drawbacks to acceptance in human practice include variations in analysis due to imprecise enzymatic degradation, variations in bioavailability, and immunogenicity. Ghandimi has reported batch variation in all products evaluated.[25] In addition, nitrogen bioavailability has been questioned in reports indicating that 30 to 45 per cent of all available nitrogen is in conjugated form or biologically unavailable dextroisomers.[25, 59] The merits of these claims are unresolved for veterinary species, as studies in growing puppies and adult dogs utilized protein

hydrolysates for the nitrogen source on a chronic basis with satisfactory results.[11, 18-21] Casein by-products have been reported to invoke mild hypersensitivity reactions in susceptible individuals.[59]

Dissatisfaction with nonuniform composition, as well as advances in protein chemistry, have led to the development of solutions with known amino acid composition. Commercial preparations are presently offered by several manufacturers. These solutions are formulated with individual crystalline amino acid components and are available in several concentrations.[59] All solutions include amino acids identified as essential by NRC requirements for the dog and cat. Products presently available include Freamine III 3.0, 8.5, and 10%*; Travasol 3.5, 5.5, 8.5, and 10%‖; and Aminosyn.† Parenteral nutrition has been used to support patients with specific metabolic diseases. Amino acid formulas for patients with renal disease are now commercially available. Essential amino acids are included to prevent endogenous catabolism. The total nitrogen intake is reduced to minimize nonprotein nitrogen imbalance in the previously compromised patient.[69] Current investigations also include clinical trials of protein formulas for individuals with hepatic disease.[69] Protein substrate in liver failure is provided by the branch chain amino acids valine, leucine, and isoleucine. These amino acids are structurally separate in that deamination and carbon skeleton fuel utilization can occur in skeletal muscle as well as at hepatic sites. In patients with hepatic injury or disease, biotransformation of these amino acids for gluconeogenesis and incorporation of amino groups into alanine and glutamine in skeletal muscle allows for continued protein homeostasis in the presence of liver disease as well as hydrocarbon chains for energy utilization.[32, 76] Nephramine 5.4%* and Aminosyn-RF‡ are formulated for patients with renal disease.[69] These products contain only known essential amino acids and have a lower total nitrogen assay than the balanced solutions noted previously. Also available commercially is a formulation for use in hepatic failure patients (Heptamine*).[69]

Lipid Sources

Currently, two sources of fatty acids are commercially available. Soybean oil–based products are marketed as Intralipid 10 and 20%§ and Travamulsion 10%.†[33, 51, 56, 70] The difference in concentrations reflects the caloric content of the solutions. Safflower oil–based preparations are available as Liposyn 10 and 20%.‡[56] Safflower oil contains a higher content of linoleic acid and a lower content of linolenic acid than soybean oil.[56] Arachidonic acid is a metabolic product of linoleic acid in the dog and cat.[53, 54] There-

*Travenol Laboratories, Deerfield, IL.
†Abbott Laboratories, North Chicago, IL.
‡Cutter Laboratories Berkeley, CA.
§McGaw Laboratories, Irvine, CA.

*McGaw Laboratories, Irvine, CA.
†Travenol Laboratories, Deerfield, IL.
‡Abbott Laboratories, North Chicago, IL.
§Cutter Laboratories Berkeley, CA.

fore, essential fatty acid deficiency is primarily dependent upon linoleic acid content.[53, 54]

Carbohydrate Sources

Glucose (dextrose) is the predominant carbohydrate component in parenteral nutrition.[69] Wide availability, low cost, primary biochemical utilization, and solution compatibility have contributed to its widespread use. Glucose is available in a wide range of concentrations (5 to 70%).[31, 69] Hypertonic solutions may induce peripheral vascular irritation and should be centrally administered.[18-21, 31] Fructose, galactose, xylitol, and sorbitol have all been successfully used as carbohydrate substrates.[24] The sugars xylitol and sorbitol are metabolized to fructose analogues and are utilized in a similar manner.[24] Fructose and glucose are preferred substrates owing to their primary biochemical utilization without biotransformation.[24] Other carbohydrate sources have been used in parenteral nutrition with some success, but undesirable side effects have been reported.[31]

Vitamin Sources

Several multivitamin preparations are commercially available. A commonly used preparation in parenteral nutrition is multivitamin infusion (MVI-12*). It is a balanced vitamin solution except for the absence of vitamin K. Separate parenteral administration of vitamin K can be added on a weekly basis.[31] Other multivitamin supplements available include M.V.C. 9 + 3,† and Multivitamin Additive.‡ All are similar in composition to MVI-12 and are administered at the same daily dose.[31]

Electrolyte Sources

Balanced electrolyte infusion is an integral component of parenteral nutrition. Solutions using individual electrolyte components may be formulated.[13] In recent years, combination electrolyte–amino acid solutions have become commercially available. Not all electrolyte requirements may be satisfied by this route, therefore supplementation may be considered for specific deficit or maintenance therapy.[69] Individual salts may be added to balance electrolyte requirements.[13]

Mineral Sources

Trace minerals should be considered in chronic diet administration. Guidelines in humans suggest the importance of the trace elements zinc, copper, chromium, and manganese.[31] These may be added as single salts or administered by commercially available multitrace mineral preparations. Preparations currently available include M.T.E.-4,* and Multiple Trace Metal Additive.† Dose requirements may be calculated from NRC tables for nutritional requirements.[53, 54]

PREPARATION OF PARENTERAL SOLUTIONS

The correct preparation of parenteral nutrition solutions is vital to the success of therapy. Rigid asepsis throughout the preparation procedure cannot be overemphasized.[28, 31] Most patients considered for parenteral nutrition have pre-existing medical or surgical conditions that may alter immunocompetence or predispose to superinfection. "Breaks" in aseptic technique may result in systemic septicemia and death. Therefore, adherence to aseptic principles is vital to success.[28, 31]

Generally, a base formula is compounded and checked for contamination.[28, 31] The addition of specific components to establish a complete diet is based on individual nutrition requirements. Currently, most basic formulas include hypertonic glucose solutions (50%) plus a protein source and electrolytes.[13, 28, 31] Individual electrolytes, minerals, and vitamins are added on a daily basis to fulfill nutritional requirements. Veterinary practice does not include high-volume parenteral nutrition services, so batch compounding is impractical. Most studies suggest that the basic formulas will remain stable for eight to ten weeks at room temperature.[31] The addition of electrolytes and vitamins decreases shelf life to 21 days at 4°C.[31] It may be practical to compound the basic formula on a weekly basis, with the daily addition of nutritional supplements prior to infusion.

Ideally, the formulas should be prepared in a low-traffic area with facilities for high-frequency air exchange in a laminar flow pattern.[28, 31, 73] A closed transfer preparation technique minimizes the need for air exchange requirements.[13] Closed transfer mixing is the preferred technique.[13, 73] The exterior surface of the polyethylene bags or glass bottles of glucose and protein source is disinfected, and each bag or bottle is connected to an arm of a Y-type administration set.[63, 73] The outflow of this administration set is connected to an empty polyethylene bag (Viaflex*) after appropriate disinfection.[63, 73] A volume of glucose and protein are then delivered. Various ratios are used, depending on protein source and concentration of glucose solution. Several authors recommend 250 gm carbohydrate plus 42 gm protein as a standard ratio.[31, 73] After filling the container, it is essential to recleanse the infusion port to maintain asepsis. Amino acid solutions with electrolytes help

*Armour Pharmaceutical Co.
†Lypho-Med, Chicago, IL.
‡Abbott Laboratories, North Chicago, IL.

*Travenol Laboratories, Deerfield, IL.
†Abbott Laboratories, North Chicago, IL.

minimize electrolyte deficiencies inherent in chronic administration. Commercially available, partially filled polyethylene bags or evacuated glass bottles containing hypertonic dextrose concentrations (10 to 50%) minimize the number of transfers required for production of a basal formula.[13] Theoretically, one transfer of amino acid base into a partially filled dextrose bag will compound a standard formulation. If specific electrolyte abnormalities are suggested by clinical evaluation or biochemical analysis, a base amino acid formula without balanced electrolytes is selected.[13, 69] Specific electrolyte supplementation may be provided by commercially available injectable solutions.

Most solution components are compatible in mixtures; however, the addition of supplemental agents may result in incompatibility. Supplemental pharmacological administration should be minimized, if not avoided, in parenteral nutrition solutions. Albumin, heparin, insulin, and hydrocortisone appear to be compatible in standard formulations and may be safely administered.[31, 73] Hypertonic dextrose may cause red blood cell clumping; therefore it is inadvisable to administer whole blood through a parenteral nutrition catheter. Sodium bicarbonate may be added to the solution for pH adjustment; however, its addition may interfere with the actions of insulin and

B complex vitamins and may induce precipitation of calcium salts.[73] Magnesium sulfate may be included for a specific deficiency. However, in combination with calcium chloride it may form a calcium sulfate precipitate. Calcium gluconate should be included when magnesium is to be administered.[73] Calcium and phosphorus salts may precipitate if added incorrectly. The addition of phosphate-containing electrolyte salts should precede the addition of calcium.[13, 31, 73] The sum of calcium and phosphorus salts should not exceed 45 mEq/L.[31]

Most glucose-based solutions are hyperosmolar and require administration by a central catheter. A base formula using 40 to 50% dextrose and 8.5% amino acid solution results in a concentration of 1,690 mOsm/L, which is far in excess of standard plasma values.[31, 69] Slow infusion by a centrally placed catheter allows for reduction of this concentration in the venous blood. Peripheral infusion does not allow rapid mixing due to lower blood flow, and tissue reaction with the solution may occur.[31]

Examples of standard formulation procedures are outlined in Table 17–3. Most pharmaceutical compounds currently marketed do not significantly differ in composition.[69] The specific component analysis should be known for each solution used in the formulation.

TABLE 17–3. Standard Formulations for Total Parenteral Nutrition

Component	Volume (ml)	Final Concentration/L
Dextrose (50%) + 5.5% amino acid with electrolytes (Travenol)		
Dextrose 50%	500	25%
5.5% amino acid + electrolytes	500	2.75%
Sodium		35 mEq
Potassium		30 mEq
Magnesium		5 mEq
Phosphate		15 mMoles
Chloride		35 mEq
Acetate		50 mEq
Calcium (gluconate 10%)	10	5 mEq
Total Kcal		960
Amino acids		27.5 gm
Osmolarity		1690 mOsm
Dextrose (50%) + 8.5% amino acid with electrolytes (Travenol)		
Dextrose 50%	500	25%
8.5% amino acid + electrolytes	500	4.25%
Sodium		35 mEq
Potassium		30 mEq
Magnesium		5 mEq
Phosphate		15 mmol
Chloride		35 mEq
Acetate		67.5 mEq
Calcium (gluconate 10%)	10	5 mEq
Total Kcal		1020
Amino acids		42.5 gm
Osmolarity		1845 mOsm

Note: Additional sodium or potassium salts may be included without adverse reactions. Salts may be chloride or acetate, depending on anion requirements of the patient. Multiple vitamin solutions are added prior to use.

ADMINISTRATION OF PARENTERAL SOLUTIONS

Central and peripheral venous sites are used to administer parenteral solutions.[16, 31, 72, 75] Peripheral veins may be used with formulations that do not exceed normal osmolality. Formulas that have low concentrations of carbohydrate (glucose) or that incorporate lipid substrates for caloric balance are amenable to peripheral vein infusion.[8, 31, 72] The increased osmolality of solutions by the addition of hypertonic glucose is associated with thrombophlebitis and vascular thrombosis.[18-21, 28, 31, 72] Solutions containing hypertonic glucose as a component should be administered by central venous catheter. Even with infusion at this site, occasional vascular thrombosis may be noted.[11]

The calculated daily requirements are administered by a continuous infusion over a 24-hour period.[28, 31] The institution of continuous infusion of a hypertonic glucose solution may be accompanied by an interim hyperglycemia.[28, 31] As infusion continues, the patient adapts through increased insulin secretion to compensate for this acute glucose "load." The addition of regular insulin to the solution regulates serum glucose levels until accommodation can occur, usually not more than 24 hours in animals with normal exocrine pancreatic function.[31] The constant infusion technique is preferred to prevent acute vacillations in serum glucose levels that may result in coma, seizures, and death.[28, 31] However, canine studies in which delivery was inadvertently interrupted did not demonstrate these complications.[11]

A side effect of the physiological elevation in serum insulin levels is an acceleration of intrahepatic lipogenesis. This frequently produces an enlarged fatty liver in patients receiving long-term parenteral nutrition.[31] To circumvent this side effect, controlled cyclic administration of parenteral solutions is currently under investigation.[31] Cyclical withdrawal of dextrose with continued infusion of amino acids and lipid solutions has been suggested. This approach was used in one veterinary clinical case report.[58] Advantages suggested with this approach include mobilization of lipids as an energy substrate, utilization of infused amino acids for visceral protein synthesis (serum albumin and serum transferrin) instead of musculoskeletal incorporation, a slight decrease in total daily caloric requirements, and a lower incidence of fatty liver development.[31] Phasic alteration in serum insulin level has been noted; however, no change in free fatty acid, ketone, or lactate levels is apparent.[31] This approach may prove beneficial in the future.

Apparatus for delivery of parenteral nutrition should include an inline filter device.[13, 31, 73] A reduced incidence of intravascular sepsis from contamination during preparation and a filtration of residues caused by glass, rubber, plastic, or protein aggregates, or microprecipitation of solution components are reported advantages. Filter size is variable. The standard inline filter (0.45 micron) allows for gravity flow and removes all particulate and infectious agents except pleomorphic forms of *Pseudomonas* and *Staphylococcus* spp.[31] A 0.22-micron filter removes all substances; however, older designs limited gravity flow of solutions. Newer designs allow for larger volume delivery by both gravity feed and mechanical pump devices.[13] Under ideal mixture preparation and delivery conditions, little benefit has been demonstrated with inline filters.[31] However, the use of filters in veterinary patients in less than optimum surroundings is to be encouraged.

Administration rates depend on calculated nutritional requirements and the size of the patient. A study using dogs weighing 7 to 11 kg tested a continuous infusion rate of 34 ml/hr.[11] Guidelines for human patients suggest initiation of parenteral nutrition at a rate of 20 to 50 ml/hr with increases to 100 to 125 ml/hr as needed.[31] The infusion rate is determined by calculating daily patient requirements and converting to an administration rate per hour basis. Lipid base infusion may be administered at a rate of 1 ml/min of a 10% solution.[31, 58] Administration of 10 to 15 ml/kg/hr has been reported in the veterinary literature for short-term (four hours) daily infusion.[58] Others have administered 10% Intralipid at a rate of 6 g/kg/day for ten weeks in the dog without major side effects.[34, 77] Current practice favors intermittent infusion of lipid products on a daily basis with constant administration of carbohydrate–amino acid mixtures. When lipid was used as a major calorie source, diet formulations were infused until daily requirements were obtained, and supplemental amino acids were infused continuously.[58] All components of parenteral nutrition appear compatible, so simultaneous infusion of each component through the same intravenous catheter should produce no adverse effects. Mixing of all three major components into one infusion reservoir was acceptable in both canine and human studies.[36] The infused mixture in canine studies was 60% lipid emulsion (10% solution), 20% amino acids (5.5% amino acid + electrolytes), and 20% dextrose injection (10% solution) and was administered seven hours per day through a peripheral vein.[36]

CHRONIC CATHETERIZATION AND INFUSION CARE

Administration of long-term parenteral nutrition requires management and care of the implanted catheter. Depending upon the composition of the mixture and the goals of parenteral nutrition, either peripheral or central implantation sites may be used. Irrespective of site selection, materials for catheter construction are the same for all commercial catheter designs, and knowledge of their biological reaction is useful in selection and use.

Presently, materials available for catheter construction are derivatives of plastic monomers (polyethylene, polyvinyl) or fluorinated hydrocarbon derivatives (Teflon) and silicone (Silastic).[57, 65, 71] All material classes are flexible and biologically inert during chronic tissue implantation. However, numerous reports suggest that intravascular catheterization can be associated with complications, some of which may be related to the thrombogenic potential of these two materials.[27, 48, 57, 61, 62, 65, 71, 75] Experimental data suggest that intraluminal introduction of either material evokes a rapid, platelet-mediated fibrin deposition on the external surface of the catheter.[57] This may be noted as soon as 15 minutes after catheter placement and may "plateau" by 40 minutes.[48, 57] The fibrin sheath remains for the duration of catheter implantation and dislodges upon removal.[48] The freed thrombi may migrate in the venous blood, resulting in subclinical pulmonary emboli. Heparin bonding to the catheter surface may briefly impede this fibrin aggregation; however, little advantage is realized with long-term implantation.[27, 48] Of the three materials, silicone has the lowest complication rate.

Peripheral veins (cephalic, lateral tarsal) may be selected as cannulation sites when isotonic solutions are used. Amino acid solutions and lipid-based preparations may be safely administered at these sites.[58] Hypertonic solutions using a dextrose base or combined dextrose, amino acids, and lipids should be given at a central venous site. Percutaneous or surgical catheter implantation of the anterior vena cava via the external jugular vein is recommended.[11, 18-21, 58]

Placement techniques for long- and short-term cannulas differ. Wound care and implantation under aseptic conditions are critical to prevent complications.[61, 62] The proposed implantation site is prepared aseptically using three successive surgical scrubs of povidone-iodine with a water rinse after each scrub. After the final scrub, povidone-iodine solution or tincture of iodine should be applied. The site is barrier draped, and aseptic surgical technique is used for catheter placement. The operator wears gloves and performs catheter venipuncture using standard technique. An occlusive dressing with povidone-iodine ointment is placed over the venipuncture site, and the catheter is secured by either single ligature fixation to the skin using monofilament suture material or incorporation into a bandage dressing. A protective cover made of materials with minimal absorption properties is applied, and continuous care is given. Every one to two days (or more frequently if gross soiling is observed), the dressing is removed and the venipuncture site is examined for erythema, induration, or other signs of infection. Using aseptic technique and surgical gloves, the skin around the wound is cleansed, and a new occlusive dressing using antibiotic or antimicrobial ointment is applied. Changing administration sets and venipuncture site may be considered at this time.[10, 29, 39-41, 62, 75]

If wound care is appropriate and no clinical signs of catheter-related sepsis are noted, sequential venous rotation on a regular basis is not mandatory.[62] Central venous placement of catheters in man has been maintained for as long as 55 days at one site with minimal complications when good catheter care was observed.[75] Catheters have been implanted in dogs for as long as 100 days with appropriate care.[18-21] Complications associated with chronic cannulation of peripheral veins have not been reported. If intimal injury from hypertonic glucose occurs, thrombophlebitis may be noted as soon as 48 to 72 hours after catheter placement.[58]

Continued nursing care is critical to maintenance of aseptic cannulation. The entire administration apparatus should be considered a "closed" system. Administration of pharmacological agents, blood sampling, and physiological measurements (CVP) from the parenteral nutrition catheter should be avoided.[31, 62] All connections and the administration set should be continuously disinfected. Each reservoir change should include cleaning of both the administration part of the bottle or bag and the coupling terminal of the administration apparatus with povidone-iodine.[29, 39-41] Each time a junction is disconnected, both ends should be cleansed prior to re-attachment.[29, 39-41] The administration set and in-line filter should be changed every 24 hours or whenever it is contaminated.[31, 62] Any accidental disconnection should be treated as a septic break, and the administration apparatus and solution must be replaced.[31] Contamination of the catheter site merits either replacement or rotation of the catheter to an alternate site.[31, 62, 63] Although these procedures may seem extreme, sepsis in the debilitated patient has extreme consequences.

MONITORING THE PARENTERAL NUTRITION PATIENT

After the decision to provide nutritional support has been made, criteria for patient response to therapy must be established. The parameters should be easily monitored, should provide good data for individual and "trend" analyses, and should not be excessively invasive to the patient. Established patient protocols have been reported in the human literature. Not all parameters are applicable or technically possible in veterinary practice owing to equipment and patient limitations. A scheme of monitoring is presented in Table 17–4, and individual procedures will be described. It should be emphasized that not all procedures may be appropriate for an individual patient; however, the stricter degree of monitoring is beneficial in assessing patient status and response to nutritional support.

Physical parameters are essential to patient evaluation as well as providing clues as to progress during therapy. Weight should be recorded daily. Human values suggest that gains of 0.2 to 0.5 kg/day lean body mass can be expected in a 70-kg adult.[28, 31] Greater daily gains suggest inaccurate weight measurement or accumulation of body fluid.[31] Fluid balance may be quantitated by measuring input and

TABLE 17–4. Monitoring Parameters During Total Parenteral Nutrition

Parameter	Monitoring Frequency
Physical Parameters	
Weight	*
Fluid measurements	
Infusate volume	*
Oral intake	*
Urine output	*
Records of calorie/protein	*
Vital signs	*
Metabolic Parameters	
Hematology	
CBC and platelet count	‡
Total protein and albumin	†
Biochemical profile	
Glucose	§
BUN	§
Creatinine	§
SGPT	‡
Alkaline phosphatase	†
Total bilirubin	†
Sodium, potassium, chlorides, bicarbonate	§
Calcium, magnesium, phosphorus	†
Prealbumin	†
Serum transferrin	‡
Triglycerides-cholesterol (if lipid infusion)	‡
Urinary profile	
Urine glucose	*(4×)
Urinary urea nitrogen (24-hr urine)	‡
Creatinine excretion (24-hr urine)	‡

Notes: * = daily.
      † = semiweekly.
      ‡ = weekly.
      § = daily for initial administration period; semiweekly after stabilization.

output of fluid volume. Records of infused volume, water ingestion, and urine output (sensible water loss) provide information regarding net water balance.[28, 31] In addition to allowing clinical evaluation of hydration status and body weight, these data allow assessment of water metabolism of the patient. Evaluation of vital parameters (temperature, pulse, respiration) may permit early detection of complications such as thrombophlebitis, sepsis, or dyscrasia to therapy.[28, 31] Records of solution composition and protein-calorie ratio provide data relative to the patient's response to current therapy.[12, 28, 31] All of these variables are semiquantitative; however, they allow patient evaluation and provide early indications of potential complications related to therapy.

Metabolic parameters aid in monitoring and quantitating progess during nutritional support. Hematology is valuable in monitoring patient response to possible sepsis and platelet numbers during therapy.[28, 31] Differential counts, leukocyte numbers, and platelet counts are especially beneficial in this re-

spect. Lymphocyte counts may indicate overall immune competence, especially the cell-mediated component.[31] Guidelines in humans suggest mild immune depletion with lymphocyte counts of 1,200 to 2,000 cells/cm³, moderate depletion with 800 to 1,200 cells/cm³, and severe depletion with fewer than 800 cells/cm³.

Biochemical evaluation is useful for assessing therapeutic response. Serum glucose levels indicate patient response to increased carbohydrate substrate during initial therapy.[12, 28, 31] Hyperglycemia is a frequent finding during initial therapy, and serum glucose values aid in preventing complications related to glucose metabolism.[28, 31] Glucose intolerance may be noted in patients with pre-existing stress, malnutrition, sepsis, or diabetes mellitus. Even low levels of glucose infusion may produce abnormal responses in these patients.[64] Creatinine and BUN are valuable in assessing parenteral nutrition. Analysis of BUN quantitates metabolism and elimination of nitrogen by-products delivered as a nutritional component.[31] In addition, BUN indicates renal competence in excretion of the administered protein and amino acid loads. Creatinine may serve a dual role. In addition to indicating renal function, creatinine is an indirect measurement of lean body mass.[31] Creatinine, a by-product of creatine metabolism, reflects hepatic biosynthesis and muscle protein metabolism. During malnutrition, creatinine excretion is proportional to skeletal muscle depletion. In man, approximately 20 mg/kg/day creatinine is excreted in the urine. Assay of urinary creatinine values over a 24-hour period may reveal somatic protein depletion.[12, 31] This analysis of total creatinine excretion can be used to calculate a creatinine excretion index as follows:

$$\text{Creatinine excretion index} = \frac{\text{Actual 24-hour creatinine excretion}}{\text{Predicted 24-hour creatinine excretion}} \times 100$$

Creatinine excretion less than 60 to 80 per cent represents mild somatic protein depletion; 40 to 50 per cent moderate depletion; and less than 40 per cent severe protein depletion. Interpretation of creatinine excretion may be variable between patients and can only be used as a guideline.

Hepatic enzyme values (SGPT, alkaline phosphatase) and total bilirubin are valuable for assessing secondary organ dysfunction from parenteral nutritional support. Monitoring of serum enzyme values provides early detection of morphological change and allows for adjustments in therapy to circumvent further complications.

Electrolyte monitoring is essential for patient assessment during therapy. Balanced amino acid solutions include an electrolyte component based on standard nutritional requirements previously established. Not infrequently, supplementation of one or more electrolytes may be considered in individual therapy. For all these reasons, frequent monitoring of electrolyte components is important during therapy.[12, 28, 31, 69]

Evaluation of visceral protein status may be provided by albumin, serum transferrin, and thyroxin-binding prealbumin levels.[31] All of these proteins are hepatically synthesized, and plasma level alterations can be associated with limitations in substrate supply associated with malnutrition. Serum transferrin is a beta-globulin with a molecular weight of 88,000 to 90,000. It functions in plasma iron transport, binding 1.25 mg ferric ion per gram of protein. Normal values in man range from 250 to 300 mg/dl. The advantage of this protein for assessment of therapy is its relatively short half-life of 8.8 days. Because of this rapid turnover, protein malnutrition is accurately profiled in its early stages and monitored during recovery of protein balance.

Thyroxin-binding prealbumin plays a major role in thyroxin transport. Its serum half-life is estimated to be 48 hours, suggesting rapid reflection of changes in protein status. However, levels may be influenced by trauma, infection, and oral protein ingestion, making its interpretation less reliable.[31] Serum albumin levels may be depressed during stress, infection, neoplasia, thermal injury, and hypothyroidism. Persistence of hypoalbuminemia for longer than seven days is suggestive of nutritional deficiency. Albumin is not useful as an early index of protein deficiency because levels fluctuate slowly with nutritional change owing to a relatively long serum half-life (20 days) and a large circulating pool. However, albumin response is indicative of protein malnutrition and therapeutic response.[31]

If lipid is used in nutritional support, serum values of by-products of lipid metabolism (triglycerides and cholesterol) should be analyzed.[12] Dogs placed on lipid therapy for ten weeks demonstrated increases in serum values of triglycerides and cholesterol as a reflection of therapy.[34] The values stabilized after the fourth week of therapy and returned to baseline after discontinuation of lipid support. Triglycerides rose by 66 per cent and cholesterol by 64 per cent, reflecting increased lipid administration. Marked deviations in these values indicate the need for recalculation of daily lipid therapy.

Biochemical analysis of urine may prove useful in monitoring trends during parenteral nutrition. Analysis of urine glucose is rapid and simple and can provide valuable information relative to patient response to carbohydrate load.[12, 28, 31] Glycosuria may be noted in cases of glucose intolerance related to severe stress, malnutrition, septicemia, diabetes mellitus, and extremes of age. Continuous glycosuria predisposes to osmotic diuresis and the development of hyperglycemic, hyperosmolar, nonketotic acidemia. It is, therefore, best to monitor urine glucose levels frequently during initiation of therapy and to adjust glucose administration accordingly. Tolerance to glucose loading occurs as insulin secretion is stimulated in the first two to three days after initiation of therapy. Adjustments to total glucose, administration rate, and administration of exogenous insulin occur during this period. Conversely, after high glucose

supplementation, tapering of glucose administration is necessary to prevent a hypoglycemic crisis.[28, 31]

Measurement of urinary urea nitrogen and creatinine aids in assessment of nitrogen balance.[31] Urea nitrogen values may provide additional data about overall nitrogen (protein) balance. Increased urea nitrogen excretion reflects increased metabolism of skeletal muscle protein and hepatic synthesis of urea. Assay by the micro-Kjeldahl method for total urinary nitrogen in a 24-hour sample can be used to calculate nitrogen balance using the following formula:

$$N_{bal} = \frac{\text{Protein intake (gm)}}{6.25} = \text{TUN} - 5 \text{ mg N/kg} - 12 \text{ mg N/kg}$$

where

$$\text{TUN} = \text{total urinary nitrogen for 24-hour period,}$$
$$5 \text{ mg N/kg} = \text{insensible N losses, and}$$
$$12 \text{ mg N/kg} = \text{gastrointestinal N losses.}$$

A positive value signifies an anabolic state. Conversely, a negative value indicates catabolism, with 5 to 10 gm/day representing mild, 10 to 15 gm/day moderate, and 15 gm/day or greater severe catabolism. This analysis, in conjunction with urinary creatinine, can provide an overview of protein metabolism in the parenteral nutrition patient.[31]

It should be re-emphasized that not all of the previously mentioned evaluations may be available, necessary, or appropriate for a particular therapeutic protocol. They represent what is available and, in most cases, reasonable for veterinary patients receiving parenteral nutrition. The greater the number of parameters one can monitor, the better the overall assessment and understanding of the patients' response to therapy.

COMPLICATIONS OF PARENTERAL NUTRITION

Catheter-related Complications

Sepsis

Chronic catheter implantation has been reported to be associated with numerous complications, many of which are preventable with good catheter care. Cannula sepsis, thrombophlebitis, air embolism, and vascular occlusion have been reported.[39-41, 61, 62] Catheter-related sepsis is the most frequent complication.[22, 29, 62, 74] Inadequate preparation or maintenance of the catheter site may result in bacterial or fungal sepsis. In the dog, gram-negative species account for the majority of contaminants in inadequately prepared venipuncture sites.[10] In man, cultures of catheters withdrawn after administration of parenteral nutrition showed fungi as the predominant catheter-related contaminant.[29, 62] *Candida* species were most frequently isolated; however, a low incidence of *Staphylococcus*, *Klebsiella*, and *Pseudomonas* spp. was also noted. Antibiotic ointments in the occlusive dressings and amino acid base solutions inhibited bacterial growth but allowed for fungal multiplication.[39] Occlusive dressings with antimicrobial agents (tame iodophor ointment) have been recommended to inhibit both bacterial and fungal sepsis.[29]

Unexplained pyrexia, leukocytosis, chills, glucose intolerance, alterations in level of consciousness, and generalized deterioration of condition are all clinical signs noted with sepsis.[61, 62] Hematogenous dissemination from a septic anatomical site may be an additional contributing factor. It should be determined whether sepsis is catheter-related or secondary to an anatomical site. Catheter-related sepsis is usually noted shortly after implantation. Fibrin sheaths surround the catheter during the first three to five days following implantation.[31, 62] After this time, bacterial colonization of the catheter from remote sites is difficult.[31] Introduction of cutaneous organisms during venipuncture and migration from the venipuncture site down the catheter shaft have been suggested as contributing to catheter sepsis.[29] If catheter-related sepsis is suspected, removal of the administration system and solution container is mandatory.

Antibiotic infusion through a contaminated catheter is not therapeutic.[31, 62] After removal, culture of the catheter, administration apparatus, and solution is suggested. In man, removal of a contaminated catheter is accompanied by remission of pyrexia in 12 to 24 hours.[31] The patient can be maintained on 5% dextrose administered by peripheral catheter during this time. If remission continues for 48 hours, a new catheter can be safely placed and parenteral nutrition re-established.[31] In cases of refractory pyrexia (greater than 24 hours) or secondary catheter sepsis from a remote anatomical site, antibiotics should be administered if not previously initiated for other reasons.[31, 62] Blood cultures should also be considered in cases of refractory fever. Total parenteral nutrition should not be discontinued in the presence of a secondary septic site; rather, the primary septic focus should be treated by appropriate medical or surgical therapy.

Thrombophlebitis

Thrombophlebitis and vascular occlusion have been associated with chronic catheterization.[11, 62, 71] Chemical and mechanical factors may predispose to the complication. Hypertonic solutions may induce endothelial irritation and stimulate platelet accumulation.[75] Peripheral veins are especially susceptible owing to the disparity between catheter diameter and venous lumen. This disparity predisposes the venous lumen to low blood flow and retarded dilution of hypertonic solutions, allowing for vascular irritation and thrombophlebitis.[75] Mechanical injury to endothelium from catheter placement may additionally create or augment this complication.[75] Central catheter placement minimizes these factors, but thrombophlebitis and vascular occlusion have been reported with central catheter placement.[18-21, 62] Canine studies using hypertonic glucose solutions with chronic catheter implantation (longer than 21 days) suggest a high incidence of complications.[11] Seven of ten dogs exhibited thrombosis of the vena cava at postmortem examination. Fibrosis of endothelium at the catheter tip was also demonstrated in four dogs. All dogs studied remained clinically normal. One study in man reports postmortem signs of vascular thrombosis in patients supported by parenteral nutrition methods.[62] However, only one patient in this study died as a result of vascular thrombosis.

Several recommendations have been proposed to minimize thrombophlebitis. A study comparing four catheter materials showed a lower incidence of complications when fluoroethylenepropylene or Silastic was used as a catheter material.[71] These materials are superior to plastic, polyvinylchloride, and tetrafluoroethylene as a catheter material. The addition of heparin (500 units) and hydrocortisone (1 mg/L parenteral solution) decreased thrombophlebitis in peripheral veins.[71] Inline filtering to prevent infusion of particulate matter was noted to decrease vascular complications. Venipuncture may also be noted to create mechanical injury and tissue thromboplastin release. This injury secondarily creates platelet aggregation and promotes thrombus formation.[71] Attention to these details as well as appropriate skin preparation decreases the incidence of thrombophlebitis in parenteral nutrition patients.[10]

Metabolic Complications

Initiation and maintenance of parenteral nutrition may be accompanied by metabolic responses different from those expected with oral nutrition. Some responses are not complications per se but patient responses to aggressive nutritional management and can be anticipated and safely managed as they become evident.

Glucose Metabolism

High-level glucose concentrations used in total parenteral nutrition require physiological accommodation to be utilized efficiently. Pancreatic responses to therapy, i.e., increased insulin release to assimilate this additional metabolic load, occur in most cases.[28] However, certain patients show intolerance to increased glucose loads owing to existing metabolic changes. Patients with severe stress, trauma, septicemia, diabetes, and chronic malnutrition may exhibit insulin-related changes that inhibit glucose assimilation.[2, 28, 31] Diminished blood levels of insulin or the presence of insulin resistance due to increased plasma levels of catecholamines, glucocorticoids, and glucagon may retard glucose uptake.[5, 66] Data for metabolic alterations in domestic animals with similar signs are currently unavailable; however, similar responses would be expected. In studies using healthy dogs supported with total parenteral nutrition, acute glucose intolerance with initiation of therapy has not been reported; however, stressed, injured, or septic animals have not been studied.[11] Alteration in patient acceptance of increased glucose administration may result in hyperglycemia, glycosuria, or hyperosmolar, nonketotic dehydration.[28, 31] These complications can be circumvented or managed if recognized early. Several precautions should be observed relative to glucose metabolism during the initial stages of total parenteral nutrition:

1. Blood and urine glucose levels should be monitored during the first 24 to 72 hours after initiation of parenteral nutrition.[28, 31, 66] Glucose oxidase (Tes-Tape) for urine glucose assessment is less influenced by the urinary presence of other drugs.[31] If blood glucose levels remain elevated (> 250 gm/dl) or 4+ urine glucose levels persist during adjustments in administration rate, changes in support should be considered, including altering the glucose concentration of the solution, adding crystalline insulin (10 IU/1000 calories dextrose), or changing calorie sources from carbohydrate to lipid.[28, 31, 66] If sudden changes in glucose levels occur in a patient during therapy after stabilization, other underlying causes, e.g., sepsis, should be suspected.[28]

2. If signs of persistent glycosuria, polyuria, dehydration, or altered states of consciousness (stupor, confusion, coma) are noted in the first 24 hours after initiation of therapy, nonketotic hyperosmolar acidosis may have developed.[31] This syndrome can be accompanied by a mortality rate of 40 to 50 per cent in man, and early diagnosis and aggressive therapy are indicated. Re-establishment of fluid balance using 0.45% NaCl with 20 mEq/L potassium should be initiated. Regular insulin should be administered at a rate of 5 to 10 units/hr to decrease glucose levels, and administration of sodium bicarbonate to treat acidemia is recommended. As glucose levels diminish, polyuria should diminish concurrently with blood and urine glucose levels. Caution should be exercised to prevent rapid fluctuations in glucose levels because hypotension, diminished intravascular volume, and cerebral edema may occur.[31] If laboratory data are available, serum osmolality may be calculated by the following formula:

$$\text{mOsm/Kg} = 1.86\,\text{Na} + \frac{\text{Glucose}}{18} + \frac{\text{BUN}}{2.8}$$

3. Refractive glucosuria during therapy may signify electrolyte imbalance. Sodium, potassium, chromium, and manganese level alterations have all been associated with glucose intolerance and should be monitored during therapy. Correction of these electrolyte levels is usually accompanied by a more normal blood glucose concentration.[31]

Abrupt discontinuation of parenteral nutrition may be accompanied by a hypoglycemic crisis.[28, 31] This is related to an increased secretion of endogenous insulin in response to an augmented glucose load.

Hypoglycemia may be noted as soon as one-half hour after interruption of nutritional support. It is advisable to "taper" glucose administration over several days to prevent this complication.[28, 31] Substitution of 5% dextrose is satisfactory for 24 hours prior to catheter withdrawal or in cases of interruption of nutritional support. Patients on lipid support do not appear to react in a similar fashion, and discontinuation of lipids is more elective.[35, 46]

Amino Acid Metabolism

Complications related to protein solutions have been described during parenteral nutrition. These complications may be resolved by altering the composition of the administered solution or by adjusting the infusion schedule.

Acidosis may be noted with infusion of chloride salts of crystalline amino acids. Metabolism of amino acid salts in the tricarboxylic acid cycle results in liberation of free hydrogen anion plus chloride cation, resulting in metabolic acidosis.[16, 28, 31, 59, 61, 66] Metabolites of the amino acids arginine, histidine, and lysine have been specifically documented as participating in this process. Formulations of amino acid solutions initially contained a high proportion of chloride salts. Newer products utilize acetate salts to minimize this effect. Guidelines for maintaining a 1:1 ratio of sodium to chloride to circumvent excessive chloride concentrations have been proposed.[31] Lactate, acetate, and phosphate salts are suggested alternatives.

In addition to acidosis related to chloride salts, both protein hydrolysates and amino acid solutions contain fixed acidity. Protein hydrolysates may have a pH of 2.5 to 3.5, thereby contributing to total acidity. Individuals with renal or pulmonary disease should be closely monitored for acid-base equilibrium when protein hydrolysates are used.[8, 31]

Hyperammonemia is an uncommon complication of protein metabolism.[25, 28, 31, 59, 61] Hyperammonemia may occur in patients with hepatic or renal disease as well as newborns with immature metabolic pathways. An altered metabolism of essential amino acids with diminished conversion of ammonia to urea is the mechanism involved. Arginine deficiency or high glycine concentration in protein solutions contributes to this complication.[25, 31] Clinical signs are similar to those seen in other syndromes with elevated blood ammonia levels and include alteration in mental state, seizures, and limb clonus. Recent research in protein metabolism suggests that branch chain amino acids may reduce hyperammonemia in patients with limited metabolic capacity.[31, 69]

Occasionally, parenteral solutions may induce prerenal azotemia.[28] Usually, correction of hydration status and reduction in administered protein levels correct this problem. All patients may experience increased BUN during parenteral nutrition; however, these values usually remain within normal limits.

Lipid Metabolism

Complications related to lipid metabolism should be categorized according to inclusion or exclusion of lipid substrates in the formula. In dietary configurations that include only nitrogen and carbohydrate substrates, essential fatty acid deficiency may be noted.[30, 43] Arachidonic, linoleic, and linolenic acids are essential fatty acids and must be supplied.[30, 43, 66] In man, provision of linoleic acid is critical, as this fatty acid may undergo biotransformation to produce arachidonic acid. The role of linolenic acid is not entirely clear in either animals or man.[30] Exclusion of essential fatty acids alters the ratio of triene:tetraene base fatty acids; analysis of this ratio has been beneficial in understanding fat metabolism.[30] In all patients surveyed, weekly assays suggest the development of an essential fatty acid deficiency by four weeks after fat free dietary support as well as a high degree of alteration in the triene:tetraene ratio by two to three weeks after initiation of lipid-free therapy. Abnormalities of the triene:tetraene may be noted as early as three days after therapy is instituted.[66] The rapid development of fatty acid deficiency is postulated to be a result of carbohydrate supplementation. Increased glucose administration stimulates insulin release. Insulin depresses lipolysis, thereby diminishing the release of free fatty acids from storage sites. Growing animals and humans may show early alteration in triene:tetraene ratios owing to growth processes and a high rate of fatty acid metabolism.[30] Lipid supplementation should be provided weekly to circumvent the development of essential fatty acid abnormalities. No correlation between alteration in the fatty acid triene:tetraene ratio and the emergence of clinical signs of essential fatty acid deficiency has been described; however, an altered triene:tetraene ratio indicated fatty acid deficiency.

Clinical signs of fatty acid deficiency are multisystemic.[31] Essential fatty acids are crucial in cholesterol ester and phospholipid components of plasma and mitochondrial lipoproteins. They play a significant role in membrane structure and transport processes. Deficiency decreases calorie utilization, dissociates oxidative phosphorylation, and decreases high-energy phosphate bond formation. Clinical signs of chronic deficiency include dermatological abnormalities of both hair follicle and skin cells, diarrhea, retardation of wound healing, immune depression, and osteoporosis. Biological changes may include decreased cholesterol levels, thrombocytopenia, platelet changes, anemia and increased red cell fragility, increased capillary permeability, and elevated hepatic enzyme levels related to hepatomegaly. Treatment is the provision of essential fatty acids through exogenous sources. Oral ingestion of corn or safflower oil (10 to 15 ml/day) is recommended, and topical application may also be considered.[31] Alternatively, lipid may be included in the dietary formulation on a therapeutic basis.[30] Since serum fatty acid levels can be altered in as little as three days after deprivation, fatty acid support should be considered from the onset of therapy.

Administration of soybean oil–based fat emulsions (Intralipid) or soyflower oil–based emulsions (Liposyn) has been extensively studied for toxicity in both humans and animals.[34, 35] Complications associated with lipid administration may be divided into acute and chronic reactions. Acute reactions are generally transient and may include tachycardia, hypotension, tachypnea, precordial pain, pyrexia, paralumbar pain, and emesis,[35] especially with older lipid preparations. Currently available sources appear to carry a significantly lower incidence of these reactions. Anaphylaxis has not been reported as an acute response to infusions.[35]

Signs may also be noted with excessive administration rates of these products. No explanation for this mechanism has been described. Chronic administration of lipid emulsions has produced several clinical and organ dysfunction syndromes. Elevation in hepatic enzymes, hepatomegaly, brown pigmentation (lipofuscin) of Kupffer cells, intrahepatic lipidosis and cholestasis, hyperbilirubinemia, thrombocytopenia, leukopenia, eosinophilia, hyponatremia, anemia, splenomegaly, and thrombophlebitis have all been reported with lipid administration.[4, 9, 34, 35] Intrahepatic lipidosis and lipofuscin deposition in reticuloendothelial tissue are generally noted with lipid infusion.[70] The significance of these findings is unclear at the present time, although one author alludes to immune competence alterations in patients supported by lipid solutions.[33]

Similar signs may be acutely noted with excessive administration rates of lipid solutions (overloading syndrome). Hemorrhage, pyrexia, emesis, altered coagulation profile, and thrombocytopenia may also be noted.[35] Most of these signs are reversible with discontinuation of lipid support; however, chronic pigmentation of RE cells remains.[33] Fat emulsions are contraindicated in patients with lipid metabolism abnormalities concurrent with diseases such as pancreatitis, hepatic disease, coagulation disorders and thrombocytopenia, diabetes mellitus, and pulmonary disease.[17]

Electrolytes and Minerals

Electrolyte abnormalities have been noted when solution preparations do not include electrolyte supplementation. This complication may be prevented by providing electrolytes as a standard solution component. Many commercially available amino acid solutions contain balanced electrolytes. However, if electrolytes are not incorporated, hypophosphatemia and magnesium imbalance may be clinically noted.[28, 31, 66]

Hypophosphatemia may develop in the patient supported by parenteral nutrition without phosphorus supplementation.[28, 31, 38, 66] With lowered serum phosphorus levels, alterations in acid-base status may affect intracellular phosphorylation of carbohydrates.

Competition may exist between phosphorus-binding drugs (magnesium and aluminum hydroxide antacids) and phosphorus, altering phosphorus bioavailability. Primary diseases in which phosphorus may be a component (hyperparathyroidism, Fanconi syndrome, renal disease) may also influence phosphorus conservation.[31] Magnesium imbalance may also be associated with altered phosphorus levels. Alterations may be noted as soon as 24 hours after initiation of parenteral nutrition and may reflect acute incorporation of phosphorus into somatic protein after conversion to an anabolic state.[28, 31] Clinical signs of hypophosphatemia are usually noted when the serum concentration of inorganic phosphorus is less than 1.0 mg/dl and is always noted when serum values are less than 0.5 mg/dl.[31] Signs include tachycardia, muscle weakness, extremity tremors, paresthesia, anisocoria, mental depression, and hyperventilation.[31, 66] Laboratory studies show diminished red cell and platelet function related to depletion of ATP and red cell membrane rigidity.[31] Shifts in the oxyhemoglobin dissociation curve due to alteration in 2,3 DPG will affect oxygen-carrying capacity.[28] White blood cell chemotaxis and phagocytosis are also impaired. Indications of decreased myocardial stroke work have also been described.[31]

The treatment of hypophosphatemia is the inclusion of phosphorus salts. Recommendations in man range from 3 to 17 mmol potassium dihydrate phosphate per 1000 Kcal.[31] Most authors recommend 7 to 9 mmol/1000 Kcal.[31] Supplementation of phosphorus should be accompanied by 0.2 to 0.3 mEq calcium per liter to circumvent tetany related to hypocalcemia.

Magnesium plays a vital role in a broad spectrum of physiological functions. Oxidative phosphorylation, stabilization of DNA and RNA, high-energy phosphate transfer, and myocardial integrity all rely on adequate magnesium levels. Hypomagnesemia (<1.0 mEq/L) due to inadequate dietary supplementation may be clinically noted by signs of musculoskeletal fasciculation, tremor, and spasticity; generalized muscle weakness; depression; nausea; vomiting; and electrocardiographic changes in the ST segment.[31] Many signs are similar to other (calcium, phosphorus) electrolyte imbalances and require laboratory confirmation. The treatment of hypomagnesemia is the inclusion of magnesium salts in the dietary formulation. Therapeutic administration of magnesium sulfate will relieve clinical signs noted with magnesium depletion.[31]

Renal failure patients may exhibit magnesium retention if parenteral nutrition is used.[31] Amino acid solutions formulated for renal patients exclude magnesium. Signs of hypermagnesemia include drowsiness, hyporeflexia, muscle paresis, and electrical conduction disturbances evidenced by prolonged QT interval, atrioventricular block, or cardiac arrest. Administration of 10% calcium gluconate is temporary therapy, however; serum levels must be reduced by improved renal function.

Chronic parenteral support may be accompanied by trace mineral deficiencies—zinc, manganese, copper, iodine, and chromate. This does not suggest that other trace elements are less important, as iron, selenium, cobalt, and others have been documented as essential. Zinc has been noted, under certain circumstances, to be deficient after one week of nutritional support.[28, 42, 66] Other trace minerals vary in time until deficiency states exist. Specific supplementation of trace elements is suggested to prevent deficiency.[66]

Vitamins

The parenteral nutrition patient should be regularly supplemented with a multiple vitamin preparation.[31] Fat-soluble vitamins (especially vitamin K) should be administered on a regular basis by parenteral injection at a tissue site.

Physiological Complications

Administration of increased carbohydrate loads and acetate salts has been documented to increase carbon dioxide production as metabolism occurs. This increased production raises the respiratory quotient from a base of 0.8 toward unity and results in increased alveolar ventilation, minute gas exchange, altered oxygenation, and increased carbon dioxide levels.[3, 5, 14] Patients without underlying respiratory disease may adapt to this alteration through central and peripheral neurogenic input and augmented ventilatory exchange. However, this augmentation increases the work of breathing and requires a greater percentage of total available energy for respiratory gas exchange. When pre-existing pulmonary disease is present, compensatory changes may not be available, and carbon dioxide retention occurs with respiratory acidosis.[3, 5, 14] The inability to satisfactorily augment minute ventilation ultimately leads to fatigue of respiratory muscles and respiratory failure, requiring ventilatory support. Reduction of nonprotein calories delivered by carbohydrate and inclusion of lipid calories have been advanced to minimize this complication.[3, 14] Altered pulmonary membrane diffusing capacity with lipid administration has also been described; however, this finding is not consistent in all studies.[51]

An alteration in hepatic enzymes may be noted with parenteral nutrition. In both human and animal studies, elevations in SGPT, SGOT, alkaline phosphatase, and bilirubin have been demonstrated.[6, 31, 47, 67] In patients and experimental animals who have demonstrated enzyme elevations and who have undergone hepatic biopsy or tissue section, periportal steatosis, fatty infiltration, intrahepatic cholestasis, bile duct proliferation, and canalicular occlusion and pigmentation were noted histologically.[6, 31, 47, 67] Most of these changes were reversible, although one patient had residual elevation in hepatic enzymes and periportal fibrosis on repeated biopsy.[67] Several theories have been forwarded for these observations. An imbalance of the amino acid:dextrose ratio may account for fatty infiltration similar to malnutrition of protein origin (kwashiorkor). Experimental studies in rats fed glucose as the sole calorie source confirm fatty changes in hepatic architecture. Deprivation of lipotrophic substances (choline) or amino acids (methionine) may impede lipid metabolism and retard hepatic redistribution of lipid.[67] The chemical interaction of tryptophan and the antioxidant sodium bisulfite present in all commercial amino acid solutions may result in toxic by-products that may produce a toxic hepatitis.[31, 67] A deficiency in essential fatty acids may damage cell membranes and produce liver function abnormalities.[67] This has been noted in dogs supported by total parenteral nutrition. It has been suggested that an incomplete understanding of all metabolic interactions occurs, and present formulations remain imperfect. Clinical improvement has been noted when decreased carbohydrate loads are administered, re-adjustment of the carbohydrate:amino acid ratio producing a beneficial response.[47, 67] Inclusion of soybean oil emulsion may also be helpful. Cyclic parenteral nutrition (16 hours per day) may also aid in reversal of signs.[31] Clinical judgment and hepatic monitoring dictate the necessary management techniques.

The ultimate complication is failure to provide adequate nutritional support.[31] Failure to achieve positive nitrogen balance, weight gain, and electrolyte balance despite administration of calculated requirements suggests inadequate support. In many cases, the patient is hypermetabolic and additional nutrition is required. However, an occasional case may require hormonal support. Insulin supplementation may be beneficial in low doses to stimulate anabolism. A high insulin:glucagon ratio favors glycogenolysis, tissue synthesis, and nitrogen retention, all favorable to anabolism. Demonstration of improved nitrogen retention as an index of anabolism during insulin supplementation has been described.

SUMMARY

Support by parenteral nutrition is in its infancy in all medical disciplines. We still do not fully understand the interaction of numerous biochemical pathways and their response to dietary supplementation. The goals of this chapter have been to introduce the topic to veterinary surgery, describe current philosophy and practice, and examine its shortcomings and potential complications. Further details may be obtained from the accompanying references.

1. Abbott, W. M.: Indications for parenteral nutrition. In Fischer, J. E. (ed.): Total Parenteral Nutrition. Little, Brown, Boston, 1976, p. 3.
2. Askanazi, J., Carpentier, Y. A., Elwyn, D. H., et al.: Influence of total parenteral nutrition on fuel utilization in injury and sepsis. Ann. Surg. 191:40, 1974.
3. Askanazi, J., Weissman, C., Rosenbaum, S. H., et al.: Nutrition and the respiratory system. Crit. Care Med. 10:163, 1982.
4. Barness, L. A., Dallman, P. R., and Anderson, H.: Use of intravenous fat emulsions in pediatric patients. Pediatrics 68:738, 1981.
5. Biebuyck, J.: Nutritional state: Implications for anesthesiologists and use of hyperalimentation. Annual Refresher Courses, Am. Soc. Anesth. 31:112, 1980.
6. Black, D. D., Suttle, A., Whitington, P. F., et al.: The effect of short-term parenteral nutrition in the neonate: A prospective randomized study demonstrating alteration of hepatic canalicular function. Pediatrics 99:445, 1981.
7. Blackburn, G. L., Bistrian, B. R., Maini, B. S., et al.: Nutritional and metabolic assessment of the hospitalized patient. J.P.E.N. 1:11, 1977.
8. Blackburn, G. L., Flatt, J. P., and Hensle, T. W.: Peripheral amino acid solutions. In Fischer, J. E. (ed.): Total Parenteral Nutrition. Little, Brown, Boston, 1976, p. 363.
9. Bryan, H., Shenna, A., Griffin, E., et al.: Intralipid—Its rational use in parenteral nutrition of the newborn. Pediatrics 58:787, 1976.
10. Burrows, C. F.: Inadequate skin preparation as a cause of intravenous catheter-related infection in the dog. J. Am. Vet. Med. Assoc. 180:747, 1982.
11. Carter, J. M., and Freedman, A. B.: Total intravenous feeding in the dog. Am. J. Vet. Res. 171:71, 1977.
12. Cerra, F. B.: Adult Parenteral Nutrition Monitoring. Univ. of Minnesota Hospitals, Form PS01-936, 1983.
13. Clinite, J.: Personnal communication, 1982.
14. Covelli, H. D., Black, W., Olsen, M. S., et al.: Respiratory failure precipitated by high carbohydrate loads. Ann. Intern. Med. 95:579, 1981.
15. Cuthbertson, D. P.: Protein requirements after injury—Quality and quantity. In Wilkinson, A. W. (ed.): Parenteral Nutrition. Williams & Wilkins, Baltimore, 1971, p. 4.
16. Daly, J. M., and Long, J. M.: Intravenous hyperalimentation: Techniques and potential complications. Surg. Clin. North Am., 61:583, 1981.
17. Das, J. B., Joshi, I. D., and Philippart, A. I.: Intralipid intolerance in pancreatitis: The role of hepatic triglyceride lipase in plasma clearance of the lipid emulsion. J. Pediatr. Surg. 16:1021, 1981.
18. Dudrick, S. J., Copeland, E. M., and MacFayden, B. V.: Hyperalimentation in infants. Z. Ernährungswiss. 15:9, 1976.
19. Dudrick, S. J., Sterger, E., Wilmore, D. W., et al.: Continuous long-term intravenous infusion in unrestrained animals. Lab. Anim. Care 20:521, 1970.
20. Dudrick, S. J., Wilmore, D. W., and Vars, H. M.: Long-term parenteral nutrition with growth in puppies and positive nitrogen balance in patients. Surg. Forum 18:356, 1967.
21. Dudrick, S. J., Wilmore, D. W., Vars, H. M., et al.: Long-term total parenteral nutrition with growth, development, and positive nitrogen balance. Surgery 64:134, 1968.
22. Freeman, J. B., Lemire, A., and MacLean, L. D.: Intravenous alimentation and septicemia. Surg. Gynecol. Obstet. 135:708, 1972.
23. Freeman, J. B., and MacLean, L. D.: Intravenous hyperalimentation: A review. Can. J. Surg. 14:180, 1971.
24. Froesch, E. R., and Keller, U.: Review of energy metabolism with particular reference to the metabolism of glucose, fructose, sorbitol, xylitol and of their therapeutic use in parenteral nutrition. In Wilkinson, A. W. (ed.): Parenteral Nutrition. Williams & Wilkins, Baltimore, 1971, p. 105.
25. Ghandimi, G. H.: Conventional amino acid solutions for parenteral use. In Ghandimi, G. H. (ed.): Total Parenteral Nutrition. John Wiley and Sons, New York, 1975, p. 373.
26. Ghandimi, G. H., and Tejani, A.: Protein and amino acid requirements. In Ghandimi, G. H. (ed.): Total Parenteral Nutrition. John Wiley and Sons, New York, 1975, p. 213.
27. Glancy, J. J., Fishbone, G., and Hanz, E. K.: Nonthrombogenic arterial catheters. Am. J. Roentgenol., 108:716, 1970.
28. Goldfarb, I. W., and Yates, A. P.: Total Parenteral Nutrition:

Concepts and Methods. Synapse Publications, Pittsburgh, 1978.

29. Goldmann, D. A., and Maki, D. G.: Infection control in total parenteral nutrition. J. Am. Med. Assoc., *223*:1360, 1973.

30. Goodgame, J. T., Lowry, S. F., and Brennan, M. F.: Essential fatty acid deficiency in total parenteral nutrition: Time course of development and suggestions for therapy. Surgery *84*:271, 1978.

31. Grant, J. P.: *Handbook of Total Parenteral Nutrition.* W. B. Saunders, Philadelphia, 1980.

32. Grant, J. P., Custer, P. B., and Thurlow, J.: Current techniques of nutritional assessment. Surg. Clin. North Am. *61*:437, 1981.

33. Grotte, G., Jacobson, S., and Wretlind, A.: Lipid emulsions and technique of peripheral administration in parenteral nutrition. *In* Fischer, J. E. (ed.): *Total Parenteral Nutrition.* Little, Brown, Boston, 1976, p. 335.

34. Hokansson, I., Holm, I., and Wretlind, A.: Studies of complete intravenous alimentation in dogs. Nutr. Diet. *8*:1, 1966.

35. Hansen, L. M., Hardie, W. R., and Hildago, J.: Fat emulsion for intravenous administration: Clinical experience with Intralipid 10%. Ann. Surg. *184*:80, 1976.

36. Hardy, G., Cotter, R., and Dawe, R.: Physical and metabolic stability of 10% lipid emulsion admixed in a total parenteral nutrition regimen. Submitted for publication, 1983.

37. Hend, W. C., MacMillan, R. W., and Winters, R. W.: Total parenteral nutrition in the pediatric patient. *In* Fischer, J. E. (ed.): *Total Parenteral Nutrition.* Little, Brown, Boston, 1976, p. 253.

38. Hyman, A. I.: Hyperalimentation and the surgical patient. Annual Refresher Courses, Am. Soc. Anesth. *32*:142, 1981.

39. Kaminski, M. V.: *Parenteral Hyperalimentation: Prevention and Treatment of Complications.* Walter Reed General Hospital Hyperalimentation Registry, Washington, D.C., November, 1972.

40. Kaminski, M. V., and Harris, D. F.: Prolonged uncomplicated intravascular catheterization. Am. J. IV Ther. *3*:19, 1976.

41. Kaminski, M. V., and Stoler, M. H.: Parenteral hyperalimentation—a quality of care survey and review. Am. J. Hosp. Pharm. *31*:228, 1974.

42. Kay, R. G., Tasman-Jones, C., Pybus, J., et al.: A syndrome of acute zinc deficiency during total parenteral alimentation in man. Ann. Surg. *183*:331, 1976.

43. Kellenberger, T. A., Johnson, T. A., and Zaske, D. E.: Essential fatty acid deficiency: A consequence of fat-free total parenteral nutrition. Am. J. Hosp. Pharm. *36*:230, 1979.

44. Ladefoged, K., Berthelsen, P., Brockner-Nielsen, J., et al.: Fructose, xylitol and glucose in total parenteral nutrition. Intensive Care Med. *8*:19, 1982.

45. Law, D. H.: Total parenteral nutrition. N. Engl. J. Med. *297*:1104, 1977.

46. Lindholm, M., and Rissner, S.: Rate of elimination of the intralipid fat emulsion from the circulation in ICU patients. Crit. Care Med. *10*:740, 1982.

47. Lindor, K. D., Fleming, C. R., Abrams, A., et al.: Liver function values in adults receiving total parenteral nutrition. J. Am. Med. Assoc. *241*:2393, 1979.

48. Lipton, M. J., Doherty, P. W., Goodwin, D. A., et al.: Evaluation of catheter thrombogenicity *in vivo* with indium-labeled platelets. Radiology 135:191, 1980.

49. Long, C. L., Schaffel, N., Geiger, J. W., et al.: Metabolic response to injury and illness: Estimation of energy and protein needs from indirect calorimetry and nitrogen balance. J.P.E.N. *3*:452, 1979.

50. Mather, G. W., and Parlin, M. A.: *Feeding Hospitalized Canine Patients.* Gaines Professional Services, White Plains, NY, 1979.

51. Meng, H. C.: Fat emulsions in parenteral nutrition. *In* Fischer, J. E. (ed.): *Total Parenteral Nutrition.* Little, Brown, Boston, 1976, p. 305.

52. Munro, H. N.: Amino acid requirements and metabolism and their relevance to parenteral nutrition. *In* Wilkinson, A. W. (ed.): *Parenteral Nutrition.* Williams & Wilkins, Baltimore, 1971, p. 34.

53. *Nutrient Requirements of Cats. Nutrient Requirements of Domestic Animals*, Vol. 13. National Academy of Sciences, Washington, D.C., 1978.

54. *Nutrient Requirements of Dogs. Nutrient Requirements of Domestic Animals*, Vol. 8. National Academy of Sciences, Washington, D.C., 1974.

55. Ota, D. M., Imbembo, A. L., and Zuidema, G. D.: Total parenteral nutrition. Surgery 83:503, 1978.

56. Pelham, L. D.: Rational use of intravenous fat emulsions. Am. J. Hosp. Pharm. *38*:198, 1981.

57. Peters, W. R., Bush, W. H., Jr., McIntyre, R. D., et al.: The development of fibrin sheath on indwelling venous catheters. Surg. Gynecol. Obstet. *137*:43, 1973.

58. Renegar, W. R., Stoll, S. G., Bojrab, M. J., et al.: Parenteral hyperalimentation—The use of lipid as the prime calorie source. J. Am. Anim. Hosp. Assoc. *14*:411, 1979.

59. Rosen, H. M.: Types of solutions available. *In* Fischer, J. E. (ed.): *Total Parenteral Nutrition.* Little, Brown, Boston, 1976, p. 15.

60. Rubecz, I., Mestyan, J., and Varga, P.: Energy metabolism, substrate utilization, and nitrogen balance in parenterally fed postoperative neonates and infants. J. Pediatr. *98*:42, 1981.

61. Ryan, J. A., Jr.: Complications of total parenteral nutrition. *In* Fischer, J. E. (ed.): *Total Parenteral Nutrition.* Little, Brown, Boston, 1976, p. 55.

62. Ryan, J. A., Jr.: Abel, R. M., Abbott, D. M., et al.: Catheter complications in total parenteral nutrition. N. Engl. J. Med. *290*:757, 1974.

63. Sauve, F. S., Sr.: Preparation of solutions for hyperalimentation. Can. J. Hosp. Pharm. 8:60, 1972.

64. Schultis, K., and Baisbarth, H.: Post-traumatic energy metabolism. *In* Wilkinson, A. W. (ed.): *Parenteral Nutrition.* Williams & Wilkins, Baltimore, 1971, p. 225.

65. Schlossman, D.: Thrombogenic properties of vascular catheter materials, in vivo. Acta Radiol. *14*:186, 1973.

66. Sheldon, G. F.: Hyperalimentation: Its rationale and effect on anesthetic management. Annual Refresher Courses, Am. Soc. Anesth. *30*:120, 1979.

67. Sheldon, G. F., Petersen, S. R., and Sanders, R.: Hepatic dysfunction during hyperalimentation. Arch. Surg. *113*:504, 1978.

68. Stein, T. P., and Buzby, G. P.: Protein metabolism in surgical patients. Surg. Clin. North Am. *61*:519, 1981.

69. Teasley, K. M.: *Parenteral Nutrition Preparations.* Pharmacology Therapeutics Conference, Univ. of Minnesota Medical School, 1982.

70. Thompson, S. W.: *The Pathology of Parenteral Nutrition with Lipids.* Charles C Thomas, Springfield, IL, 1974.

71. Turco, S. J.: Infusion phlebitis: Pathogenesis remains unclear, but preventive measures emerge from many studies. Crit. Care Monitor 2:6, 1982.

72. Walters, J. M., and Freeman, J. B.: Parenteral nutrition by peripheral vein. Surg. Clin. North Am. *61*:593, 1981.

73. White, P. L., and Nagy, M. E. (eds.): *Total Parenteral Nutrition.* Publishing Sciences Group, Acton, MA, 1974.

74. Wilkinson, A. W.: Complications of parenteral feeding. *In* Wilkinson, A. W. (ed.): *Parenteral Nutrition.* Williams & Wilkins, Baltimore, 1971, p. 242.

75. Wilmore, D. W., and Dudrick, S. J.: Safe long-term venous catheterization. Arch. Surg. *98*:256, 1969.

76. Wolfe, B. M., and Chock, E.: Energy sources, stores, and hormonal contacts. Surg. Clin. North Am. *61*:509, 1981.

77. Wretlind, A.: Modern principles of the use of fat emulsions in parenteral nutrition. *In* Wilkinson, A. W. (ed.): *Parenteral Nutrition.* Williams & Wilkins, Baltimore, 1971, p. 160.

18 Preoperative Consideration of the Surgical Patient

Roy T. Faulkner

Evaluation of the surgical patient prior to an operative procedure should not be taken lightly; it could be the most important step in the entire surgical plan. The surgeon must confirm that a surgical problem exists. In addition, the degree of urgency for surgical intervention not only affects the extent of the preoperative evaluation but also the amount of time available to institute and treat any concurrent medical problems. Although a chronic condition, such as malnutrition, may not be corrected prior to an operation, recognition of the problem is an important aspect of the preoperative evaluation. The management of the problem must be planned preoperatively so that the patient will have a successful operative and postoperative course. On the other hand, certain deficiencies vital to the successful outcome of the surgery may be corrected prior to surgical intervention.

OPERATIVE RISK

The assessment of operative risk is a significant part of the surgeon's preoperative evaluation. Factors including age of the patient, benefits of surgical intervention compared with outcome without surgery, urgency of the situation, nature of the clinical problem, anticipated duration of the surgical procedure, and concurrent medical problems must be considered in assessing operative risk. Major organ systems that influence the degree of operative risk include the cardiovascular, respiratory, renal, and gastrointestinal. Multiple organ system malfunction may be present in older patients. Impairment of more than one organ system may profoundly influence the operative risk. The effects of multiple organ system disease may be so significant as to eliminate the patient from surgical consideration. Although good clinical judgment, which is mainly gained through experience, is inherent in assessing the operative risk, the parameters involved in the decision-making process can be difficult to define. Therefore, some degree of quantification is desirable to support one's clinical impression and to provide the less experienced with a means of improving their clinical skills.

CLIENT COMMUNICATION

An important preoperative consideration is the presurgical discussion with the client. Major factors that influence the surgeon-client relationship include whether an elective or nonelective procedure is being considered, whether the client is seeking professional help, or if surgical treatment is being initiated solely by the surgeon. Both the emotional and financial aspects of a proposed surgical operation must be taken into account. The surgeon should discuss with the client the reasons for the surgery, its benefits, degree of operative risk, possible complications, prognosis, possible alternative courses of action, preoperative work-up, operative and postoperative courses, and financial responsibilities of the client. Clients seeking elective surgical procedures usually have fewer emotional and financial problems, whereas those with animals requiring nonelective surgery usually require more time and consideration. However, it should also be recognized that the final surgical recommendation may not be possible until radiographic or clinical laboratory evaluations are made. The results of such procedures may be necessary before one can determine if surgery is necessary or even feasible. Therefore, discussions may be helpful in explaining the need and costs of these presurgical evaluation procedures. The better one communicates with a client prior to initiating a course of action, the less chance there is of a misunderstanding later.

SURGICAL PLAN

Prior to any operation, the surgeon should develop a complete surgical plan that incorporates a preoperative course of action (clinical laboratory evaluation, radiographs, treatment for fluid or blood volume deficits); an intraoperative plan of action (surgical approach, material and equipment needed, technical and support personnel); and postoperative requirements (oxygen cage, nutritional and fluid support, radiographs, bandages). A surgeon should not undertake a surgical procedure that is beyond his capabilities. Referring cases to a more experienced colleague or a better-equipped institution best serves the patient and client. Referrals, if handled properly, are an integral part of the practice of high-quality medicine rather than a defeat of an individual practitioner.

PHYSICAL EXAMINATION

The physical examination is probably the most important aspect of a presurgical patient evaluation. All the specifics of a physical examination are beyond the scope of this chapter; however, guidelines to the physical examination of specific organ systems are available.[1] The completeness of the examination may depend on the urgency of the situation. For example, patients with life-threatening respiratory distress or in shock require immediate resuscitation, which may preclude certain aspects of the initial physical examination. The signalment, nature and duration of the problem, previous medical history, and a systematic approach to the physical examination are essential for proper patient evaluation. Checklists have been used to prevent oversights during the physical examination.[11] Such lists become part of the patient's permanent record and are especially helpful when the initial physical examination is performed by someone other than the surgeon. The physical examination should not focus solely on the primary problem or be limited to the examiner's primary area of interest. A thorough and systematic examination of the entire patient is needed to detect possible problems that may influence the outcome of the surgical procedure. Examples that may lead to a disastrous situation include the patient with an obvious long bone fracture that may also have a neurological deficit of the involved limb, a ruptured urinary bladder, a diaphragmatic hernia, or traumatic lung syndrome.

The physical examination should provide an initial assessment of the patient's physical state and should help define potential organ system problems that may need further radiographic, laboratory, electrophysiological, or clinical evaluation. Defining the physical status of a patient based on history and physical examination will help assess the operative risk to the patient and determine the need for additional testing procedures. A classification scheme that can help define the physical status of the surgical patient is presented in Table 18–1.[5, 11, 12] Although all cases may not accurately fit into a particular grade, an estimate of the patient's status can still be helpful in formulating the surgical plan.

LABORATORY SCREENING

The extent of clinical laboratory testing depends on factors such as the patient's age and physical status, the anticipated duration of the surgical procedure, and the availability of various clinical laboratory tests. Regardless of whether a hospital is equipped to perform certain clinical laboratory evaluations, it is important to recognize those patients that require clinical laboratory evaluations to better assess their operative risk. The appropriate samples may be sent to an outside laboratory, or the patient may be referred elsewhere. An in-depth discussion of the pertinent clinical laboratory data recommended for all possible cases is not feasible. Table 18–2 provides a classification system for several designated screening profiles and the various clinical laboratory evaluations included in each profile.[7, 11]

The mini screen, consisting of a packed cell volume (PCV), total plasma protein (TPP), and scanning of a stained blood smear, is inexpensive and easily performed and should be within the capability of any veterinary hospital. The TPP may be determined with a refractometer and the blood smear stained with new methylene blue. The laboratory procedures recommended for the general and maxi screen profiles are performed in many veterinary hospitals today or can be easily requested through an outside commercial clinical laboratory. With the availability of multistick strips, new methylene blue stain for urine sediment examination, and a refractometer for urine specific gravity determinations, a complete urinalysis can easily be performed. The additional clinical laboratory tests for the ancillary screen, which is included in the emergency screen, require expensive instrumentation and trained technical personnel. Even though these tests would most likely not be available in the majority of veterinary hospitals, they can be performed by a commercial laboratory. Patients with a grade 4 or 5 physical status, of which

TABLE 18–1. Classification of Physical Status for the Surgical Patient

Definition	Grade	Examples
Animals that are clinically healthy or that have only a localized problem without any clinically detectable systemic effects.	1	Elective procedures, e.g., castration, ovariohysterectomy, ear trim, and caudectomy; minor wound lacerations
Animals with pre-existing disease that does not interfere with normal activity or cause any systemic effects.	2	Skin tumor, obesity, simple fracture, minimal pneumothorax, uncomplicated hernias
Animals with pre-existing disease that is detectable and could affect ability to physiologically respond to a surgical procedure.	3	Low fever, slight to mild dehydration, polydipsia/polyuria, evident respiratory distress, anemia, weight loss, jaundice, cardiac murmur, moderate hypovolemia, occasional arrhythmia
Animals with pre-existing disease with significant disturbance that would be life-threatening if not corrected.	4	Severe dehydration, high fever, significant anemia, significant hypovolemia, cachexia, uremia, toxemia, cyanosis, cardiac decompensation, significant arrhythmia
Animals in a moribund condition.	5	Patients not expected to live 24 hours with or without surgery

TABLE 18–2. Patient Screening Profiles

Screening Profile	Clinical Laboratory Evaluation											
	PCV	TPP	Blood Smear Scan	WBC and Differential	BUN	Alkaline Phosphatase	SGPT	SGOT	Glucose	Serum Na, K, Cl, Ca	Acid Base	Urinalysis
Mini screen	X	X	X									
General screen	X	X		X	X		X					X
Maxi screen	X	X		X	X	X	X	X	X			X
Ancillary screen										X	X	
Emergency screen	X	X	X		X				X	X	X	X

many will be emergency cases, often have significant fluid, electrolyte, and acid-base disturbances requiring a substantial degree of preoperative management. The availability of the tests within the ancillary screen could be vital to a successful outcome. Depending on the endemic endoparasites, fecal flotations and heartworm microfilaria examinations may need to be included in the routine screening procedures.

Table 18–3 presents the recommended laboratory screening profile based on a patient's age and physical status and the duration of surgery. A surgical procedure is considered minor when the duration of surgery is expected to be no more than 30 to 45 minutes and the patient has a graded physical status of 1, 2, or 3. In contrast, a surgical procedure is considered major when the duration of surgery is expected to be longer than 30 to 45 minutes or the patient has a graded physical status of 4 or 5 regardless of the anticipated duration of surgery.

PHYSIOLOGICAL CONSIDERATIONS

Blood Volume

Normal blood volume of the dog and cat is approximately 90 and 70 ml/kg, respectively. Acute hypovolemia and chronic anemia are the most commonly encountered blood volume deficits requiring preoperative management. Treatment of acute hypovolemia is directed toward establishing a circulating blood volume that will produce the arterial blood pressure needed for adequate tissue perfusion. A complete discussion of shock, its pathophysiology and treatment, is beyond the scope of this chapter but can be found elsewhere (see Chapter 11).[3, 4]

Some patients presented in hypovolemic shock may require emergency surgical intervention to correct the underlying cause of their hypovolemia or other life-threatening injury. The fluid given for blood volume support should be a type that will remain within the extracellular space. Since sodium is the major extracellular electrolyte, isotonic sodium replacement solutions are preferred.[9] The most commonly used crystalloid fluid for blood volume support in the hypovolemic patient is lactated Ringer's solution.

Patients can be intravenously transfused at a rate of 25 to 90 ml/kg body weight over a period of 15 to 30 minutes.[9] Monitoring of central venous pressure, which is normally between 0 and 10 cm H_2O, will help detect overloading. If the arterial blood pressure can be monitored, a minimum pressure of 70 mm Hg should be maintained. Patients with pulmonary, cardiovascular, or renal disease are less tolerant of rapid fluid administration. Packed cell volume, hemo-

TABLE 18–3. Recommended Patient Screening Profiles for Minor or Major Surgery

	Physical Status	Screening Profile		
		<5*	5 to 10*	>10*
Minor Surgery	1	Mini	General	Maxi
	2	General	General	Maxi
	3	Maxi	Maxi	Maxi
Major Surgery	1	General	Maxi	Maxi
	2	Maxi	Maxi	Maxi
	3	Maxi	Maxi	Maxi
	4	Maxi, ancillary	Maxi, ancillary	Maxi, ancillary
	5	Emergency	Emergency	Emergency

*Age in years.

globin concentration, and total plasma protein should also be monitored to detect hemodilution anemia and hypoproteinemia. To maintain the oxygen-carrying capacity of the blood, a packed cell volume of 20 per cent and a hemoglobin concentration of 7 gm/dl should be maintained. Since albumin is the major plasma protein responsible for the colloidal osmotic pressure that maintains fluid within the vascular space, a plasma protein content of 3.5 gm should also be maintained. Therefore, when severe blood loss occurs, blood transfusion may be required in addition to crystalloid fluid infusion.

The major preoperative concern in the chronically anemic patient is maintenance of the patient's oxygen-carrying capacity. Hypoxemia, hypothermia, or decreased tissue perfusion can occur with anesthesia; an additive effect may result, further decreasing the oxygen-carrying capacity in an anemic patient. A packed cell volume of 27 to 30 per cent and a hemoglobin concentration of at least 7 to 10 gm/dl should be attained in the anemic patient prior to surgery. These levels should compensate for surgical blood loss, hypotensive intravascular fluid redistribution, and hemodilution needed for volume support.[9]

The only means of increasing the oxygen-carrying capacity of the patient is a blood transfusion. The amount of donor blood needed can be estimated by the following formula[8]:

$$\text{Blood needed (ml)} = \begin{matrix}\text{Recipient's} \\ \text{weight}\end{matrix} \times \left(\frac{\text{Desired PCV} - \text{Recipient's PCV}}{\text{Donor's PCV}}\right) \begin{matrix}70 \text{ [cat]} \\ \text{OR} \\ 90 \text{ [dog]}\end{matrix}$$

Since the main concern in the anemic surgical patient is the oxygen-carrying capacity of the blood, the amount of blood needed to raise the hemoglobin (Hb) to a certain level can be calculated from the following formula[16]:

$$\text{Blood needed (ml)} = \frac{\text{Recipient's wt (kg)} \times \text{Hb rise (gm/dl)} \times 70}{\text{Donor's Hb concentration (gm/dl)}}$$

Correction in the anemic patient should be gradual. It is best to raise the hemoglobin concentration over several days, thus allowing for excretion of excess plasma. Many chronically anemic patients have a normal total blood volume due to a compensating gradual increase in the plasma volume, thus allowing them to tolerate their anemic state.

Fluid and Electrolytes

Frequently, a dehydrated patient will be presented with an underlying problem requiring surgical treatment. A clinical assessment of this patient and at least a partial correction of the fluid deficit and electrolyte imbalance are required before proceeding. Detailed information for determining the degree of dehydration, classifying the nature of the water deficit, and selecting the proper fluid to use and its method of administration are available (see Chapter 9).[15] The urgency of the operation determines the time available for correction of the fluid deficit and electrolyte imbalances. Although complete correction may not be possible, a significant replacement of the total fluid deficit will be required. A maximum of 90 ml/hr/kg body weight may be administered intravenously with an isotonic fluid such as lactated Ringer's solution. This rate should not be used when concurrent cardiovascular, pulmonary, or renal disease exists. Significant correction may be obtained in many patients within one to three hours.

Dehydration may be isotonic (the losses of water and sodium are equal), hypotonic (the loss of sodium is greater than the loss of water), or hypertonic (the loss of water is greater than the loss of sodium). A normal sodium concentration with isotonic dehydration is most frequently observed in fluid loss from the gastrointestinal tract. In addition, isotonic dehydration can be observed in soft tissue injuries, intestinal obstruction, and peritonitis. Patients with hypotonic dehydration have a decreased plasma sodium concentration. This type of dehydration is frequently detected in adrenocorticoid insufficiency and when a hypotonic solution is used to treat an isotonic loss. Hypertonic dehydration, with an increased plasma sodium concentration, may be seen in diabetes insipidus, hyperosmolar diabetes mellitus, and heat stroke.

The degree of dehydration is estimated clinically by assessing skin pliability and elasticity (skin turgor), dryness of the oral mucosa, and the amount of ocular orbital depression. The fluid deficit (liters) can be estimated by multiplying the degree of dehydration (per cent) by the patient's body weight (kg). The degree of dehydration will be between 5 and 12 per cent, with 5 per cent indicating a mild degree of dehydration and 12 per cent approaching shock and death. Packed cell volume and total plasma protein determinations can also be used to evaluate a dehydrated patient. Both determinations should be performed to help detect anemic or hypoproteinemic patients that may appear to have normal values while being dehydrated but actually had low values before they became dehydrated. After the deficit is calculated, the daily water maintenance requirement (40 to 60 ml/kg), and an estimate of continuing loss must be included to determine the total 24-hour fluid requirements of the patient. Lactated Ringer's solution is the most commonly used isotonic replacement fluid for restoration of the extracellular fluid space. It also provides some correction of metabolic acidosis by hepatic conversion of lactate to bicarbonate.

Acid-Base Status

Patient history, clinical signs, and physical examination findings are helpful in identifying patients with acid-base abnormalities (see Chapter 10).[10, 13, 14] To determine the extent of such disturbances, blood pH, partial pressure of oxygen, partial pressure of carbon dioxide, and bicarbonate concentration must be measured. Ideally, an arterial blood sample should be collected for evaluation; if this is not possible, a free-flowing jugular sample may be used. The blood pH evaluation will determine if acidemia (pH < 7.4) or alkalemia (pH > 7.4) is present. Respiratory acidosis leading to acidemia is due to an abnormal increase in blood carbon dioxide; a decreased rate of carbon dioxide removal from the lungs is usually the cause. Inadequate ventilation can occur with anesthesia, pneumothorax, intrapleural fluid accumulation, or diaphragmatic hernia. Treatment is correction of the primary problem and provision of adequate ventilation.

Once adequate ventilation has been achieved, the acidemia will quickly be resolved. With chronic acidemia due to respiratory acidosis, a compensatory increase in the blood bicarbonate level will be mediated through the kidneys. A decrease in blood carbon dioxide due to increased ventilation will cause a respiratory alkalosis. Excessive carbon dioxide elimination from the lung can result from excitement, pain, or a low blood oxygen level, which may occur with pneumonia or pulmonary edema. If a low blood oxygen concentration (< 60 mm Hg) becomes the main respiratory stimulus, the hyperventilatory state created will lead to a lower blood carbon dioxide concentration. An alkalemia due to a chronic respiratory alkalosis will result in a compensatory decrease in the blood bicarbonate concentration. The primary treatment for respiratory alkalemia is elimination of the cause.

Whereas respiratory causes of acidemia and alkalemia involve blood carbon dioxide concentration, metabolic causes of acidemia and alkalemia revolve around the blood bicarbonate concentration. A metabolic acidosis will cause a decrease in the bicarbonate concentration, and a metabolic alkalosis will cause an increase in blood bicarbonate. A reduction in blood bicarbonate level can occur either as an actual loss of body bicarbonate (via the gastrointestinal tract or from the kidneys) or as a result of the accumulation of acids (inorganic or organic) within the body, which neutralizes the bicarbonate. If the metabolic acidosis is severe enough and cannot be compensated for by the blood buffers and respiratory system, acidemia will occur. Actual loss of bicarbonate occurs with diarrhea, vomiting fluid that contains bile and pancreatic secretions, and renal tubular disease. Accumulation of acid products occurs in renal failure, urinary obstruction, urinary leakage into the peritoneal cavity or body tissues, diabetic ketoacidosis, and poor tissue oxygenation causing an increase in lactic acid concentration.

Even though a rapid compensatory respiratory alkalosis occurs with a metabolic acidosis, the kidneys are ultimately responsible for correction by retaining bicarbonate and excreting hydrogen ions. However, it may take two to three days for the kidneys to reach their maximum responsive capabilities. Therefore, in addition to treating the primary cause, additional alkalinization therapy may be needed. The use of sodium bicarbonate in the treatment of acidemia due to metabolic acidosis depends on the severity of the acidemia. Generally, a mild acidemia (pH > 7.2) may be treated without bicarbonate therapy. Treating the underlying cause and administering lactated Ringer's solution may be sufficient. Lactated Ringer's solution provides one milliequivalent of bicarbonate for each milliequivalent of lactate administered. Sodium bicarbonate therapy should be considered with a marked acidemia (pH < 7.2). The amount of bicarbonate to be given can be calculated using the following formula:

Bicarbonate needed (mEq) =
　0.5 × body wt (kg) × desired bicarbonate (mEq/l) −
　　　　　　measured bicarbonate (mEq/L)

No more than one-half of the calculated amount should be given over a short period of time. One-fourth of the calculated dose may be given intravenously and the other fourth added to a liter of lactated Ringer's solution. Additional bicarbonate should not be given until the blood bicarbonate concentration is measured.

Alkalemia due to metabolic alkalosis is uncommon. An increase in the blood bicarbonate concentration is present. The major causes include iatrogenic administration of alkalizing agents and the vomiting of only acidic gastric secretions. A compensatory respiratory acidosis may be observed. Metabolic alkalosis due to vomiting may be corrected with Ringer's solution (without lactate) to replace chloride loss. If a hypokalemia is also present and renal function is adequate, potassium chloride (35 mEq/L) may be added to the Ringer's solution.

Nutritional State

The nutritional state of the patient is more critical in the chronically diseased animal than in the acute surgical patient. Although correction of nutritional imbalances should be secondary to correction of fluid, electrolyte, and acid-base abnormalities, the surgeon still needs to establish a preoperative plan that will meet the postoperative caloric requirements of the patient. The daily maintenance caloric requirement of the normal adult dog ranges between 66 and 110 Kcal/kg body weight.

Parenteral hyperalimentation with 50% dextrose and 10% amino acid hydrolysate solutions is one way of meeting the caloric requirements intravenously. These solutions are not routinely used in veterinary medicine because they are expensive, require additional clinical laboratory support to monitor their use, and can produce metabolic disturbances.

When possible, oral alimentation is preferred to parenteral administration. Feeding via stomach tube, pharyngostomy tube,[2] or gastrostomy tube[6] is probably the easiest and most economical means of ensuring adequate nutrition. When long-term force feeding is anticipated, either gastrostomy or pharyngostomy tube feeding should be considered. Each method requires some degree of wound care and bandaging where the tube leaves the patient. A possible complication of gastrostomy tube feeding is generalized peritonitis. Significant gastric leakage can occur if the catheter balloon ruptures or deflates or if a poor serosal-peritoneal seal occurs. The catheter balloon tip should be filled with a fluid and not air, which will diffuse through the rubber. Volume over-feeding may cause some degree of discomfort followed by regurgitation or vomiting. The normal gastric volume of the dog is 10 to 20 ml/kg. Therefore, frequent feedings are required to meet daily water and caloric requirements.

Pharyngostomy tubes can cause mechanical interference with the epiglottis and can lead to respiratory embarrassment and aspiration. An increase in saliva production, with drooling, is not unusual. Owing to persistent tongue manipulation by the animal, the tube may occasionally be regurgitated.

PREOPERATIVE ANTIBIOTICS

The surgeon must decide for each individual case whether to use prophylactic preoperative antibiotics. In certain situations, antimicrobial prophylaxis can be important to the successful outcome of a surgical procedure. However, their use should not be considered a substitute for asepsis or good surgical technique. Even though the obvious benefit of reducing the incidence of infection following surgery is an advantage, these drugs can produce toxic side effects either alone or by interacting with other drugs. By altering the normal microbial flora, they can also lead to the development of resistant pathogens (see Chapters 4 and 5).

SPECIAL CONSIDERATIONS

Cardiovascular System

The history and physical examination should provide enough information to detect a patient with underlying heart disease. Such patients commonly have a history of coughing, exercise intolerance, some degree of breathing difficulty, or occasional syncope. A cardiac murmur, jugular pulse, ascites, pulse deficit, and resting heart rate below 70 or above 160 beats per minute are some physical findings that may cause suspicion. Patients with heart disease should have an electrocardiographic examination to evaluate

the heart and a thoracic radiographic examination to evaluate pulmonary vasculature, lung parenchyma, and heart size. These evaluations should also be performed as a routine preoperative screen in geriatric patients and breeds, such as the Great Dane, that have a high incidence of cardiomyopathy.

Operative risk increases significantly in patients with jugular vein distension or premature atrial or ventricular contractions, especially if more than three to five per minute. Even in the absence of these findings, an increased operative risk must be anticipated when concurrent abnormalities such as low oxygen tension, elevated arterial carbon dioxide tension, abnormal potassium concentration, acid-base disturbance, elevated blood urea nitrogen concentration, or increased liver transaminases are present.

Respiratory System

Again, the history and physical examination provide an index of suspicion for patients with underlying respiratory disease. In veterinary medicine, evaluation of these patients is limited to radiographic examination of the thorax and arterial blood gas (oxygen and carbon dioxide) analysis. Since many trauma patients have some degree of traumatic lung injury, presurgical thoracic radiographs are indicated. Patients with even moderate respiratory distress should also have arterial blood gas evaluations. The patient's recovery can be monitored with serial radiographs and arterial oxygen tension measurements.

Urinary System

With clinical pathological screening for blood urea nitrogen and complete urinalysis, an absence of polydipsia or polyuria, and normal physical findings, the surgeon can feel reasonably confident about the patient's renal function. Serum creatinine concentration is a better indicator of glomerular filtration rate and is less affected by extrarenal factors than blood urea nitrogen. Thus, serum creatinine determinations should be done in patients with an elevated blood urea nitrogen. Urine specific gravity is also an important indicator of kidney function. Urine specific gravity values of 1.008 to 1.012 indicate the inability of the kidneys to dilute or concentrate urine and could be an early sign of renal failure without significant blood urea nitrogen elevation. Serum sodium, potassium, calcium, and phosphorus abnormalities are present in more advanced cases of renal failure. Water balance studies, quantitative urine protein loss, creatinine clearance, and intravenous excretory urography may be needed to better evaluate the renal patient. Ultimately, a renal biopsy may be needed to determine the underlying etiologic cause and accurately assess its reversibility.

Although not a primary renal problem, animals with lower urinary tract obstruction or leakage of urine into the peritoneal cavity have significant progressive increases in blood urea nitrogen and potassium concentration. Such patients are poor anesthetic risks owing to their uremia, acidemia, and hyperkalemia. A urethral catheter placed into the urinary bladder diverts urine in cases of bladder or urethral tears. Abdominal drains and lavage may be used to remove abdominal accumulation of urine and may provide some degree of dialysis. Supportive fluid therapy is also needed. Surgical intervention should not be attempted until blood urea nitrogen and potassium concentration values have decreased significantly.

Hepatic System

By the time hepatic dysfunction is clinically detectable (e.g., jaundice, palpable hepatomegaly, ascites), significant hepatic pathology is present. A screening profile that includes serum glutamic pyruvate transaminase (SGPT), serum glutamic oxaloacetic transaminase (SGOT), and serum alkaline phosphatase determinations is helpful in detecting patients with occult liver disease. Additional clinical pathological evaluations, such as albumin/globulin concentration, ammonia levels, bromsulphalein excretion, serum arginase, and bilirubin (conjugated and unconjugated), may be needed. Hepatic biopsy, obtained percutaneously, may be needed for a definitive diagnosis and reliable prognosis.

Of additional importance in hepatic patients is the possibility of blood coagulation abnormalities. Since the liver is the major source for protein synthesis, including those responsible for coagulation, a variety of coagulation defects may occur in parenchymal or obstructive liver disease. Parenchymal disease impairs the synthesis of coagulants such as prothrombin and fibrinogen, whereas obstructive hepatic disease prevents the absorption of vitamin K, which is needed for prothrombin synthesis. Therefore, blood coagulation studies may be needed for patients with significant hepatic disease.

Musculoskeletal System

Most orthopedic patients have encountered a significant degree of trauma and need close evaluation. A complete neurological examination must be conducted to detect possible peripheral or spinal cord trauma, especially in those patients with distal humeral (radial nerve) or pelvic (nerves from the lumbosacral plexus) fractures. Urinary bladder rupture and urethral tears must be ruled out. If the urinary bladder is not palpable, abdominal radiographs and blood urea nitrogen determinations may be helpful. If a urinary bladder or urethral tear is suspected, a positive contrast urethrogram and cystogram can be performed. Abdominal paracentesis may produce a

fluid with elevated blood urea nitrogen and creatinine levels. Intravenous excretory urography may be needed to confirm a ureteral tear. Thoracic radiographs should be taken to evaluate intrathoracic or pulmonary parenchymal trauma. Heart rate and pulse deficits may indicate traumatic myocarditis, and electrocardiographic examination should be performed to confirm and classify the arrhythmia.

CONCLUSION

The preoperative evaluation of the surgical patient must include many factors. The initial step is the history and physical examination. The urgency of the situation, age and physical status of the patient, and anticipated duration of surgery can be used as guidelines to assess the initial operative risk and to select the appropriate clinical laboratory evaluations. The operative risk is further defined following the clinical laboratory procedures and any ancillary procedures (e.g., radiography, electrocardiography). The detection of additional problems will guide the surgeon in selecting other procedures needed to better define specific organ dysfunction. With this information, the surgeon can develop a complete surgical plan that will aid in the preoperative, intraoperative, and postoperative management of the patient.

1. Bistner, S. I. (ed.): Symposium on physical diagnosis. Vet. Clin. North. Am. 11:441, 1981.
2. Bohning, R., DeHoff, W. D., McElhinney, S., and Hofstre, P. C.: Pharyngostomy for maintenance of the anorectic animal. J. Am. Vet. Med. Assoc. 156:611, 1970.
3. Brasmer, T. H. (ed.): Symposium on shock. Vet. Clin. North Am. 6:173, 1976.
4. Clark, D. R., and Adams, H. R.: Symposium on circulatory shock. J. Am. Vet. Med. Assoc. 175:77, 1979.
5. Clifford, D.: Preanesthetic evaluation. In Soma, L. R. (ed.): Textbook of Veterinary Anesthesia. Williams & Wilkins, Baltimore, 1971, p. 259.
6. Crane, S. W.: Placement and maintenance of temporary feeding tube gastrostomy in the dog and cat. Comp. Cont. Ed. 2:770, 1980.
7. Feldman, B. F.: Presurgical laboratory evaluation. J. Am. Anim. Hosp. Assoc. 10:58, 1974.
8. Greene, C. E.: Practical considerations of blood transfusion therapy. Proc. 47th Ann. Mtg. Am. Anim. Hosp. Assoc. 1980, p. 187.
9. Haskins, S. C.: Blood volume support. Vet. Clin. North Am. 6:265, 1976.
10. Haskins, S. C.: An overview of acid-base physiology. J. Am. Vet. Med. Assoc. 170:423, 1977.
11. Henry, W. B.: Presurgical evaluation of the surgical patient. Vet. Clin. North Am. 5:317, 1975.
12. Lumb, W. V., and Jones, E. W.: Veterinary Anesthesia. Lea & Febiger, Philadelphia, 1973, p. 21.
13. Sabatini, S., Arruda, J. A. L., and Kurtzman, N. A.: Disorders of acid-base balance. Med. Clin. North Am. 62:1223, 1978.
14. Schaer, M.: A practical review of simple acid-base disorders. Vet. Clin. North Am. 12:439, 1982.
15. Schaer, M. (ed.): Symposium on fluid and electrolyte balance. Vet. Clin. North Am. 12:353, 1982.
16. Webb, A. I.: Fluid therapy in hypotensive shock. Vet. Clin. North Am. 12:515, 1982.

Section

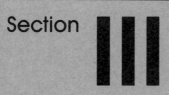

Surgical Methods

Andreas F. von Recum
Section Editor

19 Principles of Surgical Asepsis

D. M. McCurnin and R. L. Jones

Wound infections have been a major problem since surgery began. Over the years, the surgeon has developed an elaborate ritual to help prevent wound infection. Nevertheless, wound infections still occur today.

Historically, veterinary surgery (unlike human surgery) has been financially restrained in the refinement of surgical techniques. Despite these restraints, modern veterinary surgery has evolved to rival its financially unrestrained human counterpart. Wound infection continues to remain an important factor, even under aseptic conditions, owing to increased use of surgical treatments when the patient has decreased resistance (e.g., organ transplantation, old age, neoplasia, and so on).

Increased sophistication in small animal surgery has resulted in an increased number of group practices with increased concentrations of patients and microorganism populations. The increased use of antimicrobial agents tends to select for resistant organisms. Resistant microorganisms pose a serious concern to all hospitalized patients in veterinary group practice. Prevention of nosocomial (hospital-acquired) infections requires strict attention to all details of aseptic technique.

DEFINITION OF TERMS

A brief review of the more commonly used terms associated with aseptic technique is necessary. The absence of pathogenic microbes in living tissue constitutes a state of *asepsis. Sterilization* is the process of killing all microorganisms with the use of either physical or chemical agents. *Steam under pressure* is the most reliable means of sterilizing surgical supplies because of its power of penetration, antimicrobial efficiency, ease of control, and economy of operation. *Dry-heat sterilization* is commonly used for glassware or materials that resist penetration by steam, such as petroleum jelly, fats, and oils. *Gas sterilization* employs ethylene oxide as a sterilizing agent in specially designed chambers in which temperatures and humidity can be controlled and from which air can be evacuated. Gas sterilization is used for delicate surgical instruments, rubber or plastic tubing, plastic syringes, and so on. *Radiation sterilization* refers to ionizing radiation using cobalt-60 sources and electron accelerators. It is currently used commercially to sterilize disposable hospital supplies, such as plastic hypodermic syringes and sutures. *Chemical sterilization* may be achieved with a 2% aqueous solution of glutaraldehyde. This compound is an effective disinfectant for surgical, anesthetic, and dental equipment; rubber and plastic endotracheal tubes; catheters; lensed or delicate cutting instruments; and heat-sensitive hospital equipment. This solution is bactericidal and virucidal in ten minutes and sporicidal within three hours.[11]

An *antiseptic* is a chemical agent that either kills pathogenic microorganisms or inhibits their growth as long as there is contact between agent and microbe. By custom as well as by federal law, the term "antiseptic" is reserved for agents applied to the body. The antiseptic may actually be a disinfectant used in dilute solutions to avoid damage to tissues. A *disinfectant* is a germicidal, chemical substance that kills microorganisms on inanimate objects, such as instruments and other equipment, that cannot be exposed to heat. Disinfectants are essential for good housekeeping in hospitals and clinics, where they are used on floors, cages, tables, and countertops.

Antimicrobial drugs are used to alter the activity of microbial agents in the patient. A *bacteriostatic* antimicrobial agent inhibits bacterial growth; growth may resume upon removal of the agent. *Bactericidal* agents kill bacteria. Bactericidal action differs from bacteriostasis in that it is irreversible; i.e., the "killed" organisms can no longer reproduce, even after being removed from contact with the agent.

HISTORICAL ASPECTS

The two most decisive steps in bringing surgery to its present stage of development were the discovery of anesthesia and the development of antiseptic methods. In the last half of the 18th century and the first half of the 19th century, human hospitals were being built in increasing numbers and the sick and injured crowded into them. As a result, infections of all degrees of severity became of increasing concern.

Surgeons still attempted primary closure, but less frequently. Eventually, the wounds were packed open in anticipation of "laudable pus" but with the hope of eventual recovery. Only the most urgently required operations were performed. It was observed that the same danger of infection was not associated with wounds treated outside the hospital setting.

Separately and unknown to one another, two physicians theorized that infectious organisms could be transmitted from physician to patient. Ignaz Philipp Semmelweis in Vienna and Oliver Wendell Holmes in America were outraged by the high mortality caused by puerperal fever. The death of a patient from infection transmitted by a physician injured during the autopsy of an infected patient brought their attention to the fact that infection was being directly transmitted from physician to patient. Both men excluded other causes such as air, food, and so on in their final analyses. Both recognized that something was being transferred from the infected dead patient to the uninfected patient, usually by the attending physician's hands. Washing the hands, changing clothes, and staying away from other patients after attending one with puerperal fever were advocated by both.[7]

Soon after the discovery of bacteria by Pasteur, their implication in wound infections was quickly recognized by Lister. He published his first description of the "antiseptic principle" in 1867.[24] The dilute carbolic acid dressings, sprays, and soaks advocated by Lister were not readily accepted by physicians, and he repeatedly had to defend their use. The Germans were receptive, and their acceptance eventually led to the introduction of steam sterilization in 1886, followed by an elaborate aseptic ritual in 1891.[7] In America, however, Lister's theory was slow to catch on and was not fully accepted until about 1910. In 1913 the use of the surgeon's glove was described by Halsted, who also championed aseptic and meticulous technique.[7]

Owing primarily to economic concerns, aseptic veterinary surgery was not fully practiced until the late 1940s. Caps, masks, gowns, and gloves were not routinely used in small animal surgery until the 1960s.

TYPES OF SURGICAL INFECTIONS

The veterinary surgeon contends with infection in five major settings: (1) as a primary surgical disease, (2) as a complication of an operation not otherwise associated with infection, (3) as a complication of diagnostic or support procedures, (4) as an entity totally unrelated to the primary surgical disease, and (5) as a complication (short- and long-term) of prosthetic implants. Each area will be briefly described.

Infection as the Primary Surgical Disease

A significant portion of surgical treatment is directed toward the therapy of infections. These infections may be presented as abscesses, peritonitis, pleuritis, or other closed body cavity infections or as trauma that may include contamination with foreign material.

The bacterial etiology varies but is usually characteristic of the type and location of the trauma. Following penetrating trauma, the infection is characteristic of the surface penetrated by the traumatic instrument (e.g., the skin in a penetrating gunshot wound) in addition to those organisms found within organs damaged directly or indirectly (e.g., gram-negative organisms from perforation of the gastrointestinal or genitourinary tract). For example, cat abscesses are usually caused by punctures from an-

other cat's claws or teeth. The most common organisms isolated from cat abscesses are *Bacteroides* and *Pasteurella* spp., both normally found in high numbers in the cat's mouth.[25] Should the infection result from perforation of a hollow viscus without external trauma, the etiology then reflects the flora of the viscus involved. The patient is usually presented owing to the effects of the infection (anorexia, swelling, pain, and so on). Therefore, these infections are therapeutic problems requiring surgical drainage and antimicrobial therapy; prevention is not possible by surgical means.

Postsurgical Wound Infection

During most surgical procedures, the skin and fascia (the body's natural barriers to infection) are incised, altering the body's protective barrier against contamination. Great care must be exercised to avoid unnecessarily exposing deeper tissues to microorganisms both during and after the operation. Attention to aseptic technique and meticulous skin closure reduce the risk.[2] Supplementing the protection afforded by the skin and fascia, a group of tissues including the reticuloendothelial system and the leukocytes constantly combat infectious agents that do invade the body. These tissues prevent disease in two ways: (1) they nonspecifically destroy invading agents by phagocytosis, and (2) they destroy specific invading organisms through immune recognition. These tissues aid the surgeon, provided the level of contamination is not overwhelming and the systems have not been compromised by previous disease, exposure to immunosuppressive drugs, or other immunodeficiencies.

Postoperative wound infection results from bacterial contamination during or after a surgical procedure and usually involves the subcutaneous tissues.[28] The risk varies with the magnitude of bacterial contamination and the type of surgical procedure being performed. Surgical procedures can be grouped into *clean operations* (ovariohysterectomy, hip prosthesis), *clean-contaminated operations* (enterotomy, gastrotomy, pulmonary resection), *contaminated operations* (oral or anal surgical procedures), and *dirty operations* (external trauma or perforation of a viscus, e.g., gunshot injury to abdomen). The bacterial contaminants vary relative to the flora of these areas. Clean wounds are rarely infected with organisms other than gram-positive aerobic bacteria, usually of skin origin, whereas gram-negative or anaerobic bacteria usually arise from contamination from the gastrointestinal or genitourinary tract.[11]

Despite efforts to maintain asepsis, most surgical wounds are contaminated to some degree with bacteria. If the contamination is minimal, if the wound has been made without undue tissue trauma, and if there is no dead space, infection rarely develops.[13] Any factor that interferes with wound healing increases the possibility of wound infection. Unnecessary trauma from retractors, inappropriate use of electrocautery, gross ligation of bleeders, foreign bodies, and dead space all contribute heavily to postoperative wound infection.

The incidence of infection following surgery in potentially contaminated or contaminated and dirty wounds can be reduced through skillful and thoughtful improvements in surgical technique. Veterinary surgery has only recently begun to appreciate the care that must be given to tissue handling.[33] Strict aseptic technique will not make up for poor tissue handling.

Infectious Complications of Diagnostic and Support Procedures

The scope of surgical therapy has enlarged to include the very young and the very old patient and various levels of risk. It is not uncommon to perform lengthy and sophisticated procedures on the very young, severely traumatized, or malnourished patient. As the sophistication of surgical technique has increased, postoperative support methods and diagnostic monitoring techniques have become more extensive.

Continuous fluid therapy, continuous urinary monitoring, and frequent blood sampling have increased the complications associated with these techniques. A trio of support mechanisms accompanies these procedures: (1) continuous intravenous therapy, (2) endotracheal intubation, and (3) urinary catheter drainage. Each shares a common problem: if the therapy is continued long enough, infection develops, and if the device is left in place after superficial infection occurs, systemic infection follows.[28]

Natural barriers to bacterial invasion are breached by endotracheal tubes and urinary and intravenous catheters. Cautious technical insertion of these devices and careful nursing care are required to prevent infection. Injected materials must be sterile, and great care must be taken in the preparation, assembly, and maintenance of intravenous equipment to avoid gross contamination. Intravenous catheters, tubes, and needles are changed at regular and frequent intervals, probably not exceeding 48 hours. A different site is chosen for each injection. Endotracheal tubes must be handled so as to avoid additional bacterial contamination. Urinary catheters should be connected to closed drainage bags or jars.

Infections Unrelated to the Primary Surgical Disease

The surgical patient is always at risk of developing infectious diseases. Postoperative fever and depression may be a consequence of diseases such as parvovirus enteritis, canine distemper, and feline rhinotracheitis. The surgeon must keep these diseases in mind to avoid misdiagnosis of postoperative complications. A careful history must be taken at admission to ensure that the patient has been protected against infectious diseases when feasible. Postsurgical nosocomial infection may develop unrelated to the primary surgical disease.

Infection of Prosthetic Implants

The use of prosthetic implants has increased in the past 20 years. Orthopedic and vascular prostheses are used routinely in the human patient in spite of one of its most catastrophic complications, namely, infection.[5] Prosthetic infections are invariably associated with prolonged hospitalization, increased expense, and patient suffering.

A common phrase in both research and clinical situations is "infected implant." This is a misnomer, since it is the tissue surrounding the implant that is infected rather than the implant itself. Three types of infection are associated with prosthetic implants.[31] The first type is the *superficial immediate infection*, which is due to the growth of organisms on or near the skin in association with an implant. Examples include suture infections and the growth of microorganisms under burn dressings.

The second type is the *deep immediate infection*, which is a low-frequency infection commonly seen immediately after surgery. The bacteria responsible are usually skin residents carried into the implant site during the surgical procedure.

The third type is the *deep late infection*, which may occur years after the surgery in sites with no history of infection. It represents a major problem in many procedures, such as total joint replacement and heart valve implantation.

In veterinary surgery, the two most commonly infected implants are sutures and total hip joint replacements. Complications in the canine hip joint replacement are minimized if attention is paid to strict asepsis. Infection involving polymethyl methacrylate is disastrous. The cement limits the ability of medication and the body's defense mechanisms to reach bacteria. Deep infection of the hip always results in constant lameness and ultimate removal of the implant.[29]

Suture materials play an important role in postoperative wound infections, and different suture materials elicit different degrees of reaction in a contaminated wound. Steel and nylon sutures produce considerably less reaction in the presence of infection than braided nonabsorbable sutures, polyglycolic acid, or catgut.[35] Although a sinus can develop with any suture material, the likelihood is greater with braided, nonabsorbable material than with monofilament or catgut material.[10] The braided suture material protects bacteria by enabling them to hide in the interstices of the suture and multiply beyond the capabilities of the body's defenses.

Since most surgical procedures require sutures and since sutures act as a foreign body, consideration must be given to the type of suture material and the number of sutures used. Monofilament suture is less likely to harbor bacteria than multifilament suture.

When managing tissues surgically, great care must be taken in the proper handling, selection, sterilization, and placement of all prosthetic and suture materials. Poor surgical judgment in the use of suture material or prosthetic implants results in delayed healing or failure due to infection, rejection, or breakdown.

PATHOGENESIS OF SURGICAL WOUND INFECTION

The prevention of infection during surgery is the primary objective of modern aseptic surgery. The surgeon must understand the pathogenesis of surgical wound infections to be able to reduce the risks of this complication. First, the surgeon must realize that there is no such thing as *sterile* surgery. The veterinary surgeon is not presented with a germfree patient in a sterile environment. Therefore, all surgical wounds must be considered to be contaminated with bacteria. Second, by breaking the integrity of the bacteria-resistant skin, the surgical incision provides an increased risk of infection. However, surgical wounds do not always become infected when they are contaminated with bacteria. Numerous factors determine whether infection (microbial damage of tissue) will result: (1) those factors that reduce the host's resistance to bacterial infection, (2) the characteristics of the bacterial contaminants, and (3) the interaction between the host and the bacteria that results in a tissue-damaging infection.[2, 8, 26]

Host Resistance to Infection

A variety of events may predispose the patient to infection. These factors may be separated into physiological abnormalities and mechanical factors.[8] Mechanical factors are produced by surgical therapy, whereas some physiological abnormalities may pre-exist. The astute surgeon must carefully evaluate the surgical patient so that he can be aware of the increased risk of infection due to these factors.

The pathophysiological conditions that increase the risk of infection are not always completely understood.[2] Extremes in age (very old or very young), poor physical condition, and malnutrition may predispose to infection. Other conditions that may decrease resistance to bacterial infection include systemic disease such as diabetes, malignant processes such as leukemia, immunodeficiency such as hypogammaglobulinemia, suppression by corticosteroid or cytotoxic drugs, and metabolic or physiological alterations caused by anesthetics and hypothermia. Various stressful conditions such as massive blood loss or systemic shock also predispose to infection. Local

conditions at the surgical site are some of the most important factors increasing susceptibility to infection. Necrotic tissue serves as a growth medium for bacteria and is often not accessible to the host's defense mechanisms. In addition, the necrotic tissue has a reduced oxygen content that permits anaerobic bacterial growth. Phagocytosis and humoral immunity are significantly decreased when tissue integrity is interrupted during the operation. Hematomas and dead space serve as excellent locations for infection because bacteria can increase to large numbers in these areas, in which there is relatively little host response. Epinephrine in the incision may significantly reduce the animal's ability to control bacteria by reducing the blood supply.

The most obvious mechanical factor reducing resistance to infection is a skin incision. The skin is the normal primary barrier to infectious agents. When it is incised, tissues that are rarely contaminated with bacteria become contaminated. The mechanical trauma of incision and dissection is incidental to surgical therapy. The damage caused by clamps, ligatures, retractors, hemorrhage, and thrombosis tends to alter the blood supply and decrease the efficiency of host defenses. Foreign materials such as sutures and surgical implants may produce little or no inflammatory response in the tissue as long as they are sterile, but they cause a significant reduction in the size of inoculum necessary to cause infection. While physically disrupting host defenses, they provide a matrix that harbors and protects the bacteria while they significantly increase in number.

Bacterial Contamination of the Surgical Wound

Since Lister introduced his "antiseptic principle," the objective of aseptic surgery has been to reduce the level of contamination of surgical wounds by pathogenic bacteria. Knowledge of the sources and types of bacteria that may contaminate surgical wounds enables the surgeon to reduce the incidence and severity of wound infection.

The most common source of bacteria that contaminate surgical wounds is the animal's endogenous microbial flora.[4] Prevention of exposure to this flora and resulting infection is most important at the time of surgery. Preoperative preparation of the patient (i.e., clipping the hair and scrubbing the surgical site) reduces the risk of infection by these agents. The judicious use of preoperative antimicrobial agents and the careful management of the wound postoperatively are also important control measures. Modern aseptic principles of surgery can be quite effective in controlling exogenous sources of bacteria (Table 19–1). The scrubbed surgeon, wearing a gown, cap, mask, and gloves, rarely contaminates the wound unless one of these barriers fails to function as expected. Surgical equipment and instruments were

TABLE 19–1. Agents Associated With Surgical Infections

Operative Site Infections	Primary Sources
Staphylococcus aureus	Skin, mucous membranes
Staphylococcus spp. (coagulase-negative)	Skin, mucous membranes
Streptococcus spp.	Mucous membranes
Escherichia coli	Enteric flora
Proteus spp.	Enteric flora
Pseudomonas aeruginosa	Soil
Clostridium perfringens	Enteric flora
Bacteroides spp.	Mucous membranes, enteric flora
Fusobacterium spp.	Enteric flora

Surgery-Associated Infections	Site of Infection
Escherichia coli	Respiratory and urinary systems
Klebsiella pneumoniae	Respiratory and urinary systems
Staphylococcus aureus	Respiratory and urinary systems
Pseudomonas aeruginosa	Respiratory system
Proteus spp.	Respiratory and urinary systems
Pasteurella spp.	Respiratory system
Yeast (*Candida*, etc.)	Mucous membranes

once a significant source of bacterial contamination, but the variety of sterilization methods now available should eliminate this source. Air in contact with the surgical wound is the most common vehicle for delivering bacteria to the wound. The bacteria in the air are usually from the animal and nonscrubbed personnel in the operating room, and the concentration of these organisms in the air is directly related to the amount of activity within the operating room.[8]

Bacteria that infect surgical wounds utilize the opportunity offered by the weakened defense mechanisms of the host to become established and inflict tissue damage. Therefore, these opportunistic agents may not possess all of the classic virulence characteristics. They are often organisms of low virulence, unable to invade intact body surfaces, or they do not survive well in the tissues and therefore must be present in large numbers. The most common bacteria involved in these infections are the gram-positive cocci *Staphylococcus aureus* and *Streptococcus* spp. Gram-negative bacilli of fecal origin can occasionally be identified in surgical wound infections owing to the difficulty of preventing contamination of the animal's haircoat and skin. If the surgery has invaded a mucous membrane, anaerobic bacteria may be involved in subsequent infections. Most mucous membranes are normally colonized with obligate anaerobes. If these bacteria become involved, the infection is often much more serious owing to their toxic nature.[15] Most surgical wound infections result in localized necrosis of tissue accompanied by stimulation of a suppurative exudate by pyogenic bacteria such as streptococci. However, these infections may range in severity to the extreme necrotizing, gangrenous infections caused by *Clostridium perfringens* or a highly toxicogenic disease such as tetanus.

Development of Infection

Infection of "clean" surgical wounds is frequently related to some unknown gross break in aseptic technique. However, infrequent, sporadic infections indicate a more random cause. Unrecognized breaks in technique result in clusters of infection that persist until the problem is identified and corrected.

Factors that lead to the development of most surgical wound infections are a combination of the predisposing factors in the host and concurrent contamination with bacteria. The host's resistance to these infections is predominantly due to nonspecific defenses that do not depend on previous immunological experience. The development of a surgical wound infection then depends on the probability of sufficient bacteria falling on a small site where the host resistance has been decreased enough to allow sufficient bacterial growth to cause further tissue damage. All "clean" surgical wounds are contaminated with many bacteria during the surgical procedure. Bacterial infections resulting in tissue damage generally require growth of the contaminating organisms to numbers of 10^6 or greater per gram of tissue.[12] This growth can occur only when the microenvironment is favorable for bacterial survival and growth, which means that host resistance must be impaired.

Several conditions that may reduce resistance in specific foci have previously been discussed, such as necrotic tissue, capillary thrombosis, dead space, or foreign bodies. The importance of these factors in reducing host resistance and increasing the probability of infection has been demonstrated with suture material. For example, an inoculum of 10^6 or more *Staphylococcus aureus* organisms is required to produce a lesion in healthy skin, but in the presence of a silk suture, the required inoculum is reduced one-thousandfold to less than 10^3 bacteria.[12] Blood clots or pockets of serum serve as excellent growth media for bacteria. The reduced blood supply and oxygenation of the tissue provide an environment more favorable to anaerobic bacterial growth. In summary, the probability of infection developing in a surgical wound depends on the probability of virulent bacteria contaminating a portion of the surgical wound when the host's resistance has been sufficiently impaired to provide a favorable microenvironment for bacterial survival and growth to numbers that can cause further tissue damage.

PREVENTION OF SURGICAL INFECTION

Protection of the surgical patient from infection is a primary consideration throughout the preoperative, operative, and postoperative phases of surgical care. The risk of infection can be reduced by (1) proper selection and preparation of the patient, (2) surgical personnel preparation, (3) adequate sterilization of surgical equipment and materials, (4) proper maintenance of the surgical rooms, (5) attention to operative technique, (6) correct patient aftercare, and (7) proper use of prophylactic antimicrobial agents.

Proper Selection and Preparation of the Surgical Patient

Surgical patient selection and preparation require attention to a number of details that can be easily overlooked in a busy practice. The patient should always receive a complete physical examination followed by the necessary (or required) minimum laboratory work-up. A complete history from the owner will often guide the depth of the physical and laboratory examinations. The information that the owner can provide may be invaluable in solving the diagnostic problem at hand.

Some of the important historical considerations are acute or chronic corticosteroid therapy, use of long-term antimicrobials, or history and evidence of remote infection elsewhere in the patient's body (e.g., staphylococcal dermatitis when contemplating a hip prosthesis). Furthermore, during the preoperative evaluation the patient should be protected from unnecessary exposure to infectious diseases through proper immunization or isolation. The urgency of the operation will dictate some of the preoperative concerns. However, the surgeon must always balance the risk of an adverse complication with the potential benefits of the operation.

In summary, the preoperative evaluation of the patient should be comprehensive in order to assess the overall state of health, to determine the risk of the impending surgical treatment, and to guide the preoperative preparation. Most importantly, all the information gathered must be shared with the owner (including treatment options, risks, and costs) to enable both veterinarian and owner to form treatment plans. Without the consent and support of the owner, the diagnostic evaluation, surgical skills, postoperative care, and surgical facilities and equipment may not be used to full potential.

Preparation of the patient's surgical site (see Chapter 22) should ideally start the day before surgery, hair in the area of the surgical site being removed with electric clippers. A bath could also be given if time and the type of surgical procedure permit. Scrubbing and application of skin antiseptics may occur both the day before and just prior to the operation. More commonly, the surgical site is prepared immediately prior to the operation unless a specific protocol has been developed, as with an elective hip prosthesis.

Preparation of Surgical Personnel

Surgical personnel preparation will be dealt with in detail in Chapter 21. Great attention has been focused on the proper preparation of the patient, instruments, and equipment, but few benefits are received unless the same attention is given to preparation of the operating personnel. Disposable caps, masks, gloves, and gowns are economical. Some disposable items may be resterilized and used several times, thus increasing their cost effectiveness.

Prior to entering the scrub area, the surgeon should change into a conventional scrub suit, cap, mask, and clean shoes or shoe covers. Strict attention must be paid to the proper preparation of the surgeon's hands and arms with an approved method of scrubbing (see Chapter 21). Gowning and gloving techniques must be practiced to ensure aseptic results. Surgical gloves should be free from holes and changed immediately if punctured or contaminated.

Sterilization of Surgical Equipment and Materials

Surgical equipment and material sterilization is accomplished outside the surgery room (see Chapter 20). Failures of such sterilization usually result from inadequate maintenance of the equipment or attempts to modify sterilizing procedures without careful attention to all details. Penetration of the sterilizing medium in an active form for a sufficient length of time is a prerequisite of all sterilization. To ensure adequate sterility, biological sterility indicators or monitors must be used with each item being sterilized. Minimum monitoring should include both temperature and time if biological indicators are not available. Continued sterility must be assured through adequate storage, transportation, and handling.

Recently, the increased popularity of ultrasonic instrument cleaners, improved germicidal solutions, and gas sterilization have improved the cleaning and sterilizing of many surgical materials. Boiling and soaking in antiseptic solutions are now rarely used as sterilization techniques.

Maintenance of the Operating Room

Operating room maintenance is the responsibility of both the operating room personnel and the veterinarian (see Chapter 23). In spite of improvements in operating rooms, sterility remains difficult to achieve. Several factors have contributed to an improved environment in the operating room, such as isolating the surgery area from all other hospital traffic, reducing the number of observers within the room, using air conditioning that delivers air under positive pressure, and providing surgical preparation areas (for both surgeon and patient) outside the operating room.

The operating room must be strictly reserved for surgery and must not be used for any other purpose, e.g., examinations or treatments. Prior to each surgical day, the operating room should be thoroughly cleansed with an appropriate disinfectant. Disinfected surfaces should include floors, walls, tables, lights, countertops, and so on. Between operations, all flat surfaces should be wiped down with a disinfectant. If carefully cleaned, the floor, tables, lights, and other equipment are sources of few bacteria. An important operating room source of bacteria is the personnel.[16] Many bacteria are shed from the skin, particularly from the area below the waist. Care should be taken to keep scrub suits and gowns dry. In addition, face masks are crucial barriers to the transmission of bacteria from the nose and mouth.

Patient Preparation

The patient's skin cannot be completely sterilized. The transient bacteria on the skin surface can be killed with appropriate solutions, but the resident bacteria in the hair follicles and sebaceous glands cannot be destroyed. During the operation, resident bacteria come to the surface and, with the addition of bacterial fallout from the air, are a source of wound contamination.

The patient's surgical drapes (see Chapter 22) are an important barrier to the continued threat of contamination from the skin and air. Cloth drapes allow penetration by bacteria when wet. Waterproof paper drapes allow little penetration by bacteria even when wet. For additional patient safety, an adherent plastic sheet may be placed over the operative site (through which the incision is made) during prolonged orthopedic procedures. Instruments, gowns, gloves, and so on that are used during contaminated surgery should be changed and excluded from the remaining clean portions of the operation.

Operative Technique

One of the most important means of preventing infection and achieving optimal healing is through proper operative technique (see Chapter 26). Tissues should be protected from internal or external contamination as well as from drying. Fine instruments, sharp dissection, and minimal and skillful use of electrocautery, ligatures, and sutures are essential. Any factor that may interfere with wound healing enhances the possibility of wound infection.

All operations should be performed to minimize the disturbance of blood flow through the tissue involved, otherwise healing will be slowed and infection enhanced; e.g., the preservation of the blood supply is essential for the healing of an intestinal anastomosis. Sutures, whether used to interrupt blood vessels or to hold the wound in apposition to permit healing, interfere with blood flow through the tissues to some degree. Sutures that are too tightly placed or too closely positioned eventually result in wound disruption because of necrosis of the tissue

encompassed by the suture material. Since wounds swell in the early postoperative period, sutures that were tight when placed will cause necrosis from increased tissue pressure (for more details see Chapter 26).

Since sutures combine the undesirable effects of the presence of foreign bodies and interference with blood supply, as few sutures as possible should be used to close or approximate the wound. Sutures should be as fine as possible, monofilament, and nonreactive and should be tied as loosely as approximation will allow. The neophyte veterinary surgeon tends to place too many sutures too tightly, particularly in the subcutaneous layers where the blood supply is poor and the likelihood of infection is increased. Sutures within fat have no holding power and provide an optimal opportunity for infection to begin around minimal contamination in the presence of a foreign body. Furthermore, deep retention sutures are large foreign bodies, impair blood flow, and provide bacterial tracts from the exterior to the interior of the wound.

No single technical complication is as frequently associated with infection as is the presence of a hematoma (implying poor hemostasis).[30] Bleeding vessels should be clamped with as little adjacent tissue as possible and tied with the finest appropriate ligature to avoid necrosis of a large mass of tissue distal to the tie. Electrocautery must be very skillfully used. In addition, wounds made with a scalpel heal better and are less susceptible to infection than those made with an electrosurgical knife.[30]

If a hollow viscus is to be opened or other sources of contamination are to be exposed, protective towels, gauze, or plastic should be used to shield the adjacent clean tissues. Dead space should be eliminated and devitalized tissue removed, as these are potential areas of bacterial growth. Meticulous operative technique is largely a matter of respect for tissues and awareness of the healing process.

Postoperative Care

One of the most neglected areas of veterinary surgery is postoperative care (see Chapter 31). Most veterinary surgical patients remain in the hospital for observation following surgery. This phase of postoperative care is monitored through the efforts of the veterinarian and the animal health technician. Wounds must be protected from contamination during this period by bandages or appositional maintenance of wound edges. Wounds must also be protected from damage by the patient by the use of collars or other restraint devices (see Chapter 31). Drains must be maintained and protected to prevent ascending contamination.

The home convalescence period varies in length but occurs in all surgical cases. Most owners do an excellent job if properly instructed in how to care for the patient, including what areas need to be monitored or observed on a regular basis. The key to successful home convalescence is an informed owner. Either the veterinarian or animal health technician must provide the necessary explanation and information to allow the owner to function as a medical support unit. The owner must know what to observe and when to contact the veterinarian.

If postoperative wound infection occurs, local signs consist of pain, swelling, warmth, and erythema. In contrast to an infected wound, the healthy wound that is several days old usually is neither painful nor excessively swollen. The entire wound may not be infected initially. If no more than seven to ten days have elapsed since surgery, the incision may simply be spread open with a hemostat and drained. Effective drainage usually abolishes local and systemic evidence of infection and accelerates wound healing.[20] The insertion of a drain for 24 to 72 hours may be desirable if properly maintained.

If systemic evidence of infection persists (i.e., fever, depression, anorexia, and so on) after drainage, either the local drainage was inadequate or other sources of infection exist and must be identified. Blood, pus, and urine specimens should be cultured for bacterial isolation and identification. Antibiotic susceptibility testing should be performed if indicated. Meanwhile, initial antimicrobial therapy should be instituted based on the usual susceptibilities of the most likely pathogens. After the specific organism has been identified and the appropriate agents administered, therapy must continue until the majority of organisms are destroyed and clinical signs abated. Above all, the therapy should not be stopped prematurely, since early termination of therapy may permit resurgence of the infection.

NOSOCOMIAL INFECTIONS

Infections that are acquired by the patient during the course of hospitalization are known as nosocomial infections. These infections may occur in anatomical sites other than the surgical wound and may develop preoperatively, postoperatively, or even after the patient has been discharged. Although many nosocomial infections are preventable by improved techniques and patient management, the development of a nosocomial infection does not necessarily imply negligence. Nosocomial infections must be differentiated from community-acquired infections that are incubating at the time of hospitalization. The most common nosocomial infections are of the urinary tract, lower respiratory tract, and surgical wound. Most nosocomial infections can be associated with risk factors such as overuse of antimicrobials, therapeutic medical devices, diagnostic procedures, surgical procedures, advanced age, and chronic disease.

The incidence of nosocomial infections in veterinary hospitals is not well-documented but is probably similar to that seen in human hospitals, where the rate is approximately 5 per cent of hospitalized patients.[6, 9] The incidence is known to vary with the size and type of hospital and the sophistication of infection control programs. The highest incidence rates are observed in large referral or teaching institutions.[9] The most important risk factors appear to be an increased number of personnel having contact with the patient and an increased mean number of hospitalization days per patient. Therefore, these infections are an increasingly significant problem in teaching hospitals and large group practices where intensive medical and surgical care is available through a large staff. These institutions also tend to care for the more critical and chronic patients.

The individual patient risk factors include (1) the animal's susceptibility to infection, (2) the virulence of the infectious agent, and (3) the nature of exposure to the agent. Although the surgeon must be aware of the first two factors, he has little control over them. Owing to the debilitated status of hospitalized patients, they are usually more susceptible to infections. Factors that predispose to nosocomial infections may include old age, debilitating disease, diagnostic or medical procedures such as urethral or intravenous catheterization, immunosuppressive therapy (corticosteroids or cytotoxic drugs), long periods of hospitalization (especially preoperatively), antimicrobial therapy, remote infections, and surgical or body cavity drains. The surgeon can reduce the incidence of nosocomial infections by limiting the spread of the agents and controlling the sources of exposure to the patient.

Nosocomial Infectious Agents

Bacteria are the most common infectious agents involved in nosocomial infection. The bacteria commonly involved tend to be environmentally resistant, and the increasing use of antibiotic therapy precedes an increased antibiotic resistance in nosocomial agents. Before the antibiotic era, penicillin-susceptible gram-positive cocci of the genera *Streptococcus* and *Staphylococcus* were the most common infectious agents. Then penicillin-resistant *Staphylococcus* strains became important. Currently, the major problem is with extremely antibiotic-resistant gram-negative bacilli such as *E. coli*, *Salmonella*, *Klebsiella*, *Pseudomonas*, and *Serratia*. Fungi, such as *Candida albicans*, have occasionally been identified. As the nosocomial infection problem is better defined in veterinary hospitals, no doubt more fungal infections will be identified, especially with improved intensive care of the cancer patient.

Epidemiology

An understanding of the source and transmission of nosocomial agents is necessary for effective control.

The source of most agents can be classified as the endogenous flora of the patient or exogenous agents of the hospital microflora. The endogenous flora of the animal causes disease when it is able to enter normally sterile tissues through anatomical, physiological, or biochemical defects in the host defense mechanisms. Exogenous bacteria may directly contaminate tissues and cause infection. However, these agents usually colonize the body surfaces of the patient first and then cause an infection in much the same manner as the endogenous flora.

Nosocomial infectious agents are transmitted by contact exposure, contaminated vehicles, and airborne spread. Direct transmission by contact between patients or members of the hospital staff is the most prevalent method of infection. Proper hand washing technique by *all* hospital personnel before and after any contact with a patient is the most important preventive measure. The spread of infectious agents by contaminated vehicles usually indicates a breakdown in aseptic techniques or disinfection and sterilization procedures. Various medical devices, such as catheters and implants, have been incriminated in the spread of infection when inadequately cleaned and sterilized. Diagnostic equipment is commonly used in many veterinary practices without adequate disinfection between animals. Rectal thermometers and stethoscopes have been found to be contaminated with nosocomial strains of *Klebsiella*.[22] The airborne spread of bacteria in hospital air currents is generally considered to be of limited importance, although it is known to be particularly important in the transmission of viral agents such as canine distemper.

Colonization of body surfaces by nosocomial bacterial pathogens is often a prerequisite to infection. Direct contamination of exposed tissues, which results in infection, occurs less frequently. Therefore, the patient is its own major reservoir of these agents. Common reservoir sites are the lower intestinal tract, lower urinary tract, and naso-oropharyngeal area. Antimicrobial treatment is the most important predisposing factor allowing colonization with unusual organisms.[34] The suppression of normal flora by antimicrobials readily allows other agents to become established. Antimicrobial therapy is most damaging when it selectively reduces the anaerobic bacterial population. Gram-negative enterics, especially those with plasmid-mediated antibiotic-resistant factors, are then selected and allowed to increase to unusually high numbers, which in turn increases the exposure and risk of infection. These multiple drug–resistant bacteria are the most common causes of serious nosocomial infections. Orally administered antibiotics, such as ampicillin, chloramphenicol, and cloxacillin, have the greatest selective effect because the anaerobic flora is quite susceptible to these drugs. In addition, significant portions of each dose of ampicillin may not be absorbed from the intestine. Since aminoglycosides have little effect on the anaerobic

bacteria, they should be used only when absolutely necessary because they exert a very strong selective pressure for drug-resistant strains of bacteria. Other factors that predispose the patient to colonization by unusual bacteria include surgery, functional abnormalities such as ileus, increased severity of illness, increased length of preoperative hospitalization, and increased frequency and duration of diagnostic and supportive manipulative procedures such as catheterizations and endoscopic examinations.

Prevention of Nosocomial Infections

Nosocomial infections are an established problem in veterinary teaching hospitals and large group practices.[17, 19, 23] Total prevention of this problem is an unrealistic goal. Improved medical technology and owner acceptance require that the veterinarian provide intensive care for the critical animal for prolonged periods of time. Nosocomial infection is a risk that accompanies these improved services. Therefore, surveillance and control procedures must be adopted to identify nosocomial infections and reduce their incidence.

Surveillance

An effective surveillance program in a veterinary facility must be both a comprehensive and sensitive detection system. The first step is recognition of an atypical infectious disease problem. This is facilitated by timely identification of the agent and prompt reporting of infections. An efficient surveillance system defines the endemic level and type of nosocomial infection. It also must quickly identify epidemics and clusters of infections as they occur. Monitoring systems will be discussed further as part of a control program. Precise identification of the agent is required.[18] Bacteria should be identified to the species level as a minimum. In addition, an accurate antibiogram is essential. Minimum inhibitor concentration testing provides better information than agar diffusion susceptibility testing. Additional identifying characteristics that may serve as useful epidemiological markers include biotyping, phage typing, serotyping, and plasmid fingerprinting.

Clinical microbiology personnel will probably first recognize an unusual cluster of isolates of a single pathogen or unusually resistant antibiograms. Therefore, close liaison with the clinical microbiology laboratory is necessary. The identification of a possible nosocomial infection should be reported to the hospital infection control officer daily. Some cases require immediate telephone reporting. If the nosocomial infection has become established as an endemic problem, retrospective study of microbiology records may be necessary.

Scheduled or periodic microbiological sampling of the hospital environment to monitor the level of contamination with potential nosocomial agents may not be cost effective or rational.[14] However, microbiological sampling is an important epidemiological tool when used to detect a specific agent that is responsible for the appearance of a cluster of nosocomial infections. Sampling of sterilized equipment is not necessary if sterilization procedures are adequately monitored by biological testing. Environmental surfaces, air quality, and housekeeping practices are best evaluated with a "white glove" inspection. These inspections are usually less expensive and as meaningful as microbiological sampling. Cleaning, disinfection, and maintenance protocols must be established, and adherence to these protocols can best be evaluated by physical inspections.

When evaluating the microbial contamination of patient care equipment, a useful categorization is (1) critical (2) semicritical and (3) noncritical equipment. Critical equipment includes those devices introduced directly into the body, such as surgical instruments, catheters, and implants. The sterility of this equipment is absolutely essential. Semicritical equipment includes those items that come in contact with various mucous membranes. Although sterilization of these items is desirable, it is not essential. Disinfection of these items must inactivate all vegetative cells. Semicritical equipment, such as thermometers, speculums, endotracheal tubes, and various diagnostic devices, is often inadequately disinfected in veterinary hospitals and has been found to be responsible for transmission of nosocomial agents. These devices are very effective vehicles because they introduce the agent to a mucous membrane on which the organism can colonize. The actual infection may not develop for a period of days to weeks. Subsequently, the infection may not be properly recognized as a nosocomial disease. Noncritical equipment includes environmental surfaces such as cages, tables, floors, walls, and so on. Sterilization of these surfaces is impractical, and properly designed and supervised cleaning protocols are adequate. These surfaces should be periodically cleaned with a detergent and chemically disinfected.

Control

Control of nosocomial infections requires more than crisis intervention. A control program must include a systematic evaluation of the problem, application of sound management techniques, and integration of a productive educational program for all hospital personnel. The sophistication of the control program should be tailored to the needs of the hospital. A limited program may be sufficient in smaller veterinary hospitals and clinics, whereas large referral practices and teaching hospitals should consider developing a comprehensive control program,[3] which would include the following:

1. The appointment of an Infection Control Committee or Infection Control Officer.

2. The development of written standards for medical asepsis and hospital sanitation.

3. The development of a practical system of surveillance, identification, and accurate reporting of infections.

4. Facilities for the isolation of infected patients.

5. An adequate microbiology service.

6. A periodic review of the use of antimicrobial agents.

The Infection Control Committee is responsible for developing guidelines and standards for infection prevention and control, surveillance reporting, and patient management. These policies must be presented to all hospital personnel and reinforced through a continuous educational program. This committee should consist of staff members representing various hospital disciplines. A representative of the administration must be included who has authority to make major decisions concerning hospital policy and who is acquainted with medicolegal issues. Each of the major surgical and medical services must be represented as well as the microbiology laboratory and the hospital epidemiology department. Representatives of the pharmacy, central supply service, maintenance, and housekeeping staffs should be consulted and invited to attend meetings when appropriate. The policies established by this committee must be effective, efficient, and financially feasible. Current and accurate data must be available to the committee so that it can make recommendations needed to prevent and control infections. An Infection Control Officer should be appointed as the "strong arm" of the committee. This individual is responsible for assessing adherence to the committee's policies and enforcing them on a daily basis.

The committee should develop and continuously evaluate written standards for medical asepsis and hospital sanitation as well as the procedures and techniques used for meeting the standards. A system must be developed for surveillance and reporting of nosocomial infections so that the committee has the most current information available as a basis for policy decisions.

The most sensitive subject the Infection Control Committee must face is a review of the use of antimicrobial agents in the hospital. Veterinarians tend to jealously guard their prerogative to independently choose and prescribe antimicrobial agents. They often resent any attempt to influence their choice of therapy. Misuse is best corrected by careful development and presentation of educational programs. Attempts to change antimicrobial use through administrative directives usually fail. The committee must evaluate use to determine if the medical condition requires antimicrobial treatment, that the most effective and least expensive drug is chosen, and that the correct dosage and duration of therapy have been prescribed. It is estimated that at least one-half of all administrations of antibiotics to hospitalized humans do not comply with these criteria.[4] Similar misuse in veterinary medicine undoubtedly exists.

Educational programs need to be developed that will encourage veterinarians to prescribe appropriate antimicrobials only when indicated. The pharmacokinetics of the drugs should be reviewed. The mechanisms of interaction of the drug with the bacteria, or pharmacodynamics, must be emphasized. Principles of broad spectrum and combination therapy need to be included. The indications for bactericidal therapy versus bacteriostatic therapy should be defined and guidelines developed for the rational selection of appropriate antimicrobial therapy. The unnecessary cost, both in the direct expenses for the drug as well as the indirect expenses of administration, of the injudicious use of antimicrobial agents should be emphasized. In some cases, the committee should take the responsibility to issue specific restraints on antimicrobial usage. Highly potent bactericidal antimicrobials such as amikacin and third-generation cephalosporins should be restricted from general prescription. These drugs should be used only after careful case review by a committee representative and approval of such therapy.

The specific objectives of a nosocomial infection control program must be directed against the spread of agents from one patient to another. Isolation facilities must be evaluated and procedures developed that will provide physical containment of the agent. Various levels of isolation strategy may be developed that reflect the method and risk of transmission. Ventilation systems need to be evaluated as well as effective disinfection procedures established for contaminated cages and runs. All hospital personnel must adhere to prescribed hand washing procedures and wear protective clothing and gloves when necessary. The control program should recommend preferred procedures such as closed systems for urine drainage. Aseptic management techniques must be proposed and reviewed for urinary catheters, IV catheters, tracheostomies, and wounds. Specific prehospitalization immunization programs are necessary to prevent nosocomial outbreaks of viral diseases such as canine distemper and parvovirus gastroenteritis.

As medical and surgical technology for treating animals improves, techniques must also be developed to prevent associated nosocomial infections. Reducing the use of prophylactic antimicrobials in the surgical service is the most effective method of reducing the incidence of bacterial nosocomial infections. The misuse of antimicrobials is not poor practice simply because of the selection of resistant bacteria, the predisposition to superinfections, or the economic impact; it also indicates an unwillingness to apply scientific technology wisely.

1. Altemeier, W. A. and Alexander, J. W.: Surgical infections and choice of antibiotics. *In* Sabiston, D. C. (ed.): *Davis-Christopher Textbook of Surgery*, 12th ed. W. B. Saunders, Philadelphia, 1981, pp. 333–357.
2. Altemeier, W. A., et al. (eds.): *Manual on Control of Infection in Surgical Patients*. J. B. Lippincott, Philadelphia, 1976.
3. American Hospital Association, Committee on Infections Within Hospitals: *Infection Control in the Hospital*. American Hospital Assoc., Chicago, 1979, pp. 19–43.
4. Bennett, J. V., and Brachman, P. S. (eds.): *Hospital Infections*. Little, Brown, Boston, 1979.
5. Bernhart, L. M.: Management of infected vascular prosthesis. Surg. Clin. North Am. 55:1411, 1975.
6. Brachman, P. S.: Nosocomial infection control: an overview. Rev. Infect. Dis. 3:640, 1981.
7. Brieger, G. H.: The development of surgery. *In* Sabiston, D. C. (ed.): *Davis-Christopher Textbook of Surgery*, 12th ed. W. B. Saunders, Philadelphia, 1981, pp. 1–22.
8. Burke, J. F.: Factors predisposing to infection in the surgical patient. *In* Maiback, H. I., and Hildick-Smith, G. (eds.): *Skin Bacteria and Their Role in Infection*. McGraw-Hill Book Co., New York, 1965, pp. 143–155.
9. Dixon, R. E.: Control of nosocomial and other infections acquired in medical care institutions. *In* Lennette, E. H., et al. (eds.): *Manual of Clinical Microbiology*, 3rd ed. American Society for Microbiology, Washington, D.C., 1980, pp. 934–938.
10. Dulisch, M. L.: Suture reaction following extra-articular stifle stabilization in the dog. Part I: A retrospective study of 161 stifles. J. Am. Anim. Hosp. Assoc. 17:569, 1981.
11. Dunphy, J. E., and Way, L. W.: *Current Surgical Diagnosis and Treatment*, 5th ed. Lange Medical Publications, Los Altos, CA, 1981, pp. 106–112.
12. Edberg, S. C.: Methods of quantitative microbiological analyses that support the diagnosis, treatment, and prognosis of human infection. CRC Crit. Rev. Microbiol., 8:339, 1981.
13. Elek, S. D.: Experimental staphylococcal infections in the skin of man. Ann. N.Y. Acad. Sci., 65:85, 1956.
14. Favero, M. S.: Sterilization, disinfection, and antisepsis in the hospital. *In* Lennette, E. H., et al. (eds.): *Manual of Clinical Microbiology*, 3rd ed. American Society for Microbiology, Washington, D.C. 1980, pp. 952–959.
15. Finegold, S. M.: Anaerobic infections. Surg. Clin. North Am. 60:49, 1980.
16. Ford, C. R., et al.: An appraisal of the role of surgical face masks. Am. J. Surg. 113:787, 1967.
17. Fox, J. G., et al.: Nosocomial transmission of *Serratia marcescens* in a veterinary hospital due to contamination by benzalkonium chloride. J. Clin. Microbiol. 14:157, 1981.
18. Goldman, D. A.: Laboratory procedures for infection control. *In* Lennette, E. H., et al. (eds.): *Manual of Clinical Microbiology*, 3rd ed. American Society for Microbiology, Washington, D.C., 1980, pp. 939–951.
19. Glickman, L. T.: Veterinary nosocomial (hospital-acquired) *Klebsiella* infections. J. Am. Vet. Med. Assoc. 179:1389, 1981.
20. Hardy, J. D.: Surgical complications: *In* Sabiston, D. C. (ed.): *Davis-Christopher Textbook of Surgery*, 12th ed. W. B. Saunders, Philadelphia, 1981, pp. 420–438.
21. Hirschmann, J. V., and Inui, T. S.: Antimicrobial prophylaxis: a critique of recent trials. Rev. Infect. Dis. 2:1, 1980.
22. Jones, R. L.: Unpublished data, 1982.
23. Ketaren, K., et al.: Canine salmonellosis in a small animal hospital. J. Am. Vet. Med. Assoc. 179:1017, 1981.
24. Lister Centenary Conference. Br. J. Surg. 54:405, 1967.
25. Love, R. F., et al.: Characterization of bacteroides species isolated from soft tissue infections in cats. J. Appl. Bacteriol. 50:567, 1981.
26. Meakins, J. L., et al.: The surgical intensive care unit: current concepts in infection. Surg. Clin. North Am. 60:117, 1980.
27. Miles, A. A., et al.: The value and duration of defense mechanisms of the skin to the primary lodgement of bacteria. Br. J. Exp. Pathol. 38:79, 1957.
28. Nora, P. F.: *Operative Surgery—Principles and Techniques*, 2nd ed. W. B. Saunders, Philadelphia, 1980, pp. 18–24.
29. Olmstead, M. L., et al.: Technique for canine total hip replacement. Vet. Surg. 10:44, 1981.
30. Postlethwait, R. W.: Principles of operative surgery: antisepsis technique, sutures and drains. *In* Sabiston, D. C. (ed.):

Davis-Christopher Textbook of Surgery, 12th ed. W. B. Saunders, Philadelphia, 1981, pp. 317–332.

31. Rae, T.: Localized tissue infection and the influence of foreign bodies. *In* Williams, D. F. (ed.): *Fundamental Aspects of Biocompatibility*, Vol. II. CRC Press Inc., Boca Raton, FL, 1981, pp. 139–158.
32. Sandusky, W. R.: Use of prophylactic antibiotics in surgical patients. Surg. Clin. North Am. *60*:83, 1980.
33. Swaim, S. F.: *Surgery of Traumatized Skin: Management and*

Reconstruction in the Dog and Cat. W. B. Saunders, Philadelphia, 1980, pp. 237–296.
34. Van der Waaij, D.: Colonization resistance of the digestive tract: clinical consequences and implications. J. Antimicrob. Chemother. *10*:263, 1982.
35. Varma, S., et al.: Comparison of seven suture materials in infected wounds—an experimental study. J. Surg. Res. *17*:165, 1974.

Sterilization

Chapter **20**

R. John Berg and Charles E. Blass

Sterilization is defined as the complete destruction of living organisms. In the surgical sense, sterilization is the complete elimination of microbial viability, including both the vegetative forms of bacteria and spores.

Joseph Lister (1827–1912) was among the first to recognize that wound infections are caused by microorganisms. His work as well as that of others provided the body of knowledge on which the modern principles of aseptic technique are based. Sterilization of surgical equipment, implants, linens, and attire is one aspect of a series of highly regimented steps constituting aseptic technique.

The methods of sterilization can be divided into two general groups: physical and chemical. Although sterility can be achieved with certain chemicals, physical methods are generally more reliable. Thermal energy, filtration, and radiation energy are the three most commonly used physical methods of sterilizing medical and surgical materials. Chemical sterilization is usually accomplished with ethylene oxide, although formaldehyde and betapropiolactone are also used occasionally. Finally, various disinfectants can be used as cold sterilants for noncritical surgical supplies. This chapter emphasizes steam and ethylene oxide sterilization, since these are the most commonly used techniques in veterinary medicine.

PHYSICAL STERILIZATION

Sterilization by Thermal Energy

Principles of Steam Sterilization

The mechanism by which heat destroys microorganisms is not perfectly understood. The temperature range within which microorganisms are able to survive is determined largely by the thermal viability of their proteins and nucleic acids.[4] The denaturation or destruction of cellular proteins appears to be the principal means by which heat destroys microorganisms. This is most likely a gradual chemical process that occurs in a stepwise fashion and in its early stages may be reversible.

Bacteria are destroyed by either wet or dry heat, although when moisture is present death occurs at a lower temperature and in a shorter period of time. Bacterial spores also show a greater resistance to dry than to moist heat.[4] This phenomenon is directly related to the ability of moisture to hasten the coagulation of cellular proteins and is consistent with the principle that water catalyzes all chemical reactions.[4] Although the ultimate cause of death from both wet and dry heat is protein denaturation, it appears that moist heat causes death by the coagulation of critical cellular proteins, whereas death by dry heat is primarily an oxidation process.[4]

The thermal death of bacteria and spores occurs in a logarithmic fashion.[4] The velocity at which individual organisms die is directly proportional to their concentration at a given time.[4] This velocity varies for each individual type of bacteria or spore and is proportional to the death rate constant, K. The determination of the death rate constant makes it possible to compare the heat resistance of different organisms at the same temperature or the heat resistance of a given organism at different temperatures.[4] There is no one temperature at which all microorganisms in a sample are killed instantaneously, and the thermal death of bacteria and spores is always a function of a time-temperature relationship.

Moist heat in the form of saturated steam under pressure is the most dependable medium known for the destruction of all forms of microbial life.[4] Boiling water at ambient pressures attains relatively low temperatures and is best considered a disinfecting rather than a sterilizing agent. Saturated steam is vapor produced by the heating of water. If the steam is contained in a vessel from which its escape is restricted, application of additional heat to the water produces an increase in both temperature and pressure of the steam. By definition, at a given pressure there is only one possible temperature for saturated

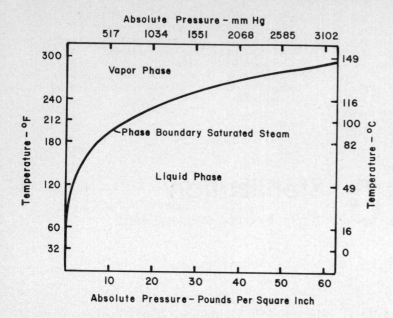

Figure 20–1. The constant temperature-pressure relationship of saturated steam. (Redrawn with permission from Perkins, J. J.: *Principles and Methods of Sterilization in Health Sciences.* Charles C Thomas, Springfield, 1969.)

steam and vice versa. This constant relationship between the temperature and pressure of saturated steam is illustrated in Figure 20–1. For sterilization, steam is maintained under pressure for the sole purpose of attaining a higher temperature. The pressure itself has no direct effect on the microbicidal properties of steam.

Steam is unique as a thermal sterilizing agent in its ability to permeate porous substances by the relatively rapid process of condensation. Unlike dry heat, which actually burns microorganisms following the slower process of heat absorption, steam gives up its heat by condensing back into the water from which it came.[4] Therefore, each item to be sterilized absorbs or contains moisture in exact proportion to the heat absorbed by the article. For sterilization, it is essential that supplies be arranged to allow rapid and complete penetration of steam. Steam penetrates each pack to be sterilized, heats the pack through condensation, and leaves the entire contents slightly moistened. Because steam sterilization is based on direct steam contact, certain materials such as oils and greases should not be sterilized using this technique. Their exterior surfaces are sterilized by steam, but the interior is inaccessible. Similarly, needles and fine instruments cannot be sterilized in test tubes with stoppered ends; the tubes should be sealed with cotton plugs.

Air in steam sterilizers is the principal factor inhibiting thorough diffusion of steam.[4] If the steam is unable to displace this air, condensation does not occur on all surfaces being sterilized. In addition to preventing thorough steam penetration, air reduces the temperature of steam at any given pressure, and because air and steam do not mix readily, the presence of air creates temperature variations in various parts of the chamber.[4] Modern steam sterilizers differ principally in the mechanisms by which they evacuate air from the sterilizing chamber.

Types of Steam Sterilizers

Several terms are used to refer to steam sterilizers, including *autoclave, pressure steam sterilizer, steam pressure sterilizer, vacuum steam sterilizer, vacuum sterilizer,* and *dressing sterilizer*. Of these, the term *autoclave* is probably used most commonly. The word autoclave means self-closing; that is, the door of the sterilizing chamber is held closed by the pressure within the chamber.

The autoclaves in use in most veterinary institutions and private practices today are *gravity displacement* or *downward displacement* sterilizers. In these autoclaves, steam is introduced under pressure into the top of the sterilizing chamber. Because the steam is considerably less dense than air, it "floats" to the top of the chamber, compressing the air to the bottom.[4] Some residual air may remain in the sterilizer, and this air eventually mixes with the steam. The air and condensate are removed from the chamber by a thermostatic valve and are discharged into the environment. Most gravity displacement sterilizers are also equipped with condensers, vacuum pumps, and ejector systems, which assist in the removal of air. The effectiveness of air removal from the chamber can be determined by measuring the temperature of the discharged air.[4] After all air has been eliminated and is replaced by steam, the indicated temperature rises to the temperature of the steam. The coldest steam, or steam with the highest air content, continues to be discharged so that the thermometer always indicates the temperature of the coldest region of the chamber. Thermometers are not placed inside the chamber because they indicate the temperature at a specific point. The design of a typical gravity displacement sterilizer is shown in Figure 20–2.

Prevacuum steam sterilizers have come into general use recently. In these autoclaves, air is evacuated

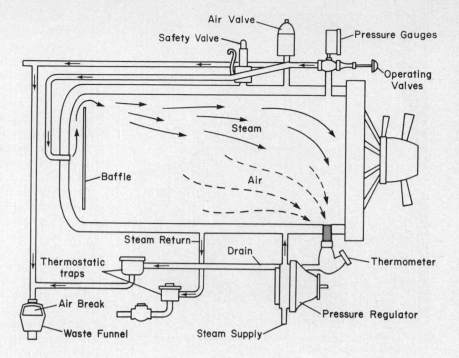

Figure 20–2. A gravity displacement sterilizer. All air in the sterilizing chamber is displaced downward by steam, and the thermometer measures the temperature of the exhausted air and steam. (Redrawn with permission from Lawrence, C.A., and Block, S.S.: *Disinfection, Sterilization, and Preservation.* Lea & Febiger, Philadelphia, 1968.)

from the chamber by means of a vacuum pump before steam is admitted to the chamber. This system eliminates the time lag required for the complete air displacement necessary in gravity displacement autoclaves. Because of this, the total sterilization time can be greatly reduced. In addition, the problem of air entrapment within the chamber is minimized. In gravity displacement sterilizers, the steam entering the surgical pack pushes air ahead of it, often resulting in a central "bubble" of air.[4] If the autoclave has been properly loaded, regions of entrapped air are slowly displaced by gravity. In prevacuum sterilizers, steam penetrates the load almost instantly, permitting the use of a high sterilization temperature and a reduced holding time.[4] As a result, these autoclaves allow the sterilization of surgical instruments and materials on an emergency basis.

Finally, *steam pulsing systems* are available that decrease the need for the development of a high prevacuum. High prevacuum autoclaves are expensive because they need sophisticated mechanical components and control devices.[4] In steam pulsing systems, a steam pulse increases the chamber pressure to a set pressure whereupon the chamber is vented to a minimal pressure preceding the next pulse. The time required to evacuate the air from the chamber depends on the amplitude or strength of each pulse and the time expended for each pulse.[4] Although the total cycle times for these autoclaves are not as fast as those for prevacuum systems, they are significantly faster than gravity displacement systems.

The Steam Sterilization Procedure

1. **Cleaning of surgical supplies prior to sterilization.** Gross contamination must be removed from surgical instruments prior to sterilization, regardless of the sterilization technique being used. Dried blood conceals microorganisms, particularly those in less accessible parts of instruments, and renders sterilization more difficult. Instruments may be cleaned manually, with washer sterilizers, or with ultrasonic cleaning equipment. Regardless of which cleaning technique is employed, instruments should be cleaned as soon as possible after use. Immediately after surgery the instruments should be rinsed in cold water to remove blood and debris. If there is a delay before the final cleaning, they should be immersed in warm water containing an effective detergent.

Manual cleaning is best achieved with a hand brush that has stiff bristles.[4] These brushes also should be washed and sterilized following their use. In cleaning instruments, ordinary soaps should be avoided because they tend to leave behind an insoluble alkaline residue. Abrasive compounds may damage the surfaces of instruments and also should be avoided. The best cleaning agents are moderately alkaline, low sudsing detergents.[4] After washing, the instruments should be rinsed in hot water and dried thoroughly.

In *washer-sterilizers*, washing is accomplished by means of an agitated detergent bath. The process is rapid, and handling of equipment contaminated by pathogenic organisms is minimized. Following the cycle, in which sterilization is provided by steam under pressure, the instruments are ready to be stored until needed. However, the instruments are unwrapped, and this procedure is not well adapted to routine sterilization of surgical supplies.

Ultrasonic cleaners use vibratory waves of a frequency higher than the upper frequency limit of the human ear to clean through *cavitation*. In cavitation, minute gas bubbles are generated by ultrasonics,

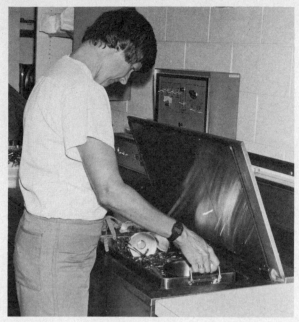

Figure 20–3. Instruments are loaded into an ultrasonic cleaner for washing prior to sterilization.

which expand until they are unstable then collapse. The implosion of these bubbles creates a minute vacuum that is responsible for the cleaning process.[4] In general, ultrasonic cleaning is capable of removing tightly bound soils that are poorly removed by other washing processes.[4] The instruments are loaded loosely in wire mesh trays with all box locks open. During the cleaning cycle, dense particles fall to the bottom of the cleaning tank, and finer soils rise to the surface of the water. Therefore, instruments must be rinsed thoroughly following ultrasonic cleaning. Following the rinse, the ultrasonic cleaner dries the instruments in warm air. A typical ultrasonic cleaner is illustrated (Fig. 20–3).

2. **Preparation of surgical packs and loading of the autoclave.** Most veterinary hospitals have an established routine for the preparation of surgical packs. In general, instruments and supplies should be segregated and packed according to their intended use. The system of packing should be standardized, and each type of pack should always contain the same material. Similar surgical instruments should be kept together, and linens should be stacked according to the order in which they are to be used.

Steam must be able to thoroughly penetrate both the material in which the pack is wrapped and the contents of the pack itself. The ideal wrapping material should be permeable to steam but not microbes, resistant to damage when handled, flexible, and easily returned to a flat position.[1, 7] Cotton muslin wraps are more durable and flexible than other wraps and have the best handling properties. Cotton muslin has a thread count of 140 threads per square inch.[4] The main disadvantage of muslin is that it provides a shorter safe storage time than do other wraps.[1] Muslin wraps should be double layered, and two wraps should be used for each pack.

A number of different types of paper are also available for the preparation of surgical packs. Crepe papers are superior to noncrepe papers because they are more flexible, more durable, and more easily handled. It is recommended that autoclave paper not be reused.[7] Paper may be used in either single or double layers, although single layers provide a shorter safe storage time. Regardless of the number of layers used, paper provides storage time superior to that of fabrics.

Materials should be positioned in packs to allow complete steam penetration. To ensure that all surfaces of instruments are exposed to steam, they should be sterilized with the box locks open. Several types of instrument pins, racks, and holders are available to allow an orderly, secure arrangement of unhinged instruments. Complex instruments such as Balfour retractors should be disassembled if possible unless they are specifically designed for steam penetration. Containers such as saline pans should be positioned in the pack so that the open end is facing either down or horizontally when the pack is in the sterilizer.

Guidelines for the preparation of instrument packs also apply to packs containing only linens, such as towels, gowns, and drapes. The procedure begins with laundering and ironing, both of which reliably remove most gross contamination from linens. Linen packs are limited in size to 12 × 12 × 20 inches and should not weigh more than 6 kg.[4] Table drapes are particularly difficult to sterilize because they are closely woven and create an extremely compact mass once ironed and folded. Therefore, drapes should be wrapped singly and should not be packaged with other equipment. Layers of linen should be alternated in their orientation to permit the least possible resistance to steam penetration.[4]

Instrument packs are positioned vertically (on edge) and longitudinally in the sterilizer. In this position they are oriented with the direction of steam flow and do not trap air. A slight amount of empty space should be present between each pack. Linen packs are loaded so that their layers are oriented vertically. If the layers are oriented horizontally, air and steam must travel downward through successive layers to escape, instead of between layers. Similarly, linen packs should not be stacked in the autoclave because this increases their effective thickness. Figure 20–4 illustrates the proper technique for loading a steam sterilizer.

3. **Autoclave operation.** Once the autoclave is loaded, the sterilization cycle is begun. A number of minimum time-temperature standards have been established for the routine sterilization of surgical packs; the guidelines used by various veterinary hospitals vary. Most authorities agree that 13 minutes exposure to saturated steam at 120°C (250°F) is a safe minimum standard.[4] In general, five to 10 minutes at this

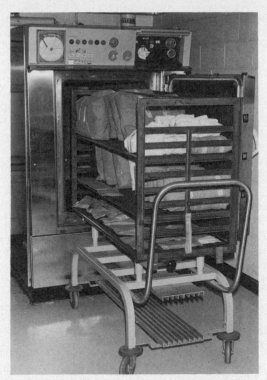

Figure 20–4. The proper arrangement of surgical packs for steam sterilization. All packs are oriented vertically, and a small amount of space separates the packs.

temperature will destroy most resistant microbes and the additional three to eight minutes provides a margin of safety. The timing of the exposure begins when the temperature in the exhaust line reaches the desired level, at which time the entire contents of the sterilizing chamber are completely exposed to steam. The time required for the sterilizing temperature to be reached is referred to as the heat-up time and is extremely short (about one minute) in prevacuum- and pulsing-type sterilizers.

Emergency sterilization of instruments is usually performed in prevacuum sterilizers. The recommended exposure time is three minutes at 131°C (270°F).[1] The instruments are sterilized in perforated metal trays that may be carried to the operating field using detachable handles.

Large linen packs require both a longer heat-up time and a longer exposure time. General guidelines for their sterilization are 30 minutes at 121°C (250°F)

TABLE 20–1. Safe Storage Time for Sterile Packs

Wrapper	Closed Cabinet	Open Shelves
Single-wrapped muslin (two layers)	1 week	2 days
Double-wrapped muslin (each two layers)	7 weeks	3 weeks
Single-wrapped crepe paper	At least 8 weeks	3 weeks

in gravity displacement sterilizers and 4 minutes at 131°C (270°F) in prevacuum sterilizers. All instrument and linen packs should be allowed to dry for a minimum of 20 minutes following the sterilization cycle. This is best achieved by opening the door of the autoclave a fraction instead of widely.

A number of indicator systems are available to monitor the effectiveness of the autoclave cycle. Regardless of the system used, the indicator is placed in the center of each pack. If a single indicator is used for the entire load, it is placed in the center of a test pack located in the front and center of the sterilizing chamber. All indicators undergo either chemical or biological changes in response to some combination of time and temperature factors.[7]

Chemical indicators most commonly are paper strips impregnated with a chemical that undergoes a color change when a certain temperature is reached. The most important drawback to these systems is that they provide no information regarding the time of exposure to a given temperature. For this reason, chemical indicators such as autoclave tape should not be overinterpreted. Their main value is in informing the surgeon that a pack has been exposed to the sterilization process, not that sterilizing conditions have been met.

Biological indicators are superior to chemical indicators, as they provide absolute proof that sterilizing conditions have been met. Numerous biological indicator systems are available. All systems employ a heat-resistant organism that is many more times resistant to the sterilization process than the organisms likely to be present as natural contaminants.[3] The most commonly used organism is the spore of *Bacillus stearothermophilus*. In one popular indicator system, these spores are contained in a liquid culture medium within a sealed glass vial. After the sterilization cycle, the vials are incubated for 24 to 48 hours and checked for turbidity or a color change, which indicates that growth is occurring. A disadvantage of this type of system is that it responds only to heat and temperature. If the steam is not properly saturated, a false indication may result.[3]

Whatever type of indicator system is employed, it should not be relied upon too heavily. Close supervision and exact standards for the preparation, packaging, and loading of supplies are the best guarantees of effective steam sterilization.

4. **Sterile pack storage.** If possible, sterile packs should be stored in closed cabinets rather than on open shelves. Safe storage times are significantly longer in cabinets, and there is less chance that the packs will come in contact with free water. All packs should be dated, preferably with an expiration date. Safe storage times for packs wrapped in commonly used materials are given in Table 20–1.[3]

Sterilization by Filtration

Filtration refers to the separation of particulate material from liquids and gases. The mechanism by which microorganisms or other particles are removed from filtered materials depends on the filter type. *Screen filters* collect all particles larger than their pore size on the surface of the filter. *Depth filters* are composed of a matrix of porous material. Microorganisms retained by depth filters may be much smaller than the pore size of the filter. Depth filters randomly trap microorganisms and particles throughout the filter matrix. The greater the depth of the filter, the more likely a particle will be entrapped while passing through the filter.

Pharmaceuticals are commonly sterilized by filtration. Filtration also has a direct application to surgery by way of the laminar flow principle of contamination control in the operating room. In this application, a bank of bacterial-retentive depth-type filters removes contaminants from the air circulating through the operating room.

Sterilization by Radiation

Certain materials sensitive to heat or chemicals are sterilized by radiation. Radiation kills organisms by producing ionization in or near the organism. Gamma rays, x-rays, and ultraviolet rays are the most common forms of radiation.

Because of their heat sensitivity, many pharmaceuticals are sterilized by radiation. Likewise, many heat-sensitive hospital and surgical materials, such as tissue grafts, are sterilized by gamma radiation. Ultraviolet irradiation has been used to destroy airborne microorganisms.

CHEMICAL STERILIZATION

Chemical sterilization refers to the use of gaseous or liquid chemicals. Chemical methods were developed to sterilize materials that are damaged by wet or dry heat. Few liquid chemicals classified as high-level disinfectants have the capability of sterilizing. However, three gaseous agents can be considered practical for sterilization: ethylene oxide, formaldehyde, and betapropiolactone.

Ethylene Oxide

Ethylene oxide is currently the most popular agent for gaseous sterilization. It is flammable and explosive except when mixed with carbon dioxide. Ethylene oxide is capable of destroying all known microorganisms, including bacteria, spores, fungi, and at least the larger viruses.[5]

Physical and Chemical Properties of Ethylene Oxide

Ethylene oxide is a simple cyclic ether. It is a colorless gas that liquefies at 10.9°C and freezes at −111.3°C. Ethylene oxide–air mixtures are flammable and explosive. As little as 3 per cent ethylene oxide supports combustion. Ethylene oxide is available in safe, nonflammable mixtures with carbon dioxide and variants of Freon.[5] Because ethylene oxide and carbon dioxide have different atomic weights, they tend to stratify in storage containers. Because of this, under certain circumstances the final 20% of the gas may not be capable of sterilization. This is not a problem with ethylene oxide–Freon mixtures.[5] Ethylene oxide diffuses and penetrates rapidly so that objects may be packaged prior to sterilization. It also rapidly diffuses from the object after sterilization. Because ethylene oxide vaporizes at 10.9°C, it is an effective sterilizing agent even at room temperature.

Ethylene oxide kills all organisms by alkylation. Labile hydrogen atoms are replaced by hydroxyethyl groups that block the reactive groups necessary for essential metabolic reactions. Moisture is necessary for the entrance of the gas into the cell.

Effects of Concentration, Temperature, Time, and Humidity

The effectiveness of ethylene oxide as a sterilizing agent depends on four variables: (1) gas concentration, (2) temperature, (3) exposure time, and (4) humidity.[5] Ethylene oxide gas is effective in concentrations of from 450 to 1,500 mg/L. Doubling the ethylene oxide concentration decreases the sterilization time by approximately one-half. Ethylene oxide sterilizers usually operate at from 21 to 60°C. The activity of ethylene oxide is slightly more than doubled with each 10°C increase in temperature. Exposure time varies from 48 minutes to several hours. Twelve hours exposure is allowed when sterilizing at room temperature. Increasing the chamber temperature to 55°C reduces the exposure time to four hours or less, assuming appropriate gas concentrations.[5] In general, an "oversterilization" period is allowed to ensure that adequate exposure has been allowed.

Ethylene oxide sterilizers operate at humidities ranging from uncontrolled ambient humidity to controlled high humidity. Optimum relative humidity is approximately 40 per cent.[1] Moisture is necessary for the lethal action of ethylene oxide. Time for the humidification of desiccated bacteria and spores is essential. Usually 30 to 60 minutes is allowed for moisture to penetrate wrappings and contact the items to be sterilized. Conversely, moisture left in tubing and needles when placed in the ethylene oxide sterilizer may slow the action of the gas below the lethal point.[5] Most ethylene oxide sterilizers operate at relative humidities of between 40 and 60%. A minimum relative humidity of 33 per cent is essential for sterilization.[5] In less automated sterilizers, moisture within the chamber can be provided by vials of water or water-soaked sponges.

Equipment and Technique

As with any method of sterilization, items should be thoroughly cleaned prior to ethylene oxide steri-

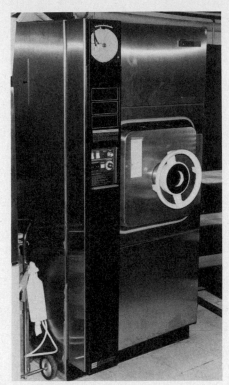

Figure 20–5. A large automated autoclave-type ethylene oxide sterilizer.

lization. Any container that can be sealed may be used. The operation of small, room temperature sterilizers is simple; the operation of large ethylene oxide sterilizers is technically more difficult (Fig. 20–5). In all cases, strict adherence to manufacturer's recommendations is essential.

The positioning of packs and packages is not as important for ethylene oxide sterilization as it is for steam sterilization, because ethylene oxide diffuses generally rather than descending vertically, as steam does. Many sterilizers operate with a vacuum to enhance penetration of ethylene oxide gas. The sterilizer should not be overloaded, as compression of

packages prevents penetration of the gas. At the end of the exposure time, the ethylene oxide gas is removed from the chamber. Air, preferably filtered, is admitted to the sterilization chamber until ambient pressure is attained.[1]

A period of aeration is allowed for diffusion of ethylene oxide gas from sterilized objects. Different objects require varying periods of time for aeration after sterilizing. Rubber and certain plastic materials trap and hold ethylene oxide gas and its by-products. Glass, stainless steel, and certain other plastics resist penetration by ethylene oxide gas, resulting in a relatively rapid eluting of ethylene oxide and its by-products. Two methods of aerating objects sterilized by ethylene oxide gas exist. The natural method is accomplished by allowing the mandatory poststerilization minimum time to elapse.[5] The second method is mechanical aeration. Mechanical aerators use high vacuum and moderately raised temperatures to reduce the time required to remove all traces of ethylene oxide gas. Recommended minimum aeration times for different materials are listed in Table 20–2. When materials are to be implanted, aeration periods as long as 10 to 15 days are desirable.[1]

Almost any material can be sterilized with ethylene oxide.[5] Ethylene oxide may form condensation products with water, which can damage rubber and plastic; hence such articles must be dry when put into the ethylene oxide sterilizer.[1] Freon dilutants, which are added to render ethylene oxide nonflammable, may damage certain plastics. Objects susceptible to heat damage may be sterilized at room temperature with exposure to ethylene oxide for 12 hours.

Several materials are available in which an object can be sterilized with ethylene oxide and remain sterile until used. Conventional packaging in muslin or paper is satisfactory for short periods, but new transparent plastics are often preferable because they allow observation of the sterile object. Some of the most commonly used wrapping materials include polyethylene, polycoated paper and Mylar, uncoated paper and Mylar, uncoated paper and nylon, poly-

TABLE 20–2. Aeration Times for Various Surgical Supplies Following Ethylene Oxide Sterilization

Material	Natural Aeration (hr)	Mechanical Aerators (hr)
Absorbent anesthesia equipment	120–168	5–8
Conductive rubber	30	16
Gloves, catheters	168	—
Items sealed in plastic	96	—
Internal pacemakers	500	—
⅛″ thick PVC	300	—
1/16″ thick PVC open heart surgery tubing	168	—
Polyethylene	48	12
Polypropylene	48	12
Red rubber	55	18
Thick rubber	24	4
Thin PVC	168	12
Thin rubber	6	1
Vinyl plastic	76	32

ethylene and nylon, and polyethylene and Mylar.[5] Generally, nylon should be avoided as a packaging material for ethylene oxide sterilization because of poor gas penetration.[5] Safe storage life is 15 to 30 days for cloth wraps, 30 to 60 days for paper wraps, 90 to 100 days for plastic wraps sealed with tape, and one year for plastic wraps that have been heat sealed.[5]

Sterilization Indicators

Only biological indicators ensure sterility, and periodic culture tests are recommended. Spores of *Bacillus subtilis* var. *globigii* are usually tested because they are more resistant to ethylene oxide than are other organisms. A disadvantage of biological methods is that results are unavailable for one to seven days. Chemical indicators that undergo color changes, indicating that sterilizing conditions have been met, are also available. Positive assurance of sterilization can be obtained only through the use of an ethylene oxide sterilization indicator placed inside each pack or package. Ethylene oxide indicator tape is useful for identifying packets that have been exposed to ethylene oxide sterilizing conditions. Such outside indicators cannot ensure that sterilizing conditions were achieved inside the package.[5]

Toxicity

Exposure to ethylene oxide gas and its by-products should be avoided. Ethylene oxide sterilizers and aerators should be located in a room that has at least ten air changes per hour. The air should be exhausted to the outside. The highest likelihood of exposure to ethylene oxide occurs at the end of the sterilization cycle.[2] The operator should open the sterilizer door as soon as possible after completion of the cycle then leave the area to allow residual ethylene oxide to dissipate and be removed by the ventilation system. The load is transferred from the sterilizer immediately to the aerator.

If the load must be handled, protective gloves should be worn, and prolonged breathing of vapors is avoided. Ethylene oxide is toxic and irritating to skin and mucous membranes. Contact with liquid ethylene oxide does not immediately irritate the skin but may produce delayed skin burns characterized by large blisters. Contact with liquid ethylene oxide causes severe eye injury; vapors are irritating to the nose and throat, and their presence is readily detected by smell. Continued exposure leads to olfactory fatigue, and the warning factor of smell is lost.[2] Clinical signs of human toxicity are nausea, vomiting, and mental disorientation.

Any object, expecially one made from polyvinyl chloride, previously sterilized by radiation should not be resterilized with ethylene oxide,[1, 5] as this may result in the formation of highly toxic ethylene chlorohydrin.[1, 5] Once ethylene chlorohydrin is formed, it is difficult to elute.

Formaldehyde

Pure formaldehyde is a white solid that gives off gaseous formaldehyde at room temperatures. Formaldehyde gas has been used to sterilize medical and surgical equipment, bedding, and other materials. Under proper conditions, vegetative bacteria are killed in one to two hours. Up to 12 hours is required to kill bacterial spores. After sterilization with formaldehyde, prolonged airing is necessary. Formaldehyde is highly irritating.

Betapropiolactone

Betapropiolactone has been used to sterilize hospital rooms and animal housing buildings. Betapropiolactone acts more rapidly than does either ethylene oxide or formaldehyde. The disadvantages of this gas are that it may damage painted and plastic surfaces. It is highly toxic and also carcinogenic.

Cold Sterilization

Cold sterilization refers to the practice of soaking instruments in disinfectant solutions. A disinfectant is an agent that destroys pathogenic organisms on inanimate objects. Disinfectants, in general, destroy all bacteria with the exception of the tubercle bacillus. Spores and viruses may not be destroyed by disinfectants, and for this reason cold sterilization should not be used for critical instruments. Critical instruments are those that potentially may be introduced beneath the surface of the body.[4] The only veterinary instruments that should be prepared by cold sterilization on a routine basis are dental supplies. Some properties of the commonly used cold "sterilants" are discussed next.

Alcohols. Ethyl alcohol and isopropyl alcohol kill bacteria by the coagulation of protein. Ethanol is generally used as a 70 per cent solution, and isopropyl alcohol is effective in concentrations of up to 99 per cent. Because alcohols evaporate more rapidly than does water, alcohol solutions fall in concentration if allowed to stand in open containers. At lower concentrations, they become bacteriostatic rather than bactericidal. Because of their poor activity against viruses and spores, alcohols should generally not be used as cold sterilants.

Aldehydes. Formaldehyde is available as formalin, a 37 per cent solution of formaldehyde and water. Although formalin is capable of killing all bacteria, viruses, and spores, it is extremely irritating to skin and mucous membranes and has limited application as a cold sterilizing agent. Glutaraldehyde in dilute concentrations is less toxic than formaldehyde and has a similar broad spectrum of activity. It is occasionally used to cold-sterilize items that cannot be exposed to steam, such as anesthetic accessories, and is the liquid disinfectant of choice for lensed instruments.[4, 7]

Chlorhexidine. This is an antiseptic agent available in detergent, tincture, and aqueous formulations. It has recently come into widespread use as an agent for the preparation of surgical patients and for surgical handscrubs because it is extremely nonirritating to skin.[6] It is immediately effective against both gram-positive and gram-negative organisms. In addition, this agent possesses residual activity, and its effectiveness increases after repeated use.[6]

Iodines. Inorganic iodines are good bactericidal agents but stain fabrics and tissue. They have good viricidal but poor sporicidal activity.[4] Concentrations greater than 3.5 per cent are toxic to tissue and do not provide additional disinfectant activity. The main disadvantage of iodines as cold sterilants is that they corrode instruments. However, they are excellent general purpose disinfectants.

Iodophors are iodines that are complexed with organic molecules such as detergents. Free iodine is released slowly from the carrier molecules and acts as a disinfectant. Iodophors have less tendency than inorganic iodines to stain fabric and tissue and are less irritating to skin. As with inorganic iodines, long-term use of iodophors may produce corrosion of instruments.

Phenols. Phenol or carbolic acid is the oldest known germicidal agent.[4] Phenolic derivatives have replaced phenol generally and may be divided into two groups. Cresols are primarily used as general disinfectants on environmental surfaces, and *bis*-

phenols are used as antiseptics.[7] Phenols are bactericidal but do not affect viruses and spores. Unlike many disinfectants, they are not adversely affected by organic materials. Phenols are commonly used as cold sterilants in combination with detergents or soaps to increase the spectrum of their activity.

Quaternary ammonium compounds. Quaternary ammonium compounds such as benzalkonium chloride are synthetic cationic detergents. These are surface-active agents that dissolve lipids in bacterial cell walls and membranes.[7] They are effective against both gram-positive and gram-negative bacteria but do not affect spores or viruses. They are very bland and nontoxic to tissues and are therefore quite popular. One limitation is that they are selectively absorbed by fabrics such as gauze, a fact that should be recognized when these compounds are used for surgical preparation.

1. Altemeier, W. A., et al.: *Manual on Control of Infection in Surgical Patients.* J. B. Lippincott, Philadelphia, 1976.
2. *Gas Sterilization/Aeration Systems.* American Sterilization Company, Erie, Pa., 1982.
3. Lawrence, C. A., and Block, S. S.: *Disinfection, Sterilization, and Preservation.* Lea & Febiger, Philadelphia, 1968.
4. Perkins, J. J.: *Principles and Methods of Sterilization in Health Sciences.* Charles C Thomas, Springfield, 1969.
5. *Principles and Practice of Ethylene Oxide Sterilization.* ATI Company, North Hollywood, 1982.
6. Rosenberg, A., Alatary, S. D., and Peterson, A. F.: Safety and efficacy of the antiseptic chlorhexidine gluconate. Surg. Gynecol. Obstet. *143*:789, 1976.
7. Tracy, D. L., and Warren, R. G.: *Small Animal Surgical Nursing.* C. V. Mosby, St. Louis, 1983.

Chapter **21** | # Preparation of the Surgical Team

Stanley D. Wagner

A primary and continuing source of aerial bacteria in surgery is the skin of surgical team members.[7, 17, 45] The surgical team consists of the surgeon, assistant surgeons, anesthetist, and calculating assistant. It is very rare that properly maintained mechanical equipment, walls, or instruments are sources of contamination. A naked individual with normal skin may desquamate 100,000 to 30,000,000 particles per minute, of which 3,000 to 50,000 are microbes.[37] Even when barriers such as scrub suits, masks, and caps are worn, particulate matter is still shed into the air.

In a clean, unoccupied room with a conventional air flow system, the numbers of airborne bacteria are as low as about 1 organism per cubic foot (Fig. 21–1). After the surgical team arrives, the airborne bacterial count increases to about 10 organisms per

cubic foot. There is a correlation between number of people in a room, degree of activity, and the airborne bacterial population[43] (Fig. 21–2). With increased activity more organisms are moved from the floor to the air, because increased activity causes friction between clothes and skin; thus, particles are shed.[3] Bacterial fluctuation in the environment can be recorded by sampling the air. Air samples can be taken in any operating room by exposing three blood agar plates to room air for 15 minutes. After overnight incubation, the colonies are counted. The number of colonies per plate is roughly equivalent to the number of particles per cubic foot of air as determined by conventional air sampling apparatus.[43]

Clean wound sepsis rates for small animal surgical services are not well-documented.[8] The orthopedic

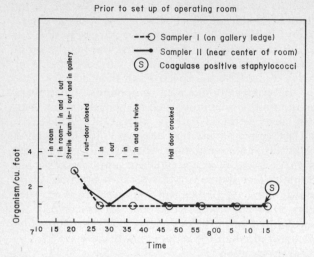

Figure 21-1. Preoperative microorganism levels in an operating room prior to surgery and arrival of patient as determined by air sampling apparatus in two different areas of the room. (Data from Ulrich, J. A.: Microbiology of surgery suites. Symposium on Clean Room Technology in Surgery Suites, Cape Kennedy Space Center, FL, May, 1971.)

services have reported on cultured wound sepsis, but these are directed toward the diagnosis and management of osteomyelitis. One of these authors suggested that the surgical team may be the source of infection.[39]

This chapter does not provide epidemiological studies to show that the surgical team is the origin of operative sepsis but reviews the barrier apparel available for separation of bacteria from the surgical wound.

SCRUB SUITS

The scrub suit is an occlusive but not impermeable barrier to microorganisms.[7] Preoperative contact cultures of the front of scrub suits that had undergone routine laundering revealed heavy bacterial contamination in 100 per cent of the suits. *Staphylococcus* species were cultured from 96 per cent of the scrub suits.[34] The scrub suit may act as a source of pathogenic bacteria for seeding and contamination of the surgical wound if the gown covering the suit is an ineffective barrier.[48] Routine laundering of the suits does not eliminate pathogenic organisms; the suits need to be steam sterilized periodically.

The majority of scrub suits consist of two pieces—shirt and trousers. A one-piece jumpsuit is available, and, although not used as frequently, it does reduce environmental bacterial shedding. Scrub suit trousers should have elastic or tie cuffs to reduce shedding of bacteria from the legs and perineum, where bacterial counts are normally higher.[12] If the trouser legs are occluded by shoe covers, there is a marked decrease in the number of bacteria shed into the environment.[3, 6] The shirt should be worn inside the trousers (Fig. 21–3).

Scrub suits should be made of material that provides lint-free wearing, comfort, durability, limited shrinkage, and convenient maintenance. Suits made from materials such as sanforized cotton, 50% polyester/50% combed cotton percale, 65% polyester/34% cotton/1% stainless steel, or disposable nonwoven material meet these requirements. When the surgeon leaves the operating room, the scrub suit should be protected by a coat to reduce contamination from

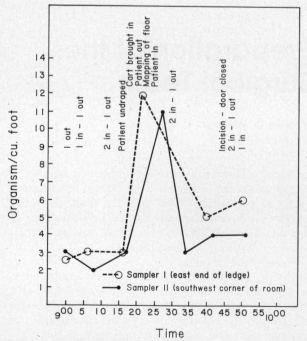

Figure 21-2. Effect of activity in operating room on microorganism levels as determined by air sampling apparatus in two different areas of the room. (Data from Ulrich, J. A.: Microbiology of surgery suites. Symposium on Clean Room Technology in Surgery Suites, Cape Kennedy Space Center, FL, May, 1971.)

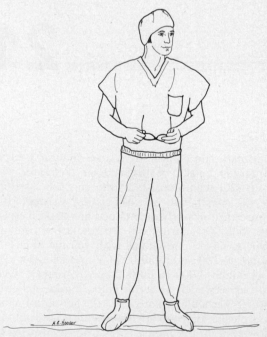

Figure 21-3. Two-piece scrub suit worn properly, with shirt inside the trousers to reduce bacterial shedding into the air. If trouser legs are occluded by shoe covers there is a further decrease of bacteria shed into the environment from the legs and perineum.

higher microorganism counts in the hallways and patient wards.

SURGICAL HEAD COVERS

Hoods (Fig. 21–4) rather than caps are recommended for all operating room personnel, because hair acquires and sheds bacteria-containing particles, although there is no statistical difference in environmental contamination in the wearing of caps, hoods, or bouffants.[25, 44] Human hair of the occipital and temporal regions harbors bacteria, including *Staphylococcus aureus*, *Escherichia coli*, and *Streptococcus viridans*. Hair carriers of *S. aureus* are now more prevalent than nasal carriers, as shown when one individual had the organism recovered from his hair but not from nasal, throat, or finger cultures.[14] Ritter states that length of hair or wearing of beards in the operating room has no effect on microbial environment.[44]

Head covers should cover occipital and temporal hair completely, be durable and comfortable to wear, and not shed lint into the wound. Three disposable head covers other than woven ones are discussed hereafter.

The least expensive of the three materials, dry-lay rayon, is a nonwoven material manufactured by a totally dry process. Dry-lay rayon is composed of many small, very short fibers. This material has directional strength, meaning that it has strength in only one direction. Dry-lay rayon is cooler to wear than wet-lay rayon, but the very short fibers are easily brushed from the surface, causing a linting problem. Wet-lay rayon is a more expensive material and is used by fewer manufacturers. The wet-lay process involves mixing the rayon fibers in a wet solution and then spreading this mixture in the desired thickness. The material is stiff and paperlike in consistency. Spun-bonded polypropylene is a material made of many long fibers that are spun together, forming a mass of fibers that are interdependent. This silklike material has adequate porosity and is lint free and flame resistant. If cloth head covers are used, they must be laundered daily.

SHOE COVERS

Shoe covers are available in many different types of re-usable or disposable materials. When properly worn, they effectively exclude bacteria from street shoes and reduce the possibility of contaminating the operating room. Shoe covers also protect the wearer's own shoes from contamination by hospital bacteria. Blood on leather shoes dries and flakes off into the environment, where it acts as nutrient medium.[25] If the pant leg of the scrub suit is forced down into the shoe cover, there is less spread of bacteria from the legs and perineum into the environment[6] (see Fig. 21–3). Newer shoe covers are made of light-weight nonwoven material that is waterproof and will not tear. These shoe covers do not retain heat or water, as plastic boots or heavy cloth shoe covers do. Shoe covers can be purchased with conductive strips to eliminate static electricity.

FACE MASKS

Of all the traditional surgical articles worn to promote asepsis in the operating room, the face mask contributes the least. Face mask is a misnomer, because it does not cover the face, only the mouth and nose. The forehead, temple, angle of the jaw, and the skin under the eye and chin normally have a high bacterial population, but these areas are not covered by the mask. When environmental bacterial colony counts are measured in identical rooms, one containing a group of people wearing face masks and the other group not wearing face masks, the colony counts are not statistically altered.[45] When human albumin microspheres are sprayed on the inner surface of a face mask worn during surgery, no microspheres are seen on the mask's exterior surface microscopically, but microspheres can be recovered from saline flushes of the wound prior to closure.[21] Masks will contain droplets and particles of microorganisms shed from the naso- and oropharynx and direct their flow to the lateral sides and bottom of the mask, ultimately reaching the surgical environment[13] (Fig. 21–4A). The major function of a face mask in surgery is to protect the wound from droplets of saliva expelled by the surgical team members when talking.[31]

Most surgical masks today rate high in filtration efficiency (90 to 99 per cent), either wet or dry, for up to eight hours of wearing time.[13, 42] Disposable nonwoven masks are made in a layered construction using a combination of natural and synthetic materials. Cloth masks vary in the number of layers of cotton muslin. There is a difference in *in vitro* and *in vivo* studies on masks. In the former, artificially

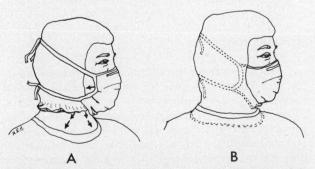

Figure 21–4. A, Nasopharyngeal organisms may escape around the edges of the face mask and enter the surgical site. *B,* Nasopharyngeal organisms can be contained when edges of the face mask are covered by the surgical head gear. (Adapted from Ha'eri, M. D., et al.: The efficiency of standard surgical face masks: An investigation using "tracer particles." Clin. Orthop. Rel. Res. *148*:160, 1980.)

A   B

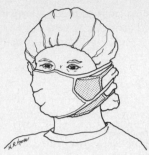

Figure 21–5. Two face masks that overlap in the front cover more surface area of the face than a single face mask.

generated droplets pass through masks held in a form-fitting frame. In the latter, droplets are generated unevenly by human breath and are subject to abrasion over an uneven surface when laughing, sneezing, and talking. The filtration efficiency of masks is greater for particulate matter larger than 3.3 microns in diameter than for particles smaller than 3.3 microns in diameter. Particles smaller than 3.3 microns in diameter do not fall easily on their own into a wound during surgery.[42] In the operating room environment, bacteria are usually carried by particles and droplets of the upper respiratory tract that are 5 to 30 microns in diameter.[21]

The structural design of a face mask is important for wearing comfort and effectiveness. Masks with a large diffusion area offer more breathing comfort to the wearer as well as cover more surface area of the face. The addition of pleats to a mask increases wearing comfort and efficacy. Stiffly contoured material keeps the mask away from the lips for clear speech but covers less area and has less efficiency. One of the criticisms of cloth masks is the billowing effect around the lateral sides of the face, which increases dispersal of bacteria (see Fig. 21–4A). Reports vary on the efficiency of filtration of cloth masks.[13, 38, 42]

Face masks should be designed to prevent the escape of bacteria from the lateral sides and to better cover the face.[21] One suggestion is to wear two masks that overlap in the front, giving ear to ear coverage (Fig. 21–5). Another is to require the wearing of surgical head hoods so that the mask edges are covered by the head gear[17] (Fig. 21–4B). Plastic, bubble-helmeted, surgeon isolator systems are impractical for veterinary use, and their relevance in human surgery is suspect.[25, 37]

PREPARATION OF THE SURGEON'S SKIN

The objectives of the surgical scrub are to (1) remove gross dirt and oil from the hands, (2) reduce the microorganism count to as close to 0 as possible, and (3) have a prolonged depressant effect on the microflora of the hands and forearms.[18] Other objectives to consider include the following: (1) the surgical scrub should not be excessively time consuming, and (2) the antiseptic and scrub method should not irritate the skin with repeated use. Monologues on the methodology of surgical hand preparation are available in textbooks on veterinary surgical techniques.[24]

Skin cleaners are used to kill transient and resident bacteria.[23] Resident bacteria are able to multiply within the skin microenvironment. Transient bacteria do not multiply and are presumed to be deposited on the skin from the mucous membranes or the environment. Washing with bar soap removes most of the transient bacteria, and the resident population is removed by antiseptic solutions. Three surgical scrub solutions used are hexachlorophene, povidone-iodine, and chlorhexidine gluconate. The use of a pour-on germicide applied by basin dip, spray, or dispenser following a scrub solution is not justified.

The surgical scrub protocol is based on either a timed anatomical scrub procedure or the counted brush stroke method. Either method assures sufficient exposure of all skin surfaces to friction and the antimicrobial solution. Individual attention to nails and subungual and interdigital areas is essential. Numerous studies indicate that there is no significant difference in bacterial populations following five- or ten-minute timed scrubs.[18, 54] No difference was noted when disposable polyurethane brush/sponges were substituted for re-usable brushes.[18] With the long-term use of stiff scrub brushes, the skin is stripped of its natural oils, which leads to bacterial colonization and dermatitis. A high-pressure pulsating water jet lavage of antiseptic solutions to the hands has been advocated as a substitute for the brush scrub.[20] One author suggests a three- to five-minute brush scrub with a detergent antiseptic for the initial surgical scrub of the day and then two- to three-minute scrubs with an antiseptic-impregnated sponge between additional surgical operations.[10] Of the three antiseptics available, all were highly effective in removing bacteria from the skin of hands and arms when the percentage of bacteria before and after scrubbing was compared. Any one of these antiseptic agents may be chosen on the basis of personnel preference or cost analysis. The advantages and disadvantages of the three are discussed.

Hexachlorophene

Hexachlorophene is combined with several moisturizing agents to lessen the effects of daily surgical preparation. Hexachlorophene is effective against gram-positive but not gram-negative bacteria. The presence of organic material will lower its efficiency. Hexachlorophene has a cumulative antibacterial action following subsequent application because it is not metabolized by skin enzymes and is bound to keratin. It passes into the blood stream unchanged. Hexachlorophene is not as effective as chlorhexidene gluconate or povidone-iodine on bacterial reduction immediately after scrubbing when used once. Hexachlorophene's cumulative antibacterial action can be nullified by alcohol. Hexachlorophene is reported to cause photosensitivity and dermatitis in individuals sensitive to halogenated phenols. Hexachlorophene oxidizes stainless steel containers and becomes discolored when exposed to direct sunlight.

Hexachlorophene is available for surgical scrubs in three forms: 3% hexachlorophene detergent, 0.25% hexachlorophene soap, and 0.23% hexachlorophene in a 46% ethyl alcohol base. Hexachlorophene toxicity has been documented after oral and topical application in man and animals. Blood levels of surgical personnel are 0.22 part per million with the detergent, 0.07 ppm with the soap, and 0.03 ppm with the foam. Histopathological changes in the brains of rats after oral ingestion of hexachlorophene are associated with a blood level of 1.21 ppm.[9] The antiseptic foam is rubbed on the hands and forearms for three minutes after washing with bar soap and water, and the arms are allowed to air dry. Low surgical sepsis rates have been maintained with this method. In addition, there is less skin irritation, less water wasted, and less time involved in scrubbing.[16, 18]

Povidone-Iodine

Povidone is a polymer that has attained wide usage because of its ability to detoxify and prolong the activity of many drugs. When combined with iodine it retains the bactericidal activity of iodine and releases the iodine slowly. Surgical scrub solutions of 7.5% povidone-iodine yield 0.75% available iodine. Other iodophors available are poloxamer iodine and nonoxynal iodine complex. Povidone-iodine is effective against gram-positive and gram-negative bacteria, fungi, viruses, yeasts, and protozoa. Iodophors have a greater immediate reduction in bacterial counts after scrubbing than hexachlorophene. Conflicting results on the depressant effect of povidone-iodine on the accelerated regrowth of bacteria under surgical gloves have been reported.[50] Glove fluid yielded higher colony counts in one- to six-hour postscrubbing samples when compared with colony counts taken immediately following povidone-iodine skin preparation.[41] Lowbury and coworkers reported a greater reduction in skin flora when sampled after glove wear for three hours than when samples were made immediately after disinfection of the skin.[33] Other authors report that the iodophors inhibit bacterial regrowth for up to two hours in the gloved hand.[16, 18, 23] Skin reactions are less frequent with the iodophors than with hexachlorophene. The presence of organic material does not affect the efficiency of povidone-iodine.

Chlorhexidine Gluconate

This surgical scrub solution has been used in Europe for many years in a 4% concentration. Chlorhexidine gluconate produced the greatest initial reduction in bacterial colonies when compared with the iodophors and hexachlorophene. Reductions in bacterial counts increased following repeated use of this product.[41, 47] Chlorhexidine gluconate in aqueous, alcoholic, or detergent solutions is effective against both gram-positive and gram-negative bacteria, including *Pseudomonas aeruginosa*. Its bactericidal activity is not reduced by the presence of blood or pus, and there is no systemic absorption. Chlorhexidine gluconate appears to equal or surpass the iodophors as a hand cleanser.[32]

GOWNS

In the 19th century, gowns were introduced to act as a barrier between the skin of the surgical members and the patient.[34] These barriers were made of woven materials, usually cotton. In 1952 it was observed that dry cloth is an aseptic barrier that loses all of its properties when it becomes wet. It was also shown that cloth used in surgery was not an effective barrier to microorganisms when either wet or dry.[2] Bacteria are transported from a nonsterile to a sterile area not by their own motility but by some vehicle such as blood, serum, or electrolyte solutions. Inasmuch as the cloth gown materials cannot be looked upon as bacterial filters, the transmission of moisture is tantamount to the transmission of contained bacteria.[26]

Since this discovery, the concept of moist bacterial penetration has been well-documented with cloth gowns. Increasing the thickness or number of layers of pervious cloth material does not make the gown a more effective barrier.

Surgical gowns should be made of material that establishes a barrier, eliminating the passage of microorganisms between sterile and nonsterile areas.[35] Criteria to be met in establishing an effective barrier are as follows:

1. Blood and aqueous fluid resistance. Liquids with a low surface tension penetrate fabrics more readily than those with a high surface tension. Surface tension of water is 72.8 dynes/cm^2, blood and body fluids range between 42 and 60 dynes/cm^2, and saline solution is 73.7 dynes/cm^2.[48]

2. Resistance to the stresses of stretch, pressure, and friction.

3. Freedom from linting to reduce the number of particles in the air. Other criteria to be considered are fire resistance, wearing comfort, economy, and accessibility.

Two terms used in gown manufacturing are *woven* and *nonwoven*. Woven fabric is produced by interlacing two yarns or similar materials so that they cross each other at right angles. The warp, or end, threads run lengthwise in the fabric, and filling threads run from side to side. The yarn is made by twisting a small number of fibers together. These fibers can be natural or man-made. Nonwoven fabrics are not made from yarn but directly from fibers. Fibers are bonded or interlocked together by mechanical, chemical, thermal, or solvent methods.[11] Nonwoven material in this discussion refers to a disposable, single-use item.

A popular material for cloth gowns is loosely woven all-cotton fabric type 140 muslin.[5] This muslin has 140 threads per square inch of material and is still used in single or double layers. Promotional materials often refer to type 140 muslin as a standard with which newer gown products are compared. Type 140 muslin is not a standard and is instantly permeable to moist bacterial penetration when wet.[26, 29]

In 1963, the textile industry introduced a re-usable woven fabric with fluid barrier capability made from the finest, longest, pima cotton stable yarn. These yarns are first subjected to a vigorous combing process to remove foreign bodies and impurities, further refining the quality of the yarn. After combing, the yarns are tightly twisted, then woven into a high-count fabric of 270 to 272 threads per square inch with a pore size of 10 microns.[3] After weaving, additional processing yields a very smooth and dense fabric, 270 pima cloth.[4] The woven fabric is treated with the water repellent Quarpel. Quarpel is a fluorochemical finish that, when combined with a pyridinium or melamine hydrophobe, produces an exceptionally durable water-repellent finish.[29] The performance and durability of the Quarpel are partially contingent upon the quality and weave of the material to which it is applied. Quarpel-treated 270 pima cotton gowns are marketed by several manufacturers under different trademarks.[11, 26, 29] Gowns made of 270 pima cotton not treated with Quarpel finish are as rapidly permeable to bacteria as ordinary 140 muslin.

Scanning electron microscopy of bacteria applied to one side of 140 muslin cotton and tightly woven pima cotton waterproofed with Quarpel demonstrated the following:

1. Type 140 muslin cotton showed bacteria on the reverse surface as well as on the applied surface (Fig. 21–6).

2. Tightly woven Quarpel-treated pima cotton halted the permeation of the bacterial solution at the surface. Cross sections and the reverse surface showed no bacteria (Figs. 21–7 and 21–8A). After 75 washing-sterilization cycles, individual fibers appeared shredded (Fig. 21–8B), and bacteria were found in all layers of cross sections as well as on the reverse surface of the woven material[27] (Fig. 21–9).

These findings indicate the need for some type of numbering system to identify when gowns have been washed and sterilized 75 times.[48] Laundering of these dense woven products is done by the conventional wash-rinse process, but some manufacturers suggest washing within 12 hours if blood is present. The construction of the pima cotton Quarpel-treated gown contributes to an unusually high moisture-holding power; for this reason an additional rinse cycle may be required to remove any detergent residue, which could adversely affect fabric life.[5] Each time a re-usable woven gown is laundered, the pores in the fabric become wider; an increased perforation size of 1 to 50 microns after only two washings has been demonstrated.[15, 44]

Woven materials need to be inspected every time they are processed for tears or punctures, which destroy their barrier quality. Woven gowns should not be repaired by sewing, because the needle holes

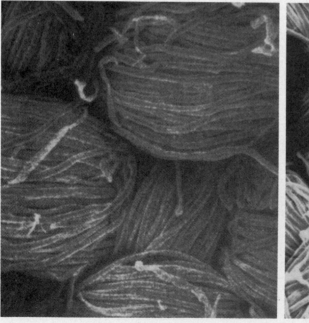 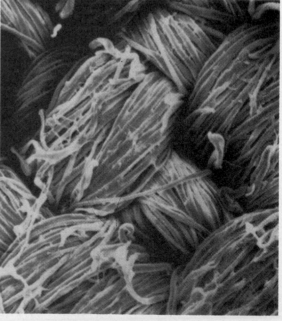

| A | B |

Figure 21–6. A, View of surface of 140-thread cotton shows comparative size of bacteria, fibers, and interstices. Application surface. ×411. B, View of reverse surface shows bacteria. ×411. (Reprinted with permission from Laufman, H., et al.: Scanning electron microscopy of moist bacterial strike-through of surgical materials. Surg. Gynecol. Obstet. *150*:165, 1980. By permission of SURGERY, GYNECOLOGY & OBSTETRICS.)

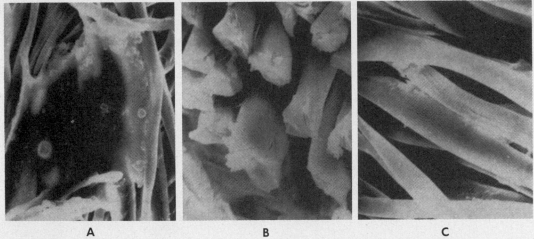

Figure 21–7. *A,* Bacteria on surface of tightly woven, 270-thread, Quarpel-treated Pima cotton, unused. ×524. *B,* Cut surface of same sample shows no penetration of bacteria. ×524. *C,* Reverse side of same sample shows no penetration of bacteria. ×524. (Reprinted with permission from Laufman, H., et al.: Scanning electron microscopy of moist bacterial strike-through of surgical materials. Surg. Gynecol. Obstet. *150:*165, 1980. By permission of SURGERY, GYNECOLOGY & OBSTETRICS.)

will cause further damage. The average diameter of microorganisms is 0.5 to 5.0 microns[25]; the hole made by a needle and thread is 20 microns, thus destroying barrier qualities. Towel clamps and suture needles also destroy barrier qualities. Holes should be repaired with heat-sealed vulcanized fabric patches reinforced with a plastic film. Patching does not interfere with steam sterilization of the woven gown if no more than 20 per cent of the gown's surface is occluded by the heat-sealed patches.[19]

Nonwoven gowns are not made from yarn but directly from fibers. By a variety of patented manu-

facturing methods, raw materials are transformed into a thick and syrupy liquid. This liquid material is extruded through a nozzle with fine holes or slits, then hardened either by air or a chemical bath into a fiber. These fibers are made of regenerated fibers (cotton or wood pulp) and man-made or synthetic fibers made from chemicals obtained from coal, air, water, sulfur, or natural gas.[11] The length, thickness, and shape of the fibers can be controlled, and these fibers may be preferentially oriented in one direction or deposited in a random manner into sheets or mats of fiber and then bonded together. Nonwoven ma-

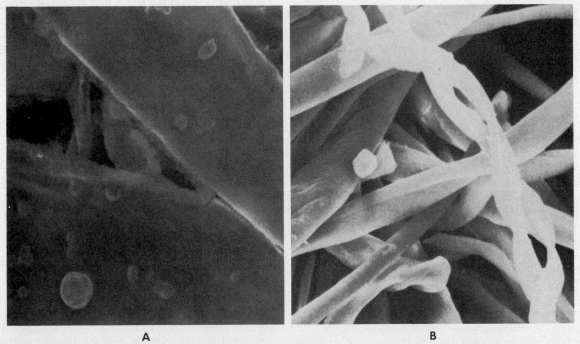

Figure 21–8. *A,* Tightly woven, 270-thread, Quarpel-treated Pima cotton, unused or less than 75 washing and sterilizing cyclings. Note smoothness of fibrils. ×86. *B,* Same material after 100 washing and sterilizing cyclings. Note relative roughness and curly appearance of fibrils as the Quarpel waterproof treatment wears off. ×86. (Reprinted with permission from Laufman, H., et al.: Scanning electron microscopy of moist bacterial strike-through of surgical materials. Surg. Gynecol. Obstet. *150:*165, 1980. By permission of SURGERY, GYNECOLOGY & OBSTETRICS.)

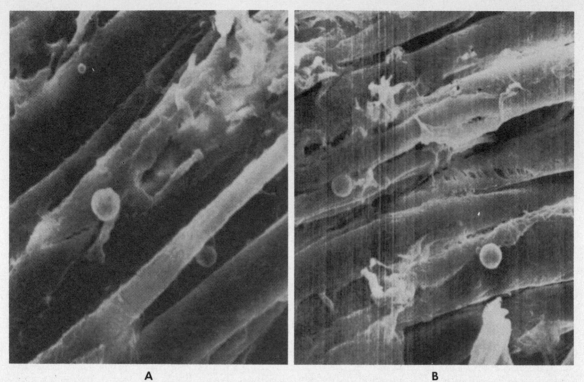

A   B

Figure 21–9. *A,* Bacteria on application surface of tightly woven, 270-thread, Quarpel-treated Pima cotton that has been through 100 or more washing and sterilization cyclings. ×449. *B,* Bacteria on the reverse surface of same sample are an indication of penetration. ×449. (Reprinted with permission from Laufman, H., et al.: Scanning electron microscopy of moist bacterial strike-through of surgical materials. Surg. Gynecol. Obstet. *150:*165, 1980. By permission of SURGERY, GYNECOLOGY & OBSTETRICS.)

terials have interstices that are so closely joined that bacteria and fluids are prevented from passing through.[14] Not all nonwoven gowns are impervious to moist bacterial contamination, and not all woven gowns are pervious, as previously noted.[26, 27] Nonwoven gowns made from a single layer of fabric exhibit great variation in bacterial permeation. When single-layer gowns are re-inforced with a layer of plastic film, the gowns are impervious, but, when re-inforced with another layer of the same material, they are still pervious.[29]

Some of the nonwoven gown materials used are olefins and polyesters (see Fig. 21–10). Olefin is a manufactured fiber in which the fiber-forming substance is any long-chain synthetic polymer composed of at least 85 per cent (by weight) ethylene, propylene, or other olefin unit (polyethylene fibers). Polyester is a manufactured fiber in which the fiber-forming substance is a long-chain synthetic polymer composed of at least 85 per cent (by weight) ester of a dehydric alcohol and terephthalic acid.[11]

The number of microorganisms isolated from the surgical environment was lowered when disposable, single-use, nonwoven materials were used by the surgical team. A 90 per cent reduction in airborne organisms was provided by the use of disposable gowns when compared with cloth.[14] Although the use of disposable nonwoven materials does not reduce the environmental contamination to 0, it does significantly improve the situation (Figs. 21–10 and 21–11). Disposable nonwoven gowns come folded in sterilized packages, which may be more economical when one considers the labor costs involved in the proper maintenance of cloth gowns.[28, 40] Disposable gowns should not be laundered and recycled for use in sterile surgery, because individual fibers may break. This is difficult to detect grossly, but the material becomes porous.

In some nonwoven gowns the seams on the sleeves, which are glued or stitched, are positioned so that they become moistened during surgery. Seams should be positioned so that they are protected.[29]

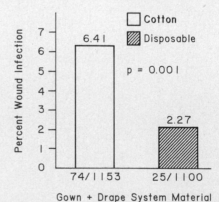

Figure 21–10. The overall postoperative wound infection rates from two different hospitals following 2,253 consecutive general surgeries. The wound infection rates are compared based on the barrier system used. (Reprinted with permission from Moylan, J. A., and Kennedy, B. V.: The importance of gown and drape barriers in the prevention of wound infection. Surg. Gynecol. Obstet. *151:*465, 1980. By permission of SURGERY, GYNECOLOGY & OBSTETRICS.)

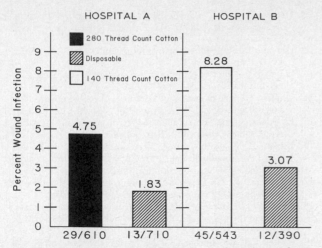

Figure 21–11. Postoperative wound infection from the two hospitals in Figure 21–11 when barrier materials of 280- and 140-thread count are compared with disposable barrier materials (Reprinted with permission from Moylan, J. A., and Kennedy, B. V.: The importance of gown and drape barriers in the prevention of wound infection. Surg. Gynecol. Obstet. *151*:465, 1980. By permission of SURGERY, GYNECOLOGY & OBSTETRICS.)

Lint has also been reported as a problem with nonwoven gowns. Peritoneal granulomas have occurred in surgical patients from cellulose lint.[28, 52] An area of permeability in both woven and nonwoven surgery gowns is the stockinette cufflet. Gown cuffs act as a wick, permitting almost immediate moist bacterial contamination without the application of a stress factor. Ideally, gown cuffs should remain covered by the surgeon's glove during an operation, therefore remaining dry. In reality, the gown cuffs often become uncovered and wet, especially when there is intraoperative manipulation.[26, 29] Manufacturers' tests for bacterial permeability in woven and nonwoven gowns should be studied from the standpoint of correlating bacterial permeation with the type of stresses encountered during actual surgical operations.[26] Laboratory studies cited by a manufacturer may show gown material impermeability to bacteria, but the material may be very permeable in wearing studies.[48] This discrepancy in bacterial penetration is thought to be due to the mechanical force generated by body motion and pressure during the operative procedure. Unopposed pressure or friction points of the surgical gown, such as those of the surgeon's forearm, elbow, or abdominal area, often transmit bacteria from the wearer to the surgical field, especially when the gown is moist.[26, 29]

Lengthy surgical operations during which surgical gowns are subjected to the stresses of stretch, shear, and pressure and come in contact with blood and other fluids have a greater risk of moisture strikethrough contamination.[25, 26] A gown should be considered a sterile field only from the surgeon's shoulder to the waist, including the sleeves. The front and lower sleeves of woven gowns should be Quarpel-treated, and this area in nonwoven gowns should be re-inforced with a polymeric film for waterproofing.[26, 29] Individually packaged disposable nonwoven

sterile replacement sleeves are available. These sleeves can be used as re-inforcement or replacement if there is a break in sterility. All surgery gowns, woven or nonwoven, should have stand-up collars for better fit, wide sleeves for freedom of movement, and overlapping back panels so that the back of the gown remains sterile.

GLOVES

Gloves were introduced in surgery to prevent contact dermatitis of a surgical team member's hands from instrument disinfectant rather than for patient protection.[49] Some gloves were made of linen, which possessed no barrier qualities.

Surgical gloves are manufactured by dipping hand-shaped molds into a film-forming liquid such as latex. Powders are placed on the inside of the glove to assist as mold release agents or as donning lubricants.[53] Lycopodium and talcum powder and magnesium silicate were used as powders until documented as a cause of foreign body reactions in all body cavities.[1, 49] In 1947, cornstarch derivatives were marketed as completely absorbable inert substances that were safe to use as a gloving powder. After initial etherification with epichlorohydrin to render the granules resistant to autoclaving, the cornstarch is mixed with magnesium oxide to prevent clumping.[51]

Starch powder is slowly absorbed from the canine peritoneal cavity by an inflammatory reaction that histologically shows starch granules. There were more adhesions in dogs two days after introduction of the powder into the peritoneal cavity than at three weeks.[30] In the rabbit it has been shown that starch is absorbed within six months after introduction into the peritoneal cavity.[36] Animals show adhesion formation with smaller amounts of gloving powder if inflammation or peritoneal defects exist prior to the addition of the gloving powder.[22] Adhesive disease may vary between species. The rate of removal depends on the amount of powder present, clumping of the starch particles, and presence of infection.[51]

When 100, 50, and 25 mg of gloving powder were introduced into a confined body cavity (canine stifle), there was a marked histopathological inflammatory response, with necrosis of the synovial lining. Evidence of synovial inflammation was present at the end of four weeks, when the larger quantities were introduced.[49]

To lessen the possibility of adhesions developing secondary to surgical gloving powders, the manufacturers place a warning label on the glove packets. Washing the gloved hands may not be sufficient to remove powder from the exterior surface, and the gloves should be wiped on a lint-free towel to remove the powder. Although no guidelines can be offered for the amount of gloving powder to be used when preparing surgical gloves for sterilization, the use of any gloving powder should be regulated. It is estimated that the amount of powder placed on a pair of surgical gloves during manufacturing is approximately

200 mg.[49] The use of any gloving powder containing talcum should be abandoned.

Several features must be considered when selecting surgical gloves. Sterility is guaranteed with disposable gloves unless the package is damaged. Gloves can be purchased with an inner lining to protect against skin irritation or with curved fingertips and extra long, beaded cuffs to prevent them from rolling down. Some glove manufacturers offer custom glove sizing based on both width and length of the surgeon's hand. Custom gloves give palm musculature the proper fit, reducing fatigue and the trampoline effect in the palm area. Special processing produces gloves with thinner fingertips for sensitivity and thicker cuffs to resist tearing. Gloves can be recycled for sterile surgery, but the processing costs may not make it economically feasible.[40]

From 1.4 to 12 per cent of new unused gloves have been reported to be defective.[40, 44, 46] Gloves alone cannot be viewed as complete barriers to microbial contamination.

In one study using one surgical glove per hand at the end of a clean surgery, 13 per cent of the gloves had holes and 31 per cent were contaminated with bacteria. Ninety-five per cent of the contaminated gloves did not have holes in them. When double gloves were worn, 44 per cent of outer gloves had holes and 36 per cent of all the gloves were contaminated. Of the inner gloves, 47 per cent were contaminated and 3 per cent had holes. The contaminant was never on the same finger as the finger with the hole in the glove.[44, 46] One-third of the punctures occurred in the thumb and index fingers. Surgeons were responsible for 46 per cent of the damaged gloves and assistants 32 per cent. In one study in which 11.6 per cent of the surgical gloves had holes in them after a clean surgical procedure, no wound infections were reported.[10] In a study of 60 glove perforations, only once were bacteria cultured from the punctured glove.[55]

1. Aarons, J., and Fitzgerald, N.: Persisting hazards of surgical glove powder. Surg. Gynecol. Obstet. 138:385, 1974.
2. Beck, W. C., and Collette, T. S.: False faith in the surgeons gown and drape. Am. J. Surg. 83:125, 1952.
3. Belkin, N. L.: Reduction of airborne contamination through operating room apparel. AORN J. 4:75, 1966.
4. Belkin, N. L.: The other side of the drape: Reusable fabrics. AORN J. 28:588, 1978.
5. Belkin, N. L.: Evaluating surgical gowning draping fabrics. AORN J. 34:499, 1981.
6. Bergman, S. E., Borgstrom, S. J. H., and Stenstrom, S. J.: Operating room outfit and the spread of bacteria. Acta Chir. Scand. 136:35, 1970.
7. Bernard, H. R., Cole, W. R., and Gravens, D. L.: Reduction of iatrogenic bacterial contamination in operating rooms. Ann. Surg. 165:609, 1967.
8. Burrows, C. F.: Inadequate skin preparation as a cause of intravenous catheter-related infection in the dog. J. Am. Vet. Med. Assoc. 180:747, 1982.
9. Butcher, H. R., Gallinger, W. F., Gravens, D. L., et al.: Hexachlorophene concentrations in the blood of operating room personnel. Arch. Surg. 107:70, 1973.
10. Cruse, P. J. E., and Foord, R.: The epidemiology of wound infection. Surg. Clin. North Am. 60:27, 1980.
11. Dembeck, A. A.: Guidebook to Man-Made Textile Fibers and Textured Yarns of the World, 3rd ed. Textile Book Services, New York, 1969.
12. Dineen, P.: Prevention of infection. Bull. Am. Coll. Surg. December, 1970, p. 18.
13. Dineen, P.: Microbial filtration by surgical mask. Surg. Gynecol. Obstet. 133:812, 1971.
14. Dineen, P.: Role of impervious drapes and gown in preventing surgical infection. Clin. Orthop. Rel. Res. 96:210, 1973.
15. Eftekhar, N. S.: The surgeon and clean air in the operating room. Clin. Orthop. Rel. Res. 96:188, 1973.
16. Eitzen, H. E., Ritter, M. A., French, M. L. V., and Gioe, T. J.: Microbiological in-use comparison of surgical hand washing agents. J. Bone Joint Surg. 61A:403, 1979.
17. Fitzgerald, R. H.: Microbiologic environment of the conventional operating room. Arch. Surg. 114:772, 1979.
18. Galle, P. C., Homesley, H. D., and Rhyne, A. L.: Reassessment of the surgical scrub. Surg. Gynecol. Obstet. 147:215, 1978.
19. Greene, V. W., Borlaug, G. M., and Nelson, E.: Effects of patching on sterilization of surgical textiles. AORN J. 33:1249, 1981.
20. Gross, A., Selting, W. J., Cutright, D. E., and Bhaskar, S. N.: Evaluation of two antiseptic agents in surgical preparation of hands by a new method. Am. J. Surg. 126:49, 1973.
21. Ha'eri, G. B., Orth, M., and Wiley, A. M.: Efficacy of standard surgical face masks: An investigation using tracer particles. Clin. Orthop. Rel. Res. 148:160, 1980.
22. Jagelman, D. G., and Ellis, H.: Starch and intraperitoneal adhesion formation. Br. J. Surg. 60:111, 1973.
23. Joress, S.: A study of disinfection of the skin: A comparison of povidone iodine with other agents used for surgical scrubs. Ann. Surg. 155:296, 1962.
24. Knecht, C. D., et al.: Fundamental Techniques in Veterinary Surgery, 2nd ed. W. B. Saunders, Philadelphia, 1981.
25. Laufman, H.: Control of operating room infection: Discipline, defense mechanisms, drugs, design and devices. Bull. NY Acad. Med. 54:465, 1978.
26. Laufman, H., Eudy, W. W., Vandernoot, A. M., et al.: Strike through of moist contamination by woven and nonwoven surgical materials. Ann. Surg. 181:857, 1975.
27. Laufman, H., Montefusco, C., Siegal, J. D., and Edberg, S. C.: Scanning electron microscopy of moist bacterial strike through of surgical materials. Surg. Gynecol. Obstet. 150:165, 1980.
28. Laufman, H., Riley, L., Badner, B., and Zelner, L.: Use of disposable products in surgical practice. Arch. Surg. 111:20, 1976.
29. Laufman, H., Siegal, J. D., and Edberg, S. C.: Moist bacterial strike through of surgical materials: Confirmatory tests. Ann. Surg. 189:68, 1979.
30. Lee, C. M., Collins, W. T., and Largen, T. L.: A reappraisal of absorbable glove powder. Surg. Gynecol. Obstet. 95:725, 1952.
31. Letts, R. M., and Doermer, E.: Conversation in the operating theater as a cause of airborne bacterial contamination. J. Bone Joint Surg. 65A:357, 1983.
32. Lowbury, E. J. L., and Lilly, H. A.: Use of 4% chlorhexidine detergent solution (Hibiscrub) and other methods of skin disinfection. Br. Med. J. 1:510, 1973.
33. Lowbury, E. J. L., Lilly, H. A., and Ayliffe, G. A. J.: Preoperative disinfection of surgeon's hands: Use of alcoholic solutions and effect of gloves on skin flora. Br. Med. J. 4:369, 1974.
34. Moylan, J. A., Balish, E., and Chan, J.: Intraoperative bacterial transmission. Surg. Gynecol. Obstet. 141:731, 1975.
35. Moylan, J. A., and Kennedy, B. V.: The importance of gown and drape barriers in the prevention of wound infection. Surg. Gynecol. Obstet. 151:465, 1980.
36. Myllarniemi, H., Frilander, M., Turunen, M., et al.: The effect of glove powders and their constituents on adhesion and granuloma formation in the abdominal cavity of the rabbit. Acta Chir. Scand. 131:312, 1966.
37. Nelson, J. P., Glassburn, A. R., Talbott, R. D., and Mc-

Elhinney, J. P.: Clean room operating rooms. Clin. Orthop. Rel. Res. *96*:179, 1973.

38. Nicholes, P. S.: Comparative evaluation of new surgical mask medium. Surg. Gynecol. Obstet. *118*:579, 1964.

39. Nunamaker, D. M.: Management of infected fractures, osteomyelitis. Vet. Clin. North Am. *5*:259, 1975.

40. Perkins, J. J.: *Principles and Methods of Sterilization in Health Sciences*, 2nd ed. Charles C Thomas, Springfield, IL, 1969.

41. Peterson, A. F., Rosenberg, A., and Alatary, S. D.: Comparative evaluation of surgical scrub preparations. Surg. Gynecol. Obstet. *146*:63, 1978.

42. Quesnel, L. B.: Efficiency of surgical masks of varying design and composition. Br. J. Surg. *62*:936, 1975.

43. Richards, G. K.: Epidemiology of sepsis. Clin. Orthop. Rel. Res. *96*:5, 1973.

44. Ritter, M. A.: Experts discuss value of various OR garments. Hospital Infection Control, April, 1980, p. 45.

45. Ritter, M. A., Eitzen, H., French, M. L. V., and Hart, J. B.: Operating room environment as affected by people and the surgical face mask. Clin. Orthop. Rel. Res. *111*:147, 1975.

46. Ritter, M. A., French, M. L. V., and Eitzen, H.: Evaluation of microbial contamination of surgical gloves during actual use. Clin. Orthop. Rel. Res. *117*:303, 1976.

47. Rosenberg, A., Alatary, S. D., and Peterson, A. F.: Safety and efficacy of the antiseptic chlorhexidine gluconate. Surg. Gynecol. Obstet. *143*:789, 1976.

48. Schwartz, J. T., and Saunders, D. E.: Microbial penetration of surgical gown materials. Surg. Gynecol. Obstet. *150*:507, 1980.

49. Singh, I., Chow, W. L., and Chablani, L. V.: Synovial reaction to glove powder. Clin. Orthop. Rel. Res. *99*:285, 1974.

50. Smylie, H. G., Logie, J. R. C., and Smith, G.: From Phisohex to Hibiscrub. Br. Med. J. *4*:586, 1973.

51. Sobel, H. J., Schiffman, R. J., Schwartz, R., and Albert, W. S.: Granulomas and peritonitis due to starch glove powder. Arch. Pathol. *91*:559, 1971.

52. Tinker, M. A., Burdman, D., Deysine, M., et al.: Granulomatous peritonitis due to cellulose fibers from disposable surgical fabrics: Laboratory investigation and clinical implications. Ann. Surg. *180*:831, 1974.

53. Tolbert, T. W., and Brown, J. L.: Surface powders on surgical gloves. Arch. Surg. *115*:729, 1980.

54. Tucci, V. J., Stone, A. M., Thompson, C., et al.: Studies of the surgical scrub. Surg. Gynecol. Obstet. *145*:415, 1977.

55. Wiley, A. M., and Barnett, M.: Clean surgeons and clean air. Clin. Orthop. Rel. Res. *96*:168, 1973.

Chapter **22**

Preparation of the Surgical Patient

Dennis L. Powers

Preparation of the animal patient for surgery may begin any time from weeks to minutes before the surgical procedure. In emergency cases in which internal cardiac massage is indicated, for example, minimal surgical preparation is indicated, whereas in nonemergency cases, numerous steps should be taken to optimally prepare the animal for surgery.

In some patients, initial medical therapy is chosen as an alternative to surgical therapy, whereas in others, some type of medical treatment is necessary to stabilize or improve the patient's condition prior to anesthesia and surgery. Examples include patients with diabetes, congestive heart failure, or uremia.

This discussion is confined to patient preparation in the immediate preoperative period, including preparing the animal for anesthesia, cleansing and reducing bacterial populations on the skin, providing and maintaining sterile barriers between the animal and the surgical wound, and properly presenting the anatomical site to the surgeon for the procedure.

DIETARY RESTRICTIONS

Dietary restrictions are often imposed to prepare the animal's gastrointestinal tract for surgery. Food intake is generally restricted 6 to 12 hours prior to anesthesia to ensure an empty stomach and to avoid postoperative emesis, which may cause undue stress on the incision or tracheobronchial aspiration of stomach contents. If adequate fasting time is unavailable or in the event of accidental feeding, emesis may be induced with apomorphine 0.04 mg/kg body weight intravenously or 0.08 mg/kg intramuscularly or subcutaneously.[3]

Large intestinal operations, as well as some small intestinal procedures, require specialized preparations, such as extended dietary restrictions (48 hours) or enteric antibiotics. Oral kanamycin, 10 mg/kg every four hours, oral penicillin G, Na, or K, 40,000 U/kg every 6 hours, and neomycin, 20 mg/kg every six hours orally, have all been recommended.[15] Neomycin has minimal effects on *Pseudomonas* anaerobes, and penicillin may promote the recurrence of bowel cancer[25]; therefore, some surgeons recommend only mechanical cleansing. The administration of oral medications in vomiting patients is also of questionable value.[15] Water is generally allowed until the anesthetic premedication is administered.

During the course of preparation and while the animal is under the care of the surgeon, administration of any medically indicated therapeutic or prophylactic medications (e.g., insulin, antibiotics, diethylcarbamazine) should be initiated or continued.

EXCRETIONS

Shortly before anesthesia the animal should be allowed to defecate and urinate. This is often best accomplished by walking the animal in a suitable environment. Colon surgeries require more thorough bowel evacuation, and rectal enemas consisting of warm, soapy water to stimulate peristalsis and defecation may be needed. Mechanical cleansing can be initiated by giving an enema the evening before surgery. In the morning, enemas can be given every two hours up to one hour before surgery. Three to four enemas are generally adequate. In addition to providing a cleaner environment for surgery, such procedures also reduce postoperative constipation and associated straining that may cause undue stress on incisions.

An empty urinary bladder is often needed for abdominal procedures, especially pelvic or large intestinal procedures. If the urine is not evacuated naturally, the bladder may be expressed under general anesthesia with gentle, manual pressure or via a urethral catheter passed into the urinary bladder. Urogenital procedures, such as feline perineal urethrostomies, repair of urethral lacerations, or urethrostomies for urethral obstructions, may require this catheterization for urethral localization and maintenance of patency. Such catheters can also be used for monitoring the urine production during the operative and postoperative periods.

These procedures as well as an anal purse-string suture are effective in preventing fecal and urine leakage, which may contaminate the operating field. These sutures are placed in a simple continuous pattern circumferentially about the anus. They are tied in a position that inhibits the passage of feces and are removed postoperatively.

TREATMENT OF HAIR

If needed and if conditions permit, it is useful to bathe the entire animal before the procedure to remove loose hair, debris, and external parasites, promoting a cleaner operating room. Some cooperative patients who are associated with a high anesthetic risk benefit from preliminary clipping of the hair at the operative site prior to anesthetic induction to reduce total anesthetic time. Scanning electron and transmission microscopic studies have shown that clippers and razors, even when carefully used, cause microlacerations of the epidermis.[16] Such trauma disrupts the body's first line of defense against bacterial invasion[23] and without the subsequent application of germicides can allow bacteria to multiply on the skin.[2, 7, 30] It is recommended that the hair is removed close to the skin only shortly before skin preparation.[2, 7, 30]

With the animal anesthetized, careful removal of the hair can commence. A liberal area around the planned incision is clipped so that, if necessary, the incision can be extended within a sterile field. A general guideline is to clip 20 centimeters on each side of the incision. The hair can be removed most effectively with an Oster-type clipper and a #40 blade. Patients with dense haircoats may be clipped first with a coarser blade. The higher the blade number, the shorter the remaining hair. A #40 blade gives the skin a shaved appearance. Sharp blades are needed to minimize skin trauma. Dull blades may pull hairs out of their follicles and cause what is commonly called "clipper burn."

Depilatory creams are considered less traumatic than other hair removal methods, although they do induce a mild lymphocytic reaction in the dermis.[16] Such creams are more costly than blades but are faster, easier to use, and sterile and eliminate the need to clean and sterilize blades.[16] Clinical trials have shown that the use of depilatory creams reduces wound infection rates in human patients.[16] These creams are not as effective in animal patients, which have higher concentrations of hair follicles.[33] Some benefit may be apparent in irregular areas (interphalangeal or intertriginous areas) where adequate hair removal is difficult.

After hair removal is completed, all the loose hair is removed with a vacuum. The incision site is then given a general cleansing scrub. The skin, ears, mouth, and rectum are flushed with povidone-iodine.* Ophthalmic antibiotic ointments or lubricants are placed onto the cornea and conjunctiva.

SKIN PREPARATION

The skin is scrubbed with germicidal soaps to remove debris and reduce bacterial populations in preparation for surgery. It is not possible to sterilize the skin without causing damage or irritation that would impair its natural, protective function and interfere with wound healing. Furthermore, hair follicles can harbor bacteria that may appear at the skin surface after scrubbing,[19] thus accounting for the persistence of 20 per cent of the skin's bacterial population.

The skin is a medium for bacteria. Normal or resident organisms live in the superficial cornified layers and the outer hair follicles. Resident canine skin flora include *Staphylococcus epidermidis*, *Corynebacterium* spp., and *Pityrosporon* spp.[21] Transient bacteria do not multiply on the skin but can be significant secondary invaders of wound epidermis. Common transient pathogens are *Staphylococcus aureus*, *E. coli*, *Streptococcus* spp., *Enterobacter* spp., and *Clostridium* spp.[21]

There are various methods of applying germicides. Recent studies in human patients have shown no significant difference in the effectiveness of scrubbing, painting, or spraying as application techniques.[28] Some hospitals use a single application of a germicidal solution either as spray or a paint to save

---
*Betadine Surgical Scrub, The Purdue Frederick Company, Norwalk, CT.

time. In a study conducted by Lowbury and Lilly,[18] it was concluded that applying skin antiseptics by rubbing with a gloved hand is superior to using applicator sticks and gauze. These methods have not been used extensively owing to hospital standards as well as fear of surgical infections.

A more traditional method involves scrubbing the skin with germicides. Mechanical scrubbing in itself has been shown to reduce bacterial counts by the washing and massaging motions.[18] Scrubbing is recommended in animals over spraying or painting owing to their greater concentration of hair follicles[33] and attached bacteria to help reduce postsurgical infection due to bacterial contamination.

The operative site is initially scrubbed with gauze sponges soaked in germicide. The area is lathered well until all dirt and oils are removed. This is a generous scrub that often encompasses the hair surrounding the operation site to secure unattached hair and dander that may be disturbed during draping.

Sterile preparation begins after transporting and positioning the animal. Gauze sponges are sterilized in a pack along with bowls into which the germicides can be poured. The sponges are handled with sterile sponge forceps or the gloved hand using aseptic technique. The scrubbing is started at the incision site, usually near the center of the clipped area. A circular scrubbing motion is used, moving from the center to the periphery as shown in Figure 22–1. Care should be taken not to return a sponge from the periphery to the center to avoid transferring peripheral bacteria onto the incision site. Sponges are discarded after reaching the periphery. Overzealous scrubbing can cause undue irritation to the skin and should be avoided.

Commonly used scrubbing solutions are hexachlorophene, iodophors, chlorhexidine, alcohols, and quaternary ammonium salts. Hexachlorophene* is often incorporated in soaps and with long contact time (three days) reduces gram-positive bacterial counts on the skin. It has the potential for neurotoxicity, especially in young animals.[6, 10, 11, 29] Hexachlorophene loses its efficiency in the presence of alcohol, and in most hospitals it is used in combination with iodophor compounds.[13] Its use as the sole germicidal

*pHisoHex, Winthrop Laboratories, New York, NY.

agent is not recommended unless the patient is sensitive to other antiseptics.[6]

Quaternary ammonium compounds are bactericidal for gram-positive bacteria and are ineffective against spores and many gram-negative bacteria.[22] They are inactivated by proteins, phospholipids, and soaps. Use of these compounds is not recommended.[9]

Iodine compounds have been used for many years with good antimicrobial effect. The occasional irritation and allergic reactions to iodine distort the skin surface and create problems when precise skin measurements must be made for plastic procedures. These reactions have been reduced by combining the iodine with a carrier, usually polyvinylpyrrolidone. These carriers are called iodophors, or povidone-iodine, and are available as scrubs or solutions. Povidone-iodine is a potent germicide that kills bacteria, fungi, and spores[24, 25] but is not effective against *Clostridia*.[25] Iodophors can be used as the sole germicidal agent or in combination with alcohols. Their sporicidal action takes 15 minutes.[25]

Alcohol (ethyl or isopropyl), although not effective against spores, produces a fast kill of bacteria[22] and acts as a defatting agent.[1, 20] The use of alcohol by itself is not recommended, but it is commonly used in conjunction with povidine-iodine.[13] A common procedure is to scrub the site alternatively with each solution three times to allow for five minutes of contact time.[8] When the final povidone-iodine scrub is washed with alcohol, a 10% povidone-iodine solu-

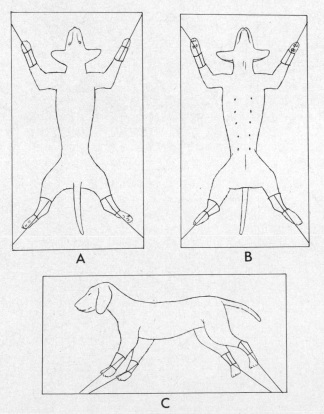

Figure 22–2. Animal positions for surgery. *A*, Ventral recumbency. *B*, Dorsal recumbency. *C*. Lateral recumbency.

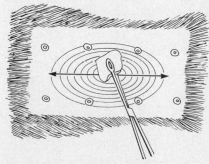

Figure 22–1. Scrubbing method, starting at the incision and moving circumferentially to the periphery.

tion is sprayed or painted on the site. Any excess solution on the table or in body "pockets" should be blotted.

More recently, chlorhexidine* has been studied in the preparation of operation sites for surgery.[13] Chlorhexidine 0.5% in 70 or 90% ethyl alcohol has been shown to be effective against gram-positive and gram-negative bacteria[5, 19, 26, 31] and to have greater residual activity than iodophors.[31] Two 30-second applications are adequate for antimicrobial activity.[26]

POSITIONING

Prior to the sterile application of the epidermal germicide, the animal is moved to the operating room. All previous preparations are performed outside the operating room. The animal is positioned so that the operative site is best presented to the surgeon. The surgeon should consider each procedure separately in choosing the animal's position. With forethought, the surgeon can avoid standing in an unusual posture that causes undue stress and premature fatigue. The flexibility of the position, such as the ability to use more than one approach or

*Nolvasan Surgical Scrub, Fort Dodge Laboratories, Inc., Fort Dodge, IA.

to alter the approach during the procedure, should also be considered. Commonly used positions are shown in Figure 22–2.

When positioning the animal, the surgeon should avoid interfering with respiratory function and peripheral circulation as well as the musculature and its innervation. Positioning pillows should be used to minimize the effect of positioning on the cardiopulmonary system and to avoid neurovascular injuries, which are often the result of ischemia. V-shaped trays are useful in dorsal and ventral recumbency. Strangulation of the distal limb should be avoided when tying the animal to the table. Vacuum-activated positioning bags provide support while conforming to the animal's shape. These plastic positioners, which resemble bean bags, are positioned under the animal and the air is evacuated with a vacuum to provide stable support.

Access to the patient must be maintained for proper anesthetic administration and monitoring. This may be achieved by using a frame that is secured to the table and extends over the front of the animal. This supports the sterile drapes and effectively separates the anesthetist from the sterile field. This type of frame may also be used to prevent undue pressure on the thorax from sterile surgical equipment or a surgeon's resting arm.

Animal contact with heat-conductive, metallic sur-

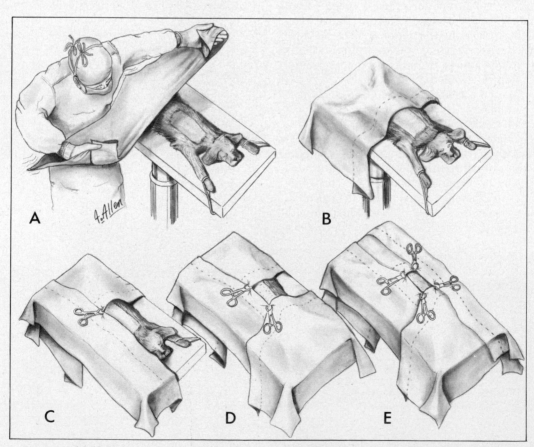

Figure 22–3. Placement of field drapes to isolate unprepared areas near the surgical site. (Reprinted with permission from Knecht, C. D., et al.: *Fundamental Techniques in Veterinary Surgery*, 2nd ed. W. B. Saunders, Philadelphia, 1981, p. 16.)

faces can contribute to hypothermia. The animal's body temperature can be more effectively controlled by interposing a thermostatically controlled water blanket between the animal and the table. When supplemental heat is required, this provides an evenly distributed heat source that avoids epidermal burns.

If not already established with the induction of anesthesia, any monitoring devices should be connected or the connections re-checked when the animal is positioned on the surgical table. As discussed in Chapter 29, urinary catheters, vascular catheters, electrocardiograph leads, blood pressure cuffs, and esophageal and rectal probes may be connected or inserted at this time.

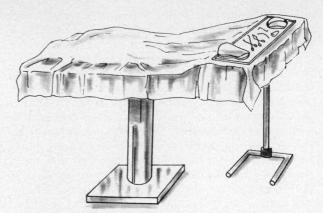

Figure 22–4. Final draping of the animal, table, and instrument stand.

DRAPING

Once the animal has been positioned and the skin prepared, the animal is ready to be draped. The purpose of drapes is to create and maintain a sterile field around the operative site.

Draping is performed by the gowned and gloved surgeon or surgical team member and begins with placement of field drapes to isolate the unprepared portion of the animal (Fig. 22–3). These towels can be placed one at a time at the periphery of the prepared area. Once the towels are placed, they should not be re-adjusted towards the incision site, as this carries bacteria onto the prepared skin. Any additional projecting areas such as limbs and tables can be appropriately covered to prevent inadvertent contamination of the surgical team during the draping procedure. These towels are secured at strategic locations with Backhaus towel clamps. The tips of the towel clamps, once placed through the skin, are considered nonsterile and should be handled appropriately. These clamps, although providing an avenue for bacterial migration, are necessary to secure the drapes in position.

With the animal and incision site further protected by the field drapes, final draping can be more effectively performed. A large drape is placed over the animal, the entire table, and the instrument stand to provide a continuous sterile field as shown in Figure 22–4. Cloth drapes should have an appropriately sized and positioned opening that can be placed over the incision site while the drape covers the remaining surfaces. Paper drapes, without a precut opening, may be placed to cover the field and a suitable opening is then created by the surgeon.

Draping of limbs requires a more specialized pro-

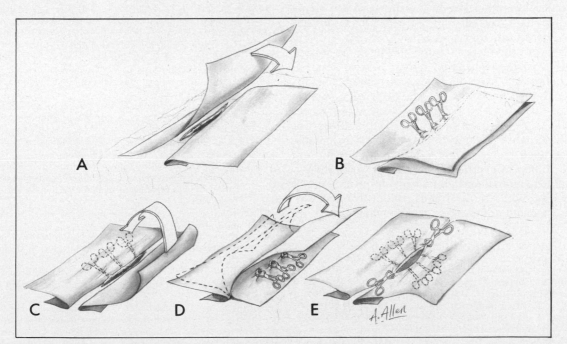

Figure 22–5. Towelling-in to reduce skin exposed to the surgical wound. (Reprinted with permission from Knecht, C. D., et al.: *Fundamental Techniques in Veterinary Surgery*, 2nd ed. W. B. Saunders, Philadelphia, 1981, p. 17.)

cedure. The hair of the leg is removed from the foot to the body around its circumference, and the leg is suspended with tape or other material that does not fray. The foot may be wrapped with tape or covered with a glove to reduce its exposure during handling. The skin is prepared while the limb is suspended. The field drapes are then placed about the unprepared portion of the body surrounding the limb as well as the table beneath it. While an assistant holds the leg with a sterile towel, the circulating nurse removes or cuts the suspending tape from the leg. A stockinette is placed over the leg and unrolled so that it can be secured to the field drapes. The leg can then rest on the field drapes until it is placed through a hole in the large drape that covers the animal, table, and instrument stand. Skin incisions are made through the stockinette.

To reduce skin exposure and subsequent contamination during the procedure, additional skin draping, or "towelling-in," can be performed after the skin incision is made. When operating on limbs, one can secure the edges of the stockinette to the skin edges with a continuous suture or Michele clips. In other areas, towels are secured on both sides of the incision with towel clamps as shown in Figure 22–5. Alternatively, plastic adhesive drapes can be applied to the skin and surrounding drapes for the same purpose. Microbial build-up beneath these drapes due to poor skin ventilation has been shown to be insignificant.[4, 12] Studies have shown significant reductions in postoperative counts of endogenous bacteria with the use of plastic drapes compared with cloth drapes.[12, 27] Their efficacy in reducing clinical postoperative infections has not been proven.[17] Proper drying of the skin with a final alcohol rinse is imperative to achieve adequate adherence to the skin. Adherence to animal skin with coarser, more abundant hair is generally less acceptable than that achieved with human patients.

The recent development and testing of antimicrobial adhesive drapes has shown them to be as effective in reducing bacterial populations as traditional scrubbing and painting methods and to have a longer duration of activity.[14, 32] Iodophor-containing films* have been used with human patients, but their use as an alternative to traditional methods in animals has not been tested. They would, however, be expected to be as effective as nonantimicrobial films.

When the animal and all nearby unsterile surfaces are covered with sterile drapes, the instrument tray can be arranged and surgery can commence.

1. Altemeir, W. A.: Surgical antiseptics. *In* Block, S. S. (ed.): *Disinfection, Sterilization and Preservation,* 2nd ed. Lea & Febiger, Philadelphia, 1977.
2. American College of Surgeons: *Manual on Control of Infection in Surgical Patients.* J. B. Lippincott, Philadelphia, 1976.
3. Bailey, E. M.: Emergency and general treatment of poisonings. *In* Kirk, R. W. (ed.): *Current Veterinary Therapy VI.* W. B. Saunders, Philadelphia, 1977.

*Ioban 2 Antimicrobial Film, 3M Co., St. Paul, MN.

4. Beck, W. C., Geffert, J. P., and Hansen, M.: The incise drape—boon or hazard: an experimental study. Am. Surg. 47:8, 1981.
5. Berry, A. R., Watt, B., Goldacre, M. J., Thomson, J. W. W., and McNair, T. J.: A comparison of the use of povidone-iodine and chlorhexidine in the prophylaxis of post operative wound infection. J. Hosp. Infect. 3:55, 1982.
6. Cox, J. E.: Hexachlorophene toxicity. J. Am. Anim. Hosp. Assoc. 10:542, 1974.
7. Cruse, P. J. E., and Foord, R.: A five year prospective study of 23,649 surgical wounds. Arch. Surg. 107:206, 1973.
8. Dineen, P.: An evaluation of the duration of the surgical scrub: five minutes versus ten minutes. Surg. Gynecol. Obstet. 129:6, 1969.
9. Dixon, R. E., Kaslow, R. A., Mackel, D. C., et al.: Aqueous quaternary ammonium antiseptics and disinfectants. J. Am. Med. Assoc. 236:2415, 1976.
10. Edds, G. T., and Simpson, C. F.: Toxicity of hexachlorophene to pups. Am. J. Vet. Res. 35:1005, 1974.
11. Fletch, A. L., Walker, G. C., and Perry, D. H.: Hexachlorophene toxicity in neonatal pups. J. Am. Vet. Med. Assoc. 165:747, 1974.
12. French, M. L., Eitzen, H. E., and Ritter, M. A.: The plastic surgical adhesive drape: an evaluation of its efficacy as a microbial barrier. Ann. Surg. 184:1, 1976.
13. Garner, J. S., Emori, T. G., and Haley, R. W.: Operating room practices for the control of infection in U.S. hospitals. October 1976 to July 1977. Surg. Gynecol. Obstet. 155:873, 1982.
14. Geelhoed, G. W., Sharpe, K., and Simon, G. L.: A comparative study of surgical skin preparation methods. Paper presented at the American College of Surgeons, Annual Meeting, 1982.
15. Grier, R. L.: Technique for intestinal anastomosis. *In* Bojrab, M. J. (ed.): *Current Techniques in Small Animal Surgery.* Lea & Febiger, Philadelphia, 1975.
16. Hamilton, H. W., Hamilton, K. R., and Lone, F. J.: Preoperative hair removal. Can. J. Surg. 20:3, 1977.
17. Jackson, D. W., Pollock, A. V., and Tindal, D. S.: The value of a plastic adhesive drape in the prevention of wound infection. A controlled trial. Br. J. Surg. 58:340, 1971.
18. Lowbury, E. J. L., and Lilly, H. A.: Gloved hand as an applicator of antiseptic to operation sites. Lancet 7926:153, 1975.
19. Lowbury, E. J. L., Lilly, H. A., and Ball, J. P.: Disinfection of the skin of operative sites. Br. Med. J. 2:1039, 1960.
20. Morton, H. E.: Alcohols. *In* Block, S. S. (ed.): *Disinfection, Sterilization and Preservation,* 2nd ed. Lea & Febiger, Philadelphia, 1977, pp. 301–318.
21. Muller, G. H., and Kirk, R. W.: Cutaneous bacteria. *In Small Animal Dermatology,* 2nd ed. W. B. Saunders, Philadelphia, 1976, p. 223.
22. Muller, G. H., and Kirk, R. W.: Topical treatment. *In Small Animal Dermatology,* 2nd ed. W. B. Saunders, Philadelphia, 1976, p. 194.
23. Polk, H. C.: Operating room acquired infection: a review of pathogenesis. Am. Surg. 45:349, 1979.
24. Polk, H. C., and Ehrenhranz, N. J. (eds.): Therapeutic advances and new clinical implications: medical and surgical antisepsis with Betadine microbials. Purdue Frederick, New York, 1972.
25. Preventing infections at the operation site. Br. Med. J. 6039:773, 1976.
26. Raahave, D.: Antisepsis of the operation site with aqueous centrimide/chlorhexidine and chlorhexidine in alcohol. Acta Chir. Scand. 140:595, 1974.
27. Raahave, D.: Effect of plastic skin and wound drapes on the density of bacteria in operation wounds. Br. J. Surg. 63:421, 1976.
28. Ritter, M. A., French, M. L., Eitzen, H. E., and Gloe, T. J.: The antimicrobial effectiveness of operation-site preparative agents. J. Bone Joint Surg. 62A:5, 1980.
29. Scott, D. W., and Bolton, G. R.: Hexachlorophene toxicosis in dogs. J. Am. Vet. Med. Assoc. 162:947, 1973.

30. Seropian, R., and Reynolds, B. M.: Wound infections after preoperative depilatory versus razor preparation. Am. J. Surg. *121*:251, 1971.

31. Smylie, H. G., Logie, J. R. C., and Smith, G.: From pHisoHex to Hisbiscrub. Br. Med. J., *4*:586, 1973.

32. Ulrich, J. A.: Antimicrobial efficacy of three surgical skin prep regimens against seeded organisms on human skin. Paper presented at the American College of Surgeons, Annual Meeting, 1982.

33. Winter, G. D.: Some factors affecting skin and wound healing. *In* Kenedi, R. M., and Cowden, J. M. (eds.): *Bedsore Mechanics.* University Park Press, Baltimore, 1966, p. 47.

Chapter **23** # Surgical Facilities and Equipment

H. P. Hobson

GENERAL CONSIDERATIONS

The surgery suite should be located near the work and intensive care areas of the hospital but away from the general flow of traffic. The operating room (OR) should have a single doorway, thus prohibiting the room from becoming a high traffic area. The door should lead to the preparation room, which usually doubles as a treatment room. The scrub sink should be outside the OR, usually in the preparation (treatment) room. Gas tanks should be located in a room in close proximity to the OR and other areas of use.

This room should have a doorway leading to the outside and quite often can double as a storage room. In larger facilities, e.g., Texas A&M University (Fig. 23–1), the surgery suite becomes a working unit in itself, away from the general hospital work areas but in close proximity to the radiology department, and includes the anesthesia–surgery preparation, recovery, and intensive care rooms. Traffic flow is kept to a minimum throughout the area and is limited to those in sterile attire anywhere along the sterile corridor or within the operating rooms.

One-way traffic flow is maintained from the patient

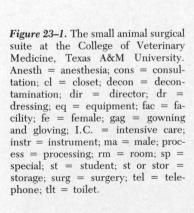

Figure 23–1. The small animal surgical suite at the College of Veterinary Medicine, Texas A&M University. Anesth = anesthesia; cons = consultation; cl = closet; decon = decontamination; dir = director; dr = dressing; eq = equipment; fac = facility; fe = female; gag = gowning and gloving; I.C. = intensive care; instr = instrument; ma = male; process = processing; rm = room; sp = special; st = student; st or stor = storage; surg = surgery; tel = telephone; tlt = toilet.

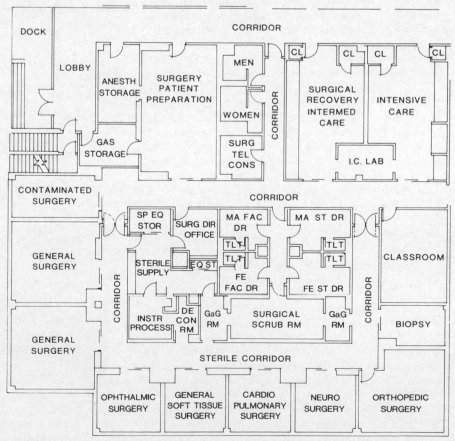

preparation area to the operating and recovery rooms. The intensive care ward is immediately adjacent to the recovery ward and communicates with it through a small emergency laboratory.

A room temperature of approximately 70°F with a relative humidity of approximately 50 per cent provides a comfortable environment for the surgeon. Lower ambient room temperatures make it more difficult to maintain the patient's normal body temperature. Airflow should move from areas of least potential contamination to areas of greatest potential contamination. Air within the OR should be under mild positive pressure so that when the surgery room door is opened air flows out of rather than into the room.[1] A minimum of 25 air exchanges per hour is recommended if the air is recirculated or 15 air exchanges per hour if the air is exhausted to the outside.[5]

Floors, walls, and ceilings should be constructed of impervious material with no seams so that they are easily cleaned and disinfected. Doors must be wide enough to permit passage of a rolling table and high enough to allow passage of large equipment such as x-ray machines. They must be well fitted and kept closed to keep contamination to an absolute minimum. There should be no open drain in the operating room, nor should a scrub sink be located there.[1] Every effort should be made to avoid areas and equipment that are difficult to keep clean.

Almost all power equipment needed in the surgery area utilizes 110-V electrical current. Special provisions should be made for any 220-V equipment being considered, including some x-ray machines. Few, if any, explosive anesthetic agents are currently used. Therefore, explosion-proof switches and electrical outlets are rarely, if ever, needed. Electrical outlets should be located waist high, if not for concern for explosion safety then certainly for convenience.

Some provision should be made for emergency lighting. Battery units, with or without automatic turn on, are usually used in smaller facilities. If automatic battery units are used, only those with automatic recharging capabilities should be relied on. Larger facilities should have an automatic generator. At least one surgery light in each operating room plus one electrical outlet should be wired into this system. Whatever auxiliary power source is used, it must be kept in good working condition and checked routinely.

Cabinets with tight-fitting doors help minimize dust accumulation. Recessed units (Fig. 23–2) or floor-to-ceiling units should be used for the same reason. Glass doors on the cabinets are quite beneficial in work areas. Pass-through cabinets from the sterile corridor to the OR improve efficiency and minimize traffic in the OR. The stainless steel and glass construction of these cabinets allows them to be cleaned and disinfected more effectively.

An operating room supervisor should always be designated. In smaller clinical facilities, this individual would undoubtedly double as the scrub nurse or

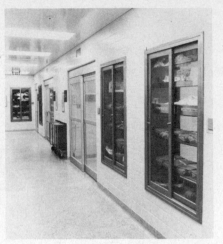

Figure 23–2. The sterile corridor immediately adjacent to the surgery room. Stainless steel and glass cabinets, mounted in the walls, open from either the operating room or the corridor. Electronically controlled sliding glass doors to the surgery rooms close automatically.

anesthetist. He would also assist in anesthetic induction, preoperative preparation of the patient, and postoperative patient supervision. In larger facilities, these positions may be filled by different individuals and may include a technician in the intensive care ward. Additional help is needed for instrument cleaning, surgical pack packing, instrument sterilization, OR cleaning and disinfecting, and so on. Written job descriptions should be maintained and should be readily accessible for each individual employed. Specific responsibilities in each area allow for maximum accountability (for more details see Chapter 24).

ANESTHESIA AND SURGICAL PREPARATION ROOM

Preparation of patients must be completed in a room separate from the OR (Fig. 23–3). The room can double as a treatment room, however.

The preparation counter surface should be imper-

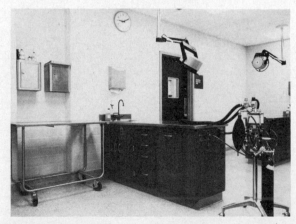

Figure 23–3. The anesthesia-surgical preparation room. The preparation cabinet should be self-contained with the pipeline outlets, lighting, and lock boxes located in a convenient manner.

vious and easily cleaned and disinfected. Units with built-in sinks are convenient for presurgical emptying of the bladder in cases of abdominal surgery and for cleansing of the surgical site. Clippers fitted with a surgical blade should be located within the surgical preparation unit or mounted on the wall or ceiling immediately adjacent. Five-gallon canister vacuum cleaners are commercially available that fit nicely in the prep cabinet and do an excellent job of picking up loose hair as the surgical site is clipped.

The cabinet should be stocked with preanesthetic agents, anesthetic agents, syringes, needles, intravenous catheters, and so on that are used on all patients.

Even in smaller facilities, installation of an oxygen pipeline should be considered, as it will probably pay for itself in a relatively short period of time (Fig. 23–4). Provisions must be made for the storage of the oxygen H tanks, preferably near an outside door. The tanks should be secured to the wall.[3] Small E tanks are necessary for the maintenance of an oxygen supply to the patient during transport. Tanks of oxygen must still be kept on hand in case of power failures.

When gas-driven surgical equipment is utilized, provisions should be made for the piping of nitrogen to the OR to supply these units. Nitrous oxide should be piped to areas of use. Vacuum lines should be run to each OR as well as to the intensive care ward. Gas scavenger negative pressure pipelines, with the appropriate outlets, should be present in all areas in which gaseous anesthetic agents are to be used.[4]

An area must be provided for the storage of anesthesia machines. A sink is required for cleaning rebreathing bags, hoses, and endotracheal tubes. A rack on which to hang the rebreathing bags and hoses while draining and drying should be provided. Provisions must be made for disinfecting anesthetic equipment, including the sterilization of endotracheal tubes and the maintenance of sterile endotracheal tubes when disposable ones are not in use.

A laryngoscope must be stored in the surgery

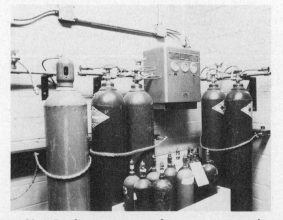

Figure 23–4. Pipeline systems provide a more economical source of gas. For safety, large H tanks should be chained to the wall. Smaller E tanks, when not mounted on anesthetic machines, should be stored in a heavy wooden box or rack.

cabinet or be otherwise immediately available for respiratory emergencies. A selection of endotracheal tubes of various sizes must also be available for this purpose. A metal stylet, slightly shorter than the endotracheal tube, can be quite useful when intubating very small dogs or cats.

Background fluorescent lighting should provide 100 to 150 foot candles of light. Spot lights, of the examination room type, should also be available and should be ceiling-mounted to allow for maximum illumination of the patient's throat during intubation. This light should provide approximately 3000 foot candles of light and should be positioned 1 meter from the examination area. Portable lights may be used but are much less convenient when other portable emergency equipment is used.

CONTAMINATED SURGERY ROOM

To minimize the spread of infection and the cleaning and disinfecting of the surgical suite, a surgery room outside the sterile surgery area for operating on known contaminated cases is most beneficial, particularly in larger facilities. Examples of these cases include pyothorax, draining sinus tracts, and perianal fistulas. With proper cleaning and disinfecting, this room may also be used for surgery on larger exotic animal patients and patients that require intraoperative radiology. It may also be used for after-hours emergency cases, such as a gastric torsion, that may contaminate the sterile surgical suite.

STERILE OPERATING ROOM

Microfilm dust pads applied to the floor outside the sterile corridor collect much of the dust from patient transport table rollers and so on.

All individuals in the sterile surgery suite should change out of or cover their street clothes. Caps, masks, and shoe covers must be worn. Anyone approaching the surgical field must wear gowns and gloves (for more details see Chapter 24).

The size of the OR depends on the ancillary equipment used in the room. In new construction, the minimum size of the OR should be 180 to 200 square feet. Operating rooms that contain specialized and large equipment, such as the cardiopulmonary bypass equipment, should be twice as large.

Surgery tables (Fig. 23–5) should be constructed of stainless steel with hydraulic raise-lower, tilt, and V trough capabilities.

Instrument tables that can straddle the operating table should be used. They should be of stainless steel construction and should be easily raised and lowered as well as easily rolled into position. Smaller instrument stands mounted on a singular pedestal are difficult to position properly and are too small for more involved procedures such as bone plating.

Even in the smaller surgical facility, provisions

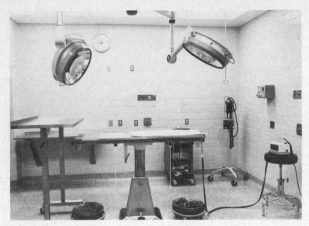

Figure 23–5. The operating room should be well lighted, easily cleaned, and well equipped.

should be made for piping oxygen and other gaseous agents used routinely. Whenever gaseous anesthetic agents are used, some provisions must be made for collecting the used gases. The outlets should be positioned approximately waist high on the most convenient wall away from the OR door. An alarm system should be installed that is activated when the oxygen pressure drops too low.

Suction capabilities must be provided. Portable suction units are adequate; however, in facilities with multiple operating rooms, the pipeline system is much more efficient. Plug-in units with disposable containers work especially well, are easily cleaned, and minimize contamination.

Flush-mounted fluorescent lights should be used to provide background lighting, which should be in the range of 70 to 130 foot candles. At a distance of 1 meter from the surgical field, the surgical lights should yield the following illumination ranges: flood, 1,600 to 3,800 foot candles; medium setting, 2,000 to 5,000 foot candles; and spot, 2,500 to 6,600 foot candles. The lights should produce a maximum of 25 microwatts per cm^2 heat to minimize tissue drying and to provide a comfortable environment for the surgeon. To provide normal tissue color, the light should be approximately 4,400° Kelvin.*

The surgery light should be mounted in the ceiling directly over the operating table and should have maximum maneuverability. Hinged arms that allow the light to be directed from nearly any angle and that are stable once positioned are imperative. Two lights, directed from different angles, are preferred when viewing internal structures at surgery. Ceiling track mountings, especially those directly over the surgical field, are undesirable because of potential contamination of the surgical field. Headlights or intraoperative fiberoptic lights worn by the surgeon may be particularly useful in specific procedures.

The patient's body temperature must be maintained during surgery, especially when the patient is small or short-haired or the surgical procedure is

*Amsco Industrial, Richardson, TX.

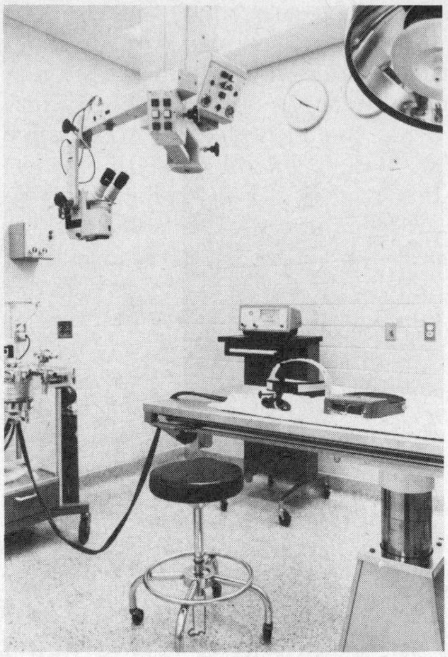

Figure 23–6. The operating microscope or some other form of magnification equipment is indispensable, especially for eye and microsurgical techniques.

unusually long. This is best accomplished with a circulating water blanket positioned between the patient and the operating table.

A kick bucket or pan, readily accessible to both the surgeon and assistant, helps to minimize the clutter and contamination of the surgical area. Plastic bag liners for these containers facilitate clean up.

Each OR must be provided with a radiographic view box, preferably flush mounted. Some provision should be made for intraoperative radiography. Portable capacitor discharge units, with or without Polaroid capabilities, are used more frequently. However, hand-held imaging devices will undoubtedly soon be used extensively for checking the presence or degree of reduction of a fracture, pin or screw placement, and so on.

A wall clock should be present in each surgery room. A time elapse clock may be quite valuable when performing certain surgical procedures, especially those involving vascular occlusion. Some type of magnification equipment (Fig. 23–6) should be available in any surgery room. Head loops of various designs are used more frequently. Operating microscopes are a valuable aid in many procedures and are essential for microsurgical techniques.

SURGICAL RECOVERY—INTERMEDIATE CARE

Patients must be monitored closely following surgery and should remain intubated with the cuff inflated until the swallowing reflex has returned. When the surgery case load is high, a separate ward should be available where these patients can be readily observed and yet kept separate from sick patients.

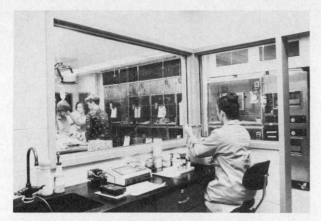

Figure 23–7. Basic clinical pathology capabilities should be available in close proximity to the intensive care ward.

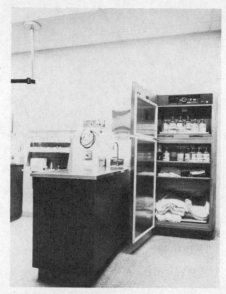

Figure 23–8. Warming cabinets provide a ready source of warm fluids or blankets for the hypothermic patient.

Cages in this ward should be easily cleaned and disinfected. It is of considerable advantage for these cages to have readily available interchangeable oxygen doors. Oxygen can be piped easily to each cage through flow meters and moisturizers mounted above the cages. The cages should have heating capabilities. A thermometer and a humidity gauge should be mounted in each oxygen door. The entire room should be kept several degrees warmer than the other wards, as nearly all surgery patients exhibit subnormal temperatures after surgery.

Monitoring equipment should be present or readily available. Patients requiring continuous monitoring should be taken directly to the intensive care ward from surgery or transferred there as the condition of the patient dictates. Minor clinical pathology laboratory facilities should be readily available (Fig. 23–7) and should include a microhematocrit centrifuge, microscope, refractometer, reflectance meter, urograph sticks, and possibly blood gas analyzing equipment.

Cleaning equipment should be readily available but stored in a separate closet equipped with a laundry sink.

INTENSIVE CARE

Patients requiring continuous monitoring should be taken directly to the intensive care ward. Those patients unable to control their own body temperature should be maintained in total environmental control units, which regulate oxygen content, temperature, and humidity. The rest of the cages should have heating capabilities with oxygen piped to them through flow meters and moisturizers.

Monitoring equipment, including electrocardiographic, arterial and central venous pressure, and respiratory arrest alarms should be immediately available for use as needed. Continuous temperature monitoring equipment may be very helpful in selected patients. Fluid infusion pumping equipment with warming, calibrated flow and positive pressure

administration capabilities should be available. Warm fluids and blankets from warming cabinets (Fig. 23–8) provide immediate aid to hypothermic patients.

The intensive care area must be readily accessible to a clinical pathology laboratory but also immediately adjacent to a small emergency laboratory. A true intensive care unit requires continuous supervision and must be staffed accordingly. Cleaning equipment and supplies must be readily available in this area, as ongoing cleaning must be performed by hand.

SUPPORT AREAS

A dressing area must be provided where individuals involved with surgery can change. In larger facilities separate dressing rooms should be provided and should include a small locker for valuables; a hanging area for street clothes; a cabinet for scrub suits, caps, masks, and shoe covers; a cabinet for

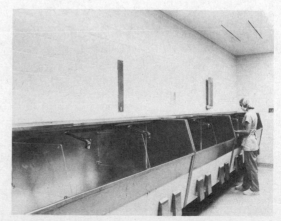

Figure 23–9. Stainless steel scrub sinks with knee-operated water valves and soap dispensers.

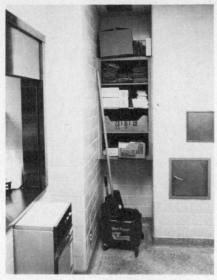

Figure 23–10. Decontamination room with trash compactor, pass-through window into the instrument cleaning and packing room, cleaning supplies, and laundry chute.

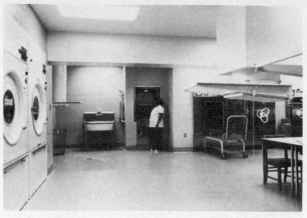

Figure 23–12. Laundry and sterilizing room with commercial washers and dryers, steam and gas sterilizers, and laundry chutes and dumb waiter communicating with the surgery area above.

dirty laundry, or, when the laundry facility is in the basement, a laundry chute; and a half bath. A separate scrub sink room is ideal (Fig. 23–9), with deep stainless steel sinks with knee-, elbow-, or foot-operated water flow and soap dispensers. Fingernail cleaner and brush dispensers must be within easy reach. When re-usable brushes are used, the dispensing container, including the cleaned brushes, must be detached and autoclaved regularly.

A separate area should be provided for gowning and gloving, although, if desired, this can be performed within the OR.

In larger facilities, a decontamination room (Fig. 23–10) should be provided in the surgery suite. Disposable paper goods, gauge sponges, and so on are placed in a trash compactor; bloody drapes are rinsed in a laundry sink and sent down the laundry chute to the basement; and dirty instruments are passed through to the washing and packing room. Amputated tissues not submitted for pathological examination are placed in plastic bags and taken to

the incinerator for proper disposal. A mop and bucket as well as cleaning and disinfecting supplies are kept in the decontamination room.

A specific area or room should be provided for the cleaning and inspecting of instruments and the packing of packs (Fig. 23–11). A small ultrasonic cleaner should be available for the cleaning of instrument hinges as necessary. Instruments may be cleaned in large ultrasonic cleaners instead of by hand.

Instruments of a given pack are identified with colored tape and packed according to a list for that particular pack. When laundry and sterilizing facilities (Fig. 23–12) are located in the basement below the surgery area, a dumb waiter provides a convenient means of transport.

A conference room should be provided where regular surgery rounds can be held.

ANCILLARY EQUIPMENT

A flash autoclave should be available in all facilities when multiple uses of a given instrument may be necessary in a short span of time.

Esophageal stethoscopes should be available to monitor each surgical patient. Apnea alarms may be used to advantage. Electrocardiographic equipment should be available and used as indicated, as should central venous pressure and systemic arterial blood pressure monitoring equipment. Body temperatures should be continuously monitored.

An emergency drug cart (Fig. 23–13) must be immediately available to the anesthesia, surgery, recovery, and intensive care areas. It should include the necessary instruments to open the chest should internal CPR be necessary.

A direct current defibrillator with a discharge capability of 350 wattseconds must also be available in these same areas. It should be equipped with external as well as at least two sizes of internal paddles.

A positive pressure ventilator should be available for internal thoracic surgical procedures, respiratory arrest, and so on.

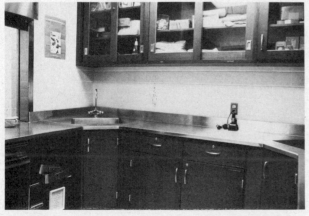

Figure 23–11. Instrument cleaning and packing room.

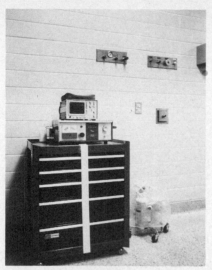

Figure 23–13. Emergency drug and equipment cart, defibrillator, and electrocardiographic monitoring equipment.

Electrosurgical equipment should be available for a wide range of surgical procedures when optimal visibility of the surgical field or control of hemorrhage is critical as well as when total surgical time may be a major factor.

Cryosurgical units should be available for use during glaucoma surgery, or removal of multiple skin neoplasms, for surgery in which the cosmetics of an area or the function of an organ may be more easily maintained with cryosurgery, and in selected other cases. Surface freezing may be accomplished with N_2O units, whereas deep freezing requires liquid nitrogen.

Endoscopic units have become essential for a definitive presurgical diagnosis in many hollow organs. Surgery through small openings into these areas with the aid of the endoscope, although not likely to reach those proportions expected in human surgery, is likely to continue to expand in veterinary surgery.

Well-constructed rolling tables are needed for patient transport. They should be made from stainless steel and should have relatively large wheels with bearings that can be readily lubricated and rubber bumpers mounted on the corners to prevent inadvertent damage to doors and walls.

An erasable surgery board should be positioned outside the surgery suite listing pending surgeries. This serves both to organize the logical order of procedures to be performed and as a ready reference of postoperative cases to be checked.

FACILITY AND EQUIPMENT CLEANING AND MAINTENANCE

In-house control of cleaning personnel, whereby specific individual accountability can be defined for specific areas of cleaning, usually results in optimal performance of duty. Contracts with cleaning companies specializing in cleaning larger hospital facilities may be quite adequate or even superior.

ORs must be cleaned superficially between each surgery and thoroughly on a daily basis. The entire room should be disinfected at least once weekly or immediately after a contaminated operation has been performed. If postoperative infections are encountered, cultures should be taken of all surfaces, including the floor, as well as from the patient's surgical site following surgical preparation, the surgeons' hands following scrubbing, and the nares of all individuals working in the surgical arena.

Cleaning equipment and solutions must be kept clean. Mop heads as well as the disinfectant solution used to clean the floors must be changed as soon as they appear dirty (at least daily).

The specific disinfectant solution used should be virucidal as well as bactericidal and nonstaining and noncorrosive. The surfaces to be disinfected should be cleaned well prior to the disinfecting procedure.

Air duct filters should be checked once a week and replaced as needed.

In larger facilities, in-house maintenance of equipment, both mechanical and electrical, undoubtedly results in a superior performance. Equipment must be cleaned and serviced regularly. Repairs can be made while the problem is still minor. More complex equipment, however, usually requires specialized service. Service contracts are often available from the sales company at the time of purchase, or service may be arranged through larger medical facilities in the area. Certain companies, when asked, will provide similar equipment on loan during down time. This type of agreement can be arranged at the time of purchase of the equipment.

1. American Animal Hospital Association: *Manual of Standards for Animal Hospitals.* American Animal Hospital Association, Sound Bend, IN, 1983.
2. Hobson, H. P.: unpublished data, 1983.
3. Lumb, W., and Jones, E.: *Veterinary Anesthesia.* Lea & Febiger, Philadelphia, 1973, p. 145.
4. Sawyer, D.: *The Practice of Small Animal Anesthesia.* W. B. Saunders, Philadelphia, 1982, p. 59.
5. U.S. Dept. of Health, Education, and Welfare: *Minimum Requirements of Construction and Equipment for Hospital and Medical Facilities.* Public Health Service, Health Resources Administration, Washington, D.C., 1982.

24 The Surgery Department

J. W. Alexander and M. P. Lavery

An organization may be viewed as a framework within which people in various groups and at various levels perform certain jobs or tasks. Formal organizational theory is based on several major principles: that the division of labor is essential for maximum efficiency, that coordination of efforts is a primary responsibility of management, that the formal structure is the main network for organizing and managing the various activities of the institution, and that the span of supervision sets outside limits on the number of subordinates a manager can effectively supervise.[4]

Efficiency, which is the key to any well-run surgery department, can be viewed as the "attainment of quality reviewed in relationship of the manpower, facilities, supplies, and equipment to the appropriateness, acceptability, and cost to the client."[2] Individuals, both professional and lay, must work together and coordinate their efforts to better accomplish the tasks necessary to achieve a common goal. In the operating room this common goal "is to provide for the safety and welfare of each and every patient admitted through the doors."[2] In order to accomplish any goal, individuals must be willing to work together as team members. This team effort must not only be between individuals in the surgery department but between all hospital departments. The activities of the surgery department must be coordinated with those of the recovery room unit, anesthesiology group, radiology department, and clinical pathology area, to name just a few. Each department will take on the personality of the individuals in it. This group personality will lead to a reputation, either positive or negative.

It is generally recognized that time is an important element in the operating room. Poor managers of people and their time will lead to a reduced efficiency of the group as a whole. The surgery department should be arranged to allow the identification of problems and a means of solving them as rapidly as possible and to have as an underlying aim the development of more efficient and economical work methods.

ORGANIZATION OF THE SURGERY DEPARTMENT

Although there are numerous organizational schemes that have been proposed, we have found the example in Figure 24–1 to be an efficient and

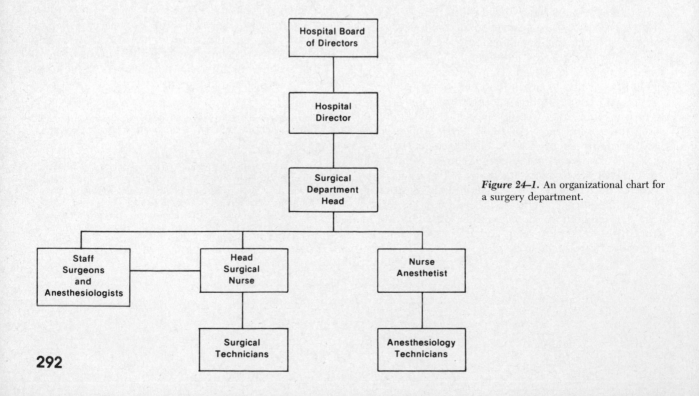

Figure 24–1. An organizational chart for a surgery department.

effective one. No matter what the organizational scheme, it should meet the following criteria:

1. Provide a climate for open communication that will lead to employee development and satisfaction. The best way for any organization to reach its goals is for the individuals within the organization to reach their goals at the same time.

2. Allow for input from all levels of the organization as to the objectives of the surgery department and standards to be maintained. The objectives of the surgery department should be practical and specific and within the accepted standards of operating room protocol. Frequently, difficulties arise between personnel in the delegation, coordination, and establishment of standards in the absence of unified objectives.[4] Whatever the agreed upon objectives and standards, they should be written down, available for review, and understood by all personnel.

3. Allow for frequent individual meetings between staff surgeons and support personnel.

Policies and Procedures

The operating room should be managed with policies and procedures that serve to outline guidelines for the provision of efficient and safe patient care.

1. Policies should be written, dated, and above all, enforceable.
2. Policies should have the support of the surgical personnel.
3. Policies should be periodically reviewed, updated, and revised and deleted when they become obsolete.
4. Policies for the operating room should include environmental control, safety regulations, disaster plans, operating room protocol, and visitor and traffic control.

5. Procedures should be established to:
   a. set standards for appraisal of operations
   b. produce predictable outcomes
   c. analyze currently used methods
   d. standardize operations
   e. reduce errors.
6. Procedures for the operating room shall include[1]:
   a. operating room sanitation
   b. care and disposal of surgical specimens, cultures, and foreign bodies
   c. care of special equipment, including maintenance contracts and repair records
   d. emergency procedures, e.g., cardiac resuscitation.

PRELIMINARY PREPARATIONS

Scheduling

Operating room scheduling must be coordinated with other hospital departments. The need for cooperation between the the departments of surgery, anesthesiology, and radiology cannot be overstressed. Scheduling of surgical cases should be the responsibility of the surgical nurse. A surgery scheduling board will help to coordinate proposed surgical procedures (Fig. 24–2). The board should include:

1. Client and patient name.
2. Patient case number.
3. Proposed procedure(s).
4. Requested table time.
5. Name of veterinary surgeon(s).

Prior to any surgical procedure, an instrument request form should be filed with the surgical nurse (Fig. 24–3). This form allows the nurse to be sure all requested equipment is available and sterile and serves as a means of recording equipment for the purposes of re-ordering and cost accounting.

Figure 24–2. A surgery scheduling board.

Anesthesia- Surgery Schedule

DATE TIME	OR	PROCEDURE	SURGEON	PATIENT NAME & NO	WARD & CAGE NO	ANESTHETIST

Surgery Request Form

Case No. _____ Surgeon _____

Client's Name _____ Asst. Surgeon _____

Patient's Name _____ Procedure _____

Species _____ Table Time _____

Date _____

Gloves (No.) 6__, 6½__, 7__, 7½__, 8__, 8½__, 9__

Instrument Sets
- ____ S.A. General
- ____ L.A. General
- ____ Orthopedic
- ____ Dental
- ____ Neuro
- ____ Cardiovascular
- ____ Thoracic
- ____ Minor (suture set)
- ____ Ambulatory
- ____ Orthopedic
- ____ Ophthalmic

Linen Packs
- ____ S.A. Major
- ____ S.A. Minor
- ____ L.A. Laparotomy
- ____ L.A. Limb
- ____ Bovine Standing Hip
- ____ Extra Towels
- ____ Extra Gowns (No.__)
- ____ Basin (sm, lg)
- ____ Other _____

Implant Trays
- ____ Intramedullary Pins
- ____ Wire size ____
- ____ Lg. Compression Set
- ____ Lg. Screw Set
- ____ Sm. Compression Set
- ____ External Fixation Set (sm, lg)
- ____ Spinal Plates
- ____ Other _____

Individual Instruments
- ____ Osteotomes
- ____ Gigli Handles and Wire
- ____ Mallet
- ____ Periosteal Elevator

Individual Instruments (Cont'd)
- ____ Pin Cutter
- ____ Chuck and Key
- ____ Bone Rasp
- ____ Bone Curettes
- ____ Ronguers
- ____ Bone Holding Forceps
- ____ Bone Cutter
- ____ Pliers
- ____ A-O Drill
- ____ A-O Oscillating Saw
- ____ Micro Wire Driver
- ____ Surgairtome II
- ____ Dremel Drill
- ____ Cautery
- ____ Suction
- ____ Retractors _____
- _____

Suture
- ____ Dexon (size ____)
- ____ Gut (size ____)
- ____ Vetafil (size ____)
- ____ Wire (size ____)
- ____ Nylon (size ____)
- ____ Umbilical tape
- ____ Skin Staples
- ____ L.A. Needle Pack
- ____ S.A. Taper Needles
- ____ S.A. Cutting Needles
- ____ Spay Hook
- ____ Hemoclip Set
- ____ Other (list)
  1. _____
  2. _____
  3. _____

Soft Goods
- ____ Stockinette (____ in.)
- ____ Penrose Drain
- ____ Culture Tube
- ____ Saline Irrigation
- ____ Steridrapes
- ____ Gelfoam
- ____ Bone Wax
- ____ Chest Tube
- ____ Heimlich Valves
- ____ Urinary Catheter
- ____ Marlex Mesh
- ____ Extra Blades
- ____ Other (list)
  1. _____
  2. _____
  3. _____
  4. _____
  5. _____

Dressings
- ____ 4x4 Gauze
- ____ Cotton Roll
- ____ Cast Padding
- ____ Elastikon
- ____ Micropad
- ____ Vet Wrap
- ____ Plaster
- ____ Mason Metasplint
- ____ Splint Rod
- ____ Other (list)
  1. _____
  2. _____
  3. _____

Figure 24–3. A surgery request form.

Preparation of the Operating Room

Proper preparation of the operating room is an essential first step in the establishment of an acceptable surgical environment. *Clean surroundings are the least that any client can expect for his animal.* A safe operating room environment should be established, controlled, and maintained. The following tasks should be performed prior to any operating day[2]:

1. Remove unnecessary tables and equipment from the operating room.

2. Damp dust the overhead operating lights, furniture, flat surfaces, and all portable or mounted equipment with a germicidal solution.

3. Wet vacuum the floors with detergent disinfectant.

4. Position operating tables under overhead operating light fixture.

5. Turn on the operating light to check focus and intensity. Pre-position the light in relation to the location of the surgeon at the operating table and that part of the animal's anatomy that will be encountered during the operation.

6. Obtain and check electrical equipment that will be needed.

7. Check gas supply in all tanks used to operate power equipment.

8. Connect and check suction device.

9. Line each kick bucket with a plastic bag and a cuff turned over the edge.

10. Put the sterile linen pack on the instrument table so that when opened the wrapper will adequately drape the table and the linen will be in its proper place.

11. Obtain a basic set of sterile instruments.

12. Select the correct size gloves for each member of the surgical team.

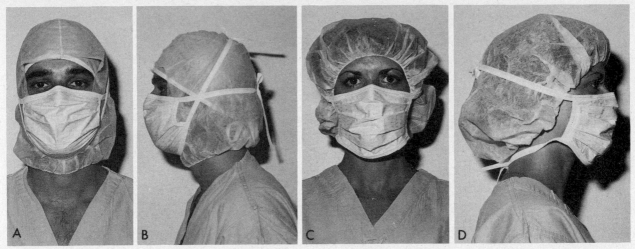

Figure 24–4. A and B, The correct way to wear a surgical hood and mask. C and D, The correct way to wear a woman's surgical cap and mask.

13. Collect additional instruments and supplies according to the instrument request form (see Fig. 24–3).

14. Adjust the height of the operating table to produce the least physical strain on the operating surgeon. The ideal height varies, but as a general rule the table should be set to place the operative field approximately at the level of the surgeon's elbow when his arm is at his side.

Traffic Control

An essential objective of any surgery department is to establish policies and protocols that reduce to a minimum the potential introduction of microbes into the operating room. Only authorized personnel are permitted to enter the restricted areas, and they must be dressed properly.

1. Everyone entering the operating room should remove street clothes or clothes worn elsewhere about the hospital and change into a surgical scrub suit.

2. Before entering the operating room, cap or hood, mask, and shoe covers should be donned. The cap should completely cover the hair. The mask must be up over the nose (Fig. 24–4).

3. Anyone who participates in an operation on an animal with an infection should wear clean operating garb before helping with or performing another operation.

POLICIES AND PROCEDURES DURING THE OPERATION

Basic Aseptic Techniques

As mentioned previously, the entire surgery team should try to prevent the introduction of microbes into the surgical field. The basic rule is that an object is considered sterile when it is completely free of all living microorganisms and incapable of producing any form of life.[4] Strict adherence to aseptic procedures minimizes sources of contamination. Certain basic principles must be observed during surgery to provide a well-defined margin of safety for the patient.

1. All materials in contact with the wound and used within the operative field must be sterile. Prior to opening any pack or package, its integrity must be checked for tears and watermarks. The expiration date and the sterilizer-indicating tape must also be checked.

2. Gowns of the operating team members are only considered sterile from shoulder to table level, including sleeves. The back of the gown is not considered sterile.

3. Motions of the surgical team are from sterile to sterile areas and from unsterile to unsterile areas. Anyone who is not scrubbed must never touch or reach over a sterile field.

4. When opening a sterile pack, it should be placed on a table and handled in such a way that only the outside cover is touched (Fig. 24–5). Alter-

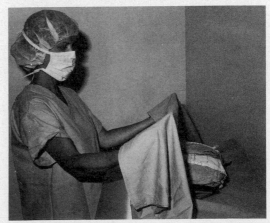

Figure 24–5. The correct way to open a sterile pack on the operating table. The pack wrapping should be handled so that only the outside portion is touched.

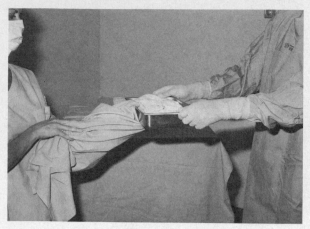

Figure 24–6.

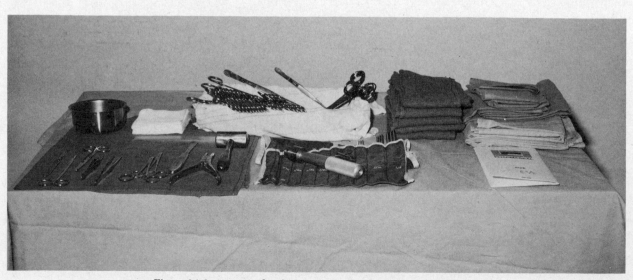

Figure 24–7.

Figure 24–6. Passing an instrument pack to a scrubbed member of the operating team.

Figure 24–7. The correct way to unwrap and place a sterile pack on the operating table. The hands should be placed under the wrapping to provide a wide margin of safety between the inside of the package and the hands.

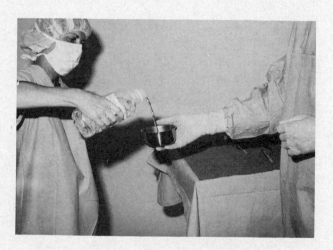

Figure 24–8. Pouring a sterile solution into a sterile receptacle so as to reduce the possibility of splashing the solution onto the operating field.

Figure 24–9. A neat and orderly manner of organizing a surgery table.

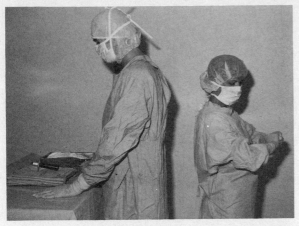

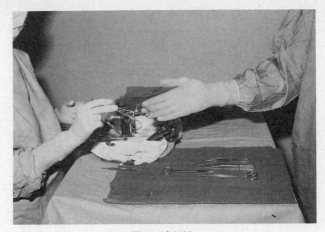

Figure 24–10.   *Figure 24–11.*

Figure 24–10. An acceptable way of changing positions during a surgical procedure.

Figure 24–11. An acceptable hand signal for a hemostat.

natively, the pack may be held in the left hand and unwrapped with the right hand (Fig. 24–6).

5. When opening a sterile package, the hands are placed under the cuff to provide a protected wide margin of safety between the inside of the package and the hands (Fig. 24–7).

6. If a solution must be poured into a sterile receptacle on a sterile table, a scrubbed person should hold the receptacle away from the table while the solution is poured into the container (Fig. 24–8), after first rotating the bottle while pouring into a bucket to clean the lip.

7. In practice, the state of sterility is an absolute—items are either sterile or unsterile.[4]

Correct Conduct at the Operating Table

Correct conduct at the operating table is important to prevent distractions and reduce possible bacterial contamination.

1. There should be no unnecessary talking unless initiated by the operating surgeon.

2. An effort must be made to keep the operating table neat and orderly (Fig. 24–9).

3. Soiled sponges should be removed from the sterile field as soon as they are used.

4. If it becomes necessary to change positions at the operating table, the scrubbed individuals should pass back to back or front to front (Fig. 24–10).

5. Instruments should be passed in a positive and decisive manner. When an instrument is properly passed, the surgeon will know he has it and will not have to look away from the operative site.

6. There are some widely accepted hand signals used at the operating table in an attempt to speed up the passage of instruments and reduce talking in certain situations[3]:

   a. Hemostat: extend the hand supinated (Fig. 24–11).

   b. Scissors: extend the index and middle fingers

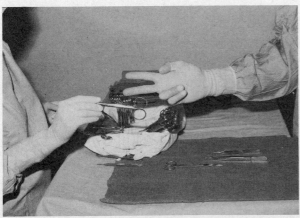

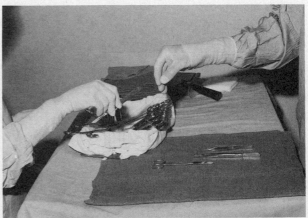

Figure 24–12.   *Figure 24–13.*

Figure 24–12. An acceptable hand signal for a pair of scissors.

Figure 24–13. An acceptable hand signal for a scalpel.

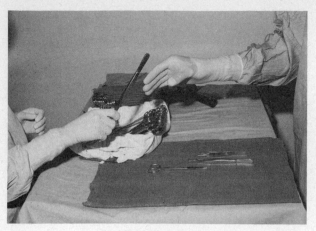

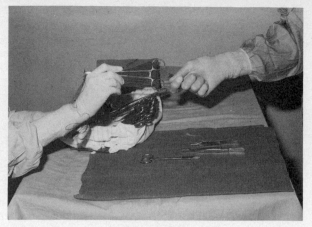

Figure 24–14.　　　　　　　　　　　　　*Figure 24–15.*

Figure 24–14. An acceptable hand signal for thumb forceps.

Figure 24–15. An acceptable hand signal for a needle holder with suture.

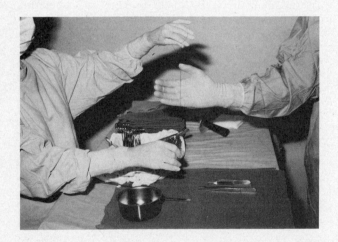

Figure 24–16. An acceptable hand signal for a ligature.

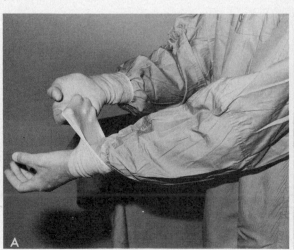

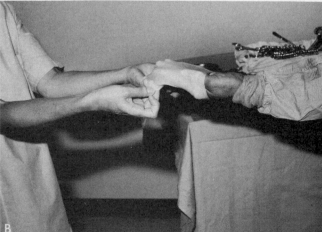

Figure 24–17. A and B, Removal of a glove during a surgical procedure.

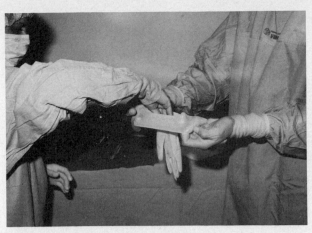

Figure 24–18. Regloving of a scrubbed member of the operating team by another scrubbed member.

and adduct and abduct the two fingers in a shearing motion (Fig. 24–12).

c. Scalpel: hold the hand pronated with the thumb against the distal phalanx of the fingers and flex the wrist to simulate holding the scalpel and performing a cutting maneuver (Fig. 24–13).

d. Forceps: hold the hand pronated and appose the thumb and index finger (Fig. 24–14).

e. Suture: extend and rotate the hand from pronation to supination. This simulates holding a needle holder and the motion used in inserting the suture (Fig. 24–15).

f. Tie: hold the hand elevated with the palm toward the assistant. The assistant grasps the tie at each end and places the mid portion in the surgeon's palm (Fig. 24–16).

Glove Changes

Should it become necessary to remove a damaged glove during the course of an operation, the surgeon should grasp the cuff from the outside and turn it down over the palm. The hand should then be held out to an unsterile assistant, who grasps the edge of the cuff and pulls the glove off (Fig. 24–17).

When regloving it is best, if possible, to allow a scrubbed person to assist in the process (Fig. 24–18).

Should it become necessary to reglove and regown during an operation, the gown is removed before the gloves. This is also the proper technique between operations.

COMPLETION OF THE OPERATION

Prior to leaving the operating room, the surgeon and all scrubbed assistants should remove their gowns

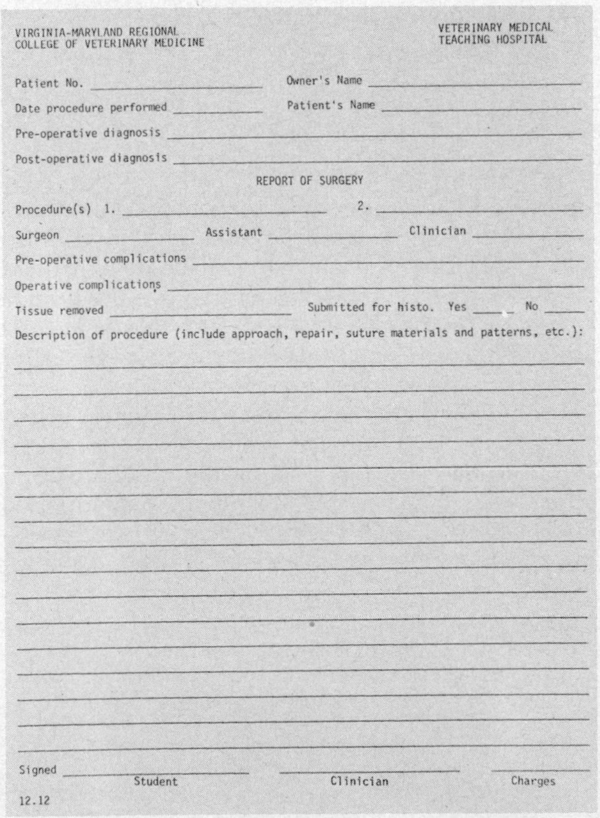

VIRGINIA-MARYLAND REGIONAL
COLLEGE OF VETERINARY MEDICINE

VETERINARY MEDICAL
TEACHING HOSPITAL

Patient No. ____________ Owner's Name ____________

Date procedure performed ____________ Patient's Name ____________

Pre-operative diagnosis ____________

Post-operative diagnosis ____________

REPORT OF SURGERY

Procedure(s) 1. ____________ 2. ____________

Surgeon ____________ Assistant ____________ Clinician ____________

Pre-operative complications ____________

Operative complications ____________

Tissue removed ____________ Submitted for histo. Yes ____ No ____

Description of procedure (include approach, repair, suture materials and patterns, etc.):

Signed ____________ ____________ ____________
Student Clinician Charges

12.12

Figure 24–19.

VIRGINIA-MARYLAND REGIONAL
COLLEGE OF VETERINARY MEDICIN.

'ERINARY MEDICAL
'.ACHING HOSPITAL

CASE SUMMARY

PATIENT NUMBER____________ OWNER'S NAME____________

CLINICIAN____________ PATIENT'S NAME/NO.____________

ADMISSION DATE: DISCHARGE DATE: SERVICE: MED SUR A U O

CODE

DIAGNOSES

CODE

OPERATIONS

ANESTHETIC AGENT USED:
Complications (specify):

VACCINE(S) GIVEN:

IN-HOSPITAL MEDICATIONS:

DIAGNOSTIC PROCEDURES:
__Clinical Exam Only __Electrophysiology
__Gross Pathology __Hematology
__Histopathology __Urinalysis
__Serology __Chemistry
__Microbiology __Parasitology
__Radiology __Ophthalmology
Other ____________

HOSPITAL COMPLICATIONS:
__None __Anesthetic Death
__Surgical Infec. __Parasitism
__Post-surgical shock or hemorrhage __Infectious disease (Non-surgical)
__Wound Dishiscence __Metabolic Disease
__Drug Idiosyncrasy __Other (state below)

DISCHARGE STATUS:
__Undetermined (Alive) __Improved __Died--Necropsy __Euthanatized--Necropsy
__Recovered __Unimproved __Died--No Necropsy __Euthanatized--No Necropsy

____________ CLINICIAN ____________ DATE

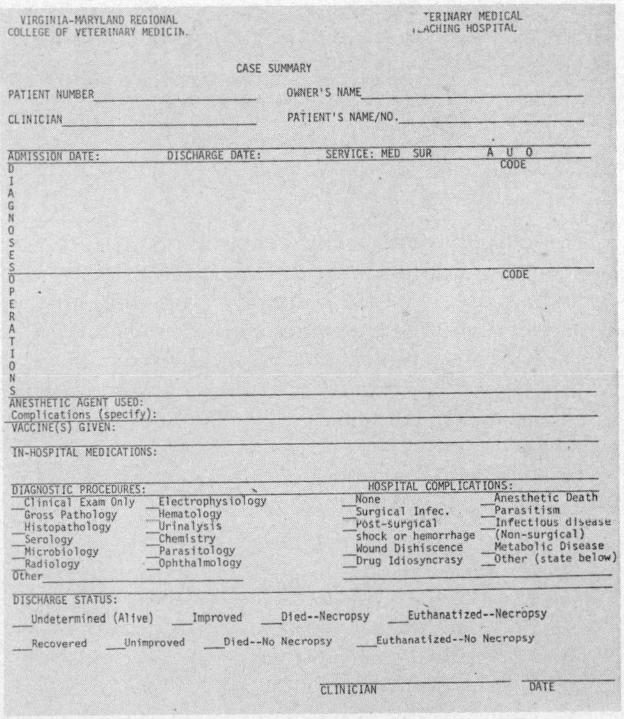

Figure 24–20.

Figure 24–19. An operating report form.
Figure 24–20. A case summary record.

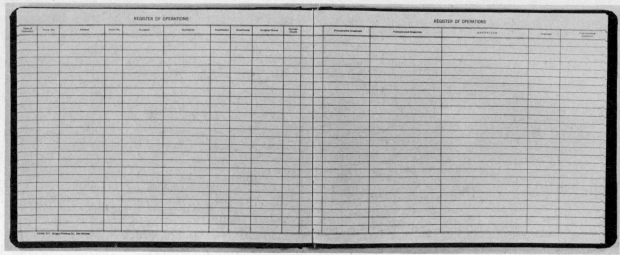

Figure 24–21. A surgical log book.

and gloves if there are no other procedures. The cap, mask, and shoe covers should not be removed until the surgical team has left the operating suite.

Postoperative clean-up procedures must be rigidly outlined and adhered to.[2]

1. Tables are thoroughly scrubbed using both mechanical friction and chemical disinfection.

2. Equipment and tanks are wiped clean.

3. Ceiling and wall-mounted fixtures are cleaned on all surfaces.

4. Kick buckets are emptied.

5. Floors and walls are checked for soil spots and cleaned as indicated.

6. Cabinets and doors are cleaned, especially around handles or push plates, where debris is likely to accumulate.

RECORDS

The surgery department's records should be both informative and meaningful. The three primary records that are generated directly from the surgery department are the treatment authorization form, the operative report, and the case summary record.

The treatment authorization form documents the client's consent to have agreed upon procedures performed.

The operative report (Fig. 24–19) and case summary record (Fig. 24–20) should include:

1. Patient and client's name.

2. Patient's hospital number.

3. Date of the procedure.

4. Preoperative diagnosis.

5. Postoperative diagnosis.

6. List of any tissue removed.

7. Name of the surgeon, assistant surgeon, and attending clinician.

8. Liberal space for a description of the operative procedure.

9. List of any operative complications.

10. Discharge status of the patient.

The latter two forms allow a documentation of surgical procedures performed and give a retrievable source for ready review for annual reports, case reviews, and the success or failure of given surgical procedures. A well-organized surgical log book can also be helpful in these areas, especially if a large number of surgical procedures are being performed (Fig. 24–21).

BUDGETING

The formulation of an accurate budget is extremely important to the surgery department. The budget predicts the number and types of surgical procedures to be performed, the income generated from these procedures, and the cost incurred in performing them. The budget should also allow for a priority listing of new equipment that the department desires to purchase as the funds become available.

It is equally important to keep an accurate inventory of all available supplies. The instrument request form can be used to help in the re-ordering of supplies used during the operation. Seldom used supplies should have a clearly marked sterilization date and, if applicable, an expiration date.

1. *Standards of Administrative Nursing Practice: Operating Room,* Assoc. Operating Room Nurses, 1976.

2. Atkinson, L. J., and Kohn, M. L.: *Berry and Kohn's Introduction to Operating Room Technique.* McGraw-Hill Book Co., New York, 1978.

3. Nealon, T. F.: *Fundamental Skills in Surgery.* W. B. Saunders, Philadelphia, 1979.

4. Rhodes, M. J., Gruendeman, B. J., and Ballinger, W. F.: *Alexander's Care of the Patient in Surgery,* C. V. Mosby, St. Louis, 1978.

Chapter 25

Surgical Instruments

David F. Merkley and Ronald L. Grier

INTRODUCTION

The veterinary surgeon has at his disposal a great variety of surgical instruments. In addition to instruments produced in the United States, many are imported from countries such as Germany, England, Sweden, Pakistan, Japan, Italy, and France. There is no governmental agency in the United States that oversees quality standards for instrument production. Thus, the control of instrument quality lies solely with the individual manufacturer.

Responsible instrument manufacturers who maintain high-quality control standards are careful to select quality materials to ensure long, trouble-free service. Most high-quality instruments today are made from various stainless steels.

The economics of veterinary practice dictate that good judgment be used when initially selecting instrument and in their subsequent handling and care. In the long run, the purchase of lesser quality (and usually cheaper) instruments may prove to be more expensive because their performance may not meet certain needs and rapid wear or corrosion may necessitate early replacement. Good quality stainless steel surgical instruments that are handled properly should last for ten years before replacement becomes necessary. An understanding of instrument production and materials and procedures accepted for their proper care and handling is necessary to ensure this durability.

INSTRUMENT METALS

Chromium-plated carbon steel surgical instruments are commonly found in veterinary hospitals. They are popular because of their low price, ease of maintenance, and highly polished finish. The plated surface, however, is susceptible to attack by low pH solutions, saline, and other chemicals. Early deterioration by pitting, rusting, and blistering of the plated surface is a very common problem, resulting in early repair or replacement.

Today, better quality surgical instruments are fabricated from stainless steel. Of the standard stainless steels produced, only a few are used in hospitals. Of these, the 300 and 400 series stainless steels are most often selected for surgical instrument production.

Stainless steels consist primarily of iron, chromium, and carbon, with other elements such as nickel combined in different proportions to achieve desired properties. The higher carbon, lower chromium 400 series (martensitic) stainless steels provide greater hardness through heat treatment. This imparts wear resistance which is especially important for cutting surgical instruments; they must maintain fine edges and exhibiting the strength and durability of stainless steel. The hard martensitic stainless steels are used most commonly in the manufacture of surgical instruments.

The austenitic, or 300 series, stainless steels are not hardenable by heat treatment but are occasionally used for surgical instrument manufacture. The lack of hardness exhibited by these alloys is offset somewhat by their higher resistance to corrosion. Austenitic steels are of greatest value when some degree of malleability in an instrument is desired.

A few surgical instruments are made primarily of titanium alloys. They are used most commonly in microsurgical instruments. They are said to have excellent corrosion resistance (comparable to that of stainless steels) and high temperature strength (comparable to that of austenitic stainless steel). The internal structure makes these alloys somewhat brittle, and this can present manufacturing problems. Its greatest use may be as a substitute for stainless steels when weight saving is important.

Tungsten carbide inserts add a new dimension to gripping and cutting surfaces. These substances are very hard and very resistant to wear. The inserts are attached to the stainless steel instruments by various means and can be removed and replaced by the manufacturer.

RESISTANCE TO CORROSION

Producing a surgical instrument that is resistant to staining and corrosion begins with selecting the proper steel. A smooth surface is desired and is achieved by buffing and polishing. Three types of instrument finishes are presently available. The highly polished finish seems most resistant to spotting and discoloration; however, it reflects light easily and can cause mild eye irritation. More recently a dull or satin finish has become popular; its greatest advantage is reduced eye strain. The dull finishes are applied by silicone or glass-bead sandblasting or by fine abrasion using various types of polishing wheels. The third type of finish, a (black) ebonizing finish, is achieved by coating the instrument in a chemical bath.

The final process instruments go through to become corrosion resistant is passivation. This process (nitric acid bath) removes any foreign particles (iron) imbedded on the instrument surface. Additionally, a thin layer of chromium oxides forms on the stainless steel surface, providing more corrosion resistance. A subsequent polishing is usually needed to produce a very smooth surface, removing any rough sites where corrosion could begin.

Once an instrument is used it can further passivate itself. Exposure of an instrument to the atmosphere or to certain oxidizing agents during its handling and use can continue this oxidation process, building and maintaining the continuity of the chromium oxide layer. Certain cleaning and handling processes can damage this protective layer and should be avoided. Abrasive cleaners and instrument marking with vibrating etching equipment can disturb the oxide layer, promoting the development of corrosion. Once the chromium oxide layer is altered and corrosion begins, repassivation and repolishing by the manufacturer become necessary.

INSTRUMENT CLEANING

Most major hospitals recognize that proper training of central supply personnel in instrument cleaning and handling techniques saves enormous sums of money in yearly instrument replacement. Proprietors of veterinary hospitals and clinics are usually aware that surgical instruments are expensive, delicate, and must be handled correctly in the operating room to ensure longevity. A sometimes forgotten fact, however, is that inappropriate cleaning and sterilizing have a significant impact on instrument life. Most instrument manufacturers provide detailed information on the cleaning and handling of their product. Their recommendations should be followed.

Manual Cleaning

Most small veterinary clinics must process their instruments by hand; the general principles for manual cleaning should be followed. Gross visible debris should be removed from the instruments *immediately* after their use. Saline solution is very corrosive to stainless steel; consequently, distilled or de-ionized water should be used for the initial removal of debris. Subsequent instrument cleaning will then be easier, as blood and tissue debris do not have a chance to dry in serrations and box locks. If further processing is not immediately possible, instruments should be submerged in warm de-ionized water that contains a mild noncorrosive, low-sudsing, neutral detergent. Adequate soaking time allows the detergent to loosen inaccessible soil films. Prolonged soaking must be discouraged, however, as detergent action on the instrument surface may cause damage.

The final cleaning process should be conducted with care. Each instrument is carefully scrubbed, including the box locks, ratchets, serrations, and other areas not easily exposed. A hand brush with stiff plastic bristles is appropriate for cleaning. Abrasive tools or cleaners should be avoided, however, as repeated cleanings can damage the instrument's surface and promote corrosion. A moderately alkaline (pH<8), low-sudsing detergent is most satisfactory. Ordinary soap should not be used, especially with hard water, as insoluble alkali earth films can form on the instruments, protecting trapped bacteria from sterilization.

The final rinse should be carried out thoroughly with distilled or de-ionized water. It has a pH of 6.7 to 7.2 and leaves a neutral surface pH as the alkaline wash water residue is rinsed away. Alkaline earth deposits (calcium, magnesium, phosphate) and metals (iron, copper, cadmium) will not deposit themselves on the surface to promote corrosion. Distilled water also contains no dissolved or undissolved solids to adhere to the instrument surface.

The instrument must be dried completely, especially if it is to be stored for a period of time prior to sterilization. The heat of hot rinse water may aid the drying process. Inadequate drying will result in rusting during storage.

Washer-Sterilizer

Institutions that process large volumes of surgical instruments have adopted mechanical methods for routine cleaning. The washing process is accomplished in an instrument washer-sterilizer by means of a vigorously agitated detergent bath, the result of a combination of high-velocity jet streams of steam and air, which produces violent underwater turbulence.[4] The machine has presoak, wash, and sterilize cycles, after which the instruments may be removed and immediately used or stored for future use. Many factors influence the effectiveness of soil removal from surgical instruments cleaned in a washer-sterilizer, including the kind of soil, quality of water, type of detergent, concentration of detergent, types of instruments to be cleaned, time the detergent solution is permitted to act, and efficiency of the washer-sterilizer.[4]

Blood, tissue fats, and other organic matter are common types of soil encountered on surgical instruments. Better cleaning in the washer-sterilizer is achieved when soil is not allowed to dry on the instruments and processing occurs shortly after use.

Water plays a major role in cleaning and alone accounts for much of the solvent action that occurs during instrument cleaning. The quality of tapwater in many areas is poor, and careful consideration should be given to matching water quality with the appropriate detergent. Softened, demineralized, or distilled water should be considered to eliminate the deposition of hard water salts on instruments.

A good, low-sudsing, neutral to slightly alkaline detergent is strongly recommended. According to Perkins, some of the common phosphate detergents recommended for mechanical dishwashers are ineffective in washer-sterilizers.[4] Cleaning of the instruments is not adequate, and the polyphosphated detergents have a solubilizing effect on internal copper in the washer-sterilizer. The result is a brassy metallic staining of the instruments due to copper deposition by electrolytic action.

The type of surgical instrument, its configuration, and its condition play a major role in cleaning effectiveness. Mostafa and Chackett demonstrated quantitatively that soil retention is greatest with instruments with a poor geometric configuration and those whose serrated tips showed visible corrosion.[3] They showed that corroded serrations and cavities near the hinges of worn joints were particularly effective in retaining soil and that there is a clear correlation between soil retention and the microscopic state of the instrument surface.

Finally, the washer-sterilizer affords a degree of protection to those who clean surgical instruments. Manual cleaning contributes to the dissemination of microorganisms by aerosols and droplets during the cleaning process, whereas automated mechanical cleaning controls this problem.[4]

Ultrasonic Cleaner

Small ultrasonic units are available that can be used conveniently in veterinary clinics. Ultrasonic cleaners can remove up to 90 per cent of instrument soil in five minutes and far surpass manual cleaning procedures. This is demonstrated by the effective removal of soil from areas that are inaccessible to brushing such as box locks, deep grooves, serrations, and even cracks in the instrument. Ultrasonic cleaners do not sterilize.

Ultrasonic instrument cleaners produce sinusoidal energy waves at either of two frequencies. If metallic transducers are used, the frequency of vibrations is 20,600 per second. If crystal transducers are used, the frequency of vibrations is 38,000 per second. The latter unit is believed to be the more efficient.[2]

The effectiveness of ultrasonic cleaning is based on a process called *cavitation*. Ultrasonic energy forms minute bubbles from gas nuclei within the cleaning solution. These minute bubbles form on every surface of soiled instruments. The size of the gas nuclei and subsequent bubbles formed depends on the surface tension of the liquid, temperature of the solution, wetting action of the detergent, and the frequency of the ultrasonic energy used.[4] These bubbles continue to expand until their surface becomes unstable. They then collapse by implosion (bursting inward). The bubbles implode as fast as they form, creating small vacuum areas. This process releases energy that breaks the bonds that hold soil to instrument surfaces. The soil and binding material are dislodged or dissolved into the solution.

The effectiveness of an ultrasonic cleaner can be altered by many variables, including temperature, gas content of the solution, and the detergent used. The temperature of the bath solution should be kept below 60°C (140°F) to prevent protein coagulation. Coagulated protein tends to absorb ultrasonic vibrations, which reduces the energy available for bond breaking and makes the soil more difficult to remove. Bath solutions containing too much dissolved gas lose cleaning effectiveness because the gas fills the cavitation bubbles. This cushions the shock due to implosion and reduces the energy released. Water can be de-aerated by running the ultrasonic cleaner for five minutes before use or letting the water stand overnight. Detergent specifically formulated for ultrasonic cleaners should be used because they decrease aeration problems.[4] In addition, the detergent is chosen for its cleaning abilities and its chemical effects on the instruments being cleaned. Highly alkaline or highly acid detergent should not be used, as they can induce corrosion or cracking, which can lead to early instrument failure. The detergent should have a neutral pH, contain a wetting agent, and be low sudsing and free rinsing. Finally, the proper concentration of cleaner should be employed, since the heat of the ultrasonic cleaner increases the strength of the cleaner. If too much detergent or heat is employed, the cleaning solution can become very caustic. This leads to removal of the chromium oxide layer, which is so important in corrosion resistance. The impassivated instrument is then susceptible to rusting and breakage.

Instruments removed from an ultrasonic cleaner must be rinsed thoroughly. The cleaner effectively removes the soil into solution or suspension, and when the instruments are removed they become covered with this finely dispersed soil. This soil, although not always visible to the eye, must be rinsed away. Rinsing also removes residual detergent that may be present.

Dissimilar metals should not be processed together in an ultrasonic cleaner. Stainless steel should not be mixed with brass, copper, or aluminum, otherwise electrolytic etching and redeposition may occur. Chrome-plated instruments that show pitting or flaking can be further damaged in an ultrasonic cleaner.

INSTRUMENT LUBRICATION

Surgical instruments with box locks often become stiff with repeated use, especially if cleaned inadequately. Dried blood, alkaline deposits, and debris can build up in box locks and serrations. Autoclaving bakes this material on the instrument, further retarding movement. Cleaning procedures, when employed properly, help to prevent this problem.

Instrument lubrication is commonly practiced but can present problems if not properly performed. Mineral oil, machine oils, grease, and some silicones must be avoided, as they leave an oily film on the instrument surface. This can prevent adequate steam contact with organisms, and spores can become trapped in the oil film during steam sterilization.[4] Continuous use of these materials can also leave undesirable residues on the instruments that become gumlike and retard box lock movement.

Instrument manufacturers recommend the routine lubrication of instruments with antimicrobial water-soluble lubricants (instrument milk). These lubricants are water-oil emulsion preparations that do not interfere with steam sterilization. Many also contain antimicrobial materials inhibiting organism growth in bath preparations. Rust-inhibiting agents provide an additional measure of protection by retarding electrolysis and preventing mineral deposition on instrument surfaces.

Mechanical instrument processing especially with ultrasonic cleaners, removes all traces of lubricant. Lubrication should therefore be carried out after cleaning. The lubricant bath should be prepared with de-ionized or distilled water at the manufacturer's recommended concentration. Instruments should be dipped in the bath for 30 seconds with box locks open. After removal from the bath, the lubricant solution should be allowed to drain away without rinsing or manual drying. The lubricant remains on the instrument during steam sterilization and storage. This gives added protection against rusting, staining, and corrosion.

INSTRUMENT IDENTIFICATION

It is common practice in veterinary hospitals and institutions to mark instruments for easy identification and to discourage theft. Impact-type marking devices and electric vibrating engravers should be avoided. These units damage the instrument's highly polished passivated outer layer and predispose to staining and corrosion. Marking of an instrument in the box lock (hinge) area can create microfaults or fractures that lead to early breakage. If instruments must be engraved use the shank and not the box lock area. Be sure the manufacturer's warranty is not voided by such practices.

Color-coded plastic autoclavable tape is preferred over engraving for instrument identification. Some manufacturers do provide a marking or etching service when you purchase or repair your surgical instruments. Electrochemical etching equipment is available that will not damage an instrument's surface when used properly. Following marking, adequate neutralization of the etching fluid is necessary, as the acid solution can continue to interact with the stainless steel, promoting corrosion.

INSTRUMENT PACKAGING

Proper instrument packaging and storage are important considerations for veterinary institutions and small clinics. Universally accepted standards for instrument packaging have not been established. Problems are compounded by manufacturers who are continually developing new and often better packaging products. Packaging materials used frequently today are classified as textiles (linen and muslin), nonwoven fabric, paper, plastic, and paper and plastic combinations.[5]

Textiles

Linen or muslin wrappers are most commonly used for instrument set packaging. Standard, double-thickness, 140-thread count linen is flexible, easy to use, memory free, and long lasting. The weave of one thickness is perpendicular to the other, and the wrap is sewn at the edges only. Linen packs are easily contaminated by contact with moisture, and the contamination becomes undetectable after the moisture dries. Laundry procedures must be carefully monitored. If harsh detergents not adequately rinsed from the fabric come in contact with stainless steel instruments, staining and corrosion can be induced.[2]

The necessity of double wrapping surgical packs with two-layer linen has been repeatedly demonstrated.[6-8] Photographs of a single-thickness standard muslin at $40 \times$ magnification demonstrate a small opening at almost every thread junction. Single wrapping with two-layer linen can allow microbial penetration of the pack within three days. Double wrapping with two-layer linen increases safe storage time to three to four weeks. Longer storage time may be obtained by using outside (dust cover) wraps of water-repellent paper drape fabrics or sterile 3-ml plastic bags.

Open shelf storage of sterile packs has been shown to allow up to ten times more viable microbial contamination of the outside of the pack than closed shelf or cabinets storage, thus reducing safe storage time.[7] Other factors also have been incriminated in surgical pack contamination. Unnecessary handling and vibration should be minimized along with rapidly changing atmospheric conditions.

Finally, double wrapping of sterile packages provides a margin of safety during package opening.[6] Microbiological contamination that has settled on a package is thrown into the surrounding air during opening making contamination of contents very likely. A second wrap greatly reduces this risk.

Consideration can be given to the use of 288-thread count linen. This material has twice the thread per inch as the standard 140-thread count general use linen. A single thickness of this material can replace the standard double-layer wrappers. This wrap is a good moisture retardant and is an improved barrier to microbiological and liquid penetration over 140-thread count linen. Good penetration of sterilants is allowed, although as a general rule the higher the thread count the less penetration by steam. The major disadvantage of this moisture-retardant linen is its higher cost.

Nonwoven Fabrics

Nonwoven wraps are a product of disposable surgical drape programs and offer some advantages over general use linen, including reduced labor and laundry costs. Nonwoven wraps are water resistant, strong, and tear resistant. Sterilants such as ethylene oxide and steam penetrate readily and do not change the handling characteristics or quality of the material for use as a wrapper or drape. Although product quality is excellent, nonwoven fabrics should be used as disposable items. Repeated sterilization can result in breakage of fibers, especially along folds in the material, which could result in pack contamination.

Nonwoven fabrics are available in light, medium, or heavy weight. The lightweight material does not withstand handling well and is not recommended for operating room packaging.[5] The medium-weight wrapper material is best suited for sterile packaging wraps.

Paper Wraps

Paper wraps have come into wide use as replacement for linen. Several disadvantages are recognized, however. Like linen, paper has good wick action and can absorb moisture and dry qucikly, making it difficult to detect a contaminated pack. Also, paper has memory and will not open flatly. The paper flips back along fold lines, often resulting in contamination during opening. Paper wraps should not be re-used, as minute cracks in the paper fabric are difficult to detect and can easily compromise sterility. Personnel should be aware of these sources of contamination when using paper drapes.

Plastic Wraps

Plastic wraps usually come in pouches presealed by the manufacturer on two or three sides. Their greatest use is in individual article packaging. Polyethylene, polypropylene, and polyvinyl chloride pouches are produced only for ethylene oxide sterilization, as they may be heat sensitive and impermeable to steam.[4, 5] Detailed opening instructions are necessary, as sterile removal of items from these pouches is difficult. Plastic wraps can also be used as dust covers on previously sterilized muslin- or paper-wrapped surgical packs that are stored for variable periods before use. Any plastic cover used for this purpose that has accumulated dust should be removed before the surgical pack is placed inside the clean zone of the operating room.

Plastic and Paper Wraps

Plastic and paper combinations are used extensively. They offer several advantages. Materials are available that withstand steam and ethylene oxide sterilization. Good steam penetration and aeration is evident through the paper backing, and the article is visible through the plastic. Peel-back opening for presentation of sterile items lessens the possibility of contamination. Sealing of the pouch can be accomplished by sterilizer indicator tape or heat.

Dating and labeling of these packages with felt-tip markers should be done on the plastic side only, as puncture or ink bleed through the paper is possible. Also, sterile indicator tape should be placed on the plastic side, as the sterilize indicating device incorporated into the paper is often overlooked during opening.[5]

SURGICAL INSTRUMENTS

The selection of surgical instrumentation is up to the individual surgeon. Variation in quality is obvious. A surgeon's skill may frequently be impaired by poor-quality or poorly conditioned instruments. Important considerations in instrument quality and care have been pointed out. Most veterinary hospitals and clinics develop surgical packs for various procedures. A basic soft tissue surgical pack is often employed; specific instruments for special procedures are packed and prepared either individually or in special procedure packs. The instruments found in a basic surgical pack for most small animal surgical procedures are listed in Table 25–1.

Needle Holders

The most common needle holder used in veterinary surgery is the Mayo-Hegar needle holder (Fig. 25–1). Various lengths (5 to 12 inches) are available. The smaller needle holders are more delicate and

TABLE 25–1. Soft Tissue Surgical Pack

Instrument	Size (inches)	Number
Backhaus towel clamp	3½	6
Adson tissue forceps (1 × 2 teeth)	4¾	1
Brown-Adson tissue forceps (9 × 9 teeth)	4¾	1
DeBakey tissue forceps (atraumatic tips)	6	1
Mayo dissecting scissors (straight)	5½	1
Mayo dissecting scissors (curved)	6¾	1
Metzenbaum dissecting scissors (curved)	5¾ or 7	1
Mayo-Hegar needle holder	5	1
Mayo-Hegar needle holder	7	1
Halsted mosquito forceps (straight)	3½ or 5	4
Halsted mosquito forceps (curved)	3½ or 5	4
Kelly or Crile hemostatic forceps (curved)	5½	2
Rochester-Carmalt hemostatic forceps (straight)	6¼	3
Ovariohysterectomy hook (Snook or Covault)	8	1
Surgical knife handle #3	4⅞	2
Allis tissue forceps (4 × 5 teeth)	6	4
Senn retractors (double-ended)	6¾	2
Weinstein instrument pack	7	1

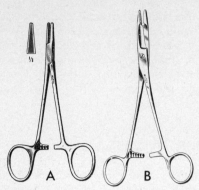

Figure 25–1. A, Mayo-Hegar needle holder. B, Olsen-Hegar needle holder. (Reprinted with permission from Miltex Instrument Co., Lake Success, NY.)

probably find greater use in small animal surgery. No surgical instrument receives greater abuse than the needle holder. Its use requires constant metal-to-metal contact. The size and weight of the needle holder selected should match those of the needle being used. Small needle holders can be damaged when used to grip large needles. If the ratchet is tightly applied the box lock or shank can be damaged. Small needles can be damaged or inadequately gripped if large needle holders are used. There is a great tendency, especially in orthopedic procedures to use the needle holder inappropriately. Using the needle holder to twist wire or as pliers leads to early failure.

The better-quality needle holders can easily be identified by the tungsten carbide inserts of their gripping jaws (Fig. 25–2). These inserts greatly increase grip and durability. Some manufacturers also identify their better-quality instruments by gold-colored handles.

Olsen-Hegar needle holders (Fig. 25–1)B) are a

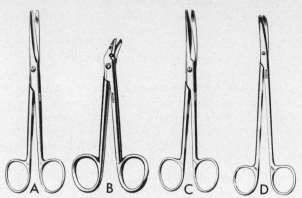

Figure 25–3. A, Straight Mayo dissecting scissor. B, Wire-cutting suture scissor. C, Curved Mayo dissecting scissor. D, Curved Metzenbaum dissecting scissor. (Reprinted with permission from Miltex Instrument Co., Lake Success, NY.)

combination needle holder and scissors. They may have an advantage for the individual who is doing surgery alone. The suture material can be cut after placement without a suture scissors. The disadvantage of accidental cutting of suture material during suturing can be troublesome. Tungsten carbide inserts are available with the needle holder portion of the instrument.

Scissors

Many types of surgical scissors are available for many different uses. Those most applicable for gen-

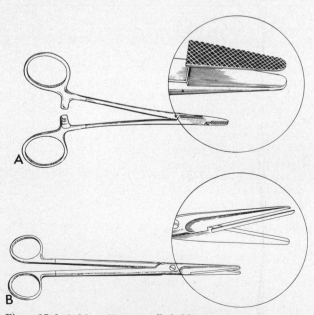

Figure 25–2. A, Mayo-Hegar needle holder with a tungsten carbide insert. B, Metzenbaum surgical scissor with tungsten carbide insert. (Reprinted with permission from Miltex Instrument Co., Lake Success, NY.)

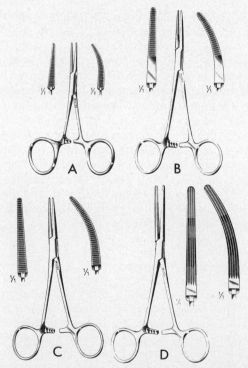

Figure 25–4. A, Halsted mosquito hemostatic forceps. B, Kelly hemostatic forceps. C, Crile hemostatic forceps. D, Rochester-Carmalt hemostatic forceps. (Reprinted with permission from Miltex Instrument Co., Lake Success, NY.)

eral surgical use in veterinary surgery are the Mayo and the Metzenbaum.

Each surgery pack should have a scissor designated as a suture scissor. Repeated cutting of suture material with delicate tissue scissors, such as the Metzenbaum, leads to dulling and/or misalignment of blades. A short (5 inches) straight Mayo dissecting scissors (Fig. 25–3A) without tungsten carbide inserts can function well. It is durable and will last a long time. Special wire-cutting scissors should be employed for orthopedic wire cutting (Fig. 25–3B).

Tissue dissecting (blunt and sharp) requires a high-quality tissue scissors. The curved Mayo dissecting scissor (Fig. 25–3C) with or without tungsten carbide inserts is excellent for connective tissue dissection and separation of tougher facial plains. The Metzenbaum tissue-dissecting scissor (Fig. 25–3D) is more delicate and should be reserved for less strenuous dissecting and cutting. It would seem inappropriate to use a fine Metzenbaum to open the linea alba. Fine, delicate cutting, as required in hollow organ surgery or controlled delicate dissecting, would be more applicable to Metzenbaums. Tungsten carbide inserts and gold-colored handles designate the finest quality surgical scissors (see Fig. 25–2B).

Forceps

Halsted Mosquito Hemostatic Forceps

Mosquito forceps (Fig. 25–4A) are available in 3½ and 5-inch lengths in both curved and straight configurations. These instruments are very delicate and should be used only for the control of point bleeders. Stump or pedicle ligations, where additional tissue is often included in the ligature, should be avoided, as damage to the instrument can result. Mosquito forceps have been recently introduced with rat tooth (1 × 2) teeth located at the very tip of the gripping blades. This modification prevents the instrument from slipping from the tissue it is holding. If the instruments are in good working order and are used for their intended purpose, this addition may be unnecessary.

Kelly or Crile Hemostatic Forceps

These two forceps are very similar in design and use. The only difference is in the extent of the transverse grooves on their gripping surfaces. The Kelly (Fig. 25–4B) has only the distal half of its tips grooved. The intended use of these hemostatic forceps is similar to that of the mosquito forceps. However, they are larger (5½ inches) and much sturdier so that they can withstand more aggressive use.

Rochester-Carmalt Hemostatic Forceps

The Rochester-Carmalt hemostatic forceps (Fig. 25–4D) is primarily used in veterinary surgery in stump or pedicle ligations. It is sturdy and the grooves on the gripping blades run longitudinally (with a few cross grooves at the tip), allowing for easy removal during ligation.

When a Carmalt clamp is placed on a pedicle of tissue for crushing prior to ligation, the tissue is forced outward in the clamp and is, in effect, spread. When ligation occurs, the clamp must be loosened before the ligature is secured or the tissue cannot be drawn together to collapse the vessel being ligated. One must also keep this spreading effect in mind when ligating close to a second Carmalt clamp that has been placed. This spreading effect on tissue by the clamp can result in loose ligatures.

Tissue Forceps

Tissue forceps of various sizes, shapes, and uses are available. Several have found extensive use as general surgical tissue forceps in small animal surgery.

Allis Tissue Forceps

Allis tissue forceps (Fig. 25–5A) are very popular in veterinary surgery. The plane of grip is perpendicular to the direction of pull. The tip of the Allis forceps has intermeshing teeth that provide a secure grip on tissue. The Allis is said to be atraumatic to tissue; however, this feature seems to be commonly

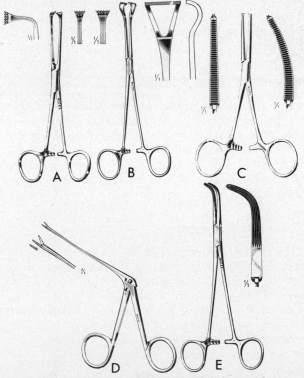

Figure 25–5. A, Allis tissue forceps. B, Babcock tissue forceps. C, Kocher-Oschner tissue forceps. D, Alligator tissue forceps. E, Right-angle tissue forceps (Lehey gall duct forceps). (Reprinted with permission from Miltex Instrument Co., Lake Success, NY.)

abused. The Allis should be used to grip connective tissue and facial planes only. It should never be used to grasp the skin or to grip hollow organs such as the stomach. The crushing effect of this grip is too traumatizing for these delicate tissues.

Babcock Tissue Forceps

The Babcock forceps (Fig. 25–5B) is similar in design to the Allis except that there are no gripping teeth. Its uses would be similar to those of the Allis. The Babcock has received some use in hollow organ surgery; however, its grip may be excessively traumatizing. The more appropriate use of stay sutures to manipulate hollow organs would seem prudent.

Kocher-Oschner Tissue Forceps

The Kocher-Oschner tissue forceps (Fig. 25–5C) is very sturdy and can withstand aggressive use. The 2×1 rat tooth tip allows secure gripping of tissue. This instrument has very limited soft tissue use; however, orthopedic surgeons find the instrument helpful in manipulating bone fragments in fracture repair.

Alligator Tissue Forceps

This special instrument is very delicate but provides a needed capability. The long shaft and pivot point near the tip or its jaws allow introduction and grasping through a small narrow opening. Removal of foreign bodies from ear canals and disc material during thoracolumbar fenestrations are appropriate applications.

Right-Angle Tissue Forceps

The right-angle tissue forceps (Lahey gall duct forceps) (Fig. 25–5E) has longitudinal grooves on its gripping surface. It is very suitable for delicate dissection, especially in hard to visualize areas. The instrument is excellent for dissecting behind a patent ductus arteriosus and is used extensively in other thoracic surgeries.

Adson Tissue Forceps

The Adson (delicate) (Fig. 25–6A) is probably the most common tissue forceps in use. The 2×1 rat tooth tips are small and provide good tissue grip with minimal pressure on the blades. It is most applicable when suturing skin and facial planes. Although it is relatively atraumatic when used properly, better tissue forceps are available for hollow organ surgery.

Brown-Adson Tissue Forceps

The Brown-Adson (Fig. 25–6B) also has extensive use. It is similar to the Adson except for its tip. Multiple intermeshing fine teeth provide a broad tip

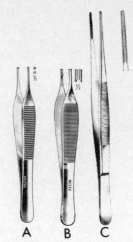

Figure 25–6. A, Adson tissue forceps. B, Brown-Adson tissue forceps. C, DeBakey tissue forceps. (Reprinted with permission from Miltex Instrument Co., Lake Success, NY.)

for secure gripping. When suturing, this feature makes gripping of a needle being pulled through tissue easier than with the Adson. The Brown-Adson is relatively atraumatic if used properly i.e., on skin and facial planes only.

DeBakey Tissue Forceps

Every surgery pack should have a delicate thumb forceps for atraumatic work. The DeBakey tissue forceps (Fig. 25–6C) was initially developed for cardiovascular surgery. The tips are slightly ribbed in a longitudinal direction. Various widths (1 to 2 mm) on the tip and weights (delicate to regular) are available. This instrument is excellent for thoracic and abdominal surgery. Very delicate handling of a tissue being sutured is possible.

Towel Forceps

The Backhaus towel forceps (Fig. 25–7) is used for securing surgical drapes to skin. It is also used to secure suction lines, electrocautery cables, and power equipment lines to drapes. Two sizes are commonly seen, and the smaller (3½ inches) is more appropriate

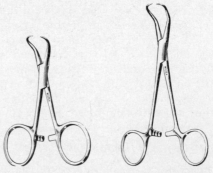

Figure 25–7. Backhaus towel forceps. (Reprinted with permission from Miltex Instrument Co., Lake Success, NY.)

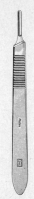

Figure 25–8. Bard-Parker #3 surgical handle. (Reprinted with permission from Miltex Instrument Co., Lake Success, NY.)

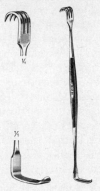

Figure 25–10. Senn retractor (hand-held). (Reprinted with permission from Miltex Instrument Co., Lake Success, NY.)

for small animal surgery. Some towel forceps (Roeder) have a metal bead or ball stop on their tips to prevent the drapes from moving up. The Jones towel forceps may be used in more delicate applications.

Surgical Knife Handles

Surgical knife handles with detachable blades are most popular. The Bard-Parker #3 medium handle (Fig. 25–8) is available with various scalpel blade attachments (#10, 11, 12, 15). This handle seems to be the most applicable for small animal surgery. The #3 handle is also available in a longer form. Fine handles (#7 and 9) receive the same blades.

The #4 Bard-Parker handle is larger and uses detachable blades #20, 21, 22. This handle-and-blade combination seems more appropriate for large animal surgery.

Ovariohysterectomy Hooks

Two ovariohysterectomy hooks (Fig. 25–9) are available. The Snook and Covault hooks are similar in shape with slight differences in the handles and

the hook tips. Both are effective for their intended use of retrieving the horn of the uterus through a relatively small incision. Which instrument to use depends on how comfortable the handle feels in a surgeon's hand.

Retractors

Many types of soft tissue retractors are available. A most useful classification would distinguish between hand-held and self-retaining retractors. The greatest disadvantage of hand-held retractors (Fig.

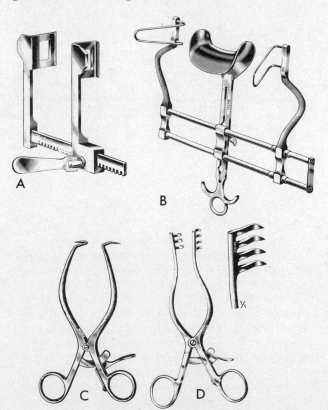

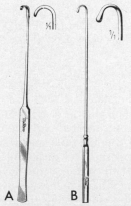

Figure 25–9. A, Snook ovariohysterectomy hook (flat tip). *B,* Covault ovariohysterectomy hook (buttoned tip). (Reprinted with permission from Miltex Instrument Co., Lake Success, NY.)

Figure 25–11. A, Finochietto rib retractor. *B,* Balfour abdominal retractor. *C,* Gelpi perineal retractor. *D,* Weitlaner retractor. (Reprinted with permission from Miltex Instrument Co., Lake Success, NY.)

25–10) is the need for an assistant to manually retract the tissue. This inconvenience is significant in veterinary surgical procedures, where extra surgical assistants are often not available.

Self-retaining retractors (Fig. 25–11) offer the advantage of maintaining tissue separation once placed without additional assistants. The Finochietto rib retractor for thoracic surgery and the Balfour retractor for abdominal surgery are sturdy and very effective. These self-retaining retractors are necessities if adequate exposure to thoracic and abdominal viscera is to be achieved and maintained. The Gelpi and Weitlaner retractors are two smaller self-retaining retractors that offer versatility in tissue separation and exposure during surgical procedures.

Preventive Maintenance

Periodic evaluation of instrument performance may indicate that preventive maintenance is needed. Instrument manufacturers stress the economics of preventive maintenance programs. Costs for restorations vary but can be as low as one-fifth replacement costs and one-half repair costs. A preventive maintenance program includes evaluating, refurbishing, adjusting, and refinishing each instrument. Carbide inserts are replaced if worn or cracked, tips of instruments are re-aligned, shanks and springs are adjusted for proper

tension and conformation, ratchets and jaws are redefined and reset, cutting edges are sharpened, and all missing parts are replaced. After this complete refurbishing each instrument is ultrasonically cleaned. Preventive maintenance programs for good-quality surgical instruments reduce costs and increase instrument longevity.

1. Hurov, L, et al.: *Handbook of Veterinary Surgical Instruments and Glossary of Surgical Terms*. W. B. Saunders, Philadelphia, 1978.
2. McElmurry, M., and Byrd, D.: Surgical instruments: manufacture and proper care. A.O.R.N. J. 19:5, 1974.
3. Mostafa, A. B., and Chackett, K. F.: Cleaning of surgical instruments: a preliminary assessment. Med. Biol. Eng. 14:524, 1976.
4. Perkins, J. J.: *Principles and Methods of Sterilization in Health Sciences*. Charles C Thomas, Springfield, IL, 1969.
5. Ryan, R.: Basics of packaging. A.O.R.N. J. 21:6, 1975.
6. Speers, R., and Shooter, R. A.: The use of double-wrapped packs to reduce contamination of the sterile contents during extraction. Lancet 2:469, 1966.
7. Standard, P. G., et al.: Microbial penetration of muslin- and paper-wrapped sterile packs stored on open shelves and in closed cabinets. Appl. Microbiol. 22:5, 1971.
8. Standard, P. G., et al.: Microbial penetration through three types of double wrappers for sterile packs. Appl. Microbiol. 26:11, 1973.
9. *The Care and Handling of Surgical Instruments*. Codman and Shurtleff Inc., Randolph, MA, 1981.
10. *The Care and Handling of Surgical Instruments*. Miltex Instrument Co., Lake Success, NY, 1982.

Chapter **26** # Operative Techniques

James P. Toombs and Dennis T. Crowe, Jr.

It is excellence of technique that distinguishes the surgical artist from the mere manipulator.

E. L. Doyen

Nearly all operative procedures, regardless of their degree of complexity, can be reduced to four basic techniques: (1) incision and excision of tissues; (2) maintenance of hemostasis; (3) handling and care of exposed tissues; and (4) use of sutures and knots to restore anatomical structure and support tissues during healing. Countless methods have been employed for the execution of each of these basic techniques. An unabridged review of them is beyond the scope and purpose of this chapter. Instead, major emphasis has been placed on the foundation skills of surgery—efficient and accurate use of basic instruments and methods to minimize the trauma associated with surgical intervention.

INCISION AND EXCISION OF TISSUES

Steel Scalpel

The "sharp scalpel" with disposable steel blades (Fig. 26–1) is the standard soft tissue cutting instrument against which all others are compared. Properly used, it allows the surgeon to divide tissues with the least amount of trauma.[31] Its major advantage is the consistent sharpness of its disposable blades, which are discarded when dull or contaminated. The practice of discarding a blade following use on the skin—"skin knife, deep knife ritual"—has been found to be unnecessary.[22] For application to and removal from

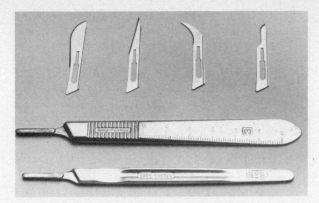

Figure 26–1. Sharp scalpel with disposable steel blades. Bard-Parker blades (from left to right) #10, #11, #12, and #15 are generally applied to either #3 or #9 Bard-Parker handles. The #7 Bard-Parker handle (not shown) is also compatible with these blades.

the scalpel handle, blades should be grasped and manipulated with a needle holder rather than the surgeon's gloved hand.

Three basic grips have been advocated for holding the scalpel: the pencil grip, the fingertip grip, and the palm grip.[1] Each grip has specific advantages and limitations.

The pencil grip (Fig. 26–2A) facilitates steadying of the hand by allowing it to rest on the patient and uses finger rather than arm movement to incise with the scalpel. Fine motor control of the intrinsic muscles of the hand makes this grip particularly advantageous for short, precise incisions.[1] The major disadvantage of this grip, compared with the others, is that the scalpel is held at a greater angle to the tissue, thereby decreasing cutting edge contact. This makes the pencil grip less suitable for long incisions than the other grips. Control of both incision depth and direction for long incisions is directly proportional to cutting edge contact.[1] Changes in cutting pressure distributed over a greater length of blade deliver less pressure to each increment of tissue, thus promoting more consistent control over depth. A greater length of tissue in contact with the blade promotes increased tissue resistance, which counteracts sudden changes in blade direction and depth.

Incisions exceeding 3 cm in length can be more efficiently executed with the fingertip grip (Fig. 26–2B) than with the pencil grip. The fingertip grip utilizes arm motion rather than finger motion to incise tissue and maximizes contact of the cutting edge of the blade with the tissue to be incised.[1] Although the index finger is placed on the upper edge of the blade for stability, it should neither touch the tissue being incised nor obstruct the surgeon's view of the incision.[23] The fingertip grip is applicable to most scalpel cutting.

The palm grip (Fig. 26–2C) provides the strongest grasp of the scalpel and is advantageous when great

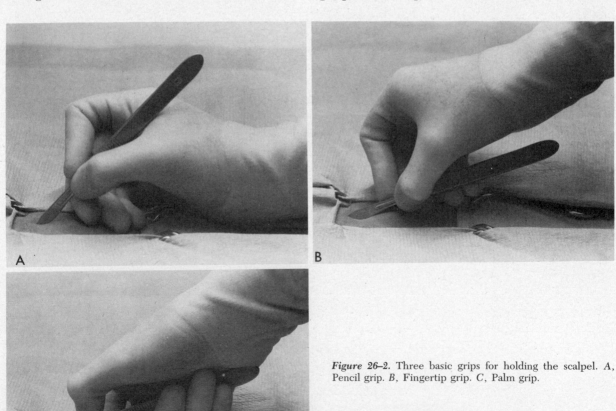

Figure 26–2. Three basic grips for holding the scalpel. A, Pencil grip. B, Fingertip grip. C, Palm grip.

pressure must be applied to incise tissue.[1] This grip is more applicable to other cutting instruments, such as the periosteal elevator, than to the scalpel. As with the fingertip grip, arm motion rather than finger motion is employed to provide incisional force.

Four motions of the cutting edge of the scalpel blade have been described for incising and excising tissues: pressing, sliding, sawing, and scraping.[1] Of these, press cutting and slide cutting are the most

applicable. Press cutting (Fig. 26–3A) utilizes the pencil grip and application of increasing pressure in the same direction as the proposed motion of the blade.[1] A stab incision results when the bursting threshold of the tissue is exceeded. Press cutting is most often used to initiate incisions in hollow, fluid-filled structures such as the urinary bladder. Once the wall has been penetrated, the fluid provides space so that the blade can decelerate without dam-

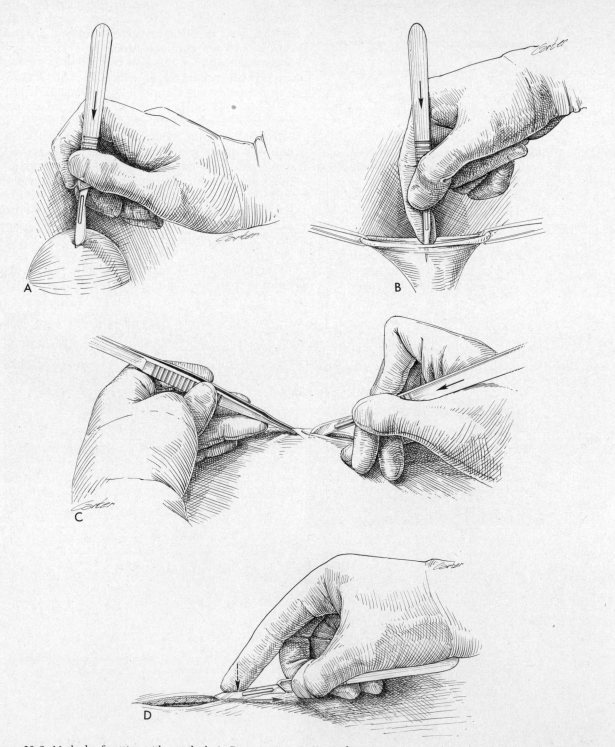

Figure 26–3. Methods of cutting with a scalpel. *A,* Press cutting. *B,* Finger-bumper press cutting. *C,* Inverted blade press cutting. *D,* Slide cutting.

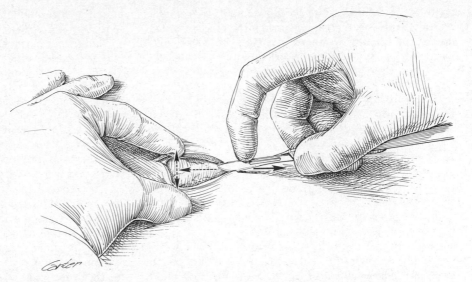

Figure 26–4. Force vectors applied by the surgeon's free hand to increase slide cutting efficiency are indicated by dashed arrows. These include longitudinal tension opposite the blade movement and lateral tension promoting separation of the wound edges.

aging deeper structures. Depth control is poor with press cutting but can be improved by using the index finger as a bumper (Fig. 26–3*B*). This effectively limits penetration of the blade to a predetermined depth. Elevation of the tissue layer to be incised and press cutting with an inverted blade (Fig. 26–3*C*) provide increased safety. This technique has been used to initiate gastrotomy, cystotomy, and ventral midline celiotomy incisions.[49]

Slide cutting (Fig. 26–3*D*) is the safest and most common method of incising tissues with a scalpel. Slide cutting utilizes the pencil grip for short incisions through delicate tissues. The fingertip grip is preferable for long incisions and for tissues requiring greater incisional pressure. The increased safety of slide cutting is attributable to application of pressure at a right angle to the motion of the blade (See Fig. 26–3*D*). This facilitates precise control of incisional depth as the blade is drawn through tissue.

The basic principles of effective slide cutting, which is applicable to most tissues, are best illustrated by a properly executed skin incision. Following identification of landmarks for the incision, the skin should be stretched with the surgeon's free hand as shown in Figure 26–4. Properly done, this exerts longitudinal tension opposite the movement of the blade and lateral tension, promoting separation of the wound edges as the incision is made. These forces immobilize the tissue being incised and allow for increased cutting efficiency and direct visualization of the depth of the blade. As the blade moves farther and farther from the assisting hand, these forces progressively decrease until the depth of the blade can no longer be seen. At this point, slide cutting is suspended until the assisting hand can be repositioned closer to the scalpel. The blade should remain in contact with the tissue throughout, to maintain single stroke action when cutting is resumed. For incisions that run parallel to the long axis of the operating table, slide cutting should progress from left to right for a right-handed surgeon. For incisions that run perpendicular to the long axis of the operating table, cutting should progress toward rather than away from the surgeon's body. The scalpel should be used with the dominant hand.

With precise depth control and accurate blade

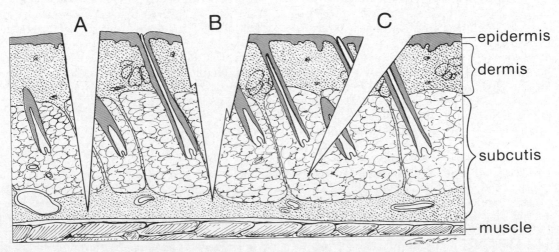

epidermis

dermis

subcutis

muscle

Figure 26–5. Incisions. *A,* Correct method of incising skin and subcutis. *B,* Jagged incision resulting from timid slide cutting. *C,* Bevelled incision resulting from inaccurate attitude of the scalpel blade.

attitude, a single pass of the scalpel completely transects the tissue layer, resulting in minimal trauma and perpendicular wound edges (Fig. 26–5A). Timid slide cutting and short paintbrushlike strokes necessitate multiple passes of the scalpel to completely transect the tissue. This results in greater trauma, jagged wound edges, and increased hemorrhage (Fig. 26–5B). There is a tendency when incising a curved surface to keep the blade perpendicular to the floor rather than to the tissue surface.[1] This produces an inaccurate blade attitude and results in wound margins with bevelled edges (Fig. 26–5C). In summary, effective slide cutting depends on stabilization of the tissue to be incised, precise depth control to facilitate complete incision with a single stroke, and maintenance of blade attitude perpendicular to the tissue surface.

Sawing or push-pull slide cutting uses the pencil grip and allows a short incision to be continued deeper than a single slide cut without removal and re-insertion of the blade into the wound.[1] This type of cutting motion demands tremendous caution because depth control is poor during the pushing phase, jeopardizing structures deep to the tissue being cut.

The fourth type of cutting motion with the scalpel is scraping and is analogous to shaving whiskers with a razor. It is most effectively accomplished by holding the scalpel with the fingertip grip to maximize blade contact. Sub-bursting pressure is applied to the tissue layer beneath the blade while moving the blade perpendicular to its cutting edge.[1] Accuracy of tissue layer separation without the risk of cutting or "buttonholing" deeper tissue layers is the major advantage of scraping. The scraping motion is useful for developing subcutaneous or fascial pouches for prosthetic devices such as cardiac pacemakers, for subperiosteal elevation of muscles, and for separation of pleural, pericardial, and peritoneal adhesions.[1]

High-Energy Scalpels

Electrosurgical, CO_2 laser, and argon plasma generator scalpels are the high-energy cutting instruments currently in clinical use.[18] Although their energy sources differ, the basic cutting mechanism is similar for all three.[19,26,44] Energy is focally transmitted to the tissue, depending on its water content. This results in vaporization of cells along the line of incision, a variable degree of thermal necrosis of the wound edges, and a so-called bloodless incision.

Advantages reported for these incisional methods over the steel scalpel include (1) reduction of total blood loss,[26] (2) decreased necessity for ligatures, reducing the amount of foreign material left in the wound,[19] and (3) reduction of operating time.[18] These advantages are acquired at the expense of a variable degree of thermal necrosis of the wound margins,[17,26,28] delayed wound healing,[24,26,28] and decreased resistance of wounds to infection.[26,28] These undesirable effects are least evident with the CO_2

laser,[17,46] intermediate with the electroscalpel,[26] and most pronounced with the argon plasma scalpel.[26]

The proper cutting technique with hand-held high-energy scalpels differs markedly from that described for the steel scalpel. The pencil grip should be used to hold the instrument nearly perpendicular to the tissue surface to minimize the energy contact area at the point of incision.[23] The instrument should be moved rapidly across the tissue so that no more than one tissue plane is transected with a single pass. This is important, because depth control with these instruments is generally less precise than with the steel scalpel. Use of the lowest energy setting capable of producing the incision is recommended. This improves depth control and reduces the amount of thermal necrosis in the incision. High-energy scalpel cutting is often contraindicated in the presence of cyclopropane, ether, alcohol, and certain bowel gases owing to the risks of fire and explosion.

High-energy cutting in small animal surgery is most often accomplished with electrosurgical instrumentation. Electrosurgery utilizes radiofrequency current to produce one or more of the following effects: incision, coagulation, dessication, or fulguration of tissues. The predominant effect depends on the wave form of the current.[19] Continuous undamped sine waves provide maximal cutting and minimal coagulation. Conversely, interrupted damped sine waves maximize coagulation and minimize cutting capability. "Blended function" (simultaneous coagulation and cutting) is accomplished with modulated, pulsed sine waves. The magnitude of the selected effect is directly proportional to the duration and power (wattage) of the applied current.[19] Frequent cleaning of the tip (active electrode) of the electroscalpel is necessary for optimal function. The accumulated charred material on the tip acts as an insulator. This results in the following undesirable effects: (1) higher power is required to incise tissues, (2) current is dispersed to a larger area of tissue, thus diminishing control, and (3) thermal necrosis of the wound margins is increased.[1]

Further discussion of CO_2 laser and argon plasma scalpel use is beyond the scope of this chapter. For additional information pertaining to these techniques, the reader is referred to other sources.[18,26,44] Similarly, for a more complete discussion of electrosurgical principles and instrumentation, the reader is encouraged to review these important aspects in other sources.[1,19,32,42]

Scissors

Dissecting scissors are available in numerous lengths, shapes, and weights. They are classified according to the type of tips (blunt versus sharp), the shape of the blades (straight versus curved), and the type of cutting edge (plain versus serrated).[23] Three types of scissors generally required for most operative procedures are shown in Figure 26–6. Metzenbaum

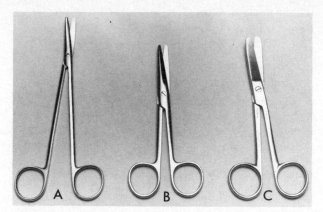

Figure 26–6. Commonly used surgical scissors. *A,* Metzenbaum scissors. *B,* Mayo scissors. *C,* General purpose scissors with blunt tips.

scissors are recommended for blunt dissection and for sharp dissection of delicate tissues. The heavier blades of Mayo scissors are better suited to sharp dissection of dense tissue layers. To avoid dulling of the blades, tissue dissecting scissors should not be used to cut sutures. General purpose scissors with blunt tips are recommended for cutting sutures.

Next to the steel scalpel, dissecting scissors are the most commonly used instruments for dividing tis-

sues.[31] Whereas the scalpel is better suited for cutting dense tissues and those that can be held under tension, scissors are best suited for flaccid tissues.[1] Properly used, scissors stabilize flaccid tissues between the blades during cutting and provide excellent control over both depth and direction of incision.

Efficient scissor cutting depends on three forces: (1) closing force, which causes the blades to come together; (2) shearing force, which pushes one blade flat against the other during closing; and (3) torque, which rolls the leading edge of each blade inward to touch the other.[1] The grip that best utilizes scissor design to maximize these forces is the wide base tripod grip (Fig. 26–7A), in which the tips of the right thumb and ring finger are placed through the rings to grasp the scissors and the right index finger is placed on the shanks near the fulcrum for support.[1,23,31] The thenar eminence–ring finger grip (Fig. 26–7B), preferred by some surgeons, provides adequate shearing force, reduced closing force, and practically no torque compared with that of the wide base tripod grip.[1]

Right-handed cutting and a wide base tripod grip are recommended for the majority of operative situations requiring scissor dissection. As most dissecting scissors are designed for the right hand, left-handed surgeons should either learn to cut with the right

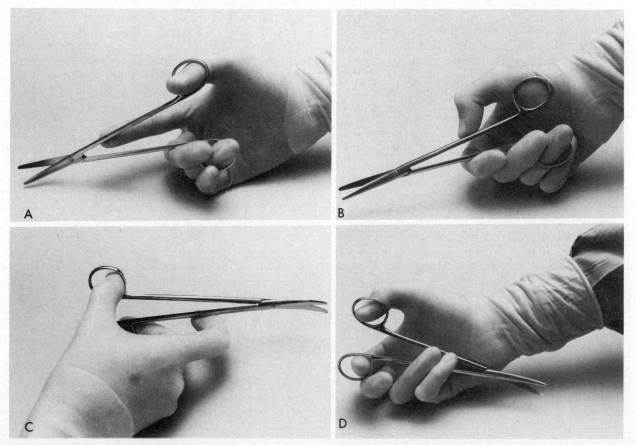

Figure 26–7. Methods of gripping dissection scissors. *A,* Wide base tripod grip. *B,* Thenar eminence–ringfinger grip. *C,* Backhand thumb–ringfinger grip. *D,* Backhand thumb–index finger grip.

hand or obtain scissors specifically designed for the left hand.[1] Alternatives to the wide base tripod grip are recommended only for the following situations: (1) when the surgeon must execute a scissor cut proceeding toward his dominant side (from left to right for a right-handed surgeon), a backhand variation of the thumb–ring finger grip (Fig. 26–7C) is more efficient; and (2) when the surgeon must perform a reverse cut across the table toward his body, a backhand thumb–index finger grip (Fig. 26–7D) is less awkward, provides better direction control, and is more efficient.

Scissor cutting, push cutting, and blunt dissection are the three basic methods of incising and excising tissues with scissors. The first two methods constitute sharp dissection and are properly executed using the cutting edges only near the tips of the scissor blades.[23,31] When scissors are opened too widely, tissues engage the blades closer to the fulcrum, where cutting forces are greatly attenuated. Attempting to cut tissues with this portion of the blades results in crushing injury to the tissue and ragged incisions.[1]

Scissor cutting is most applicable to short incisions. In order to avoid a ragged incision with this technique, only the tips are used for cutting and the blades are nearly, but not completely, closed as the scissors are advanced through the tissue with a series of consecutive short cuts.[23] Long incisions are often initiated with a scissor cut and continued by pushing the nearly closed scissor blades forward to cut the tissue in one continuous motion. This technique, termed *push cutting*, is especially useful for incising sheets of tissue such as pleura, peritoneum, pericardium, and light fascia.[1] Denser tissues such as the walls of hollow organs, tendons, muscles, and skin can be more atraumatically divided with scissor cuts or scalpel incisions. Straight scissors provide a greater mechanical advantage than curved scissors and thus are recommended for scissor cuts through dense tissue. Curved scissors offer the advantages of increased mobility and visibility and are preferred for scissor dissection in deep wounds and body cavities. Scissors with sharp tips are generally not recommended for deep dissection.

Scissors with blunt tips are preferable to other instruments for blunt dissection. Alternating sharp and blunt dissection can then be conducted with maximum control and without changing instruments.[1] Blunt dissection is accomplished by inserting the closed scissor blades between the tissue layers to be separated and opening the handles to spread the blades. Scissors are then withdrawn from the wound prior to closing the blades, thus preventing inadvertent transection of vital structures within the deeper portions of the wound. The closed blades are then re-inserted into the wound to continue further blunt dissection.

Blunt dissection is generally reserved for separating anatomical structures, such as muscle bellies, that are loosely bound together by a tissue of lesser tensile strength, such as areolar tissue or fat.[1] Blunt dissection is especially useful for exposure of structures such as major blood vessels and nerves when sharp dissection might place these structures in jeopardy. It is not recommended where old scars traverse normal dissection planes or where the tissue to be divided has greater tensile strength than the tissues it binds.[1] Sharp dissection is preferable in these situations, as it is more accurate and less traumatic.

ALTERNATIVES TO CONVENTIONAL METHODS OF EXCISION

Excision—the cutting of tissues to effect their removal for therapeutic or diagnostic purposes—is generally accomplished by dissection with scalpel and scissors. Alternative cutting methods, such as water beam dissection[33] and electrosurgery,[19,32,42] are sometimes preferable when hemostasis is difficult to obtain following conventional methods of excision. One such example involves hepatic surgery. Intralobar partial hepatectomy often results in persistent hemorrhage due to marked vascularity and friability of the tissue involved. Water beam dissection of the liver, i.e., the use of a high-pressure jet of saline solution to wash away parenchymal cells while preserving the integrity of regional ducts and blood vessels, has been found to reduce both operative time and total blood loss compared with sharp excision and finger fracture techniques.[33] Effective hemostasis can be equally difficult to obtain when access to the operative site is limited, such as in oropharyngeal surgery. For this reason, some surgeons prefer electrosurgical instruments to scalpel and scissors for the excision of tonsils or redundant portions of the soft palate.[33,42]

Electrosurgical[33,42] and cryosurgical[5,50] destruction of abnormal tissues has been used instead of or as a supplement to standard surgical excision. Appropriate biopsy procedures to confirm the diagnosis are a prerequisite to use of these methods. Electrosurgical treatment uses damped radiofrequency current to coagulate, desiccate, or fulgurate tissue, dependent upon the physical method of application. Coagulation is produced by brief passage of the current directly through the tissue. Electrodesiccation and fulguration are achieved by passage of a spark from the active electrode to the tissue. Desiccation occurs when the spark is generated within the tissue or with a gap of less than 1 mm. Fulguration occurs when the spark gap equals or exceeds 1 mm. Electrosurgical destruction of tissue has been used in the treatment of small benign growths of the skin, urinary bladder, and mucous membranes of the oral cavity and vagina.[23,32,42] Additionally, electrodesiccation and fulguration have been used to destroy remaining neoplastic or infected cells in excisional tissue beds.

Cryosurgical treatment utilizes either direct or indirect application of refrigerants such as nitrous oxide and liquid nitrogen to freeze abnormal tissues, thus destroying them. Rapid freezing to minus 60°C or lower, slow unassisted thawing, and a minimum of two freeze-thaw cycles are recommended to obtain maximal cryonecrosis.[5] Cryosurgery has been used in the treatment of perianal fistulae, lick granuloma, and certain tumors involving the skin, nasal cavity, oropharynx, rectum, and prostate.[50] The reader is referred to the oncology section of this text and other sources[5,7,31,43,50,51] for more specific information regarding the types of tumors that are amenable to cryosurgical therapy.

The potential advantages of cryosurgery over sharp excision include the following: (1) primary hemorrhage is greatly reduced; (2) freezing of tissues is associated with an analgesic effect, which minimizes the need for general anesthesia; (3) regional destruction of sensory nerve endings decreases postoperative pain; (4) abnormal tissue can be destroyed without sacrificing major vascular structures that are inseparable from the lesion; and (5) the incidence of strictures and exuberant granulation tissue is reduced for lesions in which resection precludes closure of the wound. The major disadvantages of cryosurgery are (1) imprecise control of tissue destruction, (2) sloughing of necrotic tissue for up to three weeks following the procedure, which may stress the ability of the owner to cope with the appearance and odor of the wound, and (3) tissue sloughing, which sometimes results in severe secondary hemorrhage.

All of the methods discussed as alternatives or supplements to standard excision offer the potential advantages of reduced trauma, hemorrhage, and operative time for certain procedures. Each of these techniques also has the potential to inflict extensive trauma to surrounding normal tissues, thus negating any advantage over sharp excision. The reader is strongly encouraged to review other sources[5,19,32,33,37,42] for a more complete discussion of important technical details pertaining to each of these methods.

HEMORRHAGE AND HEMOSTASIS

General Considerations

Hemostasis is a spontaneous physiological defense mechanism to arrest hemorrhage. It depends upon vascular, extravascular, and intravascular factors acting in concert to initiate effective thrombus formation at the bleeding site (Fig. 26–8). Various surgical methods (Fig. 26–9) are used to augment, facilitate, or obviate the physiological clotting mechanism to reduce blood loss and the attendant complications.

The contribution of effective hemostasis to successful surgical results cannot be overemphasized. Hemostasis is important because (1) bleeding obscures the surgical field, thereby reducing operative accuracy and efficiency; (2) blood on the field, gloves, instruments, and drapes provides an ideal medium for bacterial growth and increases the likelihood of surgical wound infection; (3) postoperative hemorrhage prevents proper coaptation of wound edges, delays healing, and encourages infection; and (4) severe or protracted hemorrhage may result in shock, progressive hypoxemia, and death of the patient.

Primary hemorrhage, i.e., that which occurs immediately following traumatic disruption of blood vessels,[2] is a predictable consequence of even the most skilled surgical dissection. Its quantity, however, is often inversely proportional to the technical and anticipatory skills of the surgeon. The experienced surgeon practices "preventive hemostasis" through careful planning of approaches and gentle, accurate dissection to minimize primary hemorrhage.

Delayed hemorrhage, termed _intermediate_ if it occurs within 24 hours of injury and _secondary_ if it occurs thereafter,[2] is often the result of inappropriate or ineffective treatment of primary hemorrhage. Slipped ligatures and necrosis or suppuration of ligated or cauterized vessels are common causes of delayed hemorrhage. Additionally, intraoperative hy-

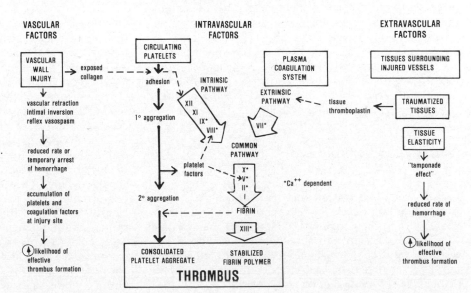

Figure 26–8. Physiological hemostasis.

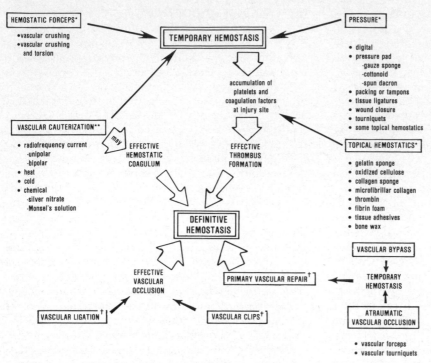

Figure 26–9. Surgical methods of hemostasis.

potension may prevent detection of vascular injury or ineffective hemostatic technique. Restoration of normal blood pressure is accompanied by delayed hemorrhage.

A "dry" surgical field and absence of delayed hemorrhage are the results of effective and atraumatic treatment of primary hemorrhage. A blind or frenzied attempt to clamp off a bleeding point—the hysterical approach to hemostasis—often results in further laceration of the vessel, increased hemorrhage, and damage to surrounding structures. Placing a finger on the point of hemorrhage and applying gentle pressure is an extremely effective method of temporary hemostasis, even for major arteries. Temporary arrest of hemorrhage then allows the surgeon to improve visibility in the field through suction, lavage, and light adjustment. If exposure is inadequate, the incision is enlarged or tissue retraction is modified to provide accurate identification and definitive treatment of the source of hemorrhage.

Pressure Pad Hemostasis

Control of low-pressure hemorrhage from small vessels can often be obtained by applying pressure to the bleeding points for several minutes with gauze sponges or similar material.[30] Hemorrhage following the incision of skin and subcutaneous tissues is frequently treated in this manner. Tissues should be gently compressed or blotted with the pressure pad rather than wiped; wiping abrades tissues and dis-

lodges blood clots that have formed. The success of this method depends upon the maintenance of pressure long enough for effective thrombus formation to occur, followed by careful removal of the pressure pad to avoid disruption of blood clots. Properly used, this method is atraumatic and leaves no foreign material in the wound. Its use on larger vessels should be considered as temporary rather than definitive treatment.

Hemostatic Forceps

When bleeding vessels are to be sacrificed rather than repaired, they can be clamped with hemostatic forceps. A wide variety of lengths, shapes, and types are available, including Halsted mosquito and Kelly forceps for small vessels and Crile, Oschner, and Carmault forceps for large tissue bundles and vessels (Fig. 26–10). In contrast to the relatively atraumatic occlusion of vessels provided by vascular forceps, hemostatic forceps crush tissue at the point of application. Each is equipped with a ratchet so that the hemostat may be applied and left in position. This occludes blood vessels, thus temporarily arresting hemorrhage, and damages the vascular wall sufficiently to activate the physiological clotting mechanism. Definitive hemostasis with vascular crushing or vascular crushing and torsion[2] is limited to small, low-pressure bleeders and requires adequate clamping time for thrombus formation to occur. For larger vessels, hemostats are applied to obtain temporary

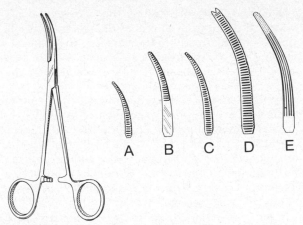

Figure 26–10. General design and comparative jaw serration patterns of commonly used hemostatic forceps. *A*, Halsted mosquito forceps. *B*, Kelly forceps. *C*, Crile forceps. *D*, Oschner forceps. *E*, Carmault forceps.

hemostasis, facilitating ligation or cauterization of the vessel.

Technical aspects of applying hemostatic forceps are summarized in the following guidelines:

1. The smallest hemostat capable of accomplishing hemostasis should be selected.

2. Curved hemostats facilitate improved visibility and are generally preferred to straight hemostats.

3. For greatest accuracy of application, a single hemostat should be grasped with the dominant hand using the wide base tripod grip (Fig. 26–11A).

4. For noncritical situations when many hemostats are being applied in succession, time can be saved by carrying multiple hemostats with the ring finger and palm (Fig. 26–11D) when a surgical assistant is not available.

5. For occluding small superficial bleeders:
   a. the tip of the hemostat should be pointed toward the vessel such that the instrument is held perpendicular to the bleeding surface during application,
   b. the tip rather than the jaw of the forceps should be used to grasp the smallest amount of tissue possible, preferably only the bleeding vessel itself (Fig. 26–11B), and
   c. forceps should be applied so that they fall lateral to the incision with the concave aspect of the curved tip facing down.

6. For occluding *deep bleeders*, *large isolated vessels*, and *vascular pedicles*:
   a. hemostatic forceps should be applied perpendicular to the vessel with the concave surface of the tip facing the transected end or proposed line of vascular transection to facilitate ligation (Fig. 26–11C),
   b. the jaw rather than the tip of the forceps should be used to grasp the vessel for greater security (See Fig. 26–11C), and
   c. large pedicles should be clamped with Carmault or a similar type of forceps to reduce slippage or laceration of the pedicle.

Cautery

Vascular cauterization can be used to obtain definitive hemostasis for arteries up to 1 mm and veins up to 2 mm. It is most often accomplished with highly damped radiofrequency current from an electrocautery unit (Fig. 26–12). Technical aspects vary depending on whether a monopolar or bipolar mode

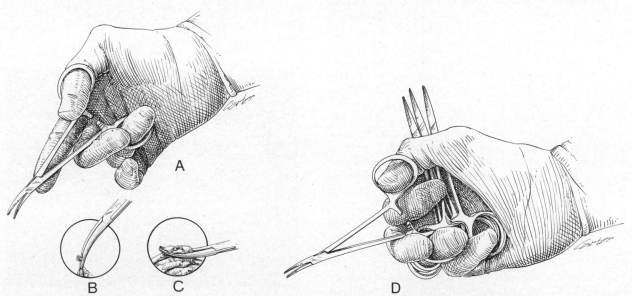

Figure 26–11. Handling and application of hemostatic forceps. *A*, Wide base tripod grip. *B*, Tip clamping method. *C*, Jaw clamping method. *D*, Method for carrying multiple hemostats.

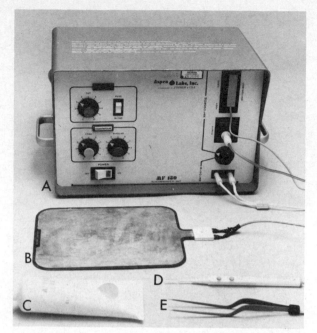

Figure 26–12. Basic electrosurgical instrumentation. A, Electrocautery unit with monopolar and bipolar modes of coagulation; B, patient ground plate; C, electrosurgical conduction gel; D, Monopolar handpiece; E, bipolar electrode forceps.

of coagulation is used. Monopolar coagulation, the more commonly used mode, involves flow of current from the handpiece (active electrode) through the patient's body to a ground plate. Bipolar electrodes, in contrast, are usually in the form of bayonet thumb forceps. When the tips are held about 1 mm apart, current passes from one tip through the tissue to the opposite tip, thus eliminating the need for a patient ground plate. The effectiveness of bipolar coagulation depends on two special requirements. For current to be effectively conducted, there must be continuity of electrolyte fluid (water, electrolytes, and tissue) between the electrode tips.[1] Also, a slight gap must be maintained between the tips as they grasp the tissue to be coagulated. If tissue is grasped so that the tips touch one another, the current short circuits without generating adequate heat for tissue coagulation. Advantages of bipolar over monopolar coagulation include (1) less current required for a similar coagulative effect,[10,23,47] (2) the risk of unintentional injury to surrounding tissues is greatly decreased and alternate pathway burns of distant tissues are precluded, as current passes through a much smaller volume of tissue,[47] and (3) effective coagulation can be obtained in a wet surgical field.[1,10,47] Bipolar cautery is most frequently used in plastic and neurosurgical procedures where precise coagulation of small vessels is required.

The major advantage of monopolar electrocautery is its ability to cut and coagulate tissues. In contrast, bipolar cautery is capable of coagulation only. Effective monopolar coagulation depends on a dry surgical

field immediately surrounding the vessel to be cauterized. Current from the tip of the electrode can be applied either directly to the vessel or to a hemostat grasping the vessel to achieve coagulation. In both methods, neither the active electrode nor the hemostat should contact the tissues except at the point where coagulation is desired. Holding the hemostat or the active electrode perpendicular to the wound during coagulation greatly decreases the likelihood of injury to surrounding tissues. Regardless of whether the monopolar or bipolar mode of coagulation is used, the minimum intensity and duration of current capable of producing hemostasis should be selected to minimize tissue trauma.

In summary, the advantages of electrosurgical coagulation over other methods of hemostasis are decreased operative time and economy of blood loss. Properly employed, this method provides definitive hemostasis without significant deterence to wound healing. Hemostatic security, although often sufficient, is lower for cauterized vessels than for those that have been ligated. Improper use of electrocautery has been associated with increased frequency of secondary hemorrhage, severe patient burns, delayed wound healing, increased rates of wound infection, and operating room fires and explosions.[1]

Alternative methods of cauterizing vessels include the direct application of heat, cold, or certain chemicals. Disposable, battery-powered cautery units with a heated filament (Fig. 26–13) provide precise and effective coagulation of extremely small vessels and are useful in certain ophthalmic and neurological surgical procedures. The use of cryoprobes can also be considered a form of cautery in that destruction of tissue by freezing is often associated with excellent hemostasis. Additionally, styptics such as silver nitrate and ferric subsulfate have an astringent action on tissues capable of producing hemostasis. Owing to the escharotic action of these substances, they must be used judiciously and only on superficial areas.

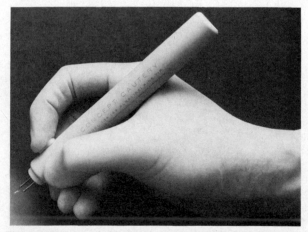

Figure 26–13. Disposable (AA battery–powered) thermal cautery unit. Resterilization with ethylene oxide gas permits repeated use of these cautery units.

CORRECT   INCORRECT

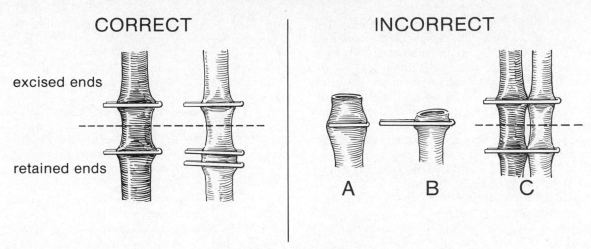

excised ends

retained ends

A   B   C

Figure 26–14. Vascular clip application.

Vascular Clips and Ligatures

The most secure method of hemostasis for severed vessels that do not require primary repair is the application of ligatures or vascular clips. Slippage of properly placed clips and ligatures is much less likely than dislodgement of the hemostatic coagulum, upon which other methods depend. The major disadvantage of clips or ligatures is the foreign material left in the wound.

Vascular clips are usually bent pieces of metal (silver, tantalum, or stainless steel) that can be easily and rapidly applied to vessels using an applicator similar in design to a needleholder. Clips and applicators are available in various lengths suitable for effectively occluding vessels up to approximately 5 mm in diameter. The basic principles of vascular clip application are summarized in Figure 26–14. Metal vascular clips offer the following advantages over ligatures: (1) clips can be applied much more rapidly than ligatures; and (2) clips can be easily and securely placed in locations inaccessible to ligation. Disadvantages associated with metal vascular clips include the following: (1) vascular clips are more frequently dislodged by continuing surgical manipulations than are ligatures[40]; (2) they persist in the wound as foreign bodies; and (3) their presence occasionally interferes with subsequent radiographic studies.[29] These problems have, to a great extent, been overcome by the recent introduction of absorbable ligating clips of polydioxanone.[40]

Ligation, the use of suture material and surgical knots to effectively occlude blood vessels, is the most commonly used surgical hemostatic method. Ligatures offer increased security over hemostatic clips and are better suited for the occlusion of multiple vessels and vascular tissue pedicles. The major disadvantage of ligatures, compared with other hemostatic methods, is the increased application time. For noncritical vessels other hemostatic methods are often employed to save time. For larger vessels, definitive hemostasis is of prime importance and the increased security provided by ligatures more than compensates for the time spent on their proper application.

Suture materials frequently used for ligation include chromic surgical gut, silk, cotton, and synthetic absorbable sutures such as polyglactin and polydioxanone.[14] The choice of suture material is often determined by individual preferences of the surgeon.

Different kinds of surgical knots are illustrated in Figure 26–15. As a general rule, ligatures should be tied with square knots, as these are least likely to loosen or untie. The simple knot, referred to in some texts as a half-hitch, is the basic component of three different types of knots. Depending on how they are thrown, two consecutive simple knots can result in a square knot, a granny knot, or a half-hitch knot. Square knots are produced by reversing direction on each successive simple knot and maintaining even tension on both strands parallel to the plane of the knot as each throw is tightened. Failure to reverse direction on successive throws results in a granny knot. Failure to maintain even tension on both strands or applying upward tension on the strands (pulling the strands away from the plane of the knot) often results in a half-hitch knot. Granny and half-

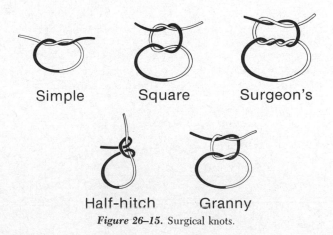

Simple   Square   Surgeon's

Half-hitch   Granny

Figure 26–15. Surgical knots.

hitch knots are not generally recommended, as both are subject to slippage. This characteristic can occasionally be used to the surgeon's advantage, however. These knots are sometimes intentionally applied and tightened to overcome tissue tension when placing deep ligatures. When this is done, the knot should be covered with several square knots to prevent loosening.

A surgeon's knot is similar to a square knot except that one strand is passed through the loop twice on the first throw. This additional twist of the suture around itself produces increased suture friction. This can be used to advantage for ligation of vascular pedicles with synthetic sutures when tissue tension precludes adequate tightening of the first throw of a square knot. This is especially helpful when tying with polyglactin or a similar material. A surgeon's knot is not recommended when using surgical gut, as increased friction tends to fray the material at the knot, thus substantially weakening it. The increased bulk and asymmetry of the surgeon's knot make it less suitable for general ligation purposes than the square knot. Additionally, its knot security is often less than satisfactory unless covered by a square knot.

Basic methods of tying knots include one hand,

two hand, and instrument ties. Numerous variations have been described for each of these methods. Step-by-step illustrated instructions for various knot tying techniques have been amply presented in other sources, which the reader is encouraged to review.[1,14,23,31,34,52] The two-hand tying method offers the following advantages: (1) it is the most reliable technique for consistently producing square knots, and (2) it enables the surgeon to maintain continuous tension on the knot throughout the entire process of tying, thus decreasing the chance that the first throw will loosen before the second is thrown. Disadvantages of the two-hand tie include the following: (1) it is the most time-consuming method of producing a knot,[52] and (2) it is awkward for deep ligatures, as it requires more working room than other techniques. In contrast, the one-hand tie promotes rapid tying, allows the surgeon to carry an instrument in one hand, and is more adaptable to application of deep ligatures. One-hand ties are, however, more susceptible to loosening of the first throw and inadvertent conversion to half-hitch knots. Instrument ties promote economy of suture material and are a reliable method of producing square knots. Additionally, they are perhaps best for application of deep ligatures.

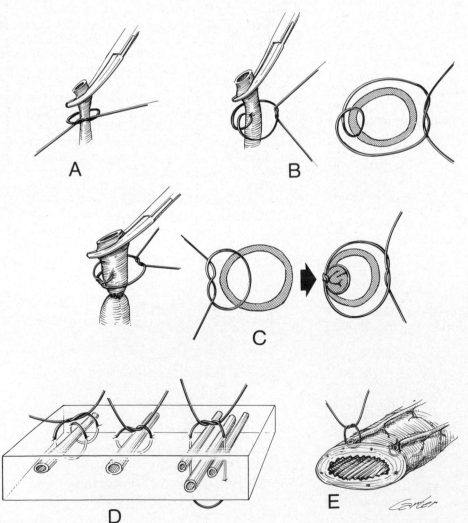

Figure 26–16. Different ligatures and ligation techniques. *A,* Simple ligature. *B,* Halsted transfixation ligature. *C,* Modified transfixation ligature. *D,* Tissue ligatures (from left to right): cruciate, simple, and mattress. *E,* Stick ties.

Complete tightening of each throw is somewhat less consistent with instrument ties, as the surgeon receives less tactile feedback than with hand ties. Each of the three basic knot tying methods provides specific advantages, making it the technique of choice for certain types of ligatures. Mastery of all these methods enables the surgeon to apply secure ligatures in a wide variety of operative situations.

Different types of ligatures and techniques that facilitate ligation are summarized in Figures 26–16 and 26–17. Many isolated vessels and small vascular pedicles can be effectively occluded with simple ligatures (Fig. 26–16A). Following its application, the hemostat is initially elevated away from the tissue to facilitate ligature passage around the clamped vessel. The hemostat is lowered parallel to the tissue and rotated so that the curved tip points up, and the ligature is effectively trapped beneath the clamp. The

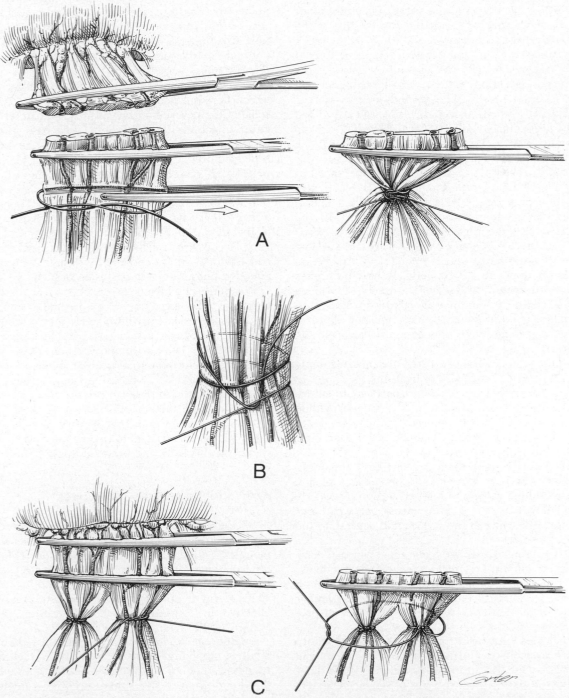

Figure 26–17. Methods of ligating vascular pedicles. A, Three forceps method. B, Modified Miller's knot. C, "Divide and conquer" method.

hemostat is gently released as final tightening of the first throw is completed. Square knots and a minimum of three throws are generally recommended. The completed ligature should lie at least several millimeters away from the cut end of the vessels to prevent slippage.

Large isolated vessels, especially arteries, should be doubly ligated. Interposition of a transfixation ligature between a simple ligature and the cut end of the vessel provides increased security over two simple ligatures. The original transfixation suture proposed by Halsted[20] is shown in Figure 26–16B. This method depends on fine suture material (4-0 or smaller), a swagged taper needle, and twisting of the vessel to prevent hemorrhage at the points where the vascular wall is penetrated. A more recent method[31] (Fig. 26–16C) utilizes double ligation and a modified transfixation ligature, which enables use of larger suture material. The second method can be easily adapted for vascular pedicles as well as isolated vessels. Bleeding vessels that are difficult to isolate can often be occluded with tissue ligatures or "stick ties" as shown in Figure 26–16D and E.

Methods of ligating vascular pedicles are shown in Figure 26–17. The "three forceps" method facilitates application of a simple ligature to a crushed line of tissue on a vascular pedicle (Fig. 26–17A). If the pedicle is too large, this method often fails to effectively occlude the contained vasculature and variable degree of hemorrhage ensues following transection and clamp removal. Large pedicles can sometimes be more effectively ligated with a modified Miller's knot (Fig. 26–17B). Another alternative involves subdivision of the pedicle with as many separate ligatures as necessary to promote effective vascular occlusion (Fig. 26–17C).

The following general principles of knot tying apply to all sutures but especially to ligatures.

1. Knot security is inversely proportional to suture diameter, thus the smallest suture material providing adequate strength should be used.[23] Sutures no larger than 3-0 for isolated vessels and no larger than 0 for tissue pedicles are recommended.

2. Inadequate tightening of each throw results in a bulkier and less secure knot. Adequate tension must be applied evenly to both strands in a carefully controlled manner to produce secure square knots and to avoid cutting of the tissues and damage to the suture material.

3. To minimize foreign body reaction, the completed knot should be small with the ends cut short, about 3 mm long for silk and synthetic sutures and 6 mm long for surgical gut.[14] Gut must be cut longer because of its tendency to swell in tissues can promote loosening of the knot.

4. Inclusion of a frayed portion of material within a suture weakens it substantially. To prevent fraying and twisting of the suture material, carry the knot down to the tissues with the tips of the index fingers and lay the strands flat by drawing them in opposite directions. Needle holders or hemostats should never

be placed on a portion of the suture that is to remain *in situ*, especially the knot.

5. Extra knots should be avoided, as they result in unnecessary suture bulk. Apply only the minimum number of throws necessary to produce a secure knot.

Primary Vascular Repair

Injuries to critical vascular structures, transplantation of organs, and many cardiovascular surgical procedures require specific hemostatic techniques that enable primary vascular repair. When successfully executed, primary vascular repair is the ideal method of hemostasis because it maintains rather than sacrifices vessels.

Primary vascular repair depends on effective regional hemostasis obtained by routine methods and reliable temporary hemostasis at the repair site. The latter is achieved using one of two basic methods depending on the anatomical site and the working time required. Procedures such as anastomosis of peripheral vessels can often be accomplished by applying atraumatic vascular occlusion using vascular tourniquets or special vascular forceps. Hemostatic forceps should never be used for this purpose because of the trauma they inflict on the vascular wall. Vascular forceps are available in numerous types, shapes, and lengths. All are specifically designed to provide effective but atraumatic occlusion of blood vessels.

Procedures involving the heart or great vessels are often of sufficient duration to preclude continuous vascular occlusion. In these cases intermittent vascular occlusion or vascular bypass techniques are employed to maintain temporary hemostasis. Heart lung bypass, intraluminal vascular bypass,[33] and extraluminal vascular[38] bypass techniques have been used successfully to perform primary vascular repairs in the dog. For further information on these special aspects of hemostasis and on primary vascular repair, the reader is encouraged to review the cardiovascular section of this book and other sources.[8,9,15,25,38,39]

Additional Hemostatic Techniques

Occasionally the surgeon is confronted with diffuse low-pressure hemorrhage that is not amenable to hemostatic methods previously discussed. The use of topical hemostatic agents, such as gelatin sponge, oxidized cellulose, microfibrillar collagen, or collagen sponge, in combination with applied pressure is effective in controlling hemorrhage from the cut surfaces of the liver and spleen.[6,11,12,21]

Another means of controlling diffuse hemorrhage involves applying pressure by various techniques. Bleeding from cut bone surfaces, sometimes encountered in decompressive spinal surgeries, can often be controlled by gently pressing small amounts of bone wax into the cancellous bone at hemorrhage points.

Umbilical tape wound packing in the nasal cavity and gauze tampons in the vaginal region have been used to reduce postoperative hemorrhage from these areas. Wound closure and external pressure bandages are additional examples of limiting hemorrhage by pressure.

HANDLING AND CARE OF TISSUES

General Considerations

Surgical manipulation of tissues by hands and instruments produces varying degrees of tissue trauma. Successful surgical results depend on keeping such injury to an absolute minimum. Inadequate incision length, poor exposure, excessive retraction, blunt dissecting instruments, failure to use normal cleavage planes in dissection, excessive undermining or blunt dissection, and unnecessary or improper handling of tissues often result in an unacceptable amount of surgical trauma. Gentle manipulation of tissues and proper respect for their blood supply, innervation, and hydration are prerequisites to "atraumatic" surgical technique. The simple gesture of washing residual talc off of one's gloves prior to entering the wound indicates a proper and necessary respect for tissues. Failure to maintain this attitude throughout the entire procedure precludes optimal results.

Tissue Forceps

The most frequently used instrument for manipulating tissues is the tissue forceps. This is a nonlocking instrument available with smooth grasping surfaces or various tooth patterns. Three of the more commonly used types of tissue forceps are shown in Figure 26–18A. Skin and other dense tissues can be adequately manipulated with any of these three. Smooth-tipped tissue forceps or DeBakey vascular tissue forceps are recommended for handling viscera and other delicate tissues.

Tissue forceps are usually held in the surgeon's nondominant hand. When in use, they should be grasped with a pencil grip (Fig. 26–18B). When temporarily not in use, tissue forceps may be carried in the palmed position, leaving the surgeon's thumb, index finger, and middle finger free to perform ties or other manipulations (Fig. 26–18C). Tissue forceps are used to stabilize tissues for incision or suturing, to retract tissues for exposure or excision, and to grasp vessels for electrocauterization. Additionally, they may be used to pass ligatures, extract needles, pack sponges, and clear blood with cotton or small sponges of a similar material. When using tissue forceps, the surgeon should grasp the minimum amount of tissue necessary to produce a secure hold, complete the intended maneuver, and release the tissue. Grasping too much tissue or repeated regrasp-

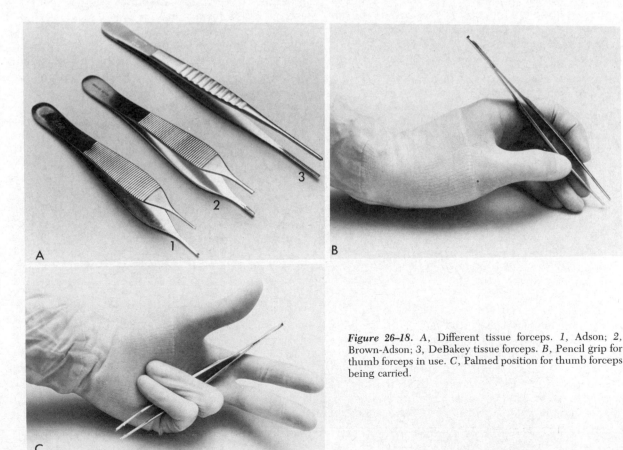

Figure 26–18. *A,* Different tissue forceps. *1,* Adson; *2,* Brown-Adson; *3,* DeBakey tissue forceps. *B,* Pencil grip for thumb forceps in use. *C,* Palmed position for thumb forceps being carried.

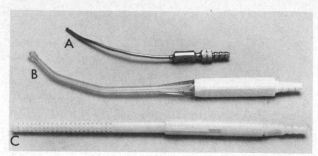

Figure 26–19. Commonly used suction tips. *A*, Frazier tip; *B*, Yankauer tip; *C*, Pool tip.

ing of the tissue produces unnecessary trauma and should be avoided. Further technical details on using tissue forceps in combination with a needle holder will be covered in the wound closure section of this chapter.

Stabilization and Retraction of Tissues

Numerous varieties of forceps with box locks are available for stabilizing tissues or occluding hollow organs during surgery. Commonly used types include Allis and Babcock tissue forceps, Rochester-Carmalt hysterectomy forceps, and Doyen intestinal forceps. These instruments may be applied with impunity to tissues that are to be excised. They must be used judiciously, however, on tissues that are to remain *in situ*, as they are capable of producing an undesirable degree of crushing trauma.

Alternative methods of stabilizing tissues include the use of stay sutures, noncrushing forceps, or the hands of surgical assistants. Hollow viscera such as the stomach and urinary bladder can easily be stabilized and manipulated with multiple stay sutures of 2-0 monofilament suture. Pericardium, dura, and similar sheets of tissue can be effectively manipulated with stay sutures of smaller diameter. For procedures such as resection and anastomosis of the small intestine, noncrushing clamps such as Glassman intestinal forceps can be used to hold viable portions of the intestine while crushing clamps such as Carmalts are used for resection. Additionally, the index and middle fingers of the assistant provide an atraumatic clamp for occluding and manipulating intestinal segments that are to be retained. In most other instances, however, manipulation of tissues with the fingers and hands is not recommended, as it results in more diffuse cellular trauma than careful manipulation with instruments.[49]

The ideal surgical exposure for a given region necessitates a variable degree of tissue retraction depending on the length of the incision. Adequate length greatly facilitates retraction and minimizes tissue trauma. Exposure can be established and maintained with stay sutures, laparotomy sponges, and various types of hand-held or self-retaining retractors. Protection of the tissue to be retracted with a moistened laparotomy sponge is often preferable to direct placement of the retractor on the tissue. This is especially true for self-retaining retractors, as these are often left in position for long periods of time.[1] Frequently used self-retaining retractors and their common applications are as follows: Balfour: abdominal procedures; Finochietto: thoracotomies; Gelpi:

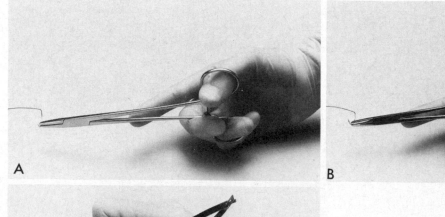

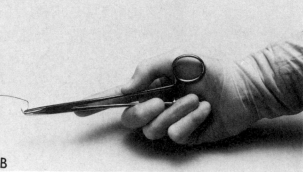

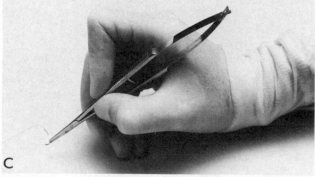

Figure 26–20. Three basic methods of grasping the needleholder. *A*, Thumb-ringfinger grip. *B*, Modified thenar eminence grip. *C*, Pencil grip.

orthopedic and neurosurgical procedures; and Weit-laner: cranial, cervical, and neurosurgical procedures. The major hazard of self-retaining retractors is trauma or ischemia at the pressure point.[1] Excessive retraction pressure is to be avoided with all types of retractors. During long procedures it is advisable to release self-retaining retractors periodically to prevent devitalization of the wound edges.

Moistened laparotomy sponges are useful for packing off structures that creep into the field (such as bowel loops) and to cover the peripheral portions of the field to prevent dehydration of tissues. Thorough isolation of the surgical repair site with laparotomy sponges is mandatory when entering a contaminated structure such as the lumen of the intestine.

Wound Irrigation and Suction

Maintaining a clear surgical field is paramount to good exposure. This is greatly facilitated by wound irrigation and suction. Wound irrigation or lavage is performed with physiological solutions (saline or Ringer's lactate), to which antibiotics are sometimes added. Lavaging and suctioning of the wound remove tissue debris, blood, and blood clots, all of which can impair visibility. In addition, wound lavage moistens tissues, counteracting the drying effects of exposure to air and the heat of surgical lights. Wound lavage has been associated with reduced rates of postoperative infection for both clean[27] and contaminated wounds[41] in direct proportion to the volume of irri-

gating solution used. This has been attributed to removal, dilution, or reduction of bacteria within the wound.[13] This effect is enhanced by moderate- and high-pressure lavage systems.[45] A simple moderate-pressure lavage system capable of delivering about 7 psi of pressure to the wound consists of a 35-ml syringe and a 19-gauge needle.[16]

Suctioning is the most efficient means of removing blood and other fluids from the wound. Suction is faster than sponges when removing large quantities of blood and permits a more accurate account of total blood loss.[1] Preferably, the unit should provide adjustable regulated vacuum in a range of 0 to 200 mm Hg. For general use, a vacuum of 80 to 120 mm Hg is recommended. Higher settings must be used cautiously to prevent aspiration injury to tissue. This is especially true when using suction tips with a single terminal opening.[1]

Three commonly used suction tips are shown in Figure 26–19. The multifenestrated sump-type design of the Pool tip makes it ideal for use in body cavities where other tips often plug or injure viscera.[31] Regular tips can be used in the peritoneal cavity provided a laparotomy sponge is placed over the top to prevent tissue from being sucked into the single opening.[31] Suctioning of delicate tissues is most safely conducted by interposing cottonoid or a gauze sponge between the tissue and the tip. Fluid is then aspirated through the material using a fine tip such as a Frazier tip and low-pressure vacuum. The Frazier tip has a finger port near the handle that can be used to vary the suction by covering and uncovering

TABLE 26–1. Ten Steps in Taking a Bite*

Step	Description	Comments
1.	Positioning the needle	Generally grasped perpendicular to the long axis of the needle holder near tip of needle for greatest driving force (dense tissue) near midpoint for general purpose suturing near eye for delicate tissue
2.	Properly grasping the needle holder	Thenar eminence grip used for suturing speed Pencil or thumb–ring finger grip for suturing precision
3.	Positioning the free end of the suture	Generally placed on the far side of the field or carried by the assistant
4.	Placing the needle point	Forehand sewing (introduction of the needle towards oneself) is easiest Distance between the needle puncture site and the wound edge should approximate the thickness of the tissue layer being sutured.
5.	Driving the needle	A single rotating motion is most efficient
6.	Releasing the needle	Use of tissue forceps to stabilize tissue layer during release reduces chance of needle dislodgement
7.	Regrasping the needle	Perpendicular regrasp is most efficient
8.	Extracting the needle	Extraction with the hand supinated often allows the next bite to be taken without having to reposition the needle Extraction with the hand pronated facilitates more precise extraction
9.	Pulling the desired length of suture through the wound	One uninterrupted motion with the needle holder is preferable to hand-over-hand pulling of the suture
10.	Tying the knot or repositioning the needle for the next bite	

*After Anderson, R. M., and Romfh, R. F.: *Technique in the Use of Surgical Tools.* Appleton-Century-Crofts, New York, 1980.

it with the index finger. Its small size and design make it well suited for use in joints and in many neurosurgical procedures.

WOUND CLOSURE

Needle Holder

Wound closure involves the placement of sutures for restoration of anatomical structure and support of tissues during healing. This is accomplished primarily with the use of two instruments, tissue forceps and the needle holder. Most needle holders are similar in design to hemostatic forceps with the following exceptions: (1) the tips are shorter, heavier, and usually grooved in a crisscross pattern; and (2) many have a longitudinal groove in the tip to aid grasping of the needle. Numerous varieties and lengths are available.

Three basic methods of grasping the needle holder are shown in Figure 26–20. Specific advantages have been stated for each. In the thumb–ring finger grip (Fig. 26–20A), the digits are used to precisely control opening and closing of the instrument.[1] When sutur-

ing delicate tissues, this precision in grasping and releasing the needle reduces inadvertent motion of the needle and needle holder, which might otherwise cause trauma. Continuous sutures can be more rapidly applied using a modified thenar eminence grip (Fig. 26–20B), as it allows the needle to be more easily grasped and extracted so that it is properly positioned for applying the next suture.[48] Imprecise release of the needle, however, makes this method poorly suited to delicate suturing.[1] Spring-opening needle holders with finger pressure release locks, such as the Castroviejo needle holder, are usually held with a pencil grip (Fig. 26–20C). Maximal needle holder control, provided by fine movements of the fingers, makes this method especially well suited for delicate work on small vessels,[1] nerves,[36] and the eye.[4]

Inefficient use of the needle holder accounts for more wasted time than poor technique with any other instrument.[1] Its proper use in taking a bite involves ten basic steps, as outlined in Table 26–1. Efficient use of tissue forceps greatly simplifies suture placement. Beginning on the far side of the wound, tissue forceps should initially grasp the tissue layer above the one being sutured and retract it upward

TABLE 26–2. Appositional Sutures*

Type	General Features	Common Uses
1. Simple interrupted (Fig. 26–21A)	Provides secure, anatomical closure Precise suture tension possible Easily applied Excessive tension may cause wound inversion	Skin, subcutis, fascia, blood vessels, nerves, GI tract
2. Gambee (Fig. 26–21B)	Modified simple interrupted suture Less susceptible to wicking of bowel contents than 1 Prevents mucosal eversion, unlike 1 Tied tightly so that suture impresses itself on the bowel	Intestinal anastomosis
3. Interrupted intradermal or subcuticular (Fig. 26–21C)	Upside down simple interrupted suture placed in dermis and subcutis	Intradermal skin closure
4. Interrupted cruciate or cross mattress (Fig. 26–21D)	Provides stronger closure than 1 Resists tension and prevents eversion Easiest of all mattress sutures to apply	Skin, especially amputation stumps of tail and digits
5. Simple continuous (Fig. 26–21E)	Saves time and promotes suture economy Provides good apposition and an air- or watertight seal Good for layers under low tension Provides less strength than 1 Excessive tension causes puckering and strangulation of skin	Skin, subcutis, fascia, blood vessels, GI tract
6. Continuous intradermal or subcuticular (Fig. 26–21F)	Modified horizontal mattress suture Saves time and promotes suture economy Provides less strength than skin closure	Intradermal skin closure
7. Continuous lock or Ford interlocking (Fig. 26–21G)	Similar to 5 except that it provides greater security if broken	Skin, diaphragm

*From Knecht, C. D., Allen, A. R., Williams, D. J., and Johnson, J. H.: *Fundamental Techniques in Veterinary Surgery.* W. B. Saunders, Philadelphia, 1981; Nealon, T. F.: *Fundamental Skills in Surgery,* 2nd ed. W. B. Saunders, Philadelphia, 1971; and Swaim, S. F.: *Surgery of Traumatized Skin: Management and Reconstruction in the Dog and Cat.* W. B. Saunders, 1980.

TABLE 26–3. Inverting Sutures*

Type	General Features	Common Uses
1. Lembert (Fig. 26–22A)	A variation of the vertical mattress suture Can be used in interrupted or continuous pattern Penetrates the submucosa but not the lumen of the bowel	Fascial imbrication or plication, closure of hollow viscera
2. Halsted (Fig. 26–22B)	A variation of 1	Second layer of closure for hollow viscera
3. Cushing (Fig. 26–22C)	Penetrates the submucosa but not the lumen of the bowel Provides less inversion than 1	Closure of hollow viscera
4. Connell (Fig. 26–22D)	Similar to 3 except penetrates bowel lumen Subject to wicking of bowel contents, unlike 1, 2, and 3	First layer of closure for hollow viscera
5. Parker-Kerr (Fig. 26–22E)	A single layer of 3 sewn over a clamp, pulled tight as clamp is removed, and oversewn with a continuous layer of 1	Closure of hollow visceral stumps
6. Purse-string (Fig. 26–22F)	A circular variation of 1 Stump must be held inverted as suture is tightened	Inversion of visceral stumps, securing of "ostomy" tubes and lavage catheters

*From Knecht, C. D., Allen, A. R., Williams, D. J., and Johnson, J. H.: *Fundamental Techniques in Veterinary Surgery.* W. B. Saunders, Philadelphia, 1981; and Nealon, T. F.: *Fundamental Skills in Surgery*, 2nd ed. W. B. Saunders, Philadelphia, 1971.

TABLE 26–4. Tension Sutures*

Type	General Features	Common Uses
1. Interrupted vertical mattress (Fig. 26–23A)	Appositional to everting Stronger in tissues under tension than Type 2 A single layer can be used for concurrent closure of skin and subcutis to eliminate dead space	Skin, subcutis, fascia
2. Interrupted horizontal mattress (Fig. 26–23B)	Appositional to everting suture depending on suture tension and whether suture penetrates tissue full or split thickness Potential for tissue strangulation can be reduced with stents	Skin, subcutis, fascia, muscle, tendon
3. Quilled (Fig. 26–23C)	A variation of Type 1 that loops over a stent on either side of the incision Everting	Combined with appositional suture for skin in areas of extreme stress
4. Near and far (Fig. 26–23D)	A variation of Type 1 Provides necessary tension for wound edge approximation without applying tension to the wound edge itself Excessive tightening causes inversion	Skin, subcutis, fascia
5. Stent (Fig. 26–23E)	Modified simple interrupted suture passed through skin, subcutis, and fascia, and tied over a gauze roll Effective obliteration of dead space	Used in combination with appositional closure of skin and subcutis in layers
6. Continuous horizontal mattress (Fig. 26–23F)	Appositional to everting suture depending on suture tension Facilitates rapid closure	Skin, subcutis, fascia
7. Locking loop or modified Kessler (Fig. 26–23G)	Provides superior apposition and equal holding strength compared with other tendon sutures Combined with simple interrupted sutures in paratenon	Tendons
8. Intraneural (Fig. 26–23H)	Centrally placed neurorrhaphy suture anchored externally with silicone buttons	Nerves

*From Aron, D. N.: A "new" tendon stitch. J. Am. Anim. Hosp. Assoc. *17:*587, 1981; Knecht, C. D., Allen, A. R., Williams, D. J., and Johnson, J. H.: *Fundamental Techniques in Veterinary Surgery.* W. B. Saunders, Philadelphia, 1981; Nealon, T. F.: *Fundamental Skills in Surgery*, 2nd ed. W. B. Saunders, Philadelphia, 1971; Raffee, M. R.: Peripheral nerve injuries in the dog (Part II). Comp. Cont. Ed. *1:*269, 1979; and Swaim, S. F.: *Surgery of Traumatized Skin: Management and Reconstruction in the Dog and Cat.* W. B. Saunders, Philadelphia, 1980.

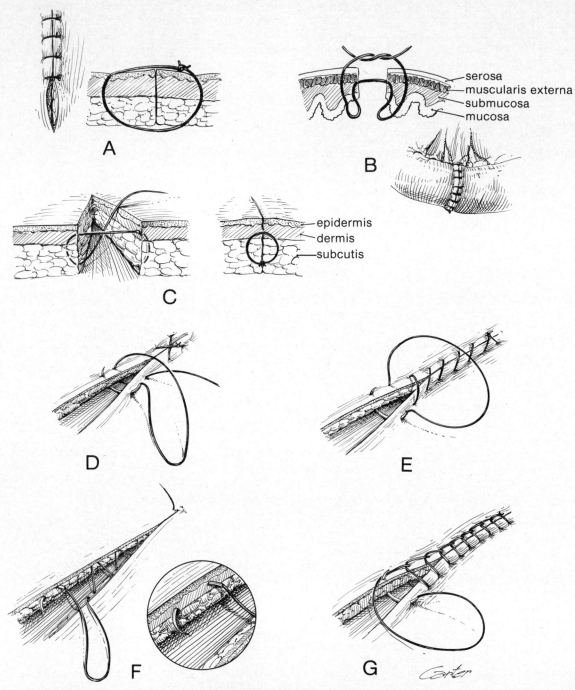

Figure 26–21. Appositional sutures.

and outward to provide exposure for needle placement. As the needle is driven, the tissue forceps is moved to the layer being sutured, which is elevated to expose the needle exit point. The forceps is then moved to the near side of the wound to expose the needle entrance site. As the needle penetrates the near side, the tissue forceps is moved to retract the layer above. In this manner, visibility of the needle is maximized throughout, thus aiding accurate suture placement. Although time can be saved by penetrating both sides of the wound with one motion of the needle, more accurate approximation of wound margins is obtained by taking separate bites on each side.

In order of descending preference, the needle can be extracted from tissue with a needle holder, smooth-tipped tissue forceps, or tissue forceps with teeth. Use of the last alternative may blunt both the needle and the teeth of the tissue forceps and is not generally recommended.

Suture Patterns

A vast number of sutures have been described for use in animals. They have been categorized according to the following factors: (1) anatomical areas in which they are routinely placed; (2) tendency to promote apposition, inversion, or eversion of tissues; (3) ability to neutralize tension forces; and (4) whether they are placed in a continuous or an interrupted fashion. Selected suture patterns, their synonyms or eponyms, general features, and common uses are summarized in Tables 26–2 through 26–4. Corresponding illustrations are provided in Figures 26–21 through 26–23.

Each suture is a separate entity in closures employing interrupted patterns. Failure of one suture in this case is often inconsequential. Suture breakage in a continuous pattern, however, frequently leads to disruption of the entire line of closure. Additional advantages of interrupted sutures include ease of placement and the ability to precisely adjust tension of each suture in accordance with variable spreading forces of the wound margins.[45] Disadvantages of interrupted patterns include increased time needed to tie multiple knots, increased volume of foreign material left in the wound when sutures are buried, and poor suture economy.

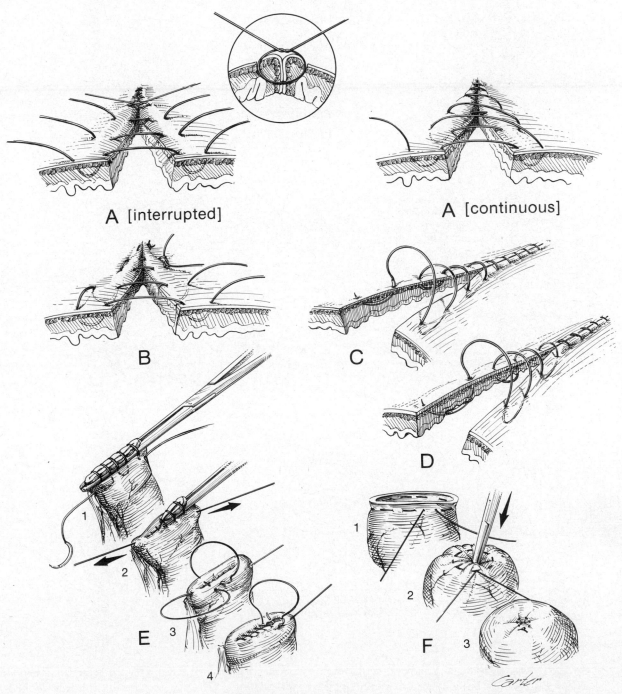

A [interrupted]

A [continuous]

B

C

D

E

F

Figure 26–22. Inverting sutures.

Continuous suture patterns, in contrast, use less suture material and minimize knots. This, in turn, reduces both operative time and the amount of suture material left in the wound. In addition, continuous patterns form a more air- or watertight seal.[23] Dis-advantages of continuous patterns include less precise control of suture tension[45] and the potentially disastrous effects of suture breakage. Accordingly, strands of suture used for continuous closures must be handled with the utmost care.

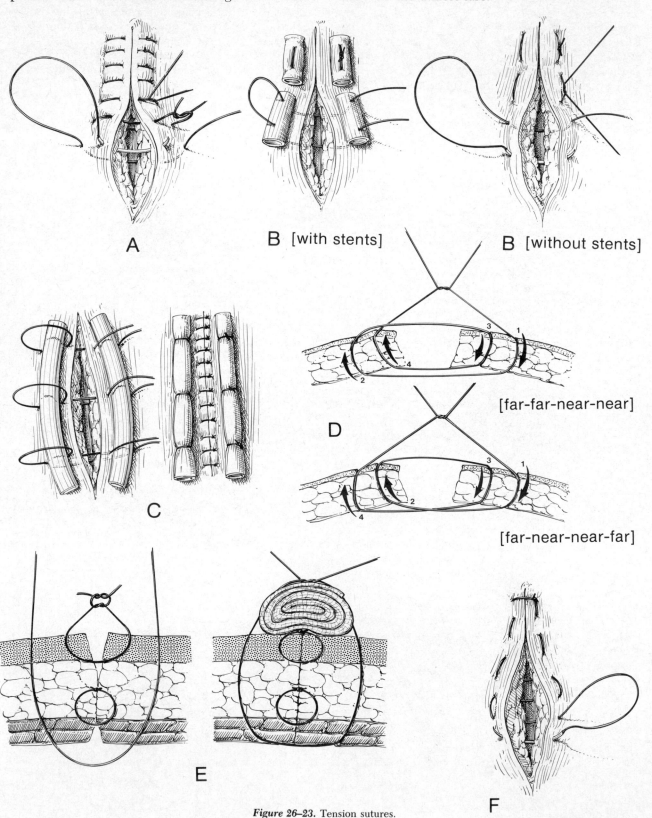

Figure 26–23. Tension sutures.

Illustration continued on opposite page

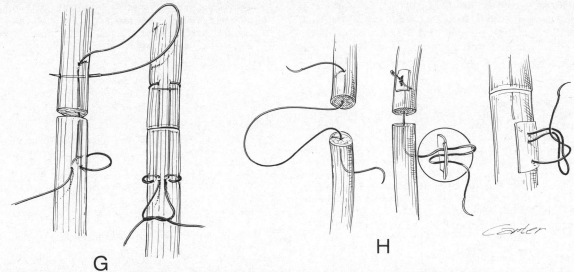

G   H

Figure 26–23 continued

The ability of a pattern to invert or evert tissues may or may not be beneficial depending on the anatomical area. Although inversion is often desirable for closure of hollow viscera, it is considered detrimental to proper healing of the skin.[45] Further information regarding wound closure factors conducive to healing in specific anatomical regions can be found in other chapters of this text and elsewhere.[3,4,15,35,36,39,45,49] Information on suture materials and tissue adhesives is provided in the next chapter.

1. Anderson, R. M., and Romfh, R. F.: *Technique in the Use of Surgical Tools.* Appleton-Century-Crofts, New York, 1980.
2. Archibald, J., and Blakely, C. L.: Surgical principles. *In* Archibald, J. (ed.): *Canine Surgery*, 2nd ed. American Veterinary Publications, Inc., Santa Barbara, CA, 1974, pp. 17–51.
3. Aron, D. N.: A "new" tendon stitch. J. Am. Anim. Hosp. Assoc. *17*:587, 1981.
4. Bistner, S. I., Aquirre, G., and Batik, G.: *Atlas of Veterinary Ophthalmic Surgery.* W. B. Saunders, Philadelphia, 1977.
5. Bojrab, M. J.: Veterinary cryosurgery: An overview. Norden News Spring: 16, 1978.
6. Borst, H. G., Haverich, A., Walterbusch, G., and Maatz, W.: Fibrin adhesive: An important hemostatic adjunct in cardiovascular operations. J. Thorac. Cardiovasc. Surg. *84*:548, 1982.
7. Borthwick, R.: Cryosurgery and its role in the treatment of malignant neoplasms. J. Small Anim. Pract. *13*:369, 1972.
8. Buchanan, J. W., and Lawson, D. D.: Cardiovascular system. *In* Archibald, J. (ed.): *Canine Surgery*, 2nd ed. American Veterinary Publications, Inc., Santa Barbara, CA, 1974, pp. 446–478.
9. Butler, H. C.: Vascular surgery. *In* Bojrab, M. J.: *Current Techniques in Small Animal Surgery I.* Lea & Febiger, Philadelphia, 1975, pp. 326–334.
10. Chehrazi, B., and Collins, W. F.: A comparison of effects of bipolar and monopolar electrocoagulation in brain. J. Neurosurg. *54*:197, 1981.
11. Collins, J. A., James, P. M., Levitsky, S. A., et al.: Cyanoacrylate adhesives as topical hemostatic aids. II. Clinical usage in seven combat casualties. Surgery *65*:260, 1969.
12. Coln, D., Horton, J., Ogden, M. E., and Buja, L. M.: Evaluation of hemostatic agents in experimental splenic lacerations. Am. J. Surg. *145*:256, 1983.
13. Committee on Trauma, American College of Surgeons: *Early Care of the Injured Patient*, 2nd ed. W. B. Saunders, Philadelphia, 1976.
14. Donawick, W. J., and Johnston, D. E.: *Veterinary Surgical Sutures.* Pitman-Moore, Washington's Crossing, NJ, 1982.
15. Eastcott, H. H. G.: *Arterial Surgery.* J. B. Lippincott, Philadelphia, 1973.
16. Edlich, R. F., Rodeheaver, G. T., Thacker, J. G., et al.: Management of soft tissue injury. Clin. Plast. Surg. *4*:191, 1977.
17. Finsterbush, A., Rousso, M., and Ashur, H.: Healing and tensile strength of CO_2 laser incisions and scalpel wounds in rabbits. Plast. Reconstr. Surg. *70*:360, 1982.
18. Glover, J. L., Bendick, P. J., and Link, W. J.: The use of thermal knives in surgery: Electrosurgery, lasers, plasma scalpel. Curr. Probl. Surg. *15*:7, 1978.
19. Greene, J. A., and Knecht, C. D.: Electrosurgery: A review. Vet. Surg. *9*:27, 1980.
20. Halsted, W. S.: Ligature and suture material. The employment of fine silk in preference to catgut and the advantages of transfixion of tissues and vessels in control of hemorrhage. J. Am. Med. Assoc. *60*:1119, 1913.
21. Harris, W. H., Crothers, O. D., Moyen, B. J.-L., and Bourne, R. B.: Topical hemostatic agents for bone bleeding in humans. A quantitative comparison of gelatin paste, gelatin sponge plus bovine thrombin, and microfibrillar collagen. J. Bone Joint Surg. *60A*:454, 1978.
22. Jacobs, H. B.: Skin knife-deep knife: The ritual and practice of skin incisions. Ann. Surg. *179*:102, 1974.
23. Knecht, C. D., Allen, A. R., Williams, D. J., and Johnson, J. H.: *Fundamental Techniques in Veterinary Surgery.* W. B. Saunders, Philadelphia, 1981.
24. Knecht, C. D., Clark, R. L., and Fletcher, O. J.: Healing of sharp incisions and electroincisions in dogs. J. Am. Vet. Med. Assoc. *159*:1447, 1971.
25. Kolata, R. J., Cornelius, L. M., Bjorling, D. E., and Mahaffey, M. B.: Correction of an obstructive lesion of the caudal vena cava in a dog using a temporary intraluminal shunt. Vet. Surg. *11*:100, 1982.
26. Kink, W. J., Incropera, F. P., and Glover, J. L.: A plasma scalpel—comparison of tissue damage and wound healing with electrosurgical and steel scalpels. Arch. Surg. *111*:392, 1976.
27. Lord, J. W., Rossi, G., and Daliana, M.: Intraoperative antibiotic wound lavage: An attempt to eliminate postoperative infection in arterial and clean general surgical procedures. Ann. Surg. *185*:634, 1977.

28. Madden, J. E., et al.: Studies in the management of the contaminated wound: IV. Resistance to infection of surgical wounds made by knife, electrosurgery, and laser. Am. J. Surg. *119*:222, 1970.

29. Marks, W. M., and Callen, P. W.: Computed tomography in the evaluation of patients with surgical clips. Surg. Gynecol. Obstet. *151*:557, 1980.

30. Murray, G.: The dry surgical incision. Can. Med. Assoc. J. *71*:439, 1954.

31. Nealon, T. F.: *Fundamental Skills in Surgery*, 2nd ed. W. B. Saunders, Philadelphia, 1971.

32. Ormrod, A. N.: Electro-surgery: Its usefulness and limitations for the small-animal surgeon. Vet. Rec. 75:1095, 1963.

33. Papachristou, D. N., and Barters, R.: Resection of the liver with a water jet. Br. J. Surg. 69:93, 1982.

34. Partipilo, A. V.: *Surgical Technique and the Principles of Operative Surgery*, 6th ed. Lea & Febiger, Philadelphia, 1957, pp. 125–142.

35. Peacock, E. E., and Van Winkle, W.: *Wound Repair*, 2nd ed. W. B. Saunders, Philadelphia, 1976.

36. Raffee, M. R.: Peripheral nerve injuries in the dog (Part II). Comp. Cont. Ed. *1*:269, 1979.

37. Rand, R. W.: *Cryosurgery*. Charles C Thomas, Springfield, IL, 1961.

38. Rawlings, C. A., and Wilson, S. A.: Intracaval repair of a persistent ductus venosus in a dog. Vet. Surg. *12*:155, 1983.

39. Rich, N. M., Hughes, C. W., and Baugh, J. H.: Management of venous injuries. Ann. Surg. *171*:724, 1970.

40. Schaefer, C. J., and Geelhoed, G. W.: Absorbable ligating clips. Surg. Gynecol. Obstet. *154*:153, 1982.

41. Singleton, A. O., and Julian, J.: An experimental evaluation of methods used to prevent infection wounds which have been contaminated with feces. Ann. Surg. *151*:912, 1960.

42. Staff Report: Can you use electrosurgery? Mod. Vet. Pract. 47:47, 1966.

43. Stone, D., Zacarian, S. A., and DiPeri, C.: Comparative studies of mammalian normal and cancer cells subjected to cryogenic temperatures in vitro. Cryosurgery 2:43, 1969.

44. Strong, M. S., Jako, G. J., Polanyi, T., and Wallace, R. A.: Laser surgery in the aerodigestive tract. Am. J. Surg. *126*:529, 1973.

45. Swaim, S. F.: *Surgery of Traumatized Skin: Management and Reconstruction in the Dog and Cat*. W. B. Saunders, Philadelphia, 1980.

46. Tauber, C., Farine, I., and Horoszowski, H.: Healing of CO_2 laser incision in the skin and fascia. Harefuah 98:1, 1980.

47. Vallfors, B., and Erlandson, B. E.: Damage to nervous tissue from monopolar and bipolar electrocoagulation. J. Surg. Res. 29:371, 1980.

48. Weiss, Y.: Simplified method of needle-holder handling. Arch. Surg. *106*:735, 1973.

49. Wingfield, W. E., and Rawlings, C. A.: *Small Animal Surgery—An Atlas of Operative Techniques*. W. B. Saunders, Philadelphia, 1979.

50. Withrow, S. J., Greiner, T. R., and Liska, W. D.: Cryosurgery: veterinary considerations. J. Am. Anim. Hosp. Assoc. *11*:271, 1975.

51. Zacarian, S. A.: *Cryosurgery of Tumors of the Skin and Oral Cavity*. Charles C Thomas, Springfield, IL, 1973.

52. Zikria, B. A.: *Manual of Surgical Knots*. Pitman-Moore, Washington's Crossing, NJ, 1973.

Chapter 27 Suture Materials and Tissue Adhesives

Harry W. Boothe

Many different types of suture materials are currently available to the veterinary surgeon. Some types have been introduced only recently, whereas others have been used for centuries. The choice of suture material has too often been governed by the training, experience, and preference of the surgeon rather than by scientific fact. Suture selection should more appropriately be based on knowledge of the physical and biological properties of suture materials, an assessment of local conditions in the particular wound, and knowledge of the healing rate of wounds of various tissues.[31]

THE IDEAL SUTURE MATERIAL

If there were one ideal suture material, the surgeon would only have to choose the appropriate size. No such ideal suture material exists; however, many of the currently available suture materials have excellent properties. Ideally, a suture material should maintain adequate tensile strength until its purpose is served; be nonelectrolytic, noncapillary, nonallergenic, and noncarcinogenic; be comfortable for the surgeon to use; have good knot security; stimulate minimal tissue reaction; be either absorbable at a dependable rate after healing is well advanced or encapsulated without postoperative complications; and be inexpensive, readily available, and easily sterilized without alteration. Also, the ideal suture material should not be corrosive or toxic or create a situation favorable to bacterial growth.[3, 33, 40]

CLASSIFICATION

Sutures are generally classified as either absorbable or nonabsorbable. Absorbable sutures are defined as those that undergo degradation and rapid loss of tensile strength within 60 days.[4, 13] Nonabsorbable sutures are those that retain tensile strength for longer than 60 days.[13] Sutures may also be further classified as natural and synthetic. Examples of natural fiber absorbable suture materials are surgical gut (catgut) and collagen. Synthetic absorbable suture materials currently available are polyglycolic acid (PGA), polyglactin 910, and polydioxanone (PDS). Examples of natural fiber nonabsorbable suture materials (including metallic sutures) are silk, cotton, stainless steel, and tantalum. Synthetic nonabsorbable suture materials include polyamides (nylon, polymerized caprolactam), polyester, and polyolefin plastics (polypropylene and polyethylene).

Absorbable Sutures of Natural Origin

Surgical Gut (Catgut)

Surgical gut is the most widely used suture today (Fig. 27–1).[22] It is prepared from either the submucosa of sheep small intestine or the serosal layer of cattle small intestine. It was originally referred to as kitstring or kitgut, meaning the string or cord on a fiddle. The term *catgut* seemingly derived from a change in the meaning of the term *kit* from fiddle to young cat.[15] Surgical gut is composed essentially of formaldehyde-treated collagen. It is a capillary multifilament suture composed of several plies that are twisted slightly, machine ground, and polished to yield a relatively smooth surface and diameter that resembles a monofilament.[13, 49] Surgical gut is sterilized by ionizing radiation. It is not autoclavable, since heat denatures the protein and causes a loss of strength.[33] The unopened inner aluminum foil package may be adequately disinfected in chemical solutions (e.g., 2% activated glutaraldehyde solution).[33] Ethylene oxide sterilization, however, prolongs the absorption time.[49]

The absorption of surgical gut following implantation is a twofold mechanism primarily involving the macrophage.[37] First, a loss of tensile strength results from the cleaving of molecular bonds by acid hydrolytic and collagenolytic activity. Second, digestion and absorption by proteolytic enzymes occur during the later stages of implantation. Because of its collagenous composition, surgical gut stimulates a significant foreign body reaction in the implanted tissue. Surgical gut exhibits a wide variation in the rate of absorption and loss of tensile strength. The wide variability in rate of loss of tensile strength is one property in which chromic gut compares unfavorably with synthetic absorbable sutures.[3] Premature absorption is observed when surgical gut is exposed to the acidic pepsin secretions of the stomach, infected environments, and highly vascularized tissue. Its absorption is also increased in protein-depleted patients. Increasing suture diameter has little influence on the time required for its absorption. As with the other absorbable sutures, absorption of surgical gut often occurs relatively long after the suture material has lost its effective strength. Medium chromic gut loses about 33 per cent of its original strength after 7 days of implantation and about 67 per cent after 28 days.[33]

Surgical gut is available in plain and chromic forms. Treatment with chromium salts results in an increase in intermolecular bonding. This crosslinking action of chromium increases tensile strength and resistance to digestion and decreases tissue reactivity.[3] Three grades of chromic gut have been developed: mild chromic (type B), medium chromic (type C), and extra chromic (type D). The rates of loss of tensile strength for these grades of chromic gut are 10, 20, and 40 days, respectively. Medium chromic gut is currently the type most commonly used. Plain gut produces such a severe tissue reaction and exhibits such a rapid loss of tensile strength that it has little use in surgery.[3]

Surgical gut generally exhibits good handling characteristics. However, when wet, surgical gut swells, weakens, and exhibits poor knot security.[20] Disadvantages of surgical gut include the inflammatory reaction it induces, the variability in rate of loss of tensile strength, its capillarity, and the occasional sensitivity reactions.[3]

Collagen

Collagen is a multifilament suture material that was introduced in 1964 (see Fig. 27–1).[43] It is processed from bovine flexor tendon and treated with formaldehyde or chromium salts or both. Its nonseptic source and simplicity of processing are advantages compared with surgical gut. Although collagen contains less noncollagenous protein than surgical gut, the rate and method of absorption of these sutures do not appear to differ.[3] Collagen sutures are currently made only in fine sizes and are used almost exclusively in ophthalmic surgery.

Absorbable Sutures of Synthetic Origin

Synthetic absorbable sutures were introduced to reduce the variability in absorption and subsequent loss of tensile strength associated with natural products.[43]

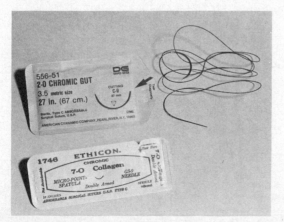

Figure 27–1. Chromic gut and chromic collagen suture material. One of these absorbable sutures is shown with needle attached. Collagen is available only in fine sizes.

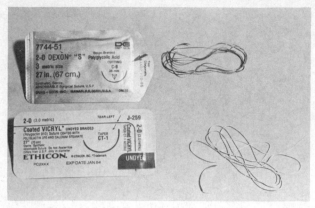

Figure 27–2. Polyglycolic acid and polyglactin 910 suture material. These sutures are available in a wide range of both suture diameters and needle sizes and types.

Polyglycolic Acid

Polyglycolic acid (PGA) is a noncollagenous synthetic absorbable suture (Fig. 27–2).[32] It is a braided multifilament polymer of glycolic acid (hydroxyacetic acid) that was first described in 1970.[3] Unlike other polyester sutures, PGA is relatively limp and pliable.[43]

The method of absorption of PGA differs from that of surgical gut. PGA is absorbed by hydrolysis—not phagocytosis—presumably through esterase activity.[3, 43] In vitro studies indicate that the suspected degradation products of PGA sutures are potent antibacterial agents.[13] Absorption is associated with a markedly reduced inflammatory process compared with surgical gut.[43] Complete absorption of PGA sutures usually occurs in 100 to 120 days.[3] Absorption is minimal until 14 days after implantation.

Hydrolysis of PGA proceeds more rapidly in an alkaline environment.[3] In vitro studies have shown PGA to be prematurely absorbed in urine.[39] PGA sutures were dissolved on the sixth day in sterile urine and on the third day in infected urine. Chromic gut dissolved on the eighth day in the infected urine and not at all in the sterile urine.[39] Despite this observation, PGA sutures have been successfully used in the closure of the urinary bladder.[1]

PGA suture is a relatively strong and ductile suture material similar to polyglactin 910 and monofilament nylon.[6] It has greater tensile strength than surgical gut, silk, and cotton.[43] PGA suture does not lose strength when immersed in saline solution.[43] Loss of tensile strength has been shown to be 33 per cent during the first seven days after implantation and approximately 80 per cent within two weeks.[32] PGA suture has a much higher initial tensile strength compared with surgical gut, but it loses its strength more rapidly. Because of its rapid loss of tensile strength, PGA may be inferior to nonabsorbable suture materials for re-apposing slowly healing tissues (e.g., ligaments, tendons, and joint capsules).[43] PGA has superior tensile strength compared with surgical gut during the most critical phases of wound repair.[43]

PGA is suitable for use in a wide variety of surgical procedures. It is well tolerated not only in clean wounds but also in situations in which gross infection is present.[11] A marked reaction to PGA sutures has been observed in the acute stages of infection, although little tissue reaction is demonstrated in later stages.[52] PGA sutures are well tolerated in infected wounds despite their surface binding of large numbers of bacteria compared with monofilament sutures (Fig. 27–3).[25, 44]

Disadvantages of PGA sutures include their tendency to drag through the tissues, to cut friable tissue, and possibly to have poorer knot security than surgical gut.[43] Friction can be reduced by wetting the suture before use. Knot security can be ensured by careful placement and selective tightening of each throw.[3, 43, 46]

Polyglactin 910

Polyglactin 910 is a braided synthetic fiber composed of glycolic and lactic acid in a ratio of 9:1 (see Fig. 27–2).[10] This suture is braided, because monofilament constructions were found to be too stiff for proper surgical handling.[3] Polyglactin 910 sutures are both more hydrophobic and more resistant to hydrolysis than PGA sutures.[10] The suture is sterilized by ethylene oxide and is available as a coated and uncoated suture. The absorbable coating compound is composed of a mixture of calcium stearate and a copolymer of lactide and glycolide in a ratio of 65:35.[7] The coated suture has been judged to have improved handling characteristics compared with the uncoated suture.[5, 7]

Polyglactin 910 is absorbed by the same mechanism as PGA, i.e., hydrolysis. Absorption occurs within 40 to 90 days after implantation.[3, 10] Polyglactin 910 shows a pattern of loss of tensile strength similar to that of PGA. This suture loses 50 per cent of its strength after 14 days and 80 per cent after 21 days.[3] Both polyglactin 910 and PGA sutures have no detectable strength by 21 days.[36] Also similar to PGA, polyglactin 910 absorption is independent of suture size.[10] Tensile strength loss is hastened in high temperatures and under alkaline conditions.[10] This suture was stronger than PGA sutures at all time periods from 0 to 35 days following implantation in the rat.[10] Like PGA, polyglactin 910 is stronger than surgical gut, and its rate of loss of strength was greater than that of surgical gut in all tissues except stomach.[3, 34] Polyglactin 910 sutures are well tolerated in many different wound conditions.[5, 7, 9, 26, 34, 36, 38] They were found to have an excellent size-to-strength ratio, were relatively easy to handle, were stable in contaminated wounds, and elicited minimal tissue reaction.[7, 10] Polyglactin 910 elicits almost no acute vascular reaction after implantation. Cellular reactions were predominantly mononuclear in character and limited to the immediate vicinity of the implanted strand.[10] Polyglactin 910 sutures exhibit less friction than PGA sutures when dry but more friction when wet.[36]

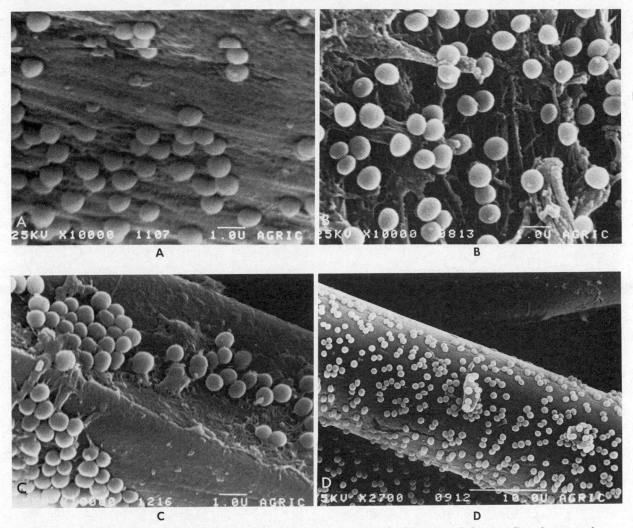

Figure 27–3. Bacterial adherence to sutures. Composite scanning electron micrographs showing staphylococci adhered to surgical sutures. *A*, Monofilament nylon. ×10,000. *B*, Chromic catgut. ×10,000. *C*, Silk. ×10,000. *D*, Dexon. ×2,700. (Reprinted with permission from Katz, S., Izhar, M., and Mirelman, D.: Bacterial adherence to surgical sutures: A possible factor in suture induced infection. Ann. Surg. *194*:41, 1981.)

Polydioxanone

This recently available synthetic monofilament suture is a polymer of paradioxanone.[35] Polydioxanone (PDS) is melt-extruded into monofilaments of variable size and is sterilized by ethylene oxide. It has a greater flexibility than either PGA, polyglactin 910, or polypropylene. The strength of PDS suture prior to implantation was greater than that of monofilament nylon and polypropylene.[35]

PDS, like PGA and polyglactin 910, is degraded by hydrolysis. Hydrolysis occurs at a regular rate and predictable manner in tissue.[35] Loss of tensile strength of PDS suture is slower than that of PGA or polyglactin 910 suture. PDS suture loses 26 per cent of its tensile strength after two weeks, 42 per cent after four weeks, and 86 per cent after eight weeks.[35] Absorption of PDS suture also occurs more slowly than with PGA or polyglactin 910 sutures. Evidence of absorption of PDS was present at 91 days, and absorption was essentially complete at 182 days after implantation. Degradation products of PDS suture were excreted primarily in the urine.[35]

Tissue reactivity of this monofilament synthetic absorbable suture material was similar to that of PGA and polyglactin 910. A minimal foreign body reaction was elicited by PDS suture during the entire time the suture remained in the tissues. Macrophages and fibroblasts were the predominant cell types observed. Upon absorption of the suture, reactions were either absent or characterized by a few enlarged macrophages or fibroblasts.[35]

Nonabsorbable Sutures of Natural Origin

Silk

Silk is obtained from the cocoon of the silk worm and is available as a twisted or braided multifilament (Fig. 27–4).[43] It is processed to remove the natural

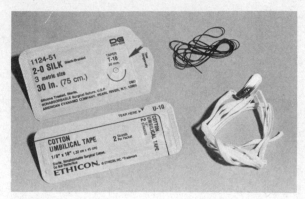

Figure 27–4. Silk and cotton suture material. The tissue reactivity of these multifilament natural-origin nonabsorbable suture materials is the greatest of that of all nonabsorbable suture materials.

waxes and gums and dyed with a vegetable dye to aid in its identification in tissues.[3] It may be treated by immersion in oil, wax, or silicone to decrease the natural capillarity. Silk was recommended as a suture to replace surgical gut by Theodor Kocher of Switzerland in the late 1880s.[17] Although classified as a nonabsorbable suture, silk slowly loses tensile strength and is absorbed after tissue implantation.[22] Silk loses 30 per cent of its tensile strength by two weeks, 50 per cent at one year, and essentially all of its tensile strength two years after implantation.[43, 49]

Silk is inexpensive and has excellent handling characteristics.[3, 43] It has been described as having the best "feel" of any available suture material.[31] Silk has been found to be distinctly inferior to many other suture materials in terms of strength and knot security.[20, 46] Wax or silicone impregnation further diminishes the knot security of silk.[20, 43] Silk also becomes 10 to 15 per cent weaker when wet.[45]

One of the disadvantages of silk is the tissue reaction that it incites.[31, 45] Although not severe, this reaction is greater than that caused by other nonabsorbable sutures.[45] Silk has a greater ability than nylon to bind gamma globulin. This binding ability eventually leads to an acute inflammatory reaction.[3] Silk has certain limitations in application including the potential to produce ulceration in the gastrointestinal tract if the suture protrudes into the lumen. Silk also may serve as a nidus for calculi formation in the lumen of the urinary bladder or gallbladder.[43] Because of these tendencies, silk should not be used in the lining epithelium of hollow viscera.

Silk should also be avoided in wounds having known or suspected bacterial contamination.[13] The many interstices between its fibers permit serum and blood to penetrate the suture and form a refuge for bacteria.[45] Silk has been shown to potentiate infection, probably related to its tissue reactivity.[45] The introduction of staphylococci on a silk suture can enhance the development of infection by as much as ten-thousandfold.[13]

Cotton

Cotton was introduced as a suture material in 1939 (see Fig. 27–4).[49] Its use became popular during World War II when silk was relatively scarce.[3] It is an inexpensive multifilament suture with capillarity. Cotton has naturally twisted fibers that tend to unravel soon after implantation in tissues.[3, 43] It can be autoclaved; however, prolonged autoclaving results in a decrease in tensile strength.[3]

Cotton gains in tensile strength and knot security when wet.[20, 43] The knot security of cotton is better than that of silk.[20] It slowly loses its tensile strength upon implantation in tissues, although it is not absorbed.[45] Cotton loses 50 per cent of its strength in six months and about 70 per cent at the end of two years.[49] It stimulates a degree of tissue reactivity similar to that seen with silk.[43]

Disadvantages of cotton include its ability to potentiate infection, its capillarity, its tissue reactivity, and its inferior handling ability.[3, 20, 40, 45, 50] Cotton has electrostatic properties that cause it to cling to gloves and surgical linen.[3, 45]

Nonabsorbable Metallic Sutures

Stainless Steel

Metal sutures have been used for centuries.[3] Presently, stainless steel is the only metallic suture that has received wide acceptance (Fig. 27–5).[43] The type suitable for sutures is austenitic stainless steel containing iron, chromium (17 per cent), nickel (10 per cent), and molybdenum (2.4 per cent).[3] It is available as a monofilament or twisted multifilament suture. Stainless steel is biologically inert, noncapillary as a monofilament, and easily sterilized by autoclaving.[3, 43] It has the highest tensile strength of all the suture materials, and it maintains this strength when implanted in tissues.[20, 43, 46] Stainless steel also has the greatest knot security of all the suture materials.[45, 46]

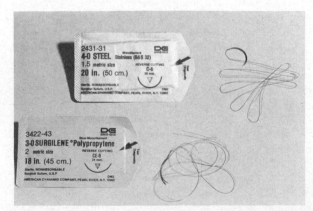

Figure 27–5. Stainless steel and polypropylene suture material. These sutures are quite nonreactive and can be used in contaminated wounds.

Stainless steel incites virtually no inflammatory reaction upon implantation.[45] It is good for suturing tissues that heal slowly.[45] The monofilament form can be used effectively in contaminated and infected wounds because it does not support infection.[45] However, the stiffness of the knot ends of stainless steel is believed to impair the wound's ability to resist infection.[13] Tissue movement against the inflexible ends of suture may cause inflammation and tissue necrosis.[3] Fragmentation and migration of implanted stainless steel suture material, particularly the multifilament form, have been observed.[3, 42]

Disadvantages of stainless steel include its tendency to cut tissues, its poor handling characteristics (especially in knot tying), and its diminished ability to withstand repeated bending without breaking.

Other Metallic Sutures

Tantalum, aluminum, and silver have been used as suture materials. They have not met with wide acceptance in surgery.[43] Tantalum is a pure metal and has been used both for sutures and as a mesh for hernia repair.[3] It has inferior tensile strength and knot security compared with stainless steel but superior ability to withstand repeated bending. Aluminum sutures increase the strength of the healing wound compared with silk and stainless steel.[43] Silver is occasionally used to repair intractable rectal prolapse in man.[43] None of these sutures is commonly used today.

Nonabsorbable Synthetic Sutures

Polyamide Sutures

Nylon and polymerized caprolactam are examples of readily available polyamide suture materials (Fig. 27–6).

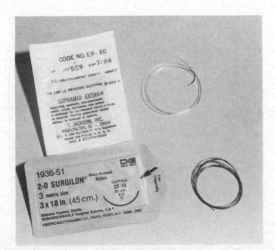

Figure 27–6. Polymerized caprolactam and nylon suture material. Both polyamide suture materials are available in a wide variety of sizes, and nylon is manufactured as both a monofilament and a multifilament suture.

Nylon

Nylon is an amine-containing thermoplastic.[3] It is derived from hexamethylenediamine and adipic acid.[43] Nylon is available as monofilament and multifilament suture materials. It is biologically inert and noncapillary in the monofilament form.[3, 43] Nylon is intermediate in tensile strength, similar to polypropylene.[20, 46]

Nylon causes minimal tissue reaction.[3] It produced the least reaction upon implantation in the canine tendon.[42] After implantation, monofilament nylon loses about 30 per cent of its original tensile strength over two years. Multifilament nylon retains almost no tensile strength after six months in tissue.[43] This loss of tensile strength is thought to be associated with chemical degradation of the nylon.[43] *In vitro* studies indicate that the suspected degradation products of nylon are potent antibacterial agents.[40]

Nylon has wide application as a suture material. The incidence of infection in contaminated tissues containing monofilament nylon is reportedly lower than the infection rate of tissues containing any other nonabsorbable suture except polypropylene.[40] The microscopic reactions to nylon in infected surgical wounds are minimal compared with those occurring with stainless steel.[51] Monofilament nylon is used effectively as a skin suture. Nylon is not recommended for use within a serous or synovial cavity, because buried sharp ends may cause frictional irritation.[3]

The main disadvantages of nylon are its poor handling characteristics and knot security.[3, 43] Monofilament nylon exhibited the most slipping of knots during *in vitro* tests.[46] It possesses "memory," which is a tendency to revert to its original configuration. This characteristic may be overcome by gentle stretching of the suture material. Knot security can be improved by careful placement of knots with four or five loops.[43] The resultant knots tend to be bulky and are time-consuming to tie.

Polymerized Caprolactam

This is a twisted multifilament polyamide suture of the nylon family.[20] It was introduced in the late 1940s and is in relatively common use in veterinary surgery.[17] Polymerized caprolactam is enclosed in a smooth sheath of "proteinaceous" material.[18] It can withstand autoclaving and is available only in relatively large diameters.[18] Chemical sterilization does not render this material sufficiently sterile for it to be safely implanted in tissues.[18] Ethylene oxide or heat sterilization is necessary prior to implantation.

Polymerized caprolactam has superior tensile strength when compared with nylon.[20] It loses about 15 to 20 per cent of its tensile strength when wet.[45] *In vitro* tests showed it to have relatively poor knot security.[46] Autoclaving increases the difficulty in handling this material.[17] Polymerized caprolactam is intermediate in tissue reactivity.[18] Skin incisions closed with polymerized caprolactam are generally more reactive and inflamed than those closed with stainless steel staple.[21] Excessive swelling with or without sinus formation has also been reported in 21 per cent of stifle surgeries using this suture material extra-articularly.[12]

Polyester Fibers

Polyester suture material is a braided multifilament available in plain and coated forms (Fig. 27–7). Coatings include polybutylate, Teflon, and silicone.[3, 43] These coatings add a lubricant-like quality, which decreases suture drag when drawn through tissue.[43] Polyester fiber sutures were introduced in the 1950s and are classified as relatively hard, brittle sutures.[6, 17] This suture is one of the strongest nonmetallic suture materials available.[22, 43] Sutures of small diameter provide high initial tensile strength with little or no loss after implantation in tissues. Once properly placed, polyester sutures offer prolonged support for slow-healing tissues.[43]

The handling characteristics of polyester sutures have considerably limited their use.[40] Noncoated polyester fibers have a high coefficient of friction.[45] Coatings generally decrease this friction, but they also reduce knot security markedly.[20] Polyester suture material has poor knot security.[43, 46] A five-throw knot with each throw tightly tied against the adjacent throw is recommended with polyester fiber.[47]

Polyester suture causes the most tissue reaction of the synthetic suture materials.[18] It produced a reaction equal to that seen with chromic gut when implanted for four weeks in a canine tendon.[42] Shedding of the Teflon coat in tissues increases the inflammatory response.[43] Implanted polyester sutures are encapsulated by fibrous tissues. The use of polyester sutures in contaminated or infected wounds has been associated with a persistent local infection and exaggerated tissue reaction.[40, 51] Coating the polyester suture with an inert material does not alter the contaminated tissue's response to the suture.[40]

Disadvantages of polyester suture material are its poor knot security, its high coefficient of friction, and its reactivity, particularly in contaminated environments. Other synthetic suture materials are recommended for use in the contaminated wound.

Polyolefin Plastics

These materials induce little tissue reaction and are distinctly hydrophobic.[23] Two readily available examples of polyolefin suture materials are polypropylene and polyethylene (see Fig. 27–5).

Polypropylene

Polypropylene suture was introduced in 1961 and is available as blue or clear monofilament suture.[22, 43] It is a polymer of propylene, a derivative of propane gas.[13, 22] Polypropylene is sterilized by ethylene oxide gas.[3] It has relatively low tensile strength but relatively high knot strength.[46] Polypropylene has lower tensile strength than nylon.[23] It is a relatively weak but ductile and tough suture material.[6] If the knots are set firmly, a flattening occurs where strands cross each other, providing a "locking" action.[3, 22, 31] Polypropylene has greater knot security than all other monofilament nonmetallic synthetic materials.[45]

Polypropylene retains its strength upon implantation in tissues.[3] It is not weakened by tissue enzymes and is the least thrombogenic suture.[22] For these reasons, polypropylene is frequently used in vascular surgery. Polypropylene, because of its high flexibility, is suitable for closing tissues having great elongation capability, such as skin and cardiac muscle.[6] It also exhibits the least potentiating effect in converting a contaminated wound to an infected wound.[40, 50]

Advantages of polypropylene suture are its strength, inertness, retention of strength after implantation, minimal tissue reactivity, and resistance to bacterial contamination. The only disadvantage of this suture is its slippery handling and tying characteristics.[3, 43]

Polyethylene

Polyethylene is a monofilament suture with excellent tensile strength but very poor knot strength.[45, 46] It can be autoclaved repeatedly without significant loss of tensile strength.[27] Polyethylene is similar to polypropylene in its minimal tissue reactivity and its resistance to bacterial contamination.[27] The major disadvantage of polyethylene suture is its poor knot security.

SELECTION OF SUTURE MATERIALS

With the many types of sutures currently available, proper suture selection may be difficult. Suture materials should be chosen on the basis of known biological properties of the suture and the particular clinical situation at hand.[49] Although there is generally not one ideal suture for every possible indication, certain suture materials are superior to others in

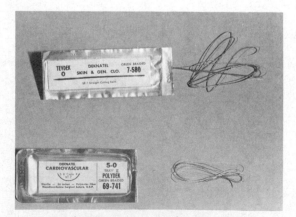

Figure 27–7. Polyester suture material. Many types of polyester sutures are available. This suture material is the strongest and most reactive of the nonmetallic synthetic nonabsorbable sutures.

different wound environments. Certain principles should be considered when choosing a suture material.

Sutures should be at least as strong as the normal tissue through which they are placed.[49] Skin and fascia are the strongest tissues, stomach and small intestine are much weaker, and the urinary bladder is weaker still.[49] A suture is not needed after a wound has healed.[31] Unfortunately, no available suture material retains strength for varying but known periods of time in different tissues and then disappears.[31] The relative rates at which the suture loses strength and the wound gains strength are important.[49] Visceral wounds heal rapidly, attaining strength within 14 to 21 days.[31] Absorbable sutures are generally adequate for these tissues. Fascia heals very slowly, and nonabsorbable sutures are more suited for its closure. Skin also heals slowly, and a nonabsorbable suture is usually indicated for its closure.[31]

If the suture biologically alters the healing process, these changes must be taken into consideration when selecting a suture.[49] One example of such alteration of the healing process is the sutured contaminated or infected wound.[13, 25, 40] Sutures are known to potentiate the development of wound infection.[25] The ability of the sutured tissue to resist infection varies, depending on the physical and chemical configuration of the sutures.[2, 13, 25, 40] Monofilament sutures withstand contamination better than multifilament sutures of the same material.[2] Synthetic sutures are superior to natural sutures.[40] Polyglycolic acid, polyglactin 910, monofilament nylon, and polypropylene reportedly have the lowest incidence of infection when used in contaminated tissues.[4, 13] However, even the least reactive suture impairs the wound's ability to resist infection. Therefore, the use of sutures should be minimized in contaminated wounds.[13] The potential calculogenic effect of silk in the urinary bladder and gallbladder is another example of alteration of the healing process by sutures.[43]

The mechanical properties of the suture should closely match those of the tissue to be closed.[6] Although information concerning mechanical properties of tissue is incomplete, one measure is the stress-strain curve. Because of similar stress-strain curves, polypropylene and nylon are judged to be most suitable for closing tissues having great elongation capability, such as skin.[6]

USE OF SUTURE MATERIALS IN DIFFERENT TISSUES

Skin. Monofilament nylon and polypropylene are the preferred sutures for skin.[3, 4, 49] Sutures that are capillary or reactive should be avoided in the skin.

Subcutis. Synthetic absorbable sutures are preferred because of their low tissue reactivity.

Fascia. Synthetic nonabsorbable suture materials are recommended for closure of fascia if prolonged suture strength is required.[4] Surgical gut and the synthetic absorbable sutures have also been used effectively in fascia.

Muscle. Synthetic absorbable or nonabsorbable sutures may be used effectively in muscle. Based on mechanical properties, nylon and polypropylene are recommended for use in cardiac muscle.[6]

Hollow Viscus. Surgical gut, PGA, polyglactin 910, and monofilament nonabsorbable sutures may be used in viscera.[4, 49] PGA may not be the ideal suture for use in the urinary bladder, since its premature absorption in urine has been observed. Multifilament nonabsorbable sutures should be avoided.

Tendon. Nylon and stainless steel are usually recommended for tendon repair.[4, 49] The newly available absorbable PDS suture may also be effective as a tendon suture because of its prolonged tensile strength.[34]

Blood Vessel. Because it is the least thrombogenic suture, polypropylene is probably the material of choice in vascular repair. Nylon and coated polyester have also been used effectively.[4, 49]

Nerve. Nonreactivity is the most important consideration in peripheral nerve repair. For this reason, nylon and polypropylene are the recommended sutures.[4, 49]

SELECTION OF THE APPROPRIATE SUTURE SIZE

Proper suture selection involves the choice of both the appropriate type and size. Suture is sized as either USP or metric. The smallest USP size is 10–0 and the largest is 7. The metric size is the suture diameter expressed in tenths of a millimeter.[3] Stainless steel wire may also be sized according to the Brown and Sharpe (B and S) wire gauge; sizes range from 41 gauge (equivalent to USP 7–0) to 18 gauge (equivalent to USP 7).[3]

Veterinary surgeons tend to choose inappropriately large suture sizes. Use of too large a suture results in an excessive amount of foreign material in the wound. It also needlessly alters the architecture of the sutured tissue. Guidelines for the selection of appropriately sized suture in small animal surgery are listed in Table 27–1.[4]

TABLE 27–1. Guidelines for Selection of Sutures in Small Animal Surgery

Tissue	Suture Size (USP)
Skin	4–0 to 3–0
Subcutis	4–0 to 3–0
Fascia	3–0 to 0
Muscle	3–0 to 0
Hollow viscus	5–0 to 2–0
Tendon	3–0 to 0
Vessel (ligatures)	4–0 to 2–0
Vessel (sutures)	6–0 to 5–0
Nerve	6–0 to 5–0

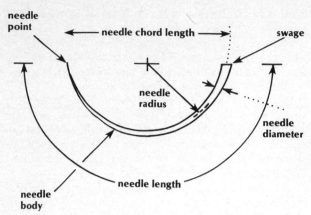

Figure 27–8. Parts of the surgical needle. (Reprinted with permission from Heath, M. M.: Needle selection in veterinary surgery. Anim. Health Tech. 4:45, 1983.)

SELECTION OF SURGICAL NEEDLES

The important factors to be considered in needle selection are the characteristics of the tissue being sutured, the wound to be sutured, and the needles themselves. There are two categories of surgical needles: swaged, or eyeless, needles and eyed needles. Swaged needles are immediately available, less traumatic to the tissue, and always sharp and their sterility is guaranteed. Eyed needles are reusable and less expensive than swaged needles.[4] Generally, the veterinary surgeon closes using one needle per suture strand (single-armed suture). In

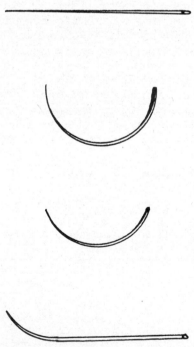

Figure 27–9. Shapes of surgical needles. Different configurations of the longitudinal shaft of a needle are shown. Straight needles (A) are usually used on or near the body surface. Curved needles (B–D) are used in either superficial or deep wounds. (Reprinted with permission from Bellenger, C. R.: Sutures part II: The use of sutures and alternative methods of closure. Comp. Cont. Ed. Pract. Vet. 4:587, 1982.)

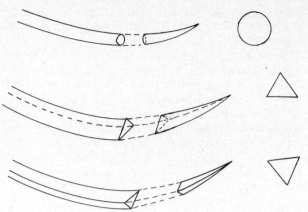

Figure 27–10. Types of needle points. The shape of the point and body of noncutting (taper) (A), conventional cutting (B), and reverse cutting (C) needles are shown. (Reprinted with permission from Bellenger, C. R.: Sutures part II: The use of sutures and alternative methods of closure. Comp. Cont. Ed. Pract. Vet. 4:587, 1982.)

cardiovascular surgery and other specialty areas, a double-armed suture may be appropriate.[19]

Surgical needles are manufactured from stainless steel wire.[48] Their design varies as to size, shape, and type of needle point. The needle length and diameter are important aspects of needle size (Fig. 27–8). The needle should be long enough to reach both sides of the incision. Too large a needle diameter results in increased tissue trauma. Surgical needles that exceed a length-to-diameter ratio of 8:1 may tend to buckle or bend easily.[19]

Needle shapes vary considerably (Fig. 27–9). The common shapes are straight, half-curved, and parts of a circle (⅜ circle, ½ circle, and so on).[4] The tissue type and the depth, size, and accessibility of the wound are determining factors in the choice of the appropriate needle shape.[19] Straight needles are best used near the surface of the body. One-half circle needles are convenient for small wounds and wounds deep within a cavity.[19]

The type of point is another consideration in needle selection (Fig. 27–10). Noncutting needles are round (taper) needles with no edges.[19] They are generally used for parenchymatous organs, fat, and muscle.[19, 48] Cutting needles are ground and honed to produce an edge that will penetrate dense tissues.[48] Three types of cutting needles are available: conventional, reverse, and tapered. Conventional curved cutting needles have the cutting edge along the concave surface. Reverse curved cutting needles have the cutting edge along the convex surface. They have two advantages over the conventional cutting needle: minimized risk of cutting out of the tissue and increased needle strength.[4, 48] Tapered cutting needles combine a round shaft with a cutting point.[19] They are used on more delicate fibrous tissue.

Certain requirements should be met when choosing a needle. First, the needle should make a hole in the tissue large enough to permit introduction of the suture material only. Second, the architecture of the sutured tissue should not be weakened. Third, microorganisms, foreign bodies, chemicals, or other substances should not be introduced into the wound. Fourth, the needle should be of such material and design so as to minimize damage and breakage. Finally, the needle should be large enough and of appropriate shape and design to permit rapid, accurate, and precise suturing.[48]

TISSUE ADHESIVES

The group of materials that have been used most extensively as tissue adhesives are the cyanoacrylates.[41] Monomers of cyanoacrylate are converted from a liquid to a solid state by polymerization,[16] a process that is catalyzed by minute amounts of water present on the surface of tissues.[4, 8, 41] The setting time ranges between 2 and 60 seconds, depending on the thickness of the film and the amount of moisture present.[8]

Tissue toxicity is a problem of some of the cyanoacrylates (especially methyl and propyl cyanoacrylate).[4, 41] The iso-butyl, *N*-octyl, and fluoro analogues appear to have the most potential for clinical use.[4, 41] Other problems that have been reported with the use of cyanoacrylate tissue adhesives are granuloma formation, severe wound infections when used in contaminated wounds, delayed healing if the wound edges are separated, and poor adhesion of the substance on excessively moist surfaces.[4, 16, 41]

Tissue adhesives have been effectively used both experimentally and clinically in oral surgery, intestinal anastomosis, management of corneal ulceration, control of hemorrhage from the cut surface of parenchymatous organs, microvascular anastomosis, and skin grafts.[4, 14, 23, 28-30, 41, 45] Their most widespread use has been in oral surgery, particularly in the grafting of mucous membrane.[4]

1. Adams, H., Barnes, R., Small, C., and Hadley, H.: Sutures and bladder wound healing in the experimental animal. Invest. Urol. *12*:267, 1975.
2. Alexander, J. W., Kaplan, J. Z., and Altemeier, W. A.: Role of suture materials in the development of wound infection. Ann. Surg. *165*:192, 1967.
3. Bellenger, C. R.: Sutures. Part I: The purpose of sutures and available suture materials. Comp. Cont. Ed. Pract. Vet. *4*:507, 1982.
4. Bellenger, C. R.: Sutures. Part II: The use of sutures and alternative methods of closure. Comp. Cont. Ed. Pract. Vet. *4*:587, 1982.
5. Blaydes, J. E., and Berry, J.: Comparative evaluation of coated and uncoated polyglactin 910 in cataract and muscle surgery. Ophthalmic Surg. *11*:790, 1980.
6. Chu, C. C.: Mechanical properties of suture materials. Ann. Surg. *193*:365, 1981.
7. Conn, J., Jr., and Beal, J. M.: Coated vicryl synthetic absorbable sutures. Surg. Gynecol. Obstet. *150*:843, 1980.
8. Converse, J. M.(ed.): *Reconstructive Plastic Surgery: Principles and Procedures in Correction, Reconstruction, and Transplantation.* W. B. Saunders, Philadelphia, 1964, pp. 9–11.
9. Corman, M. L., Veidenheimer, M. C., and Coller, J. A.: Controlled clinical trial of three suture materials for abdominal wall closure after bowel operations. Am. J. Surg. *141*:510, 1981.
10. Craig, P. H., Williams, J. A., Davis, K. W., Magoun, A. D., Levy, A. J., Bogdansky, S., and Jones, J. P., Jr.: A biologic comparison of polyglactin 910 and polyglycolic acid synthetic absorbable sutures. Surg. Gynecol. Obstet. *141*:1, 1975.
11. Dardik, H., Dardik, I., and Laufman, H.: Clinical use of polyglycolic acid polymer as a new absorbable synthetic suture. Am. J. Surg. *121*:656, 1971.
12. Dulish, M. L.: Suture reaction following extra-articular stifle stabilization in the dog—Part I: A retrospective study of 161 stifles. J. Am. Anim. Hosp. Assoc. *17*:569, 1981.
13. Edlich, R. F., Panek, P. H., Rodeheaver, G. T., Turnbull, V. G., Kurtz, L. D., and Edgerton, M. T.: Physical and chemical configuration of sutures in the development of surgical infection. Ann. Surg. *177*:679, 1973.
14. Fogle, J. A., Kenyon, K. R., and Foster, C. S.: Tissue adhesive arrests stromal melting in the human cornea. Am. J. Ophthalmol. *89*:795, 1980.
15. Goldenberg, I. S.: Catgut, silk, and silver. The story of surgical sutures. Surgery *46*:908, 1959.
16. Grabb, W. C., and Smith, J. W. (eds.): *Plastic Surgery: A Concise Guide to Clinical Practice.* Little, Brown and Co., Boston, 1973, p. 22.
17. Grier, R. L.: Surgical suture—Part I: A review. Iowa St. Univ. Vet. *33*:132, 1971.
18. Grier, R. L.: Surgical sutures—Part II: Indications for different suture materials and comparable costs. Iowa St. Univ. Vet. *34*:89, 1972.
19. Heath, M. M.: Needle selection in veterinary surgery. Anim. Health Tech. *4*:45, 1983.
20. Herrmann, J. B.: Tensile strength and knot security of surgical suture materials. Am. Surg. *37*:209, 1971.
21. Hess, J. L., DeYoung, D. W., Riley, M. G. I., and McCurnin, D. M.: Comparison of stainless steel staple and synthetic suture material on skin wound healing. J. Am. Anim. Hosp. Assoc.*15*:501, 1979.
22. Holt, G. R., and Holt, J. E.: Suture materials and techniques. Ear Nose Throat J. *60*:23, 1981.
23. Homsy, C. A., McDonald, K. E., and Akers, W. W.: Surgical suture. Canine tissue interaction for six common suture types. J. Biomed. Mater. Res. *2*:215, 1968.
24. Karl, P., Tilgner, A., and Heiner, H.: A new adhesive technique for microvascular anastomoses: A preliminary report. Br. J. Plast. Surg. *34*:61, 1981.
25. Katz, S., Izhar, M., and Mirelman, D.: Bacterial adherence to surgical sutures: A possible factor in suture induced infection. Ann. Surg. *194*:35, 1981.
26. Kobayashi, H., Tsuzuki, M., Kawano, N., Fukuda, O., and Saito, S.: Coated polyglactin 910—A new synthetic absorbable suture. Jpn. J. Surg. *11*:467, 1981.
27. Koontz, A. R., and Kimberly, R. C.: The promise of an ideal suture material—Marlex (blue linear polyethylene). Arch. Surg. *86*:162, 1963.
28. Linn, B. S., Cecil, F., Conly, P., Canaday, W. R., Jr., and Wolcott, M. W.: Intestinal anastomosis by invagination and gluing. Am. J. Surg. *111*:197, 1966.
29. Matsumoto, T.: Vienna international symposium—tissue adhesives in surgery. Arch. Surg. *96*:226, 1968.
30. Ota, K., Mori, S., Mizuno, K., and Inou, T.: Experimental and clinical use of adhesive on parenchymatous organs. Arch. Surg. *96*:231, 1968.
31. Peacock, E. E., Jr., and Van Winkle, W. (eds.): *Wound Repair.* W. B. Saunders, Philadelphia, 1976, pp. 215–231.
32. Postlethwait, R. W.: Polyglycolic acid surgical suture. Arch. Surg. *101*:489, 1970.
33. Postlethwait, R. W.: Principles of operative surgery: Antisepsis, technique, sutures, and drains. *In* Sabiston, D. C., Jr. (ed.): *Davis-Christopher Textbook of Surgery: The Biological Basis of Modern Surgical Practice.* W. B. Saunders, Philadelphia, 1977, pp. 330–334.
34. Postlethwait, R. W., and Smith, B. M.: A new synthetic absorbable suture. Surg. Gynecol. Obstet. *140*:377, 1975.
35. Ray, J. A., Doddi, N., Regula, D., Williams, J. A., and Melveger, A.: Polydioxanone (PDS), a novel monofilament synthetic absorbable suture. Surg. Gynecol. Obstet. *153*:497, 1981.

36. Rodeheaver, G. T., Thacker, J. G., and Edlich, R. F.: Mechanical performance of polyglycolic acid and polyglactin 910 synthetic absorbable sutures. Surg. Gynecol. Obstet. 153:835, 1981.

37. Salthouse, T. N., Williams, J. A., and Willigan, D. A.: Relationship of cellular enzyme activity to catgut and collagen suture absorption. Surg. Gynecol. Obstet. 129:691, 1969.

38. Saunders, R. A., and Helveston, E. M.: Coated vicryl (polyglactin 910) suture in extraocular muscle surgery. Ophthalmic Surg. 10:13, 1979.

39. Sebeseri, O., Keller, U., Spreng, P., Tscholl, R., and Zingg, E.: The physical properties of polyglycolic acid sutures (dexon) in sterile and infected urine. Invest. Urol. 12:490, 1975.

40. Sharp, W. V., Belden, T. A., King, P. H., and Teague, P. C.: Suture resistance to infection. Surgery 91:61, 1982.

41. Silver, I. A.: Tissue adhesives. Vet. Rec. 98:405, 1976.

42. Srugi, S., and Adamson, J. E.: A comparative study of tendon suture materials in dogs. Plast. Reconstr. Surg. 50:31, 1972.

43. Stashak, T. S. and Yturraspe, D. J.: Considerations for selection of suture materials. J. Vet. Surg. 7:48, 1978.

44. Sugarman, B., and Musher, D.: Adherence of bacteria to suture materials. Proc. Soc. Exp. Biol. Med. 167:156, 1981.

45. Swaim, S. F. (ed.): Surgery of Traumatized Skin: Management and Reconstruction in the Dog and Cat. W. B. Saunders, Philadelphia, 1980, pp. 247–261.

46. Tera, H.,and Aberg, C.: Tensile strengths of twelve types of knot employed in surgery, using different suture materials. Acta Chir. Scand. 142:1, 1976.

47. Thacker, J. G., Rodeheaver, G., Moore, J. W., Kauzlarich, J. J., Kurtz, L., Edgerton, M. T., and Edlich, R. F.: Mechanical performance of surgical sutures. Am. J. Surg. 130:374, 1975.

48. Trier, W. C.: Considerations in the choice of surgical needles. Surg. Gynecol. Obstet. 149:84, 1979.

49. Van Winkle, W., Jr., and Hastings, J. C.: Considerations in the choice of suture material for various tissues. Surg. Gynecol. Obstet. 135:113, 1972.

50. Van Winkle, W., Jr., Hastings, J. C., Barker, E., Hines, D., and Nichols, W.: Effect of suture materials on healing skin wounds. Surg. Gynecol. Obstet.140:7, 1975.

51. Varma, S., Johnson, L. W., Ferguson, H. L., and Lumb, W. V.: Tissue reaction to suture materials in infected surgical wounds—a histopathologic evaluation. Am. J. Vet. Res. 42:563, 1981.

52. Varma, S., Lumb, W. V., Johnson, L. W., and Ferguson, H. L.: Further studies with polyglycolic acid (Dexon) and other sutures in infected experimental wounds. Am. J. Vet. Res. 42:571, 1981.

Chapter 28 Endoscopy

David C. Twedt

Endoscopy is a procedure using special optical instruments, endoscopes, to view the interior of a body cavity or lumen. Several endoscopes are available, varying in basic type, complexity, and diagnostic capabilities. Recommendations for selection of suitable endoscopes are based on the area to be examined, techniques to be performed, and the available instruments.

An endoscopic examination should be regarded as a diagnostic technique that aids in the evaluation of a patient. The indications and limitations of each technique must be reviewed before undertaking a new endoscopic examination. To obtain useful information through endoscopy, experience in the basic instrumentation must be coupled with an accurate interpretation of the findings. The use of endoscopes in veterinary medicine will no doubt increase with experience and advances in technology. If used wisely, endoscopy becomes a less invasive alternative to exploratory surgery.

ENDOSCOPIC PRINCIPLES

There are two basic types of endoscopes: rigid and flexible. The rigid instruments have simple optical systems, are generally less expensive, and are quite durable. The flexible instrument transmits light and images through thousands of small glass fibers, enabling examination of areas not normally viewed by the rigid endoscope. Flexible endoscopes have the disadvantages of being expensive and fragile and requiring special care and maintenance. Endoscopes are also classified as to type of illumination or the means of optical transmission of images.

Illumination

Areas for endoscopic examination are usually dark and at a distance from the eye, requiring illumination and a magnifying system. Older endoscopes consisted simply of a rigid tube with a lens system and an incandescent light source at either the proximal eyepiece or the distal tip. The disadvantage of such a system lies in the considerable amount of heat dissipated for the amount of useful illumination given off. The amount of heat released and the potential for tissue damage by the incandescent lamp limit the quantity of illumination that can be used.

With the development of fiberoptics, much brighter illumination is obtained without danger from thermal damage. In this system, the light source is removed from the patient. Light, without heat, is transmitted through fiberoptic glass bundles to the endoscope. The principle of light transmission

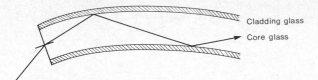

Figure 28–1. Principle of light transmission through a glass fiber. A light ray (arrow) entering a glass fiber is repeatedly reflected internally by a cladding coat of glass of a different refractive index. The reflected light ray leaves the glass fiber with almost the same intensity as when it entered.

through fiberoptics is based on total internal reflection of light through glass fibers.[2] Light entering the cut-end surface of a fiber travels through the fiber, is repeatedly reflected internally, and leaves the fiber with almost the same intensity as when it entered (Fig. 28–1). Light transmission continues through the bundles even though the glass threads may be twisted or bent. Light transmission through the glass fibers without loss through scattering of light is accomplished by an insulating coat or cladding on the exterior of each light-transmitting fiber. The cladding coat is a glass of a lower reflective index than that of the fiber that reflects the light internally. Approximately 100,000 glass fibers are combined to form a bundle that is 1/8 inch in diameter.[19] The fibers are grouped into bundles and attached at only the proximal and distal ends, allowing for greater flexibility of the fiber bundles.

Optics

Early endoscopes consisted of a simple hollow tube illuminated by an external incandescent light source. With technological developments, a magnifying lens was placed at the proximal end to aid in viewing the luminal surface. Today's proctoscopes, esophagoscopes, and many rigid bronchoscopes continue to use this basic principle. Other solid endoscopes contain a series of lenses throughout the length of the scope surrounded by a system of glass fibers for light transmission.[13] Laparoscopes, arthroscopes, and some bronchoscopes employ this optical system. Flexible fiberoptic endoscopes contain two separate fiber bundle components: one for light transmission and the other for transmission of an optical image. In contrast to those in the light-transmitting bundles, the fibers in the optic bundle must be coherently oriented at

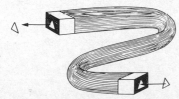

Figure 28–2. Principle of image transmission through a glass fiber. An optical image (triangle) enters a bundle of glass fibers and exits at the other end. The glass fibers must be coherently arranged at both ends so that the image conveyed is the same as the image transmitted.

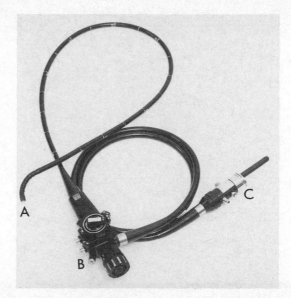

Figure 28–3. Olympus GIF-P₂ pediatric gastrointestinal endoscope with a flexible distal viewing end (A), eyepiece with control valves and four-way directional control levers (B), and light transmission cable (C) for attachment to a light source (not shown). (Reprinted with permission from Twedt, D. C., and Wingfield, W. E.: Diseases of the stomach. In Ettinger, S. J.: *Textbook of Veterinary Internal Medicine*, 2nd ed. W. B. Saunders, Philadelphia, 1983, pp. 1233–1277.)

both ends so that the image emerging at the proximal end is the same as the one entering the distal end (Fig. 28–2). The optic resolution of the flexible fiberoptic endoscope depends on the regularity, density, and compactness of the image-transmitting glass fibers at both ends.[2]

Modern flexible fiberoptic endoscopes have enhanced the examination of the respiratory and gastrointestinal systems.[5] Many areas not previously viewed by rigid instruments can now be easily observed. In addition to the flexibility of these endoscopes, the distal tip can be directed through a control knob in the handpiece. Most flexible endoscopes have a channel for the suctioning of fluids or the passage of biopsy forceps or cytology brushes. Biopsy forceps can be directed precisely through manipulation of the distal tip of the endoscope. A second channel is found on most gastrointestinal fiberoptic endoscopes for insufflation of air to distend the lumen or the addition of water, which exits the distal tip of the endoscope as a fine spray to clean away any debris over the lens. Control valves for air, water, and suction are on the handpiece of the endoscope (Fig. 28–3).

EQUIPMENT SELECTION

The following section deals with common, available equipment and recommendations for selection of endoscopes for specific examinations. There are many endoscopes similar to those described that are equally suitable. Justification in purchasing certain endoscopes should be based on the type of examination to be performed, the frequency of use, and the

TABLE 28–1.　Suggested Equipment Required for Specific Endoscopic Examinations

Endoscopic Equipment	Rhinoscopy	Nasopharyngoscopy	Tracheobronchoscopy	Thoracoscopy	Esophagoscopy	Gastroscopy	Colonoscopy	Laparoscopy	Cystoscopy-Urethroscopy	Vaginoscopy	Arthroscopy
Rigid Fiberoptic Instruments											
Esophagoscope					B		P				
Bronchoscope			B		P						
Proctoscope					P		B	P		B	
Laparoscope				B				B		B	
Arthroscope	B			P				P	B		B
Flexible Fiberoptic Instruments											
Bronchoscope	P	B	B						P	P	
Gastrointestinal scope		P	P		B	B	B			B	

B = Best selection.
P = Possible, with limitations.

purchase and maintenance costs. The versatility of instrument application must be considered when selecting equipment. Suggestions will be made regarding suitable instruments for specific examinations as well as other possible alternative uses (Table 28–1). Endoscopes are usually available in a number of lengths and diameters with specific individual features. Most are designed for use in humans. Standard adult models are frequently too large for small animals; pediatric sizes are usually better suited. Size, type of illumination, optical features, and diagnostic capabilities are important considerations when selecting an endoscope.

Respiratory System

Rhinoscopy

Examination of the nasal cavity in dogs and cats requires small, rigid endoscopes ranging in diameter from 1.7 to 3.0 mm. Such endoscopes include arthroscopes and the Needlescope. Larger-diameter laparoscopes or small flexible endoscopes are generally not suitable for examination of the nasal turbinates. Small flexible bronchoscopes (3 to 4 mm in diameter) may be suitable for rhinoscopy in some large dogs.

The nasal turbinates are quite vascular, and bleeding occurs with minimal trauma to these tissues. Endoscopes equipped with an outer cannula through which fluids can be infused during the examination are useful for flushing away blood and mucus, which may obscure the lens. Nasal foreign bodies, inflammatory lesions, and neoplasia are detectable on endoscopic inspection.

The *nasopharynx* is best viewed with a small-diameter flexible bronchoscope or pediatric endoscope with the tip bent behind the soft palate to look rostrally at the nasopharynx (Fig. 28–4).[5] This examination technique is difficult in cats and small dogs because of the space required to manipulate the endoscope into the pharynx and bend it back above the soft palate.

Tracheobronchoscopy

Examination of the larynx, trachea, and primary bronchi of small animals was first described using human rigid bronchoscopes. Rigid, either hollow or solid, bronchoscopes are 40 cm in length and range in diameter from 4 to 9 mm and are suitable for

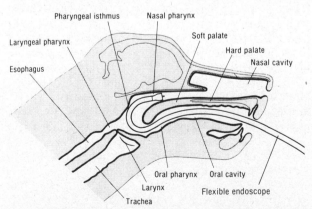

Figure 28–4. A diagrammatic representation of a flexible endoscope for examination of the nasopharynx and caudal aspects of the endoturbinates. (Reprinted with permission from Johnson, G. F., and Twedt, D. C.: Endoscopy and laparoscopy in the diagnosis and management in neoplasia in small animals. Vet. Clin. North Am. 7:77, 1977.)

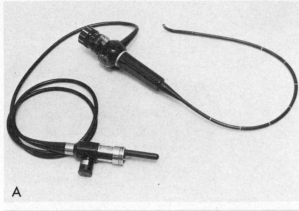

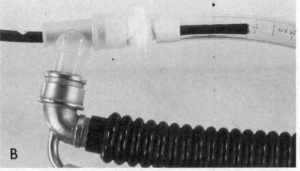

Figure 28–5. *A,* Olympus bronchofiberoscope Type B3 (5.9 mm diameter × 60 cm long). *B,* Endotracheal tube adaptor, which allows simultaneous gas ventilation and bronchoscopy.

examination of the larynx, trachea, and principal bronchi of most animals.[11, 17] The limitations are the length, which may be insufficient for some giant breeds, and the diameter, which may be too large for very small animals. Laparoscopes or small arthroscopes, may also be used to examine the larynx and trachea. All rigid instruments lack the versatility and diagnostic capabilities of flexible fiberoptic bronchoscopes, which can be selectively directed into secondary and tertiary bronchi.

Flexible endoscopic bronchoscopes range in diameter from 3 to 6 mm and are usually 40 cm long. These fiberoptic bronchoscopes can be used in all but the smallest dogs and cats.[9] General anesthesia is required, and, with a special adapter attached to an endotracheal tube, simultaneous bronchoscopy and ventilation through the endotracheal tube can be achieved (Fig. 28–5). The endotracheal tube size limits the size of the endoscope. In small dogs and cats, the bronchoscope must be directly placed down the trachea without an endotracheal tube, and assisted ventilation must be used.

Flexible bronchoscopes have a control lever that moves the distal tip in two directions and permits placement of the scope into specific bronchi.[15] Small biopsy forceps, brushes, or aspirating tubes can be passed down a biopsy channel. When required, oxygen or gas anesthesia can be passed through the same biopsy channel. Foreign bodies in the respira-

tory tree are often removed under endoscopic direction with small grasping forceps.

Pediatric gastrointestinal fiberoptic endoscopes (9 mm diameter or less) are usually adequate for tracheobronchoscopy if the patient's trachea is of sufficient size to safely accommodate the endoscope. A veterinary (small animal) endoscope (American Optical) has a small diameter and is suitable as both a bronchoscope and a gastrointestinal endoscope.

Thoracoscopy

This endoscopic technique involves the introduction of a solid rigid endoscope into the mediastinal space or pleural cavity to view and biopsy thoracic structures.[1, 4] An artificial pneumothorax must be induced, requiring general anesthesia and assisted ventilation. Standard abdominal laparoscopes have been used for thoracoscopic examination in the dog. Thoracoscopy in veterinary medicine is underutilized, and its indications and potential diagnostic capabilities must be established.

Gastrointestinal System

Esophagoscopy

Examination of the pharynx and esophagus in dogs and cats can be performed with either flexible or hollow rigid endoscopes. Flexible gastrointestinal endoscopes permit excellent examination of the esophagus and stomach. Human pediatric (9 mm diameter) endoscopes are easily passed through the esophagus of most small animals regardless of size. Flexible endoscopes are discussed in more detail under gastroscopy.

Rigid hollow esophagoscopes are used for visual examination, biopsy, and foreign body removal. These instruments are illuminated either with incandescent bulbs or through fiberoptics (Fig. 28–6). A 12-mm diameter endoscope can be passed down the esophagus of most small animals. For very large dogs, a minimum length of 75 to 80 cm is suggested.[10] An inexpensive rigid hollow veterinary gastroscope (Med-Tech, Inc.), which is powered by batteries and

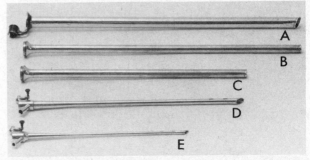

Figure 28–6. Rigid hollow endoscopes: (*A* and *B*) esophagoscopes, (*C–E*) bronchoscopes. An external incandescent light source is required for illumination.

has a hand inflation bulb, is suitable for examination of the esophagus. Standard proctoscopes can also be used for examination of the esophagus, but their usefulness is limited by their shorter length (approximately 25 cm).

Rigid esophagoscopes are generally preferred over flexible endoscopes for the removal of esophageal foreign bodies. The esophagus of dogs and cats can accommodate an endoscope of a surprisingly large diameter (10 to 30 mm). The largest possible instrument should be passed to separate the esophagus from the foreign body. Pronged grasping forceps are passed through the endoscope to the foreign body. Once the foreign body is grasped, the object and endoscope are both removed.

Gastroscopy

Gastroscopy is the endoscopic examination of the luminal surface of the stomach. Rigid endoscopes, either hollow tubes or solid optics, are of limited value in the examination of the small animal stomach. They have been useful in the removal of various gastric foreign bodies.

With the development of flexible fiberoptics, examination of the gastrointestinal system has improved. The entire stomach and proximal duodenum can now be adequately seen. With experience, the endoscope can often be passed through the pylorus into the duodenum.[16] Endoscopes used for examination of the stomach consist of a long, flexible insertion tube with a bending distal tip, an eyepiece, and a control section (see Fig. 28–3). The distal tip of the endoscope is directed through either a two- or four-way control knob in the handpiece. In addition to the fiber bundles, two channels are present. One allows a variety of endoscopic tools to be passed and fluids to be withdrawn. The other channel carries air for insufflation of the organ or water to wash away mucus and other material from the viewing window. A separate light source with a pump for instillation of fluid and air and a separate suction apparatus are required. Biopsy forceps, cytology brushes, aspirating tubes, snares, and grasping forceps are available.[5]

Most endoscopes are designed for human use, although less expensive veterinary endoscopes have been developed (American Optical). Gastroscopy is best performed with a human pediatric endoscope (see Fig. 28–3). These endoscopes have a diameter of about 9 mm and a working length of 110 cm, making them versatile for small dogs and cats as well as for giant breeds.[16] Used or rebuilt endoscopes are less expensive and can be obtained from most manufacturers. Gastrointestinal endoscopes with a diameter of greater than 12 mm have diminished flexibility and are limited to use in large dogs.

Colonoscopy

The flexible endoscopes described for gastroscopy are also suitable for colonoscopy. The advantage of flexible instruments is that the ileocolic sphincter and

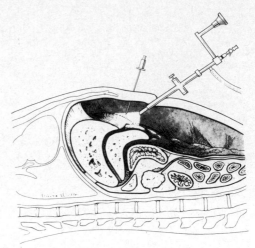

Figure 28–7. A laparoscope placed through the abdominal wall. A pneumoperitoneum is established to displace the abdominal wall from the viscera. A biopsy needle is passed through a second puncture site and guided under direct vision. (Reprinted with permission from Johnson, G. F., and Twedt, D. C.: Endoscopy and laparoscopy in the diagnosis and management of neoplasia in small animals. Vet. Clin. North Am. 7:77, 1977.)

ascending and transverse colons can be inspected and biopsied.

Rigid, distally illuminated proctoscopes or sigmoidoscopes (Welch Allyn) are used for the examination of the descending colon and rectum. Most small animals accommodate a standard human sigmoidoscope (23 mm diameter × 35 cm length). Small dogs and cats require a pediatric sigmoidoscope (11 mm diameter × 25 cm length). Since most colonic disease occurs in the descending colon and rectum, rigid endoscopes are in most cases quite suitable.[7]

Laparoscopy

Laparoscopy is an endoscopic procedure for the visual examination of the abdominal cavity and its contents. A rigid solid endoscope is introduced into the peritoneal cavity through a cannula, which has been passed through the abdominal wall with a trochar.[3] A pneumoperitoneum must first be established to raise the abdominal wall away from the viscera (Fig. 28–7). The site of introduction depends on the organs to be viewed and the specific objectives of the procedure. Frequently only sedation and a local anesthetic are required to perform laparoscopy.

Laparoscopy should not be considered an alternative to abdominal surgery; rather, it offers a less invasive technique for viewing and obtaining biopsies of certain organs. The liver, kidney, spleen, pancreas, and adrenal and prostate glands have been biopsied under laparoscopic direction.[12] Research groups in reproductive physiology find laparoscopy useful for examination and manipulation of the ovaries and uterus.[18] Certain surgical manipulations, such as splenic pulp pressure measurements, splenoportography, and cholecystocholangiography, have been performed under endoscopic direction.[5]

Standard laparoscopes range in diameter from 3 to 10 mm with a variety of viewing angles. The most

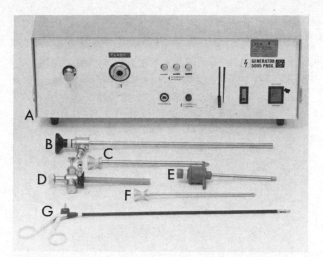

Figure 28–8. Laparoscopic equipment: (*A*) external light generator, (*B*) Wolf 180° viewing angle 8-mm diameter fiber light laparoscope, (*C*) trochar, (*D*) trochar sleeve with piston valve, (*E*) second puncture trochar sleeve and (*F*) trochar, (*G*) biopsy forceps. Not shown is a light transmitting cable.

popular instruments for use in small animals, regardless of size, are 5- to 8-mm diameter telescopes with 180° forward view. The basic laparoscopic set includes the telescope, trocar and cannula, light cable, light source, and a means for establishing a pneumoperitoneum (Fig. 28–8). Accessory equipment includes a second-puncture accessory trocar-cannula unit (3 or 6 mm in diameter) through which biopsy forceps, needles, and manipulating probes can be passed. Operating laparoscopes have an offset eyepiece and biopsy channel through which instruments can be passed. These operating laparoscopes have the disadvantage of being 10 mm or larger in diameter. A small arthroscope or Needlescope may be used in examining very small animals, but the amount of illumination given off and the small field of vision limit its use. It is possible to perform laparoscopy using a human sigmoidoscope, but the optical quality and operative capabilities are disappointing when compared with those of a standard laparoscope.[7]

Urogenital System

Endoscopic examination of the urogenital system is an uncommon procedure in small animals. Its usefulness is limited by available endoscopic equipment, small urethral diameter, and the constraints of an os penis in the male dog.

Cytoscopy and Urethroscopy

These procedures are limited to female dogs. Small-diameter rigid endoscopes or arthroscopes (1.7 to 3.0 mm in diameter) may be passed through the urethra and into the bladder of some female dogs. Cystoscopy in the bitch is limited by urethral diameter and length. Often standard arthroscopes are too short to reach the bladder in larger animals. Very

small flexible endoscopes or bronchoscopes have been passed into the bladders of some large female dogs. Human rigid cystoscopes with biopsy capabilities would be beneficial, but little clinical experience is reported with these instruments in veterinary medicine.

Vaginoscopy

Vaginoscopy is the endoscopic examination of the caudal reproductive tract in the bitch, including the mucosal aspect of the cervix, vagina, vestibule, and vulva. Successful examination of the caudal reproductive tract has been performed in dogs using either a small flexible gastrointestinal endoscope, a pediatric sigmoidoscope, or a rigid pediatric cystoscope (4.7 mm in diameter with an oblique viewing angle of 30°).[8] An outer removable cystoscope sheath that allows the introduction of gas through the sheath is required with vaginoscopy. Regardless of the endoscope type, a means of insufflating air into the vaginal canal to distend the lumen is required for complete visualization.

Examination of Joint Space

Arthroscopy is the endoscopic examination of the interior of the joint space. Small rigid arthroscopes or Needlescopes (1.5 to 2.5 mm in diameter) must be used. The usefulness of arthroscopy in small animals is limited by joint size. Visual examination of the canine stifle joint, including diagnostic evaluation of the condylar cartilage, ligaments, menisci, and joint capsule, has been reported.[14] Biopsies or surgical techniques through arthroscopic direction offer little promise because of the small joint space within which to work.

CARE AND MAINTENANCE

Properly cleaned and maintained endoscopic equipment is essential for conducting trouble-free endoscopic examinations. Poorly maintained or damaged equipment often makes a simple endoscopic examination difficult and eventually results in costly repairs. Manufacturer's instructions for care and cleaning should always be read and followed before the instrument is used.

Rigid endoscopes are more durable than their flexible counterparts. Care should be taken to keep light connections clean and protected. Fiberoptic light-carrying cables should be handled gently to avoid breakage of fiber bundles. Cleaning should be done with mild soap and sterilization with ethylene oxide or an antiseptic solution recommended by the manufacturer. Endoscopes with a solid lens system or fiberoptics should never be autoclaved.

Flexible fiberoptic endoscopes are extremely fragile. The glass fibers are protected by only a thin polyvinyl sheath. Sudden blows or acute bending of the endoscope usually results in breakage of glass fibers. Broken fibers in the optic bundles appear as black dots in the image. When damage is extensive both the light transmission and image projection are decreased. Animals should always be anesthetized and a mouth speculum used to protect the instruments. Flexible endoscopes should only be used at room temperature, because extreme cold will make the fibers brittle, resulting in breakage.

The endoscope should be cleaned after each examination. Body fluids and mucus left to dry will build up and eventually cause damage to the endoscope. The biopsy channel must be cleaned with a brush and flushed with a suitable antiseptic solution. The eyepiece and control unit should be wiped off but never immersed in any solution. The flexible shaft should be wiped down with an approved antiseptic solution or 70% alcohol. Complete sterilization of flexible endoscopes is usually not necessary but can be accomplished with ethylene oxide. The instrument should be hung in a cabinet to air dry. It is not advisable to store endoscopes in the manufacturer's storage case. Dampness or moisture retained in a closed case promotes rusting or corrosion of the parts.

SOURCE OF INSTRUMENTS

The following is a limited list of instrument sources. Additional information and possible modifications can be obtained from the manufacturers.

Arthroscopes and Laparoscopes

1. Richard Wolf Medical Instrument Corp., 7046 Lyndon Ave., Rosemont, Illinois 01801
2. Needlescope, Dyonics, Woburn, Massachusetts 01901.
3. Karl Storz Endoscopy America, Inc., 658 South San Vicente Blvd., Los Angeles, California 90048.
4. Eder Instrument Co., 5100 N. Ravenwood Ave., Chicago, Illinois 60640.

Flexible Fiberoptic Bronchoscopes and Gastrointestinal Endoscopes

1. Olympus Corp., Medical Instrument Division, 4 Nevada Dr., New Hyde Park, New York 11042.
2. Pentax Precision Instrument Corp., 55 Oak St., Norwood, New Jersey 07648.
3. American Cystoscope Makers, Inc., 300 Stillwater Ave., Stamford, Connecticut 06902.
4. Veterinary Endoscopes, American Optical Corp., Scientific Instrument Division, Buffalo, New York 14215.

Rigid Bronchoscopes, Esophagoscopes, and Proctoscopes

1. George P. Pilling & Son Co., Delaware Dr., Fort Washington, Pennsylvania 19034.
2. Richard Wolf Medical Instrument Corp., 7046 Lyndon Ave., Rosemont, Illinois 01801.
3. Welch Allyn Inc., State Street Rd., Skaneateles Falls, New York 13153.
4. Canine Gastroscope, Med-Tech, Inc., P.O. Box 338, Elwood, Kansas 66024.

Endoscopic Accessories

1. Medi-Tech, Inc., 150 Coolidge Ave., Watertown, Massachusetts 02172.

1. Bloomberg, A. E.: Thoracoscopy in perspective. Surg. Gynecol. Obstet. 147:433, 1978.
2. de Kock, M. A. (ed.): Equipment and technique. In Dynamic Bronchoscopy. Springer-Verlag, New York, 1977.
3. Harrison, R. M., and Wildt, D. E. (eds.): Laparoscopic instrumentation. In Animal Laparoscopy. Williams & Wilkins, Baltimore, 1980.
4. Hinkle, R. F.: Paratracheal mediastinotomy in the dog and cat. Vet. Med./Sm. Anim. Clin 75:1121, 1980.
5. Johnson, G. F.: Endoscopic examinations. In Anderson, N. V. (ed.): Veterinary Gastroenterology. Lea & Febiger, Philadelphia, 1980.
6. Johnson, G. F., and Twedt, D. C.: Endoscopy and laparoscopy in the diagnosis and management of neoplasia in small animals. Vet. Clin. North Am. 7:77, 1977.
7. Jones, B.: The use of endoscopy and laparoscopy as a diagnostic tool in veterinary medicine. Proc. 44th Ann. Mtg. Am. Anim. Hosp. Assoc., 1978, 241–244.
8. Lindsay, F. E. F.: The normal endoscopic appearance of the caudal reproductive tract of the cyclic and non-cyclic bitch: post-uterine endoscopy. J. Small Anim. Pract. 24:1, 1983.
9. McKiernan, B. C.: Lower respiratory tract disease. In Ettinger, S. J. (ed.): Textbook of Veterinary Internal Medicine, 2nd ed. W. B. Saunders, Philadelphia, 1982.
10. O'Brien, J. A.: Endoscopic examination. Part III. Esophagoscopy. In Anderson, N. V. (ed.): Veterinary Gastroenterology. Lea & Febiger, Philadelphia, 1980.
11. O'Brien, J. A., and Roszel, J. F.: Bronchoscopy and bronchial cytology. In Kirk, R. W. (ed.): Current Veterinary Therapy V. W. B. Saunders, Philadelphia, 1974.
12. Patterson, J. M.: Laparoscopy in small animal medicine. In Kirk, R. W. (ed.): Current Veterinary Therapy VII. W. B. Saunders, Philadelphia, 1980.
13. Prescott, R.: Optical principles of laparoscopy. In Harrison, R. M., and Wildt, D. E. (eds.): Animal Laparoscopy. Williams & Wilkins, Baltimore, 1980.
14. Siemering, G. H.: Arthroscopy of dogs. J. Am. Vet. Med. Assoc. 172:575, 1978.
15. Stradling, P.: Development of the bronchoscope. In Diagnostic Bronchoscopy. Churchill Livingstone, New York, 1981.
16. Twedt, D. C.: Diseases of the stomach. In Ettinger, S. J. (ed.): Textbook of Veterinary Internal Medicine, 2nd ed. W. B. Saunders, Philadelphia, 1982.
17. Venker-van Haggen, A. J.: Bronchoscopy of the normal and abnormal canine. J. Am. Anim. Hosp. Assoc. 15:397, 1979.
18. Wildt, D. E., Kunney, G. M., and Seager, S. W. J.: Laparoscopy for direct observation of internal organs of the domestic cat and dog. Am. J. Vet. Res. 38:1429, 1977.
19. Zimmer, J. F.: Gastrointestinal fiberoptic endoscopy. In Kirk, R. W. (eds.): Current Veterinary Therapy VII. W. B. Saunders, Philadelphia, 1980.

Chapter 29

Monitoring the Surgical Patient

Ronald J. Kolata

Introduction

Diseases, trauma, anesthesia, and surgery all have deleterious effects on a patient's ability to maintain a balanced internal environment (homeostasis). When several of these effects are combined, a patient's homeostatic mechanisms may be taxed beyond their abilities to maintain life. Monitoring of important physiological functions allows the surgeon to be aware of his patient's homeostatic state, to respond to adverse changes in it, and to prevent compensatory failure.

Monitoring involves measuring, recording, and evaluating physiological variables. Monitoring surgical patients began at the start of this century.[14] Harvey Cushing devised an "ether chart" to plot breathing and heart rates of patients during anesthesia. Not long after, T. C. Janeway began recording the breathing and pulse rates along with the systolic blood pressures of patients in hospital wards. With the development of cardiac surgery in the 1950s, monitoring of postoperative patients became highly organized and routine. In the early 1950s, the concept of monitoring surgical patients was introduced to veterinary medicine by F. P. Sattler.[48]

In the 1960s there was an explosion in the availability of electronic equipment that could convert physiological events into electronic signals that could be recorded as numerical values, e.g., arterial blood pressure and arterial blood gas values. Patient monitoring became easier to do at more frequent intervals and became more sophisticated with respect to the variables that could be monitored. The technology explosion continues, and presently recording devices are being connected to minicomputers that make computations and derive values that are more valuable than the raw data. Many new monitoring devices have built-in alarms when preset physiological limits are exceeded. Some are being connected to microprocessors programmed to make simple corrections, such as increasing or decreasing the rate of infusion of medication when preset physiological endpoints are passed. In the future, computer-controlled monitoring systems will be found in veterinary practice. But despite technological advances, there is not likely to be a combination of sensors, signal processors, microprocessors, and servomechanisms that will be able to take over in the care of a surgical patient. There will always be the need for the finely tuned senses and considered judgment of an experienced surgeon to select the variables to be monitored, to interpret the values obtained, and to adjust the treatment in light of the patient's overall condition.

GENERAL VARIABLES

Monitoring as a concept of medical care is a broad term and can include almost any repeated assessment of a patient. This chapter is confined to assessments most commonly made on the surgical patient during the operative period.

Studies have pointed to the critical role of cardiorespiratory functions with respect to survival or mortality in the operative and postoperative periods.[55] Fluid, electrolyte, and acid-base balance changes have also been shown to occur in surgical patients and to contribute to their survival or death.[60] Therefore, monitoring of surgical patients centers on assessment of cardiovascular and pulmonary functions and the status of body fluid compartments. Assessment of these physiological variables is done directly by specific observation and indirectly by measurement or observation of variables strongly influenced by the one of interest. For instance, measurement of body temperature is a direct observation, whereas measurement of urine output is often used to assess tissue perfusion. Ventilatory, blood and fluid, and circulatory variables for dogs and cats are presented in Table 29–1.

General Condition

The overall appearance of a patient is used as a nonspecific parameter of health status. It is the summation of the effects of many body functions and is a valuable part of any monitoring regimen.[46] Deviations from normal can be detected by simple observation of general condition, and, although the information it relates lacks specificity and objectivity, observation of overall condition is valuable for interpreting the significance of changes in other variables.

A patient's general condition includes variables such as alertness, muscle tone, posture, appetite, and pattern of breathing. Alertness, i.e., interest in the environment, depends largely on mental clarity, which is influenced by how well the brain is being oxygenated, by drugs, by the level of comfort the patient is experiencing, and by other undefined physiological and psychological changes accompanying illness and injury.[46] Muscle tone and posture are related and are influenced by muscle perfusion, pain, and the internal biochemical environment of the body. Although appetite is influenced by numerous factors, a normal appetite is a general sign of well being and a relatively normal internal environment. The pattern of breathing is a readily observed variable

TABLE 29–1. Normal Values For Some Physiological Variables in Dogs and Cats*

Variable	Dog	Cat†	Variable	Dog	Cat†
Ventilatory Variables			*Circulatory Variables*		
Breaths/min	16–30		Heart Beats/min	80–140	60–140
Tidal volume	10–15 ml/kg		Arterial pressure		
Pa_{O_2}	85–105		Systolic (direct)	100–156 mm Hg	
Pv_{O_2}	35–40		Systolic (indirect)	110–158 mm Hg	
Pa_{CO_2}	26–38		Mean (direct)	85–130 mm Hg	
Pv_{CO_2}	29–44		Mean (indirect)	80–110 mm Hg	
Arterial pH	7.33–7.45	7.29–7.40	Central venous pressure		
Venous pH	7.30–7.40	7.24–7.38	(mean)	1–4 mm Hg	
Hb saturation %	Arterial 95.97		(mean)	1–6 cm H_2O	
	Venous 65–75		Pulmonary artery pressure		
Blood and Fluid Variables			(systolic)	20–35 mm Hg	
			(diastolic)	8–15 mm Hg	
Sodium mEq/L (serum)	140–160		(mean)	10–16 mm Hg	
Potassium mEq/L (serum)	3.7–5.8	4.0–4.5	Pulmonary wedge pressure		
Chloride mEq/L (serum)	100–115	115–123	(mean)	6–10 mm Hg	
Bicarbonate mEq/L (serum)	16–23		(mean)	7–14 cm H_2O	
Total protein gm/dl	5.0–7.6	5.2–6.6	Cardiac index	1.8–3.5 L/m_2	
Hb gm/dl PCV	12–18	8–15	Tissue pH	7.31–7.42	
	35–49	27–45	Capillary refill time	1–2 sec	
Urine output	1.0–1.7 ml/kg/min	0.8–1.5 ml/kg/min			
Urine specific gravity	1.015–1.045	1.020–1.060			

*These variables have been gathered from many sources, the data from which have been averaged and rounded to clinically useful ranges.

†Data for cats are presented only if they differ from those for dogs. Also data for some variables are not available.

and is influenced by pulmonary function, oxygen consumption, pain, neurological state, acid-base status, drugs, and body temperature.

Body Temperature

Body temperature is controlled in the hypothalamus. Heat is produced by metabolism and heat conservation or dissipation is carried out through the ventilatory and cardiovascular systems. The body temperature of warm-blooded animals must be kept within a narrow range so that metabolic processes in tissues and organs can function optimally. Surgical patients experience changes in body temperature due to anesthesia, drugs, tissue injury, environmental exposure, and infection.[44]

Anesthetics depress the thermoregulatory center, making environmental exposure an important source of heat loss during surgery. During procedures in which body cavities are open, evaporative heat loss may be dramatic, particularly in small animals, which have a large surface area relative to body mass. Hypothermia should be avoided, as it decreases metabolic rate, slowing biotransformation of drugs and anesthetics, and thus prolonging their effects. Low body temperature during recovery from anesthesia causes the release of epinephrine and shivering, which increases oxygen consumption, placing increased demands on the cardiovascular system when it may already be taxed severely.[18]

Elevations in body temperature during anesthesia may signal the onset of malignant hyperthermia[44] or heat gain from a heating pad. Patients kept in oxygen cages, under heating lamps, or on heating pads may also have elevations in temperature. Elevations in body temperature within the first 24 hours after surgery are usually benign and due to tissue injury.

In addition to core temperature, skin temperature can be useful in monitoring the postoperative patient.[27] Since heat is carried to the extremities by blood flow and because skin vessels are under the control of the sympathetic nervous system,[31] measurement of the temperature of the skin between the third and fourth digits of the rear limb can be exploited to give information regarding peripheral perfusion.[32] With an ambient temperature of 20 to 23°C (68 to 74°F), the temperature of the toe web is 2 to 5°C (3 to 8°F) less than the rectal temperature of a dog with normal sympathetic tone, cardiac output, and local blood flow. When the difference between rectal and toe web temperature is greater than 6°C (10°F), peripheral perfusion is reduced, indicating vasoconstriction or obstruction to flow. Temperature differences greater than 20°C (35°F) indicate extreme vasoconstriction and are associated with severe shock. This measurement has been found to be of value in monitoring postoperative patients and is an accurate indicator of low cardiac output.[31,32]

Monitoring

Intraoperative temperature monitoring is most conveniently done using a thermistor probe and an electronic thermometer. During surgery, a temperature taken well down the esophagus (lower fourth) accurately reflects core temperature, as it is near the liver. Core temperature is not accurately reflected by a rectal or an esophageal probe if the abdominal or thoracic cavity, respectively, is open during surgery. After surgery, rectal temperature is most commonly monitored intermittently using a glass and mercury thermometer. Skin temperature is monitored with an electronic thermometer and thermistor or with a mercury thermometer with a scale between 20 and 40°C (60 and 110°F).

VENTILATORY VARIABLES

Breathing Pattern

The function of breathing is to exchange gases between the atmosphere and the blood. Breathing rate and character are influenced by pathological conditions and a wide range of reflexes. Breathing rate and character are not directly related to oxygen demand or the efficiency of ventilation.[39] Nonetheless, breathing rate, character, volume, and breath sounds are important indicators of changes in oxygen demand and effectiveness of breathing.[61]

Many conditions induce changes in the rate of breathing. During surgery, tachypnea can indicate a lightening of anesthesia, pain, or, if anesthesia is being maintained with a closed system, saturation of the CO_2 absorber. Bradypnea can be due to deepening anesthesia, stimulation of the vagus nerve, alkalosis, or hypocarbia. In the postoperative period, tachypnea can signal hemorrhage, pneumothorax, pulmonary edema, pneumonia, pain, or increased body temperature.

Changes in the pattern of breathing are signs of thoracic or pulmonary abnormalities. Breathing is deep and shows signs of increased effort, i.e., retraction of the thoracic inlet and intercostal muscles, if there is restriction of lung expansion by partial airway obstruction or effusion of fluid or blood. When restriction of expansion of the lungs or chest causes inspiration to become difficult and of low volume, expiration becomes active to force air out of the lungs rapidly so another breath can be taken. In this situation, ventilatory effort is obvious and an expiratory grunt may be heard. These abnormal patterns of breathing, although indicating problems within the ventilatory system, do not indicate inadequate blood oxygenation. Despite decreased tidal volume, the increases in rate may provide a great enough minute volume for adequate oxygenation.

Areas of diminished breath sounds indicating congestion, atelectasis, or effusion and wheeze and crackles indicating fluid or secretions in the airways and alveoli may be heard on auscultation. As with the patterns of breathing, abnormal breath sounds may not be associated with insufficient ventilation but are important in monitoring the course of the abnormality causing them.

Monitoring

Assessing and monitoring ventilatory efficiency is done by thoughtful observation, stethoscopy, ventilometry, and, when indicated, radiography. Table 29–1 shows the normal values for ventilatory variables.

Tidal volume can be estimated by observing the chest wall and, during anesthesia, the movement of the rebreathing bag. Placing an ear near the patient's mouth and nose to feel and hear the puff of air expired or holding a polished metal surface (e.g., mirror) in front of the nostrils so that the expired air and moisture create a haze on the polished surface is also a means of estimating tidal volume. The most objective method of assessing tidal volume is the use of a ventilometer attached by a short, ridged tube to a tight-fitting face mask or fitted tracheal tube.

Changes in the rate, character, and sounds of breathing do not correlate directly with changes in blood gas values and are only presumptive evidence of impaired ventilation. However, they are important signs and should be monitored routinely. These variables are monitored by thoughtful observation of the patient, stethoscopy, and, when indicated, thoracic radiography.

Blood Gases

Arterial blood gas measurements are used to assess the efficiency and adequacy of breathing and, in conjunction with mixed venous blood gas values, are used to assess tissue oxygenation.

Arterial CO_2 tension (Pa_{CO_2}) is used to characterize ventilatory status, elevated Pa_{CO_2} indicating hypoventilation and decreased Pa_{CO_2} indicating hyperventilation. Blood CO_2 in conjunction with blood pH is used to determine a patient's acid-base status, which is categorized as respiratory acidosis or alkalosis, metabolic acidosis or alkalosis, or mixed or compensated states. Respiratory acidosis is seen with accumulation of CO_2 through hypoventilation. Conversely, respiratory alkalosis is seen with excessive elimination of CO_2 due to hyperventilation. Metabolic acidosis is due to accumulation of nonvolatile acids such as lactic acid. Metabolic alkalosis comes about through loss of nonvolatile acids. This is seen when hydrochloric acid is lost through vomiting. Mixed states are created when the body attempts to compensate for one of these states (alkalosis or acidosis). An example is hypocarbia (respiratory alkalosis), which is the body's response to lactic acidosis in shock.

Arterial oxygen tension (Pa_{O_2}) is used to assess the efficiency of ventilation. It is only slightly influenced by the rate and depth of breathing. It is more strongly influenced by the balance between pulmonary blood flow and alveolar ventilation.[39] Problems that reduce the ratio of ventilated to perfused alveoli, such as pneumonia, pulmonary contusion, and atelectasis, cause a decrease in oxygen tension despite hyperventilation.

Blood oxygen tension informs the surgeon about the pressure gradients for the exchange of oxygen across cell membranes. Oxygen saturation informs him of the amount of oxygen held by hemoglobin (Hb). Hb concentration and saturation informs him of the amount of oxygen available to the body. Therefore, oxygen saturation of arterial and mixed venous blood is used to assess tissue oxygenation. If cardiac output and Hb concentration are known, oxygen availability and consumption can be calculated. These are extremely important variables for determining the efficiency of blood circulation and tissue metabolism.[55] Table 29–1 shows normal values of arterial and venous blood gases.

Monitoring

Blood samples for analysis are obtained from an artery. They are drawn under anaerobic conditions in heparinized syringes. If only acid-base status is of interest, venous blood is suitable. The sample should be analyzed immediately because gas exchange between the blood and the external environment proceeds through the plastic syringe wall. Samples can be stored in ice water for up to three hours without the development of clinically important changes.[23] Oxygen saturation can be measured using an oximeter. Two types are available: one monitors hemoglobin saturation intravascularly using a fiberoptic sensor, and the other has a sensor that is applied to an area with a dense superficial capillary bed uncovered by pigment, e.g., lip, tip of the tongue, or nasal septum.

Packed Cell Volume

Packed cell volume (PCV) is an important variable because of its association with oxygen transport.[11] Changes in PCV are commonly seen in surgical patients and are usually associated with blood loss or dehydration.[7]

Optimal PCV varies with the organ studied but appears to be in the range of 30 to 40 per cent at other than extreme altitudes.[14] Packed cell volumes above 45 per cent are associated with decreased oxygen transport due to decreased capillary flow. Low PCVs are tolerated if they develop slowly so that physiological compensation can be effective.[62] However, patients with abnormally low PCVs, i.e. less than 20, do not tolerate stress as well as those with normal PCVs.[7]

The oxygen demand of a postoperative patient may increase 20 to 50 per cent above baseline values.[52] If PCV is reduced by half, the patient's cardiac output must double to meet baseline requirements and must triple to meet maximum postoperative demand. Such increases may not be possible in very ill or hypovolemic patients.[6,7,47] Additionally, myocardial oxygenation is inadequate if PCV is acutely lowered to 20 per cent or less.[26] This corresponds to a Hb of 7 to 8 per cent.[26] If myocardial oxygenation is inadequate, left ventricular failure may develop, particularly when cardiac output must be elevated to meet postoperative oxygen demands.

In critically ill patients, a PCV in the range of 27 to 33 per cent (corresponding to a hemoglobin concentration of 10 to 12 per cent) has been found to be most compatible with survival.[7]

Monitoring

The color of the patient's mucous membrane is used as a crude estimate of PCV and hemoglobin content. Packed cell volume is conveniently monitored using capillary tubes and a microhematocrit centrifuge. Colorimetric methods are available to measure hemoglobin.

CIRCULATORY VARIABLES

Heart Rate

The heart is a pump. Its output depends on its rate of pumping and its stroke volume. Heart rate, although an important determinant of output, does not correlate directly with cardiac output. Nonetheless, rates outside the normal range, both high and low, are associated with reduced cardiac output.[35] Although the number of beats per minute alone does not describe cardiac function, trends in rate do reflect some changes in function. Pain and excitement cause transient elevations. A continuously high resting rate or a rate that is gradually increasing with time indicates hypoxemia, deteriorating myocardial function, or inadequate intravascular volume.[50] Bradycardia is caused by vagal stimulation during surgery, deep planes of anesthesia, and hypothermia. Bradycardia can reduce oxygen transport and allow development of dysrhythmias.

Heart rhythm is important with respect to rate and cardiac output. Dysrhythmias can be seen during anesthesia because of the effects of anesthetics, catecholamines, and myocardial hypoxia.[30] Ventricular dysrhythmias can elevate heart rate while decreasing cardiac output. Because optimal cardiac output is necessary for adequate oxygen delivery and because rate and rhythm influences output and cardiac work, these variables are important in surgical patients.

Monitoring

Heart rate can be measured by palpating the apex impulse on the chest wall or palpating the arterial pulse; by auscultation; by recording arterial pulse waves using a catheter, strain gauge, and recorder; or by electrocardiography.

Each of these methods has unique advantages and

disadvantages. Palpation of either the apex impulse or the arterial pulse detects cardiac activity but can be unreliable in obese patients and those in shock. In addition, palpation of the arterial pulse may be inaccurately low in patients with some dysrhythmias. Precordial and esophageal auscultation provides accurate assessment of rate and additionally provides some indication of the strength of cardiac activity, as the audible volume of the heart sounds roughly correlates with the strength of contraction and ejection volume.[40] Commercial amplifiers that can be connected to stethoscopes assist auscultation and make such monitoring during surgery more convenient.

An ultrasonic Doppler flow probe can be placed over a suitable artery and connected to a signal amplifier for continuous monitoring of the heart rate during surgery. The audible signal of each pulse wave can be heard and can be used to monitor heart rate and blood flow.[17] A disadvantage of this method is the probe's sensitivity to position and movement.

Electronic heart rate meters that trigger on the R wave can be used for continuous heart rate monitoring. Their usefulness is limited inasmuch as no information about the mechanical activity of the heart is obtained.

Direct recording of arterial pulse waves is highly accurate. Its disadvantages include its invasive nature and the expense of the equipment. However, it is highly desirable in critical cases when a beat-by-beat assessment of cardiac function is important, as it gives information concerning pressure and stroke volume and can detect ventricular dysrhythmias.[28] The method is described under Arterial Pressure.

Cardiac Electrical Activity

Depolarization and repolarization of cardiac muscle fibers are normally mechanical activities. During anesthesia and surgery and, under some circumstances, during recovery (e.g., after correction of gastric torsion), abnormal electrical activity is not uncommon. Factors influencing development of cardiac dysrhythmias include local myocardial injury, manipulation of the heart and other anatomical structures (e.g., trachea, abdominal viscera), hypothermia, hypoxemia, hypercarbia, acidosis, changes in potassium concentration, and the effects of drugs and anesthetics. In many instances there is a synergy between the inciting factor and the patient's sympathetic nervous system. An example is the depressing effect of halothane on the myocardium, which lowers the threshold for the arrhythmogenic effects of catecholamines. Because most of the events disposing to dysrhythmias occur during induction and recovery from anesthesia, ECG monitoring is important in all surgical patients. Seriously ill patients with problems associated with dysrhythmias, e.g., gastric dilation–torsion or myocardial contusion, require prolonged ECG monitoring through the recovery period.

Monitoring

ECG monitoring is ideally done using a recorder with an oscilloscope and a paper recorder. Since diagnostic quality recordings are not necessary and the position of the patient may preclude standard placement of electrodes, a three-lead system placed in an appropriate configuration on the chest wall and using modified alligator clips, needle electrodes, or mini towel clips can be used to obtain tracings from leads II and III. Proper grounding of the patient is important. Satisfactory grounding reduces interference due to other electrical equipment and the chance of burns when an electrosurgical instrument is used.

Arterial Pulse

The arterial pulse is a product of left ventricular contraction. Its character depends on stroke volume, rate and force of ejection, and vascular tone. Palpation of the pulse is a time-honored way to quickly and easily make a subjective evaluation of cardiovascular function. Some points regarding propagation of the arterial pulse must be kept in mind. The character of the pulse changes as it proceeds distally.[49] The amplitude increases and duration decreases from the aorta to the periphery. This means that the peripheral pulse feels sharper than a more central pulse.

Variations in the determinants of pulse character change it in definable ways. A small stroke volume ejected rapidly into a vascular tree having increased tone, as seen in patients in early shock, produces a sharp, high-amplitude, short-duration pulse in the femoral artery and an imperceptible pulse in a distal artery. Conversely, a normal volume ejected with less than normal vigor into a dilated vascular tree, as may exist during anesthesia, produces a soft, low-amplitude, long-duration pulse in the femoral artery and a weak distal pulse.

Palpation of proximal and distal artery pulses allows crude estimation of blood pressure. The weaker the proximal pulse and the more difficult it is to palpate the distal pulse, the lower blood pressure is likely to be.

Palpating the arterial pulse can also assist in detecting and monitoring some dysrhythmias, as rhythm is irregular and pulse strength varies irregularly.

Monitoring

The arterial pulse is most readily monitored by palpating a peripheral artery. The femoral artery is most commonly used, but the lingual, labial, brachial, distal ulnar, cranial tibial, plantar, and median coccygeal arteries can also be used.

To obtain the most information when palpating arterial pulses, familiarity with the character of the normal pulses of animals is necessary. Variations from the expected character or rate should initiate more objective investigation and assessment of the cardiovascular system.

Arterial Pressure

Arterial pressure depends on cardiac output and vascular tone. A range of arterial pressures can be found among normal animals, and the pressure can vary from minute to minute in an individual.[24,42] The variation is within a relatively narrow range, as pressure must be maintained to allow autoregulation of blood flow within organs. If arterial pressure is below a mean pressure of about 60 mm Hg, blood flow within organs becomes pressure-dependent, and perfusion is inadequate and organ function will begin to fail.

Monitoring

Arterial pressure can be estimated by palpation of the pulse, or it can be measured directly or indirectly. Direct measurement of arterial pressure is best accomplished using a saline-filled intra-arterial catheter, a transducer, a signal processor, and a recorder (Fig. 29–1). This method gives accurate systolic and diastolic pressures recorded as pulse waves, which can be permanently recorded for further evaluation. Alternatively, arterial pressure can be directly measured using an aneroid or mercury manometer connected to the arterial catheter by a tube with an air column in its proximal segment to prevent fluid or blood from entering the manometer. Systems with a manometer and integral air space barrier are available commercially. The signal obtained by these methods of direct measurement is damped, and only a mean value is reliable. Direct arterial pressure measurement is accurate and has the advantage of allowing access to arterial blood for blood gas analysis. However, direct measurement has the distinct disadvantage of being invasive; complications such as thrombosis, embolization, hemorrhage, and infection can occur, and frequent nursing care is required. Also, the electronic equipment is expensive and requires maintenance.

The femoral artery is commonly used for direct measurement by either percutaneous catheterization or surgical cutdown. If a cutdown is used, the cranial saphenous artery may be more suitable, as it is more superficial than the femoral artery and at a more distal position on the animal's leg, making it easier to secure the catheter by bandaging.

Blood pressure is indirectly measured most conveniently using either of two types of ultrasonic detectors. One is a flow detector that detects the movement of red cells, and the other detects movement of the arterial wall as it moves with the pulse wave. These detectors are used with a pneumatic cuff to occlude flow and an aneroid manometer to measure pressure. Both of these detectors are accurate and correlate well with direct measurements if a proper width cuff is used.[15] Two disadvantages of indirect measurement are that at low pressure, it may be difficult to find a peripheral artery over which to place a sensor and that it is least accurate at low pressures, the pressure range of most interest. Another disadvantage is that sensor location is critical and is easily disturbed by patient movements. Nonetheless, indirect blood pressure measurement is relatively inexpensive, easy, noninvasive, and safe, and, as mentioned previously, the flow detector can be used to monitor heart rate and blood flow as well as pressure. Aneroid manometers used for either direct or indirect pressure measurements should be calibrated periodically to ensure accuracy.

Central Venous Pressure

Blood pressure in the cranial vena cava and intrathoracic portion of the caudal vena cava depends on intrathoracic pressure, tone of capacitance vessels, blood volume, rate of venous return, and right ventricular function. Central venous pressure (CVP) is used clinically to monitor fluid volume infusion because of its relationship to blood volume, although this relationship is indirect. When right ventricular function is adequate, CVP is controlled by the tone of the capacitance vessels and by intrathoracic pressure. Only when blood volume or venous return exceeds the upper or lower limits of possible venous compensation is CVP outside the normal range. The ability of changes in venous tone to compensate for changes in volume makes following trends in CVP during volume therapy a more reliable guide than simply making isolated measurements.

Central venous pressure does not reflect pulmonary venous or left atrial pressure and therefore

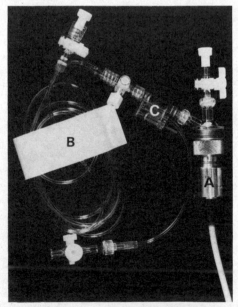

Figure 29–1. Transducer (A) and connector tubing (B) with valve for continuous flushing (C) for monitoring vascular pressures.

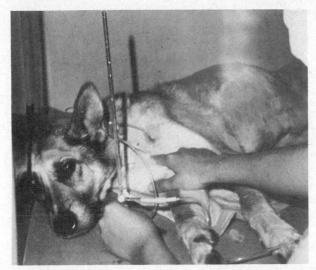

Figure 29–2. Central venous pressure monitoring. A saline manometer is being used. The zero point (manubrium) is verified before a reading is taken.

cannot reliably identify conditions disposing to pulmonary edema.[8] However, in patients without pulmonary vascular disease or left ventricular failure, these facts do not interfere with its value as a guide for fluid volume replacement.[42]

Monitoring

Central venous pressure is measured using a large-bore catheter inserted into the cranial vena cava near the right atrium. The catheter is commonly connected to a saline-filled manometer and CVP is read in cm of saline. Because of the low pressures measured, the technical aspects of CVP monitoring are crucial if accuracy and reliability are to be achieved.[20] Catheter position and 0 calibration are important and should be verified before measurements are made (Fig. 29–2). Radiography is the most accurate way of determining catheter position, but it is more convenient to assume accurate placement by seeing pressure fluctuations of about 5 mm of saline corresponding to respiratory pressure changes in the pleural cavity. The measurement reference point must be at the level of the right atrium. The system should be flushed to remove all air bubbles and clear the catheter. The position of the catheter tip and the reference point must be verified before each measurement. Pressure readings should be taken over several breathing cycles to ensure accuracy. Even though every effort is made to follow proper technique, values obtained by a saline manometer can be falsely high by as much as 2 to 4 cm H_2O owing to the slow frequency response of the system.[36] The most accurate measurement of CVP involves a transducer and electronic recorder.

Pulmonary Arterial and Wedge Pressures

Pulmonary arterial systolic pressure is the highest pressure generated by the right ventricle and is normally about one-fifth of left ventricular systolic pressure. Pulmonary arterial diastolic pressure reflects pulmonary vascular resistance and pulmonary wedge pressure, which, when correlated with pulmonary capillary pressure, reflect left atrial pressure.[42]

These pressures are used to assess right ventricular function, pulmonary vascular tone, and, in conjunction with systemic arterial pressure, left ventricular function. Key variables are pulmonary arterial diastolic pressure and pulmonary wedge pressure. These reflect pulmonary vascular resistance and left ventricular filling pressure, respectively. Wedge pressure reflects the ability of the left ventricle to pump the blood presented to it and, therefore, provides information about the likelihood of pulmonary edema formation and left ventricular function during volume replacement. These measurements are most valuable in patients whose left ventricular function is likely to fail, i.e., those with pre-existing heart disease or recovering from severe or prolonged hypotension.

Monitoring

Pulmonary arterial and wedge pressures are measured using a balloon-tipped catheter (Swan-Ganz catheter) inserted via the jugular vein (Fig. 29–3) by cutdown or percutaneously using a special introducer. The balloon allows the catheter to be carried in the stream of blood passing through the right ventricle and on into the pulmonary artery. With the catheter in the pulmonary artery as confirmed by pressure measurement (Fig. 29–4) and with the balloon still inflated, the catheter is secured, the balloon is deflated, and pulmonary arterial pressure is recorded. The balloon is re-inflated when wedge pressure is to be measured. Insertion and proper placement of the catheter require some training and are best achieved under visual control using a fluoroscope. The pressures are best measured using a transducer and recorder; however, an aneroid or

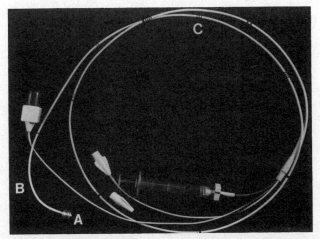

Figure 29–3. A balloon-tipped catheter with thermistor for measuring thermodilution cardiac output. There is a lumen open at the distal end (*A*), a thermistor 5 cm proximal to the balloon (*B*), and a lumen open 30 cm proximal to the balloon for injection of the indicator solution (*C*).

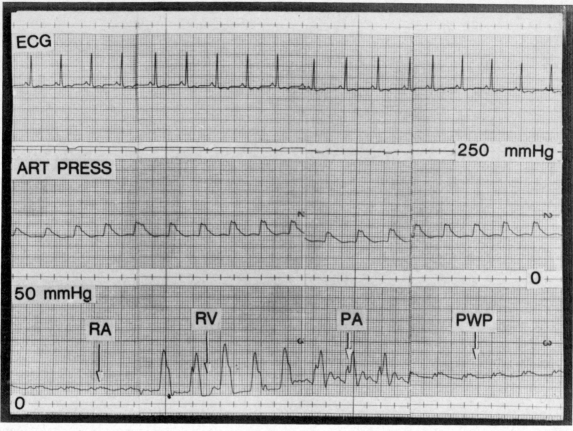

Figure 29–4. A strip chart recording of pressure measurements recorded as a Swan-Ganz catheter is advanced from the right atrium into the pulmonary artery and wedged. RA = Right atrial pressure; RV = right ventricular pressure; PA = pulmonary artery pressure; PWP = pulmonary wedge pressure.

saline manometer can be used. This monitoring method has the disadvantages of other invasive techniques plus the problems associated with balloon malfunction.

Cardiac Output

Cardiac output (CO) is the volume of blood pumped per unit time and is a product of heart rate and stroke volume and, therefore, an important determinant of oxygen transport. Cardiac output is influenced by venous return, peripheral resistance, blood volume, heart rate, stroke volume, and cardiac contractility. At rest under normal conditions, CO is approximately equal to blood volume but varies widely to maintain adequate oxygen delivery to all tissues. After moderate to major surgical stress, resting CO may be increased by 5 to 30 per cent.[2]

Perhaps the most important use of CO measurement is in combination with arterial and venous oxygen saturation values to calculate oxygen transport and consumption parameters.[55] These parameters have been found to be excellent indicators of tissue perfusion and cell metabolism. Cardiac output divided by the patient's body surface area in m^2 provides the cardiac index (CI), a frequently used variable that allows comparison between patients.

Monitoring

Cardiac output can be calculated using oxygen consumption measurements or measured using indicator dilution methods. Either dye or temperature is used as an indicator. The development of balloon-tipped catheters with thermistors at their distal ends along with minicomputers has made thermodilution cardiac output determination the most commonly used clinical method.[34] It is rapid, reliable, safe, easy, and repeatable. It can be used in small patients because it does not require removal of blood; this makes it a potentially useful technique in veterinary medicine. Presently the necessary equipment is expensive, limiting its veterinary application. Cardiac output can be estimated by measuring heart rate or pulse quality or pressure along with parameters of tissue perfusion. These are evaluated in light of their relationship to blood flow, and CO is described as adequate or inadequate.

Tissue pH

The pH of interstitial fluid is normally very near that of blood.[4] Under conditions of poor tissue perfusion, pH of the interstitial fluid (tissue pH) is less than that of arterial blood. This results from elaboration of lactic acid into tissue space because of anaerobic metabolism of the cells. The difference between arterial pH and tissue pH closely follows changes in local blood flow. As a result, measurement of tissue pH is used to assess tissue perfusion and has been found to be very useful.[12]

Monitoring

Tissue pH is monitored using a special pH electrode and a pH meter. The electrode is placed on the surface of a superficial muscle after a cutdown has been done. The electrode is secured by a bandage.[12] This method of monitoring tissue perfusion is simple and needs only relatively inexpensive equipment. Needle electrodes that do not require surgical cutdown are being developed. When needle electrodes are perfected, monitoring tissue pH will be simplified further and may be very useful in veterinary practice.[57]

Capillary Refill Time

Capillary refill time (CRT) is a simple method for assessing tissue perfusion. When arterial pressure is reduced, or, more importantly, when arterial and arteriolar vasoconstriction are present, perfusion of a capillary bed is diminished and slower than normal. Consequently, mucous membranes are pale and, if an area of membrane is blanched by pressure of a fingertip, on release of that pressure blood flow and hence return of color into the area are slower than normal. CRT reflects vasomotor tone and not blood pressure. Low pressure with vasodilation as in a deeply anesthetized or recently expired patient can result in a normal CRT, whereas an apprehensive patient with, therefore, peripheral vasoconstriction with normal blood pressure may have a prolonged CRT.

Monitoring

Capillary refill time can be assessed using accessible nonpigmented oral mucous membranes. Digital pressure is applied for a short time (one to two seconds) and rapidly released. The time needed for the blanched area to return to the color of the surrounding membrane is CRT. Using a stopwatch to time the return of color allows consistency in evaluation. However, CRT is generally judged as normal or abnormal by simple observation. The patient's PCV and the incident light affect recognition of the return of color, and changes in them should be taken into account when judging changes in CRT.

BODY FLUID VARIABLES

Urine Output

The kidneys regulate the volume, toxicity, and chemical composition of the extracellular fluid; in doing so, they receive about 20 per cent of the CO.[33] Important influences on urine output from normal kidneys are the intravascular volume, the extracellular sodium concentration, and the toxicity of extracellular fluid.

Intravascular volume is an extremely important stimulus for changes in urine output. Decreases in intravascular volume cause an increase in antidiuretic hormone secretion with a decrease in urine volume. As volume is further decreased, glomerular filtration pressure is decreased and further reduction in urine volume occurs.[38] If mean arterial pressure decreases to about 60 mm Hg, renal autoregulation fails, glomerular filtration stops, and urine production ceases. Because of these renal responses to intravascular volume and pressure changes, measuring urine output provides information about fluid volume and intravascular pressure and, by inference, tissue and organ perfusion.

Monitoring

Urine output measurement requires collection and measurement of urine produced during a preselected interval. The most effective method of collecting urine is by means of an indwelling urethral catheter that continuously empties into a closed sterile container. Intermittent drainage using an indwelling catheter can be done by occluding the catheter between collections. This method is subject to error by urine loss around the catheter if the bladder distends between collections. The catheter must be aseptically inserted and managed to avoid urinary tract infection. Measurement of the specific gravity of the urine as well as the volume collected provides additional information about intravascular volume and fluid balance. Noting the color of the urine collected can be important in the early detection of hemoglobinuria due to hemolysis during transfusion or cardiovascular surgery.

Fluid Balance

Fluid is the major constituent of the body; it bathes and passes into and out of cells, and it transports nutrients and metabolic products between tissues and organs. The volume and distribution of fluid in the three major body compartments must be normal to maintain a constant and adequate exchange of nutrients and metabolic products throughout the body. Osmotic forces maintain the volume of these compartments in a close relationship. Water is translocated from the extracellular to the intracellular compartment and back again as it is lost or gained by the body.

A common problem seen in surgical patients is the loss of extracellular fluid, which occurs through hemorrhage, loss of gastric or intestinal fluid, sequestration of fluid in injured or inflamed tissues or body cavities, and water deprivation.[53]

A less common, or perhaps less commonly recognized, problem is overhydration. This can come about through the neurohumoral response to trauma, anesthesia, surgery, and shock wherein increased amounts of antidiuretic hormone and aldosterone are secreted.[19] Water and sodium are retained despite restoration of a normal circulatory blood volume.[1] Inappropriate or careless fluid therapy can compound and exaggerate this problem.[19]

Monitoring

Fluid balance can be monitored by assessing a number of volume-dependent variables and measuring input and output.

Weighing a patient twice daily is a means of monitoring fluid balance. Body weight fluctuates rapidly with water gain or loss. In the fasting postoperative patient, a slow, constant loss of weight is expected, and sudden gains or losses can be attributed to fluid retention or dehydration.

Changes in physical signs of hydration, such as skin turgor, when assessed carefully, can provide information about fluid balance. Care should be taken in selecting a skin site for testing. Thick skin or skin under tension does not accurately reflect the state of hydration.

Since the kidney plays a key role in regulating water balance, urine output and urine specific gravity are important variables in assessing fluid balance, particularly when matched with measurement of fluid input.[33] In the absence of renal tubular disease, urine specific gravity within the normal range suggests adequate hydration; elevated specific gravity indicates conservation of water and suggests dehydration, and low specific gravity suggests the converse.[13]

Measurement of PCV and plasma or serum total solids (TS) with a refractometer is also an important means of assessing fluid balance.[56] In the absence of ongoing red cell or protein loss, PCV and TS are inversely related to intravascular water concentration and elevated levels point to dehydration.

Because they lack specificity, several of the variables discussed should be monitored concurrently and considered in relation to one another so that a fairly accurate estimate of fluid balance can be made.

Acid-Base Balance

Acid-base abnormalities are common in surgical patients. They may occur before surgery as part of the disease problem requiring treatment and may develop during anesthesia and surgery and the postoperative period. Of the four classically described acid-base states, perhaps the most commonly encountered are respiratory and metabolic acidoses along with mixed states.[3] Respiratory acidosis develops during hypoventilation, as can happen during anesthesia or due to depressant drugs, e.g., xylazine,

TABLE 29–2. Changes in Some Variables Associated with Acidemia

Variable	Respiratory Acidosis	Metabolic Acidosis	Mixed States* A	B
P_{CO_2}	> 38	< 33	> 38	< 33
pH	< 7.35	< 7.35	7.35	7.35
HCO_3	> 16	< 16	< 16	> 16

*A represents respiratory acidosis with metabolic compensation.

B represents metabolic acidosis with respiratory compensation.

morphine, or droperidol-fentanyl. Metabolic acidosis is seen in patients with poor tissue perfusion during shock and prolonged anesthesia.[22] Mixed states occur in the pre- and postoperative periods as a result of compensation for primary imbalances; e.g., metabolic alkalosis due to vomiting and pyloric obstruction stimulates a compensatory respiratory acidosis.[3,22]

Perhaps the most important effects of acid-base changes are on the heart and oxygen transport (Table 29–2). Acidosis depresses ventricular function when severe (pH 7.2), and alkalosis (pH 7.5) inhibits oxygen delivery to tissues by shifting the oxygen hemoglobin dissociation curve to the right.[10,21,58] Acid-base changes also influence the distribution of electrolytes.

Monitoring

Acid-base balance is most rapidly and accurately assessed by measuring blood pH and CO_2 tension with a blood gas analyzer. With these variables and a nomograph, acid-base status is determined.

Another method of assessing acid-base status is titrating an anaerobically obtained blood sample with acid to determine bicarbonate content. If pH is unknown, errors in interpreting the titration results occur, as the effects of metabolic alkalosis and compensation for respiratory acidosis raise plasma bicarbonate and the effects of metabolic acidosis and compensation for respiratory alkalosis decrease plasma bicarbonate.[53]

Serum Protein

Serum proteins are important components of the internal environment.[29] They have several vital functions; globulins produced by lymphocytes are active in specific immunity, and alpha globulins produced by the liver are important in nonspecific immune responses. This nonspecific response has been shown to be important after trauma or surgery.[43] The albumin component of serum protein is the single most important species.[29] Albumin is important for maintenance of plasma volume and proper hydration of tissue through its colloid osmotic effect. It is an important binding and transport system for drugs, metabolism products, and hormones, and it is a reserve of protein for catabolism and repair.

These functions are so important that patients with hypoproteinemia, particularly hypoalbuminemia, have higher complication and mortality rates than those with normal protein concentrations.[43,54] Surgical patients lose protein owing to pre-existing diseases, hemorrhage, and tissue injury and through inflamed and traumatized mesothelial membranes and tissue surfaces during surgical procedures.[25,51,54]

Monitoring

Total protein and albumin can be measured by colorimetric methods. Total protein can also be measured by a refractometer using the plasma obtained by determining PCV.

Electrolytes

Electrolyte abnormalities are linked to fluid imbalance and acid-base abnormalities and are found pre- and postoperatively. Fluid and electrolyte losses take place in the presence of conditions such as vomiting, diarrhea, gastrointestinal obstruction, and peritonitis. Each of these problems causes loss of a particular combination of electrolytes, allowing imbalances to develop.[13] Electrolyte abnormalities can be caused by inappropriate or excessive fluid therapy and chronic diuretic or steroid therapy. After surgery, electrolyte abnormalities can arise owing to lack of intake, in the case of potassium, or retention, in the case of sodium and water.[19,37]

Sodium is the major extracellular cation and is the electrolyte primarily responsible for maintaining the tonicity of extracellular fluid.[45] Sodium is lost through vomiting and diarrhea and when extracellular fluid is sequestered in injured tissues or body cavities. In these instances, sodium is lost with water and the serum or plasma concentration of sodium is normal. Hypernatremia occurs if water loss is in excess of sodium. This is rarely seen but may occur in patients with large evaporative water losses who are unable to drink. Hyponatremia occurs when water loss is less than sodium loss, as in hyperadrenocorticism. Hyponatremia may also occur in patients whose antidiuretic hormone response to anesthesia, surgery, or hypovolemia is coupled with inappropriate fluid replacement.[1,19,53]

Potassium is the other major cation. Its concentration in the extracellular fluid is low and must be kept within a narrow range to ensure normal neuromuscular and cardiac function. Potassium concentration in the extracellular fluid is affected by acid-base balance, being elevated during acute acidosis and depressed during alkalosis.[54] Therefore, patients with uremia, hypoadrenocorticism, and severe metabolic acidosis often also have hyperkalemia. Hyperkalemia can also be seen transiently after massive tissue trauma.

Hypokalemia may be the most common electrolyte abnormality to develop in surgical patients.[51] Potassium is not conserved as avidly by the kidneys as is sodium. Therefore, patients that are not eating and that have conditions predisposing to potassium loss deplete their potassium pool and develop hypokalemia, as in patients presented because of vomiting due to a gastrointestinal obstruction. Such a patient may not eat for several days after surgery and is likely to develop hypokalemia.

Chloride is the major extracellular cation, and its movements are associated with those of sodium.[54] To maintain electrochemical neutrality, chloride varies inversely with bicarbonate, and therefore changes in its concentration are associated with acid-base changes. Hyperchloremia can be seen in acidosis, and hypochloremia can be seen in alkalosis.

Monitoring

Physical signs of major electrolyte abnormalities are nonspecific and apparent only at concentration extremes. The most accurate and reliable method of determining sodium, potassium, and chloride concentrations is either flame photometry or ion-selective electrodes. Photometric and titration methods are also available for determining chloride.

Clinically important changes in potassium can be detected and monitored by interpreting the ECG.[5] Hyperkalemia tends to impair conduction from the sinoatrial nodes to the atrioventricular node. At potassium concentrations of 6.0 to 6.5 mEq/L, peaked T waves are seen. Wide QRS complexes and flattened P waves are associated with potassium concentrations of 6.5 to 7.0 mEq/L. Atrial standstill, depressed S-T segments, and wide QRS complexes are seen when potassium reaches 7.0 to 9.0 mEq/L, and cardiac arrest can occur at concentrations greater than 9.0 mEq/L.

Hypokalemia tends to increase the rate of discharge of nodal tissue and decreases conduction through the ventricle. In hypokalemia, ECG findings include bradycardia, prolonged Q-T interval, and small biphasic T waves. Hypokalemia is not as accurately detected by ECG as is hyperkalemia.

Hypoxemia causes changes in the ECG, which may be confused with changes in potassium concentration. However, hypoxemia causes peaking of T waves and elevation of the S-T segment[5] without the P wave and QRS changes seen with potassium abnormalities.

PATHOPHYSIOLOGICAL BASIS FOR MONITORING

All surgical patients require some monitoring during their course of treatment to detect complications associated with anesthesia, emergence from anesthesia, and the surgical procedure. Even the normal patient presented for a minor elective procedure must have its vital functions monitored during anesthesia and recovery. It is obvious that the patient coming to surgery needs diligent care because of preexisting abnormalities and the superimposition of the additional stresses due to anesthesia and surgery.

Stimulus response patterns affecting homeostasis among surgical patients have been defined and characterized.[59] The stimuli are tissue injury, circulating volume reduction, low blood flow and tissue hypoxia, invasive infection, and starvation. One, two, or all of these stimuli may affect a particular surgical patient. Stimulation may begin before surgery and may continue through convalescence. The physiological responses to these stimuli are neuroendocrine and metabolic and can cause sweeping changes in a patient's internal environment. The specific response pattern found in each patient varies with the intensity and nature of the stimulus. Circulating volume reduction, tissue anaerobiosis, and invasive infection, stimuli that most adversely affect cellular homeostasis, cause the most profound and intensive response. Particularly important in response to these stimuli is the outpouring of catecholamines, which should be prevented or checked as soon as possible. Prevention or reduction of high circulating catecholamine levels halts or prevents adverse circulatory and catabolic effects, thus allowing stabilizing and anabolic neuroendocrine reactions to predominate and restore homeostasis.

The underlying goal of monitoring is to ensure that the internal environment of the patient remains within limits that allow normal metabolism at least in vital organs and optimally in the entire body.[9] In general, this means there must be an adequate delivery of oxygenated blood to all organs. Consequently, surgical monitoring centers on assessing and controlling cardiovascular and ventilatory variables. Attention to variables reflecting fluid, electrolyte, and acid-base balance controls only cardiopulmonary function.

The particular monitoring regimen chosen for a patient depends on several criteria: (1) the physiological abnormalities and the severity of their deviation from normal as detected on preoperative evaluation; (2) the changes expected due to anesthesia and surgery; and (3) the magnitude of physiological change expected in the postoperative period.[16] Selection of a specific variable to be monitored depends on its specificity for signalling changes in the function of interest. If, for example, there is a need to monitor the heart because of a potential risk of dysrhythmias, monitoring ECG is preferable to monitoring heart rate because ECG has the specificity for detecting and evaluating dysrhythmias. The selection of parameters also depends on their risk-benefit ratio. For instance, direct arterial pressure monitoring is of benefit despite the risk of complications when accurate information regarding peak systolic and diastolic pressures and pulse contour is important. Indirect measurements are safer and, therefore, of less risk but of equal benefit when peak systolic or mean arterial pressures alone are needed. Finally, the selection of the monitoring regimen depends on the availability of equipment and an appropriately skilled staff to make the measurements, evaluate their significance, and take the appropriate therapeutic steps. Much of the information needed to make appropriate clinical decisions is derived from many different variables. The information they relate must be integrated and interpreted over a prolonged period before a recognizable trend becomes apparent. Rarely does a single bit of data or even continuous monitoring of a single variable give enough information to reliably guide treatment. The adequacy of blood volume and circulation, for instance, can only be determined indirectly. To obtain an accurate picture, several variables must be monitored. Heart rate, pulse character, arterial pressure, CVP, urine output, and skin temperature when monitored concurrently and evaluated according to their relationships to one another as influenced by blood volume and distribution will allow the surgeon to make valid judgments about his patient's circulating volume. Some variables are rather specific. Blood gas determination is a reliable and accurate way of determining ventilation efficiency. If this test is not available, however, the surgeon must evaluate a number of less objective variables, i.e., breathing rate, breath volume, character of breathing, heart rate, ECG, and color of peripheral tissues.

Standard Monitoring

The monitoring regimen selected for a particular patient must be tailored to individual needs and circumstances. Three groups of surgical patients and their general needs, as defined by the stimulus response patterns, can be described[63] (Table 29–3). These can be used as starting points for developing monitoring regimens for particular patients.

Category I (Low Risk)

This category includes patients with minor tissue injury and no injuries within a major body cavity. These patients experience only minimal blood or fluid losses and no hypotension. There is little chance of invasive infection developing, and the expected period of starvation is short. Most healthy patients with minor injuries and those undergoing elective surgery are in this category. The monitoring required by these patients is minimal, as their homeostatic reserves are intact and are only compromised briefly during anesthesia. The stimuli of surgery and subsequent recovery are also minimal.

The variables to be monitored include general condition, pulse rate and quality, ventilatory rate and character, CRT, and body temperature. Surveillance is frequent during surgery and recovery from anesthesia. It becomes less so as the patient's protective reflexes return to normal and body functions stabilize.

TABLE 29–3. Basic Monitoring for Patients in Categories I Through III

Variable	Category I	Category II	Category III
General condition	+	+	+
Rectal temperature	+	+	+
Breathing rate	+	+	+
Pulse rate	+	+	+
Capillary refill time	+	+	+
Packed cell volume	±	+	+
Serum total solids	±	+	+
Urine output		+	+
Skin temperature		+	+
Electrocardiogram		±	+
Central venous pressure		±	+
Systemic arterial pressure		±	+
Blood gases and pH			+
Serum electrolytes			+
Body weight			+
Pulmonary artery/wedge pressure			±
Tissue pH			±
Tidal volume			±
Cardiac output			±

Note: ± indicates that the variable may be important but not vital in that category of patients.

Category II (Moderate Risk)

These patients have moderate tissue injury with a large volume of tissue involved. Blood and fluid losses are significant but are replaced rapidly, and hypovolemia and hypotension are short-lived. A major body cavity is entered, and the chance of invasive infection is present. The anticipated period of starvation does not exceed 72 hours.

This category includes patients undergoing major elective surgery such as comminuted femoral fracture. Because of the greater deviation from normal (actual or expected owing to the more intense stimulus response pattern), monitoring for these patients must be more intense than for patients in the previous category. Variables such as CVP, urine output, and arterial blood pressure are measured in addition to the basic variables. Blood sampling for laboratory analysis of PCV and TS is often also necessary. The patient is monitored frequently during surgery and in the postoperative period for up to 48 hours, since restoration of a normal internal environment may take several days.

Category III (High Risk)

This category contains patients with massive tissue injury or severe illness. Invasion of a body cavity has occurred or is necessary in these patients. Hypovolemia and hypotension are present, and the chance of invasive infection is greater than 50 per cent. Prolonged (longer than 72 hours) starvation is anticipated.

Patients with severe preoperative illness or multiple trauma fall in this category, e.g., patients with pyometra or heart valve disease. These patients frequently require emergency surgery, for example, those with gastric dilatation-torsion syndrome. The stimulus response patterns in these patients are complex, intense, and prolonged. In order for these patients to survive surgery and the recovery period, they require intensive and often continuous intraoperative and postoperative monitoring. In addition to monitoring basic variables as for patients of Category I, variables of greater specificity, such as blood gases, CVP, arterial pressures, and electrolytes, are needed for patients in Category III. These patients need comprehensive, continued surveillance for up to several days after they are stabilized.

To summarize, the number and specificity of the variables monitored increase as the degree of physiological insult increases. The preceding three categories of patients and monitoring regimens are only models recommending a combination of variables most frequently monitored in patients within each category. The frequency of measurements is the responsibility of the surgeon and is based on his judgment of the patient's condition and the resources at his disposal. His decisions must be founded on a thorough knowledge of the involved pathophysiology.

1. Abrams, J. S., Diane, R. S., and Davis, J. H: Adverse effects of salt and water retention on pulmonary function in patients with multiple trauma. J. Trauma 13:788, 1973.
2. Clowes, G. H. A., Jr., Del Guercio, L. R., and Barwinsky, J.: The cardiac output in response to surgical trauma. Arch. Surg. 81:212, 1960.
3. Cornelius, L. M., and Rawlings, C. A.: Arterial blood gas and acid-base values in dogs with various diseases and signs of disease. J. Am. Vet. Med. Assoc. 178:992, 1981.
4. Couch, N. P., Dmochowski, J. R., Van DeWater, J. M., et al.: Muscle surface pH as an index of peripheral perfusion in man. Ann. Surg. 173:173, 1971.
5. Coulter, D. B., and Engen, R. L.: Differentiation of electrocardiographic changes due to asphyxia and to hyperpotassemia in dogs. J. Am. Vet. Med. Assoc. 160:1419, 1972.
6. Crowell, J. W.: Oxygen transport in the hypotensive state. Fed. Proc. 29:1848, 1970.

7. Czer, L. S. C., and Shoemaker, W. C.: Optimal hematocrit value in critically ill postoperative patients. Surg. Gynecol. Obstet. *147*:363, 1978.

8. DeLaurentis, D. A., Hayes, M., Matsomoto, T., et al.: Does central venous pressure accurately reflect hemodynamic and fluid volume patterns in the critical surgical patient? Am. J. Surg. *126*:415, 1973.

9. Del Guercio, L. R. M., and Cohn, J. D.: Monitoring methods and significance. Surg. Clin. North Am. *56*:977, 1976.

10. Douglas, M. E., Downs, J. B., Mantini, E. L., et al.: Alteration of oxygen tension and oxyhemoglobin saturation. Arch. Surg. *114*:326, 1979.

11. Fan, F. C., Chen, R. Y. Z., Schuessler, G. B., et al.: Effects of hematocrit variations on regional hemodynamics and oxygen transport in the dog. Am. J. Physiol. *238*:H545, 1980.

12. Filler, R. M., Das, J. B., and Espinosa, H. M.: Clinical experience with continuous muscle pH monitoring as an index of tissue perfusion and oxygenation and acid-base status. Surgery 72:23, 1972.

13. Finco, D. R.: General guidelines for fluid therapy. J. Am. Anim. Hosp. Assoc. 8:155, 1972.

14. Gedes, L. A.: Perspectives in physiological monitoring. Med. Instrument. *10*:91, 1976.

15. Glen, J. B.: The accuracy of indirect determination of blood pressure in dogs. Res. Vet. Sci. *14*:291, 1973.

16. Greenberg, A. G., and Peskin, G. W.: Monitoring in the recovery room and surgical intensive care unit. *In* Saidman, J. S., and Smith, N. T. Y. (eds.): *Monitoring in Anesthesia*. John Wiley and Sons, New York, 1978, p. 221.

17. Grunace, C. F. V.: Doppler ultrasound monitoring of systemic blood flow during CPR. J. Am. Coll. Emerg. Phys. 7:180, 1978.

18. Gump, F. E., Martin, P., and Kinney, J. M.: Oxygen consumption and caloric expenditure in surgical patients. Surg. Gynecol. Obstet. *137*:499, 1973.

19. Hall, L. W.: Preliminary investigation of the effects of injury on the body fluids of cats and dogs. J. Small Anim. Pract. *21*:679, 1980.

20. Hardy, J. D., Garcia, J. B., Hardy, J. A., et al.: Fluid replacement monitoring. Ann. Surg. *180*:162, 1974.

21. Harken, A. H.: Hydrogen ion concentration and oxygen uptake in an isolated canine hindlimb. J. Appl. Physiol. *40*:1, 1976.

22. Haskins, S. C.: An overview of acid-base physiology. J. Am. Vet. Med. Assoc. *170*:423, 1977.

23. Haskins, S. C.: Sampling and storage of blood for pH and blood gas analysis. J. Am. Vet. Med. Assoc. *170*:429, 1977.

24. Hosomi, H.: Unstable state of the arterial pressure central system after mild hemorrhage. Am. J. Physiol. *235*:R279, 1978.

25. Hoye, R. C., Bennett, S. H., Guilhoed, G. W., et al.: Fluid volume and albumin kinetics occurring with major surgery. J. Am. Med. Assoc. *222*:1255, 1972.

26. Jan, K.-M., Heldman, J., and Chien, S.: Coronary hemodynamics and oxygen utilization after hematocrit variations in hemorrhage. Am. J. Physiol. *240*:H326, 1980.

27. Joly, H. R., and Weil, M. H.: Temperature of the great toe as an indication of the severity of shock. Circulation *39*:31, 1969.

28. Jwrado, R. A., Matucha, D., and Osborn, J. J.: Cardiac output estimation by pulse contour methods: Validity for their use for monitoring the critically ill patient. Surgery 74:358, 1973.

29. Kaneko, J. J.: Serum proteins and the dysproteinemias, *In* Kaneko, J. J. (ed.): *Clinical Biochemistry of Domestic Animals*, 3rd ed. Academic Press, New York, 1980.

30. Katz, R. L., and Bigger, J. T.: Cardiac arrhythmias during anesthesia and operation. Anesthesiology 33:193, 1970.

31. Kholoussy, A. M., Sufian, S., Pavlides, C., et al.: Central peripheral temperature gradient. Am. J. Surg. *140*:609, 1980.

32. Kolata, R. J.: Significance of changes in toe web temperature in dogs in circulatory shock. Proc. 28th Gaines Vet. Symposium, 1978, pp. 21–26.

33. Leaf, A., and Cotran, R.: *Renal Pathophysiology*. Oxford University Press, New York, 1976, p. 66.

34. Levett, J. M., and Replogle, R. L.: Thermodilution cardiac output: A critical analysis and review of the literature. J. Surg. Res. *27*:392, 1979.

35. Little, R. C.: *Physiology of the Heart and Circulation*. Year Book Medical Publishers, Chicago, 1977, p. 158.

36. Mann, R. L., Graziano, C. C., and Turnbull, A. D.: Comparison of electronic and manometric central venous pressures. Crit. Care Med. 9:98, 1981.

37. Michell, A. R.: The pathophysiological basis of fluid therapy in small animals. Vet. Rec. *104*:542, 1979.

38. Osswald, H., Haas, J. A., Marchand, G. R., et al.: Glomerular dynamics in dogs at reduced renal artery pressure. Am. J. Physiol. *236*:F25, 1979.

39. Peters, R. M.: Coordination of ventilation and perfusion. Ann. Thorac. Surg. *6*:570, 1968.

40. Prys-Roberts, C.: Monitoring of the cardiovascular system. *In* Saidman, L. J., and Smith, N. T. (eds.): *Monitoring in Anesthesia*, John Wiley & Sons, New York, 1978.

41. Rabarts, W. M.: Nature of the disturbance in the body fluid compartments during and after surgical operations. Br. J. Surg. *66*:691, 1979.

42. Rice, C. L., Hobelman, C. F., John, D. A., et al.: Central venous pressure or pulmonary capillary wedge pressure as the determinant of fluid replacement in aortic surgery. Surgery 84:437, 1978.

43. Robbins, A. B., Doran, J. E., Reese, A. C., et al.: Cold insoluble globulin levels in operative trauma: Serum depletion, wound sequestration and biological activity: An experimental and clinical study. Am. Surg. *46*:663, 1980.

44. Roe, C. F.: Surgical aspects of fever. Curr. Probl. Surg. Nov.:15, 1968.

45. Rooth, G.: *Acid-Base and Electrolyte Balance*. Year Book Medical Publishers, Inc., Chicago, 1974, p. 38.

46. Rose, E. A., and King, R. C.: Understanding post-operative fatigue. Surg. Gynecol. Obstet. *147*:97, 1978.

47. Sarelius, I. H., and Sinclair, J. D.: Effects of small changes of blood volume or oxygen delivery and tissue oxygenation. Am. J. Physiol. *240*:H177, 1981.

48. Sattler, F. P., and Knowles, R. P.: The concept. *In* Sattler, F. R., Knowles, K. P., and Whittick, W. G. (eds.): *Veterinary Critical Care*. Lea & Febiger, Philadelphia, 1981.

49. Schlant, R. C., and Felner, J. M.: The arterial pulse clinical manifestation. Curr. Probl. Cardiol. 2, 1977.

50. Schroeder, J. S., and Daily, E. K.: Techniques in bedside hemodynamic monitoring. C. V. Mosby, St. Louis, 1976, p. 34.

51. Smith, J. S.: Hypokalemia in resuscitation from multiple trauma. Surg. Gynecol. Obstet. *147*:18, 1978.

52. Shoemaker, W. C.: Cardiorespiratory patterns of surviving and nonsurviving postoperative patients. Surg. Gynecol. Obstet. *134*:810, 1972.

53. Shoemaker, W. C.: Fluid and electrolyte problems in the adult. *In* Shoemaker, W. C., and Thompson, W. L. (eds.): *Critical Care: State of the Art*, Vol. 3. Society of Critical Care Medicine, Fullerton, CA, 1982.

54. Shoemaker, W. C., Bryan-Brown, C. W., Quigley, L., et al.: Body fluid shifts in depletion and post-stress states and their correction with adequate nutrition. Surg. Gynecol. Obstet. *136*:371, 1973.

55. Shoemaker, W. C., and Czer, L. S. C.: Evaluation of the biologic importance of various hemodynamic and oxygen transport variables. Crit. Care Med. 7:424, 1979.

56. Tasker, J. B.: Fluids, electrolytes, and acid-base balance. *In* Kancko, J. J. (ed.): *Clinical Biochemistry of Domestic Animals*, 3rd ed. Academic Press, New York, 1980.

57. Walters, F. J. M., Wilson, G. J., Steward, D. J., et al.: Intramyocardial pH as an index of myocardial metabolism during cardiac surgery. J. Thorac. Cardiovasc. Surg. 78:319, 1979.

58. Wildenthal, K., Mierzwiak, D. S., Myers, R. W., et al.: Effects of acute lactic acidosis on left ventricular performance. Am. J. Physiol. *214*:1352, 1968.

59. Wilmore, D. W., Long, J. M., Mason, A. D. et al.: Stress in

surgical patients as a neurophysiologic reflex response. Surg. Gynecol. Obstet. *142*:257, 1976.

60. Wilson, R. F., and Krome, R.: Factors affecting prognosis in clinical shock. Ann. Surg. *169*:93, 1967.

61. Wilson, R. F., and Gibson, D.: The use of arterial-central venous oxygen differences to calculate cardiac output and

oxygen consumption in critically ill surgical patients. Surgery *84*:362, 1978.

62. Woodson, R. D., Wills, R. E., and Lenfant, C.: Effect of acute and established anemia on O_2 transport at rest, submaximal, and maximal work. J. Appl. Physiol. *44*:36, 1978.

Chapter **30** # Drains, Dressings, and Other Surgical Materials

Kenneth R. Presnell

DRAINS

Terminology and Definitions

Drain: any device by which a channel or opening may be established and maintained for the exit of fluid or purulent material from any cavity, wound, or infected area.[8]

Drainage: the systematic withdrawal of fluid from any wound, sore, or cavity in the body.[8]

Penrose drain: the most commonly used drain, made of soft, thin-walled rubber tubing 0.64 to 2.54 cm (0.25 to 1.0 inch) in diameter.

Sump drain: a large tube with a second smaller tube in the wall or within the lumen of the larger tube. The smaller tube allows air to enter and facilitates drainage of fluid from the cavity.

Cigarette drain: originally a Penrose* drain with a gauze strip in its lumen. It may also be a Penrose drain with a rigid or semirigid rubber or vinyl tube inside to aid in drainage.

Types of Drainage Tubes, Lavage Systems, and Associated Equipment

The selection of a drain depends on the area to be drained, anticipated complications, efficiency of drainage, and the duration of required drainage. The decision is usually based on previous experience, knowledge of employment of various drains, available supplies, and cost.

The simplest method of drainage is to open the area or cavity to a dependent area of the skin and leave it open. This allows the free flow of materials. The puncture site must be kept clean and open and is usually allowed to heal by second intention. Strips of dry gauze or gauze coated with petroleum antisep-

tic or antibiotic ointment have been placed in the draining cavities and left protruding through the puncture site. These are now contraindicated because better drainage systems are available. The gauze acts as a drain only while the fabric can absorb fluid or as it is withdrawn steadily and slowly from the wound. Once it is saturated (only a few hours), the fluid clots or precipitates on the gauze and prevents further drainage.[2] Gauze strips are used primarily to maintain patency of an orifice, in which case it acts as a dressing and not as a drain.

In 1859, Chasargnac introduced the use of soft rubber tubes for drainage.[30] These rubber tubes have been replaced by Penrose drains, which are simple drains made of thin-walled, soft rubber tubing. The drains are available in various diameters from 0.635 to 2.54 cm (0.25 to 1.0 inch) and come in precut lengths in sterilized packages or unsterilized rolls. The tubes may be fenestrated with scissors prior to insertion. As drainage occurs around the tube fenestration is not essential. These tubes are relatively histocompatible and are nondegradable in body fluids and hence produce very minimal tissue reaction.

Firmer rubber, Silastic, or nylon tubes are available in many different sizes and designs and are usually perforated at the tip. They are usually employed for flushing and suction-drainage of deep wounds or excavations of the pleural cavity when negative pressure is essential for drainage. Owing to their nature and construction, these drains cause more tissue reaction than Penrose drains.

Sump drains are available commercially or can be made by inserting a small-diameter tube within a larger second tube. The smaller tube allows air or fluid to enter into the pocket to help overcome the vacuum and thus permits better drainage of the effluent material from the second, or larger, tube. A negative pressure can be applied to the larger tube to aid drainage. Some of these systems are more complex and use three or four tubes.

---

*Latex Penrose tubing, Argyle Brunswick, St. Louis, MO.

In 1882, Kehrer placed a gauze strip inside a rubber tube to enhance drainage and help decrease adhesions to the gauze—the "cigarette drain."[20] Today the gauze has been replaced by a semirigid vinyl or polyvinyl tube. The Penrose tube over the semisolid tube helps prevent soft tissue occlusion or obstruction of the drain and allows negative pressure to be applied. A sump drain may be covered with a Penrose drain.

Most drainage systems used today are modifications of the previously mentioned simple systems and range from very simple to very complex in design. The simpler designs have proved to provide the type and efficiency of drainage needed in veterinary medicine.

Continuous or intermittent suction drainage is achieved using a semisolid tube connected to a negative pressure source. Underwater drainage systems have been employed for the chest cavity and work very well. Small vacuum units* that mechanically produce a continuous mild vacuum are employed for wounds or areas that cannot be drained dependently. Tiny drains may use Vacutainers (blood-collecting tubes with a pre-established vacuum) that are connected to the drainage tube with a hypodermic needle. When the tube becomes filled it is replaced with a fresh tube. These systems establish and maintain a mild negative pressure (5 to 10 mm Hg) and can be taped to the animal's body. The application of these drains to various body systems is discussed under specific applications or body systems.

Indications

As a treatment measure drainage should be considered in patients with (1) grossly contaminated wounds of the skin and underlying tissues that cannot be completely debrided and that may still contain foreign material, and (2) well-organized abscesses.

As a prophylactic measure drainage is established to prevent formation of dead space by the accumulation of blood, serum, air, or purulent material. The drain is inserted at the time of the initial wounding or at surgery. Drains should be used prophylactically in the following situations:

1. Following surgery on an organ that lacks the serosal covering or that for other reasons has a greater than expected potential for leakage at the surgical or anastomotic site;

2. In any area where delayed or slow healing is expected; and

3. In organs such as the gallbladder, liver, ureters, bile duct, pancreas, and so on that may leak irritating material, e.g., bile.

With advances in surgical closure, improved surgery materials, meticulous care of surgically exposed tissue, and the obliteration of dead space with precise anatomical apposition of tissue, the need for and use

*Wound Suction Set, Argyle Sherwood, St. Louis, MO.

of drains have been greatly reduced. Improved asepsis, antiseptics, and antibiotics have further decreased the need for drains.

Application and Placement of Drains

Abdominal Cavity

Complete and total drainage of the peritoneal cavity is anatomically and physiologically impossible because of the anatomy of the cavity and the ability of the peritoneal membrane and the omentum to develop pockets and seal drains rapidly. Penrose-type drains are of no value in the abdominal cavity; they are promptly walled off and isolated from the peritoneal cavity, usually within six hours following insertion.[30] Peritoneal drainage is used for short-term therapy, including decreasing dead space; preventing the accumulation of blood, serum, and purulent exudate; removing irritating substances such as urine, bile, or glandular secretions; and assisting in lavage of the abdominal cavity. Permanent percutaneous peritoneal drainage for ascites is not practical owing to the high risk of infection.

The peritoneal cavity is able to encapsulate irritating stimuli so well that drains must be placed surgically to the specific area to be drained. This is especially true for the pancreas; the drain must be placed right from the pancreas to the dependent body wall. The drains are anchored in place in the abdominal cavity, because of the mobility and motility of the organ in the cavity and are usually attached with one suture of 3-0 plain gut. The drain can be removed easily when the strength of the suture has broken down (in approximately five to seven days). The drain must also be fixed to the exit site through the skin with two simple sutures, one at either edge of the drain, or with a large stainless steel safety pin running through the drain to anchor it firmly to the adjacent skin.

The most effective drains for the abdominal cavity are multiple lumen tubes, i.e., sump or tube drains enclosed in a Penrose drain and preferably with negative pressure applied. The suction tends to help the fluid drain to the area of the abdominal cavity where it is removed by the drain. Intermittent irrigation through a second soft tube (placed high into the abdominal cavity) is very beneficial for lavage and flushing. Usually, two Penrose drains are placed, without kinks, in the abdominal cavity (one anteriorly and one posteriorly just off the midline and away from both the incision and the falciform ligament). The exit holes must be large enough to allow free flow of fluid but small enough to prevent evisceration or herniation.

Pleural Cavity

Drainage of the pleural cavities requires a semirigid tube for negative pressure drainage. Many different types of tubes are available, but a sterile disposable 10 French rubber feeding tube* or the center tube from a soft vinyl esophageal stethoscope† without the cuff is adequate. The tube should be perforated over the distal 3 to 5 cm, and the holes should be less than one-half the diameter of the tube to prevent kinking and occlusion. Placement is quick and easy with local or general anesthesia. The chest drain is inserted in the jaws of a large Pean forceps through a skin incision at the dorsal third of the tenth intercostal space and passed subcutaneously and anteriorly for two rib spaces. It is then inserted through the eighth intercostal space into the chest. When the chest cavity is open the tube should be gently slid anteroventrally into the chest until it lies ventrally along the thoracic floor with the tip passing cranially. A purse-string suture is placed around it in the skin and tied securely to the tube. An ointment-saturated 3×3 gauze sponge is placed over the tube at the exit site from the skin and a bandage is applied to fix the tube to the chest to prevent slippage or air leakage. At least two clamps should be placed on the tube at all times.

Negative pressure is applied intermittently with a large syringe and three-way stopcock or continuously with an underwater drain. If the accumulation is bilateral and thick or tenacious, bilateral chest drains are necessary. When the drain is removed, the skin is sutured and a light bandage is placed over the incision to prevent further leakage.

A number of complications may occur with thoracic drains. Hemothorax, pneumothorax, or infection may be introduced by improper tube insertion. The tube itself causes some effusion by irritating the tissues (approximately 2 ml/kg body weight/day). Evaluation of the pleural effusion is a very valuable diagnostic aid.[13]

One-way valves‡ are ideally suited for continuous drainage of the thoracic cavity in active animals. Unlike the underwater drainage system, in the one-way-valve system the valve can be tightly clamped to the rubber tube. This prevents accidental air entry into the chest, and as the animal moves and breathes the one-way valve lets fluid or air escape from the chest via the tube and one-way valve.[24]

Wounds

Drainage of superficial wounds is by direct incision. However, because of problems with wound care in animals it is preferable to close the soft tissue and use a Penrose drain. It should be placed in the deepest portion of the wound using sterile surgical technique. A suture may be passed through the skin and into the deepest part of the drain and back out through the skin. This anchors the tube at the most

proximal portion and allows removal of the suture externally. Buried sutures should not be used for anchorage. If the wound is large and incorporates a number of tissue planes, several drains should be employed over the area to be drained. Multiple drains should be exited through at least two or more sites in the skin. The drain should be sutured to the skin with one suture at each edge of the Penrose drain. Mattress or purse-string sutures should be avoided, as these occlude the tube and close the skin incision. The drain is cut off, leaving 1 to 2 cm protruding through the skin. The drain should not be inserted near tendon sheaths, nerves, vessels, or other delicate organs, as it stimulates varying amounts of inflammation and may interfere with function.

Drains are left in place as long as there is sufficient drainage or evidence that the pocket is still present (from 1 to 14 days). The amount and consistency of drainage material are best evaluated by covering the ends of the drain with a soft, absorbent bandage, which can be changed as needed. The animal should wear an Elizabethan collar to prevent mutilation and premature removal of the drains.

Fractures (see Chapter 155)

Hollow Organs

Drainage is usually established by passing a catheter through normal drainage channels. The stomach is an exception; a retention catheter* is inserted through the abdominal wall to drain stomach contents and anchor the stomach to the abdominal wall. This provides a permanent gastropexy following the dilation-torsion complex.

Biliary System

Following severe trauma to the liver or surgery on the liver or biliary tract, drainage is usually employed because of the possibility of bile leakage with subsequent peritonitis.[7] The liver and anterior abdomen are drained by placing several sump or tube Penrose drains near the liver and running them out through the ventral body wall. Negative pressure is helpful, although not essential.

For repair of a ruptured common bile duct, a T-tube drainage tube has been employed in man and in dogs.[12] The tube is made of soft rubber with two short arms and one long arm. One short arm is inserted into the common bile duct distal to the rupture and the other is inserted into the gallbladder; the long arm emerges from the gallbladder through its wall and out through the abdominal wall. This T-tube allows bile drainage from the gallbladder through the abdominal cavity and hence decom-

*Feeding tube, Argyle Brunswick, St. Louis, MO.
†Esophageal stethoscope, American Hospital Supply, McGaw Park, IL.
‡Heimlich Chest Drain Valve, Bard-Parker, Rutherford, NJ.

*Foley Catheter, Bardex, Bard International Ltd., Sunderland, England.

presses the gallbladder while the duct heals. A Penrose drain is inserted from the anastomosis in the abdominal cavity and out through the abdominal wall. Once the bile duct can accommodate bile flow as evaluated radiographically (from seven to ten days), the tube is occluded and, if the patient tolerates this, the tube is extracted by removing the skin fixation suture and applying gentle, steady traction on the tube. The leakage following removal is minimal, as the connective tissue fistula that forms around the tube as it emerges usually seals within 24 hours.[9]

Urinary System

Catheter drainage is employed for nonsurgical management of ruptured urinary bladders, particularly when the rupture is dorsal and the patient is a poor surgical candidate. A retention catheter is inserted into the bladder via the urethra, and its cuff is inflated. It is used to drain the bladder for seven to ten days until the bladder heals. Similar catheters are employed after repair of a severed urethra or after prostate resection.

Small, soft catheters can be used to aid re-anastomosis of a severed or ruptured ureter. They can be passed down the ureter to the bladder and out through the urethra with the proximal end passing across the anastomosis and up toward the kidney. The anastomosis is completed over the outside of the tube, which serves as a stent. The tube is left in place and is sutured to the skin of the prepuce or vulva to allow drainage of urine and decreased leakage through the anastomotic site into the abdominal cavity. Once healing is completed (seven to ten days), the catheter is extracted by removing the fixation sutures and applying gentle traction.

Other Areas

Drains may also be used in abscesses and cysts elsewhere in the body. They are used to drain cervical mucoceles that develop after the rupture of salivary ducts, especially if they have become infected. They are placed after the affected gland has been surgically removed and the cavity drained. A Penrose tube is run from the area of the cyst out through the skin ventrally. Ranulas are usually treated with direct drainage by incising the cyst on its rostral surface and suturing it with absorbable sutures to the adjacent mucous membrane.

The middle ear may be drained by the McBride method,[2] whereby drainage is established from the tympanic bullae to the pharynx. A small fenestrated rubber tube is placed from the external ear channel through the ear and tympanic bulla into the pharynx. It is trimmed flush with the mucous membrane of the pharynx and is sutured at that point to the mucous membranes with four or five sutures. The tube is left in place for three to five days and is removed by cutting the sutures and pulling the tube out through the mouth.

Efficiency of Various Drainage Systems

The choice of drain, mode of insertion and exit, depth of the area to be drained, and number of drains inserted all have a marked effect on the efficiency of the drainage system. Comparison of four common drainage systems (Penrose drain, a semirigid fenestrated rubber or polyvinyl catheter, a sump drain, and a sump drain covered with Penrose tube) revealed a marked difference in efficiency. Evaluation of drainage of a known amount of fluid instilled into the abdominal cavity in dogs over a three-hour period revealed the following efficiency rates: catheter, 39 per cent; Penrose drain, 40 per cent; sump drain, 58 per cent; and sump covered with Penrose drain, 72 per cent. These values reflect the average amount drained compared with the initial volume introduced into the abdominal cavity. The sump or tube drain effectively removed accumulated fluid but frequently became obstructed. The Penrose drain did not appear to become obstructed, but its draining ability was markedly lower than that of the other systems. The sump covered with a Penrose drain had the advantages of both; the Penrose over the drain prevented occlusion by body tissues or secretions, and the sump provided a good drainage system.

Care of Drains

Drains should be placed aseptically if possible, exit as ventrally or dependently as possible, and be covered with absorbent gauze pads. The skin may be covered with a petrolatum dressing or ointment to prevent excoriation. The bandage helps prevent gross contamination. The bandage should be changed daily or more frequently if there is an excessive amount of drainage. Because the external portion of the drain is contaminated, flushing is not recommended because it drives bacteria and ancillary substances deeper into the tissues. As it exits from the skin, the drain should be cleaned with an iodine or chlorhexidine solution whenever the bandage is changed. An Elizabethan collar should be kept on the patient while the drain is in place to prevent licking, chewing, or pulling on the drain.

Disadvantages of Drains

Tissue damage may occur during drain insertion. The Penrose drain is the least irritating drain but is still recognized by the body as a foreign substance. Drains may damage adjacent tendon sheaths, nerves, vessels, or other delicate organs. They may erode through the serosal surface of any organ if left in place too long or if not properly placed. Drains act as a two-way conduit and allow infection to ascend in and around them. The danger of ascending infection increases directly with the length of time the drain is left in place.[18] One study in dogs with drains used after splenectomy showed a 90 per cent positive culture of the drain seven days after insertion.[18] Drains may be lost in or from the body. They should contain a radiographic marker to allow their recovery if the former occurs. Dehiscence or herniation may occur at the incision site for the insertion of the drain.

The drain is not a substitute for thorough evacuation of fluid, debridement of contaminated or vital tissues, or proper hemostasis, nor should it compensate for poor or traumatic surgical technique.

Agents for Flushing Wounds and Cavities

Washing the wound with water under pressure followed by irrigation with sterile saline or Ringer's solution is effective in removing gross contamination and tissue debris lying free on the surface.[20] Tap water causes less tissue injury than distilled or sterile water when used in this manner.[5] For peripheral wounds, sterile saline or Ringer's solution causes the least tissue damage; however, the volume needed for grossly contaminated wounds may make it expensive for initial flushing. Tap water under pressure may be used for initial clean-up followed by lavage with sterile saline or Ringer's solution. Wounds in body cavities should be treated and flushed with 500 to 1000 ml of sterile Ringer's solution or saline. Larger amounts are necessary in badly contaminated wounds.[21] Flushing causes minimal tissue damage, effectively eliminates bacterial contamination, and further dilutes the contaminants left.[15] Early lavage is more effective on loose surface materials.

Soaps or detergents damage tissues and are not recommended. Muscles, tendons, blood vessels, cartilage, and synovia are irritated by these substances, which may lead to an increased susceptibility to infection and, ultimately, delayed or inadequate wound healing.[28] Chlorhexidine and povidone-iodine surgical scrubs contain antiseptic agents and detergents. The antiseptic solution destroys bacteria and the detergent aids in removal of contaminants; however, they damage tissues and may decrease normal defenses and promote inflammation.

Povidone-iodine instilled into the abdominal cavity of dogs with active peritonitis causes death more rapidly than the instillation of Ringer's solution.[4] This may be associated with the absorption of excessive amounts of iodine. In dilutions of 1:100 iodine is less damaging to tissues.[5] There is little bacterial resistance to iodine.[16]

Chlorhexidine is less irritating to tissues when used in dilute solutions (0.5 per cent or 1:40 dilution of a 2 per cent solution) and is recommended for prophylaxis in wound infection. It is very active at low concentrations against gram-negative and gram-positive bacteria, and resistance has not been observed.[10] Alcohol, acetic acid, benzylchloride, and iodine may help protect against infection.[9] Irrigation with ethyl alcohol, chloramine-T, or carbolic acid is ineffective in treating contaminated wounds.[9]

Enzymatic debridement of wounds is indicated whenever anesthesia and surgery are considered too risky.[14,25]

Topical antibiotics are most effective when applied immediately after injury and prior to significant bacterial contamination or proliferation.[17] They may be useful initially before debridement. The antiseptics mentioned previously are cheaper and possibly more effective. Often, Ringer's solution does a better job than a small lavage with antibiotics.

Peritoneal Dialysis and Lavage Systems

Intraoperative peritoneal lavage, although initially unpopular because it dispersed contamination, is beneficial (if sufficient volume is used) because it removes contaminating debris and dilutes and disperses the remaining bacteria. By spreading them around the peritoneal cavity, the concentration of bacteria is diluted and the bacteria are in contact with more peritoneum.[19] Flushing also disperses intraperitoneal antibiotics and decreases the concentration of endotoxin. The peritoneal or pleural cavity must be lavaged with warm fluid (at least 40°C) in sufficient quantities (in animals less than 15 kg up to 500 ml and in animals over 15 kg a minimum of 1000 ml has been recommended).[19] Antibiotics may be beneficial in the flushing fluid. Penicillin (100,000 units/kg), cephalothin (50 mg/kg), or chlorhexidine (0.05 per cent dilution) has been recommended in the last flush.

If the abdominal cavity is contaminated during laparotomy or if this is suspected, the abdomen should be lavaged with copious amounts of warm Ringer's solution. For closed abdominal lavage at least two sump Penrose or Penrose tube drains are placed in the abdomen plus one tube in the dorsal abdomen through the flank. The lavage should be done two or three times daily. The fluid is instilled until the desired amount is reached or the abdomen dilates or appears tense. The fluid is allowed to drain by gravity or mild suction. Two or three days of therapy may be required, the duration depending on the effluent and the animal's condition. Complications with lavage include anemia, hypoproteinemia, hypokalemia, hyponatremia, hypothermia, and superinfection.

DRESSINGS

This section discusses dressings concerned with wound management. Dressings play a major role in veterinary medicine, as the patient is often uncooperative, and in an unhygienic environment.

Wound dressings serve four primary functions:[17] protection, absorption of drainage material, compression to decrease dead space and reduce hematoma formation, and stabilization and immobilization.

Types of Dressings and Their Application

Dry Bandages

Dry dressings are indicated in situations in which they will not adhere to underlying tissues, e.g., immediately after most fracture repairs to reduce edema and swelling. They help keep the wound edges apposed, promote healing, and provide a clean environment. Soft cotton padding,* applied initially, is covered with an elastic wide mesh gauze,† which may be covered with a more rigid covering such as adhesive‡ or nonadhesive elastic wrap.§

When the wound or traumatized tissue is discharging water-soluble fluids, a bulky dry dressing is indicated to absorb the discharge and prevent mechanical damage and excoriation of the skin. If minimal discharge is expected, a nonstick bandage or gauze coated with a water-soluble dressing is placed immediately over the wound to prevent adhesions. On large, denuded wounds nonadhesive ‖ fenestrated bandages are usually required to allow exudate to be absorbed by the bulky overdressing.

If dry gauze, particularly the large size mesh, is placed over an epithelializing wound, cells grow into the bandage material. The wound is damaged when these are stripped off. This retards healing and is not recommended unless this method is used to debride the wound.

Another indication for dry dressings is to cover a wet dressing (such as silver nitrate applied to burns). The wet dressing is covered with cellophane or wax paper to hold the fluid within the inner portion of the bandage. This is then covered with a bulky soft bandage, which acts as an occlusal dressing and provides a controlled, moist environment over the burned surface.

Dry bandages may be applied as pressure bandages to prevent swelling, edema, and dead space formation. The term *pressure bandaging* is misleading, as it is very difficult to maintain any type of pressure on a wound unless it is applied with an elastic dressing. A soft dressing material such as cotton compacts under the dressing, and the pressure applied to the wound is negligible. Pressure bandages prevent expansion rather than apply pressure.

Wet Dressings

Wet dressings are used to cover infected wounds in two ways. (1) A loose gauze dressing is placed over

the wound. Catheters are laid over or into this dressing, or one is placed into the wound. These catheters are covered with a bulky gauze bandage, which is covered with a layer of waterproof wrap, which is again covered with a dry bandage of cotton and gauze. One catheter irrigates the wound and the second allows drainage. (2) Hot, wet compresses are intermittently applied to the wound for 15 to 20 minutes two to four times a day. A warm wet dressing is more beneficial than a cold wet dressing. The dressing helps remove the water-soluble debris from the wound and decreases the viscosity of the secretion. The water has two desirable effects, both of which promote drainage:[20] (1) it transports the heat, and (2) it enhances capillary formation. The bandage also aids lymphocyte migration into the wound and sterilization of the wound environment (this mechanism is not totally understood).[20]

If wound debris is not water-soluble, is firmly attached to the underlying tissue, or is devitalized, simple hot packing is not adequate and more intensive measures such as pressure lavage or surgical debridement must be employed. Intermittent application of wet dressings is recommended, as continuous application of the same wet dressing for more than 24 hours may cause deterioration of the tissues and the wound.[22]

Biological Dressings (see also Chapter 38)

Skin isografts are the most physiologically normal dressings available. Split thickness grafts may be used for large defects and are especially useful for wounds of the extremities. Mesh grafts may be used to increase the surface area covered by the graft. Advantages of skin grafts are that (1) some or all of the wound may be closed, and (2) any take of the graft decreases the size of the remaining wound.

Biological dressings have a beneficial effect on the wound in addition to providing protective covering. They help increase phagocytosis by increasing the acidity of the wound fluids,[28] increase the temperature under the dressing, and help prevent the accumulation of fluid and debris on the wound surface. One study showed a reduction in bacterial count by 98 per cent; the wounds were considered sterile in 50 to 78 per cent of the cases by the eighth day following coverage.[28] Thus, biological dressings have been advocated as a method of sterilizing infected wounds, primarily by stimulating immunity.

Porcine skin is the most readily available xenograft dressing. It has the greatest value when superficial skin loss has occurred and skin grafting must be delayed or when there is inadequate skin for covering the wound. It may be used as a dressing to protect the wound until autologous grafting can be performed. It is used to establish a more ideal wound environment by keeping the lesion moist and clean while promoting granulation and healing. It also helps relieve pain and decrease irritation and self-mutilation. Xenograft dressings should be changed every

---

*Sof-rol Cast Padding, Johnson & Johnson, Vancouver, Canada.
†Kling Conforming Gauze, Johnson & Johnson, New Brunswick, NJ.
‡Elastoplast, Smith and Nephew Inc., Lacine, Quebec, Canada.
§Vetrap Bandaging Tape, 3M Co., St. Paul, MN.
‖Telfa Non-adherent Dressing, Kendall, Toronto, Canada.

four to five days to prevent tight adherence to "take" of the graft. Porcine skin also augments the host's immunological response, but the mechanism for this is not clearly understood.[28]

Porcine skin can be stored in three ways: (1) fresh skin can be stored at 4°C for up to 10 days; (2) the skin may be frozen at −17°C for a maximum of 30 days; or (3) in its commercially available lyophilized form it can be stored for up to two years. It is sterilized by radiation and requires rehydration before use.

Biological dressings offer many advantages for wound management but are not used extensively due to their cost.

Man-made "Biological" Dressings

Surgical dressings have been developed that mimic biological dressings. Biological and man-made "biological" dressings are used for massive skin loss, e.g., in the burn patient or those with extensive skin debridement. They diminish wound retraction, a normal phase of wound healing that is highly undesirable in large surface skin defects.

Ideally, man-made biological dressings should have the following beneficial characteristics:

1. Control fluid and electrolyte losses;
2. Protect the body tissues at the wound site;
3. Lightly adhere to or closely cover the wound to provide an optimal environment for healing;
4. Be resistant to bacterial penetration but absorbent;
5. Be nonreactive with body tissues;
6. Be readily sterilized and stable with a long shelf-life; and
7. Be economical.

Examples of this type of dressing include a nonadherent absorbent dressing* made with two layers of porous cellophane-type material sandwiching a thin layer of absorbent cotton; and a polyurethane reticulated foam† that is laminated to a porous polypropylene film. It adheres to the wound surface like a skin graft, and is thrombogenic, relatively impervious to bacteria, immunologically inert, and readily sterilized and stable. This material has been found to repair a wound for grafting in the same manner as allografts and in approximately the same amount of time.[1]

It is best to change a synthetic biological dressing daily until the granulation bed starts developing. Once the granulating bed is healthy and developing well, the dressing may be left in place for up to four days provided the condition of the wound is satisfactory. These materials do not conform to the wound well and are difficult to apply. They should not be used with ointments or creams, as this tends to decrease the intimacy of contact between the dressing and the wound.

Rigid Bandages

Some rigid bandages are designed to limit the motion of a body part, e.g., application of a splint or cast. These bandages are applied to provide pain relief, to decrease stress on the wound, and to prevent suture line dehiscence and postoperative swelling and edema.[28]

Reduced motion may allow better healing of the injury, especially in areas subject to excessive motion, e.g., the footpads or the tuber calcanei, by reducing the stress on the suture line and healing tissues. The reduced motion and associated trauma to the tissue may decrease the risk of infection.[20,22]

The wound is dressed with gauze or a nonstick pad, a small amount of cotton padding, and a conforming plaster cast. The joints above and below the site of injury are immobilized. The area may have a mild odor for five to seven days, but preferably the dressing should not be changed for two weeks. When the cast is removed the wound is cleaned and a second cast is applied over a petroleum-soaked gauze dressing. This procedure may be repeated three times.

Rigid bandages do not allow swelling. Consequently, limbs should be bandaged so that the tips of the digits remain exposed for evaluation of temperature, pain, and circulation.

Others

Metallic dressings such as silver foil or charged gold leaves have been used in man. They are expensive and have minimal usage and few advantages.

Perforated cellophane is effective for wound coverage, as cells do not readily invade it. It can be removed with minimal wound damage, as it does not adhere to the wound. This material is often used in man-made biological dressings.

Contraindications and Complications

If the material adheres to the wound too tightly, if it is left in contact with the wound for too long, or if the epithelial cells can grow into the bandage, the wound will be disrupted and healing retarded every time the bandage is removed. Careless application of the bandage can also retard healing. An uncomfortable bandage encourages the patient to mutilate the wound. If swelling occurs under a rigid bandage, circulation to the extremity is reduced, leading to avascular necrosis and tissue death. Prolonged continuous wet dressings may retard wound healing.

If the patient is not hospitalized or under the direct supervision of a veterinarian, the owner needs to be carefully instructed in the management of the band-

---

*Telfa Non-adherent Dressing, Kendall, Toronto, Canada.
†Epigard, Parke-Davis, Morris Plains, NJ.

age and alerted to the warning signs of possible problems.

OTHER SURGICAL MATERIALS

Mesh

Types of Mesh

Polyester fiber mesh* is a synthetic malleable mesh available in sheets that is used as an onlay graft. It is strong and can be cut or trimmed to size with scissors, as it does not unravel at the edges. It contours well and appears to cause minimal tissue reaction.[6]

Knitted polypropylene mesh† may be readily trimmed, as its edges resist unravelling. Granulation tissue is able to grow through the mesh itself. It is strong and relatively nonreactive.[29]

Woven plastic mesh‡ is less elastic than the other types of mesh mentioned but is much less expensive. It can be autoclaved repeatedly but tends to shrink each time. It may be trimmed to size, but, because of its woven nature, it tends to unravel along the edges.

Carbon mesh§ is well accepted by tissue, and is readily sterilized and flexible. It is available in a fiber, mesh, or felt. Connective tissue grows through the carbon mesh and the combination provides good structural support for abdominal defects. This mesh is very resistant to tearing and causes little tissue reaction.[29]

Applications of Mesh

Mesh has been used for herniorrhaphy, when the strength of the patient's own tissues is not adequate, when the tissues have been badly traumatized, when there is inadequate soft tissue to close the defect, and when the hernia has been repaired multiple times without success. In this application, the prosthetic mesh can be applied in two ways. (1) The mesh can be used to reinforce each side of the defect to be closed. In this manner it sandwiches the edges of the wound. It is sutured on both sides of the muscle. This is repeated on the opposite side, and the defect is sutured through the folded part of the prosthesis and the enclosed muscle. (2) The mesh can be used in a sheet as an onlay graft either inside or outside the muscular layers. It is advantageous to have it covered by peritoneum on the visceral side of the abdominal wall, as this causes less irritation to the serosa within the peritoneal cavity.[6,29] One layer of mesh is adequate for dogs and cats.

In bursting strength tests of rat abdominal cavity

wound repairs reinforced with an onlay graft of polyester fiber mesh, the bursting strength was significantly greater than in wounds repaired with a braided polyester suture* alone.[6] The increase was most apparent in the first week postoperatively. The mesh reinforces the wound by the strength of the mesh itself and seems to stimulate a dense ingrowth of fibrous tissue.[6]

Mesh is also used as a patch graft to reinforce or enlarge a blood vessel or cardiac outflow tract or as a 360° total replacement for a segment of blood vessel.

Hemostatic Materials

Oxidized regenerated cellulose† is an absorbable knitted fabric that is prepared by controlled oxidation of regenerated cellulose. It can be cut or sutured without fraying at the edges. It is supplied in sterile vials and should not be autoclaved, as autoclaving causes physical breakdown of the material. It accelerates clotting by a physical effect on clot formation.

Absorbable gelatin sponge‡ is a sterile, pliable, nonallergenic sponge prepared from purified gelatin solution. It is capable of absorbing and holding many times its weight in blood and is used to aid hemostasis and healing of wounds. It provides a fibrinlike framework for proliferating granulation tissue. For application it is cut to the desired size and applied dry or saturated with Ringer's solution. It is applied to the bleeding surface and held for 10 to 15 seconds until it stays in place.

---

*Mersilene, Ethicon Corp., Somerville, NJ.
†Surgicell, Surgikos, Johnson & Johnson, New Brunswick, NJ.
‡Gelfoam, The Upjohn Co., Kalamazoo, MI.

1. Alexander, J. W., et al.: Clinical evaluation of Epigard, a new synthetic substitute for hemograft and heterograft skin. J. Trauma 13:374, 1973.
2. Archibald, J., and Blakesley, C. L. (eds.): Canine Surgery, 2nd ed. American Veterinary Publications, Santa Barbara, CA, 1974.
3. Baker, M. S., et al.: Sump tube drainage as a source of bacterial contamination. Am. J. Surg. 133:617, 1977.
4. Bolton, J. S., Bornside, G. H., and Cohn, C.: Intraperitoneal povidone-iodine in experimental canine and murine peritonitis. Am. J. Surg. 137:780, 1979.
5. Branemark, P. I., et al.: Tissue injury caused by wound disinfectants. Am. J. Bone Joint Surg. 49A:48, 1967.
6. Cerise, E. J., et al.: The use of mersilene mesh in repair of abdominal wall hernias. Ann. Surg. 181:728, 1975.
7. DeHoff, W. D., et al.: Surgical management of abdominal emergencies. Vet. Clin. North Am. 2:301, 1972.
8. Dorland's Illustrated Medical Dictionary, 26th ed. W. B. Saunders, Philadelphia, 1981.
9. Edlich, R. F., et al.: Studies in management of contaminated wounds: III. Assessment of the effectiveness of irrigation with antiseptic agents. Am. J. Surg. 118:31, 1969.
10. Grant, J. C., and Findlay, J. C.: Local treatment of burns and scalds using chlorhexidine. Lancet 272:862, 1957.
11. Hanna, W. A.: Efficiency of peritoneal drainage. Surg. Gynecol. Obstet. 131:983, 1970.
12. Hoffer, R. E., Niemeyer, K. H., and Patton, M.: Common

---

*Polyester Fiber Mesh, Ethicon Inc., Somerville, NJ.
†Marlex Mesh, Deval Canada Ltd., Mississauga, Ontario.
‡Proxplast, Goshen Laboratories, Goshen, NY.
§Carbon Fiber, Dow Corning Corp., Midland, MO.

bile duct repair utilizing the gallbladder and T-tube. Vet. Med./Sm. Anim. Clin. *66*:889, 1971.

13. Holmberg, D. L.: Management of pyothorax. Vet. Clin. North Am. 9:357, 1979.

14. Hoboleek, J.: Clinical experience with a proteolytic enzyme. Vet. Med./Sm. Anim. Clin. *68*:148, 1973.

15. Hoover, N. W., and Ivins, J. C.: Wound debridement. Arch. Surg. *79*:701, 1959.

16. Houang, E. T., et al.: Absence of bacterial resistance to povidone-iodine. J. Clin. Pathol. *29*:752, 1976.

17. Jennings, P. B.: Surgical techniques utilized in the presence of infection. Arch. Offic. J. Am. Coll. Vet. Surg. *4*:43, 1975.

18. Neuman, N. B.: Management of contaminated wounds of the extremities. Vet. Med./Sm. Anim. Clin. *69*:1275, 1974.

19. Parks, J.: Peritoneal drains. J. Am. Anim. Hosp. Assoc. *10*:289, 1974.

20. Peacock, E. E., and VanWinkle, W.: *Wound Repair*. W. B. Saunders, Philadelphia, 1976.

21. Peterson, L. W.: Prophylaxis of wound infection: Studies with particular reference to soaps with irrigation. Arch. Surg. *50*:177, 1945.

22. Rausch, J. E.: Trauma to the extremities. Canine Pract. *2*:38, 1975.

23. Sabiston, D. C.: *Textbook of Surgery*, 11th ed. W. B. Saunders, Philadelphia, 1977.

24. Sauer, B. W.: Valve drainage of the pleural cavity of the dog. J. Am. Vet. Med. Assoc. *155*:1977, 1969.

25. Shelby, R. W., et al.: Enzymatic debridement with activated whole pancreas. Am. J. Surg. *96*:545, 1958.

26. Singleton, A. O., Jr., Davis, D., and Julian, J.: The prevention of wound infection following contamination with colon organisms. Surg. Gynecol. Obstet. *108*:389, 1959.

27. Starke, R. B.: *Plastic Surgery*. Harper & Row, New York, 1962.

28. Swaim, S. F.: *Surgery of Traumatized Skin*. W. B. Saunders, Philadelphia, 1980.

29. Tulleners, E. P., and Fretz, P. B.: Prosthetic repair of large abdominal wall defects in horses and food animals. J. Am. Vet. Med. Assoc. *182*:258, 1983.

30. Yates, J. L.: An experimental study of the local effects of peritoneal drainage. Surg. Gynecol. Obstet. *1*:6, 1905.

Patient Aftercare

Chapter 31

Nancy O. Brown

THE RECOVERY PERIOD

The concept of recovery room care was established soon after World War II and gained wide acceptance as surgical morbidity and mortality rates decreased. Recovery room patients are those in the initial postanesthetic and postsurgical phases of convalescence.

Definition

The recovery period begins with the termination of both anesthesia and surgery. The termination of anesthesia is marked by the return of consciousness. When the patient has regained the gag reflex, can swallow, has increased jaw tension, and responds to manipulation of the endotracheal tube, extubation occurs. The postanesthetic period ends when the sensorium has cleared and pulse and blood pressure are stable. The termination of surgery is marked by placement of the last suture or the end of surgical manipulation.

Initial Concerns

The recovery period is as critical as the operative period. It is the period in which cardiovascular and respiratory responses are diminished. The level of anesthesia may deepen when surgical stimuli are removed. Lightening of anesthesia and return to consciousness can occur long before many drugs are eliminated from the body.[34] Some drugs have side effects that should be taken into consideration. Barbiturates are more undissociated in an acid environment and have a greater effect on a patient with metabolic or respiratory acidosis.[32] The phenothiazines cause release of epinephrine, resulting in a decrease in antidiuretic hormone, an increase in ACTH, and an increase in serum glucose. Thiamylal and halothane sensitize the myocardium to the arrhythmic effect of catecholamines. Ketamine causes partial vagal blockade, sinus tachycardia, arrhythmias, and bradycardia. Zylazine increases vagal tone, interferes with cardiac conductivity, and causes sinoatrial and atrioventricular blockade.

Other factors must also be considered. Injury is produced during surgery by tissue manipulation and anesthetic agents. Psychic stress causes release of adrenocortical steroids. Afferent stimuli from the injury cause release of catecholamine and corticosteroids. Hypovolemia, if present, triggers the release of epinephrine, norepinephrine, corticosteroids, renin, aldosterone, and ADH.[45] If the postoperative period is equated with early convalescence (one to two days), it is characterized by a systemic adrenergic-corticoid response.[37]

Incisional pain or restrictive chest bandages may make the animal reluctant or unable to cough or fully expand its lungs. Tracheobronchial secretions may accumulate as a result of weak cilary activity and a depressed cough reflex. Aspiration may occur from vomiting or excessive salivation. Brachycephalic breeds are prone to partial or complete collapse of the upper airway. Since recovery is gradual, the cardiovascular homeostatic reflexes may not be fully effective. Rapid reversal of hypercapnia at the termination of surgery removes sympathetic stimulation and may precipitate hypotension.[34] Finally, the animal may be in shock if in severe pain, or if hypovolemic or hypothermic.

GENERAL CONSIDERATIONS

Patient History

The recovery period is an extension of the preoperative and operative periods. Essential to recovery management is an accurate history of the patient's condition. This includes preoperative physical and laboratory data and detailed information of the surgical procedure, anesthetic management, patient response, and any complications that might have been encountered.

General Principles

General principles of recovery room management include the following:

1. The patient is carefully and continuously observed. Temperature, pulse, and respiration should be assessed every five to ten minutes as the patient is recovering.

2. The airway is kept free of secretions, and postural drainage, sponges, and suction apparatus are used.

3. The ambient temperature is kept at 20 to 24°C (68 to 75°F), and stainless steel is covered with insulated pads. Temperature is mantained using towels, blankets, and protected heating pads.

4. The animal's position is changed frequently to prevent hypostatic congestion, atelectasis, and decubital ulcers; to remove inhalants; and to control secretions.

5. If the patient is slow to recover it may be stimulated by rubbing, flexing, and extending the limbs.

6. Tranquilizers or analgesics are used with caution if the animal is distressed or in pain.

7. Fluid therapy that has been instituted during surgery is continued.

8. Coughing is induced by palpating the larynx and trachea.

9. Respiration is assisted and oxygen given if necessary.

10. The patient is radiographed if there is any question about the status of the thoracic or abdominal cavity.

Potential Complications

Recovery should be smooth and uneventful. However, because we are dealing with a complex organ system that has been subjected to many different stimuli, complications frequently arise during the recovery period.

Shock

The most common cause of postoperative shock is hypovolemia. The normal circulating blood volume in the dog is 90 ml/kg and in the cat 70 ml/kg.[1] Signs of shock become evident when blood loss exceeds 30 per cent of the circulating blood volume.[1] Other causes of shock include respiratory insufficiency, cardiac failure, electrolyte imbalance, invasive infection, and vascular complications such as pulmonary embolism.[20]

Respiratory Insufficiency

Normal breathing (eupnea) is desired in the recovery period. Signs of respiratory distress are manifest by variations from this normal pattern. Apnea, in which respiration ceases, can be caused by airway obstruction, drugs, muscle paralysis, or hyperventilation. Dyspnea, difficulty in breathing, is more frequent. It is not always apparent and can be attributed to many causes. Evaluation of chest wall movement is insufficient for quantitative estimation of ventilatory exchange. If the volume of gas exchange through the nose can be measured, a more accurate determination of respiratory competence is possible.[22]

Many varied respiratory patterns are possible. Tachypnea, an increased rate, can be seen with pain or anxiety, fever, pneumonia, compensatory respiratory alkalosis, respiratory insufficiency, or lesions of the central nervous system respiratory centers. Bradypnea (slow respiration) can be seen with sleep, opiates, other analgesics and tranquilizers, or respiratory decompensation. Hyperpnea (deep respirations) may occur with pain, hypoxia, surgical stimulation, or hypercapnia.

Several factors predispose to inadequate exchange, respiratory insufficiency, or respiratory failure, including cardiac insufficiency, pulmonary congestion, oversedation with drugs and anesthetic agents, an unstable or damaged chest wall, pain and splinting, laryngotracheal or pulmonary edema, lung collapse, coughing, bronchospasm, pneumothorax, space-occupying lesions within the thorax, and body weight.[20] The respiratory changes occurring during surgery predispose to ventilatory inadequacy, pooling of secretions, atelectasis, and pulmonary infections. Anesthesia increases respiratory work and decreases lung compliance. It can cause respiratory acidosis from hypoventilation or diffusion hypoxia from the use of insoluble gases. Edema may result from cardiac, hypoxic, or toxic causes. Lung collapse may result from hypoventilation, recumbency, ineffective coughing, or muscle relaxants. Pneumothorax may result from ruptured alveoli. Finally, an increase in body weight of two to three times normal decreases lung compliance by one-half.[21]

Cardiac Abnormalities

Cardiac disturbances may be detected by a change in heart rate. Bradycardia may be due to drug interactions or hypothermia. Tachycardia may result from pain, apprehension, hypoventilation, or hypothermia.

Cardiac disturbances may also manifest themselves as arrhythmia patterns. Causes of cardiac arrhythmias include extubation, electrolyte disturbances, hypoxia, acidosis, increased catecholamine levels, drug interactions, and prolonged anesthesia. The incidence of arrhythmias is greatly increased if surgery is longer than three hours.[2] There are twice as many arrhythmias in spontaneously breathing patients as in patients with controlled respiration.[11] In addition, the dose of catecholamines necessary to produce an arrhythmia is decreased as much as one-tenth the normal dose in the presence of halothane and other anesthetics.[2] The most common arrhythmias associated with anesthesia in dogs are wandering sinus pacemaker, sinus bradycardia, and sinus arrhythmia.[11]

Pulse pressure may be low or high. Hypotension results from hypovolemia, cardiac depression, adrenal insufficiency, and, occasionally, pain. Hypertension is seen as the patient awakens from anesthesia and feels painful stimuli. It can also be attributed to pre-existing hypertension or the use of vasopressors during surgery.[17]

Cyanosis is an unreliable and late warning of low oxygen tension[32] and may be central or peripheral. The confirmation of cyanosis depends on the determination of blood gases, particularly decreased p_{O_2}. The presence of cyanosis may indicate right-to-left shunting, decreased cardiac output with peripheral stagnation, hypothermia, local vasoconstriction, or respiratory problems.

Electrolyte Imbalance

Electrolyte imbalance often reflects an uncorrected preoperative deficit or excess of water or electrolytes.

The normal composition of electrolytes in serum is given in Table 31–1. Electrolyte abnormalities associated with common diseases are given in Table 31–2.

Oliguria and Renal Failure

Oliguria is defined as a urinary output less than 25 per cent of normal; e.g. a patient producing less than 0.27 mg/kg/hr or 6.5 ml/kg/day is oliguric. The renal response to surgery during the first 48 hours is water and sodium retention from increased aldosterone.[54] The glomerular filtration rate can decrease by 30 per cent, returning to normal by the third or fourth day.[54] If renal problems develop after surgery one must differentiate prerenal, renal, and postrenal causes. Signs of renal disease include vomiting, weakness, depression, a decrease or increase in urine production, elevated blood urea nitrogen or creatinine levels, anemia, and aberrations in the urinalysis. Predisposing factors include hypotension with associated hypoperfusion, vasoconstriction and ischemia, abnormal heme pigments, nephrotoxic antibiotics, urinary blockage or trauma, and decompensation in an animal with previously compensated chronic renal disease.

Jaundice

Jaundice is evident when the serum bilirubin level exceeds 1.5 mg/dl and a yellow discoloration of the tissues becomes evident. The causes of postoperative jaundice include hemolysis, pre-existing liver disease, liver hypoxia, drug or anesthetic toxicity, septicemia, pulmonary embolism, and hepatic infection.[20]

Infection

Hallmarks of postoperative infection are fever, leucocytosis with a left shift, and an increased pulse rate. Bacteremia, the presence of microorganisms in

TABLE 31–1. Distribution of Body Electrolytes and Fluids*

	Dog Serum (mEq)		Cat Serum (mEq)
Na$^+$	141.0–157.0		152.0–161.0
K$^+$	4.3–5.6		4.0–5.3
Ca^{++}	9.8–11.4		8.9–10.6
Mg^{++}	1.8–2.4		2.0–3.0
Cl$^-$	98.0–116.0		115.0–123.0
HCO$_3$$^-$	17.0–24.0		17.0–24.0
	Adult Dog	**Puppy**	**Adult Cat**
Total body water	60% of body weight	75–85%	60%
Extracellular water	20% of body weight	40%	25%
Intracellular water	40% of body weight	40%	35%
Plasma volume	5% of body weight		5%
Daily water intake	50 cc/kg body weight		64 cc/kg
Daily urine output	22 cc/kg body weight		22–33 cc/kg

*Reprinted with permission from Short, C. E.: Fluid and electrolyte therapy. *In* Kirk, R. W. (ed.): *Current Veterinary Therapy VII.* W. B. Saunders, Philadelphia, 1980.

Note: Laboratory values from N.Y.S.C.V.M. Values may vary geographically or in other laboratories.

TABLE 31–2. Electrolyte Imbalances*

	Conditions Causing Increased Levels	Conditions Causing Decreased Levels
Sodium (mEq/L)	Primary water deficit Dehydration Osmotic diuresis	Severe diarrhea Chronic renal failure Diuretic administration Vomiting Congestive heart failure Malabsorption
Potassium (mEq/L)	Hemolysis Addison's disease Shock Renal dysfunction Diarrhea Respiratory (acidosis)	Diuretic administration Vomiting or diarrhea Treated diabetes Ketosis Urine loss (adrenocortical function) Inadequate intake
Chloride (mEq/L)	Dehydration Overtreatment with saline Respiratory alkalosis Complete renal shutdown Cirrhosis	Vomiting Chronic renal disease Emphysema Diuretic administration Hypoventilation (pneumonia)

*Reprinted with permission from Zaslow, I. M.: Personnel and physical requirements. *In* Sattler, F. P., Knowles, R. P., and Whittick, W. G. (eds.): *Veterinary Critical Care.* Lea & Febiger, Philadelphia, 1981, p. 23.

the blood stream, and septicemia, the systemic disease associated with microorganisms or their toxins, may occur during the recovery period. Predisposing factors to infection are devitalization of tissue, location of the injury, presence of foreign bodies, systemic factors, and the duration of surgery.[2] Local wound infection is characterized by pain, tenderness, swelling, warmth, erythema, and suppuration. Every operative wound is contaminated with bacteria. The incidence of wound infection varies from less than 1 per cent in clean primarily closed wounds to 30 per cent or more in wounds created by emergency operations or on an injured colon.[24] Serial white blood cell counts, collection and examination of exudates,

TABLE 31–3. Disturbances in Acid-Base Balance*

Respiratory Acidosis–Carbonic Acid Excess (Free CO_2)
A. Respiratory center depression
   1. Surgical anesthetics
   2. Morphine, barbiturates
B. Cardiac disease
   1. Congestive heart failure
C. Pulmonary disease
   1. Emphysema
   2. Atelectasis (chronic obstructive airway disease)
   3. Asthma
   4. Pneumonia
D. Musculoskeletal disease

Metabolic Acidosis–Bicarbonate Deficit (Combined CO_2)
A. Excessive production of organic acids (proton donors)
   1. Shock
   2. Convulsions
   3. Hypoxia
   4. Impaired liver function
   5. Endocrine disorders—diabetic ketosis
B. Excessive loss of bicarbonate
   1. Diarrhea
   2. Renal tubular insufficiency
   3. Addison's disease
   4. Vomiting

Respiratory Alkalosis–Carbonic Acid Deficit (Free CO_2)
A. Respiratory center stimulation
   1. Fever
   2. Hypoxia
   3. C.N.S. disease
B. Respirators
C. High altitudes
D. Hysterical hyperventilation

Metabolic Alkalosis–Bicarbonate Excess (Combined CO_2)
A. Endocrine disorders
   1. Cushing's disease
   2. Pancreatic fibrosis
B. Iatrogenic
   1. Excessive steroids
   2. Diuretics
   3. Enemas
   4. IV infusion therapy without potassium

*Reprinted with permission from Zaslow, I.M.: Personnel and physical requirements. *In* Sattler, F. P., Knowles, R. P., and Whittick, W. G. (eds.): *Veterinary Critical Care.* Lea & Febiger, Philadelphia, 1981, p. 23.

blood cultures, and biopsies can be used to select and monitor therapy and its response. (More details on infection are provided in Chapter 4.)

Disorders of Consciousness

Disorders of consciousness include lethargy, aggression, and coma. Seizures may be apparent in some patients. Causes of these problems include prolonged effects of anesthetics, cerebral hypoxia, embolism, intracranial hemorrhage, thrombosis, and alterations in cerebral metabolism.[20]

Alimentary Tract Dysfunction

Alimentary tract problems include aspiration, vomiting, ileus, fecal impaction, and inadequate nutritional intake. Early return to function helps to control many of these complications.

Acid-Base Abnormalities

Disturbances in acid-base balance are often undiagnosed (Table 31–3). Hypoxemia and hypercarbia, the most commonly diagnosed postsurgical problems, are often accompanied by restlessness, anxiety, tachycardia, and tachypnea. Evaluation of P_{O_2}, P_{CO_2}, and bicarbonate and correction of abnormalities are advisable for complete recovery room care.

Temperature

Patients may be hypothermic or hyperthermic. A patient's temperature may drop 2 to 3°C during a 60-minute surgical procedure.[27] Mild hypothermia is about 37°C (98°F), moderate about 35°C (95°F), and severe about 33°C (92°F). Hypothermia leads to shivering and delayed recovery. The smaller patient with a larger body surface area dissipates more heat to the environment than a larger patient and, therefore, can more readily become hypothermic. Hyperthermia leads to heat prostration.

Core and skin temperatures are used to evaluate the temperature of the patient.[33] The core temperature (rectal or esophageal) is within a few tenths of a degree of the temperature of the body core (viscera and head). The skin temperature correlates well with cardiac and peripheral blood flow and can be used to monitor response.[7, 30]

A low-grade fever is commonly seen for the first one to three days after surgery. This is attributed to trauma, low-grade infection, and tissue and protein absorption.[56] If the fever continues or becomes more elevated, a more serious physiological problem should be sought.

Pain

Incisional pain is usually not severe and can be managed easily with minimal use of narcotics. More severe pain may indicate tension, inflammation, pressure, or ischemia. There are many unknown factors in the etiology and management of pain, but recovery may be assisted if severe pain is managed therapeutically.[19]

Hemorrhage

Hemorrhage may result from blood loss or from hemostatic disorders. Disorders of hemostasis may exist prior to surgery or may result from surgical or anesthetic manipulation of the patient. Accurate assessment of all clotting parameters and control of the inciting causes may be necessary for their reversal (see Chapters 6 and 81).

General Concerns

Fluids

An intravenous catheter with direct access to the circulatory system is essential for good postoperative care and allows one to correct fluid imbalances due to insensible or obligatory fluid loss or blood loss. Since anesthetic agents depress glomerular filtration rate, renal plasma flow, and urinary output, fluid administration promotes adequate renal perfusion. A fluid line also allows one to monitor and maintain electrolyte balance, acid-base balance, and central venous pressure and to administer emergency and prophylactic medications.

Fluids should not be given in excess after surgery unless special problems exist. Assessment of preoperative fluid administration, intraoperative blood loss and continued loss at the surgical site helps determine the amount of fluids necessary.

Special fluid considerations in the postoperative period fall into several categories. Administration of excess volume causes overexpansion of the extracellular fluid space, continued water loss, and hypernatremia. Hyponatremia may develop and can be prevented by adequate replacement of extracellular fluid deficits. If the patient is oliguric, daily water requirements are reduced. Exogenous needs are further reduced by the cellular release of water from cellular catabolism and metabolic acidosis. Intracellular shifts of sodium may occur with sepsis and reduced kidney function, causing a relative decrease in serum sodium levels. Hypernatremia, on the other hand, can occur with solute loading, tubular damage, or fever. A final area of concern is high-output renal failure occurring from a less severe or modified episode of renal injury than that producing classic oliguric renal failure.[50]

Fluids are given to replace deficits, meet current needs, and replace current losses.[13, 49] The degree of dehydration can be used to calculate fluid replacement needs.[13, 51] Normal fluid losses average 40 ml/kg/day and include both extrarenal and renal losses.[13]

One ml of blood loss should be replaced with either an equal volume of blood or 3 ml of physiologically balanced solution. If the body temperature is elevated, fluid volumes should be increased.

Replacement fluids should be isotonic and polyionic. Typical intravenous fluids and their contents are listed in Chapter 9. They should be warmed to 37°C prior to administration. If one is uncertain about the rate of administration, a safe estimate is 40 ml/kg/day in the dog and 30 ml/kg/day in the cat.[7] The object is to cause a mild diuresis, which can be assessed by monitoring patient response. Signs of adequate fluid replacement include an acceptable pulse, heart rate and volume, respiratory pattern, capillary refill and color, alertness, and skin elasticity. More specific indices include packed cell volume and total solids, central venous pressure, urine output, and determination of plasma osmolarity or tonicity.[22, 51]

Bicarbonate requirements can be determined from arterial blood gas analysis. The total bicarbonate dose can be calculated as follows: HCO_3^- mEq needed = .03 kg × (25 -HCO_3 mEq deficit).[57] The first half of this deficit can be replaced rapidly intravenously and the remainder given slowly through the intravenous catheter. Bicarbonate is given slowly and to effect to prevent iatrogenic alkalosis, paradoxical cerebral acidosis, and hyperosmolarity from hypernatremia.[10] If no information on the quantity of bicarbonate needed is available but metabolic acidosis is suspected, 2.2 mEq/kg can be added to the intravenous drip.[51]

Electrolyte abnormalities are not commonly seen in the postsurgical patient. Potassium should not be given postoperatively unless a potassium deficit is documented. Since potassium is primarily an intracellular ion, serum values can be erroneous. A potassium deficit of greater than 3.5 mEq/L has been used as a guide for replacement therapy.[48] A normal daily allowance of potassium is 2.0 mEq/kg.[34]

Complications of parenteral fluid therapy are many. They include hematoma formation from laceration of the vein wall, extravasation of fluids, local infection, catheter embolus, and hemorrhage from laceration of the vessel wall.[36]

Transfusions are necessary when there is acute blood loss or reduction in effective circulating blood volume. Twenty ml/kg of blood is necessary to raise the packed cell volume 1%. Blood may be given from a fresh donor or a stored pack or by autotransfusion.[1, 5, 15, 60]

Antibiotics

Antibiotics given in the recovery period are usually an extension of those given before or during surgical intervention. Broad spectrum antibiotics are chosen because of existing or potential infection.[44] The selection of an appropriate antibiotic includes an appreciation for its need, a logical approach toward its sensitivity, and knowledge of drug interactions.[18, 42]

The aminoglycosides potentiate nondepolarizing muscle relaxants and can cause cardiac and respiratory depression or tubular necrosis, decrease the availability of calcium at the axonal terminal, and induce either auditory or vestibular disorders.[12] Chloramphenicol blocks microsomal enzyme systems, causing respiratory depression and a prolonged recovery time.[26] It has increased activity with barbi-

TABLE 31–4. Analgesics and Sedatives Used in the Dog and Cat*

| Drug | Dosage | |
	Dog	Cat
Morphine	0.5–2.0 mg/kg SQ or IM q4h	0.1 mg/kg SQ or IM q4h
Meperidine	2.5–8.0 mg/kg IM q2–4h	Same
Oxymorphone	0.02–0.1 mg/kg SQ, IM, IV	Same
Nallorphine	0.2 mg/kg IM, IV	†
Nalbuphine HCl	0.8–2.0 mg/kg IV	†
Levallorphan	0.04 mg/kg IM or IV	†
Naloxone HCl	0.01–0.02 mg/kg IM or IV	†
Pentazocine	1.0–2.0 mg/kg SQ, IM, IV	†
Aspirin	10 mg/kg q12h PO	10/mg/kg q2d
Acetaminophen	10 mg/kg q12h PO	Do not use
Phenylbutazone	9 mg/kg q8 hr PO	Same
Flunixin meglumine	0.5 mg/lb IV‡	†
Valium†	0.1–0.5 mg/kg IM or IV	Same
Promazine HCl	1.0–2.0 mg/kg IM or IV	2.0–4.0 mg/kg IM or IV
Acetylpromazine	0.04–0.1 mg/kg IM or IV	0.04–0.2 mg/kg IM or IV

*Data from Archibald, J., Holt, J. C., and Sokolovsky, V.: *Management of Trauma in Dogs and Cats.* American Veterinary Publications, Inc., Santa Barbara, 1981; Kaplan, M.: Pain. *In* Ettinger, S. J. (ed.): *Textbook of Veterinary Internal Medicine,* 2nd ed. W. B. Saunders, Philadelphia, 1983; Klide, A.: Personal communication, 1983; and Penny, B. E., and White, R. J.: Narcotic analgesics in the domestic cat. Vet. Clin. North Am. 8:317, 1978.

†Use with caution as single intravenous agent.

‡Manufacturer's recommendation.

turates and can cause cardiac depression. Penicillins and cephalosporins can cause hypersensitivity, anaphylaxis, and angioneurotic edema.

Aspiration

Aspiration of gastric contents into the tracheobronchial tree can be disastrous and can result in laryngospasm, bronchospasm, or acute hypoxia. More long-term problems include a chemical pneumonia or a lung abscess from particulate matter. Postural drainage or suction will control the final disposition of gastrointestinal contents. Suction is best done with saline flushing to ensure elimination of as much material as possible.

The use of atropine is a controversial subject. It has been used routinely in the past to prevent salivary secretions, control vomiting, and inhibit the bradycardia of vagal stimulation. It is an anticholinergic, parasympatholytic, and antispasmodic. Other effects include a mild central nervous system depression, bronchodilation, mydriasis, reduction in gastrointestinal motility, bladder and ureteral contractions, and a reduction in secretions of the respiratory tract, gastrointestinal tract, and oral and nasal cavities. Negative effects of atropine have been noted. It may produce an initial sinus bradycardia owing to stimulation of vagal nuclei in the central nervous system.

It greatly increases the incidence of cardiac arrhythmias, including second degree heart block and ventricular premature beats. It tends to induce a sinus tachycardia, thereby increasing myocardial oxygen consumption. And it decreases the level of stimulation needed to induce ventricular arrhythmias and ventricular fibrillation.[46]

Analgesics and Sedatives

Analgesics are given to relieve pain. Sedatives are given to prevent violent recovery and control seizures. Analgesics are divided into the narcotics and mild analgesics.[25] Mild analgesics produce a finite level of pain relief, but narcotics increase pain relief as the dose is increased.

Narcotics cause miosis, decreased tidal volume and respiratory rate, bradycardia, salivation, nausea, and vomiting. Morphine, the standard drug against which all potent analgesics are evaluated, is a positive inotrope and a respiratory depressant and produces hypothermia in the dog and hyperthermia in the cat.[25] Some of the semisynthetic derivatives include oxymorphone and meperidine. Some of the narcotic antagonists can also be used as analgesics. These include pentazocine, nallorphine, and nalbuphine hydrochloride. The mild analgesics include aspirin, acetaminophen, flunixin meglumine, and phenylbu-

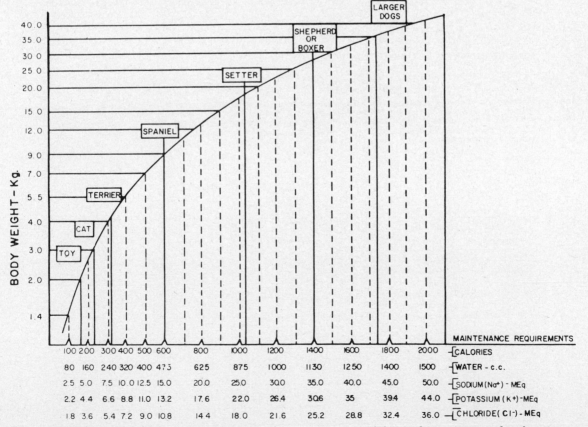

Figure 31–1. Maintenance requirements of calories, water, and electrolytes of caged dogs and cats. (Reprinted with permission from Finco, D. R.: A scheme for fluid therapy in the dog and cat. J. Am. Anim. Hosp. Assoc. 8:178, 1972. Adapted from Kirk, R. W. (ed.): *Current Veterinary Therapy VI.* W. B. Saunders, Philadelphia, 1977.)

tazone.[25] Aspirin should be used with caution because of its effect on platelets and subsequent hemorrhage.

Pentazocine (Talwin) has analgesic properties roughly equivalent to those of meperidine with relatively minor respiratory depression. Because it is also an agonist, it can be antagonized by the pure antagonist naloxone.

Diazepam (Valium) depresses the limbic system, thalamus, and hypothalamus; decreases sympathetic tone; and produces a calming effect. It is used as a muscle relaxant. It is eliminated through the liver. It has minimal side effects that include central nervous system depression, hypotension, and changes in respiratory rate and tidal volume.

The phenothiazine tranquilizers are α blockers; they reduce the activity of the reticular formation and hypothalamus and suppress the sympathetic nervous system. They produce hypotension, lower the seizure threshold, and depress the myocardium and vascular smooth muscle. A reflex tachycardia can develop from the hypotension. They protect against epinephrine-induced cardiac irregularities and are useful as antiemetics. Care must be exercised in their use because they potentiate narcotics and other drugs used to produce general anesthesia. They are detoxified in the liver and produce clinical effects for four and eight hours.

Table 31–4 lists the analgesics and sedatives that are in common use with their appropriate dosages.

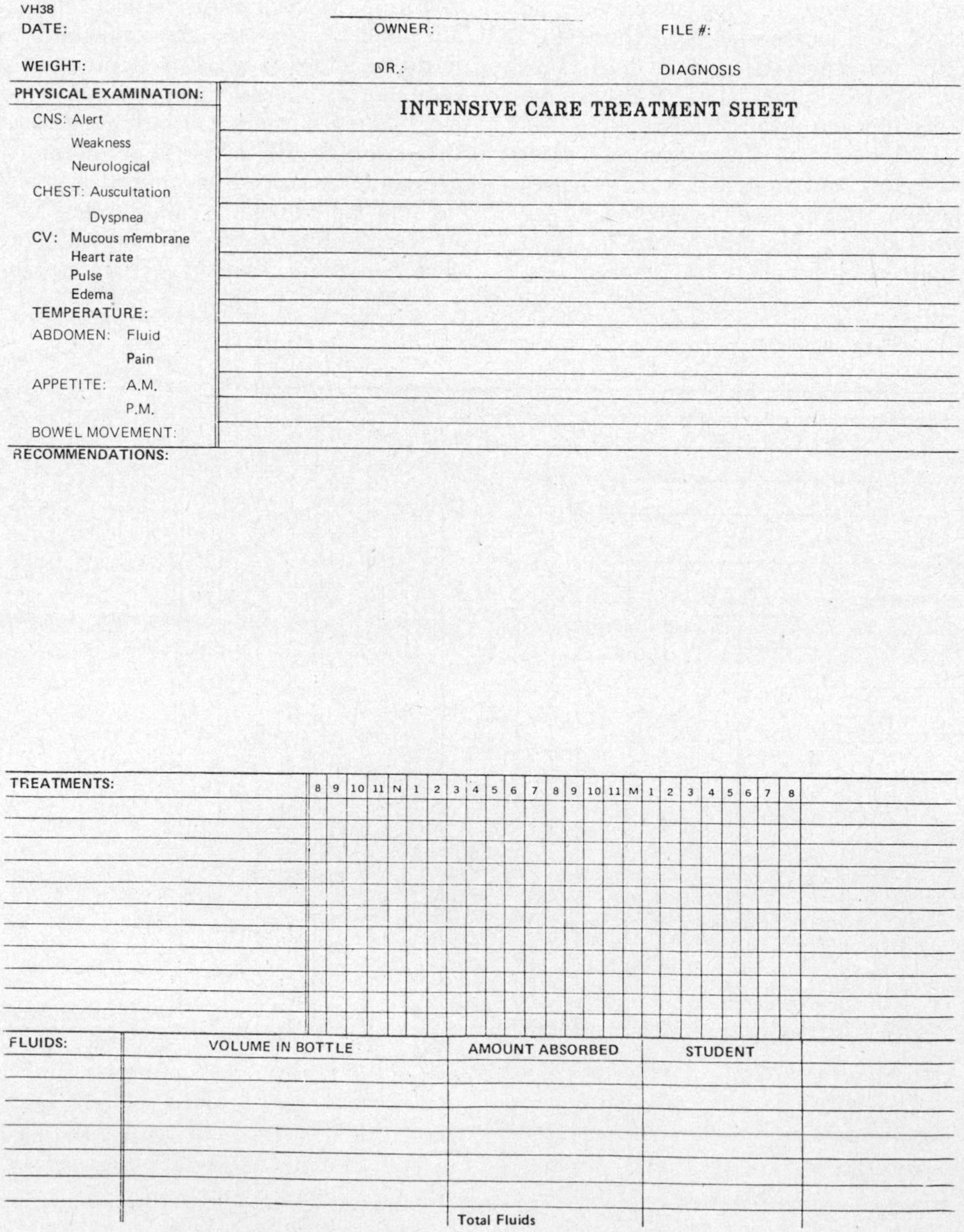
VH38
DATE: OWNER: FILE #:
WEIGHT: DR.: DIAGNOSIS
PHYSICAL EXAMINATION:
INTENSIVE CARE TREATMENT SHEET
CNS: Alert
Weakness
Neurological
CHEST: Auscultation
Dyspnea
CV: Mucous membrane
Heart rate
Pulse
Edema
TEMPERATURE:
ABDOMEN: Fluid
Pain
APPETITE: A.M.
P.M.
BOWEL MOVEMENT:
RECOMMENDATIONS:
TREATMENTS: 8 9 10 11 N 1 2 3 4 5 6 7 8 9 10 11 M 1 2 3 4 5 6 7 8
FLUIDS: VOLUME IN BOTTLE AMOUNT ABSORBED STUDENT
Total Fluids

Figure 31–2. Intensive care treatment sheet.

Nutrition

The nutritional status usually returns to normal within two or three days.[54] Nutritional supplementation is needed when there are pre-existing deficits, when the surgical condition precludes eating for more than three or four days, or when there are large demands for energy production, as with burns or sepsis. A nomogram for calories, water, and electrolytes is given in Figure 31–1. An animal requires 7 cal/kg/day to prevent most body protein catabolism and 25 cal/kg/day to prevent both protein and fat catabolism.[51] A minimum protein intake of 2.2 gm/kg/day is necessary to ensure a positive nitrogen balance. In addition, dextrose at 4.4 gm/kg/day is necessary for energy and as a protein-sparing measure to allow protein to be used for tissue repair and synthesis. Nutritional requirements can be met through oral, pharyngostomy, enteral, or parenteral techniques. Eating can be supplemented with commercial veterinary foods, homemade formulations, or hyperalimentation solutions (see Chapter 17).[1, 7, 14, 16, 31]

Positioning and Ambulation

Initial positioning techniques are used to assist respiration and control secretions. Early movement helps restore body tone and decreases intestinal distress.[56]

MONITORING IN THE RECOVERY ROOM

The Environment

Adequate recovery room care requires close surveillance and specialized equipment. Close observation must continue until the patient is physiologically stable. Patient signs must be evaluated (directly by physical examination or indirectly through the use of special aids) and interpreted. The recovery area should be clean and designed with concern for both space and time. Equipment should be clean, accessible, and in good functional condition.

Vital Signs

All vital signs should be recorded on a flow chart and noted in the patient's record. The flow chart enables one to see trends, whereas the patient record enables one to elaborate on the details of therapy and response (Figs. 31–2 through 31–4). Parameters that should be noted include heart rate and rhythm, pulse rate and quality, capillary refill, color of mucous membranes, respiratory rate and rhythm, temperature, packed cell volume and total solids, state of consciousness, mobility, and urine output. In the more critical patient, serum biochemistries, coagulation profile, electrocardiogram, central venous pressure, acid base parameters, and arterial blood pressure should also be noted.

Cardiovascular Status

Determinations of the status of the heart can be made with a stethoscope and electrocardiogram; of the capillary circulation by examination of mucous membrane color, capillary refill time, and core or local temperature; of the venous circulation through central venous pressure; and of the arterial circulation with either palpation of the pulse pressure or catheterization of an artery and direct pressure recording. The heart should be evaluated with regard to rate, rhythm, and pattern of conduction. Auscultation allows one to make general determinations about cardiac status. Use of an electrocardiogram may include an oscilloscope for rapid visual assessment and a paper trace for more accurate, permanent evaluation.[59] Capillary refill time is a better index of peripheral perfusion than mucous membrane color. After compression, color should return to the mucous membrane in 0.5 to 1.0 second. A prolonged refill time may indicate hypotension, hypovolemia, or peripheral vasoconstriction.[22]

Central venous pressure is measured by a catheter positioned near the right atrium with a saline manometer zeroed to the level of the right atrium. It indicates the capacity of the heart pump in relation to venous return and helps define the relationship between myocardial contractility, vascular resistance, and blood volume. Serial measurements are important to show trends in the general status of the patient and response to therapy. Normal CVP is -2 to $+4$ cm H_2O. An increase in CVP is seen with heart failure, venoconstriction, and hypervolemia. A decrease is seen with hypovolemia, increased peripheral resistance, and vasodilation.[1, 30]

Digital palpation of the pulse provides some indication of arterial blood pressure. It should be checked at frequent intervals and in more than one location. Changes in the pulse rate may indicate cardiac arrythmias, infection, hypoxemia, or continuing fluid losses. Blood pressure can be measured directly through percutaneous or cutdown techniques or indirectly with an occlusion cuff placed over a distal artery and attached to a sphygmomanometer. Normal mean arterial pressures in the dog are between 90 and 120 mm Hg.[6, 22, 30, 59]

Respiration

The respiratory status of the patient can be determined by observing the ventilatory rate and rhythm, auscultating the thorax, and determining the acid-base status. The average tidal volume in the dog is 15 ml/kg and in the cat 5 mg/kg.[32] The ventilatory rate is between 10 and 25 per minute. The respiratory minute volume equals tidal volume × rate/minute.

Initial postoperative concerns include management of secretions, atelectasis, pain, and bronchospasm. Secretions can be managed by tracheal suctioning, mucolytic agents, and postural drainage. Atelectasis can be prevented by achieving maximal lung expansion, turning, tracheal compression and induction of

INTENSIVE CARE UNIT — LABORATORY RECORD CHART

Name

Date								
Hematocrit								
Hemoglobin								
Red Blood Count								
White Blood Count								
Retic Count								
Platelet Count								
Sodium								
Potassium								
Total Protein								
Albumin								
Globulin								
Calcium								
Phosphorus								
Glucose								
Creatinine								
Bun								
SGPT								
Alkaline Phos								
Cholesterol								
Total Bilirubin								
Direct Bilirubin								
SAP								
Amylase								
Lipase								
BSP								
PT								
PTT								
FSP								
Urinalysis pH								
Specific Gravity								
Protein								
Glucose								
Hb.								

VH32

Figure 31–3. Intensive care unit laboratory record chart.

coughing, percussion and manual vibration of the chest wall, and slinging in an upright position. Pain can be managed by appropriate sedation. Bronchospasm can be controlled with bronchodilators (isoproterenol, theophyllines, and epinephrine), and adrenocorticosteroids.[35]

The need for oxygen therapy is determined by a state of hypoxia and proven by measurement of the partial oxygen pressure in arterial blood (Pa_{O_2}). Subjective determinations of hypoxia include cardiac abnormalities, dyspnea, depressed motor activity, drowsiness, increased excitability, cyanosis, and cold extremities. The only accurate quantitative determination is arterial blood gas analysis. The optimal inspired oxygen concentration is that which results in a Pa_{O_2} between 80 and 100 mm Hg. An inspired oxygen concentration of 30 to 40 per cent is usually adequate to meet this requirement.[7]

Oxygen can be administered through a mask, intratracheal or nasal catheter, oxygen cage, pediatric incubator, endotracheal tube, or tracheostomy tube.[30]

The mask can be attached to a self-inflating Ambu bag and an oxygen line. The mask can also be attached to a conventional anesthetic unit. Oxygen cages are used when an oxygen-rich environment is needed and the patient is able to ventilate spontaneously. Oxygen concentrations of 30 to 40 per cent can be administered.[30] A flow rate of 10 L/min maintains 37 to 40 per cent oxygen in a cage.[22] Temperature and humidity are controlled to about 40 to 50 per cent.[22]

Endotracheal tubes or tracheostomy tubes are used in more severely affected patients. Tracheostomy tubes reduce dead space, bypass obstructions of the upper airway, and facilitate control of tracheobronchial secretions but demand constant supervision. Placement involves a sterile, atraumatic surgical procedure and fixation to the patient's neck. A pliable tube is preferred over a rigid one. It should be inflated to a minimal occlusive volume. Principles of management include wound care, humidification of inspired air, and tracheal suctioning, and these tubes should be used only as long as needed.[1, 22] Compli-

INTENSIVE CARE UNIT — ELECTROCARDIOGRAM FLOW SHEET

Name _____ Date _____ Time _____ Speed _____ Voltage_____

Name _____ Date _____ Time _____ Speed _____ Voltage_____

Figure 31–4. Intensive care unit electro-cardiogram flow sheet.

Name _____ Date _____ Time _____ Speed _____ Voltage _____

Name _____ Date _____ Time _____ Speed _____ Voltage _____

VH36

cations are many and include tracheal wall effects (obstruction; tracheoarterial, tracheoesophageal, tracheopleural fistulae; stenosis; pressure necrosis; fibrosis; inflammation; ulceration; hemorrhage; tracheomalacia; tracheal dilation), esophageal injury, injury to adjacent blood vessels, subcutaneous or mediastinal emphysema, pneumothorax, aspiration, and infection.[19, 22, 59]

Air entering the trachea during nasal inspiration has a temperature of 32 to 34°C with a relative humidity of 80 to 90 per cent (water content 27 to 34 mg/L). The water content inspired during the maintenance of artificial airways should approach that of nasally inspired air (27 to 34 mg/L).[22] Humidification is needed to prevent irritation of the mucous lining of the respiratory tract and the accumulation of inspissated secretions. Humidification can be accomplished with heated humidifiers or ultrasonic nebulizers or by bubbling oxygen through water. Heated humidifiers can provide mist densities of 27 to 44 mg/L, jet nebulizers can provide mist densities of 20 to 28 mg/L, and ultrasonic nebulizers can provide a supersaturated mist.[22] The addition of mucolytic agents or alcohol helps to reduce secretions and surface tension and prevent froth formation.

Artificial ventilation is given if the patient cannot breathe adequately without assistance. The respiratory centers may be depressed from anesthesia, neuromuscular agents, drug toxicities, acidosis, coma, toxic metabolites, head trauma, or nerve trauma (edema). The patient may be unable or reluctant to expand its chest adequately owing to pain, chest trauma, thoracic surgery, abdominal distension, muscle weakness, obesity, or positioning. Inability to expand the chest may also result from pneumothorax, pleural fluid, diaphragmatic hernia, thoracic surgery, neoplasia, pneumonia, or atelectasis. The most serious reasons for ventilatory support include pulmonary edema, pulmonary insufficiency, and cardiopulmonary arrest.

Respiratory assistance can be manual or mechanical. Methods of positive pressure ventilation include blowing into the mouth, nose, or airway tube and using a self-inflating bag (Ambu bag), a T-tube, or an automatic ventilator.[22, 59] Ventilation can be assisted or controlled. In the assist mode the ventilator assures complete tidal volumes but the patient controls the ventilatory rate. This mode is indicated when the inspiratory capacity is compromised but the medullary response to chemical stimulants is normal. In the controlled mode the patient is not triggering any part of the respiratory cycle. It is indicated when the respiratory centers are depressed, when there is insufficient respiratory effort, and when there is a need to control Pa_{CO_2}. The best indicators of adequate ventilatory support are the arterial CO_2 tension (Pa_{CO_2}) and ventilometry.

Regardless of the means of ventilatory support, several principles are appropriate. The ventilatory rate should be about 12 breaths per minute. Peak airway pressure should be between 10 and 20 cm H_2O. Inspiratory/expiratory time should be in a ratio of 1:2. Inspiration should last about one second. PEEP (positive end expiratory pressure) should be considered when intermittent positive pressure ventilation (IPPV) is not improving gas exchange.[52] Tidal volume should be about 10 to 15 ml/kg.[22] Chest wall movements should be observed during ventilation. Finally, the adequacy of delivery should be assessed by observing patient signs and evaluating laboratory data.

Ventilators are either volume-cycled or pressure-cycled. The controversy over the advantages and disadvantages of each continues. The volume-cycled ventilator delivers a preset volume of gas. The pressure-cycled ventilator delivers gas during the inspiratory phase until the system reaches a preset pressure. Commonly used ventilators include North American Dräger (volume-cycled), Bird (pressure-cycled), and Metomatic (volume-cycled and pressure-limited).[22, 59]

Ventilatory support has several inherent problems.[22] When the patient is gradually disconnected from the ventilator, ventilatory support must be removed gradually. This is best done by hypoventilating with an enriched oxygen mixture and giving a deep breath every 30 seconds. Positive pressure ventilation increases airway diameter, leading to increased dead space; decreases lung compliance and lung volume, leading to atelectasis and hypoxia; and increases mean airway pressure, leading to decreased cardiac output, blood pressure, and pulmonary blood flow. Impairment of thoracic blood flow resulting in decreased cardiac output is probably the major complication to be managed with controlled ventilation.

Other respiratory complications include pneumothorax, thoracic effusions, pulmonary edema, and pneumonia. Pneumothorax can best be managed with thoracocentesis and chest drainage (see Chapter 66). Thoracic effusions are managed in a similar manner. Pulmonary edema is managed with oxygen, aspiration, nebulization, intravenous digitalis or aminophylline, reduction in fluids, diuretics, rotating phle-

botomies, vasodilators, and adrenocortical steroids.[2, 4] Pneumonia is best managed by culture and sensitivity analysis of the infective agent and appropriate antibiotic therapy.

Urinary Output

Urinary output reflects visceral organ perfusion. It should be greater than 2.0 ml/kg/hr and can be monitored subjectively by visual observation or objectively by catheterization. Catheters should be flexible, sterile, and nonreactive. Rigid metal catheters are used only in the female dog. Catheter placement demands sterile technique and fixation. A closed collection system and antibacterial flushing should be used, and catheters should be removed as soon as monitoring is no longer needed.

Temperature

Temperature should be monitored and controlled. A continuous reading thermometer is more expensive but gives a much more accurate assessment than a mercury thermometer with less distress to the patient.[30, 59]

If the patient is hypothermic, protection with blankets and towels helps to prevent dissipation of body heat. The ambient temperature should be above 21°C (70°F), and the patient should be kept clean of blood, feces, and urine. Temperature can best be increased with circulating water pads. Electric heating pads must be closely watched and are capable of overheating the adjacent skin, with local burns and tissue death resulting. Heating lamps and dryers have similar limitations. Hot water bottles lose heat rapidly and can overheat an adjacent part. Pediatric incubators are helpful for the smaller patient.

If the patient is hyperthermic, the most effective therapy is internal cooling of the viscera, e.g., gastric lavage with iced water. Surface cooling is much easier and more readily used. Cooling methods include cold baths, cold enemas, and irrigation of the nasal alar folds.

Drainage (see Chapter 30)

Wound Protection

Wound protection may be helpful when delayed or faulty wound healing is anticipated.[28] Wound healing is affected by adrenocortical steroids; phenylbutazone; aspirin; hypoproteinemia and nutritional deficiencies; dehydration; endocrine imbalances; car-

TABLE 31–5. Normal pH and Blood Gas Values

	Mean	Range
pH	7.4	7.35 to 7.45
Pa_{O_2}	95 mm Hg	80 to 110 mm Hg
Pa_{CO_2}	40 mm Hg	35 to 45 mm Hg
HCO_3	24 mEq/L	22 to 27 mEq/L

diac, renal, and liver disease; infection; hypothermia; and anemia.[40, 55] Extensive devitalization, delay before treatment, location, presence of dead tissue, foreign bodies, and systemic factors predispose to infection.

Intravenous Catheters

Intravenous catheters are used for measurement and therapy.[53, 59] Percutaneous catheters are used more frequently because they are less traumatic to introduce. They come with the catheter either over the needle or through the needle. Size ranges in dogs and cats are 14 to 22 gauge.[51] Accessible veins for catheterization include the cephalic, jugular, medial and lateral saphenous, aural, abdominal, and sublingual.[22]

The catheter should be introduced aseptically. Larger veins are chosen for prolonged use or administration of large quantities of fluids. The catheter should be fixed to the surrounding tissue, connected to a closed system, and managed with a dry dressing and topical antibiotic/antifungal ointment. It should be periodically flushed with heparin (1 unit per 10 ml saline), used only as long as necessary, and removed when problems occur.[51]

Problems associated with the use of intravenous catheters include infiltration of drugs around the venipuncture site, spasm, thrombosis, phlebitis, intimal dissection, false aneurysm, hemorrhage, stenosis, arteriovenous fistula, embolism, perforation, infection, allergic reaction, cardiac arryhthmias, pericardial tamponade, and chylothorax.[10, 22]

Acid-Base Balance (see also Chapter 10)

Normal pH and blood gas values are listed in Table 31–5. There are many causes of acid-base imbalance. Respiratory acidosis is seen with anesthesia or respiratory depressant drugs, obesity, brain damage, pulmonary disease, and thoracic trauma. Respiratory alkalosis is seen with fear, fever, pneumonia, hypoxemia, left-to-right shunts, and heart failure. Metabolic acidosis is seen with diabetes, diarrhea, vomiting, shock, trauma, and renal disease. Metabolic alkalosis is seen with acute vomiting and excessive use of diuretics.

Equipment for blood gas analysis is expensive, and analysis requires frequent evaluation and careful monitoring. It is not, therefore, a practical investment for many veterinary practitioners. Equipment for analysis of plasma bicarbonate and pH is less expensive and more feasible. Local human hospitals can also be helpful in performing blood gas analyses if prior arrangements have been made.

Sample collection should be done carefully and with regard to several principles. One should avoid negative pressure, eliminate all dead space in the needle and syringe, and rinse the syringe with heparin. Arterial blood should be used with anaerobic technique and immediate analysis. A correction factor should be used for temperature.

To interpret pH and blood gas measurements, one can follow several simple steps. Acidemia or alkalemia is determined by the pH, respiratory status by the Pa_{CO_2}, and metabolic status by the bicarbonate. The primary problem is determined by matching either the Pa_{CO_2} or HCO_3^- or both with the pH. Pa_{CO_2} is determined to evaluate compensation. Replacement therapy is determined by using the formula $0.03 \times kg \times HCO_3$ (24 − deficit mEq/L) = the amount of bicarbonate needed for replacement therapy. One-half is given rapidly and the rest is administered with utmost care, either by repeating blood gas parameters or by observing clinical signs.

POSTOPERATIVE CONSIDERATIONS— SPECIFIC BODY SYSTEMS

Thoracic—Cardiovascular System

Evaluation of patient status involves assessment of the rate and character of the pulse, the heart rate and rhythm, and the pulse deficit; palpation of the thorax to determine the point of maximal impulse; auscultation; percussion; radiography; and electrocardiography. The differential diagnosis should include the use of concurrent drugs, potentiating ventricular arrhythmias, pre-existing heart disease, myocardial irritability, hypoxemia, and oligemia. Since cardiac output and contractility are reduced with anesthetic agents and since cardiac patients are prone to develop arryhthmias, careful monitoring is essential. Some measures that should be considered with acute heart failure[3] are listed (Table 31–6).

Abdominal System

Gastrointestinal System

Physical examination includes examination of the oral cavity; abdominal palpation for pain, tone, and fluid; abdominal auscultation; rectal examination; and subjective determination of mental attitude. Additional information can be obtained from a complete blood count and serum biochemistries, analysis of electrolytes and blood gas parameters, fecal examination, abdominal paracentesis, and plain or contrast radiography.

Care of the gastrointestinal patient depends on an understanding of pre-existing disease and status. The level of obstruction, the degree of ischemia, the duration of the problem, and the alterations of fluids and electrolytes must be known.[38, 43] Hydration, acid-base status, and cardiac status of patients with gastric dilatation-volvulus complex must be assessed. Patients with pre-existing liver disease must be closely monitored both during and after surgery. Those with

TABLE 31–6. Management of Acute Heart Failure*

General Measures
Reduction of activity—cage rest
Sedation
  Morphine sulfate—0.2–0.5 mg/kg (IV, IM, SQ) (canine)
  Acepromazine—0.1–0.5 mg/kg (SQ) (feline)

Measures to Improve Gas Exchange
Oxygen therapy—40–60% (avoid > 50% for > 24 hours)
Ethyl alcohol nebulization—40% solution
Aminophylline—6–10 mg/kg (IV, SQ); can repeat q6h
Endotracheal suctioning

Measures to Reduce Capillary Pressure
Furosemide (Lasix)—2–4 mg/kg (IV, IM, SQ); can repeat q6–8h
Phlebotomy—remove 6–10 cc/kg body weight
Positive inotropes and vasodilators

Measures to Improve Cardiac Output
Digitalis glycosides:
  Digoxin
    IV: 0.01–0.02 mg/kg. Administer ½ calculated dose IV, wait 30–60 minutes and administer ¼ of dose; wait
      30–60 minutes and administer remaining dose, if necessary.
    Oral: 0.02–0.06 mg/kg. Administer ½ dose; give remainder 12 hours later.
  Digitoxin
    IV: 0.01–0.03 mg/kg. Administer as per digoxin.
    Oral: 0.06–0.1 mg/kg. Administer ⅓ dose q8h.
Dobutamine (Dobutrex)—2.5 µg/kg/min. constant rate infusion†
Dopamine HCl (Intropin)—2–8 µg/kg/min. constant rate infusion
Vasodilator therapy:
  Na Nitroprusside (Nipride)–5–20 µg/kg/min. constant rate infusion
  Nitroglycerine ointment (Nitrol 2%)—¼–¾ inch cutaneously, q6–8h
Antiarrhythmic therapy:
  Digitalis glycosides—as above
  Propranolol (Inderal)—0.04–0.06 mg/kg IV (*with caution* if diseased myocardium)
  Lidocaine (Xylocaine)—2.6 mg/kg IV bolus; 25–80 µg/kg/min constant rate infusion
  Procainamide (Pronestyl)—6 mg/kg IV, IM (hypotensive IV), 10–35 µg/kg/min constant rate infusion

Other Therapy
Aspiration of pleural effusion
Aspiration of pericardial effusion

*Reprinted with permission from Bonagura, J.: Acute heart failure. *In* Kirk, R. W. (ed.): *Current Veterinary Therapy VII*. W. B. Saunders, Philadelphia, 1980.

†Formula for CRI: $\left(\dfrac{\dfrac{\text{Infusion dose in mg}}{\text{kg}}}{\text{minute}} = \text{body weight in kg} \right) \left(\dfrac{360}{\text{minutes}} \right) = \begin{array}{l} \text{Total dosage in} \\ \text{mg given for a} \\ \text{6-hour period} \end{array}$

1 µg = 0.001 mg

decreased liver function can have difficulty metabolizing anesthetic agents and providing substances such as albumin, glucose, and fibrinogen. Relevant tests include those for ammonia, bilirubin, hepatic enzymes, total protein, albumin, and globulin (even though the half-lives are in terms of days); glucose; and clotting factors.

Postoperative problems that should be considered include vomitus, acute gastric dilatation, ileus, peritonitis, ischemia of bowel, and intussusception of inflamed bowel.[2] Persistent vomiting may be a result of obstruction, increased intracranial pressure, drug idiosyncrasies, or hepatitis. Acute gastric dilatation may result from aerophagia or delivery of oxygen from a nasal catheter that is positioned too low. Adynamic ileus results from sympathetic overactivity and increased alpha-adrenergic stimulation.[54] Parasympatholytics may prolong or exacerbate ileus. Peritonitis may result from the initiating disease or from surgery. Complications include metabolic acidosis, hyperkalemia, renal failure, pancreatitis, excessive caloric expenditure, disseminated intravascular coagulation, thoracic extension, shock, and death.

Treatment measures for the gastrointestinal patient include withholding food for several hours after operation and maintaining fluid and electrolyte balance during this period. Oral intake of low-bulk soft diets can be started 12 to 24 hours after surgery to help promote gastrointestinal motility. Decompression with a nasogastric tube and the use of alpha-blockers such as guanethidine may counter postoperative ileus. Stool softeners and low-bulk enemas may help eliminate fecal materials and promote bowel motility. Clean, uncontaminated abdomens are closed routinely without drainage. If contamination is seen or suspected, flushing, drainage, and antibiotic therapy begin after surgery and continue during the recovery period. Intermittent postoperative lavage is indicated with contamination.[1, 23, 58] Close attention to volume of fluids administered, addition of proper antibiotic concentrations, fluid temperature, and response to therapy is necessary. Monitoring parameters include packed cell volume, serum proteins, electrolytes, temperature, and local drain site reactions.

Urogenital System

Monitoring of urogenital disorders includes urine output, urinalysis, serum parameters, acid-base values, electrolyte determination, culture and sensitivity analysis, and radiography. Differentiation of prerenal, renal, and postrenal abnormalities is essential to therapy. Oliguria may result from physiologic compensation, hypovolemia, hypotension, acute tubular necrosis, postrenal obstruction, ruptured pathway, or terminal renal failure.[39] Many drugs are dependent upon renal excretion and can exacerbate renal disease. Polyuria, associated with high output renal failure or acute renal failure, must be assessed and supported. Obstruction may be corrected by sterile catheterization and flushing and urinary retention counteracted with catheterization. Infection is treated by fluid therapy and appropriate antibiotics.

The primary cause of oliguria is treated. Therapy with physiologic fluids may correct the acute oliguria. If fluid replacement is insufficient to reverse the process, osmotic diuretics, furosemide, inotropic agents, and dopamine hydrochloride may be used.[39]

Endocrine System

Animals with diabetes mellitus must be closely watched after surgery. Proper management before and after surgery should prevent any unusual problems. If an abnormality in blood glucose is suspected during the recovery period, blood and urine glucose can be determined to lower or raise serum glucose levels. Diabetics also have delayed healing capacities and susceptibility to infection.[20]

Hypothyroidism, if undetected preoperatively or compounded by surgery and anesthesia, may lead to prolonged recovery.[47] Immediate correction is difficult without adequate circulating thyroid hormones. Myxedemic coma is a controversial phenomenon in veterinary medicine.[9] If low thyroid hormone levels are suspected based on clinical history, physical signs, and poor postoperative recovery, immediate replacement can speed recovery.

Musculoskeletal System

Factors in postoperative care include pain, drainage, positioning, hemorrhage, bandaging, bracing, and physical therapy. Pain is managed through the systemic administration of analgesics. Hemorrhage may continue either from tissues that were damaged at the initial injury or from surgical manipulation. Control depends on surgical assessment but may involve replacement of blood loss with physiologic solutions or whole blood during the recovery period. Monitoring of vital signs will indicate continued blood loss. Bandaging or bracing is usually done immediately at the end of the surgical procedure. During recovery bandages are kept dry and are prevented from slipping or being chewed off. They should not be too tight. Positioning is important because of the movement limitations inherent in many orthopedic procedures. Helping the patient to move controls ventilation, urination, defecation, and pressure sore development. Drainage is performed with either soft pliable drains or a closed suction system. Maintenance of either system is essential for proper evacuation of fluids from the surgical site.

Nervous System

Neurological complications are seen during what should otherwise be a normal recovery. Problems include emergence delirium, prolonged recovery, incoordination, extensor rigidity, shivering, abnormal eye signs, motor deficits, and convulsions.[2] Many clear with general supportive care. Emergence delirium may be caused by rapid return to consciousness in the presence of pain, cerebral anoxia, or rapid elimination of carbon dioxide with resultant vasoconstriction. Sedation, restraint, oxygen therapy, and restoration of blood pressure to normal help to eliminate this problem. Convulsions are best controlled with intravenous diazepam.

Patients that are prone to disturbances because of existing or potentially related medical problems must be closely watched. These include the diabetic that has become hypo- or hyperglycemic, the epileptic that may be sensitive to anesthetics and phenothiazine tranquilizers, the young or small patient that becomes hypoglycemic, and the insulinoma patient that has a low blood sugar. Awareness of the history, knowledge of medications that were given previously, and close supervision avert many problems.

Neurological complications may be the result of surgery. An increase in intracranial pressure may result from edema, hemorrhage, or obstructive masses. Identification of this problem is difficult unless a CSF tap and manometer are used, but control can be achieved with corticosteroids and osmotic diuretics.[1] Paralysis from pre-existing medical problems or immobility from additional surgical manipulation may be managed by positional changes and control of bowel and bladder.

Ocular System (see also Chapter 100)

The most important concerns after ophthalmic surgery are ocular or periocular pain and the patient's tendency to traumatize the eye. Many patients benefit from the use of post operative analgesics, eye patches, eye bandages, Elizabethan collars, and buckets over the head to keep the patient from scratching the eye. Another important concern is the application of topical medications to reduce pain, decrease inflammation, control infection, or maintain mydriasis. Treatment must be frequent enough to obtain either continuous or intermittent effects without aggravating the patient and causing additional pain. Systemic medications can be used if additional ocular penetration is desired.

1. Archibald, J., Holt, J. C., and Sokolovsky, V.: *Management of Trauma in Dogs and Cats.* American Veterinary Publications, Inc., Santa Barbara, 1981.
2. Artz, C.: Infections in surgery. *In* Artz, C. P., and Hardy, J. D. (eds.): *Management of Surgical Complications.* W. B. Saunders, Philadelphia, 1975, pp. 1–20.
3. Bonagura, J. D.: Acute heart failure. *In* Kirk, R. W. (ed.): *Current Veterinary Therapy VII.* W. B. Saunders, Philadelphia, 1980, pp. 359–367.
4. Bonagura, J. D.: Pulmonary edema. *In* Kirk, R. W. (ed.): *Current Veterinary Therapy VII.* W. B. Saunders, Philadelphia, 1980, pp. 243–248.
5. Buening, G. M.: Transfusions. *In* Bojrab, M. D. (ed.): *Pathophysiology in Small Animal Surgery.* Lea & Febiger, Philadelphia, 1981, pp. 478–482.
6. Burrows, C. F.: Intensive care of the critically ill dog and cat—Part I: Philosophy, organization of the intensive care unit, and monitoring techniques. Comp. Cont. Ed. 4:875, 1982.
7. Burrows, C. F.: Intensive care of the critically ill dog and cat—Part II. Fluid therapy, respiratory care, and nutrition. Comp. Cont. Ed. 4:1007, 1982.
8. Butler, W. B.: Use of a flutter valve in treatment of pneumothorax in dogs and cats. J. Am. Vet. Med. Assoc. *166*:473, 1975.
9. Chastain, C. B., Graham, C. L., and Riley, M. G.: Myxedema coma in two dogs. Canine Pract. 9:20, 1982.
10. Cohen, J. S.: A summary of complications of fluid therapy. Vet. Clin. North Am. *12*:545, 1982.
11. Cohen, R. B., and Tilley, L. P.: Cardiac arrhythmias in the anesthetized patient. Vet. Clin. North Am. 9:155, 1979.
12. Conzelman, G. M.: Pharmacotherapeutics of aminoglycoside antibiotics. J. Am. Vet. Med. Assoc. *176*:1078, 1980.
13. Cornelius, L. M.: Fluid, electrolyte, acid-base, and nutritional management. *In* Bojrab, M. J. (ed.): *Pathophysiology in Small Animal Surgery.* Lea & Febiger, Philadelphia, 1981, pp. 12–32.
14. Crane, S. W.: Placement and maintenance of a temporary feeding tube gastrotomy in the dog and cat. Comp. Cont. Ed. *11*:770, 1980.
15. Crowe, D. T.: Autotransfusion in the trauma patient. Vet. Clin. North Am. *10*:581, 1980.
16. Crowe, D. T.: Enteral nutrition for the critically ill or injured patient. Paper presented, in part, at the Annual Meeting of the Veterinary Critical Care Society, April, 1982.
17. Davis, H. S.: Complications of anesthesia. *In* Artz, C. P., and Hardy, J. D. (eds.): *Management of Surgical Complications.* W. B. Saunders, Philadelphia, 1975, pp. 143–219.
18. Davis, L. E.: Antimicrobial therapy. *In* Kirk, R. W. (ed.): *Current Veterinary Therapy VII.* W. B. Saunders, Philadelphia, 1980, pp. 2–16.
19. Fitts, C. T., and Davis, J. H.: Miscellaneous complications in the pre-operative and post-operative periods. *In* Artz, C. P., and Hardy, J. D. (eds.): *Management of Surgical Complications.* W. B. Saunders, Philadelphia, 1975, pp. 220–242.
20. Hardy, J. D.: Surgical complications. *In* Sabiston, D. C. (ed.): *Textbook of Surgery.* W. B. Saunders, Philadelphia, 1977, pp. 424–442.
21. Hartsfield, S. M.: Anesthesia of the critical patient. *In* Sattler, F. P., Knowles, R. P., and Whittick, W. G. (eds): *Veterinary Critical Care.* Lea & Febiger, Philadelphia, 1981, pp. 384–394.
22. Haskins, S. C.: Standards and techniques of equipment utilization. *In* Sattler, F. P., Knowles, R. P., and Whittick, W. G. (eds.): *Veterinary Critical Care.* Lea & Febiger, Philadelphia, 1981, pp. 60–110.
23. Hoffer, R. E.: Peritonitis. Vet. Clin. North Am. 2:189, 1972.
24. Hunt, T. K.: Wound complications. *In* Artz, C. P. and Hardy, J. D. (eds.): *Management of Surgical Complications.* W. B. Saunders, Philadelphia, 1975, pp. 21–32.
25. Kaplan, M.: Pain. *In* Ettinger, S. J. (ed.): *Textbook of Veterinary Internal Medicine,* 2nd ed. W. B. Saunders, Philadelphia, 1983, pp. 39–45.
26. Kelly, M. J.: Drug interactions—indications and contraindications. Gaines Veterinary Symposium, 1981, pp. 23–29.
27. Kinney, J. M., and Caldwell, F. T.: Fever; etiology and metabolic effects and management in surgical patients. *In* Sabiston, D. C. (ed.): *Textbook of Surgery.* W. B. Saunders, Philadelphia, 1977, pp. 185–199.
28. Kinney, J. M., Egdahl, R. H., and Zuidema, G. P.: *Manual of Pre-operative and Post-operative Care.* W. B. Saunders, Philadelphia, 1971.
29. Klide, A.: Personal communication, 1983.
30. Kolata, R. J., Burrows, C. F., and Soma, L. R.: Shock, pathophysiology and management. *In* Kirk, R. W. (ed.): *Current Veterinary Therapy VII,* W. B. Saunders, Philadelphia, 1980, pp. 32–48.
31. Lewis, L. D., and Phillips, R. W.: Diarrhea. *In* Bojrab, M. J. (ed.): *Pathophysiology in Small Animal Surgery.* Lea & Febiger, Philadelphia, 1981, pp. 148–154.
32. Lumb, W. V., and Jones, E. W.: *Veterinary Anesthesia.* Lea & Febiger, Philadelphia, 1973.
33. McCurnin, D. M., and Grier, R. L.: Temperature control in the critical and surgical patient. *In* Sattler, F. P., Knowles, R. P., and Whittick, W. G. (eds.): *Veterinary Critical Care.* Lea & Febiger, Philadelphia, 1981, pp. 403–414.
34. McDonell, W.: Surgical principles. *In* Archibald, J. (ed.): *Canine Surgery.* American Veterinary Publications Inc., Santa Barbara, 1974, pp. 53–73, 82–106.
35. McKiernan, B. C.: Lower respiratory tract disease. *In* Ettinger, S. J. (ed.): *Textbook of Veterinary Internal Medicine,* 2nd ed. W. B. Saunders, Philadelphia, 1983, pp. 760–828.
36. Moncreif, J. A.: Complications of parenteral fluid therapy. *In* Surgical Complications, Artz, C. P., and Hardy, J. D. (eds.): *Management of Surgical Complications.* W. B. Saunders, Philadelphia, 1975, pp. 68–82.
37. Moore, F. D.: Homeostasis: Bodily changes in trauma and surgery. Sabiston, D. C. (ed.): *Textbook of Surgery.* W. B. Saunders, Philadelphia, 1977, pp. 27–64.
38. Palminteri, A.: Diagnosis and management of intestinal obstruction. Vet. Clin. North Am. 2:131, 1972.
39. Parker, H. R.: Renal failure. *In* Sattler, F. P., Knowles, R. P., and Whittick, W. G. (eds.): *Veterinary Critical Care.* Lea & Febiger, Philadelphia, 1981, pp. 195–237.
40. Peacock, E. E., and Van Winkle, W.: *Wound Repair.* W. B. Saunders, Philadelphia, 1976.
41. Penny, B. E., and White, R. J.: Narcotic analgesics in the domestic cat. Vet. Clin. North Am. *8*:317, 1978.
42. Powers, T. E., and Garg, R. C.: Principles of antimicrobial therapy in surgery. *In* Bojrab, M. J. (ed.): *Pathophysiology in Small Animal Surgery.* Lea & Febiger, Philadelphia, 1981, pp. 52–60.
43. Rawlings, C. A., Chambers, J. N., and Greene, C. E.: Small bowel obstruction. *In* Sattler, F. P., Knowles, R. P., and Whittick, W. G. (eds.): *Veterinary Critical Care.* Lea & Febiger, Philadelphia, 1981, pp. 167–181.
44. Riviere, J. E., Kaufman, G. M., and Bright, R. M.: Prophy-

lactic use of systemic antimicrobial drugs in surgery. Comp. Cont. Ed. 3:345, 1981.

45. Rosin, E.: The systemic response to injury. *In* Bojrab, M. J. (ed.): *Pathophysiology in Small Animal Surgery.* Lea & Febiger, Philadelphia, 1981, pp. 3–11.

46. Ross, J. N., and Breznock, E. M.: *In* Sattler, F. P., Knowles, R. P., and Whittick, W. G. (eds.): *Veterinary Critical Care.* Lea & Febiger, Philadelphia, 1981, pp. 435–466.

47. Schaer, M.: The thyroid gland. *In* Bojrab, M. J. (ed.): *Pathophysiology in Small Animal Surgery.* Lea & Febiger, Philadelphia, 1981, pp. 314–323.

48. Schaer, M.: Disorders of potassium metabolism. Vet. Clin. North Am. *12*:399, 1982.

49. Schall, W. D.: General principles of fluid therapy. Vet. Clin. North Am. *12*:453, 1982.

50. Shires, G. T., and Canizaro, P. C.: Fluid and electrolyte management of the surgical patient. *In* Sabiston, D. C. (ed.): *Textbook of Surgery.* W. B. Saunders, Philadelphia, 1977, pp. 95–118.

51. Short, C. E.: Fluid and electrolyte therapy. *In* Kirk, R. W. (ed.): *Current Veterinary Therapy VII.* W. B. Saunders, Philadelphia, 1980, pp. 49–53.

52. Short, C. E.: Therapy for respiratory emergencies. *In* Kirk, R. W. (ed.): *Current Veterinary Therapy VII.*, W. B. Saunders, Philadelphia, 1980, pp. 277–279.

53. Spencer, K. R.: Intravenous catheters. Vet. Clin. North Am. *12*:533, 1982.

54. Stahl, W. M.: *Supportive Care of the Surgical Patient.* Grune & Stratton, New York, 1982.

55. Swaim, S. F.: *Surgery of Traumatized Skin.* W. B. Saunders, Philadelphia, 1980.

56. Thorek, P.: *Illustrated Pre-operative and Post-operative Care.* J. B. Lippincott, Philadelphia, 1973.

57. Twedt, D. C., and Grauer, G. F.: Fluid therapy for gastrointestinal, pancreatic and hepatic disorders. Vet. Clin. North Am. *12*:463, 1982.

58. Withrow, S. J., and Black, A. P.: Generalized peritonitis in small animals. Vet. Clin. North Am. 9:363, 1979.

59. Zaslow, I. M.: Personnel and physical requirements. *In* Veterinary Critical Care, Sattler, F. P., Knowles, R. P., and Whittick, W. G. (eds.) *Veterinary Critical Care.* Lea & Febiger, Philadelphia, 1981, pp. 3–59.

60. Zenoble, R. D., and Stone, E. A.: Autotransfusion in the dog. J. Am. Vet. Med. Assoc. *172*:1411, 1978.

Chapter **32** # Principles of Operating Room Emergencies

Steve C. Haskins

INABILITY TO KEEP THE PATIENT ANESTHETIZED OR SUDDEN AWAKENING

As patients awaken from general anesthesia, a complex of signs is usually manifested: spontaneous muscular movement (stretching, paddling, blinking, chewing, or shivering); an increase in mandibular muscle tone; the appearance of a strong palpebral reflex; central position of the eye with a small to medium pupillary aperture; an increase in ventilation rate and volume; and an increase in heart rate, cardiac output, and blood pressure.[83, 114, 125] The response of individual patients varies considerably, and different anesthetics exhibit different characteristics.[142] It is important to evaluate as many of the signs of anesthetic depth as are available so that a reasonable assessment of the patient's level of anesthesia can be made. Care should be taken not to attribute too much significance to any one sign. An increase in ventilation rate may be caused by a number of events, including too light a level of anesthesia. A patient may fight a ventilator or attempt to breathe during thoracotomy if the anesthetic level is too light and in the presence of hypoxia or hypercapnia. A patient may move spontaneously while under the influence of some anesthetics (ketamine or enflurane) and yet be quite well anesthetized. Tachycardia may be a sign of light anesthesia or shock. Heart rate and ventilation rate are often unreliable indicators of anesthetic level.

Causes of Premature Awakening

Surgical Stimulation

The level of anesthesia that a patient exhibits is a balance between the amount of anesthetic administered and surgical stimulation. Variations in surgical stimulation cause changes in anesthetic level. The change is most dramatic with those agents that have poor analgesic properties (e.g., barbiturates, halothane).[25] A sudden lightening of anesthesia occurs with traction on the mesenteric attachments, pleural manipulation, introduction of contrast material for myelographic studies, stimulation of the meninges during laminectomies, and occasionally with extensive fracture manipulation or intraocular surgeries. The depth of anesthesia need not be increased if the surgical stimulation is temporary or if the patient is not moving at an inappropriate moment.

Postinduction Hypoventilation

Barbiturate induction followed by maintenance with a gaseous agent is a common anesthetic protocol.

Hypoventilation following barbiturate induction is common, and, as a consequence, the gaseous agent is not taken up in sufficient amounts to accommodate barbiturate redistribution. Stimuli such as moving or rolling the patient or the placement of towel clamps may suddenly awaken the patient. If postinduction hypoventilation is suspected, the lungs should be artificially inflated once every 30 seconds until the patient regains spontaneous ventilation. This assures administration of the gaseous agent and prevents development of hypoxemia or hypercapnia during hypoventilation or apnea.

Inadequate Administration of Gaseous Anesthetic

Uptake of a critical volume of anesthetic is required for general anesthesia. Relatively large doses of anesthetic are necessary to saturate the blood and visceral organs in the early phases of anesthesia.[82] As anesthesia progresses, the rate of administration is decreased. Anesthetic maintenance requirements average approximately 1.25 × MAC* but vary considerably among patients. Inadequate administration may be due to the following:

---

*MAC is the minimum alveolar concentration necessary to prevent muscular movement in response to surgical stimulation in 50 per cent of subjects.[36]

1. Vaporizer control not set high enough;
2. Decreasing the setting prior to adequate loading of visceral and muscular tissues; or
3. A fresh gas flow rate that is too low to deliver an adequate volume of anesthetic to the circuit with "vaporizer-outside-the-circuit" systems.

Appropriate flow and vaporizer settings vary among patients, anesthetic machines, and circuits (Table 32–1).

Improperly Functioning Vaporizer

An accumulation of water on the cotton wicks of in-circuit vaporizers displaces the anesthetic and decreases vaporizer efficiency. The wick should be air dried periodically. An accumulation of preservative on the copper screens in precision vaporizers decreases their efficiency. They should be cleaned and recalibrated every one to two years. Enflurane and isoflurane are stable and do not contain preservatives.

Precision vaporizers are calibrated at 23°C. Anesthetic vapor pressure and vapor output diminish as temperature decreases. Efficiency decreases when vaporizers are used in cool, air-conditioned rooms or outdoors. Glass vaporizers conduct atmospheric heat poorly and do not prevent the cooling of the anesthetic liquid caused by the vaporization process. These vaporizers are less efficient with high gas flows or large patients.

TABLE 32–1. Gas Flow Rates and Vaporizer Settings for Anesthetic Administration

	Approximate Values for Initial Loading	Approximate Values for Maintenance
Gas Flow Rates		
Circle system		
Oxygen alone	> 40 ml/kg/min	7.5–15 ml/kg/min
50% O$_2$/50% N$_2$O*	> 40 ml/kg/min	15–30 ml/kg/min
Nonrebreathing system† (regardless of the nature of the carrier gas)	> 200 ml/kg/min	100–200 mg/kg/min
Vaporizer Setting		
Halothane		
Circle system	2.0 ± 0.5%	1.0 ± 0.2% after 30–60 min‡
Nonrebreathing system§	1.5 ± 0.5%	1.0 ± 0.2% after 15–30 min
Methoxyflurane		
Circle system	1.5 ± 0.5%	0.5 ± 0.2% after 45–75 min
Nonrebreathing system	1.0 ± 0.25%	0.5 ± 0.2% after 30–60 min

*Oxygen/nitrous oxide mixtures generally require higher maintenance flows than oxygen alone to assure an adequate supply of oxygen. Both need higher initial total flows to assure an adequate delivery of anesthetic to the circuit.

†Nonrebreathing systems require higher flows than circle systems during loading and maintenance to minimize rebreathing.

‡Time from induction to maintenance vaporizer setting for the average patient. The downward titration from the loading dose vaporizer setting begins shortly after induction (5 to 15 minutes).

§Nonrebreathing systems are much more efficient than circle systems with regard to the actual percentage of anesthetic delivered to the patient compared with that delivered by the vaporizer. Therefore, initial loading doses need not be as high nor do they need to be maintained as long before titrating down to maintenance concentration.

Esophageal or Endobronchial Intubation

The only sure way to determine the presence of the endotracheal tube in the trachea is to see or feel it pass through the larynx. Coughing is good evidence of proper placement. All other techniques are progressively more fallible, depending on the skill and experience of the operator, and they should be interpreted with caution. For instance, there may be some rebreathing bag movement associated with ventilation during esophageal intubation if there is air in the esophagus; cyclic excursion of the stomach is sometimes easily confused with ventilation of the lungs during positive pressure ventilation.

Endobronchial intubation reduces the lung surface area for anesthetic uptake. Tubes should be positioned so that the cuff is beyond the larynx and the tip of the tube is rostral to the thoracic inlet. New endotracheal tubes are characteristically too long and should be shortened prior to use. Endobronchial intubation may fail to keep the patient anesthetized, as indicated by tachypnea and hyperventilation, hypoxemia and cyanosis, decreased tidal volume and pulmonary compliance, and hypercapnia. If endobronchial intubation is suspected, withdraw the tube until its proper position can be verified by palpation of the external trachea.

Insufficient Cuff Inflation

Insufficient cuff inflation allows the patient to inspire room air around the tube. This diminishes inspired anesthetic concentration. The cuff is inflated just enough to stop the leakage of air during application of positive airway pressure (15 cm H_2O). Care must be taken not to overinflate the cuff, since this predisposes to avascular necrosis of the tracheal wall.[32]

Carrier Gas Leaks

Leaks between the flowmeter and the vaporizer, such as at the upper seal of the flowmeter tube, interfere with the delivery of carrier gas to the vaporizer. Leaks between the vaporizer and the circuit, such as cracks in the rubber tubing between the machine outlet and the circuit inlet, interfere with the delivery of carrier gas and anesthetic to the circuit. Leaks within the circuit may necessitate higher than normal gas flows to provide proper bag inflation. This decreases in-circuit anesthetic concentrations with "vaporizer-inside-the-circuit" systems. Anesthetic machines should be pressure checked prior to use: with all outlets plugged, inflate the circuit to a pressure of 40 cm H_2O; if the carrier gas flow necessary to maintain this pressure exceeds 200 ml/min, the leak is excessive and should be repaired.[77] Prevention of environmental pollution with gaseous anesthetic agents is another reason to check an anesthetic machine before use.[86, 87]

Oxygen Flush

The oxygen flush bypasses the vaporizer. Refilling of the rebreathing bag by this technique decreases the in-circuit anesthetic concentration and predisposes to premature awakening. If the rebreathing bag needs to be filled rapidly with anesthetic-containing gases, use high flowmeter settings. The oxygen flush is used to fill the bag rapidly and decrease in-circuit anesthetic concentrations for terminating the anesthetic, anesthetic overdosage, or cardiac arrest.

EXCESSIVE ANESTHETIC DEPTH OR PROLONGED RECOVERY

The physical signs of excessive anesthetic depth include flaccid muscle tone and absence of all reflexes; centrally positioned eyeballs, dilated pupils, and dry corneas (owing to the absence of tear production); absence of the pupillary light reflex; and bradycardia, hypotension, and bradypnea. A patient may have bradycardia, hypotension, or apnea and yet be lightly anesthetized. A patient may have minimal muscle tone one moment and yet become excessively lightly anesthetized the next. All available signs are evaluated before a judgment of the level of anesthesia is made.

Causes of Excessive Anesthetic Depth

Individual Variation and Synergistic Events

There are individual differences in anesthetic requirements. Diseases such as hypothermia, hypotension, shock, hypoxia, hypercapnia, hypothyroidism, preanesthetic exhaustion, acid-base and electrolyte disorders, endogenous or exogenous toxemias, and brain disease have CNS depressant effects and decrease the amount of anesthetic necessary.[34] The vaporizer setting is decreased to prevent anesthetic overdosage if any of these problems develop. Preanesthetic sedatives also decrease the requirements for the primary anesthetic. Great care should be exercised when supplementing xylazine with barbiturates or gaseous anesthetics owing to the ease of anesthetic overdosage.

Nonrebreathing Circuits

Nonrebreathing circuits such as the Ayre's T-piece or Bain's circuit are much more efficient than the large reservoir circle systems because they enhance anesthetic delivery; i.e., the patient inhales anesthetic concentrations much closer to those that leave the vaporizer. Vaporizer settings that work satisfactorily with circle systems easily result in anesthetic overdosage with nonrebreathing systems (see Table 32–1).

Positive Pressure Ventilation

Positive pressure ventilation (PPV) also enhances anesthetic delivery because it provides a larger tidal volume than spontaneous ventilation. The vaporizer setting is reduced whenever PPV is instituted. Excessive administration of gaseous anesthetics may occur:

1. During controlled ventilation because the patient cannot decrease ventilatory rate as the anesthesia deepens;

2. When PPV is used with a nonrebreathing circuit;

3. When PPV is used with "vaporizer-inside-the-circuit" systems (each time the carrier gas is forced around the circuit it passes through the vaporizer and picks up additional anesthetic, rapidly increasing the inspired anesthetic concentration); and

4. When PPV is used to deepen anesthesia, especially if the vaporizer setting is simultaneously increased. It generally takes very little additional anesthetic to re-anesthetize such a patient. There is always a lag period between the time the anesthetic is delivered to the lungs and the time it affects the brain. Aggressive bagging should cease as soon as the anesthesia deepens.

Improperly Functioning Vaporizer

A vaporizer may deliver anesthetic even though the control knob is turned off.[143] If anesthesia deepens after the vaporizer has been turned off, it may be wise to smell the in-circuit gas or disconnect or change the anesthetic machine.

Postoperative Sedatives

Postoperative analgesics or tranquilizers have additive effects when anesthetic drugs are still in the patient. The dosage of postoperative sedatives should be decreased 50 to 75 per cent from premedication dosages.

TACHYPNEA, EXAGGERATED BREATHING EFFORTS, AND HYPERVENTILATION

Tachypnea is rapid breathing without regard to volume. Tachypnea may be associated with hyperventilation, normal ventilation, or hypoventilation, depending on the nature of the disturbance. Hyperventilation refers to a higher than normal alveolar minute ventilation without regard to breathing rate. These abnormalities are physiologically different but commonly occur in an overlapping fashion and have similar causes (Fig. 32–1). Normal medullary and neuromuscular responses to a respiratory stimulus are present.

Respiratory rates in normal dogs and cats vary between 10 and 40 breaths per minute (BPM).[3, 43, 130] Preoperative respiratory rates range between 15 and 40 BPM for dogs and 20 and 50 for cats; intraoperative rates range between 10 and 30 BPM for dogs and 10 and 40 for cats. Minute ventilation ranges between 150 and 350 ml/kg/min in normal dogs and cats.[3, 43, 130]

Causes of Tachypnea During Surgery

Hypercapnia (page 395), hypoxemia (page 395), hypotension (page 401), and hyperthermia (page 406) are important causes of tachypnea and should be identified early, since their consequences are severe.

Light or Deep Levels of Anesthesia

Too light a level of anesthesia may be associated with tachypnea and hyperventilation. Too deep a level of anesthesia may be associated with tachypnea, exaggerated but shallow breathing efforts, and hypoventilation; PPV should be instituted until the patient's anesthetic level is light enough so that it can maintain a coordinated and adequate minute volume. PPV support should be guided by tidal and minute volume measurements and, if possible, end-tidal or arterial carbon dioxide measurements.

Airway Obstruction

Upper airway obstruction may cause tachypnea, exaggerated breathing efforts, and hypoventilation. Extrathoracic airway obstructions may be associated with inspiratory stridor and paradoxical inspiratory thoracic collapse; intrathoracic obstructions may be associated with expiratory stridor.

Pleural Space Complications

Hydrothorax, chylothorax, hemothorax, or diaphragmatic hernia may cause respiratory difficulties even though there was no apparent preoperative respiratory distress owing to the additive adverse pulmonary effects of general anesthesia. The development of these restrictive abnormalities is heralded by increased breathing rates and decreased tidal volumes, decreased compliance, abnormal auscultatory or percussion findings, and blood gas evidence of subnormal blood oxygenation or decreased alveolar ventilation. A diagnostic thoracentesis may identify the nature of the abnormal pleural space accumulation.

Closed pneumothorax may be dramatically worsened by PPV. PPV should be avoided unless required by lung contusion, and then it should be applied with minimal pressures. Nitrous oxide should be avoided, since it will readily diffuse into the gas pocket, causing it to approximately double in size in 10 to 15 minutes.[35] General anesthesia for patients with a closed pneumothorax should be postponed if possible for several days to allow the pleural tear to heal. The chest should be prepared for chest drain insertion and the patient monitored closely for signs of pro-

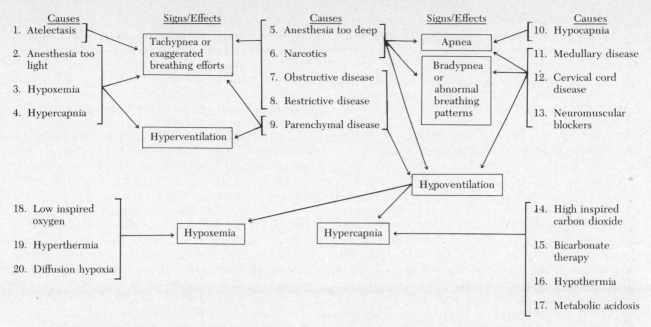

Figure 32–1. Interrelationship between causes and effects of stimulated and depressed ventilation,

gression of the pneumothorax. If early surgery is required, an indwelling chest drain* should be placed prior to or shortly after anesthetic induction.

Fluid-filling defects that cause distress should be drained prior to induction of general anesthesia or during surgery.

Obesity

Excessive obesity may restrict ventilation secondary to either mediastinal fat accumulations or extra weight on the thoracic wall and diaphragm.

Abdominal Complications

Space-occupying abdominal abnormalities such as gastric or intestinal tympany, ascites, neoplastic masses, a gravid uterus, or pyometra may restrict diaphragmatic excursions and cause tachypnea and hypoventilation.

Pulmonary Parenchymal Complications

The pulmonary and thoracic effects of general anesthesia exaggerate respiratory distress induced by parenchymal diseases such as edema, pneumonia, contusion, neoplasia, or aspiration. If surgery cannot be postponed, a rapid anesthetic induction technique followed by endotracheal intubation and PPV is indicated. PPV re-expands collapsed small airways and alveoli and maximizes the respiratory surface area of the lungs.

Atelectasis

Small airway collapse and atelectasis may cause tachypnea and are relieved by administering a few deep breaths. All anesthetized patients should be artificially ventilated at five-minute intervals to minimize the inevitable small airway and alveolar collapse that occurs during general anesthesia. More frequent sighs may be indicated if the breathing pattern is shallow or if mild to moderate parenchymal lung disease exists (once per minute or continuously).

Drugs

Narcotics occasionally cause panting owing to their effect on the thermoregulatory center.[46] The breathing pattern usually regresses spontaneously in 10 to 30 minutes. It is not possible to interrupt the process by PPV, and it is unwise to attempt to override it with excessive doses of anesthetic. The panting may be terminated by reversing the narcotic or administering a neuromuscular blocking agent. Usually, the syndrome is allowed to run its course unless it interferes with the surgical procedure. Hyperthermia has developed secondary to excessive muscular activity and could be treated by terminating the tachypneic breathing pattern. Anesthetic agents that stimulate the central nervous system (ketamine, diazepam, or narcotics) may cause tachypnea.[46] Anesthetic agents that stimulate airway irritant receptors (ether) may cause breath holding or tachypnea. The role of these receptors in producing tachypnea with modern gaseous anesthetics, which are pungent but not irritating, is not known.

Idiopathic Causes

The normal respiratory response to general anesthesia in some patients is rapid and shallow in nature.

---

*For emergency or short-term chest drainage, a fenestrated, large-bore, catheter-over-the-needle intravascular catheter with a three-way stopcock may be used.

If none of the previously mentioned complications can be documented and the patient appears to be oxygenating properly, PPV once every minute to compensate for any deficiencies that may exist in minute volume and to prevent excessive small airway and alveolar collapse and continuous monitoring for specific abnormalities are suggested.

BRADYPNEA, HYPOVENTILATION, AND APNEA

Bradypnea is slow breathing without regard to volume. Hypoventilation is a lower than normal alveolar minute volume without regard to breathing rate. Bradypnea may be associated with hypoventilation depending on the size of each tidal volume. Hypoventilation occurs with many of the disorders associated with tachypnea (airway obstruction; pleural space, pulmonary parenchymal, or abdominal complications; and obesity). Complications causing medullary respiratory center or neuromuscular depression are associated with bradypnea or apnea and hypoventilation (see Fig. 32–1).

The ranges for normal respiratory rate and minute ventilation were defined previously. PPV should be considered if the minute ventilation is measured or estimated to be below normal.

Breathing patterns of a depressed medulla include forms other than bradypnea, apnea, or hypoventilation. The diaphragm (abdomen) and thorax normally expand simultaneously. In deeper levels of anesthesia the diaphragmatic component precedes the thoracic component and dominates the inspiratory effort.

Cheyne-Stokes breathing is cyclic hyperventilation and hypoventilation. Most anesthetized patients breathe in this fashion, but it is only when the process becomes extreme that it is clinically recognizable. The breathing pattern is attributed to greater than normal delays in the medullary response to changing carbon dioxide levels. If it is associated with signs of deep anesthesia, the anesthetic depth should be lightened. If not, its effect on overall ventilation and oxygenation should be evaluated and PPV instituted if necessary.

Biot's breathing is cyclic hypoventilation and apnea and is a sign of a serious medullary disturbance. PPV should be instituted until the underlying cause can be determined and effectively treated.

Agonal gasps are characterized by periodic retraction of the hyoid apparatus and mouth gaping. There may be movement of a small amount of air associated with spasmotic diaphragmatic contraction. It is always a very serious sign and is rarely associated with successful resuscitation.

Causes of Bradypnea

Hypocapnia

Carbon dioxide is the primary chemical stimulant of the respiratory center, and hypocapnia in an an-

esthetized patient results in apnea. Most anesthetics are potent respiratory depressants, and many are given as boluses to induce anesthesia. Most patients hyperventilate just prior to induction owing to excitement and apprehension. Patients are often intubated and artificially ventilated to assure proper cuff inflation. Apnea and bradypnea are common following anesthetic induction even though the patient may be lightly anesthetized. Spontaneous breathing usually resumes when the carbon dioxide levels have increased to a level sufficient to stimulate the depressed medulla. Unless the patient is attached to a 100 per cent oxygen source, serious hypoxemia may develop before spontaneous ventilation resumes. If insufficient quantities of anesthetic are taken up, the patient awakens prematurely once the induction agent has been redistributed. It is therefore important to artificially ventilate the patient once every 30 seconds to assure adequate delivery of oxygen and anesthetic. Care must be taken not to ventilate too much, since it prevents carbon dioxide accumulation. If ventilation has not commenced within 10 to 15 minutes, full support PPV (10 to 12 BPM) is instituted for 10 minutes before the weaning process is repeated.

Medullary Complications

Depression of the respiratory centers may be caused by general anesthesia, severe metabolic disturbances, or organic lesions such as edema, hemorrhage, neoplasia, or thromboembolic phenomena.[10, 75] General anesthesia causes excessive respiratory depression in patients with pre-existing pulmonary or nonpulmonary systemic debilitation (hypothermia, shock, hypotension). The respiratory response to general anesthesia in some patients is bradypnea or hypoventilation without other abnormalities.

Neuromuscular Complications

Interference with motor efferents may occur preoperatively with disc prolapse, vertebral fractures, myasthenia, or polyradiculoneuritis or during operation with spinal cord edema secondary to needle tap or surgical trauma. Neuromuscular blocking agents may cause a residual problem if they are not adequately reversed at the end of the procedure.[90] Aminoglycoside antibiotics may cause neuromuscular blockade when administered during surgery.[90, 91]

Operative Complications

Operative maneuvers such as head-down positioning, the laying of heavy instruments on top of a small thorax, or aggressive rostral traction for anterior abdominal surgical exposure may interfere with adequate ventilation and should be avoided when possible. When avoidance is not possible ventilation should be closely monitored and supported as necessary.

HYPERCAPNIA

Hypercapnia is an arterial blood carbon dioxide partial pressure (Pa_{CO_2}) of greater than 45 mm Hg. The Pa_{CO_2} should not be allowed to exceed 60 mm Hg because of its tendency to cause excessive acidemia and progressive CNS narcosis.[99, 109] Hypercapnia causes increased cerebral blood flow and should be avoided in patients with increased intracranial pressure.[122] The Pa_{CO_2} of a blood sample may be measured with a blood gas analyzer,[1, 99] or it may be approximated by measuring the P_{CO_2} or the percentage of CO_2 of a gas sample obtained after exhalation.[99, 132]

Causes of Hypercapnia

Hypoventilation

Hypoventilation causes systemic accumulation of carbon dioxide. Pulmonary parenchymal diseases are often associated with hypocapnia due to hypoxia-induced hyperventilation.

Increased Inspired Carbon Dioxide

Hypercapnia may be associated with excessive dead space rebreathing (large face mask; nonfunctioning directional valves in the anesthetic circuit; insufficient fresh gas flows with nonrebreathing circuits; nonrebreathing circuits that are attached backwards) or exhausted soda lime within the anesthetic circuit.

Sodium Bicarbonate Administration

The administration of sodium bicarbonate increases the carbon dioxide content of the blood (carbonic acid equilibration). If a blood sample is taken soon after the administration of the bicarbonate, the measured P_{CO_2} is misleadingly elevated.[12]

Hypothermia

The increase in temperature of a blood sample taken from a hypothermic patient and measured in a warm blood gas analyzer increases the partial pressure of the measured gases. Failure to correct the measured P_{CO_2} value results in an apparently high P_{CO_2}.[42]

Compensatory Respiratory acidosis

Hypercapnia may occur as a compensatory response to metabolic acidosis. Hypoventilatory compensation is limited by concurrent hypoxemia; the P_{CO_2} is not likely to exceed 60 mm Hg by compensation alone.[121]

HYPOXEMIA

Hypoxemia is lower than normal blood oxygen content and is usually identified by a measured arterial blood oxygen partial pressure (Pa_{O_2}) of less than 80 mm Hg.

Unconsciousness occurs when the Pa_{O_2} decreases to about 36 mm Hg in the absence of other cardiovascular abnormalities.[121] Many compensatory mechanisms and hypothermia protect the brain from hypoxia; numerous cardiovascular and metabolic abnormalities lower the threshold to hypoxemia-induced brain damage.[99] Specific minimum values for Pa_{O_2} in individual patients are, therefore, variable and difficult to predict. Hypoxemia is an important respiratory stimulant at Pa_{O_2} values below 60 mm Hg.[29] Hemoglobin saturation and whole blood oxygen content are well maintained down to a Pa_{O_2} of 60 mm Hg. A Pa_{O_2} of 50 to 60 mm Hg is a commonly selected minimum value during respiratory therapy.[29, 137] Values below 60 mm Hg represent an important stress to the patient, and support procedures such as enriching the inspired oxygen concentration or ventilation therapy should be utilized to maintain the Pa_{O_2} above 60 mm Hg.

Cyanosis is a sign of pulmonary disease but should be interpreted with caution and requires an absolute amount of unoxygenated hemoglobin (5 gm/dl).[99] If a patient is moderately anemic, death from lack of oxygen could occur without cyanosis.[99] Cyanosis may also be due to peripheral stagnation of blood flow during severe shock, hypothermia, or cardiac arrest even though pulmonary function is normal. Drug-induced methemoglobinemia causes severe cyanotic discoloration[55] and reduced blood oxygen content even though pulmonary function and the measured Pa_{O_2} may be normal. We have observed methemoglobinemia in cats after spraying the larynx with concentrated benzocaine spray. PPV had no effect on the cyanosis, and 100 per cent inspired oxygen concentrations had only minimal palliative effects. The disease runs a course of several hours. The methemoglobin level may be reduced by the administration of methylene blue (1 to 2 mg/kg),[55] but its use should be monitored, since it may cause Heinz body hemolytic anemia.[124]

Causes of Hypoxemia

Hypoventilation

Hypoxemia is always associated with hypoventilation if the patient is breathing room air. When hypoxemia is due to hypoventilation, improvement of the ventilatory status of the patient, not oxygen therapy, is the treatment of choice.

Obstructive or Restrictive Pulmonary Complications

Hypoxemia may be due to airway obstruction; pleural space, pulmonary parenchymal, or abdominal complications; or obesity. If the hypoxemia is due to parenchymal lung disease, some combination of oxygen and ventilation therapy is often required to restore acceptable blood oxygen levels.[60] If 100 per cent oxygen fails to provide relief, PPV should be instituted. Therapy is continuously monitored by the observation of physical signs and, when possible, by Pa_{O_2} measurements. Pa_{CO_2} defines the ventilatory status of the patient and is used to guide ventilation therapy. Pa_{O_2} defines the oxygenating capabilities of the lung and is used to guide the inhaled oxygen concentration and the end-expired airway pressure. The combination of all techniques should be sufficient to restore the Pa_{O_2} to at least 60 mm Hg.

Decreased Inspired Oxygen

Hypoxemia may be associated with excessive dead space rebreathing or with insufficient fresh oxygen flow or excessive nitrous oxide flow into the anesthetic circuit. Oxygen flow may be decreased accidentally, or the oxygen source may be depleted.

Hyperthermia

The decrease in temperature of a blood sample taken from a hyperthermic patient and measured in a normothermic blood gas analyzer decreases the partial pressure of the measured gases. Failure to correct the measured P_{O_2} value results in an apparently low P_{O_2}.[42]

Diffusion Hypoxia

Diffusion hypoxia may occur if a patient breathing nitrous oxide is not allowed to breath 100 per cent oxygen for three to five minutes after the nitrous oxide has been turned off.[41]

UPPER AIRWAY OBSTRUCTION

Extrathoracic upper airway obstructions cause inspiratory stridor and thoracic retraction. Intrathoracic upper airway obstructions cause expiratory stridor and an expiratory abdominal contraction.[100] Patients with upper airway obstructions can be sedated with a small dosage of sedative or tranquilizer; further excitement should be avoided until the underlying disorder can be corrected.[100]

Obstructions After Endotracheal Intubation

These obstructions are invariably caused by occlusion of the lumen of the endotracheal tube.

Dried lubricating jelly from a previous preparation may occlude the tube lumen. All tubes should be checked immediately prior to insertion.

The beveled end of the tube may be occluded by the wall of the bronchus at the carina if the tube is inserted too far or by the wall of the trachea if eccentric cuff inflation forces the opening of the tube against the epithelium. Eccentrically inflating cuffs may obstruct the tube and form a ball valve. Some tubes are curved so that in certain head and neck positions the tube opening is forced against the tracheal wall. In these cases the patient is able to inhale but not exhale through the tube.

Collapse of the endotracheal tube may be caused by excessive cuff inflation, by extreme head and neck angulations, by extreme angulation of the endotracheal tube after it leaves the mouth, or by tying roll gauze too tightly around the tube.

Accumulations of exudative debris in patients with pneumonia or froth in patients with pulmonary edema impair free air flow through the tube.

When unexplained obstructions occur, the cuff should be deflated and the position of the tube changed. If the obstruction is not relieved, exchange the endotracheal tube with another that functions properly.

Obstructions After Connection to the Anesthetic Machine

These obstructions may be due to improper connection of the corrugated tubing to the anesthetic circuit, rebreathing valves that are stuck closed, occlusion of the rebreathing bag port, or collapse of the rebreathing bag.

PULMONARY EDEMA

Pulmonary edema may develop owing to excessive capillary hydrostatic pressure or increased capillary permeability. Auscultation of fluid sounds may occur with mucous accumulations in the endotracheal tube or with nasopharyngeal fluid accumulations in unintubated patients or via the esophageal stethoscope owing to fluid and air in the esophagus. The fluid sounds should be localized by careful thoracic and cervical auscultation before diagnosing pulmonary edema. Central venous pressure or pulmonary capillary wedge pressure should be monitored in patients with preoperative evidence of pulmonary edema or congestive heart failure,[19, 102] and fluid therapy should be conservative. Once pulmonary edema has developed, appropriate combinations of oxygen therapy and positive pressure ventilation should be instituted until the underlying disorder can be effectively treated.[8] All attempts should be made to lower pulmonary capillary hydrostatic pressure without causing excessive hypotension.[104, 107]

ASPIRATION OF GASTRIC CONTENTS

Consequences of Aspiration

Aspiration of acid gastric contents with a pH below 2 causes an immediate cellular necrosis.[69] Mechanical airway obstruction contributes to impaired pulmonary function. Bronchopneumonia is a common sequela of aspiration.

Preoperative Considerations

Vomition and regurgitation are minimized by preoperative withholding of food. If a patient has a full stomach, surgery should be postponed. If this is not possible, vomition is induced with apomorphine (0.04 mg/kg) or morphine (0.2 to 0.4 mg/kg). If vomition is undesirable, anesthesia is induced and the patient intubated rapidly. A patient with an esophagus full of fluid (persistent right aortic arch or esophageal achalasia) is induced and intubated in a sternal position with the head elevated.

Operative Considerations

Operative regurgitation of gastric fluid may be enhanced by head-down dorsal recumbency and by stomach compression during abdominal surgery. The pH of any regurgitated material should be checked to determine the relative danger of aspiration. Lavaging the stomach, esophagus, and mouth with an alkaline solution may be beneficial if done before aspiration. The mouth and pharynx should be cleaned prior to extubation.

Postoperative Considerations

Endotracheal intubation should be maintained as long as possible in a patient that may vomit during recovery. The patient should be extubated in a head-up sternal position after return of the swallowing reflex and monitored closely. Head-down positioning is recommended if vomition occurs. Oxygen therapy and broad spectrum antibiotics are indicated if aspiration occurs.[52] Tracheal lavage or steroids are of little value in the treatment of aspiration.

BRADYCARDIA

Bradycardia requires definitive therapy when it causes the mean blood pressure to fall below 60 mm Hg and when in the absence of a blood pressure measurement, the heart rate decreases below 60 BPM. Preoperative heart rates range between 80 and 150 BPM for the dog and 100 and 200 for the cat; during surgery rates range between 100 and 140 BPM for the dog and 140 and 180 for the cat.

Common Causes of Bradycardia

Excessive Anesthetic Depth

Excessive administration of anesthetic agent slows spontaneous pacemaker depolarization and delays conduction.

Excessive Vagal Tone

High vagal tone may cause bradycardia and atrioventricular conduction block. Vagal tone may be enhanced by endotracheal intubation, traction or pressure on the eye and extraocular muscles, visceral traction, or periosteal stimulation.[71]

Drugs

Many anesthetics and some neuromuscular blockers cause bradycardia either by increasing vagal tone (narcotics; atropine; anticholinesterase agents, e.g. neostigmine) or by decreasing sympathetic tone (xylazine, beta-receptor blocking agents).[72, 106] Some agents directly stimulate postganglionic cholinergic receptors (succinylcholine) or affect depolarizing myocardial cells directly (halothane, methoxyflurane, barbiturates, lidocaine).[106]

Hypothermia

Hypothermia decreases tissue oxygen demands and decreases heart rate, cardiac output, and blood pressure.[13] Direct cold-induced myocardial depression does not occur until the core temperature decreases below 25°C.[13]

Toxemia

Exogenous toxemia and endogenous metabolic disturbances such as hypoxia, acidosis, digitalis intoxication, hypothyroidism, visceral organ failure, hyperkalemia, hypocalcemia, and end-stage shock may also cause bradycardia.

Prevention

Atropine (0.04 mg/kg IM) is often given prior to induction to prevent vagus-mediated bradycardia. The duration of vagal blockade produced by atropine is variable. Although additional injections of atropine are usually not given during the operative period, repeat doses can be administered (0.01 mg/kg IV) if bradycardia develops. Large doses of atropine predispose the patient to tachycardia and ventricular arrhythmias.[33] Atropine causes a centrally mediated increase in vagal tone prior to peripheral vagal blockade, and bradyarrhythmias are occasionally seen before peripheral cholinergic blockade.[47]

Treatment

If the cause of the bradycardia cannot be determined and if the condition is judged to have deleterious effects on blood pressure and has not responded to atropine, beta-receptor stimulants may be indicated (see Table 32–1). Isoproterenol is a pure beta-receptor stimulant and may cause substantial peripheral vasodilation if administered to hypovolemic patients. Dopamine, dobutamine, and mephentermine cause less vasodilation (see Table 32–1).

SINUS TACHYCARDIA AND HYPERTENSION

Sinus tachycardia is defined as a heart rate above 160 BPM in the dog and 180 in the cat.[37] Hypertension is a mean blood pressure above 160 mm Hg or a systolic blood pressure above 200 mm Hg. Normal systolic blood pressures during surgery are 90 to 150 mm Hg.

Consequences of Sinus Tachycardia and Hypertension

Sinus Tachycardia. Excessive sinus tachycardia may be associated with inadequate diastolic ventricular filling and insufficient cardiac output.
Hypertension. Excessive hypertension increases the workload of the heart and may precipitate heart failure.[64] Hypertension is associated with increased capillary hydrostatic pressure, which may precipitate cerebral and pulmonary edema.[23, 64, 133]

Common Causes of Sinus Tachycardia and Hypertension

Hypertension may be caused by increased blood volume, cardiac output, or peripheral vasomotor tone.

Hypervolemia

Hypertension and an increased heart rate may be caused by the rapid administration of any fluid but is especially likely with concentrated mannitol or glucose solutions, colloidal solutions, or whole blood.

It is not possible to set any maximum dosage above which hypervolemia will occur, because individual patients start at such widely diverse points. Conservative fluid therapy is advised in patients with patent ductus arteriosus, anuric renal failure, congestive heart failure, recent lung trauma, and pulmonary or central nervous system edema. Central venous pressure[54] or pulmonary capillary wedge pressure[19, 102] should be monitored during the infusion to prevent fluid overload.

Light Anesthetic Levels

Light levels of anesthesia are often associated with tachycardia and hypertension. These two signs are not consistent findings in lightly anesthetized patients, since heart rate and blood pressure may not increase until after the patient's level of anesthesia becomes excessively light. If the patient's level of anesthesia is very light and no other causes of tachycardia or hypertension can be identified, the treatment is to increase the depth of anesthesia.

Drugs

Tachycardia and hypertension may be caused by certain sympathomimetics and anesthetics (e.g., ketamine). Xylazine causes hypertension and bradycardia. Hypertension may occur during narcotic and neuromuscular blocking techniques but is probably not due to surgical stimulation if it persists after large doses of narcotics. A small dose of diazepam may effectively decrease and stabilize blood pressure.

Adverse Physiological Response to General Anesthesia

Increasing heart rate and blood pressure may signal the development of an underlying anesthetic complication such as hypoxia or hypercapnia. Tachycardia, but not necessarily hypertension, may be associated with hyperthermia during surgery.

Pre-existing Diseases

Hypertension may be due to pheochromocytoma[18] or hyperthyroidism.[101] CNS ischemia, hypoxia, or elevated intracranial pressure may cause reflex hypertension.[11] Patients with patent ductus arteriosus or any large left-to-right shunt may be hypervolemic and may develop hypertension when the shunt is occluded.

Appendage Tourniquets

Hypertension occasionally occurs one to two hours after the application of an appendage tourniquet for orthopedic surgical procedures. The hypertension regresses immediately upon removal of the tourniquet and may be due to tourniquet or ischemic nociceptive afferent feedback.

Treatment of Sinus Tachycardia or Hypertension

Eliminate Obvious Causes

If the cause of the tachycardia or hypertension is a light level of anesthesia, hypoxia, hypercapnia, hyperthermia, appendage tourniquets, or drug administration, the underlying problem should be corrected. It is unwise to override hypertension with excessive anesthetic dosages.

Pre-existing Diseases

If the cause is a coexisting disease, therapy should be directed toward the underlying disease process.

TABLE 32–2. Vasodilators

Generic Name	Brand Name (Source)	Mechanism of Action	Dose and Method of Administration (Onset; Peak; Duration)	Important Considerations and Effects*
Morphine		Dilates primarily capacitance but also resistance vessels	0.05–0.2 mg/kg IM (10 min; 30–45 min; 2–4 hr)	CNS depression Respiratory depression Histamine-mediated hypotension (nausea, vomiting)
Acetylpromazine	Acepromazine (Ayerst)	Alpha-receptor blockade	0.02–0.1 mg/kg IM (10 min; 30–45 min; 6–8 hr)	CNS depression
Hydralazine	Apresoline (Ciba)	Direct arteriolar smooth muscle relaxant Little effect on venous capacitance vessels	0.2–0.5 mg/kg (10–20 min; 10–80 min; 2–8 hr)	With prolonged use: Systemic lupus erythematosus Neuritis Blood dyscrasias
Diazoxide	Hyperstat (Schering)	Direct arteriolar smooth muscle relaxant on primarily resistance vessels	5 mg/kg rapidly IV (Immed.; 5–10 min; 30 min to 10 hr)	Inhibits insulin release → hyperglycemia
Nitroprusside	Nipride (Roche)	Direct arteriolar and venular smooth muscle relaxant	3 μg (0.5–10.0/kg/min IV Dilute in D5W, IV with continuous blood pressure monitoring (Immed.; 1 min; 2 min)	Light sensitive; bottle must be covered with foil and kept for no longer than 4 hr Avoid in hepatic or renal failure Large doses may cause cyanide toxicity Keep total dose below 1.5 mg/kg/2 hr; treat with sodium nitrite (0.5 to 0.75 mg/kg slow IV) followed by sodium thiosulfate (0.2 gm/kg slow IV) Thiocyanate accumulation (disorientation)
Trimethaphan	Arfonad (Roche)	Postsynaptic ganglionic blocking agent (dilates resistance and capacitance vessels) Direct arteriolar smooth muscle relaxant	Dilute 50 mg in 500 ml D5W 0.4–4.0 μg/kg/min (Immed.; 5–10 min; 10–15 min)	Releases histamine Parasympatholytic effects
Phentolamine	Rigitine (Ciba)	Alpha-receptor blockade and direct smooth muscle relaxation of resistance and capacitance vessels	5–30 μg/kg/min IV (Immed.; 2 min; 5–10 min)	Sympathomimetic cardiac stimulation Parasympathomimetic gastrointestinal stimulation
Phenoxybenzamine	Dibenzyline (Smith Kline & French)	Alpha-receptor blockade	0.5–1.0 mg/kg IV diluted in saline administered over 1 hr (30–60 min; 1–2 hr; 12–24 hr)	Available only as an experimental drug

*Excessive hypotension, secondary cardiac stimulation, and renal sodium and water retention are implied adverse effects of most of the vasodilators.

Vasodilator therapy may be necessary to obtain rapid control of blood pressure until the underlying disease process can be diagnosed and effectively treated (Table 32–2).

Hypervolemia

Hypervolemic hypertension is usually treated by cessation of fluid administration, allowing time for vascular accommodation, fluid redistribution, and renal excretion. Depending on the severity of the hypervolemia, further therapy may include:

1. Administration of diuretic agents (furosemide,[5, 70, 135, 139] dopamine[44]);

2. Phlebotomy;

3. Administration of moderate vasodilators such as furosemide, morphine,[62] or small dosages of acetylpromazine[105] or clonidine[5, 70, 139] (see Table 32–2) when arterial blood pressure is not monitored; or

4. Administration of potent vasodilators such as hydrazaline, phentolamine, phenoxybenzamine, nitroprusside, diazoxide, or trimethaphan[5, 70, 139] (see Table 32–2) when arterial blood pressure is monitored.

PREMATURE VENTRICULAR CONTRACTIONS

Premature ventricular contractions (PVCs) signify an underlying complication that may lead to more serious arrhythmias or cardiac arrest if unchecked.

Recognition

PVCs should be suspected whenever auscultation reveals a triple heart sound followed by a compensatory pause. This rhythm is often irregular and associated with a pulse deficit (Fig. 32–2). The diagnosis should be confirmed by the following electrocardiographic signs: a bizarre QRS complex (the actual wave form is determined by the location of the ectopic foci); no preceding P wave or a shortened P-R interval; and an abnormal complex too closely following the preceding complex and followed by a compensatory pause.[16]

Causes of Premature Ventricular Contractions

Catecholamines

PVCs may be caused by endogenous catecholamine release during light levels of anesthesia or during any stress such as hypoxemia, hypercapnia, or hypotension. Exogenous catecholamine therapy has a high potential for producing PVCs.[5, 70, 139] Some anesthetics lower the threshold of catecholamine-induced arrhythmias (halothane, xylazine).[68, 96]

Endogenous or Exogenous Toxemias

PVCs may be caused by severe acidosis or alkalosis, hypokalemia (potentiated by alkalosis or glucose or insulin therapy), hypercalcemia (potentiated by acidosis), hypoxia, hypotension, visceral organ failure, severe hypothermia (less than 26°C), digitalis toxicity (potentiated by hypokalemia and hypercalcemia), and some anesthetics (thiamylal).[30, 98]

Direct Endocardial, Myocardial, or Epicardial Stimulation

Endocarditis, myocarditis, direct endocardial stimulation by long jugular catheters, or epicardial stimulation by surgical manipulation of the heart may cause PVCs. Myocardial stress due to excessive pre-

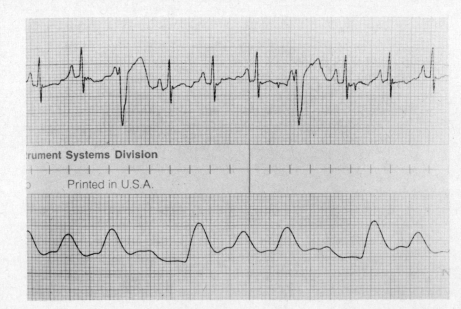

Figure 32–2. Premature ventricular contractions associated with pulse deficits.

load (high end-diastolic filling volume caused by a fluid overload or congestive heart failure) or afterload (high diastolic arterial blood pressure caused by peripheral vasoconstriction) may also cause PVCs.

Treatment of Premature Ventricular Contractions

Definitive therapy should be considered when PVCs are multifocal or are increasing in frequency or severity.[16, 30, 37] The following therapeutic regimen is suggested:

1. Evaluate the level of anesthesia and make appropriate adjustments to the vaporizer setting.
2. Maximize inspired oxygen.
3. Provide ventilatory support.
4. Check the anesthetic machine or ventilator to rule out machine-related causes of hypoxemia or hypercapnia.
5. Begin rapid fluid administration.
6. If the PVCs persist, discontinue administration of agents that may cause or lower the threshold of the arrhythmias.
7. If the PVCs persist, consider administration of antiarrhythmic agents such as xylocaine (1–5 mg/kg IV), procainamide (1–5 mg/kg IV), or propranolol (0.05–0.3 mg/kg IV) by titrating to effect with repeated small dosages and maintaining the antiarrhythmic effect with continuous infusions.

HYPOTENSION

Arterial blood pressure determines cerebral and coronary perfusion. Blood pressure depends on a proper balance between blood volume, cardiac output, and peripheral vasomotor tone. Impairment of one of these factors is usually compensated for by the other two to maintain adequate blood pressure. If the impairment is severe or if the compensatory processes are exhausted or debilitated by disease, excessive hypotension develops. Adequate cerebral and coronary perfusion requires a mean systemic blood pressure of at least 60 mm Hg.[85]

Causes of Hypotension

Hypovolemia

Hypovolemia is the most common cause of hypotension. Probably the most common cause of hypovolemia is a fluid deficit unmasked by induction of general anesthesia. Extracellular fluid losses result from such disorders as diarrhea, vomition, diuresis, third-space fluid accumulations, and inadequate intake. Vascular volume deficiencies may be due to whole blood or plasma losses or hypoproteinemia. Signs of vascular volume deficits include tachycardia,

weak pulse, and peripheral vasoconstriction. The signs of an interstitial volume deficit are decreased skin turgor and an acute loss of body weight.

Decreased Cardiac Output

Decreased cardiac output may be due to decreased venous return, decreased contractility, bradycardia, severe tachycardia, or severe arrhythmias. Decreased venous return may be caused by surgical packing, positive pressure ventilation, gastric torsion, or pericardial tamponade. Decreased contractility may be due to acute or chronic intrinsic heart failure, anesthetic drugs, or endogenous or exogenous toxemias and electrolyte disturbances (potassium, calcium, magnesium).[30, 71]

Vasodilation

Some anesthetic drugs (acetylpromazine, bolus dosages of most anesthetics, epidural or subarachnoid deposition of local anesthetics.[2]), beta-receptor stimulants (see Table 32–4), and specific vasodilator drugs (see Table 32–2) cause peripheral vasodilation and hypotension. Hypoxia, hypercapnia, hyperthermia, surface rewarming of hypothermic patients,[141] and sepsis[117] cause peripheral vasodilation and may cause hypotension. The accumulation of noxious metabolic products and hypoxia in tissues that have sustained an extended episode of inadequate perfusion (catecholamine- or shock-induced vasoconstriction or cardiac arrest) causes peripheral vasodilation and hypotension.[81]

Treatment of Hypotension

When hypotension occurs during general anesthesia, the quantity of anesthetic administered is reduced. It may be necessary to change the anesthetic to agents that have less inherent cardiovascular depressant properties.

Hypovolemia

The volume of replacement fluids is determined by the evaluation of the clinical signs of vascular and interstitial volume deficiencies. The type of fluid to administer is determined by the balance of the measured constituents of the blood (Table 32–3) (see Chapter 11).

Decreased Cardiac Output

Myocardial infarction is rare in animals. If it is suspected it should be treated as is the human disease.[15] The long-term management of congestive heart failure involves effective control of contractility, preload, and afterload.[53, 111] The immediate manage-

TABLE 32–3. Important Considerations in Replacement Fluid Therapy*†

Parameter	Applicable Measurement and Desired Level	Fluids of Choice if Measured Parameter is Outside Desired Level
Volume	Central venous pressure: 2 to 10 cm H_2O	1. Crystalloid sodium replacement solution (lactated Ringer's)*
	Arterial blood pressure: 70 to 120 mm Hg (mean)	2. Colloid expander (dextran, plasma)
	Pulse quality: strong	3. Whole blood
	Capillary refill time: <1 second	
	Mucous membrane color: pink	
	Normal skin turgor	
Oxygen carrying capacity	Packed cell volume: >20 per cent	1. Whole blood
	Hemoglobin: >7 gm/dl	
Colloid oncotic pressure	Total plasma protein: >3.5 gm/dl	1. Colloid expander (plasma, dextran)
		2. Whole blood
Osmolality	Sodium concentration: 130 to 160 mEq/L	1. Crystalloid sodium replacement solution to maintain (lactated Ringer's) or increase (saline) sodium concentration
	Serum osmolality: 270 to 330 mOsm/kg	2. Hypotonic solution to decrease osmolality (½ lactated Ringer's or saline and ½ 5 per cent dextrose in water)
Viscosity	Packed cell volume: <60 per cent	1. Crystalloid sodium replacement solution (lactated Ringer's)

*Reprinted with permission from Kirk, R. W.: *Current Veterinary Therapy VIII.* W. B. Saunders. Philadelphia, 1983.
†Potassium and bicarbonate should be added as necessary.
‡Lactated Ringer's solution or any equivalent isonatremic solution.

ment of heart failure may require sympathomimetic therapy and correction of the underlying systemic disease. An appropriate sympathomimetic is selected on the basis of desired receptor stimulating activity (Table 32–4).

Agents that cause minimal peripheral vasoconstriction should be utilized for prolonged blood pressure support (isoproterenol, dobutamine, dopamine, or mephenteramine) (see Table 32–4).[5, 70, 139] These agents may readily cause excessive hypertension and arrhythmias, and their use should be monitored (arterial blood pressure, electrocardiography) to assure that they are effective without causing adverse effects. In many respects there is little difference between these four drugs; however, there is sufficient pharmacological difference that an alternate agent should be tried if one does not have the desired effects.

Isoproterenol[5, 70, 139] can be used if bradycardia or heart failure is the cause of the hypotension. It causes vasodilation and may improve tissue perfusion but may cause excessive hypotension. Dosages of 0.01 to 0.06 μg/kg/min effectively increase contractility and cardiac output with minimal chronotropic effects in man.[118] Higher dosages are associated with tachycardia and arrhythmias without further improvement in cardiac output.

Dobutamine[5, 45, 70, 139] has minimal alpha-receptor and strong beta-receptor agonist activity. It has less effect on heart rate than isoproterenol but about the same as dopamine. It promotes less peripheral vasoconstriction than dopamine but more than isoproterenol.

Dopamine[5, 45, 70, 139] causes less vasodilation than isoproterenol and may cause vasoconstriction at higher dosages. Dopamine enhances myocardial contractility with less effect on heart rate than isoproterenol and may be preferable when the initial hypotension is not associated with bradycardia. Dopamine increases renal blood flow (dopaminergic receptors) when administered at very low dosages of 2.5 μg/kg/min and is useful for acute renal failure.[44] Its alpha-receptor agonist properties are manifested at higher dosages (above 10 μg/kg/min). A dosage that increases heart rate or blood pressure causes renal vasoconstriction.

Mephentermine[5, 70, 139] has a longer duration of action (30 minutes) than previously mentioned agents (3 to 5 minutes) and can be given as an intermittent bolus. It has much less tendency to promote ventricular arrhythmias.

Calcium may be useful in idiopathic heart failure, halothane-induced depression of myocardial contractility, and hyperkalemia-induced heart failure and may enhance the activity of other sympathomimetics.[28]

CARDIAC ARREST

Cardiac arrest may be caused by severe abnormalities in any organ system of the body. Effective treatment of these complications and prevention of cardiac arrest are considerably easier than their treatment. A comprehensive resuscitation effort requires

TABLE 32–4. Sympathomimetics Used for Cardiovascular Support*

Drug (Receptor Activity)	Trade Name (Manufacturer)	Myocardial Chronotropy and Inotropy	Peripheral Vasomotor Tone	Major Indication	Dosage (IV)
Catecholamines					
Epinephrine (α + + +; β + + +)	Adrenalin (Parke-Davis; Vitarine; Bristol)	Increased	Increased	Cardiac arrest	0.05–0.5 mg (0.5 to 5 ml 1:10,000 solution) for average-sized dog (15 kg)
Norepinephrine (β + + +; β +)	Levophed bitartrate (Breon)	Variable	Increased	Vasoconstriction	0.10–1.0 mg for average-sized dog (15 kg)
Dopamine (dopa and β + + +; α + +)	Intropin (Arnar-Stone)	Increased	Variable	Blood pressure support ↑ visceral perfusion	10–50 µg/kg/min 2.0–5 µg/kg/min 80–200 mg in 500 ml D_5W
Isoproterenol (α0; β + + +)	Isuprel (Winthrop)	Increased	Decreased	Cardiac stimulation	0.4–1.0 mg in 500 ml D_5W (to effect; start 0.01 µg/kg/min)
Noncatecholamines					
Mephentermine (α +; β + +)	Wyamine (Wyeth)	Increased	Variable	Blood pressure support	0.1–0.75 mg/kg
Metaraminol (α + + +; β +)	Aramine (Merck Sharp & Dohme) Metaraminol bitartrate (Bristol; Invenex)	Variable	Increased	Vasoconstriction	0.1–0.2 mg/kg
Methoxamine (α + + +; β0)	Vasoxyl (Burroughs Wellcome)	None	Increased	Vasoconstriction	0.1–0.2 mg/kg
Phenylephrine (α + + +; β0)	Neo-Synephrine	None	Increased	Vasoconstriction	0.01–0.1 mg/kg
Dobutamine (α +; β + + +)	Dobutrex (Lilly)	Increased	Variable	Blood pressure support	100–400 mg in 500 ml D_5W (to effect; start 5 µg/kg/min)
Ephedrine (α + +; β +)	(Vitarine)	Increased	Variable	Blood pressure support	0.05–0.5 mg/kg IV, IM
Miscellaneous					
Calcium	(Bristol; Invenex; Vitarine)	Increased	Variable	Increase contractility	10% CaCl 1.5–2.0 ml 10% CaGluc 6–8 ml for average-sized dog
Digitalis Digoxin Digitoxin	(Wellcome) (Parke-Davis)	Increased	No direct effect	Increase contractility	Loading dose: 0.1–0.2 mg/kg divided into 4 doses over 48 hours Maintenance: 0.01–0.02 mg/kg divided b.i.d.
Glucagon	(Lilly)	Increased (variable effect on heart rate)	Decreased	Increase contractility	25–100 µg/kg/hr

*Reprinted with permission from Kirk, R. W.: *Current Veterinary Therapy VIII*. W. B. Saunders, Philadelphia, 1983.

substantial preplanning and a coordinated group effort. Necessary equipment and drugs should be organized and set up in advance (Fig. 32–3). Protocols and drug dosages should be posted in plain view (Table 32–5). All persons in the area should be trained to be a functional part of the resuscitation team.

Cardiopulmonary resuscitation has two different objectives.[58] The first is effective support of the cardiopulmonary system by cardiac compression, artificial ventilation, and fluid administration. The second is to restart a normal sinus electrical rhythm and an effective mechanical contraction with drug and electroshock therapy.[112] A more detailed description is presented in Chapter 12. A cardiopulmonary resuscitation flowchart is presented on the inside front cover of this book.

METABOLIC ACIDOSIS

Diagnosis

Metabolic acidosis during surgery is usually attributed to lactic acidosis secondary to inadequate tissue perfusion and may potentiate the severity of any preexisting acidosis.[110] Ideally the base or bicarbonate deficit would be calculated from measurements made with a blood gas analyzer, a Harleco Total CO_2 Analyzer, or an Oxford Titrator.[59] If these measurements are not available, the extent of the metabolic acidosis can only be estimated by a subjective interpretation of the severity and duration of the clinical signs of inadequate tissue perfusion.

Treatment

Initial therapy in metabolic acidosis is correction of the underlying disturbance and maximization of tissue perfusion with appropriate fluid therapy. Alkalinizing therapy should be conservative and should be reserved for those patients with moderate to severe metabolic acidosis. If the base or bicarbonate deficit calculation is available, the bicarbonate dosage is calculated by the following formula: base or bicarbonate deficit $\times$ 0.3 $\times$ body weight (kg). If the base or bicarbonate deficit calculations are not available and the degree of inadequate tissue perfusion and metabolic acidosis is judged as mild to severe, 1 to 5 mEq/kg body weight of sodium bicarbonate can be administered over a minimum of 20 to 30 minutes.

HYPOTHERMIA

Hypothermia during general anesthesia is the consequence of anesthetic-induced decreases in basal metabolic rate and muscular activity coupled with increased heat loss associated with depilation, evaporation of antiseptic solutions, exposure to cold table surfaces, and open body cavities. Standard restrictive thermometers, with tags of tape attached, can be used to measure deep esophageal temperature. Nonrestrictive laboratory thermometers or electronic thermometers can also be used for temperature monitoring.

Consequences of Hypothermia

The clinical importance of hypothermia is outlined in Table 32–6.

The single largest problem with hypothermia is nonrecognition. Continued administration of normothermic quantities of anesthetics to hypothermic patients results in an anesthetic overdose. When appropriate support measures are instituted, hypothermia is safe to quite low temperatures.

Prevention of Heat Loss

Heat loss may be reduced by minimizing the duration of antiseptic preparation of the surgical site; protecting the patient from the cool environment with blankets or towels; minimizing the duration of the surgical procedure; and actively warming the patient or his immediate environment.

Methods of Applying Heat

Circulating Warm Water Blanket

A circulating warm water blanket may be placed under or over the patient. The efficiency of the blanket in maintaining or restoring core temperature is determined by surface contact area.

Electric Blankets

Electric heating may easily overheat the body surface, causing burns and extensive skin sloughs. This is most likely to occur in patients that are hypothermic or in shock owing to vasoconstricted skin vasculature. If used, blankets should be either well insulated with towels or placed around the patient so as to avoid direct contact between the skin and the blanket. The temperature between the skin and the blanket should be measured to assure that it is less than 41°C (106°F).

Hot Water Bottles

Hot water bottles may be placed around the patient and under the drapes but should not touch the patient if the water temperature exceeds 41°C (106°F). Bottles should be changed when their measured temperature is below that of core temperature because they re-absorb heat from the patient.[21]

Infrared Heat Lamps

Infrared heat lamps may be used during or after the surgery. The optimum distance between the lamp and the patient is about 75 cm; a distance of 50 cm is associated with excessive skin heating, whereas a distance of 100 cm is associated with ineffective warming.[21] Excessive drying of the tissues in the surgical field must be prevented.[113] Radiant-heat infant warmers are also available commercially.

Flushing with Warm Fluid

Open body cavities may be flushed with warm sterile saline (less than 42°C). Intravenous fluids may be warmed but cannot be administered in sufficient quantities to have much influence on core temperature.

TABLE 32–5. An Outline for Cardiopulmonary Resuscitation

Airway
  Establish and maintain an open airway via endotracheal intubation.

Breathing
  Begin intermittent positive pressure ventilation: one ventilation per five seconds.

Circulation
  Begin external cardiac compression: 60 to 80 compressions per minute. Evaluate the effectiveness of the cardiac compression procedure continuously. If the external technique is ineffective:

  1. Alter the external technique.
  2. Administer fluids rapidly.
  3. Apply a tight rear leg and abdominal wrap.
  4. Perform a thoracotomy for internal cardiac compression.

Drugs
  Epinephrine: 0.1 to 0.5 mg (average-sized dog)
  Sodium bicarbonate: 0.5 to 1.0 mEq/Kg/5 minutes of cardiac arrest.
  Calcium solution: 1.5 to 2.0 ml of 10% $CaCl_2$ (average-sized dog)
                        6.0 to 8.0 ml of 10% CaGluc
  Fluids (lactated Ringer's): 40 ml/kg (dog)
                        20 ml/kg (cat)
  Atropine: 0.005 to 0.01 mg/kg

Electrocardiographic monitoring
  Electroshock therapy (defibrillation) when necessary.

Follow-up monitoring and support
  Cardiovascular, pulmonary, and CNS function.
  CNS dehydration therapy.

Postoperative Warming

During recovery the patient's environment can be warmed by infrared heat lamps, surgical lamps, electric floor heaters, forced-air hair dryers, heating blankets, or hot water blankets. Care should be taken to avoid excessive environmental temperatures and overheating of the patient. A warm water bath may also be used, but the surgical incision must be protected from contamination.

HYPERTHERMIA

Hyperthermia occasionally occurs during general anesthesia.[26, 89, 120] High metabolic activity associated with light levels of anesthesia, large or obese patients, insulation by surgical draping, and breathing a fully humidified gas mixture all contribute to increased core temperature. Malignant hyperthermia syndrome is a rapid and progressive hyperthermia. It is often associated with the administration of halothane or succinylcholine. In humans and swine the disorder is related to a genetic functional defect within the sarcoplasmic reticulum.[49] Although the basic cause is unknown, the muscular defect is associated with abnormal calcium fluxes and increased muscle enzyme activity and heat production.[49] Muscular rigidity occurs if the cytoplasmic calcium concentration is greater than approximately 10^{-5} mM/L.[67] Lower calcium concentrations are not associated with muscular rigidity, but hyperthermia still develops owing to sarcoplasmic reticulum and cellular membrane metabolic activity.

Consequences of Hyperthermia

The harmful effects of hyperthermia are primarily related to high metabolic activity and cellular oxygen consumption. When the body temperature rises above about 41°C (106°F), oxygen utilization exceeds supply and hypoxic cellular damage occurs.[51] Hyperthermia increases metabolic activity, which further increases the hyperthermia. This vicious cycle may become self-perpetuating when the temperature exceeds 41°C.[51] All body tissues are affected by hypoxia, but the organs most likely to show insufficiencies are the brain, kidneys, liver, and blood (disseminated intravascular coagulation and hemolysis).[74]

Treatment of Hyperthermia

General Support

Hyperthermic patients should breathe an enriched oxygen mixture. Rapid administration of fluids helps restore an effective circulating blood volume and cools the patient. Corticosteroid and sodium bicarbonate therapy should be considered if the hyper-

TABLE 32–6. Clinical Importance of Hypothermia

Temperature °C(°F)	Clinical Importance
36 and above (97)	No effect except for postanesthetic shivering. Shivering increases oxygen consumption and decreases ventilatory capacity;[50] hypoxemia may be a problem in patients debilitated by anesthetic drugs or pulmonary disease.
32 to 34 (90 to 94)	Anesthetic requirements are reduced owing to the hypometabolic effects of the hypothermia. Recovery may be prolonged. Thermoregulation may be impaired, and artificial rewarming may be necessary.
28 to 30 (82 to 86)	Little or no anesthetic required for the maintenance of anesthesia. Recovery is prolonged. Patients must be artificially rewarmed. Ventilatory support should be instituted. Metabolic acidosis due to inadequate tissue perfusion occurs on rewarming.
25 to 26 (77 to 79)	Cold-induced EKG changes begin to occur (prolonged P-R interval and widened QRS complexes).[33] Increased automaticity of heart (appearance of arrhythmias such as premature ventricular contractions or fibrillation). Bradycardia in excess of the hypometabolism results in an insufficient cardiac output. Microcirculatory sludging due to excessive blood viscosity may occur.
22 and below (72)	Spontaneous ventilation ceases. Ventricular fibrillation and coagulation disorders occur.[33]

thermia is severe or prolonged. Brain, liver, kidney, gastrointestinal, and endocrine function should be monitored by appropriate clinical and laboratory tests for several days following severe hyperthermic episodes.

Enhancing Evaporative and Conductive Heat Loss

Evaporative heat loss can be enhanced by soaking the skin with water or alcohol. Conductive heat loss can be enhanced by immersing the patient in a cold water (or ice water) bath. The choice of therapy depends on the extent of the hyperthermia and the rate at which the temperature is to be decreased. Infusion of cold fluids intravascularly or into an open body cavity and ice water enemas or gastric lavage may also be used. Surface cooling techniques may have a substantial peripheral effect before much core cooling is noted. The core temperature continues to decrease as the core and peripheral temperatures equilibrate (afterdrop). Since the extent of the afterdrop is unpredictable, aggressive cooling techniques such as ice water baths should cease as soon as the core temperature decreases below 40°C (104°F). Additional cooling can be applied if necessary after the core and peripheral temperatures are equal.

Antipyretics

Antipyretics (aspirin, aminopyrine, dipyrone, phenylbutazone) may directly lower hypothalamic thermostatic settings or inhibit the release of pyrogens and lower body temperature. Dipyrone has caused excessive hypothermia in a few patients.

Malignant Hyperthermia

If malignant hyperthermia is suspected, the offending agent should be removed and aggressive attempts to lower the body temperature should be made. Procaine and dantrolene reduced mortality rates in pigs with malignant hyperthermia syndrome.[54]

ELECTRICAL, EXPLOSION, AND BURN HAZARDS IN THE OPERATING ROOM

Electrical Accidents

Electrical accidents occur when a body conducts electricity to ground. The mains circuitry of an electronic instrument is normally insulated from the instrument chassis. Even with intact insulation, however, the chassis commonly accumulates electrical charge by inductance of stray leakage currents from the mains circuitry.[79] The amount of leakage current should be periodically checked with an ammeter attached to an ungrounded instrument.[131] The chassis becomes progressively more electrified if the insulation deteriorates because of age or damage. A functional ground wire attached to the chassis minimizes the electrical hazard to the operator by dissipating the electrical charge arising from either small leakage currents or a direct mains-current contact. A broken ground wire or the complete lack thereof is one of the most common problems seen with electrical equipment. Ground wire breakage usually occurs within the plug and occurs when the plug is pulled out of the socket by the cord but may occur anywhere within a damaged cord. The integrity of the ground wire circuit should be periodically checked with an ohmmeter.[131]

Ground fault circuit interrupters (a balanced core-earth leakage device) can be used to detect the voltage difference between the live and neutral wires of the mains circuit.[65] Power to the device is interrupted if a voltage difference of sufficient size occurs, regardless of whether the leakage is vented to ground. Power isolation transformers provide an additional means of protecting operating room personnel and patients from electrocution.[38]

Electrical currents disperse over an infinite number of pathways when they pass through the body. Current density is highest at the points of entrance and exit from the body; current density through the heart is considerably less. Patients with external conductive pathways to the heart (cardiac pacemaker wire or fluid-filled catheter) are more susceptible to electrical shock because the point of current entrance or exit (and the highest current density) is at the heart. These susceptible patients may develop ventricular fibrillation at electrical thresholds far below those necessary for gross perception. They must be isolated from all sources of leakage current. All mains-operated devices must be well insulated and well grounded to a common earth (plugged into the same wall socket).[48] The patient should not be grounded. The wearing of rubber gloves when handling intracardiac leads helps minimize patient grounding via operating room personnel. The use of isolated circuits and battery-operated and ungrounded equipment is highly desirable.

Fire and Explosion Hazards

Fires and explosions occur when flammable material is exposed to heat in the presence of oxygen. Elimination of any one of the three prevents combustion.

Flammable Material

Flammable anesthetic agents are rarely used nowadays. If used, strict protocols that eliminate mains power and static electric ignition sources must be adhered to.[84] Other flammable materials still used in the operating room include alcohol, antiseptic solutions, adhesive tape, and cloth such as drapes and gauze packs.

Electrical Ignition Sources

Conventional electrical sockets, switches, nonexplosion-proof (not gastight) electrical circuits, and electrosurgical units should not be used within 25 cm of leaks in the anesthetic circuit (including around the cuff of the endotracheal tube), especially if flammable anesthetic agents are used,[136] and also in the presence of other flammable materials and oxygen. Equipment used within the breathing circuit must be electrically isolated from it and must not exceed a surface temperature of 150°C (302°F).[39]

Oxygen

The enriched oxygen mixtures and oxygen–nitrous oxide mixtures used during general anesthesia support combustion better than atmospheric air and increase the violence of conflagration. These gas mixtures should be isolated from flammable materials and sources of ignition.

Burn Hazards

Burn hazards may be associated with electrical heating blankets or hot water bottles and electrosurgical units. In electrosurgical units, the current supplied by the active electrode coagulates or cuts the

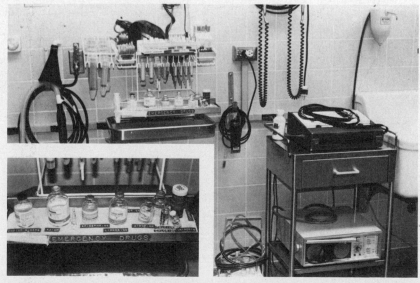

Figure 32–3. Wall-mounted emergency supplies and equipment.

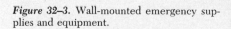

TABLE 32–7. Emergency Equipment, Supplies, and Drugs

Equipment	Supplies	Drugs
Highest Priority		
Oxygen	Intravenous catheters for peripheral and jugular veins: full assortment of sizes	Epinephrine, 10% calcium chloride
Positive pressure ventilation: anesthetic machine, automatic ventilator, or self-reinflating resuscitation bag	Administration sets (regular and pediatric; for blood and clear fluids), extension sets, and three-way stopcocks	Sodium bicarbonate
An assortment of endotracheal tubes		Atropine
		Heparin
Laryngoscope with small, medium, and large blades	Fluids Replacement solution, lactated Ringer's	Antiarrhythmic: Xylocaine Blood pressure stimulant: dopamine or mephentermine
Flashlight	5% dextrose in water 50% dextrose in water	
Portable hair clippers	Whole blood Heparinized saline	Alpha-receptor stimulant: phenylephrine or norepinephrine
Sterile surgical instruments for cutdown procedures	Needles and syringes (all sizes)	Narcotic agent: oxymorphone
Sterile towel packs	Surgical scrub solutions	Anesthetic and adjunct: thiamylal or thiopental inhalational, diazepam, ketamine, Innovar
Suction apparatus and catheters	Chest drainage equipment	
Stethoscope	Adhesive tape	
Stomach tubes: small, medium, and large	Suture material	Glucocorticoid: dexamethasone or prednisolone
	Surgical gloves	
Defibrillator with small and large internal and external paddles	Stomach tubes	Antihistamine: diphenhydramine (Benadryl)
	Tourniquet	
	Cotton-tipped applicators	
	Urinary catheters	

tissue surface and distributes itself through the body via an infinite number of pathways and exits through the ground plate. The contact between the ground plate and the body surface should be large, and the application of contact gel should be generous. Bony prominences are avoided. The ground plate should be placed as close to the operating site as possible. Proper ground plate contact should be re-affirmed if

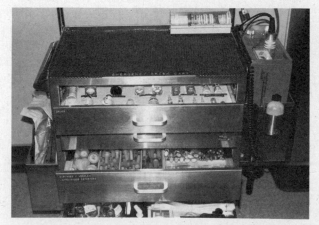 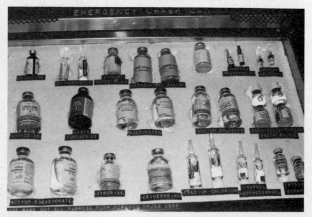

Figure 32–4. Mobile emergency cart.

TABLE 32–7. Emergency Equipment, Supplies, and Drugs Continued

Equipment	Supplies	Drugs
Not Essential but Helpful		
Hematocrit tubes and centrifuge	Low and high molecular weight dextran	Other blood pressure stimulant: Isoproterenol, dobutamine
Refractometer	Mannitol	
Face masks	Calibrated burrettes for accurate fluid infusions	Beta-receptor blocking agent: Propanolol
Blood pressure–measuring equipment	Blood collection tubes	Narcotic reversing agent: naloxone
pH and blood gas analyzer	Urinary catheters	Respiratory stimulant: doxapram
Heat block and tubes for activated clotting time	Box for disposal of contaminated or sharp expendables	Neuromuscular blocking agent: pancuronium or gallamine
		Neuromuscular blocking agent reversing agent: neostigmine
		Diuretic: furosemide
		Digitalis preparation
		Nitroprusside
		Dipyrone
		Antibiotics
		Potassium chloride
		Other antiarrhythmic: procainamide or quinidine

the patient is moved during the operative procedure. The ground plate circuit should be periodically evaluated to assure its proper performance. Prior to each use, the alarm that signals a break between the active electrode and the return circuit should be checked.

If the grounding circuit is defective, the current can leave the body via other routes to ground such as the table, the ECG electrodes, the conductive tubing of the anesthetic machine, thermistor probes, intracardiac catheters, or operating room personnel.[39, 126] These exit points are small, and excessive heat production may cause postoperative tissue necrosis. ECG electrodes should be positioned as far as possible from the operating site and should have large contact areas in the event of ground plate failure. The patient should be isolated from ground. Isolated input ECG monitors do not provide complete protection against the high-frequency currents of electrosurgical units. A high-frequency protection block can be placed in the patient lead cable.[138]

An isolated output electrosurgical unit protects against burns at monitoring sites, since current must leave the patient via the return electrode in order for current to flow at all. It will not, however, prevent burns at the site of an improperly applied ground plate.

LOSS OF POWER

Essential life support or life-saving equipment and all equipment necessary for the completion of the surgical procedure should have an emergency power source available in the event of a main power interruption or circuit breaker interruption. If a central emergency power source is unavailable, back-up equipment, such as battery-powered surgical lamps and vital monitoring equipment and compressed gas–powered ventilators, needs to be immediately available. Essential life support equipment should, perhaps, not be attached to a common ground fault circuit breaker with other instrumentation, since a fault in any of the other instruments will cause a loss of power to the life support equipment.[38]

EMERGENCY EQUIPMENT, SUPPLIES, AND DRUGS

The successful management of an emergency situation requires (1) the necessary emergency equipment and drugs, (2) adequately trained personnel to operate the equipment and administer the drugs, (3) the knowledge basic to the appropriate application of equipment, interpretation of measurements, and administration of the correct drug, (4) adequate preparation, and (5) adequate monitoring to know when the emergency is imminent or has occurred.

Table 32–7 provides a list of emergency equipment, supplies, and drugs for various emergency situations (Figs. 32–3 and 32–4). The list has been divided into two categories: those that, in my opinion, are absolutely essential and should be immediately available, and those that, although not absolutely essential, are highly desirable.

1. Adams, A. P., Morgan-Hughes, J. O., and Sykes, M. K.: pH and blood-gas analysis. Anaesthesia 22:575, 1967; 23:47, 1968.
2. Akamatsu, T. J.: Cardiovascular response to spinal anesthesia. In Bonica, J. J. (ed.): Clinical Anesthesia. F. A. Davis, Philadelphia, 1969, Chap. 5.
3. Altman, P. L., and Dittmer, D. S. (eds.): Biology Data Book, Vol. III, 2d ed. Fed. Am. Soc. Exp. Biol., Bethesda, MD, 1974.
4. Amery, A., Fagard, R., Lynen, P., and Staessen, J. (eds.): Hypertensive Cardiovascular Disease: Pathophysiology and Treatment, Developments in Cardiovascular Disease, Vol. 16. Martinus Nijhoff Publishers, Boston, 1982, pp. 629–900.
5. Angel, J. E.: Physician's Desk Reference. Medical Economics Co., Oradell, NJ, 1983.
6. Aver, L., and Bell, K.: The AB blood group system in the domestic cat. Anim. Blood Groups Biochem. Genet. 11:63, 1980.
7. Aver, L., Bell, K., and Coates, S.: Blood transfusion reactions in the cat. J. Am. Vet. Med. Assoc. 180:729, 1982.
8. Ayres, S. M.: Mechanisms and consequences of pulmonary edema: cardiac lung, shock lung, and principles of ventilation therapy in adult respiratory distress syndrome. Am. Heart J. 103:97, 1981.
9. Beatler, E., and Wood, L.: The in vivo regeneration of red cell 2,3 diphosphoglyceric acid (DPG) after transfusion of stored blood. J. Lab. Clin. Med. 74:300, 1969.
10. Berger, A. J., Mitchell, R. A., and Severinghaus, J. W.: Regulation of respiration. N. Engl. J. Med. 297:92, 138, 197, 1977.
11. Berman, I. R., and Ducker, T. B.: Pulmonary, somatic and splanchnic circulatory responses to increased intracranial pressure. Ann. Surg. 169:210, 1969.
12. Bishop, R. L., and Weisfeldt, M. L.: Sodium bicarbonate administration during cardiac arrest. JAMA 235:506, 1976.
13. Blair, E.: Hypothermia. In Soma, L. R. (ed.): Textbook of Veterinary Anesthesia. Williams & Wilkins, Baltimore, 1971, Chap. 38.
14. Bliss, J. Q., Johns, D. G., and Burgen, A. U. S.: Transfusion reactions due to plasma incompatibility in dogs. Circ. Res. 7:79, 1959.
15. Blocker, W. P., and Cardus, D.: Rehabilitation in Ischemic Heart Disease. SP Medical and Scientific Books, New York, 1983.
16. Bolton, G. R.: Handbook of Canine Electrocardiography. W. B. Saunders, Philadelphia, 1975.
17. Breivik, H., Grenvik, A., Millen, E., and Safar, P.: Normalizing low arterial CO_2 tension during mechanical ventilation. Chest 63:525, 1973.
18. Brown, B. R.: Anesthesia for pheochromocytoma. In Brown, B. R. (ed.): Anesthesia and the Patient with Endocrine Disease. F. A. Davis, Philadelphia, 1980.
19. Buchbinder, N., and Ganz, W.: Hemodynamic monitoring: invasive techniques. Anesthesiology 45:146, 1976.
20. Bull, B. S., Huse, W. M., Braver, F. S., and Korpman, R. A.: Heparin therapy during extracorporeal circulation. J. Thorac. Cardiovasc. Surg. 69:685, 1975.
21. Burrows, C. F.: Intensive care of the critically ill dog and cat. Part I. Comp. Cont. Ed. Vet. 4:875, 1982.
22. Chang, T., and Glazko, A. J.: Biotransformation and disposition of ketamine. Int. Anesthesiol. Clin. 12:157, 1974.
23. Chen, H. I., and Chai, C. Y.: Pulmonary edema and hemorrhage as a consequence of systemic vasoconstriction. Am. J. Physiol. 227:144, 1974.
24. Clark, J. M., and Lambertsen, C. J.: Pulmonary oxygen toxicity, a review. Pharm. Rev. 23:38, 1971.
25. Collins, V. J.: Principles of Anesthesiology, 2nd ed. Lea & Febiger, Philadelphia, 1976, pp. 210–214.
26. DeJong, R. H., Heavner, J. E., and Amory, D. W.: Malignant hyperpyrexia in the cat. Anesthesiology 41:608, 1974.
27. Deneke, S. M., and Fanburg, B. L.: Normobaric oxygen toxicity of the lung. N. Engl. J. Med. 303:76, 1980.
28. Denlinger, J. K., Kaplan, J. A., Lecky, J. H., and Wollman, H.: Cardiovascular responses to calcium administered intravenously to man during halothane anesthesia. Anesthesiology 42:390, 1975.
29. Don, H. F.: Ventilatory management. In Berk, J. L., Sampliner, J. E., Artz, J. S., and Vinocur, B. (eds.): Handbook of Critical Care. Little, Brown, Boston, 1976, Chap. 5.
30. Dreifus, L., and Likoff, W.: Cardiac Arrhythmias. Grune and Stratton, NY, 1973.
31. Drop, L. J., and Laver, M. B.: Low plasma ionized calcium and response to calcium therapy in critically ill man. Anesthesiology 43:300, 1975.
32. Dunn, R. C., Dunn, D. L., and Moser, K. M.: Determinants of tracheal injury by cuffed endotracheal tubes. Surg. Gynecol. Obstet. 129:1235, 1969.
33. Eger, E. I.: Atropine, scopolamine and related compounds. Anesthesiology 23:365, 1962.
34. Eger, E. I.: Anesthetic Uptake and Action. Williams & Wilkins, Baltimore, 1974.
35. Eger, E. I., and Saidman, L. J.: Hazards of nitrous oxide anesthesia in bowel obstruction and pneumothorax. Anesthesiology 26:61, 1965.
36. Eger, E. I., Saidman, L. J., and Bradstater, B.: Minimum alveolar anesthetic concentration: A standard of anesthetic potency. Anesthesiology 26:756, 1965.
37. Ettinger, S. J., and Suter, P. F.: Canine Cardiology. W. B. Saunders, Philadelphia, 1970.
38. Feldtman, R. W., Derrick, J. R., Hoxie, D., and Wire, K.: Hospital electrical safety. Am. Fam. Physician 13:127, 1976.
39. Finlay, B., Couchie, D., Boyce, L., and Spencer, E.: Electrosurgery burns resulting from use of miniature ECG electrodes. Anesthesiology 41:263, 1974.
40. Fleming, W. H., Bowen, J. C., and Petty, C.: The use of pulmonary compliance as a guide to respirator therapy. Surg. Gynecol. Obstet. 134:291, 1972.
41. Frumin, M. J., and Edelist, G.: Diffusion anoxia: A critical reappraisal. Anesthesiology 31:243, 1969.
42. Gabel, R. A.: Algorithms for calculating and correcting blood-gas and acid-base variables. Resp. Physiol. 42:211, 1980.
43. Gleysteen, J. J., and Stroud, R. C.: Respiration and Circulation. Fed. Am. Soc. Exp. Biol., Bethesda, MD, 1971.
44. Goldberg, L. I.: Cardiovascular and renal actions of dopamine: potential clinical applications. Pharmacol. Rev. 24:1, 1972.
45. Goldberg, L. I., Hsieh, Y. Y., and Resnekov, L.: Newer catecholamines for treatment of heart failure and shock: An update on dopamine and a first look at dobutamine. Progr. Cardiovasc. Dis. 19:327, 1977.
46. Goodman, L. S., and Gilman, A. G.: The Pharmacologic Basis of Therapeutics. 6th ed. Macmillan, New York, 1980.
47. Goth, A.: Medical Pharmacology: Principles and Concepts, 10th ed. C. V. Mosby, St. Louis, 1981; p. 150.

48. Grant, G. C.: A simple introduction to electrical safety. Anaesth. Intensive Care 2:164, 1974.

49. Gronert, G.: Malignant hyperthermia. Anesthesiology 53:395, 1980.

50. Gruber, V. F.: *Blood Replacement.* Springer-Verlag, New York, 1969, pp. 55–104.

51. Guyton, A. C.: Body temperature, temperature regulation and fever. *In* Guyton, A. C. (ed.): *Textbook of Medical Physiology,* 3rd ed. W. B. Saunders, Philadelphia, 1966, Chap. 68.

52. Hamelberg, W. V., and Bosomworth, P. P.: *Aspiration Pneumonitis.* Charles C Thomas, Springfield, 1968.

53. Harpster, N. K.: Feline cardiomyopathy. Vet. Clin. North Am. 7:355, 1977.

54. Harrison, G. G.: Control of malignant hyperpyrexic syndrome in MHS swine by dantrolene sodium. Br. J. Anesth. 47:62, 1973.

55. Harvey, J. W., Sameck, J. H., and Burgard, F. J.: Benzocaine-induced methemoglobinemia in dogs. J. Am. Vet. Med. Assoc. 175:1171, 1979.

56. Haskins, S. C.: Standards and techniques of equipment utilization. *In* Sattler, F. P., Knowles, R. P., and Whittick, W. G. (eds.): *Veterinary Critical Care.* Lea & Febiger, Philadelphia, 1980, Chap. 3.

57. Haskins, S. C.: Hypothermia and its prevention during general anesthesia in cats. Am. J. Vet. Res. 42:856, 1981.

58. Haskins, S. C.: Cardiopulmonary resuscitation. Comp. Cont. Ed. Vet. 4:170, 1982.

59. Haskins, S. C.: Blood gases and acid-base balance: Clinical interpretation and therapeutic implications. *In* Kirk, R. W. (ed.): *Current Veterinary Therapy VIII.* W. B. Saunders, Philadelphia, 1983, Chap. 3.

60. Haskins, S. C.: Management of pulmonary disease in the critical patient. *In* Zaslow, I. (ed.): *Veterinary Trauma and Critical Care.* Lea & Febiger, Philadelphia, 1983.

61. Haskins, S. C.: The pathophysiology and management of the circulatory collapse states (shock). *In* Kirk, R. W. (ed.): *Current Veterinary Therapy VIII.* W. B. Saunders, Philadelphia, 1983.

62. Henney, R. P., Vasko, J. S., Brawley, R. K., Oldham, H. N., and Morrow, A. G.: The effects of morphine on the resistance and capacitance vessels of the peripheral circulation. Am. Heart J. 72:242, 1966.

63. Heyl, J. T., Gibson, J. G., and Janoway, C. A.: Studies on the plasma proteins. V. The effect of concentrated solutions of human and bovine serum albumin on blood volume after acute blood loss in man. J. Clin. Invest. 22:763, 1943.

64. Hickler, R. B., and Vandam, L. D.: Hypertension. Anesthesiology 33:214, 1970.

65. Hull, C. J.: Electrocution hazards in the operating theatre. Br. J. Anaesth. 50:647, 1978.

66. Hunt, H.: Relationships between the chemical and physiochemical properties of dextran and its pharmacological effects. *In* Derrick, J. R., and Guest, M. M.: *Dextrans.* Charles C Thomas, Springfield, 1971, Chap. 1.

67. Isaacs, H., and Heffron, J. J. A.: Morphological and biochemical defects in muscles of human carriers of the malignant hyperthermia syndrome. Br. J. Anaesth. 47:475, 1975.

68. Johnston, R. R., Eger, E. I., and Wilson, C.: A comparative interaction of epinephrine with enflurane, isoflurane and halothane in man. Anesth. Analg. (Cleve.) 55:709, 1976.

69. Karetzky, M. S., and Khan, A. V.: Review of current concepts in aspiration pneumonia. Heart Lung 6:321, 1977.

70. Kastrup, E. K., and Boyd, J. R.: *Drug Facts and Comparisons.* J. B. Lippincott, Philadelphia, 1982.

71. Katz, R. L., and Bigger, J. T.: Cardiac arrhythmias during anesthesia and operation. Anesthesiology 33:193, 1970.

72. Klide, A. M., Calderwood, H. W., and Soma, L. R.: Cardiopulmonary effects of xylazine in dogs. Am. J. Vet. Res. 36:931, 1975.

73. Kopriva, C. J., Ratliff, J. L., Fletcher, J. R., Fortier, N. L., and Valeic, C. R.: Biochemical and hematological changes associated with massive transfusion of ACD-stored blood in severely injured combat casualties. Ann. Surg. 176:585, 1972.

74. Krum, S. H., and Osborne, C. A.: Heatstroke in the dog: A polysystemic disorder. J. Am. Vet. Med. Assoc. 170:531, 1977.

75. Lambertsen, C. J.: Effects of drugs and hormones on the respiratory response to carbon dioxide. *In* Finn, W. O., and Rahn, H. (eds.): *Handbook of Physiology: Respiration,* Vol. 1. American Physiologic Society, Washington, D.C., 1964.

76. Lamson, P. D., Greig, M. E., and Hobdy, C. J.: Modification of barbiturate anesthesia by glucose, intermediary metabolites and certain other substances. J. Pharmacol. Exp. Ther. 103:460, 1951.

77. Lecky, J. F.: The mechanical aspects of anesthetic pollution control. Anesth. Analg. (Cleve.) 56:769, 1977.

78. Lenaghan, R., Silva, Y. J., and Walt, A. J.: Hemodynamic alterations associated with expansion rupture of the lung. Arch. Surg. 99:339, 1969.

79. Leonard, P. F.: Characteristics of electrical hazards. Anesth. Analg. (Cleve.) 51:797, 1972.

80. Liem, S. T., and Aldrete, J. A.: Control of post-anesthetic shivering. Canad. Anaesth. Soc. J. 21:506, 1974.

81. Lillehei, R. C., Longerbeam, J. K., Block, J. H., and Manax, W. G.: The nature of irreversible shock: Experimental and clinical observations. Ann. Surg. 160:682, 1964.

82. Lowe, H. J., and Ernst, E. A.: *The Quantitative Practice of Anesthesia. Use of Closed Circuit.* Williams & Wilkins, Baltimore, 1981, pp. 194–200.

83. Lumb, W. V., and Jones, E. W.: *Veterinary Anesthesia.* Lea & Febiger, Philadelphia, 1973.

84. MacIntosh, R., Mushin, W. W., and Epstein, H. C.: *Physics for the Anaesthetist,* 3rd ed. Blackwell Scientific Publications, Oxford, 1963; Chap. 20–23.

85. MacKenzie, E. T., Farrar, J. K., Fitch, W., Gradom, D. I., Gregory, P. C., and Harper, A. M.: Effects of hemorrhagic hypotension on the cerebral circulation. Stroke 10:711, 1979.

86. Manley, S. V., and McDonell, W. N.: Recommendations for reduction of anesthetic gas pollution. J. Am. Vet. Med. Assoc. 176:519, 1980.

87. Manley, S. V., Taloff, P., Aberg, N., and Howitt, G. A.: Occupational exposure to waste anesthetic gases in veterinary practice. Calif. Vet. 9:37, 1982.

88. Marshall, B. E., Soma, L. R., Harp, J. R., Neufeld, G. R., and Wurzel, H. A.: Microaggregate formation in stored blood. I. Species differences and storage time; II. Influence of anticoagulants and blood components. Circ. Shock 2:175, 185, 1975.

89. McGrath, C. J., Rempel, W. E., Jessen, C. R., Addis, P. B., and Criml, A. J.: Malignant hyperthermia-triggering liability of selected inhalant anesthetics in swine. Am. J. Vet. Res. 42:604, 1981.

90. Miller, R. D.: Antagonism of neuromuscular blockade. Anesthesiology 41:318, 1976.

91. Miller, R. D.: Neuromuscular blocking agents. *In* Smith, N. T., Miller, R. D., and Corbascio, A. N. (eds.): *During Interactions in Anesthesia.* Lea & Febiger, Philadelphia, 1981, Chap. 18.

92. Miller, W. V. (ed.): *Technical Manual of the American Association of Blood Banks,* 7th ed. American Association of Blood Banks, Washington, D. C., 1977, Chap. 15.

93. Mollison, P. L.: *Blood Transfusion in Clinical Medicine,* 7th ed. Blackwell Scientific Publications, Boston, 1983.

94. Moore, F. P., Dagher, F. J., Boyden, C. M., Lee, C. J., and Lyons, J. H.: Hemorrhage in normal man: I. Distribution and dispersal of saline infusions following acute blood loss. Ann. Surg. 163:485, 1966.

95. Morgan, A. P.: The pulmonary toxicity of oxygen. Anesthesiology 29:570, 1968.

96. Muir, W. W., Werner, L. L., and Hamlin, R. L.: Effects of xylazine and acetylpromazine upon induced ventricular fibrillation in dogs anesthetized with thiamylal and halothane. Am. J. Vet. Res. 36:1299, 1975.

97. Mushin, W. W., Pendell-Baker, L., Thompson, P. W., and Mapleson, W. W.: *Automatic Ventilation of the Lungs,* 2nd ed. F. A. Davis, Philadelphia, 1969.

98. Musselman, E. E.: Arrhythmogenic properties of thiamylal sodium in the dog. J. Am. Vet. Med. Assoc. *168*:145, 1976.

99. Nunn, J. F.: *Applied Respiratory Physiology,* 2nd ed. Butterworths, Boston, 1977.

100. O'Brien, J. A., and Harvey, C. E.: Diseases of the upper airway. *In* Ettinger, S. J. (ed.): *Textbook of Veterinary Internal Medicine,* 2nd ed. W. B. Saunders, Philadelphia, 1983, Chap. 39.

101. Oyama, T.: *Anesthetic Management of Endocrine Diseases.* Springer-Verlag, New York, 1973, Chap. 6.

102. Pace, N. L.: A critique of flow-directed pulmonary arterial catheterization. Anesthesiology *47*:455, 1977.

103. Paine, J. R., Lynn, D., and Keys, A.: Observations on the effects of the prolonged administration of high oxygen concentration to dogs. J. Thorac. Cardiovasc. Surg. *11*:151, 1941.

104. Peters, R. M., and Hargens, A. R.: Protein vs electrolytes and all of the Starling forces. Arch. Surg. *116*:1293, 1981.

105. Popovic, N. A., Mullane, J. F., and Yhap, E. O.: Effects of acetylpromazine maleate on certain cardiorespiratory responses in dogs. Am. J. Vet. Res. *33*:1819, 1972.

106. Pratila, M. G., and Pratilas, V.: Anesthetic agents and cardiac electromechanical activity. Anesthesiology *49*:338, 1978.

107. Prewitt, R. M., McCarthy, J., and Wood, L. D. H.: Treatment of acute low pressure pulmonary edema in dogs. J. Clin. Invest. *67*:409, 1981.

108. Rarey, K. P., and Youtsey, J. W.: *Respiratory Patient Care.* Prentice-Hall, Inc., Englewood Cliffs, NJ, 1981.

109. Refsum, H. E.: Relationship between state of consciousness and arterial hypoxaemia and hypercapnia in patients with pulmolnary insufficiency, breathing air. Clin. Sci. *25*:361, 1963.

110. Rose, R. D.: *Clinical Physiology of Acid-Base and Electrolyte Disorders.* McGraw-Hill, New York, 1977.

111. Ross, J. N.: Heart failure. *In* Ettinger, S. J. (ed.): *Textbook of Veterinary Internal Medicine,* 2nd ed. W. B. Saunders, Philadelphia, 1983, Chap. 46.

112. Ross, J. N., and Breznock, E. M.: Resuscitation. *In* Sattler, F. P., Knowles, R. P., and Whittick, W. G. (eds.): *Veterinary Critical Care.* Lea & Febiger, Philadelphia, 1981, Chap. 19.

113. Sawyer, D. C.: Malignant hyperthermia. J. Am. Vet. Med. Assoc. *179*:341, 1981.

114. Sawyer, D. C.: *The Practice of Small Animal Anesthesia.* W. B. Saunders, Philadelphia, 1982.

115. Schalm, O. W., Jain, N. C., and Carroll, E. J.: *Veterinary Hematology,* 3rd ed. Lea & Febiger, Philadelphia, 1975, p. 605.

116. Schweizer, O., and Howland, W. S.: 2,3 Diphosphoglycerate levels in CPD-preserved bank blood. Anesth. Analg. (Cleve.) *53*:516, 1974.

117. Shatney, C. H., and Lillehei, R. C.: Pathophysiology and treatment of circulatory shock. *In* Zschache, P. A. (ed.): *Mosby's Comprehensive Review of Critical Care,* 2nd ed. C. V. Mosby, St. Louis, 1981, Chap. 41.

118. Shoemaker, W. C.: Pathophysiology and therapy of shock states. *In* Berk, J. L., et al. (eds.): *Handbook of Critical Care.* Little, Brown, Boston, 1976, Chap. 10.

119. Shoemaker, W. C., and Monson, D. O.: The effect of whole blood and plasma expanders on volume-flow relationships in critically ill patients. Surg. Gynecol. Obstet. *137*:453, 1973.

120. Short, C. E., and Paddleford, R. R.: Malignant hyperpyrexia in the dog. Anesthesiology *39*:462, 1973.

121. Siggaard-Andersen, O.: An acid-base chart for arterial blood with normal and pathophysiological reference areas. Scand. J. Clin. Lab. Invest. *27*:239, 1971.

122. Smith, A. L., and Wollman, H.: Cerebral blood flow and metabolism: Effects of anesthetics and drugs, Anesthesiology *36*:378, 1972.

123. Smith, C. W., Lehan, P. H., and Monks, J. J.: Cardiopulmonary manifestations with high oxygen tensions at atmospheric pressure. J. Appl. Physiol. *18*:849, 1963.

124. Smith, R. P., and Olson, M. V.: Drug-induced methemoglobinemia. Semin. Hematol. *10*:253, 1973.

125. Soma, L. R. (ed.): *Textbook of Veterinary Anesthesia.* Williams & Wilkins Co., Baltimore, 1971.

126. Spierdijk, J., Nandorff, A., and von Bijnen, A.: Burns caused by monitoring in anesthesia. Acta Anaesth. Belg. *29*:305, 1978.

127. Stormont, C., and Suzuki, Y.: Canine blood groups. *In* Shifrine, M., and Wilson, F. D. (eds.): *The Canine as a Biomedical Research Model: Immunological, Hematological, and Oncological Aspects.* Technical Information Center, US Department of Energy, Washington, D.C., 1980, pp. 127–133.

128. Sullivan, H. G., Keenan, R. L., Isrow, L., and Feria, W.: The critical importance of $PaCO_2$ during intracranial aneurysm surgery. J. Neurosurg. *52*:426, 1980.

129. Suter, P. M., Fairley, M. B., and Isenberg, M. D.: Optimum end-expiratory airway pressure in patients with acute pulmonary failure. N. Engl. J. Med. *292*:284, 1975.

130. Swenson, M. J. (ed.): *Duke's Physiology of Domestic Animals,* 8th ed. Cornell University Press, Ithaca, 1970.

131. Swift, S., and Carithers, R. W.: Electrical safety for the veterinarian: Macroshock hazards. J. Am. Vet. Med. Assoc. *172*:903, 1978.

132. Takki, S., Aromaa, U., and Kauste, A.: The validity and usefulness of the end-tidal pCO_2 during anaesthesia. Ann. Clin. Res. *4*:278, 1972.

133. Tyson, G. W., and Jane, J. A.: Pathophysiology of head injury. *In* Cowley, R. A., and Trump, B. F. (eds.): *Pathophysiology of Shock, Anoxia and Ischemia.* Williams & Wilkins, Baltimore, 1982.

134. Valeri, C. R.: Blood components in the treatment of acute blood loss: Use of freeze-preserved red cells, platelets and plasma proteins. Anesth. Analg. (Cleve.) *54*:1, 1975.

135. Vallette, H., Hebert, J. L., Raffestin, B., Lockhart, A., and Apoil, E.: Comparison of hemodynamic effects of furosemide and piretanide in normovolemic patients. J. Cardiovasc. Pharmacol. *2*:103, 1980.

136. Vickers, M. P.: Fire and explosion hazards in operating theatres. Br. J. Anaesth. *50*:659, 1978.

137. Votteri, B. A., and Wade, J. F.: Respiratory management. *In* Zschache, D. A. (ed.): *Mosby's Comprehensive Review of Critical Care,* 2nd ed. C. V. Mosby, St. Louis, 1981, Chap. 15.

138. Vyttendaele, K., Brobstein, S., and Srietz, P.: Monitoring instrumentation, isolated inputs, electrosurgery filtering, burns protection: what does it mean? Acta Anaesth. Belg. *29*:317, 1978.

139. Wade, A., and Reynolds, J. E. F.: *Martindale: The Extra Pharmacopoeia,* 27th ed. The Pharmaceutical Press, London, 1977.

140. Warren, J. V., Stead, E. A., Merrill, A. J., and Brannon, E. S.: Chemical, clinical and immunological studies on the products of human plasma fractionation. IX. The treatment of shock with concentrated human serum albumin. J. Clin. Invest. *23*:506, 1944.

141. Wickstrom, P., Ruiz, E., Lilya, G. P., Hinterkopf, J. P., and Haglin, J. J.: Accidental hypothermia; core rewarming with partial bypass. Am. J. Surg. *131*:622, 1976.

142. Winters, W. P., Ferrar-Allado, T., Guzman-Flores, C., and Alcaraz, M.: The cataleptic state induced by ketamine: A review of the neuropharmacology of anesthesia. Neuropharmacology *11*:303, 1972.

143. Wyant, G. M.: *Mechanical Misadventures in Anesthesia.* University of Toronto Press, Toronto, 1978, pp. 47–55.

144. Wylie, W. D., Churchill-Davidson, H. C.: *A Practice of Anaesthesia.* 3rd ed. Year Book Medical Publishers, Chicago 1972, Chap 30.

Chapter 33

Computers in Veterinary Surgery and Surgical Research

Stephen W. Crane and Andrew Wasilewski

INTRODUCTION

Remarkable developments in microelectronic components, microcircuitry design, and peripheral computer hardware have led to the revolution in computer applications in virtually every professional and technical field. Technological progress has caused costs of computer hardware to drop so rapidly that even seemingly trivial applications of computer technology are becoming feasible. Computers are now available for less than $100 that are capable of monitoring and regulating 8 to 32 analog-to-digital and digital-to-analog channels. Reasonably priced and "user friendly" software is another major stimulus for the rapid dispersal of computer hardware and software in the hospital setting.

The purpose of this chapter is to review developing applications of computers in the clinical sciences and practice of surgery.

EARLY HISTORICAL PERSPECTIVE

Because early computers were large and extremely expensive to purchase and operate, their use was limited to government and universities. Input into central processing units was usually through punched cards, paper tape, or other mechanical means, and processing was done in batches. Error correction procedures were complicated and often did not follow system designs. In spite of these difficulties, the collection and statistical analysis of patient variables and other biomedical research data were important and obvious early applications of computer technology. Medical billing, accounts receivable, and insurance claims processing were among the earlier hospital uses for computers.

The early literature regarding computer application in medicine reveals substantial interest in algorithms and programs to automate the diagnostic process.[21,22] Comparisons were made between a computer-assisted diagnosis and the consensus diagnosis of clinicians.

As computer size decreased and efficiency improved, human hospitals began to invest in "mainframe" computers for routine fiscal and management purposes. With the advent of complex, multi-user operating systems and the time-sharing concept, such computers also became available for clinical research. During the late 1960s, many larger hospitals installed labor-saving electronic clinical laboratory processing and reporting systems, automated infection and operative indices, and pharmacy systems utilizing computerized formulary and medication profiles.

The advent of the minicomputer initiated early trials using analog-to-digital conversion of selected physiological data such as temperature and heart rate for patient monitoring purposes. This trend has recently increased in critical care medicine.[17]

RECENT HISTORICAL REVIEW

Comprehensive, specific, and reliable total management systems for managing medical data, records, and fiscal accounting were developed for large human hospitals. MUMPS (Massachusetts General Hospital Utility Multi-Programming System) and COSTAR (COmputer STored Ambulatory Record), an applications system running under MUMPS, are examples of systems that have been embellished and reconfigured by several commercial firms. Similar systems, customized to user need, emerged in the veterinary market in the early 1980s. The pioneer institutional and private practitioners investing in these systems have reported enhanced abilities to control medical and herd health records, inventory, and fiscal records.[19,26,28]

At a lower level of hardware capacity, the advent of the "personal" microcomputer began to have major implications for personal and professional use. Although initially a machine for computer hobbyists, elegant personal computers from reliable vendors coupled with dedicated and powerful software packages are being produced on a nearly monthly basis in the 1980s. Several major applications using the eight-bit z-80 and 6502 central processor units are described in the veterinary literature of the early 1980s.[2-6,10,13,15,24,26] It appears that this inexpensive hardware, coupled with specifically designed products for the professional veterinarian, will be the primary research focus and the major portion of the commercial market.

In order to make the tabletop microcomputer capable of truly useful systems interactions, fast response times, detailed graphics, voice recognition and speech synthesis, and interactive video, three technological developments were needed: larger internal random access memories, significantly greater external storage capacity, and high rates of transfer of digital code between the two. During the early 1980s, small machines were designed to include these technological necessities. Large memory-addressing capability and extensive logic power were made possible by bank switching and the advent of 16- and 32-bit microprocessors. One edition of the latter contains 450,000 transistors on a silicon wafer less than half a centimeter square and can execute one million instruction cycles per second. Rapidly spinning hard discs became economically realistic in the early 1980s and should slowly replace other modes of memory storage such as magnetic tapes and floppy diskettes. A laser-read optically encoded disc can contain hundreds of times more information than a magnetic disc of comparable size and is capable of extremely fast rates of transfer into central processing units. The laser discs are also erasable. Because there is no contact with mechanical devices such as tape heads, wear is virtually nil.

Such technology allows the development of truly "user friendly" and integrated families of software. For example, it is possible to have one system of programs consisting of a word processor, a data base manager, an electronic spread sheet, and graphics and plotting packages. All of these subsystems can read and display data created by the others and can be integrated into a coherent and comprehensive total electronic office and research program.

COMPUTERS IN VETERINARY HOSPITALS

In 1982, the American Veterinary Medical Association reported that 4 per cent of veterinary practices in the United States had computer hardware on the premises and 9 per cent consulted with outside computer services.[28] Practices utilizing computer services were typically larger than average and used the equipment for client demographics, medical records management, accounts receivable tracing, itemized bill generation, mailing list management, inventory control, profitability and resource allocation analyses, and other applications.[27,28]

While there are substantial potential benefits, it is important to appreciate that there are also pitfalls in the adoption of any new technology.[27] These include failure to specifically identify the intended purposes and tasks of the machinery, which may result in selection of inappropriate equipment. In our opinion, the electronic replacement of manual methods of office and practice management will proliferate and withstand the test of time.

Medical-Surgical Records

The management of data within a hospital record system is one major application of computer technology that can directly influence the practice of surgery. All record systems, whether electronic or ink on paper, have in common fragments of information

brought together and filed at a central point.[25] Patient demographics and signalment, final diagnoses, medical-surgical summaries, anesthesia and drug histories including dose and reaction, clinicopathological data, radiographic interpretations, and routine health histories such as infectious disease and heartworm prophylaxis are examples of information conveniently stored in electronic files.[18,28] Maintenance of all of the daily patient progress notes is usually not practical owing to the large memory size required.

With well-designed logic algorithms and efficient programming, an electronic patient data information system can provide substantial improvements in the presentation and availability of the medical record. These improvements largely result from better organization, data integration, validation of input, and security of storage.[18,19,25] For example, an occasional problem of the medical record library is the "lost chart." This situation is largely eliminated by using electronic record storage supplemented with appropriate computer back-up files. The structure and organization of the medical record that results from coherent systems of "menu-driven" data entry tend to minimize differences between clinicians in documentation. Enhanced uniformity within the medical record library is also established in the way information is coded and formatted.[25]

COMPUTERS IN SURGERY

Computer technology will play an increasing role in veterinary surgery during the 1980s. Programs assisting in diagnosis, providing guidance for developing therapeutic options, allowing interactive and convenient continuing educational opportunities, assisting in primary surgical instruction, and allowing data management applications in veterinary surgical research are currently available and will develop rapidly.[1,4,12,13,17–24,26]

Microprocessor-controlled monitoring equipment is widely available in human surgical and critical care units and provides sophisticated monitoring capabilities for nearly every imaginable application.[5,8,9,11,17,20] The large-scale acceptance and adoption of these devices in veterinary surgery will be influenced, to some degree, by factors of cost justification, reliability, and user acceptance.

Computer-Assisted Diagnosis and Patient Management

Diagnostic acumen results from an ability to construct differential diagnostic possibilities from one or more clinical signs. This process is maximized when clinical experiences and observational skills complement an extensive mental data base that can prepare an association matrix of clinical signs with all diagnostic possibilities. The use of "free form" thought provides, of course, variable degrees of effectiveness and efficiency in solving diagnostic problems. The problem-oriented medical record has been one popular method of providing increased focus for the mental deliberations involving a particular problem or set of problems.

Higher level processes include automated analysis of the matrix considering all diagnostic possibilities from the signs presented.[21] Differential "rule-outs" are constructed from the association matrix, and the remainder of nonexcluded items constitute the differential diagnosis. Other systems might have logic branches based, conditionally, on certain findings and observations. At this point, the program might suggest certain other tests or procedures that could make the diagnostic discrimination more absolute. A probability of diagnostic correctness can also be prepared based on the presence or absence of pathognomonic signs or the clustering of typical elements of syndromes. These general schemes, and several modifications, have been used as aids in computer-assisted diagnosis.[21–24,26] Currently, many computer-assisted diagnostic programs are available in both human and veterinary medicine and are most applicable in multifaceted or complex clinical situations. Some examples include analysis of dermatoses and endocrinopathies and the radiographic interpretation of bone lesions.[7,22] When using computerized diagnostic aids it must be remembered that machines do not have observational ability, clinical experience, or "common sense." These negative features of an inanimate technology are partially offset by the advantages of rapid data processing, extensive memory, and extremely high levels of repeatability and reliability.[17,20]

As machines become more efficient and rapid data base access becomes more common, it will be possible for local systems to automatically acquire the latest references and abstracts from national and international bibliographic services related to the differential diagnostic list being promulgated. Such automated services would be an important improvement in computer-assisted diagnosis and a major link in the chain of total information management in the clinical setting.

Computer-assisted case management is a logical extension of the diagnostic process and is available in some critical care units of large human hospitals.[8,11,12,17] Totally computerized diagnosis has been a strongly sought but elusive goal of physicians and computer scientists for many years. As machines with true artificial intelligence emerge in the 1990s, the computational and "reasoning" power for making the myriad of judgments requisite in a totally automated medical diagnostic process may be at hand.

Computer-Assisted Diagnostic Instrumentation

Enhancement and averaging of electrophysiological signals from electroencephalography, electroretinog-raphy, and evoked potentials studies are important microprocessor applications.[2,6,17,22] Radiographic, digital fluoroscopic, axial tomographic, and thermal and ultrasonic image enhancement by computers are outstanding applications of computers in the diagnostic process.[5]

Computers in the Operating Room and Critical Care Unit

Continuous and automated physiological monitoring of certain postsurgical patients in the recovery room and critical care ward is well-established in human surgery.[22] Electrophysiological signal acquisition and interpretation provide automated monitoring assistance and an extra degree of the "watchful eye."[8,17,20] A variety of semiconductor-based and microprocessor-compatible transducers and sensors can be attached to or inserted in the patient to measure departures from homeostatic or other preprogrammed limits and to signal the human caretaker when such events occur. For example, computerized signal processing from electrocardiographic monitors is especially prevalent and detects cardiac rate and rhythm changes.[13,17,18,20] Transcutaneous oxygen electrodes and temperature thermistors provide indirect information regarding the flow state of the peripheral circulation.[20] Intravascular devices such as chemical sensors can provide frequent and accurate electrolyte monitoring without repeated venipuncture.[9] Machine-readable pressure and flow-tipped catheters are also important critical care monitoring tools. Depending on their placement, such instruments continuously provide valuable information regarding cardiopulmonary status, pulmonary function, and the resistance status of the peripheral circulation.[22] Microprocessor-controlled counters, servocontrolled drug and fluid infusion pumps, gas and fluid pressure regulators, weighing tools, and image enhancement devices are among other equipment used in the critical care setting.

Statistical "trending" programs for patient status are important predictive tools in the critical care and postoperative environments.[20,22] Such data management systems accumulate and group large banks of physiological and clinical data from similar general categories of patients. Computation of predictive inferences are made when departures from group averages occur. Multivariate regression analysis, pattern recognition techniques, and Bayesian statistical methods are employed in these predictions.[22]

Programmable hand-held calculators are other useful tools in clinical care. Calculators are easily used to figure the variables surrounding nutritional requirements in total parenteral nutrition, in automating the computation of blood gas and electrolyte balance data, and in calculating drug dosages when administration is based on metabolic size or body surface area.[11]

Although "smart" instrumentation offers considerable theoretical advantages, care must be taken that techniques and methods intended to save labor and promote patient safety do not have the opposite effect.[27] In fact, there is skepticism that such methods do not enhance patient care but only enhance the collection of data. If true, certain interesting medical and ethical paradoxes suggest themselves.[8]

Computers in Operative Surgery

Several advanced applications of computer technology are currently or futuristically available in operative surgery beyond patient monitoring. For example, microprocessor control of the microscopically focused and delivered infrared cutting beam of the carbon dioxide laser is available.* A constant sweep speed of the laser beam over a preprogrammed area makes uniform the energy density delivered to target tissue. The surgeon, working through the operating microscope, first outlines the perimeter of the intended field of treatment with a light beam manipulated by a joystick. The X and Y coordinates for the intended surgical surface area are digitized and stored in memory as the lesion is circumscribed. Microprocessor control of motorized mirrors then actively reflects and controls the laser beam onto the target. The Z axis, and thus depth and volume, of tissue vaporization and ablation is under the control of the surgeon, who determines the number of repetitions of the cycle.

COMPUTER APPLICATION IN VETERINARY SURGICAL RESEARCH

Computer management of information such as demographic and epidemiological data files is already a widely accepted and common element of veterinary surgical research.[14,15,18] The acquisition and reduction of laboratory data are most powerful uses of computer technology. Such data may be collected from equipment, including laboratory and patient monitoring devices, that provides any analog measurement.[3] The use of telemetry data in medical diagnosis and research will increase, and such data may be collected continuously from an animal subject or on demand from data storage cells. Observations from almost any conceivable type of biomedical research project can be digitized, catalogued, analyzed, manipulated, stored, graphically displayed in multiple forms, reproduced, and transmitted from electronic files.

One data analysis tool and organizer is the electronic "spread sheet." Once the data variables within the observational groups have been ordered into ranks and files, running summations between and within data sets are constantly available and markedly save time usually spent with a pencil and calculator. Such programs also allow the user to propose "What

if" questions regarding the projected effect of alterations in the data. The predictive extrapolations available with this simple method can facilitate experimental design and save research labor and money. It may also be possible to reduce the numbers of animals in experimental groups using such information. Multidimensional statistical testing of research observations is routinely accomplished with the aid of analysis programs available at reasonable cost for even small computers.

Modelling and simulation are other powerful applications of computer technology, which is moving rapidly from the engineering stage to the medical laboratory. Analysis, prediction, and graphic display of physical data such as force vectorgrams, joint motion, and stress and strain and other bioengineering measurements in clinical orthopedics, experimental kinesiology, and orthosis research are available. Modelling of cell and tissue morphometrics and three-dimensional mapping of normal anatomy and tumors are other potentially useful techniques. A wide variety of biochemical, physiological, pharmacological, and microbiological reactions, responses, compartmental dynamics, and systems functions may also be statistically described, experimentally projected, graphically depicted, and otherwise changed through computerized simulations.[22]

Management of bibliographical and other files of resource information is also an important aid to research. Extensive networks of information searching and sharing, such as *Medline*, are well developed and literally indispensable in literature searching. Recently, two national information services have developed low-cost access to major information search services available to users of personal microcomputers. *Knowledge Index*, from the Dialog Information Retrieval Service, and *Bibliographic Retrieval Services/After Dark* are early entrants into the information market.

1. Booth, F.: Patient monitoring and data processing in the ICU. Crit. Care Med. *11*:57, 1983.
2. Bowen, J. M.: Applications for computers in electromyography. In *Symposium on Computer Applications in Veterinary Medicine*. Mississippi State University, 1982, pp. 733–741.
3. Branch, C. E., and Marple, D. N.: Use of inexpensive personal computers with laboratory equipment. In *Symposium on Computer Applications in Veterinary Medicine*. Mississippi State University, 1982, pp. 415–427.
4. Branch, C. E., and Smith, E. P.: Interactive video. Newsletter, Am. Vet. Comp. Soc. 2:4, 1983.
5. Budinger, T. F.: Image analysis in critical care medicine. Crit. Care Med. *10*:835, 1982.
6. Cartledge, R. M.: Computer processing of the electroencephalogram in Veterinary Medicine. In *Symposium on Computer Applications in Veterinary Medicine*. Mississippi State University, 1982, pp. 743–755.
7. Denovellis, R., and Conroy, J. D.: Canine dermatology: A computerized approach to diagnosis. In *Symposium on Computer Applications in Veterinary Medicine*. Mississippi State University, 1982, pp. 815–852.
8. Eberhart, R. C.: Changing perspectives in critical care computing. Crit. Care Med. *10*:805, 1982.
9. Eberhart, R. C., et al.: Indwelling chemical sensors based on semiconductor technology. Crit. Care Med. *10*:841, 1982.

---

*Advanced Surgical Technology Inc., Schaumburg, IL.

10. Eicker, S. W.: Mark sense medical data collection. *In Symposium on Computer Applications in Veterinary Medicine.* Mississippi State University, 1982, pp. 593–600.

11. Edwards, F. H.: Computer-assisted planning of parenteral hyperalimentation therapy. Crit. Care Med. *10*:539, 1982.

12. Gardner, R. M., et. al.: Computer-based ICU data acquisition as an aid to clinical decision making. Crit. Care Med. *10*:823, 1982.

13. Hahn, A. W., et al.: Computer-assisted monitoring and record keeping in a veterinary intensive care unit. *In Symposium on Computer Applications in Veterinary Medicine.* Mississippi State University, 1982, pp. 803–813.

14. Hasman, A., and Chang, S. C.: A data storage and retrieval system for clinical research. Comp. Biomed. Res. *15*:145, 1982.

15. Janssen, D. L., and Bush, M.: The microcomputer as an aid to medical records management in a zoological park. J. Am. Vet. Med. Assoc. *181*:1381, 1982.

16. Kasvand, T., et al.: Computers and the kinesiology of gait. Comp. Biol. Med. *6*:111, 1976.

17. Osborn, J. J.: Computers in critical care medicine: Promises and pitfalls. Crit. Care Med. *10*:807, 1982.

18. Physick-Sheard, P. W.: An interactive program for on-line entry, retrieval and searching of veterinary clinical patient data: A retrospective view. *In Symposium on Computer Applications in Veterinary Medicine.* Mississippi State University, 1982, pp. 601–611.

19. Pollock, R. V. H., and Lewkowicz, J. M.: Provides: A knowledge coupler system for veterinary medicine. *In Symposium on Computer Applications in Veterinary Medicine.* Mississippi State University, 1982, pp. 315–322.

20. Prakash, O. M., et al.: Computer-based patient monitoring. Crit. Care Med. *10*:811, 1982.

21. Schoolman, H. M., and Bernstein, L. M.: Computer use in diagnosis, prognosis and therapy. Science *200*:926, 1978.

22. Siegel, J. H.: Computers and mathematical techniques in surgery. *In* Sabiston, D. C. (ed.): Davis-Christopher *Textbook of Surgery: The Biological Basis of Modern Surgical Practice.* W. B. Saunders, Philadelphia, 1981, pp. 223–249.

23. Szolovitx, P., and Pauker, S. G.: Categorical and probablistic reasoning in medical diagnosis. Artif. Intell. *11*:115, 1978.

24. Trynda, R. S.: The role of computer-assisted instruction in a veterinary medical curriculum: An overview. J. Vet. Med. Ed. *6*:113, 1979.

25. White, M. E.: A coding scheme for veterinary clinical signs. Cornell Vet. *70*:160, 1980.

26. White, M. E.: Computer-assisted differential diagnosis in veterinary medicine. *In Symposium on Computer Applications in Veterinary Medicine.* Mississippi State University, 1982, pp. 711–720.

27. Wise, J. K.: Acquiring a computer system. J. Am. Vet. Med. Assoc. *180*:1484, 1982.

28. Wise, J. K.: Market report on veterinary practice computers. J. Am. Vet. Med. Assoc. *181*:608, 1982.

Skin and Adnexa

Michael M. Pavletic
Section Editor

Chapter 34

The Integument

Michael M. Pavletic

FUNCTIONS OF THE SKIN

The skin (integument) is one of the largest body organs and contains a variety of glands, nerves, vessels, and muscles.[12] The integument of the puppy is 24 per cent of its body weight but only 12 per cent of that of an adult dog.[1] Functionally, the integument serves as the body's first line of defense against microorganisms.[6] The outer horny layer, the stratum corneum, provides protection against desiccation and hydration.[23, 38] The skin produces vitamin D and serves as a reservoir for electrolytes, water, fat, carbohydrates, and protein.[16, 38] The total cutaneous circulation has a considerable volume and can affect blood pressure.[16, 23] The skin is a sensory receptor for touch, pressure, vibration, heat, cold, and pain.[1, 23] The skin and its overlying haircoat provide a barrier against chemicals and radiation and, in combination with subcutaneous fat, provide a cushion against mechanical trauma as well as insulation against heat and cold.[1, 6, 12, 23, 38] Because no wound is healed until its epithelial, endothelial, and mesothelial surfaces are covered,[33] a basic review of the anatomy of the integument is essential if the veterinary surgeon is to manage diseases and injuries to the skin with consistent success.

SKIN STRUCTURE

The skin is composed of an outer stratified epithelium (epidermis) and an underlying fibrous dermis (corium). The epidermis is derived from embryonic ectoderm, whereas the dermis has a mesenchymal origin (Fig. 34–1).[3, 10]

Epidermis

The epidermis originates as a single layer of cuboidal ectodermal cells that become increasingly stratified and specialized as the fetus matures.[3] The epidermis of hairy skin consists of three major layers: the stratum cylindricum (stratum basale), the stratum

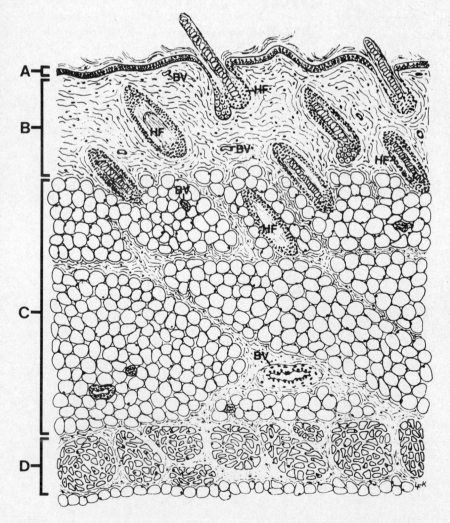

Figure 34–1. Structure of the skin from the lateral thorax of the dog. *A,* Epidermis; *B,* dermis; *C,* hypodermis; *D,* cutaneous trunci muscle. Beneath the dermis is a looser connective tissue layer called the hypodermis *(C).* The hypodermis is transformed into subcutaneous adipose tissue, forming a layer called panniculus adiposus. It is continuous with the deep fascia, which joins the cutaneous trunci muscle layer. The blood vessels (BV) are present in three layers represented in cross sections: subcutaneous or subdermal plexus, cutaneous plexus, and subpapillary plexus layer. The subpapillary plexus is composed of small capillaries that nourish the epidermis. Hair follicles (HF) are present at different depths in the dermis and in the upper part of the hypodermis. The amount of subcutaneous fat between the dermis and panniculus muscle layer is variable. (Diagram courtesy of F. Al-Bagdadi, Louisiana State University, School of Veterinary Medicine, Baton Rouge, LA.)

spinosum (stratum malpighii, prickle cell layer), and the stratum corneum.[10, 21] The stratum cylindricum and stratum spinosum are collectively termed the *stratum germinativum*. Mitotic activity in both layers is responsible for proliferation of the epidermal cells.[10] Melanocytes derived from the neural crest of the embryo are located among the cells of the stratum cylindricum and the lower layers of the stratum spinosum.[12] In a few areas of the hairy skin, the stratum granulosum and stratum lucidum are evident, but only where keratinization is retarded, such as around the hair follicle orifices. These two layers are well developed in the footpads but are absent in the other major specialized skin area, the planum nasale.[1] Epidermal pegging, which is evident in the footpads, planum nasale, and lip of the dog, is not evident in the hairy skin.[21] Rather, the dermal-epidermal junction of hairy skin is thrown into folds that parallel the contour of the skin surface.[21] Small tactile elevations (0.33- to 0.35-mm dome-shaped enlargements) termed *epidermal papillae* are noted over hairy skin surfaces of the dog and cat.[1, 21, 36] As a rule, the epidermis is thicker in areas that lack a thick haircoat and thinner in regions with a dense hair growth.[12, 38] The thickest epidermis occurs on the nose and digital pads.[1]

Dermis (Corium)

The dermis consists of collagenous, reticular (precollagen), and elastic fibers surrounded by a mucopolysaccharide ground substance. This ground substance, composed of hyaluronic acid and chondroitin sulfuric acid, is the major component of the dermis.[37] Ninety per cent of the dermal fibers are composed of collagen.[23] Fibroblasts, macrophages, plasma cells, and mast cells are present throughout the dermis but are more numerous in the superficial layer of the dermis.[10, 12] Chromatophores and fat cells are also seen on occasion.[12] The dermis contains the cutaneous capillary network, lymphatics, nerve components, and arrector pili muscles as well as ectodermally derived hair follicles and glandular structures.[10, 12, 21, 26, 39]

The dermis of the dog and cat is divided into two indistinct layers, the superficial stratum papillare and the deep stratum reticulare.[1, 10, 12, 25, 39] The stratum papillare consists of fine, densely interwoven collagenous bundles with fine elastic and reticular fibers. Reticular fibers condense along with a viscous ground substance to form the basement membrane, to which the stratum cylindricum attaches with cytoplasmic processes.[10] The stratum reticulare is composed of densely interwoven collagen bundles of a coarser nature with fewer cellular elements.[10, 12] Elastic fibers are more numerous in the reticular layer.[10, 39]

The most pliable skin regions (axilla, flank, dorsum of the neck) have smaller and more loosely woven collagen bundles in the dermis. Elastic fibers in these areas are more numerous in the papillary layer, unlike other regions of hairy skin. Elastic fibers in the inguinal region are larger than those in the superficial dermal layer. Areas where the skin is least mobile (tail, ear, digital pads) have wider, more closely packed collagen bundles with fewer elastic fibers. Collagenous fibers are roughly parallel to the skin surface in areas of thick skin (head, dorsal body surfaces).[39]

Collagen bundles in feline skin are generally coarser and denser, and the arrector pili muscles are larger than those in canine skin.[10] The stratum papillare of feline skin contains fine, more uniform collagenous fibers, which usually parallel the epidermis compared with the reticular layer. The stratum reticulare contains dense, irregularly arranged collagenous fibers three times larger than those of the papillary layer. Collagen bundles are smaller and more loosely arranged in the most flexible cutaneous areas of the cat (dorsal neck, scapular region, lateral upper forelimb, and so on).[36]

The thickness of the skin is directly related to the thickness of the dermal layer and varies according to body area, sex, breed, and species.[12] Thick skin has a dermis greater than 1 mm in thickness, whereas thin skin has a dermal thickness less than 1 mm.[39] The thickest skin of the dog and cat is located over the head, dorsum of the neck, back, and sacrum. The thinnest skin is located along the ventral body surface, the medial surface of the limbs, and the inner pinna.[12, 36, 39] I have noticed a similar distribution in the dog.

APPENDAGES OF THE SKIN

The appendages, or adnexa, of hairy skin include the hair follicles, sweat glands, and sebaceous glands, all of which are of ectodermal origin. During embryonal development, these epidermal structures extend down into the dermis and subcutaneous tissue, the epithelium of which is continuous with the epidermis (Fig. 34–2).[3, 10, 12] Other glands of ectodermal origin are the mammary glands, supracaudal (tail) gland, anal sacs, superficial circumanal glands, and perianal (deep circumanal) glands.[1, 3, 37]

Hair

The basic unit of hair production is the hair follicle. The wall of the hair follicle is continuous with the epidermis and is divided into inner and outer root sheaths.[1] During fetal development hair follicles originate from clusters of germinative cells in the epidermis. These cells sink into the dermis, forming a cylindrical epidermal peg, the base of which develops into the hair bulb, which molds around a mesenchymal papilla. These germinative cells eventually give rise to the inner epithelial root sheath and the hair shaft. Epidermal cells encircling the shaft become the outer epithelial root sheath,[3, 37] which is a contin-

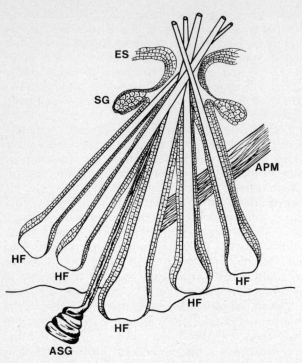

Figure 34–2. A compound hair follicle (HF) with its associated structures, the sebaceous gland (SG), apocrine sweat gland (ASG), and arrector pili muscle (APM). Note the epidermal cellular components of these cutaneous adnexa, which are continuous with the epidermal surface (ES).

uation of the stratum cylindricum (basale) (see Fig. 34–2). Hair follicles are located in the lower portions of the dermis and also extend into the subcutaneous tissue. Sebaceous glands develop as extensions of the outer root sheath at the upper part of the follicle.[3, 10, 21, 26, 37] An apocrine sweat gland develops with each hair follicle in the dog and cat and extends into the hypodermis. The duct empties into the common portion of the follicle complex between the skin surface and sebaceous gland orifice.[1, 21, 26, 36] Mesenchymal tissue adjacent to the developing hair follicles forms the arrector pili muscles.[1, 3, 21] These muscles originate in the dermal papillary layer and insert in the connective tissue of the hair follicle.[1, 12, 21] They are anchored by elastic fibers at their attachments and are innervated by the autonomic nervous system. The arrector muscles are especially well developed along the back of the dog, causing the hair to bristle upon their contraction.[12]

At birth, hair follicles in the dog develop from a simple follicle containing a single hair to a compound follicle containing seven to ten hairs emerging from a common follicle orifice at 28 weeks of age as a result of accessory buds arising from the original follicle.[21] Sebaceous glands also become compound, emptying where the hairs are contained as a single tubular follicle.[21] The compound follicle contains a main or guard hair surrounded by a number of finer, woolly lanugo, or underhairs. Although the hair shafts share the same external follicular orifice at the epidermal surface, they branch into their own respective hair

follicles below the level of the sebaceous glands. The guard hair follicle is larger and penetrates into the subcutaneous tissue (see Fig. 34–2). As a rule, compound follicles occur in clusters of three, with the center follicle slightly larger than the other two.[12, 32]

In cats, hairs are arranged in clusters of two, three, four, and five, grouped around a central guard hair. Clusters of two and three are more common on the dorsal aspect of the feline body, whereas clusters of four and five usually occur on the ventral body and lower extremities.[36] Each lateral group contains 3 primary hairs surrounded by 6 to 12 lanugo hairs.[36] Three to 15 hairs are noted in each compound follicle of the adult dog,[21] whereas 12 to 20 hairs are present in each compound follicle of the cat.[1, 36] Growth patterns, length, and type of hair vary among individuals, breeds, and species.

Siamese cats have a temperature-dependent coat color owing to an enzyme that converts melanin precursors to melanin at lower temperatures.[37] As a result, haircoats grow back darker after clipping, a fact best explained to the owner prior to a surgical procedure.

Hair growth rates vary seasonally among breeds. Hair growth in male beagles has been noted to be 0.4 mm/day in the winter and 0.34 mm/day in the summer, whereas greyhounds have a growth rate of 0.18 mm/day in the fall and 0.04 mm/day in the summer.[1] Hair growth is more rapid in the winter. As a rule, short canine haircoats take approximately 130 days to regrow. However, as long as 18 months is required for regrowth of the haircoat in long-haired breeds such as the Afghan.[37] These facts must be taken into account prior to clipping a dog.

Several characteristics of the haircoat in dogs and cats vary with the location on the body. The haircoat is usually thicker over the back and sides of the body, whereas the hair inside the ears and on the flanks, ventral abdomen, and underside of the tail is thinner.[37] Cosmetic wound closure should account for variations in growth patterns and direction of growth of the coat. However, when attempting to close major skin defects, hair growth usually plays a secondary role in choosing the method of closure. The veterinary surgeon and owner must consider the safest, simplest, and most economical method to effectively restore function to the affected area. In my experience, mild variations of hair growth after closure are not a major deterrent to the owner.

Glandular Structures of the Skin

The major cutaneous glands include the sebaceous glands, sweat glands, supracaudal (tail) glands, anal sacs, circumanal glands, and mammary glands. Like the hair follicles, these glands are ectodermally derived by downgrowth of epidermal cells into the dermis during embryonic development.[3, 12, 26]

Sebaceous glands most frequently originate from the external root sheath (see Fig. 34–2). The oily secretion produced exits through the pilosebaceous canal to keep the skin and hair soft and pliable and to protect them from excessive moisture and drying.[37] Sebaceous glands are best developed over the neck, back, and tail of the dog, particularly in the tail gland area.[1, 12] Sebaceous glands unassociated with hair follicles include the meibomian, or tarsal, glands of the eyelids and glands of the labia, vulva, anus, prepuce, glans penis, and external ear canal. These holocrine glands empty directly onto the epithelial surface.[1, 37] The sebaceous gland complex associated with the hair follicles of the cat is smaller and simpler in structure compared with that of the dog. Larger sebaceous glands are found in association with the hair follicles of the upper jaw, prepuce, and dorsal tail surface.[10]

Circumanal glands (superficial sebaceous glands) and perianal glands (deep sebaceous glands) are modified sebaceous glands located at the mucocutaneous junction of the anus. Circumanal glands have a well-defined duct, whereas perianal glands have a solid duct with no secretory activity.[1, 37] Circumanal glands contain fat, whereas the deeper perianal glands do not. Perianal gland cells are filled with proteinaceous cytoplasmic granules.[12] Perianal glandular tissue can also be found in the skin of the prepuce and groin.[26]

The mammary glands of the skin are compound tubulo-alveolar apocrine glands resembling sweat glands in their mode of development. They remain rudimentary in the male but undergo conspicuous changes during pregnancy and during and after lactation in the female.[9, 12]

Anal sacs contain both sebaceous and apocrine sweat glands and have a thin, stratified squamous epithelial lining.[1, 6, 12] Sebaceous glands tend to line the neck of the sac, whereas the apocrine glands are concentrated in the fundus.[1]

Sweat (sudoriferous) glands are apocrine and merocrine (eccrine) in nature.[12] Apocrine sweat glands of the skin are large, simple, saccular or tubular structures with a coiled secretory portion and a straight duct. The glands may be tortuous or serpentine.[12] The apocrine sweat gland duct opens at the external root sheath between the skin surface and pilosebaceous canal (see Fig. 34–2).[1, 12] Merocrine glands also are coiled, simple, tubular glands found mainly in the footpads of the dog and empty directly onto the epidermal surface.[1, 12] Sweat glands are better developed in the long, fine-haired dog breeds.[39]

Sweat glands in the hairy skin of dogs and cats do not participate actively in the central themoregulatory mechanism but protect the skin from an excessive rise in temperature.[2] This is in contrast to human beings, in whom the cutaneous sweat glands are vital for vaporizational heat loss to cool the body at high temperatures.

Dogs pant at 26 to 30°C. The heat lost by water vaporization from the respiratory passages helps maintain the dog's normal body temperature.[23] In a similar environment, cats produce copious watery saliva secondary to sympathetic stimulation of the submaxillary salivary gland. As the cat spreads this saliva over the coat by licking, vaporizational heat loss occurs.

Areas of the body that have apocrine glands of specialized structure and function include Moll's glands of the eyelids, the ceruminous glands of the external ear canal, the anal sac, and the glands of the prepuce, vulva, and circumanal region.

SURGICAL CONSIDERATIONS

Partial-thickness skin losses, in which the epidermis and a variable portion of the dermis are tangentially removed or destroyed, often heal by adnexal re-epithelialization (Fig. 34–3). As previously noted, the hair follicles, apocrine sweat glands, and sebaceous glands have a common ectodermal origin. The epithelial components of these adnexa may remain viable and serve as a source of epithelial cells to resurface the raw dermal surface (Fig. 34–4). This is in contrast to full-thickness skin losses, which rely on wound contraction and epithelialization from the viable bordering skin.[19, 32]

These glands have increased secretory function during inflammatory processes, especially where large numbers of these glands are assembled. This usually necessitates more frequent bandage changes

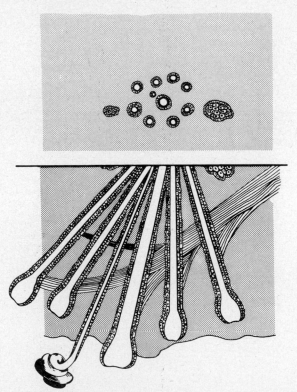

Figure 34–3. A partial-thickness skin loss resulting in removal of the epidermis and a superficial portion of the dermis. Note the epidermal components of the hair follicles and associated glands on the exposed dermal surface (top view).

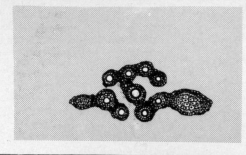

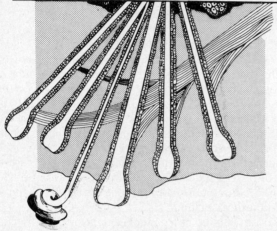

Figure 34–4. Adnexal epithelialization of the dermal surface. Note the proliferation and migration of epithelial cells over the wound surface to restore epithelial integrity to the area.

and gentle wound cleansing to prevent the development of a moist environment, which could promote infection.[37]

THE HYPODERMIS (SUBCUTIS)

The hypodermis is composed primarily of fat with loose collagenous trabeculae and elastic fibers (see Fig. 34–1).[12, 23, 25, 37] It varies in thickness in various regions of the body, being poorly developed beneath the eyelids, ears, and scrotum, and other areas where the skin is closely attached to underlying structures.[37]

The inherent elasticity of the skin; its lack of firm attachments to bone, muscle, and fascia; and the length and extensibility of the direct cutaneous vessels account for the high degree of mobility of skin over the head, neck, and trunk of the dog and cat. In one histological study, two distinct layers of the hypodermis were reported: the stratum adiposum subcutis (containing fat), and a deeper stratum fibrosum subcutis, which includes the panniculus carnosus (panniculus muscle).[25]

Although the hypodermis is not a part of the skin, it is closely associated with skin function. Direct cutaneous vessels must traverse this layer to supply the overlying skin. In this respect, the panniculus muscle plays a valuable role during surgical undermining and manipulation of the skin.[30]

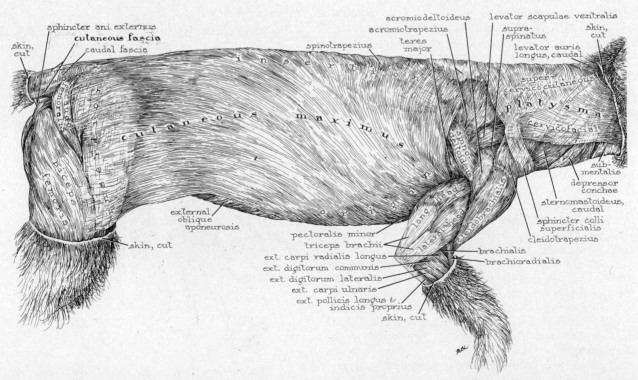

Figure 34–5. Cutaneous muscles in the cat. Note the broad cutaneous trunci muscle (cutaneous maximus) and the platysma muscle in the cervical and facial areas. The dog has a similar distribution of panniculus muscles. (Reprinted with permission from Crouch, J. E., and Lackey, M. B.: *Text-Atlas of Cat Anatomy.* Lea & Febiger, Philadelphia, 1969.)

Panniculus Muscle

The *panniculus muscle* (panniculus carnosus) is a term used to describe a collection of thin cutaneous muscles that occur in the hypodermis in the dog and cat. The panniculus muscles in the head and neck regions are the platysma, sphincter colli superficialis, and sphincter colli profundus. The cutaneous trunci is the major cutaneous muscle of the body, extending from the gluteal region cranial and ventral to the pectoral region (see Fig. 34–1).[1] Fibers from this muscle make up the preputialis muscle in the male dog and the supramammarius muscle in the female dog.[1]

The cat has a similar cutaneous muscle distribution. The cutaneous trunci (cutaneous maximus) of the cat extends over the thoracic and abdominal regions of the body (Fig. 34–5).[11] The platysma in the cat covers the head and neck. In the cervical region, the platysma can be subdivided into the supercervicocutaneous muscle and cervicofacial muscle along a line of attachment to the skin. The associated sphincter colli superficialis muscle is smaller and of irregular occurrence (Figs. 34–6 and 34–7).[11] Light microscopic studies indicate that the feline panniculus muscle is a component of the stratum fibrosum subcutis, the deep connective tissue layer of the hypodermis.[25] Panniculus muscle fibers are very irregular, tend to run transversely, and penetrate the dermis and allow voluntary movement of the skin.[12] The cutaneous trunci is used to shake the skin in response to irritating or noxious stimuli.[1, 13] Repeated contraction (shivering) of this muscle can increase heat production in cold animals.[1] The platysma muscle moves the vibrissae and gives expression to the face.[6, 13] The preputial muscle in dogs draws the prepuce over the glans penis after erection, whereas the supramammary muscle aids in the support of the mammary glands and perhaps in milk ejection in the bitch.[13]

The cutaneous trunci originates caudally in the gluteal region in the dog and cat and terminates in the axilla and caudal border of the deep pectoral muscle.[13] It is not present beneath the skin over the middle and lower portions of the limbs.[13, 31] The panniculus muscle is closely associated with the cutaneous circulation, and its preservation is vital to the survival of the skin during surgical manipulation (Fig. 34–8).[29, 31]

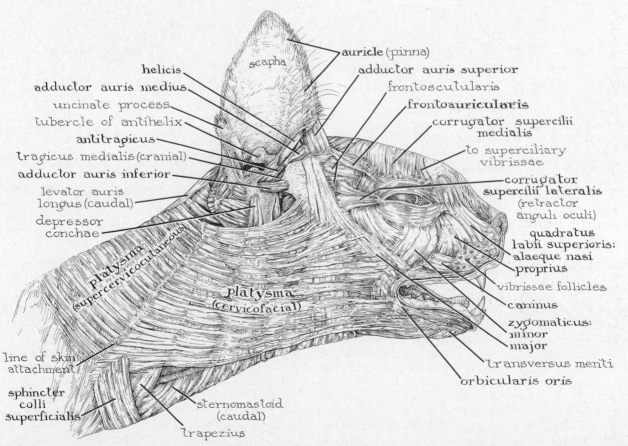

Figure 34–6. Superficial muscles of the head and face in the cat, lateral aspect. Note the distribution of the platysma muscle. (Reprinted with permission from Crouch, J. E., and Lackey, M. B.: *Text-Atlas of Cat Anatomy.* Lea & Febiger, Philadelphia, 1969.)

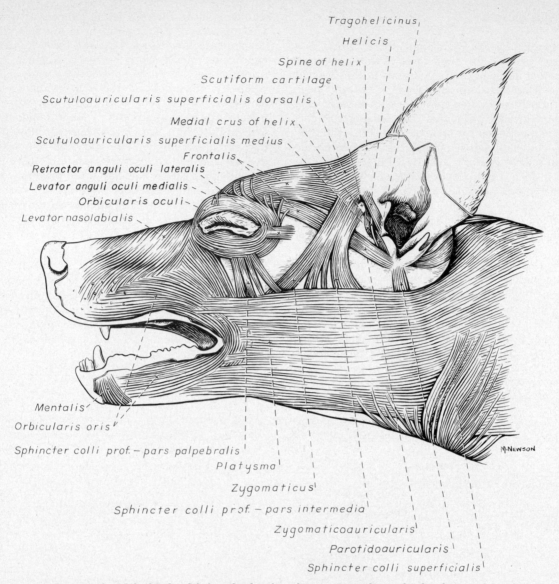

Figure 34–7. Superficial muscles of the head and face in the dog, lateral aspect. Note the similar distribution of the platysma muscle in the cat. (Reprinted with permission from Evans, N. E., and Christensen, G. C.: *Miller's Anatomy of the Dog.* W. B. Saunders, Philadelphia, 1979.)

VASCULAR SUPPLY TO THE SKIN

Capillary networks in all body regions of vertebrates develop from "blood islands" in the splanchnic mesoderm of the embryo. As these islands hollow out, peripheral cells form the vascular endothelium, whereas centrally located cells form the earliest blood cells. A primitive blood plasma forms, apparently from the cells of the blood islands. As the fetus develops, these separate vascular spaces join to form vascular plexuses. Proliferative growth of the endothelium links the simple vascular spaces into continuous channels. New vessels subsequently arise as outgrowths of pre-existing vessels once the primitive system of closed vessels is established. Definitive arteries and veins arise through the selection, enlargement, and differentiation of appropriate paths in

these networks by inherited patterns and hemodynamic factors.[3]

The cutaneous vascular system is divided into three interconnected levels: (1) the deep, subdermal, or subcutaneous plexus, (2) the middle, or cutaneous, plexus, and (3) the superficial, or subpapillary, plexus (see Fig. 34–8). This general vascular arrangement is present in the hairy skin, but variations in the arrangement are noted in the canine external ear, footpad, nipple, and the mucocutaneous junctions of the nostril, lip, eyelid, prepuce, vulva, and anus.[18, 29]

The subdermal plexus is the major vascular network to the overlying skin. The vessels of this plexus generally run in the subcutaneous fatty and areolar tissue on the deep face of the dermis of the middle to distal portions of the limbs where no panniculus muscle is present. Where there is a layer of cutaneous

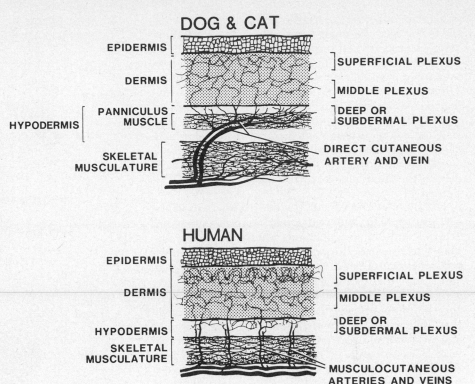

Figure 34–8. Cutaneous circulation in the dog, cat, and human. The subdermal plexus is formed and supplied by terminal branches of direct cutaneous vessels at the level of the panniculus muscle in the dog and cat. Note the parallel relationship to the direct cutaneous vessels to the overlying skin in comparison to the perpendicular orientation of musculocutaneous vessels in the human.

muscle, the subdermal plexus lies both superficial and deep to it.[18, 29] An experimental study on the misapplication of subcutaneous pedicle flaps in the dog demonstrated the vital relationship between the panniculus muscle and the overlying skin. Complete severance of the panniculus muscle results in necrosis of the island flap, whereas preservation of the muscular layer assures its survival by preserving the subdermal plexus.[31] As a result, skin should be undermined in the fascial plane beneath the cutaneous musculature to preserve the integrity of the subdermal plexus (Fig. 34–9).[29] In areas devoid of this muscle layer, one should undermine in the fascial plane well below the dermal surface to preserve it.[30]

The subdermal plexus supplies the hair bulb and follicle, tubular glands, and deeper portions of the ducts as well as the arrector pili muscle. Branches of the subdermal plexus ascend into the dermis to form the middle, or cutaneous, plexus located at the sebaceous glands. Branches from the cutaneous plexus ascend and descend into the dermis to supply the sebaceous glands and reinforce the capillary networks around the hair follicles, tubular gland ducts, and arrector pili muscle. The middle plexus shows developmental and positional variations according to the distribution of the hair follicles in the skin. Radicals from the middle plexus ascend to supply the superficial plexus. The superficial plexus lies in the outer layer of the dermis. Capillary loops from this plexus project into the dermal papillary bodies to supply the epidermal papillae and adjacent epidermis. However, the capillary loop system and papillary bodies are poorly developed in the dog and cat, unlike the human being, anthropoid ape, and pig, all

of which have well-developed capillary loops (see Fig. 34–8). This anatomical difference explains why canine skin generally does not normally blister with superficial burns.[29]

Segmental vessels arising from the aorta deep to the body muscle mass give off perforator branches, which traverse the skeletal muscles to supply the subdermal plexus. Two types of arteries supply the cutaneous circulation in the human: musculocutaneous arteries and direct cutaneous arteries. Mus-

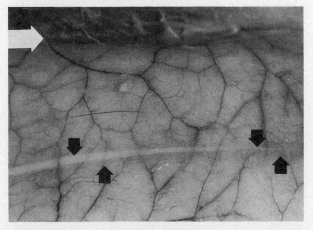

Figure 34–9. Skin reflected off the back of a cat cadaver. Blue latex has been injected into the arterial system to highlight the direct cutaneous arteries. The thin cutaneous trunci (panniculus) muscles on each side of the cat join over the dorsal midline (black arrows). A direct cutaneous artery can be seen approaching the panniculus muscle and overlying skin in parallel fashion (white arrow). As it arborizes, terminal branches "form" and supply the subdermal plexus. Note the "mirror" image formed by the direct cutaneous vasculature on each side of the midline.

culocutaneous arteries are the primary vascular supply to the skin of humans, apes, and swine. Perforator arteries send several branches to the overlying muscle mass before terminating as musculocutaneous arteries perpendicular to the skin (see Fig. 34–8). Direct cutaneous arteries arise from perforator arteries that send few branches to the overlying muscle mass before ascending to the subdermal plexus. Direct cutaneous arteries run parallel to the skin and supply a greater area of the skin compared with a single musculocutaneous artery but play a secondary role in the total cutaneous circulatory pattern in the human.[29]

Hughes and Dransfield[18] divided arteries supplying the canine skin into two groups: mixed cutaneous arteries and simple cutaneous arteries. Mixed cutaneous arteries run through a muscle mass and supply a significant number of branches to it before emerging and supplying the skin. Simple cutaneous arteries give few branches to muscles, between which they run, before supplying the skin. Despite the descriptive similarities to the perforator-musculocutaneous and perforator–direct cutaneous systems of man, all vessels in the skin of dogs and cats approach and travel parallel to the skin and are direct cutaneous

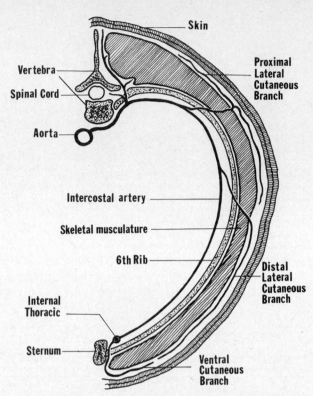

Figure 34–11. Cross section of the thoracic wall, illustrating the proximal and distal lateral cutaneous branches of the intercostal arteries in the dog. Note the parallel relationship of the direct cutaneous arteries (and veins) with the overlying skin. (Reprinted with permission from Pavletic, M. M.: Canine axial pattern flaps, using the omocervical, thoracodorsal, and deep circumflex iliac direct cutaneous arteries. Am. J. Vet. Res. *42*:391, 1981.)

arteries (Figs. 34–10 and 34–11).[29, 30] Standard anatomy texts illustrate the superficial arteries of the canine trunk (Fig. 34–12).[13]

Dogs and other loose-skinned animals lack musculocutaneous vessels (see Fig. 34–8). This has special significance to the veterinarian, who must avoid human pedicle grafting techniques, which have little or no application in the dog and cat based on these anatomical variations.[29, 30, 31]

CONGENITAL SKIN DISORDERS

Cutaneous Asthenia

Cutaneous asthenia is a congenitohereditary skin disorder reported in humans and other animals. In animals this condition is analogous to the Ehlers-Danlos syndrome (EDS) seen in human beings, an eponym for a group of collagen disorders characterized by unduly fragile connective tissue.[17, 19, 27] Other names for those diseases involving fragile hyperextensible skin include *dermatosparaxis* and *collagenous tissue dysplasia* in cattle, sheep, and cats.[22] Eight forms (types I through VIII) of this syndrome have been described in man based on variable clinical features.[27] Autosomal dominant (EDS I, II, III, VIII), X-linked recessive (EDS V), and autosomal recessive

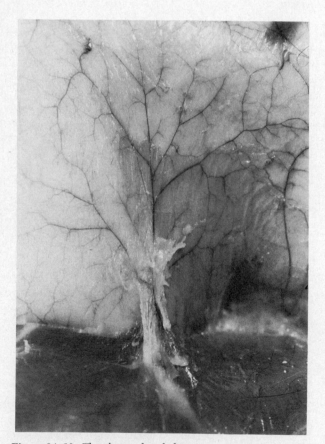

Figure 34–10. The thoracodorsal direct cutaneous artery in the cat. Blue latex has been injected to highlight the arterial branches. Note the fine terminal branches that supply the subdermal plexus (subcutaneous on deep plexus). Veins parallel the cutaneous arterial supply. Incorporating long direct cutaneous vessels into the flap will enable the surgeon to develop large pedicle grafts with less risk of skin necrosis secondary to ischemia.

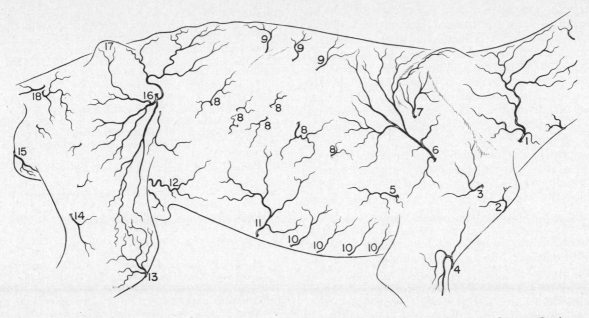

Figure 34–12. Superficial arteries of the canine trunk. *1*, Superficial cervical branch of omocervical; *2*, cranial circumflex humeral; *3*, caudal circumflex humeral; *4*, proximal collateral radial; *5*, lateral thoracic; *6*, cutaneous branch of thoracodorsal; *7*, cutaneous branch of subscapular; *8*, distal lateral cutaneous branches of intercostals; *9*, proximal lateral cutaneous branches of intercostals; *10*, ventral cutaneous branches of internal thoracic; *11*, cranial superficial epigastric; *12*, caudal superficial epigastric; *13*, medial genicular; *14*, cutaneous branch of caudal femoral; *15*, perineal; *16*, deep circumflex iliac; *17*, tubera coxae; *18*, cutaneous branches of superficial lateral coccygeal. (Reprinted with permission from Evans, H. E., and Christensen, G.: *Anatomy of the Dog*. W. B. Saunders, Philadelphia, 1979.)

(EDS VI, VII) inheritance have been noted in humans.[19] The disease is considered autosomal dominant with incomplete penetrance in mink, dogs, and cats,[17, 28] although dermatosparaxis in cattle, sheep, and some cats is a recessive trait.[22] Affected canine breeds include springer spaniels, beagles, German shepherds, dachshunds, boxers, St. Bernards, Manchester terriers, Welsh Corgis, and mixed breeds. It also has been noted in Persian, Himalayan, and domestic short-haired cats.[8, 27, 28, 34, 35] Documented biochemical disorders in humans have included a defect of type III collagen synthesis (EDS IV), a deficiency of lysyl hydroxylase (EDS VI), and a deficiency of procollagen peptidase (EDS VII).[19] These variable soft collagen disorders in human beings can manifest themselves as joint hypermobility, congenital vascular fragility, bowel ruptures, hernias, and ocular lesions.[19] However, increased skin fragility with hyperelasticity and laxity is the outstanding clinical feature of EDS in humans and cutaneous asthenia in the dog and cat (Fig. 34–13).[4, 17, 19, 20, 22, 28, 34, 35] Hyperlaxity may increase with the age of the dog and may be a more prominent feature than hyperelasticity.[15] The skin may appear excessive in quantity, hanging in folds, especially around the limbs.[15, 34] Affected animals usually have a history of lacerations, abscesses, and "tissue-paper" thin scars (onion skin scars).[34, 35] Pseudotumor formation from injury to fragile blood vessels may be noted.[20] The skin tears easily with minor trauma, but usually little bleeding is noted.[35]

Histologically, the dermis may be thick, normal, or thin, whereas the epidermis may be normal or thin. The most severe alterations noted usually are in the size, shape, and orientation of the collagen bundles. Many of the fibers appear smaller in diameter than normal, and mature and large collagen fibers may be fragmented. Collagen bundles may be dissociated and haphazardly arranged, lacking the normal characteristic interwoven appearance. In addition, the collagen may also lack normal staining uniformity.[4, 15, 17, 22, 28, 34, 35] Abnormalities in dermal collagen packing into fibrils and fibers have been recently reported in mixed breed dogs.[22] A "skin extensibility index" was employed to clinically quantitate cutaneous extensibility of affected animals. A

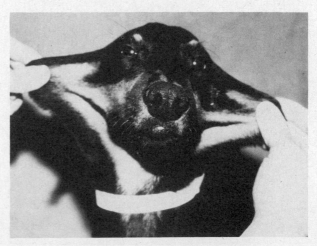

Figure 34–13. Cutaneous asthenia in a mixed breed dog. The loose elastic skin was easily demonstrated. (Picture courtesy of Drs. Stephen White and Susan Reinke.)

consistent correlation was noted between a skin extensibility index greater than 17 per cent and collagen packing defects.[22] A reduction in acid glycosaminoglycan has been reported without histological evidence of collagen fiber abnormalities.[7] Extracutaneous collagen fragility has been noted in the mesentery, intestinal wall, aorta, and muscle attachments in the dog.[4] Radiographic and microradiographic studies have also revealed subclinical involvement of bone.[22]

Surgical problems associated with EDS are proportional to the severity of the connective tissue abnormality. Hernias associated with human EDS may require reinforcement with plastic mesh. In the dog and cat, skin injuries are the primary problem. Clipping of the hair of the skin and preparation for any surgical procedure must be performed gently. Round-bodied atraumatic suture needles may be advisable to prevent skin tears during suturing.[14] Tension suture patterns may be necessary if simple interrupted sutures pull through the delicate tissue. Use of nonreactive monofilament nonabsorbable suture materials may be advisable in surgical repairs because they supply prolonged wound support in affected animals. Affected cats may require claw removal to prevent self-mutilation.[27]

Because of the likely hereditary nature of this condition in dogs and cats, breeding of affected animals should be discouraged.

Epitheliogenesis Imperfecta

Epitheliogenesis imperfecta has been reported in lambs, horses, and cats. Affected areas of the skin and mucous membranes lack an epidermis. Affected kittens are presented to the veterinarian with ulcers and are susceptible to septicemia secondary to infection of the denuded surfaces. Therapy is reported to be of little benefit, but excision and closure of the defects or skin grafting techniques may be employed in selected cases. Breeding of affected animals should be discouraged.[5, 24, 35]

1. Al-Bagdadi, F., and Lovell, J.: The integument. In Evans, H. E., and Christensen, G. B. (eds.): Miller's Anatomy of the Dog, 2nd ed. W. B. Saunders, Philadelphia, 1979.
2. Aoki, T., and Wada, M.: Functional activity of the sweat glands in the hairy skin of the dog. Science 114:123, 1951.
3. Arey, L. B.: Developmental Anatomy, 7th ed. W. B. Saunders, Philadelphia, 1966.
4. Arlein, M. S.: Generalized acute cutaneous asthenia in a dog. J. Am. Vet. Med. Assoc. 111:52, 1947.
5. Austin, V. H.: The skin. In Catcott, E. J. (ed.): Feline Medicine and Surgery II. American Veterinary Publications, Inc., Santa Barbara, 1975.
6. Ballard, W. W.: Comparative Anatomy and Physiology. The Ronald Press Company, New York, 1964.
7. Butler, W. F.: Fragility of the skin in a cat. Res. Vet. Sci. 19:213, 1975.
8. Butler, W. F.: Torn skin in a cat. Vet. Rec. 96:276, 1975.
9. Christensen, G. C.: The mammae. In Evans, H. E., and Christensen, G. C. (eds.): Miller's Anatomy of the Dog, 2nd ed. W. B. Saunders, Philadelphia, 1979.
10. Creed, R. F. S.: The histology of mammalian skin, with special reference to the dog and cat. Vet. Rec. 70:171, 1958.
11. Crouch, J. E., and Lackey, M. B.: Text-Atlas of Cat Anatomy. Lea & Febiger, Philadelphia, 1969. .
12. Dellmann, H., and Brown, E. M.: Textbook of Veterinary Histology. Lea & Febiger, Philadelphia, 1976.
13. Evans, H. E., and Christensen, G. C. (eds.): Miller's Anatomy of the Dog. W. B. Saunders, Philadelphia, 1979.
14. Fitchie, P.: The Ehlers-Danlos syndrome. Vet. Rec. 90:165, 1972.
15. Gething, M. A.: Suspected Ehlers-Danlos syndrome in a dog. Vet. Rec. 89:638, 1971.
16. Guyton, A. C.: Textbook of Medical Physiology. W. B. Saunders, Philadelphia, 1976.
17. Hegreberg, G. A., Padgett, G. A., and Henson, J. B.: Connective tissue disease of dogs and mink resembling Ehlers-Danlos syndrome in man. Arch. Pathol. 90:159, 1970.
18. Hughes, H. V., and Dransfield, J. W.: The blood supply to the skin of the dog. Br. Vet. J. 15:299, 1959.
19. Hunt, T. K., and Dunphy, J. E.: Fundamentals of Wound Management. Appleton-Century-Crofts, New York, 1979.
20. Keep, J. M.: Cutis hyperelastica in a dog. Aust. Vet. J. 45:593, 1969.
21. Lovell, J. E., and Getty, R.: The hair follicle, epidermis, dermis, and skin glands of the dog. Am. J. Vet. Res. 18:873, 1957.
22. Minor, R. R., Lein, D. H., Patterson, D. F., et al.: Defects in collagen fibrillogenesis causing hyperextensible, fragile skin in dogs. J. Am. Vet. Med. Assoc. 182:142, 1983.
23. Muller, G. H., and Kirk, R. W.: Small Animal Dermatology. W. B. Saunders, Philadelphia, 1976.
24. Munday, B. L.: Epitheliogenesis imperfecta in lambs and kittens. Br. Vet. J. 126: xlvii, 1970.
25. Nevrand, K., and Schwarz, R.: Light microscopic studies of feline skin: Epidermis, corium and subcutis. DTW 76:497, 1969.
26. Nielsen, S. W.: Glands of the canine skin—morphology and distribution. Am. J. Vet. Res. 14:448, 1953.
27. O'Neill, C. S.: Hereditary skin disease in the dog and cat. Comp. Cont. Ed. Pract. Vet. 3:791, 1981.
28. Patterson, D. F., and Minor, R. R.: Hereditary fragility and hyperextensibility of the skin of cats. Lab. Invest. 37:170, 1977.
29. Pavletic, M. M.: The vascular supply to the skin of the dog: a review. Vet. Surg. 9:77, 1980.
30. Pavletic, M. M.: Canine axial pattern flaps, using the omocervical, thoracodorsal, and deep circumflex iliac direct cutaneous arteries. Am. J. Vet. Res. 42:391, 1981.
31. Pavletic, M. M.: Misapplication of subcutaneous pedicle flaps in the dog. Vet. Surg. 11:18, 1982.
32. Peacock, E. E., and Van Winkle, W.: Surgery and Biology of Wound Repair. W. B. Saunders, Philadelphia, 1970.
33. Schilling, J. A.: Wound healing. Surg. Clin. North Am. 5:859, 1976.
34. Scott, D. W.: Cutaneous asthenia. Vet. Med./Sm. Anim. Clin. 69:1256, 1974.
35. Scott, D. W.: Congenital hereditary disorders. J. Am. Anim. Hosp. Assoc. 16:463, 1980.
36. Strickland, J. H., and Calhoun, M. L.: The integumentary system of the cat. Am. J. Vet. Res. 24:1018, 1963.
37. Swaim, S. F.: Surgery of Traumatized Skin: Management and Reconstruction in the Dog and Cat. W. B. Saunders, Philadelphia, 1980.
38. Swenson, M. J.: Duke's Physiology of Domestic Animals, 5th ed. Comstock Publishing Company, Inc., Ithaca, 1970.
39. Webb, A. J., and Calhoun, M. L.: The microscopic anatomy of the skin of mongrel dogs. Am. J. Vet. Res. 15:274, 1954.

Chapter 35

Management of Superficial Skin Wounds

Ronald M. Bright and Curtis W. Probst

Wounds are injuries produced by external forces. These forces can be accidental, due to violence, or iatrogenically caused by the surgeon's knife. All wounds differ in degree, but the nature of wounds is the same. A wound may be open, i.e., a break in the skin, or closed. Open wounds present a variable problem of contamination and infection. A laceration with a piece of glass is likely to have less tissue damage and bacterial inoculation than a wound from a dog bite.

The manner in which a wound is sustained often determines the amount of tissue damage.[8] Varying degrees of trauma result in dissipation of kinetic energy throughout the surrounding tissue. In closed injuries, a shock wave often travels deep to the skin and damages tissue in its path (Fig. 35–1). In open injuries, such as those due to gunshots, the amount of tissue damage depends primarily on the velocity, mass, and type of bullet and the tissues involved (see Fig. 35–1).[19] In low-velocity penetration, the tissues absorb the relatively weak penetrating force with minimal injury to the surrounding tissues (Fig. 35–2A). A special kind of low-velocity injury occurs when rotational stresses are applied to skin and underlying structures, as seen with avulsion injuries. The common feature is tearing of the skin and subcutaneous tissues from their blood supply, with the formation of a flap. In contrast, high-velocity missiles explode the surrounding tissues with a shock wave (Fig. 35–2B).[8] Cavitation waves set up vibrations resulting in contusion and devitalization of neighboring tissues. The severity of these wounds obviously calls for a more aggressive and energetic local treatment.

WOUND CLASSIFICATION

Closed wounds may be classified as direct or indirect (contre coup) (Fig. 35–1). These nonpenetrating

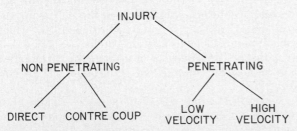

Figure 35–1. A simple classification of wounds. (Reprinted with permission from Dudley, II. A. F. (ed.): *Hamilton Bailey's Emergency Surgery.* 10th ed. John Wright and Sons, Ltd., Bristol, England, 1977.)

wounds of the skin usually result from the impact of blunt objects. The skin is intact, but a severe crushing injury can cause considerable damage to underlying tissues. A shock wave can pass deep to the skin and cause direct tissue damage to any structure in its path. Alternatively, the traumatic forces can cause indirect (contre coup) injury by throwing an abdominal organ such as liver, spleen, kidney, or bowel against a bony tissue such as a rib or vertebra. In humans, the indirect injury is most often associated with the deceleration effects associated with motor vehicle accidents.

If the crushing injury is limited to the skin and subcutaneous tissues, hemorrhage may occur at the time of injury and continue for a short period afterward.[25] Swelling eventually occurs owing to hemorrhage and edema.

Open wounds, as previously defined, are classified into four major groups[25]:

1. Abrasion—a superficial wound that consists of rubbing off of the epidermis and a variable portion of the dermis.

2. Incision—a wound made by a sharp object. The edges of the wound are smooth and large blood vessels or nerves may be severed.

3. Laceration—a wound inflicted by a dull object that is sufficiently sharp to tear the tissues. The cut is not orderly and extends to varying depths. Important underlying tissues may be damaged.

4. Stab or puncture wound—a wound resulting from penetration of the skin or mucous membrane by a sharp object. If the object enters the body but does not emerge beyond it, the injury is termed *penetrating*; if it does emerge, it is called a *perforating* wound. The amount of tissue damage caused by a small entry wound can be deceiving, because the depth of penetration may be difficult to discern. Teeth or other sharp objects may penetrate deeply and frequently carry debris and bacteria into the deeper tissues.

Combination wounds are those with penetrating (open) and crushing (contusion) components. For example, dog bites are frequently combination wounds with a tremendous amount of damage to underlying subcutaneous tissues. The tearing and crushing actions of a dog's teeth almost always result in a considerable amount of devitalized tissue.

ASSESSMENT OF THE OPEN WOUND

Wounds from small punctures are likely to develop an infection unless properly treated.[20] Because for-

431

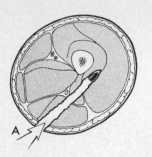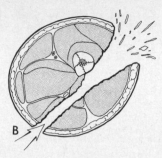

Figure 35–2. Contrast between low-velocity (a) and high-velocity (b) injuries due to missiles. (Reprinted with permission from Dudley, H. A. F. (ed.): *Hamilton Bailey's Emergency Surgery.* 10th ed. John Wright and Sons, Ltd., Bristol, England, 1977.)

eign matter and devitalized tissue cannot exit from such wounds, conditions are ideal for wound infection. Incisions from sharp objects usually cause minimal damage to surrounding structures and are less likely to become infected than lacerations or penetrating wounds.

An open wound may be classified as *clean* when it is created surgically and under aseptic conditions. Tissue trauma is minimal, and exposure to bacteria is strictly controlled. A *contaminated* wound related to trauma has a bacterial component acquired from street flora, the soil, or, in the case of a bite wound, the oral cavity of another animal. These wounds are considered *clean-contaminated* if there is minimal contamination and they can be surgically cleaned. A *dirty* wound is defined as one in which pus is encountered and infection is obvious.

Open wounds formed under nonsterile conditions are automatically considered contaminated.[8] Devitalized tissue, blood clots, foreign debris, and circulatory damage all contribute to progression from contamination to sepsis.[4]

Table 35–1 is a guide to the classification of open wounds. The nature and location of the wound, the blood supply, and the environmental circumstances under which the wound was sustained modify this classification.[4, 8] If any doubt exists when planning the management of any wound, it is safer to "downgrade" the classification from contaminated to infected.[8]

TABLE 35–1. Classification of Open Wounds*

Class	Nature	Duration	Contamination
1	Clean lacerations	0–6 hours	Minimal
2	Incised or ragged tissue damage	6–12 hours	Significant
3	Incised or ragged tissue damage	12 hours	Gross

*When doubt exists, the wound should be "downgraded." (Reprinted with permission from Dudley, H. A. F. (ed.): *Hamilton Bailey's Emergency Surgery.* 10th ed. John Wright and Sons, Ltd., Bristol, England, 1977.)

WOUND MANAGEMENT

Management of the Open Wound

Open wounds should be closed as soon as possible.[8] How closure is achieved depends on the initial classification of the wound (see Table 35–1).

Incised wounds that are seen early (within 6–8 hours) have less contamination than older wounds, in which the likelihood of infection is greater. Converting an incised wound to a clean wound usually requires minimal debridement and hemostasis. Primary closure can then be considered. If the wound is older, debridement is followed by leaving the wound open initially for three or four days and closing primarily at that time.[12] In selected cases, the entire wound can be excised for safe primary closure.

Lacerations and puncture wounds often require varying degrees of debridement. The aim of debridement is to convert a wound lined with damaged and potentially infected tissue to a surgically clean wound.[8, 32] This time-honored technique is the single most important factor in the management of the contaminated wound.[18] Debridement removes dirt and bacteria as well as devitalized tissues that impair the wound's ability to resist infection.[13] Devitalized tissue inhibits the bactericidal capacity of *in vitro* leukocytes, suggesting an inhibitory effect on leukocyte bacterial killing.[13] The growth of bacteria in devitalized tissue is similar to growth in nutrient broth at 37°C.[13] Thus, the harmful effects of devitalized tissue on wound defenses underline the importance of wound debridement in the care of the traumatic wound. Experimentally, the capacity of devitalized fat, muscle, and skin to enhance infection was comparable.[13]

Early wound management is important, but minimal interference with a wound before definitive treatment is encouraged.[32] The wound is immediately protected by any type of clean and dry occlusive dressing, to prevent further contamination and damage and to enhance hemostasis.

Just prior to definitive care of the wound, measures should be taken to protect it while preparing the surrounding area.[20] The skin edges can be apposed with skin staples, a continuous suture pattern, or towel clamps. Alternatively, it can be left open and packed with saline-moistened sterile gauze sponges or filled with a water-soluble lubricating jelly. Clipping around the wound can proceed. Scissors dipped in mineral oil can be used to trim the hair along the free edges of the wound. In instances in which subcutaneous damage may be extensive (high-velocity gunshot, dog bite), a large area of surrounding skin should be clipped and scrubbed as if for surgery.[32]

A surgical scrub using an acceptable antiseptic solution can proceed, with care taken to prevent the solution from entering the wound.[32] Following the scrub routine, the animal can be draped.

Debridement should begin with the skin and proceed to deeper structures.[8, 32] Surgical debridement should be performed under strict asepsis in the operating room. Multiple changes of gloves, gowns, and drapes may be necessary to enhance the possible conversion of a massively contaminated wound to a clean one. All damaged tissue should be removed by sharp dissection, sparing nerves, tendons, blood vessels, joint capsules, and articular surfaces.[8] If nerves, vessels and tendons are encountered, they are preserved and covered by protective tissue.[8, 20] Identification of devitalized tissue, especially muscle, is often difficult.[8] Color is of doubtful value in this determination. However, presence of bleeding and contraction following stimulation are both considered to be fairly accurate determinants of muscle viability.[4] These subjective evaluations of viability are more accurate four or five days after injury.

Skin damage may be easier to assess initially, although an apparent line of demarcation between healthy and dead tissue may take days to be clearly visible. Although intravenous fluorescein has been successfully employed in humans to assess cutaneous circulation,[22] its use is subject to interpretation and has questionable value in the dog (see "Subjective Assessment of Flap Circulation" and "Objective Assessment of Flap Circulation" in Chapter 37).

In gunshot wounds caused by high-velocity missiles, the degree of tissue damage is particularly difficult to determine.[20] Exploration for bullet fragments and other foreign objects should be limited. Invasion of tissues not adjacent to the wound is inadvisable, unless foreign matter is intra-articular or near vital structures.[2] Repeated debridement may be necessary over several days following the initial surgical treatment of high-velocity wounds, depending on the appearance of the wound.

Surgical debridement should be used with discretion. In some cases, areas of questionable viability should be spared and subsequently reexamined to determine whether further debridement is required, especially in the lower extremities, where the availability of loose skin for cover is limited.

Enzymatic Debridement

Enzymatic debridement following wound cleansing and irrigation may be used rather than surgical debridement in severely injured patients in which the anesthetic risk is too great. Likewise, it is a useful means of debriding wounds affecting the distal extremities, where surgical debridement of necrotic areas may inadvertently damage vessels, tendons, and nerves. Moreover, areas on necrotic skin can be removed without additional destruction or removal of viable cutaneous tissue. A variety of enzymatic debriding agents of variable strength are available for use in veterinary medicine.[32] Travase ointment* is

an effective debriding agent.[26] Prior to its application, the wound should be irrigated with sterile saline. Antiseptic ointments or topical antibiotics may diminish its enzymatic action and should not be used concomitantly. The wound can be bandaged as previously mentioned. Applying wet saline bandages over the wound enhances the enzymatic action of this agent. Two applications per day is ideal, and after 2 to 3 days, enzymatic debridement is usually adequate. Although enzymatic debriding agents play an effective role in wound management, they are not a substitute for surgical debridement when a significant amount of necrotic tissue is present.

Wound Irrigation

In wounds in which complete excision of specialized tissue (nerves or tendons) is not possible, high-pressure irrigation is recommended. Copious irrigation under high pressure removes tissue debris, dirt, and bacteria,[11, 35, 36] which are normally refractory to removal by low-pressure irrigation with sterile isotonic solutions.[29] Small particle removal is considerably enhanced by the high-pressure irrigating stream.[27] A marked reduction in the infection rate of grossly contaminated wounds has been demonstrated experimentally.[35] A Surgilav,* a surgical lavage unit similar to the WaterPik,† works well for high-pressure irrigation. An inexpensive high-pressure system consisting of a 19-gauge hypodermic needle attached to a 35-ml syringe is also capable of delivering an effective pressure stream. Full force of the syringe plunger delivers a fluid pressure of 8 psi when the needle is placed perpendicular to the wound as close to its surface as possible.

Crush type wounds respond particularly well to pressure irrigation. Additionally, wounds containing dirt benefit from this procedure, because infection-potentiating factors have been identified in soil. The most active factor in inorganic soil is the colloidal clay fraction.[29]

There has been some concern about the possibility that high-pressure irrigation may force bacteria and particulate matter into the deeper recesses of tissue surrounding the wound, but this is largely unfounded. There is some legitimate concern about tissue damage that accompanies the use of high-pressure lavage; thus, the use of this irrigation method should be confined to the initial treatment of heavily contaminated wounds. The advantages of this technique, however, outweigh its disadvantage.[35]

Topical Antimicrobials

Although adequate excision is the foundation of good wound care, it alone may not suffice to insure against sepsis. Adding antimicrobial agents to irriga-

---

*Travase ointment (Sutilain's ointment, U.S.P.), Flint Laboratories, Deerfield, IL.

*Surgilav, Stryker Corporation, Kalamazoo, MI.
†Telodyne, Ft. Collins, CO.

tion solutions should be considered in the initial care of grossly contaminated superficial wounds. Antibiotics and antiseptics, the most common antimicrobials used, reduce the local bacterial count. Following the initial high-pressure irrigation of wounds with or without antimicrobials,[5] low-pressure lavage with antimicrobial solutions can be used over five to seven days or longer, depending on whether primary closure is performed. The method of irrigation must ensure that the solution contacts all surfaces of the wound.

Commonly used antibiotics include neomycin, cephalothin, sodium ampicillin, and penicillin.[31] In canine and feline bite wounds, the most common microorganisms transferred from the oral cavity to subcutaneous tissues are *Pasteurella* species. The use of neomycin-bacitracin-polymyxin is effective against staphylococcal and streptococcal infections after minor skin trauma.[15]

A mixture of 4 gm. of cephalothin or carbenicillin indanyl sodium per liter of 0.9% saline is excellent for Staphylococci and Streptococci and has good results also against *E. coli*. Neomycin given at 10 gm/liter of 0.9% saline has also given excellent results against these organisms as well as *Klebsiella* and *Pseudomonas*.[14] A minimum 15-second exposure to the antibiotic solution is required.

A 25 per cent (by volume) solution of povidone-iodine solution was shown to be 100 per cent effective against all gram-positive and gram-negative bacteria.[29] Povidone-iodine, besides controlling wound sepsis, augments wound healing.[6] Other suitable antiseptic solutions include 2 per cent chlorhexidine and benzalkonium chloride; these solutions are highly effective against all bacteria and have not been associated with resistant strains of bacteria.[14]

Some antiseptics are potent drugs that injure the host tissue.[3, 30] One prospective study reported that the use of povidone-iodine in surgical wounds actually caused an increase in wound sepsis, possibly owing to tissue damage predisposing the wound to infection.[23] A recent study comparing antiseptics in dogs demonstrated little tissue reaction with chlorhexidine and povidone-iodine in clean noninfected and infected wounds.[1] This limited experimental study reports excellent control of wound sepsis using 0.5 and 1 per cent solutions of chlorhexidine and a high concentration of benzalkonium (1:2500). Slightly less effective, even at high concentrations (0.5 per cent), was povidone-iodine.[1]

Although it is generally accepted that contaminated or infected wounds benefit from irrigation with antiseptic solutions, the volume of the irrigant and the pressure under which it is applied (initially) are the most important factors.

Wound Dressings and Bandaging Techniques

Wound maintenance between the time of initial treatment and closure is an important part of wound management. The purposes of bandaging a wound are: (1) to minimize hematoma and edema formation, (2) to help obliterate dead space, (3) to protect against additional contamination or trauma, (4) to absorb drainage, and (5) to minimize excessive motion.

The ideal dressing for a wound is one that provides excellent protection and is occlusive; that is, it provides a good physical environment for wound healing. A biological dressing serves this function well but is impractical in animals in most cases. Telfa pads* and Dermicell† are two semiocclusive materials that have been developed to mimic biological dressings. These materials have good absorbency and are nonadherent. The nonadherent surface is ideal to place in direct contact with the wound, as it helps decrease wound disruption when the bandage is changed.

If a wound is discharging a large amount of low-viscosity exudate, a dry bulky dressing is indicated.[32] Early in the course of wound management, the amount of exudate may be copious, and two to three bandage changes per day may be necessary. Baby diapers work well in some wounds in which exudation is considerable and a large degree of absorbency is required.

If a wound has exudate that is thick and dry, wet wound dressings are preferred. A wet dressing helps enhance the dilution and removal of thick exudate by reducing the viscosity of the secretions.[32] It also helps in the removal of dried necrotic debris when the gauze is removed. Saline-soaked sponges are applied directly to the wound and allowed to dry. These are sometimes termed "wet to dry" dressings. When they become dry, bandage changing is indicated. Removal of the dried gauze is enhanced by saturating it with saline just prior to removal, in order to decrease the pain to the animal yet still allow debridement of the superficial necrotic debris and exudate that is present on the wound. If the gauze dries out quickly, several applications of wet to dry dressing may be necessary daily.

In the management of infected wounds, topical antimicrobial agents can be used under the occlusive bandage. Some agents actually decrease the rate of reepithelialization, whereas others enhance it or have no effect at all. Although petrolatum (Vaseline) prevents crust formation and keeps the wound surfaces moist, it retards epidermal resurfacing.[7] However, low-melting-point petrolatum (as found in Neosporin ointment) has no adverse effect on healing when used alone; when combined with the antimicrobial agents (neomycin, polymyxin, and bacitracin-zinc), it greatly enhances wound healing.[7]

Although the vehicle in Furacin‡ (in Solubase) does not affect healing, Furacin cream itself may retard epidermal migration. Pharmadine,§ a povi-

---

*Telfa Pads, The Kendall Co., Hospital Products, Boston, MA.
†Dermicell Sterile Pad, Johnson & Johnson, New Brunswick, NJ.
‡Furacin, Norwich-Eaton Pharmaceuticals, Norwich, NY.
§Pharmadine, Sherwood Pharmaceutical Co., Mahwah, NJ.

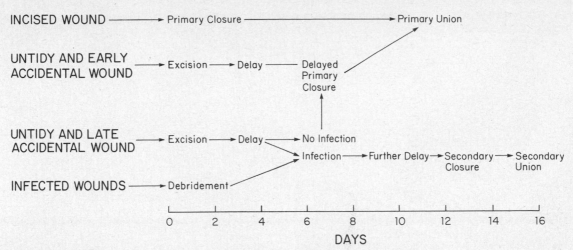

Figure 35–3. Pathways leading to wound healing are varied. When contamination of the wound is heavy or the wound is old, delayed primary or secondary closure should be considered. (Reprinted with permission from Dudley, H. A. F. (ed.): *Hamilton Bailey's Emergency Surgery.* 10th ed. John Wright and Sons, Ltd., Bristol, England, 1977.)

done-iodine solution with a water vehicle, does not alter the healing rate; its antimicrobial activity is excellent and it is an acceptable dressing material.[7]

In one study the dressing that produced the fastest healing rate was Silvadine,* a water-miscible cream containing 1 per cent silver sulfadiazine.[7] It has a broad antimicrobial activity spectrum and, compared with results in nontreated control wounds, produced a 28 per cent greater rate of healing.[7]

In wounds contaminated with *Pseudomonas*, we have successfully employed neomycin in saline at 0.25 per cent strength. Gentamicin ointment (0.1 per cent) also works well in these troublesome wounds.[32]

Wound Closure

After the completion of debridement and irrigation, closure of a wound is related to: (1) the degree of contamination, (2) the amount of devitalized tissue

*Silvadene, Marion Laboratories, Inc., Kansas City, MO.

that remains, (3) the patient's general condition, (4) hemostasis, (5) time since injury, (6) the financial status of the owner, and (7) whether the wound can be observed following closure (Fig. 35–3). Whether the wound should be closed after the initial debridement or left open is not always an easy decision. When there is any doubt, leave the wound open.[8] The development of infection in questionable wounds can be prevented by delayed primary closure (Fig. 35–4). Because of the local response in the open wound, the ability to combat infection increases, allowing primary closure to occur any time between two and five days. If residual necrotic tissue, edema, and redness of the wound margins remain, closure may be delayed even longer. It may even be necessary to debride the wound again. Quantitative bacterial counts of the tissue from the wound can be taken, and if the wound contains less than 10^6 bacteria per gram of tissue and is free of devitalized tissue, primary closure can be performed.[13]

When closure is performed more than five days after injury, it is called *secondary closure.*[15] The term

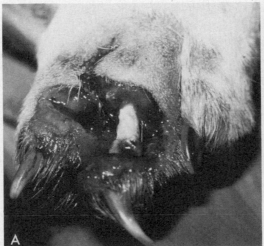
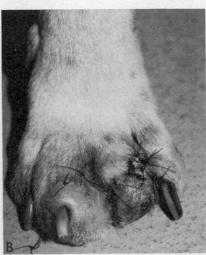

Figure 35–4. *A,* The foot of this dog was caught in a trap, causing extensive tissue damage and gross contamination. *B,* Four days after debridement and high- and low-pressure irrigation, delayed primary closure was performed with excellent results.

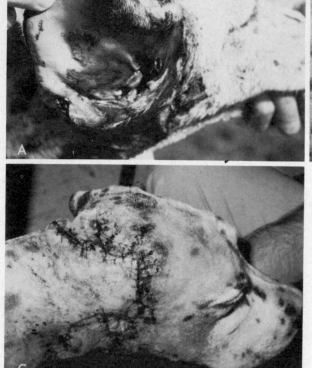

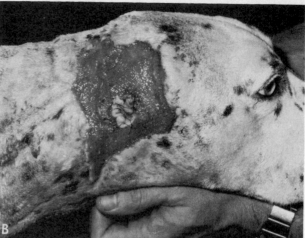

Figure 35–5. A, A gangrenous ear wound in a dog sustained five days prior to presentation and treatment. B, Extensive debridement and irrigation was performed, Eight days later a healthy granulation bed was suitable for primary closure. C, A sliding pedicle flap was placed over the defect.

implies that granulation tissue has formed in the wound (Fig. 35–5). When closure is performed, the excess granulation tissue is usually excised along with a thin rim of skin at the margin of the wound, the skin is mobilized, and primary closure is performed.[32] Undermining of adjacent skin, however, should be kept to a minimum.

When primary closure is performed, dead space should be eliminated. Sutures can assist in the elimination of dead space but the number of sutures should be kept to a minimum. The sutures should be small in diameter and properly placed to gently appose tissue layers. They should not strangle the tissue or cause a massive knot. Improper suture placement and excessive suture material can retard healing, as all suture material is a foreign body. With gut, tissue irritation is excessive and may cause exudation. Polyglycolic acid (PGA), monofilament nylon, polydioxanone, and polygactin 910 are our choices for sutures under these circumstances. On certain occasions, dead space can be eliminated with a pressure bandage carefully applied over the area without resorting to buried sutures.

A hematoma is an excellent medium for bacterial growth and must be eliminated prior to closure. Where oozing of serum or blood may continue in spite of attempts at hemostasis, an active suction apparatus (Redivacette*) can be employed. This "active" drainage system is most often used in deep wounds with muscle and tendon involvement. Redivacette drains consist of fenestrated tubes placed in the wound and allowed to surface through the skin through small puncture holes. This tubing is connected to a vacuum reservoir that can be placed under a vacuum so that a slight amount of suction is always present on the drain placed in the deeper tissues. The drains are commercially available and, when indicated, are excellent for deep wound drainage. They are usually left in place for three to five days.

When dead space cannot be closed, or postoperative tissue fluid accumulation is likely, placement of a passive drain may be necessary. Other indications for drains include those wounds in which foreign material may still be in deeper tissues and when massive contamination has occurred (e.g., wounds around the anus).[32] Latex rubber tubing (Penrose)† is soft and pliable, is relatively inert, and highly efficient (Fig. 35–11).[9, 32] Because these drains work by capillary action and gravity flow, they must always exit through a separate "stab" incision at the most

*Redivacette, Orthopedic Equipment Co., Bourbon, IN.
†Tomac Latex Penrose Tubing, American Hospital Supply Division of AHS Corp, McGraw Park, IL.

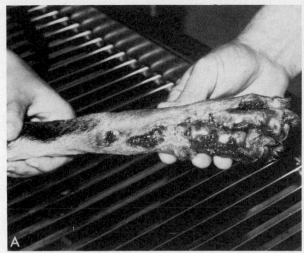

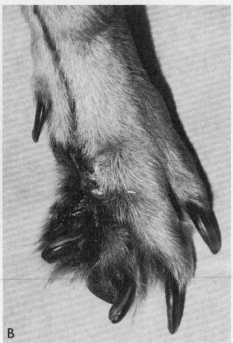

Figure 35–6. *A,* This open wound on the forelimb of a dog contained a large amount of devitalized tissue and was grossly contaminated. Several days of high- and low-pressure irrigation and enzymatic debridement was followed with long-term bandage and dressing changes by the owner. *B,* Wound contraction resulted in complete coverage of the defect. Some distortion of the second digit (contracture) necessitated an amputation at a later date.

dependent portion of the wound. Rubber or plastic tube drains can also be used in wounds in which encroachment on vital structures is minimal. Soft plastic tubes usually cause less tissue reaction than those made of rubber.

In general, a drain should be removed as soon as possible, ideally when there is little or no drainage from the wound. If possible, a bandage should always be placed over the drain to decrease the risk of an ascending infection. This practice allows the assessment of the amount of drainage, prevents the animal from chewing and possibly removing the drain, and decreases the likelihood of an ascending infection.[32] If there is a large volume of drainage, many bandage changes may be necessary. In most cases, daily bandage changes are sufficient.

Tension across the skin edges should be minimized. Tension-relieving techniques or local flaps may be necessary (see Chapters 36 and 37). The remaining defect may be left open in selected cases and protected until healing occurs by second intention.

A decision to allow a wound to heal by second intention should be made when there is an extensive amount of tissue devitalization, the effectiveness of the local tissue defenses is compromised, and a severe infection is present (Fig. 35–6). A further consideration is a large skin defect that would preclude primary or secondary closure. Financial considerations of the owners or the inexperience of the veterinarian may also influence the decision to proceed with second intention healing. Although healing time is protracted, and the cosmetic and functional results may be compromised,[17] this method of treating wounds in companion animals is a well-accepted technique.

Wounds can be large and still heal completely with a full-thickness skin cover (see Chapter 3). Linear wounds on the extremity parallel to the long axis of the limb can also heal with minimal scar (Fig. 35–7).[32]

Healing by second intention requires the formation of granulation tissue, wound contraction, and epithelialization.[32] A healthy wound enhances wound contraction by resisting infection, allowing epithelium to

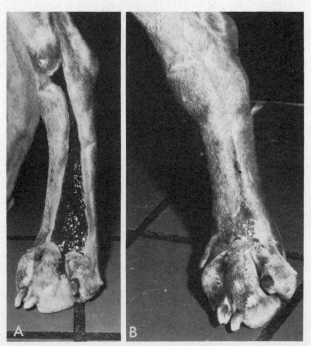

Figure 35–7. *A,* A ten day old linear defect in the rear limb of a dog, healing by wound contraction. *B,* A small defect is all that remains at 50 days. This defect eventually bridged with a full-thickness skin cover.

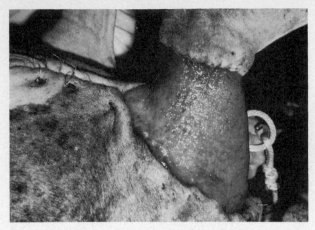

Figure 35–8. A wound approximately 30 days old underwent cessation of wound contraction. The granulation tissue was relatively smooth and pale.

migrate across its surface, and containing the factors responsible for contraction. Significant contraction is not seen until five to nine days after trauma.[38]

Adequate debridement of the wound, proper application of dressings and bandages throughout the healing period, control of infection, and the maintenance of good overall nourishment of the animal assist in the formation of healthy granulation tissue.

If wound contraction ceases and there is still some looseness in the surrounding skin, the status of the granulation tissue should be evaluated closely. A smooth and pale granulation bed indicates that it is largely composed of collagen and ground substance and lacks myofibroblasts (Fig. 35–8).[17] There is overwhelming evidence that the cellular mechanism of wound contraction involves these contractile fibroblasts (see Chapter 3). This tissue must be excised so that fresh granulation tissue can form, and the contraction process can be allowed to go to completion (see Figs. 35–6 and 35–7).

Prophylactic Use of Antibiotics

Antimicrobial prophylaxis is the administration of an antimicrobial drug in the absence of infection.[28] The causes of the wound contamination and the ability of the patient to respond are important when deciding whether to use prophylactic antimicrobials. When bacterial contamination or tissue trauma is great enough to present a serious risk of infection, supplementation of the host's natural resistance with antimicrobials should be considered.[28] Chemoprophylaxis may be a valuable adjunct to the initial management of a traumatically induced superficial wound. It should never be used, however, as a substitute for good judgment and excellent technique.[14]

A major principle in the use of chemoprophylaxis is to have the antibiotic in the tissues prior to surgical debridement and any further bacterial contamination from the hospital environment. If an animal is pre-

sented with a wound that is obviously infected, longer-term antimicrobials should be employed after a specimen is obtained for gram staining and culture and sensitivity testing.

The drug selected should be narrow in spectrum but effective against bacteria that would be expected in superficial wounds, i.e., Staphylococci, Streptococci, and *E. coli*.[16] In dog and cat bites, *Pasteurella* is most likely.

A bactericidal drug is preferred and should be given parenterally prior to debridement. In one study, oral antibiotics administered postoperatively did not decrease the incidence of infection in patients with simple lacerations.[33] If a drug is not given until debridement is under way, intravenous administration is recommended. Following surgical debridement, an additional bolus of drug is given to bolster resistance, which immediately postoperatively is lowered because of the stress response.

Drugs with chemoprophylactic efficacy include ampicillin, cephalosporins, penicillin, cloxacillin, and clindamycin. A more recent cephalosporin, cefamandole, has a wider spectrum of activity against aerobic and anaerobic soft tissue infections.[10] Presumably, this agent would be useful prophylactically as well. It can be given intramuscularly or intravenously.

When therapeutic antimicrobials are used for an established soft tissue infection, they should be continued for at least seven days. As mentioned previously, gram staining can be helpful in the initial selection of an antimicrobial. This quick and easy method of identifying the offending microorganism is probably underused and underrated in veterinary surgery. In the majority of cases, culture and sensitivity results support the initial selection based on a gram stain. To monitor the effectiveness of antimicrobial therapy, repeat culture and sensitivity testing should be performed three or four days later, and if it yields no growth, the initial therapy can be continued. However, a change in antibiotics should be considered when: (1) a culture and sensitivity test result dictates another agent, (2) there is little change in the appearance of the infected wound after two or three days, and (3) the animal's general condition worsens and septicemia is possible.

MANAGEMENT OF SPECIFIC WOUNDS

Dog Bites

The teeth of dogs can cause a tremendous amount of crushing and tearing of the skin and underlying tissues. The extent of devitalized muscle and fascia is often unnoticed at first, since the most obvious sign is one or two small puncture holes.[9] Pneumothorax must be suspected with bite wounds involving the thorax. Rib fractures and damage to the abdominal viscera are often caused by the slashing action of a dog's teeth.

Following a fight, some dogs have tremendous

tissue damage and are in shock. Attention should be directed first toward the life-threatening problem. A chest drain may be necessary to correct the respiratory distress caused by pneumothorax, followed by intravenous fluid support. Penetrating bite wounds into the abdominal cavity warrant an exploratory laparotomy to assess the integrity of the gastrointestinal tract and other viscera as soon as initial stabilization of the patient can be achieved. Rib fractures and ventral abdominal hernias may be corrected if found during surgical debridement, depending on the overall status of the patient. Liberal removal of devitalized muscle and fat should be performed, according to the protocol previously described. Nerves, tendons, fascia, and ligaments should be preserved when possible.[24]

After the debridement of extensive bite wounds, dead space cannot be eliminated simply by suturing. Drains are necessary to obliterate the dead space and prevent seroma formation. In some cases it may be advisable to treat the wound as an open wound, delaying closure for three to five days. An antiseptic solution such as chlorhexidine (0.5 to 1.0 per cent) is flushed gently over the wound; this practice is continued twice daily in open wounds. Antibiotics should be started immediately upon presentation of the patient and should be maintained for ten to 14 days. Because *Pasteurella* is the most common microorganism, penicillin or ampicillin is the initial drug of choice.

If the placement of drains and the use of antibiotics are all that is done to treat bite wounds, a poor outcome is likely. Enlargement, debridement, and irrigation of the wound are the hallmarks of successful management of dog bite wounds. In small puncture wounds in which trauma to underlying tissues is minimal, enlarging the wound to enhance drainage is helpful. Irrigation can then be performed. Penicillin or ampicillin should be administered in these cases.

Gunshot Wounds

Gunshot wounds, like bite wounds, have the potential for extensive tissue destruction and bacterial contamination.[20, 21] Damage by a low-velocity missile is usually confined to laceration and crushing of tissue immediately surrounding the perimeter of the bullet as it traverses tissue. In contrast, a high-velocity missile elicits a shock wave causing an outward displacement of surrounding tissues, with the potential for extensive destruction to tissues a considerable distance from the projectile's pathway. Because of this difference in the amount of tissue damage, the type of weapon used to inflict the injury should be determined whenever possible.[20, 21]

Handguns are considered low-velocity weapons and usually cause little tissue damage. Therefore, clipping of the hair and thorough cleansing of the superficial portions of the entry and exit wounds may be all that is necessary, followed by daily changes of sterile dressings.[20] However, an exploratory procedure is warranted for wounds penetrating the abdominal cavity, projectiles entering a joint space, or wounds involving vital structures. Patient stabilization and a thorough physical examination are warranted for all gunshot injuries before proceeding. Therapeutic antibiotics should be administered and continued if infection is likely.

There are two types of high-velocity bullets. The jacketed or military bullet usually creates a tract that is constant in diameter as the missile penetrates tissues.[32] The bullet itself undergoes little deformation. The bullet used by most hunters expands upon contact and, as it moves through soft tissues, creates a wide wound tract. The wound is conical rather than cylindrical. The skin wound at its point of exit is much larger than at its point of entrance. The tissue damage is much more extensive with the expanding bullet, especially if it also undergoes some tumbling as it passes through the tissue.[32]

A more aggressive surgical approach should be taken if a high-velocity missile injury is suspected. In high-velocity wounds, the entire missile tract should be explored, and hair and debris removed. Devitalized tissue is removed, but nerves, vessels, and tendons should be identified and preserved.[30] Exploration for bullet fragments should not invade tissues far from the wound tract unless they are intra-articular or close to vital structures.[30] Following debridement and thorough flushing of the wound with sterile saline, primary closure with a drain can be attempted or the wound can be left open for closure at a later time. Early antimicrobial therapy of these highly contaminated wounds is mandatory.[34] Bullets should be saved and identified for legal purposes and complete records must be kept.

Abscesses

An abscess, a localized collection of pus in any part of the body, can be managed several ways, depending on the stage of development. Most abscesses begin as a cellulitis that becomes localized. Although antibiotic therapy may be used successfully to treat a cellulitis due to bacteria, they may simply delay the inevitable formation of the abscess, especially if a foreign body is present. On occasion, suppuration of the subcutaneous tissue spreads along fascial planes. This condition is referred to as *phlegmon,* and it can result in extensive tissue destruction. Needle aspiration of its contents can be done with identification of the organism by culture and Gram stain. Common microorganisms associated with subcutaneous abscesses include *Staphylococcus, Streptococcus, Pasteurella,* and *E. coli.* Hot compresses can enhance abscess maturation and pointing. Antibiotic therapy should be initiated and the abscess lanced at its most dependent site. We prefer a cephalosporin, cloxacillin, or sulfadimethoxine-trimethoprim, continued for seven to ten days after draining. Evacuation of contents is followed by thorough flushing with an antiseptic solution (10 per cent povidone-iodine or 1 per cent chlorhexidine). A sterile probe is used to assure that all pockets of the abscess communicate with the opening. Necrotic tissue should be removed. For unilocular abscesses, a Penrose drain may be required. In most cases, it is not necessary if hot packing is continued for three to four days after lancing. The crusts and exudate should be removed prior to each hot packing, to promote continuous drainage and minimize local skin irritation.

Abscesses caused by anaerobes are common and often are thick-walled abscesses that seldom come to a head even with hot compresses.[32] Aspirating these abscesses often reveals a viscous exudate with a fetid odor. Lancing at the most ventral aspect of the abscess followed by irrigation and placement of a drain is recommended. Penicillin, ampicillin, or chloromycetin for seven to ten days is advisable.

Recurring or nonresponsive abscesses indicate either ineffective antibiotic selection or a more serious underlying condition (foreign body, neoplasia, immunosuppression of the patient, etc.) that warrants a more aggressive therapeutic approach.

"Degloving" Injuries

"Degloving" is a low-velocity avulsion injury resulting from rotational stresses applied to the skin and underlying structures.[8] The tire of a vehicle is the usual cause. The skin may actually be torn away from underlying tissues, forming a flap (Fig. 35–9); this is an *anatomical* "degloving" injury.[32] A *physiological* "degloving" injury occurs when the skin remains intact but has been completely disrupted from underlying fascia and from its blood supply.[32]

The principles related to skin preparation, wound debridement, irrigation, and use of drains all apply to an avulsion injury, with some special considerations. Areas of obvious necrosis should be excised, and the remaining portion of the flap sutured into position. The skin should be closely observed postoperatively for viability (see Chapter 37). A line of demarcation between viable and nonviable tissue often occurs, at which time any nonviable tissue should be excised.

Many "degloving" injuries also have associated tendon, ligament, joint capsule, and bone damage. These must be handled in accordance with the severity of the injury. When orthopedic problems exist it may be necessary to provide temporary external fixation (e.g., Kirschner-Ehmer device). Definitive orthopedic repair should be performed when infection is controlled and soft tissue structures are healthy and viable.

WOUND HEALING COMPLICATIONS

Dehiscence

Causes of dehiscence include imperfect technical closure of a wound, hematoma with or without infection, infection, underlying metabolic disorders, presence of a foreign body, and inadequate tissue strength to allow a strong closure. An impending wound dehiscence often follows the presence of necrotic skin edges, palpation of fluid deep to the skin, and serosanguinous discharge from the suture line.[30]

When the deeper layers have become disrupted, as often evidenced by serosanguinous fluid, reoperation may be advisable. If infection is not a problem and there is no underlying disease to impair wound healing, primary closure can be attempted again. A soft rubber drain may be necessary to obliterate dead space and allow the egress of accumulating fluid. If infection is a problem, a nonoperative approach may be taken, allowing the wound to heal by second or third intention. Breakdown of most superficial skin wounds that were closed primarily is usually due to technical error or error in judgment by the surgeon. Incorrect suture material, improper use of drains, inadequate debridement, and poor understanding of how to treat contaminated wounds increase the chances of wound disruption.

Hemorrhage and Seroma Formation

When blood or serum collects between tissue layers, apposition of tissue layers is less likely. A large hematoma can cause some interference of blood supply to overlying and adjacent tissues. It can also prevent or inhibit the delivery of phagocytic cells to

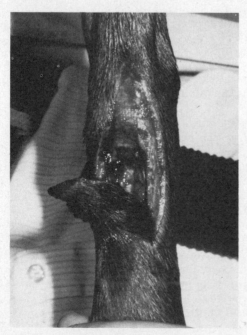

Figure 35–9. A "degloving" injury on the forelimb of a dog.

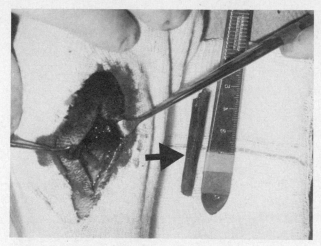

Figure 35–10. This wound of two month's duration continued to drain and did not heal. Removal of a piece of wood *(arrow)* allowed wound healing to proceed.

the area. A hematoma that is slow to be absorbed can act as an ideal culture medium for bacteria.[12] Meticulous hemostasis is mandatory before closure of any deep wound. If oozing cannot be stopped, hematoma formation can be minimized with a pressure dressing or with an active suction apparatus (Redivacette) as previously described.

If during the closure of a wound all tissues are not carefully approximated, residual dead space can soon become filled with tissue fluid. Formation of a seroma is enhanced by excess movement of the skin, indiscriminate use of suture material, the presence of foreign bodies, and excessive surgical trauma. As with hematomas, the protein-rich serum can support the growth of bacteria, with subsequent sepsis. Seromas can be prevented by use of atraumatic techniques, good hemostasis, obliteration of dead space including the use of drains, delayed wound closure, and compression bandages.

Treatment of a seroma includes the placement of drains, application of hot compresses, and needle aspiration followed by compression bandaging or removal of skin sutures to allow second-intention healing. Small seromas often resolve with no treatment.

Foreign Bodies

In traumatic wounds, not only must debridement be complete, but all foreign material should be carefully removed. Some common foreign bodies include dirt, glass, wooden splinters, tooth fragments, and metallic objects such as bullets (Fig. 35–10). Some foreign bodies may remain inert and cause little tissue reaction if not contaminated. A foreign body in a wound usually contributes to infection, which often remains until the foreign body is removed. Wound healing will not progress to completion in the presence of sepsis.

Suture material is a common foreign body. Braided nonabsorbable suture materials should not be used, because they can form a nidus for infection with resultant sinus tract formation. If ligatures are necessary for hemostasis, fine polyglycolic acid or polydioxanone sutures should be used because of their minimal tissue reaction and favorable absorption characteristics. For tissue apposition and elimination of dead space, these same materials can be used, but their diameter should be small, and short ends should be left on the suture. Monofilament nylon, polypropylene, or stainless steel is also satisfactory. Regardless of the suture selected, it is mandatory that the surgeon use the least number of sutures necessary to achieve the end result.

Contracture

Wound contraction is a basic mechanism of wound healing that often accomplishes wound closure with-

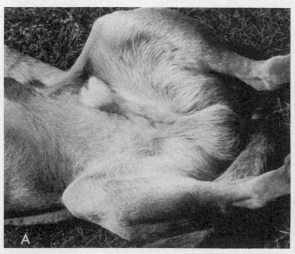
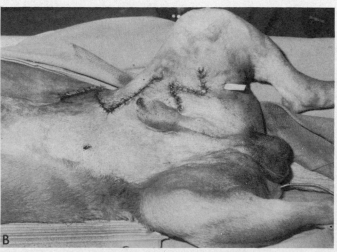

Figure 35–11. *A,* An injury near the flank of a dog resulted in a wound contracture deformity involving the left rear limb and prepuce. *B,* A Z-plasty was used to correct the problem. A penrose drain was employed to prevent seroma formation postoperatively. (Courtesy Dr. Ken Kagan.)

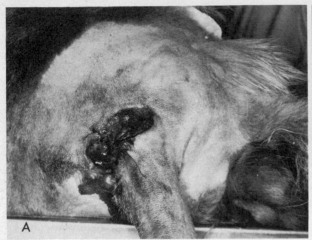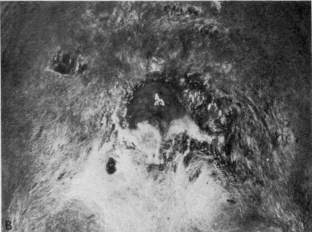

Figure 35–12. A, A severe open crushing injury to the tailhead of a dog required extensive wound debridement, including an amputation. Because of the large amount of tissue devitalization and gross contamination, management of the wound by second intention healing was chosen. B, The wound several months later. The defect is minimal but contraction has caused anal stricture.

out any additional reconstructive surgery. It can result in a deformity or even in complete loss of function of a part; this complication is called wound contracture.

Two types of contractures or deformities are associated with wound contraction seen in animals.[17] Flexion contracture is due to formation of a web of tight skin near the flexor aspect of a joint (Fig. 35–11). The second deformity is seen near body orifices, particularly the anus and eye (Fig. 35–12). Reconstructive procedures, such as Z-plasty, can correct this problem.

Infection

Factors that influence the establishment of a wound infection include: (1) pathogenicity and virulence of the organism, (2) size of the bacterial inoculum, (3) presence of a foreign body, (4) blood supply to the site, (5) general health of the animal, and (6) poor judgment in the initial handling of the wound. The last-named includes such things as inadequate debridement, poor hemostasis, rough handling of tissues, improper use of drains, poor use of dressings and bandages, and incorrect use of supportive antimicrobial therapy.

Infection retards wound healing. The number of bacteria and the wound environment are two factors that strongly influence whether a wound becomes infected.[30] Physical separation of the wound surfaces by exudate deters healing. Bacteria produce collagenases, which degrade collagen and result in decreased wound strength (see Chapter 3). Infected wounds have decreased fibroblastic activity, whereas wound pH changes due to bacteria may also affect local mediators of healing.

Other factors that can contribute to delayed or complicated wound healing include hypovolemia,

anemia, radiation therapy, chemotherapy, corticosteroid therapy, and uremia (see Chapter 3).

1. Amber, E. I., Henderson, R. A., Swaim, S. F., et al.: A comparison of antimicrobial efficacy and tissue reaction of four antiseptics on canine wounds. Vet. Surg. *12*:63, 1983.
2. Ashby, M. E.: Low velocity gunshot wounds involving the knee joint: surgical management. J. Bone Jt. Surg. *54A*:1047, 1974.
3. Branemark, P. I., Ekholm, R., Albrektsson, B., et al.: Tissue injury caused by wound disinfectants. J. Bone Jt. Surg. *59A*:48, 1967.
4. Burke, J. F.: Infection. *In* Hunt, T. K., and Dunphy, T. E. (eds.): *Fundamentals of Wound Management.* Appleton-Century-Crofts, New York, 1979.
5. Cutright, D. E., Bhaskar, S. N., Gross, A., et al.: Effect of vancomycin, streptomycin and tetracycline pulsating jet lavage on contaminated wounds. Milit. Med. 810, 1971.
6. Dedo, D. D., Alonso, W. A., and Ogura, J. H.: Povidone-iodine: an adjunct in the treatment of wound infections, dehiscences and fistulae in head and neck surgery. Trans. Am. Acad. of Ophthalmol. Otolaryngol. *84*:68, 1977.
7. Dineen, P.: *The Surgical Wound.* Lea & Febiger, Philadelphia, 1981.
8. Dudley, H. A. F.: Wounds and their management. *In* Dudley, H. A. F. (ed.): *Hamilton Bailey's Emergency Surgery.* 10th ed. John A. Wright & Sons, Ltd. Bristol, England, 1977.
9. Furneaux, R. W.: Management of contaminated wounds. Canine Pract. May-June, 1975, p. 22.
10. Glanges, E., Webber, C. E., Crenshaw, C. A., et al.: Treatment of serious skin and soft tissue infections with cefamandole. Scand. J. Infect. Dis. Suppl. *25*:69, 1980.
11. Gross, A., Cutright, D. E., and Bhaskar, S. N.: Effectiveness of pulsating water jet lavage in treatment of contaminated crushed wounds. Am. J. Surg. *124*:373, 1972.
12. Hackett, R. P.: Delayed wound closure—a review and report of use of the technique on three equine limb wounds. Vet. Surg. *12*:48, 1983.
13. Haury, B., Rodeheaver, G., Vensko, J., et al.: Debridement: an essential component of traumatic wound care. Am. J. Surg. *135*:238, 1978.
14. Hoeprich, P. D.: Chemoprophylaxis of infectious diseases. *In* Hoeprich, P. D. (ed.): *Infectious Diseases—A Modern Treatise of Infectious Processes.* Harper & Row, Hagerstown, 1977.
15. Houang, E. T., Gilmore, O. J. A., Reid, C., et al.: Absence

of bacterial resistance to povidone-iodine. J. Clin. Pathol. 29:752, 1976.

16. Hunt, T. K., Alexander, J. W., Burke, J. F., et al.: Antibiotics in surgery. Arch. Surg. 110:148, 1975.

17. Johnston, D. E.: The healing processes in open wounds. Comp. Cont. Ed. Pract. Vet. 1:789, 1979.

18. Jones, R. C., and Shires, G. T.: Principles in the management of wounds. In Schwartz, S. I. (ed.): Principles of Surgery. 2nd ed. McGraw-Hill, New York, 1974.

19. Leyden, J. J., and Sulzberger, M. B.: Topical antibiotics and minor skin trauma. Am. Fam. Physician 23:121, 1981.

20. Lipowitz, A. J.: Management of gunshot wounds of the soft tissues and extremities. J. Am. Anim. Hosp. Assoc. 12:813, 1976.

21. Liu, Y. Q., Wu, B. J., Xie, Z. C., et al.: Wounding effects of two types of bullets on soft tissues of dogs. Acta Chir. Scand. Suppl. 508:211, 1982.

22. Meyers, M. B.: Prediction and prevention of skin sloughs in radical cancer surgery. Pacific Med. Surg. 75:315, 1967.

23. McCluskey, B.: A prospective trial of povidone-iodine solution in the prevention of wound sepsis. Aust. N. Z. J. Surg. 46:254, 1976.

24. Neal, T. M., and Key, J. C.: Principles of treatment of dog bite wounds. J. Am. Anim. Hosp. Assoc. 12:657, 1976.

25. Noer, R. J.: Wounds. In Cole, W. H., and Peustow, C. B. (eds.): Emergency Care—Surgical and Medical. 7th ed. Lea & Febiger, Philadelphia, 1975.

26. Pennisi, V. R., Capozzi, A., and Friedman, G.: Travase, an effective enzyme for burn debridement. Plast. Reconstr. Surg. 51:371, 1973.

27. Probst, C. W., Peyton, L. C., Bingham, H. G., et al.: Split

28. Riviere, J. E., McCall-Kaufman, G., and Bright, R. M.: Prophylactic use of antibiotics in the surgical patient. Comp. Cont. Ed. Pract. Vet. 3:345, 1981.

29. Rodeheaver, G. T., Pettry, D., Thacker, J. G., et al.: Wound cleansing by high pressure irrigation. Surg. Gynecol. Obstet. 141:357, 1975.

30. Rodeheaver, G. T., Bellamy, W., Kody, M., et al.: Bactericidal activity and toxicity of iodine-containing solutions in wounds. Arch. Surg. 117:181, 1982.

31. Scherr, D. D., and Dodd, T. A.: In vitro bacteriological evaluation of the effectiveness of antimicrobial irrigating solutions. J. Bone Jt. Surg. 58A:119, 1976.

32. Swaim, S. F.: Management of contaminated and infected wounds. In Swaim, S. F. (ed.): Surgery of Traumatized Skin: Management and Reconstruction in the Dog and Cat. W. B. Saunders, Philadelphia, 1980.

33. Thirlby, R. C., Blair, A. S., III, and Thal, E. R.: The value of prophylactic antibiotics for simple lacerations. Surg. Gynecol. Obstet. 156:212, 1983.

34. Tikka, S.: The contamination of missile wounds with special reference to early antimicrobial therapy. Acta Chir. Scand. Suppl. 508:281, 1982.

35. Wheeler, C. B., Rodeheaver, G. T., Thacker, J. E., et al.: Side effects of high pressure irrigation. Surg. Gynecol. Obstet. 143:775, 1976.

36. Wilson, R. F., and Walt, A. J.: General principles of wound care. In Walt, A. J., and Wilson, R. F. (eds.): Management of Trauma—Pitfalls and Practices. Lea & Febiger, Philadelphia, 1975.

thickness skin grafting in the dog. J. Am. Anim. Hosp. Assoc. 19:355, 1983.

Chapter **36** Principles of Plastic and Reconstructive Surgery

Steven F. Swaim

BASIC INSTRUMENTS

An elaborate array of instruments is not necessary for uncomplicated skin closure in the dog and cat. However, certain instruments will refine the surgeon's technique. A needle holder–scissor combination, such as the Olsen-Hegar or Gillies needle holder, as well as small ophthalmic needle holders is useful. Straight, sharp-pointed scissors are useful for trimming wound margins and for careful blunt dissection. Curved, blunt-pointed scissors, e.g., Metzenbaum scissors, are used for cutting tissues as well as for undermining. A short, heavy pair of scissors with serrated blades is used for cutting all sutures, especially wire sutures. Lightweight, sharp, thin-pointed scissors with a hollowed-out cutting surface are best for removing sutures.[32, 36]

Fingers are the least traumatic instruments for manipulating skin. However, skin hooks or a sharp suture needle in needle holders can also be used to manipulate skin atraumatically. Forceps with fine teeth, such as Adson tissue forceps, will hold skin without slipping or undue pressure.[2, 7, 12, 32, 36, 46]

For marking proposed lines of incision on the skin, a sterile toothpick or splintered wooden applicator tip dipped in sterile methylene blue may be used. A Bard-Parker #3 metric scalpel handle and an assortment of blades are necessary for skin incisions (Fig. 36–1).

SUTURES

Principles of Suturing

This section covers the proper placement and tying and properties of some of the common suture patterns used in reconstructive skin surgery. The reader is

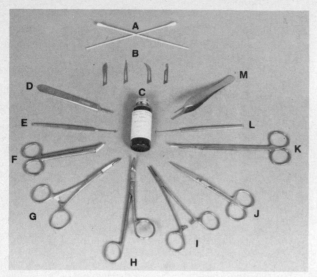

Figure 36–1. Basic instruments for plastic and reconstructive surgery. *A*, Cotton-tipped applicator sticks. *B*, Assortment of Bard-Parker scalpel blades. *C*, Methylene blue. *D*, No. 3 Bard-Parker scalpel handle. *E*, Cottle skin hook. *F*, Suture-wire scissors. *G*, Olsen-Hegar combined needle holder and scissors. *H*, Gillies combined needle holder and scissors. *I*, Derf ophthalmic needle holders. *J*, Straight, sharp, Mayo scissors. *K*, Curved Metzenbaum scissors. *L*, Converse skin hook. *M*, Brown-Adson tissue forceps, 1 × 2 delicate teeth.

referred to other sources for information on the types of suture materials as available and their properties.[4, 5, 43, 46]

Placement of Sutures

For suture placement, the skin edges are manipulated atraumatically using either fingers, skin hooks, or fine-toothed tissue forceps.[46] The goal in skin closure is square skin edges accurately apposed with no overlapping. Slight eversion of the edges helps

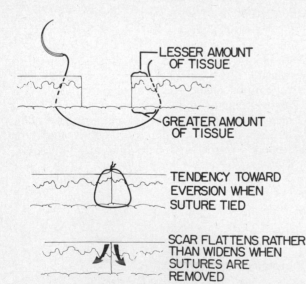

LESSER AMOUNT OF TISSUE

GREATER AMOUNT OF TISSUE

TENDENCY TOWARD EVERSION WHEN SUTURE TIED

SCAR FLATTENS RATHER THAN WIDENS WHEN SUTURES ARE REMOVED

Figure 36–2. Proper placement of a skin suture. (After McGregor, I. A.: *Fundamental Techniques of Plastic Surgery*, 7th ed. Churchill Livingstone, Edinburgh, 1980, p. 20.)

ensure good dermal apposition and avoids inversion of skin edges.[36] The surgeon should strive to maintain contact of the stratum germinativum of both wound edges to prevent a widened scar. Since the epidermis is quite thin, the skin edges should be accurately opposed.[11]

The curved needle with swaged suture attached is passed through the tissue in a rolling fashion at a slight angle so that a greater bite is taken in the deeper dermis.[36] As the needle passes through the second side of the wound, it again passes at an angle to include more tissue in the deeper part of the wound[3, 7, 11–14, 36, 46] (Fig. 36–2). This helps prevent inversion of the skin edges. In general, the distance between the needle puncture site and the wound edge should equal the skin's thickness.[7] However, sutures should penetrate the skin a minimum of 5 mm from the wound edge owing to diminished tissue strength within this area secondary to collagenolytic activity.[5]

Occasionally, it is necessary to suture wound edges of unequal thickness or wound edges that do not lie on the same level. If skin edges are of unequal thickness, both edges should be undermined at the same depth in the superficial subcutaneous tissue. A flap of subcutaneous tissue of the desired thickness can be prepared beneath the thicker side and advanced under the thinner side, where it will be sutured to bring the skin edges to the same level.[25, 46] Another technique of elevating the lower skin edge is to pass the suture needle down through the higher side and up through the lower side, catching a small amount of subcutaneous tissue with the needle to elevate the lower skin edge.[19, 46] When wound edges are uneven because of an angular cut through the skin and cannot be trimmed to lie at right angles to the surface, they can be sutured by unequal placement of the needle by passing it through the "obtuse" side of the wound near the skin edge and through the "acute" side at some distance from the skin edge.[33]

A useful rule is to place as many sutures as close together as necessary to satisfactorily appose the wound edges. Wounds along tension lines have less tension on them and need fewer sutures compared with wounds across tension lines.[7, 37] Sutures in wounds in thick skin can generally be spaced further apart.[7, 41] Therefore, the distance between sutures varies with the wound type and location and requires judgment for the best and most cosmetic closure.

Suture Knots

The square knot is the most common knot used in surgery. When tying this knot, equal tension should be placed on both suture ends, and the loops should not be twisted, thus assuring a secure square knot.[5, 20] A half-knot on top of the square knot gives added security. If the suture material has a low coefficient of friction, additional throws or a combination of a surgeon's knot and additional throws may be necessary to prevent slippage.[5, 12, 25, 26] Knots should be tied tightly enough to furnish gentle apposition of the skin edges. After the knot is tied, the surgeon should be able to gently pull it up and see a space between the suture loop and tissue, signifying that allowance has been made for normal postoperative swelling.[5]

Ideally, the knot is not placed over the incision. Knots are placed on the side of the incision *away* from (1) vital structures, (2) sources of contamination, and (3) any structure that may be irritated. Knots are placed on the side of the incision that (1) has a better blood supply, (2) is the recipient side, not the flap side, (3) is most cosmetically acceptable, (4) facilitates suture placement, and (5) facilitates leveling of skin edges.[39] Skin sutures should be left 10 to 15 mm long to facilitate removal.[5]

Sutures tied too tightly can lead to cut or torn tissues, excessive exudation, strangulation and subsequent necrosis of tissues, delayed healing, pain, infection, wound disruption, and unsightly scars.[2] There are two kinds of suture tension: intrinsic and extrinsic. Intrinsic tension is the constricting tension within the suture loop and is dependent on the tightness of the suture in relation to the encircled mass of tissue. Pressure, ischemia, necrosis, and scarred suture marks can result. The size of the suture material and the amount of tissue included in the suture also affect intrinsic tension. The heavier the suture material, the easier it is to apply greater tension. The greater the amount of tissue enclosed in the suture, the greater the force necessary to appose the wound edges.[15, 46]

Extrinsic tension is tension from outside the suture loop. These are tensions applied to cut surfaces themselves. Any forces applied to cut surfaces are transmitted through the sutures to the tissues encompassed by them.[15, 46]

To avoid excess tension on skin sutures, dead space and large tissue gaps should be eliminated by the use of subcutaneous sutures, "walking" sutures, and/or intradermal sutures prior to the placement of the skin sutures. Fine suture material should be used to close the skin, e.g., 3/0 to 4/0 in dogs.[25, 46] Instrument ties should be used for greater finesse in tension regulation and knot placement.[32, 36]

Basic Suture Patterns

Subcuticular and Intradermal Sutures

Subcuticular sutures are placed in the subcutaneous tissues. They have three essential roles: (1) elimination of dead space, (2) reduction of tension across the wound margin before placing skin sutures, and (3) approximation of wound margins.[12, 36, 46] A simple continuous subcuticular suture is placed by burying the knot and closing the subcuticular tissues in a simple continuous suture pattern. Several small bites are taken in the subcutaneous tissue on each side of the wound, with occasional bites being taken in underlying tissues to close dead space[32] (Fig. 36–3A).

The subcuticular suture is related to the intradermal suture, which is placed in the lower dermis or in the area where dermis and subcutis blend.[2] Intradermal sutures may be interrupted with buried knots or they may be continuous. The first bite of the interrupted suture is placed from deep to superficial in the subcutis and deep dermis. The direction of needle passage is reversed for the second bite on the opposite side of the wound. When tied, the suture is basically upside down and the knot is buried in the subcutaneous tissue[5, 12–14, 32, 41, 46] (Fig. 36–3B).

With the continuous intradermal suture, the needle is passed horizontally through the dermis, taking small bites alternately from each side. The entrance site of each bite is slightly behind the previous point of exit to prevent the two sites from being directly opposite one another[5, 12, 25, 32, 46] (Fig. 36–3C). If this suture is to be removed at a later date, removal can be facilitated by passing the suture

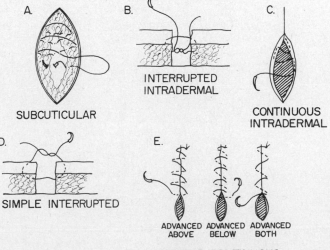

Figure 36–3. Basic suture patterns for skin surgery. *A*, Continuous subcuticular. *B*, Interrupted intradermal. *C*, Continuous intradermal. *D*, Simple interrupted. *E*, Simple continuous sutures that advance above the skin, below the skin, or both.

through the skin to the outside at intervals along its length.[7, 14, 25, 46]

Simple Interrupted Sutures. The most common pattern for skin closure is the simple interrupted suture. Each suture is a single loop of suture material passed perpendicular to the plane of the tissues, with the ends emerging on opposite sides of the wound (Fig. 36–3D).

Simple Continuous Sutures. The simple continuous suture pattern is a progressive series of sutures inserted perpendicular to the plane of the tissues without interruption, with only the two ends of the suture tied. These sutures can be placed so that the suture advances above or below the skin or both (Fig. 36–3E). This suture pattern provides adequate rapid closure of subcutaneous tissue.[2, 5, 32, 46] This suture can also provide rapid skin closure, which is useful for closing extensive skin defects; however, continuous sutures are not as secure as interrupted sutures.

Vertical Mattress Sutures. A vertical mattress suture is a loop of suture material placed perpendicular to the tissue plane with both suture ends emerging on the same side of the wound (Fig. 36–4A). It is useful as both a tension suture and an everting skin suture. In the presence of minor skin tension, it can be used in combination with simple interrupted sutures to close a wound. Vertical mattress sutures are generally removed three to four days postoperatively when used in this fashion. These sutures are indicated after considerable skin loss, for wounds over joints, when wounds are liable to swell, and when delayed healing is expected.[2, 5, 7, 18, 25, 32, 46]

Interrupted Horizontal Mattress Sutures. These sutures are placed in the same plane as the tissue, with both ends of the suture emerging on the same side of the wound (Fig. 36–4B). They evert skin edges, close dead space, and relieve tension. Owing to their geometric configuration, they may tend to cut through the skin and impair the blood supply to the wound edges.[5, 7, 11, 13, 18, 25, 32, 46] A half-buried horizontal mattress suture is effective in closing the point of a V-shaped wound or skin flap. The portion of suture in the point of the V passes intradermally in a horizontal plane to help prevent necrosis in the tip of the V[12, 18, 25, 36] (Fig. 36–4C).

Continuous Lock Sutures. The continuous lock suture pattern is a progressive series of sutures inserted in the same plane as the tissue, with the needle passing over the unused suture material after each suture (Fig. 36–4D). This suture pattern has the advantage over simple continuous sutures of greater stability in the event of partial failure.[32, 36, 46] It has the additional advantage of allowing rapid skin closure.

Staples

Tissue stapling devices,*† have been used for skin closure.[5, 21, 27, 40, 46] A disposable skin stapler* provides an everted, accurate skin closure, is easily mastered, and is faster and more convenient than conventional suturing.[21, 40] However, the high cost of the equipment and sutures is a significant disadvantage.

Although the manufacturer does not recommend resterilization of the staple device, an activated dialdehyde solution of isopropyl alcohol can be successfully used to disinfect the staples and stapler if all the staples are not used at one surgery.[40] Microscopic comparison of canine skin wounds closed with stainless steel staples and with synthetic woven sutures revealed less reaction and inflammation in stapled incisions. Granulation tissue was more mature and epithelial regeneration was greater in stapled wounds.[27]

Undermining and Advancing Skin

Undermining Techniques

Undermining is indicated when a wound is too large to close with tension sutures and stents alone but is not large enough to warrant the use of a skin flap. The procedure frees skin from its subcutaneous attachments and allows the use of its full elastic potential in stretching it to cover a defect.[11, 48, 51] Blunt undermining can be accomplished with the blunt end of a scalpel handle or by opening blunt-pointed scissor blades under the skin. Snipping the subcutaneous tissues with scissor blades as they move through the tissues and cutting the subcutaneous tissues with a scalpel blade are examples of sharp undermining.[46, 48, 51] Undermining on the trunk and

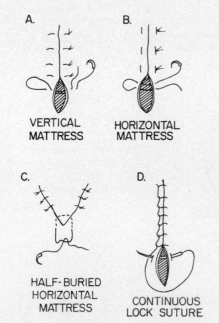

Figure 36–4. Basic suture patterns for skin surgery (continued). *A,* Interrupted vertical mattress. *B,* Interrupted horizontal mattress. *C,* Half-buried horizontal mattress. *D,* Continuous lock suture.

---

*Proximate, Ethicon Inc., distributed by Pitman-Moore, Washington's Crossing, NJ.

†Autosuture, U.S. Surgical Corp., Norwalk, CT.

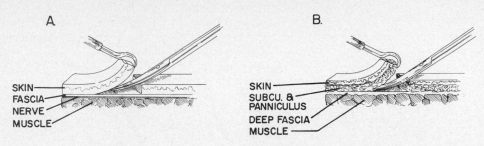

Figure 36–5. Undermining techniques. *A*, Undermining on the face should be just under the dermis and platysma muscle to avoid damage to the facial nerve and vessels. *B*, Undermining on the trunk should be under the panniculus carnosus muscle. (After McGregor, I. A.: *Fundamental Techniques of Plastic Surgery*, 7th ed. Churchill Livingstone, Edinburgh, 1980, p. 13.)

limbs should be relatively deep between the subcutaneous tissue and deep fascia. On the face, undermining should be just beneath the dermis (and associated platysma muscle) to avoid damage to branches to the facial nerve and vessels (Fig. 36–5*A*). On the trunk, undermining should be under the panniculus carnosus muscle[36, 46, 48, 51] (Fig. 36–5*B*). Direct cutaneous vessels coming from underlying tissues to supply the skin are left intact when undermining. Skin around a wound should be undermined the width of the wound on each side of the wound. If the edges still cannot be apposed, undermining should be extended another 50 per cent.[11] Undermining one-half the wound's length on either side of a fusiform defect has been advocated to facilitate closure.[24]

Walking Sutures

Walking sutures are indicated for closing both large and small wounds in dogs and cats. They are particularly useful in areas where the skin is loosely attached (i.e., on the trunk). The skin is undermined around the wound, leaving intact any large blood vessels coming from underlying tissues to the dermis. Using 2-0 or 3-0 absorbable suture material, the first walking suture is placed near the junction of the

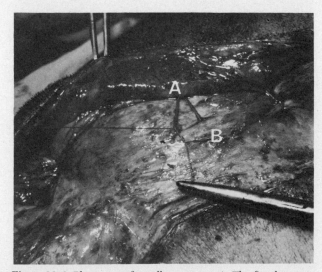

Figure 36–6. Placement of a walking suture. *A*, The first bite is in the deeper dermis. *B*, The second bite is in the underlying fascia toward the center of the wound. (From Swaim, S. F.: *Surgery of Traumatized Skin: Management and Reconstruction in the Dog and Cat.* W. B. Saunders Co., Philadelphia, 1980, p. 303.)

undermined skin with the underlying tissue. Each suture is placed by passing the needle in the deeper portion of the dermis first, followed by a second bite in the underlying tissue *toward* the center of the wound. Tying the suture advances the skin slightly toward the wound's center (Fig. 36–6). Walking sutures are placed in rows, which gradually advance the skin over the wound. After placing two or three rows of walking sutures, the skin has usually been advanced halfway across the defect. The same procedure is repeated on the opposite side of the wound, with the final result almost complete wound closure. A simple continuous subcuticular suture of 2-0 or 3-0 absorbable suture material is placed along the wound edge, and simple interrupted skin apposition sutures complete the skin closure. Walking sutures have the advantages of (1) moving skin from the area around the defect to cover the defect, (2) obliterating dead space, and (3) evenly distributing tension to the tissues around the wound rather than concentrating tension at the wound's edge.[45, 46, 48, 49, 51]

Cosmetic Closure of Variously Shaped Wounds

Fusiform Defects

Most skin lesions can be corrected by fusiform excision. The proposed excision is outlined around the lesion with methylene blue so that the sides are of equal length and in a 4:1 length:width ratio. After incision, one end of the tissue to be removed is elevated with a layer of subcutaneous tissue, and the tissue is dissected away from its bed.[7, 9, 25, 49, 51] If undermining of surrounding skin is necessary for easier closure, it is performed as previously described, and the wound is closed in two layers (Fig. 36–7).

Fusiform excisions are made parallel to skin tension lines if possible. When uncertain of the direction of tension lines, the surgeon should excise the lesion in a circular pattern. After noting the direction of the long axis of the defect created by the pull of adjacent tension lines, the defect can be remodeled to a fusiform shape with its long axis in the direction of tension.[46] An alternative is to excise the lesion in a circle, close the defect along the lines of least tension, and remove redundant skin at the ends of the closure as needed. The amount of normal skin removed may be less and the resultant scar smaller when using this technique.[17]

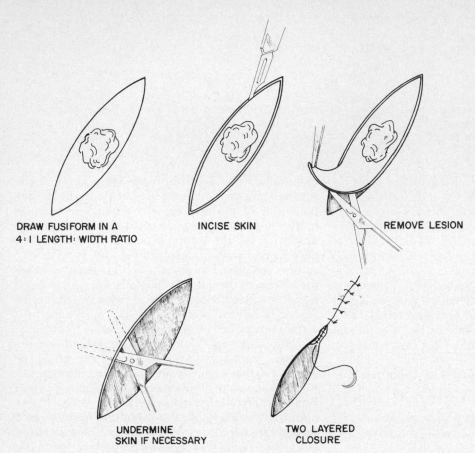

DRAW FUSIFORM IN A
4:1 LENGTH: WIDTH RATIO

INCISE SKIN

REMOVE LESION

Figure 36–7. Fusiform excision of a skin lesion. (Reprinted with permission from Swaim, S. F.: Plastic and reconstructive surgery. *In* Archibald, J. (ed.): *Surgery of the Dog and Cat,* 3rd ed. American Veterinary Publications, Inc., Santa Barbara, CA, in press.)

UNDERMINE
SKIN IF NECESSARY

TWO LAYERED
CLOSURE

If the long axis of a fusiform defect is too short, skin bunches up at the end of the suture line as closure progresses, resulting in a "dog-ear." A dog-ear also forms if one side of the defect is longer than the other. Many dog-ears tend to flatten with time but can be removed at the time of surgery for a more cosmetic closure.[25, 46] Correction techniques for dog-ears resulting from closure of a broad, short ellipse include (1) extending the incision and removing two small triangles of skin,[46] (2) incision along one side of a large dog-ear's base and removal of one large skin triangle,[29a, 36] (3) extension of the fusiform excision,[25]

(4) removal of an arrowhead-shaped piece of skin and closure in the shape of a Y,[25] and (6) a half-Z correction[22] (Fig. 36–8). Dog-ears can be corrected without excision by folding the center of the dog-ear back toward the wound and suturing the two smaller side arms that are created. However, this often results in two smaller dog-ears rather than one large

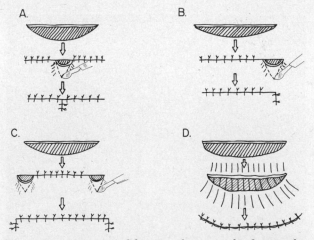

Figure 36–9. Correction of dog-ears when one side of a wound is longer than the other. *A,* Suturing from the ends to the center with the central dog-ear removal. *B,* Suturing from one end to the other with dog-ear removal at one end. *C,* Suturing from the center to the ends with dog-ear removal on both ends. *D,* "Fudging" technique for placing sutures to eliminate dog-ears when discrepancy between sides is small. Sutures are further apart on the longer side of the wound.

Figure 36–8. Techniques for correcting dog-ears. *A,* Removal of small triangles. *B,* Removal of one large triangle. *C,* Extension of the fusiform excision. *D,* Removal of an "arrowhead"-shaped piece of skin. *E,* Half-"Z" correction.

dog-ear. These can be treated in a similar manner, producing four even smaller dog-ears.[22]

Dog-ears that form when closing a defect with one side longer than the other (i.e., a crescent-shaped defect) can be corrected by (1) suturing toward the center and removing a dog-ear in the center of the suture line, (2) suturing toward one end and removing the dog-ear by L-plasty, or (3) suturing from the center to the ends with removal by a double L-plasty.[9, 12, 23, 25, 36, 46, 51] If the discrepancy between the wound edges is small enough such that removal of the dog-ears can be avoided, the "fudging" technique can be used. Sutures are placed closer together on the short side of the wound and farther apart on the long side of the wound[23] (Fig. 36–9). To help equalize the lengths of the sides of an incision when there is little discrepancy between the length of the sides, a skin hook can be placed at each end of the wound and traction applied while suturing.[3]

Triangular, Rectangular, and Square Defects

When located in an area where there is movable skin on all sides of a triangular, rectangular, or square defect, the defect should be closed from the corners toward the center. Suturing progresses around the defect from corner to corner. The result is a Y-shaped scar for triangular closure (Fig. 36–10A), a double Y-shaped scar for rectangular closure (Fig. 36–10B), and an X-shaped scar for square closure[11, 41, 42, 46, 47, 49, 51] (Fig. 36–10C).

Various types of rotation and advancement flaps (i.e., rotation flaps and H-plasty) have been described for closing triangular, square, and rectangular defects (see Chapter 37).[11, 41, 46, 47]

Crescent-Shaped Defects

Closure of crescent-shaped defects entails suturing two skin edges of unequal length, necessitating the removal of dog-ears at some point during the surgery. These defects can be closed as described for fusiform defects (see Fig. 36–9).

Chevron-Shaped Defects

With V-shaped wounds, part of the skin flap may have been lost or will be trimmed with debridement.

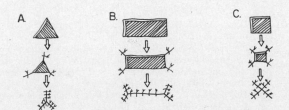

Figure 36–10. Techniques for closing. *A,* Triangular defects. *B,* Rectangular defects. *C,* Square defects. Closure is from the corners to the center of the defect.

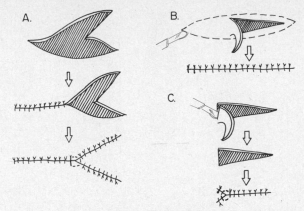

Figure 36–11. Closure of chevron-shaped defects. *A,* Closure from the base with final closure of the two resulting arms. *B,* Conversion of a long narrow flap to a fusiform defect followed by routine closure. *C,* Amputation of the flap followed by Y-shaped closure. (*A* after Dixon, A. C.: The secondary closure of wounds. Vet. Rec. 75:1140, 1963. *B* and *C* after Pullen, C. M.: Reconstruction of the skin. *In* Bojrab, M. J. (ed.): *Current Techniques in Small Animal Surgery.* Lea & Febiger, Philadelphia, 1975, p. 283.)

The resulting chevron-shaped defect is closed in the shape of a Y. Starting at the point of the chevron, suturing is continued until wound tension begins to develop; then the two arms of the Y are closed. A half-buried horizontal mattress suture is placed at the tip of the skin flap to join the three suture lines.[46, 49, 51] (Fig. 36–11A).

Long, narrow, V-shaped flaps may be amputated and the resulting defect transformed to a fusiform shape for closure (Fig. 36–11B). An alternative is to amputate the flap and suture the triangular defect in a Y shape[41, 46, 49] (Fig. 36–11C).

Circular Defects

A technique for closing circular defects so as to avoid dog-ears involves converting the defect to a fusiform shape by removing two triangle-like pieces of skin on opposite sides of the circle with the base of each triangle incorporated into the circle's edge. The defect is then closed as a fusiform defect.[1, 46, 49, 51] The height of each triangle should be equal to the diameter of the circle.[1] With these measurements, there may be one hundred and fifty-six per cent or more normal skin removed[1] (Fig. 36–12A). To obtain a fusiform excision with a 4:1 length:width ratio, the height of the two triangles would have to be one and one-half times the diameter of the circle.

Two similar modifications of the fusiform technique are the double S incision[1] and the bi-winged excision[28] techniques. Only one-half of the triangle-like skin segment is removed from opposite sides of the defect. These techniques require the removal of less normal tissue than that removed in the fusiform closure technique for circular defects. When closing the defect, dog-ear correction may be necessary, as there will be some discrepancy between the lengths of the sides of the wound (Fig. 36–12B).

The bow tie and combined V incision techniques

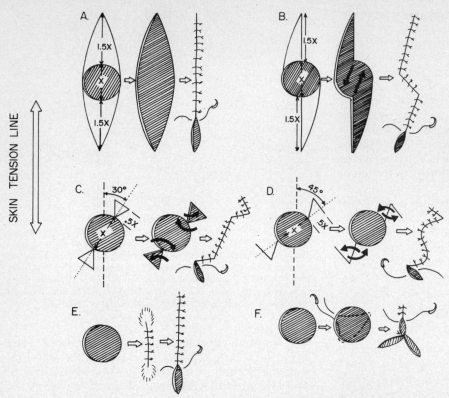

SKIN TENSION LINE

Figure 36–12. Techniques for closing circular wounds. *A*, Fusiform correction. *B*, Double "S" incision. *C*, Bow tie incision. *D*, Combined "V" incision. *E*, Closure along the lines of least tension with removal of dog-ears as needed. *F*, Three-point closure. (*A*, *B*, *C*, and *D* after Alvarado, A.: Reciprocal incisions for closure of circular defects. Plast. Reconst. Surg. 67:484, 1981. *F* after Dixon, A. C.: The secondary closure of wounds. Vet. Rec. 75:1139, 1963.)

also allow closure of circular defects.[1] The bow tie method removes less normal tissue than the fusiform excision and the double S incision. To perform a bow tie closure, two equilateral triangles equal in height to one-half the diameter of the defect are removed from the skin adjacent to the defect. These triangles are on opposite sides of the defect, and their centers are 30° from the axis of skin tension on the circular defect. After removal of the triangles, the defect assumes the shape of a bow tie. The flaps of skin are moved and sutured to shorten the sides of the circle (Fig. 36–12*C*).

The combined V incision requires removal of no normal tissue to close the circular defect. The technique for a combined V incision is the same as that for the bow tie closure, except that the centers of the two equilateral triangles are 45° from the axis of skin tension on the circular defect. Only two sides of the triangle are incised so that the angle created by the incisions points toward the axis of the skin tension. The resulting flaps of skin are moved and sutured to shorten the sides of the circle (Fig. 36–12*D*).

The bow tie and combined V incision procedures work best on smaller defects. There are no dog-ears with the bow tie technique and there is only a slight tendency to form dog-ears with the combined V incision. The larger the defect, the greater the tendency to form dog-ears.

Circular defects may also be closed without modification along the lines of least tension with the removal of dog-ears at the ends of the closure as necessary[17] (Fig. 36–12*E*). This technique generally works best on smaller defects; however, it can be used on larger defects. The tendency to form dog-ears becomes greater with the size of the lesion.

Circular defects may be closed in the shape of an X or Y. Three or four points are selected around the circle and drawn together with an intradermal suture.

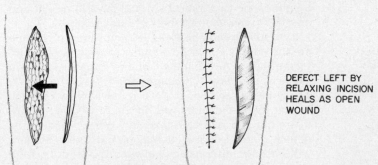

DEFECT LEFT BY RELAXING INCISION HEALS AS OPEN WOUND

Figure 36–13. A simple relaxing incision has been made in the skin adjacent to a defect. The skin between the defect and incision has been moved to close the defect. The new defect heals as an open wound. (Reprinted with permission from Swaim, S. F.: Plastic and reconstructive surgery. *In* Archibald, J. (ed.): *Surgery of the Dog and Cat*, 3rd ed. American Veterinary Publications, Inc., Santa Barbara, CA, in press.)

SIMPLE RELAXING INCISION

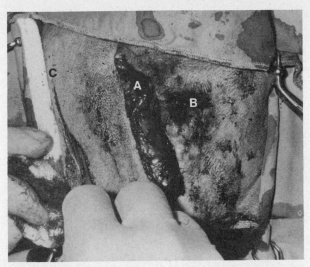

Figure 36–14. Elongated defect (A) adjacent to the anus (B). Closure would have resulted in a slight deviation of the anus. A relaxing incision (C) is being made in the loose skin on the lateral aspect of the leg. (Reprinted with permission from Swaim, S. F.: Management of skin tension in dermal surgery. Comp. Cont. Ed. 2:763, 1980.)

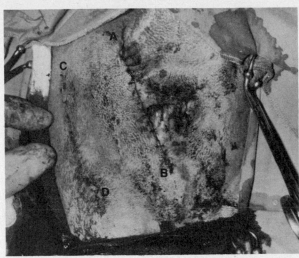

Figure 36–16. Final closure of both defects. A to B, Perianal closure. C to D, Bipedicle flap defect closure. The bipedicle flap defect closed easily because it was in loose skin. (Reprinted with permission from Swaim, S. F.: Management of skin tension in dermal surgery. Comp. Cont. Ed. 2:763, 1980.)

The three or four short arms that are created are sutured with simple interrupted sutures. It may be necessary to remove normal tissue in correcting dog-ears that develop when the points of the circle are drawn together[19, 46, 49, 51] (Fig. 36–12F).

Tension-Relieving Techniques

Relaxing Incisions and Bipedicle Flaps

Simple Relaxing Incision. A simple relaxing incision is made parallel and adjacent to a wound to

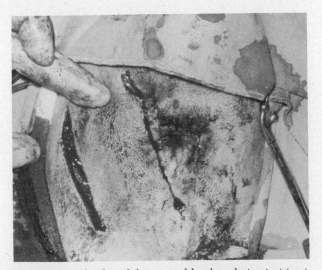

Figure 36–15. The flap of skin created by the relaxing incision in Fig. 36–14C is wider than the original lesion. The flap is undermined and moved to close the perianal defect. (Reprinted with permission from Swaim, S. F.: Management of skin tension in dermal surgery. Comp. Cont. Ed. 2:763, 1980.)

advance the skin between the wound and the incision over the defect. Because of the lack of loose elastic skin in the area, the relaxing incision is left to heal as an open wound. These incisions should be used to close wounds that are too large to close with extensive undermining and yet do not require more involved reconstructive procedures.[11] When relaxing incisions are created on both sides of a defect, the width of each flap should equal the widest part of the defect. The flaps are undermined, advanced over the lesion, and closed with some form of tension suture. Two smaller defects are left in the healthy skin adjacent to the closed defect to heal as open wounds.[11] When only one relaxing incision is used, the defect left after closing the original wound is about as large as the original wound; however, it is in healthy skin and usually heals uneventfully[48, 51] (Fig. 36–13).

Bipedicle Flap. A bipedicle flap is similar to the relaxing incision, but the defect left after closing the original wound is closed because it is in loose, elastic skin (see Chapter 37). These flaps are indicated for chronic wounds surrounded by fibrotic, immovable skin (e.g., chronic decubital ulcer) and for wounds near structures that would be distorted by closure under tension (e.g., eye or anus)[48, 51] (Figs. 36–14, 36–15, and 36–16). When the flap is created in loose elastic skin adjacent to a chronic fibrotic lesion, the incision is parallel to the edge of the lesion with a slight curve toward the lesion.[46, 49, 51] The width of the flap is not as critical if the flap is being created in areas with loose skin. However, the flap is as wide as the defect to be covered. The undermined flap is advanced to close the defect. The secondary defect created after closing the original wound is easily closed because it was made in loose, elastic skin.[48]

V-Y Plasty. This procedure is indicated when there

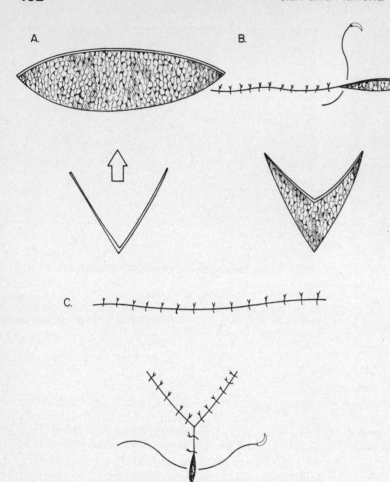

Figure 36–17. V-Y plasty used as a relaxing incision. *A*, "V"-shaped incision with the point of the "V" away from the defect. *B*, The skin flap is undermined and advanced for closure of the defect. *C*, Closure of the "V"-shaped incision in the shape of a "Y". (Reprinted with permission from Swaim, S. F.: Management of skin tension in dermal surgery. Comp. Cont. Ed. 2:764, 1980.)

is sufficient skin adjacent to a wound to allow a Y-shaped closure of a V incision. A V incision is made in the loose elastic skin adjacent to the area where relaxation is needed, with the point of the V away from this area. The skin between the V and the area of needed relaxation is undermined and advanced. The remaining chevron-shaped defect is closed in the shape of a Y[25, 46, 48] (Fig. 36–17).

Z-Plasty

Although Z-plasty is a tension-relieving technique, it will be discussed more thoroughly under Z-Plasty and W-Plasty (see hereafter).

Tension Sutures

Simple Interrupted Tension Sutures. These sutures are indicated for closing wounds with minimal tension. The size of the bite of tissue is alternated when placing the skin approximation sutures (i.e., wide bite, narrow bite, wide bite).[2, 46, 48] If skin edges cannot be apposed with thumb forceps and mild tension, simple interrupted sutures should not be used. Likewise, if a simple interrupted suture causes blanching of the skin beneath the suture when it is tied, it should not be placed[11] (Fig. 36–18A).

Horizontal Mattress Sutures. Horizontal mattress sutures are placed well away from the skin edge in the manner previously described to serve as tension sutures. Placing stents of rubber tubing or buttons under the sutures helps to overcome the tendency of these sutures to cut through the skin and impair circulation at the wound edges.[5, 11, 46, 48] Simple interrupted skin apposition sutures can be used in conjunction with horizontal mattress tension sutures (Fig. 36–18B).

Vertical Mattress Sutures. Vertical mattress sutures are placed at a distance from the wound margin as tension sutures. When wound closure results in significant tension, stents of firm or soft rubber or buttons can be placed under the suture loops.[2, 5, 30, 46, 48] These sutures have less tendency to compromise the circulation at the wound edges than do horizontal mattress sutures[46, 48] and can be used with simple interrupted skin apposition sutures (Fig. 36–18C).

Cruciate Sutures. These tension sutures provide strength and prevent eversion of the wound edges. The needle is inserted from the wound edge on one side and is directed to the opposite side of the wound like a simple interrupted suture. The needle is advanced and crosses the wound without penetrating the tissue. The needle is passed a second time through the tissue parallel to the first passage. The

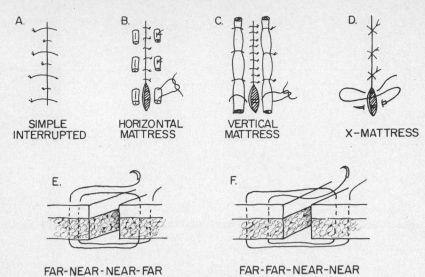

Figure 36–18. Basic tension sutures for skin surgery. *A*, Simple interrupted tension sutures. *B*, Horizontal mattress tension sutures over rubber tubing. *C*, Vertical mattress tension sutures over rubber tubing. *D*, X-mattress tension sutures. *E*, Far-near–near-far suture. *F*, Far-far–near-near suture.

suture ends, which are on opposite sides of the wound, are tied together to form an X on the skin surface[32] (Fig. 36–18D).

Far-Near–Near-Far Sutures. These sutures are placed in the order that their name implies and serve as both approximating and tension sutures.[34, 41, 46, 48] The *far* component serves as the tension suture, and the *near* component serves as the approximating suture. The *far* component of the suture is placed first so that the knot will not lie on the suture line. The *near* component is placed 1 to 2 mm from the *far* component.[41] More suture material is placed in the wound than with other suture patterns, and the surgeon must be careful not to tie the suture too tightly, preventing suture line inversion[32] (Fig. 36–18E).

Far-Far–Near-Near Sutures. This suture is also placed in the order of its name and serves as both a tension and approximating suture. It has also been called a plastic surgeon's suture pattern and is considered a very cosmetic tension suture pattern[11, 46, 48] (Fig. 36–18F).

Z-Plasty and W-Plasty

Dynamics and Design of a Z-Plasty

Z-plasty is the transposition of two interdigitating triangular flaps of skin. The geometric configuration is composed of a central limb and two arms, all of equal length, positioned in the shape of a Z. The angles can vary from 30 to 90°, with 60° being the most common and most workable angle in the skin (Fig. 36–19). The angle sizes are usually equal but can differ.[3, 12, 14, 18, 24, 25, 36, 46, 51]

When the flaps of a Z-plasty are transposed, there is a gain in length in the original direction of the central limb of the Z as the result of a shortening of the skin along the opposite sides of the Z-plasty. There is also a rotation of the axis of the tissues included in the flaps of the Z and a change in the direction of the central limb of the Z[3, 12, 18, 23–25, 36, 46, 48] (Fig. 36–20).

Theoretically, as the angle size of the Z increases, the length along the direction of the original central

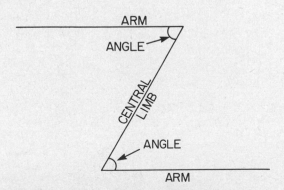

Figure 36–19. Components of a Z-plasty. (From Swaim, S. F.: *Surgery of Traumatized Skin: Management and Reconstruction in the Dog and Cat.* W. B. Saunders Co., Philadelphia, 1980, p. 395.)

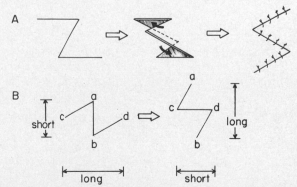

Figure 36–20. *A*, Dynamics of a Z-plasty. *B*, There is gain in length in the direction of the central limb of the "Z". When the flaps are transposed, distance a-b gets longer at the expense of distance c-d. There is a rotation tissue axis included in each flap of the "Z". (Reprinted with permission from Swaim, S. F.: Plastic and reconstructive surgery. *In* Archibald, J. (ed.): *Surgery of the Dog and Cat*, 3rd ed. American Veterinary Publications, Inc., Santa Barbara, CA, in press.)

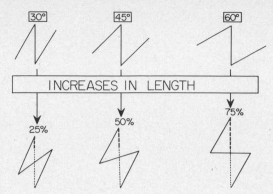

Figure 36–21. Percentage increase in length with various angle sizes. (After Grabb, W. C.: Basic techniques of plastic surgery. *In* Grabb, W. C., and Smith, J. W. (eds.): *Plastic Surgery*, 3rd ed. Little, Brown and Co., Boston, 1979, p. 60.)

limb increases. With a 60° equal angle Z-plasty, the gain in length is 75 per cent (Fig. 36–21). The actual gain in length with a Z-plasty is governed by the length of the central limb of the Z. The longer the tral limb of the Z, the greater the gain in length.[12, 23, 25, 36, 46] The actual gain from a Z-plasty is determined by the skin and scar tissue where it is performed.[14]

Uses of Z-Plasty

Tension Release Along a Web-Like Scar. Z-plasty can be used to release tension along a linear web-like scar across a curved flexor surface, thereby limiting extension of the surface.[16, 24, 25, 31, 36, 41, 46, 48] The Z is designed with the central limb along the linear contracture, and the two arms are usually at 60° angles off opposite sides of this limb. After the Z is incised, the flaps are undermined, transposed, and sutured into their new position (Fig. 36–22). If a band or web of tissue underlies the central limb of the Z, it should be incised.[14, 36]

In some instances in which the tissue of the web-like scar is extensive, e.g., severe burns, it is best to

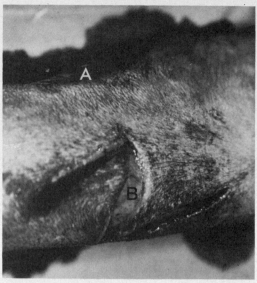

Figure 36–23. *A*, An open wound on a dog's forelimb. *B*, Z-plasty incisions have been made adjacent to the wound. The central limb of the "Z" is in the direction in which relaxation is needed.

remove the scar and use a graft or flap to reconstruct the area rather than use a Z-plasty.[25]

Relaxing Incision. Z-plasty can be used as a relaxing incision to aid in the closure of large defects.[7, 46, 48, 51] Prior to using a Z-plasty in this manner, the skin around the defect is manipulated to determine if there is sufficient skin in one plane to allow relaxation in the perpendicular plane. A Z-plasty with 60° angles is designed adjacent to the defect with the central limb of the Z in the direction in which relaxation is needed. The Z is incised; its flaps and the skin between the Z and the defect are then undermined. The skin can be advanced toward the center of the defect because of the relaxation (gain in length along the direction of the central limb of the Z) provided by the Z-plasty. The original defect is

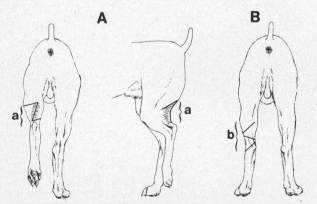

Figure 36–22. *A*, A linear cicatricial contracture (a) across a flexion surface. A Z-plasty is outlined over the contracture. *B*, After transposition of the Z-plasty flaps (b), the contracture is released. (From Swaim, S. F.: *Surgery of Traumatized Skin: Management and Reconstruction in the Dog and Cat.* W. B. Saunders Co., Philadelphia, 1980, p. 396.)

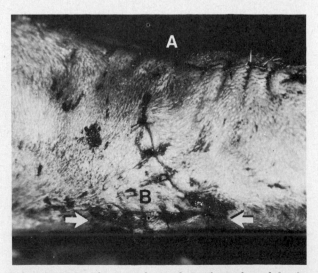

Figure 36–24. *A*, The sutured wound. *B*, The Z-plasty defect has been sutured. The central limb of the "Z" (arrows) has rotated 90°.

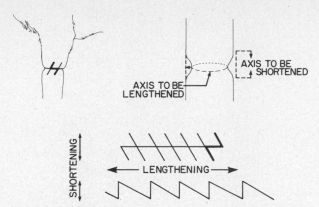

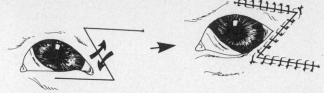

Figure 36–25. Multiple Z-plasties to enlarge the circumference of a constricting scar. (After McGregor, I. A.: The Z-plasty. Br. J. Plast. Surg. 19:86, 1966.)

Figure 36–27. Relocation of the lateral canthus of an eye using a Z-plasty. (After Borges, A. F.: *Elective Incisions and Scar Revision.* Little, Brown and Co., Boston, 1973, p. 47.)

closed followed by closure of the Z-plasty defect[46, 48] (Figs. 36–23 and 36–24).

Relieving Constriction of Circular Scars. The circumference of an encircling constricting scar can be increased (lengthened) by multiple small Z-plasties. The circumference is increased at the expense (shortening) of the tissue on either side of the stricture. A circular incision is made at the depth of the stricture to serve as the central limb of the Z, along which lengthening will occur as the Z-plasty flaps are transposed. Multiple arms are constructed off this central limb to form multiple Z-plasties. As the individual Zs are incised and transposed, the overall length of the central limb is increased, increasing the circumference of the area of constriction[35, 46] (Fig. 36–25).

Z-plasties may be used to enlarge the circumference of an orifice constricted by scar tissue. Double, opposing Z-plasties are applicable in such instances.[10, 14, 38, 51] Two opposing Zs are designed at the periphery of the constricted orifice. The Zs are incised, the flaps are reflected, underlying constricting scar tissue is removed, and the Z-plasty flaps are transposed and sutured (Fig. 36–26).

Alignment of Displaced Structures. Certain structures (e.g., lateral canthus of an eye) that have been distorted because of traumatic scarring or congenital malalignment may be realigned with a Z-

plasty.[7, 16, 25, 46] If the lateral canthus has been displaced by contraction of underlying scar tissue, it may be returned to its natural position by inclusion in one of the Z-plasty flaps. As the flaps are transposed, the canthus is moved back into position[46, 51] (Fig. 36–27).

Changing the Direction of Wounds or Scars. Z-plasty can be used to change the direction of widened linear scars resulting from tension and nonhealing linear wounds. Wound healing is enhanced when the direction of some nonhealing linear wounds is changed. These are wounds in which skin tension or movement of underlying tissues (i.e., bones and joints) has caused poor healing.[46] The direction of the wound can be changed so that it runs parallel to skin tension or runs at a different direction in relation to an underlying bony prominence or joint by making the scar the central limb of a 60° angled Z-plasty. Transposition of the Z-plasty flaps aligns the new central limb of the Z with skin tension lines or changes its direction over a bony prominence or joint (Figs. 36–28 and 36–29; see Fig. 36–32).

W-Plasty

Indications and Principles. A linear scar that has widened because of skin tension can be revised by W-plasty. As with the use of a Z-plasty in realigning

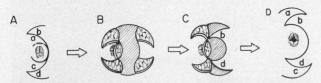

Figure 36–26. Use of two Z-plasties to enlarge a stenotic anal orifice. *A,* Design of the two "Z's" (a, b and c, d). *B,* Lines of the Z-plasties have been incised and the resulting flaps have been reflected. *C,* Transposition of one flap of each of the Z-plasties (b and d). *D,* Transposition of the remaining flap of each of the Z-plasties (a and c). (After Converse, J. M.: Introduction to plastic surgery. *In Reconstructive Plastic Surgery: Principles and Procedures in Correction, Reconstruction and Transplantation,* Vol. 1, 2nd ed. W. B. Saunders Co., Philadelphia, 1977, p. 60.)

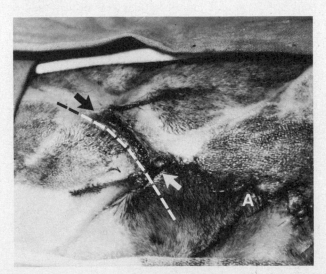

Figure 36–28. A Z-plasty designed with the central limb (arrows) along a linear nonhealing wound on the dorsal border of the scapula (broken line). *A,* A W-plasty correction of a widened scar that connected with one end of the nonhealing wound.

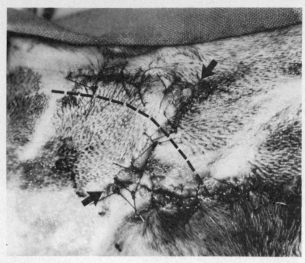

Figure 36–29. After transposition of the Z-plasty flaps, the central limb of the "Z" (arrows) lies perpendicular to the dorsal border of the scapula (broken line).

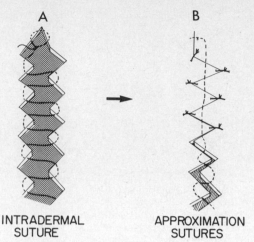

INTRADERMAL   APPROXIMATION
SUTURE   SUTURES

Figure 36–31. *A,* Proper placement of the continuous intradermal suture. *B,* The simple interrupted skin approximation sutures. (After Borges, A. F.: *Elective Incisions and Scar Revision.* Little, Brown and Co., Boston, 1973, p. 188.)

a nonhealing linear wound or scar, the principle of the W-plasty is to realign the scar so that it runs parallel to the lines of skin tension.[3, 7, 8, 14, 25, 29a, 46, 50] The difference is that the W-plasty breaks the scar up into many small segments, whereas the Z-plasty rotates the entire scar.

The ideal scar on which to use a W-plasty is a linear scar that is not depressed or raised above the surrounding skin but crosses lines of skin tension. It should not be used on scars that follow skin lines of tension or that are webbed, grooved, or circularly constricting. The technique should not be used in areas where skin is extremely taut.[29a, 46, 50]

Technique. A W-plasty template made from processed x-ray film is used to trace the W-plasty on either side of the scar (Fig. 36–30). The small triangles of the template are equilateral, and the sides are 7 mm in length. After removing the scar, a simple continuous monofilament suture (polypropylene)* is

*Prolene, Ethicon, Inc., Somerville, NJ.

passed alternately from one side of the wound to the other through each triangular flap so that the flaps pull together in an interdigitating fashion. Final closure is accomplished by placing interrupted sutures through the tip of each triangle[46, 50] (Fig. 36–31). The end result is usually a more cosmetically pleasing scar that is narrower than the original scar[50] (Fig. 36–32).

BANDAGES AND DRESSINGS

The reader is referred to other chapters for information about the bandaging of open wounds. This

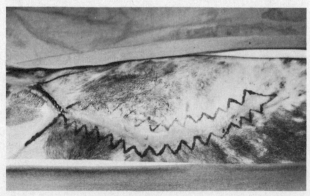

Figure 36–30. A W-plasty has been marked around a widened scar with a Z-plasty on the nonhealing cranial aspect of the lesion. (Reprinted with permission from Swaim, S. F., Faircloth, J. C., and Sutton, H. H.: Evaluation of W-plasty for revision of unesthetic wide scars in small animals. J. Am. Anim. Hosp. Assoc. *18*:305, 1982.)

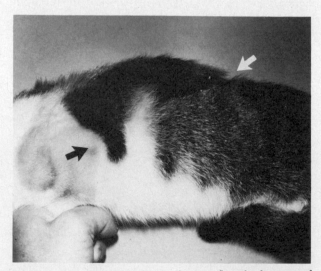

Figure 36–32. Appearance of revised scar and nonhealing wound from Fig. 36–30 six months postoperatively. W-plasty area (arrows) is discernable but not as wide as original scar. The Z-plasty (dorsal to the black arrow) has healed. (Reprinted with permission from Swaim, S. F., Faircloth, J. C., and Sutton, H. H.: Evaluation of W-plasty for revision of unesthetic wide scars in small animals. J. Am. Anim. Hosp. Assoc. 18:305, 1982.)

section deals with bandaging closed skin wounds. The purposes of a bandage are (1) to protect the wound from contamination, (2) to prevent tension on wound margins, (3) to obliterate dead space, (4) to supply sufficient pressure to minimize postoperative hemorrhage and edema, (5) to restrict motion, and (6) to prevent trauma to the wound.[7, 31, 32, 44, 46]

One technique for bandaging wounds into which drains have been placed consists of applying a nonadherent absorbent pad* held in place with a tertiary dressing. If an abundant amount of discharge is expected from the wound, more absorbent dressings† should be placed over the wound prior to placing an outer dressing. These dressings should be changed daily until drainage stops and the drains are removed.[6]

For bandaging closed wounds from which little or no drainage is expected, a nonadherent pad‡ is placed over the suture line, followed by circumferential wrapping of the body part with some type of soft, rolled bandage material§ and a final application of adhesive tape to cover the bandage and anchor it to the hair at either end of the bandage.

Pressure bandages are occasionally indicated to obliterate minor dead space and prevent hematoma or seroma formation.[32, 46] However, such bandages are not a substitute for good surgical technique in closing dead space with sutures. Pressure bandages also provide immobility and splinting. Pressure bandages should be carefully applied to accomplish their purpose and yet not impede circulation, which could lead to severe edema, soft tissue damage, gangrene, and sloughing. A cardinal rule is to avoid pressure rings and pressure points when applying pressure bandages.[32, 46]

Depending on the patient's habits and activities as well as the type and location of the wound, it may be necessary to incorporate a splint into a bandage or cover a bandage with a cast to immobilize an area to improve wound healing. The statement "The younger and more irresponsible the patient, the larger and more secure the bandage must be"[44] also applies to animals.

Frequent examination of bandages is necessary, and they should be changed as necessary. This is especially true when bandages become wet with excreta, since these bandages provide a favorable medium for bacterial growth. Urine on and in bandages is a source of irritation for both the wound and the veterinarian. In my opinion, a bandage with dirt on the outer layer of tape that is clean and dry from that point inward docs not pose as great a threat of infection as does a wet bandage.[46] Although techniques are described using wet saline bandages to treat open infected wounds,[6] bandages on closed wounds should be kept dry.

Attempts may be made to waterproof bandages by applying rubber or plastic sheeting (i.e., rubber glove or plastic bag) over the bandage. Unless these materials are made watertight, they will retain moisture that does enter. A bandage placed inside a plastic or rubber bag should be removed periodically, since normal body moisture accumulates in the bag and moistens the bandage.[46] Rubber bands should not be used to secure rubber or plastic bags over a bandage. They can slip off the bag and up under the patient's hair, remaining unnoticed until their constricting effects become visible.[46]

1. Alvarado, A.: Reciprocal incisions for closure of circular skin defects. Plast. Reconst. Surg. 67:482, 1981.
2. Archibald, J., and Blakely, C. L.: Sutures. In Archibald, J. (ed.): Canine Surgery, 2nd ed. American Veterinary Publications, Inc., Santa Barbara, Cal., 1974.
3. Barron, J. N., and Saad, M. N.: An introduction to operative plastic and reconstructive surgery: General principles and basic techniques. In Barron, J. N., and Saad, M. N. (eds.): Operative Plastic and Reconstructive Surgery. Churchill Livingston, Edinburgh, 1980.
4. Bellenger, C. R.: Sutures, Part I. The purpose of sutures and available suture materials. Comp. Cont. Ed. 4:507, 1982.
5. Bellenger, C. R.: Sutures, Part II. The use of sutures and alternative methods of closure. Comp. Cont. Ed. 4:587, 1982.
6. Bojrab, M. J.: A Handbook on Veterinary Wound Management. The Kendall Co., Boston, 1981.
7. Borges, A. F.: Effective Incisions and Scar Revision. Little, Brown and Co., Boston, 1973.
8. Borges, A. F.: W-plasty. Ann. Plast. Surg. 3:153, 1979.
9. Borges, A. F.: Dog-ear repair. Plast. Reconst. Surg. 69:707, 1982.
10. Bowman, K. F., Swaim, S. F., and Vaughan, J. T.: Double opposing Z-plasty for correction of stenotic nares in a horse. J. Am. Vet. Med. Assoc. 180:772, 1982.
11. Braden, T. D.: Plastic and reconstructive surgery of the canine torso. Vet. Clin. North Am. 9:285, 1979.
12. Chang, W. H. J.: Wound management. In Chang, W. H. J. (ed.): Fundamentals of Plastic and Reconstructive Surgery. Williams and Wilkins, Baltimore, 1980.
13. Chernosky, M. E.: Scalpel and scissors surgery as seen by the dermatologist. In Epstein, E. H., and Epstein, E., Jr. (eds.): Skin Surgery, 4th ed. Charles C Thomas, Springfield, IL., 1977.
14. Converse, J. M.: Introduction to plastic surgery. In Converse, J. M. (ed.): Reconstructive Plastic Surgery: Principles and Procedures in Correction, Reconstruction and Transplantation, Vol. 1, 2nd ed. W. B. Saunders Co., Philadelphia, 1977.
15. Crikelair, G. F.: Skin suture marks. Am. J. Surg. 96:631, 1958.
16. Davis, J. S., and Kitlowski, E. A.: The theory and practical use of the Z-incision for relief of scar contractures. Ann. Surg. 109:1001, 1939.
17. Davis, T. S., Graham, W. P., and Miller, S. H.: The circular excision. Ann. Plast. Surg. 4:21, 1980.
18. Dingman, R. O.: General principles of skin surgery. In Epstein, E. H., and Epstein, E., Jr. (ed.): Skin Surgery, 4th ed. Charles C Thomas, Springfield, IL., 1977.
19. Dixon, A. C.: The secondary closure of wounds. Vet. Rec. 75:1133, 1963.
20. Flinn, R. M.: Knotting in medicine and surgery. Practitioner 183:322, 1959.
21. Georgiade, G., Riefkohl, R., Serafin, D., et al.: Use of skin staples in plastic surgery. Ann. Plast. Surg. 5:324, 1980.
22. Gillies, H., and Millard, D. R.: The Principles and Art of Plastic Surgery, Vol. I, Little, Brown and Co., Boston, 1957.

---

*Telfa Wet-Pruf pads, The Kendall Co., Boston, MA.
†Kerlix sponges, Wet-Pruf pads, The Kendall Co.
‡Telfa nonadherent strips, The Kendall Co.
§Kerlix rolls, The Kendall Co.

23. Gorney, M.: Tissue dynamics and surgical geometry. *In* Kernahan, D. A., and Vistnes, L. M. (eds.): *Biological Aspects of Reconstructive Surgery.* Little, Brown and Co., Boston, 1977.

24. Gourley, I. M., and Snyder, C. C.: Fundamentals of shifting tissues in plastic and reconstructive small animal surgery. Proc. 45th Ann. Mtg. Am. Anim. Hosp. Assoc., 1978.

25. Grabb, W. C.: Basic techniques of plastic surgery. *In* Grabb, W. C., and Smith, J. W. (eds.): *Plastic Surgery,* 3rd ed. Little, Brown and Co., Boston, 1980.

26. Hermann, J. B.: Tensile strength and knot security of surgical suture material. Ann. Surg. 37:209, 1971.

27. Hess, J. L., DeYoung, D. W., Riley, M. G. I., et al.: Comparison of stainless steel staple and synthetic suture material on skin wound healing. J. Am. Anim. Hosp. Assoc. 15:501, 1979.

28. Hirshowitz, B., Kaufman, T., and Amir, I.: Biwinged excision for closure of rounded defect. Ann. Plast. Surg. 5:372, 1980.

29. Hughes, N. C.: Scar excision. *In* Watson, J., and McCormack, R. M. (eds.): *Operative Surgery: Fundamental International Techniques: Plastic Surgery,* 3rd ed. Butterworths, Boston, 1979.

29a. Hughes, N. C.: Excision of tumors with direct closure of defect. *In* Watson, J., and McCormack, R. H. (eds.): *Operative Surgery: Fundamental International Techniques, Plastic Surgery,* 3rd ed. Butterworths, Boston, 1979.

30. Johnston, D. E.: Hygroma of the elbow in dogs. J. Am. Vet. Med. Assoc. 16:213, 1975.

31. Johnston, D. E.: The healing process in open wounds. Comp. Cont. Ed. 1:789, 1979.

32. Knecht, C. D., Allen, A. R., Williams, D. J., et al.: *Fundamental Techniques in Veterinary Surgery,* 2nd ed. W. B. Saunders Co., Philadelphia, 1981.

33. Knowles, R. P.: Injuries to skin, muscle and tendon. *In* Some Techniques and Procedures in Small Animal Surgery. Veterinary Medicine Publishing Co., Inc., Bonner Springs, KS., 1963.

34. Larsen, J. S., and Ulin, A. W.: Tensile strength advantage of the far-and-near suture technique. Surg. Gynecol. Obstet. 131:123, 1970.

35. McGregor, I. A.: The Z-plasty. Br. J. Plast. Surg. 19:82, 1966.

36. McGregor, I. A.: *Fundamental Techniques of Plastic Surgery,* 7th ed. Churchill Livingstone, Edinburgh, 1981.

37. McGuire, M. F.: Studies of the excisional wound: I. Biomechanical effects of undermining and wound orientation on closing tension and work. Plast. Reconst. Surg. 66:419, 1980.

38. Muhlbauer, W. D.: Elongation of mouth in post-burn microstomia by a double Z-plasty. Plast. Reconst. Surg. 45:400, 1970.

39. Noe, J. M.: Where should the knot be placed? Ann. Plast. Surg. 5:145, 1980.

40. Porter, D. B.: A clinical evaluation of the Proximate stapling system for closing skin incisions. Vet. Med./Sm. Anim. Clin. 76:320, 1981.

41. Pullen, C. M.: Reconstruction of the skin. *In* Bojrab, M. J. (ed.): *Current Techniques in Small Animal Surgery.* Lea & Febiger, Philadelphia, 1975.

42. Spreull, J. S. A.: The principles of transplanting skin in the dog. J. Am. Anim. Hosp. Assoc. 4:71, 1968.

43. Stashak, T. S., and Yturraspe, D. J.: Considerations for selection of suture materials. Vet. Surg. 7:48, 1978.

44. Straith, R. E., Lawson, J. M., and Hipps, J. C.: The subcuticular suture. Postgrad. Med. 29:164, 1961.

45. Swaim, S. F.: A "walking" suture technique for closure of large skin defects in the dog and cat. J. Am. Anim. Hosp. Assoc. 12:597, 1976.

46. Swaim, S. F.: *Surgery of Traumatized Skin: Management and Reconstruction in the Dog and Cat.* W. B. Saunders Co., Philadelphia, 1980.

47. Swaim, S. F., Henderson, R. A., and Sutton, H. H.: Correction of triangular and wedge shaped skin defects in dogs and cats. J. Am. Anim. Hosp. Assoc. 16:225, 1980.

48. Swaim, S. F.: Management of skin tension in dermal surgery. Comp. Cont. Ed. 2:758, 1980.

49. Swaim, S. F.: Trauma to the skin and subcutaneous tissues of dogs and.cats. Vet. Clin. North Am. 10:599, 1980.

50. Swaim, S. F.: Evaluation of W-plasty for revision of unesthetic wide scars in small animals. J. Am. Anim. Hosp. Assoc. 18:299, 1982.

51. Swaim, S. F.: Plastic and reconstructive surgery. *In* Archibald, J. (ed.): *Surgery of the Dog and Cat.* American Veterinary Publications Inc., Santa Barbara, Calif., in press.

Chapter 37   Pedicle Grafts

Michael M. Pavletic

INTRODUCTION

Plastic and reconstructive surgery deals with the repair of defects and malformations of a congenital or acquired nature.[4, 14] Pedicle grafts (skin flaps) play an instrumental role in this expanding area of veterinary surgery.

A pedicle graft is a portion of skin and subcutaneous tissue with a vascular attachment moved from one area of the body to another. The word *flap* denotes a tongue of tissue, whereas the term *pedicle* denotes its base or stem. Thus, the term *pedicle flap* is redundant and is best avoided.[14, 35, 36]

Properly developed flaps survive because of their intact circulation, unlike free grafts, which depend on revascularization from the recipient bed. Flaps with intact pedicles are also capable of improving circulation to ischemic areas.[35, 36] As a result, pedicle grafts can be used to cover defects with poor vascularity, areas difficult to immobilize, holes overlying cavities, and areas where padding and durability are essential (see Fig. 37–17).[14, 35, 36] They are equally valuable for the immediate coverage and protection of nerves, vessels, tendons, and other structures susceptible to exposure and trauma.[87] A skin flap has even been used to reconstruct the cervical esophagus in a dog.[80]

The loose, elastic skin over the head, neck, and trunk of the dog and cat permits its mobilization for wound closure. Large flaps can often be elevated without creating a secondary defect not amenable to primary closure.[6, 77, 79, 85] This is in contrast to humans, in whom a free skin graft is usually required to close the donor bed after major flap transfer.[14, 35, 36]

Cosmetic results in the dog and cat depend on the transfer of hairy skin with a color and pattern of hair growth similar to that of the recipient area. In comparison, cosmetic results in man depend on matching skin of similar color, texture, and thickness without transplanting hairy skin into non–hair-bearing areas.[14, 35, 36] Unfortunately, cost is a major consideration when selecting the method of wound closure in veterinary medicine, with the simplest (and, therefore, least expensive) means of closure to restore function to the area often a more important consideration than appearance. Fortunately, hair growth variations usually do not deter owners from choosing pedicle grafts; any hair growth is more acceptable than no hair growth in fur-bearing animals.

Pedicle grafts from areas adjacent to the recipient bed remain the most practical method of closing wounds not amenable to direct closure. This differs from human reconstructive surgery, in which a free graft is generally preferable to local and distant flaps.[14, 35, 36] As a rule, major skin losses of the lower extremities in the dog and cat are not readily amenable to local flaps owing to a lack of loose skin.[87, 102] Other options for lower limb restoration include the direct or indirect transfer of distant flaps and free grafts.[2, 5–7, 52, 59, 87, 99, 102–105, 114] It must be emphasized, however, that healing by second intention (contraction and epithelialization) remains a valuable and practical method of closing major contaminated and infected wounds in small animals.[79, 102] When used properly, flaps can bypass many of the potential problems associated with contraction and epithelialization, including prolonged healing time and wound care, nonhealing, excessive scarring, a fragile epithelialized surface more prone to re-injury, wound contracture, compromised venous return distal to the injury, and the direct exposure of important underlying structures until healing occurs (see Fig. 37–19).[79, 81, 83, 87, 102] The choice of the method employed ultimately rests with the judgment and experience of the veterinarian. Economic considerations, however, do not give the veterinarian license to select a closure technique contrary to sound surgical principles.

The dog and rabbit were the first experimental animals employed to study vascular changes in tubed flaps.[30, 110] Further research with dogs, rats, rabbits, and swine has been subsequently utilized to study skin circulation.[35] In recent years, significant differences have been noted between species.[19, 35, 36, 78, 82] Researchers currently use swine for most human-related research in plastic surgery because of similarities in their cutaneous circulation and their lower cost compared with primates.[19, 35, 36, 66, 67, 78] Discretion is required before the veterinary surgeon extrapolates surgical techniques and research data between species.[19, 35] For example, although the successful clinical use of subcutaneous pedicle flaps has been reported in the dog, experimental and anatomical studies have indicated that this human pedicle grafting technique carries an unreasonably high incidence of necrosis in dogs unless a portion of the panniculus muscle layer or a direct cutaneous artery and vein maintain circulation to the island of skin. Therefore, subcutaneous pedicle flaps have no practical clinical advantage in the dog over simpler, safer flap techniques that make use of the loose skin available for wound closure.[82]

This chapter covers the major flaps available to reconstruct skin defects of various sizes in the dog and cat. Not all the pedicle grafts discussed in the literature are presented in this chapter. I have selected the common and advanced pedicle grafting techniques most relevant to the veterinary surgeon.

FLAP CLASSIFICATION

In general, flaps can be categorized according to (1) circulation, (2) various forms of compound or composite flaps, and (3) location in relation to the recipient bed.[14, 35, 36, 86, 102] In man, flaps are also classified according to the anatomical region to which the flap is moved.[14, 35, 36]

Flap Classification Based on Blood Supply

Most pedicle grafts employed in the dog and cat are elevated without including a direct cutaneous artery and vein. Flap survival is dependent on the deep or subdermal plexus entering the base of the flap. I have termed this a *subdermal plexus flap* to distinguish it from the *random or cutaneous flap* in humans and swine, which is dependent upon musculocutaneous vessels perpendicular to the skin (Figs. 37–1 and 37–2).[78, 79] The subdermal plexus in the dog and cat is fed by terminal branches of direct cutaneous arteries, both of which are associated with the panniculus muscle layer (panniculus carnosus).[78, 79] However, in the middle to distal portions of the

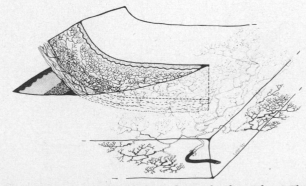

Figure 37–1. The subdermal plexus flap in the dog and cat. This flap is analogous to the random or cutaneous flap in persons. The flap is nourished by the subdermal plexus and attenuated branches of the direct cutaneous vessels some distance away. (Reprinted with permission from Pavletic, M. M.: Canine axial pattern flaps, using the omocervical, thoracodorsal, and deep circumflex iliac direct cutaneous arteries. Am. J. Vet. Res. *42*:391, 1981.)

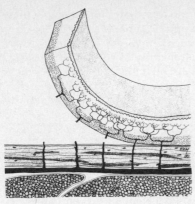

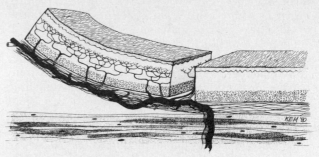

Figure 37–2. The random or cutaneous flap in man. Note the musculocutaneous vessels at the base of the flap (pedicle) supplying the circulation to the length of the flap. (Reprinted with permission from Pavletic, M. M.: Canine axial pattern flaps, using the omocervical, thoracodorsal, and deep circumflex iliac direct cutaneous arteries. Am. J. Vet. Res. 42:391, 1981.)

Figure 37–4. Island arterial flap or island axial pattern flap in the dog. Note that the graft is nourished solely by the direct cutaneous artery and vein. Island flaps have greater mobility than axial pattern flaps. Vessels have the potential to be severed and re-anastomosed with microvascular surgery at a distant recipient site. (Reprinted with permission from Pavletic, M. M.: Canine axial pattern flaps, using the omocervical, thoracodorsal, and deep circumflex iliac direct cutaneous arteries. Am. J. Vet. Res. 42:391, 1981.)

extremities where the panniculus muscle is lacking, they are associated with the undersurface of the dermis.[24, 82, 87]

A pedicle graft incorporating a direct cutaneous artery and vein is termed an *axial pattern flap* (arterial pedicle graft) (Fig. 37–3).[14, 35, 36, 77–79, 81, 85] Axial pattern flaps have an excellent blood supply and a surviving area approximately 50 per cent greater than that of subdermal plexus flaps of comparable dimension in the dog.[78, 79] A "delay procedure" required to enhance the circulation to long subdermal plexus flaps prior to transfer is rarely indicated with properly developed axial pattern flaps.[79] A delay procedure, however, may be employed to enhance circulation to the terminal or dependent portion of an extremely long axial pattern flap to assure its survival.[35, 38, 40, 108]

Variations of the axial pattern flap include the *island arterial flap* (island axial pattern flap) (Fig.

37–4), the *secondary axial pattern flap*, and the *free flap*. An island arterial flap is a segment or island of skin nourished only by a direct cutaneous artery and vein.[14, 35, 36, 64, 77–79] Secondary axial pattern flaps are created by positioning skin flaps over tissue that includes a major artery or vein.[14, 22, 35, 36, 41, 95, 112] The skin can be transferred once healing and vascularization occur between the skin and its new blood supply. A free skin flap is formed by dividing the direct cutaneous vessels of an island arterial flap or vessels of the secondary axial pattern flap and re-anastomosing their vascular pedicle to an artery and vein at the recipient site.[14, 19, 32, 35, 36, 60, 64, 79]

Another variation of the axial pattern flaps is the canine reverse saphenous conduit flap (see Fig. 37–28).[87] Saphenous arterial branches and associated branches of the medial saphenous vein are elevated along with the direct cutaneous vessels that supply and drain the overlying skin. Distal arterial and venous anastomotic connections maintain a reversal of arterial and venous flow through the flap's saphenous conduit, thus enabling the flap to be elevated and rotated to skin defects at or below the tarsal joint.[87]

Compound and Composite Flaps

A *compound flap* or *composite flap* denotes the elevation and transfer of flaps that incorporate skin with other tissues including muscle, fat, bone, and cartilage.[14, 35, 36, 60] Compound flaps created by the submuscular elevation of a muscle segment and overlying skin as a unit (*myocutaneous* or *musculocutaneous flaps*) have been effectively employed in human reconstructive surgery (Fig. 37–5).[14, 35, 36, 79] The resultant flap may be transferred without resorting to a *delay procedure* to enhance its cutaneous circulation as long as the muscle's blood supply is preserved to nourish the skin through the musculocutaneous vessels.[14, 35, 36]

Musculocutaneous flaps based on the submuscular

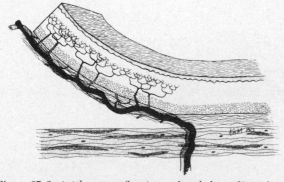

Figure 37–3. Axial pattern flap (arterial pedicle graft) in the dog and cat. A flap created over the direct cutaneous vessels has an intact blood supply capable of supporting a flap of considerable size. An axial pattern flap in humans is similar with the exception of their poorly developed panniculus muscle. (Reprinted with permission from Pavletic, M. M.: Canine axial pattern flaps, using the omocervical, thoracodorsal, and deep circumflex iliac direct cutaneous arteries. Am. J. Vet. Res. 42:391, 1981.)

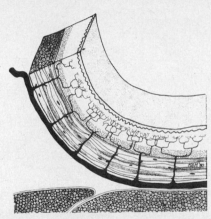

Figure 37–5. Myocutaneous flap in man. The skin is nourished by musculocutaneous vessels, which receive circulation from the intact skeletal muscle vasculature (Reprinted with permission from Pavletic, M. M.: Canine axial pattern flaps, using the omocervical, thoracodorsal, and deep circumflex iliac direct cutaneous arteries. Am. J. Vet. Res. *42*:391, 1981.)

elevation of the gracilis muscle and a portion of the latissimus dorsi muscle with the overlying skin have been used for microvascular studies in dogs.[42, 96, 107] Secondary or revascularized musculocutaneous flaps have also been developed in research dogs by suturing skin to portions of the adductor and sartorius muscles.[23, 95] Vascularization subsequently occurs between the muscle-dermal interface, allowing the successful transfer of the muscle and attached island of skin to another region as a free flap.

Other examples of composite flaps in the dog include the labial advancement flap for full thickness

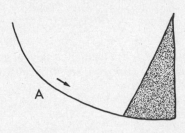

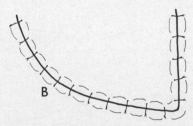

Figure 37–6. The rotation flap is a semicircular pedicle graft for triangle-shaped defects (recipient beds). Two rotation flaps could be developed on each side of a large triangular defect to facilitate closure.

rostral labial defects (see Fig. 37–29) and the composite mucocutaneous subdermal plexus flap for complete lower eyelid reconstruction (see Chapter 101).[83, 84] By strict definition, skin flaps elevated in the dog and cat with subcutaneous fat and panniculus muscle could be considered composite flaps.[42, 60]

The routine elevation of major skeletal muscles to transfer the overlying skin is fortunately unnecessary in the dog and cat. The ample amount of loose, elastic skin available and the comparable ease of elevating axial pattern flaps preclude their routine clinical use.[79]

Flap Classification Based on Location with the Recipient Bed

Pedicle grafts developed adjacent to the recipient bed are termed *local flaps*, whereas flaps transferred from a distant region are termed *distant flaps*.[14, 35, 36, 86, 91, 102, 114]

Local Flaps

Techniques employing local flaps are the most practical method of closing defects that cannot be approximated by simple undermining and suturing.[86] The effective use of these flaps usually depends on forming a flap in a neighboring area where loose, elastic skin prevails. Thus, any secondary defect created by the shifting of a flap to the defect can be closed. Local flaps are both simple and economical. They are more able to maintain a similar pattern of hair growth and color than distant flaps. Local flaps are of two basic types: (1) flaps that rotate about a pivot point (rotating flaps), and (2) flaps that travel in a forward direction without lateral movement (advancement flaps).[14, 35, 36, 86, 102]

Rotating Flaps

Rotation flaps, transposition flaps, and interpolation flaps are the three basic flaps that rotate on a pivot point.[14, 35, 36, 102]

The rotation flap is a semicircular flap that rotates into the adjacent recipient bed (Fig. 37–6). Single or paired flaps can be employed to close triangular defects.[102] As a general rule, no secondary defect is created with the rotation flap in the dog and cat.

The transposition flap is a rectangular pedicle graft elevated and rotated into defects, usually within 90° of the wound's axis (Fig. 37–7; see Fig. 37–16).[14, 35, 36, 59, 86, 91, 102] Transposition flaps can be rotated up to 180° of a defect, but considerable shortening of the flap occurs the more the flap is rotated, a fact that must be kept in mind during planning.[14, 35, 36, 86, 102] The transposition flap is the most useful of the rotating flaps. Z-plasty, a modification of the transposition flap, is discussed in Chapter 36.

The interpolation flap is a rectangular flap rotated into a nearby, but not immediately adjacent, defect (Fig. 37–8). A portion of the flap must pass over the

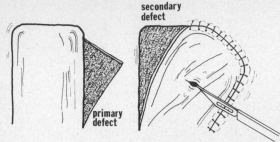

Figure 37–7. Transposition flap adjacent to the primary defect. The secondary defect is closed by undermining the skin edges for closure. If the dimensions have been misjudged, a stab incision may be made along the "line of greatest tension" to allow graft expansion without undue tension. The hole is allowed to heal by second intention. (Redrawn from Grabb, W. C., and Smith, J. W.: *Plastic Surgery*, 3rd ed. Little, Brown, Boston, 1979.)

skin between the donor and recipient beds. The exposed subcutaneous surface is either left exposed or covered temporarily with a free graft.[14, 35, 36, 102] The redundant portion of the flap is usually excised after healing to the recipient defect is complete.

Advancement Flaps

The single pedicle advancement flap, bipedicle advancement flap, and the V-Y advancement flap are examples of pedicle grafts moved forward into a wound without lateral movement (Fig. 37–9).[14, 35, 36, 102] The single pedicle advancement flap (sliding flap) is probably the most common local flap employed in veterinary medicine because of its simple design and because there is no secondary defect requiring closure.[86] Paired single pedicle advancement flaps can be employed to close square or rectangular defects, resulting in an H closure design (H-plasty) (see Fig. 37–18).[14, 35, 36, 86, 102]

The bipedicle advancement flap is constructed by making a skin incision parallel to the long axis of the defect, with a flap width generally equal to the width of the defect (Fig. 37–10). The undermined skin segment is advanced into the recipient bed. The bipedicle advancement flap has the advantage of two sources of circulation to maintain a longer flap body.[14, 35, 36, 81, 102] The *relief incision* used to aid wound closure is a bipedicle advancement flap (see Chapter 36).

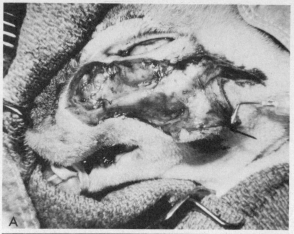

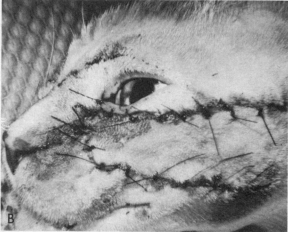

Figure 37–9. *A*, Elevation of a single pedicle advancement flap to reconstruct the cutaneous surface of the lower eyelid after resection of a large skin tumor. The flap width is determined by the width of the defect. *B*, Postoperative view. Healing was uncomplicated. The normal direction of hair growth was maintained with excellent cosmetic and functional results. Note that the base (pedicle) of the flap is slightly wider than the width of the flap end to prevent its accidental narrowing intraoperatively.

V-Y advancement is a triangular advancement technique primarily employed to relieve tension (see Chapter 36).

Distant Flaps

Distant flaps are pedicle grafts constructed at a distance from the recipient bed.[14, 35, 36, 86, 102] They are

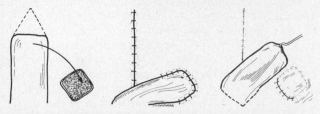

Figure 37–8. Interpolation flap. The flap is developed and rotated from a position that is not immediately adjacent to the defect. A portion of the flap must pass over the skin between the donor and recipient beds. The redundant portion of the flap is eventually excised to complete the transfer. (Redrawn from Grabb, W. C., and Myers, M. B.: *Skin Flaps*. Little, Brown, Boston, 1975.)

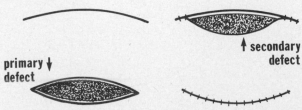

Figure 37–10. Bipedicle advancement flap. The flap width generally equals the width of the defect. The secondary defect (donor bed) is closed by direct apposition. (Redrawn from Grabb, W. C., and Myers, M. B.: *Skin Flaps*. Little, Brown, Boston, 1975.)

used almost exclusively for major skin losses involving the extremities.[2, 5–7, 52, 59, 86, 99, 102–105, 114] Distant flaps can be transferred to the defect (1) directly (direct flaps) or (2) indirectly (indirect flaps).[14, 15, 36, 86, 102]

Direct Flaps

Direct flaps include the single pedicle design (hinge flap) (Fig. 37–11) and the bipedicle design (pouch flap) (Fig. 37–12) developed on the middle or lower lateral surface of the thorax or abdomen.[2, 6, 52, 59, 86, 91, 99, 102, 104, 105, 114] The affected limb is lifted and the *recipient bed* is sutured to the elevated flap. The pedicles are eventually divided in stages to complete the transfer. Direct flaps are used successfully in small animals, although cats are better suited to this technique than dogs because of their size, flexible limbs, and the ample loose, elastic skin available over the trunk. However, some animals tolerate poorly the immobilization of their limbs in an elevated position.

Direct flaps have the disadvantage of requiring prolonged immobilization of the affected limb to assure flap survival and healing to the wound.[2, 6, 52, 59, 86, 91, 99, 102, 104, 105, 114] I have noticed mild muscle atrophy of the limb until normal use of the leg is regained. Because multiple stages are required to complete their transfer, the cost to the owner is moderate. The transplanted skin assumes the same hair growth characteristics despite its new location on the limb.

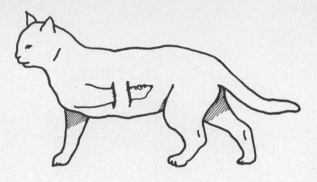

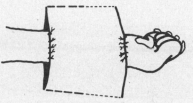

Figure 37–12. Distant bipedicle direct flap. Two incisions equal to the width of the skin defect are made. The flap is undermined below the panniculus muscle. The affected limb is secured beneath the pedicle graft, and the edge of the recipient bed is sutured to the edges of the graft. When the flap "takes," the two pedicles are severed in four stages (one-half is severed every two days) to avoid vascular compromise.

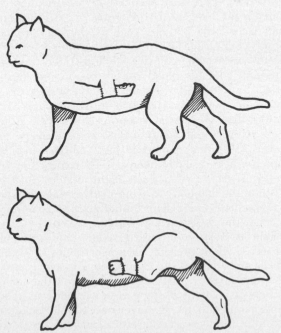

Figure 37–11. Single pedicle direct flaps for closure of lower fore- and hind limb defects. A ventrally based pedicle graft can also be employed depending on the location of the skin defect (see Fig. 37–19). The pedicle is eventually severed in stages to avoid sudden vascular compromise to the established graft.

Indirect Flaps

Indirect flaps are almost entirely of tubed flap design, in whch a bipedicle flap is sutured into a tube prior to its eventual transfer to the recipient bed (Fig. 37–13).[5–7, 50, 51, 86, 99, 102, 103] Tubing the flap prevents the flap from healing to the donor bed, minimizes infection, and facilitates eventual transfer to the recipient bed.[35, 110] Most long tubed flaps require a two- or three-week "delay" to enhance their circulation before one pedicle can be severed and advanced toward the defect.[6, 7, 46, 50, 91, 102, 103] Although tubed flaps can be "walked" great distances by periodically severing each pedicle alternately and advancing the freed end toward the recipient bed at two-week intervals,[6] it is both time-consuming and impractical. Each successive step required increases the likelihood of partial flap necrosis from an ineffective delay period, accidental kinking or twisting of the intact pedicle, trauma, or infection. As a result, tubed flaps are best developed close enough to the recipient bed to allow their immediate application to the wound after the initial delay period. Tubed flaps "shrink" or contract prior to their transfer and should be made larger than the recipient bed and longer than the length required to reach the defect. Like direct flaps, the color and quality of hair growth after transplantation of the flap are maintained despite its new location. The use of delayed tubed flaps is no

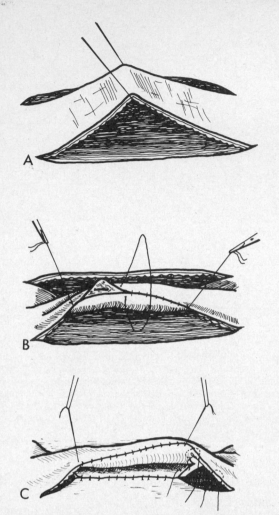

Figure 37–13. Tubed (indirect) flap in the dog. *A,* Elevation of the bipedicled flap. *B,* Suturing into a tube. *C,* Completion of the tubed flap and closure of the underlying donor bed. The flap should be created 2 or 3 cm longer and wider than measured to offset flap shrinkage during the delay period. After a three-week delay, one pedicle is severed in stages and the remaining pedicle serves as the sole source of blood supply until the graft heals to the recipient bed. The transfer pedicle can eventually be severed in stages once the graft has taken (see Fig. 37–20). (Redrawn from Converse, J. M.: *Reconstructive Plastic Surgery: General Principles.* W. B. Saunders, Philadelphia, 1977.)

longer popular in veterinary medicine and has been replaced by other techniques.

PLANNING THE FLAP

The simplest method of satisfactorily closing a skin defect prevails because of cost considerations. Fortunately, the local pedicle graft is the easiest and often the most cosmetic method for closing large wounds of the head, neck, and trunk in the dog and cat.

The surgeon should consider all possible flap designs and combinations of designs. Skin tension and pliability are assessed by manually lifting or pushing the adjacent skin toward the center of the wound. Ideal donor areas have ample skin available to elevate a flap without creating a secondary defect (donor bed) unamenable to simple closure. It is best to avoid donor sites subject to excessive motion and stress to avoid wound dehiscence or compromise to local mobility. Exceptions include cases in which closure of a wound for the protection of exposed structures has priority over the creation of a secondary defect.[14, 35, 36, 87] In this situation, the secondary defect can be closed by a second flap or a free graft or by wound contraction and epithelialization.

The shape and size of the wound naturally influence the selection of the pedicle grafts.[14, 35, 36, 102] Triangular defects are frequently closed with single or paired rotation flaps or transposition flaps, whereas square or rectangular defects are frequently closed with single or paired single-pedicle advancement flaps.[14, 35, 36, 102] However, all local flaps reviewed have potential application for variable geometric designs.[102] Irregularly shaped defects can be trimmed to a simpler geometric design for closure.[14, 35, 36, 102]

Factors that maximize the circulation to a pedicle graft should be considered during flap planning. Increasing the width of a pedicle graft does not increase its total surviving length. Flaps created under the same conditions of blood supply survive to the same length regardless of flap width. Increasing the width of the pedicle graft only permits the chance of including direct cutaneous vessels in the flap.[29, 35, 36, 66, 67, 76, 79, 100] Moreover, the cutaneous circulation differs regionally and a set length:width ratio is not applicable.[78, 79] Narrowing of a pedicle can reduce the perfusion to the body of the flap and increase the likelihood of necrosis.[14, 35, 36] Procedures that narrow the pedicle, such as the backcut technique (counterincisions), are best avoided (see Fig. 37–15). However, Wexler demonstrated that the musculocutaneous blood supply of random flaps in swine branches like a tree and narrowing of the cutaneous pedicle is possible in small flaps. Axial pattern flaps are also an exception to this rule as long as the direct cutaneous artery and vein are preserved.[67, 79] Creating unduly long subdermal plexus flaps can also result in necrosis. Therefore, I recommend (1) flaps with a base slightly wider than the width of the flap body to avoid inadvertent narrowing of the pedicle and (2) flaps limited to the size required to cover the recipient bed without tension.

Skin is best undermined below the panniculus carnosus, when present, to preserve the subdermal plexus and adjacent direct cutaneous vasculature (see Chapter 34).[78, 79] Flaps developed over the middle and lower portions of the extremities lack an underlying panniculus muscle layer and should be undermined in the loose areolar fascia between the dermis and skeletal muscle fascia.[82, 87] Skin flaps developed over areas where the skin is more closely associated with the muscle fascia (e.g., skin overlying the superficial pectoral muscle) may require the inclusion of a portion of the muscle with the elevated flap to preserve the subdermal plexus. Large flaps should include a direct cutaneous artery and vein when possible.[14, 35, 36, 77, 79, 81, 85] Unfortunately, the consistent development of axial pattern flaps requires predictable anatomical landmarks and proper patient positioning.[77, 79] Because axial pattern flap development is not possible or necessary for the coverage of all recipient beds, it may be beneficial to position the base of the flap in the direction of known direct cutaneous vessels arborizing in their general vicinity to improve the perfusion pressure to the pedicle graft.[78]

Two or more small flaps may be preferable to a single large flap whose effective circulation is questionable. The surgeon should consider the use of bipedicled flaps when longer flaps are required.[14, 35, 36, 102] A delay procedure should be considered when there is a concern regarding the flap's circulation and survival if transferred in a single stage to the recipient site.[6, 7, 14, 16, 30, 35, 36, 45, 50, 51, 73, 86, 91, 99, 102, 103, 110] Careful planning and meticulous, atraumatic surgical technique are necessary to prevent excessive tension, kinking, pressure, hematoma, circulatory compromise, and infection of the flap.[14, 35, 36, 86, 102]

All measurements of the defect and proposed flap are recorded in centimeters. A cloth template of the flap is made to represent the dimensions of the defect and the additional skin required for the flap to reach the recipient bed from the proposed donor site. The flap template is positioned over the defect, and the base of the flap model is held in a fixed position as the model is transferred to the proposed donor site. This procedure is repeated until the template is an accurate model for successful flap transfer. The final template is usually slightly larger than required to assure proper coverage. (Any excess tissue can be trimmed prior to closure.) The flap template is drawn onto the skin with a marking pen and serves as reference lines for the skin incision.[14, 35, 36, 86, 102]

Distant flaps for covering defects of the middle or lower portions of the limb also require careful planning. Indirect tubed flaps generally require a surgical delay to ensure that the flap circulation is adequate prior to transfer.

The Delay Phenomenon

Large flaps raised in two or more stages prior to transfer are more likely to survive than pedicle grafts transplanted at the first operation. This method of augmenting flap survival is called the "delay phenomenon."[14, 15, 35, 36, 45, 51, 86, 97, 102] The improved circulation after a delay procedure can help offset the hazards of torsion and tension on flap transfer.[45, 97]

Studies have focused on the microcirculatory mechanisms that account for delay and the optimal timing of flap transfer. Selective division of the nerve, artery, and vein in neurovascular island flaps of rats has demonstrated that both denervation (sympathectomy) and ischemia play major roles in the delay

phenomenon.[18, 27, 35, 36, 54, 97] Although the exact delay mechanism is unclear, sustained vasodilation is currently believed the cause of improved flap survival.[27, 36, 72] Delay is a two-phase response, the second phase being vasodilation of the microcirculation from causes other than changes in the flap's sympathetic innervation.[72]

Angiography and functional studies employed to examine the developing circulation within canine tubed flaps (8 to 10 cm long, 3 to 3.5 cm wide)[30] as well as tubed flaps in rabbits[15] have demonstrated that vessels in the subcutaneous tissue (corresponding to the subdermal plexus) increased in size and number with parallel re-orientation of main vascular channels to the long axis of the flap.[15, 30, 97] The researchers concluded that tubed flaps in dogs can be safely transferred with a seven-day delay.[30] Other researchers, however, note that although delayed flaps often have larger, straighter arteries, there are exceptions.[15, 30, 35] Some delayed flaps do not demonstrate these vascular changes, whereas some freshly elevated flaps demonstrate vascularity similar to that seen in delayed flaps on angiographic studies.[35] The longitudinal vascular arrangement in delayed flaps is most evident in loose-skinned research subjects (dog, rat, rabbit) compared with swine.[15, 30, 35] As a result, angiographic studies suggest but do not prove that delay leads to improved circulation in the skin.[35]

A later study in dogs employed Na^{24} to assess circulation in delayed single pedicled and bipedicled flaps.[45] Clearance of radioisotopes is a measure of capillary circulation and nutrient blood flow in the dermis.[90, 113] The papillary region of the dermis has the greatest isotope clearance and has been proposed as the most active region in flap vascularization.[113] Circulation fell approximately 40 per cent below normal immediately after elevating bipedicled flaps, with a gradual increase to 120 per cent at about two and one-half weeks.[45] The circulation rapidly fell to normal one to three days later. Single-pedicle flaps demonstrated an immediate drop in circulation (approximately 10 per cent of normal) with a gradual rise to 150 per cent of normal three weeks later (Fig. 37–14). The circulation thereafter maintained a short plateau and fell to normal three to five days later.[45, 97] A subsequent study revealed that elevated single-pedicle flaps in dogs, after a three-week delay, had a drop in circulation to 90 per cent of normal compared with a fall to 10 per cent of normal after their initial elevation.[46, 97] These data indicated that transfer of a delayed flap in the dog within a week of elevation is dangerous to the flap.[45] Circulatory efficiency, after initial flap elevation, can decline immediately or over a period of three to seven days.[45] This suggests that the increased tubed flap vascularity noted after one week in the previous study[30] is not a reliable guideline for tubed flap transfer. Moreover, some researchers consider *survival* upon transfer as the only meaningful test of adequate circulation for the delayed flap.[35]

Although two other reports suggest that a one-week delay is satisfactory in the dog, others recom-

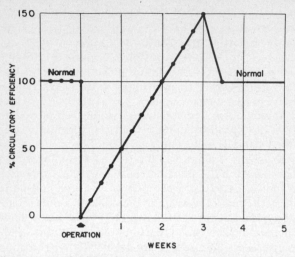

Figure 37–14. The fall and gradual rise in circulatory efficiency of a single pedicle flap after a surgical delay. Note a peak of 150 per cent in the circulatory efficiency of the flap at three weeks. (Based on data reported by Hoffmeister, F. S.: Plast. Reconstr. Surg. *19*:283, 1957. Redrawn from Grabb, W. C., and Smith, J. W.: *Plastic Surgery: A Concise Guide to Clinical Practice*, 2nd ed. Little, Brown, Boston, 1973.)

mend a two-week interval.[5, 6, 50, 91, 99, 102, 103] Other time intervals have been reported.[7, 51, 102, 103] If ischemia and denervation are the stimuli for effective delay, tubed flaps of variable length, located in different regions of the body, and on different animals have variable circulatory efficiency. Flaps with adequate circulation do not benefit appreciably from a surgical delay compared with ischemic flaps.[27, 38] As a result, the variable tubed flaps employed clinically and experimentally suggest that the shorter delay periods employed for small tubed flaps (two weeks or less) may be insufficient for long tubed flaps with greater ischemia. The optimal time for transfer varies between species. The maximum delay effect in rabbits and swine occurred in eight to ten days, whereas rats required up to six weeks.[15, 35, 73] A three-week delay is the safest interval for the dog based on Hoffmeister's research. At 18 days, I divide one-half of the pedicle; the second half is severed three days later to complete the delay. Long tubed flaps may also require staged elevation to avoid an ischemic

crisis from immediately tubing the bipedicle flap (see Fig. 37–20).[35, 36, 102]

Failure of delayed tube flaps is not always a result of a single dramatic event but often of the accumulation of minor misadventures.[101] In one study in humans, failures most frequently occurred during the initial tube elevation or extension.[101] Eight-inch tubes were all successful in this study, but staged elevation was advised with long tubed flaps. All failures occurred with 10-inch tubed flaps in this report.[101]

Physiological delay has been employed to "train" a tube to rely on vascular support from one pedicle by applying a sphygmomanometer cuff, rubber-padded intestinal clamp, or Penrose drain tubing around the opposite pedicle.[52, 102] Compression is applied for progressively longer periods of time until the tubed flap circulation can survive on the unclamped pedicle.[102]

PREPARING THE RECIPIENT BED

The recipient bed should be free of debris, necrotic tissue, and infection.[14, 35, 36, 102] Flaps properly developed and transferred can survive on avascular beds.[14, 35, 36] Distant flaps require the establishment of circulation from the defect in order to eventually divide the pedicles for completion of flap transfer.[109] Vascular tissue, such as healthy muscle, periosteum, and the paratenon, is capable of vascularizing an overlying skin flap.[14, 35, 36, 102] Chronic granulation tissue is excised to re-establish a healthy granulation bed. Epithelialized borders on the wound are also removed to cover the entire wound with skin.

GUIDELINES FOR LOCAL FLAP DEVELOPMENT AND TRANSFER

Rotation Flap

The rotation flap is a semicircle sharing a common border with the triangular defect (Fig. 37–15). In humans, the incision arc is four times the length required to rotate the flap into the defect.[35, 36, 102] In practice, a curved incision is created in a stepwise

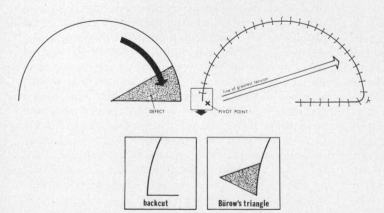

Figure 37–15. Rotation flap demonstrating the line of greatest tension from the pivot point of the flap to the most distant point of the flap (or defect). Methods suggested to relieve tension on an improperly designed flap include a backcut and Bürow's triangle. The backcut narrows the flap pedicle and is not recommended for the subdermal plexus flap. Bürow's triangles are minimally useful. A stab incision along the line of tension is a reasonable alternative (see Fig. 37–7). (Redrawn from Grabb, W. C., and Smith, J. W.: *Plastic Surgery: A Concise Guide to Clinical Practice*, 2nd ed. Little, Brown, Boston, 1973.)

fashion and the flap is undermined until it covers the wound without excessive tension. Paired rotation flaps can be employed to close wider triangular defects.[102] Similarly, two rotation flaps can be employed to correct rectangular defects by closing the two triangular areas formed by a diagonal line across opposing corners of the defect.[102] Properly planned rotation flaps in the dog and cat rarely create a donor defect unamenable to primary closure. Excessive tension can be relieved with a small stab incision perpendicular to the line of greatest tension (see Fig. 37–6).[35, 36] Bürow's triangles are minimally effective for relieving tension and are rarely employed.[86] Any small dog-ears usually resolve but may be excised at surgery as long as the flap pedicle is not compromised. Monofilament nylon (3/0) or polypropylene sutures are routinely used in a simple interrupted pattern for closure.

Transposition Flap

The transposition flap is a rectangular pedicle graft usually created within 90° of the long axis of the defect. An edge of the defect comprises a portion of the flap border. The width of the flap normally equals the width of the defect. The flap length from the pivot point of the flap to the most distant point of the flap should be equal to or greater than the distance between the pivot point and the most distant point of the defect (Fig. 37–16; see Fig. 37–7).[14, 35, 36, 86, 102]

Transposition flaps decrease in length as the arc of rotation increases. A dog-ear also develops the more the flap is rotated. The greater the angle at which the flap is taken, however, the less the tension on the primary repair (Fig. 37–17).[14, 35, 36, 102]

In general the transposition flap is most effective when directly adjacent to the wound and at a 45 or 90° angle to the long axis of the defect. Secondary defects are usually closed directly after the cutaneous borders are undermined. A second local flap may be

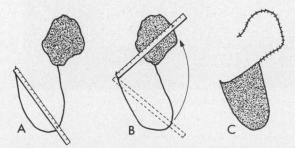

Figure 37–16. Transposition flap at 90° to the long axis of the defect. *A*, Removal of defect and outline of intended flap incision. *B*, Rotation and alignment of flap. *C*, Closure. Note that the ruler measurement from the pivot point to the tip of the flap must equal the distance between the pivot point and the most distant point of the defect (recipient bed). The secondary defect created is sutured after local undermining. (Redrawn from Converse, J. M.: *Reconstructive Plastic Surgery: General Principles.* W. B. Saunders, Philadelphia, 1977.)

employed to close the donor bed if necessary. Mild tension along the line of greatest tension can be relieved with a small perpendicular stab incision (see Fig. 37–7).[35, 36] Monofilament nylon (3/0) or polypropylene sutures are routinely used in a simple interrupted pattern.

Interpolation Flap

The interpolation flap is a rectangular flap lacking a common border with the skin defect (see Fig. 37–8).[14, 35, 36, 102] As a result, a portion of the flap must cross the skin between the donor and recipient beds. The resultant exposed surface is either left open or covered with a split thickness graft in man.[14, 35, 36] Large skin segments can be tubed to avoid the drawbacks of these two techniques. An easier alternative is the creation of a "bridge incision" between the donor and recipient bed, the skin edges of which are sutured to the overlying margins of the flap (see Fig. 37–28D–F).[83, 87] The donor bed is closed directly and the redundant portion of the flap can be excised after healing is complete. Interpolation flaps must be carefully planned and measured similar to transposition flaps. Interpolation flaps are rarely employed in veterinary surgery.

Advancement Flap

The single-pedicle advancement flap is one of the local flaps most commonly employed in animals.[80] Advancement is accomplished by taking advantage of the elasticity of the skin.[102] Two single-pedicle advancement flaps (H-plasty) may be more effective than a longer single advancement flap to close a large square or rectangular wound (Fig. 37–18). A variety of techniques have been employed to improve the mobility of advancement flaps. The use of Bürow's triangles has been advocated to prevent dog-ear formation and improve flap mobility.[6, 99, 102] They are rarely required to prevent dog-ears and are minimally effective in relieving tension.[86]

To create a single-pedicle advancement flap, two skin incisions equal to the width of the defect are made in progressive fashion. The distant edge of the flap borders the defect. The two incisions diverge slightly to assure that the flap pedicle is not narrowed as it is developed. The flap is undermined and is advanced into the defect (see Fig. 37–9A and B). Monofilament nylon (3/0) or polypropylene sutures are routinely used with a simple interrupted pattern.

Bipedicle Advancement Flap

Bipedicle advancement flaps are constructed by making an incision parallel to the long axis of a defect, the width of the flap being equal to the width of the adjacent defect.[14, 35, 36, 102] Advancement may be facil-

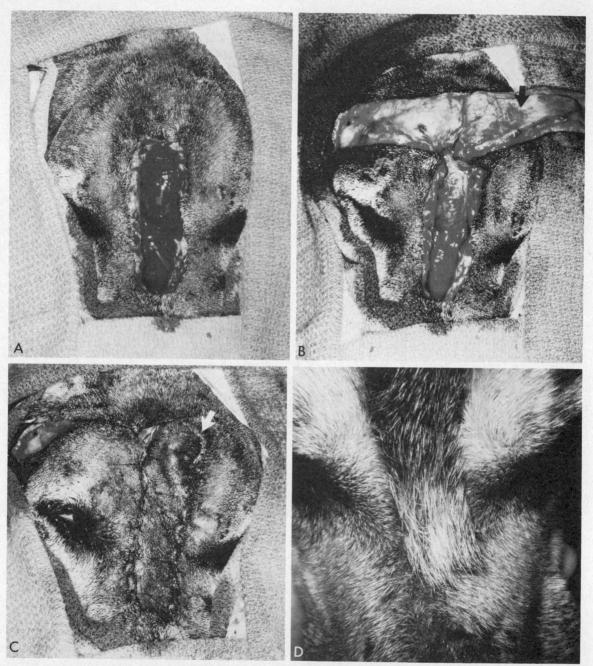

Figure 37–17. *A,* Hole overlying the nasal cavity of several months duration, the result of wound dehiscence secondary to a nasal exploratory for aspergillosis. Repeated attempts at re-opposing the skin edges failed to close the opening. The edges have been debrided, permitting slight overlapping of the flap borders. *B,* Elevation of a 90° transposition flap. A portion of the frontalis muscle was included with the skin flap for additional bulk. The proposed flap was carefully measured and drawn onto the skin with a marking pen prior to surgery (see Fig. 37–16). *C,* The flap was sutured in place with 3–0 monofilament nylon and the donor bed closed after undermining the skin edges. A small dog-ear formed (arrow). *D,* Cosmetic results after healing. Note the rostral direction of hair growth. The dog-ear was not noticeable.

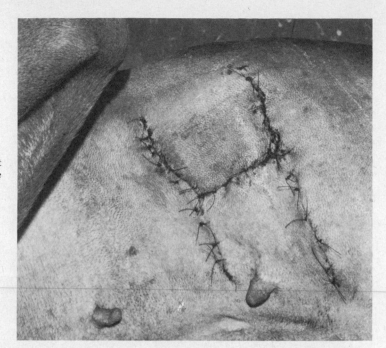

Figure 37–18. H-plasty. Two single pedicle advancement flaps were employed to close a rectangular defect of the lateral abdominal wall.

itated if the relaxing incision is curved with the concave side toward the defect.[35] The flap is undermined and sutured into the defect (see Fig. 37–10). The secondary defect is usually closed by undermining and suturing the adjacent skin edge. Two pedicles allow longer flaps to be created. Necrosis can occur at the vascular interface between the two pedicles.[35] This does not necessarily correlate with the center of the flap unless the circulatory perfusion pressure from each pedicle is equal.[35] The relief incision, which is occasionally used to close wounds, is a bipedicle advancement flap (see Chapter 36).

GUIDELINES FOR DISTANT FLAP DEVELOPMENT AND TRANSFER

Direct Flap

Direct flaps include the single-pedicle flap (hinge flap) (Fig. 37–19; see Fig. 37–11) and the bipedicle flap (pouch flap) (see Fig. 37–12).[2, 6, 52, 59, 86, 99, 102, 104, 105, 114] The affected limb is elevated to the flap and secured beneath it until each pedicle can be divided to complete the transfer.

The donor area is generally located over the lateral surface of the thorax or abdomen, depending on the size and location of the defect. The width of the flap equals the width of the defect, whereas the length of the flap is determined by the length of the defect plus that additional portion required to position the flap over the recipient bed. The flap base may be positioned dorsally or ventrally, depending on the location of the limb defect. Lateral limb defects are the easiest to cover, whereas wounds on the medial aspect of the limb are the most difficult to close with a direct flap. Circumferential defects of the limbs can

be closed by wrapping the severed pedicles of a distant flap around the remaining (medial) defect. The survival of the freed end of the flap depends on the new circulation established from the portion of the flap that has healed to the lateral recipient bed. Bipedicle flaps are occasionally impossible to use for proximal limb defects (especially in the dog) because the elbow and carpus cannot be flexed enough to rotate and extend the limb beneath the flap. In this case, a single-pedicle flap is used (see Fig. 37–19).

Pedicles are divided 10 to 14 days after the initial transfer[52, 86, 102, 114] in stages, one-half to one-third every two or three days to avoid ischemia (see Fig. 37–19D).[14, 35, 36, 86] Although it is possible to sever the base of the flap earlier by omitting the staged division, the few additional days minimize the risk of necrosis.

Direct flaps have been used successfully in the dog and cat but require a cooperative patient and owner. The donor sites are easily closed by undermining the skin edges prior to suturing.

Direct flaps require thoughtful preoperative planning and postoperative care. Bandages are required to secure the limb to the trunk, minimize movement between the flap and recipient bed, prevent shifting of the limb resulting in tension on the pedicles, and protect the surgical site from external trauma. Tight bandages can compromise flap circulation and should be avoided. Elastic tape and "stay sutures" between the limb and trunk are useful to minimize shifting of the limb until healing occurs (see Fig. 37–19B). Light padding between the elevated limb and trunk is required to prevent the development of a moist dermatitis. Ventral drainage is necessary to allow tissue fluid and purulent material to drain.

Bandages are usually changed every three days until completion of the transfer. The patient is se-

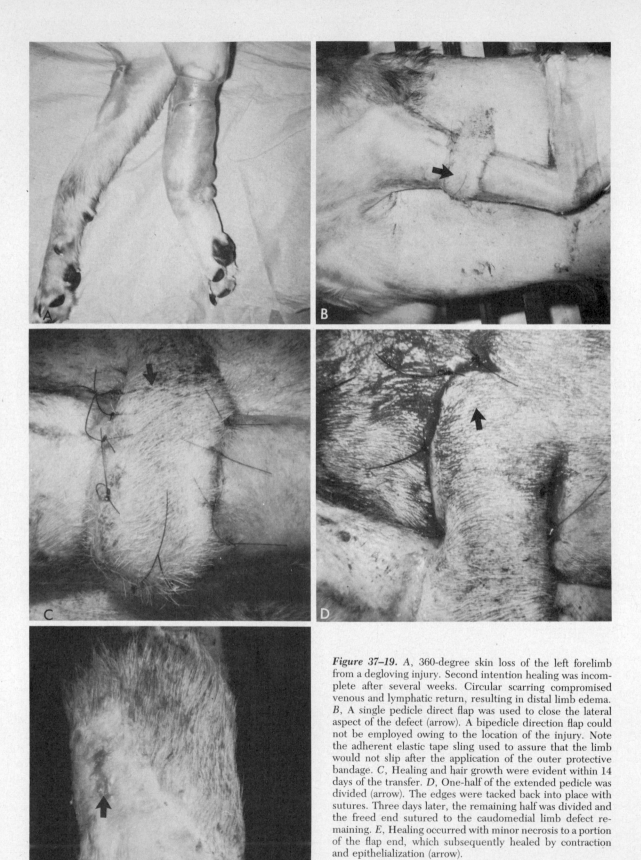

Figure 37–19. A, 360-degree skin loss of the left forelimb from a degloving injury. Second intention healing was incomplete after several weeks. Circular scarring compromised venous and lymphatic return, resulting in distal limb edema. B, A single pedicle direct flap was used to close the lateral aspect of the defect (arrow). A bipedicle direction flap could not be employed owing to the location of the injury. Note the adherent elastic tape sling used to assure that the limb would not slip after the application of the outer protective bandage. C, Healing and hair growth were evident within 14 days of the transfer. D, One-half of the extended pedicle was divided (arrow). The edges were tacked back into place with sutures. Three days later, the remaining half was divided and the freed end sutured to the caudomedial limb defect remaining. E, Healing occurred with minor necrosis to a portion of the flap end, which subsequently healed by contraction and epithelialization (arrow).

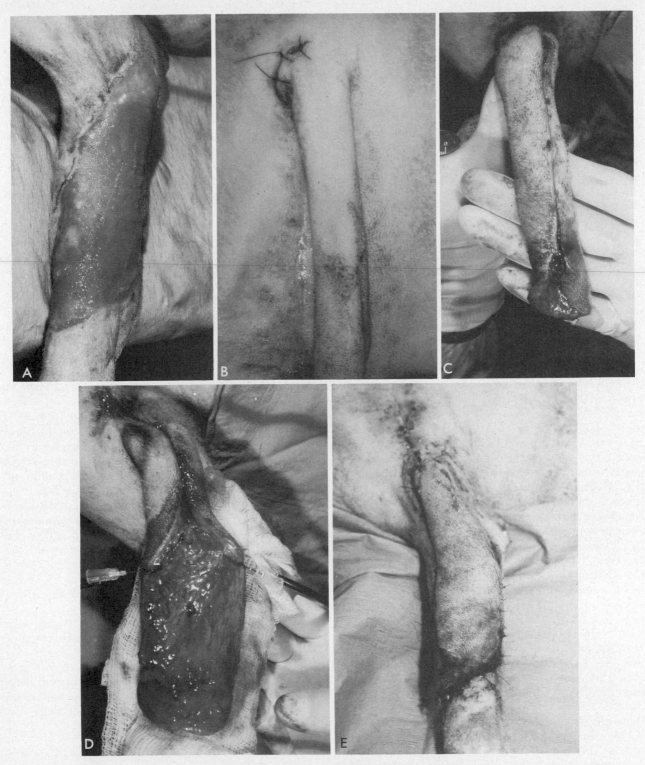

Figure 37–20. *A*, Large skin loss over the left forelimb, a result of a degloving injury. A healthy granulation bed was prepared to receive the flap. *B*, Tubed flap development over the left humerus and scapula. This long tubed flap was partially raised and replaced on its original bed for seven days, after which time it was re-elevated and sutured into a tube. One-half of the dorsal pedicle was divided and sutured to its original position 11 days later (day 18). *C*, The remaining half of the pedicle was severed three days later (day 21) and the tube rotated down to the recipient bed. *D*, The tubed flap was opened along the original seam. Curved, 20-gauge hypodermic needles held with hemostats served as skin hooks to apply traction to the flap while the tube was opened by gentle blunt dissection using Metzenbaum scissors. *E*, Seven days after transfer. The lower 1 to 2 cm of the flap underwent necrosis. This area sloughed and healed by second intention uneventfully. The tubed pedicle nourishing the flap was divided in stages beginning 14 days after the initial transfer. (A tubed thoracodorsal axial pattern flap could have been employed for immediate coverage of this large wound, bypassing the time, cost, and problems associated with delayed tubed flaps.)

dated and manually restrained or lightly anesthetized to avoid struggling during the procedure. Distant flaps are surprisingly successful, although the cosmetic results depend on the donor skin and the direction of hair growth after transplantation.

Indirect Flap

Delayed tubed flaps are used to transfer skin to a distant donor site if there is no immediate need to cover an area (see Fig. 37–13). They are employed only if simpler methods of skin transfer are unable to close a defect.[5–7, 86, 99, 102, 103]

The length and width of tubed flaps are determined by the size of the deficit and the additional portion of flap required to reach the recipient bed without tension. The length and width of the proposed flap are increased 2 to 3 cm longer and wider than measured to offset flap shrinkage, which results from loss of skin elasticity and build-up of fibrous connective tissue during a delay procedure.[16] The flap must be wide enough to suture into a tube without tension. Although removal of subcutaneous fat has been advocated to facilitate the tubing of flaps in obese human patients,[14, 16, 35, 36] this is usually unnecessary in small animals. Moreover, the removal of subcutaneous fat[14, 16] and the associated panniculus muscle[78, 82] can inadvertently damage the subdermal plexus and the associated vasculature, significantly compromising flap circulation. If adipose tissue may impair tubing, the flap should be designed so that it is wide enough to avoid this problem.[16] The proposed flap also must be designed to "swing" into its next position without excessive twisting or kinking of the remaining pedicle.

In general, tubing the flap is easily accomplished by elevating the bipedicled flap and suturing its edges together.[14, 35, 36] The donor bed is undermined and closed directly. Modifications to this simple design include staggering the parallel incisions to facilitate closure of the tubed extremities.[102] This design is reported to decrease shortening of tubed flaps, although the resultant linear scar formed may interfere with the later development of a "pancake" of skin on the end of the tube.[102] The donor site can also be closed by converting one edge into an advancement flap (the Bunnell method).[102] Long tubed flaps may require staged elevation to avoid ischemia during their construction by maintaining a central pedicle for several days until the circulation improves enough to tube the flap.[35, 36, 102, 103]

Postoperatively, the tube must be protected from trauma and supported with a soft cotton bandage, depending on its position. Soft cotton rolls are usually taped on each side of the tubed flap, followed by a soft cotton bandage over the area, until the flap is transferred.[102] The bandage should place no pressure on the flap.

Delays of two or three weeks are most commonly employed to improve flap circulation prior to the staged division of one pedicle to complete the transfer.[5–7, 50, 51, 99, 102, 103] One-third to one-half of the pedicle is severed and resutured every two or three days to avoid ischemia (Fig. 37–20A and B).[35, 36, 86] Each pedicle does not necessarily have the same circulatory contribution to the flap body. The "dominant" pedicle, which has greater perfusion, is best preserved whereas the "nondominant" pedicle can be divided with less danger of distal flap necrosis after the delay procedure.[35] Tube necrosis occurs at the vascular interface between the two pedicles.[35] This does not occur at the center of a tubed flap unless the circulatory contribution of each pedicle is equal.[35]

Tubed flaps are moved by migration in dogs and cats by one of three techniques: "caterpillaring," "waltzing," or "tumbling."[14, 35, 36, 102] Caterpillaring entails moving one end of the flap close to the other, in essence doubling the flap on itself. After a second delay procedure, the other pedicle is severed and the freed end is extended toward the defect. Waltzing requires the alternate movement of each pedicle in a lateral motion, whereas tumbling entails severing one pedicle and extending it forward, thereby advancing the flap directly toward the defect. Of the three, tumbling is the most direct method of transfer, especially when it is developed close to the defect, thus enabling immediate application of the flap to the area after a single delay period.

To cover the recipient site, the flap is divided along its original seam and opened by careful blunt dissection with Metzenbaum scissors. Skin hooks are employed to apply mild traction to the skin edges during the procedure. Surgical trauma should be minimized to preserve circulation to the flap (Fig. 37–20C–E). An alternate technique of covering the defect is the delayed development of a round skin segment (pancake) attached to the freed end of the flap.[35, 102, 103] The "pancake" is used to cover the recipient site, whereas the tubed pedicle serves as a vascular conduit to the area. Hair growth in either case is determined by the donor skin and its position on the recipient bed.

The remaining pedicle is divided in stages once the flap has healed to the area, 10 to 14 days after its application.[7, 50, 51, 86]

The multiple stages required to complete the procedure increase the likelihood of surgical complications and flap necrosis. Careful planning minimizes the technical pitfalls associated with tubed flaps.

GUIDELINES FOR AXIAL PATTERN FLAPS

Although it is not possible to include a direct cutaneous artery and vein in every pedicle graft elevated, axial pattern flaps enable the surgeon to transfer large skin segments in a single stage safely without the necessity of a delay procedure. The four major direct cutaneous arteries of the dog employed for axial pattern flaps include the caudal superficial epigastric artery, the cervical cutaneous (superficial

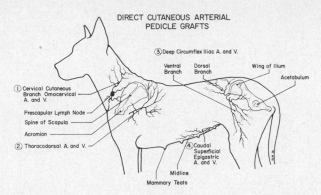

Figure 37–21. Four major direct cutaneous arteries are illustrated in relation to their anatomical landmarks. (Reprinted with permission from Pavletic, M. M.: Canine axial pattern flaps using the omocervical, thoracodorsal, and deep circumflex iliac direct cutaneous arteries. Am. J. Vet. Res. *42:*391, 1981.)

cervical) branch of the omocervical artery, the thoracodorsal artery, and the deep circumflex iliac artery (Fig. 37–21).[77, 79, 81, 85, 86]

Anatomical landmarks reference incisions, and potential uses for each are summarized (Table 37–1) (Fig. 37–22). The guidelines presented enable closure of the donor defect without excessive tension. However, wider flaps are possible in dogs and cats with ample loose skin at the donor site.

Careful positioning of each patient is necessary

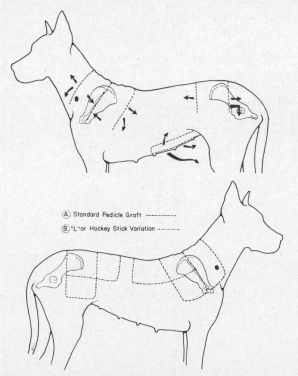

Figure 37–22. Reference lines for the omocervical, thoracodorsal, deep circumflex iliac, and caudal superficial epigastric axial pattern flaps. Flaps may be created in the standard peninsula (dashed lines) or "L" or hockey-stick (dashed and dotted lines) configuration. (Reprinted with permission from Pavletic, M. M.: Canine axial pattern flaps using the omocervical, thoracodorsal, and deep circumflex iliac direct cutaneous arteries. Am. J. Vet. Res. *42:*391, 1981.)

prior to outlining the proposed flap on the dog. Skin distortion in relation to the anatomical landmarks may result in failure to include the direct cutaneous vessels in the pedicle graft.[79, 85]

Axial pattern flaps can be rotated into adjacent defects or to distant sites of the lower trunk and extremities. A portion of the flap can be tubed to traverse the skin between the donor and recipient beds or a bridge incision may be employed to avoid tubing the flap.[83, 87] The flap body can be elevated as the standard (peninsular) or the "L" ("hockey stick") design (see Fig. 37–22).[79, 85] Peninsular flaps have the advantage of greater total length compared with the hockey stick design but may encroach upon the contralateral axillary or flank regions. The hockey stick design bypasses this problem, but the flap will not extend the full length of the peninsular configuration. This flap, however, has the major advantage of conforming to wide and irregularly shaped defects.[79, 85]

The cutaneous circulation of the cat and the placement of the direct cutaneous vessels are similar to those of the dog. Axial pattern flaps have been successfully developed and transferred in the cat.[81]

Omocervical Flap[79, 86]

The hair is completely clipped from the neck and cranial half of the canine trunk. The dog is placed in lateral recumbency with the forelimb in relaxed extension. The cervical and thoracic skin are grasped, lifted, and allowed to spontaneously retract to normal position. A felt-tipped marking pen is used to draw a line over the spine of the scapula. The cranial shoulder depression is palpated and the approximate location of the prescapular lymph node is located. The cranial incision is drawn on the skin parallel to the caudal incision site, equal to the distance between the cranial shoulder depression and caudal incision line. The reference lines are extended to the dorsal midline and down the opposite side to the contralateral scapulohumeral joint (see Fig. 37–22). The flap is elevated below portions of the sphincter colli superficialis muscle and rotated into the adjacent defect. The flap may also be partially tubed to reach a distant defect or sutured to a "bridge incision" to traverse the interposing skin.

Thoracodorsal Flap[79, 86]

The hair is completely clipped from the neck and cranial half of the canine trunk. The dog is placed in lateral recumbency with the forelimb in relaxed extension. The lateral cervical and thoracic skin are grasped, lifted, and allowed to spontaneously retract to a normal position. A felt-tipped marking pen is used to draw a line over the spine of the scapula, forming the cranial border of the flap. The caudal shoulder depression is palpated, and the caudal in-

TABLE 37–1. Anatomical Landmarks, Reference Incisions, and Potential Use for Axial Pattern Flap Development

Artery	Anatomical Landmarks	Reference Incisions	Potential Uses*
Cervical cutaneous branch of the omocervical artery	Spine of the scapula Cranial edge of the scapula (cranial shoulder depression) Dog in lateral recumbency, skin in natural position, thoracic limb placed in relaxed extension Vessel originates at location of the prescapular lymph node	Caudal incision: spine of the scapula in a dorsal direction Cranial incision: parallel to caudal incision equal to the distance between the scapular spine and cranial scapular edge (cranial shoulder depression) Flap length: variable; contralateral scapulohumeral joint	Facial defects Ear reconstruction Cervical defects Shoulder defects Axillary defects
Thoracodorsal artery	Spine of the scapula Caudal edge of the scapula (caudal shoulder depression) Dog in lateral recumbency, skin in natural position, thoracic limb in relaxed extension Vessel originates at caudal shoulder depression at a level parallel to the dorsal point of the acromion	Cranial incision: spine of the scapula in a dorsal direction Caudal incision: parallel to the cranial incision equal to the distance between the scapular spine and caudal scapular edge (caudal shoulder depression) Flap length: variable; can survive ventral to contralateral scapulohumeral joint	Thoracic defects Shoulder defects Forelimb defects Axillary defects
Deep circumflex iliac artery	Cranial edge of wing of ilium Greater trochanter Dog in lateral recumbency, skin in natural position, pelvic limb in relaxed extension Vessel originates at a point cranioventral to wing of the ilium	Caudal incision: midway between edge of wing of ilium and greater trochanter Cranial incision: parallel to caudal incision equal to the distance between the caudal incision and cranial edge of the iliac wing Flap length: dorsal to contralateral flank fold	Thoracic defects Lateral abdominal wall defects Flank defects Lateral/medial thigh defects Defects over the greater trochanter
Caudal superficial epigastric artery	Midline of abdomen Mammary teats Base of prepuce	Medial incision: abdominal midline In the male dog, the base of the prepuce is included in the midline incision to preserve the adjacent epigastric vasculature Lateral incision: parallel to medial incision at an equal distance from the mammary Flap length: variable; may safely include the last four mammary glands and adjacent skin	Flank defects Inner thigh defects Stifle area Perineal area Preputial area

*Major defects only.

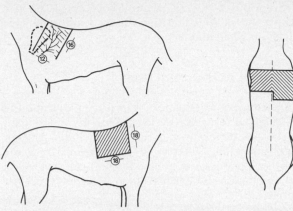

Figure 37–23. Three views of preoperative outline of the left hockey stick thoracodorsal axial pattern flap to reconstruct the left axilla and inner brachium of a dog. Measurements are in centimeters. (Reprinted with permission from Pavletic, M. M., and MacIntire, D.: Phycomycosis of the axilla and inner brachium in a dog: Surgical excision and reconstruction with a thoracodorsal axial pattern flap. J. Am. Vet. Med. Assoc. *180*:1197, 1982.)

cision is drawn on the skin parallel to the cranial incision, equal to the distance between the cranial incision and caudal shoulder depression. The reference incision lines extend to the dorsal midline. At this point, the standard "peninsula" or "hockey stick" ("L") configuration can be created, depending on the location and size of the defect (Fig. 37–23; see Fig. 37–22). Flaps are elevated below the cutaneous trunci muscle beginning at the distant border of the flap and are rotated into the adjacent defect. The flap may also be partially tubed to reach a distant defect or sutured to a bridge incision to traverse the interposing skin (Fig. 37–24).

Deep Circumflex Iliac Flap[79, 86]

The hair is completely clipped from the caudal half of the trunk. The dog is placed in lateral recumbency with the hind limb in relaxed extension. The lateral thoracic and abdominal skin are grasped, lifted, and allowed to spontaneously retract to a normal position. A felt-tipped marking pen is used to draw the caudal reference incision line between the cranial border of the wing of the ilium and the greater trochanter. The cranial incision is drawn parallel to the caudal reference incision line equal to the distance between the iliac border and the caudal incision line. The reference lines are extended to the dorsal midline. At this point, the standard "peninsula" or "hockey stick" ("L") configuration can be created, depending on the location and size of the defect (see Fig. 37–22). Flaps are elevated below the level of the cutaneous trunci muscle and fascia beginning at the distant border of the flap. Once elevated, the flap is transferred in a fashion similar to that previously described for axial pattern flaps. Although the ventral branch of the deep circumflex iliac artery can be employed for flap elevation, it has limited use owing to its flank location.

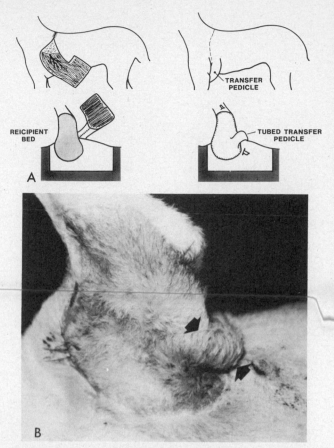

Figure 37–24. A, Diagram illustrating thoracodorsal axial pattern flap elevation, tubing of the proximal portion of the graft, and application to the recipient bed after the excision of a large granulomatous mass (phycomycosis) from the left axilla and inner brachium in a dog. *B*, The tubed transfer pedicle (arrows) and the graft body have healed in place. (Reprinted with permission from Pavletic, M. M., and MacIntire, D.: Phycomycosis of the axilla and inner brachium in a dog: Surgical excision and reconstruction with a thoracodorsal axial pattern flap. J. Am. Vet. Med. Assoc. *180*:1197, 1982.)

Caudal Superficial Epigastric Flap[79, 86]

The ventral abdomen and thorax are clipped. The animal is placed in dorsal recumbency. A midline abdominal incision is drawn with a felt-tipped pen beginning caudal to the last mammary teat and continued in a cranial direction (Fig. 37–25A). In male dogs, the midline incision must incorporate the base of the prepuce to preserve the epigastric vasculature (Fig. 37–25B). The reference incision line is drawn between glands 1 and 2 or glands 2 and 3 (depending on the length required) and continued as the lateral incision parallel to the medial incision line at an equal distance from the mammary teats. The flap is undermined below the supramammarius muscle and above the aponeurosis of the external abdominal oblique muscle progressively in a caudal direction. Wider flaps are possible if adequate skin remains to close the donor bed. The flap is transferred to the defect in the fashion previously described for the omocervical, thoracodorsal, and deep circumflex iliac axial pattern flaps (Fig. 37–26; see Fig. 37–25A).

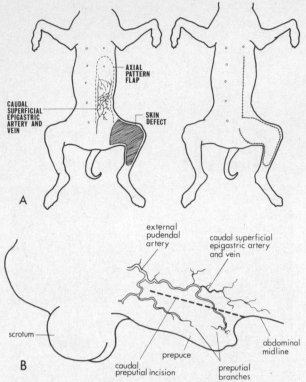

Figure 37–25. *A*, Outline of the caudal superficial epigastric flap and transfer to the medial thigh. The flap can be transplanted within 180° provided that care is taken to avoid twisting or kinking of the direct cutaneous artery and vein. *B*, In the male, care is taken to avoid transection of the caudal superficial epigastric artery and vein by including the base of the prepuce in the medial incision. (Reprinted with permission from Pavletic, M. M., and Peyton, L. C.: Plastic and reconstructive surgery in the dog and cat. *In* Bojrab, M. I. (ed.): *Current Techniques in Small Animal Surgery*, 2nd ed. Lea & Febiger, Philadelphia, 1983.)

The origin of the cranial superficial epigastric vessels precludes their effective use for most cutaneous defects in small animals.

Secondary Axial Pattern Flaps

A secondary axial pattern flap is a modification of the axial pattern flap design.[22, 36, 41, 95, 112] Skin flaps can be positioned over tissue that includes a major artery and vein. Once healed and vascularized, the cutaneous pedicle can be divided and can survive on the circulation established from the new vascular source four to five weeks later. Examples include secondary axial pattern flaps based on an omental pedicle that includes the gastroepiploic artery and vein.[36, 41, 112]

Secondary axial pattern flaps have also been developed in rabbits by implanting the central auricular artery and vein or femoral artery and vein into skin flaps.[22, 41, 112] Secondary axial pattern flaps are usually developed for eventual microvascular transfer as a free flap to distant defects and cannot be employed for immediate reconstruction to an area. Such flaps have potential in veterinary medicine if long vascular pedicles can be employed for secondary axial pattern flap development, enabling eventual flap rotation into an adjacent defect without the routine need for microvascular transplantation.

Island Arterial Flaps

Island arterial flaps can be developed in each of the canine axial pattern flaps by dividing the cuta-

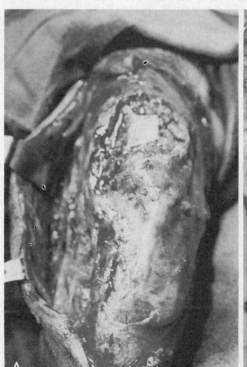

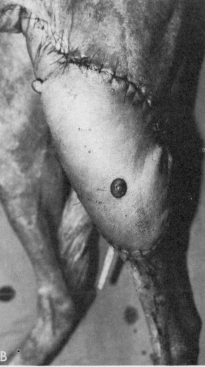

Figure 37–26. *A*, Extensive injury to the left knee of a male dog with large skin loss, the result of an automobile accident. The wound was cleaned, debrided, and treated with wet saline dressings on a daily basis for the first week. *B*, Rapid and complete restoration of the stifle area with a caudal superficial epigastric axial pattern flap including the last four mammary glands. A bridge incision was employed eliminating the need to tube a portion of the flap (see Fig. 37–28*D* and *E*).

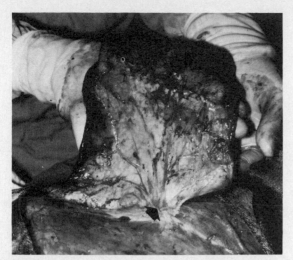

Figure 37–27. Island arterial flap in the dog over the cervical cutaneous (superficial cervical) branch of the omocervical artery and vein. The arrow marks the entry of the direct cutaneous artery and vein. Island arterial flaps have potential application for free flap transfer with microvascular surgical anastomosis at a distant location.

neous pedicle below the entry of the respective direct cutaneous artery (Fig. 37–27).[77, 79]

Island arterial flaps are dependent on a single direct cutaneous artery and vein. Although island arterial flaps are more mobile than conventional axial pattern flaps, they have limited clinical use at the present time. The similar survival area of axial pattern flaps and island arterial flaps[67] indicates that a backcut procedure at the pivot point of a skin flap can be performed to improve flap mobility with a considerable degree of safety in an axial pattern flap as long as the direct cutaneous artery and vein are preserved.

A neurovascular island flap has been employed to cover small trophic ulcers of the paw in dogs.[34]

Free Flaps

Free flap transfer (both skin and myocutaneous flaps) has been successful in humans and experimental animals by dividing the major supplying artery and vein and re-establishing circulation by microvascular anastomosis to an artery and vein at the recipient site.[14, 19, 32, 35, 36, 41, 42, 60, 64] Its use in the dog is almost entirely experimental,[32, 41, 60] and its widespread clinical use is presently unlikely owing to the microsurgical equipment, surgical skills, and postoperative care required for consistent success.[79] Fortunately, the loose skin available in the dog and cat, skin flaps, and free grafts can be effectively employed for wound coverage without the time and expense of microvascular surgery.[79]

Reverse Saphenous Conduit Flaps[87]

Reverse saphenous conduit flaps with pedicles incorporating the cranial and caudal branches of the saphenous artery and medial saphenous vein have been successfully elevated after division of their femoral vascular connections. Blood flow was maintained in reverse by distal anastomotic arterial and venous connections between (1) the cranial branch of the saphenous artery and the superficial branch of the cranial tibial artery as well as the cranial tibial artery; (2) the caudal branch of the saphenous artery and the perforating metatarsal artery via the medial and lateral plantar arteries; (3) the cranial branch of the medial saphenous vein and the cranial branch of the lateral saphenous vein; and by other venous connections with the cranial and caudal branches of the medial saphenous veins distal to the tibiotarsal joint.

Circulation to the overlying skin was maintained via direct cutaneous vessels branching off the saphenous vasculature. The reverse saphenous conduit flap is not a true axial pattern flap but a variation that incorporates the saphenous artery, a "vascular" conduit to the overlying skin and lower extremity.

The resultant flap has potential use for major cutaneous defects at or below the tibiotarsal joint as long as the saphenous vessels and the collateral circulation are preserved. When the reverse saphenous conduit flap is considered for skin defects secondary to extensive trauma, angiography should be considered to ensure that anastomotic connections are intact and that the saphenous artery and medial saphenous vein are not the major routes of circulation to the lower limb.

Measurements are taken to determine the length of the flap needed to reach and cover the lower limb defect. The flap width is tapered distally owing to the limited skin available for flap development. A skin incision is made across the central third of the inner thigh, at or slightly above the level of the patella. Metzenbaum scissors are used to expose the underlying saphenous artery, medial saphenous vein, and nerve prior to their ligation and division. Two incisions are extended distally in converging fashion, 0.5 to 1 cm cranial and caudal to the borders of the cranial and caudal branches of the saphenous artery and medial saphenous vein, respectively. The flaps are undermined beneath the saphenous vasculature. To avoid injury to the caudal branch of the saphenous artery and medial saphenous vein during progressive raising of the pedicle graft, a portion of the medial gastrocnemius muscle fascia is included with the flap. Below this point, the tibial nerve merges with the descending caudal branches of the saphenous artery and medial saphenous vein and is preserved by meticulous dissection between these structures. Ligation and division of the peroneal (fibular) artery and vein are necessary for flap mobility (Fig. 37–28A). Flap raising is completed proximal to the anastomosis between the cranial branch of the medial saphenous vein and the cranial branch of the lateral saphenous vein. The donor bed is initially closed with interrupted subcuticular sutures, then with simple interrupted skin sutures, using 3-0 monofilament nylon at the end of the transplantation. The "transfer

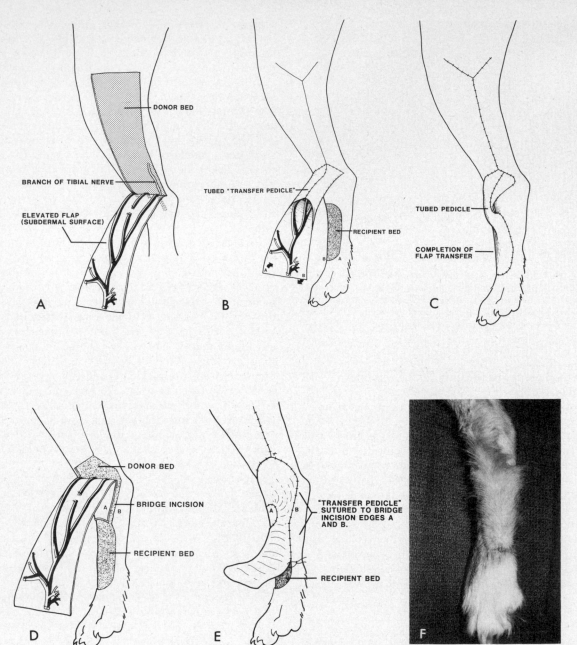

Figure 37–28. A, The reverse saphenous conduit flap raised from the donor bed. Notice the division of the peroneal artery and vein and the tibial nerve merging with the caudal branch of the saphenous artery and medial saphenous vein. *B,* After suturing the proximal segment of the flap into a skin tube (tubed transfer pedicle), the distal portion of the graft is rotated into the recipient bed. *C,* Completion of the transfer. *D,* Flap transfer using a bridge incision. After elevation of the flap, an incision is made, connecting the donor and recipient beds. Care is taken not to sever any underlying vessels. *E,* The proximal portion of the flap is rotated and sutured to edges A and B of the bridge incision. The distal portion of the flap is sutured to the recipient bed with a simple interrupted pattern. *F,* Transplantation of a reverse saphenous conduit flap over the craniomedial metatarsal surface, 75 days after surgery. A bridge incision was used. (Reprinted with permission from Pavletic, M. M., Watters, J., Henry, R., and Nafe, L.: Reverse Saphenous Conduit Flap in the dog. J. Am. Vet. Med. Assoc. *182:*380, 1983.)

pedicle" can be tubed or sutured to a "bridge incision" connecting the donor and recipient beds (Fig. 37–28*B–F*). Care is taken that the tubed transfer pedicles are not under undue tension with extension of the tibiotarsal joint.

COMPOUND AND COMPOSITE FLAP DEVELOPMENT AND TRANSFER

Compound and composite flaps play a limited clinical role in veterinary surgery.[23, 42, 95, 96, 107] Myocu-

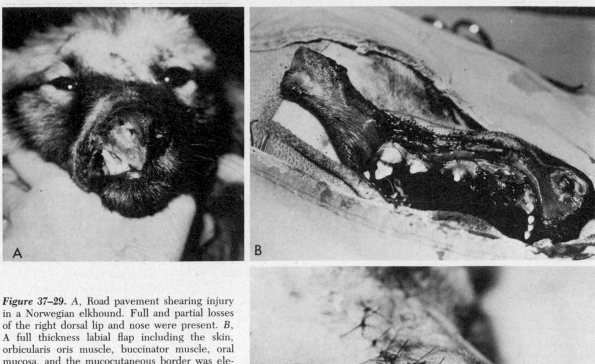

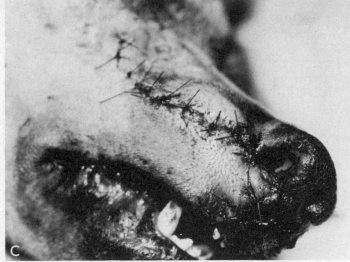

Figure 37–29. *A,* Road pavement shearing injury in a Norwegian elkhound. Full and partial losses of the right dorsal lip and nose were present. *B,* A full thickness labial flap including the skin, orbicularis oris muscle, buccinator muscle, oral mucosa, and the mucocutaneous border was elevated and advanced forward to restore the rostral labial defect. The dorsal labial artery and vein included in this composite flap assured its survival. *C,* Completion of the procedure. Complete restoration of the cutaneous and mucosal epithelial surfaces was accomplished while maintaining a natural mucocutaneous border. (Reprinted with permission from Pavletic, M. M.: Nasal and rostral labial reconstruction in the dog. J. Am. Anim. Hosp. Assoc., *19*:913, 1983.)

taneous flaps (primary and secondary) have limited clinical use in the dog and cat owing to the generous amount of loose skin available for wound closure and axial pattern flap development.[79] They may be useful in adding "bulk" or padding to depressions after trauma or tumor removal. Composite flaps employed on a clinical basis include the canine mucocutaneous subdermal plexus flap for complete lower eyelid restoration (see Chapter 101) and the full thickness labial advancement flap for rostral labial defects[83, 84] (Fig. 37–29)

FLAP REVASCULARIZATION AND PEDICLE DIVISION

When a skin flap is raised, the inherent vascular supply may be insufficient to maintain flap viability. Vascular growth in ischemic areas of swine flaps is first noted three to four days after surgery, and the whole flap has a collateral blood supply in seven to ten days.[113] The greatest functional changes are in the ischemic areas.[12, 113] Ischemia is an important factor in revascularization.[12, 113] Revascularization is sufficient to maintain the flap by six or seven days in rats and four to five days in pigs.[109] Revascularization from the wound bed is of greater importance than from the wound edges.[109] Beds with a high vascular density vascularize a flap more rapidly, especially ischemic areas of the flap. Staged division of the pedicle may stimulate vascularization from the bed so that complete division of the pedicle can be accomplished earlier.[12] Division of the neurovascular bundle of axial pattern flaps in rats four days after elevation improved flap survival when the pedicle was completely divided on the seventh day.[12] Flaps that had the direct cutaneous vessels and cutaneous pedicle divided simultaneously on day 7 had a decreased survival rate. Thus, staged division of axial pattern flaps can enhance the size and density of vessels entering the flap from vascular recipient beds.[12] Moreover, staged division of pedicles in axial pattern flaps or distant flaps without direct cutaneous vessels can (1) avoid sudden ischemia and (2) enhance revascularization of the flap by staged ischemia.[12] Initial division of direct and indirect flaps is usual in

10 to 14 days to ensure that healing and vascularization between the flap and recipient bed have occurred.

FLAP NECROSIS

Causes of Flap Necrosis

Although flap necrosis can result from infection and toxic agents, an inadequate blood supply is the cause in most cases.[35] The fate of a skin flap is determined by the ability of its circulation to meet the metabolic needs of its tissues.[13] Acidosis, increased glucose comsumption, changes in cellular enzymes of intermediary metabolism, and a shift to anaerobic metabolism have been demonstrated in ischemic flaps.[13, 31, 49, 58]

Sufficient perfusion pressure is necessary to drive blood into the distant portion of the flap to avoid necrosis. As little as 10 per cent of the total circulation is necessary for nutrient support of the skin, whereas 90 per cent of the total circulation is employed for thermoregulation.[35, 36] Although the skin of fur-bearing animals does not play a significant role in thermoregulation,[3] Hoffmeister's study of the delay phenomenon in dogs demonstrated that flaps can survive after a significant decrease in circulation, with a subsequent increase in flow with an average three-week delay.[45] In this ischemic condition, the flap can little afford further compromise.

Labelled radioactive microsphere measurement of skin flow in dogs demonstrated flow rates of 0.02 to 0.24 ml/gm/min, with an average flow of 0.07 ml/gm/min.[76] Flap elevation resulted in a marked fall in cutaneous blood flow, especially in the most distant region of the flap. Blood flows were only 5 per cent of control flows in most cases, with some flows falling to less than 1 per cent in distal regions of the flap.[76] Kane and Grim reported blood flow to the skin of the canine pelvic limb by employing ^{42}K and ^{86}Rb clearance as 0.08 ml/gm/min with a drop in flow to 0.04 ml/gm/min after exercise.[53] Similarly, flows of 0.046 to 0.053 ml/gm/min occur in elevated canine caudal superficial epigastric island arterial flaps with a flow of 0.041 to 0.048 ml/gm/min after re-anastomosis as a free flap.[64]

Complete arterial or venous compromise to a flap causes necrosis.[74] Pure arterial obstruction caused pale flaps in experimental rabbits without obvious signs of necrosis for over three days. Pure venous obstruction resulted in venous engorgement, ecchymosis, and cyanosis within 24 hours with variable degrees of necrosis. Experimentally, it was extremely difficult to produce flap necrosis in rabbits by venous obstruction alone unless all visible veins were ligated. Even then, only 50 per cent of the flap necrosed. It was concluded that combined arterial and venous occlusion is the most common cause of flap necrosis, with cyanosis in the rabbit flap by one hour and a clear demarcation of necrosis by three days.[74] Other work suggests that flap necrosis is primarily due to arterial insufficiency.[56] Canine flap necrosis was not visually apparent for five or six days in some flaps, and a minimum of one week was required to determine whether all portions of a flap survived.[79] This may be explained, in part, by a progressive decline in circulation over a three- to seven-day period.[45] Darkly pigmented skin is also difficult to assess for color changes associated with circulatory embarrassment.

Excessive wound tension is one cause of flap necrosis. A skin tension of 25 gm applied to each side of experimental skin flaps is sufficient to cause an elevation of interstitial fluid pressure resulting in flap necrosis from circulatory compromise.[70] Wound tension retards wound healing. Skin wounds under marked tension in dogs often separated, although no sloughing occurred if skin circulation was maintained.[70] As a result, flap circulation should be preserved and excessive tension, kinking, and twisting of the flap should be minimized to avoid necrosis and dehiscence.[35]

Underlying hematomas have been implicated as a cause of flap necrosis from pressure generated beneath the flap. Experimental studies in rats suggested that a high molecular weight component in the hemolysate had a toxic effect on skin flaps.[68] Evacuation of the hematoma within 12 hours of its formation may improve flap survival, although a flap delay of one week protected pedicle grafts in rats against necrosis associated with hematoma.[68]

The effect of gravity on the arterial supply and venous drainage of skin flaps has also been a concern in flap survival.[47, 97] Venous return was augmented by elevating the free end of the flap higher than the base, whereas the reverse improved arterial blood flow.[47, 97] Studies in swine and rabbits indicated that gravity did not promote necrosis in nondelayed flaps, whereas delayed flaps in a dependent position had a smaller area of survival.[11, 75] Flap studies utilizing canine axial pattern flaps and reverse saphenous conduit flaps placed in a dependent position have not demonstrated any adverse effects from gravity.[79, 87]

Infection is more likely to occur in tissue with poor circulation.[86, 102] Studies in germ-free rats suggest that endogenous bacterial flora may play a role in flap necrosis.[61]

An obstruction to blood reflow in peripheral tissues, caused by various periods of tourniquet ischemia, has been assigned the term *no-reflow phenomenon*.[8, 62] Two explanations for this phenomenon have emerged: (1) vascular and parenchymal edema and swelling causing a narrowing of the capillary lumen and trapping the formed blood elements; and (2) sludge or thrombus formation in the stagnant blood within the vascular tree of the ischemic flap.[8, 62]

Experimental studies in denervated free epigastric flaps in rabbits demonstrated the progressive nature of this obstruction after prolonged periods of ischemia, reaching a point of irreversibility after 12 hours, leading to flap necrosis.[62] Findings were consistent with the hypothesis that the no-reflow phenomenon is caused by cellular swelling, intravascular aggregation, and leakage of intravascular fluid into the interstitial space.[62]

Previous research in the rat indicated that halothane anesthesia has an adverse effect on flap survival.[35, 102] Studies with axial pattern flaps as well as numerous clinical cases with subdermal plexus flaps with halothane anesthesia have failed to demonstrate any significant problem with flap necrosis.[77, 79, 80–83, 85, 87] Halothane anesthesia probably has no adverse effect on canine and feline cutaneous pedicle grafting procedures.[79]

The multiple factors that contribute to poor circulation underscore the importance of atraumatic surgical technique, asepsis, hemostasis, and careful planning of the flap transfer. Surgical trauma and unnecessary division of cutaneous vascular channels, excessive edema, kinking or twisting of the flap pedicle, hematoma formation, infection, and improper postoperative bandaging techniques all have a cumulative negative effect on flap survival.

Subjective Assessment of Flap Circulation

Color, warmth, pain sensation, and bleeding are used to assess the viability of damaged skin. Unfortunately, all are deceptive and subject to inaccurate interpretation.

Skin color after trauma is deceptive. Contused skin often survives if no additional circulatory compromise occurs. Portions of flaps with severe circulatory compromise have been noted to pass through changes in color: from red, (inflammation) to lavender, to deep purple, and finally to black after one to six days.[79, 87] Pigmented skin may initially show no obvious color changes[58] until fissuring occurs between viable and nonviable areas within a week of the initial flap elevation.[87] Portions of flaps pass from red to lavender with eventual resolution without necrosis.[79, 87] As a result, color changes in the early stages of circulatory compromise can have variable outcomes.

Temperature measurements of skin flaps under controlled conditions are necessary to accurately assess circulation.[58] Because most flaps are partially nervated when elevated, a lack of pain sensation in a responsive animal is not an accurate reflection of flap survival. Although bleeding along the skin margins is considered a desirable intraoperative clinical sign of adequate flap circulation, it does not give any information about venous return. Vasospasm may cause a temporary drop in circulation with a misleading decline in bleeding from the wound edge.[79, 87] The presence of circulation within a flap is also no assurance that trauma, edema, infection, venous compromise, or progressive thrombosis will not subsequently destroy the circulation.[37, 87]

Digital pressure and blanching of the skin with color return within four seconds is a primitive test to evaluate flap circulation in man.[35] Because the skin of the dog and cat does not readily blanch, this test has little or no practical application for the veterinarian.[58]

Hair growth has been associated with circulatory adequacy.[15, 35, 102] Hair growth was sparse with poor circulation in tubed rabbit flaps with good hair growth seen by day 12.[15] Unfortunately, the rate of hair growth is of little use when assessing flap survival in the early postoperative period.

Objective Assessment of Flap Circulation

A number of clinical tests have been devised in humans to evaluate the viability of skin flaps by assessing their circulation to determine the "optimum" time to transfer a flap following a delay procedure. Liquid crystallometry, photoplethysmography, infrared thermography, mass spectrometry, blood pressure studies, and radioactive isotope clearance studies have been employed with varying degrees of accuracy but are of little clinical use to the veterinary practitioner.[15, 35, 36, 97, 102] The saline wheal test, atropine absorption test, and histamine scratch test are simple methods that have been employed in humans and rely on a response within a measurable time period.[15, 35, 36, 97, 102] Results give the surgeon a general idea of the circulatory efficacy of the flap. No information is available on the effective clinical use of those tests in veterinary medicine; extrapolating results from man may be inaccurate owing to major cutaneous differences between species.

Fluorescein dye has been used to assess circulation in skin, bowel segments, and areas compromised by peripheral vascular disease.[15, 17, 20, 33, 35, 36, 48, 69, 79, 87, 89, 98, 102, 106] Fluorescein is currently the most widely accepted agent for predicting flap survival. Intravenous fluorescein dye is a simple, safe, and relatively effective means of estimating flap survival in humans, swine, rats, and rabbits. A strong ultraviolet or blue light source can demonstrate a yellow-to-green fluorescence in areas of adequate cutaneous circulation. Areas lacking circulation do not fluoresce, whereas areas of spotty fluorescence in human patients are indicative of poor circulation, although such areas may survive.[36] Nonfluorescent areas often undergo necrosis; excision of nonfluorescent and poorly fluorescent areas is often performed in human patients during a surgical procedure to avoid complications associated with necrosis.[35, 36]

A clear delineation between fluorescent and nonfluorescent regions of flaps has been reported in swine, rats, and humans.[35, 36] This was also noted in two reports with dogs.[20, 23] However, I have not noticed a well-defined line of fluorescence in canine flap studies. Rather, the fluorescent pattern was mottled and irregular, and false-negative and false-positive results with fluorescein occurred intraoperatively and in the immediate postoperative period.[79, 87]

Nonfluorescent areas of canine flaps do survive in some cases.[79, 87] A false-negative result was also reported in another canine study.[20] Temporary vasospasm of the direct cutaneous vessels is one explanation for this phenomenon.[79, 87] False-negative results after fluorescein administration are commonly found on visual examination with an ultraviolet light. Because fiberoptic dermofluorometers are able to detect discrete fluorescence, they have been advocated to minimize false-negative results.[98]

Flaps areas with poor fluorescence also undergo necrosis.[87] Indeed, one cannot predict circulatory deterioration by use of fluorescein after thermal injuries.[37] The development of postoperative edema and other factors promoting flap necrosis can negate positive fluorescein fluorescence. Repeated fluorescein dye studies are required to assess circulatory compromise in the postoperative period.[58]

Disulphine blue[66, 67, 113] and patent blue[54] dye have also been employed in experimental flap studies and may be more useful in pigmented skin. However, fluorescein is safer, with fewer adverse reactions than disulphine blue,[35] and is readily available for clinical use.

Kerrigan and Daniel recently reported obtaining blood samples from swine flaps with small cutaneous stab wounds using a No. 11 scalpel blade to assess blood pH, blood gas measurements, and the hematocrit with heparinized hematocrit tubes.[58] The hematocrit and pH were accurate guidelines to determine circulatory compromise. Threatened pedicle grafts had a rise in the hematocrit to 54% compared with 35% in control flaps, whereas the pH readings were 0.4 unit below the control. These two measurements proved to be more accurate than intermittent surface temperature readings. Stab wound analysis is repeatable at any time in the postoperative period, unlike fluorescein studies, which require an interval of eight hours before the test can be repeated.[58] This test may have practical clinical application in veterinary institutions and large private practices, pending studies to confirm its accuracy in the dog and cat.

Salvaging the Failing Flap

While much research is directed at developing flaps with a built-in blood supply that permits large flap elevation with little likelihood of necrosis (axial pattern flaps, free flaps, and myocutaneous flaps), other research has been directed at changes occurring in the flap microcirculation and methods to prevent necrosis once circulatory compromise to the skin is evident. Studies of the delay phenomenon may help us understand the pathophysiology of flap failure, its prevention, and its successful treatment.[27, 35, 36, 54, 90]

Denervation, partial devascularization (ischemia), and inflammation contribute to the delay phenomenon.[27, 36, 72] One study suggested that arteriovenous shunting occurs as a result of denervation and ischemia, diverting blood from the nutrient circulation of the pedicle graft.[90] Shunting became lethal only in areas of impaired circulation.[90] If sufficient circulation remained to maintain the flap during the delay, skin shunts would close, resulting in improved flap circulation.[90]

Other researchers have rejected the arteriovenous shunting theory.[27, 36, 39, 72] A subsequent study using swine failed to correlate arteriovenous shunts with surgical delay.[39] Many researchers currently feel that vascular relaxation occurs during surgical delay, resulting in improved flap circulation from sustained vasodilation.[27, 36, 72] Controlling the diameter of blood vessels may be a major determinant in blood flow and its distribution. If so, chemical vasodilators may be selected to replace the time and expense associated with surgical delays and may be employed to salvage failing flaps. A variety of drugs have been employed in experimental animals and human clinical patients with variable results.[1, 9, 17, 18, 21, 25, 26, 29, 43, 44, 55, 56, 65, 72, 93, 94, 115]

Isoxsuprine, a direct smooth muscle relaxant, has been effectively employed to improve survival of neurovascular island flaps in rabbits, island myocutaneous flaps in swine, myocutaneous flaps in humans, and skin flaps in rats.[9, 25, 26, 28, 29, 56, 71] Isoxsuprine has also been reported to have little influence on cutaneous blood flow in man and rats.[9, 56, 93] As a result, isoxsuprine may be beneficial in those skin flaps that include the underlying panniculus carnosus or myocutaneous flaps.[9] However, controlled research is required in the dog and cat before its clinical use can be recommended especially when a subsequent study in rats failed to demonstrate isoxsuprine's efficacy.[93]

Corticosteroids are beneficial in improving flap survival in rabbits and pigs.[56, 65] They may be useful in sustaining anoxic cells, may have a vasodilating action, and may stimulate alternate metabolic pathways. Prednisolone was reported to be more beneficial in porcine axial pattern flaps than in random pattern flaps and appears to be effective in improving the afferent blood supply provided by small arteries, such as those found in the panniculus carnosus of rabbits.[65] Neurovascular island flap studies of the rabbit pinna demonstrated that prednisolone sodium succinate dramatically reduced edema. The intensity of inflammatory response was greatly reduced and resolved in a shorter period of time compared with untreated rabbits. Minimizing postoperative edema may be valuable in preventing circulatory compromise due to swelling. Prednisolone is best given preoperatively to reach compromised tissues after the blood supply has shut down.[65]

The mechanical elevation of skin flaps may result in the release of certain prostaglandin compounds that may cause vasoconstriction and thrombus formation.[94]

Prostaglandin inhibitors increase flap survival in rats and may be beneficial by causing vasodilation with increased blood flow, decreased thrombus formation, decreased inflammation, and stabilization of lysosomes.[94] Prostaglandins (PGs) and thromboxane (TxA_2) are synthesized and released by blood vessels and many other tissues in response to a wide variety of stimuli (hormones, trauma, enzymes, inflammation, pyrogens, and immune and allergic reactions). PGE compounds are known to produce vasodilation, whereas F series PGs produce vasoconstriction in most mammalian species. Other arachidonic acid metabolites, such as prostacyclin (PGI_2), also influence vascular smooth muscle tone. PGI_2 is synthesized in blood vessels and is a potent inhibitor of platelet aggregation and is also a smooth muscle relaxant. TxA_2 is produced by platelets and has the opposite effects of prostacyclin. Both steroidal and nonsteroidal (aspirin, ibuprofen, indomethacin) antiinflammatory drugs are nonspecific inhibitors of prostaglandins and TxA_2 synthesis at different stages of metabolic pathways of arachidonic acid.[94] Imidazole and its l-methyl analogue are specific inhibitors of TxA_2 synthesis. Rat flaps treated with the prostaglandin inhibitors indomethacin and ibuprofen (Motrin) alone and with the vasodilator PGE_2 had a significantly higher survival rate than controls. Flaps treated with indomethacin and PGF_2-alpha had significantly lower areas of survival. The combination of PGE_2 and prostaglandin inhibitors had the most beneficial results. The low viability of flaps treated with a prostaglandin synthesis inhibitor and PGF_2-alpha suggests that certain arachidonic acid metabolites produced during flap elevation may be detrimental to flap survival.[94]

Altering the rheology of blood improves flap survival. Anemia in dogs and rabbits and protein depletion in rats were useful in decreasing blood viscosity with improved flap survival. However, inducing anemia and hypoproteinemia to improve flap survival is not a logical option.[57]

Additional controlled studies are required in the dog and cat to determine the effectiveness of agents reported to be useful in other species.

Topical dressings (antibiotic creams) improve the surviving length of rat flaps by diminishing the depth of tissue loss from desiccation of the deeper ischemic portions of the flap until revascularization can occur.[63] Similar experimental flaps in rats have been protected in a similar fashion by covering the pedicle graft with a semipermeable membrane or a "tunnelling procedure" (by suturing the adjacent wound edges over the top of the flap).[92]

Hypothermia can prolong survival of free flaps.[57, 96, 107] Under normothermic conditions, rat skin is able to tolerate ischemia for 6 to 9 hours, rabbit free skin flaps more than 8 hours, and island flaps in swine between 8 and 13 hours.[57] Delayed flaps can withstand only four hours of normothermic ischemia, apparently owing to depleted metabolic stores. In humans, free skin flaps and amputated digits are able to tolerate six to eight hours of normothermic ischemia.[57] At 3 to 4°C, skin grafts can tolerate up to three weeks of complete ischemia. Storage of experimental free skin flaps in rats at 4°C can prolong ischemia time for over 72 hours. Rabbit free flaps stored in 6 to 7°C can tolerate up to 3.8 days of complete ischemia. Flaps in the human have been maintained after 30 hours of hypothermia and human digits after 28 and 36 hours.[57]

Free groin flaps in rabbits have been supported for up to 72 hours with hypothermia, whereas successful experimental limb implantation has been supported for up to 108 hours with supplemental hypothermia.[107] Latissimus dorsi free flap research in the dog demonstrated prolonged survival for up to 96 hours when stored at 4°C. Only flaps perfused with Collins' solution demonstrated viability beyond this point.[107] Canine latissimus dorsi myocutaneous flaps were better able to withstand hypothermia than epigastric flaps, most likely owing to the higher flow per gram of tissue.[96] Hyperbaric oxygen, tissue perfusion, and hypothermia either alone or in combination are accepted methods of reducing the effects of anoxia.[57, 107]

MANAGEMENT OF THE NECROTIC FLAP

In the event of flap necrosis, excision is best performed within one week. Healing is slowed by necrotic skin by mechanically delaying wound contraction. The deeper layer of the flap dermis may also heal to the underlying bed and delay formation of granulation tissue. Wound healing was accelerated in this study if the slough was left on the wound for a couple of days.[88] However, the surgeon must weigh the risk of infection by retaining the slough against the minor benefit gained in wound healing.

It is unusual for the entire pedicle graft to undergo necrosis. Variable portions of the proximal flap usually survive. The next option for wound closure depends on the remaining portion of the recipient bed that requires coverage. Small areas may close satisfactorily by contraction and epithelialization. Otherwise, development of a second flap or use of free grafts may be considered.

1. Aarts, H. F.: Regional intravascular sympathetic blockade for better results in flap surgery. An experimental study of free flaps, island flaps, and pedicle flaps in the rabbit ear. Plast. Reconstr. Surg. 66:690, 1980.
2. Alexander, J. W., Hoffer, R. E., and MacDonald, J. M.: The use of tubular flap grafts in the treatment of traumatic wounds on the extremity of the cat. Feline Pract. 6:29, 1976.
3. Aoki, T., and Wada, M.: Functional activity of the sweat glands in the hairy skin of the dog. Science 114:123, 1951.
4. Archibald, J.: Procedures in plastic surgery. J. Am. Vet. Med. Assoc. 147:1461, 1965.
5. Arnall, L.: Repair of an extensive brachial slough by a cervical pedicle flap graft. J. Small Anim. Pract. 1:286, 1961.

6. Cawley, H. J., and Archibald, J.: Plastic surgery. *In* Archibald, J. (ed.): *Canine Surgery*, 2nd ed. American Veterinary Publications, Inc., Santa Barbara, CA, 1974.

7. Cawley, A. J., and Francis, S. M.: Pedicle graft in a dog. A case report. Cornell Vet. *48*:12, 1958.

8. Chait, L. A., May, J. W., O'Brien, B. M., and Hurley, J. V.: The effect of the perfusion of various solutions on the no-reflow phenomenon in experimental free flaps. Plast. Reconstr. Surg. *61*:421, 1978.

9. Cherry, G. W.: The differing effects of isoxsuprine on muscle flap and skin flap survival in the pig. Plast. Reconstr. Surg. *64*:670, 1979.

10. Cherry, G. W.: Discussion: Pharmacologic treatment of the failing skin flap. Plast. Reconstr. Surg. *70*:549, 1982.

11. Cherry, G. W., Phil, D., Myers, M. B., Ardran, G., and Ryan, F. J.: The effects of gravity on delayed and transplanted delayed tubed flaps. Plast. Reconstr. Surg. *64*:156, 1979.

12. Cohen, B. E.: Beneficial effect of staged division of pedicle in experimental axial pattern flaps. Plast. Reconstr. Surg. *64*:366, 1974.

13. Cohen, B. E., Harmon, C. S., and Phizackerley, B. M.: Glucose metabolism in experimental skin flaps. Plast. Reconstr. Surg. *71*:79, 1983.

14. Converse, J. M.: *Reconstructive Plastic Surgery*, Vol. 1. W. B. Saunders, Philadelphia, 1977.

15. Conway, H., Stark, R. B., and Docktor, J. P.: Vascularization of tubed pedicles. Plast. Reconstr. Surg. *4*:133, 1949.

16. Crawford, B. S.: The management of tube pedicles. Br. J. Plast. Surg. *18*:387, 1965.

17. Crismon, J. M., and Fuhrman, F. A.: Studies on gangrene following cold injury. IV. The use of fluorescein as an indicator of local blood flow. Distribution of fluorescein in body fluids after intravenous injection. J. Clin. Invest. *26*:259, 1947.

18. Cutting, C., Bumsted, R., Bardach, J., Mooney, M., and Johnson, S.: Changes in quantitative norepinephrine levels in delayed pig flank flaps. Plast. Reconstr. Surg. *69*:652, 1982.

19. Daniel, R. K., and Williams, H. B.: The free transfer of skin flaps by microvascular anastomoses. Plast. Reconstr. Surg. *52*:16, 1973.

20. Dingwall, J. A., and Lord, J. W.: The fluorescein test in the management of tubed (pedicle) flaps. Bull. Johns Hopkins Hosp. *73*:129, 1943.

21. Edstrom, L. E.: Discussion: A study of the pharmacologic control of blood flow to acute and delayed skin flaps using xenon washout. Parts I and II. Plast. Reconstr. Surg. *71*:409, 1983.

22. Erol, O. O., and Spira, M.: New capillary bed formation with a surgically constructed arteriovenous fistula. Plast. Reconstr. Surg. *66*:109, 1980.

23. Erol, O. O., and Spira, M.: Secondary musculocutaneous flap: An experimental study. Plast. Reconstr. Surg. *65*:277, 1980.

24. Evans, H. E., and Christensen, G. C.: *Miller's Anatomy of The Dog*. W. B. Saunders, Philadelphia, 1979.

25. Finseth, F.: Clinical salvage of three failing skin flaps by treatment with a vasodilator drug. Plast. Reconstr. Surg. *63*:304, 1979.

26. Finseth, F., and Adelberg, M. G.: Experimental work with isoxsuprine for prevention of skin necrosis and for treatment of the failing flap. Plast. Reconstr. Surg. *63*:94, 1979.

27. Finseth, F., and Cutting, C.: An experimental neurovascular island skin flap for the study of the delay phenomenon. Plast. Reconstr. Surg. *61*:412, 1978.

28. Finseth, F., and Zimmerman, J.: Prevention of necrosis in island myocutaneous flaps in the pig by treatment with isoxsuprine. Plast. Reconstr. Surg. *64*:537, 1979.

29. Finseth, F., Zimmerman, J., and Liggins, D.: Prevention of muscle necrosis in an experimental neurovascular island muscle flap by a vasodilator drug, Isoxsuprine. Plast. Reconstr. Surg. *63*:774, 1979.

30. German, W., Finesilver, E. M., and Davis, J. S.: Establishment of circulation in tubed skin flaps. Arch. Surg. *26*:27, 1933.

31. Glinz, W., and Clodius, L.: Measurement of tissue pH for pedicting viability in pedicle flaps: experimental studies in pigs. Br. J. Plast. Surg. *25*:111, 1972.

32. Goldwyn, R. M., Lamb, D. L., and White, W. L.: An experimental study of large island flaps in dogs. Plast. Reconstr. Surg. *31*:530, 1963.

33. Goode, R. L., and Linehan, J. W.: The fluorescein test in postirradiation surgery. Arch. Otolaryngol. *91*:526, 1970.

34. Gourley, I. M.: Neurovascular island flap for treatment of trophic metacarpal pad ulcer in the dog. J. Am. Anim. Hosp. Assoc. *14*:119, 1978.

35. Grabb, W. C., and Myers, M. B.: *Skin Flaps*. Little, Brown, and Co., Boston, 1975.

36. Grabb, W. C., and Smith, J. W.: *Plastic Surgery*. Little, Brown, and Co., Boston, 1973.

37. Grant, T. D.: The early enzymatic debridement and grafting of the deep dermal burns to the hand. Plast. Reconstr. Surg. *66*:185, 1980.

38. Guba, A. M.: Study of the delay phenomenon in axial pattern flaps in pigs. Plast. Reconstr. Surg. *63*:550, 1979.

39. Guba, A. M.: Arteriovenous shunting in the pig. Plast. Reconstr. Surg. *65*:323, 1980.

40. Guba, A. M., and Callahan, J.: Nutrient blood flow in delayed axial pattern skin flaps in pigs. Plast. Reconstr. Surg. *64*:372, 1979.

41. Harii, K., and Ohmori, S.: Use of the gastroepiploic vessels as recipient or donor vessels in the free transfer of composite flaps by microvascular anastomoses. Plast. Reconstr. Surg. *52*:544, 1973.

42. Harii, K., Ohmori, K., and Sekiguchi, J.: The free musculocutaneous flap. Plast. Reconstr. Surg. *57*:294, 1976.

43. Hendel, P. M., Lilien, D. L., and Buncke, H. J.: A study of the pharmacologic control of blood flow to acute skin flaps using xenon washout. Part I. Plast. Reconstr. Surg. *71*:387, 1983.

44. Hendel, P. M., Lilien, D. L., and Buncke, H. J.: A study of the pharmacologic control of blood flow to delayed skin flaps using xenon washout, Part II. Plast. Reconstr. Surg. *71*:399, 1983.

45. Hoffmeister, F. S.: Studies on timing of tissue transfer in reconstructive surgery: I. Effect of delay on circulation in flaps. Plast. Reconstr. Surg. *19*:283, 1957.

46. Hoffmeister, F. S.: Timing of transfer of flaps in reconstructive surgery. Surg. Gynecol. Obstet. *108*:68, 1959.

47. Hynes, W.: The blood vessels in skin tubes and flaps. Br. J. Plast. Surg. *3*:165, 1950.

48. Hynes, W., and Macgregor, A. G.: The use of fluorescein in estimating the blood flow in pedicled skin flaps and tubes. Br. J. Plast. Surg. *2*:4, 1949.

49. Im, M. J., Su, C. T., Hoopes, J. E., and Anthenelli, R. M.: Skin flap metabolism in rats: Oxygen consumption and lactate production. Plast. Reconstr. Surg. *71*:685, 1983.

50. Jensen, E. C.: Skin grafting in the dog. Iowa State College Vet. *19*:163, 1957.

51. Jensen, E. C.: Canine autogenous skin grafting. Am. J. Vet. Res. *20*:898, 1959.

52. Johnston, D. E.: The repair of skin loss on the foot by means of a double-pedicle abdominal flap. J. Am. Anim. Hosp. Assoc. *12*:593, 1976.

53. Kane, W. J., and Grim, E.: Blood flow to canine hind-limb bone, muscle, and skin. J. Bone Joint Surg. *51*:309, 1969.

54. Kay, S. R., and LeWinn, L. R.: Neural influences on experimental flap survival. Plast. Reconstr. Surg. *67*:42, 1981.

55. Kennedy, T. J., Pistone, G., and Miller, S. H.: The effects of reserpine on microcirculatory flow in rat flaps. Plast. Reconstr. Surg. *63*:101, 1979.

56. Kerrigan, C. L., and Daniel, R. K.: Pharmacologic treatment of the failing skin flap. Plast. Reconstr. Surg. *70*:541, 1982.

57. Kerrigan, C. L., and Daniel, R. K.: Critical ischemia time and the failing skin flap. Plast. Reconstr. Surg. *69*:986, 1982.

58. Kerrigan, C. L., and Daniel, R. K.: Monitoring acute skin flap failure. Plast. Reconstr. Surg. 71:519, 1983.

59. Krahwinkel, D. J.: Reconstruction of skin defects by the use of pedicle grafts. J. Am. Anim. Hosp. Assoc. 12:844, 1976.

60. Krizek, T. J., Tani, T., Desprez, J. D., and Kiehn, C. L.: Experimental transplantation of composite grafts by microsurgical vascular anastomoses. Plast. Reconstr. Surg. 36:538, 1965.

61. Macht, S. D., and Frazier, W. H.: The role of endogenous bacterial flora in skin flap survival. Plast. Reconstr. Surg. 65:50, 1980.

62. May, W. M., Chait, L. A., O'Brien, B. M., and Hurley, J. M.: The no-reflow phenomenon in experimental free flaps. Plast. Reconstr. Surg. 61:256, 1978.

63. McGrath, M. H.: How topical dressings salvage "questionable" flaps: experimental study. Plast. Reconstr. Surg. 67:653, 1981.

64. McKee, N. H., Clarke, H. M., Nigka, C. A. L., and Manktelow, R. T.: A study of blood flow and pressure in the vessels supplying a free flap. Plast. Reconstr. Surg. 69:68, 1982.

65. Mes, L. G. B.: Improving flap survival by sustaining cell metabolism within ischemic cells: a study using rabbits. Plast. Reconstr. Surg. 65:56, 1980.

66. Milton, S. H.: Pedicled skin flaps: the fallacy of the length:width ratio. Br. J. Surg. 57:502, 1970.

67. Milton, S. H.: Experimental studies on island flaps, I. The surviving length. Plast. Reconstr. Surg. 48:574, 1971.

68. Mulliken, J. B., and Healey, N. A.: Pathogenesis of skin flap necrosis from underlying hematoma. Plast. Reconstr. Surg. 63:540, 1979.

69. Myers, M. B.: Prediction of skin sloughs at the time of operation with the use of fluorescein dye. Surgery 51:158, 1962.

70. Myers, M. B.: Wound tension and vascularity in the etiology and prevention of skin sloughs. Plast. Reconstr. Surg. 56:945, 1964.

71. Myers, M. B.: Commentary-clinical salvage of three failing skin flaps by treatment with a vasodilator drug. Plast. Reconstr. Surg. 63:546, 1979.

72. Myers, M. B.: Discussion: A study of the pharmacologic control of blood flow to acute and delayed skin flaps using xenon washout. Parts I and II. Plast. Reconstr. Surg. 71:408, 1983.

73. Myers, M. B., and Cherry, G.: Augmentation of tissue survived by delay: An experimental study in rabbits. Plast. Reconstr. Surg. 39:397, 1967.

74. Myers, M. B., and Cherry, G.: Causes of necrosis in pedicle flaps. Plast. Reconstr. Surg. 42:43, 1968.

75. Myers, M. B., Cherry, G., and Bombet, R.: On the lack of any effect of gravity on the survival of tubed flaps. Plast. Reconstr. Surg. 51:428, 1973.

76. Nathanson, S. E., and Jackson, R. T.: Blood flow measurements in skin flaps. Arch. Otolaryngol. 101:354, 1975.

77. Pavletic, M. M.: Caudal superficial epigastric arterial pedicle grafts in the dog. Vet. Surg. 9:103, 1980.

78. Pavletic, M. M.: Vascular supply to the skin of the dog: a review. Vet. Surg. 9:77, 1980.

79. Pavletic, M. M.: Canine axial pattern flaps, using the omocervical, thoracodorsal, and deep circumflex iliac direct cutaneous arteries. Am. J. Vet. Res. 42:391, 1981.

80. Pavletic, M. M.: Reconstructive esophageal surgery in the dog: A literature review and case report. J. Am. Anim. Hosp. Assoc. 17:435, 1981.

81. Pavletic, M. M.: Combined closure techniques for a large skin defect in a cat. Feline Pract. 12:16, 1982.

82. Pavletic, M. M.: Misapplication of subcutaneous pedicle flaps in the dog. Vet. Surg. 11:18, 1982.

83. Pavletic, M. M.: Mucocutaneous subdermal plexus flap from the lip for lower eyelid restoration in the dog. J. Am. Vet. Med. Assoc. 180:921, 1982.

84. Pavletic, M. M.: Nasal and rostral labial reconstruction in the dog. J. Am. Anim. Hosp. Assoc. 19:913, 1983.

85. Pavletic, M. M., and MacIntire, D.: Phycomycosis of the axilla and inner brachium in a dog: Surgical excision and reconstruction with a thoracodorsal axial pattern flap. J. Am. Vet. Med. Assoc. 180:1197, 1982.

86. Pavletic, M. M., and Peyton, L. C.: Plastic and reconstructive surgery in the dog and cat. In Bojrab, M. J. (ed.): Current Techniques in Small Animal Surgery II. Lea & Febiger, Philadelphia, 1983.

87. Pavletic, M. M., Watters, J., Henry, R. W., and Nafe, A.: Reverse saphenous conduit flap in the dog. J. Am. Vet. Med. Assoc. 182:380, 1982.

88. Pers, M.: Healing after necrosis of pedicle flaps. Plast. Reconstr. Surg. 27:303, 1961.

89. Prather, A., Blackburn, J. P., Williams, T. R., et al: Evaluation of tests for predicting the viability of axial pattern skin flaps in the pig. Plast. Reconstr. Surg. 63:250, 1979.

90. Reinisch, J. F.: The pathophysiology of skin flap circulation. Plast. Reconstr. Surg. 54:585, 1974.

91. Ross, G. E.: Clinical canine skin grafting. J. Am. Vet. Med. Assoc. 153:159, 1968.

92. Sasaki, A., Fukuda, O., and Soeda, S.: Attempts to increase the surviving length in skin flaps by a moist environment. Plast. Reconstr. Surg. 64:526, 1979.

93. Sasaki, A., and Harii, K.: Lack of effect of isoxsuprine on experimental random flaps in the flap. Plast. Reconstr. Surg. 66:105, 1980.

94. Sasaki, G. H., and Pang, C. Y.: Experimental evidence for involvement of prostaglandins in viability of acute skin flaps: effects on viability and mode of action. Plast. Reconstr. Surg. 67:335, 1981.

95. Schechter, G. L., Biller, H. F., and Ogura, J. H.: Revascularized skin flaps: A new concept in transfer of skin flaps. Laryngoscope 79:1647, 1969.

96. Schlenker, J. D.: Discussion: The effect of hypothermia and tissue perfusion on extended myocutaneous flap viability. Plast. Reconstr. Surg. 70:453, 1982.

97. Seitchik, M. W., and Kahn, S.: The effect of delay on the circulatory efficiency of pedicled tissue. Plast. Reconstr. Surg. 33:16, 1964.

98. Silverman, D. G., et al.: Quantification of tissue fluorescein delivery and prediction of flap viability with the fiberoptic dermofluorometer. Plast. Reconstr. Surg. 66:545, 1980.

99. Spreull, J. S. A.: The principles of transplanting skin in the dog. J. Am. Hosp. Assoc., 4:71, 1968.

100. Stell, P. M., and Green, J. R.: The viability of triangular skin flaps. Br. J. Plast. Surg. 28:247, 1975.

101. Stranc, M. F., Labandter, H., and Roy, A.: A study of 196 tubed pedicles. Br. J. Plast. Surg. 28:54, 1975.

102. Swaim, S. F.: Surgery of Traumatized Skin: Management and Reconstruction in the Dog and Cat. W. B. Saunders, Philadelphia, 1980.

103. Swaim, S. F., and Bushby, P. A.: Principles of bipedicle tube grafting in the dog. J. Am. Anim. Hosp. Assoc. 12:600, 1976.

104. Swaim, S. F., and Bushby, P. A.: Correction of skin defects of the stifle of dogs and cats. J. Am. Anim. Hosp. Assoc. 17:445, 1981.

105. Sykes, G. P.: Pouch graft: Resurfacing the distal extremity in the dog. Canine Pract. 7:28, 1980.

106. Thorvaidsson, S. E., and Grabb, W. C.: The intravenous fluorescein test as a measure of skin flap viability. Plast. Reconstr. Surg. 53:576, 1974.

107. Tsai, T. J., Jupiter, J. B., Serratoni, F., Seki, T., and Okubo, K.: The effect of hypothermia and tissue perfusion on extended myocutaneous flap viability. Plast. Reconstr. Surg. 70:444, 1982.

108. Tsuchida, Y., Tsuya, A., Uchida, M., and Kamata, S.: The delay phenomenon in types of deltopectoral flap studied by xenon-133. Plast. Reconstr. Surg. 67:34, 1981.

109. Tsur, H., Daniller, A., and Strauch, B.: Neovascularization of skin flaps: route and timing. Plast. Reconstr. Surg. 66:85, 1980.

110. Webster, J. P.: The early history of the tubed pedicle flap. Surg. Clin. North Am. 39:261, 1959.

111. Wexler, M. R.: An arbor flap. The tree pattern flap, or how narrow may the base of a skin flap be? An experimental study. Plast. Recontr. Surg. 68:185, 1981.

112. Yao, S. T.: Vascular implantation into clinical skin flap: Experimental study and clinical application: A preliminary report. Plast. Reconstr. Surg. 68:404, 1981.

113. Young, C. M.: The revascularization of pedicle skin flaps in pigs: A functional and morphologic study. Plast. Reconstr. Surg. 70:455, 1980.

114. Yturraspe, D. J., Creed, J. E., and Schwach, R. P.: Thoracic pedicle skin flap for repair of lower limb wounds in dogs and cats. J. Am. Anim. Hosp. Assoc. 12:581, 1976.

115. Zarem, H. A., and Soderberg, R.: Tissue reaction to ischemia in the rabbit ear chamber: effects of prednisolone on inflammation and microvascular flow. Plast. Reconstr. Surg. 70:667, 1982.

38 Skin Grafts

Chapter 38

Steven F. Swaim

INSTRUMENTATION

In addition to the basic instruments for plastic and reconstructive skin surgery discussed in Chapter 36, other instruments are available for skin grafting. Some grafting procedures require no special instruments, whereas others do. Full thickness skin grafts, full thickness mesh grafts, seed grafts, and strip grafts can be performed with the basic instruments described in Chapter 36. However, split thickness grafts and split thickness mesh grafts require special instruments.

Split thickness grafts can be harvested freehand using a knife, scalpel blade, or safety razor. Humby, Bodenham, Watson, Braithwaite, Marcks, Caltagirone, and other types of freehand knives have some depth control on the knife to regulate the thickness of skin that is cut. The Blair and Ferris-Smith freehand knives do not have such depth control devices.[4, 10, 16, 26] A small Goulian-type Weck knife can be used to cut small split thickness grafts.[50] Practice and experience are necessary to use these instruments effectively.[60, 62] Although somewhat tedious, a #10 Bard-Parker scalpel blade can be used to cut a split thickness graft.[34] However, these blades are hard to control, and holes may be cut in the skin when cutting the graft.[50] Split thickness grafts can also be cut with an unmodified Schick injector razor[58] or a Gillette safety razor that has had the central strut of the safety guard filed out.[51, 55] The electric or pneumatic Brown Dermatome* has been described for cutting split thickness grafts in veterinary surgery. Although expensive, it requires little skill or experience to use and rapidly yields a uniform split thickness graft.[10, 13, 16, 21, 26, 38, 39, 60, 62]

A disposable dermatome is also available.†[10, 16, 60] Although early models of this instrument were difficult to use,[60, 63] the instrument has been improved by increasing the length of the blade travel and the number of cutting strokes per minute[63] (Fig. 38–1).

A piece of skin can be meshed with a scalpel blade, or a split thickness segment of skin can be laid on an aluminum block that contains numerous staggered parallel rows of notched cutting blades.* As a Teflon roller is passed over the graft, numerous slits are cut in the skin, producing a mesh graft[30, 60–62] (see Fig. 38–1).

Seed grafts can be cut with a scalpel blade and suture needle. However, a disposable skin biopsy punch† may also be used to harvest small plugs of skin (see Fig. 38–1).

Various disposable tissue stapling devices‡ are available that provide a rapid, effective means of closing large incisions and fixing grafts in place.[24, 36, 60]

DEFINITION AND CLASSIFICATION

A skin graft is a segment of epidermis and dermis that is completely removed from the body and transferred to a recipient site. Its survival at the recipient site is dependent upon the absorption of tissue fluid and the development of a new blood supply.[9, 10, 16, 26, 38, 45, 60, 62] Grafts are classified as follows: (1) autografts (autogenous grafts)—the recipient and donor sites are on the same animal; (2) allografts (homografts)—the recipient and donor sites are on genetically different animals of the same species; (3) xenografts (heterografts)—the recipient and donor sites are on animals of different species; and (4) isografts—a graft between identical twins or between F_1 hybrids produced by crossing inbred strains.[13, 16, 26, 34, 60] Clinically, autografts are the most successful type of graft, since the graft and host are antigenically identical.[3] This chapter deals with autografts.

Grafts may be either full thickness (composed of epidermis and the entire dermis) or split thickness

---

*Zimmer Manufacturing Co., Warsaw, IN 46580.

†Davol Dermatome, Davol, Inc., Providence, RI 02901.

*Mesh-Skin Graft Expander, No. P-160, Padgett Instruments, Kansas City, MO 64111.

†Baker's Biopsy Punch, Chester A. Baker Laboratories, Inc., Subsid. of Key Pharmaceuticals, Miami, FL 33169.

‡Proximate, Ethicon Inc., Distributed by Pitman-Moore, Washington Crossing, NJ 08560; Autosuture, U.S. Surgical Corp., Stanford, CT 06902.

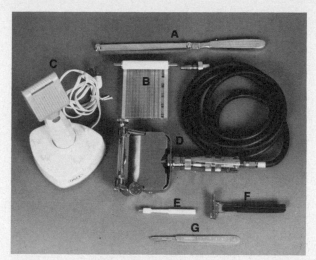

Figure 38–1. Instruments for grafting skin. *A,* Freehand skin graft knife; *B,* Aluminum block with numerous staggered parallel rows of cutting blades and a Teflon roller for making mesh grafts; *C,* disposable dermatome; *D,* pneumatic Brown dermatome; *E,* skin biopsy punch; *F,* Schick single-edge injector razor; *G,* Bard-Parker scalpel handle and blade.

(composed of epidermis and varying thicknesses of the dermis). Split thickness grafts may be thin, of intermediate thickness, or thick, depending on the amount of dermis included.[4, 10, 13, 16, 26, 38, 50, 60, 62]

INDICATIONS AND FACTORS TO CONSIDER

Skin grafts are indicated when there has been a major loss of skin as the result of either trauma or other factors that cause skin defects (e.g., tumor removal).[60, 62] In dogs, skin grafting is primarily indicated for injuries to the skin of the extremities where skin immobility precludes tissue shifting and the construction of local flaps for repair.[33, 39, 60, 67] However, they are occasionally employed to resurface full thickness burns after major thermal injuries.

The general condition of the patient should be considered before grafting is performed. Grafts are generally more successful in young individuals; however, the difference between the young and the aged in terms of graft survival is not marked. Debilitated individuals with chronic disease are more subject to infections than normal patients. Deficiencies should be corrected prior to grafting, especially anemias with low hemoglobin levels, which can adversely affect a graft's survival.[3, 60]

Local factors should also be considered prior to grafting, including the type and condition of the graft bed (recipient bed), the nature of the tissue lost, and the type of skin to be used for grafting. A graft bed should be healthy, uninfected, and well vascularized. The tissue that is lost should be replaced with tissue that has similar characteristics.[60] Since transplanted skin maintains its original characteristics,[26, 50] the skin selected for a graft ideally should match the surrounding skin as closely as possible.[10, 19]

Although skin grafting techniques for humans are applicable in dogs and cats, bandaging and postoperative care in veterinary grafting differ markedly from those in human grafting. Patient restraint, effective bandaging, and contamination are major problems in canine grafting.[33, 60, 62]

GRAFT BEDS

Where Grafts Will Take

A graft "take" is defined as that situation in which the graft has established arterial connections and adequate venous drainage with the graft bed.[44] To accomplish this, the graft bed must be capable of furnishing adequate vasculature for the graft. In general, grafts should be placed on either healthy granulation tissue or a fresh surface that is vascular enough to produce granulation tissue.[26, 38, 60, 62] The latter type of surface may be a surgically created raw surface or a surgically clean surface.[38] Such surfaces include healthy muscle, fascia, pleura, vascular fat, meninges, bare dermis, de-epithelialized scar tissue, and peritoneum.[4, 16, 26, 35, 50] A slightly contaminated wound that is seen early may be cleaned, irrigated *thoroughly,* debrided, and grafted at the same time.[60, 62] However, some allowance should be made for drainage. Clean abrasion or avulsion wounds may also be grafted immediately.[50]

A preference for a fresh, well-vascularized graft bed free of granulation tissue has been reported in the veterinary literature.[41, 46, 49, 67] In general, the blood supply of the wound should be ample enough to support granulation tissue, although the presence of a healthy granulation bed is not a prerequisite for grafting.[26] Moreover, studies on both horses[22, 23] and dogs[33] have indicated that grafts revascularize faster when placed on a fresh, nongranulating surface than when placed on granulation tissue. When epithelial tissue is noted migrating from the wound edges over a healthy granulation bed, it may be interpreted as a sign that the wound will support a skin graft.[50]

Where Grafts Will Not Take

Grafts will not take over stratified squamous epithelial surfaces.[26] Bone, cartilage, tendon, or nerve denuded of overlying connective tissue cannot support a skin graft.[4, 16, 26, 35, 38, 50, 67] An exception is the bridging phenomenon, in which a small area of graft over an avascular surface (about 1 cm diameter) will survive as a result of circulation from the pre-existing vessels in the graft as well as from newly ingrown vessels.[4, 26, 38, 50, 60, 69] A greater portion of a full thickness graft can survive by this phenomenon than a split thickness graft.[25]

Infected wounds and crushed tissues are poor recipient beds for grafts. Crushing injuries may be less vascular and thus more likely to promote early bacterial proliferation.[50] These wounds should be debrided, irrigated, and treated with antibacterial agents until a healthy granulation tissue base is formed.[60] Similarly, heavily irradiated tissues, avascular fat, long-standing granulation tissue, hypertrophic granulation tissue, and the exposed surfaces of chronic ulcers are relatively poor graft beds.[38, 50] It is advisable to excise unfavorable tissue from the wound and allow new granulation tissue to form prior to grafting. Daily compression bandages, hypertonic (3%) saline soaks, and surgical excision have been suggested as means of reducing hypertrophic granulation tissue.[50]

Grafts do not take well on irregular surfaces and wounds that are difficult to immobilize. They will "tent" across depressions in the recipient bed.[4, 38, 60, 62] The use of tie-over bandages, mesh grafts sutured to the wound surface, seed grafts, and strip grafts help to overcome these problems.[60, 62] These graft designs provide excellent drainage and can survive on beds with low-grade infections.

ACCEPTANCE OF GRAFTS ("GRAFT TAKE")

Adherence

A graft adheres to its bed early after placement via a fibrin network which is later invaded by fibroblasts, leukocytes, and phagocytes and converted to a fibrous tissue attachment between the graft and the bed.[9, 13, 20, 26] The bond between graft and bed becomes stronger over time, and by ten days the union of graft and bed is usually complete and firm. The amount of collagen increases in the graft-bed area at the expense of the fibroblasts as time passes. During subsequent days and weeks the collagen matures in the area between the graft and bed. This maturation is responsible for any graft contraction that occurs; contraction is more marked in thin split thickness grafts than in thick split thickness grafts.[13]

Plasmatic Imbibition

After a graft is removed from the donor area, its blood vessels undergo spasm and expel most of the hemic elements from the severed ends of the vessels.[5, 32] During the first 48 to 72 hours after placement, a graft takes on an edematous blue appearance, indicating that the dermal vessels and lymphatics in the graft are absorbing a fibrinogen-free serumlike fluid, which contains erythrocytes and other cells[5, 15, 16, 20, 26, 27, 50] (Fig. 38–2A). This fluid moves to and fro but does not circulate and nourishes the graft cells as well as keeps the graft vessels open for revascularization.[5, 16, 18, 50] Edema of the graft may persist for as long as five days,[45] after which time it starts to subside as the newly established blood and lymphatic flow carry the absorbed fluid away from the graft.[15, 16, 26]

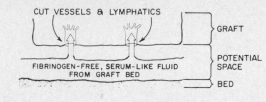

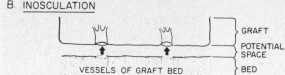

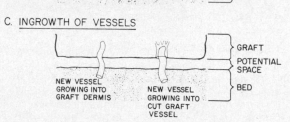

Figure 38–2. Stages of maintenance and revascularization of skin grafts. *A*, Plasmatic imbibition. *B*, Inosculation. *C*, Ingrowth of vessels. (Reprinted with permission from Swaim, S. F.: *Surgery of Traumatized Skin: Management and Reconstruction in the Dog and Cat.* W. B. Saunders, Philadelphia, 1980, p. 428.)

Inosculation

Between 24 and 48 hours after grafting, vascular buds grow from the bed into the fibrin network holding the graft on the bed.[12, 14, 57] Revascularization of a graft begins with the formation of anastomoses between the vessels of the graft bed and vessels within the graft[6, 15–17, 20, 26, 27, 38, 56] (Fig. 38–2B). In some instances graft and bed vessels are joined as they open into common "lakes" or interstices within the fibrin matrix joining the graft and bed.[12]

Many vessels may make contact and anastomose, but few survive and develop.[17] Vessels within the graft may also actively proliferate to establish host and graft connections.[5, 42] It has been suggested that blood vessels in grafts attract bed vessel growth.[43]

The development of anastomoses between bed and graft vessels and the flow of blood into graft vessels have an inhibiting effect on further proliferation of vascular buds in the graft bed. If a seroma or hematoma separates the graft from its bed, the inhibiting effect is slower in occurring, and proliferation of granulation tissue continues.[56]

Ingrowth of Vessels

Grafts are also revascularized by the ingrowth of new vessels from the bed into the graft.[6, 16, 17, 20, 26, 38] These vessels may grow into the dermis or they may grow along the paths of old vessels, which serve as conduits for new ingrowing vessels[5, 6, 16, 17, 20, 26, 27, 38, 50, 56, 70] (Fig. 38–2C). Studies in dogs have shown that most of the revascularization of a free full thickness graft occurs owing to the ingrowth of vessels.[20] The stimulus for vessel ingrowth into a graft may be a diffusible substance from the graft's dead or damaged cells or, more probably, hypoxia of the area.[68] Vessels can also invade a graft from the surrounding skin margins to a limited degree.[47] Vessel ingrowth *may* start as early as 6 to 12 hours after grafting,[17] and the circulation may be completely re-established from 4[17] to 12[20] days after transplantation.

GRAFT LOSS AND ITS PREVENTION

Three main factors are responsible for graft loss: (1) accumulation of blood or serum under a graft, (2) bacterial infection, and (3) improper immobilization of the graft.[10, 19, 26, 38, 49]

Hematomas and Seromas

A hematoma under a graft is a barrier to capillary ingrowth from the graft bed and interferes with revascularization and plasmatic imbibition.[9, 10, 16, 20, 35, 38] Likewise, serum under a graft separates the graft from its bed. Such a graft survives only by plasmatic imbibition and will not revascularize until it contacts the graft bed.[19, 38] Adequate hemostasis and provision for drainage are thus very important for graft survival. The following is a summary of the various techniques that can be used to ensure adequate hemostasis on a graft bed:

1. Prepare the graft bed before harvesting the graft to allow time for hemostasis in the graft bed.[26, 38]
2. Apply gentle pressure on the bed with saline-soaked sponges, and apply continual digital pressure on the graft while suturing.[3, 9, 41, 46, 49]
3. Clamp bleeding vessels.[46]
4. Ligate bleeding vessels.[3, 9, 26, 38]
5. Cauterize bleeding vessels.[26, 38]
6. Apply 1:100,000 epinephrine topically with a moistened sponge to diminish bleeding from small vessels. Inject 1:500,000 epinephrine into the proposed surgical site.[26]
7. Apply thrombin, gelatin foam, or gelatin film topically. These should be *removed* prior to graft application.
8. Make "pie crust" stab incisions in a graft to provide for drainage.[46, 49]
9. Apply a tourniquet prior to preparation of the graft bed, but release it prior to placing the graft.[26] Apply an Esmarch bandage to a limb prior to preparing the graft bed, and unwrap the bandage from distal to proximal to expose the surgical site, leaving the proximal portion of the bandage wrapped.

The following is a summary of the techniques that can be used to remove a hematoma or a seroma from under a graft if one should form during or shortly after application of a graft.

1. Flush sterile saline or thrombin solution under the graft before placing the final anchoring sutures or after removing a few anchoring sutures.[16, 26, 38]
2. Gently swirl a cotton-tipped applicator under the graft to remove a hematoma.[16, 26, 38]
3. Roll a gauze sponge over the graft prior to placing the final sutures or after making an incision in the graft, thus removing any blood clots.[35]
4. Use an eyedropper or sterile applicator stick to remove clots through an incision made in the graft.[16, 26]

Any incisions made in a graft after it has been applied should be made carefully to prevent damage to the graft bed, which could cause more hemorrhage.[26, 60] After a seroma or hematoma is removed, grafts should be inspected daily.[16, 26] Two or three anchor sutures can be omitted at the most dependent part of the graft to allow for drainage or to allow the introduction of a cotton-tipped applicator to remove clots. The use of minimally expanded or unexpanded mesh grafts has also been effective in providing drainage from a grafted wound.

Infection

Sepsis slows the migration of cells into a wound and thus delays revascularization of a graft. Bacteria cause cell death in both the graft and the recipient bed. In some infections, the fibrin film that adheres the graft to the bed is dissolved.[9] Therefore, grafting should not be undertaken until wound infection is controlled.[3, 59] Adequate debridement, lavage, drainage, and antimicrobials should be employed to obtain an infection-free wound that is ready for grafting.

Granulation tissue is never sterile but has a resident bacterial flora, and most of these bacteria are harmless; however, the presence of some bacteria is disastrous to skin grafts.[50] The fibrin that initially "glues" a graft to its bed has antibacterial properties under an adherent autograft.[65] The total number of bacteria per gram of tissue in a wound, although important, is not a critical factor in graft survival. The ability of the organisms to produce plasmin and proteolytic enzymes is the primary factor in bacterial infection causing skin graft loss. The plasmin and proteolytic enzymes dissolve the fibrin scaffolding between the graft and its bed. With the fibrin dissolved, the antibacterial activity of the graft is gone, and the organisms can reproduce. Therefore, if the various types of bacteria in a wound are efficient producers of plasmin and proteolytic enzymes, the chances of graft loss are great.[65] It is generally accepted that β-hemolytic streptococci are quite detrimental to graft survival. It is interesting to note that wounds infected with these organisms and pseudomonads have high levels of plasmin and proteolytic activity.[65]

Some of the organisms of concern in skin grafting are *Streptococcus pyogenes*, *Staphylococcus aureus*, *Pseudomonas aeruginosa*, *Proteus vulgaris*, and *Escherichia coli*. β-hemolytic streptococci (*S. pyogenes*) may cause complete dissolution of a graft by interfering with the normal fibrinous attachment of the graft to its bed.[19, 26, 38, 50, 59, 65] Systemic penicillin has been recommended for treating such infections.[38, 50] Topical chlorhexidine can be used to treat wounds infected with streptococcus and staphylococcus.[38] A 0.05% aqueous solution of a 2% concentration of chlorhexidine* is recommended for treatment.[60] *Pseudomonas aeruginosa* may cause loss of a graft, as its exudate tends to float a graft from its bed.[60] This is undoubtedly related to the dissolution of fibrin. Various agents have been described for the control of this organism prior to grafting, including wet dressings of 0.5% silver nitrate, topical application of 10% mafenide acetate (Sulfamylon), application of 0.5% acetic acid, and the early application of polymixin B sulfate.[60, 62]

Staphylococcus aureus, *Escherichia coli*, and *Proteus vulgaris* are also found in wounds, and the latter two are usually found in combination with *Pseudomonas aeruginosa*. A 0.1% gentamicin ointment†[60] or a 0.1% aqueous solution prepared from injectable gentamicin sulfate‡ has been effective in the treatment of infections caused by these gram-negative organisms.

Dakin's solution can be used to clean a wound of residual tissue after gross necrotic tissue has been debrided. This solution also stimulates the formation of healthy granulation tissue. Dakin's solution is a 0.5% solution of sodium hypochlorite,§ which releases chlorine and oxygen. It reduces the bacterial count of wounds and liquefies necrotic tissue. Dakin's solution should be used at half-strength (0.25%) to reduce discomfort. It should be applied as a wet bandage, and the bandage should be changed before it dries.[50]

The treatment of grafts with antibiotics prior to placement has been found beneficial to graft survival. Soaking autografts, allografts, and xenografts in 1 million units of aqueous penicillin and 1 gm of streptomycin 15 minutes before placing them on infected wounds has resulted in a marked increase in the ability to obtain a sterile wound.[2] In this study the bacterial counts in 96 per cent of the contaminated wounds were unaltered four days after placement of untreated grafts; however, only 8 per cent of the wounds were still contaminated four days after placement of antibiotic-soaked grafts.[2] Soaking grafts in 5% neomycin for 15 minutes prior to placement has also been reported to increase the percentage of graft survival.[71]

It has been stated that systemic antibiotics do not alter the quantitative level of bacteria in a granulating wound. In addition, systemic antibiotics begun more than three to four hours after wounding are of no value. However, topical antibiotics have been shown to decrease bacterial growth in open wounds.[26] Even so, the earlier the treatment of wounds is performed, the better the results. Failure of antibiotics to be effective when applied topically four hours or more after wounding is due to the protein coagulum that covers the wound and prevents contact of the antibiotic with the bacteria.[11] Topical proteolytic enzymes may be effective in breaking down the coagulum so that topical antibiotics can reach the bacteria.[11, 48]

Provision for drainage of fluid and exudate from under a graft also helps prevent graft loss due to infection.[26] The use of mesh, strip, or seed grafts allows escape of fluids so they do not lift a graft from its bed.

Improper Immobilization

One of the primary reasons grafts do not take is inadequate immobilization of the graft against its bed. Immobilization is necessary to allow revascularization of the graft from its bed. Until the graft is firmly adhered to the bed and vascular connections are adequately established, movement between the graft and bed breaks down the developing vascular connections (i.e., the inosculating and ingrowing vessels).[60] Techniques for immobilizing a graft against its bed are covered in more detail in the section on bandaging grafts.

Desiccation

Desiccation is detrimental to a graft. To prevent desiccation, the recipient bed should be prepared first, followed by harvesting and placing of the graft. Preparing the bed first allows time for hemostasis on the bed while the graft is being harvested. By harvesting the graft immediately before placing it, desiccation by surgery lights and evaporation is prevented. Physiological saline can be used to help keep a graft moist during harvesting and application procedures. The donor site should be closed after the graft is sutured in place, or an assistant surgeon can close the donor site while the surgeon sutures the graft in place.[26, 59, 60] Application of a thin coating of antibiotic ointment over the graft during bandaging helps prevent graft desiccation and infection.

TYPES OF GRAFTS

Full Thickness Grafts

These grafts are composed of epidermis and full thickness dermis. After they take, they resemble normal skin in color, texture, elasticity, and hair growth.[26, 38, 59, 60, 62] With regard to cosmetic appear-

---

*Nolvosan, Ft. Dodge Laboratories, Inc., Ft. Dodge, IA 50501.
†Garamycin Ointment, Schering Corp., Kenilworth, NJ 07033.
‡Gentocin, gentamicin sulfate solution, Schering Corp., Kenilworth, NJ 07033.
§Clorox, The Clorox Co., Oakland, CA 94612.

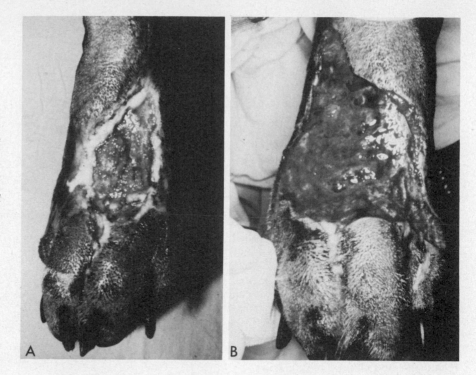

Figure 38–3. *A*, Chronic lesion on the top of a dog's foot prior to excision. *B*, The lesion after excision of the granulation tissue and peripheral epithelium. (Reprinted with permission from Swaim, S. F.: *Surgery of Traumatized Skin: Management and Reconstruction in the Dog and Cat.* W. B. Saunders, Philadelphia, 1980, p. 436.)

ance, full thickness grafts are more frequently indicated in veterinary surgery than in human surgery because they support hair growth better than split thickness grafts.[23, 39] Since the veterinarian deals with a completely hirsute patient, hair growth is an important factor. Full thickness grafts are indicated for closing large lesions on flexor surfaces to prevent contraction and traumatic defects on the distal aspect of the limbs.[33, 60, 62] Because of the relative thinness of their skin, full thickness grafts take better on cats than on dogs.

Full thickness grafts should be taken from an area where the skin is loose and abundant. Ideally, the hair should be of the same color, texture, and thickness as the hair surrounding the defect.[46] The lateral thoracic wall is a common donor site on the dog.[46, 49, 59, 60, 67] If avulsed skin is available and relatively normal, it may be worthwhile to remove any remaining subcutaneous fat and re-apply it to the lesion after proper preparation of both the graft and bed.[37] Soaking the graft in an antibiotic solution prior to grafting is indicated in this situation.

The defect is prepared to accept a graft; i.e., chronic granulation tissue is excised, the top of healthy granulation tissue is scraped, or a clean wound is debrided and thoroughly lavaged (Fig. 38–3). A piece of sterile absorbent material (e.g., sterile towel) is placed on the defect. A pattern is cut to fit the lesion based on the blood or tissue fluid imprint left on the material.[60, 62] The lesion can be traced by direct vision on a piece of clear developed x-ray film; however, a cloth is preferred, since it fits into the irregularities of the defect better.

The pattern is taken from the defect to the donor area so that the direction of hair growth on the graft is the same as that of the recipient area. If the defect is irregular in shape, care should be taken so that the pattern is not turned over during transfer from the defect to the donor site, resulting in a useless mirror image of the defect. A sterile skin-marking pen or a

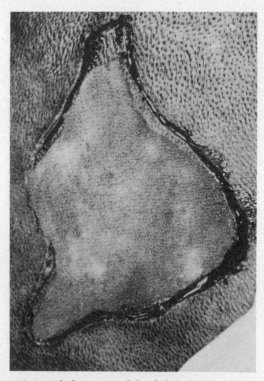

Figure 38–4. A cloth pattern of the defect shown in Figure 38–3 has been placed on the donor site so that the direction of hair growth on the graft will be like that on the foot where it will be placed. An incision has been made around the pattern. (Reprinted with permission from Swaim, S. F.: *Surgery of Traumatized Skin: Management and Reconstruction in the Dog and Cat.* W. B. Saunders, Philadelphia, 1980, p. 437.)

sterile toothpick dipped in methylene blue can be
used to trace the pattern.[26, 50, 60, 62]

A #15 scalpel blade is used to cut around the
outline[60, 62] (Fig. 38–4). All subcutaneous tissue is
removed from the dermis, since it would interfere
with revascularization of the graft. The subcutaneous
tissue can be removed as the graft is elevated from
the donor site. One edge of the graft is elevated with
stay sutures, skin hooks, or thumb forceps. As elevation continues, a sharp scalpel blade is used to cut,
rather than scrape, subcutaneous tissue from the
dermis (Fig. 38–5). The graft may be rolled over a
gauze roll or the surgeon's finger to keep it taut while
removing subcutaneous tissue.

Another technique for graft preparation is to remove the graft completely, leaving the subcuticular
tissue on the dermis and removing it later using
sharp scissors and thumb forceps. If small, the graft
may be stretched over the surgeon's index finger,
dermal side up, for subcutaneous tissue re-
moval.[3, 4, 8, 13, 22, 26, 38, 49, 50, 59, 67] If the graft is large, it
can be stretched out, dermal side up, on a piece of
sterile cardboard using 2-0 silk sutures pulled through
slits in the edges of the cardboard.[60, 62] Silk is preferred because of ease of handling.

The graft is placed on the defect so that the
direction of hair growth is the same as that of the
skin surrounding the defect. Several nonabsorbable
stay sutures are placed at key points around the graft,
and definitive suturing is done with 3-0 or 4-0 nonabsorbable (i.e., nylon* or polypropylene†) simple
interrupted sutures placed 3 to 4 mm apart (Fig. 38–
6). The sutures may be placed in a three-point pattern
in which the needle passes through the graft, the

---

*Ethilon, Ethicon, Inc., distributed by Pitman-Moore, Wash-
ington Crossing, NJ 08560.
†Prolene, Ethicon, Inc.

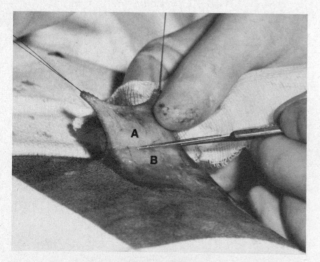

Figure 38–5. Stay sutures elevate the graft as a sharp scalpel blade
is used to cut (not scrape) the graft between, *A*, the dermis and,
B, the subcuticular fat. (Reprinted with permission from Swaim,
S. F.: *Surgery of Traumatized Skin: Management and Reconstruction in the Dog and Cat.* W. B. Saunders, Philadelphia, 1980, p.
438.)

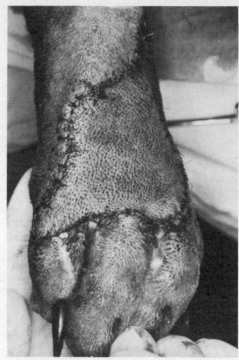

Figure 38–6. Simple interrupted sutures of 4-0 polypropylene have
been used to suture the graft. (Reprinted with permission from
Swaim, S. F.: *Surgery of Traumatized Skin: Management and
Reconstruction in the Dog and Cat.* W. B. Saunders, Philadelphia,
1980, p. 440.)

subcutaneous tissue at the wound edge, and then the
wound edge.[13] Two or three sutures may be omitted
from the most dependent portion of the graft to allow
for drainage or blood clot removal if necessary.[60] The
donor site, which has been kept moist with a saline-
soaked sponge, is closed by undermining the surrounding skin and closing the wound with deep and
superficially placed sutures.

Full thickness grafts have several advantages. (1)
They appear more like normal skin in color, texture,
elasticity, and hair growth than split thickness
grafts.[33, 49, 59] (2) Postoperative contraction is minimal.[16] (3) Full thickness grafts provide good protection for an area.[16, 49] (4) No expensive equipment or
technical help is needed.[3, 59]

Full thickness grafts also have several disadvantages. (1) Preparing the pattern, cutting the graft,
and removing subcutaneous fat are all time-consuming.[19] (2) The survival of a full thickness graft is not
as good as that of a split thickness graft, especially in
the presence of infection.[33–35] (3) There is a decrease
in hair growth when compared with skin flaps, owing
to damage to the bases of some hair follicles located
in the subcutaneous tissue that is removed.[60]

Split Thickness Grafts

These grafts are composed of epidermis and a
variable portion of dermis. The grafts may be thin,
of intermediate thickness, or thick depending on the

amount of dermis included.[16, 26, 38] The primary indication for this type of graft in the dog is the reconstruction of defects following burns in which extensive areas of skin have been lost.[33]

The lateral thoracic wall, because of its relative abundance of skin and large size, is a good donor area for split thickness grafts.[21, 62] However, the lateral neck region has also been used as a donor site.[39] After preparing the area for aseptic surgery, aliquots of sterile physiologic saline are injected in the subcutaneous tissues to push the skin away from the underlying ribs. Sterile mineral oil or water-soluble gel can be used to lubricate the skin. Using the fingertips or a sterile tongue depressor, the assistant pulls the skin in one direction while the surgeon pulls it in the opposite direction. The surgeon uses the remaining free hand to cut the graft with a graft knife. The lubricated knife blade is placed at about a 30° angle against the skin, and a few back-and-forth strokes are made to start the knife cutting the skin. The angle of the blade is changed to about 15° as the knife is moved back and forth about 3 to 5 cms behind the hand that is pulling tension on the skin.[13, 16, 26, 38, 59, 60, 62] Skill is necessary to cut a good graft of uniform thickness with a freehand knife. This should be considered before such a knife is used for the first time on a clinical case.[60, 62]

Freehand cutting may also be done with a scalpel blade.[10, 34, 50, 60, 62] The procedure works best on the thick skin over the back or shoulder area. Since the blade becomes dull rather easily, several blades may be necessary to complete the task. Some holes may be inadvertently cut in the graft as it is being raised; however, these will heal and will allow for drainage from beneath the graft.[34, 60] Scalpel blades with a curved leading edge should not be used except to harvest small grafts. A curved blade is difficult to control when cutting a graft larger than 1 cm.[50] A Weck blade or an ordinary razor blade can also be used to cut a skin graft.[26]

An unmodified Schick single-edged injector razor and blade have been used to cut grafts 1.25 inches wide × 0.012 to 0.014 inches thick.[58] The grafts can be cut in long strips or small squares. After preparing the lateral thoracic area as previously described, the single-edged razor is lubricated with sterile mineral oil and held like a pencil as it is firmly pressed against the skin and moved with a swinging motion. The blade should cut at its ends. Cutting should not be stopped once it is started until the desired length of graft is attained. The graft obtained is quite thin and has a very sparse hair growth after it takes[60, 62] (Fig. 38–7).

A Gillette single-edged safety razor can be modified to cut a split thickness graft by filing out the central strut of the safety guard.[51, 55] The thickness of the graft can be varied by inserting additional blades that have their cutting edges broken off into the razor as shims. Grafts are about 0.010 to 0.012 inches thick × 1.25 inches wide. Each shim adds another 0.004 inch of thickness to the graft.[55]

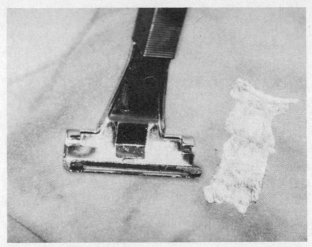

Figure 38–7. Single-edge Schick injector razor and strip of skin. (Reprinted with permission from Swaim, S. F.: *Surgery of Traumatized Skin: Management and Reconstruction in the Dog and Cat.* W. B. Saunders, Philadelphia, 1980, p. 445.)

Dermatomes used to harvest split thickness grafts in humans can be used on dogs as well. One type that works nicely is the electric or pneumatic dermatome (Brown Dermatome), which looks and operates like a large hair clipper.[7, 21, 39, 60, 62] The instrument has a disposable blade that is locked into position. Graft width is adjusted by a knob on the side of the dermatome, and graft thickness is determined by a second knob, which is calibrated in thousandths of an inch. Grafts of various thicknesses have been described in the veterinary literature. I and others[30] prefer to cut grafts 0.015 and 0.030 inch thick. The accuracy of the thickness setting can be checked. The dermatome should be set at 0.015 inch (about the thickness of a Bard-Parker #15 scalpel blade). If such a blade just fits in the opening between the adjustable platform and the dermatome blade, the setting is correct.[50, 66] The rapidly oscillating blade, which has been lubricated with mineral oil, is

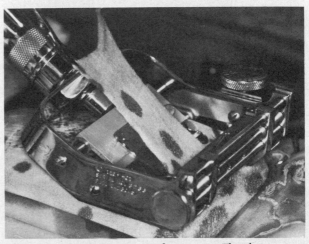

Figure 38–8. Pneumatic Brown dermatome. The dermatome is advanced as the oscillating blade splits the skin.

advanced along the donor site, which is held taut by the surgeon and assistant surgeon. The instrument removes a long strip of split thickness skin (Fig. 38–8). These instruments are easy to use and require little skill; however, their cost makes them impractical for the general practitioner.[10, 13, 16, 21, 26, 38, 50, 60, 62]

A disposable dermatome is available. It cuts a graft 0.15 inch thick × 1.5 inches wide. The disposable cutting head comes in a sterile plastic bag. The motor is an Oral B rechargeable toothbrush motor that can be placed in a sterile plastic bag and sealed. The sterile cutting head is pushed through the bag onto the motor.[10, 16, 50, 60] Early models of this instrument were difficult to use; however, recent modifications have corrected some of the earlier problems.[63]

Split thickness grafts are usually placed over the wound so that they overlap the wound edge by 0.25 to 0.50 inch. Simple interrupted sutures are placed through the graft and surrounding skin in sufficient numbers to hold the graft in place. Within a few days, the overlapped portion of the graft will die and can be excised if necessary[4, 13, 16, 21, 33, 34, 38, 41, 60, 62] (Fig. 38–9). Edge-to-edge suturing of grafts can be done[4, 16, 33]; however, a graft's edges may roll inward, producing an unsightly scar.[38]

The thicker the split thickness graft, the more abundant the hair growth on the graft and the less abundant the hair growth on the donor site. The opposite is true of thinner grafts. Since hair growth on the donor site is usually thinner and in an obvious area where skin is quite movable (e.g., lateral thorax), the donor site can be excised completely and the wound edges carefully closed with sutures to give a cosmetic appearance.[9, 59, 60, 62] The donor site may be treated as an open wound using a sterile nonadherent dressing and antibiotic ointment or gauze impregnated with scarlet red ointment and petroleum jelly.[21, 60] Dressing changes are more painful for the patient with this technique than when the donor site is excised and closed primarily. The donor site heals by re-epithelialization from the cut ends of hair follicles, sebaceous glands, and sweat glands as well as from the wound's edges.[13, 19, 26, 38, 41, 60]

The main advantage of split thickness skin grafts is that they take more successfully than full thickness grafts. This is related to the more abundant network of capillaries exposed on the dermal surface of the grafts compared with full thickness grafts. These vessels can more readily inosculate with vessels in the recipient bed. In addition, ingrowing vessels have less distance to grow in split thickness skin grafts, and the grafts can survive longer by plasmatic imbibition.[9, 16, 26, 33, 38, 39, 50, 60]

The following are some of the disadvantages that I have observed with split thickness grafts:

1. The grafts are less durable and more subject to trauma, making their use questionable on canine limbs.[33, 46, 67]

2. Hair growth is absent or sparse.[8, 19, 33, 34, 41, 59, 67]

3. If left to heal on its own, the donor site will have either a sparse hair coat or none at all.[9, 59]

4. The grafts may have a scaly appearance and may lack sebaceous glands.[33]

5. Graft harvesting may require the use of special and sometimes expensive equipment.[34, 46]

6. There may be difficulty in finding a firm flat

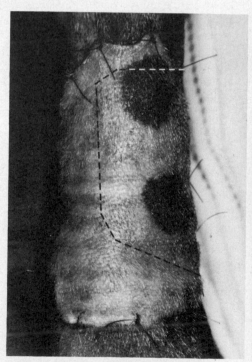
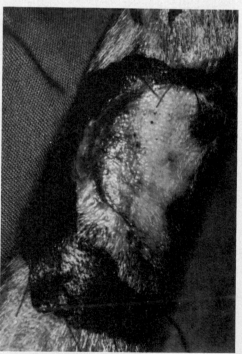

A   **B**

Figure 38–9. A, Split thickness skin graft sutured into place. Note the underlying wound edge (dotted line). B, Overlapped skin edge has sloughed and the remainder of the graft has taken over the lesion. (Reprinted with permission from Swaim, S. F.: *Surgery of Traumatized Skin: Management and Reconstruction in the Dog and Cat.* W. B. Saunders, Philadelphia, 1980, p. 448.)

area on which to operate a large dermatome on a small dog.[33]

7. There is rapid dulling of any blade used to cut a split thickness graft.[60, 62]

8. Some skill and practice are required to use freehand knives and safety razor–type dermatomes.[60, 62]

If a surgeon is interested in having a good graft take and is not concerned about the final cosmetic appearance, a split thickness graft should be considered. However, the disadvantages of the procedure should be noted.

Mesh Grafts

A mesh graft is a piece of split or full thickness skin in which numerous slits have been cut in parallel rows, allowing the graft to expand in two directions to increase its size. There are three indications for mesh grafts: (1) to graft a wound that is less than ideal, e.g., one with exudate, blood, or serum present; (2) to cover a large skin defect when there are inadequate donor sites, such as on extensively burned patients; and (3) to reconstruct irregular (i.e., concave or convex) surfaces that are difficult to immobilize.[10, 16, 28–30, 40, 52, 53, 60–62, 64]

Mesh skin grafts for animals may be made from full thickness or split thickness skin.[7, 29, 30, 60–62] If split thickness skin is used, it is taken with a free hand knife or a dermatome.[7, 28, 30, 60–62]

After a split thickness graft is cut, it is laid dermal side down on an aluminum block that contains many staggered parallel rows of small cutting blades. A

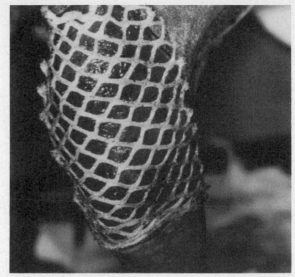

Figure 38–11. An expanded mesh graft over a lesion on the cranial aspect of a dog's stifle. (Reprinted with permission from Swaim, S. F.: *Surgery of Traumatized Skin: Management and Reconstruction in the Dog and Cat.* W. B. Saunders, Philadelphia, 1980, p. 454.)

Teflon roller is passed over the graft in the direction of the blades to cut slits in the graft. This type of graft covers three times the original width of the graft[7, 28, 30, 60–62] (Figs. 38–10 and 38–11).

A more cosmetic mesh graft can be obtained using full thickness skin. An elliptical piece of skin is cut between one-third and one-half the width of the defect and about one-third longer than the defect, or a piece of donor skin may be cut in the same shape and size as the defect using a pattern of the defect. The graft is meshed by fixing the skin dermal side up to a piece of sterile cardboard. Peripheral silk stay sutures are pulled through slits in the edge of the cardboard to stretch it. All subcutaneous fat and

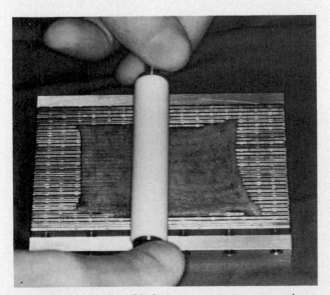

Figure 38–10. Aluminum block contains numerous staggered parallel rows of small cutting blades. The Teflon roller is rolled with moderate pressure over the split thickness graft in the direction of the blades, which slit the graft. The dermal side of the graft is against the blades. (Reprinted with permission from Swaim, S. F.: *Surgery of Traumatized Skin: Management and Reconstruction in the Dog and Cat.* W. B. Saunders, Philadelphia, 1980, p. 453.)

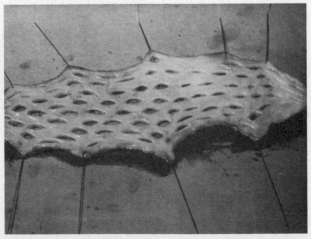

Figure 38–12. A full thickness piece of skin has been fixed dermal side up to a piece of cardboard using silk stay sutures pulled through slits in the edge of the cardboard. A #11 scalpel blade has been used to cut staggered parallel rows of slits in the skin to create a mesh graft.

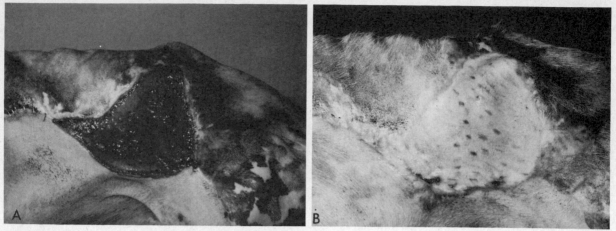

Figure 38–13. *A*, Lesion in a dog's flank to be grafted with a partially expanded full thickness mesh graft. *B*, Two weeks postoperatively there is a complete take of the graft and some of the mesh openings are almost indistinguishable, whereas others are becoming less distinct. Hair regrowth has not started. (Reprinted with permission from Swaim, S. F.: Principles of mesh skin grafting. Comp. Cont. Ed. 4:198, 1982.)

fascia are removed from the graft using thumb forceps and scissors, and numerous staggered parallel rows of short incisions (1.0 to 1.5 cm long) are made in the skin with a #11 scalpel blade[29, 60–62] (Fig. 38–12).

The grafts may be applied to fresh graft beds or graft beds that have formed granulation tissue. Grafts can be placed on wounds that are somewhat less than ideal, since the meshing allows for wound drainage. Mesh grafts are most functional and cosmetic if they are placed with the slits parallel to the direction of skin tension lines, with the hair growth in the same direction as that of the surrounding skin, and so that the mesh can expand to cover the wound.[29, 30, 60–62] Nonabsorbable suture material is used to suture the edges of the graft to the wound edge in a simple interrupted pattern. Some tacking sutures may be placed through the meshes to help hold the graft against the bed, especially if the bed is not level and if the graft is over an area that has some mobility.[61]

If a mesh graft is to be used more for drainage than for expansion to cover a large wound, it may be cut to the exact shape of the defect, meshed, sutured to one side of the wound, and stretched *slightly* to overlap the opposite side of the wound by 2 to 3 mm. The overlapped skin is excised, and the remaining graft edge is sutured to the wound edge.[61] This opens the mesh just enough to allow drainage, yet provides rapid cosmetic healing (Fig. 38–13).

Mesh grafts usually heal in place in 12 to 18 days, and hair regrowth begins at about 30 days in the dog.[64] The open areas of the mesh graft heal by epithelialization from the cut edges of the mesh. The grafts may appear unsightly because of these areas, especially if the graft has been greatly expanded. However, the grafts take on a more cosmetic appearance as they mature[29, 30, 60–62] (Fig. 38–14). In my experience, full thickness, minimally expanded or nonexpanded mesh grafts provide a good final cos-

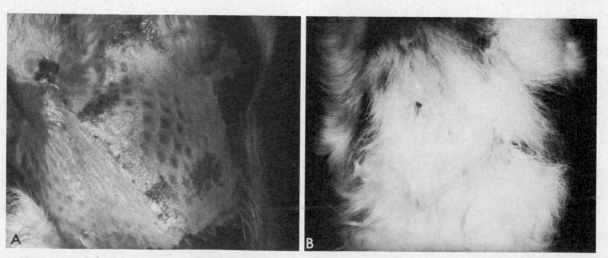

Figure 38–14. *A*, Healed mesh graft with epithelialization covering the open spaces left by the mesh. *B*, Hair regrowth on the graft two years after surgery. (Reprinted with permission from Swaim, S. F.: Principles of mesh skin grafting. Comp. Cont. Ed. 4:197, 1982.)

metic appearance, there is good regrowth of hair, and the mesh openings heal nicely (see Fig. 38–13*B*).

The advantages of mesh grafting are related to the indications previously mentioned. (1) They allow coverage of large areas with a small amount of skin if their expansion property is utilized. (2) They allow drainage of wounds and can be used for grafting less than ideal wounds (i.e., those with exudate, blood, or serum). (3) They allow grafting of irregular surfaces that are difficult to immobilize.

Seed Grafts

Seed grafts are small pieces of skin that are placed in or on a granulation tissue bed with regular spacing between them.[60] These grafts are indicated for the reconstruction of (1) granulating wounds, especially if they are large; (2) contaminated and infected wounds; and (3) wounds that can be bandaged securely for long periods of time (e.g., lower limb wounds), especially when grafts have been laid *on* rather than *in* the granulation tissue.[1, 3, 49, 60, 62]

In the dog and cat, seed grafts may be cut from the ventral abdomen, inner surface of the thigh, or flank.[1, 3, 33, 49, 60, 62] After preparing the donor area for aseptic surgery, a hypodermic needle, straight intestinal needle, curved suture needle, or Adson forceps may be used to elevate, or tent, the skin. A sharp scalpel blade is used to cut the tip off of the tent at a right angle to the direction of traction. This results in a piece of skin 2 to 4 mm in diameter.[1, 31, 33, 49, 54, 60, 62] A full thickness graft may be taken as previously described, and a 5-mm biopsy punch can be used to harvest the plugs of skin from the skin segment.[1]

Seed grafts may be placed *on* or *in* a granulation tissue bed. When placed *on* the granulation tissue, they can be placed directly on the granulation tissue

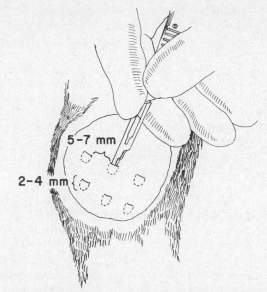

Figure 38–16. Creating pockets in the granulation tissue parallel to the wound's surface. Pockets are 2 to 4 mm deep and 5 to 7 mm apart. Each pocket will receive one seed graft. (After Hoffer, R. E., and Alexander, J. W.: Pinch grafting. J. Am. Anim. Hosp. Assoc. *12*:645, 1976.)

or in small depressions cut in the granulation tissue to accommodate the grafts (Fig. 38–15). The area must be bandaged snugly to hold the grafts in place.[8, 49, 60, 62] The most practical means of placing seed grafts *in* granulation tissue is to cut small slit-like pockets in the granulation tissue almost parallel to the surface of the wound with the openings upward. A #15 scalpel blade is used to cut the pockets. The pockets are 2 to 4 mm deep and 5 to 7 mm apart, and the grafts are placed in the pockets (Fig. 38–16). If hemorrhage tends to float a graft out of its pocket, forceps may be used to hold the graft in place for one to two minutes, or direct digital pressure

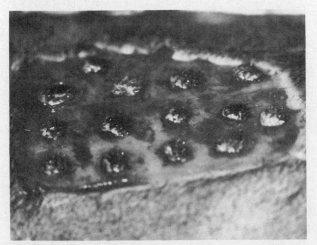

Figure 38–15. Placement of seed-type grafts on the graft bed after scarifying areas for their placement. Such placement requires snug bandaging. (Reprinted with permission from Swaim, S. F.: *Surgery of Traumatized Skin: Management and Reconstruction in the Dog and Cat.* W. B. Saunders, Philadelphia, 1980, p. 458.)

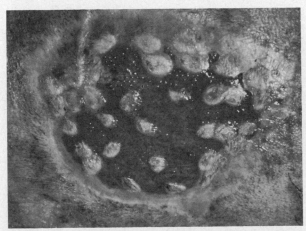

Figure 38–17. Epithelialization occurs from the edge of each seed graft and from the wound's edge. (Reprinted with permission from Swaim, S. F.: *Surgery of Traumatized Skin: Management and Reconstruction in the Dog and Cat.* W. B. Saunders, Philadelphia, 1980, p. 460.)

may be applied to the outside of the pocket.[1, 31, 34, 60, 62] When placing a graft into its pocket, it may be difficult to ascertain if the hair growth is in the proper direction.[62]

Graft donor sites may be left to heal as open wounds or closed with a simple interrupted suture in each site, or the entire area can be excised and closed primarily.[60, 62]

As the grafts take, epithelial tissue grows from each graft edge and spreads over the granulation tissue until the epithelial edges coalesce. There is also epithelialization from the wound edges[1, 31, 34, 60, 62] (Fig. 38–17).

Seed grafts have the following advantages: (1) they are simple, (2) they are resistant to infection, and (3) when placed in pockets, they withstand movement better without jeopardizing the grafts.[1, 31, 60, 62] Unfortunately, these grafts have a cobblestone appearance, give a poor epithelial coverage, and are susceptible to movement and friction if they are placed *on* the granulation tissue surface.[1, 31, 33, 49, 59, 60, 62]

Strip Grafts

These grafts are full thickness strips of skin that are placed in parallel linear grooves that have been cut in the granulation tissue of the recipient site.[34, 60, 62] After each strip is cut from the donor site (lateral thoracic wall) and placed in a groove, it is anchored with a simple interrupted suture at the ends of the groove. A few interrupted sutures can also be used to anchor the strips to the sides of the groove where indicated. These grafts are indicated for grafting wounds that have formed granulation tissue and are most applicable for reconstructing defects on the limbs[62] (Fig. 38–18).

When strip grafts are used, the grooves are cut in the granulation tissue first. By doing this, the final

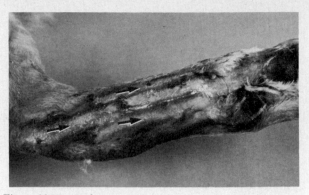

Figure 38–19. Healing strip grafts *(arrows)*. Epithelium has covered the area between grafts and the grafts are becoming wider. (Reprinted with permission from Swaim, S. F.: *Surgery of Traumatized Skin: Management and Reconstruction in the Dog and Cat.* W. B. Saunders, Philadelphia, 1980, p. 462.)

width of the groove can be seen and a suitable width graft can be cut to fit the groove. When cutting the graft, the surgeon should consider the primary skin contraction that will occur when the graft is removed from the donor site. Therefore, a graft should be cut wide enough to fit snugly into its groove. All subcutaneous fat should be removed from the strip.[62]

Strip grafts usually take well owing to their narrowness, their placement *in* the granulation tissue, and their allowance for wound drainage. Epithelial tissue spreads from the graft edges to cover the exposed granulation tissue between the strips. With time, the grafts widen out, grow some hair, and become more normal-appearing[60, 62] (Fig. 38–19).

The main advantages of strip grafts are that they require no special equipment, the technique is easy to perform, and the grafts take well. The primary disadvantage is the appearance early after placement. The healed surface lacks the durability of wounds that are completely covered with skin.

Stamp Grafts

Stamp grafts (chessboard grafts) follow the same principle as seed grafts. They are generally made from split thickness skin that is cut into patches ranging from 5 sq mm to postage-stamp size. The grafts are placed on the recipient bed with 1 mm to 1 cm of space between grafts. This allows for drainage if infection occurs. The area between grafts heals by epithelialization, resulting in a delicate and rough surface at first; however, stability and cosmesis gradually improve. The problem of movement of the graft on its bed is avoided to some extent by cutting the granulation tissue so that the graft fits into it.[26, 38, 60]

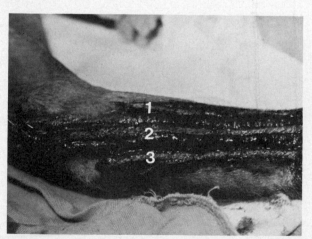

Figure 38–18. Three strip grafts (1, 2, and 3) have been placed in grooves cut in a granulation tissue bed. (Reprinted with permission from Swaim, S. F.: Plastic and reconstructive surgery. *In* Archibald, J. [ed.]: *Canine and Feline Surgery*, 3rd ed. American Veterinary Publications, Inc., Santa Barbara, in press.)

AFTERCARE OF GRAFTS

When bandaging a full thickness or a split thickness graft, antibiotic ointment may be placed around the

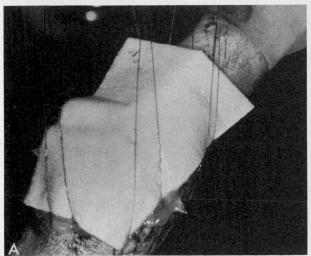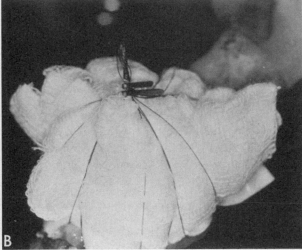

Figure 38–20. Construction of a tie-over bandage. *A,* Antibiotic ointment and a nonadherent pad are placed over the graft. Tie-over sutures are preplaced around the periphery. *B,* Sterile gauze is placed over the pad and the tie-over sutures are twisted down over the pad and fixed with metal clips. (*A* reprinted with permission from Swaim, S. F.: Reconstruction of problem skin defects on the limbs. Am. Anim. Hosp. Assoc. Sci. Proc. 1982, p. 475. *B* reprinted with permission from Swaim, S. F.: Plastic and reconstructive surgery. *In* Archibald, J. [ed.]: *Canine and Feline Surgery,* 3rd ed. American Veterinary Publications, Inc., Santa Barbara, in press.)

graft edges, or gauze pads impregnated with petrolatum may be placed over the grafted area. If antibiotic ointment is applied at the graft edges, a nonadherent pad* is laid over the graft. The area is then wrapped with an absorbent, conforming mesh gauze.† Finally, an immobilizing combined bandage-splint or a bandage and a cast are applied. Immobilization is necessary so that vascular connections can take place between the graft and bed. Immobilization should be maintained until fibrous tissue anchorage is strong enough to take a shearing strain without rupturing capillaries.[38] Pressure bandages for immobilization should be applied carefully, since too much pressure can impede normal blood flow to the graft and result in necrosis.[9, 13, 41, 44, 62]

A tie-over bandage provides good local immobilization and conformity of graft and bed. A nonadherent pad is placed over the graft, followed by the placement of several 2–0 or 3–0 monofilament nylon sutures in the host's tissues around the graft, about 1 cm from the graft margin. The ends of these sutures remain long (Fig. 38–20*A*). A bolus of sterile cotton or gauze is placed over the nonadherent pad. All ends of the preplaced sutures are drawn together over the bolus and twisted together until they pull the bolus gently down against the graft. One or two metal clips can be used to fix the twisted sutures near the bolus (Fig. 38–20*B*). Gauze, tape, and a splint or cast should be used in addition to a tie-over bandage for additional immobilization and protection.[60, 62] The metal clips can be removed for graft examination and re-applied without replacing the tie-over sutures.

Alternate methods of applying a tie-over bandage involve using staples to affix the graft to the wound edge. Some of these staples are placed over long segments of silk suture that lie across the graft. The sutures do not invade the graft or skin; the staple anchors it over the graft edge. After applying a bolus over the graft, the ends of the long silk sutures are drawn up over the bolus and tied to produce a tie-over bandage.[36]

The frequency of bandage changes depends on the temperament of the animal and the cleanliness of the bandage. The longer a bandage can go without being changed the better, since bandage changes risk contamination and movement of the graft on its bed. However, frequent (i.e., daily) bandage changes may be necessary if the animal urinates or defecates on or molests the bandage or if there is some indication of infection. In the presence of infection, bandages should be changed daily to keep exudate away from the area.

Bandage changes should be done carefully to protect the wound from movement and contamination.[60, 62] Physical or chemical restraint is usually required to prevent patient movement during bandage changes. Such movement could result in movement of the graft on its bed, which is detrimental to its survival. By using nonadherent pads and antibiotic ointment over a graft, elevation of the graft from its bed may be prevented when the dressings are lifted from the wound.

Bandaging is usually continued for 21 days after surgery. If a tie-over bandage is used, it is usually removed on the third or fourth postoperative day, followed by continued protective bandaging and immobilization until 21 days after surgery.[60, 62]

Since mesh grafts allow drainage, tie-over bandages are not used with them. The bandage-splint combination is applied to the area and changed daily or

*Telfa pad, The Kendall Co., Boston, MA 02101.
†Kerlix Rolls, The Kendall Co.

every other day to keep wound drainage fluid away from the graft. The tacking sutures help immobilize the graft to the bed during bandage changes.[62] For seed grafts that have been placed *in* pockets, bandage changes every three to five days have been advocated.[1, 31] If seed grafts have been placed *on* the wound surface, 14 days of immobilization have been advocated before the initial dressing change.[49] Strip grafts lie in grooves that help immobilize them; therefore, tie-over bandages are not used on these grafts. As this type of graft allows wound drainage, bandages are changed often.

1. Alexander, J. W., and Hoffer, R. E.: Pinch grafting in the dog. Canine Pract. 3:27, 1976.

2. Allen, H. E., Edgerton, M. T., Rodeheaver, G. T., et al.: Skin dressings in the treatment of contaminated wounds. Am. J. Surg. 126:45, 1973.

3. Archibald, J.: Procedures in plastic surgery. J. Am. Vet. Med. Assoc. 147:1461, 1965.

4. Barron, J. N., and Saad, M. N.: An introduction to operative plastic and reconstructive surgery: General principles and basic techniques. In Barron, J. N., and Saad, M. N. (eds.): Operative Plastic and Reconstructive Surgery. Churchill Livingstone, Edinburgh, 1980.

5. Birch, J., and Branemark, P. I.: The vascularization of a free full thickness skin graft: I. A vital microscopic study. Scand. J. Plast. Reconst. Surg. 3:1, 1969.

6. Birch, J., Branemark, P. I., and Lundskog, J.: The vascularization of a free full thickness skin graft: II. A microangiographic study. Scand. J. Plast. Reconst. Surg. 3:11, 1969.

7. Booth, L. C.: Split-thickness autogenous skin transplantation in the horse. J. Am. Vet. Med. Assoc. 180:754, 1982.

8. Boyd, C. L.: Equine skin autotransplants for wound healing. J. Am. Vet. Med Assoc. 151:1618, 1967.

9. Cawley, A. J., and Archibald, J.: Plastic surgery. In Archibald, J. (ed.): Canine Surgery, 2nd ed. American Veterinary Publications, Inc., Santa Barbara, 1974.

10. Chang, W. H. J.: Wound management. In Chang, W. H. J. (ed.): Fundamentals of Plastic and Reconstructive Surgery. Williams & Wilkins, Baltimore, 1980.

11. Clark, C. H.: Use of antibiotics in wounds. Mod. Vet. Pract. 61:4, 1980.

12. Clemmesen, T.: The early circulation in split-skin grafts. Restoration of blood supply to split skin autografts. Acta Chir. Scand. 127:1, 1964.

13. Converse, J. M.: Plastic surgery and transplantation of skin. In Epstein, E., and Epstein, E., Jr. (eds.): Skin Surgery, 4th ed. Charles C Thomas, Springfield, 1977.

14. Converse, J. M., and Ballantyne, D. L., Jr.: Distribution of diphosphopyridine nucleotide diaphorase in rat skin autografts and homografts. Plast. Reconst. Surg. 30:415, 1962.

15. Converse, J. M., Ballantyne, D. L., Jr., Rogers, B. O., et al.: "Plasmatic circulation" in skin grafts. Tranplant. Bull. 4:154, 1957.

16. Converse, J. M., McCarthy, J. G., Brauer, R. O., et al.: Transplantation of skin: Grafts and flaps. In Converse, J. M. (ed.): Reconstructive Plastic Surgery: Principles and Procedures in Correction, Reconstruction, and Transplantation, 2nd ed. W. B. Saunders, Philadelphia, 1977.

17. Converse, J. M., Smahel, J., Ballantyne, D. L., Jr., et al.: Inosculation of vessels of skin graft and host bed: A fortuitous encounter. Br. J. Plast. Surg. 28:274, 1975.

18. Converse, J. M., Uhlschmid, G. K., and Ballantyne, D. L., Jr.: "Plasmatic circulation" in skin grafts: The phase of serum imbibition. Plast. Reconst. Surg. 43:495, 1969.

19. Conway, H.: Skin graft. In Cooper, P. (ed.): The Craft of Surgery, 2nd ed. Little, Brown and Co., Boston, 1971.

20. Davis, J. S., and Traut, H. F.: Origin and development of the blood supply of whole thickness skin grafts: An experimental study. Ann. Surg. 82:871, 1925.

21. Fox, S. M., and Probst, C. W.: Split-thickness autogenous skin transplantation in a dog. Vet. Med. Sm. Anim. Clin. 77:782, 1982.

22. Frankland, A. L.: Autologous, split skin transplantation on the lower limbs of horses. Vet. Rec. 104:590, 1979.

23. Frankland, A. L., Morris, P. G. D., and Spreull, J. S. A.: Free, autologous, skin transplantation in the horse. Vet. Rec. 98:105, 1976.

24. Georgiade, G., Riefkohl, R., Serafin, D., et al.: Use of skin staples in plastic surgery. Ann. Plast. Surg. 5:324, 1980.

25. Gingrass, P. J., Grabb, W. C., and Gingrass, R. P.: Rat skin autografts over silastic implants: A study of the bridging phenomenon. Plast. Reconst. Surg. 55:65, 1975.

26. Grabb, W. C.: Basic techniques of plastic surgery. In Grabb, W. C., and Smith, J. W. (eds.): Plastic Surgery, 3rd ed. Little, Brown and Co., Boston, 1980.

27. Haller, J. A., and Billingham, R. E.: Studies of the origin of the vasculature in free skin grafts. Ann. Surg. 166:896, 1967.

28. Hanselka, D. V.: Use of autogenous mesh grafts in equine wound management. J. Am. Vet. Med. Assoc. 164:35, 1974.

29. Hanselka, D. V.: Inexpensive mesh grafting technique in the horse. Proc. Ann. Conv. Am. Assoc. Equine Pract. 21:191, 1975.

30. Hanselka, D. V,. and Boyd, C. L.: Use of mesh skin grafts in dogs and horses. J. Am. Anim. Hosp. Assoc. 12:650, 1976.

31. Hoffer, R. E., and Alexander, J. W.: Pinch grafting. J. Am. Anim. Hosp. Assoc. 12:644, 1976.

32. Hynes, W.: The early circulation in skin grafts with consideration of methods to encourage their survival. Br. J. Plast. Surg. 6:257, 1954.

33. Jensen, E. C.: Canine autogenous skin grafting. Am. J. Vet. Res. 20:898, 1959.

34. Johnston, D. E.: Wound healing and reconstructive surgery. Am. Anim. Hosp. Assoc. Sci. Proc. 2:383, 1975.

35. Kountz, S. L.: Autotransplantation. In Sabiston, D. C. (ed.): Davis and Christopher: Textbook of Surgery, 11th ed. W. B. Saunders, Philadelphia, 1977.

36. Larson, D. L.: rapid application of skin grafts over large areas. Ann. Plast. Surg. 5:244, 1980.

37. McGregor, I. A.: Degloving injuries: Hand. J. Br. Soc. Surg. Hand 2:130, 1970.

38. McGregor, I. A.: Fundamental Techniques of Plastic Surgery, 7th ed. Churchill Livingstone, Edinburgh, 1981.

39. McKeever, P. J., and Braden, T. D.: Comparison of full- and partial-thickness autogenous skin transplantation in dogs: A pilot study. Am. J. Vet. Res. 10:1706, 1978.

40. McMillan, B. G.: The use of mesh grafting in treating burns. Surg. Clin. North Am. 50:1347, 1970.

41. Meagher, D. M., and Adams, O. R.: Split-thickness autologous skin transplantation in horses. J. Am. Vet. Med. Assoc. 159:55, 1971.

42. Mirwin, R. M., and Algire, G. H.: The role of graft and host vessels in the vascularization of grafts of normal and neoplastic tissue. J. Natl. Cancer Inst. 17:23, 1956.

43. O'Donoghue, M. N., and Zarem, H. A.: Stimulation of neovascularization: Comparative efficacy of fresh and preserved skin grafts. Plast. Reconst. Surg. 48:474, 1971.

44. Peacock, E. E., and Van Winkle, W.: Wound Repair, 2nd ed. W. B. Saunders, Philadelphia, 1976.

45. Psillakis, J. M., DeJorge, F. B., Vilardo, R. A., et al.: Water and electrolyte changes in autogenous skin grafts. Plast. Reconst. Surg. 43:500, 1969.

46. Pullen, C. M.: Reconstruction of the skin. In Bojrab, M. J. (ed.): Current Techniques in Small Animal Surgery. Lea & Febiger, Philadelphia, 1975.

47. Rees, T. D., Ballantyne, D. L., Jr., Hawthorne, G. A., et al.: Effects of silastic sheet implants under simultaneous skin autografts in rats. Plast. Reconst. Surg. 42:339, 1968.

48. Rodeheaver, G., Marsh, D., Edgerton, M. T., et al.: Proteolytic enzymes as adjuncts to antimicrobial prophylaxis of contaminated wounds. Am. J. Surg. 129:537, 1975.

49. Ross, G. E.: Clinical canine skin grafting. J. Am. Vet. Med. Assoc. 153:1759, 1968.

50. Rudolph, R., Fisher, J. C., and Ninnemann, J. L.: *Skin Grafting*. Little, Brown and Co., Boston, 1979.

51. Sahu, S., and Rao, P. H.: Preparation and use of a double edged razor dermatome. Indian Vet. J. 55:827, 1978.

52. Salisbury, R. B.: Use of the mesh skin graft in treating massive casualty wounds. Plast. Reconst. Surg. 40:161, 1967.

53. Salisbury, R. B.: The mesh skin graft in trauma: History and preliminary report on acute wound coverage. J. Trauma 11:348, 1971.

54. Self, R. A.: Skin grafting in canine practice. J. Am. Vet. Med. Assoc. 84:163, 1934.

55. Shoul, M. I.: Skin grafting under local anesthesia using a new safety razor dermatome. Am. J. Surg. 112:959, 1966.

56. Smahel, J.: The healing of skin grafts. Clin. Plast. Surg. 4:409, 1977.

57. Smith, J. W., Ringland, J., and Wilson, R.: Vascularization of skin grafts. Surg. Forum 15:473, 1964.

58. Snow, J. W.: Safety razor dermatome. Plast. Reconst. Surg. 41:184, 1968.

59. Spreull, J. S. A.: The principles of transplanting skin in the dog. J. Am. Anim. Hosp. Assoc. 4:71, 1968.

60. Swaim, S. F.: *Surgery of Traumatized Skin: Management and Reconstruction in the Dog and Cat*. W. B. Saunders, Philadelphia, 1980.

61. Swaim, S. F.: Principles of mesh skin grafting. Comp. Cont. Ed. 4:194, 1982.

62. Swaim, S. F.: Plastic and reconstructive surgery. *In* Archibald, J. (ed.): *Canine and Feline Surgery*, 3rd ed. American Veterinary Publications, Inc., Santa Barbara, in press.

63. Swartz, B. E., and Spira, M.: The new Davol dermatome. Plast. Reconst. Surg. 67:77, 1981.

64. Tanner, J. C., Vandeput, J. J., and Olley, J. F.: The mesh graft. Plast. Reconst. Surg. 34:287, 1964.

65. Teh, B. T.: Why do skin grafts fail? Plast. Reconst. Surg. 63:323, 1979.

66. Vecchione, T. R.: A technique for obtaining uniform split-thickness skin grafts. Arch. Surg. 109:837, 1974.

67. Wallace, A. B., Spreull, J. S. A., and Hamilton, H. A.: The use of autologous free full thickness skin graft in the treatment of a chronic inflammatory skin lesion in a dog. Vet. Rec. 74:286, 1962.

68. Williams, R. G.: Experiments on the growth of blood vessels in thin tissue and in small autografts. Anat. Rec. 133:465, 1959.

69. Wright, J. K., and Brawer, M. K.: Survival of full-thickness skin grafts over avascular defects. Plast. Reconst. Surg. 66:428, 1980.

70. Zarem, H. A., Zweifach, B. W., and McGhee, J. M.: Development of microcirculation in full-thickness autogenous skin grafts in mice. Am. J. Physiol. 212:1081, 1967.

71. Zietkiewicz, W.: Influence of antibacterial defense of skin grafts on the degree of graft taking. Pol. Med. J. 7:863, 1968.

Chapter **39**

Surgical Management of Specific Skin Disorders

D. J. Krahwinkel and David L. Bone

Certain skin disorders in veterinary practice can only be successfully treated by surgery. Many of these surgical procedures involve skin folds that lead to specific diseases, some of which are related to certain breeds and sizes of animals. Many are of unknown etiology. Other surgeries are purely for cosmetic reasons and have no medical basis. These specific problems and their surgical correction will be dealt with individually in this chapter.

THE LIP

Cheiloplasty

Cheiloplasty is performed for a variety of reasons including lip-fold pyodermatitis, tumors, lacerations, and congenital cleft lip. Since cosmetic results are less crucial in veterinary surgery than in human surgery, the surgeon is more concerned with function than appearance. Several features of animals' lips make surgery relatively uncomplicated. The lips have an abundant blood supply, which greatly aids the healing process.[52] Most animals have abundant tissue forming the lips, which, along with its elastic nature, enables the surgeon to remove large portions of the lip successfully. Up to one-half of the human lip can be excised and still be closed directly without the use of flaps;[11] the same can be done in animals without deformity.

Lip-Fold Excision

Cheiloplasty is commonly employed to correct pyodermatitis in cocker spaniels, St. Bernards, schnauzers, and other breeds secondary to excessive labial tissue.[8] When saliva and food accumulate in a furrow or skin fold on the lower lip caudal to the canine tooth, a moist environment develops within the fold, resulting in chronic pyodermatitis (Fig. 39–1) and a fetid odor about the mouth and head. Medical treatment with topical antibiotics, steroids,

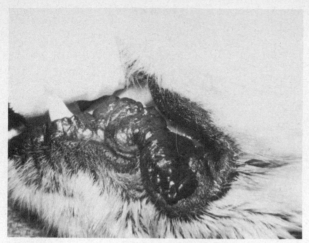

Figure 39–1. Lip folds in a cocker spaniel. These arise caudal to the lower canine tooth and run in a caudoventral direction across the ventral lip.

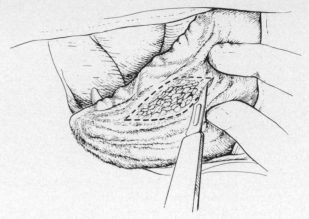

Figure 39–2. Excision of lip folds is accomplished by opening up the fold and making an elliptical incision around its margins (dashed line). The skin fold is removed and the defect closed.

and astringents helps control the disease, but only surgical excision is curative.[38]

The anesthetized dog is placed in dorsal recumbency so that the folds can be excised bilaterally without repositioning. An incision is made near the mucocutaneous junction and continued around the entire fold in an elliptical fashion (Fig. 39–2). The incision is made several millimeters away from the inflamed area to reduce bleeding. The skin fold is elevated and removed by blunt dissection of the subcutaneous tissue, and hemorrhage is controlled by pressure, ligation, or electrocoagulation. The subcutaneous tissues are closed with 3-0 absorbable sutures and the skin with 4-0 monofilament sutures. Systemic antibiotics are administered preoperatively and continued for five days after surgery owing to the inflamed and possibly contaminated condition of the surgical field. Sutures are removed in ten days.

Excision of Tumors of the Lip

The lips may be the site of malignant or benign tumors arising from the skin, subcutaneous tissues, or mucosa. Tumors can extend into all layers of the lip, necessitating a full thickness resection. Following surgical preparation, a full thickness wedge of the lip is excised, including 1 cm of normal tissue on either side of the lesion (Fig. 39–3). After hemorrhage has been controlled, the muscular and subcutaneous tissues are apposed using 3-0 or 4-0 absorbable sutures followed by closure of the skin with fine monofilament sutures. Some surgeons prefer not to close the buccal mucosa,[52] whereas others recommend a loose closure.[11]

Cheiloplasty following Mandibulectomy

When a portion of the mandible is removed as a result of neoplasia or nonresponsive osteomyelitis, the tongue commonly protrudes from the corner of

the mouth. Cheiloplasty is performed to help maintain the tongue within the oral cavity. The mucocutaneous junction is excised from the upper and lower lip beginning at the commissure and extending cranially approximately half way along each lip. The mucous membrane and skin of the upper lip are sutured to the corresponding layers of the lower lip. This procedure advances the oral commissure rostrally and provides support for the tongue previously provided by the mandible and lower dental arcade.

Traumatic Injuries to the Lip

Fresh lacerations of the lips are surgically managed like other fresh wounds. Owing to their vascular nature, lip injuries may result in severe blood loss. Debridement is indicated for any devitalized tissue prior to wound closure. The mucocutaneous border is initially apposed to ensure that "notching" of the lip margin does not occur. If accurate closure is impossible as a result of severe trauma, a wedge

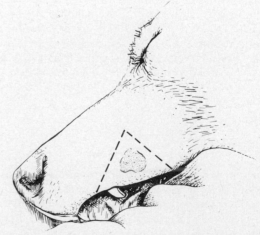

Figure 39–3. Lip tumors are removed by cheiloplasty in which a full thickness wedge excision of the lip is performed (dashed line).

resection of the entire damaged area is usually performed.

Cleft Lip (Harelip, Cheiloschisis, Primary Cleft)

A cleft cranial to the incisive foramen and involving the lip is termed a *primary cleft* (cleft lip), whereas a cleft caudal to the foramen is considered a secondary cleft (cleft palate).[25] Cleft lips are caused by a lack of fusion of a single central prolabium with one or both lateral mesodermal masses.[11] This is an uncommon anomaly in animals but is most often seen in the brachicephalic breeds.[52] Cleft lip with or without cleft palate has been reported in a variety of animal species.[12] Although genetic factors are often considered responsible for the majority of cases in animals,[12] environmental factors, toxins, teratogenic agents, hormonal factors, and mechanical factors have been implicated.[19] In man, only 10 per cent of clefts of the primary and secondary palate are inherited.[19]

Cleft lip may occur in combination with or as an extension of cleft palate.[7] Cleft lip in children is often associated with cleft palate; however, as a solitary defect, cleft lip occurs three times more frequently than cleft palate.[11] In animals, cleft palate appears more frequently than cleft lip. Cleft lip alone is more common in males in both children and puppies.[25] Some puppies with a cleft lip also show a residual scar as a result of delayed closure of the palate. The cleft lip may be located centrally or paramedially as a unilateral or bilateral lesion. Clefts of the lower lip are rare in children but do occur as median lesions.[11] Lower lip clefts in animals have not been reported.

In children, in whom cosmetic reconstruction of the vermilion border and "cupid's bow" is so crucial, multiple Z-plasty flaps are employed to meticulously reconstruct the lip.[11] These flap procedures have also been performed in puppies[25] but are probably unnecessary.[7, 52] Because dogs have a surplus of labial tissue, direct appositional closure usually renders excellent cosmetic and functional results. Surgery for

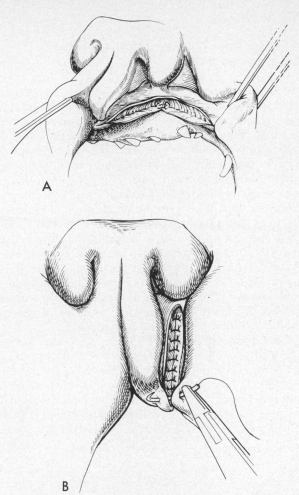

Figure 39–5. The edge of the split cleft forms inner mucous and outer cutaneous layers. *A,* The mucous membrane layer is closed water tight beginning at the dorsal extent of the cleft. *B,* The skin is closed beginning at the mucocutaneous junction to prevent notching.

primary clefts alone is usually delayed until the animal is of sufficient size to be safely anesthetized and when the lip structures are larger.

The lip is surgically prepared and the mucous membranes of the oral cavity rinsed with povidone iodine solution. The margins of the cleft are carefully incised, being careful to leave as much labial tissue as possible for the subsequent closure (Fig. 39–4). The two incised margins are bisected to a depth of 2 to 3 mm to produce an inner mucosal layer and an outer cutaneous layer. The inner layer is carefully closed with interrupted 4-0, synthetic absorbable sutures beginning at the most dorsal aspect of the cleft and extending to the lip margin. Closure should be water tight. The cutaneous layer is closed with interrupted 4-0 monofilament sutures (Fig. 39–5). The first suture is placed at the lip margin to prevent notching. The entire procedure must be performed atraumatically to ensure optimal healing and good cosmetic results. Special feeding procedures or antibiotics are usually unnecessary, and skin sutures are removed in seven to ten days.

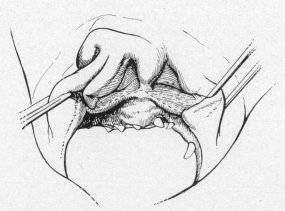

Figure 39–4. The margin of the cleft lip is incised (dashed line) to provide two layers for the subsequent closure.

THE TRUNK

Pilonidal Sinus (Pilonidal Cyst, Dermoid Sinus, Dermoid Cyst)

Pilonidal sinus is a thick-walled fibrous tissue tube lined with stratified squamous epithelium containing hair follicles, hair, sebaceous glands, and sebaceous material (Fig. 39–6).[22, 38, 51] Embryologically there is incomplete separation between the skin and spinal cord in the vicinity of the midline, resulting in an epithelium-lined sinus or cyst.[10, 22, 35] It is seen almost exclusively in Rhodesian ridgebacks and their crosses. Pilonidal sinus occurs on the dorsal midline between the neck and sacrum either cranial or caudal to the ridge but not on the ridge itself.[34, 36, 38, 53] The lesion extends from one or more openings on the skin surface to varying depths as far down as the dura mater, where it may communicate with the subarachnoid space.[33, 34, 38] It is often attached to the supraspinous ligament or connected to it by a fibrous band.[36] Multiple sites may be involved.[38]

Data from Ridgeback breeders in Great Britain revealed that 57 of 423 offspring were affected in 25 of 55 litters studied.[36] The condition is congenital and most likely inherited, but the mode of inheritance is not understood.[6, 24, 34, 36] Although no case of acquired pilonidal sinuses has been reported in the dog, their appearance is similar to that of sebaceous cysts, abscesses, epidermal inclusion cysts, follicular retention cysts, interdigital cysts, and intracutaneous cornifying epitheliomas, which are seen in any breed.

Similar lesions have been seen in other parts of the body at the junction of the skin and the subcutaneous tissue and have been referred to as dermoid cysts. They may be the result of a developmental skin defect or tramuatic inclusion of epidermis into deeper layers.[22]

Diagnosis

The diagnosis of pilonidal sinus can often be made at a very young age. All litters of Ridgebacks should be examined for the condition by lifting the skin on the dorsal midline and palpating for a thin cord of tissue extending toward the spine. A small opening in the skin with a tuft of hair protruding is usually present. If infection is present, the area may be swollen and painful with drainage from the opening. Neurological signs may be present if the sinus communicates with the dura. Histologically the sinus is lined with stratified squamous epithelium and dermal structures.

Radiology may be helpful in determining the extent and depth of the lesion and the presence of any vertebral defects. A radiopaque dye infused into the sinus produces a fistulogram. The material used should be compatible with neural tissue in the event the sinus penetrates the dura.

Treatment

Surgical excision is the treatment of choice. A longitudinally oriented elliptical skin incision should be made around the outside of the lesion, which is excised by dissecting completely around the tract. Penetration of the tract is avoided, since infection is frequently present. A dorsal laminectomy may be necessary if the tract extends to the dura. Closure should consist of absorbable sutures to eliminate dead space, followed by standard subcutaneous and skin closure. Drains and appropriate antibiotics are used if contamination or infection is present. The excised sinus should be cultured if an infection was present or contamination occurred during the surgical procedure. The tract should also be submitted for histological examination.

Prognosis depends largely on the presence or absence of infection and the depth of the lesion. A completely excised, sterile lesion has a good prognosis. Infection is the main complication, and the prognosis worsens with the presence of infection, myelitis, or meningitis.[34, 35, 38] Owners should be advised against breeding affected animals because of the potential inheritance of this disorder.

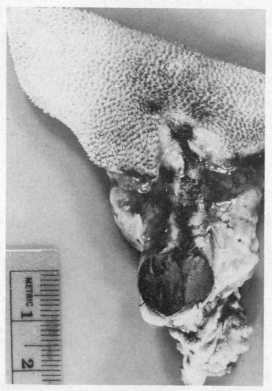

Figure 39–6. A surgically resected pilonidal sinus from a one-year-old Rhodesian ridgeback. The epithelium-lined sinus contains hair and sebaceous material. (Reprinted with permission from Wykes, P. M.: Cutaneous sinus tracts of the dog. Comp. Cont. Ed. *4*:296, 1982.)

Mastectomy

Mastectomy in the dog and cat involves the removal of one or more mammary glands. Neoplasia is the primary indication for mammary excision, although mastectomy is occasionally required for trauma or infection of the glands. For a detailed discussion of mammary neoplasia see Section 19.

Anatomy

A knowledge of the anatomy of the mammary glands, including their glandular arrangement, blood supply, and lymphatic drainage, is needed prior to surgery (Fig. 39–7). The mammary glands of the dog and cat are located subcutaneously on the ventral thorax and abdomen, and the two chains of glands extend from the cranial thoracic area to the vulva. There are normally five glands on each side of the dog, but this number may vary from four to six. Cats normally have four per side.[9, 13, 20, 49, 58] In the dog the glands are numbered 1 to 5 from cranial to caudal and are named according to region: cranial thoracic (1), caudal thoracic (2), cranial abdominal (3), caudal abdominal (4), and inguinal (5).[14, 50]

Glands 1 and 2 receive their arterial blood supply from sternal branches of the internal thoracic arteries as well as branches from the intercostal and lateral thoracic arteries. Gland 3 is primarily supplied by the cranial superficial epigastric artery, which arises from the cranial epigastric artery, a branch of the internal thoracic artery. This artery terminates by anastomosing with branches of the caudal superficial epigastric artery, which arises from the external pudendal artery and supplies glands 4 and 5. However, perforating branches of the cranial deep epigastric arteries, segmental abdominal arteries, labial arteries, and deep circumflex iliac arteries also contribute circulation to the abdominal and inguinal mammary glands to a lesser extent.[59, 60] Venous drainage generally follows the same course as the arterial supply.[14] Blood from glands 1 and 2 drains primarily into the cranial superficial epigastric and internal thoracic veins, whereas glands 3, 4, and 5 are drained primarily by the caudal superficial epigastric veins. Small veins occasionally cross the midline to the opposite chain.[49, 59, 60]

The axillary lymph node lying beneath the pectoral muscle receives lymphatic drainage from glands 1 and 2. The superficial inguinal lymph node near the external inguinal ring receives drainage from glands 4 and 5. Gland 3 drains most often to the axillary node but may drain caudally as well in the dog.[14, 50] However, there are no lymphatic connections between the second and third mammary glands when only four pairs of glands are present.[58]

Surgical Technique

A complete physical examination, CBC, chemistry panel, and radiographs are recommended when evaluating a surgical candidate, especially for the possibility of metastasis secondary to mammary neoplasia (see Section 19). The status of the patient and the

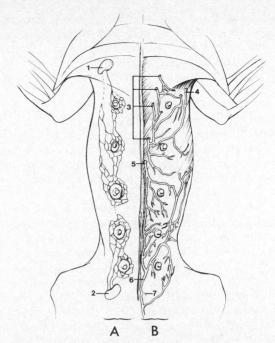

Figure 39–7. A, Lymphatic drainage of the mammary glands. 1, Axillary lymph nodes; 2, superficial inguinal lymph node. B, Major arterial supply to mammary glands. 3, Sternal branches of internal thoracic artery; 4, lateral thoracic artery; 5, cranial superficial epigastric artery; 6, caudal superficial epigastric artery; 7, external pudendal artery.

nature of the disease influence the method of surgical excision. Surgical excision of the affected gland may involve one of four methods: (1) single: removal of only one mammary gland; (2) regional: removal of known affected glands and those glands with common lymphatic drainage; (3) unilateral: removal of the entire chain of glands on one side; or (4) bilateral: removal of all glands (Fig. 39–8).

The skin incision varies with the method used. For a single, regional, or unilateral mastectomy, an elliptical incision is made to encompass all glandular tissue to be removed. The lateral incision should be lateral to the underlying glandular tissue, and the medial incision should be on the ventral midline. For

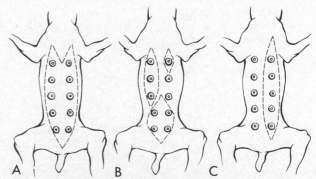

Figure 39–8. Location of skin incisions for bilateral (A), single and regional (B), and unilateral (C) mastectomies.

gland 1 the incision should extend cranially to the axillary region, and for gland 5 it should extend caudally to the level of the vulva. For a bilateral mastectomy a Y-shaped cranial incision is necessary to avoid undue tension during closure of the caudal thoracic area.[4, 54]

Following skin incision, the major blood vessels should be isolated and ligated before proceeding with deeper dissection. This is especially important for the caudal superficial epigastric artery and vein. Glands 1 and 2 are closely adherent to the pectoral muscle fascia, so careful dissection is required to free them. Caudally the glands are more loosely attached and are easily separated from the abdominal muscle fascia by blunt dissection. If a tumor has invaded the body wall, the involved portion of fascia and muscle must be excised. Unless they are enlarged or involvement is suspected, the axillary lymph nodes are not routinely removed owing to their deep location near the brachial plexus. The superficial inguinal lymph node is in close association with the inguinal mammary gland and is routinely removed along with adjacent inguinal fat. All excised tissue should be submitted for histopathological evaluation.

Skin margins should be closely examined to assure that all mammary tissue has been excised before closure. Skin closure may be the most challenging part of the surgical procedure, especially following bilateral mastectomy. The large skin defect created may require tension-relieving techniques for apposition. Skin on both sides of the wound should be undermined only enough to enable the two edges to be apposed. Undermining should be performed carefully to avoid damage to the cutaneous blood supply. Walking sutures can be used to distribute tension away from the incision line and to help alleviate dead space (see Chapter 36).[54] Various types of stent sutures can also be used but are unnecessary if walking sutures are placed properly. Surgical drains may be placed in the surgical site if excess dead space is present, especially in the inguinal area. Closure is completed with simple continuous subcutaneous and interrupted skin sutures.

Postoperatively, a sterile dressing should be applied for one to three days to eliminate dead space, prevent seromas/hematomas, prevent contamination and self-inflicted damage to the suture line, and prevent premature removal of drains. Preoperative antibiotics are advised, particularly in an older patient or if the glands were infected. If a drain is used it should be removed in two to three days.

Potential complications associated with mastectomy include infection, seromas, suture line dehiscence, and recurrence of the tumor. These complications can be kept at a minimum by paying strict attention to aseptic technique, proper tissue handling, alleviation of tension at the suture line, obliteration of dead space, wide tumor resection, and proper postoperative care.

THE LIMBS

Elbow Hygroma

Elbow hygromas occur in large and giant breed dogs as a result of trauma to the soft tissues overlying the olecranon. The trauma is usually due to the animal lying on hard surfaces. In mature dogs, repeated trauma produces a protective skin callus over the caudolateral aspect of the elbow, which helps prevent the formation of hygromas. If no callus is present, repeated trauma can produce an inflammatory response, which results in a dense-walled, fluid-filled cavity. The fluid is characteristic of a serum transudate, being yellow to red and less viscid than synovial fluid.[40] The hygroma is a false bursa and is not associated with the synovial bursa, which lies under the tendon of the triceps muscle.[26] One or both elbows may be affected.

Early in the disease, a painless fluctuant swelling is present over the olecranon process. As inflammation becomes more severe and ulceration occurs, the area becomes infected and fistulae develop.[38] Pain becomes a predominant sign, and the dog resists getting up and lying down. Occasionally the skin and underlying soft tissues may show localized areas of calcification.[42]

If hygromas are diagnosed early and while they are small, conservative medical management may be successful. Aseptic needle drainage of small hygromas followed by elimination of the elbow trauma can be successful early in the disease.[37] Soft bedding is imperative to prevent further trauma and enlargement of the hygroma. Padded "breeches" have been fitted to the dog to arrest the disease process.[38] The use of intrahygromal injection of steroids is controversial. Some authors recommend their use,[7] whereas others do not.[40]

Surgical Treatment

When conservative medical therapy does not arrest the hygroma or when ulceration has occurred, surgery is the treatment of choice. Large nonulcerated hygromas are treated by surgical drainage. Although early reports advocated the dissection and removal of the sac in toto,[7, 42] this extensive and difficult surgery is probably not necessary. Following aseptic surgical preparation, stab wounds are made into the hygroma at its most proximal and distal boundaries. Fibrin masses and loculi are digitally removed through the stab wounds. Penrose drains (¼ inch) are placed through the hygroma and exited dorsally and ventrally at the stab wounds. The drains are sutured at both exits and left in place for two to three weeks. A bulky, well-padded bandage is placed over the elbow and changed weekly until the skin has firmly adhered to the subcutaneous tissue and the pocket is obliterated (usually three to four weeks).

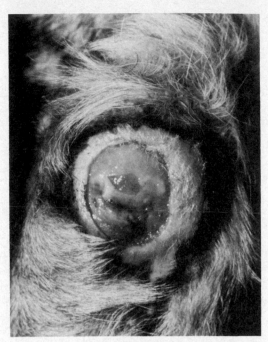

Figure 39–9. An ulcerated elbow hygroma in an Irish wolfhound.

This technique does not excise any skin and saves any protective callus that may have developed over the olecranon. Other techniques involve incising the hygroma and removing the redundant skin.[40] When this is performed, the resulting wound may break down, resulting in a large dehiscence and a more severe problem than was present originally.

Advanced cases of hygroma have large ulcerations

and granulating wounds over the olecranon (Fig. 39–9). These ulcerated wounds occur as a result of wound dehiscence, necrosis secondary to repeated trauma, or infection due to repeated needle aspirations. Complete resection of large ulcerated areas is the treatment of choice.[26, 29] The wound should be placed under an antibiotic dressing for one week preoperatively to clear any infection. The elbow is surgically prepared and an elliptical incision made around the ulcerated area (Fig. 39–10). Normal skin should be preserved to prevent undue tension on the wound closure. The entire ulcerated area is excised and the surrounding skin undermined.

Hemorrhage is often profuse owing to the chronic inflammatory nature of the disease, making electrocoagulation highly desirable. Penrose drains are placed at the excision site to prevent the development of postoperative hematomas or seromas. To promote healing, reduce tension on the sutured incision, and minimize wound dehiscence, the skin closure is positioned medial or lateral to the point of the elbow. Stent sutures can be placed through tubing to relieve tension on the primary suture line. The skin is closed with simple interrupted sutures of monofilament material. The wound is covered with a padded bandage and immobilized with a Schroeder-Thomas splint or a Robert-Jones bandage. Drains and stent sutures are removed in five days. The skin sutures are removed after 14 days. The elbow should remain immobilized for a total of four weeks.

The inciting cause must be corrected postoperatively to prevent recurrence. The dog must be kept off hard surfaces and elbow pads used if necessary to prevent further trauma.

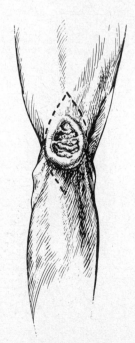

Figure 39–10. An ulcerated elbow hygroma is removed by making an elliptical incision (dashed line) around the entire lesion.

Acropruritic Granuloma (Lick Granuloma, Acral Pruritic Nodule)

Acropruritic granulomas are thickened, firm plaques and erosions on the distal surfaces of the front and rear legs of dogs that result from constant licking of the affected area (Fig. 39–11). Large breed dogs over five years of age are most commonly affected.[38] Persistent licking may occur following disease or injury to the skin, cutaneous adnexa, or underlying tissues including bone. Foreign bodies can also initiate and propagate licking of the area. Deep pyodermas have also been implicated as a cause of lick granulomas.

In most cases there is a single lesion, but multiple lesions occasionally occur on front and rear limbs. The carpus and metacarpus are the most common sites for this insidious and persistent disease.[38] The early lesion is confined to the skin but if left uncontrolled can extend by self-multilation through the subcutaneous tissue and muscle until bone is exposed.

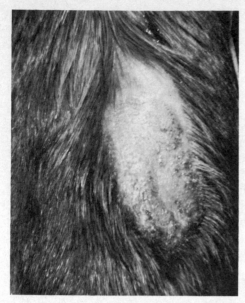

Figure 39–11. An early acropruritic granuloma on the front foot of an Irish setter.

Treatment

A complete history and physical examination are indicated in each patient. Radiographs of the affected areas are indicated to rule out bone injuries and disease such as osteomyelitis. Radiographs occasionally reveal radiographic foreign bodies amenable to surgical removal. A biopsy and deep culture of the wounds further define the disease and guide the clinician in selecting the best method of treatment.

When discovered and treated early, some lesions may respond to conservative therapy using intralesional injection of long-acting corticosteroids.[45] Other superficial granulomas may resolve following topical application of steroid-antibiotic ointments.[2] However, the area must be protected from further mutilation by the dog with the use of bandages, splints, Elizabethan collars, and sedatives.

The use of intralesional and perilesional cobra venom has been successful in the treatment of lick granulomas.[38, 45] Up to 50 mouse units (total dose) mixed with 1:1000 epinephrine has resulted in six to eight months of regression and, in some cases, a permanent cure. Weekly treatments for two to three weeks are usually required.

Intralesional and intramuscular injection of orgotein* has been reported to be highly successful in the treatment of canine lick granuloma.[39] Injection of 5 mg repeated in one week was reported to cause regression of the lesions, which had failed to respond to other modalities.

Radiation therapy has produced favorable responses in approximately 50 per cent of cases.[17] Acupuncture has also been used in the treatment of acropruritic granuloma.[5]

Small lesions that can be surgically removed and

closed without excessive tension may respond favorably. Careful suturing of the defect, using stent sutures when needed, is imperative for good results. Skin grafts or flaps can be used to cover a defect too large for primary closure. The wound must be protected from motion and trauma during the healing process by bandaging, splinting, or casting. Elizabethan collars are also useful in preventing the dog from mutilating the wound and aggravating the problem. Even after healing is complete, the animal should be watched carefully, since boredom or compulsion to lick the area may cause a recurrence at the same site or a new location.

Some lick granulomas may be attributed to a deep pyoderma.[15] For this reason antibiotic therapy with either erythromycin or lincomycin has been curative in some cases. However, a deep wound culture is necessary to assure that the correct antibiotic is selected.

Cryosurgery has also been advocated as a treatment for lick granuloma.[32, 61] Liquid nitrogen applied by either a probe or spray in a double freeze-thaw pattern to $-20°C$ can result in regression of some lesions. Cryonecrosis results in a slough of the lesion and healing by contraction and epithelialization. The mode of action is unknown but may be a result of regional analgesia secondary to freezing. Unfortunately, some cases that responded initially and healed recurred four to eight months later.

Recurrence has been noted regardless of the mode of treatment. The key to successful treatment, re-

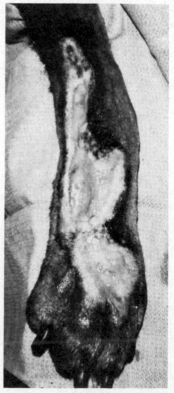

Figure 39–12. An advanced acropruritic granuloma that had been active for several years.

*Palosein, Diagnostic Data Inc., Mountain View, CA.

gardless of the modality, is early detection and treatment. Lesions that are ignored may become so extensive that even heroic measures are unsuccessful (Fig. 39–12). Although treatment for acropruritic granuloma is often unpredictable and frustrating for the owner and the clinician, persistence, patience, and a variety of therapies can frequently control or cure this perplexing disease.

THE DIGITS

Feline Onychectomy (Declawing)

Onychectomy in the cat involves removal of the distal phalanges and claws, usually from the front feet only. Although it is ordinarily an elective procedure requested by owners to protect them or their household belongings from sharp claws, it is occasionally performed on a single claw that has been badly traumatized or infected. It is a relatively quick and simple procedure, but if not done properly regrowth and other complications occur. The preferred time for declawing is between 6 and 12 weeks of age. At this age, hemorrhage and postoperative morbidity are minimal. Declawing outside cats removes their primary means of self-defense and greatly reduces their climbing ability.

Anatomy

The claw is made up of the third phalanx and a modified layer of the epidermis called the horny claw. The proximal end of the third phalanx articulates with the second phalanx by a synovial joint. The distal end is composed of an ungual process, which is a curved projection situated within the horny claw. The ungual crest encircles the base of the phalanx and serves as the insertion for the digital flexor and extensor tendons, the collateral ligaments, and the dorsal ligaments. The dorsal ligaments are two elastic structures that passively keep the claws retracted except when overcome by the deep digital flexor (Fig. 39–13).[14, 21, 46]

The stratum basale contains the germinal cells of

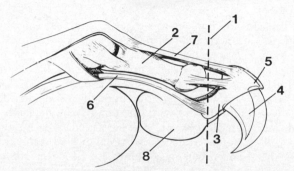

Figure 39–13. The cat's distal phalanx and structures important to onychectomy. 1, Line of excision; 2, second phalanx; 3, third phalanx; 4, ungual process; 5, ungual crest; 6, flexor tendon; 7, dorsal ligaments; 8, digital pad.

the claw and extends into the ungual crest. It is most active in the dorsal area, which must be removed during the declawing procedure to prevent regrowth of the claw.

Surgical Technique

The entire foot is prepared with a surgical scrub; hair removal is usually unnecessary. A broad, flat tourniquet is placed above the elbow. The claw can be removed with sterilized nail trimmers* or with a number 11 scalpel blade. In my opinion a nail trimmer is preferable, but whatever instrument is used, the level of the cut is important (see Fig. 39–13). The nail is extended by placing a hemostat on the claw or pushing upward on the footpad. The nail trimmer is positioned with one blade dorsally in the notch between the ungual crest and the second phalanx and the other blade against the distal edge of the footpad. The blade should be closed with a firm clean motion, cutting through all tissues with a single stroke. The digital pads must be preserved to minimize bleeding and postoperative discomfort. The wound should then be examined. The entire articular surface of the second phalanx should be clearly visible. The only part of the distal phalanx that may remain is a small triangular portion on its palmar aspect where the flexor tendon inserts. Regrowth occurs if a greater portion of the third phalanx is retained. Skin closure using absorbable sutures is occasionally used to reduce postsurgical hemorrhage, especially in large cats.

A snug-fitting bandage covering the paw up to the mid radius is applied to reduce bleeding when the tourniquet is removed. However, caution must be used to avoid tight bandages, which may compromise circulation to the paw. The bandages should be removed in 24 hours and the toes checked for hemorrhage. If bleeding is present the feet are rebandaged for another 24 hours. Sedation is occasionally required for active cats. For the first postoperative week the cat should be kept indoors with shredded papers used in place of the normal litter to minimize contamination to open wounds.

Few complications are seen if the technique and aftercare are performed properly. However, if a portion of the dorsal ungual crest is retained partial regrowth may occur, necessitating a second operation to remove the fragment. Infections may occur with poor surgical technique and improper wound care. Infected fragments of the third phalanx require removal.

Dewclaw Removal

By definition, the dewclaw is the first digit of the rear paw in the dog. It may show varying degrees of development when present. At times the first and

---

*Resco or White, Haver-Lockhart, Birmingham, AL.

second phalanges are missing and a rudimentary claw is attached only by skin and fibrous tissue. Occasionally two claws are present. The first digit of the forefoot is always present and is sometimes referred to as a dewclaw. It consists of a proximal phalanx that articulates with the first metacarpal bone and a distal phalanx but no midline phalanx.[14]

Removal of the first digit is primarily an elective procedure. In hunting dogs it is done to prevent trauma, and in other dogs it facilitates clipping and grooming. The American Kennel Club has published standards for most breeds regarding dewclaw removal.[1]

The optimum time for removal is in the first five days of life. At this time no anesthesia, clipping, and suturing are necessary, and the surgery is usually performed as an outpatient procedure. After this age it is best to wait until at least three to four months of age when aseptic surgery is done under general anesthesia.

Surgical Technique

Dewclaw removal is a minor procedure in the neonate. A surgical disinfectant and sterile instrument should be used, but clipping and draping are unnecessary. The distal web of skin between the digit and the metacarpus or metatarsus is incised with sterile Mayo scissors. The digit is then abducted and transected at the level of the metacarpus or metatar-

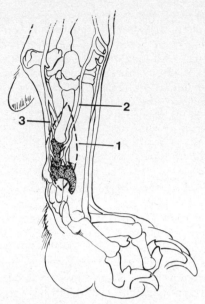

Figure 39–15. Removal of first digit, or dewclaw, in a mature dog. 1, Site of skin incision; 2, dorsal common digital artery; 3, palmar proper digital artery. The shaded area represents the structures to be resected.

sus (Fig. 39–14). A single absorbable suture can be placed to help control hemorrhage. Bandaging is unnecessary.

The procedure is more involved in an older dog. General anesthesia and routine surgical preparation are required. An elliptical incision is made around the base of the digit, and dissection is continued to the level of the metacarpophalangeal or metatarsophalangeal joint. The dorsal common digital artery and the palmar proper digital artery should be ligated and the joint disarticulated with a scalpel (Fig. 39–15). If the first and second phalanges on the hind paw are missing, only skin incisions are required to remove the claw. The skin is closed with a simple interrupted pattern. Stainless steel sutures may be necessary to discourage excessive licking. The foot is bandaged postoperatively for two to three days. Sutures are usually removed in ten days.

Digit Amputation

Toe amputations in the dog are most commonly indicated for traumatic injuries such as fractures, sprains, luxations, or severe wounds. Other common indications are neoplasia, chronic osteomyelitis, and arthritis.

The level of the amputation depends on the site of the lesion and the reason for amputation. Usually the metacarpophalangeal or metatarsophalangeal joint level is preferred, but the proximal and occasionally the distal interphalangeal joints are used for some conditions. The surgical procedure is the same for both the front and rear feet. The two most proximal sites involve removal of the respective digital pad, but the pad can be spared with a distal amputation.

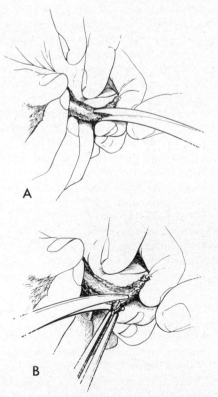

Figure 39–14. Removal of the first digit, or dewclaw, of a neonatal puppy. *A*, The first incision cuts the toe web. *B*, The second cut transects the digit at its base.

Surgical Technique

A tourniquet is helpful in controlling hemorrhage. For a distal interphalangeal amputation, a transverse skin incision is started dorsally proximal to the base of the nail, continued around the base of the nail on both sides, and jointed ventrally just cranial to the digital pad. The joint space is transected and the distal phalanx is removed. Hemorrhage is controlled with electrocoagulation or ligation. The distal condyles of the second phalanx should be removed with bone cutters to prevent direct contact with the pad. The pad is sutured to the skin with simple interrupted sutures to complete the procedure.

For more proximal amputations of the third or fourth digits, a Y-shaped incision is made with the stem of the Y on the dorsal aspect of the digit (Fig. 39–16). The two arms of the Y extend distally, encircling the base of the toe. For the second or fifth digit, the stem of the Y is made on the side of the foot, extending distally to encircle the toe. The skin is reflected to expose the joint to be disarticulated. The extensor tendons, collateral ligaments, and flexor tendons are incised along with the joint capsule, and the toe is removed. The proper digital arteries should be ligated along with any other sites of hemorrhage. If the first or second phalanx is left in place, the distal condyle of the most distal remaining phalanx should be removed. Subcutaneous sutures are used to oppose the remaining soft tissue, and the skin is closed with a simple interrupted pattern.

Padding should be placed between and around the toes postoperatively and the entire foot bandaged. The foot is kept bandaged for two to four days and sutures are removed at ten days.

Dogs function very well after removal of one or two toes, especially if the third and fourth digits are preserved. If more than two toes on one foot are removed they are usually lame.

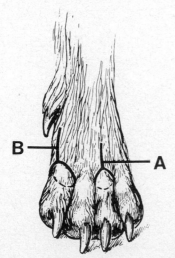

Figure 39–16. *A,* Location of skin incision for amputation of third or fourth digit at metacarpophalangeal, metatarsophalangeal, or proximal interphalangeal joint. *B,* Location of skin incision for amputation of second or fifth digit.

Interdigital Cysts (Interdigital Pyoderma, Interdigital Granuloma, Interdigital Acne, Furunculosis, Bacterial Interdigital Granuloma)

Interdigital cysts are chronic inflammatory lesions reported to develop in approximately 1.6 per cent of the canine populaton.[57] Predisposed breeds include boxers, dachshunds, German shepherds, great Danes, English bulldogs, German short-haired pointers, Pekingese, West Highland white terriers, and Scottish terriers.[38, 44, 57] Any breed may be affected, but poodles and border collies are reported to have the lowest incidence.[44, 57] The average age of onset is approximately two and one-half years, but they may occur in dogs as young as six months of age.[44]

The lesions are not actually cysts but rather granulomatous lesions containing pustules and sinus tracts.[27, 38, 48, 57] They can present as a thin-walled abscess but more commonly appear as a firm thickening in the toe web.[57] These nodules bulge above the skin surface and have a thin, purulent exudate draining from the sinus opening. Frequently there is matted hair and ulcerated skin surrounding the lesion.

The third and fourth interdigital spaces of the forefeet are the most frequently affected sites, but any of the spaces on any foot may be involved.[3, 22, 38, 44, 57] Two or more feet are usually affected.[3] The most common presenting complaints are pain and lameness in the affected foot with licking and chewing.

The etiology is quite speculative and the pathogenesis uncertain. Predisposing and etiological factors include bacterial infection of hair follicles,[44, 57] obstructed sebaceous glands,[38] bacterial or other hypersensitivity,[3, 28, 48] contact allergy,[38] foreign bodies (hair, grass awns, seeds, and so on),[3, 22, 38, 44, 48] immunodeficiency,[38] toe web conformation,[57] immune complex disease,[43] and chronic irritation (stones, briars, debris, short bristly hair, and so on).[38, 44, 57]

Staphylococcus aureus is most frequently incriminated in this condition but is probably not the primary etiologic agent. Positive cultures occur with about the same frequency as normal dog's skin.[44] Experimental interdigital infections using staphylococcal organisms from acute lesions do not produce the same clinical condition.[44] Other organisms frequently isolated from interdigital cysts are betahemolytic streptococci, *E. coli, Bacillus* sp., *Proteus vulgaris,* and *Pseudomonas aeruginosa.*[3, 44, 57] It is not completely known why the interdigital area of affected dogs is more favorable for bacterial growth than that of normal dogs.

Although the pathogenesis is unclear, it is stated that the disease is basically a pedal dermatitis and folliculitis with a secondary bacterial infection.[57] The earliest detectable change is a chronic dermatitis with acanthosis and hyperkeratosis, which causes keratinized epithelial cells to accumulate in hair follicles and kill the hair from lack of nutrition. Drainage from the sebaceous glands lining the follicle is impeded, resulting in cystic dilation and atrophy. Thus, an environment is created in which skin bacteria can produce a follicular abscess that either opens and drains or ruptures into the dermis. Eventually a granulomatous lesion is formed with fibrous tissue encapsulation and sinus tracts to the skin.[27, 57]

Treatment

Owing to the multiple etiological factors, numerous modes of therapy have been advocated.[22, 28, 38, 44, 48, 57] Treatments that have produced at least limited or temporary success include excision of cystic and inflamed skin,[22, 38, 44, 48] systemic and local antibiotics,[3, 22, 28, 38, 44, 48] cryosurgery,[18, 41] corticosteroids,[28, 38, 44] vaccination (staphylococcal toxoid),[38, 44, 48] chemotherapy,[44] autoserotherapy,[44] and radiation therapy.[44] When lesions are due to a foreign body such as a grass awn or seed (Fig. 39–17), surgical removal of the foreign body and excision of the fistulous tract are usually curative. Chronic lesions that fail to respond to medical and conservative surgical therapy are best managed by complete surgical excision of the affected interdigital web.

After surgical preparation of the entire foot, dorsal and ventral skin incisions are made at the junction of the interdigital web and each adjacent toe. A tourniquet is helpful to temporarily control hemorrhage. The entire interdigital web should then be excised. All tissue should be submitted for histopathological evaluation to rule out neoplasia. Hemorrhage should be controlled with electrocautery or ligation. Small absorbable simple interrupted sutures should be used to close dead space, but care should be taken to avoid injury of the blood supply to the toes. Nonabsorbable simple interrupted sutures should be used to appose the skin edges. The end result is two adjacent toes in close apposition without an intervening web of skin.

Postoperatively the foot should be padded and bandaged to prevent licking and swelling until the skin is healed. Taping the two adjacent toes together reduces tension on the suture line during weight bearing. Sutures should be removed in approximately ten days.

Because of the high recurrence rate with most forms of therapy, a guarded prognosis should be given for complete recovery unless the definitive etiology can be identified and corrected (e.g., foreign body). Even with complete surgical removal of the interdigital web, the condition may develop in any of the remaining interdigital spaces.

THE TAIL

Ingrown Tails (Tail Folds, Screw Tail)

In many naturally short-tailed dogs and cats the coccygeal vertebrae deviate ventrally and may ankylose in a cork-screw fashion. This has been termed *screw tail*[38] or *corkscrew*[31] and has been reported to occur in the Boston terrier, English bulldog, Schipperke, pug, and Manx cat.[38] The ventral deviation with or without the corkscrew results in deep skin folds lateral and ventral to the tail (Fig. 39–18). The folds accumulate sebum, apocrine sweat, and fecal material, resulting in a moist pyoderma. The pressure of the ingrown tail on the perineum and the itching of the pyoderma cause the animal to scoot and lick the area of the folds. Because medical treatment of this problem is of little or no value, surgery is the treatment of choice.[38] Removal of the tail may render the animal unsuitable for show purposes, and the owner must be fully aware of this before surgery is performed.

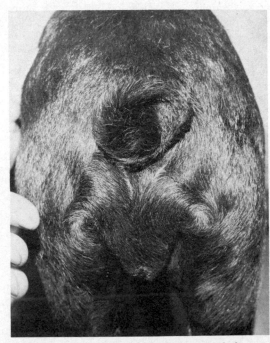

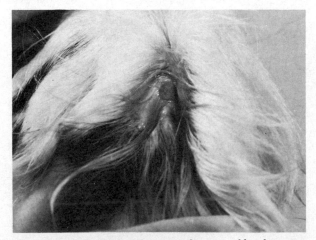

Figure 39–17. An interdigital cyst in a four-year-old male springer spaniel. Surgical exploration revealed a grass awn deep in a sinus tract.

Figure 39–18. An English bulldog with ventral deviation, or corkscrewing, of the coccygeal vertebrae, which has resulted in tail folds.

Excision of Tail Folds

Some authors recommend excising only the skin folds, but most feel that excision of the ingrown coccygeal vertebrae is also necessary.[31, 38, 47] A procedure for removing the coccygeal vertebra but leaving the boneless skin flap for cosmetic purposes has been described.[47] The dog is anesthetized and a purse-string suture is placed in the anus to include the anal sac openings. With the dog in ventral recumbency, an elliptical incision is made from the sacrum, continuing lateral to the tail, and ending above the anus. The incision is carried through the subcutaneous tissue until the tail can be identified digitally. The coccygeal and levator ani muscles are severed close to their attachment on the coccygeal vertebrae (Fig. 39–19). The loose fascial attachment of the rectum to the ventral side of the vertebrae is separated by blunt dissection. Bone cutters or a gigli wire is used to transect the vertebrae where they deviate ventrally. The coccygeal vessels are ligated, and any hemorrhage from the cut bone is controlled with sterile bone wax. Penrose tubing is placed into the depths of the wound for postoperative drainage and exits ventral to the primary incision. The roof of the pelvic canal is reformed by apposing the severed muscles and the deep fascia. The subcutaneous tissue is closed with absorbable sutures and the skin closed with monofilament sutures in a routine fashion. The purse-string suture is removed at the completion of the procedure. The drain is removed at two to three days and the skin sutures at ten days.

Tail Amputation

Tails are removed for a variety of medical reasons, such as neoplasia and trauma, but more commonly

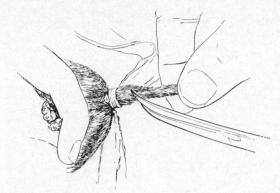

Figure 39–20. Tail amputation on puppies is accomplished by making a pair of angled cuts to create skin flaps, which are sutured over the amputated stump.

for "cosmetic" purposes. When performed for cosmetic purposes, it is best done within the first few days of life when hemorrhage and stress are minimal. Surgery on older animals becomes more complicated and aftercare more extensive. Length requirements often vary to suit individual preferences and breed standards. The owners must be consulted and the amputation performed according to their wishes. Recommendations can be obtained from the appropriate kennel club and from published tables.[7]

The tail is a common site for skin tumors, for which amputation is the preferred method of treatment. In these instances the tail should be removed at least one vertebra proximal to the tumor. Trauma resulting in extensive loss of skin or fracture of a vertebra with paralysis or deformity of the tail also necessitates amputation.

Surgical Technique

When puppies are only a few days of age the tail is removed without anesthesia. The tail is cleansed with an acceptable disinfectant and the puppy restrained in the palm of the hand. A piece of gauze is

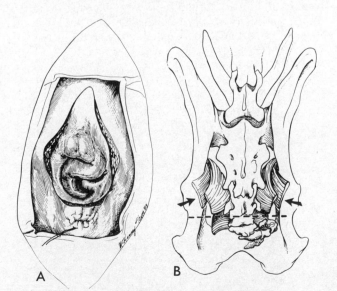

Figure 39–19. A, Tail folds along with the deviated vertebrae are removed by making an elliptical incision around the ingrown tail. B, The coccygeal muscle attachments are severed (arrows) and the bone transected (dashed line).

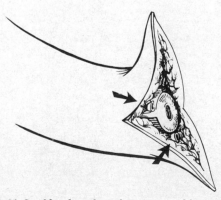

Figure 39–21. In older dogs the tail is amputated by creating skin flaps, which are reflected, and the intervertebral space is disarticulated. The paired lateral and ventral vessels are ligated (arrows).

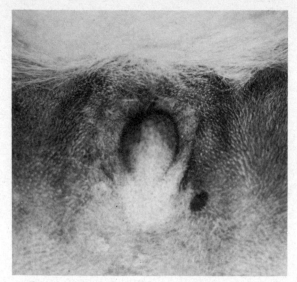

Figure 39–22. Vulvar folds in an older, obese bitch.

tied snugly at the base of the tail to serve as a tourniquet. The amputation site is selected and the tail removed with scissors. Since the coccygeal vertebrae are soft at this young age, no attempt is made to amputate between vertebra. The first cut is made halfway through the tail to create a lateral flap of skin (Fig. 39–20). The second cut is made opposite the first, which removes the tail and creates a second, proximally based flap. One interrupted absorbable suture is used to appose the two flaps over the amputated stump. This suture helps to control hemorrhage and prevents a hairless scar, which is esthetically unpleasant, especially in short-haired dogs. The tourniquet is removed in 10 to 15 minutes and the suture remains until absorbed or licked out by the mother.

In older dogs and cats the surgery is done under general or epidural anesthesia with strict aseptic technique. A tourniquet is placed at the base of the tail. The tail length is determined and the closest intervertebral space located by palpation. Skin flaps are incised dorsally and ventrally at the amputation site. The flaps are based over the appropriate intervertebral space. Following reflection of the skin flaps the paired lateral vessels and ventral vessels are ligated just proximal to the proposed amputation site. A scalpel is used to transect the coccygeal musculature and intervertebral space (Fig. 39–21). The transection may also be accomplished through a coccygeal vertebral body if necessary, using bone cutters or a gigli wire. The tail is removed and the tourniquet temporarily loosened to check for additional bleeders. Hemorrhage from the bone is controlled with bone wax. The skin flaps are pulled over the amputated stump and shortened if needed. The flaps should cover the end of the tail to prevent hematoma or seroma but without undue tension. On large dogs two to three absorbable subcutaneous sutures are placed to obliterate dead space, and skin is closed with interrupted monofilament sutures. Stainless steel skin sutures may be used to discourage licking of the surgical site. A bandage on the amputated stump for 24 to 48 hours may help to prevent hematoma formation. The skin sutures are removed at ten days.

THE VULVA

Vulvar Folds

In older, obese bitches skin folds tend to develop dorsal and lateral to the vulva (Fig. 39–22). There is no breed predilection, but the condition is more severe in bitches spayed at an early age.[16, 38] Accumulation of moisture and urine results in an intertriginous irritation and a perivulvar pyoderma. A reduction in body weight helps to reduce the severity of the disease. Topical cleansing and the use of protective lotions and powders are helpful as pallia-

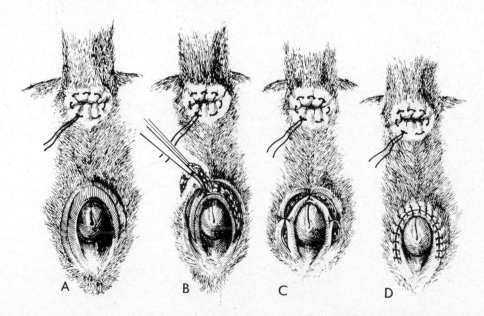

Figure 39–23. *A*, Vulvar folds are excised utilizing a pair of crescent-shaped incisions around the vulva. *B*, The intervening skin and fat are removed. *C*, Skin sutures placed at the 9, 12, and 3 o'clock positions. *D*, Subcutaneous sutures and additional skin sutures are added if the excision is adequate.

A   B   C   D

tive treatment or preoperative preparation of the patient.[7, 38, 56] The bitch usually exhibits scooting, licking, and discomfort, and the owners often complain of a foul odor from the vulvar area.

Surgical Technique: Episioplasty

The treatment of choice is to excise the redundant skin folds and excess fat and reconstruct the perineum to lift the vulva out of its recessed position. Surgery is performed under general anesthesia with the dog in ventral recumbency and a purse-string suture in the anus to prevent fecal contamination of the surgical site. An estimate is made of the amount of skin to be removed to eliminate the folds.[22] A pair of crescent-shaped incisions are made from the 8 o'clock position around the redundant skin fold, extending dorsally and ending at the 4 o'clock position. The inner incision is approximately 5 mm away from the vulva and the outer one at a sufficient distance to eliminate all the redundant folds.[22, 56] The isolated skin segment is elevated and excised with close attention to hemostasis. Sufficient subcutaneous fat is removed to ensure that the vulva does not rest in a recessed position. Simple interrupted skin sutures of monofilament nylon are initially placed at the 9, 12, and 3 o'clock positions to ascertain if sufficient skin and fat have been removed. If not, these sutures are removed and additional tissue excised. If the excision is adequate, 3-0 absorbable interrupted sutures are placed in the subcutaneous area to help relieve skin tension, and the skin is closed with additional monofilament sutures (Fig. 39–23).

Possible postoperative complications include seroma formation, wound dehiscence, and infection.[22] An Elizabethan collar may be used to prevent licking at the wound, and parenteral antibiotics may be administered for five days to control infection. Sutures are removed at ten days.

1. American Kennel Club: *The Complete Dog Book*. New York, Howell Book House, 16th ed., 1979.
2. Bagnall, B. G.: Lick granuloma—a self-inflicted skin problem. Pedigree Digest 4:4, 1977.
3. Baker, B. B.: Canine pyoderma. *In* Kirk, R. W. (ed.): *Current Veterinary Therapy V*. W. B. Saunders, Philadelphia, 1974.
4. Bartels, K. E., Ferguson, H. R., Gillette, E. L., and Ferguson, H. L.: Simultaneous bilateral mastectomy in the dog. Vet. Surg. 7:97, 1978.
5. Bullock, J. E.: Acupuncture treatment of canine lick granuloma. Calif. Vet. 32:14, 1978.
6. Burns, M., and Fraser, M. N.: *Genetics of the Dog*. J. B. Lippincott, Philadelphia, 1966.
7. Cawley, A. J., and Archibald, J.: Plastic surgery. *In* Archibald, J. (ed.): *Canine Surgery*. Santa Barbara, American Veterinary Publications, Inc., 1974.
8. Clifford, D. H., and Clark, J. J.: Mouth and teeth. *In* Archibald, J. (ed.): *Canine Surgery*. Santa Barbara, American Veterinary Publications, Inc., 1974.
9. Crouch, J. F.: *Text-Atlas of Cat Anatomy*. Lea & Febiger, Philadelphia, 1969, pp. 182–183.
10. Dwight, R. W., and Maloy, J. K.: Pilonidal sinus experience with 449 cases. N. Engl. J. Med. 249:926, 1953.
11. Edgerton, M. T., and Williams, G. S.: The mouth, tongue, jaws and salivary glands. *In* Sabiston, D. C. (ed.): *Textbook of Surgery*. W. B. Saunders, Philadelphia, 1977.
12. Edmonds, L. A., Stewart, R. W., and Selby, L.: Cleft lip and palate in Boston terrier pups. Vet. Med./Small Anim. Clin. 67:1219, 1972.
13. Ellenport, C. R.: Carnivore urogenital apparatus. *In* Getty, R. (ed.): *Sisson and Grossman's The Anatomy of the Domestic Animals*. W. B. Saunders, Philadelphia, 1975.
14. Evans, H. E., and Christensen, G. C. (eds.): *Miller's Anatomy of the Dog*. W. B. Saunders, Philadelphia, 1979.
15. Fadok, V. A.: Personal communication, 1983.
16. Furneaux, R. W.: Surgical disorders of the canine vagina and vulva. Vet. Ann. 19:245, 1979.
17. Gillette, E. L.: Radiation therapy. *In* Carlson (ed.): *Veterinary Radiology*. Lea & Febiger, Philadelphia, 1977.
18. Goldstein, R. S.: Nitrous oxide cryosurgical units: Their use in veterinary practice. Vet. Med./Small Anim. Pract. 72:1587, 1977.
19. Hammer, D. L., and Sacks, M.: Clefts of the primary and secondary palate. *In* Bojrab, M. J. (ed.): *Current Techniques in Small Animal Surgery I*. W. B. Saunders, Philadelphia, 1975.
20. Harvey, J. H.: General principles of veterinary oncologic surgery. J. Am. Anim. Hosp. Assoc. 12:335, 1976.
21. Herron, M. R.: De-clawing the cat. Mod. Vet. Pract. 48:40, 1967.
22. Hoffer, R. E.: Skin and its adnexa, burns. *In* Archibald, J. (ed.): *Canine Surgery*. Santa Barbara, American Veterinary Publications, Inc., 1974.
23. Hoffer, R. E.: *Atlas of Small Animal Surgery*, 2nd ed. St. Louis, C. V. Mosby, 1977.
24. Hofmeyr, C. F. B.: Dermoid sinus in the Ridgeback dog. J. Small Anim. Pract. 4:5, 1963.
25. Howard, D. R., Merkley, D. F., Lammerding, J. J., Ford, R. B., Bloomberg, M. S., and Davis, D. G.: Primary cleft palate (harelip) and closure repair in puppies. J. Am. Anim. Hosp. Assoc. 12:636, 1976.
26. Johnston, D. E.: Hygroma of the elbow in dogs. J. Am. Vet. Med. Assoc. 167:213, 1975.
27. Jubb, K. V. F., and Kennedy, P. C.: The skin and appendages. *In* Jubb, K. V. F., and Kennedy, P. C. (eds.): *Pathology of Domestic Animals*. Academic Press, New York, 1963.
28. Kirk, R. W.: The pyodermas. *In* Kirk, R. W. (ed.): *Current Veterinary Therapy IV*. W. B. Saunders, Philadelphia, 1968.
29. Krahwinkel, D. J., Jr.: Correction of specific skin defects. *In* Swaim, S. F. (ed.): *Surgical Management of Traumatized Skin*. W. B. Saunders, Philadelphia, 1980.
30. Krahwinkel, D. J., Jr., and Howard, D. R.: Reconstructive surgery. Proc. Am. Anim. Hosp. Assoc. 1975.
31. Krahwinkel, D. J., Jr., and Merkley, D. F.: Surgical correction of facial folds and ingrown tails in brachycephalic dogs. J. Am. Anim. Hosp. Assoc. 12:654, 1976.
32. Krahwinkel, D. J., Jr., Merkley, D. F., and Howard, D. R.: Cryosurgical treatment of cancerous and noncancerous diseases of dogs, horses, and cats. J. Am. Vet. Med. Assoc. 169:201, 1976.
33. Leyh, R., and Carithers, R. W.: Dermoid sinus in a Rhodesian Ridgeback. Iowa State Univ. Vet. 1:36, 1979.
34. Lord, L. H., Cawley, A. J., and Gilray, J.: Mid-dorsal dermoid sinus in Rhodesian Ridgeback dogs—a case report. J. Am. Vet. Med. Assoc. 131:515, 1957.
35. Mahaley, M. S.: Congenital abnormalities. *In* Sabiston, D. C. (ed.): *Textbook of Surgery*. W. B. Saunders, Philadelphia, 1972.
36. Mann, G. E., and Stratton, J.: Dermoid sinus in the Rhodesian Ridgeback. J. Small Anim. Pract. 7:631, 1966.
37. McCurnin, D. M.: Surgery of the canine elbow joint. Vet. Med./Small Anim. Clin. 71:909, 1976.
38. Muller, G. H., and Kirk, R. W.: *Small Animal Dermatology*. W. B. Saunders, Philadelphia, 1976.
39. Neibert, H. C.: Orgotein treatment of canine lick granuloma. Mod. Vet. Pract. 56:529, 1975.

40. Newton, C. D., Wilson, G. P., Allen, H. L., and Swenberg, J. A.: Surgical closure of elbow hygroma in a dog. J. Am. Vet. Med. Assoc., *164*:147, 1974.
41. Norsworthy, G. D., Miller, D. C., Radicle, L. E., and Limmer, B. L.: Cryosurgery in small animal practice. Canine Pract. *4*:18, 1977.
42. Piermattei, D. L.: Surgery of the skin and adnexa: Hygroma of the elbow. Proc. Am. Anim. Hosp. Assoc. 1973.
43. Plechner, A. J.: Canine immune complex diseases. Mod. Vet. Pract. 57:917, 1976.
44. Quadros, E.: Furunculosis in dogs: Aetiology, pathogenesis and treatment, a clinical study. Acta Vet. Scand 52(Suppl.):1, 1974.
45. Reid, J. S.: Acropruritic granuloma. *In* Kirk R. W. (ed.): *Current Veterinary Therapy V.* W. B. Saunders, Philadelphia, 1974.
46. Reighard, M. R., and Jennings, H. S.: *Anatomy of the Cat.* Rinehart and Winston, New York, 1963.
47. Rubin, L. D.: Surgical correction of tail-fold dermatitis in the English Bulldog. Vet. Med./Small Anim. Clin. 74:1623, 1979.
48. Schwartzman, R. M.: Canine dermatology. Adv. Sm. Anim. Pract. *3*:39, 1962.
49. Silver, I. A.: Symposium on mammary neoplasia in the dog and cat. J. Small Anim. Pract. 7:689, 1966.
50. Stalker, L. K., and Schlotthauer, C. F.: Neoplasms of the mammary gland in the dog: The surgical treatment of mammary tumors, report of two cases and a study of the lymphatic drainage of the mammary glands. North Am. Vet. *17*:33, 1936.
51. Steyn, H. P., Zuinlan, J., and Jackson, C.: A skin condition seen in Rhodesian Ridgeback dogs: Report on two cases. J. S. Afr. Vet. Med. Assoc. *10*:170, 1939.
52. Stoll, S. G.: Cheiloplasty. *In* Bojrab, M. J. (ed.): *Current Techniques in Small Animal Surgery I.* Lea & Febiger, Philadelphia, 1975.
53. Stratton, J.; Dermoid sinus in the Rhodesian Ridgeback. Vet. Rec. 76:846, 1964.
54. Swaim, S. F.: A "walking" suture technique for closure of large skin defects in the dog and cat. J. Am. Anim. Hosp. Assoc. *12*:597, 1976.
55. Swaim, S. F.: Etiology of skin trauma and defects. *In* Swaim, S. F. (ed.): *Surgery of Traumatized Skin.* W. B. Saunders, Philadelphia, 1980.
56. Welser, J. R.: Episioplasty. *In* Bojrab, M. J. (ed.): *Current Techniques in Small Animal Surgery I.* Lea & Febiger, Philadelphia, 1975.
57. Whitney, J. C.: Some aspects of interdigital cysts in the dog. J. Small Anim. Pract. *11*:83, 1970.
58. Wilkinson, G. T.: The treatment of mammary tumors in the bitch and a comparison in the cat. Vet. Rec. 89:13, 1971.
59. Wilson, G. P.: Mammary glands: Their development and disease. *In* Bojrab, M. J. (ed.): *Pathophysiology in Small Animal Surgery.* Lea & Febiger, Philadelphia, 1981.
60. Wilson, G. P., and Fowler, E. H.: Mammary tumors. *In* Bojrab, M. J. (ed.): *Current Techniques in Small Animal Surgery I.* Lea & Febiger, Philadelphia, 1975.
61. Withrow, S. J., Greiner, T. R., and Liska, W. D.: Cryosurgery: Veterinary considerations. J. Am. Anim. Hosp. Assoc. *11*:271, 1975.

Chapter **40** # Burns; Electrical, Chemical, and Cold Injuries

Dudley E. Johnston

BURNS

The pathophysiology and treatment of burn injuries have been poorly understood for hundreds of years. In 500 B.C., the burn wound was covered with mud, honey, and fresh meat. Obviously, systemic therapy was not applied, and the outcome was known later.[15] Prior to 1950, the pathophysiology of burn injury was centered around nebulous "burn toxins." Local treatment consisted of many procedures and applications, many of which did not fulfill the adage for therapy—"above all, do no harm."

Much of our present knowledge of burn pathophysiology was obtained after 1945, when it became apparent that future wars could involve thermonuclear weapons with mass burnings and that a much more sophisticated knowledge of burn physiology was needed. We now have a good understanding of burn toxins, of the role played by bacteria and infection, of fluid shifts and losses, and of local therapy.

Veterinary information on burns is scarce. Much information on human burns has been obtained from animal experimentation. Therefore, a study of the voluminous human literature is necessary to understand burn injuries in animals. However, great care is needed to avoid complete comparisons between animal and human burns. Animal skin is covered by hair that acts as an insulating material, and does not burn readily; human skin is directly exposed to heat and to burning clothing. Human skin forms blisters; animal skin, other than pig skin, tends not to do so. It is difficult to demarcate burn areas in animals and to estimate the percentage of skin area involved. Accordingly, all formulas for fluid and colloid therapy that are an integral part of the management of human burn wounds have limited application in animals. Finally, the most important aspects of burn wound management in humans, and most reports in the literature, are concerned with management of the patient with over 50 per cent body surface burns, and include consideration of antibiotic-resistant infection from long hospitalization and replacement of lost

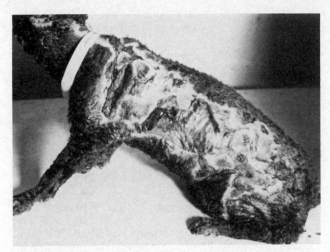

Figure 40–1. Severe third-degree skin burns in a dog that was placed on a heating pad during a surgical procedure. This injury is two months old, and the dry eschar is still attached firmly. Treatment was by total wound excision and primary closure using sliding skin flaps.

skin. The financial costs are enormous. In animals with severe burns over 50 per cent or more, immediate euthanasia should be considered.

Causes of Burns

Severe burns occur in grazing farm animals, particularly in winter rainfall areas of the world, because of the presence of tall dry grass in summer.[108] Horses are burned in stable fires. Dogs and cats rarely have this type of injury; thermal injuries in these species are usually caused by explosions and fires in homes, scalding by hot water, and accidental burning from heating pads. Anesthetized and debilitated animals on heating pads tend to be immobile, so that the tissues adjacent to the heating pad are compressed and relatively avascular and remain so for long periods. Also, skin has low heat conductance and releases heat slowly. As a result, severe burns can be sustained from low-temperature pads (Fig. 40–1).

Pathophysiology of Burns

Immunosuppression

Infection by bacteria and fungi is a serious factor in burn therapy. This infection can be enhanced by immunosuppression that accompanies burn trauma, any traumatic incident, and surgical procedures.[29, 40, 86] Impaired cellular immunity with severe thermal injury has been reported in humans and experimental animals.[18, 42, 89] An immunosuppressive factor has been isolated from serum taken immediately from severely burned humans that inhibits the migration of peripheral leukocytes and causes the lysis of peripheral lymphocytes from burned patients.[35] Thymosim (thymic hormone) enhances certain in vitro T-lymphocyte functions in burned pa-

tients, and its administration to burned patients may restore decreased cell-mediated immunity.[42] Early excision of the burn wound does not reverse the severe depression of cell-mediated immunity after thermal injury in experimental animals.[31]

Inhalation Injury

Dogs and cats in house fires can be found dead with little, if any, evidence of thermal injury. Also, burned animals commonly develop signs of respiratory distress. Pulmonary injury secondary to inhalation of noxious products of combustion is seen in 15 to 22 per cent of all human burn patients.[1, 103]

Lung injury due to inhalation of smoke was not recognized as a major threat to fire victims until 1942.[5] There have been few advances in knowledge of this subject since, partly because variables such as fluid resuscitation and pulmonary infection greatly complicate clinical investigation. Dogs exposed to smoke from burning kerosene have insignificant injury to the lungs and tracheobronchial tree immediately and for up to 21 days after exposure. However, smoke from burning wood causes severe respiratory problems. In one experiment in which ten anesthetized dogs were exposed to wood smoke, six had respiratory arrest within ten minutes, which was corrected by artificial respiration. In all ten dogs, lung weights and lung sodium contents were significantly greater than for corresponding dogs exposed to kerosene smoke and for control dogs. Lungs from all ten dogs showed pulmonary edema microscopically. In two dogs that died, the lungs showed vascular congestion, interstitial edema, and atelectasis.[112]

Analysis of the toxic agents in wood smoke has shown that the substances giving smoke its visible characteristics do not cause pulmonary damage.[79] Wood smoke contains approximately ten times the amount of carbon monoxide found in kerosene smoke. The carbon monoxide is partially responsible for some of the toxicity of smoke, although it is not irritating to lung parenchyma. Wood smoke also contains 20 times the quantity of total aldehyde gases found in kerosene smoke. Aldehyde gases are also present in high concentrations in smoke from burning household materials such as furniture and cotton. The most toxic of these aldehydes is acrolein, which causes pulmonary edema and death in a concentration of 5.5 ppm in experimental animals. The concentration of acrolein in burning wood is 50 ppm, and in burning cotton, 60 ppm.[112] The mechanism of activity of acrolein in the lung is most likely a denaturation of protein similar to the irreversible reaction between formaldehyde and amino acids.

The clinical characteristics of the respiratory distress syndrome in burned animals change with time after the burn. Within the first 24 hours, typical "smoke poisoning" or heat inhalation is seen. There are dyspnea and increased lung sounds, particularly rales. Microscopically, bronchiolitis and pulmonary edema are present. The prognosis is relatively good if the animal is not burned; however, the prognosis is very poor if a significant burn is present. Within a period of one to five days after burning, a syndrome of pulmonary edema is present. The cause is probably a combination of the direct lung injury from aldehydes, as in the "smoke poisoning," and the action of bacterial toxins. Microscopically, congestion, edema, and pneumonia are present. Pneumonia is the most common problem five days after the burn. In experimental animals, pulmonary edema associated with burn injury is not caused or augmented by excessive intravenous fluid therapy but by too little fluid therapy.[110]

In humans, improved early resuscitation after burn injury has reduced burn shock and renal failure as an early cause of death, and inhalation injury has become the primary determinant of survival in the early post-burn period. A similar situation may exist in animals.

Burn Shock

Immediately after a burn, sudden and dramatic changes in circulatory dynamics result in burn shock. There has been considerable speculation about this condition, and nebulous "burn toxins" have been implicated. It is now known that the cause is a complex of changes related to fluid loss and fluid shifts, electrolyte imbalances, blood protein losses, myocardial depression, marked increase in peripheral vascular resistance, increased blood viscosity, and other factors. A drop in cardiac output to about 50 per cent of normal precedes any measurable change in blood or plasma volume. It is followed by a rapid decrease in plasma and blood volume and a further decrease in cardiac output.[31]

Myocardial-Depressant Factor. The presence of myocardial-depressant factor is suggested by the fall in cardiac output without concurrent changes in blood volume. A circulating factor that leads to myocardial depression and ultrastructural alterations has been demonstrated in humans and in experimental animals. The substance does not appear to be any known kinin or amine and has no currently known antidote.[17, 18] It probably is not a highly significant clinical factor except in severe thermal injury.

Fluid Losses and Shifts. An extremely important clinical aspect of burns is the tremendous loss of circulating fluid. Some of this loss can be attributed to evaporation of water and loss of blood and serum from the burn. The most significant cause is fluid shift from vascular spaces to tissue spaces. The speed with which this shift of fluid occurs can be readily appreciated clinically as the rapid development of edema. Two main factors lead to this fluid shift: increased permeability of blood vessels in the burn area and loss of blood proteins.

Animal studies using dextran of various molecular sizes show that in burn injury, blood vessels in the area become permeable to dextran of a molecular weight of 125,000 daltons and below.[20] This loss of plasma proteins into the extracellular space can result in a concentration of protein as high as 3 gm/dl of extracellular fluid, a concentration adequate to hold large volumes of fluid.[21] In the first four days in burns of moderate degree, an amount of albumin equal to twice the total plasma pool can be lost from the vascular compartment, and half of this is sequestered in the tissue spaces in the burn area for three or more weeks before being returned to the blood. The other half of the albumin lost from the vascular compartment is, in fact, lost from the body through the burn wound.[19]

In addition to the effect of protein loss, the destruction of the capillary as a semipermeable membrane negates Starling's law as a significant factor in maintaining plasma volume, because colloid oncotic pressure cannot be exerted effectively across such a freely permeable membrane.

Red blood cell loss is not a significant factor in the immediate post-burn period, and the loss of circulating volume is related not to blood loss but to fluid loss and fluid shifts. Plasma volume decreases rapidly after a 40 per cent body surface burn to approximately 25 per cent below normal. The extracellular fluid volume deficit can be even greater, and measurements showing a loss of 40 to 50 per cent have been recorded.[10] The greatest losses of both plasma and extracellular fluid occur within the first 12 hours after injury, and the loss continues at a much slower rate for only six to 12 hours longer. After recovery from the acute burn shock and return of protein to circulating blood, excess fluid in tissue is reabsorbed into the circulation, a factor that together with vigorous fluid replacement therapy can lead to circulatory fluid overloading. The loss of protein externally and into tissue spaces should be monitored, and protein replacement may be needed.

Electrolyte Changes. In thermally damaged cells, low oxygen tension and lack of carbohydrate due to hormonal influences severely impair metabolism. The cell membrane is also affected, and the sodium pump is less effective. Potassium is lost from the cell and is replaced by hydrogen ions, with the development of intracellular acidosis. This loss of potassium from anoxic cells, together with an increased secretion of mineralocorticoids, results in a considerable increase in renal potassium excretion. Sodium is retained, and the urinary Na-K ratio is reversed. If this situation is not corrected, a severe potassium deficit frequently develops between the third and fifth days after a major thermal injury.

Several investigators in human burn care have argued that the net load of sodium, rather than the load of water, is critical in obtaining normal cardiovascular function and that the increase in total body weight and water, particularly lung water, is undesirable. These investigators are using hypertonic sodium solutions containing up to 300 mEq of sodium per liter for burn resuscitation.[83] The amount of sodium in routine replacement solutions is 130 to 140 mEq/liter. The use of hypertonic solutions ignores the large evaporative water loss in the burn patient and the fact that the patient retains sodium in large quantities.[23, 83] Hypertonic sodium solutions are not recommended in animals.[69]

Red Blood Cell Loss. In the early post-burn period, there is immediate red cell destruction, but the degree is rarely clinically significant. The loss of red cells is directly proportional to the extent of the burns, particularly deep burns, and is related to immediate destruction of the cells by heat. There is, however, a continuing red cell loss that has been measured in moderate to severe burns as 8 to 12 per cent loss of red cell mass per day in the first five to seven days. This continuing loss is the result of increased red cell fragility and of morphological changes that cause the cells to have a shorter life span, resulting in either intravascular or intrasplenic destruction. The continuing loss can necessitate replacement of red cells, although rarely in the first one to three days after the injury. In general, infusion of red cells in the immediate post-burn period can be detrimental to the animal because of the increased blood viscosity and high hematocrit during this time. In humans, burns exceeding 30 per cent of the body surface always require blood transfusions to avoid anemia.[11]

The factors in burn patients leading to continuing red cell destruction have been investigated. Old red cells are more resistant to heat-induced morphological changes than younger cells. A burn injury is likely to affect a larger proportion of the younger cells and leave in the circulation a high concentration of older red cells.[8] The chemical factors that lead to morphological changes in red cells in burn patients are probably substances such as lysolecithin, prostaglandins, proteases, norepinephrine, catecholamine metabolites, and free fatty acids.[37] The morphological changes induced in red cells by these substances include multiple budding, thinner than normal discocytes with membrane roughness, and thickened protruding areas.[9]

Renal Failure. Renal failure is a common concomitant of the deterioration of all body systems in a dying animal, although renal problems are not a major factor in the early post-burn period. There is no primary renal injury associated with thermal injury. However, in the presence of inadequate fluid therapy, cardiac output is lowered, peripheral resistance is increased, and renal blood flow is diminished.[73] Human burn patients most likely to develop renal failure are those who have high-voltage electrical injuries or associated trauma such as crush injuries, those in whom treatment is delayed (particularly fluid therapy), and those with extensive burns who have received estimated fluid therapy and additional fluids and remain oliguric.

Liver Damage. Clinical and laboratory evidence of liver disease is present in more than 50 per cent of humans within 24 hours of cutaneous thermal injury.[22] Severe liver damage has also been seen by the author in dogs following thermal injury. The cause of this acute liver disease is not known, but it is probably related to acute anoxic liver damage, associated with reduction in cardiac output, increased blood viscosity, and splanchnic vasoconstriction before successful resuscitation. Histologically, centrilobular necrosis of the liver parenchyma is seen. Increases in cardiac output and splanchnic blood flow are expected after fluid therapy.[6]

In humans, the magnitude of the initial liver enzyme derangements does not differentiate survivors from nonsurvivors, although jaundice is associated with a very poor prognosis. In one survey, there was a mortality rate of 90 per cent in human patients who developed jaundice.[22] The most severe liver injury in humans occurs with burns of 50 per cent of the total body surface and with septic foci.

Disseminated Intravascular Coagulation. The syndrome of diffuse hemorrhage and formation of microthrombi in organs including the lung and kidney is well known in severe trauma as well as conditions such as pancreatitis and gastric dilation and has been reported in humans and experimental animals after thermal injury. Generalized bleeding from the burn wound, from venipuncture sites, or from mucous membranes in a burned animal is a clinical sign of a coagulation disorder, and coagulation studies and thrombocyte counts should be done.[61] Decreased blood levels of thrombocytes have been observed in humans after burns; increased peripheral consumption by aggregates and microthrombi is the suggested cause.[38] Microthrombi have been found in lungs and kidneys of burned humans.[26] ADP-induced platelet aggregation is increased 24 to 48 hours after burning in experimental animals.[27] Fibrin-platelet microaggregates, which are formed in burned experimental animals, may lead to post-burn lung damage and hypoxemia after their subsequent embolization to the pulmonary vascular tree.[90]

Burn Toxins

Many of the complications of thermal injury can be readily explained by the presence of burn shock and sepsis. Severe local and systemic infection after thermal injury is probably related to the presence of devitalized tissue and immunosuppression in the burned animal. A specific burn toxin from burned tissue cannot be ruled out, however. A toxic factor has been isolated from burned skin extracts in experimental animals; it has been partially identified as a lipoprotein (40 per cent lipid and 60 per cent protein) and is a polymerization product of a precursor present in normal skin.[37]

The Burn Wound

The general parameters used to describe a burn wound are its depth and surface area. In a first-degree burn, only the epidermis is involved, the basal layer of the epidermis is not destroyed, and the wound heals in three to six days without scarring. A first-degree burn is present in sunburn in humans and in some thermal injuries in dogs caused by gas explosions and hot liquids.

In a second-degree burn, the epidermis and part of the dermis are destroyed. Some epidermal appendages and hair follicles are spared, allowing for re-epithelialization. In humans, both first- and second-degree burns characteristically contain blisters, but these are not usually seen in animal skin, except in pigs. A second-degree burn can be readily converted into a full-thickness, or third-degree, burn by inappropriate therapy, especially when bacterial infection occurs.

In a third-degree burn the entire thickness of the skin and all skin structures are destroyed. In general, the third-degree burn wound has an insensitive surface, unlike first- and second-degree burns. In dogs and cats, considerable difficulty can be experienced in determining the depth of a fresh burn. The skin surface in all three types can be covered by dry coagulum and the surface has a leathery consistency. In first- and second-degree burns, if the surface is elevated and bent, the surface coagulum usually splits so that the underlying epidermis or dermis is visible. In third-degree burns, the elevating and bending procedure produces either no split in the surface or a complete split down to the subcutaneous tissues. As stated previously, the first- and second-degree burn wounds are more painful than third-degree burns.

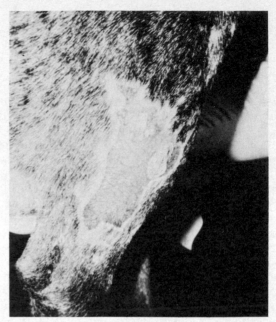

Figure 40–3. The thermal injury shown in Figure 40–2, three weeks later. Spontaneous sloughing of dead skin has occurred, to reveal a third-degree burn with small islands of second-degree burn.

It can be very difficult in dogs and cats to determine the area of a burn wound. This determination is generally easy in humans because there is little, if any, hair covering, and color and texture changes are apparent. In dogs and cats the area of second- and third-degree burns (the area of first-degree burns is not important in prognosis) can be determined more accurately by palpation than by sight because a surface coagulum is present and can be palpated.

Thermal trauma generally results in a nonuniform wound, and at the time of injury, some tissues are totally coagulated, other tissues are seriously damaged and will probably be eventually destroyed, and still others are only transiently affected (Figs. 40–2 and 40–3). In addition, the depth of the burn wound is composed of three concentric zones, an important consideration in burn management. The innermost zone, the "zone of hyperemia," is least affected and heals completely by the seventh day. The outermost zone, the "zone of coagulation," is destroyed from the outset, and therefore its status is obvious at the time of injury. Between these two zones is the "zone of capillary stasis," representing an area of intermediate injury that initially resembles the innermost zone but, by the end of 24 hours, it usually becomes indistinguishable from the zone of coagulation.[43, 72] The progression of damage in this intermediate zone during the first 24 hours is due not only to the physical effects of the heat but also to the release of proteolytic and hydrolytic enzymes, prostaglandins, and vasoactive substances.[92]

An important therapeutic aspect of the burn wound is the alteration in its blood supply. Studies by Order and Moncrief[74] demonstrated the vascular occlusive nature of thermal injury. Immediately after a full-

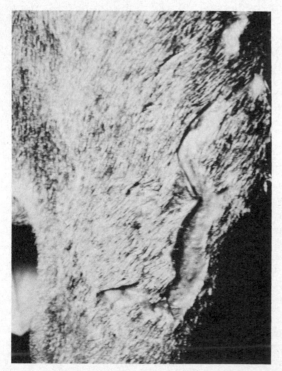

Figure 40–2. Thermal injury on the lateral aspect of the shoulder in a dog. The area and the depth of the burn wound are difficult to determine; however, most of the wound is covered by a dry eschar and is third-degree.

thickness burn the vascular supply to the area is completely occluded, and the avascular zone continues to expand for up to 24 hours. There is no agreement as to whether vascular occlusion is a function of arteriolar or venous occlusion.[60] However, no appreciable circulation is re-established for about three weeks, and circulation persists only in the granulation tissue beneath the dead tissue. The large volume of dead tissue provides an excellent medium for bacterial growth, and the occlusion of local blood supply impairs the delivery of humeral and cellular defense mechanisms and of systemic antibacterial drugs to the burn area.

In the first 24 hours after burn, many burn wounds are sterile or have only superficial bacterial colonization. Within the first two to three days, the surface colonization increases rapidly, and proliferation of microorganisms in hair follicles and other deep structures is a prominent feature. By the fourth or fifth day, extensive bacterial involvement of the entire wound, including the tissues under the eschar, is obvious. Most organisms are initially noted to be gram-positive cocci. Later, these organisms tend to be gram-negative, primarily the enteric organisms such as coliforms and pseudomonads. By the end of the first week, the eschar can be thoroughly infiltrated by tremendous numbers of organisms, and invasion of the adjacent, unburned tissue begins. This sequence of events ultimately culminates in burn wound sepsis.

Some of the important aspects of local treatment of burn wounds can be determined by an understanding of these phenomena. Systemic antibiotics penetrate poorly into burn wounds, and their use generally has disappointing results. Local antibacterial dressings are needed, preferably those that can penetrate eschars. The unaffected tissues adjacent to a thermal wound respond slowly to produce a barrier of granulation tissue and to mobilize phagocytic cells. In fact, an effective antibacterial barrier deep to a burn wound cannot be expected before three weeks. The advantages of total excision of all devitalized tissue early in the management of burn wounds are obvious. Finally, effective local therapy is needed early in burn wounds to minimize the progression of damage in the intermediate zone and to prevent conversion of second-degree burn wounds into full-thickness wounds.[25]

Nutritional Needs After Burns

Following major thermal injury there is an acceleration of whole body protein synthesis and breakdown proportional to the size of the burn.[47] There is a marked increase in calorie requirements, and if they are not met, an obligatory weight loss occurs and host defense mechanisms against infection are impaired. The mechanism of weight loss is not fully understood. It may be related to evaporative water loss, which involves obligatory calorie expenditure

and increased metabolic rate, which in turn is probably under endocrine influence and could be generated by the burn wound itself.[109] In animals not receiving sufficient calories to meet their increased metabolic demands, provision of increased dietary protein without associated increase in calories results in an apparent diversion of the additional amino acids to energy-yielding pathways.

The energy and amino acid requirements of burned humans have been studied, and much information is available about dogs from studies in beagles.[65, 101, 102] Care is needed in calculating the nutritional needs of the burned animal to take into account the requirement for total calories, the replacement of evaporative water loss, the distribution of nutrients among protein, carbohydrate, and fat, and the requirement for vitamins and minerals. Formulas are used in humans to calculate daily calorie requirement, but the accuracy of these in dogs is not known.[21]

Keeping burned experimental animals at an environmental temperature of 31°C significantly reduces mortality compared with keeping them at 25°C. It is likely that the thermal trauma produces a significant increase in heat loss, mainly owing to the evaporation of water from the surface of the burn. The increased heat loss leads in turn to a high expenditure of calories to maintain body temperature.[58]

Management of Thermal Injuries

First Aid and Initial Evaluation

The value of cold applications after burning has been well established. The benefits are two-fold. Cold stops the pain of a burn, and its immediate application stops the burning insult and can minimize the depth of injury.[36, 67] Cold is usually applied by use of wet towels soaked in ice water or submersion of the burned area in cold soapy water. Most dogs and cats are in pain and apprehensive and must be given an analgesic and a sedative. Commonly used agents include a narcotic such as morphine or oxymorphone and a tranquilizer such as acetylpromazine in dogs or ketamine plus diazepam in cats.

A general examination of the animal is needed as soon as possible to determine whether (1) thermal injury is minor and requires only local wound treatment, (2) local wound care and systemic treatment, particularly fluid therapy, are needed, or (3) the animal has lost a significant amount of skin and therefore should be euthanized (Fig. 40–4). In my opinion, if it is obvious that more than 30 per cent of the total surface area has suffered a third-degree burn, attempts at resuscitation probably should not be instigated and euthanasia should be seriously considered. In all severe thermal injuries, the animal should be evaluated continuously to determine whether resuscitation and eventual skin replacement are practical. Nursing problems alone present monumental challenges in the presence of extensive

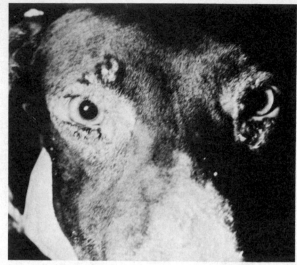

Figure 40–4. Thermal injury in a dog caused by a gas explosion in a home. Generalized first- and second-degree burns occurred over the body. Note sparing of haired areas on the face.

burns, and the expense and suffering of the animal must be considered. A human patient with second-degree thermal burns on more than 30 per cent of total body surface or third-degree burns on more than 10 per cent must be admitted to a specialty burn center for critical care.[71] In addition, the mortality and morbidity rates from burns rise sharply when the patient is more than 50 years old.[85]

Treatment of Burn Shock

Infusion of fluids and electrolytes in appropriate quantities and at appropriate rates is important. In humans, guides such as Evan's, Brook's, and Parkland's formulas are used to determine the volumes of electrolyte solutions and colloids needed; however, the use of these formulas is not practical in dogs and cats and they must be used only as rough guides in humans. A more acceptable method in animals is to administer fluids and to monitor the type and amount and rate of administration by measurement of physiological parameters.

Blood samples are obtained to measure the hematocrit, serum protein levels, hemoglobin, and, if possible, levels of the electrolytes sodium, potassium, and chloride. A central venous catheter is inserted into the jugular vein, the central venous pressure is measured, and a balanced electrolyte solution of the replacement type or lactated Ringer's solution is given. A urinary catheter is inserted, the bladder is emptied, and hourly urine output is monitored.

The amount of fluid administered and the rate of administration are determined by measurement of urine output and central venous pressure response. Urine output should be kept above 1 ml/kg body weight/hour. It can be expected that fluid input will exceed urine output by approximately three to four times in the first 48 hours and that equal volumes of

a replacement fluid and a maintenance fluid are required, up to approximately 3 to 4 ml/kg body weight/hour. An increase or a decrease in central venous pressure indicates the need to slow or increase the rate of fluid administration.

One of the important considerations in fluid and electrolyte therapy is the control of potassium. Minimal to moderate elevation of serum potassium is common in the first 24 hours after burn injury in animals with extensive burns because of thermal destruction of tissue cells and red cells. Therefore, in this period, the use of potassium-containing solutions should be minimized.[84] After 24 hours, catabolism, the loss of potassium from anoxic and heat-damaged cells, and increased secretion of mineralocorticoids all result in a considerable increase in renal potassium excretion. Sodium tends to be retained and the urinary Na-K ratio is reversed. If this condition is untreated, a potassium deficit frequently develops between the third and fifth day after burn, and serum potassium levels can fall to lethal levels. Loss of potassium can be monitored accurately by collection of 24-hour urine samples, and the level of serum potassium can be measured. The latter measurement is not necessarily an accurate assessment of total body potassium.

The loss of potassium can be minimized by the use of potassium-containing solutions after the first 24 hours after burn. In general, commercially available replacement solutions are low in potassium (4–5 mEq/l), so they can be administered early, when kidney function may be reduced and hyperkalemia is present. If kidney function is adequate, supplemental potassium can be given. For example, the potassium concentration of these replacement solutions can be raised to 15 to 20 mEq/l when measured serum potassium is within the range of 3.5 to 4.5 mEq/l. This potassium concentration can be increased to up to 80 mEq/l if measured serum potassium is below 2.5 mEq/l.

Another way to ensure adequate potassium is to use a mixture of commercial replacement and maintenance fluids for resuscitation. As stated previously, these replacement fluids usually contain 4 to 5 mEq/l of potassium and commercially available maintenance fluids contain 13 to 35 mEq/l of potassium. Therefore, it is desirable to provide approximately half the animal's daily fluid needs with a replacement solution and the remaining half with a maintenance fluid. Even with this regimen, supplemental potassium may be needed.

Animals with severe burn injury are usually acidotic, and blood gas monitoring is advised. Mild to moderate degrees of acidosis are usually corrected or controlled by the bicarbonate precursors in electrolyte solutions (lactate, gluconate, acetate, etc.). In severe injury, it is probably advisable to add up to 5 mEq/kg body weight of sodium bicarbonate to the solution so that it is administered over 30 to 60 minutes, not given as a bolus.

In severe burn injury in humans, the intracellular

anoxia, impaired carbohydrate metabolism, and acidosis together with its sequelae can often be corrected by infusion of blood with glucose and insulin (1 unit soluble insulin per gram of glucose). This infusion increases oxygen availability and combats the diabetagenic effects of the increased glucocorticoid secretion. Intracellular metabolism is improved, the sodium pump begins to work again, and extracellular respiratory alkalosis resolves.[94]

Loss of Protein and Red Blood Cells

Colloid-containing solutions and red blood cells for resuscitation are rarely indicated in the first one to two days after burning. However, serum proteins and hematocrit should be monitored and plasma and whole blood given as needed. Serum protein should be kept between 3.5 and 6.5 gm/dl and red blood cells should be given if the hematocrit falls below 25 per cent. The need for protein and red blood cells is usually at a maximum after two to five days.

Treatment of Inhalation Injury

The extent of injury to the respiratory tract should be monitored continuously. In some animals, all that is required is to turn the animal several times daily so that neither lung is overly dependent. Aspiration of fluid from the trachea and bronchi may be needed. Some severely injured animals require assisted respiration and oxygen, and injury to the nose, larynx, and trachea may necessitate a tracheotomy.

There is considerable evidence that administration of corticosteroids is not beneficial in reducing lung complications, although the administration of systemic antibiotics such as penicillinase-resistant penicillin for five days is recommended.[52]

Local Wound Therapy

Many aspects of local wound care are the same as for any accidental wound. Hair on the burn surface and surrounding skin is removed, and these areas are gently washed with water and mild soap or a detergent antiseptic such as povidone-iodine or chlorhexidine. All debris, shreds of tissue, and loose necrotic material are removed. Then the area is irrigated thoroughly with warm isotonic saline solution. A surface burn, that is, a first- or second-degree burn wound, is covered with a suitable antiseptic or antibiotic cream, and the wound is bandaged if it needs to be protected from the patient or from external trauma. The wound is cleansed daily with warm saline solution and the cream is applied. Healing should occur rapidly, and injured epithelium regenerates completely.

Third-degree burns are treated in a similar manner. A decision must be made, however, about when to remove eschars and when to close the wound. Eschars will separate spontaneously, but such separation can be a lengthy process and some eschars

persist for one to two months. The process can be hastened if edges are lifted during each dressing change, within the limits of the patient's tolerance without anesthesia. After spontaneous separation of the eschar, a wound with a granulating surface is exposed. A decision is then made whether to excise and close this wound, to close it with a reconstructive procedure, or to allow it to close by contraction and epithelialization.[57] A burn wound covered by an eschar cannot contract, so spontaneous wound closure does not occur during the eschar phase. After the eschar separates, the granulating bed produces myofibroblasts, and contraction occurs. The phase of eschar separation can occupy one to two months and the contraction phase can require one to two more months, severely prolonging the treatment period. Early eschar excision and closure may be preferred.[77]

Enzymatic debridement of burn eschars provides a satisfactory way to rapidly remove eschars. Sutilains ointment (Travase ointment)*, a sterile preparation of proteolytic enzymes elaborated by *Bacillus subtilis* in a hydrophobic ointment base, is one product used commonly to remove burn eschars. It is incompatible with some topical products such as iodine-containing creams and furazolium, but it can be used with silver sulfadiazine and most antibiotics. Debridement is usually complete in two to three weeks. The use of enzymes should be restricted to small wounds, as there can be increased fluid loss in large burns and a higher incidence of bacterial colonization and sepsis.

Excision of dead tissue followed by skin grafting, a reconstructive procedure, or healing by contraction and epithelialization is needed in many burn wounds. Excision can shorten the healing period and reduce burn wound sepsis.

Several methods are available for removal of burn eschars in humans and many are applicable to animals. *Tangential excision* refers to the excision of the outermost zone, the necrotic surface of a second-degree burn, by removing shavings of eschar until a pattern of pin-point dermal bleeding in the intermediate zone is reached.[44] This surface is immediately autografted in humans. This method is applicable in deep second-degree burns in dogs and cats to hasten removal of dead tissue, to protect the viable elements in the zone of capillary stasis, and to reduce the possibility of growth of organisms in dead tissue that would lead to sepsis. After tangential excision, the wound can be (1) autografted immediately, (2) allowed to heal as an open wound with application of a porcine xenograft (an expensive procedure) or a dressing impregnated with antibiotic or silver sulfadiazine, changing to Vaseline gauze when infection is controlled, or (3) closed by a reconstructive procedure immediately or after a period of contraction.

Tangential excision is applicable to full-thickness burns when the excision extends to clean viable

---

*Travase ointment, Flint Laboratories (Division of Travenol Laboratories, Inc.), Deerfield, IL 60015.

tissue, again in the intermediate zone of capillary stasis. This procedure is particularly recommended in the presence of grossly infected necrotic tissue. Once clean viable tissue is reached, the wound can be managed as described previously.

Burn wound excision to the deep fascia is indicated in humans for rapid reduction of wound size in massive wounds, for excision of integument in which invasive burn wound sepsis is present, and for localized deep burns.[78] Dogs and cats with massive wounds are usually euthanized, although burn wound excision can be a valuable procedure in the second and third situations just described. The fascial plane is generally easy to follow, and blood loss is minimized. The wound can be closed immediately by a reconstructive procedure, particularly in localized deep burns. In other cases, it can be autografted or allowed to heal as an open wound.

Eschars can be removed by tangential excision and total burn excision can be done by means of a cold scalpel, but bleeding can be excessive. An alternative procedure is to use electrosurgery by means of a filtered, fully rectified current.[54] The current cuts tissue cleanly, with minimal coagulation and a reduction in blood loss. In human surgery, carbon dioxide lasers and plasma scalpels have been used to minimize tissue trauma and blood loss.[28, 55, 100]

Topical wound therapy is essential to reduce burn wound sepsis. Systemic antibiotics penetrate poorly into the burn wound and eschar. Although local medications do not eradicate infection, they can reduce numbers of bacteria. Commonly, a population of 10^7 to 10^9 organisms/gm of tissue is seen in burn wound sepsis, and topical therapy can reduce the bacterial count to a median range of 10^4 bacteria/gm of tissue.

A variety of topical agents is available for use in burns. All are used to some extent in human patients, but many have little application in animals.[64]

A common agent in humans is 0.5 per cent silver nitrate solution. This silver salt was first used in 1934 in burn therapy as a 10 per cent solution combined with tannic acid. However, this mixture lost popularity because of the systemic toxicity of tannic acid and the local toxicity of the strong silver nitrate solution. The use of 0.5 per cent aqueous silver nitrate was introduced in 1965 with the specific purposes of reducing the amount of evaporative water loss from the burn wound and of providing an antibacterial agent that would control the burn wound flora.[62, 68] Both these objectives were met and the method is widely used in human burns. Dressings must be moistened with the 0.5 per cent solution every two hours, to prevent the solution from becoming more concentrated and, therefore, irritating to the wound. In addition, dressings are changed daily. The silver nitrate solution is messy, and all dressings and flesh are stained. This treatment can be associated with significant trans-eschar loss of potassium. Because of the 24-hour dressing changes and the need for wound

care every two hours, the use of 0.5 per cent silver nitrate solution is probably not practical in animals.

Mafenide (Sulfamylon)* is widely used for human burns. A methylated sulfonamide, mafenide is used at a 10 per cent concentration in a water-miscible cream. The drug has a wide spectrum of activity for both gram-positive and gram-negative organisms, and significant bacterial resistance does not develop. The drug in the water-miscible base rapidly penetrates to the subeschar space (in 30 minutes), and within five hours after application, 80 to 90 per cent of the applied drug enters and acquires a concentration of 1.5 mg/100 ml in the wound, a concentration four to five times that required for inhibition of bacterial flora.

The drug is rapidly absorbed into the body, where it is deaminated by amine oxydase to its paracarboxy breakdown product and excreted principally by the kidney. Both mafenide and its breakdown product are strong carbonic anhydrase inhibitors. There is a heavy hydrogen ion load to the body, and the buffering capability of the renal tubule is impaired by the carbonic anhydrase inhibition. The respiratory system must compensate for this acid load, and a characteristic tachypnea and hyperpnea result. This reaction can become so severe that the use of the drug must be discontinued. In addition, severe renal losses of potassium are commonly associated with mafenide therapy.

Mafenide cream is applied twice daily to the wound without dressings. Unfortunately, there is pain of varying intensity on application, and this factor, together with the carbonic anhydrase–inhibiting action, renders the drug unsuitable for use in animals.

Silver sulfadiazine (Silvadene),† introduced into burn care in 1969 to obviate the known difficulties encountered with the use of mafenide and silver nitrate, is probably the most popular topical agent. The substance is formed by the reaction of the weak acid sulfadiazine with silver nitrate and is supplied as a 1 per cent cream in a water-miscible base. When it is applied to the burn wound, approximately 10 per cent of the total amount is absorbed, resulting in blood levels from 1.5 to 4 mg/100 ml, depending on the size of the burn. Absorption of silver from the burn wound apparently does not occur.

There have been sporadic reports of gram-negative bacterial resistance, but the development of bacterial resistance during therapy is not a serious problem, and the drug has a wide spectrum of activity. The drug is applied twice daily to the wound, with no or light dressings. The application of silver sulfadiazine cream is painless, and local toxicity has not been encountered. Although leukopenia has been reported following therapy with silver sulfadiazine in humans, it has not been seen in animals, and a causative

---

*Sulfamylon cream, Winthrop Laboratories, New York, NY 10016.

†Silvadene cream, Marion Laboratories, Inc., Pharmaceutical Division, Kansas City, MO 64137.

relationship with the application of the drug in humans is questionable. The product is extremely useful in animal burns but must be used sparingly because of its cost.

Antibiotic creams and ointments are available for topical application, including gentamicin and combinations of antibiotics such as polymyxin, neomycin, and bacitracin. Preparations with a water-miscible base are preferred but are generally not available. The rapid development of resistant bacterial strains has been a serious deterrent to the long-term use of these products in humans, and in addition, aminoglycosides can be ototoxic and nephrotoxic after systemic absorption. These products are probably useful in treatment of burns in small animals if treatment is not prolonged beyond one or two weeks.

A myriad of other topical antibacterial agents have been tried in animals and humans for local burn therapy. Two prominent products are the furazolium derivatives and iodine-PVP complex. Furazolium chloride possesses a wide spectrum of activity, but in clinical use in humans, a significant number of positive *pseudomonas* cultures can be obtained from burn wounds treated with it. The product is generally more irritating than silver sulfadiazine or most antibiotic preparations and its use cannot be recommended.

Povidone-iodine (Betadine)* is available in a water-miscible cream and can be applied almost painlessly; however, it cannot be relied upon to control staphylococci in wounds. The product is extremely hyperosmolar and its use can lead to severe hypernatremia and acidosis because of free water loss from the wound.[95]

The use of local analgesic creams to reduce pain in burn wounds cannot be recommended because of the high risk of excessive absorption of the drug and systemic toxicity. Convulsions have been seen in dogs following local application of lidocaine cream on burn wounds.

Considerable attention has been given to the development of artificial burn wound coverings to control water loss and prevent infection. The general properties of a successful burn wound covering are that it must be a readily available material, have no antigenic properties, be strong and flexible, prevent microbial invasion from the environment, be capable of being sterilized, and have a water vapor transmission rate that will allow the proper moisture in the repairing wound.

Physiological dressings include autografts, allografts, and xenografts. Autografts in the form of split-thickness grafts, mesh grafts, or linear grafts can be applied in dogs and cats, but only after the wound bed is sufficiently prepared. There is little if any application for allografts, and the only practical xenograft is the use of lyophilized pig skin; this material adheres well, controls water loss, and produces a healthy granulating bed. Unfortunately, it is very expensive. Other materials used in humans include fetal membranes, collagen-based dressings, synthetic dressings of various polymers, foams, laminates, sprays, and gels. All artificial dressings are still far short of being consistently effective in management of burn wounds.[76, 87]

In dogs and cats, many uncomplicated burn wounds can be satisfactorily covered with petrolatum gauze, then a layer of an absorbent material, held in place with an outer bandage.

Control of Infection

Topical chemotherapy is the most important aspect of the prevention of infection in the burned animal.[63] Other aspects include routine care to reduce contamination from the environment and in particular to prevent infection from potentially resistant hospital pathogens. With regard to diagnosing infection in burn wounds, surface cultures are unreliable because they give no indication of the extent of wound invasion and often represent contaminating organisms. Clinical decisions should be based on quantitative measurement of organisms in the burn wound. This measurement is done by obtaining a small piece of eschar and underlying granulation tissue and subjecting it to homogenization, serial dilution, and plating. Bacterial counts of 10^5 organisms/gm or more, when taken in conjunction with clinical evidence, can indicate that the burn wound is the actual or potential source of sepsis.

Considerable controversy exists concerning the role of systemic antibiotics in burn wound care.[34] There is strong evidence that indiscriminate prophylactic antibiotic use for prolonged periods leads to rapid emergence of resistant strains and does not reduce the incidence of burn wound sepsis and septicemia.[7, 56] Therefore, systemic antibiotics should be given in the first three to five days after burning to prevent hemolytic streptococcal invasion of the burn wound and to prevent development of lung infection. Then systemic antibiotics should be given at the time of surgical manipulation, usually surgical excision, of the burn wound and if sepsis in the burn wound and septicemia develop.[71]

Gastric and Duodenal Ulceration

The incidence of the so-called Curling's ulcer in humans, once a major life-threatening complication in burn patients, has diminished markedly over the last 10 years, probably because of the rise in popularity of tube feedings that buffer gastric acid secretion. Although gastric and duodenal ulceration is seen in stressful conditions in animals, it is not known whether it is a significant problem in burn patients. It is advisable to consider the possibility of ulceration in severely burned animals and to administer an H_2-receptor antagonist such as cimetidine if clinical signs suggestive of ulceration are present. There is ade-

---

*Betadine ointment, The Purdue Frederick Company, Norwalk, CT 06856.

quate documentation in animal experiments to indicate that cimetidine is effective in the prevention of stress ulceration.[104]

Use of Anticoagulant Drugs

No information exists on the incidence of pulmonary embolism and other coagulation disorders in burned animals. In human burn patients, the reported evidence of pulmonary embolism ranges from 2 to 29 per cent,[19] and the use of anticoagulants such as coumarin derivatives and heparin is controversial.[71] In humans, universal prophylactic anticoagulation cannot be recommended, and its use in animals is not advisable.

ELECTRICAL INJURIES

The first human death from electrical injury in Lyons, France, in 1879 is well documented, but very little is known of the effects of electrical injury in animals.[46]

Electrical current of 1,000 volts or less is considered low-tension current, and above 1,000 volts, high-tension current. All household current is alternating current, which is much more dangerous than direct current. Domestic 60-cycle alternating current seriously affects the heart and respiratory center, accounting for the high incidence of fatal household accidents in humans.[105]

Types of Electrical Injury

In general, three types of electrical injury are seen in humans and can occur in dogs and cats.

In the first type, when electrical current, such as low-tension household current, passes through the body so that there are diffuse entry and exit contact areas and these areas have low resistance, e.g., wet skin, sudden death can occur. Ventricular fibrillation is caused by the effect of the alternating current on the myocardial conduction system. In addition, there are convulsive effects of the electrical current, leading to massive muscle contraction and respiratory paralysis. Usually current is insufficient to cause local heating, so electrical burns may not occur. This type of electrical injury is seen in dogs and cats that are electrocuted in a faulty animal dryer or are standing in water when they contact a live wire.

Generally, dogs and cats that are electrocuted in this manner become unconscious immediately and die rapidly. Some may recover spontaneously or after cardiopulmonary resuscitation, and some of these survivors may have local electrical injury. In humans, there are reports of transient nerve injury and cataracts long after systemic electrical injury. Permanent brain damage, despite the occurrence of unconsciousness or deep burns of the scalp, is rare. If damage to brain cells does occur, compensatory mechanisms appear to render it undetectable.[16] There is no consistent evidence that the viscera of the thorax or abdomen suffer permanent damage unless directly burned.

The second type of injury is from high-tension electrical wires, which are commonly contacted by humans in both work and play. This injury rarely happens with dogs and cats. High-tension electrical injury is characterized by severe systemic disturbances and massive local injury. In addition, the victim can be thrown away from the contact and acquire fractures, brain hemorrhages, rupture, and other severe injuries.

Seventy per cent of human victims are rendered unconscious, whether or not the current passes through the head, but recover within a few hours. Some mild changes in personality and mental capacity have been reported to occur later. Injury to internal organs, other than the heart, is rarely seen. The heart can suffer fatal disturbance of the pacemaker mechanism, and sudden death at the time of the accident can result from ventricular fibrillation.[99]

High-tension contact burns are usually very severe, with total destruction of tissue, even whole limbs. Extensive burns are caused by arcing of the current as well as passage through the limb. The extremely high temperature of the arc, up to 4,000°C, can melt bone and volatilize metal. High-tension electrical injuries are very rare in animals, and if they occur, they are fatal.

In the third most common type, low-tension electrical injury, the current touches one point on the body. There may or may not be exit points. This can produce a severe but mainly local injury. The usual cause of local low-tension electrical injury in dogs and cats is chewing live electrical cords, which has been reported in 29 dogs and seven cats.[48] Almost invariably, young animals are involved, and in the reported series, the dogs ranged in age from five weeks to 1½ years, and the cats from two months to two years.

An electrical burn varies from a small localized punctate lesion to a major injury with deep tissue destruction and remote vascular damage. This variation is determined by many factors, but the duration of contact and the voltage are primarily responsible. The injury occurs either at the point of the body's contact with the electrical current or at the location of the current's exit to the ground. In dogs and cats, the injury is invariably present in the mouth and there is no exit injury unless the animal is wet or is touching a conductor that acts as an earth contact.

Local injury in the mouth is caused by two mechanisms. First, there is arcing of the low-tension current, which produces local temperatures up to 3,000°C, and the victim's tissues are charred. Generally, in dogs and cats, the local lesion caused by this mechanism is small, often only a few millimeters in diameter. Second, the electrical current passes into the tissue, where it is converted into heat, according to Joule's law. In addition, the current can flow preferentially along blood vessels, producing damage to these vessels beyond the limits of other soft tissue injury. The tissue that is injured by this mechanism surrounds the small charred area, and the extent of this injury can be difficult to define. In many dogs and cats, the tissue appears normal. However, local ischemia is present, and demarcation and sloughing are obvious in two to three weeks. In general, the local electrical injury consists of the central zone of complete necrosis, a zone of necrosis in which tissues are intact, a zone of partial coagulation necrosis in which some tissue can survive unless destroyed by later infection, and a zone of partial coagulation of vessels from heat produced as current passes along vascular channels. The important feature of this wound is that the full extent of tissue destruction is rarely apparent before two to three weeks. Because blood vessels are thrombosed in electrical burns and, therefore, are included in the sloughing tissue, spontaneous arterial bleeding can occur during separation of the devitalized tissue.

In addition to local mouth injury in dogs and cats, severe pulmonary edema is usually present. In one report of 29 dogs, dyspnea was evident in 23 dogs and moist pulmonary crackles were heard in 20 dogs. Thoracic radiographs in 15 dogs showed characteristic pulmonary changes of lung edema.[48] Dyspnea was present in four of seven cats known to have bitten or chewed an electrical cord.[48] The cause of this lung condition is not known, and a similar condition has not been reported in humans.[75] It has been speculated that the lung edema is of centroneurogenic origin, following direct electrical stimulation of the CNS. The pathogenesis of experimentally induced centroneurogenic pulmonary edema involves a chain of events culminating in pulmonary hypertension and extravasation of blood and fluid into the pulmonary interstitial space.[48] The pulmonary edema following electrical mouth burns is very severe in dogs and can lead to death, whereas cats are less severely affected.

Clinical Signs of Electrical Injury

Dogs and cats that chew electrical cords generally are found unconscious in a tonic state or have a period of generalized tonoclonic activity.[39, 41] Vomiting and defecation can occur. Most unconscious animals regain consciousness quickly. The mouth lesion varies, depending on the severity of the injury and the period from the electrical burn. Immediately after the injury, there are punctate or larger areas of complete necrosis, which may be surrounded by a grayish necrotic zone or a reddened zone of coagulation necrosis. After one to two days, local swelling is usually present (Fig. 40–5). In two to three weeks, signs of demarcation and sloughing are present (Figs. 40–6 and 40–7). Later, there are open granulating wounds in the mouth or lips or fistulae into the nose.

Respiratory distress with dyspnea and moist pulmonary crackles occurs in most dogs and cats within

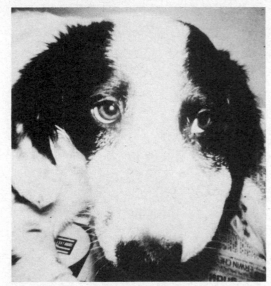

Figure 40–5. Marked local edema of the lips and cheeks following electrical injury in the mouth.

one hour of electrical contact, and pulmonary edema can be confirmed by radiographs (Fig. 40–8).

Treatment of Electrical Injury

In humans with severe electrical injury, fluid requirements are much greater than for the patient with flame burns, owing to the greater depth of injury and the common occurrence of hemoglobinuria

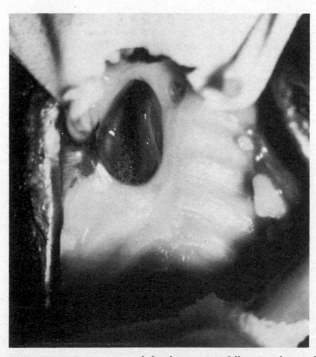

Figure 40–6. Large oronasal fistula in a cat following electrical burn of the hard palate. This fistula was closed by a sliding flap (see Figure 40–7).

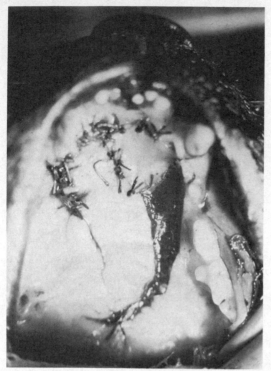

Figure 40–7. Closure of the oronasal fistula in the cat in Figure 40–6.

and myoglobinuria. The local wound often requires decompression by fasciotomy and local excision.[93] Local medications such as mafenide and silver sulfadiazine are used for the electrical burn. In dogs and cats, severe electrical injuries are rarely treated, so further discussion concerns only electrical burns to the mouth and lips.

In treating humans with electrical burns of the mouth and lips, it is important to recognize the critical role that the mouth plays in the esthetic unity of the face and its oral function. Accordingly, there is considerable discussion concerning the repair of these burn injuries. The majority of oral surgeons do not recommend debridement of burn wounds in the mouth in the first few days, because it is difficult to differentiate viable from nonviable tissue. By the 12th to 14th day after the burn, the eschar has separated, and it is possible to accurately identify the viable tissue. The majority of oral surgeons prefer to debride and reconstruct the wound at this time.[75] They claim that total healing by contraction and epithelialization can lead to microstomia, dental deviation, obliteration of the buccal sulcus, and increased amounts of scar tissue. Some surgeons, however, prefer to allow this total healing by contraction and epithelialization and to perform appropriate reconstruction five to six months later.

Other surgeons believe that in children with electrical burns of the mouth, early exploration of the path of the current in the first few days is needed. Devitalized tissue is identified and removed and this process is repeated until only viable tissues remain. This process ultimately saves tissues in the zones of partial coagulation necrosis that are capable of recovery, and serious hazards of infection are avoided. The problem with this approach is identifying cellular injury at an early stage.[81]

The situation in dogs and cats is different. In these animals, minor deformities are not usually as important, because cosmetic appearance and oral function, particularly for sound, have less significance than in humans. Also, the lips and cheeks are loose and may not be deformed by wound contraction.

In most mouth and lip injuries in dogs and cats, no specific treatment is needed. The full extent of devitalized tissues is difficult to determine, and the tissue can be allowed to separate spontaneously in two to three weeks. Then the wound should be

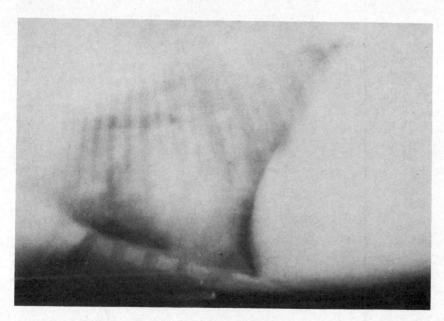

Figure 40–8. Pulmonary edema in a dog following electrical injury to the mouth.

examined to determine whether it will heal by contraction and epithelialization or a reconstructive procedure is necessary. In general, fistulae into the nasal cavity through the hard palate should be closed surgically. Animals must be monitored carefully during the period of eschar separation to detect bleeding from thrombosed and sloughing blood vessels.

Pulmonary edema in cats is rarely severe, and most cats should recover spontaneously, but edema in dogs responds poorly to treatment. In one series, ten of 26 dogs died, presumably as a direct result of pulmonary edema, in spite of therapy; the interval between injury and death ranged from 2½ hours to 12 hours.[48] No specific therapy can be recommended in dogs. Usual therapy in humans and animals includes measures to decrease pulmonary hydrostatic pressure, such as furosemide to decrease plasma volume, morphine to produce sympatholytic and vasodilatory effects, and aminophylline to cause vasodilation and bronchodilation. Phlebotomy with removal of 10 per cent of the calculated blood volume has also been recommended.[111] The alpha blocker phentolamine, which reduces vascular pressure, and corticosteroids have been recommended in dogs, together with fluid and electrolyte therapy and positive-pressure ventilation.[48]

LIGHTNING INJURIES

Lightning injuries are uncommon, being reported much more frequently in farm animals than in dogs and cats. Only one human out of three who are hit by lightning is killed.[107]

The sequence of natural events leading to lightning discharge has been described.[3] In general, large amounts of static electricity build up in clouds from the collision between particles of ice carried by updrafts and downdrafts, resulting in the development of a large negative charge at the bottom of the cloud that is, then discharged to earth.

When an animal is struck by lightning, the body becomes highly charged. If the body is grounded, the current passes through it and is discharged into the ground. Violent muscular contraction can occur and throw the victim several feet. As a result of the current passing through the body, typical injuries are produced at entrance and exit points and in any of the body organs.

Skin Lesions

Second- and third-degree burns occur on the skin in a spidery, arborescent pattern because the electrical current follows pathways of skin dampness where resistance is lowest. Healing and wound care are similar to those in thermal and electrical injuries. In general, the skin burns are minor and heal with routine wound care and do not need reconstructive procedures.

Central Nervous System Lesions

Unconsciousness, coma, or restlessness and disoriented behavior are commonly seen in the initial phase of lightning injury. Late sequelae have not been reported in animals; however, in humans, psychiatric illness, hemiplegia, cataracts, and optic atrophy have been reported.

Peripheral Nervous System Lesions

Early effects include severe vasoconstriction with loss of pulse, loss of sensation, and paralysis due to ischemia of peripheral nerves. These effects usually disappear, although late sequelae including neuritis with painful neuralgia have been reported in humans.

Cardiac Injury

Acute myocardial damage with atrial and ventricular arrhythmias is seen in the acute phase of injury. Most of these abnormalities revert to a normal pattern.

Treatment of Lightning Injuries

Sudden death in lightning injuries is the result of paralysis of the respiratory center, apnea, ventricular fibrillation, or cardiac arrest. Specific treatment includes cardiopulmonary resuscitation, which must be applied early and should be prolonged. Cardiac arrhythmias should be corrected. Fluid and electrolyte administration as in thermal injuries, with monitoring of central venous pressure and urine output, is essential. Skin burns are generally minor and are treated with topical agents such as silver sulfadiazine. Muscle necrosis as seen in electrical burns is rarely present.

CHEMICAL BURNS

More than 25,000 products capable of producing chemical burns are marketed for use in industry, agriculture, military activities, and the home. No comprehensive reports concerning the management of chemical injuries appear in the veterinary literature. In humans, chemicals produce injury by ingestion and inhalation and by local application to the skin. This discussion is limited to local application of chemicals to the skin of animals. In dogs, chemical burns are seen following accidental spillage and following malicious application, particularly to the heads of large dogs.

Nature of Chemicals that "Burn"

These chemicals can be divided into oxidizing agents, reducing agents, corrosives, protoplasmic poisons, desiccants, and vesicants.[45]

Oxidizing Agents. Chromic acid, used in metal cleaning, produces protein coagulation with ulceration after skin contact. Chlorox (sodium hypochlorite) is commonly present in the home, and skin burns from this agent have been seen in dogs. The released free chlorine coagulates cutaneous proteins. Potassium permanganate, a powerful oxidizing agent, produces a thick, brownish-purple eschar of coagulated protein on contact with skin.

Reducing Agents. These agents produce their effect much as oxidizing agents do and cause protein denaturization. Common agents are alkyl mercuric compounds, hydrochloric acid, and nitric acid. All three agents form a coagulum over a shallow ulcer and continue to "burn" until the active agent is neutralized.

Corrosives. Corrosive agents are those substances that cause extreme denaturization of tissue protein, producing a soft eschar with shallow, indolent ulcers. They include the phenols, which are used as deodorants and disinfectants, dichromate salts, and corrosive alkalis including potassium, sodium, ammonium, lithium, barium, and calcium hydroxides.

Protoplasmic Poisons. This group of agents produces its detrimental effects either by forming salts with proteins or by binding or inhibiting calcium or other inorganic ions necessary for tissue viability and function. Among these poisons are the "alkaloidal" acids such as picric and tannic acids, acetic acid, formic acid, oxalic acid, and hydrofluoric acid. The "alkaloidal" acids form homologous proteinates on contact with skin, producing thin, hard eschars, and if absorbed will produce hepatotoxicity or nephrotoxicity.

Desiccants. These agents produce their deleterious effects by causing dehydration damage or by creating excessive heat. Examples are sulfuric acid and hydrochloric acid, both commonly found in the home and industry (toilet bowl cleaners, metal cleansers in plumbing, etc.). They produce very severe injury, characterized by a hard eschar under which an indolent, deep ulcer forms.

Vesicants. Damage caused by vesicants is produced by a series of physiological changes. They frequently liberate histamine or serotonin, the result of which is the production of ischemia with anoxic necrosis at the site of contact. Important vesicants are cantharides and dimethyl sulfoxide.

Treatment of Chemical Injury

In the early treatment of chemical "burns" and in the treatment of injuries caused by chemicals that have a persistent action, specific neutralization of the injurious agent can be important. Specific antidotes include mild alkalis such as soda lime for agents such as hydrochloric acid, and a weak acid for lye burns. In general, the most important early treatment for all chemical burns consists of dilution of the chemical agent by wound irrigation with copious amounts of water or saline and debridement of separating necrotic tissue. By decreasing the concentration of and partially removing the agent, water dilution decreases the rate of chemical reaction and the hygroscopic action of the chemical. Although some heat of dilution is produced, it can be rapidly dissipated by the use of constant water flow.[14, 91] Because time is critical in preventing full-thickness injury, water dilution is suggested as an immediate first-aid measure.

Following thorough irrigation, the wound is treated like a thermal burn. Local medication, as used in thermal injuries, is important because of the presence of the eschar and considerable coagulation necrosis with thrombus formation in the microvasculature of the lesion, which lead to local bacterial growth and low tissue levels of antibiotics with systemic administration. The wound can be excised or the eschar can be allowed to demarcate and slough. The surgeon may have difficulty determining the full depth and extent of an early wound, and therefore, early excision can be incomplete or excessive.

Further tissue destruction secondary to continued chemical penetration can occur over 24 to 72 hours, resulting in underestimation of the magnitude of injury and inadequate fluid resuscitation, which can lead to hypotension and acute tubular necrosis. Therefore, in severe cases, frequent observation of vital signs and monitoring of central venous pressure and urinary output should be used to guide fluid and electrolyte therapy.

COLD INJURIES

Body Hypothermia

In humans, accidental hypothermia denotes a body temperature of less than 34°C (93.2°F) produced by exposure to cold. Animals respond to cold in a number of ways. Atrial fibrillation is the most common cardiac rhythm disturbance. It generally reverts to a normal sinus rhythm with rewarming. Fatal cardiac rhythm disturbances can occur, including profound bradycardia and ventricular fibrillation.[13]

Severe systemic hypothermia in humans of less than 88.0°F (31.1°C) can produce progressive paralysis of the central nervous system with loss of consciousness and abolition of reflexes.[82] At lower temperatures, because medullary centers are paralyzed, the pulse rate decreases and the respiration rate slows to fatal levels.[98]

Metabolically, decreases in cellular activity and physiological processes during hypothermia reflect changes in temperature-dependent biochemical reactions. Cell metabolism in general follows the van't Hoff–Arrhenius rule, which states that the rate of chemical reaction is increased or decreased two or three times for each 10.0°C rise or fall in temperature. Important factors that are affected by hypothermia are renal function, glucose metabolism, acid-base balance, and the concentration of circulating hemoglobin. The results can be glucosuria, diminished excretion of creatinine, decreased resorption of water by the kidney, dehydration, azotemia, acidosis, hypoxemia, and rapid fall in hemoglobin and hematocrit levels.

The important consideration in treatment of hypothermia is rapid rewarming in water heated to 40.0 to 42.2°C (104.0 to 108.0°F).[51] Routine fluid and electrolyte infusions are usually needed.

Frostbite

Cold injury to extremities involves either the supporting tissues, the primary circulation, or both.[30, 49, 53] There is undoubtedly damage to local blood vessels, which can be primary or secondary to damage to surrounding structures. The end result is ischemia, with dry gangrene (mummification). Infection can occur in the ischemic tissue, leading to moist gangrene.

In experimental frostbite in the feet of rabbits, swelling from edema and redness of the skin began soon after thawing and reached a maximum about 24 hours after freezing; at this time, the feet were bright red. The red discoloration and edema persisted for the next two days. It was not possible to estimate the degree and depth of injury at this time, and subsequent changes and future tissue loss could not be predicted from external appearance. Severely damaged feet began to shrink on the fourth and fifth day, and mummification was present by the seventh to tenth day. The black, shrunken tissue was clinging to the devitalized bones. Separation of the dead tissue required 30 to 40 days. In less severely affected feet, the appearance up to the third day was similar to that of severely injured feet, but after this time there was a rapid restoration to normal in most tissues. Major obstruction to blood flow in the affected feet was detected by fluorescein injection and by arterial perfusion with barium sulfate.[32]

The most accepted treatment for frostbite is rapid rewarming of the affected part in warm water at 42°C. Following this rapid thawing, endothelial cells in blood vessels remain attached to the intima and are actively proliferating after three days, the internal elastic lamina remains intact, and medial cells are minimally distorted. The opposite findings are present after slow thawing. With rapid thawing, tissue appears less severely affected and repair is initiated earlier than with slow thawing.[17]

The local treatment of the cold injury should be conservative. Local medication is not needed unless infection, manifested by moistness, occurs. Then preparations used for thermal injury can be applied. Amputation is usually delayed until the dry gangrene has completely mummified.

In humans, sympathectomy by a translumbar extraperitoneal approach seems to be beneficial in severe frostbite for relieving pain, promoting the resolution of edema, hastening the process of demarcation, and preventing harmful late sequelae.[50] This benefit has been confirmed in experimental animals.[26, 33] Probably, sympathectomy relieves arterial spasm, closing arteriovenous shunts and promoting collateral circulation.[59] The value of low-molecular-weight dextran and anticoagulants in treatment of frostbite is doubtful.[70, 80]

1. Achauer, B. M., Allyn, P. A., Furnas, D. W., et al.: Pulmonary complications; the major threat to the burn patient. Ann. Surg. 177:311, 1973.
2. Allgower, M., Cueni, I. B., Stadtler, K., and Schoenenberger, G. A.: Burn toxin in mouse skin. J. Trauma 13:95, 1973.
3. Apfelberg, D. B., Masters, F. W., and Robinson, D. W.: Pathophysiology and treatment of lightning injuries. J. Trauma 14:6, 1973.
4. Arturson, G.: Pathophysiological aspects of burn syndrome: with special reference to liver injury and alterations of capillary permeability. Acta Chir. Scand. (Suppl.) 274:1, 1961.
5. Aub, T. C., Pittman, H., and Brues, A. M.: The management of the Cocoanut Grove burns at the Massachusetts General Hospital: the pulmonary complications; a clinical description. Ann. Surg. 117:834, 1943.
6. Aulick, L. H., Goodwin, C. W., Becker, R. A., and Wilmore, D. W.: Visceral blood flow following thermal injury. Ann. Surg. 193:112, 1981.
7. Ayliffe, G. A. J., Green, W., Livingston, R., and Lowbury, E. J. C.: Antibiotic-resistant Staphylococcus aureus in dermatology and burn wards. J. Clin. Pathol. 30:40, 1977.
8. Baar, S., and Arrowsmith, D. J.: Thermal damage to red cells. J. Clin. Pathol. 23:572, 1970.
9. Baar, S.: Mechanisms of delayed red cell destruction after thermal injury. An experimental in vitro SEM study. Br. J. Exp. Pathol. 55:187, 1973.
10. Baxter, C. R., and Shires, T.: Physiological response to crystalloid resuscitation of severe burns. Ann. N.Y. Acad. Sci. 150:874, 1968.
11. Birdsell, D. C., and Birch, J. R.: Anemia following thermal burns: a survey in 109 children. Can. J. Surg. 14:435, 1971.
12. Birke, G., Liljedahl, S.-O., Plantin, L. O., et al.: Studies on burns. IX: The distribution and losses through the wound of 131I-albumin measured by whole-body counting. Acta Chri. Scand. 134:27, 1968.
13. Brauer, R. W., and Behnke, A. R.: Hypothermia and cold injury. In Harrison, T. R. (ed.): Principles of Internal Medicine. McGraw-Hill Book Co., New York, 1966.
14. Bromberg, B. E., Song, I. C., and Waldren, R. H.: Hydrotherapy for chemical burns. Plast. Reconstr. Surg. 35:85, 1965.
15. Bryan, C. P.: The Papyrus Ebers. D. Appleton and Co., New York, 1931.
16. Burke, J. E., Quinby, W. C., Brondoc, C. et al.: Patterns of high tension electrical injury in children and adolescents and their management. Am. J. Surg. 133:492, 1977.
17. Carpenter, H. M., Hurley. I. A., Hardenbergh, E., et al.: Vascular injury due to cold: effects of rapid rewarming. Arch. Pathol. 92:153, 1971.
18. Casson, P., Converse, J. M., and Rappaport, F. T.: Delayed hypersensitivity status in burned patients. Surg. Forum 17:268, 1966.
19. Coleman, J. B., and Chang, F. C.: Pulmonary embolism: an

unrecognized event in severely burned patients. Am. J. Surg. 130:697, 1975.

20. Curreri, W. P., Asch, M. J., and Pruitt, B. A.: The treatment of chemical burns: specialized diagnostic, therapeutic and prognostic considerations. J. Trauma 10:8, 1970.

21. Curreri, W. P., Richmond, D., Marvin, J., and Baxter, C. P.: Dietary requirements of patients with major burns. J. Am. Diet. Assoc. 65:415, 1974.

22. Czaja, A. J., Rizzo, T. A., Smith, W. R., Jr., and Pruitt, B. A., Jr.: Acute liver disease after cutaneous thermal injury. J. Trauma 15:887, 1975.

23. Davies, J. W. L.: The fluid therapy given to 1,027 patients during the first 48 hours after burning. II: The inputs of sodium and water and the tonicity of the therapy. Burns 1:331, 1975.

24. Day, C., and Leape, L. L.: Tissue sodium concentration after thermal burns. J. Trauma 12:1063, 1972.

25. De Camara, D. L., Raine, T. J., London, M. D., et al.: Progression of thermal injury: a morphologic study. Plast. Reconstr. Surg. 69:491, 1980.

26. Eeles, G. H., and Sevitt, S.: Microthrombosis in injured and burned patients. J. Pathol. Bacteriol. 93:275, 1967.

26a. Ervasti, E.: Frostbite of extremities and their sequelae. Acta Chir. Scand. (Suppl.) 299:5, 1962.

27. Eurenius, K., and Rothenberg, J.: Platelet aggregation after thermal injury. J. Lab. Clin. Med. 83:355, 1974.

28. Fidler, J. P., Law, E., Rockwell, R. J., Jr., and MacMillan, B. G.: Carbon dioxide laser excision of acute burns with immediate autografting. J. Surg. Res. 17:1, 1974.

29. Foley, F. D., Greenwald, K. A., Nash, G., et al.: Herpes virus infection in burned patients. N. Engl. J. Med. 282:652, 1970.

30. Fontaine, R., Klein, M., Bollack, C., et al.: Clinical and experimental contribution to the study of frostbite. J. Cardiovasc. Surg. 2:449, 1961.

31. Fried, D. A., and Munster, A. M.: Does immunosuppression by thermal injury depend on the continued presence of the burn wound? J. Trauma 15:482, 1975.

32. Gage, A. A., Ishikawa, H., and Winter, P. M.: Experimental frostbite: the effect of hyperbaric oxygenation on tissue survival. Cryobiology 7:1, 1970.

33. Golding, M. R., Mendoza, M. E., Hennigar, G. R., et al.: On settling the controversy on the benefit of sympathectomy for frostbite. Surgery 56:221, 1964.

34. Haburchak, D. R., and Pruitt, B. A.: Use of systemic antibiotics in the burned patient. Surg. Clin. North Am. 58:1119, 1978.

35. Hakim, A. A.: An immunosuppressive factor from serum of thermally traumatized patients. J. Trauma 17:908, 1977.

36. Hardy, J. D., Stolwijk, J. A. J., and Hoffman, D.: Pain following step increase in skin temperature. In Shalo, K. (ed.): The Skin Senses. Charles C Thomas, Springfield, 1961.

37. Harris, R. L., Cottam, G. I., Johnston, J. M., and Baxter, C. R.: The pathogenesis of abnormal erythrocyte morphology in burns. J. Trauma 21:13, 1981.

38. Hergt, K.: Blood levels of thrombocytes in burned patients: Observations on their behavior in relation to the clinical condition of the patient. J. Trauma 12:599, 1972.

39. Holliman, C. J., Saffle, J. R., Kravits, M., and Warden, G. D.: Early surgical decompression in the management of electrical injuries. Am. J. Surg. 144:733, 1982.

40. Howard, R. J., and Simmons, R. L.: Acquired immunologic deficiencies after trauma and surgical procedures. Surg. Gynecol. Obstet. 139:771, 1974.

41. Hunt, J. L., McMannus, W. E., Haney, W. P., and Pruitt, B. A.: Vascular lesions in acute electrical injuries. J. Trauma 14:461, 1974.

42. Ishizawa, S., Sakai, H., Searles, H. E., et al.: Effect of thymosin on T-lymphocyte functions in patients with acute thermal burns. J. Trauma 18:48, 1978.

43. Jackson, D.: Diagnosis of the depth of burning. Br. J. Surg. 40:588, 1953.

44. Jackson, D. M., and Stone P. A.: Tangential excision and grafting of burns. Br. J. Plast. Surg. 25:416, 1972.

45. Jelenko, C.: Chemicals that burn. J. Trauma 14:1, 1974.

46. Jex-Blake, A. J.: The Goulstonian lectures on death by electrical currents and by lightning. Br. Med. J. 1:425, 1913.

47. Kien, C. L., Young, V. R., Rohbaugh, D. K., and Burke, J. E.: Increased rates of whole body protein and breakdown in children recovering from burns. Ann. Surg. 187:383, 1978.

48. Kolata, R. J., and Burrows, C. F. The clinical features of injury by chewing electrical cords in dogs and cats. J. Am. Anim. Hosp. Assoc. 17:219, 1981.

49. Kulka, J. P.: Microcirculatory impairment as a factor in inflammatory tissue damage. Ann. N.Y. Acad. Sci. 116:1018, 1964.

50. Kyosola, K.: Clinical experiences in the management of cold injuries: a study of 110 cases. J. Trauma 14:1, 1974.

51. Lapp, N. L., and Juergens, J. L.: Frostbite. Mayo Clin. Proc. 40:932, 1965.

52. Levin, B. A., Petroff, P. A., Slade, C. L., and Pruitt, B. A.: Prospective trials of dexamethasone and aerosolized gentamicin in the treatment of inhalation injury in the burned patient. J. Trauma 18:188, 1978.

53. Lewis, R. B.: Local cold injury. Am. J. Phys. Med. 34:538, 1955.

54. Lewis, R. J., and Quinby, W. C., Jr.: Electrosurgical excision of full-thickness burns. Arch. Surg. 110:191, 1975.

55. Link, W. J., Zook, E. G., and Glover J. L.: Plasma scalpel excision of burns: an experimental study. Plast. Reconstr. Surg. 55:657, 1975.

56. Lowbury, E. J. L., Lilly, H. A., and Kidson, A.: "Methicillin-resistant" Staphylococcus aureus: reassessment by controlled trial in burn unit. Br. Med. J. 2:1054, 1977.

57. MacMillan, B. G.: Closing the burn wound. Surg. Clin. North Am. 58:1205, 1978.

58. Markley, K., Smallman, E., Thornton, S. W., and Evans, G.: The effect of environmental temperature and fluid therapy on mortality and metabolism of mice after burn and tourniquet trauma. J. Trauma 13:145, 1973.

59. Martinez, A., Golding, M. R., Sawyre, P. N., et al.: The specific arterial lesions in mild and severe frostbite: effect of sympathectomy. J. Cardiovasc. Surg. 7:495, 1966.

60. Massiha, H, and Monafo, W. W.: Dermal ischemia in thermal injury: the importance of venous occlusion. J. Trauma 14:705, 1974.

61. McManus, W. F., Eurenius, K., and Pruitt, B. A.: Disseminated intravascular coagulation in burned patients. J. Trauma 13:416, 1973.

62. Monafo, W. W., and Moyer, C. A.: The effectiveness of dilute aqueous silver nitrate in the treatment of burns. Arch. Surg. 91:200, 1965.

63. Monafo, W. W., and Ayvazian, V. H.: Topical therapy. Surg. Clin. North Am. 58:1157, 1979.

64. Moncrief, J. A.: Topical antibacterial therapy of the burn wound. Clin. Plast. Surg. 1:563, 1974.

65. Moncrief, J. A.: Burns. N. Eng. J. Med. 288:444, 1973.

66. Moncrief, J. A.: Effect of various fluid regimens and pharmacologic agents on the circulatory hemodynamics of the immediate postburn period. Ann. Surg. 164:723, 1966.

67. Moserova, J., Behounkova, E., and Prouza, Z.: Subcutaneous temperature measurements in thermal injury. Burns 1:267, 1975.

68. Moyer, C. A., Brentano, L., Gravens, D. L., et al.: Treatment of large human burns with 0.5% silver nitrate solution. Arch. Surg. 90:812, 1965.

69. Moylan, J. A., Jr., Reckler, J. M., and Mason, A. D., Jr.: Resuscitation with hypertonic lactate saline in thermal injury. Am. J. Surg. 125:580, 1973.

70. Mundth, E. D., Long, D. M., and Brown, R. B.: Treatment of experimental frostbite with low molecular weight dextran. J. Trauma 4:246, 1964.

71. Munster, A. M.: The early management of thermal burns. Surgery 87:29, 1980.

72. Noble, G. H. S., Robson, M. C., and Krizek, T. J.: Dermal ischemia in the burn wound. J. Surg. Res. 23:117, 1977.

73. O'Neil, J. A., Pruitt, B. A., Jr., and Moncrief, J. A.: Studies

of renal function during the early post-burn period. *In* Matter, P., Barclay, T. L., Korvicfora, Z., et al. (eds.): *Research in Burns; Transaction of the Third International Congress on Research in Burns, Prague.* Hans Huber Publishers, Bern, 1971.

74. Order, S. E., and Moncrief, J. A.: The Burn Wound. Charles C Thomas, Springfield, 1965.

75. Ortiz-Monasterio, F., and Factor, R.: Early definitive treatment of electric burns of the mouth. Plast. Reconstr. Surg. 65:169, 1980.

76. Park, G. B.: Burn wound coverings—a review. Biomater. Med. Devices Artif. Organs 6:1, 1978.

77. Parks, D. H., Carvajal, H. E., and Larson, D. L.: Management of burns. Surg. Clin. North Am. 57:875, 1977.

78. Parks, D. H., Linares, H. A., and Thompson, P. D.: Surgical management of burn wound sepsis. Surg. Gynecol. Obstet. 153:374, 1981.

79. Pattle, R. E., and Cullumbine, H.: Toxicity of some atmospheric pollutants. Br. Med. J. 2:914, 1956.

80. Penn, I., and Schwartz, S. I.: Evaluation of low molecular weight dextran in the treatment of frostbite. J. Trauma 4:784, 1964.

81. Peterson, R. A.: Electrical burns of the hand; treatment by early excision. J. Bone Jt. Surg. 48A:407, 1966.

82. Pickening, G.: Regulation of body temperature in health and disease. Lancet 1:59, 1958.

83. Pruitt, B. A.: Fluid resuscitation of burn patients: does clinical "success" necessitate "excess"? South. Med. J. 69:1399, 1976.

84. Pruitt, B. A.: Fluid and electrolyte replacement in the burned patient. Surg. Clin. North Am. 58:1291, 1978.

85. Pruitt, B. A., Mason, A. D., and Hunt, J L.: Burn injury in the aged high risk patient. *In* Siegel J. H., and Chudoff, D. D. (eds.): *The Aged and High Risk Surgical Patient.* Grune & Stratton, New York, 1975.

86. Pulaski, E. J.: *Infection and Burn Illness. Bahama International Conference on Burns.* Philadelphia, Dorrance, 1961.

87. Quinby, W. C., Hoover, H. C., Scheflan, M., et al: Clinical trials of amniotic membranes in burn wound care. Plast. Reconstr. Surg. 70:711, 1982.

88. Raffa, J., and Trunkey, D. D.: Myocardial depression in acute thermal injury. J. Trauma 18:90, 1978.

89. Rappaport, F. T., Milgrome, F., Kario, K., et al.: Immunologic sequelae of thermal injury. Ann. N.Y. Acad. Sci. 150:1004, 1968.

90. Rappaport, F. T., Nemirovsky, M. S., Bachvaroff, R., and Ball, S. K.: Mechanisms of pulmonary damage in severe burns. Ann. Surg. 177:472, 1973.

91. Rensburg, L. C. van: An experimental study of chemical burns. S. Afr. Med. J. 36:754, 1962.

92. Robson, M. C., Kucan, J. O., Paik, K. I., and Erikson, E.: Prevention of dermal ischemia after thermal injury. Arch. Surg. 113:621, 1978.

93. Rouse, R. G., and Dimick, A. R.: The treatment of electrical injury compared to burn injury: a review of pathophysiol-ogy and comparison of patient management protocols. J. Trauma 18:43, 1978.

94. Sanders, R.: The burnt patient: a general view. Br. Med. J. Aug 17, 3:460, 1974.

95. Scoggin, C., McClellan, J. R., and Cary, J. M.: Hypernatraemia and acidosis in association with topical treatment of burns (letter). Lancet 1:959, 1977.

96. Shimazaki, S., Yoshiola, T., Tanka, N., et al.: Body fluid changes during hypertonic lactated saline solution therapy for burn shock. J. Trauma 17:38, 1977.

97. Shoemaker, W. G., Vladeck, B. C., Bassin, R., et al.: Burn pathophysiology in man. I: Sequential hemodynamic alterations. J Surg. Res. 14:64, 1973.

98. Simpson, S., and Herring, R. J.: The effect of cold necrosis on reflex actions in warm blooded animals. J. Physiol. 32:305, 1950.

99. Scogg, T.: Electrical injuries. J. Trauma 10:816, 1970.

100. Stellar, S., Levine, N., Ger, R., and Levenson, S. M.: Laser excision of acute third-degree burns followed by immediate autograft replacement: an experimental study in the pig. J. Trauma 13:45, 1973.

101. Stinnett, J. D., Alexander, W. J., Watanabe, C., et al.: Plasma and skeletal muscle amino acids following severe burn injury in patients and experimental animals. Ann. Surg. 195:75, 1982.

102. Stinnett, J. D., Ogle, C. K., Alexander, J. W., et al.: Alterations of immunologic function in experimental animals following severe thermal injury; lack of effect of altering protein quality and quantity in hypocaloric diets. J. Burn Care Rehab. 2:150, 1981.

103. Stone, H. H., Martin, J. D.: Pulmonary injury associated with thermal burns. Surg. Gynecol. Obstet. 129:1242, 1969.

104. Strauss, R. L., Stein, T. A., and Wise, L.: Prevention of stress ulcerations using H_2 receptor antagonists. Am. J. Surg. 135:120, 1978.

105. Sturim, H. S.: The treatment of electrical injuries. J. Trauma 11:959, 1971.

106. Sudarsky, R. D.: Ocular injury due to formic acid. Arch. Ophthal. (Chicago) 74:805, 1965.

107. Taussig, H. B.: Death from lightning; and the possibility of living again. Ann. Intern. Med. 68:1345, 1968.

108. Wilson, R. L.: Assessment of bush fire damage to stock. Aust. Vet. J. 42:101, 1966.

109. Wilmore, D. W., and Aulick, L. H.: Metabolic changes in burned patients. Surg. Clin. North Am. 58:1173, 1978.

110. Zawacki, B. E., Jung, R. C., Joyce, A. S., and Rincon, E.: Smoke burns and the natural history of inhalation injury in fire victims; a correlation of experimental and clinical data. Ann. Surg. 185:100, 1977.

111. Zelis, R., and Cross, C. E.: Management of pulmonary edema. Rational Drug Therapy 8:8, 1974.

112. Zikria, B. A., Ferrer, J. M., and Floch, H. F.: The chemical factors contributing to pulmonary damage in "smoke poisoning." Surgery 71:704, 1972.

Section V

Body Cavities

Melvin L. Helphrey
Section Editor

ANATOMY

Thirteen pairs of ribs and costal cartilages, thirteen vertebrae, and nine sternebrae compose the bony thorax of dogs and cats. Each rib forms two synovial costovertebral joints with its corresponding vertebra (Fig. 41–1). The first nine costal cartilages form a synovial articulation with the sternum (Fig. 41–2). The movement afforded by these synovial joints in conjunction with the curvolinear shape of the ribs and costal cartilages results in expansion of the thoracic cavity when the ribs are moved in a craniodorsal direction (i.e., "bucket handle" movement).

The deep thoracic wall is completed by the internal and external intercostal muscles between each rib (Fig. 41–3). The remaining thoracic musculature includes the serratus dorsalis, serratus ventralis, scalenus, external abdominal oblique, latissimus dorsi, and pectoralis muscles (see Fig. 41–3).

The intercostal arteries and veins arise from the aorta and azygous vein, respectively. The intercostal nerves arise from the ventral branches of the thoracic nerves and, together with the intercostal vessels, course ventrally on the caudal border of each rib (Fig. 41–4). The intercostal arteries are continuous with the internal thoracic artery located lateral to the sternum and internal to the costal cartilages. Each rib also has an intercostal artery and nerve on its cranial border, which arise from a collateral branch of the main intercostal artery and nerve at the midlateral thorax (see Fig. 41–4).

PHYSIOLOGY AND PATHOPHYSIOLOGY

The thoracic wall is composed of both passive elastic structures and an active musculature. Together, these passive and active elements influence the "bucket handle" motion of the ribs, which allows expansion and contraction of the thoracic cavity.

The passive elements of the thoracic wall possess a characteristic compliance defined as the change in thoracic volume over the change in pressure across the thoracic wall (pleural pressure). The passive elements of the thoracic wall produce either an inward or outward recoil, depending on the thoracic volume. The unstressed volume (V_O) of the thorax is defined as the volume at which the passive elastic structures of the thoracic wall are relaxed (Fig. 41–5). Thoracic volumes of less than V_O result in a passive outward recoil of the thoracic wall; conversely, thoracic volumes of greater than V_O result in a passive inward recoil of the thoracic wall. The thoracic wall and lungs are functionally linked by a thin layer of pleural fluid; therefore, total pulmonary compliance represents the additive compliances of the thoracic wall and lungs (see Fig. 41–5). Abnormalities in pulmonary compliance may therefore result from changes in either lung or thoracic wall compliance.

The lung volume at which the passive elastic structures of the entire pulmonary system (lungs, diaphragm, thoracic wall) are in equilibrium is the functional reserve capacity (FRC) and is achieved following a passive expiration. At FRC, the inward elastic recoil of the lungs exactly balances the passive outward elastic recoil of the relaxed thoracic wall (see Fig. 41–5). (FRC is therefore always less than V_O.) The transthoracic pressure (tracheal pressure) at FRC is zero (see Fig. 41–5). Pulmonary diseases that

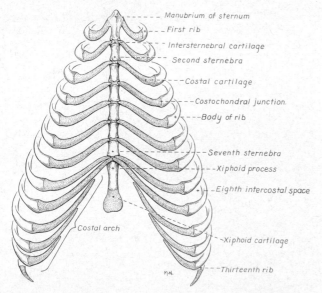

Figure 41–1. Ribs and sternum, ventral aspect. (Reprinted with permission from Evans, H. E., and Christensen, G. C.: *Miller's Anatomy of the Dog,* 2nd ed. W. B. Saunders, Philadelphia, 1979.)

Manubrium of sternum
First rib
Intersternebral cartilage
Second sternebra
Costal cartilage
Costochondral junction
Body of rib
Seventh sternebra
Xiphoid process
Eighth intercostal space
Costal arch
Xiphoid cartilage
Thirteenth rib

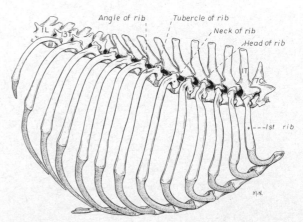

Figure 41–2. Ribs and sternum, lateral aspect. (Reprinted with permission from Evans, H. E., and Christensen, G. C.: *Miller's Anatomy of the Dog,* 2nd ed. W. B. Saunders, Philadelphia, 1979.)

Angle of rib
Tubercle of rib
Neck of rib
Head of rib
1st rib

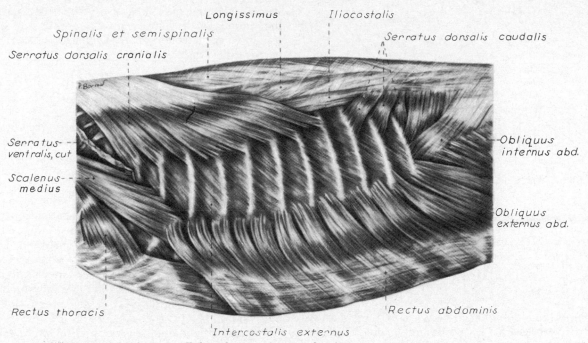

Figure 41–3. Musculature of the thoracic wall, lateral aspect. (Reprinted with permission from Evans, H. E., and Christensen, G. C.: *Miller's Anatomy of the Dog*, 2nd ed. W. B. Saunders, Philadelphia, 1979.)

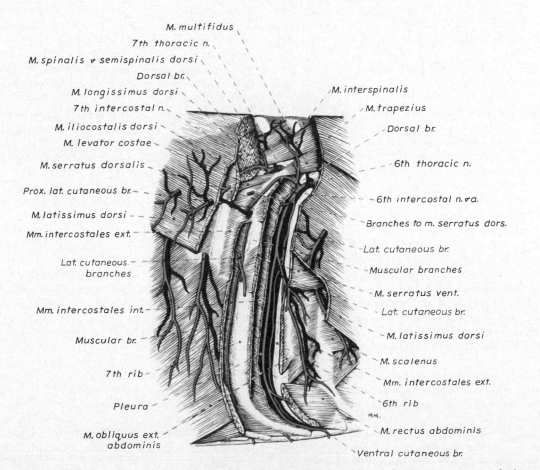

Figure 41–4. Intercostal arteries and thoracic nerves, lateral aspect. (Reprinted with permission from Evans, H. E., and Christensen, G. C.: *Miller's Anatomy of the Dog*, 2nd ed. W. B. Saunders, Philadelphia, 1979.)

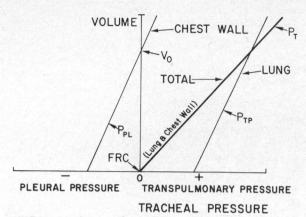

Figure 41–5. Compliance curves of the lung and thoracic wall, and the series compliance curve of the lung plus thoracic wall. P_T = tracheal pressure, P_{TP} = transpulmonary pressure, P_{PL} = pleural pressure, and V_o = volume of the unstressed thoracic cavity. (Reprinted with permission from Green, J. F.: *Cardiovascular and Pulmonary Physiology.* Lea & Febiger, Philadelphia, 1982.)

decrease lung compliance (e.g., acute respiratory failure) decrease FRC by increasing the inward elastic recoil of the lung. Diseases that decrease thoracic wall compliance (e.g., ankylosing costovertebral arthritis) increase FRC by increasing outward recoil of the thoracic wall. Loss of functional attachment between the lungs and thoracic wall results in inward recoil and collapse of the lungs and outward recoil of the thoracic wall to its V_O position. The latter explains the "sprung" appearance of the rib cage seen with pneumothorax.

The thoracic wall and the diaphragm form the active respiratory bellows. Contraction of the diaphragm and inspiratory thoracic muscles generates a negative transthoracic pressure, which results in air flow into and expansion of the lungs. Transthoracic pressures generated by the inspiratory musculature must be sufficient to overcome both airway resistance to airflow and inward elastic recoil of the lungs and thoracic wall. The passive elastic structures of the thoracic wall assist inspiration until the inspiratory volume exceeds V_O. Diseases that increase inspiratory airway resistance or decrease lung or thoracic wall compliance require generation of higher transthoracic pressures by the active respiratory bellows and therefore increase the work of respiration.

Passive expiration is driven by the elastic recoil of the lungs and thoracic wall. Pulmonary diseases that impair expiratory air flow may require active expiratory efforts by the expiratory musculature of the thoracic wall, resulting in increased work of respiration.

Paradoxical movement of the thoracic wall may result from paralysis of the thoracic wall musculature (e.g., low cervical fractures). Negative pleural pressures generated by the contracting diaphragm overcome passive outward recoil of the thoracic wall, resulting in inward movement of the thoracic wall during inspiration. Paradoxical movement of the thoracic wall reduces the effectiveness of ventilation.

Paradoxical movement may also occur in segments of the thoracic wall that are unstable as the result of trauma (e.g., flail chest) or congenital anomalies (e.g., pectus excavatum).

PREOPERATIVE DIAGNOSIS

Diagnosis of diseases involving the thoracic wall is based mostly on history and physical examination. Additional information is gained by radiographic examination, aspiration cytology, and limited pulmonary function testing.

A written history should contain information regarding age, breed, sex, origin of the patient, present environment, prior medical problems, and vaccination status. Duration, progression, previous treatments for, and present status of specific problems involving the thoracic wall are also specifically discussed. Information regarding the nature of injury in trauma patients (e.g., blunt, crush, penetrating, or bite wound) is a primary concern.

Physical examination includes observation of the pattern of breathing and inspection and palpation of the thoracic wall. The presence of a restrictive breathing pattern (i.e., rapid and shallow respirations) together with an expanded thoracic cavity suggests pleural effusion or pneumothorax. A restrictive breathing pattern in conjunction with a tightly drawn in thoracic wall suggests restrictive lung disease. An obstructive breathing pattern (i.e., slow and forced respirations) with exaggerated efforts of the thoracic wall musculature during inspiration suggests upper airway obstruction. An obstructive breathing pattern associated with exaggerated respiratory efforts by the thoracic wall during expiration suggests lower airway obstructive disease. Paradoxical breathing patterns resulting from thoracic wall paralysis, paralysis or rupture of the diaphragm, or flail segments are always significant when present.

The thoracic wall should be closely inspected for the presence of contusions, punctures, lacerations, open chest wounds, or fistulous tracts or masses. Palpation of the thoracic wall may reveal fractured ribs, intercostal muscle ruptures, subcutaneous emphysema, or thoracic wall masses.

Thoracic radiographs are indicated when history and physical examination suggest abnormalities of the thoracic wall. Intrathoracic and cranial abdominal structures should be carefully evaluated to determine the degree of concurrent involvement. Displacement of rib fractures is evaluated to determine the need for internal repair. Thoracic wall masses are evaluated for the degree and nature of rib involvement and the extent of protrusion into the thoracic cavity. Extrapleural thoracic wall masses are typically characterized by a smooth transition between the parietal pleura and the mass.[15, 16] The extent of fistulous tracts may be evaluated by infusion of contrast media into the fistula.

Information regarding thoracic wall masses may be

gained by fine needle aspiration cytology. Thoracic wall problems leading to inadequate ventilation may be quantified by arterial blood gases. A p_{CO_2} of > 45 mm Hg in conjunction with a p_{O_2} < 80 mm Hg is diagnostic of significant hypoventilation. Tidal volumes may also be readily measured in animals with a Wright's respirometer.

SURGICAL APPROACHES TO THE THORAX

Intercostal Thoracotomy

An intercostal thoracotomy is the standard approach to the thorax when exposure of a defined region of the thorax is desired. It affords good access to structures in the immediate region of the thoracotomy, may be rapidly opened and closed, and is associated with a minimum of postoperative complications. Intercostal thoracotomy provides limited access to structures not in the immediate region of the thoracotomy.

The site of an intercostal thoracotomy may be the third to the tenth intercostal space depending on the structures to be exposed (Table 41–1). A lateral thoracic radiograph should be taken to determine the intercostal space that best exposes a desired thoracic

TABLE 41–1. Location of Thoracic Structures via Intercostal Thoracotomy*

Thoracic Structure	Intercostal Space	
	Left	*Right*
Heart and pericardium	4,5	4,5
Ductus arteriosus (PDA, PRRA)	4 (5)	
Pulmonic valve (pulmonic stenosis)	4	
Lungs	4–6	4–6
Cranial lobe	(4) 5	(4) 5
Intermediate lobe		5
Caudal lobe	5 (6)	5 (6)
Esophagus		
Cranial		3,4
Caudal	7–10	7–10
Caudal vena cava	(6–7)	7–10
Diaphragm	7–10	7–10
Thoracic duct		
Dog	(8–10)	8–10
Cat	8–10	(8–10)

*( )indicates alternative surgical site.

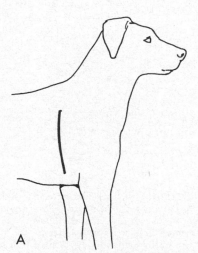

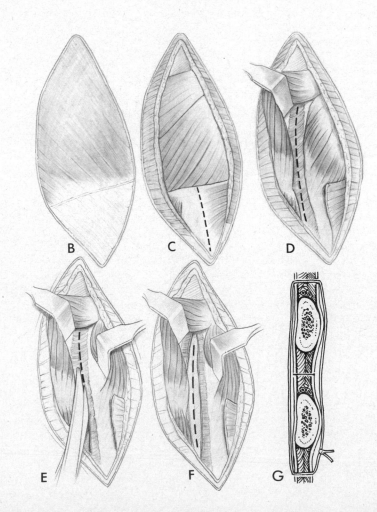

Figure 41–6. A, Site of cranial intercostal thoracotomy. B, Incision of skin and cutaneous trunci muscle, exposing the latissimus dorsi muscle and lateral thoracic nerve. C, Incision of the latissimus dorsi muscle, exposing the serratus ventralis, scalenus, and external abdominal oblique muscles. D, Incision and retraction of the serratus ventralis and scalenus muscles, exposing the fourth intercostal space. E, Incision of the intercostal muscles with scissors. F, Incision of the intercostal muscles, exposing the parietal pleura. G, Cross section of deep thoracic wall, indicating placement of circumcostal sutures for closure of intercostal incision.

structure. The cranial abdomen may be approached by a combined caudal intercostal thoracotomy and diaphragmatic incision.

Intercostal thoracotomy begins with an incision in the skin and cutaneous trunci muscle parallel to the ribs extending from the costovertebral junction to the sternum (Fig. 41–6A and B). The latissimus dorsi muscle is incised across the muscle fibers parallel to the skin incision (Fig. 41–6C). The intercostal spaces can easily be counted at this level. The fifth rib is recognized, as it marks the end of the muscular portion of the scalenus and the beginning of the external abdominal oblique muscle (see Fig. 41–3). Either the scalenus or external abdominal oblique muscle is incised, depending on the intercostal space desired. Cranial intercostal thoracotomies require incision of the serratus ventralis muscle (Fig. 41–6D). The curvilinear shape of the intercostal space usually allows the serratus ventralis muscle to be separated between its muscle bellies to expose the intercostal space (see Fig. 41–6D). The intercostal muscles are incised in the middle of the space to avoid damage to the intercostal vessels (Fig. 41–6E). Intercostal thoracotomy is completed by bluntly puncturing and opening the pleura with scissors (Fig. 41–6F). The intercostal incision is extended dorsally to the tubercle of the rib and ventrally past the costochondral arch to the internal thoracic artery. The ribs may be widely spread with a chest retractor.

Closure is accomplished by placing heavy interrupted circumcostal sutures around the ribs immediately cranial and caudal to the incision (Fig. 41–6G). The sutures are preplaced and passed bluntly through the intercostal spaces to avoid damage to the intercostal vessels. The preplaced circumcostal sutures may be used by an assistant to approximate the ribs while the surgeon ties the adjacent suture. The serratus ventralis, latissimus dorsi, scalenus, external abdominal oblique, and cutaneous trunci muscles and skin are closed using standard techniques. Each layer of muscle is closed tightly to prevent the thoracotomy from leaking air.

Rib Resection Thoracotomy

A rib resection thoracotomy offers increased exposure over an intercostal thoracotomy; however, it takes longer. Rib resection may be associated with fewer postoperative lung adhesions to the thoracotomy site and may be preferred if multiple thoracotomies are anticipated.

Exposure of the rib cage for rib resection is the same as that for intercostal thoracotomy (Fig. 41–7A). The periosteum of the rib to be resected is

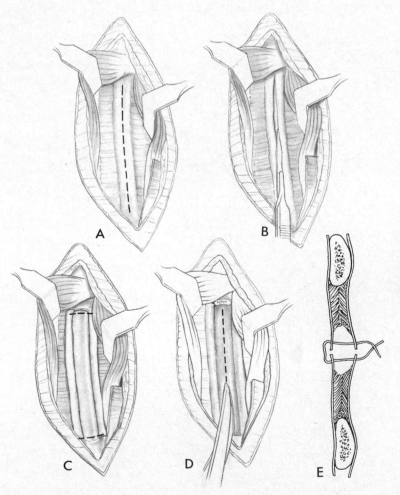

Figure 41–7. A, Incision and retraction of the serratus ventralis and scalenus muscles, exposing the fourth rib for rib resection. B, Incision of the periosteum of the fourth rib. C, Elevation of the periosteum of the fourth rib. D, Incision with scissors of the medial periosteum and parietal pleura. E, Cross section of the deep thoracic wall indicating placement of sutures for closure of the parietal pleura and rib periosteum.

incised over the midlateral surface of the rib (Fig. 41–7B). The periosteum is bluntly elevated from the rib over its lateral and medial surfaces (Fig. 41–7C). Elevation is most difficult at the intercostal muscle attachments on the cranial and caudal borders of the rib. The rib is excised with a bone cutter (Fig. 41–7C). The medial periosteum and parietal pleura are bluntly opened, and the incision is extended with scissors to complete the thoracotomy (Fig. 41–7D).

Interrupted sutures preplaced in the medial and lateral periosteal surfaces of the cranial and caudal edges of the incision are used to close the site (Fig. 41–7E). The remainder of the closure is similar to that used with an intercostal thoracotomy.

Median Sternotomy

Median sternotomy is the only thoracic approach that provides access to the entire thoracic cavity. Structures in the dorsal thoracic cavity such as the great vessels and bronchial hilus, however, may be difficult to manipulate in deep-chested dogs. Median sternotomy is associated with a higher degree of postoperative pain and an increased incidence of postoperative pleurocutaneous air leakage, particularly if the sternotomy is inadequately stabilized during closure. Median sternotomy may be combined with a ventral midline celiotomy or a ventral midline cervical incision if a combined approach to the abdomen or neck, respectively, is desirable.

Median sternotomy is performed with the patient in dorsal recumbency. The skin and subcutaneous tissues are incised on the ventral midline over the sternum (Fig. 41–8A). The pectoral musculature is sharply incised and bluntly elevated from the sternabrae (Fig. 41–8B). The sternum is incised on its midline with an oscillating bone saw, osteotome, or sternum splitter (Fig. 41–8C). A #10 scalpel blade may be used to split the sternum in young or small dogs and cats. Care is taken to protect thoracic organs during the sternotomy. Depending on the section of the thoracic cavity being exposed, it is preferable to leave either the manubrium or the xiphoid intact to increase stability of the sternotomy postoperatively. Caudal median sternotomies combined with a ventral midline celiotomy require partial incision of the diaphragm to gain complete retraction (Fig. 41–8D).

Stable closure of the sternotomy is imperative to avoid postoperative pain, pneumothorax, and nonunion of the sternum. A figure-eight orthopedic wire passed around each sternabrae that incorporates a costosternal junction within the figure-eight gives a stable closure in most instances (Fig. 41–8E). The pectoral muscles, subcutaneous tissues, and skin are closed in separate layers using standard techniques.

Transsternal Thoracotomy

The exposure of an intercostal thoracotomy may be dramatically increased by extending the thoracotomy through the sternum to connect it with an intercostal thoracotomy on the opposite side of the chest (Fig. 41–9A). A transsternal thoracotomy is indicated when extensive exposure to a specific region of the thorax is desirable, such as in open cardiac surgery. Transsternal thoracotomy at the seventh

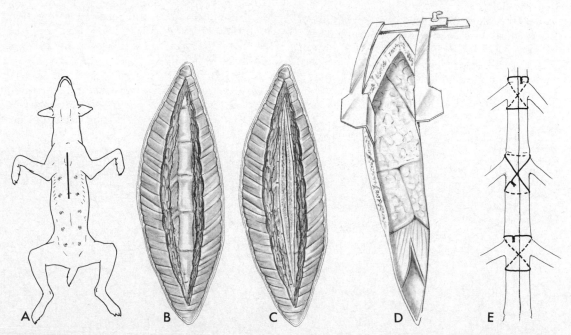

Figure 41–8. A, Site of median sternotomy. B, Incision and elevation of the pectoralis muscles, exposing the sternum for osteotomy. C, Osteotomy of the sternum. D, Retraction of a combined median sternotomy and cranial ventral midline celiotomy. The diaphragm is incised to facilitate retraction. E, Placement of orthopedic wire in a cruciate pattern for closure of median sternotomy. Note that cruciate pattern alternates with each wire to increase stability.

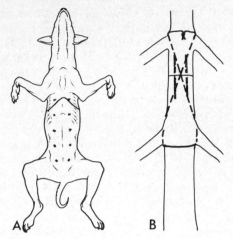

Figure 41–9. *A,* Site of transsternal thoracotomy. *B,* Closure of transverse sternotomy with small intramedullary pins and orthopedic wire.

intercostal space has been advocated for diaphragmatic hernia repair.[8]

The technique of transsternal thoracotomy is similar to that of intercostal thoracotomy. Bilateral intercostal thoracotomies are extended to the sternum, requiring ligation of the internal thoracic arteries. The intercostal thoracotomies are then made continuous by a transverse osteotomy of the sternum.

The sternal osteotomy is stabilized at closure with small intermedullary pins and orthopedic wire (Fig. 41–9B). The intercostal incisions are closed in the manner previously described.

Cranial Thoracic Wall Flap

A cranial thoracic wall flap may be created when extensive exposure to structures in the cranial mediastinum and caudal cervical regions is required (Fig. 41–10A). The approach allows access to the entire trachea, the cranial great vessels, and the cranial thoracic esophagus.[17]

The patient is positioned in dorsolateral recumbency with the upper forelimb sharply abducted dorsally. A standard fifth intercostal thoracotomy is extended to the sternum. This requires ligation and incision of the internal thoracic artery. A median sternotomy is then extended from the level of the intercostal incision cranially through the manubrium using an osteotome or bone saw. The incisions are connected by a transverse sternotomy at the juncture of the intercostal and median sternotomy incisions. Closure is accomplished as previously described for a median sternotomy and intercostal thoracotomy. The juncture of the thoracic wall flap may be stabilized with a figure-eight orthopedic wire that encircles the adjacent costosternal articulations (Fig. 41–10B).

SURGICAL CONDITIONS OF THE THORACIC WALL

Pectus Excavatum

Pectus excavatum is an uncommon congenital deformity characterized by an inward displacement of the caudal sternum and costal cartilages. The displacement results in a concave funnel deformity of the caudoventral thoracic wall (Fig. 41–11). Pectus excavatum has been reported in three puppies[18] and one adult cat.[3] Signs associated with severe defects include retarded growth, exercise intolerance, and respiratory distress.[1, 3, 18, 20] Respiratory distress results from either restrictive ventilation or paradoxical movement of the deformity during inspiration. Cardiac murmurs, arrhythmias, and mechanical cardiac tamponade have been reported in human patients with pectus excavatum.[1, 18, 20] Adults with pectus excavatum may have chronic respiratory infections.[1, 3, 20] A chronic respiratory infection was reportedly resolved by surgical correction of a pectus excavatum in a three-year-old cat.[3]

A consistent method of surgical correction of pectus excavatum in small animals has not been reported. Surgical correction of pectus excavatum by excision of the caudal sternum and costal cartilages has been

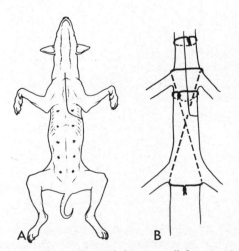

Figure 41–10. *A,* Site of cranial thoracic wall flap. *B,* Closure of sternotomy from cranial thoracic wall flap with orthopedic wire.

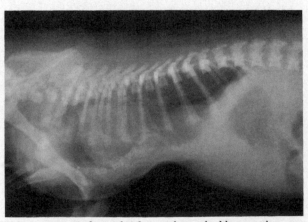

Figure 41–11. Radiograph of an eight-week-old cat with pectus excavatum.

reported in a cat.[3] Attempts at surgical repair are only indicated if cardiopulmonary impairment is significant. The principles of surgical correction of pectus excavatum in humans are (1) multiple chondrotomy or excision of malformed costal cartilages, (2) release of soft tissues contributing to sternal displacement including the diaphragm, and (3) the use of internal struts (e.g., K-wires) or external splints to maintain the position of the sternum.[1, 20]

Rib Deformities

A variety of deformities of the ribs, including missing ribs, fused ribs, extra ribs, and malformed ribs, may occur in small animals. Surgical correction of such deformities is not indicated unless the deformity results in restricted ventilation or paradoxical movement of the chest wall.

Severe kyphoscoliosis may result in malformation of the thoracic cavity. Surgical correction of such deformities is generally not recommended.

Metabolic Bone Diseases

Metabolic bone diseases such as hyperparathyroidism, hypervitaminosis D, and multiple cartilaginous exostosis are occasionally manifested in the bony thorax.[2, 9] Therapy is directed toward correction of the underlying cause of the metabolic disease.

Infections

Infections of the thoracic wall may result from penetrating foreign bodies, lacerations, bite wounds, or postoperative wound infections. The basic treatment principles of surgical drainage, debridement, and antibiotic therapy are applicable to infections of the thoracic wall. Pyothorax should be excluded in patients presented for thoracic wall infection. Osteomyelitis of the ribs or sternum is treated in a similar manner to osteomyelitis in other regions. Excision of infected ribs or costal cartilages often expedites treatment. Fistulous tracts from sequestered foreign materials occasionally erupt in the thoracic wall. A contrast fistulogram often provides information regarding the extent of the fistula. Meticulous excision of all fistulous tracts is often the only successful treatment.

Trauma

The resilient nature of the thoracic wall renders it resistant to blunt trauma. Therefore, absence of injury to the thoracic wall does not rule out significant injuries to internal organs of the thorax and cranial abdomen following blunt trauma to the thorax. Blunt trauma that does result in thoracic wall injury is likely to be associated with severe damage to internal viscera. Penetrating trauma usually causes minimal thoracic wall damage other than an open chest wound. The primary concern in penetrating thoracic injuries is the status of internal structures. Bite wounds (e.g., big dog, little dog syndrome) generally represent a combination of crush and penetrating trauma that often results in severe thoracic wall injury, usually with significant internal injuries.

Simple open wounds and lacerations of the thoracic wall are treated utilizing standard principles of open wound management. Open wounds that are continuous with the pleural cavity should be immediately sealed with a sterile petroleum-based ointment and gauze pack. Definitive management of open chest wounds should await pleural evacuation and patient stabilization.

Intercostal muscle rupture may occur as a result of blunt trauma or bite wounds. Herniation of isolated lung lobes occasionally accompanies intercostal muscle rupture. Ruptured intercostal muscles associated with pneumothorax may cause a paradoxical movement of the skin that may be mistaken for a flail chest. Isolated intercostal ruptures associated with lung herniation are closed in a manner similar to an intercostal thoracotomy. Multiple consecutive intercostal ruptures may require a series of overlapping circumcostal sutures (i.e., "basket weave" pattern) to approximate the ribs. The intercostal spaces are sealed by suturing intercostal muscles and patching defects with latissimus dorsi and external abdominal oblique muscles. In patients in whom trauma has rendered local musculature unsuitable for suturing, an omental pedical flap may be mobilized from the abdomen to seal the defect.[7]

Fractured ribs may result from blunt or crushing trauma to the thorax. Rib fractures are usually associated with contusion of thoracic musculature and laceration of the intercostal vessels. Disruption of an intercostal vessel may produce an extrapleural hematoma or a hemothorax.

Simple nondisplaced rib fractures are managed with cage rest. Intercostal nerve blocks reduce pain and may improve ventilatory efforts.[12] Chest bandages will also reduce pain; however, great caution is taken to avoid impairment of ventilation with a bandage if concomitant pulmonary injuries are present.

Multiple unstable rib fractures usually require internal fixation. Internal fixation should ideally await cardiopulmonary stabilization of the patient. If, however, a stable condition cannot be attained owing to excessive thoracic wall injury, then surgery should not be delayed. Fixation of rib fractures is accomplished using standard orthopedic techniques with orthopedic wire and small intramedullary pins (Fig. 41–12).[1, 14] The thoracic wall is further stabilized and sealed with soft tissues available in the area.

Multiple rib fractures producing a free-floating segment of thoracic wall result in a flail chest. The paradoxical movement of the flail chest segment causes significant reductions in ventilation. Hypoxemia is accentuated by ventilation-perfusion mismatching associated with pulmonary contusions that invariably accompany flail chest.[4, 10, 22] Initial management of flail chest should be directed toward elimination of paradoxical respiration and medical management of pulmonary contusion.[4, 14, 22] Chest bandages placed tightly enough to reduce paradoxical motion of a flail segment often restrict expansion of the lungs. An external splint eliminates paradoxical motion without restricting ventilation.[14] The flail chest segment is secured to an aluminum frame or polyvinylorthoplast splint using large circumcostal sutures (Fig. 41–13). External splinting may be utilized as a definitive repair or as temporary immobilization to allow patient stabilization prior to internal fixation.

Sternebral luxations are occasionally seen associated with thoracic trauma. Internal fixation is accomplished using orthopedic wire and small intramedullary pins.

Neoplasia

Neoplasms such as lipomas and benign cutaneous neoplasms commonly arise from subcutaneous tissues and skin of the thorax. Large "dissecting" lipomas are occasionally seen in the loose connective tissues between muscles of the thoracic wall. Benign neoplasms of the thorax are managed by local excision,

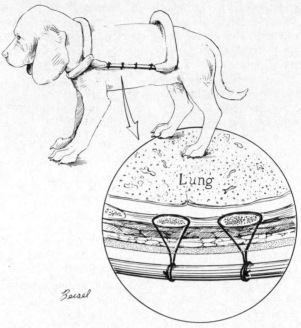

Figure 41–13. External aluminum frame for stabilization of a flail chest. The ribs are secured to the aluminum frame with circumcostal sutures. (Reprinted with permission from Kolata, R. J.: Management of thoracic trauma. Vet. Clin. North Am. *11*:103, 1981.)

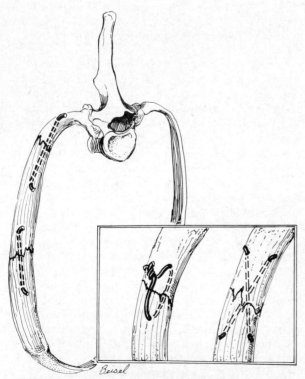

Figure 41–12. Technique of internal fixation of rib fractures with intramedullary pins or orthopedic wire. (Reprinted with permission from Kolata, R. J.: Management of thoracic trauma. Vet. Clin. North Am. *11*:103, 1981.)

ensuring that a sufficient margin of normal tissue is removed with the neoplasm to prevent recurrence.

Malignant neoplasms of the thoracic wall include chondrosarcoma, osteosarcoma, fibrosarcoma, mast cell sarcoma, and hemangiosarcoma.[11, 19] Metastasis of squamous cell carcinoma to a rib is reported in the cat.[15] Tumors that are intimately fixed to the deep thoracic wall should be considered malignant until proven otherwise. Thoracic radiographs often allow definitive diagnosis of primary bone sarcomas involving the ribs.[15, 16]

Malignant neoplasms of the thoracic wall are removed by en bloc resection of the involved thoracic wall. Wide resections are recommended to ensure complete excision of local neoplasia. Margins of the resected tissue should be examined by the pathologist for the presence of neoplasia.

RECONSTRUCTION

Reconstruction of the thoracic wall following a radical resection must be rigid to prevent paradoxical movement during respiration and airtight to prevent pneumothorax. The need for a rigid reconstruction may be circumvented in resections involving the caudal thoracic wall by transposing the diaphragm cranial to the defect.[5] Standard reconstruction of the thoracic wall is accomplished with polypropylene mesh (Fig. 41–14).[5, 6] Polypropylene mesh is tightly sutured intrapleurally across the defect using interrupted sutures. The mesh is attached to the remain-

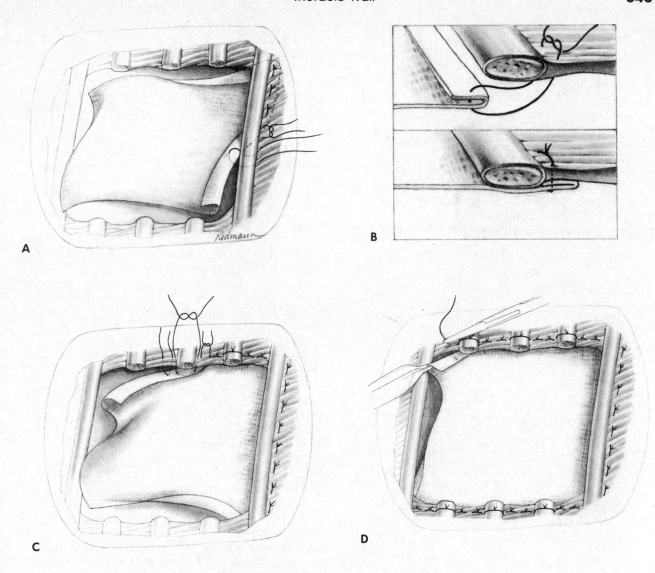

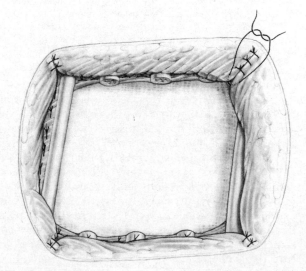

Figure 41–14. Reconstruction of *en bloc* resection of thoracic wall. *A,* Polypropylene mesh is sutured, assuring intrapleural placement. *B,* Paracostal interrupted sutures are placed adjacent to intact rib. *C,* Suture placement along the dorsal border is continued as along the side. The cut ribs are incorporated into alternate sutures to increase stability. *D,* The mesh is pulled tightly as the opposite side is sutured. *E,* The musculature is closed in a cruciate pattern. (Reprinted with permission from Bright, R. M.: Reconstruction of thoracic wall defects using Marlex mesh. J. Am. Anim. Hosp. Assoc. *17*:415, 1981.)

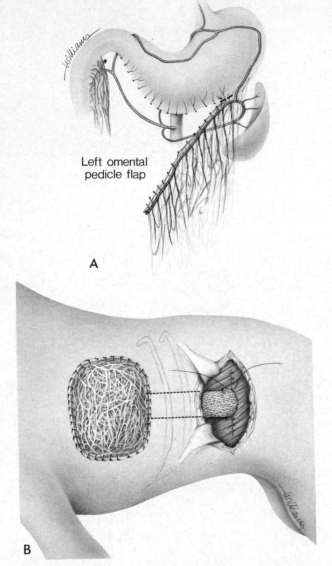

A

B

Figure 41–15. Omental pedicle flap. *A,* Mobilization of left omental pedicle flap by ligation of the right gastroepiploic artery. *B,* Transfer of the omental pedicle flap to the thoracic wall defect via a paracostal incision and subcutaneous tunnel. (Reprinted with permission from Bright, R. M.: Repair of thoracic wall defects in the dog with an omental pedicle flap. J. Am. Anim. Hosp. Assoc. *18*:277, 1982.)

ing ribs wherever possible. The mesh can generally be sutured tight enough to prevent significant paradoxical movement in resection of five ribs or less. Reconstructions involving more than five ribs may be given additional support by wiring autogenous splint rib grafts, allogenous free rib grafts, or plastic spinal plates to the ends of resected ribs.[11] Local musculature, particularly the latissimus dorsi and external abdominal oblique muscles, is then mobilized and sutured over the defect to seal the reconstruction. In patients in whom insufficient musculature is available to cover the reconstruction, an omental pedicle flap may be mobilized from the abdomen to effect an airtight seal (Fig. 41–15).[7] The omental pedicle flap may be exteriorized through a

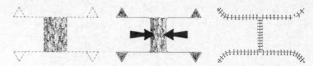

Figure 41–16. H-plasty. (Reprinted with permission from Swaim, S. F.: *Surgery of Traumatized Skin.* W. B. Saunders, Philadelphia, 1980.)

paracostal abdominal approach and then brought to the reconstruction via a subcutaneous tunnel or may be mobilized through a diaphragmatic incision. The skin is closed by a four-corner pattern that results in a cruciate incision or by an H-plasty (Fig. 41–16). A thoracostomy tube should always be placed following thoracic wall reconstruction to aid in the management of postoperative pneumothorax.

POSTOPERATIVE MANAGEMENT

The immediate recovery period is often the most critical period faced by a thoracic surgery patient. Hypoventilation, hypothermia, acid-base disorders, shock, and oliguria are among the problems that may arise following thoracic surgery. Ventilation may be depressed by anesthetic drugs, postoperative pneumothorax, or somatic pain arising from the thorax wall. Hypoventilation results in hypoxemia and respiratory acidosis, neither of which is well tolerated by the postoperative patient. Suspected hypoventilation in the recovery period is confirmed by an arterial p_{CO_2} greater than 45 mm Hg. Tidal volumes less than 10 ml/kg measured with a Wright's spirometer also suggest inadequate ventilation. Ventilation may be supported by intermittent positive pressure ventilation until the patient is capable of normal ventilation postoperatively. Ventilation with room air restores nitrogen to the lungs and decreases the degree of absorption atelectasis following surgery.

Hypothermic postoperative patients should be slowly surface-warmed with warm-water bottles or circulating water blankets. Hypothermia, hypovolemia, anesthetic drugs, and postoperative pain may produce varying degrees of circulatory shock during the recovery period. Crystalloid fluid therapy should be carefully titrated during recovery to ensure adequate venous return to the heart. Plasma is administered when total protein values approach 2.5 gm/dl. Whole blood or washed erythrocytes are indicated if the packed cell volume falls to 20 per cent. The patient should be carefully evaluated for acid-base and electrolyte disorders. Urine production should be monitored to assure adequate renal function. Hypothermia and hypotension perpetuate oliguria and therefore must be corrected early in the postoperative period.

Analgesia is indicated in most thoracic surgery patients owing to somatic pain arising from the thoracic wall. Narcotics administered in low doses provide analgesia but may also significantly depress ventilation.[12] Narcotics also suppress the coughing reflex, induce emesis, and may produce bronchoconstriction.[12] Analgesia may alternatively be provided by selective intercostal nerve blocks, thus avoiding some of the undesirable side effects of narcotics. Intercostal blocks with bupivacaine 0.75% with epinephrine provide 24 to 36 hours of analgesia.

Chest bandages aid in sealing the thoracotomy incision and reduce the development of incisional emphysema. However, the routine use of chest bandages in thoracic surgery patients should be avoided, as bandages often restrict ventilation. Routine placement of a thoracostomy tube during thoracic surgery allows the surgeon to closely monitor the pleural cavity for the presence of air or blood during the recovery period. The thoracostomy tube may often be removed within a few hours of surgery; however, in the patient that develops pneumothorax or hemothorax, the presence of a routinely placed thoracostomy tube can be life-saving.

1. Adkins, P. C.: The chest wall. *In* Effler, D. B. (ed.): *Blade's Surgical Diseases of the Chest,* 4th ed. C. V. Mosby, St. Louis, 1978.
2. Alexander, J. W.: Selected skeletal dysplasia: craniomandibular osteopathy, multiple cartilaginous exostosis, and hypertrophic osteodystrophy. Vet. Clin. North Am. *13*:55, 1983.
3. Bennett, D.: Successful surgical correction of pectus excavatum in a cat. Vet. Med. *68*:936, 1973.
4. Bjorling, D. E., Kolata, R. J., and DeNoro, R. C.: Flail chest: review of clinical experience and new method of stabilization. J. Am. Anim. Hosp. Assoc. *15*:269, 1982.
5. Brasmer, T. H.: Thoracic wall reconstruction in dogs. J. Am. Vet. Med. Assoc. *159*:1758, 1971.
6. Bright, R. M.: Reconstruction of thoracic wall defects using Marlex mesh. J. Am. Anim. Hosp. Assoc. *17*:415, 1981.
7. Bright, R. M., Birchare, S. J., and Long, G. G.: Repair of thoracic wall defects in the dog with an omental pedicle flap. J. Am. Anim. Hosp. Assoc. *18*:277, 1982.
8. Butler, H. C.: Transthoracic approach for diaphragmatic hernia repair in cats and dogs. J. Am. Vet. Med. Assoc. *131*:167, 1957.
9. Capen, C. C., and Martin, S. L.: Calcium-regulating hormones and diseases of the parathyroid glands. *In* Ettinger, S. J. (ed.): *Textbook of Veterinary Internal Medicine,* 2nd ed. W. B. Saunders, Philadelphia, 1983.
10. Craven, K. D., Oppenheimer, L., and Wood, L. D. H.: Effects of contusion and flail chest on pulmonary perfusion and oxygen exchange. J. Appl. Physiol. *47*:129, 1979.
11. Ellison, G. H., Trotter, G. E., and Lumb, W. V.: Reconstructive thoracoplasty using spinal fixation plates and polypropylene mesh. J. Am. Anim. Hosp. Assoc. *17*:613, 1981.
12. Gilman, A. G., Goodman, L. S., and Gilman, A.: *The Pharmacological Basis of Therapeutics,* 6th ed. Macmillan Publishing Co., New York, 1980.
13. Kagan, K. G.: Thoracic trauma. Vet. Clin. North Am. *10*:641, 1980.
14. Kolata, R. J.: Management of thoracic trauma. Vet. Clin. North Am. *11*:103, 1981.
15. Lord, P. F., Suter, P. F., Chan, K. F., Appleford, M., and Root, C. R.: Pleural, extrapleural and pulmonary lesions in small animals: A radiographic approach to differential diagnosis. J. Am. Vet. Rad. Soc. *13*:4, 1972.
16. Myer, C. W.: Radiography review: the extrapleural space. Vet. Radiol. *19*:157, 1978.
17. Nelson, A. W.: Personal communication, 1983.
18. Pearson, J. L.: Pectus excavatum in the dog. Vet. Med. *68*:125, 1923.
19. Pool, R. R.: Tumors of bone and cartilage. *In* Moulton, J. E. (ed.): *Tumors in Domestic Animals.* University of California Press, Berkeley, 1978.
20. Ravitch, M. M.: Disorders of the chest wall. *In* Sabiston, D. C. (ed.): *Textbook of Surgery,* 11th ed. W. B. Saunders, Philadelphia, 1977.
21. Russell, R. G., and Walker, M.: Metastatic and invasive tumors of bone in dogs and cats. Vet. Clin. North Am. *13*:163, 1983.
22. Trinkle, J. K., Richardson, J. D., Franz, J. E., et al.: Management of flail chest without mechanical ventilation. Ann. Thorac. Surg. *19*:355, 1975.

Chapter **42** **Pleura and Pleural Space**

E. Christopher Orton

ANATOMY

The thoracic cavity is lined entirely by a serous membrane known as pleura. The pleura is divided into a visceral portion, which covers the lungs, and a parietal portion, which covers the remaining thoracic cavity (Fig. 42–1). The parietal pleura is further divided into costal, diaphragmatic, and mediastinal portions (see Fig. 42–1). The mediastinal pleura on each side of the thoracic cavity combines to form an anatomically complete mediastinum in the dog and cat.[25, 54] Fenestrations in the mediastinum are postulated on the basis of bilateral distribution of saline experimentally infused into the thoracic cavities of dogs.[49, 68] The typical bilateral nature of pleural effusions in small animals gives further evidence for an incomplete mediastinum. It is unclear whether the mediastinum is truly incomplete or simply disrupted by the pleural effusion. The latter postulate is supported by reports of unilateral hemothorax, pyothorax, and pneumothorax.[65]

The caudal right hemithorax contains a pleural fold known as plica vena cava, which invests the caudal vena cava and right phrenic nerve. The plica vena

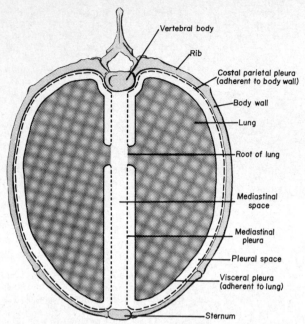

Figure 42–1. Cross-section of the thoracic cavity showing the relationship of the visceral and parietal pleura. (Reprinted with permission from Losonsky, J. M., and Prasse, K. W.: Dyspnea in the cat. Part I: Radiographic aspects of intrathoracic causes involving the pleural space. Feline Pract. 8:35, 1978.)

cava forms a medial cul-de-sac within the right hemithorax, which contains the accessory lung lobe. The pulmonary ligaments are triangular folds of pleura between the mediastinum and caudal lung lobes. The cranial portions of the parietal pleura extend through the thoracic inlet into the base of the neck to form the pleural cupula. The left pleural cupula is larger and extends further cranially than the right.

The pleura is histologically composed of a single layer of mesothelial cells supported by a delicate network of connective tissue rich in elastic fibers.[54] Elastic fibers allow local stretching of the pleura, which is important in pleural fluid dynamics.[1, 2, 5] The visceral and parietal pleura contain rich capillary networks that arise from the pulmonary and systemic circulations, respectively; in addition, the parietal pleura contains a rich lymphatic network largely responsible for lymphatic drainage of the pleural space.[1, 2, 5] Communication between the pleural space and parietal lymphatics occurs by temporary dehiscence of mesothelial cells resulting from pleural stretching.[1]

PHYSIOLOGY AND PATHOPHYSIOLOGY

Under normal conditions, the pleural space is only a potential cavity. The visceral and parietal pleura are separated only by a thin layer of pleural fluid, the average volume of pleural fluid in a 10-kg dog being 2.35 ml.[1, 5] The liquid coupling between the thoracic wall and the lungs provides instantaneous

and complete transmission of thoracic volume changes to the lungs and yet allows low-friction sliding between the pleural surfaces.

The dynamics of pleural fluid formation and absorption are controlled by Starling's forces (i.e., capillary hydrostatic pressure and colloid osmotic pressure).[1, 2, 5] The pleural space is continuous with the interstitial fluid component of the thoracic wall and lungs because of the permeability of the pleura. The hydrostatic pressure in the systemic capillaries that supply the parietal pleura is 30 cm H_2O. Pleural fluid hydrostatic pressure at functional reserve capacity is -5 cm H_2O, owing to the opposing elastic recoils of the thoracic wall and lungs. The net hydrostatic pressure for movement of fluid from the parietal pleura to the pleural space is therefore 35 cm H_2O. The movement of fluid from the parietal pleura to the pleural space is opposed by the colloid osmotic pressure of the capillaries (34 cm H_2O), which is aided by the colloid osmotic pressure of the pleural fluid (8 cm H_2O). Thus, there is a net pressure of 9 cm H_2O (35 − 34 + 8 cm H_2O) encouraging fluid movement from the parietal pleura into the pleural space (Fig. 42–2). The hydrostatic pressure of the pulmonary capillaries that supply the visceral pleura is 11 cm H_2O. Thus the net hydrostatic pressure between the visceral pleura and pleural space is only 16 cm H_2O (11 + 5 cm H_2O). The net colloid osmotic pressure encouraging fluid absorption from the pleural space remains at 26 cm H_2O as for the parietal pleura. Therefore, a net pressure of 10 cm H_2O favors fluid absorption from the pleural space by the visceral pleura (see Fig. 42–2). Thus, pleural fluid is formed by the parietal pleura and absorbed by the visceral pleura.

Complete absorption of the pleural fluid is prevented by the ability of the pleura to stretch.[1, 2, 5] As pleural fluid levels become minimal, the pleura begins stretching. The elastic deformation further lowers (i.e., more subatmospheric) the hydrostatic pressure of the pleural space below −5 cm of H_2O, thus establishing a new equilibrium of Starling forces that prevents complete absorption of pleural fluid. There-

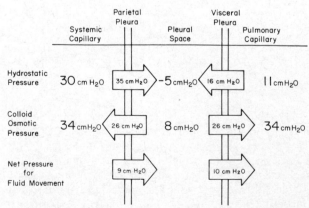

Figure 42–2. Hydrostatic, colloid osmotic, and net Starling pressures that influence the movement of fluid into and out of the pleural space.

fore, the essential coupling and sliding actions of the pleural fluid are preserved.

Pleural fluid and protein are also absorbed from the pleural space by parietal pleural lymphatics.[1, 2, 5] Lymphatic drainage of the pleural space becomes particularly important when the protein content of the pleural fluid increases, since increases in the colloid osmotic pressure of the pleural fluid reduce absorption of pleural fluid by the visceral pleura. Because parietal lymphatic vessels pass through the diaphragm and intercostal muscles, lymphatic flow from the pleural space is encouraged by normal respiratory movements. Pleural disease results when either air or excess pleural fluid (pleural effusion) enters the pleural space.

Air enters the pleural space via open wounds in the thoracic wall, perforations of the esophagus, or rupture of the trachea, bronchus, or lungs. The visceral and parietal pleura separate, the lungs collapse, and the chest wall expands. Hypoventilation results from reduced lung volumes and a lack of complete coupling between the lungs and thoracic wall. In addition, ventilation-perfusion mismatching due to partial lung collapse exacerbates the hypoxemia.

The total gas pressure of atmospheric air within the pleural space is approximately 70 cm H_2O greater than the total gas pressure of venous blood.[1, 2, 5] Because the pleura is permeable to gas, a constant gradient removes gas from the pleural space. This gradient keeps the pleural space free of gas under physiological conditions and accounts for the spontaneous resolution of a closed pneumothorax.

Pleural effusion results when factors controlling pleural fluid dynamics are altered. Increased parietal capillary hydrostatic pressure associated with right-sided congestive heart failure results in increased pleural fluid formation. Conversely, reduced pleural fluid absorption results from increased visceral capillary hydrostatic pressure secondary to left-sided congestive heart failure. Increased formation and decreased absorption of pleural fluid also result from reductions in capillary colloid osmotic pressure secondary to hypoproteinemia. Lymphatic absorption of pleural fluid and protein is reduced by inflammatory thickening of the pleura, neoplastic obstructions of the thoracic duct or lymph nodes, or lymphatic hypertension associated with right-sided congestive heart failure. Inflammation of the pleura increases both local blood flow (i.e., capillary hydrostatic pressure) and capillary permeability to protein. Elevations in protein concentration of pleural fluid encourage formation of pleural fluid.

Pleural effusions may also arise from accumulation of fluids of other than pleural origin. Examples include hemothorax, chylothorax, and liver incarceration secondary to diaphragmatic hernia. As with pneumothorax, pleural effusions result in varying degrees of hypoxemia both by reducing ventilation and by increasing ventilation perfusion mismatching in the lungs.

DIAGNOSIS

Clinical Findings

The history and clinical signs of patients with pleural effusion depend upon the cause, quantity, and rapidity of fluid accumulation. Small quantities of noninflammatory effusion are difficult or impossible to detect clinically, whereas moderate to large quantities of pleural fluid or air cause acute respiratory distress. Chronic pleural effusions associated with slow fluid accumulation are often insidious and escape observation by the owner. Affected patients may suddenly decompensate and show apparent acute respiratory distress.

Respiratory distress resulting from pleural effusion or air is restrictive. Pleural fluid or air reduces functional reserve capacity, tidal volume, and compliance of the lungs. The patient compensates with a rapid and shallow breathing pattern. The patient may exhibit increased respiratory distress in lateral recumbency (orthopnea) and a preference for a sternally recumbent or sitting position. Elbows are usually abducted, the head and neck are extended, and mouth breathing is commonly observed. Restlessness and apprehension accompany the respiratory distress. The stress associated with handling may easily induce respiratory arrest due to a limited respiratory reserve.

Inflammatory pleural effusions may induce a nonproductive cough. Patients with pleuritis and minimal effusion display pain with coughing or sudden respiratory movement. Large amounts of pleural fluid or pleural air result in an expanded appearance of the thoracic wall owing to loss of pleural coupling.

Auscultation of patients with pleural effusion reveals muffled heart sounds. Breath sounds are variable with pleural effusion, being surprisingly well preserved dorsally but distant or absent ventrally. Pleuritis with minimal pleural effusion may produce a pleural friction rub on auscultation. Pleural friction rubs, typically nonmusical grating sounds, are loudest on inspiration.

Percussion is an invaluable diagnostic tool for evaluation of the pleural space. Dull, flat, hyporesonant percussion suggests the presence of pleural fluid. Systematic percussion of the patient in a standing position may demonstrate a horizontal fluid line. Pleural air results in a characteristic hyperresonant "ping" on percussion.

Radiographic Findings

Thoracic radiographs confirm the presence of pleural effusion, particularly of small amounts of fluid that may be difficult to demonstrate clinically. As little as 100 ml of pleural fluid may be detected in a medium-sized dog on standard recumbent lateral, ventrodorsal, and dorsoventral views of the thorax (Fig. 42–3).[49] Small amounts of pleural fluid are first detected on a recumbent lateral view of the thorax

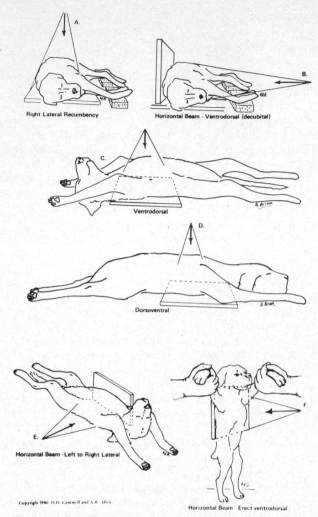

Figure 42–3. Patient positions for thoracic radiography. *A*, A recumbent lateral view; *B*, horizontal beam—decubital view; *C*, recumbent ventrodorsal view; *D*, recumbent dorsoventral view; *E*, horizontal beam—lateral view, dorsal recumbency; *F*, horizontal beam—erect dorsoventral view. (Reprinted with permission from Cantwell, H. D., Rebar, A. H., and Allen, A. R.: Pleural effusion in the dog: principles for diagnosis. J. Am. Anim. Hosp. Assoc. *19*:227, 1983.)

amounts of pleural fluid collect in the paravertebral gutters, obscuring the cardiac silhouette and cardiophrenic angle on a ventrodorsal view of the thorax. Accumulation of fluid adjacent to the cranial lung lobes gives the cranial mediastinum a widened appearance. Collapse of lung lobes associated with pleural effusion is uniform; thus, a partially collapsed lung lobe appears as a smaller version of its original shape. This tendency is called form elasticity.[49, 56] The deposition of a heavy, fibrinous layer on the visceral pleura may cause a loss of form elasticity, giving the lungs a rounded appearance that suggests a chronic inflammatory process and indicates that the lungs may be difficult to re-expand.

Pleural effusions are classified radiographically as free or encapsulated.[49, 56] Free pleural effusions move without restriction throughout the pleural space under the influence of gravity, usually also across the mediastinum. Free pleural effusions are occasionally restricted to a single hemithorax owing to either an intact mediastinum or sealing of the mediastinum with fibrin. Encapsulated pleural effusions are restricted to specific portions of the pleural space by fibrinous or fibrous adhesions and are thus only minimally influenced by gravity. Encapsulated pleural effusions are most commonly associated with

as a fluid-dense wedge that forms at the junction of the sternum and interlobar fissures of the lungs (Fig. 42–4).[18, 49, 50, 56] As fluid accumulates, these "wedges" coalesce to give the ventral borders of the lungs a scalloped appearance (Fig. 42–6). Large amounts of pleural fluid obscure the cardiac and diaphragmatic silhouettes as well as the cardiophrenic angle. Fluid eventually collects dorsally, giving the appearance of "floating lungs." The cranial and middle lung lobes may collapse and disappear on a recumbent lateral radiograph.[49, 56] Blunting of the costophrenic angle on the ventrodorsal and dorsoventral views is a sensitive sign of small amounts of pleural fluid (Figs. 42–5 and 42–6).[18, 49, 56] Fluid-dense wedges may be seen on the interlobar fissures of the lungs (see Figs. 42–5 and 42–6). An entire interlobar fissure is occasionally seen if the radiographic beam strikes the fissure tangentially.[18, 49, 50, 56] This occurs most often between the middle and caudal lung lobes.[49, 50] Moderate to large

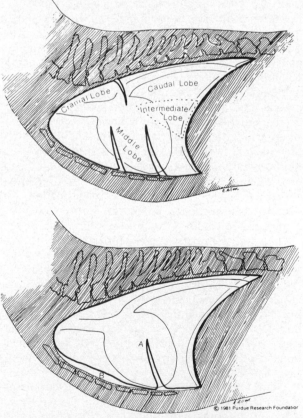

Figure 42–4. Position of right side interlobar fissures on a right recumbent lateral view of the thorax. Small amounts of pleural fluid are commonly observed at the interlobar fissures *(A)* and ventrally along the sternum *(B)*. (Reprinted by permission from Cantwell, H. D., Rebar, A. H., and Allen, A. R.: Pleural effusion in the dog: principles for diagnosis. J. Am. Anim. Hosp. Assoc. *19*:227, 1983.)

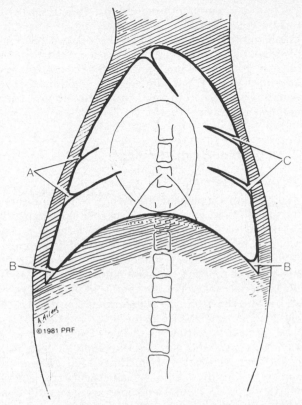

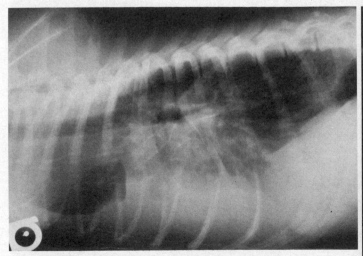

chronic exudative processes such as chronic pyothorax. Encapsulated pleural effusions may be difficult to distinguish radiographically from intrapleural masses.

Gravitational movement of pleural fluid achieved by horizontal beam radiography provides diagnostic information by: (1) demonstrating free *versus* encapsulated pleural effusion, (2) allowing visualization of thoracic structures by moving fluid away from structures of interest and (3) detecting small amounts of pleural fluid.

Standing lateral views allow estimation of the volume of pleural fluid present. A distinct fluid line will not be seen unless pleural air is also present. The standing lateral view is associated with a minimum of stress and may be preferred in orthopneic animals. The erect ventrodorsal position (see Fig. 42–3) moves pleural fluid toward the costophrenic angles, making this view highly sensitive for detecting small amounts of fluid. Rounding of the costophrenic angle is seen with as little as 50 ml of fluid in a 15-kg dog.[49] The erect ventrodorsal view also allows assessment of the cranial mediastinum for masses. The lateral decubitus views (see Fig. 42–3) are useful for detecting small amounts of pleural fluid and allow evaluation of specific lung lobes for intrapulmonary lesions (Fig. 42–7).

Radiographic diagnosis of pneumothorax depends on demonstration of free pleural air. As air fills the pleural space, the lungs retract from the parietal pleura, becoming relatively more radiopaque than

Figure 42–5. Small amounts of pleural fluid are often observed on a ventrodorsal view of the thorax at the interlobar fissures (*A* and *C*) and the costophrenic angles (*B*). (Reprinted with permission from Cantwell, H. D., Rebar, A. H., and Allen, A. R.: Pleural effusion in the dog: principles for diagnosis. J. Am. Anim. Hosp. Assoc. *19*:227, 1983.)

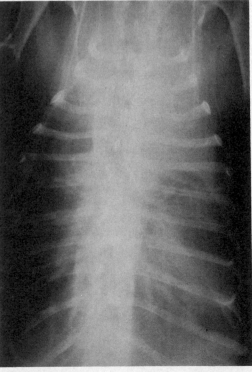

Figure 42–6. Recumbent lateral and dorsoventral thoracic radiographs of a dog with moderate pleural effusion.

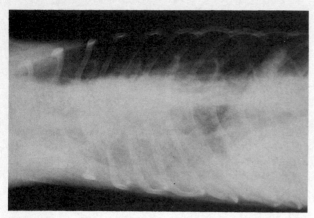

Figure 42–7. Horizontal beam—lateral decubitus thoracic radiograph of a dog with pleural effusion.

the free pleural air (Fig. 42–8). The subtle difference in contrast between free pleural air and lung is aided by careful evaluation of the peripheral pleural space for pulmonary vascular patterns. The contrast between free pleural air and collapsed lung is enhanced by expiratory radiographs.[55] The presence of free pleural air allows the heart to shift in a recumbent lateral view, making it appear to be elevated from the sternum (see Fig. 42–8). This elevation of the heart is not seen on a standing lateral view. Small amounts of free pleural air are best detected by evaluation of the costophrenic angles on the dorsoventral view or the lateral thoracic wall on a lateral decubitus view.

Combined pneumothorax and pleural effusion produce a distinct fluid line on a standing lateral radiograph, allowing assessment of the relative amounts of air and fluid within the pleural space.[55] Differential diagnoses for combined pneumothorax and pleural effusion include traumatic hemopneumothorax, traumatic chylopneumothorax, pyopneumothorax, and emphysematous pyothorax.

Clinical-Pathological Findings

Once pleural effusion is demonstrated either clinically or radiographically, thoracocentesis is indicated to remove fluid for diagnostic as well as therapeutic purposes. Diagnostic procedures performed on the pleural fluid include, in order of priority: (1) preparation of appropriately stained direct smears for cytological examination, (2) submission of fluid for aerobic bacterial, anaerobic bacterial, and fungal cultures and sensitivity testing, (3) determination of physical and biochemical characteristics (e.g., specific gravity, total protein, clotting characteristics, presence of chylomicrons), and (4) determination of total cell counts and preparation of centrifuged cell concentrate smears from fluid anticoagulated with EDTA.[18, 24, 58, 82] Pleural effusions are generally classified into one of six pathophysiological patterns: transudative, modified transudative, chylous, exudative, hemorrhagic, and neoplastic.[18, 23, 24, 58–60, 82] Although it is helpful for purposes of diagnosis to categorize pleural effusions into one of these patterns,

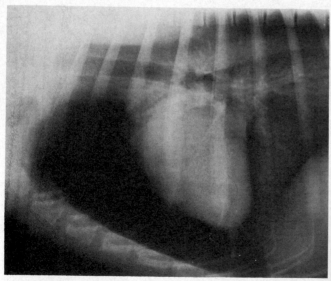

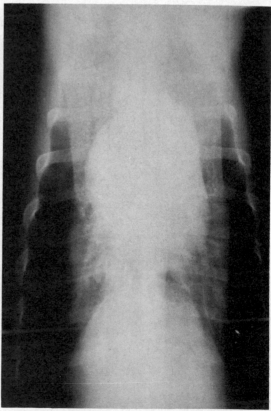

Figure 42–8. Recumbent lateral and ventrodorsal thoracic radiographs of a dog with pneumothorax.

there is considerable overlap of cytological and physiochemical characteristics between patterns. It is not uncommon for a pleural effusion to have distinct characteristics of more than one pattern. An understanding of the pathophysiological mechanisms responsible for each cytological and physiochemical finding is more useful in establishing the cause of a pleural effusion.

Transudative effusions result from disruption of the balance between capillary hydrostatic and colloid osmotic pressures responsible for pleural fluid formation and absorption. Hypoproteinemia and congestive heart failure favor transudate accumulation within the pleural space.[18, 24, 31, 33, 37, 58, 59, 82] Transudative effusions demonstrate characteristics similar to those of normal pleural fluid: specific gravity less than 1.018, total protein concentration less than 3.0 gm/dl, and nucleated cell count less than 3,000 cells/μl.[18, 31, 37, 58, 59, 82] Large (5–20 μ), pale-staining mesothelial cells predominate, usually constituting 70 per cent of the nucleated cell count.[59, 82] Single mesothelial cells are most common; however, multicellular clusters of mesothelial cells are occasionally observed and must be differentiated from neoplastic cells.[58, 82] Macrophages and lymphocytes account for the remaining nucleated cells.

As a transudative effusion becomes long-standing, mesothelial cells degenerate and attract neutrophils to the pleural space.[18, 58] The neutrophils start a mild inflammatory process, which alters the transudate. Total nucleated cell counts may approach 5,000 cells/μl, with a significant percentage of the cells being neutrophils.[18, 23, 37] These effusions are generally termed modified transudates. Transudative effusions that result from obstructive phenomena such as lung lobe torsion, diaphragmatic hernia with liver incarceration, and, occasionally, congestive heart failure usually present a distinctive picture on fluid analysis. Because the obstructive process commonly involves lymphatic as well as venous obstruction, the effusions generally have a total protein concentration of 3 to 5 gm/dl.[18, 23, 24, 59, 60, 82] Red blood cells and lymphocytes are generally present in higher numbers than in a transudate.[23, 24, 59, 82] Pleural effusions that result from obstructive phenomena are also considered modified transudates.[58–60, 82] However, some authors refer to these effusions separately as *obstructive effusions*.[23, 24]

Chylous effusion results when lymph from the thoracic duct enters the pleural space. Chylous effusions are opaque and milky white to yellow. Chyle retains its milky appearance on standing and may form a creamy top layer. Physiochemical properties of chylous effusions are similar to those of obstructive modified transudates, because hepatic lymph composes a large portion of thoracic duct chyle.[59] Specific gravity is greater than 1.012, and total protein concentration ranges from 3 to 5 gm/dl.[9, 60, 62, 82] Cytological examination of Wright's-stained smears reveals a predominance of small and large lymphocytes.[9, 23, 24, 47, 60, 62, 82] Chronic chylous effusions mod-

ify with time, showing progressive increases in the number of neutrophils, macrophages, and mesothelial cells.[23, 24, 60] Total cell counts generally do not exceed 10,000 cells/μl.[9, 60]

Demonstration of chylomicrons within a pleural effusion confirms its chylous nature. Chylomicrons can often be seen on direct smears or may be demonstrated with supravital stains such as Sudan III or IV.[24, 47, 62, 82] Clearance of an opaque fluid with ether indicates chylomicrons.[9, 24, 47, 60] An ether clearance test is performed with two equal aliquots of pleural fluid alkalinized with one or two drops of 1N NaOH. Equal volumes of ether and water are added to the aliquots. A chylous effusion clears on addition of ether. The presence of chylomicrons is most reliably confirmed by determination of triglyceride and cholesterol levels.[79] Chylous fluids show high triglyceride and low cholesterol levels compared with serum. In evaluation of chylous effusions for chylomicrons, consideration must be given to the nutritional status of the patient. A recently fasted patient with chylous effusion may have a greatly reduced level of chylomicrons. Pleural fluid from such a patient may easily be mistaken for a modified transudative or obstructive effusion. The feeding of a fatty meal will demonstrate the chylous nature of a pleural effusion in these patients.

Pleural effusions high in cholesterol or lecithinglobulin complexes appear grossly similar to *chylous effusions*. Such effusions are due to degeneration of cells associated with chronic inflammatory or malignant processes and are termed *pseudochylous effusions*. Pseudochylous effusions will not completely clear with ether and show high cholesterol and low triglyceride levels. The term pseudochylous effusion has been incorrectly used to describe milky effusions associated with feline cardiomyopathy[51, 60]; these effusions are chylous even though they do not originate directly from a thoracic duct rupture.

Exudative effusions result from inflammation of the pleura and characteristically exhibit a total protein greater than 3.0 gm/dl, a specific gravity greater than 1.018, and a total cell count greater than 3,000 cells/dl.[23, 24, 58–60, 82] Inflammatory exudates may be nonseptic or septic.

Nonseptic exudates usually have a serofibrinous or serosanguineous appearance. The distinction between modified transudates and nonseptic effusions may be difficult. Feline infectious peritonitis (FIP) produces a nonseptic exudative pleural effusion. The fluid is yellow, translucent, and viscous on gross examination. Total protein values approach serum levels, ranging from 4 to 8 gm/dl.[23, 60] Electrophoresis reveals an elevated gammaglobulin fraction. The high protein value often gives smears a faint eosinophilic granular background. The predominant cell types are nondegenerative neutrophils and macrophages, although total cell counts are generally not high, ranging from 5,000 to 15,000 cells/μl.[23, 24, 60]

Septic effusions are generally purulent. The fluid is viscous, opaque, and either white, yellow, green, or red. The fluid may clot or exhibit fibrinous debris and often has a foul odor. Cell counts range from 30,000 to 200,000 cells/µl, although accurate cell counts are difficult because of extensive cellular degeneration.[24, 60, 82] Degenerate neutrophils predominate, and bacteria are often present.[23, 24, 60, 82] Gram stains may give an early indication of the types of bacteria present. Fluids should always be submitted for aerobic and anaerobic bacterial culture. Macrophages and plasma cell increase in relative number as an exudative process becomes long-standing.

Hemorrhagic effusions are the result of hemorrhages into the pleural cavity, which are usually secondary to trauma or thoracic surgery. Specific gravity, total protein, total cell counts, and cytologic evaluation are similar to those in the peripheral blood. The myeloid-erythroid ratio is approximately one to 100, similar to that in peripheral blood. Like transudates, long-standing hemorrhagic effusions undergo inflammatory modification. The myeloid-erythroid ratio decreases owing to an influx of inflammatory cells. Protein values and cell counts decrease because of serous exudation.

The term hemorrhagic effusion is reserved for pleural hemorrhage rather than effusive processes in which cells may be present. Even long-standing hemorrhagic effusions have a hemoglobin level greater than 25 per cent of hemoglobin levels in blood, whereas serosanguineous effusions rarely have hemoglobin values exceeding 1 gm/dl.[31] Blood within the pleural cavity undergoes rapid mechanical defibrination and does not clot after aspiration.[24, 62] Platelets are present for only a short period immediately following an acute hemorrhage. Therefore hemorrhagic effusion specimens that clot immediately following thoracocentesis are probably a traumatic tap.

Neoplastic effusions may have either a basic exudative or a transudative patter and are identified by the presence of neoplastic cells on cytological examination. Any primary or metastatic neoplasm within the thoracic cavity may produce a neoplastic effusion. Thymic lymphosarcoma is the most common neoplastic effusion in cats.[23, 37] Neoplastic lymphocytes are usually prolymphocytes or lymphoblasts. These cells are large and variable in size and have intensely basophilic cytoplasm and multiple nucleoli. Metastatic carcinomas and occasionally sarcomas induce neoplastic effusions. Differentiation of neoplastic cells from reactive mesothelial cells is often difficult even for experienced cytologists. Therefore, care must be used in diagnosing neoplasia on cytological examination alone. Cytological findings must be correlated with other findings on physical and radiographic examination.

PLEURAL DRAINAGE

Once a diagnosis of pleural effusion or air is established, needle thoracocentesis is indicated to remove fluid for diagnostic as well as therapeutic purposes.

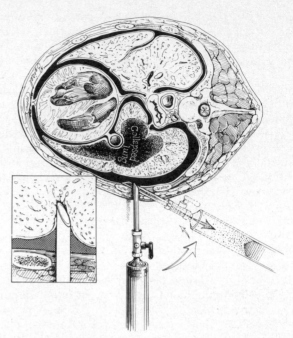

Figure 42–9. The needle for thoracocentesis is directed into the pleural space with the bevel of the needle toward the patient and parallel to the body wall. Insertion of the needle at a right angle to the thoracic wall is avoided to reduce the risk of lung laceration *(inset)*. (Reprinted with permission from Kolata, R. J.: Management of thoracic trauma. Vet. Clin. North Am. Small Anim. Pract. *11*:103, 1981.)

Needle thoracocentesis carries an inherent risk of lung laceration, which is minimized only by careful and proper technique. The needle is slowly advanced into the pleural space at a 45-degree angle with the bevel toward the patient (Fig. 42–9). Advancement of the needle is stopped as soon as it enters the pleural space. A hemostat may be placed on the needle to steady it and to prevent overpenetration. An extension tube placed between the syringe and needle allows manipulation of the syringe without potentially damaging manipulation of the needle after

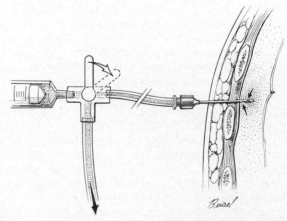

Figure 42–10. The risk of lung laceration during thoracocentesis can be reduced by using a teat cannula and an extension tube between the cannula and syringe. (Reprinted with permission from Crowe, D. T.: Thoracic drainage. *In* Bojrab, M. J. (ed.): *Current Techniques in Small Animal Surgery.* Lea & Febiger, Philadelphia, 1983.)

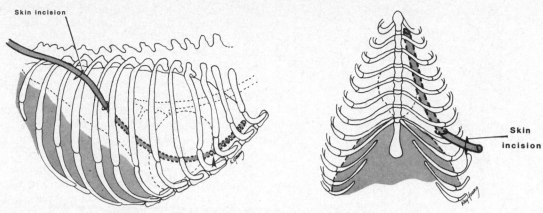

Figure 42–11. Proper placement of thoracostomy tube within the pleural space. (Reprinted with permission from Crowe, D. T.: Thoracic drainage. *In* Bojrab, M. J. (ed.): *Current Techniques in Small Animal Surgery.* Lea & Febiger, Philadelphia, 1983.)

it is in place (Fig. 42–10). A three-way stopcock is helpful if more than a single aspiration of the syringe is anticipated. Substitution of a teat cannula for the hypodermic needle also greatly reduces the risk of lung laceration (Fig. 42–10). Fluid is most efficiently collected in the ventral third of the fourth to seventh intercostal space with the patient standing or sternally recumbent. Air is collected at the highest point in the chest (i.e. mid-thorax if the patient is in lateral recumbency or the dorsal one-third of the chest if the patient is standing or sternally recumbent).

A thoracostomy tube (i.e., chest tube) is indicated if there is sufficient accumulation of pleural effusion to warrant repeated pleural drainage and is often necessary to completely evacuate the pleural space. Tubes for thoracostomy should be flexible but resistant to collapse. Red rubber feeding tubes are more reactive than commercially available thoracostomy tubes but are a practical and economic alternative to commercial tubes when long-term pleural evacuation is not anticipated. The size of a thoracostomy tube should approximate the diameter of a mainstem bronchus as estimated from a thoracic radiograph. The tube should have three to five holes to allow sufficient drainage. If the thoracostomy tube has a radiopaque line, the last hole should interrupt that line so that one may identify its position on a thoracic radiograph.

A thoracostomy tube may often be placed without anesthesia in critically ill animals. Local intercostal nerve blocks may be used in those animals requiring anesthesia. A generous portion of the lateral thorax is clipped, and strict aseptic technique is used. A small skin incision in the dorsal one-third of the lateral thoracic wall is made at the level of the tenth to 12th intercostal space. A subcutaneous tunnel is bluntly developed in a cranioventral direction over three to four intercostal spaces. With a stylet or large hemostatic forceps, the tube is introduced into the seventh or eighth intercostal space with a brisk but controlled thrust directed towards the opposite shoulder. The tube is fed into the cranial ventral pleural space (Fig. 42–11). The tube is directly sutured to the skin (Fig. 42–12). Adhesive-tape butterflies sutured to the skin often allow slippage of the chest

tube when the butterfly is wet. A liberal amount of antiseptic ointment around the entry site helps prevent leakage of air and migration of bacteria along the tube. The tube should be covered with a loose bandage. The position of the thoracostomy tube is confirmed with a thoracic radiograph. Thoracostomy tube placement following thoracotomy is performed while the chest is still open to ensure safe and proper placement.

Once a thoracostomy tube is placed, pleural drainage may be either intermittent or continuous. Intermittent pleural drainage is generally adequate when accumulation of a pleural effusion or air is not life-threatening. Intermittent pleural drainage also allows

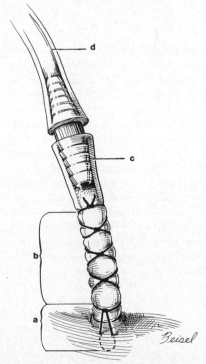

Figure 42–12. A "Chinese finger cuff" suture is used to secure the thoracostomy tube to the thoracic wall. (Reprinted with permission from Crowe, D. T.: Thoracic drainage. *In* Bojrab, M. J. (ed.): *Current Techniques in Small Animal Surgery.* Lea & Febiger, Philadelphia, 1983.)

Expiration   Inspiration

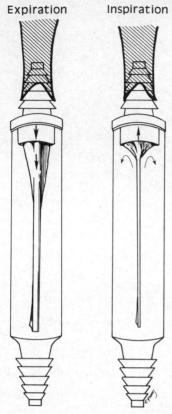

Figure 42–13. Heimlich valves may be used to evacuate a closed pneumothorax. The valve allows air to escape during expiration when positive pleural pressure develops, but prevents air from entering the pleural space during inspiration. (Reprinted with permission from Crowe, D. T.: Thoracic drainage. *In* Bojrab, M. J. (ed.): *Current Techniques in Small Animal Surgery.* Lea & Febiger, Philadelphia, 1983.)

quantitation of both fluid and air volumes. Intermittent pleural drainage allows the thoracostomy tube to be incorporated entirely into a bandage, thus reducing the chances of removal of the tube by the patient.

A Heimlich valve may be placed on a thoracostomy tube to evacuate pneumothorax in large dogs. Such a one-way valve allows air to be expelled from the chest when positive pressure is developed during expiration and prevents air from entering the pleural space during inspiration (Fig. 42–13). Problems arise when such a valve is misused or depended on too much. Heimlich valves were developed strictly for the evacuation of air from the pleural cavity. A Heimlich valve cannot be effectively used when pleural effusion is also present, as the flutter valve quickly becomes obstructed by fluid. Attempts to autoclave Heimlich valves have also resulted in obstruction of the mechanism. Because Heimlich valves were developed for human patients, small animals (less than 15 kg) often have insufficient pleural pressures and tidal volumes for Heimlich valves to be effective.

Continuous closed suction is indicated when accumulation of pleural effusions or air is life-threatening. Intermittent suction often cannot keep up

with the rapid accumulations of fluid or air associated with trauma. Continuous suction also has the advantage of keeping pleural surfaces in contact, sealing pleuropulmonary fistulas or hemorrhage. Many commercial systems are now available for continuous pleural evacuation. All are based in principle on the original underwater bottle system. Bottle systems and their descendants are best understood by reducing them to their component parts. A one-bottle system is simply a water seal that functions as a one-way valve. The end of the thoracotomy tube is submerged in 3 to 5 cm of water (Fig. 42–14). This arrangement allows excess air or fluid to escape from the pleural cavity whenever pleural pressures exceed 3 to 5 cm H_2O. The water seal prevents air or liquid from being drawn into the pleural cavity as long as the bottle is kept well below the patient (> 20 cm).

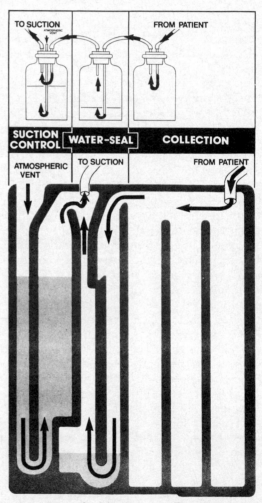

Figure 42–14. *Top,* A three-bottle system allows continuous suction to be applied to a thoracostomy tube. The bottles function as a collection reservoir, a water-seal, and a suction control. The amount of negative suction applied to the thoracostomy tube is determined by subtracting the centimeters of water of tube submersion in the water-seal bottle from the centimeters of water of tube submersion in the suction control bottle. *Bottom,* Convenient plastic systems such as the Pleur-E-Vac system are based on the same principles as the three-bottle system. (Reprinted with permission from Kurtz, L. D.: *Underwater-Seal Drainage of the Pleural Cavity.* New York, KRALE: Division of Deknatel, Inc., 1975.)

This bottle also serves as a reservoir for collection of pleural fluids.

A two-bottle system adds the ability to apply regulated suction to the water-seal bottle. The second bottle is sealed and contains a simple manometer (see Fig. 42–14). The amount of negative suction is determined by submerging the manometer to the desired number of centimeters of water. The absolute negative pressure is calculated by subtracting the number of centimeters of water in the water-seal bottle from the number of centimeters of water in the regulating bottle. A negative pressure of 10 to 20 cm H_2O is generally recommended for continuous pleural drainage. A potential disadvantage of the two-bottle system is that as liquid collects in the water-seal bottle, progressively smaller amounts of negative pressure are applied to the pleural cavity. This disadvantage is negated by the addition of a separate collection bottle proximal to the water-seal bottle in a three-bottle system (see Fig. 42–14).

Reusable bottle systems are inexpensive and work well in most instances. More convenient one-piece plastic systems based on the same principles are also readily available (see Fig. 42–14). The disadvantage of continuous suction systems is that they require constant monitoring, because the connecting tube to the patient is susceptible to removal or damage by the patient. Continuous suction systems do not allow for measurement of the air removed from the pleural cavity. Despite these disadvantages, continuous suction systems can at times be life-saving.

Thoracostomy tubes are removed as soon as they are no longer productive. The presence of the tube induces an effusion of 50 to 100 ml in 24 hours. If intermittent suction and thoracic radiographs confirm accumulations of less than 100 ml in 24 hours, the tube may be safely removed by rapid withdrawal.

HYDROTHORAX

Hydrothorax is a transudative effusion of the pleural space that results from a disturbance in the balance of Starling forces responsible for pleural fluid formation and absorption. Diagnosis of hydrothorax is based on identification of a pleural effusion as a transudate or modified transudate.

Hypoproteinemia reduces capillary colloid osmotic pressure, allowing fluid to remain in interstitial compartments, including the pleural space. Hydrothorax resulting from hypoproteinemia is often associated with other transudative processes such as ascites and dependent edema. Causes of hypoproteinemia include protein-losing nephropathy, protein-losing enteropathy, hepatic failure, malnutrition, and extensive inflammatory effusion.

Right-sided, left-sided, or biventricular congestive heart failure may induce hydrothorax by disturbing pulmonary or systemic capillary hydrostatic pressures.[24, 31, 33, 37, 82] Right-sided congestive heart failure increases pleural fluid formation, whereas left-sided congestive heart failure decreases pleural fluid absorption.

Hydrothorax also results from obstructive effusions such as occur with long lobe torsion or incarcerations of liver associated with diaphragmatic hernias. These effusions result from transudation of fluid through organ capsules due to obstruction of venous and lymphatic drainage.[23] Obstructive transudates characteristically contain high protein levels that approach serum levels.[23] Red blood cells are also usually present. These effusions quickly develop an inflammatory component if organ necrosis occurs.

The treatment of hydrothorax includes pleural drainage if respiratory distress is present as well as correction of its underlying cause.

PLEURITIS AND PYOTHORAX

Inflammatory conditions of the pleura may be dry, serofibrinous, pyogranulomatous, or purulent. An initial period of dry pleuritis often precedes inflammatory pleural effusions.[82] Causes of dry pleuritis include bacteria, viruses, and trauma. A diagnosis of dry pleuritis is suggested by clinical findings of a rapid and shallow respiratory pattern, obscure thoracic pain, nonproductive cough, and auscultation of a pleural friction rub. Therapy is directed toward prevention of pyothorax by appropriate systemic antibiotics.

Dry pleuritis is rarely recognized clinically and often proceeds to serofibrinous pleuritis. Serofibrinous pleuritis is reported with canine hepatitis, canine leptospirosis, canine distemper, and canine and feline upper respiratory viruses.[82] Bacterial pleuropneumonia is also a cause of serofibrinous pleuritis in dogs and cats.[85] Parasitic diseases such as *Aeleurostrongylus* spp. in cats and *Spirocerca lupi* in dogs occasionally induce serofibrinous pleuritis.[34, 82] Simultaneous traumatic rupture of the biliary system and diaphragm and canine tuberculosis are unusual causes of severe serofibrinous pleuritis.[8, 68, 69] Therapy is directed toward correction of the inciting cause and prevention of progression to pyothorax.

Pyogranulomatous pleuritis is specifically associated with feline infectious peritonitis.[23, 24, 82] The effusion is secondary to a virus-induced vasculitis affecting all serous membranes. Diagnosis is suggested by characteristic findings on analysis of the pleural effusion. Abdominal effusion, elevated serum globulins, and uveitis are common associated findings.[24, 82] The prognosis for feline infectious peritonitis is poor.

Purulent pleuritis, also referred to as pyothorax or empyema, is invariably the result of bacterial or fungal sepsis of the pleural space.[22, 24, 40, 77, 82, 85, 88] Sources of bacterial contamination include penetrating thoracic wounds, extension from bacterial pneumonia, migrating foreign bodies, esophageal perforations, extension of cervical, lumbar, or mediastinal infections, and hematogenous spread. Thoracic bite wounds are a frequently implicated cause of feline pyothorax.[30, 77] Inhalation and migration of a grass awn is often suspected in hunting dogs with pyothorax.

Anaerobic bacteria (Fusobacterium) and *Nocardia asteroides* are most commonly isolated from dogs with pyothorax.[82] *Pasteurella multocida* and anaerobes are the most prevalent isolates in cats.[77, 85, 88] Other microorganisms reported include *Actinomyces* spp., *Streptococcus* spp., *Entamoeba coli, Staphylococcus* spp., *Bacteroides spp., Klebsiella* spp., *Proteus* spp., *Corynebacterium* spp., *Enterobacter* spp., *Psuedomonas* spp., Spirochetes, *Aspergillus* spp., and *Cryptococcus* spp.[3, 10, 20, 24, 77, 82, 85, 88]

Pyothorax frequently has an insidious course, and presentation is often delayed. Moderate to severe respiratory distress is usually present. The patient shows signs of systemic infection characterized by anorexia, weight loss, malaise and fever. Physical and radiographic findings are those of pleural effusion, and analysis of pleural fluid shows a septic exudate. The degree of neutrophilic degeneration and the number of bacteria give an early indication of the severity of the infection. The lungs, esophagus, thoracic wall, and cervical region are evaluated to rule out possible sources of the infection.

Treatment of pyothorax must be prompt and aggressive. The prognosis is guarded but not hopeless. Dramatic results are obtained with proper therapy. The initial goal of therapy is relief of respiratory embarrassment by thoracocentesis, preferably under minimal restraint with the patient in sternal recumbency or standing. Supportive care with intravenous fluids is necessary to correct dehydration and acid-base and electrolyte imbalances. Systemic antibiotics are started once fluid is collected for aerobic and anaerobic bacterial culture. Sodium penicillin G (40,000 units/kg every 6 hours) and gentamicin (2.2 mg/kg every 8 hours) are good choices of drug to use until culture results are available.

Local treatment of pyothorax involves pleural drainage and lavage by tube thoracostomy.[17, 22, 77, 85, 88] Once the patient is stable, a thoracostomy tube is placed using local narcotic or general anesthesia. Bilateral thoracostomy tubes are occasionally necessary. Following complete evacuation of the thoracic cavity, pleural lavage is instituted. The pleural space is lavaged twice daily with 20 ml/kg of warmed saline or Ringer's solution. The lavage solution remains in the chest for one hour. Approximately 25 per cent of the lavage solution is absorbed by the patient.[40, 77, 88] The patient must be closely monitored for respiratory distress during lavage.

The addition of antibiotics to the lavage solution or local infiltration of antibiotics immediately following lavage at one-half systemic doses has been advocated.[17, 22, 40, 77, 88] The value of local antibiotics administered in addition to systemic antibiotics is unproven. In addition to antibiotics, chymotrypsin (50,000 NF units/100 ml of lavage) or streptokinase-streptodornase may be added to the lavage solution to aid mobilization of exudative debris.[24, 40, 77, 82, 85, 87]

The value of proteolytic enzymes is not universally accepted. Addition of heparin (1500 units/100 ml of lavage) to the lavage solution is recommended to reduce clotting, fibrin deposition, and fluid loculation.[22, 77] Addition of heparin to peritoneal lavage solutions has been shown to decrease the mortality of experimental bacterial peritonitis in dogs.[39]

Lack of significant clinical improvement within 48 to 72 hours or radiographic demonstration of undrained encapsulated fluid is an indication for surgical exploration of the thoracic cavity.[22, 30, 40, 77, 85] Radiographic evidence of lung lobe consolidation with pneumothorax suggests a ruptured pulmonary abscess and is a relative indication for surgery. Exploratory thoracotomy should be by median sternotomy, which gives access to both hemithoraces. Adhesions and loculated pockets of fluid are carefully broken down. The ventral mediastinum is excised, because it is invariably thickened and filled with small abscesses. Consolidated lung lobes that cannot be reinflated are excised by partial or complete lobectomy. Large lung lacerations created by adhesion breakdowns must be repaired or excised. Before closure, the thoracic cavity is vigorously lavaged with copious amounts of warmed isotonic solution. Closed pleural lavage is continued postoperatively for two or three days.

Constrictive pleuritis, a serious sequel to pyothorax, is signified by inability to inflate the lungs following resolution of the pyothorax. If the constriction is diffuse, surgical *decortication* of the fibroelastic layer from the visceral pleura is necessary. Decortication in small animals, particularly in cats, is often a difficult procedure that results in numerous pulmonary lacerations.[22] It should be attempted as early as possible because delay allows progressive fibrosis.[66]

CHYLOTHORAX

Chylothorax develops when chyle from the cisterna chyli–thoracic duct system gains access to the pleural space. An understanding of the functional anatomy of the cisterni chyli and thoracic duct is useful in diagnosing and treating chylothorax. Considerable variability exists not only between species but also and particularly between individuals of the same species.[12, 32, 43, 44, 47, 78]

The cisterna chyli is an elongated saccular reservoir receiving lymph from the lumbar and mesenteric lymphatic trunks. The cisterna chyli in the dog is sublumbar (L1–L4), dorsal to and to the right of the aorta, and bordered laterally by the crura of the diaphragm.[54] The cisterna chyli in the cat is bipartate with a large saccular portion dorsal to the aorta and a plexiform portion ventral to the aorta.[47] In the cat, the cisterna chyli is ventral to vertebrae T13–L3 and is closely associated with the diaphragmatic crura.

The thoracic duct continues cranially from the cisterna chyli through the aortic hiatus of the diaphragm. The caudal thoracic duct in the dog courses

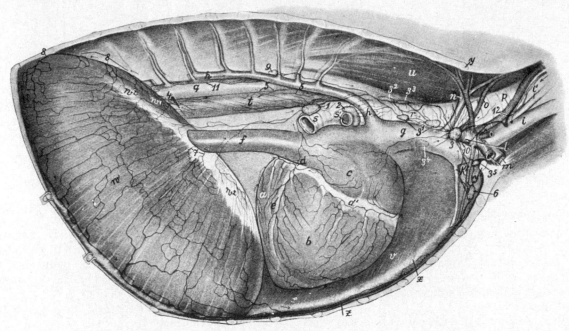

Figure 42–15. Drawing of the right hemithorax indicating the relative position of the thoracic duct (11) to the aorta, intercostal arteries and azygous vein. (Reprinted with permission from Miller, M. E., Christensen, G. C., and Evans, H. E.: *Anatomy of the Dog,* 2nd ed. W. B. Saunders Co., Philadelphia, 1979.)

to the right and dorsally on the aorta, lateral to the intercostal arteries and ventral to the azygos vein (Fig. 42–15).[44, 54] The duct crosses to the left side of the aorta ventral to the body of T5 (Fig. 42–15). The duct continues cranioventrally across the left side of the esophagus to empty at the junction of the left jugular vein and cranial vena cava (Fig. 42–16).[54]

Although the preceding description of the thoracic duct is considered "normal," few dogs exhibit this pattern without some variation (Figs. 42–17 and 42–18). In one study, only one of 20 dogs demonstrated the "normal" pattern on aqueous lymphangiography.[44] Variations include multiple collaterals of the caudal and middle portions of the duct and double

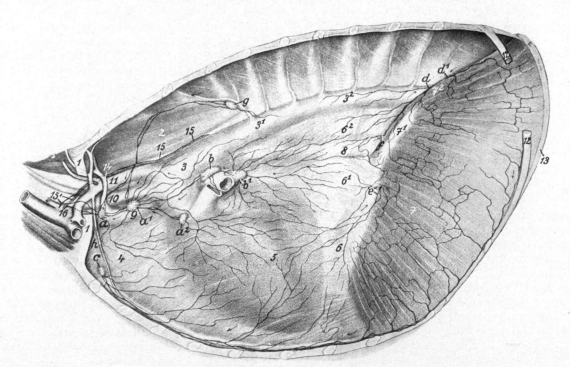

Figure 42–16. Drawing of the left hemithorax showing the course and termination of the cranial thoracic duct (15). (Reprinted with permission from Miller, M. E., Christensen, G. C., and Evans, H. E.: *Anatomy of the Dog.* 2nd ed. W. B. Saunders Co., Philadelphia, 1979.)

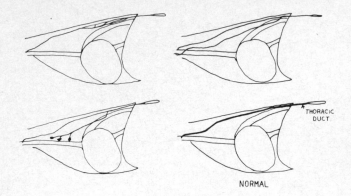

Figure 42–17. Variations of the thoracic duct on a lateral thoracic radiograph following rapid aqueous lymphangiography. (Reprinted with permission from Kagan, K. G., and Breznock, E. M.: Variations in the thoracic duct system and the effects of surgical occlusion demonstrated by rapid aqueous lymphangiography using an intestinal lymphatic trunk. Am. J. Vet. Res. 40:948, 1979.)

duct systems.[44] Collateral vessels cross from the right to left mediastinum at a single level in some individuals and at multiple levels in others.[44] Termination of the thoracic duct also varies; terminations on the right jugular vein, azygos vein, and mediastinal lymph nodes, and combinations of these, have been seen.[44, 54]

The thoracic duct in the cat passes from the dorsal left aspect of the aorta caudally to terminate on the left jugular vein.[47] The thoracic duct invariably shows multiple collaterals in the cat.[32, 47] Although the thoracic duct lies predominantly on the left surface of the aorta in the cat, collateral branches invariably pass between and to the right of the intercostal arteries.[32, 47]

The etiology of chylothorax is poorly understood in the dog and cat. Congenital abnormalities of the thoracic duct resulting in chylothorax are documented in humans.[11, 70] Congenital causes of chylothorax are speculated on but not proven in the dog or cat.[38, 81] Chylothorax in Afghans and other sight hounds is disproportionately high.[82] Congenital abnormalities of the thoracic duct may predispose the Afghan to chylothorax in later life.[81]

Trauma is the best documented cause of chylothorax in dogs and cats. Thoracic duct rupture may result from blunt as well as penetrating injuries. Inadvertent disruption of the thoracic duct during thoracic surgery is a commonly reported cause of chylothorax in humans.[11, 14, 19, 45] Although not well documented, postoperative chylothorax certainly occurs in dogs and cats. The location of the cisterna chyli and thoracic duct between the crura of the diaphragm predisposes the duct to rupture during severe coughing or vomiting in humans; a similar mechanism is proposed but not proven in animals. Rupture of the thoracic duct is reported with traumatic diaphragmatic hernia in cats.[52] Rupture of the thoracic duct from vigorous postprandial stretching of the spine is suspected in humans.

Nontraumatic causes of chylothorax are the most difficult to understand and demonstrate. Malignancies, particularly of the cranial mediastinum, may result in chylothorax. Invasion and subsequent erosion of the thoracic duct may be a cause.[9, 11, 70] Impaired healing due to the tumor may prevent ruptures from spontaneously closing.[11]

Whether or not simple obstruction of the thorax can result in chylothorax is controversial. Experimental obstruction of the thoracic duct rarely results in chylothorax.[6] Within two weeks, lymphaticovenous anastomoses to the caudal vena cava and azygos veins bypass thoracic duct obstructions.[12, 16, 57, 72, 83, 90] Multiple terminations of the thoracic duct may also bypass distal thoracic duct obstructions. However, experimental ligation of the cranial vena cava results in a high incidence (> 50 per cent) of chylothorax in dogs and cats.[6] Obstruction of the cranial vena cava likely completely arrests thoracic duct flow during the period before lymphaticovenous anastomoses develop. Speculation exists that dilation of the lymphatic ducts resulting from such an obstruction allows extravasation of chyle through the lymphatic vessel wall.

Neoplasms that occlude the cranial vena cava may induce chylothorax. Thrombosis of the cranial vena cava is also associated with chylothorax in humans.[70] Elevated venous pressures associated with right-sided congestive heart failure may explain chylothorax associated with cardiomyopathy, tricuspid dysplasia, and experimental heartworm disease in cats.[28, 51] Elevated venous pressures secondary to congestive heart failure not only inhibit lymph drainage but discourage formation of lymphaticovenous anastomoses.

Pathophysiological alterations associated with chylothorax primarily result from a loss of chyle from the body, particularly when pleural drainage is instituted. Water and electrolyte losses are sufficient to induce dehydration and electrolyte imbalance. Loss of lipid and protein rapidly leads to protein-calorie malnutrition and hypoproteinemia. Malnutrition is compounded by the loss of fat-soluble vitamins. Immunocompetence is compromised owing to loss of antibodies, lymphopenia, and malnutrition.[42]

Diagnosis of chylothorax is based on recognition of characteristic clinical and radiographic findings of pleural effusion, followed by demonstration of chylomicrons on fluid analysis. Once a chylous effusion is demonstrated, some attempt to determine its cause is necessary. Clients should be carefully questioned regarding the possibility of recent trauma or thoracic surgery. Thoracic radiographs taken after complete pleural drainage should be evaluated for the presence

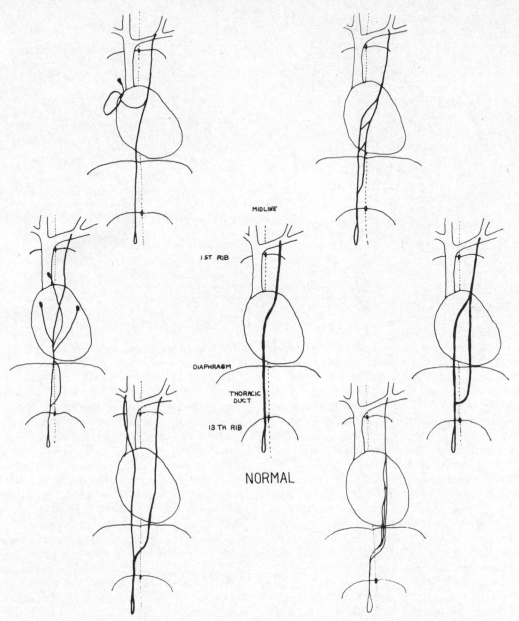

MIDLINE

1ST RIB

DIAPHRAGM

THORACIC
DUCT

13TH RIB

NORMAL

Figure 42–18. Variations of the thoracic duct on a ventrodorsal thoracic radiograph following rapid aqueous lymphangiography. (Reprinted with permission from Kagan, K. G., and Breznock, E. M.: Variations in the thoracic duct system and the effects of surgical occlusion demonstrated by rapid aqueous lymphangiography using an intestinal lymphatic trunk. Am. J. Vet. Res., *40*:948, 1979.)

of masses, particularly in the cranial mediastinum. Cytological examination of the chylous effusion for the presence of neoplastic cells may confirm neoplasia. Concurrent cardiac disease should be ruled out through physical examination, thoracic radiographs, and electrocardiogram.

Often a diagnostic work-up does not reveal the cause of a chylothorax. Direct lymphangiography is a method of determining both the presence and site of rupture or obstruction of the thoracic duct.[21, 61, 78] Direct lymphangiography involves the cannulation of a lymphatic vessel followed by injection of a contrast medium to outline the thoracic duct. Injection of Evan's blue dye into the foot pad of a pelvic limb aids in identification of a lymphatic vessel for can-

nulation. Oily and aqueous contrast media have been advocated for lymphangiography. Oily contrast media require slow injection, do not completely outline the thoracic duct, and cause pulmonary embolization.[12, 15, 21, 44, 63] Aqueous contrast media are currently preferred because their improved mixing with lymph allows rapid injection and complete filling of lymphatic vessels.[12, 44, 63]

Rapid injection of an aqueous contrast medium into an intestinal lymphatic trunk produces complete and detailed lymphangiograms of the thoracic duct.[12, 44] An intestinal trunk from the ileocecocolic region is cannulated proximal to the mesenteric lymph node via a celiotomy (Fig. 42–19). Location and cannulation of the lymphatic vessel is aided by

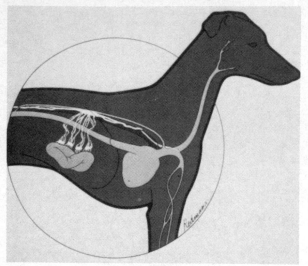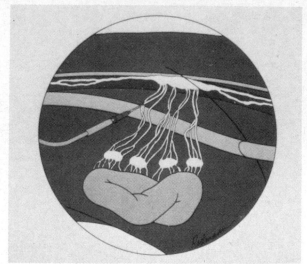

Figure 42–19. Diagram indicating the location for cannulization of an intestinal lymphatic trunk proximal to the mesenteric lymph nodes for rapid aqueous lymphangiography of the thoracic duct. (Reprinted with permission from Birchard, S. J., Cantwell, H. D., and Bright, R. M.: Lymphangiography and ligation of the canine thoracic duct: a study of normal dogs and three dogs with chylothorax. J. Am. Anim. Hosp. Assoc. 18:769, 1982.)

feeding 1 ml/kg of corn oil one hour preoperatively.[12, 44] Thoracic radiographs are taken immediately following an infusion of 5 to 15 ml of aqueous contrast medium.

Treatment of chylothorax may be medical or surgical. Formation of a therapeutic plan for chylothorax is based on a consideration of its etiology, an evaluation of the nutritional status of the patient, and an understanding of the advantages and limitations of the various treatments available. Rigid adherence to either a medical or surgical approach is inappropriate and likely to be unsuccessful.

Because spontaneous closure of a thoracic duct fistula is possible, initial medical management of chylothorax is recommended.[11, 24, 70, 82] Medical management is directed at reducing the formation of chyle and draining the pleural space. The formation of chylomicrons is reduced by eliminating fat from the diet. Diets high in protein and carbohydrate and low in fat are therefore recommended.[24, 82] The energy content of such a diet may be boosted by medium-chain triglycerides, which are absorbed directly into the portal system without formation of chylomicrons.[24, 82] Dietary manipulation does not influence the flow of lymph from other areas drained by the thoracic duct such as the liver or pelvic limbs. Therefore, no-fat diets primarily reduce the fat content of chyle rather than its volume. Parenteral hyperalimentation has been advocated for medical management of chylothorax in humans but does not have a clear advantage over no-fat diets with medium-chain triglycerides.[64] Patients on no-fat diets should receive regular supplementation with fat-soluble vitamins and essential fatty acids.

Pleural drainage is indicated during medical management of chylothorax in order to relieve respiratory distress. Pleural drainage may either be intermittent or continuous. Continuous pleural drainage has the advantage that it maintains pleural surfaces in contact, which may encourage healing of thoracic duct fistulas.[9]

Surgical management of chylothorax involves transthoracic ligation of the caudal thoracic duct.[12, 80] The rationale behind ligation of the thoracic duct is based on formation of lymphaticovenous anastomoses observed following experimental occlusion of the thoracic duct.[6, 12, 57, 72, 83, 84, 90] These lymphaticovenous anastomoses, which appear five to 14 days following thoracic duct occlusion, divert chyle flow away from the thoracic duct. Absolute indications for surgical intervention are not established in animals but the following indications for surgery are suggested on the basis of clinical experience in humans: (1) failure of the flow of chyle to significantly diminish after 14 days of medical management, (2) losses of chyle exceeding 20 ml/kg/day over five days, or (3) imminent protein-calorie malnutrition and hypoproteinemia.[76]

Transthoracic ligation of the thoracic duct is accomplished through a right ninth intercostal thoracotomy in the dog and a left ninth intercostal thoracotomy in the cat. Failure to ligate all collateral branches of the caudal thoracic duct is probably the most common cause of operative failure. Preoperative and immediately postoperative lymphangiograms are currently recommended to ensure complete ligation of the thoracic duct.[12] Serosanguineous pleural effusions may persist for a period following successful thoracic duct ligation because of pleuritis induced by chyle.[12] Despite vigorous attempts at medical and surgical management, some patients with chylothorax fail to respond. Chemical pleurodesis has been successfully used to treat refractory chylothorax in humans.[36] In addition, chemical pleurodesis is used to alleviate patients with chylothorax of neoplastic origin. Pleurodesis using infusions of tetracycline into the pleural space is currently undergoing clinical evaluation as a potential treatment of chylothorax in animals.

HEMOTHORAX

Hemothorax is accumulation of blood in the pleural cavity. Pleural effusions of a variety of causes often have a significant sanguineous component; however, the term hemothorax is reserved for effusions resulting from direct hemorrhage into the pleural space.

The most common cause of hemothorax is trauma, particularly blunt thoracic trauma involving fractured ribs. Hemothorax can also be a sequel to thoracic surgery. Inadvertent laceration of an intercostal artery during thoracotomy should be considered when hemothorax complicates the post-thoracotomy period. Coagulopathies, including thrombocytopenia, warfarin toxicity, and disseminated intravascular coagulation, occasionally manifest hemothorax.[24, 31, 33, 46, 82] Infiltration of thoracic vessel walls by neoplasia can result in vessel rupture and spontaneous hemothorax. Pathological changes in the walls of the aorta and pulmonary artery induced by *Spirocerca lupi* and *Dirofilaria immitis*, respectively, are also associated with rupture and spontaneous hemothorax.[35, 82] Spontaneous hemothorax without apparent cause is reported in dogs.[53]

Hemorrhagic effusions within the pleural space generally do not clot. Mechanical defibrination and activation of fibrinolytic mechanisms rapidly render pleural blood unable to clot even after its removal from the chest. Clotting is also impaired by the disappearance of platelets from pleural blood within eight hours of hemorrhage. Occasionally, blood from severe thoracic trauma clots in the pleural space owing to release of tissue thromboplastin.[61] Clotted pleural hemorrhage usually undergoes complete fibrinolysis within seven to ten days.[61] However, organization of pleural clots and fibrin deposits into a fibrous pleural layer is reported in dogs.[61] Fibrous layers prevent pulmonary re-expansion and encourage pleural effusion.

Diagnosis of hemothorax is based on demonstration of blood in the pleural space with cellular characteristics similar to those of peripheral blood. Hemorrhagic effusions should not clot following thoracocentesis. Clotting of the sample suggests a traumatic tap or recent hemorrhage.

Treatment of hemothorax depends on the volume and flow of hemorrhage into the pleural space. The dog is capable of complete resorption of 30 per cent of its blood volume from the pleural space within 90 hours.[87] Approximately 70 to 100 per cent of red cells are absorbed intact without hemolysis.[87] Therefore, hemothorax that is not of a great enough volume or flow to induce significant respiratory distress is managed conservatively without pleural drainage. The patient is given crystalloid volume replacement and supportive care until physiological autotransfusion can occur.

Occasionally, pleural hemorrhage is sufficient to require pleural drainage for relief of respiratory embarrassment. The patient often requires blood trans-

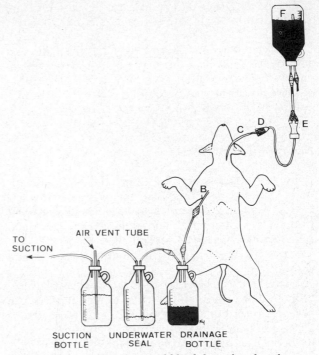

Figure 42–20. Autotransfusion of blood from the pleural space. (Reprinted with permission from Crowe, D. T.: Autotransfusion in the trauma patient. Vet. Clin. North Am. *10*:581, 1980.)

fusion in addition to crystalloid volume replacement to maintain adequate packed cell volume and total serum protein. Autogenous autotransfusion of blood removed by pleural drainage provides a readily available source of compatible blood in patients with severe hemothorax. Pleural blood collected in heparinized 60-ml syringes from a cat or small dog can be reinfused directly back into the patient. In a larger dog, blood collected in the drainage bottle of a three-bottle pleural drainage system is returned to the patient by standard gravitational infusion (Fig. 42–20). The blood is anticoagulated with 100 ml of citrate phosphate dextrose (CPD) or 60 ml of anticoagulant citrate dextrose (ACD) per 800 ml of blood.[26, 27] Filtration of autotransfused blood with a micropore filter is currently recommended to remove platelet aggregates and other microthrombi; however, studies in dogs have not demonstrated complications when filters were not used.[26]

Problems associated with autotransfusion include microembolization of platelet aggregates, hemolysis and coagulopathies due to thrombocytopenia, hypofibrinogenemia, and disseminated intravascular coagulation.[7, 26] Despite these potential problems, the practicality and life-saving potential of autotransfusion during severe traumatic hemothorax cannot be denied.

Continuous pleural drainage offers some advantage in patients with severe pleural hemorrhage because it provides a tamponade effect associated with keeping pleural surfaces in contact. Occasionally, pleural hemorrhage is of sufficient flow that continuous pleural drainage and autotransfusion cannot keep ahead of accumulation. Exploratory thoracotomy is indicated to prevent hemorrhage. Exploratory thoracotomy in animals with severe hemothorax is rarely successful.

Decortication of a pleural layer has been successfully performed in a dog with an organizing hemothorax.[66] Decortication is ideally performed within five weeks of the inciting injury, before fibrous infiltration of the visceral pleura has occurred.[66]

NEOPLASTIC EFFUSION

Pleural effusion may be associated with any primary or metastatic neoplasm involving the thoracic cavity. Common examples include lymphosarcoma, pulmonary carcinoma, metastatic carcinomas, and hemangiosarcomas.[24, 67] Mesotheliomas are rare but are associated with marked pleural effusion when present.[13, 67]

Neoplastic effusions are suspected when physical, radiographic, and laboratory findings suggest the presence of a thoracic neoplasm. Cytological identification of neoplastic cells within an effusion confirms its neoplastic origin. A pleural punch biopsy is indicated when pleural neoplasia is suspected.[67] Neoplastic pleural effusions may have an underlying transudative, exudative, chylous, or hemorrhagic pattern, depending on the mechanism by which it was induced.

Treatment of a neoplastic pleural effusion is directed at the causative neoplasm. The prognosis for animals with neoplastic effusions is poor, with the exception of an effusion associated with lymphosarcoma. Intermittent pleural drainage may give temporary relief from respiratory distress. Chemical pleurodesis has been successfully used to palliate neoplastic effusions in human patients.

PNEUMOTHORAX

Pneumothorax results when atmospheric air gains access to the pleural space. The source of pleural air is either a pleurocutaneous, pleuroesophageal, or pleuropulmonary leak.

Pleurocutaneous air leakage resulting from penetrating trauma to the thoracic wall produces an open pneumothorax. Specific causes include stab wounds, gunshot wounds, and bite wounds inflicted by larger animals. Open pneumothorax can also result from inadequate closure of a thoracotomy incision.

Esophageal perforation, generally the result of a foreign body, may permit formation of a closed pneumothorax. Pneumothorax is not an invariable result of an esophageal perforation, because of the airtight nature of the upper esophageal sphincter. Pneumothorax was reported in only two of 12 dogs with esophageal perforation secondary to foreign bodies.[73] Conditions that allow air to gain access to the esophagus, such as forced inspiratory efforts, anesthesia,

and diffuse esophagitis, increase the likelihood of pneumothorax secondary to esophageal perforation.

Pleuropulmonary air leaks originate from the trachea, bronchi, or lungs. Pneumothorax arising from pulmonary rupture may be traumatic or spontaneous. Traumatic pulmonary rupture most commonly results from blunt thoracic trauma. Iatrogenic trauma associated with diagnostic, therapeutic, and surgical procedures is also a possible cause.

Spontaneous pneumothorax occurs in dogs without evidence of trauma. Spontaneous pneumothorax is primary when the patient shows no clinical evidence of pulmonary disease and secondary when obvious pulmonary disease exists. Primary spontaneous pneumothorax resulting from rupture of pulmonary blebs or bullae have been reported in dogs.[10, 75] Pulmonary blebs are localized collections of air within the visceral pleura, and pulmonary bullae represent confluent alveoli. The cause of pulmonary bleb and bulla formation in dogs is not known. Some evidence suggests that bullae may be a latent complication of trauma.[4, 10]

Secondary spontaneous pneumothorax is linked with several pulmonary diseases in humans, including bacterial pneumonia, chronic obstructive lung disease (emphysema and chronic bronchitis), asthma, tuberculosis, and pulmonary carcinoma.[31, 33] Spontaneous pneumothorax is a rarely reported complication of bacterial pneumonia in dogs.[29, 75] Pneumothorax also results from rupture of pulmonary abscesses secondary to aspirated plant foreign bodies. Rupture of *Paragonimus* spp. or tapeworm cysts in the lungs cause pneumothorax in dogs.[89] Pulmonary arterial thromboembolism secondary to canine dirofilariasis can also result in formation of a pleurobronchial fistula.[74]

Pathophysiological alterations associated with pneumothorax are predominantly associated with inadequate ventilation. Reductions in functional residual capacity and tidal volume cause hypoxemia and respiratory acidosis. Hypoventilation is most evident in patients with a large open pneumothorax. Increases in $(A-a)P_{O_2}$ difference observed in pneumothorax patients suggest that ventilation-perfusion mismatching with increases in physiologic dead space and shunting contribute to hypoxemia.[31, 33] Decreases in cardiac output associated with pneumothorax may eventually reduce pulmonary perfusion and physiological shunting.[31, 41]

Pleural pressure generally remains subatmospheric in a closed pneumothorax except at the end of expiration. Positive pleural pressures develop when a pleuropulmonary fistula functions as a one-way valve, producing a condition known as tension pneumothorax. Tension pneumothorax collapses both the lungs and great veins, causing severe and rapidly fatal reductions in both ventilation and cardiac output.

Diagnosis of pneumothorax is based on characteristic physical and radiographic findings already discussed. Pneumothorax secondary to traumatic rupture of a large airway is often associated with subcutaneous emphysema and radiographic evidence of pneumomediastinum. Pneumothorax resulting from esophageal perforation is likely to show concurrent inflammatory pleural effusion. Open pneumothorax is readily recognized by the presence of a "sucking" thoracic wound. An open abdominal wound may also result in pneumothorax if a diaphragmatic rupture is also present. Pulmonary parenchymal disease is often evident in spontaneous pneumothorax.

Management of traumatic pneumothorax depends on the source, volume, and flow of air into the pleural space. Open thoracic wounds are quickly sealed with an occlusive dressing, and the pleural space is then promptly evacuated of air. Definitive repair of the thoracic wound can usually await stabilization of the patient. A closed pneumothorax that is not causing significant hypoventilation can often be managed by close observation, because pleural air is eventually absorbed. However, if respiratory distress is present, intermittent thoracocentesis or tube thoracostomy is indicated, depending upon the rate of air accumulation. There is no proven advantage to leaving the lungs collapsed if respiratory function is poor. Unresolved pneumothorax can only contribute to the hypoxemia and reduced cardiac output caused by concurrent pulmonary contusion and shock.

Accumulation of pleural air is occasionally so rapid that continuous underwater suction is required to maintain ventilation. Severe pneumothorax often resolves rapidly when managed by continuous underwater suction. Failure to significantly reduce the flow of a pleuropulmonary fistula after five days of continuous suction is an indication for exploratory thoracotomy. Spontaneous pneumothorax is managed by intermittent thoracocentesis or tube thoracostomy, depending on its severity. Spontaneous pneumothorax that either fails to resolve or recurs is an indication for exploratory thoracotomy. Isolated pulmonary lesions creating pleuropulmonary fistulas should be excised by partial or complete lobectomy. When exploratory surgery demonstrates multiple pulmonary bullae or blebs, operative abrasion of the pleural surface with dry gauze is advocated to achieve pleural coaptation.

1. Agostoni, E.: Mechanics of the pleural space. Physiol. Rev. 52:57, 1972.
2. Agostoni, E., and Mead, J.: Statics of the respiratory system. In Fenn, W. O., and Rahn, H. (eds.): The Handbook of Physiology. Sec. 3: Respiration. Vol. 1. American Physiology Society, Washington, D.C., 1964.
3. Armstrong, J.: Nocardial pleuritis in a cat. Can. Vet. J. 21:189, 1980.
4. Barber, B. L., and Hill, D. L.: Traumatically induced lung lesions in the dog: a radiographic report of three cases. J. Am. Vet. Med. Assoc. 169:1085, 1976.
5. Black, L. F.: The pleural space and pleural fluid. Mayo Clin. Proc. 47:493, 1972.
6. Blalock, A., Cunningham, R. S., and Robinson, C. S.: Experimental production of chylothorax by occlusion of the superior vena cava. Ann. Surg. 104:359, 1936.
7. Bell, W.: The hematology of autotransfusion. Surgery 84:695, 1978.
8. Bellenger, C. R., Trim, C., and Sumner-Smith, G.: Bile pleuritis in a dog. J. Small Anim. Pract. 16:575, 1975.
9. Berg, J.: Chylothorax in the dog and cat. Comp. Cont. Educ. 4:986, 1982.
10. Berzon, J. L., Rendano, V. T., and Hoffer, R. E.: Recurrent pneumothorax secondary to ruptured pulmonary blebs: a case report. J Am. Anim. Hosp. Assoc. 15:707, 1979.
11. Bessone, L. N., Ferguson, T. B., and Burford, T. H.: Chylothorax. Ann. Thorac. Surg. 12:527, 1971.
12. Birchard, S. J., Cantwell, H. D., and Bright, R. M.: Lymphangiography and ligation of the canine thoracic duct: a study in normal dogs and three dogs with chylothorax. J. Am. Anim. Hosp. Assoc. 18:769, 1982.
13. Breeze, R. G.: Pleural mesothelioma in a dog. Vet. Rec. 96:243, 1975.
14. Brewer, L. A.: Surgical management of lesions of the thoracic duct. Am. J. Surg. 90:210, 1955.
15. Bron, K. M., Baum, S., and Abrams, H. L.: Oil embolism in lymphangiography. Radiology 80:194, 1963.
16. Bruna, J.: Types of collateral lymphatic circulation. Lymphology 7:61, 1974.
17. Campbell, B., and Scott, D. W.: Successful management of nocardial empyema in a dog and cat. J. Am. Anim. Hosp. Assoc. 11:769, 1975.
18. Cantwell, H. D., Rebar, A. H., and Allen, A. R.: Pleural effusion in the dog: principles for diagnosis. J. Am. Anim. Hosp. Assoc. 19:227, 1983.
19. Cevese, P. G., Vecchioni, R., D'Amico, D. F., et al.: Postoperative chylothorax. J. Thorac. Cardiovasc. Surg. 69:966, 1975.
20. Collins, J. D., Grimes, T. D., Kelly, W. R., et al.: Pleuritis in the dog associated with acinomyces-like organisms. J. Small Anim. Pract. 9:513, 1968.
21. Cox, S. J., and Kinmonth, B. J.: Lymphography of the thoracic duct. J. Cardiovasc. Surg. 16:120, 1975.
22. Crane, S. W.: Surgical management of feline pyothorax. Feline Pract. 6:13, 1976.
23. Creighton, S. R., and Wilkins, R. J.: Thoracic effusions in the cat. J. Am. Anim. Hosp. Assoc. 11:66, 1975.
24. Creighton, S. R., and Wilkins, R. J.: Pleural effusions. In Kirk, R. W. (ed.): Current Veterinary Therapy VII. W. B. Saunders Co., Philadelphia, 1980.
25. Crouch, J. E.: Text-Atlas of Cat Anatomy. Lea & Febiger, Philadelphia, 1969.
26. Crowe, E. D. T.: Autotransfusion of the trauma patient. Vet. Clin. North Am. 10:581, 1980.
27. Davidson, S. J.: Emergency unit autotransfusion. Surgery 84:703, 1978.
28. Donahoe, M., Kneller, S. K., and Thompson, P. E.: Chylothorax subsequent to infection of cats with Dirofilaria immitis. J. Am. Vet. Med. Assoc. 164:1107, 1974.
29. Farrow, C. S.: Exercise in diagnostic radiology. Can. Vet. J. 22:182, 1981.
30. Fellenbaum, S.: A surgical approach to pyothorax in the feline. J. Am. Anim. Hosp. Assoc. 8:259, 1972.
31. Fishman, A. P.: Pulmonary Diseases and Disorders. McGraw-Hill, New York, 1979.
32. Forsythe, W. B.: Surgical anatomy of the thoracic duct in the cat. Feline Pract. 10:38, 1980.
33. Fraser, R. G., and Pare, J. A. P.: Diagnosis of Diseases of the Chest. 2nd ed. W. B. Saunders Co., Philadelphia, 1977.
34. Geary, J. C.: Chronic pleuritis: a sequela to spirocercosis. A case report. Auburn Vet. 20:136, 1964.
35. Giles, R. C., and Hildebrandt, P. K.: Ruptured pulmonary artery in a dog with dirofilariasis. J. Am. Vet. Med. Assoc. 163:236, 1973.
36. Gingell, J. C.: Treatment of chylothorax by producing pleurodesis using iodinized talc. Thorax 20:261, 1965.
37. Gruffydd-Jones, T. J., and Flecknell, P. A.: The prognosis and treatment related to the gross appearance and laboratory characteristics of pathological thoracic fluids in the cat. J. Small Anim. Pract. 19:315, 1978.

38. Harbert, W. B.: Dyspnea due to cystic thoracic duct in a cat. J. Am. Vet. Med. Assoc. *144*:46, 1964.

39. Hau, T., Payne, W. D., and Simmons, R. L.: Fibrinolytic activity of the peritoneum during experimental peritonitis. Surg. Gynecol. Obstet. *148*:415, 1979.

40. Holmberg, D. L.: Management of chylothorax. Vet. Clin. North Am.: Small Anim. Pract. 9:357, 1979.

41. Huber, G. L.: *Arterial Blood Gas and Acid-Base Physiology.* Upjohn Company, Kalamazoo, 1978.

42. Irvin, G. L.: Immunosuppression with lymph depletion in man. Surg. Gynecol. Obstet. *124*:1283, 1967.

43. Jacques, S., Shelden, C. H., Stansbury, R., et al.: The anatomy of the thoracic duct in cats. Feline Pract. 8:46, 1978.

44. Kagan, K. G., and Breznock, E. M.: Variations in the canine thoracic duct system and the effects of surgical occlusion demonstrated by rapid aqueous lymphography using an intestinal lymphatic trunk. Am. J. Vet. Res. *40*:948, 1979.

45. Lampsen, R. S.: Traumatic chylothorax. J. Thorac. Surg. *17*:778, 1948.

46. Legendre, A. M., and Krehbiel, J. D.: Disseminated intravascular coagulation in a dog with hemothorax and hemangiosarcoma. J. Am. Vet Med. Assoc. *171*:1070, 1977.

47. Lindsay, S. E. F.: Chylothorax in the domestic cat: a review. J. Small Anim. Pract. *15*:241, 1974.

48. Liu, S., Weitzman, I., and Johnson, G. G.: Canine tuberculosis. J. Am. Vet. Med. Assoc. *177*:164, 1980.

49. Lord, P. F., Suter, P. F., Chan, K. F., et al.: Pleural, extrapleural and pulmonary lesions in small animals: a radiographic approach to differential diagnosis. J. Am. Vet. Radiol. Soc. *13*:4, 1972.

50. Losonsky, J. M., Prasse, K. W., and Thrall, D. E.: Dyspnea in the cat. Part I: Radiographic aspects of intrathoracic causes involving the pleural space. Feline Pract. 8:35, 1978.

51. McConnell, M. F., and Huxtable, C. R.: Pseudochylous effusion in a cat with cardiomyopathy. Aust. Vet. J. *58*:72, 1982.

52. Meineke, J. E., and Clark, R. E.: Two cases of idiopathic hemothorax in the dog. J. Am. Vet. Med. Assoc. *152*:1776, 1968.

53. Meineke, J. E., Hobbie, W. V., and Barto, L. R.: Traumatic chylothorax with associated diaphragmatic hernias in the cat. J. Am. Vet. Med. Assoc. *155*:15, 1969.

54. Miller, M. E., Christensen, G. C., and Evans, H. E.: *Anatomy of the Dog.* 2nd ed. W. B. Saunders Co., Philadelphia, 1979.

55. Myer, W.: Pneumothorax: a radiographic review. J. Am. Vet. Radiol. Soc. *19*:12, 1978.

56. Myer, W.: Radiology review: pleural effusion. J. Am. Vet. Radiol. Soc. *19*:75, 1978.

57. Neyazaki, T., Kupic, E. A., Marshall, W. H., and Abrams, H. L.: Collateral lymphaticovenous communications after experimental obstruction of the thoracic duct. Radiology *85*:423, 1965.

58. Perman, V., Osborne, C. A., and Stevens, J. B.: Laboratory evaluation of abnormal body fluids. Vet. Clin. North Am. *4*:255, 1974.

59. Perman, V.: Transudates and exudates. *In* Kaneko, J. J., and Cornelius, C. E. (eds.): *Clinical Biochemistry of Domestic Animals.* 2nd ed. Academic Press, New York, 1971.

60. Prasse, K. W., and Duncan, J. R.: Laboratory diagnosis of pleural and peritoneal effusions. Vet. Clin. North Am. 6:625, 1976.

61. Prier, J. E., Schaffer, B., and Skelley, J. S.: Direct lymphangiography in the dog. J. Am. Vet. Med. Assoc. *140*:943, 1962.

62. Quick, C. B.: Chylothorax: a review. J. Am. Anim. Hosp. Assoc. *16*:23, 1980.

63. Quick, C. B., and Jander, H. P.: Aqueous lymphangiography of the canine thoracic duct. J. Vet. Res. *19*:178, 1978.

64. Ramzy, A. I., Rodriguez, A., and Cowley, R. A.: Pitfalls in the management of traumatic chylothorax. J. Trauma *22*:513, 1982.

65. von-Recum, A. F.: The mediastinum and hemothorax, pyothorax, and pneumothorax in the dog. J. Am. Vet. Med. Assoc. *171*:531, 1977.

66. Reed, R. A.: Successful treatment of organizing hemothorax by decortication in a dog: a case report. J. Am. Anim. Hosp. Assoc. *17*:167, 1981.

67. Reif, J. S.: Lung and pleural biopsy. Vet. Clin. North Am. 4:383, 1974.

68. Rigby, M., Zylak, C. J., and Wood, L. B. H.: The effect of lobar atelectasis on pleural fluid distribution in dogs. Radiology *136*:603, 1980.

69. Robins, G., Thornton, J., and Mills, J.: Bile peritonitis and pleuritis in a dog. J. Am. Anim. Hosp. Assoc. *13*:55, 1977.

70. Ross, J. K.: A review of the surgery of the thoracic duct. Thorax *16*:12, 1961.

71. Roudebush, P., and Burns, J.: Pleural effusion as a sequela to traumatic diaphragmatic hernias: a review of four cases. J. Am. Anim. Hosp. Assoc. *15*:699, 1979.

72. Roxin, T., and Bujar, H.: Lymphographic visualization of lymphaticovenous communications and their significance in malignant hemolymphopathies. Lymphology 3:127, 1970.

73. Ryan, W. W., and Green, R. W.: The conservative management of esophageal foreign bodies and their complications: a review of 66 cases in dogs and cats. J. Am. Anim. Hosp. Assoc. *11*:243, 1975.

74. Saheki, Y., Ishitani, R., and Miyamoto, Y.: Acute fatal pneumothorax in canine dirofilariasis. Jap. J. Vet. Sci. *43*:315, 1981.

75. Schaer, M., Gamble, D., and Spencer, C.: Spontaneous pneumothorax associated with bacterial pneumonia in the dog: two case reports. J. Am. Anim. Hosp. Assoc. *17*:783, 1981.

76. Selle, J. G., Snyder, W. H., and Schreiber, J. T.: Chylothorax: indications for surgery. Ann. Surg. *177*:245, 1973.

77. Sherding, R. G.: Pyothorax in the cat. Comp. Cont. Ed. *1*:247, 1979.

78. Skelley, J. F., Prier, J. E., and Koehler, R.: Applications of direct lymphangiography in the dog. Am. J. Vet. Res. *106*:747, 1964.

79. Staats, B. A., Ellefson, R. D., Budahn, L. L., et al.: The lipoprotein profile of chylous and nonchylous pleural effusions. Mayo Clin. Proc. *55*:700, 1980.

80. Stonesifer, C. A., and Moffett, W. F.: Successful treatment of chylothorax in a dog by thoracic duct ligation: a case report. J. Am. Anim. Hosp. Assoc. *10*:286, 1974.

81. Suter, P. F., and Greene, R. W.: Chylothorax in a dog with abnormal termination of the thoracic duct. J. Am. Vet. Med. Assoc. *159*:302, 1971.

82. Suter, P. F., and Sinkl, J. G.: Mediastinal, pleural and extrapleural thoracic diseases. *In* Ettinger, S. J. (ed.): *Textbook of Veterinary Internal Medicine.* W. B. Saunders Co., Philadelphia, 1983.

83. Takashima, T., and Benninghoff, D. L.: Effects of experimental thoracic duct obstruction in the dog. Invest. Radiol. *1*:450, 1966.

84. Takashima, T., and Benninghoff, D. L.: Lymphaticovenous communications and lymph reflux after thoracic duct obstruction. Invest. Radiol. *1*:188, 1966.

85. Tomlinson, J.: Review of pyothorax in the feline. Feline Pract. *10*:26, 1980.

86. Wilkinson, J. G.: Exudative pleurisy in the cat. Vet. Rec. *68*:456, 1956.

87. Wilson, J. L., Herrod, C. M., Searle, G. L., et al.: The absorption of blood from the pleural space. Surgery *48*:766, 1960.

88. Withrow, S. J., Fenner, W. R., and Wilkins, R. J.: Closed chest drainage and lavage for treatment of pyothorax in cats. J. Am. Anim. Hosp. Assoc. *11*:90, 1975.

89. Yoshioka, M. M.: Management of spontaneous pneumothorax in 12 dogs. J. Am. Anim. Hosp. Assoc. *18*:57, 1982.

90. Zajac, S.: Natural lymphaticovenous communications between the cisterna chyli and inferior vena cava. Polish Med. J. *11*:1271, 1972.

Chapter 43

Surgical Approaches to the Abdomen[1,2]

Melvin L. Helphrey

ANATOMY

Surgical entry to the abdominal cavity requires a thorough knowledge of the anatomical structures. The muscles of the abdomen from superficial to deep are the external abdominal oblique, internal abdominal oblique, rectus abdominis, and transversus abdominis (Fig. 43–1). Ventrally, the tendons of the oblique muscles cross the rectus muscle superficially, and the tendon of the transversus abdominis muscle crosses deeply. This forms the rectus sheath. The abdominal muscles are covered superficially by the cutaneous trunci muscle (Fig. 43–2).

The external abdominal oblique muscle covers the ventral half of the thoracic wall and the lateral part of the abdominal wall. Its fibers run caudoventrally and form a very broad, thin aponeurosis in the inguinal region. The muscle is divided into two parts, the pars costalis and the pars lumbalis. The pars costalis is serrated and arises from the last rib and, along with the internal abdominal oblique, forms the primary portion of the thoracolumbar fascia.

The abdominal aponeurosis is large, extending over the rectus abdominis muscle to the pubis and uniting at the linea alba. Caudally it is separated from the pelvic aponeurosis by the inguinal ring. At the inguinal ring, the superficial fascia contains strong fibers that cross the linea alba and pass to the direction of the pectineus muscle of the opposite side. The pelvic aponeurosis is also fused with the deep trunk fascia and forms the lateral wall of the inguinal canal. From the ilium, the inguinal ligament passes over the lateral surface of the iliopsoas muscle and joins the prepubic tendon, forming the caudal borders of the inguinal canal.

The internal abdominal oblique muscle lies medial to the external abdominal oblique, and its fibers run cranioventral. It is divided into the pars costalis and the pars abdominalis. The pars abdominalis has a broad aponeurosis to the lateral border of the rectus abdominis muscle. It merges with the tendon of the external abdominal oblique to form the superficial fascia of the rectus sheath.

The transversus abdominis muscle lies medial to the internal abdominal oblique and is the deepest muscle. The pars lumbalis arises from the transverse processes of all the lumbar vertebrae. The pars costalis arises from the medial aspect of the caudal four ribs. The ventral aponeurosis forms the inner fascia of the rectus sheath and unites at the linea alba with the external rectus sheath.

The rectus abdominis muscle is a long flat muscle that lies between the internal and external rectus sheaths. The fibers run caudally from the first costal cartilage to the pubis. Caudally it forms the medial wall of the inguinal canal.

The preputial muscles radiate from the xiphoid cartilage to the prepuce in the male. Near the umbilicus the paired muscles form a flat band, which attaches to the prepuce near the glans penis. The corresponding muscle in the bitch is a more delicate structure called the supramammarius muscle.

SURGICAL TECHNIQUE

The celiotomy site should be draped in a four-quadrant pattern. The lateral drapes are positioned so that a minimum of skin is exposed to safely perform the celiotomy. A large patient drape covers the entire operating table. All too often, the surgical drape material lining the incision retracts from the wound

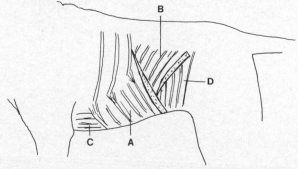

Figure 43–1. Abdominal muscles. *A,* External abdominal oblique; *B,* internal abdominal oblique; *C,* rectus abdominis; *D,* transverse abdominis.

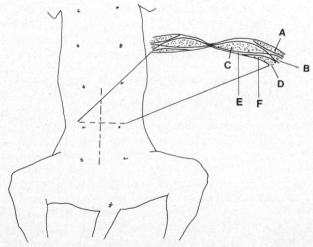

Figure 43–2. *A,* External abdominal oblique; *B,* internal abdominal oblique; *C,* rectus abdominis; *D,* transverse abdominis; *E,* rectus sheath; *F,* peritoneum.

margin after prolonged surgical manipulations of structures in the abdominal cavity. Either more towel clamps may be used to secure the drape every 10 cm along the incision or a water-repellent adhesive surgical drape may be used in celiotomies in which infected or contaminated organs are to be manipulated (e.g., gastrointestinal tract, prostate, abdominal abscesses). For long surgical procedures or when abdominal structures such as the small intestines are retracted from the abdominal cavity, such a drape helps prevent contamination of the abdomen.

The length of a celiotomy incision varies based on the surgical procedure performed. Although it has been accurately stated that wounds heal from side to side, it has also been noted that they are closed from end to end. The incision should be long enough to accomplish the surgical procedure safely; excessively long incisions create a larger wound and are unnecessary.

After the skin incision is made, subcutaneous vessels should be ligated or cauterized to prevent postoperative seroma or hematoma formation. Undermining of the subcutaneous tissue should be avoided for the same reason. The linea alba is lifted with a pair of thumb forceps cranial to the umbilicus, and a blade, positioned with the sharp side upward, is used to penetrate the abdominal wall. Unless there are adhesions to the ventral abdominal wall this is a safe way to enter the abdominal cavity. A finger may be inserted into the incision to examine for abdominal adhesions before completing the incision. Also, a grooved director may be used to protect the abdominal tissues from damage if the blade is positioned downward to penetrate the linea alba.

The falciform ligament may be removed if it improves exposure. If proper technique is used, the falciform ligament is not needed to prevent wound dehiscence.

Balfour abdominal retractors can be invaluable in retracting the abdominal wall when operating alone. Moist laparotomy sponges should be placed on the wound edges to protect the soft tissues from the pressure of the retractors. Warm saline solution should be used liberally to keep the exposed abdominal tissues moist. Hot surgery lights can cause tissue damage through dessication. The talc from surgery gloves can be very irritating to the tissues and should, therefore, be rinsed off with lavage solution prior to making the incision.

There are no absolute rules regarding the type of suture material or pattern to be used in closure of an abdominal wound. A simple interrupted pattern of absorbable suture is generally considered standard procedure. If nonabsorbable suture is used it should be monofilament to avoid capillary action. The monofilament nonabsorbable materials (except stainless steel) do not hold knots well; therefore at least four knots should be used. In geriatric patients or animals with low serum proteins or poor nutrition, it is better to use a nonabsorbable material that will last long enough to protect the suture line from dehiscence.

Monofilament stainless steel wire or synthetic nonabsorbable suture should be used.

The choice of continuous or interrupted suture pattern is left to the surgeon. A continuous pattern should be used if the patient's health is in immediate danger and if the time saved using a continuous pattern will save the animal's life. Complications of using the continuous pattern include wound dehiscence due to breakage of the suture. If the suture breaks before the wound heals, the entire suture line is subject to failure.

Ventral Midline Approach

The ventral midline approach is most frequently used for a celiotomy (Fig. 43–3). Surgery of most abdominal organs may be adequately accomplished with this approach. However, proper evaluation and manipulation of the biliary system and liver may be more easily accomplished through a paracostal or combination ventral midline and paracostal incision.

A ventral midline incision is carried caudal to the umbilicus in the male and is then made lateral to the prepuce. The preputial incision is made far enough lateral to prevent undue postoperative tissue swelling of the prepuce. The skin incision is made where the preputial skin is firmly attached to the body wall and is slightly longer than the celiotomy incision to facilitate adequate visualization and closure of the linea alba. The preputial myotomy must be made anterolateral to the prepuce. A branch of the caudal superficial epigastric artery is evident in the area of the preputial muscle. The prepuce is reflected to the opposite side of the incision and the subcutaneous dissection carried to the linea alba. The subcutaneous tissue should not be unnecessarily undermined while trying to locate the linea alba. There should be minimal bleeding if the surgeon stays on the linea alba.

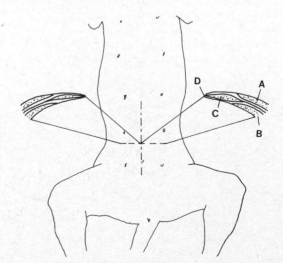

Figure 43–3. The ventral midline approach. A, External abdominal oblique; B, transverse abdominis; C, rectus abdominis; D, linea alba.

Closure consists of simple interrupted sutures through the linea alba. Care must be taken to close the fascial sheath if the incision was inadvertently made lateral to the linea alba (a paramedian incision). If the incision was made on the linea alba, the closure automatically secures the fascia and peritoneum. Research has demonstrated that closure of the peritoneum is not necessary for prevention of abdominal wound dehiscence.[3] This does not mean there should not be an attempt to close the peritoneum, but if it is not included in the closure the abdominal incision will heal as long as the abdominal fascia is securely apposed. After the abdominal muscles are approximated, the preputial muscle is sutured before any subcutaneous sutures are placed. This provides more accurate alignment of the prepuce and penis.

Paramedian Approach

The paramedian approach allows better examination of one side of the abdomen than the other. It is made parallel, but lateral, to the linea alba. The incision is made through the skin, fascia of the external abdominal oblique muscle, belly of the rectus abdominis muscle, fascia of the transversus abdominis muscle, and peritoneum. If the incision is made just off midline, only the rectus abdominis muscle will be penetrated (Fig. 43–4). Because the belly of the rectus abdominis muscle must be cut, the paramedian incision results in more bleeding than the ventral midline incision. Closure consists of apposing the peritoneum and inner fascia and then muscle with simple interrupted sutures.

Flank Approach

The flank approach is used to gain entry to the lateral abdomen. This may be used for surgery of the

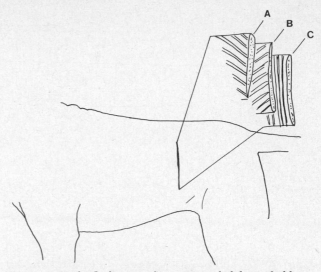

Figure 43–5. The flank approach. *A,* External abdominal oblique; *B,* internal abdominal oblique; *C,* transverse abdominis.

kidney or for an ovariohysterectomy. Because the cat has such a narrow abdomen, this approach allows easy access to the ovaries and uterus through a small incision. Most owners are reluctant to have the side of their animal shaved just for an ovariohysterectomy. The skin is incised ventral to the lumbar spine in a dorsoventral direction. The fascia of the external abdominal oblique, internal abdominal oblique, and transversus abdominis muscles are incised longitudinally and the muscle fibers bluntly dissected (Fig. 43–5). The peritoneum in this area is a thin structure that is penetrated by the transversus abdominis muscle. Biopsy of the kidney and other minor procedures may be accomplished safely through this approach. If the surgical procedure requires better exposure, a ventral midline approach is preferred.

Individual muscular layers of the incision are closed with simple interrupted absorbable suture. Adequate hemostasis is important to prevent hematoma or seroma formation postoperatively.

Paracostal Approach

The paracostal approach is used to gain lateral exposure to the anterior abdomen. This approach may be useful in surgery of the thoracic duct, portal and hepatic veins, caudal vena cava, and adrenal glands.

With the animal in lateral recumbency, a curvilinear skin incision is made 1 cm caudal to the last rib from the ventral spinal column to within 1 cm of the ventral midline. The incision is made 1 cm caudal to the last rib to assure ample tissue for a secure closure. The incision is carried through the internal abdominal oblique muscle dorsally and the external abdominal oblique, internal abdominal oblique, and rectus abdominis muscles ventrally (Fig. 43–6). The peritoneum is easily penetrated with a blade or sharp scissors. This approach provides access to the liver

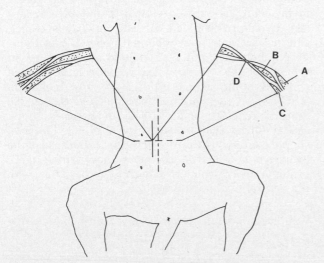

Figure 43–4. The paramedian approach. *A,* External abdominal oblique; *B,* rectus abdominis; *C,* transverse abdominis; *D,* linea alba.

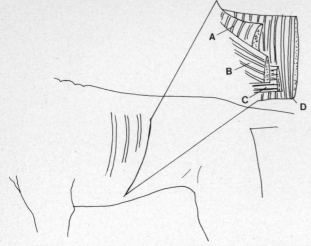

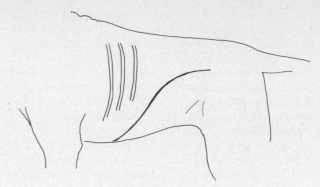

Figure 43–8. The paralumbar-paracostal approach.

Figure 43–6. The paracostal approach. *A*, Internal abdominal oblique; *B*, external abdominal oblique; *C*, rectus abdominis; *D*, transverse abdominis.

and structures dorsal, cranial, and caudal to it. From a right paracostal incision the thoracic duct may be seen by incising the muscular diaphragm and reflecting the medial portion caudally. This exposes the caudal thoracic structures.

Closure of the surgical approach consists of single layers of simple interrupted absorbable sutures. The peritoneum need not be closed separately.

Ventral Midline–Paracostal Approach

During a routine celiotomy via a ventral midline incision, adequate visualization or manipulation of the described organ, for instance the liver, may not be possible. A paracostal incision may be combined with the ventral midline approach (Fig. 43–7). A curvilinear incision is made dorsally from the xiphoid 1 cm caudal to the last rib. The incision is carried

dorsally to provide adequate exposure. Surgery of the liver and biliary system may occasionally require such an extensive approach.

Closure begins with approximation of the triangle formed by the combined incisions at the xiphoid. This will give proper alignment to the incisions, each of which are closed with simple interrupted sutures. The paracostal incision is closed in single layers, whereas the ventral midline is closed in one layer along the linea alba.

Paralumbar-Paracostal Approach

The paralumbar-paracostal incision, when combined with a transdiaphragmatic approach, is used to enter the thoracic and abdominal cavities from a lateral approach. This allows access to the caudal thoracic structures. When performed on the right side, this approach allows exposure of the portal vein, abdominal vena cava, intestines, liver, thoracic vena cava, and azygous vein. Therefore this approach may be used when exploring such anomalies as portal-azygous shunts or when exposure of the thoracic and abdominal structures may be more easily accomplished from a lateral approach. The incision is started in the flank and carried cranial to the last rib in a lazy S pattern (Fig. 43–8). The cutaneous trunci, external and internal abdominal oblique, and transversus abdominis muscles and peritoneum are incised separately. The paracostal incision can be carried ventrally to the xiphoid if necessary. The diaphragm is incised in the muscular portion, and the medial aspect is reflected caudally. This allows access to the caudal thorax. Closure consists of single layers of simple continuous absorbable sutures. Because of the extensive muscle trauma, dogs may exhibit more postoperative discomfort with this approach than with the ventral midline approach.

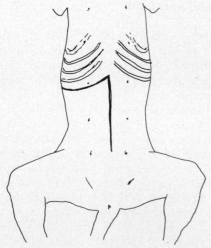

Figure 43–7. The ventral midline–paracostal approach.

1. Archibald, J., et al.: *Canine Surgery*, 2nd ed. American Veterinary Publications, Inc., Santa Barbara, 1974, pp. 51–53.
2. Lipowitz, A. J., and Schenk, M. P.: Surgical approaches to the abdominal and thoracic viscera of the dog and cat. Vet. Clin. North Am. 9:169, 1979.
3. Ward, G. W.: Abdominal wound disruption in the dog. Masters Thesis, Washington State University, 1967.

44 Peritoneum and Peritoneal Cavity

Dennis T. Crowe, Jr. and Dale E. Bjorling

The peritoneum is the serous membrane that lines the abdominal cavity. This chapter discusses surgical management of diseases of the peritoneum and peritoneal cavity including peritonitis, peritoneal defects, hemoperitoneum, urine peritoneum, chylous peritoneum, pneumoperitoneum, adhesions and abscesses, and peritoneal tumors.

EMBRYOLOGY[38, 78]

The embryonic coelom is formed by division of lateral mesoderm into splanchnic and somatic layers. The intraembryonic coelom is the precursor of the body cavities (pericardial, pleural, and peritoneal) of the adult. The splanchnic membrane swings to the midline surrounding the gut and forms the primary mesentery, which divides the coelom into right and left halves. The liver develops from the gut and pushes into the ventral mesentery. The pancreas also develops from the gut in the dorsal mesentery of the rudimentary duodenum. The spleen is formed in the dorsal mesogastrum. As the embryo enlarges, the dorsal mesentery remains to suspend the gut from the dorsal body wall, but the ventral mesentery disappears except for the falciform ligament, lesser omentum, and suspensory ligaments of the bladder. The septum transversum arises from mesenchymal tissue of the ventral body wall and eventually forms the ventral portion of the diaphragm. Rupture of the septum in embryonic life has been postulated as the most probable explanation for the common congenital pericardial-peritoneal hernia in which there is a defect in the central tendinous region of the diaphragm.

As the embryo continues to develop, the foregut rotates, bringing the spleen and greater curvature of the stomach to the left and the duodenum and pancreas to the right. The remnant of the ventral mesentery containing the developing liver shifts to the right, forming the lesser omentum. Other organs develop intraperitoneally, carrying the peritoneum, which covers them inwardly. The visceral peritoneum lies on the surface of intra-abdominal organs, and the parietal peritoneum lines the inner walls of the abdominal, pelvic, and scrotal cavities. Ligaments connecting intra-abdominal organs are formed as organs shift and peritoneal surfaces contact each other.

Final closure of the central areas of the diaphragm by the pleuroperitoneal and pericardioperitoneal membranes completes the division between the thoracic and abdominal cavities. Contributions to this final closure come from the development of diaphragmatic muscles innervated by the phrenic nerve. Congenital defects may result if the normal sequence of events during embryonic growth is disturbed or if development stops prior to completion.

ANATOMY[23, 39]

Gross Anatomy

The abdomen extends from the diaphragm to the pelvis. It contains the abdominal cavity, the largest cavity in the body. Caudally, the abdominal cavity is continuous with the pelvic cavity, the division between them being a transverse plane through the pelvic inlet (apertura pelvis cranialis) or brim of the pelvis. Cranially, the abdominal cavity is limited by the diaphragm. The lateral and ventral walls are formed by the abdominal muscles and the eighth through the thirteenth ribs. The vertebral column (from T_{13} caudally) and the muscles associated with it form the dorsal wall. It is lined internally by the *transversalis fascia*, which is covered by the parietal peritoneum.

The peritoneal cavity formed by the peritoneum is contained largely but not exclusively within the abdominal cavity. In both sexes of the dog and cat, the pelvic cavity contains the pelvic portion of the peritoneal cavity. Vaginal processes, represented as peritoneal outpouchings investing the round ligament in the female and the spermatic cord and testicle in the male, also exist as "extra-abdominal portions" of the peritoneal cavity.

The abdominal cavity and its wall may be divided by two sagittal and two transverse planes (Fig. 44–1A). A more practical division divides the abdomen into four quadrants by one transverse and one sagittal line through the umbilicus, thus creating the cranial right, cranial left, caudal right, and caudal left quadrants (Fig. 44–1B). The terms *right* and *left paravertebral gutters* are used to designate the troughlike regions in the dorsal abdominal cavity to the right and left of the vertebral column. They appear as "gutters" where fluid collects when viewing the abdominal cavity from a ventral approach with the patient supine.

Natural Openings

In the cat and dog there are three unpaired openings leading into the abdominal cavity through the diaphragm: the *esophageal hiatus*, for passage of the

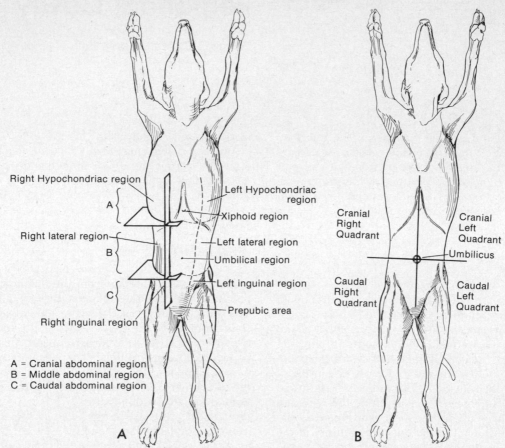

Figure 44–1. *A*, The abdominal cavity divided by two sagittal and two transverse planes. (Modified from Evans, H. E., and Christensen, G. C. (eds.): *Miller's Anatomy of the Dog*, 2nd ed. W. B. Saunders, Philadelphia, 1979.) *B*, The abdominal cavity divided by one sagittal and one transverse plane intersecting at the umbilicus and resulting in four quadrants: cranial and caudal right and cranial and caudal left.

esophagus, vagus nerve trunks, and esophageal vessels; the *vena caval hiatus*, for passage of the caudal vena cava; and the *aortic hiatus*, for passage of the aorta, lumbar cistern of the thoracic duct, and the azygos and hemiazygos veins. Paired slit like openings, dorsal to the diaphragm, are formed ventrally by the dorsal edge of the diaphragm (arcus lumbocostalis) and dorsally by the psoas muscles. At these sites the pleura and peritoneum are separated only by a thin layer of fused endothoracic and transversalis fascia. This has clinical importance in the understanding of how certain disease processes in the thoracic cavity (pneumothorax, pyothorax) can, by direct extension, lead to similar entities within the abdominal cavity (pneumoperitoneum, purulent peritonitis). The sympathetic trunk and splanchnic nerves enter the abdominal cavity in the same area, dorsal to the lumbocostal arch on each side.

Umbilicus

In the fetus, the umbilical aperture, a relatively large opening, is located midventrally. Two umbilical arteries and the single umbilical vein; the small vitelline (omphalomesenteric) duct, artery, and vein; and the stalk of the allantois pass through it. The opening becomes smaller as the fetus develops, with growth and migration of the abdominal musculature and fascia originating from the somatopleure and lower thoracic and upper lumbar somites. After the umbilical cord is disrupted at birth, the umbilical aperture rapidly closes, forming a faint *umbilical scar* on the ventral midline.

Inguinal and Pelvic Canals

The fissure between the abdominal muscles and their aponeuroses on each side of the caudal ventral part of the abdominal wall is called the inguinal canal. This contains the vaginal process and associated intraperitoneal structures. In both sexes the external pudendal artery and vein and the genital nerve pass through the caudal portion of each canal. Another pair of abdominal openings in the caudal part of the abdominal wall are the right and left *vascular lacunae*. The femoral artery and vein, lymphatics, and saphenous nerve surrounded by a short projection of transversalis fascia pass through each lacuna.

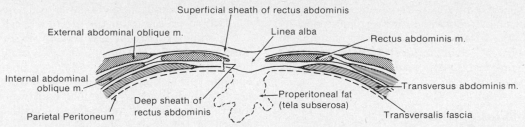

Figure 44–2. A sagittal section through the cranial portion of the ventral abdominal wall and peritoneum. Note the properitoneal fat in the falciform ligament and the reflection of the peritoneum on the inner aspect of the falciform.

Caudally, the abdominal cavity communicates freely with the pelvic cavity at the pelvic inlet. The pelvic cavity, a division of the abdominal cavity, is bounded dorsally by the sacrum and first coccygeal vertebra, laterally by the ilia, and cranially and caudally by the coccygeus, levator ani, and middle gluteal muscles. The pelvic cavity ends at the pelvic outlet (apertura pelvis caudalis), which is bounded dorsally by the first coccygeal vertebra and accompanying sacrococcygeal muscles, ventrally by the ischial arch, and bilaterally by the middle gluteal muscles. In the dog, the sacrotuberous ligament (absent in the cat) also contributes to the lateral boundary. Normally in the dog and cat the pelvic cavity contains the rectum and urethra in both sexes, the vagina and part of the vestibule in the female, and part or all of the prostate in the male.

Transversalis Fascia

The abdominal and pelvic cavities are lined by fascia throughout. In most places this fascia attaches to muscles or bone peripherally and blends with the subserous areolar tissue centrally. The fascia can be named according to the region or parts covered (e.g., diaphragmatic, iliac, internal spermatic, and pelvic fascia). The term *transversalis fascia* is used to include all of these fascial divisions. The subserous areolar tissue (tela subserosa) forms the medium whereby the peritoneum is united with the transversalis fascia (Fig. 44–2). Fat is commonly deposited between the peritoneum and transversalis fascia in this tela subserosal layer. This is particularly evident on the ventral midline when an incision through the ventral fascia, including the transversalis fascia, reveals a large accumulation of *properitoneal* fat within the falciform ligament. The peritoneal cavity in this instance has not been entered, even though all of the ventral muscle and fascial layers have been divided and the "abdomen opened." This can commonly be done along the entire length of the falciform ligament from the xyphoid to the umbilicus (Fig. 44–3). Large accumulations of fat in the subserous layer are also common in the pelvis and around the kidneys and the inguinal rings.

Retroperitoneum

Retroperitoneal organs lie against the walls of the abdominal or pelvic cavities and are covered on only one surface by parietal peritoneum. In the dog and cat these structures include the kidney, ureter, aorta, adrenal glands, lumbar (para-aortic) lymph nodes, vena cava, and diaphragm. In a strict sense the entire gastrointestinal tract and its derivatives are retroperitoneal in position. However, it is customary to speak of those structures that are almost completely enfolded by peritoneum as intraperitoneal. There are

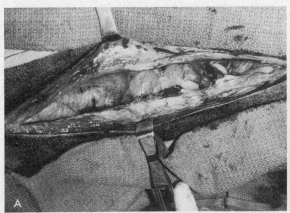
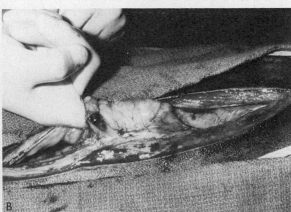

Figure 44–3. A, An incision has been made through the ventral midline linea alba including the transversalis fascia. The abdominal wall is opened, revealing the properitoneal fat (tela subserosa) of the falciform ligament. The peritoneal cavity is not open. B, Opened peritoneal cavity with finger inserted under the properitoneal fat.

important species differences regarding which organs are intraperitoneal and which are retroperitoneal by these definitions; for example, in the nonhuman primate, pancreas, duodenum, urinary bladder, and uterus are considered retroperitoneal. This is not the case in the dog or cat.

Greater and Lesser Sacs

The peritoneal cavity is divided into the general peritoneal cavity, or greater sac, and the lesser sac, which has the epiploic foramen as its only natural opening. The lesser sac, also known as the omental bursa or lesser peritoneal cavity, is completely collapsed in life. This potentially large cavity is mainly enclosed by the omentum. The other boundaries, located cranially, are the visceral wall of the stomach, the caudate lobe of the liver, and the left lobe of the pancreas.

The *epiploic foramen*, bounded dorsally by the caudal vena cava and ventrally by the portal vein, has surgical significance. By placing a finger through the epiploic foramen into the lesser sac just cranial to the pylorus of the stomach and then curling the finger around the structures ventral to it, the entire blood supply to the liver (hepatic artery and portal vein) is occluded. This technique can be used successfully to temporarily arrest bleeding resulting from life-threatening hemorrhage from the liver.[21] Loops of small intestine can also migrate through the epiploic foramen, leading to strangulation.

Microscopic Anatomy[2]

The peritoneum is a serous membrane made up of a single layer of squamous cells of mesothelial origin and a deeper, loose, connective tissue layer containing collagen and elastic fibers, fat cells, reticulum cells, and macrophages. The connective tissue layer is histologically the largest component of the peritoneum. In most areas of the peritoneal cavity, the mesothelial cells form a carpet of closely packed, flattened squamous cells with indistinct boundaries covered with numerous microvilli. On the diaphragm, however, special lymphatic collecting vessels (lacunae) are present just beneath the mesothelial basement membrane. Small stomata (8 to 12 μm in diameter) are found between the mesothelial cells and serve as openings and channels by which lymph from the peritoneal cavity enters the lacunae and efferent ducts.

Macroscopically or with low magnification, the peritoneum is a thin, transparent membrane that can be easily disrupted by digital pressure. The parietal and visceral peritoneum forms a closed sac except in females. In the bitch and queen there is an opening at the abdominal end of each uterine tube through the genital tract to the outside. This has clinical

importance because the opening is an avenue by which bacteria can enter the peritoneal cavity.[77]

No organs or tissues are actually located in the peritoneal cavity. The peritoneal cavity itself is almost nonexistent in the normal animal, containing only enough lubricating fluid to moisten the apposed peritoneal surfaces (< 1 ml/kg body weight). The fluid is clear and slightly yellowish, with a specific gravity of less than 1.016 and less than 3 gm/dl of protein, predominantly albumin. Fibrinogen is not present, and the fluid does not clot.[2] Normal peritoneal fluid contains 2,000 to 2,500 cells/mm³. The majority of these are macrophages (approximately 50 per cent). Forty per cent are lymphocytes. A few are eosinophils, mast cells, and desquamated mesothelial cells. There are usually very few polymorphonuclear neutrophils, but the number of granulocytes greatly increases with inflamation.[85]

The peritoneal fluid also contains fibrinectin, a nonspecific bacteria-opsonizing protein. Solute concentrations are nearly the same as those seen in plasma.

PHYSIOLOGY[2, 46, 69]

The surface area of the peritoneum is roughly one to one and one-half times that of the skin. Unlike the skin, however, the peritoneum is a highly permeable membrane. Most of this membrane behaves as a passive, semipermeable lining for the *diffusion* of water and low molecular weight solutes. This explains why peritoneal dialysis is an effective treatment for chronic renal failure. Peritoneal fluid is constantly being formed and absorbed. Water, electrolytes, and urea are rapidly transported across the peritoneal membrane along with detrimental agents such as bacterial toxins. During peritoneal dialysis, hyperosmolar solutions can induce a net flow of 300 to 500 ml $H_2O/h/m^2$ surface area into the peritoneal space.[2] The intensity of fluid flow can be increased by agents that increase local splanchnic blood flow or vascular permeability. Inflammatory processes have a similar effect, so that hypovolemic shock rapidly becomes an important cause of death in patients with peritonitis.

Red blood cells, bacteria, and particulate matter can be absorbed via the special lympatic collecting vessels (lacunae). Passive stretching of the peritoneum, particularly that associated with the diaphragm, results in an influx of cells and particles through the stomata into the lacunae. Contraction of the diaphragm empties the lymphatic fluid containing the red cells and other materials into efferent ducts. A simultaneous drop in intrathoracic pressure assists in the process. During exhalation reverse flow is prevented by one-way valves in the thoracic lymphatics. Red blood cells are absorbed intact by this process and can be found in the circulation within 20 minutes after their placement into the peritoneal cavity. The size of the stomata of the lacunae determines the maximum size of particles that are readily absorbed. Only a few particles 20 μm in diameter can be absorbed, but those 10 μm in diameter pass easily.[3]

Bacteria, which average 0.5 to 2 μm in size, are cleared rapidly from the peritoneal cavity by the lymphatic absorption process. Following their placement into the peritoneal cavity of dogs, they have been recoverable from the right thoracic lymph duct within 6 minutes and from the blood within 12 minutes.[93]

Many other substances are readily absorbed through the peritoneum by passive diffusion. Some of these substances include drugs that have been used intraperitoneally, including antibiotics, antibacterial agents such as providone iodine, barbiturates, and iron dextran.[84] In the same manner that protein collects in the interstitial spaces owing to leakage out of capillaries, so does it accumulate in the peritoneal cavity. This protein, predominately albumin, must be removed constantly to prevent the accumulation of fluid and electrolytes within the peritoneal cavity secondary to a colloid osmotic gradient. The majority of this protein is removed by the lymphatics. Fluid averaging 2 gm of albumin per dl passes through the peritoneal cavity in this dynamically active process[2] at the rate of approximately 80 ml/kg body weight/day.[2] Increased capillary permeability, increased capillary pressure, decreased plasma osmotic pressure, and blockage of the peritoneal lymphatics can lead to accumulations of fluid within the peritoneal cavity.

Lymphatic Drainage

Lymph drains from the peritoneal cavity of the dog through four routes.[51] Sternal lymph nodes receive about four-fifths of the total lymphatic effluent arising from the peritoneal cavity. The lymphatic vessels extend cranially through the ventral portion of the diaphragm to lymph nodes in the region of the second rib. Mediastinal lymph nodes receive lymphatic vessels from the cranial part of the peritoneal cavity, especially the peritoneal surface of the diaphragm. Many of these vessels enter the chest near the esophageal hiatus. Dorsal abdominal lymphatic vessels empty into the cisterna chyli and thoracic duct. Several retroperitoneal lymphatic vessels converge dorsally and unite with the thoracic duct. These vessels drain the region of the kidney and adrenal glands. The mesenteric lymphatics chiefly drain the intestine and not the peritoneal cavity. The omental lymphatics hold and isolate foreign material in the peritoneal cavity and transport smaller particles from the peritoneal cavity into larger channels.

Lymphatic drainage from the diaphragmatic peritoneum is the major means of keeping the peritoneal cavity from filling with fluid. The diaphragm acts as a muscular pump, contracting to drive the fluid into the lymphatics, as in particulate absorption. Fluid and particulate clearance from the peritoneal cavity can be increased by factors that increase diaphragmatic lymph flow, including hyperventilation, hyperperistalsis, increased intra-abdominal pressure, and placing the animal in a head-down position.

Blockage of the lymphatics from the peritoneum is a common cause of the accumulation of fluid in the peritoneal cavity. Other causes include an increase in capillary permeability or pressure and a decrease in plasma colloid osmotic pressure. The fluid is generally a transudate unless it is associated with inflammation. Inflammation, with the attendant increase in leukocytes and debris, leads to blockage of the lymphatics. This results in a build-up of protein in the peritoneal cavity with increases in colloid osmotic pressure of peritoneal fluid. This leads to the attraction of further fluid from the intravascular and interstitial spaces.

Capillary-Peritoneal Pressure

The peritoneal cavity is more susceptible to accumulation of excessive quantities of fluids than most of the other body cavities because the pressure in the capillaries of the visceral peritoneum is higher than that seen elsewhere. This is caused by the resistance to portal blood flow through the liver. Normal portal vein pressure is 10 to 14 mm Hg, compared with 2 to 5 mm Hg in the caudal vena cava. The high resistance offered by the liver frequently results in the formation of ascites when liver lesions, such as cirrhosis, are present. When the portal system is blocked, or even partially occluded, the return of blood from the intestines, stomach, pancreas, and spleen to the systemic circulation is impeded. Capillary pressure may rise as much as 20 to 30 mm Hg, and death may ensue within a few hours because of excessive fluid loss from the capillaries into the lumen of the intestines and into the peritoneal cavity.

Considerable distension of the peritoneal cavity is necessary before an increase in pressure within the abdomen itself is seen. The addition of 20 ml/kg body weight of fluid to the peritoneal cavity of a normal dog elevates pressure from 0 to a maximum of 5 mm Hg.[28] Normal pressure in the peritoneal cavity averages about 2 mm Hg (range − 5 to 7 mm Hg).[27] A relative negative pressure in the cranial portion of the peritoneal cavity is present when compared with the caudal portion. This is due to the removal of fluid and protein via the diaphragmatic lymphatics. Ascites or large intra-abdominal tumors or cysts may cause an increase in peritoneal pressure. Increased pressure acts as an extravascular compressive force on the caudal vena cava. With increased intra-abdominal pressure, femoral vein pressure must also increase to allow venous drainage from the pelvic limbs. Collateral venous drainage through the vertebral and epigastric veins helps prevent venous engorgement and limb edema.[28]

Innervation of the Peritoneum

Although the visceral peritoneum has little sensory innervation, the afferent fibers may detect stimuli that are sufficiently strong or prolonged, particularly in the presence of pre-existing inflammation. *The root of the mesentery is quite sensitive to traction*.

Most visceral afferent nerve fibers for *pain* run in the *splanchnic* nerves to the same cord segments that receive somatic afferent fibers. Visceral afferent nerve endings are most responsive to tension, which may be the result of increased tissue pressure from inflammation.

It is believed that most "painful" responses exhibited by animals during examination are due to stimuli perceived by the somatic afferent nerve endings in the parietal peritoneum. The ability of the parietal peritoneum of the ventral abdominal wall to initiate the sensation of pain in response to an adjacent inflammatory or irritating focus and permit localization of its origin is important in the diagnosis of acute abdominal conditions. In addition to causing the sensation of pain, stimulation of the parietal peritoneum may cause involuntary rigidity of the abdominal musculature.

Sympathetic (splanchnic) and parasympathetic visceral efferent nerve fibers primarily innervate the intra-abdominal organs, but they also supply the visceral and parietal peritoneum to a lesser degree. The efferent signals in the parasympathetic system come via the vagus and pelvic nerves and ganglia. The sympathetic nerves to the cranial abdominal viscera are from the greater and lesser splanchnic nerves. The caudal abdominal viscera receive fibers from the lumbar splanchnic nerves. The nerve fibers follow arteries leading to the abdominal viscera. With irritation of the peritoneal cavity, certain responses in the dog and cat are prominent.

Vomiting

This is often due to peritoneal irritation. It is a response that may be transmitted by the splanchnic or vagus nerves. In dogs, sectioning of the vagi or splanchnic nerves alone does not abolish vomiting associated with peritonitis. However, when both are cut in the same animal, peritonitis does not cause vomiting. Pain is also abolished.[69]

Almost all of the pain fibers in the abdominal viscera join the sphanchnic nerves.[39] The vagus nerves carry no impulses for pain. When the vagi are cut in the thorax, gastric retention and atony may result, but obscure abdominal pain is not relieved. For this, celiac and cranial mesenteric ganglionectomy is necessary.[69]

Hiccough

Hiccoughing (spasmotic contractions of the diaphragm) is a distressing effect of peritoneal irritation and is seen rarely. Its mechanism is unknown.

Ileus

Paralytic or adynamic ileus is one of the major effects of stimulation of the splanchnic nerves. Intraperitoneal manipulation generally abolishes intestinal peristaltic movements. The length of time the movements stop is directly related to species, amount of peritoneal irritation, and continuaton of peritoneal irritation. In dogs and cats, ileus primarily affects the stomach and colon.[75] It lasts a few hours with moderate visceral handling during laparotomy. The peristaltic activity of the small intestines following laparotomy usually resumes quickly.[69]

In awake dogs, the intraperitoneal instillation of gastric juice (5 ml/kg) resulted in the cessation of mechanical intestinal activity in the immediate post-instillation period. Inhibition lasted several hours, but intestinal motility was nearly normal the following day. Instillation of gastric juice was repeated for four consecutive days and did not cause progressive deterioration or delay in the return of bowel function.[1] Experimentally created gastric perforation and leakage almost completely inhibited intestinal activity within 24 hours.[75] If significant peritoneal irritation persists, as with bacterial peritonitis, intestinal ileus generally is prolonged in both cats and dogs, lasting as long as the peritonitis continues. However, active bowel motility may occur with severe peritonitis.

HEALING OF PERITONEAL INJURY AND DEFECTS

The mesothelium of the peritoneal cavity is so easily damaged that it sloughs even after exposure to air or saline.[108] Regeneration is rapid, and the healing of denuded or debrided peritoneum is usually complete within five to seven days regardless of the defect's size. This healing has been termed *reperitonealization*. A few hours after creation of a defect, round cells are observed covering the denuded subserosal surfaces.[108] Reperitonealization can also occur by spontaneous adherence of nearby structures that have a mesothelial surface.

Healing of debrided parietal peritoneum without adhesion formation was first described in 1888.[104] Reperitonealization in this case occurs by (1) mesothelial cell deposition onto the denuded surface or (2) proliferation of mesothelial cells from the depths of the wound.[66] Because peritoneal healing occurs with equal speed regardless of the size of the original defect, healing by epithelial cell migration from the edges of the defect, like that of skin, is not common.[50] Monocytes or submesothelial macrophages may also be deposited onto the denuded surface and differentiate into mesothelial cells. Wound fibroblasts may also be a source of mesothelial cells seen on peritoneal wounds.

Abdominal wounds with loss of transversalis fascia have been studied. Macroscopically, two days after injury the surface of the defect is glistening and irregular. At five days the surface is a transparent gray and smooth and homogeneous. Tissues glide across the wound without friction. As time passes the gray color gradually becomes more opaque and the wound becomes difficult to distinguish from the rest of the peritoneum. An occasonal white streak of scar tissue below the smooth surface or an indentation indicating where a muscular defect was is often the only persistent sign of previous injury.[2] Microscopically, the healing of peritoneum may be divided into stages similar to the healing stages of other wounds, i.e., lag, inflammatory, fibroblastic, and maturational stages.

Healing of denuded or debrided peritoneum or wounds involving loss of underlying transversalis fascia may also involve reperitonealization by a spontaneous or deliberate creation of an adherence of a nearby serosa-lined structure. This adherent type of peritoneal healing occurs spontaneously if the inflammatory phase of healing is accentuated by bacteria, devitalized tissue, or foreign materials. Suturing of peritoneal defects or intentional reperitonealization also increases adherent healing.[35] Localized tissue hypoxemia caused by the placement of sutures in the peritoneum has been implicated as the main reason adherence occurs in peritoneal wounds that are intentionally closed.[35] Serosal injury during the placement of sutures and the presence the suture itself are also implicated. Because adherent healing is not ideal in the healing of ventral abdominal incisions, numerous investigators have examined the healing achieved if the parietal peritoneum is intentionally not sutured.[24, 86, 89]

In ventral abdominal incisions, the majority of support for closure comes from the external rectus sheath and abdominal fascia. Less support is contributed by the internal rectus sheath, which includes the transversalis fascia. The peritoneum does not provide any strength to the wound. The results of the investigations have revealed that it is unnecessary to suture the peritoneum. If left unsutured, there is less adherent peritoneal healing and no increase in dehiscence or poor wound healing.[24, 86, 89] If closure of the deeper abdominal fascia, e.g., internal rectus sheath, is necessary, as in the closure of a large abdominal defect or in large obese patients, the suture chosen should be a nonreactive type and as little peritoneum as possible should be incorporated.

In special situations adherent peritoneal healing is sought and has been found very useful. With diseases or injury involving large defects in the deep abdominal fascia and parietal peritoneum, omental covering speeds peritonealization and prevents adherence of other intra-abdominal visceral structures. The omen-

tum also produces significant vascular ingrowth and assists in treatment of ischemic tissues.[36] In situations requiring vascular support or peritoneal coverage, the omentum is used as a pedicle graft and sutured over the area involved. The omentum may also migrate spontaneously and adhere to denuded areas without surgery.

Adhesions

Adhesions are fibrinous or fibrous bands that form abnormal unions between two or more surfaces that are normally lined with serosa. The process of adherent peritoneal healing involves the formation of adhesions. Adhesions may also occur with no mechanical interruption of the serosal surface.[50] Following peritoneal injury, fibrinous adhesions can be observed within 24 to 48 hours during the inflammatory stage of healing. Fibrin adheres the two structures involved. Often the omentum or mesothelium of the urogenital pelvic fat becomes loosely attached to the inflamed area. The attachment may break down in 48 to 72 hours as the inflammatory phase dissipates. This attachment is termed *reversible adhesion.* If the inflammatory phase persists and the fibrin network becomes replaced with capillaries and fibroblasts, *irreversible adhesions* are formed. Adhesions are termed *fibrinous* or *fibrous* depending on the make-up of the adherence between the two structures. Fibrinous adhesions that remain through the fifth day contain fibroblasts and usually persist as permanent fibrous adhesions even though there is little collagen deposited until 7 to 14 days. The keys to dissolution of reversible fibrinous adhesions are (1) the presence of adequate oxygen and a nutritious environment for the mesothelium, (2) normal mesothelial and submesothelial cells that liberate a plasminogen-activating substance, and (3) a lack of continued or severe inflammation. Three main causes of adhesion formation have been sited:[50] (1) tissue anoxia, (2) serosal injury, and (3) foreign material.

Adhesions are classified clinically as *restrictive* or *nonrestrictive.* Restrictive adhesions are firm in consistency and tightly bind the structures involved. Clinically they are more important than nonrestrictive adhesions because they are generally more apt to be involved with complications associated with visceral strangulation or obstruction. Nonrestrictive adhesions involve more compliant connections between structures. Often adhesions involving the omentum are considered nonrestrictive because of the compliant nature of the omentum even though the adhesion binding the omentum itself may be quite firm. Usually nonrestrictive adhesions are involved with fewer complications but strangulation and obstruction are still possible.

Postoperatively, adhesions may result from excessive drying of serosal surfaces; traumatic handling of serosal tissues; contamination with foreign materials such as gauze lint, glove powder, talc (magnesium silicate) crystals, and antibiotic powders; and infection. Excessive use of electrocoagulation and suture materials or the use of reactive or contaminated suture materials may also cause adhesions. Suture closure of the parietal peritoneum is another cause of adhesions.

The formation of adhesions always involves some form of peritoneal irritation and inflammation. Some inflammation is an inevitable consequence of any surgery or injury involving the abdomen. The amount of fibrin produced is proportional to the degree of chemical, mechanical, or infectious destruction and the resulting inflammation. The more fibrin produced the greater the chance of fibrous adhesions. Whole blood also potentiates adhesion formation because it provides more fibrinogen for potential fibrin conversion.

Dogs and cats have a very active fibrinolytic mechanism within their peritoneal cavities. This often prevents the development of serious restrictive fibrous adhesions by decreasing the amount of fibrin adhering to various surfaces. The fibrinolytic mechanism is stimulated naturally by plasminogen-activating substances that are present in mesothelial cells and submesothelial blood vessels. Plasminogen activation is depressed by peritoneal injury *only* in the local areas of injury and inflammation. Fibrinolytic activity must be present continuously for several days to prevent adhesions.

Among individual animals there can be great variation in the ability to form or break down (lyse) intra-abdominal adhesions. Some may have a tendency to form multiple, firm, restrictive adhesions, whereas others may have difficulty in forming even a few unrestrictive ones. Fortunately these extremes are uncommon. In untreated peritonitis, adhesion formation may be lifesaving by sealing a perforated viscus or by loculating bacteria away from the abdominal lymphatics, where they would be absorbed and cause bacteremia. In individuals that are hypoproteinemic and hypofibrinogenemic there may be difficulty in generating enough fibrin to seal accidental or surgical wounds within the abdominal cavity. This may ultimately lead to leakage and generalized peritonitis. Animals that have protein-losing diseases, severe liver disease, uremia, or malnutrition are examples. Special nutritional support such as intravenous or enteral hyperalimentation should be used preoperatively if possible in these individuals. Nutritional support not only helps reverse the tendencies toward wound dehiscence and leakage but reduces the risk of secondary bacterial infections as well. Animals that have lost more than 10 per cent of their lean body mass or have not eaten for over five days have a decrease in both humoral and cellular immunity. Feeding for two to three days reverses this decrease and helps protect them from acquiring infections. If their gastrointestinal tract is functional feeding is best done enterally.[29]

Where bowel perforation and leakage have oc-curred, an adhesion may be planned and created surgically over the perforated area to prevent further leakage.[30] This commonly involves creation of a viscerovisceral adhesion in which a "serosal patch" is constructed. An example would be the suturing of a loop of small intestine over a colonic defect. Serosal patching has been lifesaving in animals with generalized peritonitis. Often because of an intensely activated fibrinolytic system and a poor fibrin-producing system, conventional suture closure is unsuccessful in stopping leakage. The fibrin seal needed between sutures in these cases is lysed or not formed sufficiently, leading to persistent leakage.

Adhesions between adjacent bowel loops can also be surgically created to prevent intestinal intussusception or strangulation from recurring.[71, 113] Adhesions are also created between the stomach and abdominal wall to prevent recurrent gastric volvulus or between the colon and abdominal wall to prevent recurrent rectal prolapse.[67]

Intestinal obstruction or strangulation due to unintentional fibrous adhesions usually occurs within weeks after abdominal surgery or disease. Restricting fibrous adhesions that form over several weeks of maturation and contraction may lead to lumen or vessel obstruction. Unintentional adhesions following surgery, e.g., following reaction to ligatures placed during ovariohysterectomy, have also obstructed the ureter or colon.[6]

Rarely, abdominal adhesions form sheets of fibrous tissue interconnecting all abdominal organs and spanning one side of the abdominal wall to the other. These generalized adhesions are impossible to remove surgically. Clinical signs are most frequently absent. When present they are usually associated with partial or complete bowel obstruction. The etiology is unknown; a history of previous abdominal surgery or disease is not always present. A lack of peritoneal fibrinolytic enzymes is proposed as part of the pathogenesis. Differential diagnosis includes unusual forms or causes of granulomatous peritonitis, e.g., by Actinomyces sp., Nocardia sp., Candida sp., Pityrosporum sp., and foreign materials.[2]

There is no reliable way to prevent the formation of adhesions. Gloving powder and lint from surgical drapes are commonly implicated. Unretrieved threads from cotton gauze pads are important sources of irritation.[20] The various suture materials are about equal in their capacity to induce adhesions.[97] In my experience, multiple-filament materials including chromic gut and silk are most commonly associated with adhesions causing complications.

Drying of serosal surfaces and the presence of coagulated blood are important potentiating factors in the pathogenesis of adhesions following surgery.[83] Suturing areas denuded of peritoneum promote adhesion formation by two to three times.[20] In areas in which adhesions are inevitable or highly possible (such as intestinal anastomosis sites), it is best to cover the suture line with omentum, creating less rigid, unrestricting omental adhesions.[34] With other adhesions unrelated to surgery, formation is best controlled by reducing peritoneal inflammation.

A number of secondary chemical measures to prevent adhesions have been suggested. Promising materials include heparin and trypsin or heparin alone,[4] protoporphyrin,[57] oxyphenbutazone,[59] and glucocorticoids.[55] Some of these compounds have been effective but have also produced adverse secondary effects such as delayed wound healing, increased spreading of peritoneal infection, and bacterial and toxin absorption into the circulation.[37] Because of these side effects, most surgeons have abandoned their use.

Extensive adhesions may be safely inhibited to some extent by infusing the abdominal cavity four times daily with saline in a daily amount approximating 10 per cent of body weight.[117] The infused fluid is drained from the peritoneal cavity as well as possible after every treatment. Lavaging the abdomen dilutes and decreases the amount of fibrinogen, thromboplastin, and clotting factors that are required for the formation of fibrin. Without fibrin, adhesion formation is inhibited. The lavage fluid also dilutes and decreases biologically active substances liberated with mesothelial cell injury and causes decreased fibrin deposition.

PERITONITIS

Inflammation of the peritoneum may be classified by its extent, nature, and source and subclassified as (1) *primary,* or infections of the peritoneum, or (2) *secondary,* or inflammation due to peritoneal involvement subsequent to contamination. Peritonitis can also be subclassified by the amount of peritoneum involved: (1) *local,* or regional peritonitis limited to one specific and localized anatomical area, or (2) *diffuse,* or generalized peritonitis that involves a greater proportion of the peritoneal lining. Because of widespread peritoneal involvement and the absorption of toxic products into the circulation, diffuse peritonitis often leads to serious systemic illness.

Primary Peritonitis

Primary peritonitis, often termed *idiopathic,* is very uncommon, generally constituting less than 1 per cent of all cases of peritonitis. The causative agents, either bacteria or viruses, presumably gain access to the peritoneum by a hematogenous route. Examples include feline infectious peritonitis (FIP) and the occasional case of bacterial peritonitis associated with a recognizable infection elsewhere due to the same causative organism. Patients with impaired host defenses can develop a primary intraperitoneal infection without an obvious source of sepsis.

Hematogenous spread is the most likely source of infection in cases associated with a noncontiguous infection or an intravascular infection. A second means by which bacteria may gain entrance into the peritoneal cavity is via the ovarian bursa and uterus. A third source is the contiguous spread of infection. Frequently a simultaneous infection of the lungs or pleura or urinary tract may be found. The spread may have come from a hematogenous route; however, it is difficult to disprove the contiguous spread of infection across the pleural peritoneal junction.

A fourth possible route of infection is via the transmural migration of endogenous intestinal bacteria. Bacteria often cross the bowel wall during localized ischemia or systemic shock states. In humans, documented association with hepatic malfunction suggests that diminished clearance of enteric bacteria by the liver may contribute to the pathogenesis of primary peritonitis. Because this route of bacterial peritonitis is often associated with a pathological process within the peritoneal cavity, this form takes on characteristics of a secondary peritonitis and is more appropriately termed a *secondary peritonitis*.

Unlike secondary bacterial peritonitis, which often has an acute onset and serious systemic signs, primary peritonitis usually develops over a period of days to weeks. FIP signs may take months to become clinically evident. The gradual development of weakness, infected ascites, and abdominal distension is common. Fever, abdominal pain, vomiting, and severe depression can also occur but are less common.

Diagnosis is best and most easily done by analysis of ascitic fluid obtained by paracentesis with or without peritoneal lavage. An ascitic fluid leukocyte count of greater than 300/mm^3 with more than 30 per cent neutrophils is diagnostic of intraperitoneal inflammation. A specimen is centrifuged and the sediment is Gram's and Wright's stained and examined microscopically. The fluid is also cultured. The finding of only one type of organism is often seen with primary peritonitis. In primary peritonitis caused by virus infection, e.g., FIP, no organisms are found, but a moderate peritoneal neutrophilic leukocytosis is evident. If more than one type of organism is recovered, a perforated viscus and secondary peritonitis are highly suspected. In certain cases of secondary peritonitis only one organism may be found. The finding of one organism does not rule out a surgically correctable lesion.

Any patient in whom a surgically correctable lesion cannot be excluded should undergo exploratory laparotomy. This is especially true when gram-negative or multiple types of organisms are seen. Increased morbidity and mortality occurs in patients with primary peritonitis that undergo exploratory surgery. Surgical exploration should be avoided in cats with FIP. These animals frequently have wound infections and poor healing postsurgically.

Treatment for bacterial forms of primary peritonitis often requires laparotomy to remove intra-abdominal exudate and bacteria. An alternative is peritoneal lavage with the addition of appropriate antibiotics to the irrigation fluid. Systemic antibiotics should be begun as early as possible and given in high doses. Initially an aminoglycoside, such as gentamicin, and ampicillin is recommended. The antibiotic therapy is adjusted on the basis of culture and sensitivity results.

Secondary Peritonitis

Secondary peritonitis, which is much more common than primary peritonitis, is defined as peritoneal inflammation secondary to disruption of the abdominal cavity or a hollow viscus. It may be associated with a surgical procedure or may occur following trauma or disease. Because the normal gastrointestinal tract contains in excess of 10^{12} bacteria at any given time, it is the most common source of secondary peritonitis. Although this type of peritonitis, occurring subsequent to contamination, is properly termed *secondary peritonitis*, it is often simply referred to as peritonitis.

Peritonitis, while no longer the overwhelming problem it once was, is still one of the most common fatal complications of abdominal surgical treatment and diseases involving the abdominal organs. In the dog and cat, diffuse bacterial peritonitis commonly results in septic shock and, often, death. All causes of secondary peritonitis may be grouped under four broad categories: (1) mechanical and foreign body, (2) chemical, (3) infectious, and (4) other, which includes allergy, collagen-vascular diseases, and those related to neoplasms and cysts.[66] This discussion is limited to surgically related causes of secondary peritonitis.

Aseptic Peritonitis

Aseptic peritonitis results from mechanical and chemical irritants. A variety of sterile materials gaining entry to the peritoneal cavity are irritants and are associated with aseptic inflammatory reactions.

Mechanical and Foreign Body Peritonitis

Foreign bodies may reach the peritoneal cavity as a result of operative procedures. Sponges (Fig. 44–4), suture material, powder from gloves, lint and other debris from drapes, and instruments (Fig. 44–5) may be deposited in the abdomen during surgery. *Some degree of localized inflammatory reaction is produced every time the peritoneal cavity is entered surgically.* This is primarily associated with mechanical trauma. There is inevitable contamination by foreign materials and bacteria from room air, the patient's skin, minimal spillage during manipulation of viscera, and so on. However, contamination is usually minimal and can be controlled by protective mechanisms of the peritoneum.

Penetrating injuries may deposit foreign bodies in

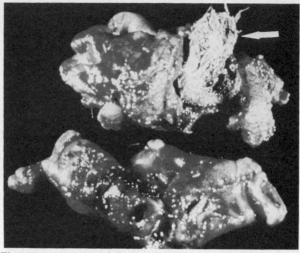

Figure 44–4. A surgical sponge (*arrow*) left in the abdomen of a dog six months previously. An enterocystic fistula and chronic localized peritonitis resulted. Approximately one-third of the urinary bladder and 12 cm of small intestine had to be resected. The sponge caused an erosive communication between the urinary bladder and small intestine and also contributed to significant adhesions.

the peritoneal cavity. Penetration of the abdominal wall and peritoneum by animal bites, missiles, or sharp objects often results in the implanation of hair and dirt into the peritoneal cavity. The gastrointestinal tract may also be the source of bones, wood splinters, toothpicks, needles, and vegetable material. Septic peritonitis usually results.

Peritoneal foreign bodies are acted upon by the body and lead to one of the three situations: (1) if small enough, phagocytosis removes the foreign material; (2) if phagocytosis cannot remove it, an attempt to wall it off may occur; this may lead to a granulomatous peritonitis or the formation of localized granuloma formation; (3) a draining fistula to the outside of the body may form in an attempt to expel the material. The relative amounts of exudate and fibrous tissue vary greatly with the nature of the foreign body present. Natural materials usually involve an intense tissue reaction. These include wood, cotton, plant fibers, and hair. Bacteria associated with the foreign materials further intensify reactions.

The clinical manifestations of an intraperitoneal foreign body vary, depending on the type of foreign body and whether bacteria are involved. Foreign bodies with smooth surfaces and made of nonreactive materials may remain clinically undetected. An example of such a foreign body is a hemostat accidentally left in the abdomen following surgery three years previously (see Fig. 44–5). An abscess may develop due to bacterial contamination and proliferation in the interstices of a sterile surgical sponge or laparotomy pad left in the abdominal cavity (see Fig. 44–5). Bacterial contamination of the foreign body may occur during surgery. With foreign body abscesses, a mass may be palpated and abdominal pain may be detected. Fever, vomiting, and signs of sepsis

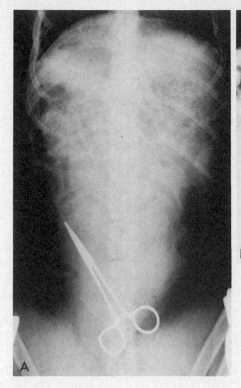

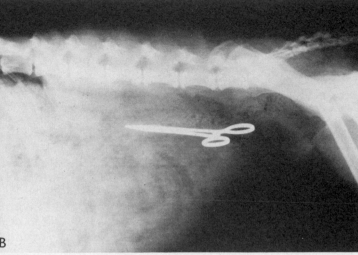

Figure 44–5. Ventrodorsal *(A)* and lateral *(B)* radiographs of an eight-year-old mixed breed dog revealed the hemostat. Ovariohysterectomy had been done three years previously. There were no abdominal problems during this three-year period or during the subsequent six months until the dog was euthanized for mammary tumors.

can also develop. Other signs related to specific organ involvement, such as jaundice with hepatic abscesses that block the common bile duct, may develop.

Foreign bodies associated with signs of specific organ involvement, intra-abdominal abscesses, or sinus tracts must be removed. Extensive adhesions resulting from attempts to isolate foreign objects in the abdominal cavity often involve local viscera. The adhesions, in turn, can cause serious complications, e.g., ureteral obstruction secondary to an intense suture reaction. Removal of the foreign body and associated mass of connective tissue may necessitate removal of attached viscera (see Fig. 44–5).

Starch Granulomatous Peritonitis

Talcum powder, commonly used on surgery gloves in the 1950s, produces granulomatous peritonitis, localized peritoneal granulomas, fecal fistulae, delayed wound healing, and even death.[33] Talcum powder, composed mainly of hydrated magnesium silicate, incites a very intense fibroblastic reaction that may cause dense adhesions within a few weeks to months.[33]

As a result, powdered corn starch and rice starch were introduced as glove powders.[64] Both of these starch powders may also cause a foreign body reaction, although not as severe and with less frequency than that seen with talcum powder.[63] For this reason, surgical gloves should always be washed and wiped off before hands are put into the peritoneal cavity, and care should be taken to avoid spillage of glove powder should a glove be torn during an operation.

The reaction associated with the retained starch particles in the peritoneal cavity and the accompanying clinical signs are dose dependent.[63] Fortunately, most cases involve a low dose of starch; consequently, the granulomatous lesions are limited, and clinical signs are mild if they occur at all. Although clinically recognized as a distinct problem in human surgery, reports in the veterinary literature are lacking. With sufficient intra-abdominal starch implantation in humans, a granulomatous peritonitis usually appears within 14 days to one month after the abdominal surgery. There usually is dull general abdominal pain. Associated wounds are frequently indurated. Skin edges may be separated.[92] Diffuse abdominal tenderness is a frequent finding. In dogs in which starch powder was purposely implanted, microscopic sections of the thickened peritoneal surfaces revealed fibrosis accompanied by a foreign body giant cell granulomatous reaction.[64]

With glove starch granulomatous peritonitis following surgery, re-operation is usually required to rule out other causes of peritonitis. The diagnosis requires the absence of other causes of peritonitis and the identification of intracellular starch granules in macrophages, multinucleated giant cells, and microabscesses associated with an intense granulomatous peritonitis. Occasionally severe adhesions are involved with the small intestine, ureter, and so on, which require lysis. This has occurred in one cat in my experience. In humans, the use of corticosteroids have been recommended once the diagnosis is definitely established. Corticosteroids hasten resolution of the symptoms.[18] Clinical signs usually subside gradually over a period of a few weeks.

Chemical Peritonitis

Bile, gastric juices, pancreatic juice, urine, anti-septics, antibacterial powders, and enema and barium sulfate solutions can cause peritonitis.

Bile reaches the peritoneal cavity from biliary tract ruptures or as a sequela to operations on or near the biliary system. The bile salts in sterile bile are mildly irritating.[106] Bile not associated with cholehepatic disease is usually sterile. Sterile bile peritonitis experimentally induced in germ-free dogs via a biliary fistula does not lead to septic peritonitis. Death from biliary peritonitis requires bacteria.[16] Following placement of sterile bile into the abdominal cavities of normal dogs, bacterial proliferation occurs within the abdominal fluid. The bacteria cultured generally include *Staphylococcus aureus*, *Clostridium welchii*, and, to a lesser extent, *Streptococcus* sp. and coliforms.[82]

Bacteria associated with naturally occurring bile peritonitis invade the peritoneal cavity as a result of permeability changes within the bowel wall due to the action of bile on the bowel's serosal surface.[82] Antibiotics given to dogs with surgically induced bile peritonitis substantially prolong their life.[19, 90]

Gastric and pancreatic juice are very irritating and produce more intense chemical peritonitis than bile. Contact with these chemical irritants produces immediate cellular damage similar to that seen with a chemical burn. Damage to the mesothelial cells causes the release of vasoactive substances, superoxides, and other cellular toxins. Capillary dilation and leakage result in a rapid and massive fluid shift and loss of plasma protein and red blood cells into the peritoneal cavity. The lymphatics become swollen and blocked with white blood cell–platelet aggregates, impeding fluid and protein return to the circulation.

Approximately three hours after the onset of the chemical irritant damage, intestinal bacteria and accumulated bacterial toxins cross damaged intestinal barriers and enter the peritoneal cavity. This converts the chemical peritonitis into both a chemical and bacterial peritonitis. At this same time, enteric bacteria also enter the blood stream, producing a bacteremia. The accumulation of bacterial hyaluronidase within the intestinal lumen aids in bacterial migration through the wall into the peritoneum and circulation.[5] Other endogenous materials that may cause some peritoneal irritation include urine, chyle, and blood itself. However, this irritation is usually minor.

Septic Peritonitis

Etiology

Although death can occur from chemical peritonitis alone, the most rapidly developing and dangerous form of peritonitis is bacterial. Septic peritonitis is a secondary peritonitis associated with virulent organisms, particularly enterobacteria. The cultured bacteria are usually a mixture of organisms, both anaerobes (*Clostridium* sp., *Peptostreptococcus* sp., and *Bacteroides* sp.) and aerobes (*E. coli*, *Klebsiella* sp., and *Proteus* sp.).

Ischemic bowel, either from strangulation or secondary to mechanical obstruction and distension, is an important source of virulent bacteria commonly associated with septic peritonitis. The bowel may still be grossly intact, yet enterobacteria enter the peritoneal cavity because of altered permeability.

Septic peritonitis following an operation is usually bacterial in nature and is commonly due to breakdown of a suture line in a hollow viscus. The integrity of the suture line is endangered by tension, ischemia, hemorrhage, mucosal eversion, infection, excessive free peritoneal fluids, and such systemic factors as hypoproteinemia and anemia. Postoperative bacterial infection extending from significant exogenous contamination of the peritoneal cavity at the time of surgery is possible. Exogenous bacteria may also enter via an abdominal wound or peritoneal drain.

Pathophysiology

Diffuse septic peritonitis can be looked upon as a large thermal "burn." Significant quantities of fluid, electrolytes, and plasma proteins along with red blood cells can be lost into the peritoneal cavity owing to peritoneal vascular dilation and increased capillary permeability. These vascular changes are secondary to bacterial effects on the host's leukocytes and platelets. Endotoxin and cellular proteases liberated from the lysed bacteria and leukocytes both activate the coagulation cascade and cause platelet activation, aggregation, and degranulation in the presence of complement. Platelet degranulation results in the liberation of many vasoactive substances. Endotoxin also activates the complement cascade. Activation of C3a through C5a causes intense increased capillary permeability.

With increases in vascular permeability, interstitial fluid accumulates rapidly. The accumulation of fluid in abdominal tissues ultimately leads to the accumulation of free peritoneal fluid. Initially the peritoneal fluid is clear, but it rapidly becomes turbid and purulent. Lymphatics are blocked with fibrin and cellular debris, leading to further accumulation of fluid within the peritoneal cavity. Eventually, the loss of circulating fluid volume leads to hypovolemic shock. Further absorption of bacterial endotoxins and exotoxins from the peritoneum into the circulation leads to signs of progressive septic shock.[39]

Phagocytosis of virulent organisms is a prime mechanism in peritoneal defense. Peritoneal polymorphonuclear leukocytes rapidly accumulate in large numbers following contamination. In dogs, various types of chemical irritants (gastric juice, pancreatic juice, urine) or septic material (stomach contents, small bowel contents, feces) placed in the peritoneal cavity stimulate a significant peritoneal leukocytosis within three hours.[85]

If peritoneal defenses, aided by appropriate therapeutic measures, contain the inflammatory process, the disease may be controlled without surgery. Exudate and fibrin associated with the localized peritonitis may eventually be degradated and absorbed. Firm fibrous adhesions may remain or become resolved as inflammation subsides. Essentially all traces of inflammation may be removed within a few weeks.

A mixed bacterial flora occurs in most cases of peritonitis secondary to contamination from the gastrointestinal tract. There is synergistic action within this mixed bacterial population, so that the total virulence is greater than the sum of its parts. In laboratory studies, mixtures of gastrointestinal bacteria resulted in a significantly more lethal peritonitis than a single species of bacteria.[98]

Certain substances, such as hemoglobin and mucus, enhance the virulence of intraperitoneal organisms. If a pure culture of E. coli containing 10^9 live organisms/dl is injected into dogs or cats at 5 ml/kg, all animals survive. If 3 to 4 grams of hemoglobin are combined with each 100 ml of the bacterial suspension and the same dose of organisms is injected, lethal peritonitis is produced in over 90 per cent of the animals.[9] Although the mechanism by which the added hemoglobin enhances the virulence is not clear, it appears that the hemoglobin retards the clearance of bacteria. Hemoglobin in the peritoneal cavity interferes with the response of leukocytes to chemotactic stimuli normally produced with bacterial peritonitis.[49]

Liquids containing bacteria rapidly disseminate throughout the peritoneal cavity. The volume, rate of infusion, and viscosity of these liquids are critical factors. When a pure suspension of bacteria is injected into the peritoneal cavity of an experimental animal, the bacteria begin to disappear almost immediately, even before the influx of phagocytic cells.[48] The first defense of the peritoneal cavity against bacterial contamination is physical removal of bacteria by the intraperitoneal circulation and absorption, primarily by the diaphragmatic lymphatics. An experimental intraperitoneal injection of bacteria and liquid radiopaque media at one locus spreads throughout the entire peritoneal cavity within two hours.[17] This spread is produced by diaphragmatic, intestinal, and abdominal wall movement.

With increased contamination of bacteria into the peritoneal cavity, other aspects of the host's defense mechanisms become vitally important. An acute inflammatory response leads to an outpouring of peritoneal fluid rich in complement and serum opsonins that bind the bacteria. The opsonized bacteria are neutralized and either pass into the regional lymph nodes or are engulfed by migrating phagocytic cells. Fibrin deposits isolate the concentrated areas of contamination and retard bacterial absorption that might lead to septic shock.[96] The fibrin deposits may also isolate the source of continued contamination and prevent persistent bacterial leakage.

The duration of leakage of contaminated fluid into the peritoneal cavity is an important factor relative to the generation of diffuse peritonitis. Continued leakage over several hours to several days can have the same effect as one massive spill in a relatively short period of time.[96] If the source of the contamination persists, the outcome is often fatal despite vigorous antibiotic and supportive therapy. If the source of contamination is stopped by natural defense mechanisms, such as fibrin sealing, or is treated appropriately with surgical intervention, even though diffuse infection is already present, many patients respond favorably.[7]

The omentum is an important means of defense against continued peritoneal contamination. Because of its great mobility the omentum contributes significantly by adhering to the site of continued contamination and walling it off. Because of its good blood supply and accessible vessels, the omentum also contributes collateral blood supply and raises local oxygen tension. In experimental studies, if a segment of bowel is devascularized and wrapped in a viable pedicle of omentum, collaterals form to maintain bowel viability. In the dog survival of up to 13 inches of devascularized small intestine occurred when omentum was wrapped around an ischemic segment.[10] The omentum also participates directly in bacterial and foreign material absorption and in the influx of phagocytic cells into the peritoneal cavity.

Intraperitoneal sepsis may be disseminated and augmented by surgical errors. Failure to drain inflammatory fluids or remove contaminated blood clots can lead to progressive complications. Inflammatory fluids are often rapidly depleted of bacterial opsonins and complement. Bacteria within the fluid, therefore, cannot be phagocytosed. Lowered oxygen tension within the fluid also contributes to ineffectual killing by neutrophils and favors the growth of anaerobic organisms.[2] The fluid is also very rich in exotoxins and endotoxins liberated by the bacteria.[7] Failure to remove the fluid may lead to progressive toxin absorption. Failure to remove contaminated clots allows the bacteria, protected from neutrophils, opsonins, and antibiotics by the surrounding fibrin, to replicate rapidly. Experimentally, contaminated clots always produce abscesses and contribute to peritonitis.[2]

Other surgical errors include the breaking down of a partially walled-off area. This thwarts the body's attempt to localize the infective process and contributes to the peritoneal spread of microorganisms and toxic products. The placement of large quantities of suture material in the abdominal cavity or inadequate debridement of devitalized tissue may promote bacterial proliferation. Failure to thoroughly lavage the peritoneal cavity may also be a serious surgical error.

Unremoved irrigating fluid also appears to play an adjuvant role in peritonitis. Saline infused intraperitoneally with nonlethal numbers of E. coli renders the combination lethal in direct proportion to the volume of saline infused.[2] Saline's effect is due to interference with two host defenses against bacteria: the opsonic proteins, which are diluted by the saline, and surfaces on which phagocytes can trap and ingest bacteria. Fluid left within the peritoneal cavity suspends the bacteria, isolating them from neutrophils on the peritoneal surface and allowing them to proliferate in lethal numbers.

Clinical Signs

The signs of septic peritonitis depend on the cause and location of the inflammation and the condition of the patient. The history of patients with peritonitis is often vague. Unless the owner reports recent trauma or abdominal surgery, the history may only indicate general depression, dysorexia, vomiting, or other nonspecific signs of illness. Occasionally an owner may describe an unusual posture, e.g., a "praying" position or kyphosis.[101] In the "praying position" the animal extends his front legs and attempts to touch his sternum to the floor while keeping his rear legs extended (Fig. 44–6). Other animals simply appear "tucked up" and show abdominal tenderness on palpation.

The signs that follow septic complications of abdominal surgery or abdominal injury usually are acute in onset and reflect a localized peritonitis, which may become diffuse. They usually appear from several hours to a few days after the operation or injury and may be accompanied by fever and tachycardia. However, fever and tachycardia may be absent in animals being treated with prostaglandin inhibitors or steroids. Physical findings that may be suggestive of peritonitis include wounds or bruises in the caudal thorax or abdominal region, abdominal discomfort, vomiting on palpation, intra-abdominal mass, injected mucous membrane (indicative of hemoconcentration and sepsis), and slow capillary refill time. Gastrointestinal ileus, another sign commonly seen with peritonitis, results in abdominal distension and hyperresonance. Bowel sounds are usually diminished or absent. Body temperature may be elevated early, but in some individuals, especially those that are old or debilitated, it may remain normal until

later in the course of the disease. Subnormal temperature often occurs as dehydration, hypovolemia, and hypodynamic septic shock ensue. The animal may initially be mentally alert or have a degree of depression that is only detectable by individuals who know how the animal normally acts. As the disease progresses, depression and lethargy are apparent. The animal often dies owing to depletion of extravascular volume.

Diagnosis

Radiographs may reveal free gas or fluid in the abdomen. This is quite common following rupture of the gastrointestinal tract. The gas may also be produced by gas-forming organisms or, rarely, from penetrating injuries that allow air to enter via a skin opening or pneumothorax. Air is normally introduced into the peritoneal cavity during surgery and can be radiographically detectable for at least one week postoperatively. This should be considered when viewing abdominal radiographs of animals that have had recent surgery. Fluid in the abdomen is seen as a lack of normal detail or gives a "ground glass" appearance. Generalized intestinal ileus is a frequent observation.

Specific contrast studies of the urinary system may be useful in determining if it is involved. Because of generalized paralytic ileus, barium placed in the stomach may remain there for many hours. From a practical point of view, it is my belief that time is better spent preparing the patient for surgery and performing an early exploratory laparotomy both for diagnosis and treatment of peritonitis. A second problem with the use of barium or hyperosmolar iodinated contrast materials in the evaluation of the gastrointestinal tract is possible contamination of the peritoneal cavity with these agents if perforation is present. Both types of agents contribute to the lethality of peritonitis.

Most cases of septic peritonitis can be accurately diagnosed by the cytological examination of fluid obtained by paracentesis or lavage.[31] It is recommended that a multiholed catheter be used for the paracentesis. If no fluid is collected, 22 ml/kg body weight of saline is infused through the catheter. The animal is gently rotated to disperse and mix the fluid. A sample is collected and examined microscopically. Toxic degenerative neutrophils with intracellular and extracellular bacteria are indicative of septic peritonitis and the necessity of exploration (Fig. 44–7). In animals that have had recent surgery, an increase in neutrophil numbers is commonly seen in the lavage fluid (up to 10,000 cells/mm^3), but none of the cells are degenerate or contain bacteria. Degenerate or bacteria-containing cells indicate a major suppurative and septic postoperative complication requiring re-exploration.[8] In intraperitoneal infection where loculation is efficient, peritoneal lavage may not be diagnostic. However, the leukocyte count of the

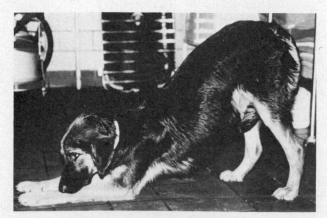

Figure 44–6. The praying position, or "position of relief." The dog had a ruptured bladder and urine peritonitis.

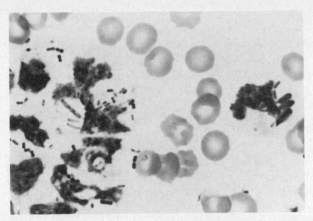

Figure 44–7. Sediment from peritoneal lavage in a dog with dehiscence of an intestinal suture line. Multiple bacteria are observed both intracellularly and extracellularly. Degenerate neutrophils predominate. Wright's stain × 900.

lavage fluid is generally over 4000/mm³. Lavage fluid leukocyte counts in normal, unoperated animals are usually less than 1000/mm³.[31]

Treatment

Every patient with peritonitis is potentially critically ill and requires adequate monitoring of vital functions. Repeated and systematic clinical examinations yield the greatest amount of information and are the most important monitoring tools available. Laboratory determinations such as urine specific gravity, hematocrit, total protein, peripheral leukocyte count and differential, serum electrolytes, serum creatinine, blood glucose, and arterial blood gases may help in making appropriate decisions about supportive therapy.

The definitive treatment of septic peritonitis depends on the cause, severity, and duration and whether it is diffuse or localized. Ultimate success in treatment is related to treatment of the primary condition. Diffuse peritonitis causes a rapid change in the fluid-electrolyte balance, and correction of this functional hypovolemia and any changes in electrolyte balance should be considered first. A balanced electrolyte solution should be administered unless contraindicated by laboratory findings. The monitoring of central venous pressure, urine output, toe web temperature, and capillary perfusion time provides important information concerning the amount and rate that should be used. The rate of administration may initially be as high as 45 ml (cats) and 80 ml (dogs) per kg body weight per hour in a severely depleted patient. The rate of fluid administration is adjusted according to changes in physiological parameters. The use of whole blood or plasma is reserved for those patients anemic on presentation or who during treatment develop a hematocrit below 20 per cent or total plasma proteins below 3.5 gm/100 ml.

The patient's acid-base status should be corrected, if necessary. In the severely dehydrated patient, metabolic acidosis can be profound. Sodium bicarbonate is best added to the electrolyte solution and given according to plasma bicarbonate and pH determinations. However, if these laboratory determinations are not available, sodium bicarbonate 2 to 4 mEq/kg body weight may safely be added and given over the first 24 hours.

Antibiotics

Appropriate antibiotics should be given intravenously in high doses as soon as the diagnosis of bacterial peritonitis is made or is suspected prior to surgery. Selection of the type of antibiotic is based on a knowledge of the organisms present. Aerobic and anaerobic bacterial cultures of the peritoneal fluid and antibiotic sensitivity testing are useful and should be done carefully at the time of paracentesis-lavage or surgery.

Gram's staining results and microscopic examination of peritoneal fluid guide the initial selection of antibiotics. Almost all antibiotics reach therapeutic levels in normal intraperitoneal fluid. The aminoglycosides, ampicillin, and cephalosporins reach intraperitoneal levels equivalent to serum levels. The level of clindamycin in intraperitoneal fluid is approximately one-half that of the serum concentration.[43] Antibiotics that are presently recommended include combinations of penicillin, ampicillin, or clindamycin with kanamycin, amikacin, tobramycin, or gentamicin.[2, 72] The broad spectrum cephalosporins and chloramphenicol have also been recommended as single agents. Of the available bactericidal agents, I prefer the combination of gentamicin, ampicillin, and clindamycin or at least gentamicin and ampicillin. Although there are several reports citing the effectiveness of single drug therapy in peritonitis,[95] I believe that double- or triple-drug treatment eliminates the maximum number of bacteria in the preoperative periods before antibiotic sensitivity tests are available. Following laparotomy, the redox potential greatly increases so that the use of anaerobic bactericidal agents such as clindamycin may not be necessary.[94] The goal of reducing the bacterial population in the peritoneum as rapidly as possible is further accomplished by the use of appropriate intraperitoneal antibiotics. Just as systemic antibiotic administration achieves high peritoneal levels, intraperitoneal administration of most antibiotics yields high systemic levels. Some studies have suggested greater survival when antibiotics are administered intraperitoneally (IP) rather than intravenously (IV).[54] Clinically, combination therapy (IV and IP) gives the most beneficial effect.[79, 80, 91] As a general rule, the same antibiotic should be used intraperitoneally and intravenously. Only antibiotics approved for intravenous use are safe for intraperitoneal use.[91]

Corticosteroids

Intravenous corticosteroids are advocated preoperatively for their positive inotropic effect on the heart owing to the liberation of ATP from the mitochondria of the myocardial muscle cells.[110] Other beneficial effects of corticosteroids include stabilization of lysosomal membranes, blockage of complement activation, and normalization of cellular metabolic derangements. These lead to decreased capillary permeability, protection against endotoxins, and restoration of normal permeability of the intestinal wall.[72] Recently, the use of flunixin meglumine as a cyclooxygenase inhibitor and blocker of prostaglandin production has been effective, in conjunction with antibiotics (gentamicin), in prolonging the life of dogs subjected to septic peritonitis.[48] Damage to cell membranes leads to activation of the arachidonic acid pathways and production of prostaglandins and toxic-free radicals. High levels of certain prostaglandins (thromboxane A_2, PGF_2, and so on) are seen in conjunction with abdominal sepsis and are associated with major organ failure (lung, kidney, liver). Decreasing the generalized production of prostaglandins appears to be beneficial.

Surgery

After appropriate supportive measures have been instituted and the patient is hemodynamically improved, surgery is recommended to treat the inciting condition and manage the peritonitis. The aims of the operation are to stop ongoing contamination, remove foreign and purulent material, and provide drainage of peritoneal exudate. An additional goal may be the establishment of tube gastrostomies and enterostomies for decompression of the gastrointestinal tract and fluid and for nutritional support.[22, 103] In these animals, intestinal function often returns prior to normal gastric motility and function. The animals are often still anorexic in this stage, which may last for several days. Nutritional support is vital to the recovery of humans with abdominal sepsis.[53] Presumably this applies to seriously ill animals as well.

Intravenous glucose prior to surgery may be required if blood glucose levels are low. This can occur in septic peritonitis and is associated with increased cellular metabolism and lack of hepatic glucose production. Blood glucose levels have been recorded as low as 20 mg/dl in dogs with peritonitis. Because hyperglycemia may also be seen with early sepsis, the need for glucose is determined by blood glucose determinations. If blood glucose cannot be determined, 2.5 to 5 per cent dextrose solution is suggested.

Exploratory laparotomy using the ventral midline approach is recommended. Care should be taken to avoid incising intestine or other structures that may be adhered to the linea alba. Temporary control of each source of contamination is undertaken as it is found.

Control of a leak in a hollow viscus is handled in a variety of ways, depending on the extent and nature of the leak and the viscus involved. These may include simple debridement and closure, resection, or the use of a nearby healthy loop of bowel as a patch to seal an involved area. Because of the tremendously active peritoneal fibrinolytic enzymes present in peritonitis, simple suturing of a perforated lesion may not successfully eliminate leakage. Serosal patching with a loop of bowel over a defect is effective in providing a serosal seal.[30, 58]

All foreign material, necrotic tissue, and blood clots should be removed from the operative field. Copious peritoneal irrigation with isotonic saline solution or Ringer's lactate solution significantly reduces the mortality and morbidity of acute diffuse peritonitis.[54] Well-formed adhesions are left intact, but otherwise, no attempt is made to keep the irrigating solution localized, and irrigation is continued until the fluid returns clear. In an average-sized dog this may take several liters of fluid. Peritoneal irrigation with warm fluids removes necrotic tissue, blood clots, fat droplets, and bacteria and decreases the total load of endogenous and bacterial toxins. It disperses intraperitoneal antibiotics and antiseptics and may help in the reduction of peritoneal adhesions. Warm irrigating fluids in the abdominal cavity are effective in treating and preventing hypothermia.[73] This is particularly true in small patients, which have a greater proportion of peritoneal surface area per kilogram body weight.

Whether antibiotics should be included in peritoneal irrigating fluid has been vigorously debated. The inclusion of water-soluble antibiotics in irrigation fluids initially increases intra-abdominal levels of antibiotics; however, concomitant intravenous administration is often necessary to maintain therapeutic levels in the serum and peritoneal fluid in the postoperative period. Adverse effects of intra-abdominal antibiotics include peritoneal irritation and the formation of adhesions (tetracycline, neomycin, streptomycin); intensified catabolic state (tetracycline, neomycin, streptomycin); allergic reactions (penicillins); and respiratory arrest and hypotension due to calcium binding and neuromuscular blockage (aminoglycosides, amikacin, tobramycin, neomycin, kanamycin, gentamicin).[62]

When cephalosporins are administered intraperitoneally, higher levels are achieved in the peritoneal cavity than by intravenous administration.[111] Furthermore, it has been claimed that therapeutic levels are maintained in the peritoneum for a longer period.[80] The use of cephalosporins intraperitoneally may promote healing of anastomotic leaks, but no mechanism for this action has been proposed.[91] Other drugs used singly with favorable results have included kanamycin, gentamicin, penicillin, ampicillin, sulfanilamide, chloramphenicol, bacitracin, streptomycin, and neomycin.[76] Intraperitoneal antibiotic combinations such as kanamycin and ampicillin are also effective.[79] The advantages of intraperitoneal administration of selected antibiotics in animals far outweigh the disadvantages.

Addition of antiseptics such as povidone iodine or chlorhexidine to irrigating fluids is effective in the treatment of peritonitis in animals and humans.[62, 70]

Both iodine and chlorhexidine have a broader spectrum than most currently available single antibiotics. Povidone iodine is as effective as cephalothin or kanamycin in the control of *E. coli* peritonitis in rats and does not result in adhesion formation or bacterial resistance.[62] Ten ml of povidone iodine stock solution (1% titratable iodine) to 100 to 150 ml of warm saline for a 12-kg dog has been recommended.[44] It is important that irrigating solutions containing antiseptics be removed from the abdominal cavity.

The abdomen may be closed at this time[68] with nonabsorbable or monofilament suture through the external rectus sheath. It is not necessary to include the peritoneum with the closure. Polypropylene in a continuous suture pattern has been used successfully in patients with septic peritonitis.[24]

Drainage

Drainage of the abdominal cavity is impossible with drainage tubes alone. Within six hours of insertion, drains are sealed from the general peritoneal cavity by fibrin and adhesions.[116] Continued drainage is important in the treatment of peritonitis.

There are two means by which sufficient drainage can be achieved: (1) continuous or intermittent lavage of the peritoneal cavity; and (2) a free-draining open peritoneal cavity protected against evisceration by sterile absorbent pads. Both of these methods have been used successfully in dogs and cats.[52, 79, 105]

When continuous or intermittent lavage is used, peritoneal lavage solutions must be effectively removed. Although research on the effectiveness of various types of abdominal drains is continuing, very few published reports are available.[47] The most efficient drain is a sump Penrose drain, made by placing a double lumen (sump) drain inside a fenestrated latex Penrose drain (Fig. 44–8). Because it is softer and more pliable than the sump drain, the outer Penrose drain helps protect the delicate viscera as well. Other types of drain tubes have been used in conjunction with peritoneal lavage, but their effectiveness has not been sufficiently tested (see Fig. 44–8).

The location of the drain within the peritoneal cavity also influences its effectiveness. Gravity causes pooling of free peritoneal fluid, and placement of drains in those areas increases their effectiveness. Usually, one or two drains are placed along each lateral wall of the peritoneal cavity. Following closure of the abdomen, infusion and collection are done with the animal in lateral recumbency. The irrigation fluid is infused through the dorsal drain and collected through the ventral drain (Fig. 44–9). Infusion and collection are reversed when the animal is rotated.

Continuous peritoneal lavage is difficult to achieve if the animal is not cooperative. However, it can be done in the early postoperative period or when the animal is sedated. Continuous low suction (40 to 60 mm Hg) is applied to the ventral sump drain as warmed physiologic salt solution containing antibiotics or povidone iodine is infused (see Fig. 44–9). With sump drains, air flows through a micropore

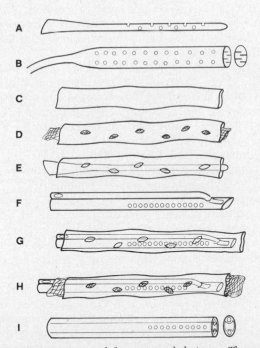

Figure 44–8. Drains used for peritoneal drainage. Those tested have the percentage of effectiveness listed.[47] Others are listed in increasing order of effectiveness according to our experience. *A*, Tube drain (fenestrated red rubber tube), 39 per cent. *B*, Silicone wound drain (Jackson-Pratt drain), resists clot formation. *C*, Penrose drain (thin Latex rubber tube), 40 per cent. *D*, Cigarette drain (gauze sponge inside a fenestrated Penrose drain). *E*, Penrose tube (double lumen) drain. Homemade sump drain. (The tube inside the fenestrated Penrose drain should also be fenestrated.) *F*, Sump (double lumen) drain. The smaller lumen is for air, 58 per cent. (This is one example of a number of commercially available types.) *G*, Penrose sump drain (sump drain inside a fenestrated Penrose drain), 72 per cent. *H*, Cigarette sump drain (sump drain inside a gauze sponge within a fenestrated Penrose drain). *I*, Triple lumen or dual sump drain (Axiom drain), made of silicone, resists clot formation.

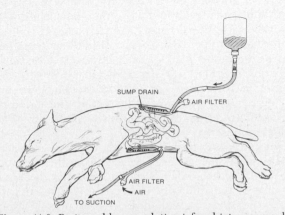

Figure 44–9. Peritoneal lavage solution infused into a sump drain and collected by a closed suction system. The sump drain is in a gravity-dependent position, and, while active low suction is continuously applied, air is pulled into the drained area through a micropore air filter. The air displaces the fluid, allowing more effective drainage. Fenestrated Penrose drains inserted over the sump drains, sterile dressings, and bandages have been omitted for clarity.

filter and into the peritoneal cavity as suction is applied. This air displaces the fluid in the peritoneal cavity and allows fluid to drain out more easily.

Intermittent lavage, two or four times per day, is a successful alternative.[52] Patients under 15 kg receive 500 ml of the peritoneal lavage solution (Ringer's or saline), and heavier animals receive 1 liter.[112] One to two grams of cephalothin per liter of lavage solution has been advocated.[44] Simple tube, sump, or sump Penrose drains can be attached to closed collection systems. Penrose drains alone cannot be attached to closed systems. For this reason, Penrose drains have become less popular for drainage of the abdominal cavity when lavage is added. Lavage is usually required for two to five days.

Complications with lavage and drainage include (1) anemia from loss of red cell mass from the peritoneal cavity; (2) hypoproteinemia from loss of large amounts of protein from the peritoneal cavity (this has been one of the most common and most serious complications in my experience); (3) hyponatremia, hypocalcemia, and hypokalemia from electrolyte loss through the peritoneal cavity; (4) hypothermia if the lavage fluids are not warmed sufficiently; (5) ascending infection from bacteria migrating up the drain, with resultant peritoneal or wound infection; and (6) blockage, malfunction, or dislocation of the drain.

Anemia, hypoproteinemia, or electrolyte disturbances may be treated by giving blood, plasma, or supplemental electrolytes intravenously. Ascending infection can be prevented by using sterile occlusive dressings and povidone iodine ointment around exit wounds. Prolonged postoperative care and monitoring are often necessary in patients requiring postoperative peritoneal lavage.

The omission of abdominal closure following laparotomy and peritoneal irrigation can also be used to drain the peritoneal cavity.[68, 105] Sterile pads cover the open peritoneal cavity, and the animal's abdomen is protected by bandages. Recumbency, standing, or sitting is encouraged for gravity drainage. Highly absorbent pads to lift and store the abdominal fluids are important. Sterile dressings are changed as often as necessary to prevent leakage of fluid and penetration of the outer bandage (usually two to four times daily for the first few days). Drainage usually decreases by the third day. When dressings are not soaked through after a 24-hour period, the abdomen can be irrigated and closed (usually on the third to fifth postoperative day).[105]

Complications associated with bandage displacement and evisceration can occur during this therapy. The caudal third to half of the incision may be closed because of the difficulty in keeping it covered with sterile dressings. In male dogs a closed urinary drainage system must also be used to prevent the dressings from becoming urine-soaked.[105]

Prognosis

The outcome of secondary peritonitis is determined by the timing of the operation, adequacy of repair and debridement, lavage and closure, choice and administration of antibiotics, and nutritional and hemodynamic support. Mortality is higher in very young or old patients and with higher or more virulent contamination. In humans the highest incidence of death is in patients with peritonitis after abdominal operations (60 to 80 per cent), attributed to a delay in diagnosis. In addition, many patients have received antibiotics which may have selected out pathological resistant strains of bacteria. Decreased host resistance, following previous injury or illness and major surgery, may decrease local peritoneal resistance to contamination.

Prior to 1965, death in patients with peritonitis was primarily due to fluid and electrolyte imbalances. The causes of these early deaths are now much less common. Since the 1970s a syndrome of major or multiple organ failure (MOF) has been noted in animals with secondary peritonitis and is attributed to septic complications.[87] Organ systems involved include the liver, kidney, lungs, and heart. Insidious and progressive failure of these organ systems, usually in the order mentioned, is not uncommon, and mortality approaches 100 per cent in affected animals. Overall mortality from secondary peritonitis is believed to be over 50 per cent. Ulceration of the gastrointestinal tract and disseminated intravascular coagulopathy are frequent complications seen in the terminal phases.

In 1979, Saba proposed that many of the distant organ system changes and terminal complications were due to toxic effects from by-products of sepsis.[87] Normally these are opsonized for phagocytosis by a plasma protein (fibronectin) and removed by the fixed reticuloendothelial systems. In infected patients these opsonins can become depleted. Preliminary data suggest that replacement therapy with whole blood or cryoprecipitate may be beneficial.[87]

The prognosis for recovery from secondary peritonitis is guarded, with response to therapy the best prognostic indicator. Other useful indicators include physical and laboratory parameters associated with complications commonly seen in septic or hypovolemic shock: (1) toeweb temperature: the lower the temperature the deeper the shock state and the poorer the prognosis; (2) activated coagulation time: prolonged times indicate consumption of coagulation factors and a poor prognosis; and (3) blood glucose: low glucose levels generally indicate liver failure and a poorer prognosis.

OTHER PERITONEAL DISORDERS

Urine Peritonitis

In small amounts, the escape of sterile urine into the peritoneal cavity is of little consequence. Prolonged leakage causes abdominal distension and peritonitis. "Third spacing" of electrolytes, proteins, and extracellular fluid into the peritoneal cavity occurs, and uremia is also a sequela to the absorption of urinary constituents from the abdominal cavity. If a bacterial infection involving the urinary tract was present before the urine began escaping into the peritoneal cavity, septic peritonitis may develop.[15] If the urine was sterile, aseptic peritonitis will occur.[15] Diagnosis is by paracentesis, lavage, or contrast radiography. Concentrations of creatinine or urea in abdominal fluid that exceed those of the peripheral blood indicate extravasation of urine into the abdominal cavity. Positive contrast radiographic studies of the upper urinary tract (excretory urography) or lower urinary tract (retrograde urethrocystography) will identify the location of urine leakage. Negative contrast studies of the lower urinary tract are less reliable and have been associated with fatal air embolism.[100]

Treatment is abdominal exploration and correction of the urinary leakage. If the animal is severely uremic and suffering from significant fluid and electrolyte depletion, surgery should be postponed until the animal's condition is improved. This requires intravenous fluid and electrolyte therapy dictated by clinical and laboratory parameters and peritoneal dialysis or preoperative peritoneal lavage to remove urine.[15] Most animals respond dramatically to 24 hours of this fluid support and urine drainage and are much better surgical and anesthetic candidates following this preoperative care. Following surgical correction of the urinary leakage, copious peritoneal irrigation is recommended. Unless overwhelming septic peritonitis is present, continued postoperative lavage or nonclosure of the abdomen is unnecessary. Parenteral antibiotic therapy with a single agent effective against gram-negative coliforms is recommended pending Gram's staining and culture results.

Chylous Peritonitis

This inflammatory process is caused by chyle in the peritoneal cavity from (1) rupture or chylous discharge arising from a lymphatic-chylous mesenteric cyst (Fig. 44–10),[66] (2) intestinal obstruction with distension and weeping of the lacteals,[66] (3) injury of the cisterna chyli or major mesenteric lymphatic vasculature,[44] or (4) blockage of chyle flow with exudation through a thin or ruptured, dilated lymph vessel.[66] The condition is rare in dogs and cats, and those reported have been associated with a history of trauma.[11, 41]

Free chyle is sufficiently irritating to produce signs of peritoneal irritation. The most significant clinical sign is progressive abdominal effusion. Diagnosis is made by abdominal paracentesis, which yields an odorless milky fluid, which on microscopic examination shows fat globules and lymphocytes but no bacteria.

Treatment varies with the etiology. Chyle is removed periodically from the abdomen by centesis to allow easier breathing. A medium-chain triglyceride diet and rest may also be used. If conservative

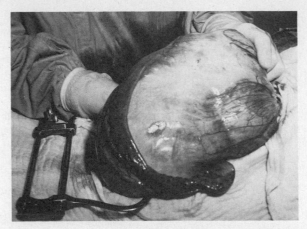

Figure 44–10. A large, thin-walled mesenteric cyst that allowed the escape of chylous fluid into the peritoneal cavity. The dog developed abdominal pain and ascites.

treatment is not successful, surgery may be necessary to identify the cause of the leakage and correct it. Because of the difficulty in isolating the leakage, a guarded prognosis must be given in cases that do not resolve spontaneously. In one report, both chylothorax and chylous peritonitis were present in the same individual.[12] Trauma was suspected as the cause. The chylothorax was treated successfully with surgery, but the chylous peritonitis was not. The chylous effusion returned despite ligation of supposedly torn lymphatic vessels. Chylous effusion causes serosal thickening and a granulomatous peritoneal inflammation, and, uncommonly, adhesions.[11]

Intra-Abdominal Abscesses

Intra-abdominal abscesses are localized collections of purulent fluid separated by a wall from surrounding tissues. Abscesses usually contain necrotic debris and neutrophils. Viable bacteria are usually present, but abscesses may be sterile. Intra-abdominal abscesses arise in three ways: (1) as a complication of generalized peritonitis, (2) adjacent to an inflamed viscus without intervening peritonitis, or (3) as postoperative or posttraumatic complications with localized leakage of gastrointestinal contents.

Pathogenesis

Owing to effective clearance of bacteria from the peritoneal cavity, it is difficult to establish intraperitoneal abscesses by injecting bacteria alone. Bacterial counts fall immediately after intraperitoneal inoculation in dogs.[40] Secondary local inflammation disrupts clearance of bacteria. Fibrin binds adjacent viscera and walls off the area of local inflammation and contamination. This slows lymphatic uptake of bacteria and foreign material that might otherwise produce a lethal bacteremia or anaphylactoid reaction.

Although these acute inflammatory mechanisms are initially protective, they lead to abscess formation. The fibrinous exudate impedes the influx of macrophages and neutrophils. Complement, opsonins, and antibodies cannot reach the bacteria, and antibiotics penetrate poorly. Because of a slow rate of bacterial growth, bactericidal antibiotics are less effective. Virulent anaerobic bacteria previously unable to grow because of too high a redox potential now proliferate owing to lower oxygen tensions.

Neutrophils are required for the formation of abscessation. They are end-stage cells that do not return to the systemic circulation after entering the tissues or peritoneal cavity. As they engulf bacteria and other foreign substances, they produce potent lysozymic enzymes and superoxides. Extracellular release of lysozymic enzymes and superoxides normally occurs to a limited extent during phagocytosis but is markedly exaggerated during attempted phagocytosis of large particles such as particulate intestinal contents. Neutrophils moving along fibrin strands that have trapped activated complement components also degranulate prematurely and release intracellular products. When neutrophils die and undergo membranolysis and release potent enzymes and superoxides, the released products lyse bacteria, nearby neutrophils, and normal tissues. The neutrophilic enzymes released are normally neutralized by plasma inhibitors, such as alpha-1 antitrypsin. Sufficient neutralizing plasma inhibitors are unavailable around the lysed neutrophils. Continued digestion of host tissue produces a rich medium for the fibrin-protected bacteria.

Neutrophils alone are sufficient to produce an intra-abdominal abscess. If sites of experimental bacterial inoculation are completely sterilized by antibiotics after the tissues have been infiltrated by large numbers of neutrophils, abscesses still develop. It is not the presence of bacteria alone but the neutrophil and its contents that ultimately lead to abscess development. Without the neutrophils, no abscessation occurs.[74]

As abscessation continues, the hypertonicity within the cavity results in an influx of fluid and gradual expansion. This hypertonic environment allows survival of bacteria, even in the presence of antibiotics that would normally kill them by disrupting cell wall formation. These bacteria lack cell walls but persist as L-forms.[2]

The systemic effects of abscess formation include fever, tachycardia, lethargy, anorexia, leukocytosis, and generalized discomfort. Some of these signs are due to the liberation and uptake of endogenous central-acting pyrogens from the surrounding inflamed tissues. Absorption of neutrophil-liberated pyrogens from the organizing abscess also contributes to the signs. Bacterial endotoxins and exotoxins also serve as exogenous pyrogens and cause centrally mediated fever. The importance of increased prostaglandin production in the development of systemic signs is an area of vigorous investigation. Nonsteroidal anti-inflammatory and antipyretic drugs inhibit generalized prostaglandin synthesis. The inhibition of prostaglandin synthesis in the hypothalamus has been

proposed as one reason fever is reduced by aspirin. After administration of endotoxin or endogenous pyrogen, prostaglandin levels increase in the cerebrospinal fluid proportional to the increase in temperature and heart rate.[2] Late manifestations of intra-abdominal abscessation are associated with the continued and increased systemic absorption of bacterial and endogenous toxic products. Sepsis and distant major organ failure are the final results and may cause death.

Clinical Signs

Intra-abdominal abscesses may cause acute abdominal pain, fever, lethargy, and signs of intestinal obstruction.[114, 115] Such abscesses may be intraperitoneal, retroperitoneal, or visceral. Anatomical boundaries of each abscess are important in determining the source of infection and possible complications. The anatomical spaces that collect intraperitoneal fluid and become the sites of abscess formation are the right and left subdiaphragmatic regions, the lesser sac, and the periuterine, pericolonic region where a cul-de-sac of parietal peritoneum reflects onto structures in the pelvic canal. Abscesses also form around diseased viscera, including the spleen, liver, gallbladder, pancreas, prostate gland, and between loops of bowel or mesentery.[114, 115, 118] Intra-abdominal abscesses may also be associated with peritoneal or retroperitoneal foreign bodies such as suture, hair, or pieces of wood.

The formation and progression of an intra-abdominal abscess is often not dramatic and may only become clinically apparent gradually. Very small abscesses may not show any clinical signs, whereas larger ones under pressure may lead to signs of sepsis rapidly. Clinical signs are often obscure and insidious in onset. Dysorexia, emesis, vague abdominal tenderness and pain, and fever and chills are common. Femoral pulse is usually strong and rapid unless shock develops, at which time it becomes weak and thready. Intra-abdominal abscesses that rupture, allowing diffuse seeding of purulent material throughout the abdomen, may develop signs of hypodynamic septic shock and cause early death. Intestinal obstruction by a mesenteric abscess has been reported.[114] Well-encapsulated abscesses may be detected by palpation of a mass or discrete areas of abdominal tenderness.

Diagnostic Aids

Radiographic evidence of abscess formation depends on the extent and location of infection and the organs involved. Localized intraperitoneal abscesses generally result in ill-defined areas of decreased abdominal detail. A localized intra-abdominal gas pattern or generalized pneumoperitoneum may be seen.[96] Retroperitoneal abscesses may result in discrete areas of thickening of the body wall, loss of the outline of the psoas muscles or the retroperitoneal fat pads, and renal displacement. Visceral abscessation may alter the radiographic appearance of involved organs.

Laboratory aids helpful in diagnosis include peripheral white blood cell counts and cytological examination of peritoneal fluid. Peripheral and lavage fluid white cell counts are elevated, with the majority of the increase due to neutrophils. Aerobic and anaerobic culturing and antibiotic sensitivity testing of the collected peritoneal lavage fluid should be done. The method of sample collection profoundly affects the ability to culture anaerobic bacteria.[94] In one study, anaerobic culture collection using a swab was one-fifth as effective as aspiration.[74] Even when the best techniques for collection and culturing of anaerobic organisms are employed, a certain percentage is missed. Therefore, Gram's staining should always be performed.

Abdominal ultrasonography and nuclear radiography using gallium-67 citrate– or chronium-51–labelled autologous leukocytes are sophisticated tests that have been used successfully in the diagnosis of intra-abdominal abscesses.[65] Ultrasonic examination of abdominal abscesses may allow differentiation from hematomas and lymphoceles, which cannot be differentiated radiographically.[99]

Intra-abdominal abscesses are often diagnosed at exploratory laparotomy when physical signs, radiography, and laboratory tests have indicated the need for abdominal exploration.

Treatment

Treatment involves the preoperative, intraoperative, and postoperative use of antibiotics, surgical drainage, and partial to complete removal of the abscess. Experimental evidence suggests that certain antibiotics are especially efficacious in treating abscesses, including cefoxitin, carbenicillin, clindamycin, and cefamandole. Others that have been useful include those listed in the treatment of secondary bacterial peritonitis. The ultimate choice of antibiotic is determined by Gram's staining and culture and sensitivity tests.

Surgical treatment may require resection of portions of abdominal viscera with the abscess. A bypass procedure may be required to relieve intestinal obstruction when the severity and location of the abscess prevent its removal. Complete drainage of abscesses and copious irrigation are important.

Pneumoperitoneum

Pneumoperitoneum is rarely of any physiological consequence. If enough air collects in the peritoneum, it may build up pressure. This rare condition is referred to as tension pneumoperitoneum. With pressures over 20 mm Hg, significant interference with breathing and venous return occurs.[56] Pneumoperitoneum more commonly is of medical significance as a radiological sign indicating rupture of a hollow viscus, bacterial peritonitis due to a gas-forming organism (e.g., *E. coli, Clostridium perfringens*), a penetrating wound, or, occasionally, pneumothorax or pneumomediastinum in which air has dissected caudally through the dorsal area of the diaphragm into the peritoneal cavity.[66, 115] Pneumoperitoneum is also expected following paracentesis or peritoneal lavage and abdominal surgery. Air may be radiographically detectable for several days following an abdominal operation. Radiographic evidence of air within the peritoneal cavity, without a history of recent abdominal surgery, indicates probable hollow visceral disruption or peritonitis. Treatment of pneumoperitoneum involving emergency decompressive paracentesis is required only when intra-abdominal pressure is elevated.

Hemoperitoneum

Most cases of hemoperitoneum are associated with traumatic rupture of the spleen, liver, kidney, or major abdominal vessels;[21] as a complication of abdominal surgery; or spontaneously in animals with neoplasia, ulceration, or clotting abnormalities. Small amounts of blood in the peritoneal cavity are difficult to detect by any means other than peritoneal lavage.[31] Larger amounts of blood may be indicated by a circular area of red discoloration in the skin around the umbilicus, the presence of a fluid wave on ballottement, or shifting dullness on auscultation.[25] Generalized loss of contrast and an increase in density in abdominal radiographs also indicate significant peritoneal fluid.

The diagnosis of hemoperitoneum by paracentesis with a hypodermic needle is often plagued by false negative results because the lumen is occluded by omentum or other viscera.[31] Use of a peritoneal dialysis catheter with multiple perforations increases reliability. If fluid cannot be directly obtained from the abdominal cavity with a multiholed catheter, 22 ml/kg body weight of sterile balanced electrolyte solution is infused rapidly by catheter into the abdomen. The animal is gently rolled from side to side to distribute the fluid, and a sample (10 to 20 ml) of fluid is obtained by gravity. If the fluid is red, an hematocrit is determined. If the fluid is red and so dark that newsprint cannot be read through it, a significant amount of blood is present in the abdomen. An hematocrit of 5% or greater indicates significant hemorrhage. The catheter may be left in place and periodic samples obtained. A steady rise in hematocrit of the fluid indicates continued intra-abdominal bleeding.

Treatment of hemoperitoneum depends on the animal's clinical state. Most cases are seen shortly after the onset, with clinical signs of hypovolemic shock, and treatment is directed at replacing blood loss (see Chapter 11).

Autotransfusion, in which the patient's blood is

aspirated from the abdominal cavity and transfused intravenously, may be useful when autologous blood has been depleted.[26] Before infusion of blood, it should, if possible, be filtered (pore size of 20 μ) to remove platelet and WBC-RBC microaggregates. Several animals have been successfully resuscitated by autotransfusion of greater than 240 ml of blood/kg body weight before the bleeding was controlled.[27] In humans, autotransfusion of abdominal blood has been used in more than 1000 cases with few complications.[60] Fatalities have been associated with the use of blood that had been in the abdomen for over 72 hours and re-infusion of grossly contaminated blood without proper filtration.[45, 102]

Deterioration of clinical signs and rising hematocrit values of serial *lavage* fluid samples are reliable criteria for the diagnosis of continued intra-abdominal hemorrhage. Peripheral blood hematocrit levels are not reliable indicators of acute hemorrhage.

Externally applied counterpressure with a pneumatic tourniquet, antishock garment, or abdominal and pelvic limb circumferential bandages is helpful in the treatment of hypotension unresponsive to rapid fluid and blood infusion.[28] Counterpressure raises blood pressure, primarily by increasing peripheral resistance.[42] In dogs there is an increase in venous return due to cranial displacement of venous blood from the compressed area of the body.[107] Blood flow to the pelvic limbs and abdominal organs is reduced.[28]

Whenever evidence of continuing intra-abdominal hemorrhage is present, counterpressure should be applied until surgery is begun. Antishock garments for dogs and cats have been developed but are not commonly available.[28] These pneumatic garments, when inflated, compress the pelvic limbs and lower abdominal region. Compressive abdominal and pelvic limb bandages are currently the best alternative. Abdominal bandages alone may interfere with diaphragmatic movement and obstruct venous return from the pelvic limbs.[28]

Intra-abdominal pressure may be increased by intraperitoneal infusion of sterile balanced electrolyte solution (up to 50 ml/kg body weight), thereby slowing down but not stopping intra-abdominal hemorrhage.[28]

During exploratory celiotomy, arterial hemorrhage may be temporarily controlled by digital pressure to the abdominal aorta near the celiac artery. Most other types of hemorrhage can be controlled by pressure with laparotomy pads. These are systematically removed while accumulated blood is aspirated and sources of hemorrhage are identified and controlled.

NEOPLASIA

Primary Neoplasm

Primary mesotheliomas of the peritoneum are rare.[13] They cause ascites, weight loss, and palpable abdominal masses. Abdominal mesotheliomas can also spread to the pleural cavity via a direct extension through the diaphragm or by hematogenous or lymphatic routes.[12] Pleural effusion in these cases is common.

Mesothelioma is diagnosed by cytological evaluation of the ascitic fluid, exploratory laparotomy, and biopsy. By the time the diagnosis is made, the tumor has usually spread diffusely within the peritoneal cavity. In one report, numerous scattered firm white nodules, 1 to 5 mm in diameter, were on the omentum, intestinal mesentery, and abdominal surface of the diaphragm.[81] Masses up to 7.5 cm in diameter were found on the lesser curvature of the stomach and splenic hilus. Surgical treatment by excision may be carried out if the tumor is found early and confined to one area. No reports of the use of adjuvant chemotherapy or radiation therapy in dogs or cats are presently available, but their use in humans has not been encouraging.

Secondary Neoplasms

Most secondary neoplasms of the peritoneum are metastatic carcinomas or sarcomas. Malignant tumors reach the peritoneal surface by penetration of the wall of an involved viscus, hematogenous or lymphatic spread, or inoculation at surgery. Metastatic tumors may be widely disseminated over the serosal surfaces by transperitoneal seeding. The gross appearance of secondary tumors varies widely, depending on the primary lesion and the mode of spread. The main clinical features are ascites and tumor nodules. The ascitic fluid usually contains some blood and may contain exfoliated tumor cells. Ascites develops by obstruction of peritoneal lymphatics with neoplastic tissue. The presence of ascitic fluid implies dissemination of the tumor throughout the peritoneal cavity. Occasionally, conversion of the omentum to a hard mass by infiltration with tumor known as an "omental cake" is observed.

Clinical signs of secondary peritoneal tumors are weight loss, weakness, abdominal distension, anorexia, abdominal pain, and palpable abdominal masses. Occasionally, a metastatic tumor nodule is present at the umbilicus as a firm mass.[32] Radiographs of the abdomen are helpful in the early detection of neoplastic disease. If neoplasia is suspected, radiographs of the thorax are indicated preoperatively to rule out macroscopic pulmonary metastasis.

1. Abe, H., Appert, H. E., and Howard, J. M.: Hemodynamic observations of adynamic ileus in the conscious dog. Ann. Surg. *179*:332, 1974.
2. Ahrenholz, D. H., and Simmons, R. L.: Peritonitis and other intra-abdominal infections. *In* Simmons, R. L., and Howard, R. J. (eds.): *Surgical Infectious Diseases.* Appleton-Century-Crofts, New York, 1982.
3. Allen, L., and Weatherford, T.: Role of fenestrated basement membrane in lymphatic absorption from the peritoneal cavity. Am. J. Physiol. *197*:551, 1959.

4. Alusia, B., Gazzaniga, M., and Beretta, T.: The effect of a fibrinolytic substance in the prevention and treatment of post-operative peritoneal adhesions. Panminerva Med. 8:432, 1966.

5. Barnett, W. O., and Hardy, J. D.: Observations concerning the peritoneal fluid in experimental strangulated intestinal obstruction: The effects of removal from the peritoneal cavity. Surgery 43:440, 1958.

6. Barnett, W. O., and Little, B. R.: Obstruction of the large bowel. South. Med J. 58:1493, 1962.

7. Barnett, W. O., Oliver, R. I., and Elliot, R. L.: Elimination of the lethal properties of gangrenous bowel segments. Ann. Surg 167:912, 1968.

8. Bjorling, D. E., Latimer, K. S., Rawlings, C. A., Kolata, R. J., and Crowe, D. T., Jr.: Diagnostic peritoneal lavage before and after abdominal surgery in dogs. Am. J. Vet. Res. 44:816, 1983.

9. Bormside, S. H.: Enhancement of *Escherichia coli* infection and endotoxic activity by hemoglobin and furic ammonium citrate. Surgery 68:350, 1970.

10. Bost, T. C.: Mesenteric injuries and intestine viability. Ann. Surg. 89:218, 1929.

11. Bradley, R., and DeYoung, D. W.: Chylothorax with concurrent chyloabdomen in a dog. Vet. Med./Small Anim. Clin. 72:1024, 1977.

12. Breeze, R. G., and Launder, I. M.: Pleural mesothelioma in a dog. Vet. Rec. 96:243, 1975.

13. Brunner, P.: Papillary-polypour mesothelioma of the pericardium of a dog (at the same time a contribution to the questions as to primary tumors arising from serous cover cells). Virchows Arch. [Pathol. Anat.] 357:275, 1972.

14. Burdick, J. F., Warshaw, A. L., and Abbott, W. M.: External counterpressure to control postoperative intraabdominal hemorrhage. Am. J. Surg 129:269, 1975.

15. Burrows, C. F., and Bovee, K. C.: Metabolic changes due to experimentally induced rupture of the canine urinary bladder. Am. J. Vet. Res. 35:1083, 1974.

16. Cain, J. L., Labat, J. A., and Cohn, I.: Bile peritonitis in germ-free dogs. Gastroenterology 53:600, 1967.

17. Cochran, D. Q., Armond, C. H., and Shucart, W. A.: An experimental study of the effects of barium and intestinal contents on the peritoneal cavity. Am. J. Roentgenol. Rad. Ther. Nucl. Med. 89:883, 1963.

18. Coder, D. M., and Olander, G. A.: Granulomatous peritonitis caused by starch glove powder. Arch. Surg. 105:83, 1972.

19. Cohn, I., Jr., Cothar, A. M., and Atik, M.: Bile peritonitis. Ann. Surg. 152:827, 1960.

20. Conolly, W. B., and Stephens, F. O.: Factors influencing the incidence of intraperitoneal adhesions. Surgery 63:976, 1978.

21. Crane, S. W.: Evaluation and management of abdominal trauma in the dog and cat. Vet. Clin. North Am. 10:655, 1980.

22. Crane, S. W.: Placement and maintenance of a temporary feeding tube gastrostomy in the dog and cat. Comp. Cont. Ed. 11:770, 1980.

23. Crouch, J. E.: *Text-Atlas of Cat Anatomy.* Lea & Febiger, Philadelphia, 1969.

24. Crowe, D. T., Jr.: Closure of abdominal incisions using a continuous polypropylene suture: Clinical experience in 550 dogs and cats. Vet. Surg. 7:74, 1974.

25. Crowe, D. T., Jr.: Evaluation of abdominal trauma. Proc. 42nd Ann. Mtg. Am. Anim. Hosp. Assoc. 2:277, 1975.

26. Crowe, D. T., Jr.: Autotransfusion in the trauma patient. Vet. Clin. North Am. 10:581, 1980.

27. Crowe, D. T., Jr.: Autotransfusion: Clinical experience with 10 cases. Paper presented at Southeastern Veterinary Surgical Association, 1981.

28. Crowe, D. T., Jr.: Internal and external abdominal counterpressure in the dog for control of intraabdominal hemorrhage: A preliminary report. Paper presented at Ann. Mtg. Vet. Critical Care Soc., 1982.

29. Crowe, D. T., Jr.: Enteral nutrition for the critically ill or injured patient: Part I. J. Vet. Crit. Care 5:8,. 1982.

30. Crowe, D. T., Jr.: Serosal patching and jejunal onlay grafting. In Bjorab, M. J. (ed.): Current Techniques in Small Animal Surgery, 2nd ed. Lea & Febiger, Philadelphia, 1983.

31. Crowe, D. T., Jr., and Crane, S. N.: Diagnostic abdominal paracentesis and lavage in the evaluation of abdominal injuries in dogs and cats: Clinical and experimental investigations. J. Am. Vet. Med. Assoc. 168:700, 1976.

32. Crowe, D. T., Jr., and Toderoff, R. J.: Umbilical masses and discolorations as signs of intraabdominal disease. J. Am. Anim. Hosp. Assoc. 18:295, 1982.

33. Eiseman, B., Seeling, M. G., and Womack, N. A.: Talcum powder granuloma: A frequent and serious postoperative complication. Ann. Surg. 126:820, 1947.

34. Ellis, H.: The aetiology of post-operative abdominal adhesions, an experimental study. Br. J. Surg. 50:10, 1963.

35. Ellis, H.: The cause and prevention of post-operative intraperitoneal adhesions: A collective review. Surg. Gynecol. Obstet. 133:497, 1971.

36. Ellis, H.: Wound repair. Reaction of peritoneal injury. Ann. R. Coll. Surg. Eng. 60:219, 1978.

37. Eskeland, G.: Prevention of experimental peritoneal adhesions in the rat by intraperitoneally administered corticosteroids. Acta Chir. Scand. 125:91, 1963.

38. Evans, H. E.: Reproduction and prenatal development. In Evans, H. E., and Christensen, G. C. (eds.): *Miller's Anatomy of the Dog,* 2nd ed. W. B. Saunders, Philadelphia, 1979.

39. Evans, H. E., and Christensen, G. C.: *Miller's Anatomy of the Dog,* 2nd ed. W. B. Saunders, Philadelphia, 1979.

40. Filler, R. M., Sleeman, H. K., Hendry, W. S., and Pulaski, E. J.: Lethal factors in experimental peritonitis. Surgery 60:671, 1966.

41. Frye, F. L., Hoelt, D. J., Hardy, R. J., and Cucuel, J. P. E.: Surgical repair of a ruptured ileocecolic lymph node in a cat. J. Am. Vet. Med. Assoc. 157:75, 1970.

42. Gaffney, F. A., Thal, E. R., Taylor, W. F., Bastian, B. C., Weigelt, J. A., Atkins, J. M., and Blomquist, C. G.: Hemodynamic effect of the medical antishock garment. J. Trauma 21:931, 1981.

43. Gerding, D. N., Hall, W. H., and Schierl, E. A.: Antibiotic concentrations in ascitic fluid of patients with ascites and bacterial peritonitis. Ann. Intern. Med. 86:708, 1977.

44. Grier, R. L.: Intestinal antisepsis and treatment of peritonitis. Arch. Am. Coll. Vet. Surg. 5:10, 1976.

45. Griswold, R. A., and Ortner, A. B.: Use of autotransfusion in surgery of serous cavities. Surg. Gynecol. Obstet. 77:167, 1943.

46. Guyton, A. C.: *Textbook of Medical Physiology,* 5th ed., W. B. Saunders, Philadelphia, 1971.

47. Hanna, E. A.: Efficiency of peritoneal drainage. Surg. Gynecol. Obstet. 131:983, 1970.

48. Hardie, E. E.: Flunixin meglumine in the treatment of septic shock in dogs. Paper presented at the 17th Ann. Mtg. Am. Coll. Vet. Surg., 1982.

49. Hau, T., Hoffman, R., and Simmons, R. I.: Mechanisms of the adjuvant effect of hemoglobin in experimental peritonitis. I. *In vitro* inhibition of peritoneal leukocytosis. Surgery 83:233, 1978.

50. Henderson, R. A.: Controlling peritoneal adhesions. Vet. Surg. 11:30, 1982.

51. Higgins, G. M., and Graham, A. A.: Lymphatic drainage from the peritoneal cavity in the dog. Arch. Surg. 19:453, 1929.

52. Hoffer, R. E., Prange, J. R., O'Neil, J. G., Niemeyer, K. H., and Knipsel, E. V.: Treatment of acute peritonitis in dogs by intermittent peritoneal lavage. J. Am. Anim. Hosp. Assoc. 6:182, 1970.

53. Hoover, H. C., Ryan, J. A., and Anderson, E. J.: Nutritional benefits of immediate postoperative jejunal feeding of an elemental diet. Am. J. Surg. 139:153, 1980.

54. Hornanian, A. P., and Saddowi, N.: An experimental study

of the consequences of intraperitoneal irrigation. Surg. Gynecol. Obstet. *134*:575, 1972.

55. Hubay, C. A., Weckesser, E. C., and Holden, W. D.: The effect of cortisone on the prevention of peritoneal adhesions. Surg. Gynecol. Obstet. *96*:65, 1953.

56. Hutchinson, G. H.: Fatal tension pneumoperitoneum due to aerophagy. Postgrad. Med. J. *56*:657, 1980.

57. Iijima, N., Yamamoto, T., and Inoue, K.: Prevention of intraabdominal adhesions by protoporphyrin, an experimental study. Jap. J. Exp. Med. *39*:311, 1969.

58. Jones, S. A., Gazzaniga, A. B., and Keller, T. B.: The serosal patch. A surgical parachute. Am. J. Surg. *126*:186, 1973.

59. Kapur, M. L., Talwar, J. R., and Gulati, S. M.: Oxyphenbutazone—anti-inflammatory agent in prevention of peritoneal adhesions. Arch. Surg *98*:301, 1969.

60. Klebanoff, G., Phillips, J., and Evans, W.: Use of a disposable autotransfusion unit under varying conditions of contamination. Am. J. Surg. *125*:273, 1973.

61. Lacroix, J. V., and Hoskins, H. P.: Surgical principles. *In* Lacroix, J. V., and Hoskins, H. P. (eds.): *Canine Surgery*, 1st ed. The North American Veterinarian, Inc., Evanston, IL, 1939.

62. Lavigne, J. E., Brown, C. S., Machiedo, G. W., Blackwood, J. M., and Rush, B. F., Jr.: The treatment of experimental peritonitis with intraperitoneal Betadine solution. J. Surg. Res. *16*:307, 1974.

63. Lee, C. M., Jr., Collins, W. T., and Largen, T. L.: A reappraisal of absorbable glove powder. Surg. Gynecol. Obstet. *95*:725, 1952.

64. Lee, C. M., Jr., and Lehman, E. P.: Experiments with nonirritating glove powder. Surg. Gynecol. Obstet. *84*:689, 1947.

65. Lopez-Majano, V., Sansi, P., Stankievicz, S., and Tison, J.: Gallium 67 scintigraphy in abdominal diseases. Eur. J. Nucl. Med. *4*:185, 1980.

66. Macbeth, R. A., and Mackenzie, W. B.: The abdominal wall and peritoneum. *In* Sabiston, D. C. (ed.): *Christopher's Textbook of Surgery*, 10th ed. W. B. Saunders, Philadelphia, 1972.

67. MacCoy, D. M., Sykes, G. P., Hoffer, R. E., and Harvey, H. F. : A gastropexy technique for permanent fixation of the pyloric antrum. J. Am. Anim. Hosp. Assoc. *18*:763, 1982.

68. Maetani, S., and Tobe, T.: Open peritoneal drainage as effective treatment of advanced peritonitis. Surgery *90*:804, 1981.

69. Markowitz, J., Archibald, J., and Downie, H. G.: *Experimental Surgery*, 4th ed., Williams & Wilkins, Baltimore, 1959.

70. Matyaskin, I. M., and Romankov, T. R.: Chlorhexidine bigluconate in the prevention and treatment of purulent complications in a surgical clinic. Sov. Med. *34*:55, 1979.

71. Mayo, C. W.: *A Handbook of Operative Surgery—Surgery of the Small and Large Intestine*, 2nd ed. Year Book Medical Publishers, Chicago, 1962.

72. McCoy, D. M.: Peritonitis. *In* Kirk, R. W. (ed.): *Current Veterinary Therapy VI*. W. B. Saunders, Philadelphia, 1977.

73. McCurnin, D. M., and Grier, R. L.: Temperature control in the critical and surgical patient. *In* Sattler, F. P., Knowles, R. P., and Whittick, W. G. (eds.): *Veterinary Critical Care*. Philadelphia, Lea & Febiger, 1981.

74. Miles, A. A., Miles, E. M., and Burke, J.: The value and duration of defense reactions of the skin to the primary lodgement of bacteria. Br. J. Exp. Pathol. *38*:79, 1957.

75. Mishra, N. K., Appert, H. E., and Howard, J. M.: Studies of paralytic ileus: Effects of intraperitoneal injury on motility of the canine small intestine. Am. J. Surg. *129*:559, 1975.

76. Moukhtar, M.: Continuous intraperitoneal antibiotic lavage in the management of purulent sepsis of the pelvis. Surg. Gynecol. Obstet. *150*:548, 1980.

77. Nelson, R. W., and Feldman, E. C.: Treatment of canine pyometra with prostaglandin E2 alpha. Proc. 31st Gaines Vet. Symp. 1981, p. 10.

78. Norden, D. M., and de Lahunta, A.: *The Embryology of Domestic Animals—Normal Development and Congenital Malformations*. Williams & Wilkins, Baltimore, in press.

79. Parks, J., Gahring, D., and Greene, R. W.: Peritoneal lavage for peritonitis and pancreatitis in 22 dogs. J. Am. Anim. Hosp. Assoc. *9*:442, 1973.

80. Peloso, O. A., Floyd, V. T., and Wilkinson, L. H.: Treatment of peritonitis with continuous postoperative peritoneal lavage using cephalothin. Am. J. Surg. *126*:742, 1973.

81. Ralflo, C. P., and Nuernberger, S. P.: Abdominal mesothelioma in a cat. Vet. Pathol. *15*:781, 1978.

82. Rewbridge, A. G., and Hardina, A. M.: The etiological role of bacteria in bile peritonitis. An experimental study in dogs. Proc. Soc. Exp. Biol. Med. *27*:528, 1929.

83. Richardson, E. H.: Studies on peritoneal adhesions. Ann. Surg. *54*:758, 1911.

84. Robinson, S. C.: Observations on the peritoneum as an absorbing surface. Am. J. Obstet. Gynecol. *83*:446, 1962.

85. Root, H. D., Keizer, P. J., and Perry, J. F.: Peritoneal trauma, experimental and clinical studies. Surgery *52*:679, 1967.

86. Rosen, E.: Continuous closure of the abdominal wall using the external rectus fascia. Paper presented at 15th Ann. Mtg. Am. Coll. Vet. Surg., 1980.

87. Saba, T. M.: Reticuloendothelial defense: Its relevance to cardiopulmonary function in septic surgical, trauma, and burn patients. Contemp. Surg. *14*:64, 1979.

88. Shear, L., Shinaberger, J. H., and Barry, K. G.: Peritoneal transport of antibiotics in man. N. Engl. J. Med. *272*:666, 1965.

89. Sheeran, E. T.: Must parietal peritoneum be sutured after abdominal surgery? Ohio State Med. J. *66*:1022, 1970.

90. Shelby, J. S., Cothar, A. M., and Maesari, M.: Antibiotics in experimental bile peritonitis. Surg. Forum *11*:305, 1960.

91. Smith, E. G.: A rationale for intraperitoneally administered antibiotic therapy. Surg. Gynecol. Obstet. *143*:561, 1976.

92. Soderberg, C. H., Low, T. Y., and Randall, H. T.: Glove starch granulomatous peritonitis. Am. J. Surg. *125*:455, 1973.

93. Steinberg, B.: *Infections of the Peritoneum*. Hoeber Co., New York, 1944.

94. Stone, H. H., Kolb, L. D., and Gehebar, B. S.: Incidence and significance of intraperitoneal anaerobic bacteria. Ann. Surg. *181*:705, 1975.

95. Stone, H. H., Morris, E. S., Kolb, L. D., and Geheber, C. E.: Management of peritonitis: Cefamandole vs. gentamicin. Contemp. Surg. *15*:21, 1979.

96. Storer, E. H.: Peritonitis and intraabdominal. *In* Schwartz, S. I. (ed.): *Principles of Surgery*, 2nd ed. McGraw-Hill, New York, 1974.

97. Storey, B. G., Lawrenson, K. B., Chant, S., and Stephens, F. O.: Factors influencing the incidence of postoperative abdominal adhesions: an experimental study. Aust. N. Z. J. Surg. *40*:338, 1971.

98. Targan, S. R.: Role of anaerobic bacteria in spontaneous peritonitis of cirrhosis. Am. J. Med. *62*:397, 1977.

99. Taylor, K. J., Sullivan, D. C., and Wasson, J. F.: Ultrasound and gallium for the diagnosis for abdominal and pelvic abscesses. Gastrointest. Radiol. *3*:281, 1978.

100. Thayer, G. W., Carrig, C. B., and Evans, A. T.: Fatal venous air embolism associated with pneumocystography in a cat. J. Am. Vet. Med. Assoc. *176*:643, 1980.

101. Thrall, D. E., Bovee, K. C., and Biery, D. N.: Demonstration of a position of relief in dogs with lesions of the stomach and small intestine. J. Am. Anim. Hosp. Assoc. *14*:343, 1978.

102. Tiber, L.: Ruptured ectopic pregnancy. Calif. Western Med. *41*:16, 1934.

103. Torosian, M. H.: Feeding by tube enterostomy. Surg. Gynecol. Obstet. *15*:918, 1980.

104. Von Dembowski, T.: Ueber die Ursachen der peritonealen

Adhasionen mach chirurgischen Engriffen mit Rucksicht auf die frage des Ileus nach laparotomieen. Arch. Klin. Chir. 37:745, 1888.

105. Walshaw, R., and Crowe, D. T.: Discussion: The treatment of peritonitis in small animals. Presented at 9th Ann. Vet. Surg. Forum, 1981.

106. Wangensteen, O.: On the significance of the escape of sterile bile into the peritoneal cavity. Ann. Surg. 8:691, 1962.

107. Wangensteen, S. L., Ludewig, R. M., and Eddy, D. M.: The effects of external counterpressure on the intact circulation. Surg. Gynecol. Obstet. 127:253, 1968.

108. Watters, W. B., and Buck, R. C.: Scanning electron microscopy of mesothelial regeneration in the rat. Lab. Invest. 26:604, 1972.

109. Weiss, R. C., and Scott, F. W.: Feline infectious peritonitis. In Kirk, R. W. (ed.): Current Veterinary Therapy VII. W. B. Saunders, Philadelphia, 1980.

110. White, B. C.: Incidence, etiology and outcome of pulseless idioventricular rhythm treated with dexamethasone during advanced CPR. J. Am. Coll. Emerg. Phys. 8:168, 1979.

111. Wilson, D. E., Chalmers, T. C., and Madoff, M. A.: The passage of cephalothin into and out of ascitic fluid. Am. J. Med. Sci. 253:449, 1967.

112. Withrow, S. J., and Black, A. P.: Generalized peritonitis in small animals. Vet. Clin. North Am. 9:363, 1979.

113. Wolfe, D. A.: Recurrent intestinal intussusceptions in the dog. J. Am. Vet. Med. Assoc. 171:553, 1977.

114. Wolfe, D. A., and Meyer, C. W.: Obstructing intestinal abscess in a dog. J. Am. Vet. Med. Assoc. 166:518, 1975.

115. Wong, P. L.: Pneumoperitoneum associated with splenic necrosis and clostridial peritonitis in a dog. J. Am. Anim. Hosp. Assoc. 17:463, 1981.

116. Yates, J. L.: An experimental study of the local effects of peritoneal drainage. Surg. Gynecol. Obstet. 1:473, 1905.

117. Zinkia, B. A.: Experimental prevention of adhesion. In Zuidema, G. D., and Skinner, D. B. (eds.): Current Topics in Surgical Research. Academic Press, New York, 1971.

118. Zolton, G. M., and Greiner, T. P.: Prostatic abscesses—a surgical approach. J. Am. Anim. Hosp. Assoc. 14:698, 1978.

Chapter **45**

The Canine Retroperitoneal Space

Dudley E. Johnston and Bruce A. Christie

The retroperitoneal space and retroperitonitis are well-recognized entities in man.[9, 10, 11] The retroperitoneal space in humans is a potential space lying between the peritoneum and the transverse fascia, lining the posterior portion of the abdominal cavity. It extends from the diaphragm, above, to the brim of the pelvis, below. Its lateral margins correspond to the lateral borders of the lumbar epaxial muscles. The retroperitoneal space is divided into an anterior space containing parts of the colon, duodenum, and pancreas, and a posterior space containing kidneys, adrenal glands, aorta, vena cava, and ureters. The posterior space is further subdivided into anterior and posterior compartments by the renal fascia.[11]

In animals, the retroperitoneal space is described indirectly, as in the description, "organs which lie against the wall of the abdominal or pelvic cavity, and which are covered only on one side by peritoneum, are said to be retoperitoneal".[3] An understanding of the anatomy of the retroperitoneal space and abdominal wall fascial planes is important in determining the extent and direction of spread of an infection that originates in the space.

ANATOMY

The common dorsal mesentery is the peritoneal fold that leaves the dorsal abdominal wall and reflects directly or indirectly around most of the freely movable organs of the abdominal cavity. The parts of the common dorsal mesentery attached to the different parts of the digestive tract are the mesogastrium, mesoduodenum, mesojejunoileum, mesocolon, and mesorectum. The right lobe of the pancreas lies in the mesoduodenum, and the left lobe of the pancreas lies in the deep (dorsal) leaf of the greater omentum,

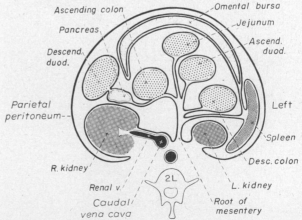

Figure 45–1. In the dog, the potential space between the apposed surfaces of peritoneum that form the mesenteries is equivalent to the anterior retroperitoneal space in humans. (Reprinted with permission from Evans, H. E., and Christensen, G. C. (eds.): *Miller's Anatomy of the Dog*, 2nd ed. W. B. Saunders Co., Philadelphia, 1979.)

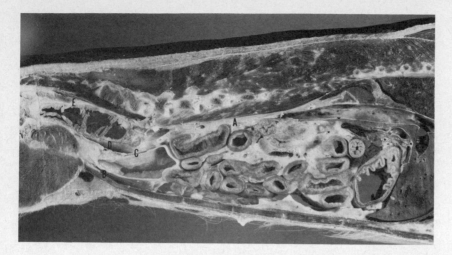

Figure 45–2. A sagittal section of a spayed female dog, just to the right of the median plane. The retroperitoneal space (*A*) extends from the diaphragm to the pelvis. *B*, Pubovesical pouch; *C*, vesicogenital pouch; *D*, rectogenital pouch; *E*, pararectal fossa.

which is derived from the mesogastrium. The spleen is attached to the greater curvature of the stomach by the gastrosplenic ligament, part of the greater omentum. The potential space between the apposed surfaces of the peritoneum that form the mesenteries is equivalent to the anterior retroperitoneal space in man (Figs. 45–1 and 45–3).

In the dog, the significant retroperitoneal space lies between the peritoneum and the muscles and bones of the back. Equivalent to the posterior retroperitoneal space in humans, it contains fat, loose

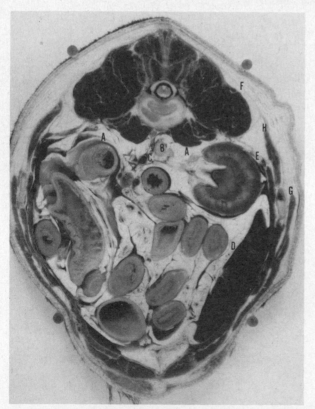

Figure 45–3. A transverse section through the abdomen at the level of the left kidney. The retroperitoneal space is large and contains much fatty tissue. *A*, Retroperitoneal space; *B*, aorta, containing latex; *C*, vena cava; *D*, spleen; *E*, transverse fascia; *F*, lumbodorsal fascia; *G*, external abdominal oblique muscle; *H*, internal abdominal oblique muscle.

connective tissue, blood vessels and nerves (aorta, vena cava, and lesser vessels), and organs (ureters, adrenal glands, and kidneys). It extends from the diaphragm rostrally to the anus caudally, and is continuous rostrally with the retropleural space and mediastinum (Fig. 45–2). Its lateral limits correspond to lateral borders of the quadratus lumborum muscles (Fig. 45–3). For practical purposes, the retroperitoneal space, from rostral to caudal, can be regarded as being the prerenal space, the perirenal space, the pararectal space, and the intra-pelvic space (see Fig. 45–2).

In the perirenal space, the kidneys are held in place by extraperitoneal connective tissue. In humans, this fibroareolar tissue, which surrounds the kidney and perirenal fat, is the renal fascia.[11] It has two layers. The anterior layer merges with tissue around the great vessels. The posterior layer is attached to the fascia of the quadratus lumborum and psoas muscles. Anterior and posterior layers are attached to each other at the hilus, preventing perirenal effusion from crossing to the other perirenal space. Cranial to the adrenal gland, the two layers fuse to connect with the fascia of the diaphragm. Caudal to the kidney the two layers remain separated.

To determine the limits of the retroperitoneal space in the dog, colored dyes were fused into the space at specific sites.[6] Green dye was infused into the perirenal space at the hilus of the left kidney, and yellow dye into the prerenal space at the esophageal hiatus of the diaphragm. The green dye extended only a small distance cranially, into the perirenal area, but passed easily to the pelvis caudally and to the lateral border of the quadratus lumborum muscle laterally. It did not cross the midline. The yellow dye passed caudally to the region of the left kidney but did not mix with the dye in the perirenal space. The yellow dye crossed from the left side to the right side. These findings agree with the description of the renal fascia and perirenal space in man.

When this experiment was repeated in another dog by infusing a large amount of blue dye into the perirenal space at the level of the caudal pole of the left kidney, the dye extended to the anus caudally,

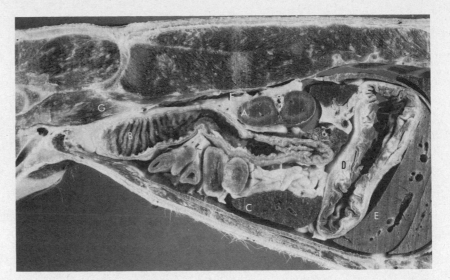

Figure 45–4. Sagittal section of a dog to the left of the midline. *A,* Left kidney; *B,* descending colon; *C,* spleen; *D,* stomach; *E,* liver; *F,* retroperitoneal space; *G,* iliopsoas muscle passing from the sublumbar position to the femur.

crossed from left to right sides, and, in addition, surrounded the kidney by spreading to the perirenal space. The dye also extended into the caudal mediastinum, past the diaphragm.

These observations may indicate a natural barrier around the kidney in the dog. The barrier is not absolute, as it is in humans, because of the spread of dye throughout the retroperitoneal space when larger volumes of dye were injected. It can be concluded that there are natural compartments surrounding the kidneys in the dog; however, the subdivision of the renal fascia to create distinct compartments in the

perirenal space is not as strongly developed in the dog. This conclusion is supported by the apparent inability of infections in the retroperitoneal space to spread into the perirenal space.

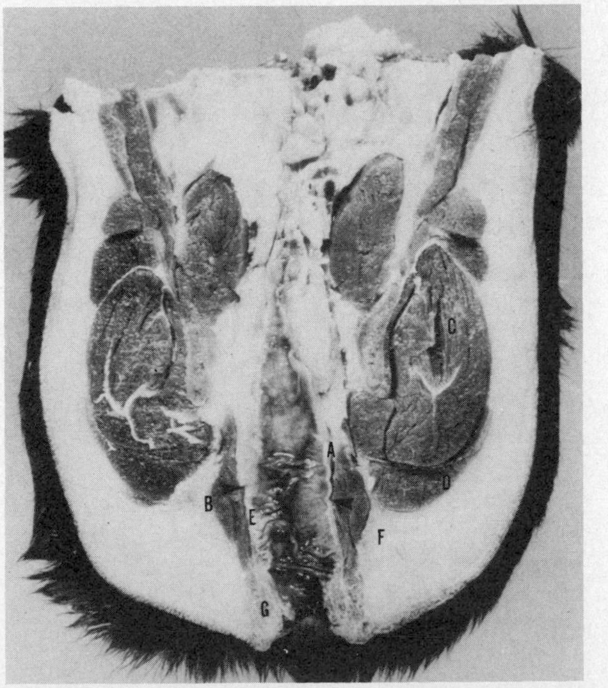

The pararectal space extends from the perirenal space into the pelvis to the peritoneal reflections (Fig. 45–2 and 45–4).

The intra-pelvic retroperitoneal space lies within the pelvis between the pelvic bones and the contained viscera, caudal to the reflections of the peritoneum. A sagittal section of the body of a spayed female dog just lateral to the median plane shows, in the caudoventral position, the peritoneum reflected dorsally from the sheath of the rectus muscle onto the neck of the bladder to form the pubovesical pouch (see Fig. 45–2). The stump of the uterus has adhered to the bladder, obliterating most of the vesicogenital pouch but leaving a large rectogenital pouch. Dorsally, the rectum is attached to the ventral surface of the sacrum by a short broad mesorectum. The mesorectum ends at a point usually opposite the second coccygeal vertebra and reflects cranially at an acute angle at the peritoneal reflection, forming in the process the pararectal fossa (Fig. 45–2 and 45–5). Retroperitoneal effusions can reach as far caudally as the anus, as shown by spread of dye injected into the retroperitoneal space.[6]

SURGICAL APPROACHES VIA THE RETROPERITONEAL SPACE

Adrenalectomy in the dog via the retroperitoneal space has been recommended (Fig. 45–3, 45–6, and 45–7).[5] The advantages over the abdominal approach are direct access to the adrenal glands, lack of trauma to abdominal organs, especially the pancreas, and lack of weight-bearing on the abdominal incision, healing of which may be delayed because of high circulating steroid levels. The retroperitoneal approach has the disadvantage that both adrenal glands cannot be examined and compared before removal.

Figure 45–5. A frontal section of the pelvis of a dog. *Arrows* point to the peritoneal reflections. *A,* Peritoneal cavity; *B,* coccygeus and levator ani muscles; *C,* gluteus medius muscle; *D,* gluteus superficialis muscle; *E,* fat in pararectal fossa; *F,* fat in ischiorectal fossa; *G,* sphincter ani externus muscle.

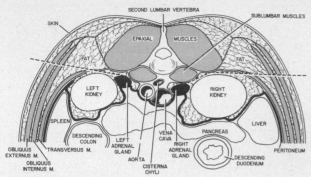

Figure 45–6. Cross-section of the dog at the 2nd lumbar vertebra. The surgical approach for adrenalectomy via the retroperitoneal approach is indicated by the broken lines. (Reprinted with permission from Johnston, D. E.: Adrenalectomy via retroperitoneal approach in dogs. J. Am. Vet. Med. Assoc. *170*:1092, 1977.)

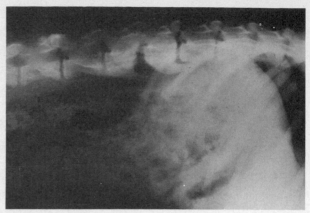

Figure 45–8. Lateral radiograph of a dog showing severe osteomyelitis of L2 and L3 and retroperitonitis. A grass awn was present in the abscess between L2 and L3.

In the removal of large kidney tumors, access to the renal vessels via a ventral midline incision is extremely difficult.[2] These vessels can be approached directly via the retroperitoneal space and can be ligated and divided. Then, the large kidney tumor can be removed by extending the retroperitoneal incision ventrally into a flank incision.

RETROPERITONITIS

Retroperitonitis is an infective process originating in the retroperitoneal space. Twenty-nine confirmed cases of retroperitonitis with four causative agents have been reported.[6]

Causes

The most common type of retroperitonitis occurs in female dogs that have been spayed prior to the development of clinical signs (see Table 45–1). The period between spaying and development of signs varied in one report from four months to four years, with a median period of six months. Only two dogs

were seen more than one year after spaying. In all cases, ligatures of silk, multifilament nylon, or braided synthetic material had been used to ligate the ovarian pedicle and uterine stump.[6]

Severe spreading retroperitonitis is seen in dogs in association with grass awns involving the lumbar vertebrae (Fig. 45–8).[7] Such cases are seen only in geographic areas where sharp grass awns are present. Retroperitonitis has been seen in hunting dogs that have access to penetrating grass awns and other foreign bodies of plant origin. No foreign bodies may be found; however, organisms identified as *Actinomyces* species can be isolated from the infected tissue.[6]

Retroperitonitis has been seen in association with other retroperitoneal foreign bodies and with perforation of the pelvic urethra with a catheter and passage of the catheter cranially into the retroperitoneal space. In one of our patients, a foreign body, identified as the top 2 cm of a branch from a pine tree, was found in an abscess in the retroperitoneal space (Fig. 45–9).

Clinical Signs

The clinical signs of retroperitonitis seen in 29 dogs are summarized in Table 45–1.[6] Pyrexia, changes in

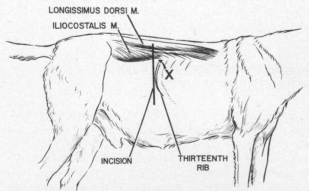

Figure 45–7. Site of skin incision for adrenalectomy via the retroperitoneal approach. The site for entry into the retroperitoneal space is indicated (x). (Reprinted with permission from Johnston, D. E.: Adrenalectomy via retroperitoneal approach in dogs. J. Am. Vet. Med. Assoc. *170*:1092, 1977.)

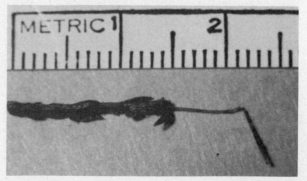

Figure 45–9. A foreign body, the end of a branch from a pine tree, found in a retroperitoneal abscess in a dog.

TABLE 45-1. Clinical Recognition of Retroperitonitis in 29 Dogs

Total No. Dogs	Cause	History	Clinical Signs and Symptoms					
			Fluctuating Abscess and Sinus in Flank	Firm Swelling and Sinus in Flank	Osteomyelitis	Pyrexia	Pain	Increased Soft Tissue Density on X-rays
18	Spay complications	Spayed female up to 4 years after spaying	18/18	0/18	0/18			
6	Grass awns	Specific geographical areas	5/6	0/6	6/6			
1	Foreign body	—	1/1	0/1	0/1	During development of abscess	Marked during development of abscess; suggestive of disc pain; pain subsided if abscess ruptured in flank	Present in all dogs
3	Actinomycosis	Hunting dogs	1/3	2/3	0/3			
1	Ruptured urethra	Catheterization	0/1	0/1	0/1			

(Modified from Johnston, D. E., and Christie, B. A.: The retroperitoneal space and retroperitonitis in dogs. Comp. Cont. Ed. (in press.)

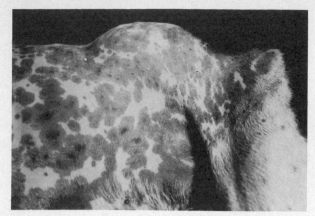

Figure 45–10. Retroperitonitis presenting clinically as a large granulomatous mass protruding from the lumbodorsal triangle. Discharging sinuses were present, and *actinomyces* organisms were isolated from the infection in the retroperitoneal space.

white blood cells, and pain are present consistently, although these signs are pronounced during the period prior to rupture of an abscess. In one study, fluctuating abscess or a firm swelling in the flank occurred in 27 of 29 dogs (Fig. 45–10).[6]

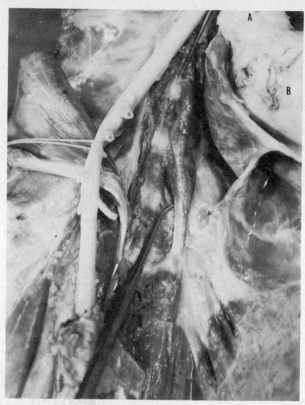

Figure 45–12. Ventral view of the abdomen of the dog shown in Figure 45–11. Muscle has been reflected from the bodies of T1, L1, and L2 vertebrae. The angled probe passes beneath a portion of the quadratus lumborum muscle. *A,* Esophagus; *B,* stomach.

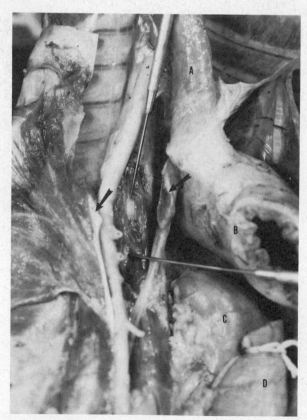

Figure 45–11. Ventral view of the abdomen of a dog. The peritoneal investment around the esophageal hiatus and the pyloric region of the stomach have been removed. *Arrows* point to the cut edges of the apposed left and right crura of the diaphragm between the esophageal and the aortic hiatuses. The aorta has been retracted slightly to the right. The two probes mark the limits of the body of the last thoracic vertebra. The left kidney and ligated descending colon are visible. *A,* Esophagus; *B,* stomach; *C,* left kidney; *D,* descending colon.

Pathogenesis

There has been speculation concerning the pathogenesis of vertebral body abscess and flank sinus associated with grass awns.[4, 7]

The pathogenesis postulated for this condition has an anatomical basis. Soon after the terminal esophagus passes through the hiatus of the diaphragm, it makes a pronounced left turn before entering the stomach (Fig. 45–11). Immediately adjacent to the dorsal surface of the terminal esophagus is the left crus of the diaphragm (Fig. 45–11). A sharp foreign body such as a grass awn could penetrate the terminal esophagus, pierce the left crus, and come to lie ventral to the vertebral body of T13 or L1. From the disposition of the sublumbar muscle fibers (Fig. 45–12), activity of these muscles would encourage caudal migration of the awn. Purulent material in the abscess cavity surrounding the foreign body could work its way dorsal to the quadratus lumborum and psoas muscles, to reach the fascial plane between the transverse and internal abdominal oblique muscles and from there to the lumbar triangle and the exterior, either to the flank or across the back (Fig. 45–13). In humans and dogs, pus in the retroperitoneal space points to the lumbodorsal triangle of Petit.[6, 10]

There are no strong natural barriers to the spread of infection within the retroperitoneal space. The

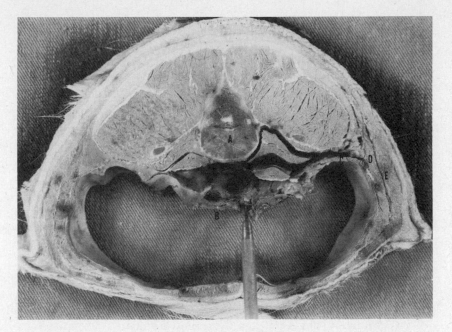

Figure 45–13. Transverse section of the abdomen of a dog through L1 vertebra. The retroperitoneal space is opened with a probe. Transverse fascia passes to the vertebral hypaxial muscles. Fluid can readily pass dorsal to these muscles to reach the abdominal wall fascial planes. *A,* L1; *B,* retroperitoneal space; *C,* transverse abdominal muscle; *D,* internal abdominal oblique muscle; *E,* external abdominal oblique muscle.

space is limited by peritoneum ventrally and fascia dorsally. Within the space, however, there is only fat and loose connective tissue. Therefore, infection can spread from one lateral limit of the space to the other lateral limit and from the diaphragm to the pelvis. It can readily extend into the fascial planes in the body wall.[6]

In addition, the retroperitoneal space lacks the resistance to infection that is found in the peritoneal cavity. In the peritoneal cavity, the peritoneum, the mesenteries, and the omentum react to localize and eliminate infective processes. These mechanisms do not exist in the retroperitoneal space.

Meyer, in 1934, showed that infection in the retroperitoneal space causes a different and more serious illness from that caused by the same infection in the peritoneal cavity.[8] Cultures of *Staphylococcus aureus* and *Pseudomonas aeruginosa* were injected into the peritoneal cavity of ten dogs and into the retroperitoneal space in 15 dogs. In the first group, the characteristic feature of the resulting illness was its acute nature, followed by rapid death or complete recovery. Five dogs died and five recovered. In the second group, with retroperitoneal injections, the resulting illness was characterized by lack of an immediate reaction of acute toxemia, apparent recovery, then a chronic illness resulting in death in 11 of the 15 animals. No abscesses were seen in any of the dogs receiving intraperitoneal injection but ten of the 15 dogs with retroperitoneal injection developed abscesses.[8]

It is unknown whether infective organisms are present in the ligature materials used in spaying procedures or whether local sterile irritation is caused by the ligature material and blood-borne organisms localize in the area of lowered resistance. It is speculated that the area of local peritonitis around the ligature material is "walled-off" from the peritoneal cavity and that the ligature material with any enclosed infection becomes retroperitoneal. Then the infective process spreads throughout the retroperitoneal space. The abscess extends to the skin in the lumbodorsal triangle.[6]

Diagnosis

Infections involving the retroperitoneal space can be difficult to diagnose because of the indefinite signs and a general lack of awareness of the nature of these infections. The clinical history and signs can be highly suggestive of retroperitonitis, and generally the diagnosis can be confirmed by radiographs. The history varies, depending on the cause, and includes spaying, access to penetrating grass awns (only in the geographic areas where these awns exist, such as Australia, Florida, and western United States), use of the dog for hunting, or passage of a urethral catheter. There is generally a history of long-standing illness with remissions and exacerbations of clinical signs. A typical history is the development of a flank abscess followed by a sinus in the area. The dog is extremely ill and in pain during the development of the abscess and improves considerably in a few weeks. The abscess recurs after a period varying from three weeks to months.

Fever is invariably present during the development phase of the infection and regresses if the abscess ruptures. Changes suggestive of a chronic infection are present in the differential and total white blood cell counts. Pain can be elicited by deep palpation of the lumbar area. The pain suggests lumbar disc disease or a painful process in the abdomen.

A definitive clinical sign is the presence of a painful swelling or a discharging sinus in the flank in the lumbodorsal triangle.[6] It is likely that an abscess and a sinus will be present in all dogs if the disease process is not halted by treatment. (In a study of retroperitonitis in humans, the retroperitoneal abscesses that spread to the lumbodorsal triangle of Petit were reported to be rare since the advent of antibiotics.[10]) Abscess formation and discharging sinus were present in 27 of the 29 dogs.[6] The abscesses fluctuated in 25 dogs and were firm granulomatous masses in two dogs with actinomycosis.

The site of the abscess and sinus is in the lumbar triangle. In seven dogs in the cited report, an abscess developed on one side of the dog, the sinus eventually healed, and, subsequently, an abscess developed on the opposite side of the body.[6]

In two dogs in which *Actinomyces* species were isolated, a large firm granulomatous mass was present over the lumbodorsal triangle.[6] Discharging sinuses were present in the mass, and characteristic "sulfur granules" were seen in the discharge. A case of actinomycotic peritonitis was reported in a dog in 1976.[1] Two interesting aspects of this case were that a draining tract was present on its left paralumbar region and that anorexia and lethargy had been present for four months. A likely pathogenesis of the actinomycotic peritonitis in this case was that it followed an actinomycotic retroperitonitis in which the infective process later invaded the peritoneum and entered the peritoneal cavity. The large mass was described as being "tightly adhered to the gastrosplenic ligament and to all surrounding peritoneal surfaces."[1]

Radiographs can be used to confirm the diagnosis. Osteomyelitis or periostitis of lumbar vertebrae may be seen, although usually only in cases of grass awn penetration (see Table 45–1).[6] In all cases, the low radiographic density of the retroperitoneal fat is not present in the radiograph. Instead, a fluid density is present that obscures the outline of the kidney.

Treatment

Treatment of retroperitonitis by administration of antibiotics has not been successful. Surgical exploration, debridement, and drainage are necessary.

Treatment of retroperitonitis caused by spaying is complex. The most satisfactory surgical approach is a lateral approach into the retroperitoneal area.[7] The ligature that is directly involved in the retroperitoneal abscess is usually found within the wall and lumen of the abscess (Fig. 45–14). After exploration of the abscess cavity, removal of the ligature, and debridement of all necrotic tissue, the incision is extended ventrally by splitting of the transverse abdominal and abdominal oblique muscles in the direction of their fibers. After the abdomen is entered, the remaining ligatures at the ovary and uterine stump (often embedded in a mass of granulation tissue), are removed (Fig. 45–15). A Penrose drain is inserted in

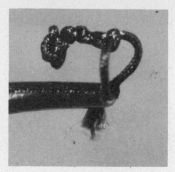

Figure 45–14. A ligature of braided nylon found in a retroperitoneal abscess in a dog after spaying. Note the numerous knots that produced a large mass of foreign material.

the abscess cavity, and the abdominal wall and skin are closed. Antibiotics are given and changed later, if necessary, when results of culture and sensitivity testing are available. Drains are removed in five to seven days.

This procedure is usually successful, although retroperitonitis has recurred in animals in which silk ligatures were used. In these cases, the material was disintegrating and difficulty was experienced in removing all pieces of ligature.[6] The recurrence should be treated surgically in the same manner.

Treatment of grass awn penetration includes removal of the grass awn, curettagae of the infected bone, debridement of necrotic tissue, insertion of a drain for five to seven days, and administration of antibiotics selected after culture and sensitivity testing. Recovery is usually rapid and complete.[7]

Treatment of dogs with *Actinomyces* infection of the retroperitoneal space can be frustrating. Following exploration, debridement, drainage, and antibiotic therapy, there can be apparent recovery and

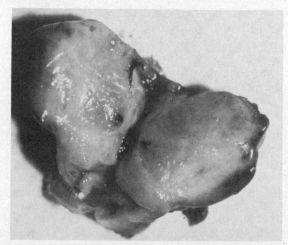

Figure 45–15. Remnants of a silk ligature embedded in a mass of granulation tissue, found at the ovarian pedicle. Particles of a silk ligature from the other ovarian pedicle were found in a retroperitoneal abscess.

then recurrence of the infection in one to two months. In one dog in which *Actinomyces* organisms were isolated, there were four recurrences of the infection, despite antibiotic therapy for up to 60 days after four surgical procedures.[6] A small sinus tract, but not generalized retroperitonitis, persisted in the dog. In other dogs, successful treatment was achieved after three recurrences. Obviously, chronicity and persistence of infection are features of these retroperitoneal infections, and long-term therapy is needed.

1. Chastain, G. B., Grier, R. L., Hogle, R. M., et al.: Actinomycotic peritonitis in a dog. J. Am. Vet. Med. Assoc. *168*:499, 1976.
2. Christie, B. A.: Incidence and etiology of vesicoureteral reflux in apparently normal dogs. Invest. Urol. 9:184, 1971.
3. Evans, H. E., and Christensen, G. C.: *Miller's Anatomy of the Dog*. 2nd ed. W. B. Saunders, Philadelphia, 1979.
4. Horne, R. D.: Grass awn migration in the dog. Canine Pract. 8:21, 1981.
5. Johnston, D. E.: Adrenalectomy via retroperitoneal approach in dogs. J. Am. Vet. Med. Assoc. *170*:1092, 1977.
6. Johnston, D. E., and Christie, B. A.: The retroperitoneal space and retroperitonitis in dogs. Comp. Cont. Ed. (in press).
7. Johnston, D. E., and Summers, B. A.: Osteomyelitis of the lumbar vertebrae in dogs caused by grass-seed foreign bodies. Aust. Vet. J. *47*:289, 1971.
8. Meyer, H. I.: The reaction of the retroperitoneal tissues to infection. Ann. Surg. 99:246, 1934.
9. Neuhof, H., and Arnheim, E. E.: Acute retroperitoneal abscess and phlegmon: a study of sixty-five cases. Ann. Surg. *119*:741, 1944.
10. Stevenson, E. O. S., and Ozeran, R. S.: Retroperitoneal space abscesses. Surg. Gynecol. Obstet. *128*:1202, 1969.
11. Warwick, R., and Williams, P. L.: *Gray's Anatomy*. 35th ed. Landau, Longman's, 1973.

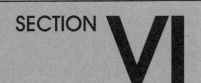

SECTION **VI**

Alimentary System

Eberhard Rosin and Colin E. Harvey
Section Editors

Chapter 46 The Oral Cavity and Pharynx

Anatomy

John Grandage

THE ORAL CAVITY

Many regard the mouth as the most specialized part of the carnivore's body. It has a unique anatomy that is predisposed to unique problems.

Lips and Cheeks

The lips of cats and dogs have few functions. They are lean, relatively immobile, and long, with an extensive rima oris between them. Because they extend far back, they do not restrict the jaws from opening widely, but they do encroach on the cheeks. The pendulous upper lip needs little support; it is weakly tethered by a small median frenulum, which is sometimes double in the dog.[118] The lower lip is thin and is prevented from everting by a close attachment to the lower jaw near the canine tooth; this allows the upper canine to pass on its outside. Even so, poor support caudal to this site encourages the lower lip of soft-mouthed dogs to fold and evert; saliva may then drool chronically from the fold.

Most of the oral cavity is obliterated when the jaws close, leaving the vestibular part the more capacious. The small buccal vestibule forms a pouch that can be useful for the administration of liquids, which can flow into the oral cavity via the interdental spaces. The environment within the buccal vestibule differs from that within the oral cavity proper because it exclusively receives the secretions of the parotid and zygomatic glands. This, in turn, may influence the variable distribution of pellicle, plaque, or calculus on the teeth.

The muscles of the lips and cheeks develop from the primitive sphincter of the neck and include the platysma, orbicular, mental, buccinator, zygomatic, canine, nasolabial, and incisive muscles. They consist mostly of flimsy strands, which are difficult to see and even more difficult to distinguish. They are all innervated by the facial nerve, paralysis of which is likely to present only subtle signs, especially in the cat. Sensory innervation is conveyed by several branches of the trigeminal (including the buccal, mental, myelohyoid, and auriculotemporal branches of the mandibular and the infraorbital branch of the maxillary[59]). Blood vessels include branches of the facial and infraorbital, and lymphatic drainage is primarily to the mandibular lymph nodes.

The Tongue

Because the carnivore's tongue participates in a number of vital functions such as lapping, sucking, and swallowing, only slight dysfunction can be tolerated.

The thick mucous membrane that covers the dorsum is roughened with papillae. The filiform variety are less numerous in cats than in dogs but are more heavily cornified with backwardly pointed hooklike tips; grooming by licking inevitably combs out hair, which is swallowed and predisposes to hairballs; threadlike foreign bodies are difficult to release. A fringe of marginal papillae sprouts from the edge of the blade of the tongue of the newborn and probably helps make an airtight seal around the nipple during sucking.[45] The gustatory papillae (fungiform, vallate, and foliate) are of little clinical significance.

The mucous membrane of the ventral surface of the tongue is thin and glistening. Paired sublingual veins are conspicuous beneath it and may be useful for venipuncture in the anesthetized animal. They lie midway between the median lingual frenulum and the curious fimbriated fold (plica fimbriata) found more laterally. The lyssa is visible in the midline on the ventral surface of the tongue's apex. In dogs it is a pale stiff tube of connective tissue about 4 cm long containing muscle, fat, and cartilage.[2] It is less well developed in cats.[118] The lyssa elongates under hypoglossal stimulation,[20] but no convincing function has been demonstrated. It was formerly removed as a prophylactic measure against rabies.[114]

The mucous membrane is bound down tightly to the lingual aponeurosis, which, in turn, is firmly attached to the underlying muscular and fatty tissues. There are three pairs of extrinsic muscles (genioglossus, styloglossus, and hyoglossus) and roughly an equal volume of intrinsic muscles whose fibers run in three planes at right angles to one another. Such architecture makes blunt dissection difficult. The tongue can be parted, however, along the fascial planes, which receive extrinsic muscles from the outside. Of these, the lingual septum is most easily divided as it runs vertically between the two genioglossi.

All the muscles receive motor innervation from the hypoglossal nerve. Its stimulation on one side causes the tongue to protrude and deviate toward that side.[111] The very apex may start to twist back again.[21]

The hypoglossal nerve sweeps down from the occipital bone, passes over the pharyngeal constrictors, and runs lateral to the hyoglossus muscle. The lingual nerve is the principal sensory nerve to the tongue with the chorda tympani, glossopharyngeal, and vagus conveying a number of sensory modalities.

The tongue is highly vascular, with about 30,000 arteriovenous anastomoses beneath the dorsum, probably serving a thermoregulatory function.[36, 126] The large lingual arteries are sinuous to allow excursions of the mobile tongue. Lymph drains to the mandibular lymph nodes.

The Teeth

The carnivore's teeth have relatively thin enamel, probably because it eats nonabrasive food and chews little. The enamel has a lower inorganic content (90 per cent) than human teeth, a factor that makes the teeth more opaque and accounts for their particularly white appearance.[15]

The permanent dentition of the dog is $2(I\frac{3}{3}\text{-}C\frac{1}{1}\text{-}P\frac{4}{4}\text{-}M\frac{2}{3}) = 42$, and that of the cat is $2(I\frac{3}{3}\text{-}C\frac{1}{1}\text{-}P\frac{3}{2}\text{-}M\frac{1}{1}) = 30$. The fewer cheek teeth of the cat reflect its more carnivorous nature, with sectorial teeth predominating.[64] The additional molars of the dog are bunodont and designed for crushing. In both cat and dog the largest sectorial tooth, the carnassial, is the last premolar of the upper jaw and the first molar of the lower jaw. Shearing by the carnassials is accomplished by closing the narrower lower dental arch inside the wider upper one; the action is assisted by a mobile mandibular symphysis, which allows each half of the mandible to twist about a longitudinal axis.[130, 137]

The deciduous dentition of the dog is $2(Di\frac{3}{3}\text{-}Dc\frac{1}{1}\text{-}Dp\frac{3}{3}) = 28$, and that of the cat is $2(Di\frac{3}{3}\text{-}Dc\frac{1}{1}\text{-}Dp\frac{3}{2}) = 26$. Most of the deciduous teeth begin to calcify during the last two to three weeks of gestation[8, 172] and erupt between three and six weeks postnatally. The upper canine teeth are usually the first to erupt, followed by the incisors. Except caudally, upper teeth usually erupt before lower ones.[15] The dog is unusual, but not unique, in having no deciduous precursor for PM1 (or arguably no permanent successor), a single tooth erupting here at about five months.[59] As the permanent teeth develop they bring about the resorption of the roof of the bony crypts in which they are housed and of the roots of the overlying deciduous teeth.[105] They cause the shedding (exfoliation) of the deciduous teeth and emerge through the gums between three and seven months in both the cat and the dog.

Various tables of eruption times have been published from which it is evident that there is considerable variability and unreliability; only coarse estimates of age may be made based on tooth eruption.[23, 38, 95, 145] Not infrequently both temporary and permanent canines may be present simultaneously and remain so for several weeks.[15] In such circumstances the permanent canines emerge medial and rostral to the reluctant temporaries.[6] The lower first molar begins calcifying prenatally, but all the other permanent teeth do so after birth.[8, 59] Disease or insult at any time in the first three months of life may affect the development of the tooth, especially the enamel. Although permanent teeth have usually fully erupted by seven months, they continue to mature for many months more. The wide pulp cavity at six months of age gradually becomes filled over the next year with dentine until it is a narrow thread that communicates with the tissues around the root by a small apical foramen.

Variations in numbers of teeth are common but probably inconsequential.[5] About half of all dogs have some anodontia, with the first or second premolars of both jaws being the teeth most often absent.[9] Brachycephalic breeds may have fewer teeth, but surprisingly they sometimes have an excess.[1] Their teeth are always crowded, and the premolars tend to rotate to lie transversely.[150]

The teeth of carnivores have one, two, or three roots (Fig. 46–1). In the dog a single root supports the incisors, canines, first premolars, and lower molar 3; the remaining lower teeth have two roots, as do the upper premolars 2 and 3. The remaining teeth (upper P4, M1, and M2) each have three roots, two vestibular and one large lingual, per tooth. The vestibular roots are often palpable over the maxilla. Only the upper carnassial tooth of the cat has three roots. Each tooth is housed in its own alveolus within the alveolar processes of the jaws. The bone is mostly cancellous, but around the wall of each alveolus it

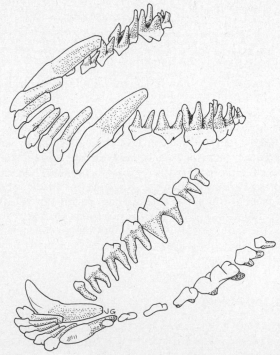

Figure 46–1. Sketch prepared from a radiograph of a Great Dane skull to show the roots of the teeth. Only the caudal upper cheek teeth possess three roots.

becomes less porous and so shows up conspicuously on radiographs as the lamina dura.[185] This plate of bone anchors the obliquely disposed fibers of the periodontal membrane, which suspend the tooth.

The teeth are innervated by alveolar nerves that run in tunnels through the alveolar processes of the jaws. Access to these nerves is difficult; local anesthesia is only readily accomplished by blocking the parent nerve from which the alveolar branches arise. The inferior alveolar nerve is a branch of the mandibular and gives off sensory branches within the mandibular canal to supply the lower teeth. Three sets of superior alveolar nerves, caudal, middle, and rostral, are given off the infraorbital nerve to supply the upper teeth. Other sensory nerves supply the adjacent regions of the gum and jaw.

The Hard Palate

The palate allows independent functioning of the respiratory and digestive systems and is especially important during the neonatal period when sucking requires an airtight oral cavity. The palate develops by the inward growth of two horizontal ledges, the palatine processes, which ultimately meet and fuse in the midline with the downwardly growing nasal septum. Abnormal growth of one or more of these processes may result in uni- or bilateral cleft palate; the consequent communication between one or both nasal fossae and the oral cavity creates difficulties in feeding. Whereas the hard palate forms a rigid partition between the respiratory and digestive systems, the soft palate forms a valve. When elevated, it closes off the nasopharynx, and when depressed it closes off the oropharynx.

THE PHARYNX

There is a basic flaw in the design of the respiratory system of air-breathing animals—the airway arises from the ventral surface of the digestive tube, where it is in constant danger of being flooded or choked by ingesta. The pharynx has evolved to cope with this danger and is an ingenious crossroads or "pharyngeal chiasma" between nasal chambers, larynx, oral cavity, and esophagus. It is equipped with valves to direct the flow, is dilatable so that it can receive large boluses of food, and is muscular so that it can pass them on quickly. Dysfunction may result in such serious consequences as inability to swallow or bronchial aspiration.

The Soft Palate

The soft palate stretches like a canopy across the front of the pharynx, dividing it into oral and nasal parts. Its free, curved, caudal edge is formed by the right and left palatopharyngeal arches (caudal pillars), which merge with the sides of the pharynx; these

arches form the rim of the intrapharyngeal ostium. The three parts of the pharynx meet at the ostium: nasopharynx above, oropharynx below, and laryngopharynx behind. A palatopharyngeal muscle within the arch acts as a sphincter for the ostium. The epiglottis usually projects through the ostium to rest on the dorsal surface of the palate, but in dogs and cats this relationship is not obligatory and the epiglottis may frequently be found beneath the soft palate.

The fibers of the palatini muscles are longitudinal and shorten the relatively long soft palate of the dog. Even brachycephalic dogs have a long soft palate;[59] radiographs reveal that their soft palate is thickened too, suggesting that these animals have sustained contractions of their palatini to maintain a patent airway. Paired tensor and levator muscles stretch and lift the soft palate, respectively, with the aponeurosis of the tensor also serving as a structural support for the palate.[59] Because the palatini and pharyngeal muscles are innervated directly from the pharyngeal plexus (IX and X), they may retain their functional integrity when the larynx is paralyzed.[69] Numerous small palatine glands keep the dorsal mucous membrane moist.

The Tonsils

Lymphoid tissue encircles the pharynx in the so-called ring of Waldeyer, or Bickel's ring. Much of it is diffuse nodular tissue, but some is organized into encapsulated tonsils. The dog and cat possess palatine tonsils on the lateral walls of the oropharynx (the fauces), pharyngeal tonsils on the roof of the nasopharynx, tonsils of the soft palate on its ventral surface, and occasionally paraepiglottic tonsils but no lingual or tubal tonsils.[118, 167] Of these, only the palatine tonsils are conspicuous as large, ovoid, discrete bodies, each partly concealed in its own tonsillar fossa by a tonsillar fold derived from the soft palate. The palatine tonsil of the dog is relatively larger and less spherical than that of the cat. It is attached by an elongated hilus to the lateral wall, through which it receives two or three tonsillar arteries and through which the efferent lymphatics depart for the medial retropharyngeal lymph node. (Like all tonsils, there are no afferent lymphatics.) In addition, there is an inconspicuous portion of tonsil found in the depths of the fossa that forms the rostral part of its lateral wall.[59] It is easy to overlook during tonsillectomy.[69]

The larynx projects up into the cavity of the laryngopharynx, creating a trough or gutter around it. The trough is partly subdivided by low membranous folds into two piriform recesses at the sides and two valleculae beneath the epiglottis.

The Pharyngeal Wall

The sides and roof of the pharynx are made up of an elastic mucous membrane, which lines a series of

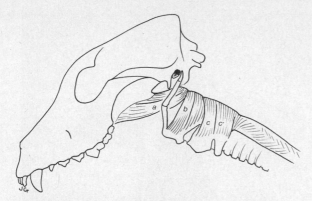

Figure 46–2. The pharyngeal constrictors: *a*, rostral; *b*, middle; *c*, caudal. Each constrictor can be subdivided into component muscles. The caudal part of the caudal constrictor, *c′*, is the cricopharyngeal muscle, which serves as a sphincter for the start of the esophagus.

three horseshoe-shaped constrictor muscles. They arise from the hard palate, the hyoid, and the larynx and are known as the rostral, middle, and caudal pharyngeal constrictors, respectively (Fig. 46–2). They fan out as they arch upward to meet their fellows in the midline along a raphe. Each constrictor can be subdivided into two. The caudal constrictor is subdivided into thyropharyngeal and cricopharyngeal parts, which arise from the thyroid and cricoid cartilages, respectively. Although these muscles are not readily separable in the dog,[44, 57] they can still be distinguished enough to perform a myotomy on the cricopharyngeus.[133] This muscle merges with the thyropharyngeus in front and the esophagus behind. It marks the caudal limit of the pharynx. Under most circumstances the cricopharyngeus acts as a sphincter (see hereafter) that keeps the esophagus closed and guards against reflux from the alimentary canal. Its location is usually betrayed on radiographs by a small bubble of gas trapped in the very first part of the esophagus whose rostral margin marks the pharyngoesophageal lumen (L = threshold).

Loose connective tissue surrounds much of the pharynx and allows it to dilate unimpeded. Many important vessels and nerves course within this connective tissue, especially over the dorsolateral wall. These include the glossopharyngeal, vagal, hypoglossal, and sympathetic nerves and their appropriate branches to the pharyngeal plexus, larynx, and esophagus; the common, internal, and external carotid arteries and their branches and companion veins; the hyoid apparatus; retropharyngeal lymph nodes; and the mandibular and parotid salivary glands.

Diseases of the Oral Cavity and Pharynx

Colin E. Harvey

Examination of the Oral Cavity

In a cooperative animal, most of the oral cavity can be examined visually and by palpation. However, because of temperament or pain associated with oral disease, many dogs and cats are reluctant to allow their mouths to be examined in detail. Gentleness and patience may make sedation or anesthesia unnecessary. A general glimpse of the oral cavity is often possible by arching the head dorsally, causing the mandible to open. Panting also affords an opportunity to see the palate, tongue, and gingiva.

The normal oral mucosa of the cheeks, gingiva, and sublingual areas is smooth and glistening. Salivary secretions are clear, and there should be no inflammation or ulceration of the mucosal surface. The location of abnormalities is of clinical significance, particularly because of the very high incidence of periodontal disease in middle-aged and old dogs. When the cheek is reflected, lesions may appear as free-standing ulcerations, even though they result from lying on severely diseased gingiva.

A thorough oral examination requires inspection and palpation of the entire mucosal surface, including the furrow under the tongue. Periodontal probing to assess the extent of gingival and periodontal disease is rarely possible without sedation. If sedation is required, consider delaying the procedure until the animal is examined drinking water and eating a small amount of food to evaluate swallowing.

Radiographs are useful for assessing the presence and extent of bony abnormalities secondary to soft tissue inflammation or neoplastic disease. Sedation or anesthesia, fine detail nonscreen films, and occlusal or oblique positioning are essential for the best results.[184] Absence or distortion of the radiolucent periodontal ligament and the normally radiodense lamina dura that surrounds the ligament is a useful radiographic sign. The size of the pulp cavity of the tooth reduces rapidly to a narrow channel as dogs approach skeletal maturity.

DISEASES OF THE TEETH

Congenital Anomalies

Absence of teeth or the presence of supernumerary teeth is common in mature animals. These abnormalities may be congenital. They are rarely cause for surgical treatment; in an occasional animal, excess teeth may require extraction if they distort occlusion.

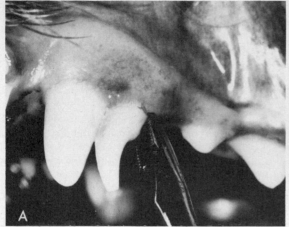
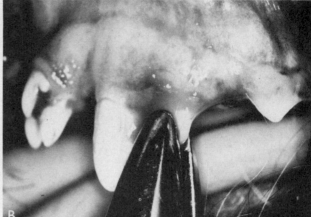

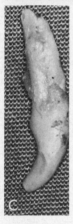

Figure 46–3. Retained deciduous teeth. *A,* Retained deciduous upper canine and incisor teeth in an eight-month-old puppy. A root elevator is cutting the periodontal ligament, separating the tooth from the surrounding bone. *B,* Once the tooth is loose, it is grasped with dental forceps, twisted, and rocked until it can be pulled free. *C,* The extracted deciduous canine tooth with intact root (compare with Figure 46–11*D*).

Retained Deciduous Teeth

Retention of the canine or incisor deciduous teeth is a common finding in toy breeds (Fig. 46–3). The condition occurs occasionally in cats as well.[173] The permanent teeth usually erupt by six months of age; when a deciduous tooth does not shed, it may cause distortion of the position or direction of growth of the permanent tooth, which in turn may cause malocclusion.[28] For this reason, deciduous teeth that are still present during eruption of the permanent teeth should be extracted. Occasionally, the attached gingiva is compressed, and food becomes compacted between the deciduous and permanent tooth; extraction of the deciduous tooth is also recommended in this case, even if occlusion is normal, to prevent gingival recession and potential loss of the permanent tooth.

Extraction of a deciduous tooth is usually easy because the root is thin and short compared with the permanent teeth (see Fig. 46–3*C*). Root fragments are unlikely to be left. Extraction techniques are described on pages 620–623. An alternative to the usual extraction techniques is to crush or snap the tooth close to the gingival margin with a dental forceps; anesthesia is not necessary.[170] This technique is not recommended when there is already evident malocclusion of the adjacent permanent teeth, as the root remains and may exacerbate the abnormality before being shed.

Impacted Teeth

Impacted teeth are rarely seen in the dog. Impaction occurs when the tooth does not erupt from the bone or through the gingiva. This is only observed if the absence of the tooth is noted by the owner; if partial eruption occurs, allowing entry of bacteria to tissue spaces below the gingiva and causing a periodontal abscess; or if an associated dentigerous cyst forms.[61] Esthetically important teeth that are impacted may be allowed to erupt by uncovering the tooth surgically, although this is rarely done.

Upper canine teeth that are impacted may cause nasal discharge. Extraction is curative but may require extensive removal of overlying bone.

Abnormalities in the Shape of Teeth

Derangement during development may result in fusion of teeth or distortion of the shape of a tooth or may cause surface irregularities, such as enamel hypoplasia. Distemper causes damage of this type. Abnormalities of this type rarely need treatment. Severely pitted teeth can be restored with a resin material if the appearance of the tooth is important. Tetracycline administration during the first two to three months of life stains the teeth of dogs and cats yellow. The shape of the tooth is not affected. Treatment by bleaching the teeth is rarely successful.

Acquired Diseases

Dental Caries

Caries is destruction of tooth structure caused by carbohydrate-fermenting bacteria. The bacteria produce acids that attack the surfaces of the tooth, either the enamel on the crown or the cementum on roots exposed by periodontal disease. Caries is uncommon in dogs and cats. The site most often affected in dogs is the crown of the upper first molar tooth. In cats it is most commonly seen in exposed roots of molar or canine teeth, although this may be confused with progressive subgingival osteoclastic resorption.[140]

Clinical signs are associated with pain as food or fluid touches the lesion; reluctance to eat, dropping of food from the mouth during eating, chattering of the teeth, and screaming or grunting during eating or drinking may be seen. Sedation or anesthesia is usually necessary for diagnosis because the animal is reluctant to open its mouth, and the lesion is often covered by plaque or dental calculus. The lesion usually has a brown discoloration, and the enamel or cementum surrounding it may form a crater. Diagnosis is confirmed with a sharp-pointed dental explorer: the surface is soft, and the explorer point can embed itself in the lesion, which differentiates caries from stained but intact enamel. A diagnosis of root caries may be difficult because of the overlying gingiva. In some animals, a reflex chattering of the jaws occurs when the exposed nerve endings are touched by the dental explorer.

Caries can be treated by extraction of the tooth or removal of the diseased tooth substance with a dental handpiece and bur and filling of the cavity with an inert substance such as dental amalgam. If the caries lesion or cavity formed during treatment extends into the pulp cavity, endodontic therapy is necessary prior to restoration.

Fracture of Teeth

Fractured teeth are common in dogs and cats and rarely cause clinical signs. Fractures result from external trauma, such as automobile accidents, or from biting on hard objects such as stones or sticks. The fracture may extend into the pulp cavity. Pain (and thus unwillingness to eat), dropping of food from the mouth, or screaming when drinking cold fluids is more likely when the fracture extends into the pulp cavity, although a fracture that does not extend into the pulp may become a focus for cariogenic activity, and endodontic disease may thus develop subsequently. Fractures that extend into the dentin but not into the pulp are partially repaired by the laying down of reparative dentin by odontoblasts on the inner surface of the dentin.

The teeth most often fractured are the canine and upper carnassial teeth. Most fractured teeth do not require treatment and are observed as incidental findings. When the fractured tooth has a jagged edge that may traumatize adjacent soft tissues, the tooth can be extracted or smoothed off with a dental drill and bur. If the tooth is functionally or esthetically important, retention of the tooth can be assured by endodontic treatment to seal off the pulp cavity; the crown can be restored by one of several methods described hereafter. Fractures that split a tooth parallel to its long axis and into the pulp cavity are less common but more difficult to treat, particularly when the fracture extends into the root of the tooth, as some of the stability of the tooth is lost; such teeth are probably best extracted, although treatment by small pin restoration has been used successfully.[90]

Avulsion of Teeth

Trauma occasionally causes avulsion of a tooth from the alveolar bone without fracturing the tooth. If desired by the owner, an attempt can be made to save the tooth by reimplanting it in the alveolus as soon as possible. In an immature dog with a large pulp cavity, pulp may regenerate. Where the periodontal ligament has lost its vitality, ankylosis of the bone to the cementum may occur. In mature animals, endodontic therapy (see hereafter) is performed to prevent subsequent pulp necrosis and root abscessation; some root resorption usually occurs, but the tooth remains firmly in place.[3] Attached remnants of periodontal ligament should not be removed from the root surface prior to reimplantation.[146]

Disease of the Pulp Cavity (Endodontic Disease)

Exposure of the pulp cavity from any cause can result in infection or injury of the pulp (Fig. 46–4A). Inflammatory swelling results in necrosis because the pulp is contained in a defined space surrounded by a rigid shell. This may be followed by the development of a root abscess (Fig. 46–4B) and loss of the tooth. Causes of endodontic disease are fracture, caries, and severe peridontal disease with exposure of the root apex. The frequency with which endodontic disease follows these conditions in the dog is not known. When retention of the tooth is desired for functional or esthetic reasons, endodontic therapy should be performed.

Diagnosis of endodontic disease may be difficult, as not all fractures or pulp exposures cause endodontic disease. Pain on eating or drinking or swelling associated with an abscess may be seen. Pain usually disappears as the pulpal tissues become necrotic. Pulp exposure can be differentiated from attrition (in which the tooth has been worn down to the pulp cavity slowly enough so that reparative dentin has formed to protect the pulpal tissues) by inserting a dental explorer into the exposed pulp recess: the explorer penetrates the cavity only if reparative dentin has not formed. Radiographs will demonstrate a root abscess (seen as loss of the dense lamina dura and surrounding alveolar bone, causing a radiolucent pocket around the affected root) but may not show any abnormality immediately following injury.

Endodontic Therapy

Treatment of endodontic disease is either extraction or endodontic therapy to save the tooth. The object is to remove the source of infection and seal off the root canal so that there is no channel from the oral environment to the bone. Treatment immediately following injury may be possible with a limited procedure; the dental pulp is removed from the coronal portion of the tooth, and calcium hydroxide paste is placed over the remaining pulp tissue and covered by a zinc oxide and eugenol dental cement. A filling of dental amalgam is inserted into the remaining defect in the crown, compacted into place, and smoothed off with a dental bur. A long-term failure rate of 20 per cent has been reported with this procedure in dogs;[93] the full endodontic treatment can be completed as one procedure, takes a

little longer than vital amputation, and is less likely to fail.

If the pulp canal has been exposed for more than a few hours, more radical treatment is necessary. The entire pulp canal is cleaned out, which requires greater access than that required for the treatment previously described. The site of exposure is enlarged with a dental bur to allow access. In a large tooth with a long root, such as a canine tooth, an additional access cavity may be necessary. In a canine tooth this additional access site is usually made on the rostral surface of the crown just above the gingiva to allow straight access to the pulp canal in the root. The pulpal tissues are cleaned out with endodontic reamers (Fig. 46–4C and E). Standard human instruments are too short to be effective on a long tooth, so adapted instruments are necessary, including reamers at least 55 mm long. The reamers are advanced into the canal and twisted to shave off some of the dentin. The canal is flushed copiously, alternating sodium hypochlorite and hydrogen peroxide to both clean and sterilize the canal. Reaming is continued

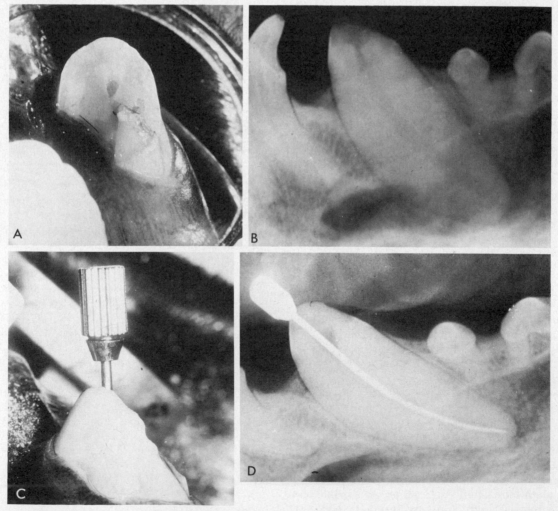

Figure 46–4. Endodontic treatment. *A*, Fractured canine tooth in a German shepherd. *B*, Radiograph of the tooth; periapical radiolucency indicates root abscess. *C*, Endodontic reamer in place. *D*, Radiograph determining tooth length.

Illustration continued on opposite page

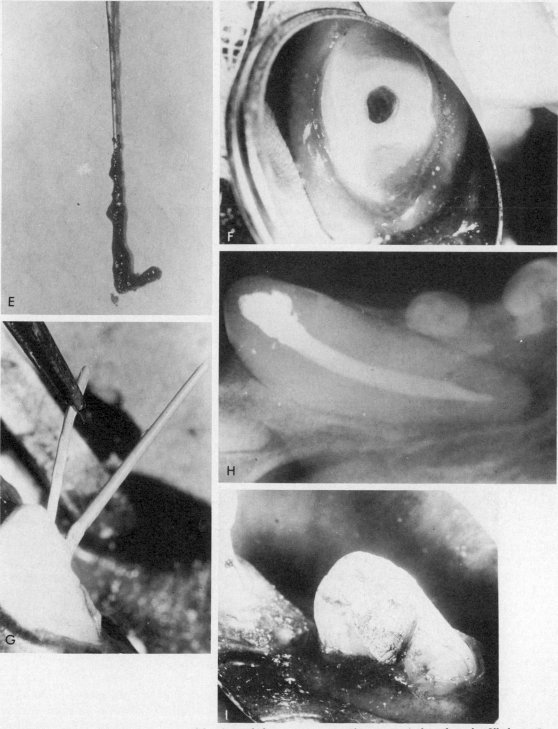

Figure 46–4 Continued. E, Pulpal tissue removed by the endodontic reamer. *F,* Clean root canal ready to be filled. *G,* Gutta percha filling material inserted into canal. *H,* Radiograph of the filled root canal covered by amalgam. *I,* Amalgam restoration of the opening into the pulp canal. (Reprinted with permission from Harvey, C. E., et al.: Oral, dental, pharyngeal, and salivary gland disorders. *In* Ettinger, S. J. (ed.): *Textbook of Veterinary Internal Medicine,* 2nd ed. W. B. Saunders, Philadelphia, 1983.)

until only clean white dentin shavings are removed and the reamer cannot be extended further into the canal. A radiograph is taken at this point to ensure that the entire canal is exposed; a reamer is left in the canal at maximum penetration and should be visible at the end of the canal against the apical delta (Fig. 46–4D).

The debrided canal is dried with sterile paper points and then sealed with gutta percha points and root canal cement (Fig. 46–4F–H). In a large canine tooth, several human-size points can be rolled together to save time. The points are condensed into the canal with a large root canal spreader. Additional points are inserted until the whole canal is filled. Excess gutta percha is removed with a heated instrument, and the access site is sealed with silver amalgam, which is compacted into place and smoothed off (Fig. 46–4I). Zinc oxide and eugenol root cement can also be used by slow injection to fill the debrided pulp canal; the material is gently compacted and then covered with an amalgam filling. Composite resin material can be used on the surface of the amalgam filling to match the color of the tooth. Restoration techniques for large crown defects are described hereafter.

If the radiograph shows that the entire root has not been cleaned, further attempts to ream the canal from the coronal access site are made. If this is impossible because of blockage of the canal by reparative dentin or severe curvature of the root or if there is a lytic area surrounding the root suggesting a root abscess, an apicoectomy is indicated.

Apicoectomy is performed by incising the gingiva directly over the root, reflecting the mucoperiosteum, and removing bone with a dental bur to expose the root. Adjacent roots are avoided. The apex of the root is removed with a dental bur to gain access to the pulp canal. The canal is reamed, cleaned, and sealed as for the coronal access site. The oral soft tissues are sutured. Extensive soft tissue infection should be drained if present. Antibiotic therapy is not necessary following apicoectomy.

The necessity for apicoectomy in endodontic treatment in dogs is controversial.[18, 19, 134, 159] Thorough reaming of the root canal to the apex of the tooth and coronal sealing are the most critical factors in the prevention of reinfection.[24, 49] Following endodontic reaming without apicoectomy, filling of 48 infected roots of 36 teeth in three experimental dogs with zinc oxide, eugenol, and formaldehyde followed by an amalgam coronal seal resulted in a 10 per cent failure rate after one year; the same author using the same technique treated 92 teeth in 75 clinic patients with 95 per cent success at a mean follow-up period of two and one-half years.[25] A failure rate of 30 per cent following conventional nonapicoectomy endodontic treatment has been mentioned but not documented.[104] A 20 to 25 per cent failure rate was reported on an unstated number of dogs at 18 to 24 months following endodontic treatment, apicoectomy, and filling of the canal with zinc oxide and eugenol.[135] No failures occurred in 20 dogs treated by apicoectomy, retrograde amalgam filling, zinc oxide and eugenol filling of the root canal, and amalgam crown restoration.[135] Most of this controversy concerns the treatment of canine teeth of military or other working dogs, which have such a long pulp canal and often an apical delta that complicates debridement of the apex. A tear drop-shaped coronal access has been advocated for instrumentation without apicoectomy.[19] Extended follow-up results of large series of cases are not available. Clinical experience suggests that apicoectomy is probably necessary only when the apical area cannot otherwise be cleaned thoroughly. Conservative endodontic treatment in large dogs requires specially adapted instruments[19] and considerable patience and attention to detail to minimize failures.

RESTORATIVE DENTISTRY

Restoration of the appearance or function of a tooth can be a simple or complex process, depending on the amount of tooth structure that has been lost. When very little of the crown is present or when the root is fractured, restoration is often not practical. The first decision is whether restoration is necessary. Generally, restoration is only considered for teeth that are esthetically or functionally important. In most dogs and cats, this restricts consideration of restoration to the canine and incisor teeth.

Composite Resin Restoration

If the pulp cavity is intact, restoration can be performed immediately. Examples are enamel hypoplasia, dental abrasion, and slab fractures limited to the enamel. In these circumstances, crown height usually is normal, and the purpose of the procedure is to restore the surface appearance of the tooth. This can be achieved most easily by using a composite resin material,[10, 17, 112] which comes in a variety of shades to match the color of the adjacent normal tooth surface. The damaged surface of the tooth is thoroughly cleaned and polished with pumice, then etched with 20% phosphoric acid for one minute, washed with water, and dried. The resin and hardener are supplied as pastes, as a powder and paste, or as a light activated paste. The composite is activated, applied to the surface of the tooth, and smoothed into place. Setting takes from 30 seconds to a few minutes, depending on the system used. The restoration is finished by removing excess resin and smoothing the surface with a dental bur (Fig. 46–5). This same technique can be used to restore normal surface color to a tooth that has been treated endodontically and has an amalgam filling that may be in an esthetically displeasing place. A cast metal cap can be cemented in place over a fractured crown where no pulp is exposed,[81, 138] although this is rarely necessary even in working dogs.

Crown Restoration

When the pulp cavity has been exposed, endodontic treatment is necessary prior to restoration to prevent subsequent development of a root abscess. The technique has been described previously. When crown height has been lost and restoration is desired,

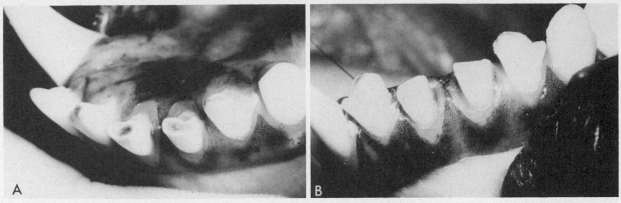

Figure 46–5. Composite resin restoration. *A*, Exposed pulp canals in lower central incisors of a dog. *B*, Following endodontic treatment and composite resin restoration. (Courtesy of L. E. Rossman.)

other factors to be considered in addition to the need for endodontic treatment include the occlusive force that the tooth and restoration will bear and whether the crown needs to be restored to its former height. A simple alternative to restoration in some dogs is to smooth off the crown to conform to a normal appearance; the opposite tooth can also be reduced to obtain symmetry. Smoothing off is done by a dental bur. Jagged edges of enamel that would otherwise lacerate the cheek or tongue can be treated in this way.

Crown height can be restored by a combination of pins and composite resin or by a cast crown. The former is simple and relatively cheap to perform and often successful[53, 91, 182] but will not provide a tooth that is capable of withstanding high occlusal stresses; this technique is therefore not practical for canine or carnassial teeth of large breed dogs. Cast crowns are more difficult and expensive to prepare properly but are usually successful when performed by experienced personnel.[91, 138]

Composite restoration reinforced with one or more threaded pins is performed as a single procedure and is usually done during the same anesthetic episode as endodontic treatment. The pins are twisted into holes drilled with a fine dental drill bit and cut off so that they protrude slightly less than the proposed crown height. The tooth is cleaned and etched with phosphoric acid, then the composite resin is activated and tooled between and around the pins to build up the crown. Final shaping is done by a dental burr when the resin has set. This procedure may be used for incisor teeth and has been used successfully to repair fractures that extend into the root of the tooth.[90]

Cast crown restoration requires at least two anesthetic episodes. During the first procedure, endodontic treatment is completed with the exception of the amalgam restoration. The obturated root canal is prepared for a post by removing some of the filling material. The crown of the tooth is prepared for the prosthesis, and an impression of this preparation is made (Fig. 46–6A). The defect in the tooth is filled temporarily with zinc phosphate cement. Particularly

with canine teeth in working dogs, it is useful to make an impression of the occlusion of the canine teeth to ensure that the cast crown will fit into normal occlusion. The crown is cast from the impression in a dental laboratory (Fig. 46–6B). Gold and stainless steel can be used, although stainless steel is both stronger and cheaper. At additional expense, a porcelain veneer can be attached to the surface of the tooth if appearance is as important as function.

During a second anesthetic episode, the temporary filling material is removed, the crown is fitted in place, and the occlusion is checked (Fig. 46–6C). Because this procedure is done under general anesthesia with an endotracheal tube usually in place, testing of occlusion is often awkward; even if the endotracheal tube is temporarily removed, the relaxed tongue must be pushed back into the mouth, risking asphyxiation. To avoid these difficulties, the endotracheal tube can be placed through a tracheotomy or pharyngotomy incision, thus allowing occlusion to be checked easily. When the fit of the prosthesis and the occlusion are acceptable, the crown is cemented in place with zinc phosphate cement. Procedures of this sort are best performed by an experienced restorative dentist to ensure that the occlusive forces can be met without fracture at the root-crown interface.

Restoration of missing teeth is theoretically possible but rarely practical in the dog and cat, as there are fewer adjacent teeth available and/or suitable for anchoring the prosthesis than in humans. There are isolated reports of the use of both fixed and removable dentures in veterinary patients.

PERIODONTAL DISEASE

Periodontal disease is common in dogs and less common but often severe in cats. It includes gingivitis, periodontitis (inflammation of the attachment apparatus: the cemental surface of the tooth, the alveolar bone, and the periodontal ligament that

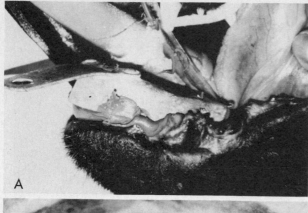

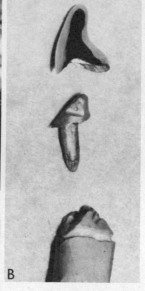

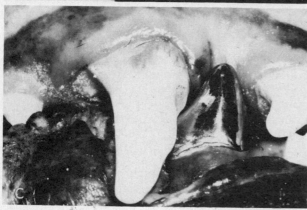

Figure 46–6. Crown restoration of a lower canine tooth. *A*, Dental impression tray in place following endodontic treatment and preparation of remaining crown. *B*, Model made from impression tray (bottom), post to be cemented into prepared root (middle), and stainless steel crown prosthesis (top). *C*, Prosthetic crown cemented in place (note that natural crown had abraded enamel of upper canine tooth prior to fracture but that prosthesis fits in normal occlusion). (Courtesy of D. Garber.)

normally joins them and holds the teeth in position), and periodontal abscess.

Gingivitis is caused by plaque,[108] and gingivitis leads to periodontal disease.[148] Plaque is the bacteria-rich soft layer that forms on the surface of teeth. The organisms predominating in the dog are gram-negative anaerobes, which produce a polysaccharide-protein complex. Plaque is more common on the teeth of dogs fed soft food, but diet is only a minor contributing factor in plaque formation. Dietary additives such as hard biscuits or oxtails significantly reduce calculus buildup;[37] however, hard foods are less successful in abrading plaque from the surface of the tooth. A more dramatic effect of diet on gingival health has been demonstrated in cats; dry cat food prevents the development of periodontal disease and can reverse some gingival disease resulting from the feeding of moist food for several months.[155] Tooth brushing starting at a young age will prevent periodontal disease in dogs;[108] however, the value of tooth brushing without using a plaque retardant is still controversial.[33, 72]

Clinical Signs and Diagnosis

Periodontal disease varies considerably in its appearance. Gingivitis may be acute, with reddening and edema of the gingival margin, or chronic, with recessed or hyperplastic gingiva. Where the condition has progressed to involve the periodontal ligament, there may be deep pus-filled pockets or abscesses beneath the gingiva. The final stage of the

disease is loss of teeth. The paramount clinical sign is halitosis, which can be sickening to the owner and veterinarian in severe cases. Other signs are bleeding from the mouth, and, infrequently, loss of appetite, although inability to manage hard food is more common.

Gingivitis or gingival hyperplasia is diagnosed by inspection of the mouth. A detailed examination requires sedation or anesthesia so that periodontal pockets can be evaluated with a blunt periodontal probe; pocket depth is normally 1 to 3 mm. Gingival hyperplasia and periodontitis both cause increased pocket depth. Radiographs demonstrate bone loss. In most dogs and cats, periodontal disease affects several areas of the gingiva; isolated gingival lesions should be biopsied because of the high incidence of oral neoplasia in the dog. Many diseases can coexist with periodontal disease and may mimic or exacerbate the clinical signs. Autoimmune and immune-suppressive diseases, chronic kidney disease, and diabetes are important examples. The examination of a dog or cat with halitosis should include serum creatinine and glucose determinations. Other examinations that are useful include a complete blood count and staining of plaque with a disclosing solution. With severe periodontitis or periodontal abscess, the white blood cell count is usually increased, and a left shift may be present with periodontal abscess. If treatment under anesthesia is considered, with the likelihood of bacteremia, the heart should be auscultated carefully.

Treatment

The objects of treatment are to return the periodontal tissues to as nearly normal as possible and to control the plaque long term to prevent or slow the development of the disease. In some dogs with mild gingivitis and no significant accumulation of dental calculus, initial treatment under anesthesia may not be necessary if the owner is able to brush the dog's teeth daily with 0.2% chlorhexidine solution. This conservative approach is rarely successful in animals presented because of halitosis.

Whether antibiotics are necessary at the time of periodontal examination or teeth cleaning has been the subject of much debate. There is evidence that invasion of the periodontal pocket with instruments causes a transient bacteremia[26, 80] and that periodontal disease is common in dogs with clinically obvious bacterial endocarditis;[40] however, there is no direct evidence that treatment of dental disease in dogs causes endocarditis. Normal dogs clear circulating blood of oral bacteria within 20 minutes of the onset of bacteremia.[147] When circumstances suggest that there is a greater than usual risk, such as a dog with chronic valvular disease on auscultation, clinical signs of cough or reduced exercise tolerance, and purulent debris in deep periodontal pockets, a single dose of a broad spectrum bacteriocidal antibiotic given im-

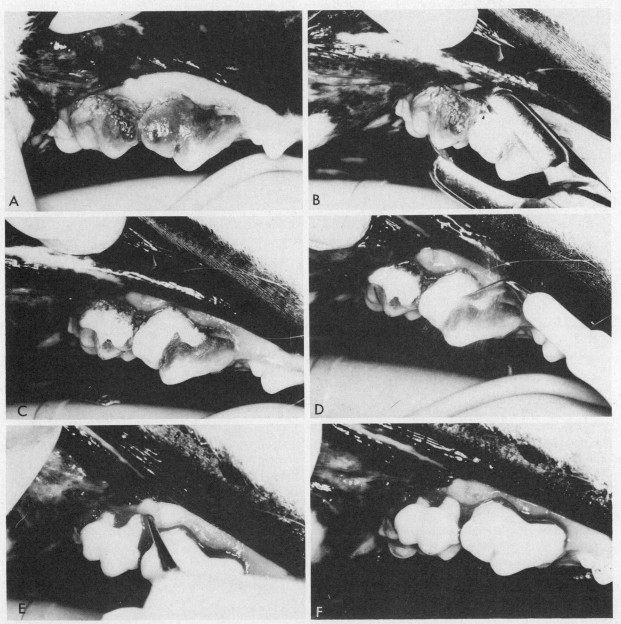

Figure 46–7. Teeth cleaning. *A,* Upper carnassial and first molar teeth with extensive calculus formation and gingival recession. *B* and *C,* Dental forceps are used to crack off large accumulations of calculus. *D,* Ultrasonic teeth scaler is used to remove remaining calculus (note plentiful cooling water spray). *E,* Roots as well as crown are scaled to remove calculus. *F,* Following cleaning and polishing, the crown and exposed root surfaces are less prone to accumulation of plaque.

mediately prior to treatment seems prudent. In general, the temptation to clean the teeth of an animal under anesthesia should be resisted if the major procedure performed creates dead space in tissue planes in an otherwise clean wound, as the bacteremia associated with the teeth cleaning may seed infection in the blood clots within the tissue spaces.[174]

The operative treatment of periodontal disease consists of one or more of the following: removal of plaque and calculus from the crowns of the teeth; removal of plaque and calculus from the roots of the teeth; gingival curettage; resection of hyperplastic gingiva; gingival flap surgery; and tooth extraction. Treatment in the past has often been less than adequate and simply consisted of removal of calculus from the crown, leaving the area of most active disease, the periodontal pocket, untreated. Effective treatment can be planned only if the extent of disease is known. Pocket depth, as measured with a periodontal probe, is the most useful indicator. It must be combined with identification of the cementoenamel junction so that increased pocket depth due to gingival hyperplasia can be distinguished from that due to loss of periodontal attachment. With thorough treatment and conscientiously applied follow-up care, even severe periodontal disease in dogs can be controlled and teeth retained.

Teeth Cleaning

Teeth can be superficially cleaned under sedation, or even in an awake dog in some instances; however, this does not allow any work to be done on the subgingival part of the teeth and is a waste of time and money in animals with established periodontal disease. Therefore, general anesthesia is recommended for all teeth cleaning procedures in dogs and cats. Considerable time and effort can be saved by using an ultrasonic teeth scaler;[97] however, hand instruments are necessary in all animals to complete the process. The ultrasonic scaler causes the tooth to vibrate very rapidly, and the calculus separates. It is sometimes difficult to dislodge large, densely mineralized calculus deposits; in this circumstance, extraction forceps are positioned with one jaw at the gingival margin and one at the coronal edge of the calculus deposit, and the forceps are then closed, cracking the calculus between the jaws (Fig. 46–7A to C). The ultrasonic scaler is moved rapidly over the surface of the tooth to prevent damage due to heat transfer. For the same reason, the cooling water supply must always be functioning during use (Fig. 46–7D). Ultrasonic scalers cause considerable contamination of the surrounding environment with water droplet–borne oral organisms;[186] for this reason, procedures to be performed under aseptic conditions should not be performed immediately following teeth cleaning procedures. Use of a face mask is recommended during ultrasonic teeth cleaning. The ultrasonic scaler can be gently inserted into subgingival pockets to loosen calculus that is attached to the

roots; however, to avoid damaging the periodontal attachment, it should not be pushed into the depths of the pocket.[51]

Following removal of major areas of calculus with the ultrasonic scaler, hand-held root scalers and periodontal curettes are used. The scaler is placed below the level of any remaining calculus and drawn toward the crown (Fig. 46–7E). This is repeated over the exposed surface of the root in any periodontal pockets that are present until the root and crown both feel smooth (Fig. 46–7F). To be effective, dental scalers and curettes should be sharp. When the tooth is finally smooth down to remaining periodontal attachment, it is helpful to polish the teeth with a mild dental abrasive polish, applied on a rubber cup rotated by a dental engine; this helps to prevent or slow down the accumulation of plaque and calculus, as it eliminates the minor grooves and other plaque-retentive features that are inevitably left following teeth scaling.[51]

Gingival Curettage

Inflamed and diseased sulcular epithelium or other soft tissue where the epithelium has been lost is removed with gingival curettes to allow healthy epithelium to reform and reattach to the tooth. The cutting edge is inserted to the depth of the pocket, directed toward the epithelium, and pulled toward the crown of the tooth. This procedure is inevitably accompanied by hemorrhage, although this usually stops within a few minutes.

Gingivectomy

When the gingiva is hypertrophied, the tooth substance is at least partially covered, preventing removal of plaque or calculus during normal occlusive abrasion or tooth brushing (Fig. 46–8A). Treatment is resection of the excess gingiva at the time of teeth scaling. Gingivectomy can be performed with a scalpel, a periodontal knife, or an electroscalpel. The pocket depth is assessed with a periodontal probe, and the gingiva is resected to form a new gingival margin at the edge at the alveolus. Hemorrhage is often brisk when a cold scalpel is used but is usually controlled with pressure from a sponge. Dilute epinephrine can be applied but is rarely necessary and is best avoided when halothane is the anesthetic agent employed, particularly in older dogs with known cardiac disease. The electroscalpel is useful, particularly for removal of extensive lesions (Fig. 46–8B). Following gingivectomy, periodontal pockets are more thoroughly cleaned, and the teeth are polished.

Gingival Flap Surgery

When increased pocket depth is due to bone loss, simple gingivectomy is not sufficient to eliminate the pocket. Pockets larger than 5 mm (that are not due

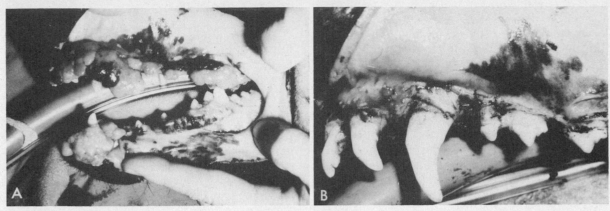

Figure 46–8. Gingivectomy. *A,* Extensive generalized gingival hyperplasia. *B,* Gingiva overlying the teeth has been removed with the electroscalpel.

to gingival hyperplasia) require more definitive surgery (Fig. 46–9).[66] Incisions are made in the gingiva perpendicular to the long axis of the tooth on either side of the tooth involved (Fig. 46–9*B* and *C*). The gingiva is reflected apically with an elevator (Fig. 46–9*D* and *E*), and the exposed root surfaces are thoroughly scaled until clean (Fig. 46–9*F*) and then smoothed with a mild dental abrasive. The alveolar surface of the pocket must also be thoroughly cleaned and freed of all soft tissue with a curette. The gingiva is resected on a line so that it is level with the alveolar crest (Fig. 46–9*G*), and sutured between teeth to adjacent epithelium to hold it in place (Fig. 46–9*H* and *I*). When there is uneven bone loss around the tooth, the bone should be removed with a bone curette or rongeur to form an even alveolar process. Nonabsorbable sutures and periodontal packs are generally not used following gingival flap surgery in dogs or cats to avoid the need for further anesthesia or sedation. Tooth brushing should be delayed for a week to allow the epithelium and periodontal tissues to adhere to the bone. Complications following this procedure include hemorrhage, which is controlled during surgery with pressure, and recurrence, which is most likely due to failure to sufficiently clean the pocket during surgery or to insufficient follow-up care.

Tooth Extraction

Extraction is a "last resort" technique for the treatment of periodontal disease in dogs and cats, although under some conditions extraction may be the treatment of choice. Examples are dogs that are not willing to allow the owner to brush their teeth and animals whose owners for any other reason are not willing to brush the teeth. Extraction may be limited to one or a few teeth, or, in occasional cases, all of the teeth are removed (Fig. 46–10). If the owner is unwilling or unable to brush all of the animal's teeth, the premolars and molar teeth can be removed, leaving the canine and incisor teeth, which are esthetically the most important and which are

more easily reached with a toothbrush. Unfortunately, the narrow single-rooted incisors are often loose and beyond saving in dogs with severe periodontal disease. Extraction techniques are described on pages 620–623.

Follow-up Care

The procedures described previously are of temporary value if not accompanied by a conscientiously applied program of aftercare. The most important part of this program is some form of daily removal of plaque from the teeth. The most efficient way to accomplish this is to brush the teeth. A soft child's toothbrush can be used, preferably in combination with a plaque retardant such as 0.2% chlorhexidine. The teeth are brushed so that all surfaces are reached, and the brush is made to squeeze the gingival margin against the tooth to clean the gingival pocket. This is best achieved by a regular rotation of the brush as it is moved over the surface of the teeth and gingiva. Ideally, this should be done following eating. If the owner is unwilling or unable to use the toothbrush, chlorhexidine can be applied as a gel or ointment with good results.[78, 183] Regular use of hard foods or chewing materials such as rawhide strips is beneficial. The plaque retardant follow-up care must be continued for the duration of the animal's life, but by doing so, the need for regular teeth-cleaning episodes under anesthesia can often be avoided.

Prognosis for Animals with Periodontal Disease

Periodontal disease is a progressive disease that affects almost all dogs and many cats older than five years. The disease can often be held in check by treatment and follow-up care as previously described.[56, 183] If the treatment does not address disease in the periodontal pockets or is not followed by the appropriate aftercare, the disease will progress, with gradual loss of teeth. Fortunately, animal patients can manage well without teeth, as the owner has control of the animal's diet.

Periodontal disease almost always resolves completely in dogs treated by total edentulation; however, this is not always the case in cats, in which soft tissue inflammatory lesions often persist, particularly at the commissures of the pharynx. These persistent lesions in cats cause pain on eating, as the inflamed tissue is separated when the jaws are opened. Chronic intermittent treatment with prednisolone is helpful in some cats.[82] These lesions in cats have been associated with feline leukemia virus infection,[13] although it is not common for the leukemia virus test to be positive in a cat presented because of oral disease.[82]

TOOTH EXTRACTION

Teeth require extraction for many reasons. Regardless of the reason, the technique is the same. The tooth is loosened with a root elevator before extraction forceps are placed or wedge leverage is applied. Particularly in small dogs or cats, in which the jaw can be fractured by excessive force, care should be taken to use as much contact as possible between the hand and jaw to spread out the force applied to the jaw. Even teeth with a considerable amount of root exposure are often adhered firmly to the jaw; this is particularly true of canine and carnassial teeth. The narrow teeth of cats are particularly prone to fracture during extraction. The use of a narrow-pointed scalpel

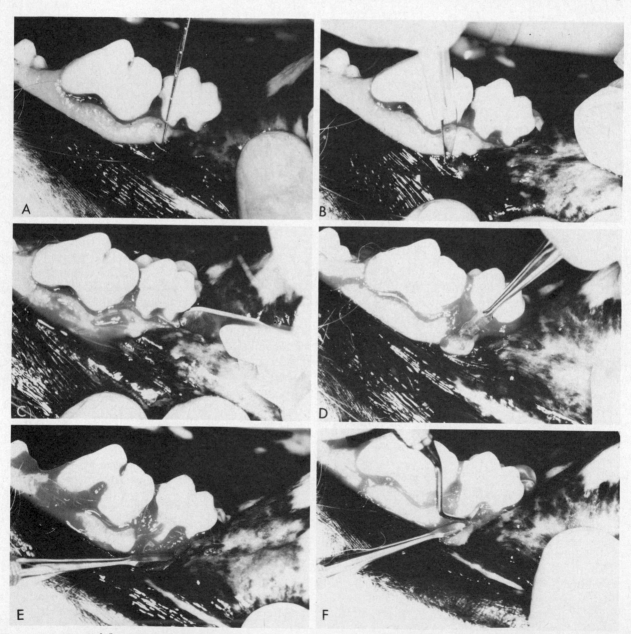

Figure 46–9. Gingival flap surgery. *A,* A periodontal probe is used to assess gingival pocket depth. *B* and *C,* The attached gingiva overlying a deep pocket is incised with a scalpel. *D* and *E,* The gingival flap is raised with a periosteal elevator or chisel, exposing the root in the pocket. *F,* The root is thoroughly scaled.

Illustration continued on opposite page

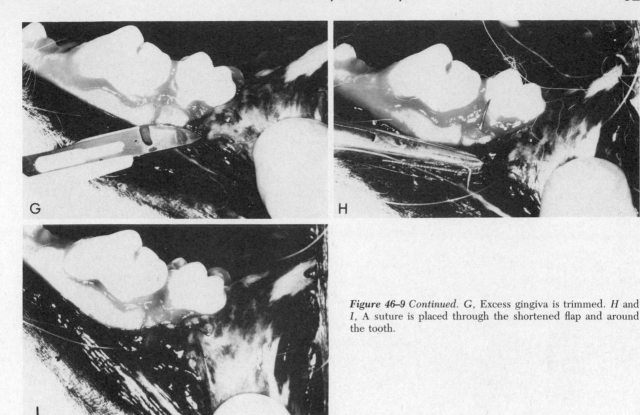

Figure 46–9 Continued. G, Excess gingiva is trimmed. *H* and *I,* A suture is placed through the shortened flap and around the tooth.

blade to sever the periodontal fibers has been suggested.[98]

Single-root teeth (incisors, canines, first premolars in both jaws, and third lower molar teeth in dogs; incisors, canines, and upper first premolar and molar teeth in cats) are removed by inserting the root elevator between the gingival margin and the crown or exposed root and applying pressure while rotating the elevator through a small arc. The instrument should be kept at a 30 to 45° angle to the long axis of the root to avoid allowing the instrument to slip off and injure the gingiva. A finger is kept extended

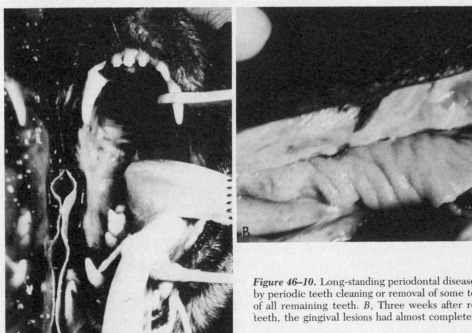

Figure 46–10. Long-standing periodontal disease in a dog not controlled by periodic teeth cleaning or removal of some teeth. *A,* Before removal of all remaining teeth. *B,* Three weeks after removal of all remaining teeth, the gingival lesions had almost completely resolved.

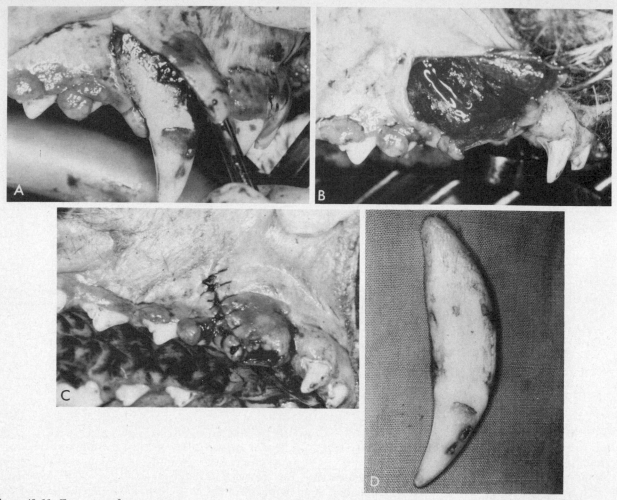

Figure 46–11. Extraction of a permanent upper canine tooth. *A*, The gingiva has been incised and bone removed, exposing the lateral surface of the root. A root elevator is separating the tooth from the alveolar bone rostral to the tooth. *B*, The tooth has been removed, leaving the medial alveolar plate of bone intact. *C*, Synthetic absorbable sutures have been placed to close the original gingival incision. *D*, Extracted canine tooth. Note length of crown (bottom) compared with root (top) (compare with Figure 46–3C).

along the blade of the elevator to act as a stop should the instrument slip. Considerable force is necessary to break down the periodontal ligament. This process is used on all available surfaces of the tooth until it begins to loosen. At that point, it is grasped with appropriately sized extraction forceps and removed by rotating the forceps while pulling.

The canine teeth have massive roots (Fig. 46–11D). In large dogs, it is often quicker and less traumatic to incise and reflect the mucoperiosteum on the lateral surface of the tooth, then to resect the alveolar bone overlying the root with a bone chisel or orthopedic or dental bur (Fig. 46–11A). The root is freed further with a root elevator, allowing the tooth to be pried from its niche (Fig. 46–11B). The gingival flaps are sutured back into place with simple interrupted absorbable sutures (Fig. 46–11C). An alternative technique is to create a mucoperiosteal flap so that, following extraction, the suture line is not located over the space left by the resected bone.[30, 127]

Two-root teeth (second and third upper premolars,

second, third, and fourth lower premolars, first and second lower molars in the dog; second and third upper premolars, first and second lower premolars, and first lower molar in the cat) can be removed in a similar fashion, or the tooth can be separated into single root sections by sawing or fracturing the crown into two pieces. Each piece is then taken out as a separate one-root tooth.

The three-root tooth most frequently extracted is the upper fourth premolar (carnassial) tooth. This tooth has roots second only to the canine tooth in size. It can be removed intact by using the root elevator to free as much of the periodontal attachment as can be reached, including making a passage through the furcation between the roots. The root elevator is passed through the channel between the roots and rotated, forcing the angled handle of the instrument into the bifurcation as a wedge, thus forcing the intact tooth from its sockets.[121] An alternative is to saw or fracture the tooth into two or three sections, using a tooth cutter, hack saw, wire saw, or dental cutting disc,[48, 89] and remove each root separately; this technique works most easily if the entire crown is removed, as each root is then exposed, allowing accurate placement of the root elevator. When working on the upper carnassial and first molar teeth, the elevator should be kept under firm control to prevent the instrument from dislodging and slipping into the facial tissues or eye. With any tooth, an effort should be made to search for fractured root fragments if the roots do not come out intact.

Following extraction, the alveolus is left empty. If hemorrhage does not stop within one minute of removal of the tooth, gauze sponge can be inserted into the alveolus; this will fall out in a day or two.

A gas-driven oscillating forceps can be used to remove teeth in dogs, requiring less time and causing less alveolar bone trauma than standard techniques.[115]

Dogs and cats tolerate extraction of teeth very well. Sedation may be necessary during the recovery stage from anesthesia, but most animals are eating without pain the next day. New bone fills the empty socket in 21 to 28 days in dogs; packing the socket with gauze delays healing considerably.[76]

Complications of tooth extraction include the following:

1. Hemorrhage, which could be severe in animals with chronic kidney disease or undetected clotting abnormalities. Some bleeding often continues for a day or two following extraction; the owner should be warned to expect some blood mixed with water in the animal's bowl.

2. Fracture of the mandible, particularly in old, small breed dogs. This can be prevented by careful extraction technique, as dogs with the highest risk of fracture of the jaw during tooth extraction are also those with the least desirable conditions for fracture healing.

3. Retention of part of a root that was fractured during extraction. This may cause no obvious abnormality or may lead to a root abscess, with subsequent fistula formation (Fig. 46–12A). Extraction of a diseased retained root (Fig. 46–12B and D) follows radiographic location of the root and may require surgical removal of overlying bone.[27] Isolated normal vital roots that are below the level of surrounding bone will be covered by bone and gingiva.[124]

4. Necrosis of bone around the extraction site occurs occasionally (Fig. 46–13A). The socket does not heal, fills with food, and becomes an area of potent bacterial activity. Osteomyelitis may spread from the original site, although this is rare. Conservative treatment is unlikely to be effective. Surgical treatment is removal of the affected bone with a rongeur until healthy bleeding bone is reached (Fig. 46–13B). The surgical site is left uncovered.

5. Oronasal fistula. Extraction of the upper canine teeth, and occasionally other upper jaw teeth, can

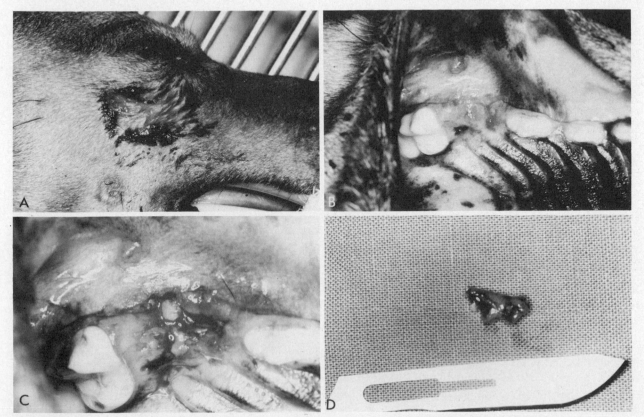

Figure 46–12. Carnassial abscess following fracture and retention of root of upper carnassial tooth. A, Draining lesion on face. B, Epithelium has healed over previous extraction wound. C, Incision over site of carnassial tooth reveals retained root. D, Extracted root fragment.

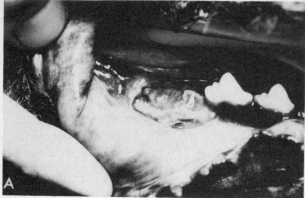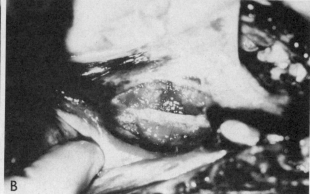

Figure 46–13. Localized mandibular necrosis following tooth extraction. *A*, Section of dead bone without epithelial cover. *B*, Following curettage of the necrotic area.

result in loss of alveolar bone. The nasal and oral epithelia heal together to form a permanent fistula. This is particularly common in narrow-nosed small dogs with extensive periodontal disease. Treatment is closure of the fistula by creating a flap of buccal epithelium (see Section 8).

6. Functional abnormalities following extraction of teeth are rare, even if all the teeth are removed. Both dogs and cats adapt well and learn to grasp food of varying consistency with the tongue. The owner should provide several types of food to see which the animal can manage best. If both mandibular canine teeth are removed, the tongue may hang out of the mouth on one side when relaxed.

THE JAWS

The shape and length of the jaws and the position of the teeth in the jaws determine the occlusion. There is considerable variation in the occlusion of dogs and less variation in cats. Any condition that changes the shape or position of the jaw may result in clinically obvious malocclusion, where the jaws are unable to close because teeth, particularly the canine or carnassial teeth, collide. Fractures and dislocations cause malocclusion of this severity. Other conditions that may prevent the jaws from closing are tumors or protuberant hyperplastic disease of the tissues that form the jaws. Buildup of dental calculus may be sufficient to prevent jaw closure in cats.

Inability to open the jaws is less common than inability to close the jaws. Causes include craniomandibular osteopathy, traumatic scarring of the lips, eosinophilic or atrophic myositis, and tetanus.

If the animal is unable to occlude the teeth sufficiently, particularly when the condition causing the malocclusion is painful, saliva dribbles from the mouth; the animal may be unable to swallow and loses condition rapidly. It is not necessary to restore occlusion to a perfect scissors bite to treat malocclusion effectively; restoration of prehension and swallowing function and relief of pain are much more important. Thus, simple treatment methods such as removal of one or more teeth may be effective in managing an animal with complex malocclusion.

If an animal is unable to manage a normal diet because of malocclusion and is on a total soft-food diet, natural teeth cleaning and gum massaging are absent. Thus, periodontal disease occurs more rapidly. The owner should be instructed to brush the animal's teeth daily.

Congenital Causes of Jaw Abnormalities

Craniomandibular osteopathy is a proliferative disease of unknown etiology that causes excessive new bone formation of the base of the skull and caudal end of the mandible. It is most common in West Highland white puppies, but several other breeds are also affected.[4, 141] Clinical signs of swelling or difficult prehension usually commence at four to six months of age. The jaw is able to open less and less because new bone wedges between the mandible and the skull. Surgery may occasionally be indicated to allow a dog to reach maturity, at which time new bone formation ceases and remodelling may occur. The procedure consists of removal of the excess bone that is most limiting the movement of the mandible, using the approach described for ventral bulla osteotomy. This is rarely performed because of the extent of disease present; dogs with less severe disease do not show clinical signs of sufficient severity to warrant treatment. Overall, results of both conservative treatment with prednisolone and surgical treatment are very poor in dogs with clinical signs caused by this disease.[4]

Temporomandibular subluxation or dysplasia occurs in young Irish Setters, basset hounds, cocker spaniels, and St. Bernards.[46, 75, 83, 94, 130, 153] The coronoid process of the mandible can become locked lateral to the zygomatic arch when the mouth is opened fully so that the dog is unable to close its mouth. In some dogs, the locking corrects itself spontaneously. If this is not the case, or to prevent further occurrences in a dog with multiple episodes, the ventral aspect or full thickness of the zygomatic arch is removed to provide space so that the abnormally mobile coronoid process does not engage the zygoma. The zygoma is approached through an incision on the side of the face. The buccal nerves and parotid salivary gland duct are located and avoided. The periosteum of the lateral aspect of the zygoma is incised and reflected ventrally, taking with it the aponeurosis of the masseter muscle. The periosteum of the medial side of the zygoma is also reflected, and the ventral half or full thickness of the zygoma is resected with a rongeur or osteotome. After controlling hemorrhage, the incision is closed by placing sutures to appose the dorsal and ventral incised edges of the periosteum. Results are usually excellent if sufficient bone is removed. Degenerative changes within the temporomandibular joint may occur subsequent to the dysplasia but have not been reported. Overlapping of the lateral joint capsule of the temporomandibular joint was attempted in one dog; locking episodes were reduced but not eliminated.[160]

Jaw Length and Teeth Position Abnormalities

Dental malocclusion is very common in dogs. The scissors bite is considered to be normal, but there are many breeds that are required to have other than a scissors bite according to the breed specifications. Brachycephalic breeds, with prominent prognathism, are obvious examples. These breed characteristics are compatible with normal prehension and jaw function. Much less frequently, congenital abnormalities occur that result in abnormal teeth positioning that prevents normal jaw function. The most common examples involve the canine and lateral incisor teeth; slight malpositioning causes the upper canine to occlude against the lower canine or lateral incisor to the point that one of these teeth develops at an abnormal angle.

Teeth can be moved or turned in their sockets to correct abnormalities of position by banding or surgery. Orthodontic procedures can produce excellent results;[132, 144] however, these procedures are unethical if the purpose is to correct an abnormality that would otherwise prevent or interfere with the show potential of a particular dog. Extraction is a simple, effective, but esthetically displeasing alternative. When the abnormality results from an acquired condition, such as a fracture, correction is not unethical.

When the abnormality is minor, collision of teeth can be prevented by removing part of the crown with a dental drill, avoiding the pulp cavity if possible. The normal occlusive pressure during growth may correct an abnormality in a dog that is only 6 to 8 months old; orthodontic correction should be put off until the dog is 10 to 12 months old unless the abnormality continues to worsen as the dog grows.

Orthodontic procedures usually require an initial anesthetic episode to obtain a dental impression of the defect and adjacent teeth. A model is made from the impression so that a suitable device can be fashioned. The animal is reanesthetized to cement or bond the device in place. Further sedation or anesthesia may be necessary to assess progress and adjust the device and finally to remove it. The device is kept in position for about two months in most dogs. Acid-etched bonding materials have made orthodontic procedures much easier and simpler to perform. Unfortunately, the wide diastema or space between dog teeth does not provide the convenient mounting available in human orthodontics. The position of teeth can be changed within very wide limits by applying pressure that causes bone resorption on the compression side and new bone formation on the tension side. The cortical surface in the direction that the tooth is being moved is also strengthened by new bone formation. Orthodontic pressure also affects the periodontal tissues; teeth undergoing orthodontic treatment should be brushed daily. Pressure sufficient to cause one tooth to move may cause the tooth to which the device is anchored to move also.

The need for orthodontic pressure can be avoided by surgically preparing the bone to create space for the tooth to move into, then levering the tooth to its new position, leaving the root apex untouched. The tooth must be stabilized by wiring it to adjacent teeth for about ten days.[3] Multiple incisor teeth abnormalities can be corrected by mandibular wedge osteotomy.[180]

A simple, though generally less useful alternative to banding, wiring, or surgical recontouring is the use of an inclined plane. To move a lower canine away from the midline, a plastic device that forces the tooth outward each time the mouth is closed is wired in place on the maxilla. In a growing puppy, ten days may be sufficient to correct the abnormality.[88]

The jaws can be lengthened or shortened surgically.[32] To shorten the mandible, a section of bone is removed caudal to the root of the canine tooth. One or more premolar teeth may have to be removed. The fractured ends are held in apposition with small bone plates. By careful use of an air drill, the neurovascular bundle within the mandible can be preserved; the canal at the osteotomy site must be enlarged to accommodate these structures prior to fracture reduction.[106] To lengthen the mandible, a step osteotomy and plate fixation are performed. Similar procedures can be performed on the maxilla but are complicated by the nasal cavity and contents. The nose can be lengthened by up to 1 cm in puppies by incising the palate, maxilla, and nasal bones and spreading the incision edges apart with a calibrated screw-driven plate system.[39]

As with some restorative dentistry procedures, the equipment, supplies, and experience needed for a successful orthodontic procedure are usually not available to or practical for veterinarinans not specializing in dentistry. If a veterinary dentist is not conveniently available for referral, human orthodontists are often interested and willing to collaborate.

Acquired Diseases of Occlusion

Mandibular Symphyseal Separation

The most commonly diagnosed "fracture" of the jaws is separation of the mandibular symphysis, often resulting from landing on the point of the jaw after falling from a height. Midline palate fracture and pneumothorax may coexist. Sufficient fixation to achieve fibrous union can be obtained by wiring the two sides together caudal to the canine teeth, using a hypodermic needle or suture passer to feed the wire subcutaneously.[71] Alteration of the angle of the canines can be prevented by forming a loop of wire around the canine teeth and a separate loop ventrally.[89] Use of nylon tie bands has been advocated, also placed through a subcutaneous tunnel and around the jaw caudal to the canine teeth.[181] A single cross pin, or double cross pins, can be used to maintain apposition at the symphysis of the mandible; the pins are placed caudal to the roots of the canine teeth. A combination of circum-mandibular wire and acrylic splint has also been suggested.[149] The simple circum-mandibular wire technique works well, particularly in cats, in which this injury is common; if the wire causes distortion of the angle of the canine teeth, additional stabilization with a cross pin or Kirschner wire is indicated. The fixation device can usually be removed in two to three weeks.

Mandibular and Maxillary Fractures

Many fractures of the mandible and maxilla do not need surgical fixation, particularly those in which the fracture lines are contained within the areas of attachment of the masticatory muscles, as these muscles effectively splint the fracture during healing. A simple external device, such as a bandage around the muzzle placed just loose enough so that the tongue can extend through to allow lapping of liquids, is often sufficient.[175] The jaws are not weight bearing, and healing by formation of a false joint is usually satisfactory; rigid fixation is thus rarely necessary.

Mandibular Fractures

Fractures of the mandible can be repaired by many means. Access to fractures of the horizontal ramus can be through the oral mucosa or ventrolaterally through a skin incision, extending the incision caudally by displacing the digastricus muscle medially.[123] Orthopedic wire used in a simple loop through holes made in the mandible with a Kirschner wire or in a figure-eight pattern is simple to place and works well;[136] two or more wires can be used to prevent overriding. The mandible has a medullary cavity that will accept small Steinmann pins or Kirschner wires. The flat surface of the mandible provides space for plate fixation.[156, 157] Cross pinning to the other mandible can be used successfully, either by itself or combined with tension wires. Tension wires can be used alone.[43, 107] If cross pinning and external fixation are used, the weight of the external fixation device can be reduced by using an acrylic side bar. A variation on the use of an external fixation device is to form a sublingual rod; a Steinmann pin is bent into a U-shape with right-angle projections at either end and placed so that the points fit into holes prepared in the mandible caudal to the last molar tooth and the rod sits comfortably just rostral to the tongue. The fractured segments are held in alignment with wires placed around the intraoral splint.[12]

An alternative external fixation device is wiring of teeth. A quick-setting acrylic splint can be fashioned to fit on the lingual surface of the mandible and can be held in place with wires around adjacent teeth.[58, 103, 161] In a fresh simple fracture, retention grooves can be cut in the cortex across the fracture site, and the acrylic material can be cured directly in the grooves.[85]

Fractures of the vertical ramus that are not splinted in satisfactory occlusion by the masticatory muscles can be held in fixation by wiring the mandibular teeth to the maxillary teeth in normal occlusion. Alimentation through a pharyngostomy or gastrostomy tube is necessary for the four-week duration of wire placement. The jaws are wired by placing and twisting 24- to 28-gauge wire subgingivally around several incisor and premolar teeth, placing the jaws in occlusion, and then twisting the wires together leaving 1 to 2 mm of movement available.[42] Interdental wire may stretch or break if fixation consists of a single wire placed on each side at the level of the carnassial teeth.[100] A similar reduction of overriding fractures can be obtained by placing screws in the maxilla and mandible and connecting them with elastic bands.[117]

From the list of techniques discussed previously, it can be concluded that no one simple technique is always satisfactory and that many techniques are satisfactory in some circumstances. The choice of fixation system depends on the equipment available, the type of fracture (horizontal or vertical ramus, overriding or acceptable occlusion), and, often, the experience and preference of the surgeon. The ability to open and close the mouth without difficulty is the primary consideration. Principles of application of orthopedic devices are described in Section XVIII. Complications of mandibular fracture fixation or failure to repair an overriding fracture include malocclusion,[41] bone resorption and subsequent nonunion, periodontal disease and tooth loss, and mandibular osteomyelitis.

When a healed mandibular fracture has resulted in locking of teeth to the point that the animal cannot close its jaws completely, extraction of one or more teeth is often sufficient to restore normal ability to eat.

If nonunion or delayed union causes malocclusion, a rigid fixation device is required. Transfixation splints with acrylic bridges[131] or biphase external fixation splints[65, 169] are tolerated by dogs for several months if necessary. The biphase external fixation splint is not suitable for small dogs because of its weight. When bone loss has occurred, grafts of rib or ilium can be used, with a good likelihood of acceptance on the mandible or maxilla,[162] although at least 18 mm of mandibular length can be replaced if a bridging bone plate is left in place for up to four months.[77]

Maxillary Fractures

Fractures of the maxilla are often more complex to manage. The maxilla is a relatively thin bone supporting the teeth and framing the nasal cavity. Rigid fixation of these thin plates of bone is rarely possible. An additional complication is that the nasal cavities may be exposed as a result of the fracture, and there is often damage to intranasal structures that may reduce or prevent air movement through the nose following the injury. Maxillary fractures are often left untreated. If the nasal cavity is exposed, the palate must be repaired to close off the airway to prevent aspiration during eating or drinking; in some animals, sutures in the mucoperiosteum are sufficient to achieve this, whereas in others the fracture must be held in fixation or the oronasal defect must await later reconstructive surgery if the damage to the maxilla is extensive. Primary fixation of large fragments of the premaxilla and maxilla is achieved with wire sutures or tension wires.[136] A severely deformed maxilla may be returned to normal occlusion and held in fixation with Kirschner wires or small Steinmann pins placed through the fractured segments and adjacent normal bone and attached to an external fixation frame. Rapidly curing acrylic bridges are light in weight and can be conformed to the shape required.[151] Maxillary and nasal fractures are discussed in Section VIII; reconstruction of missing segments of the maxilla is discussed later in this chapter.

Chronic Maxillary and Mandibular Infections

Fortunately, generalized maxillary or mandibular osteomyelitis is uncommon. This condition usually results from chronic periodontitis. During periodontitis, most or all of the teeth on the affected jaw will have fallen out or been removed. Large areas of necrotic bone, with reactive new bone surrounding it, are seen on examination of the mouth. The maxilla or mandible may be grossly swollen. Nasal discharge is not common. Medical treatment of osteomyelitis in this location is often ineffective, although drugs that are particularly effective against the spectrum of bacteria associated with severe periodontitis, such as tetracycline (20 mg/kg t.i.d. PO for four weeks) or metronidazole (50 mg/kg daily PO, five days on and five days off, repeated twice), should be tried before resorting to radical surgery. Conservative surgical treatment, such as limited curettage of necrotic bone

followed by a prolonged course of antibiotics, is usually only temporarily successful. Radical resection of affected tissue back to normal bone is much more likely to cure the condition. These techniques are discussed under management of oral neoplasms.

Carnassial Abscess

The most common form of chronic osteomyelitis of the maxilla is carnassial abscess (facial sinus, malar abscess). This condition affects the upper carnassial (fourth premolar) tooth and, less often, the upper first molar tooth. A similar syndrome occurs much less often around the first molar tooth in the mandible.[74] The condition is rare in cats.[158]

The maxillary bone is eroded over the root of the tooth, and a swelling results on the side of the face that often goes on to rupture (see Fig. 46–12A). Typically, the swelling is ventral and slightly rostral to or level with the medial canthus of the eye. Occasionally the fistula may open into the conjunctival sac.[116] The discharge produced is rarely purulent, more often being serosanguineous. Crown fracture, root abscess, or periodontal disease is obvious on some but not all affected teeth.[179] It has not yet been established whether the condition results from periodontal disease, endodontic disease, or both; pressure necrosis from occlusive trauma has been suggested as a cause.[98] When a mandibular tooth is affected, the fistula opens either into the buccal fold or onto the skin surface.

Treatment of carnassial abscess is by extraction of the tooth immediately beneath the lesion. Endodontic treatment has also been used successfully.[63] Carnassial abscess is a localized condition that can be successfully treated in almost all affected animals.

Temporomandibular Joint Disease

Temporomandibular subluxation or dysplasia was described previously.

Dislocation of the temporomandibular joint is not common in the dog or cat, probably because the joint permits tremendous crushing force to be applied but only limited movement in directions other than opening and closing of the jaws. Because of this arrangement, the temporomandibular joint can only be dislocated if the mandible is hit when the jaws are open. Where the jaw is dislocated without fracture, the condyle is repositioned by levering the jaws apart. This is done under anesthesia. A wooden rod is placed between the lower and upper carnassial teeth on the affected side, and the jaws rostral to the rod are closed firmly together. When the jaws have been closed, thus disengaging the dislocated condyle from its abnormal position, the mandible on the affected side is pushed caudally as the pressure on the jaws is relaxed, allowing the condyle to reseat in the joint. When the dislocation cannot be reduced by this simple method, more successful leverage can be obtained by placing a Steinmann pin through both mandibles at the level of the molar teeth; the chuck is left attached to the pin to provide a handle for manipulation of the jaw.[16] Chewing of hard objects should be discouraged for about two weeks to permit repair of ligaments around the condyle. Chronic dislocation is rare and results from fracture of the condyle or skull causing disruption of the joint.

Degenerative temporomandibular joint disease is rare and probably results from trauma that either was not observed by the owner or was insufficient to cause immediate clinical signs. Trauma may result in fracture of the structures forming the temporomandibular joint rather than dislocation; in cats, fractures in this area may be seen with mandibular symphyseal separation.[163] Treatment of chronic diseases of the temporomandibular joint that are not managable conservatively (i.e., soft-food diet and analgesics as needed) is condylectomy; one or both condyles can be removed in the dog and cat with little or no resulting abnormality in prehension.[101, 165] The approach is made through the masseter muscle, avoiding the buccal nerves and parotid duct and exposing the meniscotemporal and meniscomandibular joints.[123] The condyle and meniscus are removed with rongeurs or a wire saw, and the masseter muscle aponeurosis incisional edges are apposed. Dogs are able to eat normally the day after surgery.

Mandibular Neuropraxia

Mandibular neuropraxia ("dropped jaw") may mimic mandibular fracture or temporomandibular joint dysfunction. The dog is unable to close the mouth, but the owner can close the mouth easily and without pain. There are no radiographic abnormalities. The cause of this syndrome is presumed to be stretching of trigeminal nerves. A history of carrying heavy logs or stones in the mouth can be obtained in some, but not all, cases. Treatment is placement of a loose muzzle over the snout and mandible for two to three weeks; there is rarely involvement of the hypoglossal nerve, so tongue function is normal and the dog can lap fluids through the muzzle. Normal function almost invariably returns within four weeks.[79, 129]

Eosinophilic-Atrophic Myositis

Eosinophilic infiltration and subsequent fibrous replacement affect the muscles of the head and neck of some dogs, usually of large breeds such as German shepherds and Samoyeds. The cause is not known. Clinical signs are pain on opening the mouth, progressing to inability to open the mouth more than 1 to 2 cm in severely affected dogs. There may be swelling of the temporal area initially with exophthalmos, and temporal atrophy is seen. The muscles supplied by the trigeminal nerve are most often affected, although the tongue and neck muscles may show electromyographic abnormalities. Definitive diagnosis is by temporal muscle biopsy, although eosinophilia of peripheral blood and serum creatine phosphokinase levels are useful adjuncts.

Treatment in most cases is prednisolone, commencing at 1 mg/kg twice daily for several days, then gradually reducing the dosage to 0 over four to five weeks. Intermittent prednisolone is necessary in some dogs to maintain adequate ability to open the mouth. In some dogs, fibrous replacement progresses to the point that prednisolone does not result in clinical improvement and manual opening of the jaws is not possible even under anesthesia. In this case, the jaws must be pried open with a lever system, distributing the force over both sides of the jaws and protecting the teeth from fracture; overzealous treatment can cause jaw fracture. Forceful opening of the mouth must be followed by prednisolone therapy for at least a month to prevent reformation of fibrous tissue.

Mandibular symphysiotomy is described under Pharynx.

ORAL SOFT TISSUES

Healing of incisional wounds in oral mucosa is more rapid than in skin: phagocytic activity is greater, occurs earlier, and is mostly due to monocytes rather than polymorphonuclear leukocytes; epithelial migration occurs earlier; and epithelialization is completed earlier. The higher metabolic activity and higher mitotic rate of oral mucosa are believed to be responsible for these differences and may be due to the richer blood supply and higher temperature of oral mucosa.[142] In dogs, silk and Mersilene (Dacron) sutures cause a similar leukocytic infiltration; surgical gut causes a significantly greater cellular response.[22] Most sutures with knots on the mucosal surface, whether absorbable or nonabsorbable, are sloughed out within two to three weeks. Based on clinical observations, synthetic absorbable sutures appear to last somewhat longer than surgical gut and are preferred for that reason.

The Tongue

Congenital Anomalies

Congenital anomalies of the tongue are rarely amenable to surgical repair. Lateral protrusion of the tongue without hypoglossal nerve damage has been described; repair by plication has been attempted, with limited success.[50] Macroglossia has been treated by resection of the rostral section of the tongue, with good clinical results. Many brachycephalic dogs have tongues that seem grossly long compared with their jaw length, although they have good control of function, and the tongue does not become traumatized from exposure. A short frenulum causing difficulty in eating and drinking in a dog was treated by incising the frenulum for 2 cm.[178]

Trauma

The injuries most frequently observed are lacerations caused by licking sharp surfaces, penetrating foreign bodies such as chicken bones or wood splinters, electrical cord burns, and mucosal ulceration from infection or ingestion of caustics. Clinical signs are bleeding, drooling of saliva, inability or unwillingness to eat, and pawing at the mouth. Diagnosis is by inspection of the mouth, which may require sedation if painful. It is particularly important to inspect the sublingual area to ensure that no foreign bodies are embedded in the tongue or wrapped around its root.

Clean lacerations are sutured with absorbable material, both to control hemorrhage and to appose the epithelial edges. Jagged lacerations require debridement prior to suturing. Barbed foreign bodies, such as fish hooks, porcupine quills, and some bone chips or wood splinters, require incision of overlying tissue to prevent more severe damage by blunt removal.

Dogs with electrical burn injuries are examined and auscultated carefully for signs of shock or pulmonary edema.[92] The tongue injury rarely requires definitive management and is best left to slough so that the maximum amount of tongue tissue is retained. Use of a pharyngostomy or gastrostomy tube may be necessary for feeding for several days. Once the necrotic portion has sloughed, the remaining stump is covered rapidly by epithelium. Dogs and cats that have lost the entire free portion and some of the root of the tongue often manage well by sucking in food and water or by tossing chunks of food to the back of the tongue. Cats, which are more fastidious groomers than dogs, may develop a poor haircoat if the length of tongue available for grooming is insufficient.[152]

Hyperplastic and Neoplastic Lesions

Masses are less common on the tongue than on other areas of the oral mucosa. Non-neoplastic lesions include eosinophilic granuloma in cats,[119] seen as raised firm nodules, often with white streaks or whorls visible on the surface; a similar condition was recognized recently in huskies,[110, 125] although the lesions are generally more diffuse in dogs than in cats. Because these lesions are benign and usually controllable medically with corticosteroids, it is essential that mass lesions on the tongue be biopsied and diagnosed prior to radical treatment. Another benign lesion occasionally found on the tongue is calcinosis circumscripta.[54]

Neoplasms that occur on or in the tongue include squamous cell carcinoma, melanoma, fibrosarcoma, reticuloendothelial cell tumors, rhabdomyosarcoma, and leiomyoma. These infiltrating and often ulcerating lesions occasionally are amenable to total surgical excision, particularly when located on the rostral free part of the tongue or superficially on the dorsal surface. Surgical resection of part of the tongue is usually bloody. Electrosurgery is useful, and temporary occlusion of both carotid arteries through an incision in the neck should be considered if extensive surgery is likely, particularly in an animal that may have already lost blood because of ulceration of the surface of the tumor. Ideally, tongue tissue is removed as a wedge so that the mucosa can be apposed with synthetic absorbable sutures. (Treatment of particular tumor types is described in Section 19.)

Lips and Cheeks

Congenital Abnormalities

The most obvious abnormality affecting the lips is harelip, in which the two sides of the primary palate fail to fuse normally. This condition is described in the Respiratory section. The most frequent congenital abnormality affecting the lips and cheeks is the abnormal lip fold confromation seen in some spaniels. The lips form a channel, causing saliva to flow onto the skin of the lip. The result is chronic, foul-smelling moist dermatitis. Diagnosis is by inspection of the lips (Fig. 46–14A). The major differential diagnosis is halitosis caused by periodontal disease. Treatment is by resection of the folds, making a V-shaped incision through the skin and mucosa (Fig. 46–14B and C). The two layers are sutured separately (Fig. 46–14D). Results are usually excellent—the incision is clean and dry at suture removal, showing that the purpose of the surgery has been achieved.

Giant breed dogs that slobber a great deal can be treated by bilateral mandibular–sublingual gland resection or by cheiloplasty. In this latter technique, a flap of the lower lip is isolated and sutured to a defect created in the upper lip, thus eliminating the channel or pocket that allows saliva to accumulate.[154]

Trauma

Traumatic lesions affecting the lips and cheeks include bite wounds (which, particularly in cats, can cause rapidly developing abscesses), avulsion or laceration from external trauma, and necrosis following electrical injury.[92] Simple lacerations are sutured with separate layers on the mucosal and skin surfaces. Abscesses are lanced and drained, avoiding the parotid duct as it passes over the side of the face.

Necrosis of part of the lip may result in stricture of the oral commissure and inability of the dog to open its mouth (Fig. 46–15A). This can be corrected by incising the scar at the commissure and closing the mucosa and skin as two layers to lengthen the commissure (Fig. 46–15B and C); this procedure can be improved by performing a Z-plasty (see Section

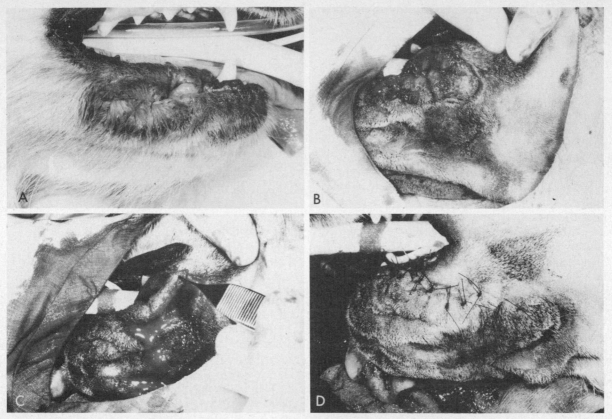

Figure 46–14. Surgical treatment of lip fold dermatitis. *A*, Moist dermatitis around the lip fold prior to surgery. *B*, Incision around the lip fold. *C*, The flap is elevated, and the incision is extended through the buccal mucosa. *D*, The incision is closed in two layers.

IV) so that the healing incision is not located at the new commissure.

Avulsion injuries may cause severe skin loss. Because the mandible is an exposed prominence, where skin is not freely available for covering bare areas, every effort is made to retain skin at the rostral end. This can be done by reattaching the avulsed skin to the gingival attachment if the skin is healthy or by rotating a flap of skin from the intermandibular area, with repair of the defect created left for a later procedure. Skin of the lip can be held in place at its rostral end by placing sutures through the skin and around adjacent teeth;[14] plastic tubing has been used to form tension-relieving sutures.[60]

Avulsion of the upper lip is less common but more spectacular if the nasal cavity is exposed. Disrupted tissues are debrided and kept in normal apposition by sutures placed through the avulsed lip and anchored to one or more incisor or canine teeth.[120]

Neoplastic and Hyperplastic Lesions

The lips and cheeks are lined by mucosal and skin epithelium, with connective tissue between. The range of neoplasms affecting the lips is therefore wide. Squamous cell carcinoma of the gingiva may invade the lip or, less often, may arise from the lip mucosa itself. Fibrosarcomas are common in the connective tissue covering the maxilla but probably arise from the periodontal connective tissue. Skin tumors affecting this area include squamous cell carcinoma, basal cell carcinoma, and mast cell sarcoma (Fig. 46–16A). Principles of surgical resection of lip and cheek lesions are: biopsy of all lesions suspected of being malignant; wide excision of known malignant lesions (Fig. 46–16B and C); maintenance of a functional commissure so that the mouth can open (this may require rotation flaps); separate closure of the incisions in the mucosa and the skin where the resection is full thickness (Fig. 46–16D); and avoidance of the parotid salivary duct when possible or ligation or transposition when avoidance is not possible. Management and prognosis of specific tumors are described in Section 19.

Lesions that appear neoplastic but are hyperplastic include lip (eosinophilic) granuloma of cats and occasional single or multiple masses in the skin of the lip that are probably chronic granulomas from foreign body penetration. Eosinophilic granulomas of cats are treated medically when possible,[143] using prednisolone or megestrol acetate. Radiation therapy is an alternative that gives excellent results in most cats.[113] Surgical resection or cryosurgical destruction[171] provides the least cosmetically acceptable results. Recurrence is possible with all treatment methods described.

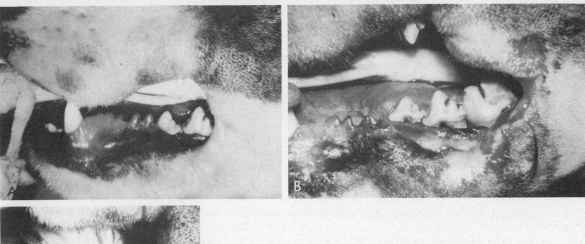

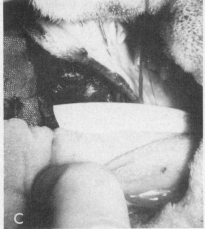

Figure 46–15. Traumatic lip stricture. *A*, Extent of ability to open the mouth following electrical cord burn of commissure of lip in a dog. *B*, The commissure is incised. Necrotic section of mandible and exposed roots of lower teeth are visible. *C*, Extent of ability to open the mouth on completion of lip incision closure.

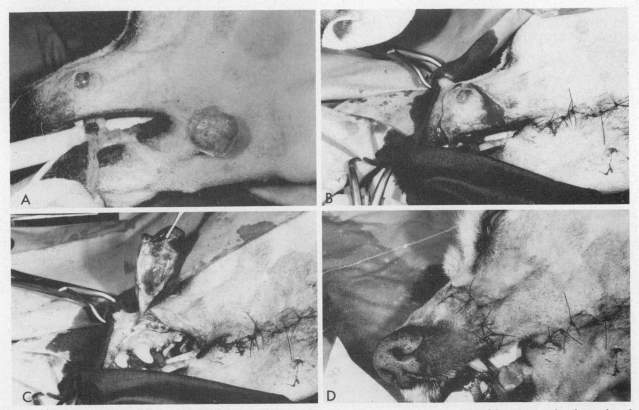

Figure 46–16. *A*, Basal cell carcinomas on the lip of a dog. *B*, The large superficial lesion was resected by incising the skin only. The smaller, rostral lesion required incision into the oral mucosa as well. *C*, The lesion is isolated by full thickness resection of lip tissue. *D*, The oral mucosa and skin edges are sutured as separate layers to reform the lip.

ORAL NEOPLASIA

Tumors of the oral cavity are common and often difficult to treat. Early diagnosis is an important part of sound management. There are also many lesions that appear malignant but are hyperplastic, or that are neoplastic but benign; the nomenclature of some oral proliferative lesions of dogs and cats is confusing.[55] Gross appearance is a useful indicator of likely diagnosis, but major treatment decisions should not be made on the basis of gross appearance alone.

Cystic lesions may be congenital in origin[7, 61] or neoplastic.[99] Other lesions arising from the tooth-forming structures in young dogs may consist of multiple odd-shaped dental structures or bony proliferation.[35, 62]

Diagnosis of some oral neoplasms, particularly squamous cell carcinoma, can be made by contact smears of the mass. In general, it is best to obtain a piece of tissue for histopathological examination. The mass is usually accessible, and a specimen of appropriate size can be obtained with biopsy forceps or scissors. Minimal restraint and local analgesic spray are often sufficient. Other essential steps prior to definitive treatment are examination of thoracic radiographs for signs of lung metastasis, which is common with some oral malignancies,[164] and radiographs of the involved jaw to determine the extent of bone invasion.

Management and prognosis of animals with specific malignancies are discussed in Section 19.

Surgical Management of Mass Lesions in the Mouth

Lesions confined to the gingival mucosa are removed by shaving off the abnormal tissue with a scalpel or electroscalpel. The epithelial defect is left uncovered. Bleeding vessels are controlled by pressure or electrocoagulation. Lesions on the mucosa of the hard palate can be removed in a similar fashion. This superficial method of excision is applicable only to hyperplastic or benign lesions that have not penetrated the basement membrane. It is often not sufficient treatment of even benign lesions such as fibromatous epulis. When there has been recurrence of a benign lesion following conservative resection, consideration should be given to radiation therapy or radical surgery, although intermittent conservative resection is also possible.

Maxillectomy

Invasive or recurrent lesions of the maxilla or palate can be cured surgically only by radical resection. Radical partial maxillectomy and palatectomy are practical and cause few or no long-term problems for the animal. Since the cheek is not resected, it is available to cover the lesion. The cosmetic defect is a sunken-in appearance on one side of the face, which is not noticeable in long-haired dogs. Partial maxillectomy is easier to perform for lesions located in the middle third of the hard palate because of the desirability of maintaining a bony platform for the nasal cartilages at the rostral end of the nose. Where possible, a 1-cm margin of grossly normal tissue is removed with the tumor.

The procedure commences with an incision in the palatal, gingival, and buccal mucosa to outline the extent of resection, staying at least 1 cm away from gross margins of the lesion. The epithelium is reflected to expose the underlying bone. Hemorrhage is often profuse, particularly when the palate is incised. This can usually be controlled by pressure until the resected tissue is lifted out, at which time the vessels themselves can be located and ligated or electrocoagulated. Temporary occlusion of one or both carotid arteries through an incision in the neck should be considered in animals with a low PCV prior to surgery. The maxilla and palate are fractured along the incision lines with an osteotome or oscillating bone saw (Fig. 46–17A and B). The line of incision may include the infraorbital canal; if so, the infraorbital artery must be ligated. The tissue to be resected is levered up, the remaining attachments are separated, and the section, usually including several teeth *in situ*, is removed en bloc (Fig. 46–17C–E). The nasal cavity will normally be exposed if the resection is adequate. Hemorrhage is controlled, blood clots are removed, and the remaining tissues are examined. If there are areas of turbinate that were partially severed or traumatized during the resection, they are cut with scissors to leave a clean edge. Hemorrhage that cannot be controlled by ligation or pressure may respond to a topical application of 0.5% cocaine solution.

The defect between the nose and mouth is covered with a buccal flap that is created by incising the buccal mucosa and undermining it until sufficient tissue is formed to cover the defect without tension. A section of palate mucosa is removed from the edge adjacent to the bone incision so as to leave a shelf of bone to support the buccal flap. The flap is sutured into position with a combination of vertical mattress and simple interrupted sutures (see Fig. 46–17D). A wide variety of materials can be used; I prefer synthetic absorbable sutures. Wire is more likely to cut through the mucosa because of its smaller diameter compared with other materials; it will not prevent the dog or cat from licking the sutures and has no advantage in this location. Drains are not necessary.

The site may be painful during the immediate recovery period, but the animal is usually able to eat without difficulty the following day. If the sutures holding the flap in place break down two to three days following surgery, the animal is reanesthetized and the flap resutured. Feeding the animal through a pharyngostomy or gastrostomy tube is of doubtful value in preventing dehiscence. Antibiotics are not

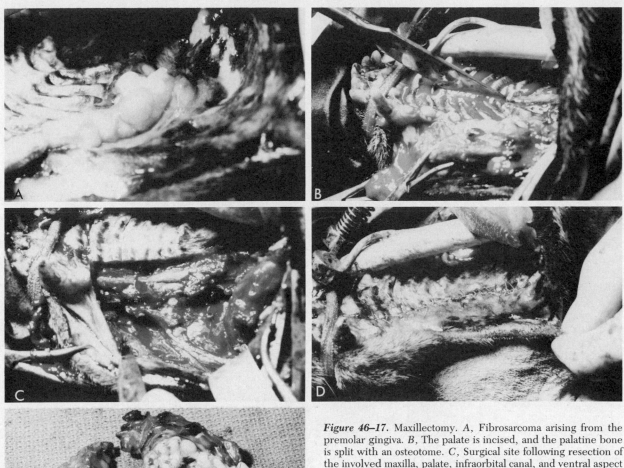

Figure 46–17. Maxillectomy. *A*, Fibrosarcoma arising from the premolar gingiva. *B*, The palate is incised, and the palatine bone is split with an osteotome. *C*, Surgical site following resection of the involved maxilla, palate, infraorbital canal, and ventral aspect of the orbit. The nasal mucosa can be seen immediately below the incised edge of the palate. *D*, A buccal flap has been formed and sutured in place to close off the nasal cavity from the mouth. *E*, Surgical specimens include the palate and maxilla as a unit and (on left) the infraorbital canal contents and zygomatic salivary gland.

necessary. The animal is fed a soft-food diet and is prevented from chewing hard objects for the next several weeks to protect the flap while it heals.

This procedure can be adapted for lesions penetrating the orbit by extending the resection to include the entire infraorbital canal and adjacent bone. The zygomatic salivary gland can be resected through this approach (see Fig. 46–17), and the tissues forming the medial wall of the orbit are available for resection if necessary. The eye remains in a normal position with the normal ability to rotate following this extensive resection.

Unilateral or bilateral radical premaxillectomy can also be performed on dogs with good results (Fig. 46–18 *F–H*).[177] The lesion is outlined by incision in the oral mucosa, and the palate and premaxilla are removed en bloc with an osteotome or bone saw, exposing the nasal vestibule (Fig. 46–18*A*, *B*, *D*, and *E*). Hemorrhage is controlled. The oral and nasal cavities are kept separate by creating unilateral or bilateral buccal mucosal advancement or rotation flaps (Fig. 46–18*C*). If bilateral surgery is performed,

the flaps are placed so that both cover the oronasal defect when sutured together, one with the epithelial surface facing dorsally to form the floor of the nasal vestibule and the other with the epithelium facing ventrally to form the new palate surface.

Lesions on the lateral aspect of the upper canine tooth can be removed by resecting only the lateral alveolar plate and canine tooth (Fig. 46–19). Suturing is not necessary if the nasal cavity is not penetrated (Fig. 46–19*F*).

Mandibulectomy

Invasive mandibular lesions can be dealt with in a similarly radical fashion. Rostral mandibulectomy has been performed for many years with excellent functional results. If the procedure is confined to the incisor and canine teeth area and the mandibular symphysis is not completely separated, no supportive procedures are necessary (Fig. 46–20). The skin can be retracted following the initial incision through the free gingiva and reattached to the shortened mandi-

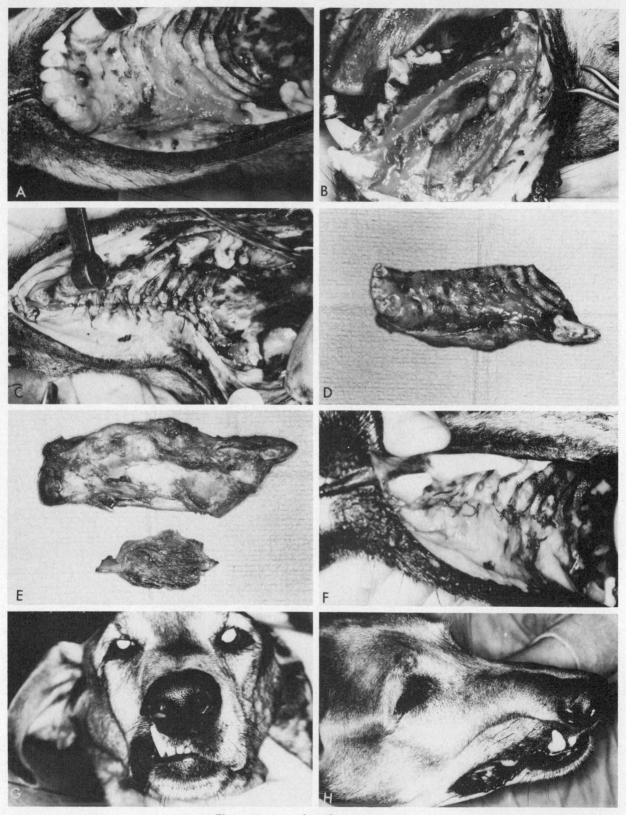

Figure 46–18. See legend on opposite page

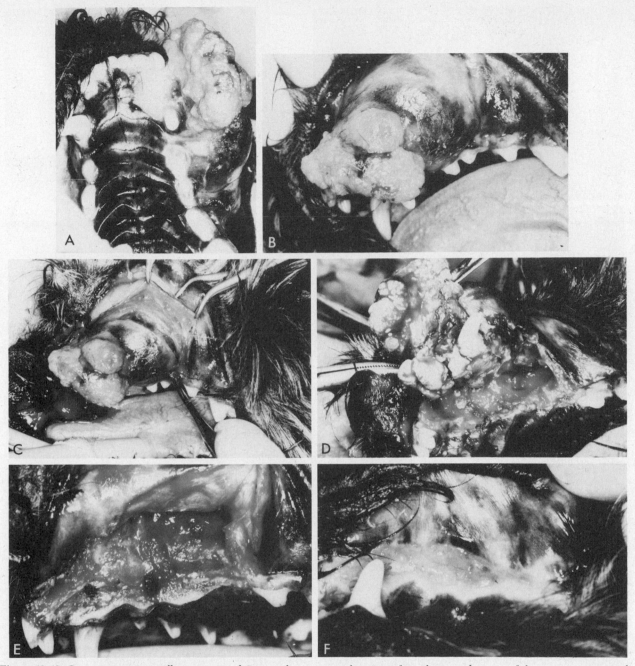

Figure 46–19. Conservative premaxillectomy. *A* and *B*, Acanthomatous epulis arising from the periodontium of the upper canine tooth. *C*, Incision in the buccal mucosa dorsal to the mass. *D*, The mass and canine and incisor teeth are elevated after incising and fracturing the premaxilla and palate. *E*, Surgical site following excision. The nasal cavity was not penetrated, and the wound was left to heal by granulation. *F*, Three weeks later, most of the wound is covered by epithelium, and the remainder has granulated and is undergoing epithelialization. The dog ate readily the day following surgery.

Figure 46–18. Premaxillectomy. *A*, Recurrent fibrosarcoma arising from the gingiva lateral to the canine and premolar teeth, which have been removed. *B*, Surgical site following resection of the premaxilla and part of the maxilla. The nasal mucosa in the nasal vestibule and rostral nasal cavity is visible. *C*, A buccal flap has been formed and sutured to close off the nasal cavity from the mouth. *D*, Surgical specimen, ventral aspect, showing the four incisor teeth and carnassial tooth that were removed in situ. The specimen extends across the midline. *E*, Surgical specimens, dorsal aspect, showing the premaxilla and maxilla (top) and ventral nasal concha (bottom), which was removed to provide space for air flow in the rostral part of the nasal cavity that was narrowed following surgery. *F*, Surgical site two weeks postoperatively. The flap has healed, and the dog is eating well and breathing comfortably through his nose. *G* and *H*, External appearance two weeks following surgery.

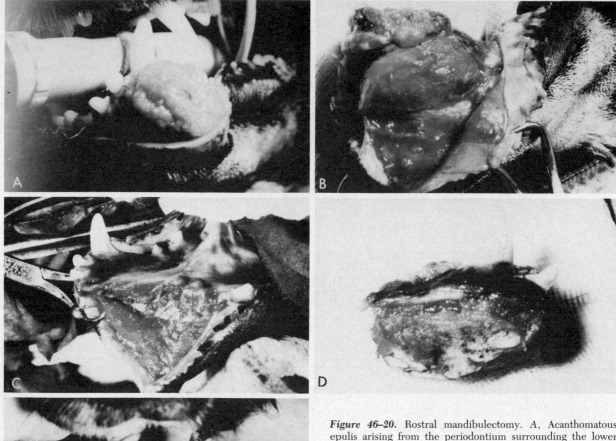

Figure 46–20. Rostral mandibulectomy. *A*, Acanthomatous epulis arising from the periodontium surrounding the lower canine tooth. *B*, Incision in normal buccal mucosa around the lesion. *C*, The mandible has been resected, including the canine tooth root. The symphysis is intact. The wound was allowed to heal by granulation. *D*, Surgical specimen including incisor and canine teeth. *E*, Surgical site two weeks following surgery. Healing is almost complete, and the dog is eating without difficulty.

ble. If necessary, excess skin can be resected. For more extensive lesions caudal to the canine teeth, the symphysis must be resected. The line of resection should be at least 1 cm away from grossly or radiographically visible lesions. The horizontal rami of the mandible are stabilized with cross pins prior to cutting bone. The mucosa around the lesion is incised, the bone is transected with bone cutters or oscillating saw, and bleeding vessels are ligated. Excess skin is resected, leaving the mucocutaneous junction intact if possible, and a flap of skin is created to cover the reformed point of the jaw.[166]

Recovery from the effects of surgery is rapid, and most animals learn to drink and eat normally in a few days. Because the canine teeth have been removed, the tongue may tend to hang out of that side of the mouth when relaxed, but this does not interfere with normal prehension and swallowing.

For lesions located in the premolar or molar area, hemimandibulectomy can be performed.[31, 176] This is particularly well tolerated in cats. Incisions are made well away from the lesional tissue in the free gingiva

(Fig. 46–21A and B), and the mandible is undermined by blunt dissection. The symphysis is separated by bone cutters or scissors (see Fig. 46–21B), and the lateral attachments of the tongue are separated (Fig. 46–21C), leaving the mandibular and sublingual gland ducts intact if they can be identified. This frees the mandible so that it can be swung independently, facilitating dissection of the masseter and pterygoid muscles from their attachments. These muscles are reflected laterally and medially, respectively, exposing the vertical ramus of the mandible. Exposed or incised vessels are ligated, the mandible is cut with a bone cutter, and the digastric muscle is transected, allowing the jaw to be removed from the surgical site. Alternatively, the entire hemimandible can be removed by continuing blunt and sharp dissection to separate muscular and tendinous attachments from the mandible; the temporomandibular ligaments are exposed by rotating the mandible (Fig. 46–21D and H) and incised.

A drain can be placed in the cavity beneath the suture line, exiting through the skin (Fig. 46–21E).

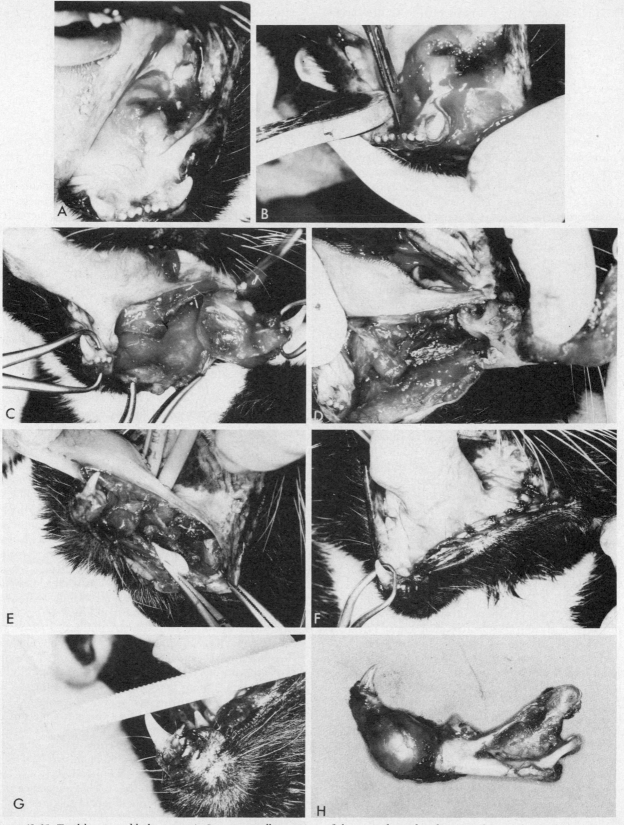

Figure 46–21. Total hemimandibulectomy. *A*, Squamous cell carcinoma of the premolar and molar area of a cat. *B*, The buccal mucosa has been incised, and the mandibular symphysis is separated with a scalpel. *C*, The mylohyoid muscle is incised, and the mandible is separated from the lingual structures. *D*, The pterygoid muscles have been separated from the mandible, which is twisted laterally to expose the temporomandibular joint. *E*, A soft rubber drain is placed in the surgical site following removal of the mandible. *F*, The buccal mucosal incised edge has been sutured to the sublingual mucosa. *G*, The remaining lower canine tooth is shortened using a steel file. The cat was able to swallow without difficulty the next day and was prehending and swallowing normally within ten days. *H*, Surgical specimen showing the large neoplastic mass and extent of dissection of the mandible possible with this technique.

The incision is closed with absorbable sutures apposing the incised oral mucosal edges (Fig. 46–21F). The opposite mandible will swing over toward the midline, which may result in the remaining mandibular canine tooth impinging on the palate when the mouth is closed; the canine tooth should be removed or shortened (Fig. 46–21G) to prevent this. A soft-food diet will probably be necessary for the duration of the animal's life.

Lesions of the coronoid process of the vertical ramus of the mandible can be resected through an approach through the zygomatic arch and masseter muscle. The periosteum of the zygoma is incised and reflected, the zygoma is resected full thickness with an osteotome or rongeur, and the temporal, masseter, and pterygoid muscles are reflected from the coronoid process, which can then be removed partially or completely with a rongeur or osteotome. The incision is closed by apposing the periosteum of the zygomatic arch to the orbital fascia. Soft rubber drains can be placed through the masseter muscle, avoiding the parotid duct, if muscle dissection was extensive.

Dogs and cats can usually eat and swallow adequately, or even normally, following the radical maxillary and mandibular procedures previously described, although some animals require a period of 10 to 14 days to adapt to the changed conditions in their mouth. Short-term complications are mainly mucosal wound breakdown. This is less likely to occur if there is minimal tension on the flap and if the flap incision is located over some supporting tissue. If the flap becomes necrotic, the epithelium is allowed to heal to form an oronasal fistula, and then another flap is created and sutured in place (see Section 8). Long-term complications are most often due to recurrence of disease. Protocols for managing particular tumor types are described in Section 19.

Cryosurgical Treatment

Cryosurgical treatment of oral tumors with liquid nitrogen has been used for several years. Results are most satisfactory for squamous cell carcinoma.[70] After the diagnosis has been microscopically confirmed and chest and lesional radiographs have been obtained, treatment is begun. Adjacent uninvolved areas are protected with petrolatum jelly–impregnated sponges or by application of a plastic cup cut to fit the lesion. Loose teeth near the lesion are removed, and tissue temperature thermocouples are inserted with the points at the deepest part of the tumor. The tumor is either frozen *in situ* or is reduced first, and remaining tumor tissue is then frozen. Using either the probe or spray, the tumor tissue temperature is lowered to at least −25°C, allowed to thaw, and then refrozen. There is usually no hemorrhage during the procedure.

Cryosurgery of tumors of the caudal oral cavity or pharynx may cause sufficient edema to result in airway obstruction requiring tracheotomy.[70] In a series of 149 dogs treated, 5 died during or immediately following the procedure, including 2 deaths from gas embolism caused by nitrogen sprays;[70] delayed hemorrhage occurred in 2 dogs.

Hyperthermic Treatment

Tissue temperatures of 50°C or more generated by radiofrequency waves, combined with standard radiotherapy, have been used to treat oral fibrosarcomas in dogs. Complications, including septicemia and death, oronasal fistula, and local infection, occurred more frequently at higher treatment temperatures. It was concluded that this form of therapy was not particularly useful in the treatment of fibrosarcomas in dogs.[34]

DISEASES OF THE PHARYNX

Congenital defects of the pharynx, such as cleft soft palate and overlong soft palate, are described in Section 8.

Tonsillar Disease (See Chapter 85)

Retropharyngeal Abscess

The mouth or pharynx of the dog and cat is frequently penetrated by chicken bones, fish hooks, sewing needles, or wooden sticks.[67] These may be retained within the sublingual, retrobulbar, or pharyngeal soft tissues, leading to a localized infection or acute abscess. When presented because of acute disease, the animal is usually pyrexic, and the pharyngeal tissues are hot, painful, and firm; are surrounded by edema (particularly rostrally); and may have a soft area that may burst if left untreated. Acute pharyngeal abscess is treated by lancing, flushing, and draining the abscess under sedation; the abscess cavity is explored digitally to break down loculations and palpate for a foreign body. The pharynx should be examined through the mouth for evidence of foreign body penetration. Antibiotics are often given but are unnecessary if drainage is thorough. It is common not to find the causative foreign body.

Chronic pharyngeal abscess develops when antibiotic therapy or local defense mechanisms effectively sterilize a foreign body in the connective tissues. The body continues to react to the foreign substance, and a serosanguineous effusion collects in the area. As for a salivary mucocele, this fluid takes the path of least resistance and appears as a firm or soft, although usually painless, swelling in the neck. Aspiration is usually sufficient to differentiate chronic pharyngeal abscess from a mucocele; if doubt exists, some of the aspirate can be stained with a mucopolysaccharide-specific stain. Radiographs are made of the neck to check for the presence of a radiodense foreign body, and the pharynx is examined. The swelling is incised, loculations are broken down, and the walls are thoroughly scraped. If a foreign body is not found, the incision is left open and the cavity is packed with antiseptic-soaked sponges to encourage granulation but prevent the skin edges from sealing. The packing is replaced daily until the swelling has been obliterated by granulation and contraction; this usually takes two to three weeks.

Diagnosis and treatment of retro-orbital abscess are described in Chapter 109.

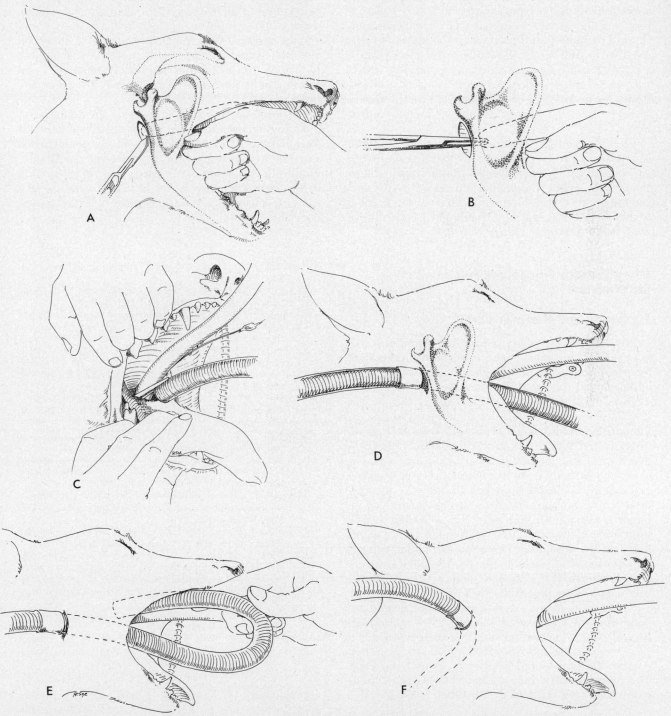

Figure 46–22. Pharyngotomy. *A,* With a finger in the mouth deflecting the hyoid apparatus and mandibular salivary gland, an incision is made in the skin caudal to the mandible. *B,* A hemostat is inserted into the incision and pushed into the pharynx. *C* and *D,* A feeding or endotracheal tube is placed between the jaws of the hemostat and withdrawn through the incision. *E* and *F,* The tube is turned and inserted into the esophagus or larynx. (Reprinted with permission from Burrows, C. F., Miller, W. H., and Harvey, C. E.: Oral medicine. *In* Harvey, C. E., (ed.): *Veterinary Dentistry.* W. B. Saunders, Philadelphia, 1985.)

Differential Diagnosis of Swellings in the Neck

There are many possible causes of cervical swelling. The most common are salivary mucocele (Chapter 47), chronic pharyngeal abscess (see previous discussion), and neoplasms.

In a young dog or cat, a firm, nonpainful swelling is most likely to be lymphosarcoma. Likely causes of firm masses in older animals are lymphosarcoma, thyroid tumors, and lymphatic metastasis from a tonsillar or oral tumor. Reactive lymphadenopathy is a possible cause of a palpable mass; a primary lesion, such as severe periodontal disease, is usually obvious from the history or results of physical examination. Needle aspiration or surgical biopsy provides a diagnosis.

Fluid-containing swellings are rarely anything other than salivary mucocele or pharyngeal abscess. An occasional cystic thyroid tumor appears as a fluctuating mass. Congenital causes of cystic neck swellings are extremely rare in dogs. If there is any question of the origin of a swelling, a section of the wall is submitted for biopsy.

Miscellaneous Procedures Performed on the Pharynx

Pharyngotomy-Pharyngostomy

Incision into the pharynx from the skin of the neck is a useful technique for several purposes, particularly for placement of an esophageal feeding tube[29] or an endotracheal tube that bypasses the oral cavity.[68]

The lateral neck area on one side is clipped and prepared for surgery. Under general anesthesia, an index finger is inserted through the mouth into the pharynx and is then flexed to palpate and deflect the hyoid arch and mandibular salivary gland. The skin is incised directly over the finger tip (Fig. 46–22A), and a large hemostat is pushed through the incision, intervening muscle, and the mucosa, guided by the finger in the mouth (Fig. 46–22B). A flexible feeding tube (or endotracheal tube) of suitable size is placed between the jaws of the hemostat and pulled through the incision (Fig. 46–22C and D). The tube is turned in the mouth (Fig. 46–22E) and inserted into the esophagus or trachea (Fig. 46–22F).

Esophageal feeding tubes should not extend beyond the midthoracic esophagus;[11] the appropriate length can be marked on the tube with tape prior to placement. The tube is attached to the skin with sutures through a tape butterfly around the tube. The pharyngotomy incision is left to close by granulation following removal of the tube.

Mandibular Symphysiotomy

Surgical access to the caudal oral cavity, pharynx, and ventrocaudal nasal cavity can be enhanced by mandibular symphysiotomy.[47]

The entire mandibular and cranioventral neck area is clipped and prepared for surgery. A midventral skin incision is made rostrally from the basihyoid bone, splitting the skin of the mandible. The mandibular symphysis is exposed, and the mylohyoid muscle is incised and separated and reflected laterally, exposing the genioglossus muscles. The mucosa rostral to the tongue is incised from the oral side lateral to the mandibular and sublingual salivary ducts. The symphysis is split with a scalpel and spread, allowing the genioglossus muscle to be tensed and incised about 1 cm from the midline. The mucosa is incised, the mandibles are widely separated, and the tongue is retracted ventrocaudally to expose the pharynx.

Closure is commenced by suturing the oral mucosa in a simple continuous pattern using absorbable suture material. The incised edges of the genioglossus and mylohyoid muscles are apposed. The mandibular symphysis is closed with cross pins or encircling wires. This procedure causes little postoperative discomfort, and no complications were observed in ten dogs and cats studied.[47]

1. Aitchison, J.: Changing incisor dentition of bulldogs. Vet. Rec. 75:153, 1963.
2. Al-Baghdadi, F.: Macro- and microscopical study of the lyssa. Iraqi Med. J. 15:1, 1967.
3. Albrecht, D. T.: Surgical positioning of maloccluded teeth in the dog. Proc. Ann. Mtg. Am. Vet. Med. Assoc., pp. 180–181, 1963.
4. Alexander, J. W.: Craniomandibular osteopathy. Canine Pract. 5:31, 1978.
5. Andrews, A. H.: A case of partial anodontia in a dog. Vet. Rec. 90:144, 1972.
6. Annis, J. R.: Teeth. In Archibald, J. (ed.): Canine Surgery. American Veterinary Publications, Inc., Santa Barbara, 1965, Chap. 14.
7. Arenzo, A. R., and Glauser, G. F. J. O.: Quiste dentigero en un perro. Rev. Med. Vet. Brazil 44:349, 1963.
8. Arnall, L.: Some aspects of dental development in the dog: I. Calcification of crown and root of the deciduous dentitions. J. Small Anim. Pract. 1:169, 1960.
9. Arnall, L.: Some aspects of dental development in the dog: III. Some common variations in the dentitions. J. Small Anim. Pract. 2:195, 1961.
10. Ashton, A. P., and Howard, D.: Repair technique for dental abrasion in the dog. Vet. Rec. 101:372, 1977.
11. Balkany, T. J., Baker, B. B., Bloustein, P. A., and Jafek, B. W.: Cervical esophagotomy in dogs: Endoscopic, radiographic, and histopathologic evaluation of esophagitis induced by feeding tubes. Ann. Oto. Rhino. Laryngol. 86:1, 1977.
12. Barchfeld, W. P.: A mandibular splint for a dog. J. Am. Vet. Med. Assoc. 133:209, 1958.
13. Barrett, R. E., Post, J. E., and Schulz, R. D.: Chronic relapsing stomatitis in a cat associated with feline leukemia virus infection. Feline Pract. 5:34, 1975.
14. Bartels, P.: Kurzbericht zur naht von skalpierwunden am unterkiefer. Kleinter. Prax. 22:171, 1977.
15. Bartley, M. H., Taylor, G. N., and Webster, S. S. J.: Teeth and mandible. In Andersen, A. A. (ed.): The Beagle as an Experimental Dog. Iowa State University Press, Ames, 1970, Chap. 9D.
16. Beattie, I. E. J.: Treatment of dislocated feline mandible. Vet. Rec. 111:493, 1982.
17. Bedford, P. G. C., and Heaton, M. G.: A repair technique for dental abrasion in the dog. Vet. Rec. 101:327, 1977.

18. Bellizzi, R.: Veterinary endodontics. J. Am. Vet. Med. Assoc. *180*:6, 1981.

19. Bellizi, R., Worsing, J., Woody, R. D., Keller, D. L., and Drobotij, E.: Nonsurgical endodontic therapy, utilizing lingual coronal access on the mandibular canine tooth of dogs. J. Am. Vet. Med. Assoc. *179*:370, 1981.

20. Bennett, G. A.: The lyssa of the dog. Anat. Rec. *88*:422, 1944.

21. Bennett, G. A., and Hutchinson, R. C.: Experimental studies on the movements of the mammalian tongue: II. The protrusion mechanism of the tongue (dog). Anat. Rec. *94*:57, 1946.

22. Bergenholtz, A., and Isaksson, B.: Tissue reaction in the oral mucosa to catgut, silk, and Mersilene sutures. Odontol. Rev. *18*:237, 1967.

23. Berman, E.: The time and pattern of eruption of the permanent teeth in the cat. Lab. Anim. Sci. *24*:929, 1974.

24. Bhaskar, S. N., and Rappaport, H. M.: Histologic evaluation of endodontic procedures in dogs. Oral Surg. *31*:526, 1971.

25. Bigler, B.: Experimentelle und klinische untersuchung zur frage der endodontischen therapie des hundegebisses. Zentralbl. Veterinarmed. *25*:794, 1978.

26. Black, A. P., Crichlow, A. M., and Saunders, J. R.: Bacteremia during ultrasonic teeth cleaning and extraction in the dog. J. Am. Anim. Hosp. Assoc. *16*:611, 1980.

27. Blogg, R.: Exodontia in the dog. Aust. Vet. J. *39*:57, 1963.

28. Bodingbauer, J.: Milchzahnpersistenz beim hund. Kleinter. Prax. *23*:339, 1978.

29. Bohning, R. H., DeHoff, W. D., McElhinney, A., and Hofstra, P. C.: Pharyngogostomy for maintenance of the anorectic animal. J. Am. Vet. Med. Assoc. *156*:611, 1970.

30. Boulton, J.: Dental flap operation for tooth extraction. Can. Vet. J. *1*:167, 1960.

31. Bradley, R. L., MacEwan, G., and Loar, A.: Forty cases of mandibular surgery for oral tumors in the cat and dog. Proc. Ann. Mtg. Am. Coll. Vet. Surg., 1980.

32. Brass, W.: Zur Korrektur von zahnstellungs und kieferanomalien des hundes mit dehnungsplatten und durch kieferchirurgische masnahmen. Kleinter. Prax. *21*:79, 1976.

33. Brayer, L., Rennert, H., and Gedalia, L.: Effect of brushing teeth with a fluoride-containing and fluoride-free dentifrice on the gingiva of dogs. J. Dent. Res. *55*:825, 1976.

34. Brewer, W. G., and Turrel, J. M.: Radiotherapy and hyperthermia in the treatment of fibrosarcomas in the dog. J. Am. Vet. Med. Assoc. *181*:146, 1982.

35. Brodey, R. S., and Morris, A. L.: Odontoma associated with an undifferentiated carcinoma in the maxilla of a dog. J. Am. Vet. Med. Assoc. *137*:553, 1960.

36. Brown, M. E.: The occurrence of arteriovenous anastomoses in the tongue of the dog. Anat. Rec. *69*:287, 1937.

37. Brown, M. G., and Park, J. F.: Control of dental calculus in experimental Beagles. Lab. Anim. Care *18*:527, 1968.

38. Cahill, D. R., and Marks, S. C., Jr.: Chronology and histology of exfoliation and eruption of mandibular premolars in dogs. J. Morphol. *171*:213, 1982.

39. Calabrese, C. T., Winslow, R. B., and Latham, R. A.: Altering the dimensions of the canine face by the induction of new bone formation. Plast. Reconstr. Surg. *54*:467, 1974.

40. Calvert, C. A.: Valvular bacterial endocarditis in the dog. J. Am. Vet. Med. Assoc. *180*:1080, 1982.

41. Cechner, P. E.: Malocclusion in the dog caused by intramedullary pin fixation of mandibular fractures: two case reports. J. Am. Anim. Hosp. Assoc. *16*:79, 1980.

42. Cerny, J.: The repair of comminuted fractures of the vertical ramus of the mandible in a cat and dog. Aust. Vet. Pract. *9*:147, 1979.

43. Chaffee, V. W.: Technique for fixation of bilateral mandibular fractures caudal to the canine teeth in the dog. Vet. Med. Small Anim. Clin. 73:907, 1978.

44. Chauveau, A., and Arloing, S.: *The Comparative Anatomy of the Domesticated Animals*. J. & A. Churchill, London, 1873.

45. Chibuzo, G. A.: The digestive apparatus and abdomen. *In* Evans, H. E., and Christensen, G. C. (eds.): *Miller's Anatomy of the Dog*, 2nd ed. W. B. Saunders, Philadelphia, 1979, Chap. 7.

46. Culvenor, J. A.: What is your diagnosis? J. Am. Vet. Med. Assoc. *172*:719, 1978.

47. Curley, B. M., Nelson, A. W., and Kainer, R. A.: Mandibular symphysiotomy in the dog and cat: a surgical approach to the nasopharynx. J. Am. Vet. Med. Assoc. *160*:981, 1972.

48. Currey, J. R.: Canine exodontia. Proc. Ann. Mtg. Am. Vet. Med. Assoc., pp. 178–180, 1963.

49. Davis, M. S., Joseph, S. U., and Bucher, J. F.: Periapical and intracanal healing following incomplete root canal fillings in dogs. Oral Surg. *31*:667, 1971.

50. Dent, R. S. C.: Operation for correction of lateral protrusion of the tongue in the dog. Vet. Rec. *64*:276, 1952.

51. Dietrich, U. B.: Dental care: prophylaxis and therapy. Canine Pract. 3:44, 1976.

52. Dimic, J., Andric, R., and Milivojevic, J.: Zur frage der pathologie und therapie der tonsillenerkrankungen der hunde. Kleinter. Prax. *17*:77, 1972.

53. Dorn, A. S.: Crown restoration of canine teeth with composite bonding. Proc. Ann. Mtg. Am. Coll. Vet. Surg., 1983.

54. Douglas, S. W., and Kelly, D. F.: Calcinosis circumscripta of the tongue. J. Small Anim. Pract. 7:441, 1966.

55. Dubielzig, R. R.: Proliferative dental and gingival diseases of dogs and cats. J. Am. Anim. Hosp. Assoc. *18*:577, 1982.

56. Durr, U. M., and Reichart, P.: Gingivitis der katze—medikamentose und chirurgische therapie. Kleinter. Prax. *23*:231, 1978.

57. Dyce, K. M.: The muscles of the pharynx and palate of the dog. Anat. Rec. *127*:497, 1957.

58. Estrada, E.: A simplified method for repair of mandibular fractures in the dog. J. Am. Vet. Med. Assoc. *136*:560, 1960.

59. Evans, H. E., and Christensen, G. C. (eds.): *Miller's Anatomy of the Dog*, 2nd ed. W. B. Saunders, Philadelphia, 1979.

60. Farrow, C. S.: Surgical treatment of lower lip avulsion in the cat. Vet. Med./Small Anim. Clin. 68:1418, 1973.

61. Field, E. A., Speechley, J. A., and Jones, D. E.: The removal of an impacted maxillary canine and associated dentigerous cyst in a Chow. J. Small Anim. Pract. *23*:159, 1982.

62. Figueiredo, C., Barros, H. M., Alvares, L. C., and Damante, J. H.: Composed complex odontoma in a dog. Vet. Med./ Small Anim. Clin. *69*:268, 1974.

63. Franceschini, G.: Traitement des fistulaires dentaires chez le chien par obturation des canaux. Rec. Med. Vet. *150*:675, 1974.

64. Gaunt, W. A.: The development of the deciduous cheek teeth of the cat. Acta Anat. *38*:187, 1959.

65. Greenwood, K. M., and Creagh, G. B.: Biphase external skeletal splint fixation of mandibular fractures in dogs. Vet. Surg. 9:128, 1980.

66. Grove, K.: Periodontal therapy. Comp. Cont. Ed. Pract. Vet. 5:660, 1983.

67. Hallstrom, M.: Surgery of the canine mouth and pharynx. J. Small Anim. Pract. *11*:105, 1970.

68. Hartsfield, S. M., Gendreau, C. L., Smith, C. W., Rouse, G. P., and Thurmon, J. C.: Endotracheal intubation by pharyngotomy. J. Am. Anim. Hosp. Assoc. *13*:71, 1977.

69. Harvey, C. E.: Personal communication, 1983.

70. Harvey, H. J.: Cryosurgery of oral tumors in dogs and cats. Vet. Clin. North Am. *10*:821, 1980.

71. Hinko, P. J.: A method for reduction and fixation of symphyseal fractures of the mandible. J. Am. Anim. Hosp. Assoc. *12*:98, 1976.

72. Hock, J., and Tinanoff, N.: Resolution of gingivitis in dogs following topical applications of 0.4% stannous fluoride and toothbrushing. J. Dent. Res. 58:1652, 1979.

73. Hofmeyer, C. F. B.: Indications for and technique of tonsillectomy in the dog. J. South Afr. Vet. Med. Assoc. 26:9–14, 1955.

74. Holmberg, D. L.: Abscessation of the mandibular carnassial tooth in the dog. J. Am. Anim. Hosp. Assoc. *15*:347, 1979.

75. Hoppe, F., and Svalastoga, E.: Temporomandibular dysplasia

in American Cocker Spaniels. J. Small Anim. Pract. *21*:675, 1980.

76. Huebsch, R. F., and Hansen, L. S.: A histopathologic study of extraction wounds in dogs. Oral Surg. *28*:187, 1969.

77. Huebsch, R. F., and Kennedy, D. R.: Healing of dog mandibles following surgical loss of continuity. Oral Surg. *29*:178, 1970.

78. Hull, P. S., and Davies, R. M.: The effect of a chlorhexidine gel on tooth deposits in Beagle dogs. J. Small Anim. Pract. *13*:207, 1972.

79. Humphreys, G. U.: Dropped jaw in dogs. Vet. Rec. *95*:222, 1974.

80. Jackson, D. A., Huse, D. C., and Kissil, M. T.: Bacteremia following ultrasonic scaling in the dog. Proc. Ann. Mtg. Am. Coll. Vet. Surg., 1981.

81. Jirava, E., Krepleka, V., and Fagos, Z.: Uber die behandlung von frakturierten zahnen bei hunden. Berl. Munch. Tierarztl. Wochenschr. *12*:235, 1966.

82. Johnessee, J. S., and Hurvitz, A. I.: Feline plasma cell gingivitis pharyngitis. J. Am. Anim. Hosp. Assoc. *19*:179, 1983.

83. Johnson, K. A.: Temporomandibular joint dysplasia in an Irish Setter. J. Small Anim. Pract. *20*:209, 1979.

84. Jones, R. S., and Thordal-Christensen, A.: Extraction of the upper carnassial tooth in the dog. Mod. Vet. Pract. *48*:68, 1962.

85. Kangur, T. T., Tolman, D. E., and Jowsey, J.: The use of methylmethacrylate in the fixation of mandibular fractures in dogs: experimental results. Oral Surg. *41*:578, 1976.

86. Kaplan, B.: A technic for tonsillectomy in the dog. Vet. Med./Small Anim. Clin. *64*:805, 1969.

87. Kataura, A., Doi, Y., and Narimatsu, E.: Histological research concerning cryotonsillectomy in dogs. Arch. Otorhinolaryngol. *209*:33, 1975.

88. Kind, R. E., and Mays, R. A.: Use of an inclined plane for correction of ectopic mandibular canine tooth in a dog. Vet. Med./Small Anim. Clin. *71*:52, 1976.

89. Kitto, H. W.: A technique of manbibular fixation in cat symphyseal fractures. Vet. Rec. *91*:591, 1972.

90. Klein, H.: Schienung einer caninus langsfraktur beim hund. Kleinter. Prax. *24*:144, 1970.

91. Klein, H.: Vergleich verschiedener uber kronungstechniken am kunstlich frakturierten caninus des hundes. Diss. Tierarztl. Hochscule Hannover, 1979, pp. 1–88.

92. Kolata, R. J., and Burrows, C. F.: The clinical features of injury by chewing electrical cords in dogs and cats. J. Am. Anim. Hosp. Assoc. *17*:219, 1981.

93. Kostlin, R., and Schebitz, H.: Zur endodontischen behandlung der zahnfraktur beim hund. Kleinter. Prax. *25*:187, 1980.

94. Kostlin, R., and Waibl, H.: Zur dislokation des processus coronoideus mandibulae beim Basset. Kleinter. Prax. *25*:169, 1980.

95. Kremenak, C. R., Jr.: Dental eruption chronology in dogs: deciduous tooth gingival emergence. J. Dent. Res. *48*:1177, 1969.

96. Kutschmann, K., Schafer, R.: Zur tonsillitis und tonsillektomie beim hund. Monatsschr. Veterinarmed. *30*:381, 1975.

97. Lane, J. G.: Small animal dentistry and the role of ultrasonic instruments in dental care. J. Small Anim. Pract. *18*:787, 1977.

98. Lane, J. G.: Small animal dentistry. In Pract. *3*:23, 1981.

99. Langham, R. F., Mostosky, U. V., and Schirmer, R. G.: Ameloblastic odontoma in the dog. Am. J. Vet. Res. *30*:1873, 1969.

100. Lantz, G. C.: Interarcade wiring as a method of fixation for selected mandibular injuries. J. Am. Anim. Hosp. Assoc. *17*:599, 1981.

101. Lantz, G. C., Cantwell, H. D., VanVleet, J. F., and Cechner, P. E.: Unilateral mandibular condylectomy: experimental and clinical results. J. Am. Anim. Hosp. Assoc. *18*:833, 1982.

102. Lantz, G. C., Cantwell, H. D., VanVleet, J. F., Blakemore, J. C., and Newman, S.: Pharyngostomy tube induced

esophagitis in the dog: an experimental study. J. Am. Anim. Hosp. Assoc. *19*:207, 1983.

103. Latimer, K. S., Kemp, W. B., Taylor, L. A., and Barton, R. A.: Emergency stabilization of jaw fractures in a dog using acrylic splints. Vet. Med./Small Anim. Clin. *72*:1029, 1977.

104. Lawer, D. R.: Root canal with retrograde amalgam filling. Calif. Vet. *33*:11, 1979.

105. Lawson, D. D., Nixon, G. S., Noble, H. W., and Weipers, W. L.: Development and eruption of the canine dentition. Br. Vet. J. *123*:26, 1967.

106. Leighton, R. L.: Surgical correction of prognathous inferior in a dog. Vet. Med./Small Anim. Clin. *72*:401, 1977.

107. Leiberman, L. L.: Open reduction of fractures of the mandible of dogs and cats. J. Am. Vet. Med. Assoc. *132*:334, 1958.

108. Lindhe, J., Hamp, S. E., and Loe, H.: Plaque induced periodontal disease in Beagle dogs. J. Periodont. Res. *10*:243, 1975.

109. MacMillan, R., Withrow, S. J., and Gillette, E. L.: Surgery and regional irradiation for treatment of canine tonsillar squamous cell carcinoma. J. Am. Anim. Hosp. Assoc. *18*:311, 1982.

110. Madewell, B. R., Stannard, A. A., Pulley, L. T., and Nelson, V. G.: Oral eosinophilic granuloma in Siberian Husky dogs. J. Am. Vet. Med. Assoc. *177*:701, 1980.

111. Malek, Abd-El: Movements of the cat tongue. J. Anat. *73*:15, 1938.

112. Marvich, J. M.: Repair of enamel hypoplasia in the dog. Vet. Med./Small Anim. Clin. *70*:697, 1975.

113. McClelland, R. B.: X-ray therapy in labial and cutaneous granulomas in cats. J. Am. Vet. Med. Assoc. *125*:469, 1954.

114. Merlen, R. H. A.: *De Canibus. Dog and Hound in Antiquity*. J. A. Allen & Co., London, 1971.

115. Mumaw, E. D., and Miller, A. S.: The application of a frequency oscillation method for tooth extraction in dogs. Lab. Anim. Sci. *25*:228, 1975.

116. Neuman, N. B.: Chronic ocular discharge associated with a carnassial tooth abscess. Can. Vet. J. *15*:128, 1974.

117. Nibley, W.: Treatment of caudal mandibular fractures. J. Am. Anim. Hosp. Assoc. *17*:555, 1981.

118. Nickel, R., Schummer, A., Seiferle, E., and Sack, W. O.: *The Viscera of the Domestic Mammals*. Verlag Paul Parey, Berlin, 1973.

119. Ochs, D. L., Irving, G. W., and Casey, H. W.: Eosinophilic granuloma in the cat: two cases involving the tongue. Vet. Med./Small Anim. Clin. *73*:1275, 1978.

120. Olmstead, M. L., Stoloff, D. R., and O'Keefe, C. M.: Correction of traumatic avulsion of the upper lip in two dogs. Vet. Med./Small Anim. Clin. *71*:1228, 1976.

121. Peddie, J. F.: Extraction of a dog's carnassial tooth. Mod. Vet. Pract. *62*:129, 1981.

122. Petrick, S. W.: Ectopic tonsil in a dog. J. South Afr. Vet. Med. Assoc. *49*:378, 1978.

123. Piermattei, D. L., and Greeley, R. G.: *Atlas of Surgical Approaches to the Bones of the Dog and Cat*, 2nd ed. W. B. Saunders, Philadelphia, 1979.

124. Plata, R. L., Kelln, E. E., and Linda, L.: Intentional retention of vital submerged roots in dogs. Oral Surg. *42*:100, 1976.

125. Potter, K. A., Tucker, R. D., and Carpenter, J. L.: Oral eosinophilic granuloma of Siberian Huskies. J. Am. Anim. Hosp. Assoc. *16*:595, 1980.

126. Prichard, M. M. L., and Daniel, P. M.: Arteriovenous anastomoses in the tongue of the dog. J. Anat. *87*:66, 1953.

127. Richman, S., and Schunick, W.: Flap operation for removal of the canine tooth. *In* LaCroix, J. V., and Hoskins, H. P. (eds.): *Canine Surgery*. North American Veterinarian, Evanston, 1939, pp. 46–48.

128. Rickards, D. A.: Tonsillectomy and soft palate resection. Canine Pract. *1*:29, 1974.

129. Robins, G. M.: Dropped jaw—mandibular neuropraxia in the dog. J. Small Anim. Pract. *17*:753, 1976.

130. Robins, G. M., and Grandage, J.: Temporomandibular joint

130. dysplasia and open mouth jaw locking in the dog. J. Am. Vet. Med. Assoc. *171*:1072, 1977.

131. Robins, G. M., and Read, R. A.: The use of a transfixation splint to stabilize a bilateral mandibular fracture in a dog. J. Small Anim. Pract. 22:759, 1981.

132. Roe, B. C.: Animal dentistry offers practice opportunities. Norden News *56*:24, 1981.

133. Rosin, E., and Hanlon, G. F.: Canine cricopharyngeal achalasia. J. Am. Vet. Med. Assoc. *160*:1496, 1972.

134. Ross, D. L.: Canine endodontic therapy. J. Am. Vet. Med. Assoc. *180*:356, 1981.

135. Ross, D. L., and Myers, J. W.: Endodontic therapy for canine teeth in the dog. J. Am. Vet. Med. Assoc. *157*:1713, 1970.

136. Rudy, R. L.: Fractures of the maxilla and mandible. *In* Bojrab, M. J. (ed.): *Current Techniques in Small Animal Surgery*. Lea & Febiger, Philadelphia, 1975, p. 364.

137. Scapino, R. P.: The third joint of the canine jaw. J. Morphol. *116*:23, 1965.

138. Scheffler, V. K. H.: Restitution des dens caninus beim diensthund. Munch. Vet. Med. *34*:504, 1979.

139. Schneck, G.: Eosinophiles granulom bei einer katze. Deutsche Tierarztl. Wochenschr. *82*:162, 1975.

140. Schneck, G., and Osborn, J. W.: Neck lesions in the teeth of cats. Vet. Rec. *99*:100, 1976.

141. Schulz, S.: Ein Fall von kraniomandibulärer Osteopathie bei einem Boxer; einige neue Aspekte. Prak. Tierarztl. *60*:972, 1979.

142. Sciubba, J. J., Waterhouse, J. P., and Meyer, J.: A fine structural comparison of the healing of incisional wounds of mucosa and skin. J. Oral Pathol. 7:214, 1978.

143. Scott, D. W.: Observations on the eosinophilic granuloma complex in cats. J. Am. Anim. Hosp. Assoc. *11*:261, 1975.

144. Selhorst, F.: Orthodontische behandlungen an hunden. Tierarztl. Umschau. *20*:166, 1965.

145. Shabestar, L., Taylor, G. N., and Angus, W.: Dental eruption patterns in the beagle. J. Dent. Res. *46*:276, 1967.

146. Sherman, P.: Intentional replantation of teeth in dogs and monkeys. J. Dent. Res. *47*:1066, 1968.

147. Silver, J. G., Martin, L., and McBride, B. C.: Recovery and clearance rates of oral microorganism following experimental bacteraemias in dogs. Arch. Oral Biol. *20*:675, 1975.

148. Soames, J. V., Entwisle, D. N., and Davies, R. M.: The progression of gingivitis to periodontitis in the Beagle dog: a histological and morphometric investigation. J. Periodont. *47*:435, 1976.

149. Spellman, G.: Reduction of fractures of the mandibular symphysis using acrylic splints with circumandibular wiring. Vet. Med./Small Anim. Clin. *67*:1213, 1972.

150. St. Clair, L. E., and Jones, N. D.: Observations on the cheek teeth of the dog. J. Am. Vet. Med. Assoc. *130*:257, 1957.

151. Stambaugh, J. E., and Nunamaker, D. M.: External skeletal fixation of comminuted maxillary fractures in dogs. Vet. Surg. *11*:72, 1982.

152. Stauffer, V. D.: Loss of the tongue in a cat and the resulting skin problem. Vet. Med./Small Anim. Clin. *68*:1266, 1973.

153. Stewart, W. C., Baker, G. J., and Lee, R.: Temporomandibular subluxation in the dog. J. Small Anim. Pract. *16*:345, 1975.

154. Stoll, S. G.: Cheiloplasty. *In* Bojrab, M. J. (ed.): *Current Techniques in Small Animal Surgery*. Lea & Febiger, Philadelphia, 1975, pp. 286–292.

155. Studer, E., and Stapley, R. B.: The role of dry foods in maintaining healthy teeth and gums in the cat. Vet. Med./Small Anim. Clin. *68*:1124, 1973.

156. Sumner-Smith, G., and Dingwall, J. G.: The plating of mandibular fractures in the dog. Vet. Rec. *88*:595, 1971.

157. Sumner-Smith, G., and Dingwall, J. G.: The plating of mandibular fractures in giant dogs. Vet. Rec. *92*:39, 1973.

158. Teague, H. D., and Toombs, J. P.: Infraocular fistula secondary to an upper canine tooth abscess. Feline Pract. *9*:32, 1979.

159. Tholen, M.: Veterinary endodontics. J. Am. Vet. Med. Assoc. *180*:4, 1981.

160. Thomas, R. E.: Temporomandibular joint dysplasia and open mouth jaw locking in a Bassett Hound. J. Small Anim. Pract. *20*:697, 1979.

161. Thomas, D. L., McAlister, C. R., and Dawe, J. R.: A technique of repair of multiple mandibular fractures in a dog. J. Am. Vet. Med. Assoc. *132*:161, 1958.

162. Thompson, N., and Casson, J. A.: Experimental onlay bone grafts to the jaws: Preliminary study in dogs. Plast. Reconstr. Surg. *46*:341, 1970.

163. Ticer, J. W., and Spencer, C. P.: Injury of the feline temporomandibular joint: radiographic signs. Vet. Radiol. *19*:146, 1978.

164. Todoroff, R. J., and Brodey, R. S.: Oral and pharyngeal neoplasia in the dog: retrospective survey of 361 cases. J. Am. Vet. Med. Assoc. *175*:567, 1979.

165. Tomlinson, J., and Presnell, K. P.: Mandibular condylectomy: effects in normal dogs. Vet. Surg. *12*:148, 1983.

166. Vernon, F. F., and Helphrey, M.: Rostral mandibulectomy: Three case reports in dogs. Vet. Surg. *12*:26, 1983.

167. Vollmerhaus, B.: Zur vergleichenden Nomenklatur des lymphoepithelialen der Haussaugetiere und des Menschen. Zentralbl. Vet. Med. 1978; cited by Nickel et al.

168. von Scupin, E.: Tonsillitis-endocarditis syndrom beim hund. Deutsche Tierarztl. Wochenschr. *85*:313, 1978.

169. Weigel, J. P., Dorn, A. S., Chase, D. C., and Jaffrey, B.: The use of the biphase external fixation splint for repair of canine mandibular fractures. J. Am. Anim. Hosp. Assoc. *17*:547, 1981.

170. Whitney, G. D.: Removal of retained deciduous teeth in dogs. Mod. Vet. Pract. *5*:46, 1973.

171. Willemse, A., and Lubberink, A. A. M. E.: Eosinophilic ulcers in cats. Tijdschr. Diergeneeskd. *103*:1052, 1978.

172. Williams, R. C., and Evans, H. E.: Prenatal dental development in the dog *Canis familiaris*: chronology of tooth germ formation and calcification of deciduous teeth. Zentralbl. Vet. Med. C. Anat. Histol. Embryol. 7:152, 1978.

173. Wisdorf, H., and Hermanns, W.: Persistierende milchhakenzahne im oberkiefer einer hauskatze. Kleinter. Prax. *19*:14, 1974.

174. Withrow, S. J.: Dental extraction as a probable cause of septicemia in a dog. J. Am. Anim. Hosp. Assoc. *15*:345, 1979.

175. Withrow, S. J.: Taping of the mandible in treatment of mandibular fractures. J. Am. Anim. Hosp. Assoc. *17*:27, 1981.

176. Withrow, S. J.: Mandibulectomy as a treatment for malignant disease: technique and followup. Proc. Ann. Mtg. Am. Coll. Vet. Surg., 1981.

177. Withrow, S. J.: Premaxillectomy in the dog. Proc. Ann. Mtg. Am. Coll. Vet. Surg., 1983.

178. Wolff, A.: Tongue-tie in a dog? Canine Pract. 7:6, 1980.

179. Wright, J. G.: Some observations on dental disease in the dog. Vet. Rec. *51*:409, 1939.

180. Yamagata, J.: Dental malocclusion and odontorthosis in dogs. J. Jap. Vet. Med. Assoc. *32*:194, 1979.

181. Zagraniski, M. J.: Reduction of a mandibular symphyseal fracture with nylon cable tie bands. Feline Pract. *10*:45, 1980.

182. Zetner, K.: Die prosthetische versorgung von zahnfrakturen mit adhasivkunstoffen. Kleinter. Prax. *21*:271, 1976.

183. Zetner, K.: Atiologie, pathogenese und therapie von zahnbettkrankheithen beim kleinter. Wien. Tierarztl. Monat. *68*:130, 1981.

184. Zontine, W. J.: Dental radiographic technique and interpretation. Vet. Clin. North Am. *4*:741, 1974.

185. Zontine, W. J.: Canine dental radiology: radiographic technique, development and anatomy of the teeth. J. Am. Vet. Radiol. Soc. *16*:75, 1975.

186. Zontine, W. J., Sims, S., and Donovan, M. L.: Bacterial environmental contamination associated with ultrasonic dental procedures in dogs. J. Am. Anim. Hosp. Assoc. 5:150, 1969.

Anatomy

John Grandage

Carnivores intermittently secrete copious amounts of saliva, mainly to lubricate their bulky food. In addition to the four or five large glands traditionally described as salivary (parotid, mandibular, sublingual, zygomatic), there are scores of tiny ones such as the lingual, labial, buccal, and palatine, each of which secretes a small quantity of mucus or serous fluid to keep the area moist. The larger glands are of more clinical significance (Fig. 47–1).

The V-shaped parotid gland fits snugly behind the jaw and temporomandibular joint and beneath the conchal part of the ear. Although it lies superficially, its borders are difficult to distinguish by palpation. One of the thin ear muscles (parotidoauricularis) runs over it, and the parotid lymph node is partly covered by its rostral border. Several important structures run deep to it (superficial temporal artery and vein, external carotid and maxillary arteries, facial nerve), and a few run over or through it. The patterns of these vessels and nerves vary. In the dog the maxillary vein runs ventral to the parotid, but in the cat it runs through it.[56] The gland itself is supplied by the parotid artery, a small branch off the external carotid that enters the deep face of the gland.

The parotid duct forms from the union of several tributaries at the rostral border of the gland, the pattern being variable.[51] The single duct courses over the ventral third of the masseter muscle, to which it is firmly attached. It resembles a branch of the facial nerve but is distinguished by its deeper location, narrower diameter, more translucent appearance, small companion artery, and its lack of mobility.[61] Its identity may be confirmed by cannulation with stiff suture material. The duct becomes mobile in front of the masseter dorsal to the buccinator muscle. It then runs downward and finally inward to open into the buccal vestibule on a small parotid papilla situated on a low mobile ridge of mucosa above the caudal end of the upper carnassial tooth (PM4). At this point its epithelium changes from stratified columnar to stratified squamous.[58] The two terminal curves may be largely straightened by pulling rostrally on the papilla[61] or rostromedially from just behind the papilla,[27] techniques that assist cannulation. Accessory parotid glands may be located along the course of the duct.[19]

The mandibular gland is larger, more compact, more rounded, and more yellowish than the parotid.[7] It shares a common connective tissue capsule with part of the sublingual gland and is a readily palpable landmark behind the angle of the jaw. Its lobules are less distinct than those of other salivary glands because of the scant connective tissue within the body of the gland.[50] In the dog it is lodged between the linguofacial and maxillary veins, whereas in the cat these veins unite over its lateral surface.[12, 56] The mandibular duct emerges from the deep surface of the gland. It courses forward, gradually becoming more medial as it runs on the inside of the jaw, sandwiched between the myelohyoid (ventrolaterally) and styloglossus (medially) and later the genioglossus (medially). It opens on a small papilla, the sublingual caruncle, at the foot of the frenulum of the tongue; the opening, a red slit about 1 mm long,[27] is often partly concealed because it is found on the ventral surface of the sublingual fold (a small flap of mucous

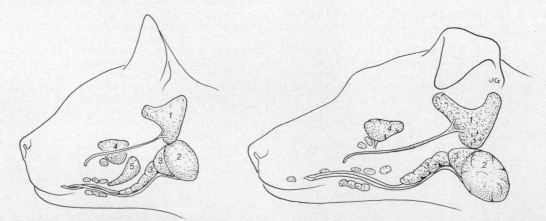

Figure 47–1. The major salivary glands of the cat (left) and dog (right). *1,* The parotid; *2,* the mandibular, which shares its capsule with part of the sublingual gland; *3,* the monostomatic part of the sublingual gland; *4,* the zygomatic; *5,* the molar. Other glands, not labelled, include the dorsal and ventral buccal and the polystomatic sublingual gland.

membrane attached to the caruncle). A survey revealed that in about 30 per cent of dogs the mandibular duct shared a common opening with the sublingual duct.[47] It is lined with two-layered cuboidal epithelium, which becomes stratified squamous on entry into the mouth.[58]

The sublingual gland is smaller and pinker than the mandibular;[7] it is clinically important because salivary mucoceles may result from leakage of saliva from a defect in its major duct.[23] The gland is divided into monostomatic and polystomatic parts. The monostomatic part consists mostly of loose lobules that cluster along the sublingual and mandibular ducts near the root of the tongue for about 3 cm. These lobules, plus a more substantial one enclosed in the mandibular gland capsule, all discharge into the major sublingual duct. The duct courses with the mandibular duct, usually dorsal to it, and opens either 1 to 2 mm caudal to it or in common with it on the sublingual caruncle. The smaller, scattered polystomatic parts of the sublingual gland discharge by several minor sublingual ducts into the lateral sublingual recess, the space between the tongue and mandible. In the cat the sublingual gland is smaller and the polystomatic part may sometimes be absent.[1]

The zygomatic gland (formerly the orbital or upper molar gland) is an enlarged member of the dorsal buccal gland series. It is well developed in carnivores but is relatively inaccessible, lying concealed deep to the rostral end of the zygomatic arch ventral to the periorbita. In the cat the gland lies ventral to the maxillary nerve, whereas in the dog it lies lateral to it.[59] One major and up to four minor ducts course over the maxillary tuberosity to open into the buccal vestibule.[10, 19] The major duct opens about 1 cm behind the parotid papilla opposite the last upper molar;[1] it is about one-half the diameter of the parotid. The minor ducts open caudal to the major one and appear as red dots.[27]

The molar gland, a modified ventral buccal gland, is well developed in the cat and lies sandwiched between the orbicularis oris muscle and the mucous membrane of the lower lip at the angle of the mouth. It opens by several short ducts into the neighboring buccal vestibule.[12]

Physiology

Michael Pass

Saliva contains water, electrolytes, mucus, a number of bactericidal substances, and, in some species, amylase. Only very small amounts of amylase are present in the saliva of dogs and cats. The organic constituents are secreted by the cells lining the salivary acini, and the electrolyte concentrations of this fluid are similar to those of plasma. Sodium and chloride ions are absorbed and replaced by potassium and bicarbonate ions as saliva passes through the salivary ducts.

Salivary secretion is controlled by the salivary nuclei located at the junction of the medulla and pons.[17] There is a continuous basal flow of saliva, and the flow is increased when the glands are stimulated by parasympathetic impulses arising from the salivary nuclei. Afferent impulses to the salivary nuclei originate when tactile and taste receptors are stimulated by food in the mouth. The sight and smell of food also stimulate salivation.

Sympathetic stimulation of the salivary glands may cause an increase in the flow of saliva into the mouth by contraction of the myoepithelial cells, which squeeze saliva from the lumen of the acini and ducts.[18] In some species, particularly the cat, sympathetic stimulation also increases secretion of fluid by the acinar cells of some salivary glands.[18]

Saliva has several important functions, including lubricating food for swallowing and dissolving food so it can react with taste chemoreceptors. Saliva contains a number of bactericidal agents, such as a protein-thiocyanate complex and lysozymes, that help prevent oral infections.[17] The continuous flow of saliva also protects against oral infections and dental decay by continuously washing the mouth and teeth. Absence of saliva rapidly results in tooth decay.[48] In dogs and cats saliva evaporates from the mouth and pharynx during panting and is therefore important in control of body temperature.

Diseases

Colin E. Harvey

HISTORY AND METHODS OF EXAMINATION

Swelling is the most common sign of disease of the salivary glands and is due to swelling of the gland itself or to an abnormal accumulation of salivary secretions. Drooling of saliva is usually the result of oral or pharyngeal pain or swelling that restricts or prevents swallowing. The mouth and pharynx should be examined carefully in drooling dogs, including watching the animal eat and drink.

The parotid and mandibular glands are easily palpable; examination of the sublingual and zygomatic glands requires sedation or anesthesia. Function of the glands and ducts can be evaluated by placing a drop of topical ophthalmic atropine solution on the tongue; in a normal dog or cat, saliva will flow copiously, although with the exception of the parotid duct it is rarely possible to distinguish flow from particular ducts. Parotid saliva is serous, compared with the mixed seromucous saliva from the other salivary glands of dogs and cats.

Plain film radiography is rarely useful in investigating salivary gland disease, except for the rare sialolith. Contrast radiography (sialography) is performed under anesthesia. A water-soluble radiopaque dye, such as that used for intravenous urography, is injected into a salivary duct through a blunt small-gauge needle at a dose of 1 ml/10 kg.[11, 27, 45] The parotid and zygomatic duct openings usually are easy to find on the buccal mucosa opposite the upper fourth premolar tooth and first molar tooth, respectively. The cannula slides directly into the zygomatic duct. The parotid duct makes a right-angle bend just before opening onto the mucosal surface at the papilla; cannulation is made easier by grasping the mucosa just caudal to the duct opening and pulling it rostrally to straighten out the bend.

The mandibular and sublingual duct openings are recognized as slits on the lateroventral surface of the lingual caruncles, which lie at the ventral end of the frenulum of the tongue. The mandibular duct is the larger and more rostral of the two and is usually easy to cannulate once identified. The sublingual duct is sometimes difficult to cannulate; in 20 to 40 per cent of dogs there is no separate opening as the sublingual duct joins the mandibular duct along its course.[20, 22, 47]

SURGICAL DISEASES OF THE SALIVARY GLANDS

Congenital Anomalies

Because there is such an abundance of functional salivary tissue compared with the minimum amount required, congenital atresia of salivary ducts or absence of one or more salivary glands is not likely to be noted.

Hypersialism (drooling) was the clinical sign noted in two dogs with congenital enlargement of the parotid salivary glands.[4, 30] Treatment by parotid duct ligation was successful in both dogs.

Drooling of saliva from a young age is usually due to abnormal conformation of the lips; this is discussed under Lips.

Salivary Gland and Duct Injury

If injury to a salivary gland or duct results in stenosis of the duct or diversion of salivary flow to a new opening into the mouth, there will be no long-term clinical consequences. For this reason, trauma to the face that may involve the salivary glands does not require any initial management directed at the salivary glands. Long-term consequences of salivary gland or duct injury include sialocele or fistula formation.

Parotid Gland and Duct Injury

The parotid gland or duct may be injured by bites or blunt trauma, during surgery on the side of the face, or as a result of adjacent disease such as carnassial abscess. If the duct is severed and saliva escapes through the subcutaneous tissues to the skin, a fistula results.[29] The fistula typically leaks a clear thin fluid, which may be more noticeable or even copious during eating. The fluid accumulates in a soft, nonpainful pocket on the side of the face if the skin is not damaged.[27, 36] Sialography is diagnostic, although the pattern varies; the distal duct may be completely obstructed, in which case dye is injected into the fistulous opening. Treatment may be divergence[36] or reconstruction of the duct,[29] although simple ligation of the duct is quick and effective.[29]

Parotid Duct Ligation. Monofilament nylon (00) suture is inserted into the duct opening in the mouth or into the fistula if the openings are not connected. Through a skin incision on the side of the face, the duct is located between the buccal nerves, lying on the surface of the masseter muscle aponeurosis. The proximal duct is undermined, the suture material in the duct is removed, and two or three ligatures are placed, tying the caudal (proximal) one less tightly so as to spread out the back pressure that follows ligation.[29]

Zygomatic Gland and Duct Injury

Trauma to the face may cause leakage of saliva from a damaged zygomatic salivary gland.[43, 55] Dogs with zygomatic mucocele show exophthalmos. A diagnosis is made by aspiration of mucoid material from the ventral aspect of the orbit and is confirmed by sialography. Treatment is either surgical resection of the gland[43, 55] or marsupialization of the swelling into the mouth.[46] The gland should be examined microscopically following resection, as zygomatic gland carcinoma may cause a large mucocele.[8]

Mandibular Gland and Duct Injury

Because the mandibular gland is contained within a firm fibrous capsule, clinically obvious long-term effects of trauma to this gland in the dog are uncommon.[14, 35] The mandibular gland is rarely the cause of a salivary mucocele.[3]

Sublingual Gland and Duct Injury

Salivary Mucocele

The most common condition of the salivary glands of the dog and cat is salivary mucocele, which is a collection of mucoid saliva that has leaked from a damaged salivary gland. Based on small sample populations, both toy and miniature poodles and German shepherds have been suggested as having an abnormally high incidence of this disease;[28, 42] other studies showed no breed predisposition.[20, 57] The sublingual gland is most frequently affected.[11, 21, 22, 26, 57] As with any fluid in body tissues, saliva takes the path of least resistance. The most common sites for collection of the extravasated saliva are the subcutaneous tissues of the intermandibular or cranial cervical area ("cervical mucocele") and the sublingual tissues on the floor of the mouth ("ranula"). A less common site is the pharyngeal wall.[31] The cause of the damage, which can occur anywhere in the gland or duct,[20] is rarely known, although occasionally a foreign body is found penetrating the sublingual gland;[2, 27] blunt trauma caused by bones or sticks chewed by the animal are likely causes, as they may crush the sublingual gland against the mandible. Grass seeds may penetrate oral mucosa and cause disruption of the duct system and mucus accumulation.[15] Cervical mucoceles and ranulas occasionally occur in cats.[25, 52, 62] Mucoceles formed in 44 per cent of 27 experimental cats following ligation of the sublingual duct rostral to the lingual nerve.[24]

Clinical Signs

The clinical signs depend on the position of the mucocele. A cervical mucocele may commence with an acute period when the swelling is firm and somewhat painful, followed by a reduction in the swelling as the initial inflammatory response to the saliva[35] subsides; however, this initial period is not often observed by the owner, and the usual presenting complaint is gradual enlargement of a soft, nonpainful mass. A ranula may be seen by the owner or may become obvious because it is damaged by the teeth, causing bleeding around the mouth or into the water bowl. A pharyngeal mucocele can cause more significant disease by obstructing the pharyngeal airway; emergency treatment involving lancing of the mucocele may be necessary occasionally to relieve respiratory distress.

Diagnosis

Palpation and aspiration of the swelling, which may require sedation if the lesion is oral or pharyngeal, aid in diagnosis. Golden or blood-stained mucus is obtained. The mucus is invariably viscid enough to form strings when exuded from the syringe through a needle. It is occasionally difficult to distinguish between a mucocele and the serosanguineous fluid found with a foreign body. Examination of smears of the cells in the fluid is not likely to be helpful; however, staining a smear of the fluid with a mucus-specific stain, such as PAS, effectively confirms the diagnosis. Although sialography can be used to confirm the diagnosis, it is time-consuming and may be unrewarding because the conjoined mandibular and sublingual ducts often prevent cannulation of the sublingual duct. A mucocele can be differentiated from the very rare congenital branchial cleft cyst by microscopic examination of the wall of the swelling, which in the case of a mucocele is composed of inflammatory or connective tissue cells, with occasional areas of epithelium at the junction with the gland or duct.[35] Occasionally, a mucocele contains hard, round objects that initially appear as calculi; these are mineralized folds of the inflammatory lining that have sloughed into the lumen.[53]

Treatment

Definitive treatment is removal of the salivary gland that is damaged to prevent further accumulation of mucus and drainage of the mucocele. However, in many cases, particularly when the animal may be a severe anesthetic risk, periodic drainage of the mucocele may be more appropriate. Periodic drainage is not recommended for pharyngeal mucoceles or some ranulas when the mucocele is causing respiratory distress or difficulty in eating or swallowing.

If conservative treatment is selected, drainage can usually be accomplished without anesthesia using a 20-gauge needle and a 10- to 50-ml syringe. In most cases, the mucocele will recur to its former size in six to ten weeks, although in a few dogs scar tissue seals the area of leakage and no further saliva accumulates.

As an alternative to resection of salivary glands, redirection of salivary flow has been suggested, particularly for ranula or pharyngeal mucocele.[6] This process is known as marsupialization. A section of the mucocele wall is removed with a scalpel or scissors, and the lining of the mucocele is sutured to the oral or pharyngeal mucosa. This is not likely to provide satisfactory long-term results, because the lining of the mucocele is fibrous or inflammatory tissue. Stainless steel sutures have been suggested as a means of maintaining the patency of the fistula.[54] Since anesthesia is necessary to perform marsupialization, it is more appropriate to perform salivary gland resection, as this provides a much greater chance of preventing recurrence.

When an animal is presented in respiratory distress because of a pharyngeal mucocele, immediate relief of the distress can be obtained by aspirating or lancing the swelling. When the diagnosis is in doubt, a diagnostic tap should be performed first. Definitive treatment can be performed during the same anesthetic episode.

Resection of a cervical salivary mucocele is possible, but tedious and may result in damage to vascular or neural structures in the area. More important, it will not prevent recurrence,[13] as the cause of the mucocele has not been dealt with. Therefore, resection of a mucocele is not recommended. In an exceptional case in which the mucocele is very large, the dependent skin can be resected following salivary gland resection.[60]

Resection of the sublingual gland without resection of the mandibular gland is not practical because of the close apposition of the two glands; thus, even though the sublingual gland is almost always the gland affected, treatment is removal of the mandibular-sublingual gland complex. Removal of both of these glands does not affect the animal adversely, even if the procedure is performed bilaterally.[22] Generally, the affected side is obvious from the clinical history or physical examination. When this is not the case, palpation and observation with the animal under anesthesia and in dorsal recumbency are helpful. Sialography may determine which side is affected but is time-consuming and may not be successful because of the frequency of combined mandibular-sublingual duct openings. A practical alternative to determine the side involved is to incise the mucocele and palpate the wall from the lumen; the unaffected side is usually rounded and smooth, whereas the affected side has a tunnel or tract that descends dorsally into the deeper tissues of the intermandibular area. When the side affected cannot be determined by one of the methods described previously, the mandibular-sublingual gland complex can be removed from both sides.

Mandibular-Sublingual Gland Resection

With the animal in dorsolateral recumbency under general anesthesia, the intermandibular and cranial neck area is clipped and prepared for aseptic surgery. A skin incision is made over the mandibular salivary gland, which can be palpated caudal to the mandible (Fig. 47–2A). The maxillary and linguofacial veins should be avoided; they can be identified by digitally occluding the jugular vein. The thin platysma muscle is penetrated and the incision is continued more deeply until the fibrous capsule covering the mandibular gland is reached and penetrated. The capsule is identified by its silvery color and by observing the salmon pink lobulated character of the gland, which is visible when the capsule is penetrated. The capsular incision is extended, and the gland is separated from the capsule by blunt dissection, commencing at the caudal and ventral edges. The gland is grasped with Allis tissue forceps and prolapsed from the capsule (Fig. 47–2B). Blunt dissection is continued to free the gland further. An artery and vein are often seen entering the medial aspect of the gland; they are clamped and ligated. The attachment of the

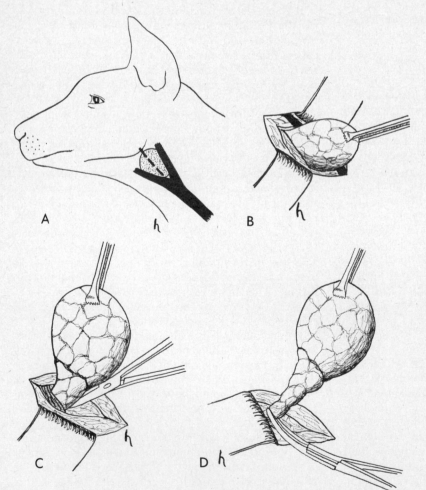

Figure 47–2. Mandibular-sublingual salivary gland resection. *A*, Lateral view of the head and neck showing the position of the jugular vein, mandibular salivary gland (dotted area), and skin incision (dashed line). *B*, The mandibular gland is prolapsed through an incision in its capsule. *C*, The sublingual gland is dissected deep to the digastric muscle. *D*, The sublingual gland is retracted caudally with a hemostat.

Figure 47–3. Resection of the rostral part of the sublingual gland. *A,* Incision in the oral mucosa lateral to the root of the tongue. *B,* The sublingual gland (stained dark by methylene blue) is dissected free.

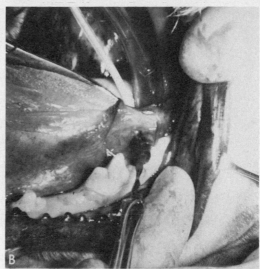

capsule to the cranial end of the gland must be penetrated without damaging the ongoing sublingual gland; this is achieved by directing the dissection parallel to the axis of the mandibular duct and sublingual gland as they disappear beneath the digastric muscle. A branch of the lingual artery that curves backward to supply the salivary glands is often visible at this point; this branch is dissected free, clamped, and ligated.

Blunt dissection is continued rostrally with scissors or a finger (Fig. 47–2C). By tunnelling the sublingual gland and duct underneath the digastric muscle or transecting the muscle, more complete removal of the rostral polystomatic part of the sublingual gland can be achieved;[33] however, this is very rarely necessary clinically. Particular care is required to prevent separation of the lobules of the sublingual gland, as the sublingual duct is small and the lobules of the gland are loosely connected. Dissection of the sublingual gland is continued as far rostral as possible, then a hemostat is placed across the most rostral part of the dissected gland and pulled caudally (Fig. 47–2D). Another hemostat is placed across newly exposed gland. This process is continued until the sublingual gland and duct finally tear. No ligatures are needed when this retraction technique is used. The incision is closed by apposing the capsule edges and subcutaneous tissues with absorbable sutures, followed by skin sutures.

The mucocele is drained following resection of the glands; a stab incision is made into the lumen and the contents are milked out. A soft rubber drain is placed in a cervical mucocele to encourage elimination of remaining fluid. Ranulas and pharyngeal mucoceles are allowed to drain into the oral or pharyngeal cavity. Antibiotics are not necessary following salivary gland surgery.

Prognosis and Management of Recurrence

Some dogs show slight swallowing abnormalities following surgery.[22, 26]

Recurrence following mandibular-sublingual gland

resection is less than 5 per cent in reported series of cases.[22, 26, 38, 57] In the occasional case where recurrence is obvious, there are two possible causes: failure to resect all of the affected gland (or resection of the wrong gland), and damage to the sublingual gland on the opposite side. Where salivary gland resection has been performed previously, sialography is particularly useful to determine the extent of glandular tissue remaining, thus allowing more exact treatment.

Where part of the sublingual gland remains in place and is known or suspected to be the site of leakage, treatment is resection of the remaining glandular tissue. Location and removal are facilitated if methylene blue is injected through a blunt cannula into the sublingual duct immediately prior to dissection. An incision is made in the oral mucosa between the tongue and the vertical ramus of the mandible (Fig. 47–3A). The gland is identified by its salmon pink color and lobular structure or by the blue color if dye has been injected. The gland lies beneath the oral mucosa, between the styloglossal and mylohyoid muscles. The gland is freed by blunt and sharp dissection, proceeding caudally as far as is necessary to remove it completely (Fig. 47–3B). The oral mucosa is sutured with absorbable suture material.

Miscellaneous Salivary Gland Diseases

Sialoliths

Sialoliths are stones in a salivary duct. They are occasionally seen in the parotid salivary ducts of dogs.[9, 49] They may cause obstruction of the duct and present because of the resulting painful swelling. Foreign bodies are possible causes.[5] They do not cause salivary mucoceles. The sialolith may be palpable or may be visible on survey radiographs or sialograms. Treatment is incision of the duct over the sialolith through the oral mucosa and expression of the sialolith (Fig. 47–4). The duct is flushed to ensure that the obstruction has been cleared. Because the

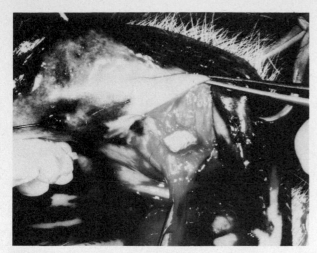

Figure 47–4. A sialolith (white structure) in the parotid duct shown through an incision in the oral mucosa.

incision is made into the mouth, there is no need to suture the incision.

Mandibular Gland Necrosis

Inflammatory diseases of the salivary glands are rarely recognized in the dog and cat. The one exception is mandibular gland necrosis. Because the mandibular gland is enclosed within a tight and strong capsule, any rapid increase in size of the gland can lead to necrosis. The cause of the inflammation in this syndrome is not known, although viral infection is a likely possibility.[39, 40]

Dogs are presented because of exquisite pain on swallowing or palpation of the mouth and neck. There is no obvious swelling of the mandibular gland, although the mandibular lymph nodes are usually swollen to some extent. Conservative treatment with antibiotics and corticosteroids has no beneficial effect. Surgical resection of the mandibular glands may provide relief for some dogs, although more often the pain persists following surgery and the dog is euthanized. Pathological examination of the resected gland shows necrosis and acute inflammation.[39]

Salivary Gland Neoplasia

Neoplasms of the salivary glands occur occasionally, usually being presented because of a palpable mass. Adenocarcinomas of the parotid and mandibular glands are most common and occur in dogs and cats with a mean age of ten years.[32, 37, 44] Unilateral firm masses in a salivary gland should be biopsied. Distant metastasis may occur; thoracic radiographs should be examined prior to definitive treatment. Lesions confined to the salivary gland itself may be amenable to surgical treatment. The mandibular gland is particularly convenient to resect because of the firm, easily recognizable capsule and the compact shape of the gland. The gland is dissected rostrally

until normal sublingual gland is reached. A ligature is placed at that point, and the mandibular and caudal sublingual glands are resected. The other salivary glands are more difficult to resect.

Parotid gland resection requires tedious dissection of the poorly defined gland, with identification and preservation of the facial nerve branches and blood vessels that traverse under and through the gland. Because of the diffuse nature of the parotid gland, complete resection of an infiltrating mass arising from this gland is rarely possible.

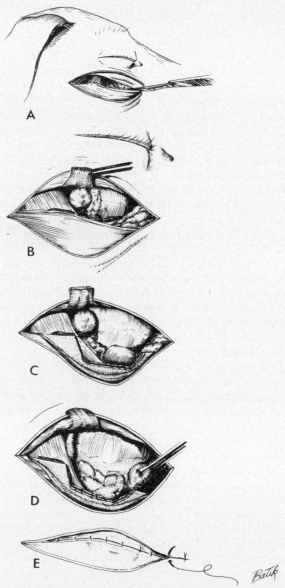

Figure 47–5. Zygomatic salivary gland resection. *A*, Incision over the zygomatic arch. *B*, The orbital ligament and fascia are incised and reflected. *C*, The dorsal section of the zygomatic arch has been resected, revealing the zygomatic salivary gland beneath the orbital fat. *D*, The gland is retracted dorsally and dissected free. *E*, Closure is by apposing the masseter aponeurosis and orbital fascia. (Reprinted with permission from Bistner, S. I. Aguirre, G., and Batik, G.: *Atlas of Veterinary Ophthalmic Surgery*. S. I. Bistner, G. Aguirre, and G. Batik, W. B. Saunders, Philadelphia, 1977.)

Zygomatic gland resection is complicated only by the protected position of the gland behind the zygomatic arch. The skin is incised directly over the dorsal rim of the zygomatic arch (Fig. 47–5A), and the periosteum is incised and reflected, taking with it the orbital fascia dorsally and masseter muscle aponeurosis ventrally (Fig. 47–5B).[41] The dorsal half of the zygomatic arch is removed with a rongeur or bone saw (Fig. 47–5C), or a bone flap is created by rostral and caudal incisions in the zygoma,[55] exposing the orbital fat. The zygomatic gland is found beneath the orbital fat, which is removed by gentle blunt dissection. The gland is lifted out, dissected free from the loose connective tissue surrounding it (Fig. 47–5D), and removed. The incision is closed with interrupted absorbable sutures in the periosteum and orbital fascia (Fig. 47–5E). For a large mass in the orbital area, the entire zygoma can be resected (see Chapter 109).

1. Barone, R.: *Anatomie Comparee des Mammiferes Domestiques.* Tome 3, Fasc 1, Splanchnologie. Lab. d'Anatomie, Ecole Nationale Veterinaire, Lyon, 1976.
2. Battershell, D.: What is your diagnosis? J. Am. Vet. Med. Assoc. *158*:256, 1971.
3. Beaumont, P. B.: Atypical cervical sialocele in a dog. Canine Pract. *7*:56, 1980.
4. Bedford, P. G. C.: Unilateral parotid hypersialism in a Dachshund. Vet. Rec. *107*:557, 1980.
5. Bell, D. A.: Grass seed in the parotid duct of a dog. Vet. Rec. *102*:340, 1978.
6. Bennett, D.: Canine salivary mucoceles. J. Small Anim. Pract. *13*:669, 1972.
7. Bradley, O. C., and Graham, T.: *Topographical Anatomy of the Dog,* 5th ed. Oliver & Boyd, Edinburgh, 1948.
8. Buyukmihci, N., Rubin, L. F., and Harvey, C. E.: Exophthalmos secondary to zygomatic adenocarcinoma in the dog. J. Am. Vet. Med. Assoc. *167*:152, 1975.
9. Chastain, C. B.: What is your diagnosis? J. Am. Vet. Med. Assoc. *164*:415, 1974.
10. Chauveau, A.: *The Comparative Anatomy of the Domesticated Animals,* 2nd ed. Fleming G. Churchill, London, 1873.
11. Christoph, H. J.: Zur erkrankung der speicheldrusen und deren ausfuhrungsgange beim hund. Berl. Munch. Tierarztl. Wochenschr. *69*:227, 1956.
12. Crouch, J. E.: *Text-Atlas of Cat Anatomy.* Lea & Febiger, Philadelphia, 1969.
13. Denis, D.: Kistes salivaires et des kistes brachiaux chez le chien. Thesis, Alfort, 1973, pp. 1–53.
14. DeYoung, D. W., Kealy, J. K., and Kluge, J. P.: Attempts to produce salivary cysts in the dog. Am. J. Vet. Res. *39*:185, 1978.
15. Durtnell, R. E.: Salivary mucocele in the dog. Vet. Rec. *101*:273, 1977.
16. Ellison, S. A.: Proteins and glycoproteins in saliva. *In* Code, C. F. (ed.): *Handbook of Physiology.* American Physiological Society, Washington, D.C., 1967, pp. 531–559.
17. Emmelin, N.: Nervous control of salivary glands. *In* Code, C. F. (ed.): *Handbook of Physiology.* American Physiological Society, Washington, D.C., 1967, pp. 595–632.
18. Emmelin, N.: Nervous control of mammalian salivary glands. Philos. Trans. R. Soc. Lond. *296*:27, 1981.
19. Evans, H. E., and Christensen, G. C.: *Miller's Anatomy of the Dog,* 2nd ed. W. B. Saunders, Philadelphia, 1979.
20. Gill, M. A.: Diseases of the salivary glands of the dog. Thesis, Glasgow University, 1980.
21. Glen, J. B.: Salivary cysts in the dog: identification of sublingual duct defects by sialography. Vet. Rec. *78*:488, 1966.
22. Glen, J. B.: Canine salivary mucoceles: results of sialographic examination and surgical treatment of fifty cases. J. Small Anim. Pract. *13*:515, 1972.
23. Habel, R. E.: *Applied Veterinary Anatomy.* Published by the author, Ithaca, 1975.
24. Harrison, J. D., and Garrett, J. R.: Experimental salivary mucoceles in the cat: a histochemical study. J. Oral. Pathol. *4*:297, 1975.
25. Harrison, J. D., and Garrett, J. R.: Ultrastructural and histochemical study of a naturally occurring salivary mucocele in a cat. J. Comp. Pathol. *85*:411, 1975.
26. Harvey, C. E.: Canine salivary mucocele. J. Am. Anim. Hosp. Assoc. *5*:155, 1969.
27. Harvey, C. E.: Sialography in the dog. Vet. Radiol. *10*:18, 1969.
28. Harvey, C. E.: Letter to the Editor. J. Am. Vet. Med. Assoc. *158*:1454, 1971.
29. Harvey, C. E.: Parotid salivary duct rupture and fistula in the dog and cat. J. Small Anim. Pract. *18*:163, 1977.
30. Harvey, C. E.: Hypersialosis and parotid gland enlargement in a dog. J. Small Anim. Pract. 22:19, 1981.
31. Harvey, H. J.: Pharyngeal mucoceles in dogs. J. Am. Vet. Med. Assoc. *178*:1282, 1981.
32. Head, K. W.: Tumors of the upper alimentary tract. Bull. WHO 53:3427, 1976.
33. Hoffer, R. E.: Surgical treatment of salivary mucocele. Vet. Clin. North Am. 5:333, 1975.
34. Hulland, T. J.: Salivary mucoceles. Proc. Ann. Mtg. Am. Vet. Med. Assoc., p. 152, 1964.
35. Hulland, T. J., and Archibald, J.: Salivary mucoceles in dogs. Can. Vet. J. 5:109, 1964.
36. Hurov, L.: Surgical correction of blocked parotid duct. Can. Vet. J. 2:348, 1961.
37. Karbe, E., and Schiefer, B.: Primary salivary gland tumors in carnivores. Can. Vet. J. 8:212, 1967.
38. Kealy, J. K.: Salivary cyst in the dog. Vet. Rec. 76:119, 1964.
39. Kelly, D. F., Lucke, V. M., Denny, H. R., and Lane, J. G.: Histology of salivary gland infarction in the dog. Vet. Pathol. 16:438, 1979.
40. Kelly, D. F., Lucke, V. M., Lane, J. G., Denny, H. R., and Longstaffe, J. A.: Salivary gland necrosis in dogs. Vet. Rec. *104*:268, 1979.
41. Knecht, C. D.: Treatment of diseases of the zygomatic salivary gland. J. Am. Anim. Hosp. Assoc. 6:13, 1970.
42. Knecht, C. D., and Phares, J.: Characterization of dogs with salivary cyst. J. Am. Vet. Med. Assoc. *158*:612, 1971.
43. Knecht, C. D., Slusher, R., and Guibor, E. C.: Zygomatic salivary cyst in a dog. J. Am. Vet. Med. Assoc. *155*:625, 1969.
44. Koestner, A. and Buerger, L.: Primary neoplasms of the salivary glands in animals compared to similar tumors in man. Pathol. Vet. 2:201, 1965.
45. Leonardi, L.: La scialografia nel cane. Gaz. Vet. *18*:20, 1965.
46. Martin, C. L.: Zygomatic salivary mucocele in a dog. Vet. Med./Small Anim. Clin. 66:36, 1971.
47. Michel, G.: Beitrag zur topographie der ausfuhrungsgange der gl. mandibularis und der gl. sublingualis major des hundes. Berl. Munch. Tierarztl. Wochenschr. 69:132, 1956.
48. Morris, G. C. R.: Pathological physiology of salivary glands. *In* Code, C. F. (ed.): *Handbook of Physiology.* American Physiological Society, Washington, D.C., 1967, pp. 679–703.
49. Mulkey, O. C., and Knecht, C. D.: Parotid salivary gland cyst and calculus in a dog. J. Am. Vet. Med. Assoc. *159*:1774, 1971.
50. Nickel, R., Schummer, A., Seiferle, E., and Sack, W. O.: *The Viscera of the Domestic Mammals,* Verlag Paul Parey, Berline, 1973.
51. Ortner, Z.: Sialografija kod psa. Veterinarski. Arhiv. Zagreb. *15*:202, 1945.
52. Pantel, M., and Wissdorf, H.: Anatomische und klinische aspekte zur ranula bei einer katze. Kleinter. Prax. *21*:277, 1976.
53. Preibisch, J.: Kamienie slinowe u psa. Med. Wet. *16*:277, 1960.

54. Prescott, C. W.: Ranula in the dog—a surgical treatment. Aust. Vet. J. *44*:382, 1968.

55. Schmidt, G. M., and Betts, C. W.: Zygomatic salivary mucoceles in the dog. J. Am. Vet. Med. Assoc. *172*:940, 1978.

56. Schummer, A., Wilkens, H., Vollmerhaus, B., and Habermehl, K.-H.: *The Anatomy of the Domestic Animals*, Vol. 3, The Circulatory System, the Skin, and the Cutaneous Organs of the Domestic Mammals. Verlag Paul Parey, Berlin, 1981.

57. Spreull, J. S. A., and Head, K. W.: Cervical salivary cysts in the dog. J. Am. Vet. Med. Assoc. 8:17, 1967.

58. Stinson, A. W., and Calhoun, M. L.: Digestive system. *In* Dellman, H.-D., and Brown, E. M. (eds.): *Textbook of*

Veterinary Histology, 2nd ed. Lea & Febiger, Philadelphia, 1981.

59. Taylor, J. A.: *Regional and Applied Anatomy of the Domestic Animals*, Vol. 1, Head and Neck. Oliver & Boyd, Edinburgh, 1955.

60. Teague, H. D.: Surgical correction of a large sialocele in a dog. Canine Pract. 6:11, 1979.

61. Testoni, F. J., Lohse, C. L., and Hyde, R. J.: Anatomy and cannulation of the parotid duct in the dog. J. Am. Vet. Med. Assoc. *170*:831, 1977.

62. Wallace, L. J., Guffy, M. M., Gray, A. P., and Clifford, J. H.: Anterior cervical sialocele (salivary cyst) in a domestic cat. J. Am. Anim. Hosp. Assoc. 8:74, 1972.

Chapter 48 Esophagus

Anatomy

John Grandage

CAPACITY

The carnivore esophagus must cope with gluttonous behavior and must be able to convey unchewed chunks of meat, including bone fragments, from pharynx to stomach. Accordingly it must have a tough, slippery mucous membrane, an efficient muscular coat, and the ability to dilate to an extraordinary degree; it must be located in a site that can accommodate that dilation. The collapsed esophagus of the average dog is some two centimeters in diameter, yet it can easily double or even triple during swallowing.[9] Radiographs of anesthetized dogs in left lateral recumbency often show a passively dilated esophagus inflated with regurgitated stomach gas. No reliable figures detail the normal maximum diameter, so care is needed to distinguish normal transient dilation from the chronic distension of megaesophagus. Beagles have an esophageal capacity of 60 ml.[5] Several dogs with megaesophagus have been found to have esophageal diameters within normal limits.[68] The more fastidious habits of the cat suggest that it has less need for its esophagus to be so distensible.

The carnivore esophagus is narrowest near its origin, near its termination, and by the thoracic inlet; an inflated esophagus also reveals a fourth constriction over the base of the heart (where it passes between the azygos vein on the right and the aorta on the left). Movement of the esophagus is most restricted at these four sites. The short distances between them do not allow the remainder of the esophagus to wander far. In the caudal part of the neck the esophagus drops away from the longus colli

muscle to rest on the left of the trachea; in the caudal thorax the surrounding structures are soft and yielding, giving the esophagus maximum freedom.

The esophagus is, curiously, invisible on most radiographs, except when its lumen contains some contrast agent (gas, food, barium); the laterally flattened, tapered esophagus does not allow the lungs to provide adequate contrast in lateral projections.

MUCOSA

An ample mucosa thrown into several deep longitudinal folds allows the stellate lumen to dilate. Barium swallows leave trails of medium within the troughs of these folds. In cats the terminal esophageal mucosa is also folded in transverse ripples, which create a herringbone pattern on radiographs.[66] The mucosa bears a white, stratified squamous epithelium that is not keratinized in carnivores.[2, 42] It becomes continuous with the mucosa of the pharynx at the limen pharyngoesophageum, an annular fold formerly called the esophageal isthmus. As the esophagus passes through the diaphragm, the epithelium changes abruptly from stratified squamous in the thoracic part to columnar in the short abdominal part.[193] In both the dog and cat, irregular mucosal folds line the cardia and may enhance its closure. The mucosal surface is lubricated by mucus from simple branched tubuloacinar glands, of which there are many thousands opening every square millimeter or so along the esophagus of the dog,[52] but which are restricted to the pharyngeal end in the cat.[9, 174]

SUBMUCOSA

A thick submucosa allows the mucosa and muscle coats to slide somewhat independently of one another.[154] It acts as a flexible skeleton and as a vehicle to convey blood vessels, glands, and an abundance of elastic tissue. Some claim that it contains nerves (the submucosal plexus of Meissner),[42, 52] whereas others positively deny their presence.[117]

MUSCULARIS

The muscular tunic of the carnivore esophagus is mostly striated. In the dog it is striated throughout, but in the cat it changes to smooth muscle in the terminal few centimeters.[42] The esophagus may therefore appear slightly redder on its external surface than the rest of the alimentary canal, which is clad in pale smooth muscle.[9, 15] The muscle is made up of two poorly defined coats whose individual fascicles wind along the esophagus in left- and right-handed spirals, crossing each other at right angles and changing from a superficial position on one side to a deep position on the other.[21, 52] To do this, the fascicles decussate dorsally and ventrally except at the two extremities, where the decussations peter out. The esophageal muscle arises partly as a direct continuation of the cricopharyngeus and partly from the cricoesophageal tendon; this tendon arises from the median crest of the cricoid cartilage, runs caudally for about one centimeter, and seems to be an important anchor for the esophagus. A number of additional longitudinal muscle bundles have been described at the cranial end of the esophagus.[52] At the caudal end the esophageal muscle merges with the muscle of the stomach in a complex manner. Essentially, the outer layers continue as the longitudinal muscle of the stomach and the deeper, more transverse layers merge with the circular and oblique layers of the stomach.

SPHINCTERS

The esophagus is undoubtedly equipped with functional sphincters,[157] although in the dog and cat these are difficult to identify anatomically.[14]

At the proximal end there is no obvious thickening of the pharyngoesophageal junction. It seems that the cricopharyngeus or an even broader bundle of muscle performs the sphincter function.[98, 116]

At the distal end the so-called caudal esophageal or cardiac sphincter of the dog seems to be located over the terminal two centimeters of the esophagus. A slight thickening of the inner circular muscle around this site has been variously described;[21, 117, 151] it probably incorporates some of the sling fibers (ansa cardiaca), which loop over the terminal stomach from the lesser curvature of the esophagus.[56, 146] The evidence for a similar sphincter in the cat is, at least anatomically, less persuasive.[194]

The fissure-like esophageal hiatus through the lumbar part of the diaphragm has been claimed to act like a sphincter,[153] but the so-called pinchcock effect it is supposed to exert is unconvincing.[14]

ADVENTITIA

This outermost layer of the esophagus allows some mobility within the neck; within the thorax the flimsy mediastinal pleura is directly adherent to it. A closed pouch of pleura exists on the right side of the esophagus just cranial to the diaphragm. Known as the cavum mediastinum serosum (formerly as the esophageal or infracardiac bursa), it is a thoracic remnant of the omental bursa.[129] It sometimes extends through the esophageal hiatus and may assist the passage of large boluses through the diaphragm. The esophagus is only loosely attached to the diaphragm by a phrenoesophageal membrane rich in elastic tissue.[14]

VESSELS AND NERVES

A myenteric plexus (of Auerbach) exists between the muscle coats. The ganglion cells retain their normal numbers in the young and old and in dogs affected with so-called achalasia (megaesophagus)[27]. The striated muscle of the esophagus is presumably innervated by special visceral efferent fibers conveyed along various branches of the vagus, beginning with the pharyngoesophageal nerve, followed by the recurrent laryngeal nerve and its paralaryngeal companion, and concluding with the dorsal and ventral vagal trunks in the caudal thorax. Cell bodies of these nerves are topographically arranged in the nucleus ambiguus of the myelencephalon (medulla). There is slender evidence that the number of cell bodies in this nucleus may be diminished in megaesophagus. Smooth muscle fibers in the terminal esophagus are innervated by general visceral efferents whose cell bodies are found in a separate nucleus (the tenth motor nucleus), which is a little dorsal to the nucleus ambiguus.[41] Most authors claim that a sympathetic innervation, derived from the sympathetic trunk, is also present.[129]

The thyroid arteries and esophageal branches of the carotids supply much of the cervical esophagus, and the bronchoesophageal artery supplies most of the thoracic part. Esophageal branches straight off the aorta usually supply the terminal segment in conjunction with the esophageal branch of the left gastric; a variable number of other arteries may also contribute to this part.[21, 52, 104]

The tiny embryonic pharynx is completely encircled by a succession of gill (aortic) arches. Normally these are little more than capillary-sized vessels. Many segments quickly disappear or become inconsequential, allowing the structures they encircled to expand. Sometimes, unusual segments of the aortic arches persist until after birth, resulting in vascular rings that encircle and constrict the esophagus and occasionally the trachea. The most common of these anomalies is a persistent right aortic arch. In this condition the esophagus becomes trapped on the left of the aortic arch (instead of lying free on the right as it does normally) and compressed by a normally placed ligamentum arteriosum. A number of other anomalies, such as double aorta and right ligamentum ateriosum, can produce similar effects.[99, 112]

Veins leaving the cervical esophagus drain into the external jugular veins, and those from the thoracic esophagus drain mostly into the azygous vein. Portocaval anastomoses exist at the gastroesophageal junction; in humans they are the site of varices associated with portal hypertension, and in dogs too when the portal vein has been experimentally occluded.[188]

Lymphatics drain into most of the large number of lymph nodes that cluster around the proximal part of the alimentary tract. They include the retropharyngeal, cervical, mediastinal, bronchial, portal, gastric, and splenic lymph nodes.[52]

Surgical Diseases

Richard E. Hoffer

PRINCIPLES OF ESOPHAGEAL SURGERY

The esophagus has an incomplete serosal covering; thus, the fibrin seal that helps to prevent leakage in the other hollow viscera may be unavailable.[82, 118, 122, 133, 134, 148, 154] The lack of serosa necessitates more careful apposition of the esophagus to prevent dehiscence. The sturdy stratified squamous epithelium and submucosa (Fig. 48–1) hold sutures well.[82, 132, 134, 142, 197]

Segmental esophageal blood supply may be a factor in poor healing following esophageal anastomosis,[8, 82, 114, 133, 154] but well-developed intramural vascular anastomoses are capable of supporting the entire esophagus, even if the blood supply from the stomach is removed.[132, 197] It is more likely that ischemic necrosis of the anastomotic suture line is the result of impairment of intramural esophageal vascular anastomoses.[132, 197]

Tension and motion at the suture line are factors that contribute to leakage or dehiscence of esophageal repair.[8, 114, 132, 134, 154, 197] Factors that can contribute to likelihood of increased leakage of an esophageal anastomosis are impairment of intramural blood supply; lack of omentum; difficulty of exposure; general debilitation of patient; poor nutritional state; and movement of saliva and food through the esophageal anastomosis.[82, 131, 132, 134, 148]

The esophageal lumen is contaminated at the time of surgery. Administration of preoperative antibiotics decreased the incidence of anastomotic leakage and lowered mortality significantly in cats in which a 3-cm segment of esophagus was resected.[134] Stricture of the esophagus may follow surgical repair, although documented cases are rare.[85, 108, 173]

The technique of choice for esophageal repair is two-layer closure: the first layer apposes the mucosa and submucosa, and the second layer apposes the muscular layer.[11, 109, 114, 130, 134, 142, 154, 173] Everting one-layer suture techniques have been successfully used for esophageal closure in dogs.[8, 85, 130, 154] When tension is anticipated, the mucosa and submucosa are apposed with a simple interrupted suture pattern with knots in the lumen (Fig. 48–2A and B). The last two sutures are preplaced (Fig. 48–2C). When tension is not likely, as with esophagotomy, the mucosa and submucosa may be closed with a simple continuous pattern (Fig. 48–2D). The sutures with either pattern should be placed 2 to 3 mm apart and 3 mm from the cut mucosal edge (see Figs. 48–1 and 48–2).[80, 82] I prefer nonabsorbable sutures such as Prolene or nylon for closing the mucosa and submucosa. One study suggested that surgical gut gives better results than Teflon-impregnated polyester fiber in growing dogs.[11] Other studies demonstrated that gut or silk produces the same results.[109, 132, 134, 142]

Before the esophageal muscles are closed, the mucosal closure can be checked by injecting saline into the lumen of the esophagus under pressure; leaks are closed with simple interrupted sutures. The esophageal musculature may be closed with a simple interrupted pattern of absorbable suture.[80, 82, 109, 122, 173] although silk has frequently been used experimentally for closing the muscle.[122, 142]

Various techniques to reinforce or reduce tension on the suture line have been described. Circular myotomy reduces tension at the suture line by 66 per cent following resection of one-third to one-half

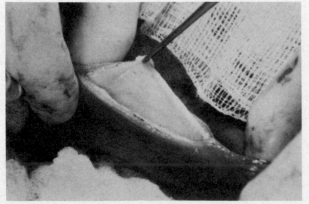

Figure 48–1. The esophagus has been incised and the white mucosal-submucosal layer is well exposed.

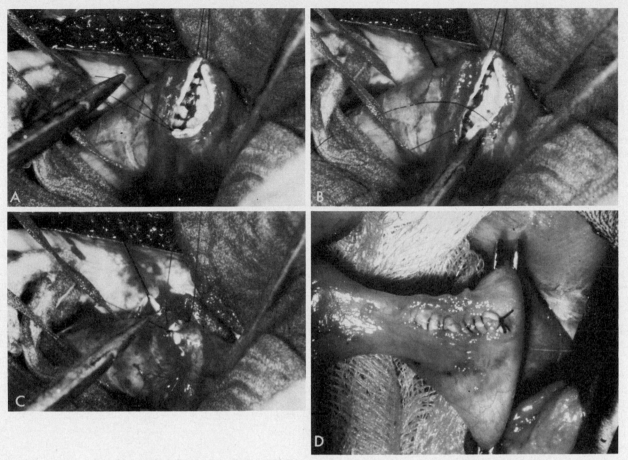

Figure 48–2. An esophageal resection is demonstrated. *A,* The sutures have been placed in the far side of the esophagus. The far side was sutured from inside the lumen. *B,* The esophagus is sutured so the knot is inside the lumen. The left side was sutured by placing the needle from inside the lumen to the outside. The right side is sutured by placing the needle from outside to inside. *C,* The last two sutures have been preplaced, and one has been tied. The second suture is tied. This may be placed as a simple interrupted suture. *D,* The esophageal mucosa and submucosa has been closed with a simple continuous suture. Note that the sutures completely close the end of the mucosal-submucosal incision.

of the thoracic or cervical esophagus in piglets.[114] Circular myotomy resulted in a higher survival rate following resection of 60 per cent of the thoracic esophagus in dogs; distal myotomy was more effective than proximal myotomy.[6] In another study in dogs, circular myotomy allowed 51 per cent of the esophagus to be resected with the same mortality as a 27 per cent resection without myotomy.[122] In both of these studies in dogs, only a partial circular myotomy was done; if the myotomy is full-thickness, the submucosal arterial network may be damaged and ischemic necrosis may result. The thickness of the muscular layers may be determined by injecting saline to separate them. Partial myotomy is as effective as full-thickness myotomy in reducing tension.[122] Combined myotomy gives the highest survival rate, and distal myotomy gives a higher survival rate than proximal myotomy.[6] Long-term follow-up 13 months after operation did not demonstrate stricture or dilation at myotomy sites, nor did cine-esophagrams and motility studies demonstrate esophageal dysfunction.[6] Partial circular myotomy directly reduces tension at the suture line to decrease the incidence of

suture line disruption when resection of a long segment of the esophagus is necessary.

Suture Line Reinforcement Techniques

These techniques bring other tissues to support and seal the suture line.

Placement of a vascularized omental graft brought through the diaphragm and wrapped around an incompletely closed esophageal anastomosis allowed ten of 12 dogs to heal without complications.[60]

Esophageal anastomoses have been reinforced with autogenous, free 2- to 3-cm-wide pericardial grafts, and bursting pressures of the anastomotic sites were compared with those in nonreinforced esophageal anastomosis. The grafted anastomoses were significantly stronger than the controls. There was no evidence of stricture in the grafted dogs by the 16th postoperative day.[92] Omental or pericardial reinforcement can be used at any level in the thoracic esophagus, although omental reinforcement does require an abdominal incision.

An intercostal pedicle graft containing the neurovascular bundles and intercostal muscles from the fourth right intercostal space was used to reinforce poorly constructed esophageal anastomoses in ten dogs; nine grafted animals survived, compared with four of the controls. There was no evidence of stricture, but motility was reduced and esophageal diameter was fixed at the anastomotic site.[17]

Pedicled diaphragmatic grafts have been used clinically in humans to reinforce esophageal surgical sites with good results.[139] The muscle grafts and the particular muscles used depend upon the location of the lesion. There are muscles that can be used as pedicle grafts at almost any area of the cervical or thoracic esophagus. The lung was utilized in a human case to replace an extensive muscular defect of the esophagus.[125] A pedicled jejunal patch (with the mucosa removed) was used successfully in five dogs to reinforce a repaired esophageal perforation of four hours' duration.[123]

Esophageal Patch Grafting

Repair following loss of esophageal tissue may require patch grafting techniques. In the cervical region, the sternothyroideus muscle in the dog was used successfully to repair a strictured area of the esophagus; the stricture was incised, and the open esophagus sutured to the muscle using a two-layer suture pattern.[93] The muscle graft must be well-mobilized and wide enough to prevent stenosis following healing of the graft.[86, 93]

A pedicle flap from the diaphragm may be used to repair perforations or strictures of the distal esophagus. Studies in dogs demonstrated good healing of the pedicle flap to the esophagus in large defects: all the defects were epithelialized with esophageal mucosa eight weeks postoperatively, and normal esophageal function was demonstrated seven months postoperatively.[110]

Intercostal pedicle grafts have been used to repair full-thickness esophageal defects without primary esophageal closure in dogs, with an uneventful recovery, and complete epithelialization without stricture formation at three to six months.[17]

Vascularized omentum has been used to close full-thickness esophageal defects.[121] The omentum seals the defect while the defect closes by contraction; a small plug of epithelialized omentum may prevent complete contraction of the defect.[121] Pericardium has been used successfully to patch graft an esophageal stenosis in nine of 11 normal dogs[36] and in humans.[180]

A gastric antrum or fundus patch produced good healing without esophageal stenosis in dogs and clinically in humans.[180] Some dogs developed esophagitis when stimulated with histamine following fundic patching; dogs with antral patches did not develop esophagitis.[94] A vascularized gastric flap from the greater curvature of the stomach was used successfully to repair pharyngoesophageal defects in 15 of 16 dogs.[129]

Esophageal Replacement

Methods for complete replacement or bypass of an obstructed area are esophagogastrostomy, jejunal or colon interposition, use of isoperistaltic gastric tube, and use of reversed gastric tube.[12, 35, 55, 65, 67, 69, 79, 101, 142, 143, 175]

Esophagogastrostomy has been used clinically in dogs, but complications are common.[55, 65, 79] Other techniques have been used experimentally but not clinically.[131] The use of pedicled intestinal grafts is not appropriate for the distal third of the esophagus because of the short vascular arcade in the dog.[118, 148, 197] The gastric tube can be used to avoid the complications of esophagogastrostomy; however, this procedure is also not without complications.[118, 131] Free jejunal segments and an inverted tube graft of skin have been used experimentally in dogs.[131, 163]

All of the techniques of esophageal replacement are technically difficult and have high morbidity and mortality rates; they should be regarded as salvage procedures. The use of prostheses for permanent esophageal replacement is still in the investigative stage.[81]

SURGICAL DISEASE OF THE ESOPHAGUS

Esophageal diseases cause obstruction, leakage, or neuromuscular malfunction. The most common abnormality is esophageal obstruction: Fluids and foods are unable to pass from the mouth into the stomach as a result of blockage or narrowing of the lumen or diversion of the bolus. Obstruction results from esophageal foreign body, esophageal diverticulum, esophageal neoplasia, hematoma or granuloma, esophageal stricture or stenosis, and vascular ring anomaly.[80, 82, 148]

Leakage of ingesta may result from esophageal perforation, esophageal laceration, and tracheal or bronchoesophageal fistula.[81, 82, 83]

Neuromuscular abnormalities prevent food from passing from the mouth to the stomach as the result of a deficiency in the neuromuscular synchronous function of the oropharynx, body of the esophagus, and esophageal sphincters. Diseases in this category may be primary or secondary. The diseases with secondary esophageal effects include Addison's disease, myasthenia gravis, lupus erythematosus, scleroderma, polymyositis, and inherited canine giant axonal neuropathy.[46, 47, 80, 82, 148] These conditions cannot be corrected surgically.

Primary esophageal neuromuscular diseases include hiatal hernia, oropharyngeal dysphagias, gastroesophageal intussusception, idiopathic megaesophagus, and acquired achalasia.[80, 82, 148]

Some diseases may cause more than one abnormality. Clinical signs are often similar. Foreign bodies may produce esophageal perforation, and vascular rings results in a neuromuscular defect of the dilated portion of the esophagus.

Obstructive Esophageal Disease

The most common clinical sign of obstructive esophageal diseases is regurgitation. The characteristics of regurgitation vary depending on the size, type, and location of the obstruction, and on the extent of preobstructive dilation.

Esophageal obstruction may be partial or complete, depending upon the cause. Complete obstruction results in regurgitation of all ingested food. If solid food is regurgitated, but semisolid or liquid foods are not, obstruction is partial. The consistency of the food that is retained indicates the degree of luminal occlusion.

The interval between ingestion of food and regurgitation is determined by the location of the obstruction and by the degree of dilation proximal to the obstruction. Generally, the lower the obstruction the longer the delay between ingestion and regurgitation. With a high cervical obstruction the patient may be presented because of dysphagia, as the material is regurgitated during swallowing. This high obstruction must be differentiated from oropharyngeal dysphagia.

Chronic partial esophageal stenosis or obstruction (whether from a foreign body or stricture) results in dilation of the esophagus proximal to the lesion. The longer the stenosis is present and the narrower the esophageal lumen, the greater the dilation. The interval between ingestion and regurgitation is longer when there is esophageal dilation proximal to a stenosis or obstruction. In addition, the history usually indicates a change in the interval between ingestion and regurgitation when esophageal dilation is secondary to stricture; the interval becomes longer as ingesta pools in the dilated esophagus before regurgitation occurs.

The character of the regurgitated material is also affected by the degree of dilation. The longer ingesta remains in the dilated esophagus, the more mucus and saliva are added to it. With large dilations, fermentation of the ingested material occurs, causing it to smell foul. Generally, regurgitant material from a nondilated stenosed esophagus is tube-shaped and of the same consistency as when ingested.[80, 82]

The diagnosis of esophageal obstruction can be suspected on the basis of the history, results of physical examination, and observation of the animal's eating patterns. The identification of the obstructing lesion and confirmation of the diagnosis are made radiographically or endoscopically. Endoscopic and radiographic examinations are necessary to determine treatment.

Surgical Exposure of the Esophagus

The surgical approach to the esophagus depends on the location of the lesion, rather than the diagnosis. The cervical esophagus is exposed through a ventral midline incision, by separation of the sternohyoideus muscles (Fig. 48–3). Extending the incision caudally to the manubrium allows the esophagus to be exposed to the second rib.

The thoracic esophagus from the second rib to the diaphragm may be exposed by a right thoracotomy. The intercostal space over the lesion is incised. The esophagus cranial to the seventh rib and caudal to the third rib in the normal dog is approached by a right thoracotomy. From this approach the great vessels are to the left of the esophagus. In the dog with a persistent right aortic arch, the cranial esophagus is approached by a left thoracotomy, since the aorta is to the right of the esophagus. A right eighth or ninth intercostal incision exposes the distal esophagus and the esophageal hiatus. Thoracotomy is discussed in Chapter 41.

An indirect technique to remove an esophageal foreign body under direct observation can be used.[179] A left eighth intercostal thoracotomy is made, and the central tendinous portion of the diaphagm is incised. The greater curvature of the stomach is elevated and incised, and the foreign body is removed. Then the stomach, diaphragm, and thorax are closed. This technique permits direct esophageal examination and manipulation without requiring esophageal incision, but does require thoracotomy.

Esophageal Foreign Bodies

Despite a very distensible esophagus, the dog and cat are susceptible to esophageal foreign bodies. Dogs, being indiscriminate eaters, have a higher incidence of esophageal obstruction by bones or materials such as metal, plastic, wood, or rubber; cats, as a result of their tendency to play and hunt, have a higher incidence of needle or fishhook inges-

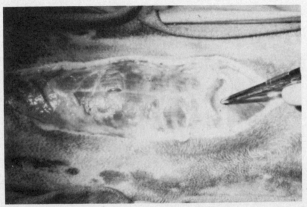

Figure 48–3. A ventral cervical incision has been made, exposing the sternohyoidius muscles. They are separated at the median raphe to expose the esophagus.

tion, resulting in perforation rather than obstruction. The type of foreign body ingested determines the signs and pathophysiologic changes that occur. Changes resulting from mechanical obstruction of the esophagus are discussed here. Esophageal perforations were discussed previously.

The esophagus narrows at the thoracic inlet, the base of the heart, and the diaphragmatic hiatus. Foreign bodies lodge at these sites, most commonly in the thoracic esophagus.[82, 109, 138, 156]

Most foreign bodies are sharp and impinge on the esophageal mucosa.[138] Bolus type foreign bodies produce a mechanical obstruction resulting in regurgitation, which may be consistent or intermittent depending upon the degree of the obstruction. Most bones allow the passage of some liquid or semisolid food around or through them, so the animal can survive for a prolonged period. Dilation may occur proximal to a foreign body, resulting in an increasing interval between ingestion and regurgitation with fermentation and mucous accumulation. Complete obstruction results in regurgitation after ingestion of any type of food and a very rapid loss of condition.[138] Some animals with obstruction have respiratory signs because of aspiration or esophageal perforation. These signs may be severe enough to mask signs of esophageal obstruction.[54, 138]

As a foreign body remains in contact with the esophagus, local changes occur. The larger and sharper the object, the more rapid and severe the local damage, with spasm of esophageal muscle and necrosis of the mucosa. Necrosis over a pointed object may extend through the entire esophageal wall, resulting in perforation with escape of intraluminal contents. The necrotic area may be sealed by adnexal tissue such as lung, and a bronchoesophageal fistula may result.[13, 105, 112] If the object is round or smooth, pressure necrosis can produce a circumferential loss of mucosa, subsequently resulting in stricture formation.[82] Death from foreign body obstruction is usually the result of pleuritis, mediastinitis, cervical cellulitis, or aspiration pneumonia. Diagnosis is based upon history and signs of regurgitation and is confirmed by radiography, with or without contrast studies, and endoscopy.

The object of treatment is to remove the foreign body without subsequent stricture formation or esophageal perforation. Direct surgical intervention allows evaluation of the entire esophagus, including depth of penetration through the esophageal wall, viability of the esophageal tissue, and involvement of adnexal tissues. It enables immediate repair of esophageal or periesophageal damage and removal of the object without surgical damage to other areas of the esophagus. Disadvantages of surgical intervention are: the need for thoracotomy; incision of the esophagus with the subsequent risk of dehiscence, infection, and stricture, longer hospitalization period, and greater expense. The decision may be based on duration of the problem: if the foreign body has been present for more than two days or there is clinical or radiographic evidence of perforation or laceration of the esophagus, I recommend direct surgical intervention.

Conservative Treatment of Esophageal Foreign Bodies

Colin E. Harvey

If equipment is available, an attempt should be made to remove any esophageal foreign body with forceps. The equipment necessary is an esophagoscope, or other long tube with a lighting system, and an appropriate set of forceps. Flexible fiberoptic diagnostic endoscopes are not suitable for forceps removal of foreign bodies; they provide a clear view of the object, but the small size of the flexible biopsy forceps available for use through fiberoptic systems is not adequate for the large foreign bodies most commonly found in dogs. The esophagus is capable of accommodating a very large tube relative to the animal's size; with a larger tube, more light is available, and observation for control of instruments is improved. In cats and small or medium-sized dogs, a rigid proctoscope provides a practical combination of length and diameter. For larger dogs, rigid esophagoscopes of 50 to 60 cm with a minimum diameter of 10 mm are necessary. The most useful forceps for removing bones from dogs are the pin forceps, originally designed to close on the ring at one end of a safety pin (which is a common foreign body in children); the blunt pointed ends can obtain a solid grip on bone that is often impossible to obtain with the usual alligator forceps found in veterinary hospitals. The forceps must be long enough to reach through the length of the tube with some working room at the end; they should not be much longer than the tube, as the additional length prevents the eye from staying close to the end of the tube.

The animal is anesthetized and placed in left lateral recumbency so that the esophagus lies above the aorta. The tube is lubricated and gently inserted through the pharynx into the esophageal opening. There is often a collection of food and saliva cranial to the foreign body; this is removed through a suction tube placed through the tube. The foreign body is examined and grasped, using any available prominence. One should avoid including part of the esophageal wall in the grip of the forceps. The forceps are gently pulled cranially. If the foreign body does not move, the forceps are twisted one-quarter or one-half turn, first one way, then the other, in an effort to disengage the foreign body from the esophageal wall. Once the foreign body can be moved by the forceps, the tube, forceps, and foreign body are removed as a unit with one gentle motion. Following removal, the tube is reinserted so that the esophageal wall can be examined; clean lacerations that do not extend through the full thickness of the esophageal wall (as judged by gently pushing the tip of the tube against the laceration) can be left to heal. Full-thickness tears or areas of necrotic esophageal wall require surgical management; for this reason, forceps removal of esophageal foreign bodies should not be attempted unless facilities and personnel for thoracotomy are available.

The foreign body should not be grasped with maximum force; if it does not disengage with one or two attempts using moderate to firm force, attempts at forceps removal are abandoned, and surgery is performed. It is possible to avulse an esophagus from its attachments, pulling the cranial esophagus out through the pharynx along with a foreign body, if too much force is applied.

Sharp foreign bodies may penetrate the esophageal wall. Poorly planned forceps removal may result in severe laceration of the esophagus. The foreign body should be examined to determine the direction of penetration, as the first step in removal is to pull the foreign body back into the lumen. This may require grasping the visible section, then pushing the foreign body caudally to disengage it. The tube is advanced to cover the tip of the object, in order to prevent repenetration as the tube, forceps, and foreign body are removed as a unit. Clean lacerations from penetration of a sharp foreign body usually do not require surgical repair.

Foreign bodies that can be seen at esophagoscopy but cannot be removed by forceps can sometimes be pushed into the stomach by the forceps or esophagoscope. Bones usually will be decalcified by digestive juices and will pass without further trouble. Metallic or other foreign materials can be removed through a gastrotomy incision at laparotomy, avoiding thoracotomy.

If esophagoscopy equipment is not available but fluoroscopic equipment is, an attempt at forceps removal under indirect visualization can be made. With the animal under general anesthesia, the forceps are advanced until they touch the foreign body. They are opened and moved farther to grasp the foreign body. The forceps are retracted or twisted while the fluoroscope screen is viewed for evidence of movement of the object. If the object cannot be grasped successfully, the forceps are pushed against the object in an attempt to move it into the stomach. This method is less satisfactory than esophagoscopy, in that the esophageal epithelium cannot be seen before and after the application of the forceps, and one cannot be sure that a fold of esophageal wall is not included in the grip of the forceps.

Dogs and cats are usually able to drink within 24 hours of foreign body removal. Soft or slurried food is given the next day. The major complication is mediastinitis. If thoracic radiographs made 12 and 24 hours following removal show no mediastinal thickening, and the animal is eating and not pyrexic, the animal can be discharged.

Used judiciously as described, forceps removal of foreign bodies is both safe and effective; 60 of 66 esophageal foreign bodies in dogs and cats were removed by forceps or pushed into the stomach at esophagoscopy in one reported series, with 98 per cent recovery.[156]

Esophagotomy

The esophagus is exposed, all adhesions are separated, and hemorrhage is controlled. The area is packed off with drapes. The esophagus is carefully examined. If primary healing appears doubtful because of the presence of devitalized tissue, reinforcing procedures, patch grafting, or resection and anastomosis may be necessary.

If the esophageal tissues are viable, the esophagus is occluded with atraumatic forceps or digital compression above and below the foreign body and is incised cranial to the foreign body. The object is removed and the esophagus is closed.

Food is withheld for 24 to 72 hours, depending upon the extent of damage. If patch grafting is necessary, oral intake should be withheld for up to 72 hours. Hydration is maintained by parenteral fluids for one to two days, or for a longer period through a gastrostomy tube placed at the time of surgery. Broad-spectrum antibiotics are given, preferably starting prior to surgery. The patient should be on normal feeding by the seventh postoperative day.

Esophageal Diverticulum

Esophageal diverticula in the dog are located in the distal esophagus.[39, 53, 78, 100, 108, 111, 137, 147, 149] They are referred to as epiphrenic diverticula and result from protrusion of the esophageal mucosa through a defect in the musculature (pulsion diverticulum), probably as a result of damage by foreign body obstruction. There may be no history or clinical evidence of foreign body obstruction, causing speculation that in dogs epiphrenic diverticulum may be congenital in origin.[78, 100, 108, 111, 137, 147] Esophageal motility disturbances have been reported in one case.[53, 78, 100, 108, 111, 137, 147] A congenital diverticulum may predispose the dog to foreign body obstruction.

The presenting signs in dogs with esophageal diverticula are regurgitation of ingesta, gagging, gulping of food, dysphagia, and coughing after ingestion of food. Emaciation may be a long-term result.[78, 100, 108, 111, 137, 147]

Diagnosis is made by radiography. On plain thoracic films, a dilated esophagus is seen in the epiphrenic area. Barium swallow demonstrates the diverticulum (see Fig. 48–4). The diverticulum may be unilateral or bilateral. Esophageal motility and gastroesophageal function should be evaluated fluoroscopically. Although epiphrenic diverticulum is usually associated with abnormal esophageal motility in humans,[39, 95, 104] this has not been the case in the dog.[53, 78, 100, 108, 111, 137]

Treatment of esophageal diverticulum is directed at removing the foreign body if present and correcting the diverticulum, usually by excision. This is more

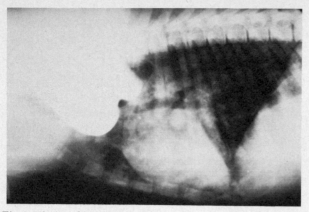

Figure 48–4. A lateral view with contrast material demonstrates the enlarged cranial portion of the esophagus. The contrast material stops abruptly at the heart, where the ligament crosses the esophagus.

easily done when there is a single diverticulum.[53, 78, 100, 111, 137, 147] For a double diverticulum, it may be necessary to resect the involved esophagus, possibly requiring mobilization of the stomach through the diaphragm as an esophagogastrostomy or esophageal substitution.[12, 34, 35, 55, 65, 67, 79, 101, 143, 175]

The lesion is approached via a thoracotomy, and the diverticulum is dissected free. If there is a bilateral defect, the decision as to whether to resect or not is based on the amount of functional esophageal tissue that will remain following resection. The esophagus is isolated, packed off, and occluded above and below the defect with Masters intestinal forceps.* The pouch is partially resected, being sure to leave enough tissue to suture the esophagus closed without compromising the lumen. The esophageal tissue is closed in two layers.

Esophageal Neoplasia

Neoplasms of the esophagus of the dog and cat are rare in the United States except in areas where the parasite *Spirocerca lupi* is endemic.[23, 34, 37, 38, 82, 97, 112, 149, 175, 182, 186] In a necropsy study of 5,854 canine neoplasms, only 19 involved the esophagus. Metastatic esophageal neoplasms are more common than primary tumors in the dog.[149] In one study of cats, 11 of 74 neoplasms included the esophagus,[166] although a higher incidence has been reported in Britain.[37, 38, 112] The primary tumor types identified are leiomyoma, squamous cell carcinoma, and fibrosarcoma.

Spirocerca lupi and associated esophageal tumors have been reported from many different countries, and several areas of the United States.[97] *Spirocerca lupi* is a nematode parasite. Eggs are found in canine feces and ingested by copraphageous beetles where they encyst. The dog may become infected by eating the beetle or a host that has ingested the beetle. The larvae penetrate the stomach wall and pass to the upper thoracic aorta where the majority migrate to the esophagus, producing nodules containing the adult worms, which may become large and protrude into the esophagus. These granulomas may undergo neoplastic transformation to osteogenic sarcoma or fibrosarcoma in the dog.[169] The diagnosis of *Spirocerca lupi* infestation is made by finding the eggs in the feces or vomitus, but the parasite must have established communication with the lumen of the esophagus before this can occur.[69, 169] If the adult worms are dead or have not penetrated the lumen, *Spirocerca lupi* appears as an esophageal mass.[7, 34, 69, 169, 182]

The predominant clinical signs of esophageal neoplasia are regurgitation, dysphagia, and weight loss, the classic signs of obstructive esophageal disease. The obstruction may result from protrusion of a large mass into the lumen, compression of the esophagus by a large external mass, or stricture of the esophagus due to intramural disease.

Often the mass develops slowly, allowing the esophagus to accommodate to the tumor encroachment; an animal showing clinical signs may improve, with later recurrence of signs. The degree of regurgitation depends on the extent of lumen obstruction. The dog may show progressive inability to swallow solid, semisolid, or liquid food as the tumor increases in size. Respiratory distress and cough or aspiration pneumonia are seen if pulmonary metastases are present.[7, 23, 34, 37, 38, 69, 79, 82, 97, 112, 142, 149, 166, 171, 182]

Radiographic contrast studies usually delineate a filling defect in the esophagus. Endoscopy may also be useful in demonstrating esophageal stenosis and permitting biopsy of a mass lesion. Care must be taken to obtain a deep enough sample of the mass to be diagnostic.[69, 112] If an esophageal mass is present, feces should be checked for *Spirocerca lupi* eggs. Because the incidence of metastatic tumors of the esophagus is higher than that of primary tumors, the patient should be closely examined for primary disease.[112, 149] Leiomyomas occur in the esophagus of the dogs but are usually asymptomatic.[82, 112, 149]

Treatment of a primary esophageal neoplasm is resection of the mass and reconstruction of the esophagus.[23, 69, 82, 112] If the mass is metastatic, treatment is dictated by the primary tumor. Usually, esophageal neoplasms are large by the time of diagnosis and require extensive resection: gastric mobilization is often necessary to reconstruct the esophagus. The results of surgical excision depend on the degree of involvement of the esophagus and adnexal tissue by the primary mass and on whether there are metastases. The best results have been obtained when the mass could be excised without having to resect the esophagus,[34, 69, 79] such as for uncomplicated *Spirocerca lupi* nodules.[34] One report of resection of a fibrosarcoma resulted in recurrence of the mass ten weeks postoperatively.[69] Results of surgical excision in the dog are not good.[34, 69, 79, 82, 97, 112, 142, 149, 166, 182]

---

*Masters Intestinal Forceps, Codman Company, MA.

Miscellaneous Esophageal Obstruction

Esophageal obstruction by an intramural hematoma has been reported in a dog. The condition was presented as a possible neoplasm, and the diagnosis was made at necropsy.[183]

Periesophageal lesions may also produce signs of esophageal obstruction and must be considered in differential diagnosis. Cervical abscess, carotid body tumor, thymic lymphosarcoma, and bronchial nodes enlarged by infection or neoplasia can produce partial esophageal obstruction.[112] Chronic papillomatous esophagitis has been reported in a cat.[196]

Esophageal Stricture

Esophageal stricture in the dog and cat is not common. Congenital esophageal stricture is extremely rare: one case has been reported in a 3½-week-old Boston terrier.[158] There is some question about whether this represented a congenital stricture, as the pup had been ingesting liquids normally just prior to presentation.

Corrosive esophageal strictures have been reported in dogs but are rare.[8, 126, 131] Caustic strictures are usually the result of ingestion of caustic medications for treatment of other medical conditions.[8, 126, 185] However, malicious feeding of caustic substances to animals can occur.

Acquired esophageal stricture resulting from foreign bodies, esophageal trauma, or esophageal surgery does occur but is not as common as previously suggested.[8, 82, 93, 170] The incidence of postoperative stricture following experimental and clinical esophageal surgery in dogs and cats is low, with the exception of a higher incidence of stricture following surgical resection and anastomosis in animals with esophagitis stricture. This type of stricture, also referred to as ulcerative esophagitis or reflux esophagitis with stricture,[70, 93, 126, 135] is believed to occur secondary to gastric reflux,[64, 69, 72, 135, 198] which produces epithelial erosion resulting in ulceration with subsequent stricture. The deeper the inflammation into the esophageal wall, the more severe the stricture. The reflux is often related to an anesthetic period and results are seen within one to eight weeks. The incidence of acquired stricture cannot be correlated with any specific factor such as use of atropine, position of the animal during anesthesia, manipulation of the abdomen, or use of an esophageal stethoscope or endotracheal tube, although all of these factors have been suggested as predisposing causes of reflux.[70, 72, 126, 137, 198]

The effects on the esophagus of reflux may be intensified during anesthesia by absence of the swallowing reflexes and suppression of secondary peristalsis.[135, 198] Some animals have a history of vomiting immediately following recovery from anesthesia.[135] Pooling of gastric contents in the thoracic inlet may also help to concentrate the effect of reflux in the area, and in many cases of postanesthetic stricture there are lesions in this region.[69, 72, 93, 126, 135] Other cases have been reported in which the area of stricture involved was not confined to the thoracic inlet.[135] The location of the lesion could be influenced by the position of the animal during anesthesia.[126, 135]

Postanesthetic esophagitis and stricture is basically a corrosive type of esophagitis that differs only in that the esophageal epithelium is destroyed by gastric acid and enzymes rather than by an external chemical substance. Given the frequency of anesthesia use in dogs and cats, the incidence of this condition is low.

The major clinical sign of acquired esophageal stricture is frequent dysphagia and regurgitation manifested by decreasing ability to eat solid food. During the first or second day after anesthesia, the dog may appear depressed and lethargic and show some discomfort and a mild fever or may be clinically normal. Aspiration pneumonia may develop, with cough and dyspnea. Progressive weight loss occurs as the inability to swallow and retain food becomes worse. Some animals are depressed and drool excessively, and others regurgitate but are otherwise normal. There may be frequent attempts to clear the pharynx of accumulated fluid.[72, 82, 126, 131, 135]

The diagnosis is made by barium contrast radiography and endoscopy. A barium swallow demonstrates segmental narrowing of the esophageal lumen. Barium contrast studies are necessary to determine the length of the stricture and usually require fluoroscopy.

Endoscopy allows diagnosis of the stricture and evaluation of the appearance and pliability of the esophageal wall. The endoscope is often too large to pass through the strictured area, so the length of the stricture cannot be determined.[70, 72, 93, 126, 135]

Esophageal stricture may be surgically treated by increasing the size of the lumen by reconstructive procedures, such as patch grafting, by resection, or by bougienage. The last-named technique offers the most satisfactory results.[69, 126, 135] Short esophageal strictures in the cervical regions (2–3 cm) can be excised with slight risk. Resection and anastomosis of a lesion located in the thoracic region or more than 3 cm in length are more difficult and may require use of suture line reinforcement or esophageal substitution techniques. Patch grafting techniques have been successful in the cervical region of the dog.[93] The cervical esophagus has been reconstructed with inverse tube graft of skin in a dog for treatment of a corrosive stricture.[109]

Conservative Treatment of Acquired Esophageal Stricture

Colin E. Harvey

Treatment by dilating the esophagus at the strictured area (bougienage) can be used as an alternative to surgery. For success with this method, it is essential to recognize that the dilation of a stricture inevitably causes further damage to the esophageal wall. Satisfactory healing occurs only if the epithelium is allowed to heal before the inflammatory response reforms the stricture. This can be achieved by two methods: repeated dilation (weekly or bi-weekly for as long as three months, with each dilation episode requiring sedation or anesthesia) or use of a lathyrogenic agent to slow collagen formation as the epithelium is healing. The most common drug used is prednisolone or another anti-inflammatory corticosteroid, although more specific lathyrogenic agents such as beta-aminoproprionitrile are currently under investigation.[22, 40] The agent must be used for at least four weeks to reduce the likelihood of stricture recurrence.[40]

Advantages of this method of treatment are that thoracotomy and esophageal surgery are avoided and that the method can be used for strictures involving a considerable length of the esophagus and not amenable to treatment by simple esophageal surgical techniques. Disadvantages are the need for special equipment to treat the range of esophageal sizes met in cats and dogs and the need for repeated treatment in some patients.

The esophagus can be dilated by any long, semirigid, blunt-tipped object of the correct size. For strictures in the cervical esophagus, endotracheal tubes are useful because they are often available in a range of sizes. Rigid esophagoscopes have been used but are likely to damage the esophagus further unless used gently and under direct vision. The ideal instruments are esophageal dilators (bougies), either steel stem or mercury-filled rubber, ranging in gauge up to 60 French.

The animal is anesthetized and placed in left lateral recumbency. The strictured area is examined through an esophagoscope, and any food or mucus accumulating there is removed. Lubricated dilators of gradually increasing diameter are passed gently through the stricture until the fit is too tight to permit passage. The esophageal diameter is enlarged by application of gradually increasing pressure while a tight-fitting dilator is slowly rotated. There are no clear guidelines as to how much a particular strictured area can be enlarged. As a rule of thumb, I force through a dilator one size larger than the one that could not be passed initially, although the esophagus should be examined for signs of tearing before a larger dilator is applied. Cats and small dogs manage well with an esophageal diameter of 1 cm or a little less if diet is restricted to soft or slurried foods. A minimum esophageal diameter of 1 to 1.5 cm should be aimed for in medium-sized or large dogs.

Prednisolone should be given (0.5 mg/kg daily by mouth initially, reducing to 0.2 mg/kg daily after 1 or 2 weeks) for four to six weeks. Beta-aminoproprionitrile cannot be recommended for use in clinical patients until more information is available from toxicologic and effective-dose studies.

Patients that are kept on a permanent diet of slurried or soft food develop periodontal disease much more readily than those on a varied-consistency or dry diet. Tooth brushing or another effective plaque control system is recommended.

Conservative treatment has been used with good results in 75 per cent or more of dogs and cats treated,[64, 72, 126, 135] compared with improvement in less than 50 per cent of animals treated surgically.[64, 72, 135]

Esophageal Resection and Anastomosis

Strictures following resection and anastomosis for postanesthetic stricture are more common than those following esophageal surgery for other causes, perhaps owing to incomplete excision of the diseased esophageal tissue or to tension on the suture line. If, following resection, the defect is too large to close by anastomosis without excess tension, a tension-relieving, esophageal reinforcement, or esophageal substitution procedure should be done. The surgeon should decide whether the lesion is operable before resection and, if it is not, should use other means of therapy.

The esophageal lesion is approached as previously described, evaluated, dissected free, and packed off. Masters clamps are placed above and below the area to be resected. The lesion is resected, and the ends of the esophagus are approximated as described earlier. Tension-relieving myotomy or suture line reinforcement is used if necessary. The surgical site is lavaged and then closed. I prefer to place a feeding gastrostomy tube during this period. Oral feeding is withheld for seven postoperative days.

Vascular Ring Anomalies

Vascular rings are congenital malformations of the embryonic aortic arch system resulting in entrapment and constriction of the esophagus by the ligamentum or ductus arteriosus, trachea, and great vessels.[18, 82, 112, 113, 184, 199] The condition occurs in dogs and cats[113, 126] and usually results from the persistence of the right fourth aortic arch instead of the left fourth arch.[126] Normally, the left fourth arch and the dorsal aortic root persist to form the permanent aortic arch, with the left sixth arch becoming the ductus arteriosus, and the right fourth arch forms part of the right subclavian artery. This arrangement normally places the aortic arch, the ductus, and the pulmonary artery to the left of the esophagus.[18, 112, 200] The most common anomaly is a right aortic arch, which results from the formation of the aortic arch from the right fourth arch and the right dorsal aortic root and the ductus formed from the left sixth arch. The esophagus is thus encircled by the ligamentum or patent ductus on the left, the base of the heart and pulmonary artery ventrally, and the aortic arch on the right.[18, 112, 184] Variations of this basic pattern of right aortic arch and left ligamentum include obliterated left subclavian artery originating cranial to the left ligamentum, and left subclavian artery arising from the brachiocephalic trunk. Other basic malformations that are less common include double aortic arch, and left aortic arch with right ductus arteriosus.[18, 19, 112, 184]

All of these malformations result in dilation of the esophagus cranial to the site of stenosis.

Esophageal deviation in four English bulldogs resulting in gastrointestinal and respiratory signs has been reported. The cause of the deviation was thought to be vascular compression of the esophagus at the level of the first and second ribs. The vascular anatomy was normal, but compression of the esophagus was demonstrated by thoracotomy in two of the dogs. The deviation and signs were corrected in two of the dogs by transecting the left subclavian artery and anastomosing it to the internal thoracic artery. There was no abnormal esophageal dilation in any of these animals.[199]

Stenosis produced by esophageal entrapment results in esophageal dilation cranial to the base of the heart. The dilation may become very large and resembles a diverticulum in appearance. It generally does not regress after separation of the constricting vessels, as demonstrated in dogs followed for up to three years after surgery.[18, 57, 126] The dilated segment of esophagus does not demonstrate normal peristaltic contraction on fluoroscopic contrast examination; myenteric ganglion cells are decreased in the dilated portion of the esophagus compared with the same region in normal dogs.[28] The esophagus continues to show a lack of normal motility in the dilated portion following separation of the obstructing vascular ring, even though there is clinical improvement.[18, 82, 112] Occasionally in a vascular ring anomaly, the esophagus is dilated along its entire length, possibly because of idiopathic megaesophagus in addition.[18, 82, 112, 126] These cases respond less well to vascular ring separation than uncomplicated vascular ring anomaly. Treatment by vascular ring separation combined with cardioplasty may give better results.

Use of dilating esophagoplasty of the stenosed area of the esophagus resulted in elimination of the esophageal dilation in two dogs.[57] Resection or enfolding of the dilated cranial esophagus does not produce better results than separation of the vascular ring alone.

Patent ductus arteriosus as part of the constricting ring occurs frequently enough that the surgeon should assume that the ligamentum is patent and take appropriate action.[18, 112, 118, 126, 170, 189] Regurgitation is usually first seen at weaning. The regurgitation initially occurs soon after ingestion, but as the cranial esophagus dilates, regurgitation occurs later. There may also be secondary respiratory signs such as coughing and dyspnea as the result of aspiration pneumonia. Most animals are thin or emaciated, depending upon the degree of obstruction.[18, 19, 112, 126, 172] The thoracic inlet and caudal neck area bulge when the chest is compressed. This sign indicates esophageal dilation and is seen in vascular ring anomalies as well as generalized esophageal dilation.

Barium swallow demonstrating stenosis of the esophagus at the base of the heart confirms the diagnosis (Fig. 48–4). Esophageal function distal to the heart is usually normal. Angiography may be helpful[189] but generally is not necessary for diagnosis.

Treatment of a vascular ring anomaly is to free the esophagus from the vessels and ligament trapping it, making sure that all the constricting connective tissue is separated to completely free the esophagus. The longer the obstruction persists, the greater the degree of dilation. It appears that the greater the duration of dilation, the more ganglion cells in the esophageal wall are lost.[28] Thus, early surgical intervention is advised.

The vascular ring is approached by a left fourth intercostal incision (Fig. 48–5A). The mediastinum is dissected carefully from the stenosed area of the esophagus. Hemorrhage is controlled. The ligament is exposed and undermined (Fig. 48–5B), and two silk ligatures are passed under the ligament and tied to control bleeding if the ligament is patent (Fig. 48–5C). The ligament is divided. Usually, additional connective tissue beneath the ligament constricts the esophagus (Fig. 48–5D) and must be dissected away so that the esophagus can expand (Fig. 48–5E). The thoracotomy incision is closed. Postoperatively, the dog is fed gruel and water within 24 hours and should be on full feed by the third postoperative day. Antibiotics are given if aspiration pneumonia is present. Dogs with a moderate to severe dilation require careful diet regulation, including feeding in an elevated position if regurgitation persists.

Esophageal Diseases with Leakage

Esophageal Perforation and Laceration

Esophageal perforation and laceration may occur as sequelae of chronic foreign body obstruction and its removal or of ingestion of a sharp foreign body with or without obstructive signs.[54, 80, 82, 156] Direct penetrating cervical or thoracic trauma or cervical bite wounds may also result in esophageal perforation or lacerations. Perforation of the esophagus may also result from endoscopic examination.[105, 112, 156] Lacerations of the esophagus may be of considerable length.

With esophageal perforation, saliva and food escape into the adnexal tissues, resulting in contamination with subsequent infection, the extent of which is determined by the size of the defect, the duration of leakage, and the condition of the tissues. Small (6 mm) perforations made in the distal esophagus of normal dogs rarely cause infection.[13, 105] Clinical perforations may be larger or may be surrounded by areas of inflamed, damaged, or necrotic tissue, and more likely to produce infection.[54, 138]

Perforation of the thoracic esophagus may result in pleuritis, mediastinitis, or mediastinal abscess. Perforation of the cervical esophagus may give rise to cervical cellulitis or abscess as well as extension through the fascial planes into the mediastinum, resulting in mediastinitis.[80, 112, 132, 133, 148] The signs of infection due to perforation may mask the primary signs of esophageal obstruction.[54, 138]

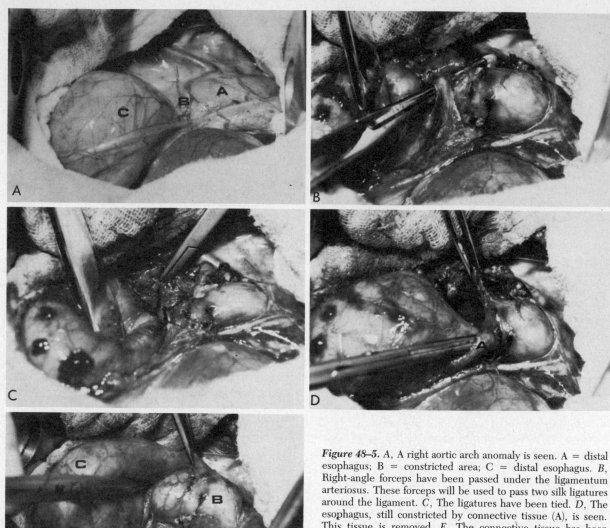

Figure 48–5. *A,* A right aortic arch anomaly is seen. A = distal esophagus; B = constricted area; C = distal esophagus. *B,* Right-angle forceps have been passed under the ligamentum arteriosus. These forceps will be used to pass two silk ligatures around the ligament. *C,* The ligatures have been tied. *D,* The esophagus, still constricted by connective tissue (A), is seen. This tissue is removed. *E,* The connective tissue has been dissected from the constricted area. Note that the esophagus distal to the ligament (B) is of normal diameter, whereas the esophagus cranial to the ligament (C) is dilated.

The clinician should strongly suspect esophageal perforation when a patient has signs suggestive of esophageal obstruction and exhibits fever, elevated WBC count, cough, dyspnea, or cervical soft tissue swelling and heat.[54, 80, 82, 130, 138, 156]

The diagnosis of esophageal perforation is confirmed by esophagoscopy or by demonstration on contrast studies of a leak in the esophagus. The use of contrast material allows assessment of the size of the defect. Barium should be used only if any perforation that is observed will be surgically explored. Iodine-based contrast media provide less radiographic contrast but are rapidly absorbed if they leak into adjacent soft tissues.[101, 181]

Leaking esophageal perforations should be surgically repaired.[73, 82, 123, 130, 132] If there is no demonstrable leakage, conservative medical therapy, con-

sisting of antibiotic administration and withholding of oral fluids for three to five days, may be used.

The use of a pharyngostomy tube has also been suggested[156] but in my experience is contraindicated, as it interferes with healing of the esophageal suture line or perforation.[86]

Acute esophageal perforation or laceration of the esophagus may be repaired with a two-layer closure. Necrotic and severely damaged tissue should be debrided. If the lesion is of more than 12 hours' duration, if there is infection in the area, or if the suture line is likely to be under tension, it may be reinforced. Patch grafting techniques may be used if debridement will compromise lumen size. In severe cases, it may be necessary to resect and anastomose the esophagus, using tension-relieving techniques when indicated.

Perforation or laceration of the cervical esophagus with leakage and infection may be treated by establishing cervical drainage, controlling the infection, and repairing the injury two to three days later. The surgeon must be careful to prevent spread of infection through the fascial planes to the mediastinum.

Esophageal Fistula

Esophageal fistula is the result of chronic leakage through the esophageal wall. The cause of the defect is usually traumatic perforation or laceration, usually by foreign bodies, but may be secondary to esophageal surgery.[10, 24, 45, 138, 181] Congenital esophageal atresia and tracheoesophageal fistula have not been reported in the dog or cat. Whether the fistula occurs into the trachea or the bronchus depends on where the perforation occurs.[10, 137] The majority of esophageal foreign bodies occur in the distal esophagus.[138] Bronchoesophageal fistula is more common than tracheoesophageal fistula in the dog,[13, 24] usually occurring between the esophagus and the right diaphragmatic lung lobe. In the cat, bronchoesophageal fistulas have been reported in the accessory lobe and the left diaphragmatic lobe.[149] Epiphrenic diverticula may be of congenital origin and are occasionally associated with bronchoesophageal fistulas.[10, 45, 137]

The communication of the pulmonary system with the esophagus results in aspiration of esophageal or gastric contents into the lung, causing pneumonia, although some animals tolerate the fistula for considerable periods.[24, 137, 181] Other complications are septicemia, lung abscess, and abdominal distension.[24, 181]

Cutaneous esophageal fistula occurs occasionally in the dog or cat. Clinical signs such as coughing and respiratory distress may not be seen until a foreign body is removed.[53] Most animals with esophageal fistula and cough after ingestion of liquid.[10, 24, 137, 181]

Diagnosis is made by radiographic evaluation or esophagoscopy. A foreign body is sometimes present.[137] Radiographic signs may vary from slight pulmonary interstitial infiltration suggestive of mild aspiration pneumonia to patchy consolidation of the lungs. Pleural thickening or fluid accumulation may be present. Contrast studies are necessary to demonstrate the communication between the esophagus and airway.[24, 137]

Treatment by ligation or closure from within the esophageal lumen is not likely to be successful. Best results are obtained by surgically separating the esophagus and involved lobe or trachea and closing the defect. If a foreign body is still present, an esophagotomy is performed and the foreign body is removed.[24] The esophagotomy incision may incorporate the esophageal defect, which is then debrided and closed as for an esophagotomy. If the fistula is associated with an epiphrenic diverticulum, the diverticulum must also be treated. If the lung is involved, it is best resected.[24] A major complication during surgery is accumulation of anesthetic gas in the stomach secondary to the positive-pressure ventilation if the fistula is located caudal to the end of the endotracheal tube. This complication is prevented by gastrostomy or endobronchial intubation.[45] Postoperative management is as for esophagotomy.

Primary Neuromuscular Disease of the Esophagus

Swallowing is a series of coordinated, precisely timed reflex contractions and relaxations of the pharynx and esophagus that result in the transport of a bolus from the mouth to the stomach.[192] It may also be defined as the synchronous passage of a bolus from the mouth to the stomach.[58, 115] Swallowing may be divided into three primary stages: oral-pharyngeal, esophageal, and gastroesophageal. These three stages are interrelated and necessary for normal swallowing. A bolus is necessary for the propagation of a peristaltic contraction through the cervical esophagus.[102, 103, 115] Diffuse esophageal spasm and caudal esophageal sphincter dysfunction may produce dysphagia in humans.[75]

The oral-pharyngeal stage may be divided into 3 phases. The oral phase includes prehension of food and collection of the bolus at the base of the tongue (Fig. 48–6A); during this phase, the pharynx contains air and is relaxed. The second phase consists of the peristaltic contraction of the pharynx and the propulsion of the bolus to the laryngopharynx (Fig. 48–6B); this is accomplished by a series of very rapid, progressive, well-synchronized reflex movements of the tongue, palatopharyngeal arch, epiglottis, larynx, and hyoid apparatus. In the third phase, the peristaltic contraction of the pharynx is synchronized with momentary opening of the cricopharyngeal sphincter, allowing the bolus to pass directly into the esophagus (Fig. 48–6C). The size of the sphincter opening varies with the size and consistency of the bolus. The third phase is ended when the cricopharyngeal sphincter closes and the pharynx relaxes[191, 192] (Fig. 48–6D).

The esophageal stage of swallowing begins when the bolus enters the esophagus. The passage of the bolus into the cervical esophagus initiates a primary peristaltic contraction that carries the bolus to the gastroesophageal junction, where the caudal esophageal sphincter (CES) is located. As a bolus enters the esophagus, (1) it may initiate a primary peristaltic contraction that carries it to the CES, (2) the bolus may remain in the proximal esophagus until two or three more swallows occur and the combined bolus is carried by a primary peristaltic contraction, (3) the bolus may pause temporarily in the esophagus until it stimulates a secondary peristaltic contraction, or (4) two or three boluses may accumulate before a secondary peristaltic contraction is initiated.[115, 192] Two types of progressive peristaltic contractions therefore normally occur in the esophagus, a primary wave initiated by a swallow, and a secondary wave

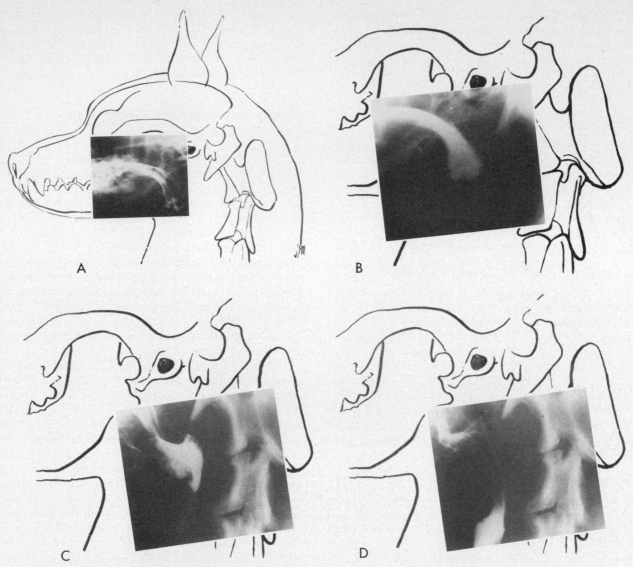

Figure 48–6. The stages of the oral-pharyngeal stage of swallowing. *A*, The oral phase is demonstrated. The bolus is in the mouth, and the tongue is pushing it into the pharynx. *B*, The bolus has accumulated in the pharynx, and the cricopharyngeal sphincter is open. *C*, The bolus is passing through the cricopharyngeal sphincter, which is beginning to close. *D*, The bolus is in the cranial esophagus. The cricopharyngeal sphincter has closed.

initiated by a bolus in the esophagus. The reflexes appear identical on manometric examination.[58, 82, 102, 115, 192]

The gastroesophageal stage follows the esophageal stage and consists of the passage of the bolus through the CES at the gastroesophageal junction.

Figure 48–7 is a manometric tracing of a primary peristaltic contraction initiated by a bolus. The measurements were made with a triple-lumen catheter with the ports 5 cm apart. Three separate waves represent progression of the bolus. The waves are progressive and are synchronous as they progress. A secondary peristaltic contraction would look identical. This tracing represents the esophageal stage of swallowing.

Figure 48–8 represents the gastroesophageal stage of swallowing. The triple-lumen catheter is positioned so the first port *(C)* is in the stomach, the second *(B)* in the CES, and the third *(A)* in the distal esophagus.

This tracing demonstrates the synchronous action of the esophagus, CES, and distal esophagus as a peristaltic contraction passes through the gastroesophageal junction. At the time the bolus is in the distal esophagus *(A)*, the CES *(B)* has already relaxed and opened to allow the bolus to enter the stomach without delay. The CES *(B)* then contracts after the bolus passes through it to prevent reflux of gastric contents. After contracting, the CES returns to a resting pressure, which prevents gastric reflux.[58, 75, 102, 103, 115, 157]

The oral-pharyngeal, esophageal, and gastroesophageal stages of swallowing are integrated synchronous functions that depend on one another. A defect in any portion of these integrated functions, from interruption of prehension, passage of food through the oral pharynx, failure of progressive peristalsis, or failure of receptive relaxation of the CES, results in esophageal disease.[75, 82, 115, 157]

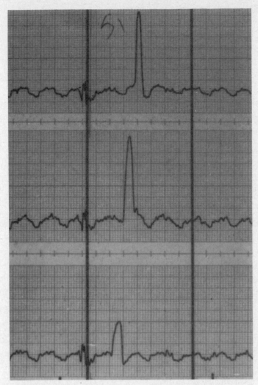

Figure 48–7. A primary peristaltic wave is demonstrated manometrically as it passes down the esophagus. Note that the swallow is progressive. The top tracing is closest to the mouth, and the bottom to the stomach.

Oral-Pharyngeal Stage Swallowing Disorders

These conditions have been reported in dogs but not in cats. Because of the rapidity with which a bolus passes through the oral-pharyngeal stage, dysphagia must be evaluated by cineradiography or cinefluoroscopy to determine which phase is involved. The veterinarian should be able to differentiate clinically an oral-pharyngeal problem from an esophageal or gastroesophageal problem but will not be able to determine what phase is involved without functional studies.[162, 178]

Oral-pharyngeal dysphagia can result from malfunction of any of the swallowing reflex nerves (V, VII, IX, X, XII), their nuclei, the swallowing center, or the structures involved in swallowing. The disorders may be functional or structural. They may be primary, such as cricopharyngeal achalasia, or secondary to other disease processes, such as cerebral trauma.

Neurologic, neuromuscular, and muscular diseases manifest themselves as functional disorders resulting in failure, spasticity, or incoordination of the muscular contractions necessary to produce synchronous esophageal function.[162, 178, 191]

Structural changes that interfere with oral and pharyngeal stages of swallowing are discussed in Chapter 46. The clinical signs of oral phase disorders

result from the inability to prehend food, to form a bolus, or to force the bolus into the pharynx. The dog may exhibit difficulty in lapping water, may lose food from the mouth because of decreased tongue movement, or may chew excessively. Movements to help force the food into the pharynx, such as tilting the head backwards, are common. Cinefluorographic signs of oral phase dysphagia are decreased plunger action of the tongue, resulting in deficient bolus formation, and retention of contrast material in the oropharynx.[147, 148, 162, 191]

The clinical and cinefluorographic signs of pharyngeal phase dysphagia are less consistent and more difficult to interpret. The most common finding is coughing with repeated attempts to swallow and aspiration pneumonia. The dog may spit out masticated food, or food may be misdirected into the nasopharynx, resulting in regurgitation two to 2½ hours after eating.[162, 178, 191] Regurgitation occurred in all cases.[178] Pharyngeal phase disorders are slowly progressive; compensatory modification of eating habits, as seen with oral phase disorders, is not common.[178, 191] Cinefluorographic study demonstrated that when the peristaltic contraction was induced, it progressed from the rostral to the caudal pharynx

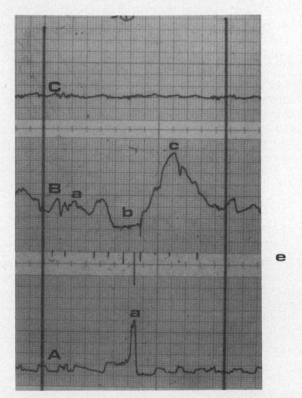

Figure 48–8. A primary peristaltic contraction is demonstrated as it passes through the CES. Note that the resting pressure of the CES (*Ba*) is higher than the gastric pressure (*C*). The CES (*B*) is located 5 cm closer to the stomach than the distal esophageal post (*A*). Therefore the CES (*B*) has relaxed (*b*) to admit a bolus, before the esophageal peristalic wave (*Aa*) has reached it. After the bolus (*Aa*) has entered the esophagus, the CES contracts (*Bc*) to prevent reflux of gastric contents.

more slowly. Contrast medium was retained in the intrapharyngeal opening and piriform recess, and there was aspiration of contrast, although cricopharyngeal sphincter function was normal. Primary esophageal peristaltic waves may not form normally.[162]

Cricopharyngeal phase dysphagia varies in its clinical signs, depending upon whether there is complete failure of relaxation of the cricopharyngeal sphincter or incoordination between the cricopharyngeal sphincter and pharyngeal contractions; the latter is more common.[162, 178, 190, 191] Cricopharyngeal dysphagia has been referred to as cricopharyngeal achalasia.[61, 144, 154, 161, 162, 178] The cause of this failure of normal relaxation of the cricopharyngeal muscles has not been identified,[144, 154, 178] although hypertrophy and neurogenic atrophy of the cricopharyngeus muscle have been suggested.

Dogs with cricopharyngeal dysphagia have a history of persistent dysphagia usually since weaning, although the disease has also been reported in a ten-year-old dog.[154, 190] Expulsion of food from the mouth by forward movement of the tongue with repeated re-eating of the food that is lost, frequent coughing and gagging, and some nasal reflux are seen.[61, 154, 190, 191] The signs of cricopharyngeal dysphagia and pharyngeal dysphagia are very similar and must be differentiated radiographically.[144, 162]

Cineradiography or fluorography demonstrates either a consistent failure of opening of the cricopharyngeal sphincter with forceful pharyngeal contractions[144, 162, 178, 190, 191] or a lack of synchronization between pharyngeal contraction and the sphincter. Some of the bolus reaches the esophagus but the rest is retained in the pharynx. The result of both types of cricopharyngeal dysphagia is aspiration of the retained bolus with subsequent coughing.[178, 190] Failure of sphincter relaxation is seen as a dorsal indentation of the bolus as it passes through the sphincter.[144, 162, 191]

The treatment of choice for cricopharyngeal phase dysphagia is cricopharyngeal myotomy.[162, 178] However, cricopharyngeal myotomy was not of value in oral stage dysphagia and it makes pharyngeal phase dysphagia worse by producing cricopharyngeal chalasia.[162, 178, 191] Oral phase and pharyngeal phase dysphagias should be treated by first treating or eliminating any underlying disease. Dietary management may be attempted by altering the consistency of foods and feeding the dog in an elevated position. Elevated feeding seems to be helpful with oral phase dysphagia. Feeding by stomach tube or feeding gastrostomy are other methods that could be used until any underlying disease is treated.[162, 178, 191]

In humans, cricopharyngeal myotomy is successful as treatment for any type of oral-pharyngeal dysphagia.[3, 51, 95, 119, 195] This is not so in the dog, probably because of differences in posture and eating habits. Cricopharyngeal myotomy could be considered as a salvage procedure for oral-pharyngeal stage dysphagias that do not respond to conservative forms of therapy.

Cricopharyngeal Myotomy

The esophagus is approached by a ventral cervical incision cranial to the larynx and extending caudally 8 cm. The incision should extend above the hyoid venous arch. The sternohyoideus muscles are separated on the midline to expose the trachea and cricothyroideus muscles (Fig. 48–9A). The larynx is grasped and rotated 180 degrees, exposing the dorsal aspect of the larynx (Fig. 48–9B). Connective tissue is dissected, exposing the cricopharyngeus and thyropharyngeus muscles (Fig. 48–9C). The median raphe between the cricopharyngeus muscles is incised to the submucosa (Fig. 48–9D), beginning caudally on the esophagus and continuing cranially to the level of thyropharyngeus muscles. Care is taken not to perforate the esophageal or pharyngeal mucosa; if perforation occurs, the defect is closed with a simple interrupted suture. The larynx is returned to its normal position, and the sternohyoid muscles are apposed with simple interrupted sutures. The skin is closed. The dog may be fed a soft diet and given water the first day if the mucosa was not penetrated. If the mucosa was penetrated, oral intake should be withheld for 72 hours.[61, 144, 154, 168]

Primary Esophageal and Gastroesophageal Stage Swallowing Disorders

Most primary neuromuscular disorders of the second or third stage of swallowing involve both stages either primarily or secondarily.[88, 190]

The most common neuromuscular swallowing disorders of the esophageal and gastroesophageal stages are acquired achalasia (AA) and idiopathic megaesophagus (IME). These have been referred to as cardiospasm, congenital achalasia, esophageal hypomotility, congenital megaesophagus, acquired megaesophagus, acquired esophageal hypomotility, and esophageal dilation.[190] Some of the confusion in the veterinary literature arises from attempts in the past to correlate these conditions with the human disease known as achalasia. Confusion has also been produced by the failure of early investigators[25, 32, 44, 71, 89, 90, 91, 154, 167] to recognize that there are two distinct disease entities in the dog. Many of the early veterinary reports grouped these two conditions together, so there are marked differences in data interpretation in all aspects of the diseases.

The final factor contributing to the confusion of primary neuromuscular esophageal disease interpretation in dogs and cats is a lack of sufficient hard data upon which to make assumptions. There have been manometric and radiographic studies of normal canine swallowing.[58, 157, 190–192] There are a few published results of manometric findings in dogs with idiopathic megaesophagus.[43, 44, 48, 89, 152, 176] These studies are simplistic, however, and do not address the complexity of second and third stages of swallowing, especially as it relates to normal components of CES functions.[58]

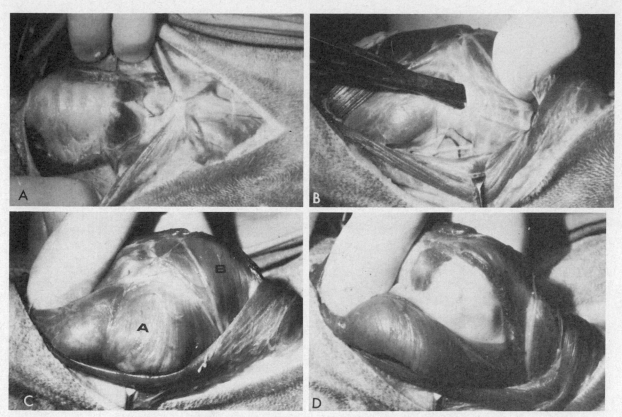

Figure 48–9. Cricopharyngeal myotomy. *A,* The sternohyoideus muscles have been separated. The larynx is seen. *B,* The larynx has been rotated 180 degrees, and the connective tissue is being removed from the dorsal aspect of the larynx. *C,* The cricopharyngeus (A) and thyropharyngeus (B) muscles have been exposed. *D,* The cricopharyngeus muscles have been incised in the median raphe, and the submucosa is seen.

The only report of manometric studies of acquired achalasia in the dog assessed only whether the sphincter responds to a swallow, not whether all the functional components of the CES are normal.[152] Radiographic studies have been reported for idiopathic megaesophagus[48, 190, 191, 192] and acquired achalasia.[88, 192] These studies indicate that the conditions often can show similar signs on fluoroscopic studies. Until there are more complete manometric data accumulated on esophageal body and CES function in idiopathic megaesophagus and acquired achalasia, discussion and characterization of primary esophageal neuromuscular disease must be based upon interpretation of available manometric and radiographic data, clinical characteristics of the disease, response to therapy, and personal experience.

It is my opinion, based on clinical experience and published and unpublished studies, that there are two distinct entities in the dog, which I will refer to as idiopathic megaesophagus (IME) and acquired achalasia (AA).[82, 88, 190, 191] Each entity has its own signs, presentation, biologic behavior, and documented response to therapy.[82, 88, 190, 191] The major clinical difference is the age of onset of signs; dogs with IME regurgitate at or soon after weaning, and dogs with AA do not regurgitate until they are mature.

IME and AA both have the same basic pathophysiologic alterations, a lack of synchronous function of the body of the esophagus and CES resulting in failure of a bolus to be transmitted through the esophagus and CES into the stomach. Figure 48–10 is a manometric recording from a dog with IME. Note that the swallow is not progressive, as it was in Figure 48–7. The rises in pressure at the three different points occurred simultaneously, indicating that a single contraction occurred rather than the progressive peristaltic passage of a bolus. This finding is in agreement with another study.[48] Diamant and colleagues[43, 44] found that the CES resting pressure was not significantly different in dogs with IME and normal dogs. They also reported that all six of their dogs had complete relaxation of the CES associated with a swallow. Rogers and associates[152] reported the same findings in dogs with IME and AA. These studies did not, however, evaluate the normal time sequences that occur between the different phases of esophageal body function and the CES function. Gaynor and co-workers[58] demonstrated a definite time sequence in which the CES was open, the time it took for the CES to open before the bolus arrived, the time it took for the CES to close after a bolus passed through it, as well as pressure variation of the different phases in normal dogs (Fig. 48–11).[142] Dia-

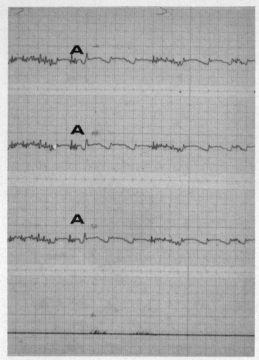

Figure 48–10. Manometric tracing of a dog with IME in the body of the esophagus. Note that there are no progressive peristaltic contractions. The only contraction occurs (A) simultaneously at all three sites.

mant and colleagues[43, 44] and others[152, 162, 172, 190] concluded that because the sphincter resting pressure was normal and the sphincter relaxed, its function was "normal." Earlam and associates[48] reported that in a dog with IME the sphincter had a normal pressure profile but relaxed poorly and infrequently. When the sphincter relaxed it was incomplete because of premature contraction. Fluoroscopically, the sphincter relaxed only three times during a ten-minute period even though the esophagus was full of contrast medium. Another study of IME demon-

strated a normal resting pressure zone that was of shorter length than in normal dogs; fluoroscopically, the CES did not completely relax in the nine dogs studied.[90] A fluoroscopic study of 12 dogs, six with IME and six with AA, demonstrated identical lack of esophageal body and CES relaxation except in two dogs with IME that spontaneously recovered.[84]

Because IME and AA are diseases of asynchronous function of the body of the esophagus and the CES, all phases of sphincter function must be evaluated. Figure 48–12 is a manometric recording of a mature dog with idiopathic megaesophagus. Note that there is no esophageal contraction in association with the CES. Therefore, a bolus has not reached the CES. The CES is showing some relaxation but it is not normal (compare with Fig. 48–8). There is also a lack of the closing contraction seen in the normal esophagus. If a bolus does not reach the CES when it is relaxed, as a result of lack of primary or secondary peristalsis, or if the CES relaxes too soon or too late or its duration of opening is not long enough, the bolus is not able to enter the stomach. The function of the esophageal body and CES must be addressed as a unit to completely evaluate whether it is normal. The fact that dogs with IME and AA regurgitate indicates that the function of the esophagus and CES is not normal. The concept is further borne out by radiographic studies that demonstrated a build-up of a barium column in the diseased esophagus even when the animals were fed with the food dish elevated.[84, 88, 90, 152, 167] Radiographs with the animals in an elevated position demonstrate the narrowed segment of the CES and barium accumulation (Fig. 48–13). If the CES functioned normally, the column of barium would not accumulate, because every time the dog swallows there is a period of 4.38 seconds during which the sphincter is open to allow the barium to empty into the stomach, especially while the dog is elevated.[58] In my experience, numerous swallows may occur while the barium is given and the sphincter remains closed in dogs with either

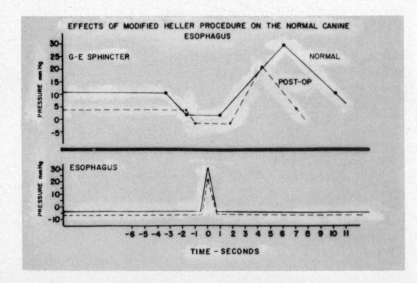

Figure 48–11. Normal swallowing complex and the effects of a modified Heller procedure. Note that there are time sequences between opening, closing, and contracting of the sphincter. Note also that the modified Heller procedure affects time sequence as well as the pressure parameters of the CES.

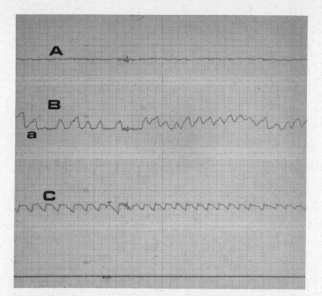

Figure 48–12. A manometric tracing of the stomach (A), CES (B), and distal esophagus (C) in a dog with idiopathic megaesophagus. Note that the esophageal pressure (C) does not change nor does the gastric pressure (A). There are variations in the pressure signs of the CES (B), but never does the pressure reach 0 (a) nor is there a contraction of the CES in relation to the swallow.

disease. Because some dogs with IME recover normal esophageal function, the confusing difference reported in esophageal function could represent different stages of recovery from IME.[82]

The debate as to whether failure of the CES to relax adequately is a function of the failure of primary and secondary peristalsis or is a problem of both body and CES is academic, since the basic element in both IME and AA is failure of coordinated synchronous function of the esophageal (second) and gastroesophageal (third) stages of swallowing.[80, 157, 162, 178, 190, 192]

The etiology of IME has not been identified. Studies in the dog have suggested that the defect producing the esophageal muscle reflex function is not in the motor innervation but rather in the afferent innervation.[63, 176, 177] Diamant and colleagues[43, 44] suggest that the problem in IME is failure of developmental maturity of the innervation or musculature of the esophagus.

Studies of the myenteric ganglia of the esophagus of the dog[25, 89, 90, 159] are not very helpful because the muscle of the esophageal wall is striated; the myenteric ganglia supply the esophageal blood vessels and the functionally unimportant muscularis mucosae. Studies in humans suggest that the primary site of the disease known as achalasia is the dorsal motor nucleus of the vagus. This nucleus innervates the predominantly smooth muscle of the esophagus. The predominantly striated muscle of the canine esophagus receives its motor innervation from the nucleus ambiguous.[27, 177, 190] Two studies in the dog demonstrated a marked reduction of the ganglion cell population in the rostral portion of the nucleus ambiguous but no change in the dorsal motor nucleus.[27] In

ten dogs, experimental bilateral lesions were placed in the rostral portion of the nucleus ambiguous; five dogs regurgitated after every feeding and died of aspiration pneumonia within three to 23 days.[77] Manometric and radiographic studies of the esophagus appeared similar to those reported for IME and AA. The other five dogs did not have any signs of esophageal dysfunction. The degree of disease could be correlated with the degree of damage to the nucleus ambiguous.[77]

Idiopathic Megaesophagus (IME). This is a disease of young dogs that is seen first at weaning but may be noticed earlier. The inherited nature of the disease has been shown in certain breeds, such as wire-haired fox terriers. Other breeds commonly affected are miniature schnauzers and German shepherds. The disease has been seen in many other breeds.[16, 43, 44, 48, 71, 82, 88, 128, 167, 170] Some dogs spontaneously recover.[43, 44, 71, 82, 89, 106, 167]

Dogs with IME have a history of regurgitation that is usually associated with feeding, although if the disease has been present for awhile the regurgitation may occur up to six hours after ingestion of food. In the early stages of the disease the vomitus may consist of a sausage-shaped bolus of undigested food. As the interval between ingestion and regurgitation lengthens, the food becomes fermented and foul-smelling and contains much mucus.[16, 31, 71, 82, 88, 106, 167]

On physical examination, the dog is usually smaller than its littermates and often emaciated. Esophageal dilation can be demonstrated by compression of the chest with the mouth and nares held closed; ballooning of the thoracic inlet, often accompanied by gurgling sounds, is noted. Most dogs have some evidence of aspiration pneumonia.

Plain radiographs demonstrate a markedly dilated esophagus usually containing air or fluid.[190–192] A barium contrast study confirms the presence of dilated esophagus. Barium studies done with fluoros-

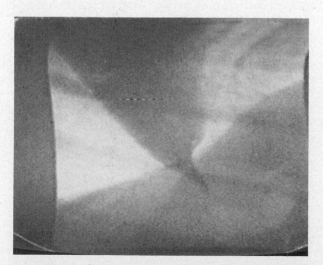

Figure 48–13. A barium contrast study of a dog with IME. The radiograph is a lateral view with the dog elevated. Note the narrowed segment, the unopened CES, and the accumulation of barium within the esophageal lumen.

copy allow the clinician to determine the presence or absence of peristalsis, the type of peristalsis, the frequency and extent of CES relaxation, and whether the esophageal body and CES function are coordinated. Dogs with IME may show a variety of esophageal functional patterns ranging from complete lack of peristalsis with failure of the CES to relax to normal synchronous function.[82, 84] Dogs whose disorder will not respond to conservative treatment continue to show an aperistalic esophagus with asynchronous CES function. Dogs with IME that become clinically normal showed higher-amplitude esophageal contractions, improved frequency of esophageal body motor response to swallowing, and a decrease in the length of the portion of nonfunctioning esophagus.[43, 44] The esophageal functional patterns seen on fluoroscopy with nonresponding IME look identical to those seen with AA, and unless the clinician is aware of the age of onset of the disease, IME in a mature dog cannot be differentiated from acquired achalasia radiographically.[82, 84]

The recommended therapy for the treatment of IME is conservative. Feeding the dog in an elevated position and manipulating the food consistency help prevent aspiration and regurgitation while waiting for spontaneous recovery. Most animals that are going to recover seem to do so by 12 months of age.[43, 44, 82, 106, 167]

One study suggests that a cholinergic anticholinesterase agent may stimulate motor activity.[43] A course of therapy using metoclopramide has been suggested, but there have been no clinical trials.[162] Aspiration pneumonia, if present, should be treated by appropriate therapy and antibiotics.

The modified Heller procedure has not been successful in treating IME.[71, 82, 88, 91, 162] The reason the surgery is effective with AA and not with IME is awaiting investigation. I suggest that we not wait too long with IME before proceeding with surgery in order to allow spontaneous recovery. If a modified Heller procedure were done at three months instead of eight to 12 months in dogs with IME, results might be improved. Because dogs that spontaneously recover from IME regain normal esophageal function, it would be easy to determine whether the surgery was beneficial; the dog with nonresponding IME would show clinical improvement without improvement of esophageal and CES function, and the dog that spontaneously recovers from IME would show normal CES function.

Acquired Achalasia (AA). This disease occurs in the mature dog without previous history of esophageal disease as a pup. Dogs with AA do not recover esophageal function spontaneously. Once present, the esophageal dysfunction remains, even though some clinical improvement can occur with dietary management and surgery.[71, 82, 88, 91]

The primary sign at presentation is regurgitation that occurs at least once a day but usually more frequently. Regurgitation is not always associated with ingestion of food, and frequently may only produce a white foam with mucus. The weight loss and severity of aspiration pneumonia are a function of the frequency and duration of regurgitation, although frequency often varies from week to week.[82, 88] The duration of signs in one study from onset to presentation varied from five months to 18 months; seven of nine dogs were presented within six months of the onset of regurgitation.[88]

On physical examination, the dogs range from being emaciated to being in poor condition. Thoracic inlet bulging can be demonstrated with this disease, as with IME and vascular ring anomaly.[82, 88]

A large dilated esophagus is present on plain films. Fluoroscopic barium studies demonstrate esophageal dilation extending the entire length from the thoracic inlet to the diaphragm. There are no primary or secondary peristaltic contractions, but there may occasionally be a tertiary contraction that is nonprogressive. The lateral projection with the dog's front elevated demonstrates a build-up of a column of barium within the esophagus even with repeated swallows. The narrowed gastroesophageal area, the CES, can be observed (see Fig. 48–25). There may be some passage of small amounts of barium through the CES into the stomach, but most of it remains in the esophagus. When the intraluminal pressure exceeds the pressure of the closed CES and the animal is in an upright position, the esophagus evacuates into the stomach rapidly, as with IME. Evacuation may be hastened by administration of a carbonated beverage. IME and AA may have an identical appearance. The differentiation is based on the age of onset of the disease and its biologic behavior; AA will not regress spontaneously.[82, 88] The functional esophageal defect persists, resulting in continued regurgitation that eventually leads to nutritional problems as well as inhalation pneumonia.[82, 88, 190]

Therapy should be directed at easing the passage of food from the mouth to the stomach. Initially, elevated feeding may be attempted as described for IME.[82, 88, 155] Most dogs with AA are not benefited by elevated feeding.[82, 88] However, it is of value to feed the dog in an elevated position while determining whether the esophageal dysfunction is secondary to some other disease process. Elevated feeding is an attempt to use gravity to force the CES to open sooner than if the dog were in a horizontal position. Ingesta accumulating in the esophagus may result in regurgitation or opening of the CES. Regurgitation results if ingesta accumulation exceeds a certain limit. If the CES resting pressure can be made less competent, the CES will open with less accumulation of ingesta, allowing the food to enter the stomach rather than be regurgitated. However, if the CES is made incompetent, reflux of gastric contents and esophagitis result.[50, 59, 75, 87]

In one study of 11 mature dogs with AA, seven were treated conservatively and four were treated surgically using a modified Heller procedure. Marked clinical improvement occurred in three of the operated dogs. Of the unoperated dogs, five died of the disease and two showed no clinical improvement.[88] In another study of 18 dogs, 11 of which could be interpreted as having AA on the basis of age of onset of regurgitation, seven of 11 mature dogs showed clinical improvement following surgery, two died of disease unrelated to the esophageal problems, and two died as a result of the procedure.[82, 88, 91]

The modified Heller procedure does not eliminate the esophageal dysfunction, in that there is still lack of peristalsis and asynchronous CES function. It does allow the esophagus to empty with a lower intraluminal esophageal pressure and thus reduces the frequency of regurgitation. A postsurgical fluoroscopic study of a dog with AA demonstrated that the intraluminal accumulation of barium was less than before operation; this finding was consistent with reduced regurgitation frequency and weight gain in spite of unchanged esophageal dysfunction.[88]

There are reports in the literature of esophageal neuromuscular diseases that do not fit the clinical picture of IME or AA.[82, 106, 159] The most common example is the mature dog that presents with classic signs of AA and is normal one month later.[82] Mature dogs should be managed by elevated feeding for at least a month after presentation before surgery is performed, unless clinical signs have been present for three months or the dog is in poor clinical condition.

Modified Heller Procedure

A modified Heller procedure, or esophagomyotomy at the esophagogastric junction, will produce a less competent CES without eliminating its function, thus preventing reflux.[32, 50, 59, 62, 87] The effect of the surgery is to lower the resting pressure and the peak contraction pressure without markedly affecting the length of the CES or its synchronized functions during swallowing (see Fig. 48–11).[50]

The esophagus is approached by a left ninth thoracotomy (Fig. 48–14A). The mediastinum, with the vagus nerves, is dissected and reflected off the esophagus, and the esophagus is mobilized. An umbilical tape is passed around the esophagus cranially, and traction is applied to it; this tents the phrenoesophageal ligament as it reflects from the diaphragm on the esophagus. Two stay sutures of 3-0 nonabsorbable material are placed 4 mm apart over the lateral aspect of the diaphragm phrenoesophageal junction (Fig. 48–14B). The phrenoesophageal ligament is incised longitudinally between the stay sutures cranial to its reflection onto the esophagus (Fig. 48–14C and D). The fingers are placed under the esophagus, and light cranial traction is applied to the umbilical tape. The esophageal muscle is incised laterally down to the submucosa, beginning 1 to 2 cm cranial to the attachment of the phrenoesophageal ligament onto the esophagus and caudally past the oblique fibers of the stomach (Fig. 48–14E and F). Care must be taken not to perforate the mucosa, especially at the esophagogastric junction. Hemorrhage is controlled by pressure rather than ligation or cautery, in order to avoid perforating the mucosa. The muscle is best incised with scissors. The final muscle fibers may be removed using a sponge to make sure the esophageal and gastric submucosa is completely exposed (Fig. 48–14G). If the esophageal mucosa is perforated, the procedure is converted to a cardioplasty (although this carries a higher risk of reflux), or a patch graft of omentum is applied over the sutured mucosal perforation.

After the myotomy is completed, the esophageal hiatus must be reconstructed. A 3-0 suture of nonabsorbable material is placed through the cranial end of the esophageal muscularis incision. This suture is then placed between the two diaphragmatic stay sutures and tied (Fig. 48–14H). This maneuver places the incised portion of the esophagus into the abdomen and successfully repositions the abdominal segment of the CES (Fig. 48–14I). The phrenoesophageal ligament is then sutured to the diaphragm with a simple interrupted pattern. Following completion of the hiatal reconstruction, the thorax is closed (see Chapter 41).

Postoperatively, food and fluid are withheld for 24 hours. The dog is then started on minimal oral intake, with the amount fed being increased until the dog is on full feed by the seventh postoperative day. It is important to prevent vomiting by dietary management, since the tremendous pressure generated could "blow out" the reconstructed hiatal region.

Following surgery, it is usually necessary to continue to feed the dog in an elevated position. It is also necessary to adjust the consistency of the diet. Some dogs do well on a soft diet whereas others do well on dry food; dietary response may change with time.[88]

Cardioplasty

The esophagus is exposed as described for the modified Heller procedure. The esophageal muscle is incised as for a Heller procedure, and the mucosa is incised for the length of the muscular incision. If the cardioplasty is being done primarily, the incision extends from the oblique fibers of the stomach and stops caudal to attachment of the phrenoesophageal ligament to the esophagus. A double-armed nonabsorbable 4–0 suture is placed from the cranial to the caudal aspect of the mucosal incision and is tied. The mucosa medial to the tie is sutured to the end with a simple continuous pattern; the mucosa lateral to the tie is sutured with a simple continuous pattern. The esophageal muscle is apposed with 3–0 absorbable sutures in a simple interrupted pattern. All the mucosa is covered by muscle. The suture patterns are similar to those used for a Heinke-Miculiz pyloroplasty.

The hiatus is reconstructed by placing the first sutures through the esophageal attachment of the phrenoesophageal ligament and the diaphragm, and closure is continued by suturing the phrenoesopha-

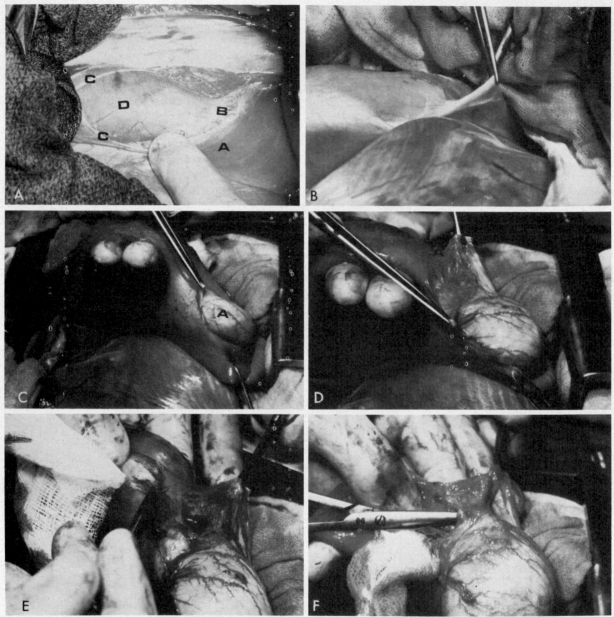

Figure 48–14. Modified Heller procedure. *A,* A left ninth thoracotomy has been done. The diaphragm (A), phrenoesophageal ligament (B), vagus nerves (C), and esophagus (D) are visible. *B,* The phrenoesophageal ligament and esophageal junction have been grasped by thumb forceps and elevated. Two stay sutures are placed at the level of the forceps, 4 mm apart and through the diaphragm. *C,* The phrenoesophageal ligament has been incised, and the cardia of the stomach (A) is seen. Allis forceps are on the diaphragm and the phrenoesophageal ligament. *D,* The phrenoesophageal ligament has been incised to the level of its reflection on the esophagus (A). *E,* The esophageal muscle has been incised beginning 2 cm cranial to the phrenoesophageal ligament attachment to the esophagus. The incision is carried through the muscle to the submucosa. *F,* Scissor dissection is used to dissect under the oblique fibers of the stomach, which are then incised. Care must be taken at this point not to perforate the mucosa.

Illustration continued on opposite page

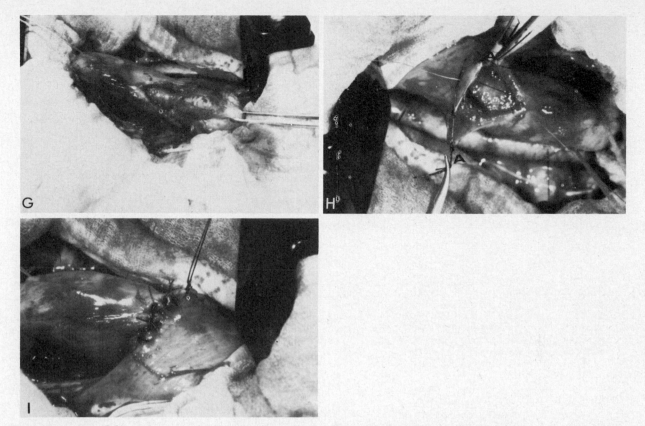

Figure 48–14 Continued. *G*, The mucosal incision has been completed. The Allis forceps are on the gastric submucosa. Any remaining muscle fibers are removed by wiping with a sponge. *H*, The esophageal hiatus is being closed. The first suture of nonabsorbable material is placed in the cranial end of the esophageal muscle incision to a midpoint between the two diaphragmatic stay sutures (A), which were placed before the phrenoesophageal ligament was incised. *I*, The esophageal hiatus has been reconstructed with simple interrupted sutures of nonabsorbable material. This procedure has placed the incised esophageal muscle within the abdomen.

geal ligament to the diaphragm. Postoperative care is the same as for esophagotomy.

Gastroesophageal Intussusception

Gastroesophageal intussusception is an uncommon condition in which the stomach invaginates into the distal esophagus.[4, 82, 107, 140, 155] The cause of this condition is not known, but a functional defect of the gastroesophageal or esophageal phase of swallowing must be considered.[82, 107] It has been demonstrated experimentally that vomiting occurring in young dogs is normally accompanied by dilation of the distal esophagus and intussusception of gastric rugae through the CES into the distal esophagus.[165] Two dogs had a radiographic diagnosis of esophageal dilation prior to onset of intussusception.[4, 140, 155] One dog did not have a history of vomiting prior to presentation with gastroesophageal intussusception.[89]

The condition occurs in young dogs, although one case has been reported in a nine-year-old dog.[155] A history of vomiting or regurgitation usually precedes presentation; dogs usually show acute dyspnea and impending shock. Progression of the signs is very rapid. Radiographically, an epiphrenic mass is seen in the distal esophagus, resembling a hiatal hernia.

In all reported cases, the dogs died during therapy. Treatment should be aimed at treating shock and restoring the normal anatomic position of the stomach. It may be necessary to perform a gastropexy to maintain the stomach in normal position.[162] Hiatal hernias and esophageal reflux are discussed elsewhere.

Feline Neuromuscular Disease

Neuromuscular esophageal diseases of the cat are less frequently reported than those of the dog. The feline esophagus contains smooth muscle in the distal one half to one third of the esophagus.[29] A condition resembling IME of dogs occurs in kittens and in mature cats with a history of vomiting as kittens.[30, 136, 190] The same number of ganglion cells were found in both normal cats and cats with hereditary esophageal neuromuscular disease resembling IME.[33]

In 13 adult cats, experimental lesions placed in the dorsal motor nucleus of the vagus produced varying results. In nine cats, regurgitation occurred and manometric study showed progressive peristalsis to be absent; however, the CES had a lower resting pressure. Radiographically, the body of the esophagus was dilated and atonic, and barium was held up at the CES. Of the other four cats, one showed a relaxed CES with reflux and the other three were normal.[77]

The therapy used in the dog may be attempted in the cat. A modified Heller procedure used in one cat was unsuccessful.[30]

Megaesophagus was associated in eight of 13 cats with pyloric stenosis. When the pyloric stenosis was treated by pyloromyotomy, three were cured, one improved clinically, and four others died or were euthanized. Whether the esophageal problem was secondary to the pyloric problem or whether the presence of both conditions is related to an autonomic nervous dysfunction has not been determined.[136]

1. Aanes, W. A.: The diagnosis and surgical repair of diverticulum of the esophagus. Proc. 21st Am. Assoc. Equine Pract., 1975.
2. Adam, W. S., Calhoun, M. L., Smith, E. M., and Stinson, A. W.: *Microscopic Anatomy of the Dog.* Charles C Thomas, Springfield, 1970.
3. Akl, B. F., and Blakeley, W. R.: Late assessment of results of cricopharyngeal myotomy for cervical dysphagia. Ann. J. Surg. 128:818, 1974.
4. Alcantara, P.: The clinical diagnosis of oesophageal invagination of the stomach in the dog. J. South Afr. Vet. Med. Assoc. 42:265, 1971.
5. Anderson, A. C. Digestive system. *In: The Beagle as an Experimental Dog.* Iowa State University Press, Ames, 1970.
6. Attum, A. A., Hankins, J. R., Ngangana, J., and McLaughlin, J. S.: Circular myotomy as an aid to resection and end-to-end anastomosis of the esophagus. Ann. Thorac. Surg. 28:126, 1979.
7. Bailey, W. S.: Parasites and cancer; sarcoma in dogs associated with *Spirocerca lupi.* Ann. N.Y. Acad. Sci. 108:890, 1963.
8. Baker, G. J., and Hoffer, R. E.: Surgical correction of esophageal stenosis in the dog. J. Am. Vet. Med. Assoc. 148:44, 1966.
9. Barone, R.: *Anatomie Comparée des mammifères domestiques.* Tome 3, Fasc 1, *Splanchnologie.* Lab. d'Anatomie, École Nationale Veterinaire, Lyon, 1976.
10. Beitzel, C., and Brinker, W. O.: Surgical removal of an esophageal foreign body which had penetrated the trachea. J. Am. Vet. Med. Assoc. 129:241, 1956.
11. Belin, R. P., Lieber, A., and Segnitz, R. H.: A comparison of techniques of esophageal anastomosis. Am. Surg. 38:533, 1972.
12. Belsey, R.: Reconstruction of the esophagus with colon. J. Thorac. Cardiovasc. Surg. 49:33, 1965.
13. Bombeck, C. T., Boyd, D. R., and Nyhus, L. M.: Esophageal trauma. Surg. Clin. North Am. 52:219, 1972.
14. Botha, G. S. M. A note on the comparative anatomy of the cardioesphageal junction. Acta Anat. 34:52, 1958.
15. Bourdelle, E., and Bressou, C.: *Anatomie régionale des animaux domestiques.* IV: *Carnivores: Chien et Chat.* J-B Bailliere, Paris, 1953.
16. Breshears, D. E.: Esophageal dilation in six-week-old male German shepherd pups. Small Anim. Clin. 60:1034, 1960.
17. Bryant, L. R.: Experimental evaluation of intercostal pedicle grafts in esophageal repair. J. Thorac. Cardiovasc. Surg. 50:626, 1965.
18. Buchanan, J. W.: Symposium: Thoracic surgery in the dog and cat. III: Patent ductus arteriosus and persistent right aorta arch surgery in dogs. J. Small Anim. Pract. 9:409, 1968.
19. Buergelt, C.-D., and Wheaton, L. G.: Dextroaorta, atopic left subclavian artery, and persistent left cephalic vena cava in a dog. J. Am. Vet. Med. Assoc. 156:1026, 1970.
20. Burke, T. J., and Froehlich, P. S.: Congenital esophageal disease in two kittens. Feline Pract. 8:18, 1978.
21. Busch, C.: Zur Struktur der Spieserohre des Hundes. Acta Anat. 107:339, 1980.
22. Butler, C., Madden, J. W., Davis, W. M., and Peacock, E. E. Morphologic aspects of experimental lye strictures. II. Effect of steroid hormones, bougienage, and induced lathyrism on acute lye burns. Surgery 81:431, 1977.
23. Carb, A. V., and Goodman, D. G.: Oesophageal carcinoma in the dog. J. Small Anim. Pract. 14:91, 1973.
24. Caywood, D. D., and Feeney, D. A.: Acquired esophagobronchial fistula in a dog. 18:590, 1982.
25. Clifford, D. H., and Gyorkey, F.: Myenteric ganglial cells in dogs with and without achalasia of the esophagus. J. Am. Vet. Med. Assoc. 150:205, 1967.
26. Clifford, D. H., and Pirsch, J. G. Myenteric ganglionic cells in dogs without hereditary achalasia. Am. J. Vet. Res. 32:615, 1971.
27. Clifford, D. H., Pirsch, J. G., and Maudlin, M. L.: Comparison of motor nuclei of the vagus nerve in dogs with and without esophageal achalasia (37136). Proc. Soc. Exper. Biol. Med. 142:878, 1973.
28. Clifford, D. H., Ross, J. N., Jr., Waddell, E. D., and Wilson, C. F.: Effect of persistent aortic arch on the ganglial cells of the canine esophagus. J. Am. Vet. Med. Assoc. 158:1401, 1971.
29. Clifford, D. H., Soifer, F. K., and Freeman, R. G.: Stricture and dilation of the esophagus in the cat. J. Am. Vet. Med. Assoc. 156:1007, 1970.
30. Clifford, D. H., Soifer, F. K., Wilson, C. F., et al.: Congenital achalasia of the esophagus in four cats of common ancestry. J. Am. Vet. Med. Assoc. 158:1554, 1971.
31. Clifford, D. H., Waddell, E. D., Patterson, D. R., et al.: Management of esophageal achalasia in miniature schnauzers. J. Am. Vet. Med. Assoc. 161:1012, 1972.
32. Clifford, D. H., Wilson, C. F., Waddell, E. D., and Thompson, H. G.: Esophagomyotomy (Heller's) for relief of esophageal achalasia in three dogs. J. Am. Vet. Med. Assoc. 151:1190, 1967.
33. Clifford, D. H.: Myenteric ganglial cells of the esophagus in cats with achalasia of the esophagus. Am. J. Vet. Res. 134:133, 1973.
34. Colgrove, D. J.: Transthoracic esophageal surgery for obstructive lesion caused by *Spirocerca lupi* in dogs. J. Am. Vet. Med. Assoc. 158:2073, 1971.
35. Collis, J. L.: Surgical treatment of carcinoma of the esophagus and cardia. 58:801, 1971.
36. Coran, A. G.: Pericardioesophagoplasty; a new operation for partial esophageal replacement. Am. J. Surg. 125:294, 1973.
37. Cotchin, E.: Further examples of spontaneous neoplasms in the domestic cat. Br. Vet. J. 112:263, 1956.
38. Cotchin, E.: Neoplasms in small animals. Vet. Rec. 63:67, 1951.
39. Davis, W. M., Madden, J. W., and Peacock, E. E.: A new approach to the control of esophageal stenosis. Ann. Surg. 176:469, 1972.
40. Debas, H. T., Payne, W. S., Cameron, A. J., and Carlson, H. C.: Physiopathology of lower esophageal diverticulum and its implications for treatment. Surg. Gynecol. Obstet. 151:593, 1980.
41. DeLahunta, A.: *Veterinary Neuroanatomy and Clinical Neurology.* 2nd ed. W. B. Saunders Co., Philadelphia, 1983.
42. Dellman, H.-D.: *Veterinary Histology.* Lea & Febiger, Philadelphia, 1971.
43. Diamant, N., Szczepanski, M., and Mui, H.: Manometric characteristics of idiopathic megaesophagus in the dog: an unsuitable animal model for achalasia in man. Gastroenterology 65:216, 1973.
44. Diamant, N., Szczepanski, M., and Mui, H.: Idiopathic megaesophagus in the dog: reasons for spontaneous improvement and a possible method of medical therapy. Can. Vet. J. 15. 66, 1974.

45. Dodman, N. H., and Baker, G. J.: Tracheo-oesophageal fistula as a complication of an oesophageal foreign body in a dog—a case report. J. Small Anim. Pract. 19:291, 1978.

46. Duncan, I. D., Griffiths, I. R., Carmichael, S., and Henderson, S.: Inherited canine giant axonal neuropathy. Muscle Nerve 4:223, 1981.

47. Duncan, I. D., and Griffiths, I. R.: Canine giant axonal neuropathy; some aspects of its clinical, pathological and comparative features. J. Small Anim. Pract. 22:491, 1981.

48. Earlam, R. S., Zollman, P. E., and Ellis, F. H., Jr.: Congenital oesophageal achalasia in the dog. Thorax 22:466, 1967.

49. Ellis, F. H., Jr.: The esophagus. In Sabiston, D. C., Jr. (ed.): Textbook of Surgery. 12th ed. W. B. Saunders Co., Philadelphia, 1981.

50. Ellis, F. H., Kiser, J. C., Schlegel, J. F., et al.: Esophagomyotomy for esophageal achalasia: experimental, clinical, and manometric aspects. Ann. Surg. 166:640, 1967.

51. Ellis, F. H.: Upper esophageal sphincter in health and disease. Surg. Clin. North Am. 51:553, 1971.

52. Evans, H. E., and Christensen, G. C.: Miller's Anatomy of the Dog. 2nd ed. W. B. Saunders Co., Philadelphia, 1979.

53. Faulkner, R. T., Caywood, D., Wallace, L. J., and Johnston, G. R.: Epiphrenic esophageal diverticulectomy in a dog: a case report and review. J. Am. Anim. Hosp. Assoc. 17:77, 1981.

54. Faulkner, R. T., Harrington, D. G., Sammons, M. L., et al.: A case of esophageal foreign body with mediastinal abscess formation in a dog. J. Am. Anim. Hosp. Assoc. 12:70, 1976.

55. Fisher, R. D., Brawley, R. K., and Kieffer, R. F.: Esophagogastrostomy in the treatment of carcinoma of the distal two-thirds of the esophagus. Clinical experience and operative methods. Ann. Thorac. Surg. 14:658, 1972.

56. Friedland, G. W., Kohatsu, S., and Lewin, K.: Comparative anatomy of feline and canine sling fibres. Digest. Dis. 16:495, 1971.

57. Funquist, B.: Oesophago-plasty as a supporting measure in the operation for oesophageal constriction following vascular malformation. J. Small Anim. Pract. 11:421, 1970.

58. Gaynor, F., Hoffer, R. E., Nichols, M. F., et al.: Physiologic features of the canine esophagus: effects of tranquilization on esophageal motility. Am. J. Vet. Res. 41:727, 1980.

59. Geever, E. D., and Merendino, K. A.: An evaluation of esophagitis in dogs following the Heller and Gröndahl operations with and without vagotomy. Surgery 34:742, 1953.

60. Goldsmith, H. S., Kirby, A. A., and Randall, H. T.: Protection of intrathoracic esophageal anastomoses by omentum. Surgery 63:464, 1968.

61. Gourley, I. M., and Leighton, R. L.: Surgical treatment for cricopharyngeal achalasia in the dog. Pract. Vet. 44:10, 1972.

62. Gourley, I. M. G., and Leighton, R. L.: Esophagomyotomy and pyloromyotomy in the dog. Pract. Vet. 43:19, 1971.

63. Gray, G. W.: Acute experiments on neuroeffector function in canine esophageal achalasia. Am. J. Vet. Res. 350:1075, 1974.

64. Grier, R. L.: Esophageal disease as a result of improper patient positioning. Arch. Am. Coll. Vet. Surg. 4:4, 1975.

65. Griffen, W. O., Daugherty, M. E., McGee, E. M., and Uttley, J. R.: Unified approach to carcinoma of the esophagus. Ann. Surg. 183:511, 1976.

66. Guffy, M. M. Radiographic examination of the esophagus of the dog and cat. J. Am. Vet. Med. Assoc. 161:1429, 1972.

67. Gunnlaugsson, G. H., Wychulis, A. R., Roland, C., and Ellis, F. H.: Analysis of the records of 1,657 patients with carcinoma of the esophagus and cardia of the stomach. Surg. Gynecol. Obstet. 130:997, 1970.

68. Hackett, R. P., Dyer, R. M., and Hoffer, R. E.: Surgical correction of esophageal diverticulum in a horse. J. Am. Vet. Med. Assoc. 173:998, 1978.

69. Hankes, G. H., and Henderson, R. A.: Radiography in the diagnosis and intensive care of a dog with esophageal fibrosarcoma. J. Am. Anim. Hosp. Assoc. 9:358, 1973.

70. Harvey, C. E., Chiapella, A. M., and Dubielzig, R. R.: Palato-pharyngeal fusion, laryngeal necrosis and esophageal stricture caused by gastric reflux in a dog: a case report. J. Am. Anim. Hosp. Assoc. 17:213, 1981.

71. Harvey, C. E., O'Brien, J. A., Durie, V. R., et al.: Megaaesophagus in the dog: the clinical survey of 79 cases. J. Am. Vet. Med. Assoc. 165:443, 1974.

72. Harvey, H. J.: Iatrogenic esophageal stricture in the dog. J. Am. Vet. Med. Assoc. 166:1100, 1975.

73. Hatafuku, T., and Thal, A. P.: The use of the onlay gastric patch with experimental perforations of the distal esophagus. Surgery 56:556, 1964.

74. Heimlich, H. J.: Reversed gastric tube (RGT) esophagoplasty for failure of colon, jejunum and prosthetic interpositions. Ann. Surg. 182:154, 1975.

75. Henderson, R. D.: Motor Disorders of the Esophagus. Williams & Wilkins, Baltimore, 1976.

76. Henderson, R. D.: Motor Disorders of the Esophagus. Baltimore, Williams & Wilkins, 1976.

77. Higgs, B., Kerr, F. W. L., and Ellis, F. H.: The experimental production of esophageal achalasia by electrolytic lesion in the medulla. J. Thorac. Cardiovasc. Surg. 50:613, 1965.

78. Hill, F. W. G., Christie, B. A., Reynolds, W. T., and Lavelle, R. B.: An oesophageal diverticulum in a dog. Aust. Vet. J. 55:184, 1979.

79. Hoffer, R. E.: Replacement of the distal esophagus by mobilization of the stomach in the dog. Masters thesis, Auburn University, 1963.

80. Hoffer, R. E.: Diseases of the esophagus. In Kirk, R. W. (ed.): Current Veterinary Therapy VI. Philadelphia, W. B. Saunders Co., 1977.

81. Hoffer, R. E.: Development of an esophageal prosthesis: N.I.H. proposal submitted 1980. Polymer Implant Center, Univ. Utah, Salt Lake City.

82. Hoffer, R. E.: Surgical diseases of the esophagus. In Bojrab, M. S. (ed.): Pathophysiology in Small Animal Surgery. Lea & Febiger, Philadelphia, 1981.

83. Hoffer, R. E.: Surgery of the esophagus. In Jones, B. (ed.): Canine and Feline Gastroenterology. W. B. Saunders Co., Philadelphia, in preparation.

84. Hoffer R. E.: Radiographic comparison of idiopathic megaesophagus and acquired achalasia, in preparation.

85. Hoffer, R. E., and Hunt, C. E.: A practical suture technique for esophageal closure in the dog. Small Anim. Clin. 3:75, 1963.

86. Hoffer, R. E., Barber, S. M., Kallfelz, F. A., and Petro, S. P.: Esophageal patch grafting as a treatment for esophageal stricture in a horse. J. Am. Vet. Med. Assoc. 171:350, 1977.

87. Hoffer, R. E., MacCoy, D. M., Gaynor, F., et al.: Physiologic features of the canine esophagus: effect of modified Heller's esophagomyotomy. Am. J. Vet. Res. 41:723, 1980.

88. Hoffer, R. E., MacCoy, D. M., Quick, C. B., et al.: Management of acquired achalasia in dogs. J. Am. Vet. Med. Assoc. 175:814, 1979.

89. Hoffer, R. E., Valdes-Dapena, A., and Baue, A. E.: Dog achalasia and the lower esophageal sphincter. Surg. Forum 17:334, 1966.

90. Hoffer, R. E., Valdes-Dapena, A., and Baue, A. E.: A comparative study of naturally occurring canine achalasia. Arch. Surg. 95:83, 1967.

91. Hofmeyr, C. F. B.: An evaluation of cardioplasty for achalasia of the oesophagus in the dog. J. Small Anim. Pract. 7:281, 1966.

92. Hopper, C. L., and Howes, E. L.: Strength of esophageal anastomoses repaired with autogenous pericardial grafts. Surg Gynecol. Obstet. 117:83, 1963.

93. Howard, D. R., Lammerding, J. J., and Dewevre, P. B.: Esophageal reinforcement with sternothyroideus muscle in the dog. Canine Pract. Surg. 2:30, 1975.

94. Hugh, T. B., Lusby, R. J., and Coleman, M. J.: Gastric patch esophagoplasty: an experimental study. Am. J. Surg. 137:226, 1970.

95. Hurwitz, A. L., Nelson, J. A., and Haddad, J. K.: Oropharyngeal dysphagia. Digest. Dis. 20:313, 1975.

96. Hurwitz, A. L., Way, L. W., and Haddad, J. K.: Epiphrenic diverticulum in association with an unusual motility disturbance: report of surgical correction. Gastroenterology 68:795, 1975.

97. Ivoghli, B.: Esophageal sarcomas associated with canine spirocercosis. Vet. Med./Small Anim. Clin. Jan:47, 1978.

98. Ingelfinger, F. J.: Esophageal motility. Physiol. Rev. 38:533, 1958.

99. Ingh, T. S., Va Den, G. M., and Linde-Sipman, J. S. van.: Vascular rings in the dog. J. Amer. Vet. Med. Assoc. 164:939, 1974.

100. Iwasaki, M., De Alvarenga, J., and DeMartin, B. W.: Esophageal diverticula in a dog. Mod. Vet. Pract. 58:606, 1977.

101. Jackson, J. W., Cooper, D. K., Guvendik, L., and Reece-Smith, H.: The surgical management of malignant tumors of the oesophagus and cardia: a review of the results in 292 patients treated over a 15-year period (1961–75). Br. J. Surg. 66:98, 1979.

102. Janssens, J., Velembois, P., Vantrappen, G., and Pelemons, W.: Is the primary peristaltic contraction of the canine esophagus bolus dependent? Gastroenterology 65:750, 1973.

103. Janssens, J., Velembois, P., Vantrappen, G., and Pelemons, W.: Studies on the necessity of a bolus for the progression of secondary peristaltics in the canine esophagus. Gastroenterology 67:245, 1974.

104. Jordan, P. H., Jr.: Dysphagia and esophageal diverticula. Postgrad. Med. 61:155, 1977.

105. Killen, D. A., and Pridgen, W. R.: Tolerance of the dog to esophageal perforation. J. Surg. Res. 1:315, 1961.

106. Kipnis, R. M.: Megaesophagus: remission in two dogs. J. Am. Anim. Hosp. Assoc. 14:247, 1978.

107. Klopfer, U., and Heller, E. D.: Invagination of the stomach into the esophagus in a dog. Vet. Med./Small Anim. Clin. 66:820, 1971.

108. Knecht, C. D., Small, E., Slusher, R., and Reynolds, H. A.: Epiphrenic diverticula of the esophagus in a dog. J. Am. Vet. Med. Assoc. 152:268, 1968.

109. Knight, G. C.: Transthoracic oesophagotomy in dogs: a survey of 75 operations. Vet. Rec. 75:264, 1963.

110. Lammerding, J., Howard, D. R., and Noser, G. A.: Diaphragmatic pedicle flaps for repair of distal esophageal defects in dogs. J. Am. Anim. Hosp. Assoc. 12:588, 1976.

111. Lantz, G. C., Bojrab, M. J., and Jones, B. D.: Epiphrenic esophageal diverticulectomy. J. Am. Anim. Hosp. Assoc. 12:629, 1976.

112. Lawson, D. D., and Pirie, H. M.: Conditions of the canine esophagus. II: Vascular rings, achalasia, tumours and perioesophageal lesions. J. Small Anim. Pract. 7:117, 1966.

113. Lawther, W. A.: Diagnosis and surgical correction of persistent right aortic arch and oesophageal achalasia in the dog and cat. Aus. Vet. J. 46:326, 1970.

114. Livaditis, A., Rodberg, L., and Odensjö, G.: Esophageal end-to-end anastomosis. Scand. J. Thorac. Cardiovasc. Surg. 6:206, 1972.

115. Longhi, E., and Jordan, P. H.: Necessity of a bolus for propagation of primary peristaltics in the canine esophagus. Am. J. Physiol. 220:609, 1971.

116. Lund, W. S. The functions of the cricopharyngeal sphincter during swallowing. Acta Otolaryngol. 59:497, 1965. (Cited by Rosin and Hanlon, 1972.)

117. Mann, C. V., and Shorter, R. G. Structure of the canine esophagus and its sphincters. J. Surg. Res. 4:160, 1964.

118. Markowitz, I., Archibald, J., and Downie, H. G.: Experimental Surgery. 5th ed. Williams & Wilkins Co., Baltimore, 1964.

119. Mitchell, R. L., and Armanini, G. B.: Cricopharyngeal myotomy: treatment of dysphagia. Ann. Surg. 18:262, 1975.

120. Moldoff, D. L., and Gordon, R. P.: Acquired esophageal dilation in a dog. Canine Pract. 3:26–30, 1976.

121. Moore, T. C., and Goldstein, J.: Use of intact omentum for closure of full thickness esophageal defects. Surgery 45:900, 1959.

122. Muangsombut, J., Hankins, J. R., Mason, G. E., and Mc-

Laughlin, J. S.: The use of circular myotomy to facilitate resection and end-to-end anastomosis of the esophagus. J. Thorac. Cardiovasc. Surg. 68:522, 1974.

123. Mutton, T., Goco, I., and Pennell, T.: Management of esophageal perforation with a pedicled jejunal patch. Curr. Surg. 38:318, 1981.

124. Nickel, R., Schummer, A., Seiferle, E., and Sack, W. O.: The Viscera of the Domestic Mammals. Verlag Paul Parey, Berlin, 1973.

125. Nissen, R.: Bridging of esophageal defect by pedicled flap of lung tissue. Ann. Surg. 129:142, 1949.

126. O'Brien, J. A., Harvey, C. E., and Brodey, R. S.: The esophagus. In Anderson, N. V. (ed.): Gastroenterology. Lea & Febiger, Philadelphia, 1980.

127. Orringer, M. B., Appleman, H. D., Argenta, L., et al.: Polypropylene suture in esophageal and gastrointestinal operations. Surg. Gynecol. Obstet. 144:67, 1977.

128. Osborne, C. A., Clifford, D. H., and Jessen, C.: Hereditary esophageal achalasia in dogs. J. Am. Vet. Med. Assoc. 152:572, 1967.

129. Papachristow, D. N., Trichilis, E., and Fortner, J. G.: Experimental use of free gastric flaps for the repair of pharyngoesophageal defects. Plast. Reconstr. Surg. 64:336, 1979.

130. Pass, M. A.: Surgical repair of esophageal defects. J. Am. Vet. Med. Assoc. 159:1453, 1971.

131. Pavletic, M. M.: Reconstructive esophageal surgery in the dog: a literature review and case report. J. Am. Anim. Hosp. Assoc. 17:435, 1981.

132. Payne, W. S., and Ellis, F. H., Jr.: Complication of esophageal and diaphragmatic surgery. In Arty, C. P., and Howdy, J. D. (ed.): Management of Surgical Complications. 3rd ed. W. B. Saunders Co., Philadelphia, 1975.

133. Peacock, E. E., Jr., and VanWinkle, W. Jr.: Wound Repair. 2nd ed W. B. Saunders Co., Philadelphia, 1976.

134. Pearlstein, L., Azneer, I. B., Polk, H. C., Jr.: An experimental assessment of esophageal anastomotic integrity. Surg. Gynecol. Obstet. 146:545, 1978.

135. Pearson, H., Darke, P. G. G., Gibbs, C., et al.: Reflux oesophagitis and stricture formation after anaesthesia: a review of seven cases in dog and cats. J. Small Anim. Pract. 19:507, 1978.

136. Pearson, H., Gaskell, C. J., Gibbs, C., and Waterman, A.: Pyloric and oesophageal dysfunction in the cat. J. Small Anim. Pract. 15:487, 1974.

137. Pearson, H., Gibbs, C., and Kelly, D. F.: Oesophageal diverticulum formation in the dog. J. Small Anim. Pract. 19:341, 1978.

138. Pearson, H.: Symposium on conditions of the canine esophagus. I: Foreign bodies in the oesophagus. J. Small Anim. Pract. 7:107, 1966.

139. Petrovsky, B. V.: The use of diaphragm grafts for plastic operations in thoracic surgery. J. Thorac. Cardiovasc. Surg. 41:348, 1961.

140. Pollock, S., and Rhodes, W. H.: Gastroesophageal intussusception in an Afghan hound: a case report. J. Am. Vet. Radiol. Soc. 11:5, 1970.

141. Postlethwait, R. W., Deaton, W. R., Jr., Bradshaw, H. H., and Williams, R. W.: Esophageal anastomosis: types and methods of suture. Surgery 28:537, 1950.

142. Postlethwait, R. W.: Surgery of the Esophagus. Appleton-Century, New York, 1979.

143. Postlethwait, R. W.: Technique for isoperistaltic gastric tube for esophageal bypass. Ann. Surg. 189:673, 1979.

144. Quick, C. B., Hankes, G., Womer, R., and Kueven, K.: Cricopharyngeal achalasia. Auburn Vet. Spring; 90, 1977.

145. Rao, K. V. S., Mir, M., and Cogbill, C. L.: Management of perforations of the thoracic esophagus. Am. J. Surg. 127:609, 1974.

146. Rayl, J. E., Balison, V. R., Thomas, H. F., and Woodward, E. R. Combined radiographic, manometric, and histologic localisation of the canine lower esophageal sphincter. J. Surg. Res. 13:307, 1972.

147. Reed, J. H., and Cobb, L. M.: The diagnosis, radiographic study and surgical relief of a case of oesophageal diverticulum. Can. Vet. J. 1:323, 1960.

148. Reed, J. H.: The esophagus. *In* Archibald, J. (ed.): *Canine Surgery.* 2nd ed. American Veterinary Publications, Santa Barbara, 1974.

149. Reif, J. S.: Solitary pulmonary lesions in small animals. J. Am. Vet. Med. Assoc. *155*:717, 1969.

150. Ridgway, R. L., and Suter, P. F.: Clinical and radiographic signs in primary and metastatic esophageal neoplasms of the dog. J. Am. Vet. Med. Assoc. *174*:700, 1979.

151. Rinaldo, J. A., Levey, J. F., Smathars, H. M., et al.: An integrated anatomic, physiologic, and cineradiologic study of the canine gastroesophageal sphincter. Digest Dis. *16*:556, 1971.

152. Rogers, W. A., Fenner, W. R., and Sherding, R. G.: Electromyographic and esophagomanometric findings in clinically normal dogs and in dogs with idiopathic megaesophagus. J. Am. Vet. Med. Assoc. *174*:181, 1979.

153. Romanes, G. J. (ed.): *Cunningham's Textbook of Anatomy.* 10th ed. Oxford University Press, London, 1964.

154. Rosin, E.: Surgery of the canine esophagus. Vet. Clin. North Am. Small Anim. Pract. 2:17, 1972.

155. Rowland, M. G., and Robinson, M.: Gastroesophageal intussusception in an adult dog. J. Small Anim. Pract. *19*:121, 1978.

156. Ryan, W. W., and Greene, R. W.: The conservative management of esophageal foreign bodies and their complications: a review of 66 cases in dogs and cats. J. Am. Anim. Hosp. Assoc. *11*:243, 1975.

157. Schlegel, J. F., and Code, C. F.: Pressure characteristics of the esophagus and sphincter in dogs. Am. J. Physiol. *183*:9, 1958.

158. Schnelle, G. B.: Congenital stricture of the esophagus. J. Am. Vet. Med. Assoc. 78:552, 1931.

159. Schwartz, A., Ravin, C. E., Greenspan, R. H., et al.: Congenital neuromuscular esophageal disease in a litter of Newfoundland puppies. *In: Advances in Veterinary Surgery: Proceedings of the 11th Annual Meeting, American College of Veterinary Surgeons.* Michigan State University, Lansing, 1976.

160. Shating, A., and Clifford, D. H.: Canine achalasia with special reference to heredity. Southwest. Vet. *19*:33, 1966.

161. Shaw, D. G., and Dodd, R. R.: Cricopharyngeal achalasia. Canine Pract. 4:33, 1977.

162. Shelton, G. D.: Swallowing disorders in the dog. Comp. Con. Ed. 4:607, 1982.

163. Siedenberg, B., Rosenak, S. S., Hurwitt, E. S., and Som, M. L.: Immediate reconstruction of the cervical esophagus by a revascularized isolated jejunal segment. Ann. Surg. *149*:162, 1959.

164. Simic, V., and Joic, D. Anatomische-roentgenologische Untersuchungen der arteriellen Vaskularisation der Speiserohre bei den Hunden. Acta vet Beogr. *17*:27, 1967. (Cited by Busch, 1980.)[21]

165. Smith, D. M., Kirk, G. R., and Shepp, E.: Maturation of the emetic apparatus in the dog. Am. J. Vet. Res. *35*:1281, 1974.

166. Smith, H. A., and Jones, J. C.: *Veterinary Pathology.* Lea & Febiger, Philadelphia, 1966.

167. Sokolovsky, V.: Achalasia and paralysis of the canine esophagus. J. Am. Vet. Med. Assoc. *160*:943, 1977.

168. Sokolovsky, V.: Cricopharyngeal achalasia in a dog. J. Am. Vet. Med. Assoc. *150*:281, 1967.

169. Soulsby, E. J. L.: *Helminths, Arthropods and Protozoa of Domesticated Animals.* 6th ed. Williams & Wilkins Co., Baltimore, 1976.

170. Spy, G. M.: Megaesophagus in a litter of greyhounds. Vet. Rec. *75*:853, 1963.

171. Stableforth, A. W.: Neoplasms in cats. Proc. Roy. Soc. Med. *45*:671, 1952.

172. Sternberg, J. C.: Megaesophagus caused by congenital heart disease. Vet. Med./Small Anim. Clin. 72:196, 1977.

173. Stick, J. A., Janver, D. K., Kunze, D. J., and Wortman, J. A.: Esophageal healing in the pony: comparison of sutured vs. nonsutured esophagotomy. Am. J. Vet. Res. *42*:1506, 1981.

174. Stinson, A. W., and Calhoun, M. L.: Digestive system. *In* Textbook of Veterinary Histology. Lea & Febiger, Philadelphia, 1981.

175. Stone, R., Rangel, D. M., Gordon, H. E., and Wilson, S. E.: Carcinoma of the gastroesophageal junction. A ten year experience with esophagastrectomy. Am. J. Surg. *134*:70, 1977.

176. Strombeck, D. R., and Troya, L.: Evaluation of lower motor neuron function in two dogs with megaesophagus. J. Am. Vet. Med. Assoc. *169*:411, 1976.

177. Strombeck, D. R.: Pathophysiology of esophageal motility disorders in the dog and cat. Vet. Clin. North Am. 8:229, 1978.

178. Suter, P. F., and Watrous, B. J.: Oropharyngeal dysphagias in the dog: A cineradiographic analysis of experimentally induced and spontaneously occurring swallowing disorders. Oral stage and pharyngeal stage dysphagias. Vet. Radiol. *21*:1980, 24–39.

179. Taylor, R. A.: Transdiaphragmatic approach to distal esophageal foreign bodies. J. Am. Anim. Hosp. Assoc. *18*:749, 1982.

180. Thal, A. P., Hatafuku, T., and Kuntzman, R.: New operation for distal esophageal stricture. Arch. Surg. 90:464, 1965.

181. Thrall, D. E.: Esophagobronchial fistula in a dog. J. Am. Vet. Radiol. Surg. *14*:22, 1973.

182. Turnwald, G. H., Smallwood, J. E., and Helman, R. G.: Esophageal osteosarcoma in a dog. J. Am. Vet. Med. Assoc. *174*:1009, 1979.

183. van Bree, H., DeRick, A., and Vandenberghe, J.: Partial esophageal obstruction by an intramural hematoma in a dog. Vet. Radiol. 22:267, 1981.

184. van den Ingh, TSGAM, and van der Linde-Sipman, J. S.: Vascular rings in the dog. J. Am. Vet. Med. Assoc. *164*:939, 1974.

185. Vaughn, J. T., and Hoffer, R. E.: An approach to correction of cervical esophageal stricture in the equine (a case report). Auburn Vet. Winter;63, 1963.

186. Vernon, F. F., and Roudebush, P.: Primary esophageal carcinoma in a cat. J. Am. Anim. Hosp. Assoc. *16*:547, 1980.

187. Vidne, B., and Levy, M. S.: Use of pericardium for esophagoplasty in congenital esophageal stenosis. Surgery 1970 68:389, 1970.

188. Vitums, A. Portosystemic communications in the dog. Acta Anat. *39*:271, 1959.

189. Walker, R. B., and Littleworth, M. C. G.: Angiography in the pre-operative assessment of vascular ring obstruction of the oesophagus in the dog. Vet. Record 76:215, 1964.

190. Watrous, B.: Esophagus diseases. *In* Ettinger, S. J. (ed.): *Veterinary Medicine Disease of the Dog and Cat.* 2nd ed. W. B. Saunders, Co., Philadelphia, 1983.

191. Watrous, B. J.: Clinical presentation and diagnosis of dysphagia. Vet. Clin. North Am. *133*:437, 1983.

192. Watrous, B. J., and Sutter, P. F.: Normal swallowing in the dog: a cinefluorographic study. Vet. Radiol. *20*:99, 1979.

193. Watson, A. G.: Structure of the canine oesophagus. N. Z. Vet. J. *21*:195, 1973.

194. Whillis, J.: The lower end of the oesophagus. J. Anat. 66:132, 1931.

195. Wilkins, S. A.: Indications for section of the cricopharyngeal muscle. Am. J. Surg. *108*:533, 1964.

196. Wilkinson, G. T.: Chronic papillomatous oesophagitis in a young cat. Vet. Rec. 87:355, 1970.

197. Williams, D. B., and Payne, W. S.: Observations on esophageal blood supply. Mayo Clin. Proc. 57:448, 1982.

198. Wilson, G. P.: Ulcerative esophagitis and esophageal stricture. J. Am. Anim. Hosp. Assoc. *13*:180, 1977.

199. Woods, C. B., Rawlings, C., Barber, D., and Walker, M.: Esophageal deviation in four English bulldogs. J. Am. Vet. Med. Assoc. *172*:934, 1978.

200. Wysong, R. L.: Embryology of persistent right aortic arch. Vet. Med./Small Anim. Clin. 64:203, 1969.

201. Youngs, J., and Nicoloff, D.: Management of esophageal perforation. Surgery 65:264, 1969.

Anatomy

John Grandage

CAPACITY

When should a full stomach be regarded as overdistended? The beagle stomach holds 400 to 500 ml easily,[2] whereas that of an "average dog" is comfortably full when containing about 700 ml.[6] In large dogs the stomach has been estimated to carry three,[6] seven,[6] or even eight[17, 40] liters of water, but these higher records may be unphysiological. Regardless, the stomach is highly distensible. Whereas the empty organ is palpably inaccessible beneath the ribs, the laden stomach bulges beyond the costal arch, pushing and crowding the intestines behind it. Zeitschmann showed a greatly distended stomach of an adult dog extending caudal to the umbilicus and remarked that the abdomen resembled that of a ruminant.[147] Such enlargement is unlikely to be experienced by normal adult dogs but may be achieved by puppies, in which stomach capacity is greater.[23, 40] Pressure within the stomach does not rise inordinately as the stomach expands but plateaus owing to receptive relaxation, especially of the fundus.[143] The feline stomach is less variable in size and can accept 300 to 350 ml of fluid,[6] a capacity two to three times that of the rest of the gut.[17]

REGIONS

There are only a modest number of terms that have been coined to describe the gross form of the stomach; unfortunately these have been applied in a number of different ways by the gross morphologist, the histologist, and the comparative anatomist. Descriptions based on gross form and luminal characteristics should be clearly distinguished from those based on glandular distribution (Fig. 49–1). The *fundus* of the stomach is that part dorsal to the cardiac ostium and refers to either its lumen or its wall. The cranial surface of the fundus pushes against the upper left half of the diaphragm. Although it is relatively small in carnivores, especially the cat,[6] it is relatively easy to identify on radiographs of standing (or prone) animals because it is typically gas-filled. In other postures the fundic gas bubbles to the new elevated part of the stomach where it can highlight the mucosa.[50] The fundus is relatively larger in the empty stomach, in which the ratio of gas to residual fluid may be 6:1.[106] After a meal of solid food the fundic gas bubble is usually temporarily lost. A horizontal plane passing through the cardia marks the ventral limit of the fundus and often corresponds to the surface of liquid contents. The fundus may be a true functional division of the stomach; evidence is accumulating that it may control the emptying of liquids, whereas the more distal parts are concerned with the trituration of ingesta, the mixing of gastric juices, and the retention of solids.[72]

The *body* of the stomach (corpus ventriculi) is pushed against the left lobes of the liver and makes up the middle third of the organ. It is succeeded by the pyloric part, from which it is arbitrarily distinguished by a plane passing through the angular notch (the acute bend at the ventral limit of the lesser curvature).

The *pyloric part* makes up a little less than one-third of the stomach. It is found ventrally and mostly on the right and surrounds a funnel-shaped pyloric antrum, which opens into a narrower pyloric canal that ends at the pyloric ostium, the orifice into the duodenum. The pylorus consists of a sphincter and its associated serosal and mucosal coats. It consistently lies on the right, pushed against the liver, a little more cranial than the cardia; it is easy to distinguish from the softer duodenum by palpation, from which it is usually marked off by a constriction.

The full and empty stomach differ in shape. The empty organ adopts a variety of J-shapes, whereas the full organ is a more constant C-shape. As the empty stomach fills, uneven expansion causes the greater curvature to increase in length from two and one-half to four times longer than the lesser curvature.[13] Shapes are further modified by various muscular activities, such as systolic contractions of the pyloric canal, general contractions of the whole body, and peristalsis, the waves of which create annular constrictions and hourglass forms, particularly over the distal half. A growing vocabulary ("beaks," "pyloric tits") describes the appearance of these shapes in the barium-filled stomach. A typical cycle of gastric motility lasts 10 to 12 seconds, during which a wave of constriction moves toward the pylorus with increasing amplitude. The pyloric ostium is reputedly open except for the last third of this cycle.[106]

FIXATION

The stomach's motility and its need to fill and empty prevent it from being firmly fixed. However, the cardia is held by the relatively immobile esophagus, and the pylorus and duodenum are anchored to the liver so that the stomach is loosely anchored

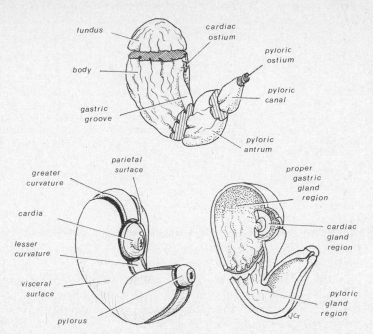

Figure 49–1. The principal regions and subdivisions of the stomach: the lumen (top), the wall (left), and the mucosa (right).

in the midline. The cardia and pylorus (and the lesser omentum between them) form an axis about which the stomach rotates as it fills. The greater curvature slides further and further caudally along the left abdominal wall while the cardia and pylorus remain stationary. In the process the parietal surface changes from facing cranially and dorsad to facing cranially and ventrad.[147]

The greater omentum arises mostly from the greater curvature of the stomach and clings around the intestines. The intestines can always be exposed by drawing the omentum cranially toward the stomach. The pulsation of the arteries within it and the squirming of the adjacent intestines automatically assist repositioning of the omentum. The omentum serves a number of functions but none of them are vital; it is most often quoted that it increases the serosal surface area for fluid production and absorption.[78] It may prevent the intestines from insinuating themselves between the stomach and liver where they could become trapped. As the stomach expands it balloons into the omental bursa, thus avoiding the danger of overriding the intestines.[51] The short but loose lesser omentum stretches from the lesser curvature to the liver.

A stout fold of mesentery conveys the portal vein to the liver; it restricts the lesser curvature moving far to the right. Pathological torsion of the stomach may involve some twisting around this mesentery and its contained portal vein.[51]

COATS OF THE STOMACH

The *muscular coat* of the stomach accounts for one-third of its weight.[27] It is made up of three layers (unlike most other parts of the alimentary tract). The outer layer (longitudinal layer, external oblique layer) runs longitudinally around the curvatures and more obliquely over the surfaces. A deeper circular layer is present over the pyloric part but is thin over the body and absent from the fundus. It is thickened to form the pyloric sphincter and may contribute some fibers to the less well-defined cardiac sphincter. Some regard its presence over the antrum as a form of prepyloric sphincter.[6]

The deepest, internal oblique layer (Gavard's muscle) is only present over the fundus and body. Some of its longest fibers are hairpin-shaped (sling fibers, ansa cardiaca) and course along the lesser curvature where they flank the gastric groove and loop over the cardia[43] (Fig. 49–2). They may contribute to the cardiac sphincter by acting like a sluice valve. Morphologically it has not been possible to identify a pacemaker amidst these muscles, although physiologically one seems to be present over the greater curvature of the body of the stomach near the junction with the fundus.[73]

The *mucosa* accounts for one-half of the weight of a canine stomach.[27] It is glandular throughout, although the nature of the glands varies from one region to another. A narrow region of cardiac glands around the cardia produces a serous secretion.[102] The proper gastric glands, which secrete both acid and enzymes from their parietal and chief cells, occupy about half of the stomach. They are disposed in two zones: a light zone occupying the fundus and body where the mucosa is thin and only a few parietal cells are present; and a dark zone occupying the body and extending almost to the pyloric region where the mucosa is thick and proper gastric glands are abundant.[128] Pyloric glands that only liberate mucus are found not only in the pyloric region but also in some of the body (see Fig. 49–1).[102] The pyloric mucosa also secretes gastrin. The various glandular zones are not easy to differentiate by gross inspection, although

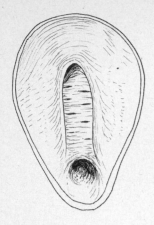

Figure 49-2. The interior of the canine stomach after removal of the mucosa. Oblique fibers flank the gastric groove and loop over the cardia (top). Lacunae in the circular muscle transmit vessels from the lesser curvature. Oblique and circular fibers unite at the beginning of the pyloric part (bottom), prompting the name prepyloric sphincter for this ill-defined ring.

the region of proper gastric glands is pinker and more mottled.[102]

A thick lamina muscularis and a loose submucosa allow the mucous membrane to be thrown into abundant transient folds, the plicae gastricae (commonly referred to as *rugae*), which can be up to 1 cm high and which do not become obliterated until the stomach is well filled. They are found throughout the stomach, are irregularly longitudinal, are particularly well developed in the body, and are less numerous in the pyloric part and less salient around the cardia and gastric groove.[17, 40, 102] The folds may be seen radiographically using appropriate agents, postures, and projections to highlight the particular region. In the nondistended, gas-filled stomach, a ratio of rugal height to interrugal space is usually greater than 2:1.[106] The form of the folds changes with inflammation, but, because they are so naturally variable, caution should be exercised in accounting any apparent increase in thickness to a inflammatory response.

VESSELS AND NERVES

The arteries to the stomach are all derived from the celiac and course along, or close to, the omental attachments (Fig. 49-3). Right and left gastrics run along the lesser curvature and right and left gastro-epiploics along the greater curvature with a couple

of branches from the splenic artery supplying the fundus.[40] Gastric branches are given off at right angles to the two curvatures to supply the adjacent stomach wall; their initial course is subserosal, but later these vessels run in the submucosa. Near the middle of the parietal and visceral surfaces there is a slender band approximately equidistant from the two curvatures that is relatively free from large blood vessels and is the site of choice for gastrotomy.[78] Eighty per cent of the arterial flow is to the mucosa, and the remainder is to the submucosa and the muscularis.[26]

The arteries are mostly accompanied by satellite veins, which unite into gastrosplenic and gastroduodenal tributaries of the portal vein. Some portocaval anastomoses occur at the cardia between the veins of the stomach and of the esophagus.[140]

Parasympathetic nerves are derived from the dorsal and ventral vagal trunks, which supply branches to the stomach immediately where they pierce the esophageal hiatus. Sympathetic nerves are ultimately derived from the splanchnic nerves; these first course to the celiacomesenteric ganglion and thence to the stomach by gastric nerves running with branches of the celiac artery.[40] Both types of autonomic fibers contribute to the myenteric and submucous plexuses.[120]

Lymph nodules are scattered throughout the mucosa, and the gastric lymphatics drain into hepatic lymph nodes.[40]

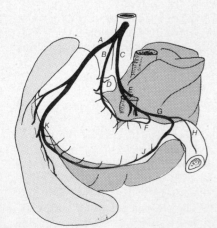

Figure 49-3. The arteries to the stomach of the dog are all branches of the celiac artery. *A*, Splenic (also supplies the pancreas); *B*, left gastric; *C*, hepatic; *D*, esophageal; *E*, right lateral hepatic (typically three branches supply left, right, and medial lobes); *F*, right gastric; *G*, gastroduodenal; *H*, cranial pancreaticoduodenal; *J*, right gastroepiploic; *K*, left gastroepiploic.

Physiology

Michael A. Pass

The stomach holds food after a meal and regulates its delivery into the small intestine to maximize the efficiency of digestion and absorption. While food is in the stomach it is mixed with gastric secretions and physically broken down into small particles by contractions of the stomach wall.

The major constituents of gastric secretions are hydrochloric acid, proteolytic enzymes (pepsins), intrinsic factor, and mucus. Gastric acid plays an important role in breaking down connective tissue to release nutrients into solution. It also activates gastric pepsins and kills ingested bacteria. Pepsins hydrolyze proteins to peptides. They are secreted as inactive proenzymes (pepsinogens), which are activated by hydrochloric acid. Once activated, the pepsin molecules can activate other pepsinogen molecules.[74] Secretion of the proteolytic enzymes as inactive precursors is an important mechanism to protect the stomach against self-digestion during enzyme secretion.

Mucus is secreted by all parts of the stomach. It lubricates the food to aid in its passage along the digestive tract. Mucus, together with bicarbonate secreted by the gastric mucosa, protects the stomach against damage by gastric acid and pepsins.[117]

The main stimulants of gastric secretion are the vagus nerves and the gastrointestinal hormone gastrin. Gastrin is a peptide released into the portal blood from G-cells in the pyloric antrum that circulates to reach the body of the stomach, where it stimulates the secretion of hydrochloric acid and gastric enzymes.[141] Secretion of gastrin is stimulated by distension of the pyloric antrum and by alkaline solutions and nutrients such as amino acids and proteins in the pyloric antrum.[141] Stimulation of the vagus nerves also stimulates the release of gastrin.[141]

Secretion has been described as occurring in three phases.[52, 74] During the cephalic phase, the vagus nerves stimulate secretion directly and through the release of gastrin. It is initiated by the sight, smell, or taste of food. The gastric phase is stimulated by food distending the stomach and is mediated by local and vagal reflexes together with the release of gastrin. The intestinal phase of gastric secretion occurs if gastric contents with a higher than normal pH enter the duodenum and cause the release of gastrin from G-cells in the duodenal wall. Usually, however, gastric secretion is inhibited by food in the duodenum. Inhibition is mediated by an enterogastric reflex and by the release of gastrointestinal hormones such as cholecystokinin and secretin from the wall of the small intestine.[68, 74]

The stomach stores and mixes food and propels it into the small intestine. When food is swallowed the stomach relaxes to receive the food[81] and then stores it. Three major types of contractions have been observed in the stomach: tonic, peristaltic, and terminal antral contractions.[20] Tonic contractions occur over a 5- to 10-cm segment of the stomach and change the capacity of that portion of the stomach. Peristaltic contractions begin proximally in the stomach and sweep along the stomach, pushing ingesta toward the antrum. Some of these contractions sweep along the antrum and propel food into the duodenum. Others fade out as they pass along the antrum. Many peristaltic contractions end in a terminal antral contraction; when this occurs, food cannot pass into the duodenum but is returned to the body of the stomach. During this process the food is forced through the ring of contracted muscle involved in peristalsis, breaking up large pieces of food.[20]

Motility is stimulated by distension of the stomach acting through local neural pathways and by the release of gastrin from the pyloric antrum. Acids, fats, and ingesta of high osmolality in the duodenum inhibit gastric motility through a local enterogastric reflex and by releasing gastrointestinal hormones.[5]

The rate of gastric emptying is related to the degree of gastric distension, the viscosity of gastric contents, and the presence of chyme in the duodenum. Emptying is faster with increased distension of the stomach, and liquids are emptied faster than solids.[63, 114] Emptying of the liquid portion of a meal may occur as a result of contractions of the proximal stomach, which increase the gastroduodenal pressure gradient so that liquid material flows into the small intestine.[72] However, before digestible solid food can pass through the pyloric sphincter it must be ground into particles less than 1 mm in diameter by antral contractions. It then becomes mixed with liquid in the stomach and is emptied with the liquid.[72] Indigestible solids are emptied last, when the pattern of gastric motility changes to that characteristic of the fasting state. Typically in this state there are periods of quiescence lasting for about one hour followed by peristaltic activity for 15 to 20 minutes.[72] Indigestible solids are emptied from the stomach during the first period of peristaltic activity that occurs after digestion has been completed.

Gastric motility is coordinated by electrical activity in the longitudinal and circular muscle layers of the stomach. A basic electrical rhythm consisting of regular periods of depolarization and repolarization has been recorded from the stomach.[24] The basic rhythm is propagated from the proximal regions of the stomach and synchronizes contractile activity. Contractions are initiated by second potentials or periods of prolonged depolarization in the muscle.[24]

VOMITING

Vomiting is the forceful expulsion of the gastrointestinal contents through the mouth. It is a reflex act integrated in the medulla oblongata. Afferent impulses that stimulate vomiting arise from many areas, and many are transmitted in the vagus or sympathetic nerves to the vomiting center.[16] Efferent impulses from the vomiting center stimulate a coordinated sequence of events, including closure of the glottis, elevation of the larynx, and contraction of the thoracic wall to increase intrathoracic pressure. Impulses to the abdomen cause relaxation of the stomach and esophagus and then a sharp contraction of the abdominal muscles to expel the gastric contents.

Vomiting is often preceded by retching. Several retches usually occur and during each retch the intra-abdominal pressure increases and intrathoracic pressure decreases.[88] Retching forces the abdominal esophagus and cardia through the diaphragm to overcome the normal antireflux mechanisms of the stomach. The retching is followed by expulsion of gastric contents, and during expulsion the intrathoracic and intra-abdominal pressures become positive.[88]

Several areas have been identified in which stimulation of appropriate receptors evokes vomiting.[16] A trigger area in the floor of the fourth ventricle is sensitive to drugs such as morphine and apomorphine. Stimulation of touch receptors in the pharynx induces vomiting, but no such receptors have been found in the esophagus.[16] Thus, obstruction of the lower esophagus by foreign bodies and megaesophagus are not always characterized by frequent vomit-

ing. In these cases vomiting is not likely to occur until sufficient fluid accumulates proximally or is regurgitated proximally to stimulate pharyngeal receptors.[64] Distension or the presence of noxious stimuli in the pyloric antrum or duodenum, but not in the body of the stomach, stimulates vomiting.[16, 49] Thus, the presence of a foreign body in the stomach often causes intermittent vomiting because receptors are not stimulated until the object is forced into the pyloric antrum. High intestinal obstructions are characterized by persistent vomiting because of continual distension of the duodenum and pyloric antrum by gastrointestinal secretion. In contrast, vomiting does not occur until late in the course of a low intestinal obstruction because it takes some time for sufficient fluid to build up proximal to the obstruction to distend the duodenum. Impulses arising from the vestibular apparatus induce motion sickness in some individuals.[16] Vomiting is also stimulated by pain in many areas of the body.

Important consequences of vomiting that may threaten an animal's life include uncorrected dehydration, acid-base imbalance, and electrolyte deficiencies leading to shock and death. Aspiration of vomitus can cause severe pneumonia.

Surgical Diseases

Frederik J. van Sluijs
and Reinier P. Happé

GASTROESOPHAGEAL REFLUX DISEASE

Gastroesophageal (GE) reflux disease (synonym, reflux esophagitis) is an inflammation of the esophagus caused by reflux of gastric or duodenal contents.

Incidence

Gastroesophageal reflux disease is a rare condition that may occur in dogs and cats of all breeds and ages.[1, 47, 56, 90, 112, 119, 129] It may be associated with congenital hiatal hernia, in which case the signs develop at a young age.[1, 47, 90] It has been described in dogs with hypersecretion of gastric acid and non-beta–islet cell tumors of the pancreas (Zollinger-Ellison syndrome)[56, 129] and may occur as a complication of general anesthesia.[112]

Pathophysiology

Gastroesophageal reflux commonly occurs in man without producing symptoms. Usually GE reflux does not cause esophagitis, because the refluxed material is quickly removed from the esophagus by normal peristalsis. However, if reflux increases or peristalsis

decreases, esophagitis may develop as a result of prolonged exposure of the esophageal mucosa to gastric contents. If there is concomitant duodenogastric reflux the injury may be more severe, since bile salts make the mucosa of the esophagus more susceptible to inflammation by increasing its permeability to hydrogen ions.[122]

In the asymptomatic animal GE reflux is minimized by a variety of mechanisms. The presence of a lower esophageal sphincter (LES) and an abdominal segment of the esophagus are the most important. Other mechanisms are the diaphragmatic pinchcock effect, the cardioesophageal angle of His, the phrenoesophageal membrane, and the gastric mucosal rosette, but these are thought to play only a minor role.

The LES lies between the crura of the diaphragm and is partially exposed to positive intra-abdominal pressure. It has a constant resting tone and relaxes only in response to swallowing or esophageal distension. If intragastric pressure increases, the LES responds by raising its resting pressure, thus offering an effective protection against GE reflux. The importance of the sphincter in the prevention of GE reflux is illustrated by the measurement of resting LES pressures in man.[8] Most patients have a lower mean resting LES pressure than asymptomatic control subjects. However, there is a considerable overlap between these two groups. The resting LES pressure of patients with reflux esophagitis may be normal or even elevated, whereas that of asymptomatic persons may be lowered. This suggests that the LES pressure is not the only determinant in the pathogenesis of reflux esophagitis and that other factors may play an important role. One of these factors is the mechanical valvelike function of the abdominal segment of the esophagus.[28]

Positive intra-abdominal pressure acts on both the stomach and the esophagus. As a consequence, the LES pressure that is needed to prevent GE reflux equals the intragastric pressure produced by gastric muscle tone. According to Laplace's law, the pressure in a hollow viscus is inversely related to its radius. Since the esophageal radius is consistently smaller than the gastric radius, it is difficult for gastric pressure to overcome the intrinsic esophageal pressure produced by the LES. The sphincter therefore remains competent as long as gastric pressure does not reach extreme values. However, if the abdominal segment of the esophagus becomes displaced into the thoracic cavity, as in hiatal hernia, this mechanism no longer works. The LES now has to withstand both intragastric and intra-abdominal pressure, both of which may rise dramatically when abdominal muscles contract during exercise, coughing, or barking. If the LES fails to increase its resting pressure accordingly, it becomes incompetent and esophagitis develops owing to increased GE reflux. The frequently noted association between reflux esophagitis and hiatal hernia may be explained in this way. Once esophagitis has developed it may become self-aggravating. Experiments have shown that inflammation of the esophageal wall may decrease both esophageal motility[58] and resting LES pressure,[37] which may result in an increase of GE reflux and a worsening of esophagitis. This process may be initiated by general anesthesia, since most anesthetics tend to lower resting LES pressure. This may explain the occasionally noted association between reflux esophagitis and general anesthesia.[112]

Clinical Signs

Characteristic signs are regurgitation, vomiting, and salivation. The last-named presumably is a response to the sour or bitter taste of regurgitated fluid. Dysphagia may be present as a result of abnormal esophageal motility or stricture formation in severe, long-standing esophagitis. Retrosternal pain ("heartburn") is a predominant sign in man and may occur in small animals. Eructation may occasionally be present. Physical examination is usually unremarkable, but weight loss may be considerable.

Laboratory Findings

There are no characteristic laboratory findings. There may, however, be secondary changes, reflect-ing the seriousness of the condition. These include leukocytosis and left shift due to inflammation, electrolyte imbalance due to vomiting, and hypoproteinemia and anemia associated with malnutrition and esophageal bleeding.

Radiographic Findings

Signs of esophagitis on survey radiographs include increased density of the terminal thoracic esophagus, retention of gas within the lumen, and altered density of the mediastinum.[106] Contrast radiography usually yields more information, as it permits evaluation of mucosal pattern and esophageal motility. In acute esophagitis, the mucosal surface may be irregular and the esophagus may have a stringy appearance due to spastic contractions. Contrast medium adheres to the mucosal surface and may accumulate between thickened longitudinal folds. In cats transverse folds in the caudal thoracic esophagus may disappear owing to submucosal edema. In chronic esophagitis the mucosal surface tends to be smooth. There may be segmental narrowing due to stricture formation and decreased motility.

As stated previously, GE reflux disease may be associated with hiatus herniation. In this abnormality the stomach is partly dislocated into the thorax. It can be classified as (axial) hiatus herniation, paraesophageal hiatal herniation, diaphragmatic herniation, or GE invagination[106] (Fig. 49–4). The first two abnormalities are difficult to diagnose. In large axial or paraesophageal hernias plain films may show a rounded mass of soft tissue density in the caudal mediastinum. The base of the mass is continuous with the left crus of the diaphragm. Small hernias are difficult to diagnose and require contrast radiography for identification of the gastroesophageal junction and gastric mucosal pattern above the esophageal hiatus (Fig. 49–5).

Diagnosis

The diagnosis of reflux esophagitis comprises four separate steps: (1) diagnosing esophagitis, (2) diagnosing GE reflux, (3) screening for hiatal herniation, and (4) measuring resting LES pressure.

Esophagitis is diagnosed by endoscopy. In our clinic we use a flexible endoscope designed for human colonoscopy.* The apparatus has a fiberoptic probe that is 1,865 mm long and 17.5 mm in diameter and can be angled in two perpendicular planes $\pm$ 240° from its neutral position. The examination is carried out with the animal under anesthesia induced by intravenous administration of a barbiturate† and maintained with inhalation anesthesia. Food should

---

*Olympus Model CF-LB2, Olympus Optical Co. (Europe), GmbH, Hamburg, FRG.

†Nesdonal, Specia, Paris, France.

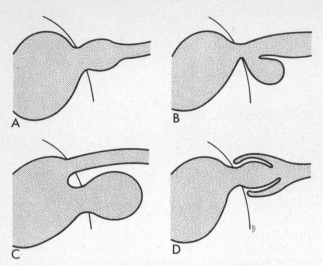

Figure 49–4. Classification of hiatal hernia. *A,* Axial hiatal hernia. *B,* Paraesophageal hiatal herniation. *C,* Diaphragmatic herniation. *D,* Gastroesophageal invagination.

be withheld for approximately 36 hours prior to the examination. The endoscope is introduced with the animal in left recumbency.

In normal animals the mucosa lies in longitudinal folds, or plicae, that join in the cardiac region. The mucosal surface is smooth and has a pale color. In animals with esophagitis the mucosal surface may appear irregular and red. Discoloration is always worse on the tops of the plicae.[55] In chronic esophagitis strictures may develop that cannot be passed by the endoscope.

Mucosal biopsies may be helpful in assessing the severity of inflammatory changes and in ruling out neoplasia. In our experience, however, the toughness of the canine esophageal mucosa makes it difficult to take biopsies with flexible endoscopic instruments. For further details on endoscopic examination of small animals the reader is referred to a recent report on this subject.[55]

GE reflux can be detected with fluoroscopy, barium cineradiography, scintigraphy, or continuous intraesophageal pH monitoring. Fluoroscopy and barium cineradiography are the least sophisticated techniques and for this reason are preferable in small animal medicine. Their major disadvantages are the relatively low sensitivity and the need to "trap" GE reflux, which usually is not a constant phenomenon but a periodic one. As a consequence, one may have to wait for GE reflux to occur, which can be distressing to both the animal and the medical personnel involved in the examination. Scintigraphy is much more sensitive than radiography and allows an exact quantification of volume and duration of GE reflux.[86] However, the equipment needed is expensive and one has to wait for reflux to occur, as in radiography. For these reasons scintigraphy is not applicable to small animal medicine, and the interested reader is referred to specialized texts on this subject.[86]

Continuous pH monitoring implies the introduction of a pH probe in the distal esophagus with the tip lying 5 cm above the LES. The probe is connected to a pH meter and a strip chart recorder and remains in the esophagus for 24 hours. The measurements obtained give an accurate summary of the frequency and duration of reflux episodes and allow a detailed prognosis.[67] However, the instrumentation is complicated and no reports have been published on the use of this technique in small animals. The diagnosis of hiatal herniation is discussed in the section on radiographic findings.

The measurement of resting LES pressure requires the introduction of a probe into the stomach, from which it is gradually withdrawn until it passes the LES. Because the LES pressure is radially asymmetrical in man it is usually measured at three recording sites subtending uniform radial angles of 120°. Two recording systems are currently used in human medicine: infused catheter systems, in which the pressure transducers are placed outside the body, and intraluminal strain-gauge systems, in which pressures are recorded directly in the esophagus.[32, 33, 127] In small animal medicine little experience has been gained using either of these systems.[48, 121]

Antireflux Surgery

Surgical treatment for GE reflux is indicated if hiatal herniation is present or if resting LES pressure is markedly decreased. In all other cases medical therapy should be tried first. Several drugs decrease the severity of symptoms in humans with reflux esophagitis. These include cimetidine,*[, 9] which reduces gastric acid production, and metoclopramide,†[, 146] which increases LES pressure. In the dog

---

*Tagamet, SK&F LAB CO., Carolina, PR. Subsidiary of Smith Kline Beckman Corporation.

†Primperan, Delagrange, Paris, France.

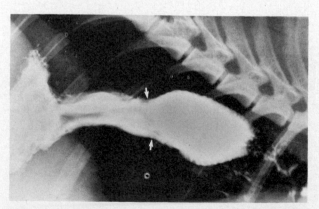

Figure 49–5. Lateral radiograph of the thorax of a cat with axial hiatal hernia. Barium outlines herringbone pattern of esophageal mucosa and longitudinal folds of gastric mucosa. The gastroesophageal junction is situated cranial to the diaphragm (arrow). (Courtesy of W. Th. C. Wolvekamp.)

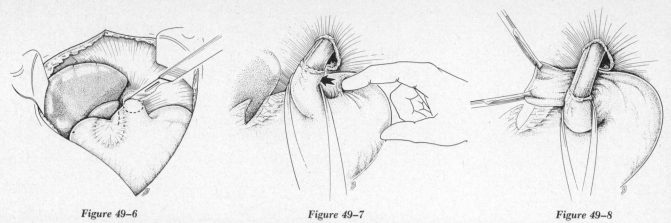

Figure 49–6   Figure 49–7   Figure 49–8

Figure 49–6. Nissen fundoplication. Incision of the phrenoesophageal membrane just below the hiatus.

Figure 49–7. Nissen fundoplication. The fundus of the stomach is passed underneath the retracted esophagus. The ventral vagal nerve is visible at the displaced thoracic part of the esophagus.

Figure 49–8. Nissen fundoplication. The displaced fundus of the stomach is held in position with tissue forceps. The ventral vagal nerve is visible at the displaced thoracic part of the esophagus.

these drugs have similar pharmacological effects,[107, 115] but their effectiveness in clinical cases has not been established. Cimetidine and metoclopramide have few side effects and can be given alone or in combination to break the vicious cycle of GE reflux and decreasing LES pressure described in the section on pathophysiology. Recommended doses are 15 mg/kg orally three times daily for cimetidine[107] and 0.2 mg/kg orally three times daily for metoclopramide.

The aims of antireflux surgery are to restore the abdominal segment of the esophagus and to create a high pressure zone at the gastric inlet that will generate a pressure comparable to normal resting LES pressures. Correction of hiatal herniation by narrowing of the hiatus alone is not sufficient and leads to recurrences in humans.[61]

Several techniques have been developed to create an intra-abdominal high pressure zone in humans. Two of these techniques have been applied successfully to small animals with GE reflux: the Nissen fundoplication[47, 90] and the Belsey fundoplication.[90] The Nissen technique is the simplest procedure and the method of choice in small animals. In large, deep-chested dogs exposure of the GE junction by an abdominal approach may be difficult. The Belsey technique may be preferable in such cases, as it allows excellent exposure of the GE junction and easy identification of the vagal nerves.

Fundoplication: the Nissen Technique

In this technique, which was first described in 1956[104] and modified in 1959,[105] the fundus of the stomach is wrapped around the distal esophagus and sutured to the right or lesser curvature side of the esophagus (see Fig. 49–10). The procedure is performed via a cranial midline abdominal approach. Prior to the operation the stomach should be intubated with an 18 French gauge Levin tube.

The hernia is corrected by manual traction on the stomach, after which the phrenoesophageal membrane is incised just below the hiatus (Fig. 49–6). The esophagus is freed from its attachments to the diaphragm and mobilized with care to protect the vagal nerves that lie directly dorsal and ventral to the esophagus. The cardia is retracted downward with a Penrose drain or a sling of umbilical tape, after which the cranial wall of the fundus is passed with one or two fingers underneath the esophagus toward the right side of the animal (Fig. 49–7). It is grabbed and held in position with two Babcock or Allis tissue forceps (Fig. 49–8). If necessary, the upper gastric vessels and a part of the lesser omentum may be divided. The fundus of the stomach should comfortably form a cuff around the lower part of the esophagus without excess tension on either of the displaced stomach walls. Seromuscular sutures of 2-0 nonabsorbable material are placed to hold the cuff in position (Fig. 49–9). Usually four to eight sutures are needed to create a cuff of sufficient length (Fig. 49–10). The Penrose drain (or the umbilical tape) is removed after the first two sutures have been tied. All sutures should include a small bite of the esophagus without perforating it. In addition to the Nissen procedure, the hiatus may be narrowed dorsally.

Fundoplication: the Belsey Mark IV Technique

In this technique, which was first introduced in 1967,[126] fundoplication is combined with herniorrhaphy by a transthoracic approach. Prior to the operation the stomach should be intubated with an 18 French gauge Levin tube. The thorax is entered through the right tenth intercostal space. The distal part of the esophagus is mobilized to the point where the vagal nerves join it from the lung roots. The phrenoesophageal membrane is divided and the car-

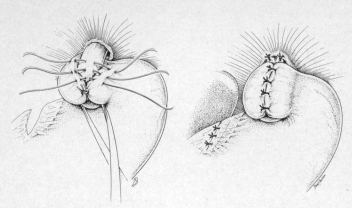

Figure 49–9. Nissen fundoplication. Seromuscular sutures are passed through the stomach and esophagus. Retraction is maintained until the first two sutures have been tied.

Figure 49–10. Nissen fundoplication. Completed fundic wrap around the esophagus.

Figure 49–9   *Figure 49–10*

dia is carefully freed so that the fundus and a part of the body of the stomach can be drawn up to the hiatus (Fig. 49–11). Care should be taken to protect the vagal nerves that lie directly dorsal and ventral to the esophagus.

The esophagus is retracted cranially with a Penrose drain or a sling of umbilical tape. Sutures of 2-0 nonabsorbable material are passed through the margins of the hiatus at its dorsal side. The sutures should be placed in the more fibrous parts of the diaphragm to avoid strangling muscle fibers. More sutures are inserted than may ultimately be necessary to approximate the two sides of the hiatus. These sutures are left untied until the end of the procedure, when the redundant sutures are removed and the remaining ones tied (see Fig. 49–14).

The fundus of the stomach is wrapped around the ventral two-thirds of the distal esophagus and held in place by two or three equidistant horizontal mat-

tress sutures of 2-0 nonabsorbable material between the seromuscular layer of the stomach and the muscle layer of the esophagus, 1.5 cm above the cardia (Fig. 49–12). The sutures are tied only tightly enough to obtain tissue apposition without disrupting the muscle fibers of the esophagus. A second row of sutures is inserted 1.5 to 2.0 cm higher. Using a spoon-shaped retractor passed through the hiatus to hold abdominal contents away from the undersurface of the diaphragm, each suture is passed first through the diaphragm from above downward at the point where the central tendon meets the muscle (Fig. 49–13). The suture is placed through the seromuscular layer of the stomach and muscle layer of the esophagus. The sequence is then reversed and the suture is finally passed through the diaphragm again from below upward with the help of the spoon, emerging 0.5 cm from the point of entry (see Fig. 49–13). Three sutures are passed in this manner. The

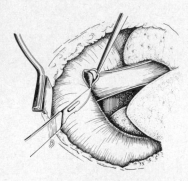

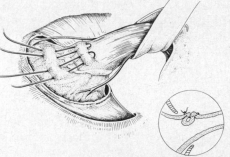

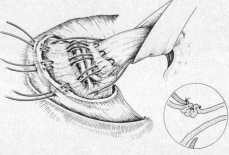

Figure 49–11   *Figure 49–12*   *Figure 49–13*

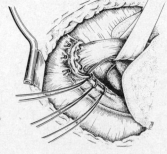

Figure 49–11. Belsey fundoplication. Incision of the phrenoesophageal membrane. The vagal nerves are visible dorsal and ventral to the esophagus.

Figure 49–12. Belsey fundoplication. Horizontal mattress sutures are passed through the stomach and esophagus.

Figure 49–13. Belsey fundoplication. A second row of horizontal mattress sutures is passed through the diaphragm, stomach, and esophagus. Sutures are tied after the reconstructed cardia has been manually placed downward through the hiatus.

Figure 49–14. Belsey fundoplication. Narrowing of the hiatus following fundoplication.

Figure 49–14

reconstructed cardia is manually placed downward through the hiatus. It must not be dragged below the diaphragm by pulling on the sutures passing through the diaphragm, as the object of these sutures is only to hold the reduction once it has been accomplished. The sutures of the second row are also tied gently to avoid damage to the esophageal muscle.

Finally, the hiatus is narrowed by tying the previously placed sutures (Fig. 49–14). These sutures will build up the buttress against which the intraabdominal segment of esophagus will be compressed. On digital exploration, the remaining hiatal opening should have similar resistance to the normal anal sphincter. Any redundant sutures are cut out, as it is better to have the hiatus slightly loose than too tight.

Aftercare and Complications

It is advisable to leave the stomach tube in place for two to five days to prevent gastric dilation which has been reported following Nissen fundoplication in a dog.[47] A pharyngostomy should be performed to keep the tube in position in the awake animal. Postoperative gastric dilation has also been reported in man and may occur as a combined effect of difficult eructation due to fundoplication and a transient decrease of gastric motility caused by surgical manipulation.[61] The condition is usually self-limiting and does not require specific treatment.

Pneumothorax has also been reported as a complication of Nissen fundoplication in the dog.[47] It is a logical consequence of severing the phrenoesophageal membrane and may occur in all fundoplication procedures.

Prognosis

Little is known regarding the prognosis of antireflux surgery in small animals owing to the limited number of case reports. The Nissen technique has been reported in three dogs.[47, 90] One dog improved following surgery and was clinically normal three months later. Another dog did not improve and suddenly died one month after surgery as a result of prolapse of the stomach. A third dog did not improve following Nissen fundoplication and was reoperated on using the Belsey technique.[90] The second surgery was successful in returning the dog to an asymptomatic state, but the animal died approximately six months later when cimetidine was withdrawn. The only significant finding at necropsy was a necrotic stomach wall with generalized ulceration through the mucosa and gastric musculature. The esophagus was grossly normal, and all surgery had healed. These findings suggest that gastric acid hypersecretion may have been a problem in this animal.

THE GASTRIC DILATION-TORSION SYNDROME

The gastric dilation-torsion syndrome is an acute, life-threatening condition characterized by distension of the stomach. Two forms can be distinguished: dilation without torsion (simple dilation), and dilation with torsion. If the degree of torsion is more than 180°, it is frequently referred to as volvulus.

Incidence

Simple dilation occurs in all breeds and at any age but is most frequently seen in the young puppy after overeating.[23, 131] In our clinic it is frequently seen in Irish setters, where it seems to be secondary to aerophagia. Gastric dilation with torsion occurs most frequently in large, deep-chested dogs.[10, 44, 46] It has, however, also been reported in the dachshund,[10, 134] the Pekingese,[10] and the domestic cat.[60, 135] Gastric torsion can occur at any age but is more frequent in older dogs.[46] Male dogs are affected more often than female dogs.[10] The overall incidence of the gastric dilation-torsion syndrome is relatively low (Strombeck reports an incidence of 13 per 10,000 cases).

Pathophysiology

In gastric torsion the stomach may rotate in a clockwise or a counterclockwise direction, seen from behind the standing animal. The clockwise rotation is also referred to as torsion to the right (Fig. 49–15) and counterclockwise rotation as torsion to the left (Fig. 49–17). Clockwise rotation is by far the most common type of gastric torsion in the dog. It is initiated by a downward displacement of the relatively undistended distal part of the stomach (pyloric antrum and canal) from the right abdominal wall to the ventral midline (Fig. 49–15B). The pylorus crosses the midline and passes underneath the distending proximal part of the stomach (fundus and corpus) to move upward along the left abdominal wall to a position next to the esophagus (Fig. 49–15C and D). The fundus moves in a ventral direction along the right abdominal wall and becomes located in the ventral part of the abdominal cavity.

The continuing dilation of the stomach induces a backward displacement of the greater curvature in addition to its rotation in the sagittal plane. The combined effect of these two movements results in the greater curvature being positioned against the left abdominal wall and the dorsal border of the abdominal cavity, where it may run parallel to or obliquely cross the axis through the vertebral column. The dorsal leaf of the greater omentum may not withstand the pressure of the distending fundus and may rupture next to the splenic artery, in which case the fundus herniates into the omental bursa through a ring formed by the left crus of the diaphragm, the splenic artery, and the short gastric arteries.[45] The

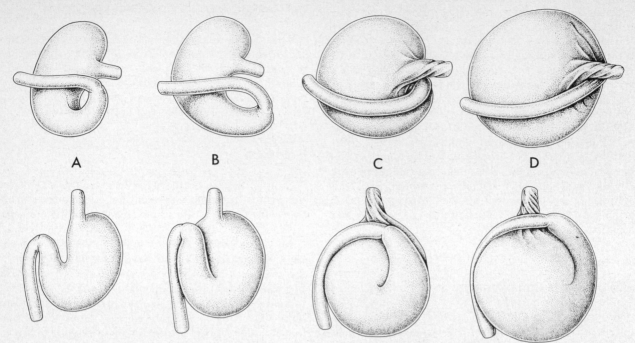

Figure 49–15. Position of the stomach at various stages of clockwise torsion as seen from right lateral (upper figures) and ventral (lower figures) positions. *A*, The normal position of the pylorus is against the right abdominal wall just cranial and ventral to the cardia. *B*, Torsion is initiated by a downward displacement of the pyloric antrum. *C*, The pylorus traverses the midline ventral to the esophagus and *(D)* moves upward along the left abdominal wall to a position dorsal to the cardia.

ventral leaf of the greater omentum is forced to follow the greater curvature and covers most of the ventral aspect of the dilated stomach (Fig. 49–16). The degree of torsion is usually expressed as the degree of rotation of the axis through pylorus and cardia in the sagittal plane. The maximum reported value in clockwise rotation is 270°.[12]

Counterclockwise rotation is seen only rarely in the dog. In this type of torsion the distal part of the stomach moves upward along the right abdominal wall until the pylorus is located next to the esophagus (Fig. 49–17). The greater curvature undergoes only little displacement in an upward and backward direction. As a consequence, the ventral leaf of the greater omentum is not pulled over the ventral aspect of the stomach. The maximal degree of torsion in counterclockwise rotation is limited to 90°.[59]

Regardless of direction and degree of torsion, gastric distension has dramatic systemic effects. The portal and caudal caval veins are compressed, which results in stasis of blood in abdominal organs and severe enlargement of the spleen. In areas with stagnant circulation, local acidosis and increased blood viscosity may initiate disseminated intravascular coagulation. Venous return decreases, leading to a fall in cardiac output and arterial tension, which results in poor tissue perfusion and organ hypoxia.[91, 92, 145]

In the heart, focal myocardial ischemia and hypoxia may cause cardiac arrhythmias that are frequently

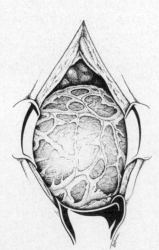

Figure 49–16. Clockwise gastric torsion. The ventral aspect of the stomach is covered by the greater omentum.

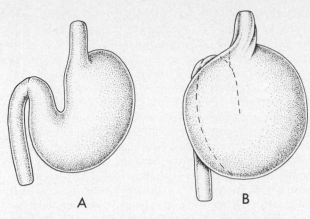

Figure 49–17. Position of the stomach in counterclockwise torsion as seen from a ventral position. The pylorus moves from its normal position against the right abdominal wall *(A)* to a position next to the esophagus at the right side of the midline *(B).*

Clinical Signs

The most characteristic signs are restlessness, salivation, retching with inability to vomit, and abdominal distension. The signs usually develop within three hours after feeding and are often related to postprandial exercise.

Physical examination reflects the seriousness of the condition. Most animals are depressed, but stress and abdominal discomfort may cause excitation. Respiration is rapid and labored. Peripheral pulse is usually rapid and weak owing to shock. In addition it may become irregular, inconsistent, and asynchronous if cardiac arrhythmia is present. Mucous membranes may be white, red, or cyanotic with a normal or prolonged capillary refill time. The abdomen is distended and tympanic on percussion.

associated with gastric dilation-torsion.[97, 99] In the lung, decreased perfusion is combined with mechanical restriction of ventilation by the distended stomach, resulting in poor oxygenation and aggravation of tissue hypoxia. In severe cases pulmonary edema, hyperemia, and hemorrhage may arise[14, 145]—often referred to as "shock lung." In the intestinal tract hypoxia causes a decrease in intestinal motility that may lead to paralytic ileus.[106]

Liver and kidney damage may become apparent as elevations of serum glutamic pyruvate transaminase (SGPT) activity and blood urea nitrogen[92] after gastric dilation-torsion has been relieved. However, the most severely injured organ is the stomach. If dilation-torsion is not relieved necrosis will occur, usually beginning at the fundus, where circulation is most seriously impaired. Ultimately the animal dies from perforation, sepsis, and shock.

Laboratory Findings

The most common findings are metabolic acidosis and hypokalemia,[98] but sometimes there is alkalosis.[67, 98] In experimentally induced acute gastric dilation, elevations were found in serum glutamic pyruvate transaminase (SGPT) activity, serum oxaloacetic transaminase (SGOT) activity, blood urea nitrogen, and creatinine.[92] These changes reflect secondary hepatic and renal damage, which may also occur in spontaneous gastric dilation-torsion.[131]

Radiographic Findings

In simple dilation the stomach appears as a large sack filled with gas and fluid. In dilation with torsion different parts of the stomach may appear separated from one another by a tissue-dense line, resulting in compartmentalization (Fig. 49–18). Depending on

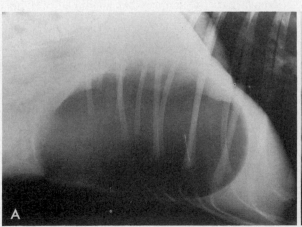
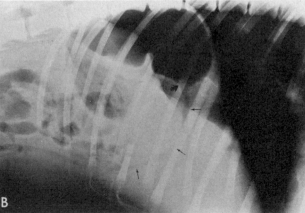

Figure 49–18. Lateral abdominal radiographs of a dog with gastric dilation-torsion before *(A)* and after *(B)* gastric decompression. Prior to intubation the stomach is greatly distended and filled with gas and fluid. Reduction of stomach size following aspiration of gastric contents clearly outlines the abnormal position of the stomach, with the pylorus located dorsally (large arrow) and the duodenum running in a ventral direction (small arrows). The position of the greater curvature suggests clockwise torsion, which was confirmed at surgery. (Courtesy of W. Th. C. Wolvekamp.)

the direction and degree of torsion, the pylorus may be located at various heights to the left or dorsally to the right of the midline (see Fig. 49–18). The gastric wall is thin and may contain small amounts of gas, indicating necrosis of the stomach wall.[106] There is splenomegaly with variable location of the body of the spleen. The vena cava and cardiac silhouette are small, and there may be ileus secondary to pain.[106]

Diagnosis

The diagnosis "gastric dilation-torsion syndrome" is made based on clinical signs. However, clinical signs alone do not allow discrimination between simple dilation and dilation with torsion. Radiography may be helpful in this respect but should not be undertaken if nonsurgical decompression fails because it delays necessary surgical intervention. Successful gastric intubation is not a very helpful criterion either, as the cardia may not be completely obstructed if torsion is less than 180°.[42] This means that there are situations in which the final diagnosis has to be made during surgery. The following landmarks can be used to arrive at a correct operative diagnosis: (1) The position of the greater omentum indicates the direction of torsion. If the greater omentum covers the ventral aspect of the stomach, torsion is clockwise (see Fig. 49–16). If the greater omentum does not cover the ventral aspect of the stomach, rotation is counterclockwise or there is simple dilation. (2) The localization of the pylorus indicates the degree of torsion.

Normally, the pylorus is localized within the costal arch at the right side of the body. It is always more cranial and ventral than the cardia.[94] In clockwise torsion the pylorus positioned at the left side of the body just dorsal to the cardia indicates a torsion of approximately 180°. If the pylorus lies more dorsally, torsion is more than 180°; if it is located more ventrally, torsion is less than 180°. In counterclockwise torsion and simple dilation the pylorus is localized at the right side of the body. A position dorsal to the cardia indicates counterclockwise torsion, whereas a position ventral to the cardia indicates simple dilation.

Preoperative and Anesthetic Management

Shock therapy should be started as early as possible. A large-bore catheter is positioned in the external jugular vein so that its tip is within the thorax. If a pharyngostomy is planned to maintain a semipermanent gastric decompression tube following surgery, it should not be performed at the same site as the venipuncture, because this enhances the risk of infection of the intravenous catheter. For right-handed surgeons the most convenient procedure is to insert the catheter into the right external jugular vein and perform the pharyngostomy at the left side of the

animal. Lactated Ringer's solution is infused at up to 80 ml/kg within the first hour.[116] Glucocorticoids may be given in large doses as intravenous bolus injections (prednisolone sodium succinate* at 10 to 20 mg/kg or dexamethasone† at 2 mg/kg), but their efficacy has not been proved in clinical studies. Correction of acid-base imbalances should be based on blood gas analysis, as both acidosis and alkalosis may occur.[70, 98]

Anesthesia should be induced and maintained with agents that have minimal effects on the cardiovascular system. Thiobarbiturates, halothane, and enflurane should be avoided because they may produce cardiovascular depression.[30, 82] Neuroleptanalgesia is a good alternative, because it is safe and produces cardiovascular stability.[30] In the dog it is mainly used for analgesic sedation and premedication, but it can also be used to induce and maintain general anesthesia.[53, 75] Controlled ventilation is mandatory to compensate for respiratory depression. Small amounts of nitrous oxide lower the dose that is needed to induce full unconsciousness but should not be given until the stomach has been decompressed, because nitrous oxide increases the distension of gas pockets in the gastrointestinal tract.[82] Bradycardia is a common phenomenon that can be treated with small doses of atropine.[30, 53, 75, 82]

Cardiac arrhythmias may occur during anesthesia. Occasional ventricular depolarizations (less than 16/min) and slow idioventricular rhythm disturbances should not be considered extremely dangerous as long as arterial pressure is maintained, but paroxysmal ventricular depolarizations and ventricular tachycardia are indications for antiarrhythmic therapy.[99] If needed, lidocaine‡ is given as a slow intravenous bolus injection in a dose of 4 to 8 mg/kg, which may be followed by a 0.2% intravenous drip in a dose of 0.05 mg/kg/min.[15, 39]

Surgical Methods

Nonsurgical decompression should always be attempted prior to surgical correction of gastric dilation-torsion. The stomach should be intubated with a soft, pliable tube of large diameter (Fig. 49–19). The tube should have large side holes in its distal part to allow aspiration of gastric contents if intubation is successful. If gastric intubation fails, gastrocentesis should be performed. After surgical preparation of the skin the stomach is punctured dorsally in the left flank with a large-bore trocar needle of sufficient length to prevent slipping of the stomach from the needle during decompression. If gastrocentesis results in marked decompression, gastric intubation and subsequent aspiration of gastric contents should be tried again, as decompression may resolve minor degrees of gastric dislocation.

---

*Solu-Delta-Cortef, The Upjohn Co., Kalamazoo, MI.
†Azium, Pitman-Moore Inc., Washington Crossing, NJ.
‡Xylocaine, Astra Pharmaceutical Products, Worcester, MA.

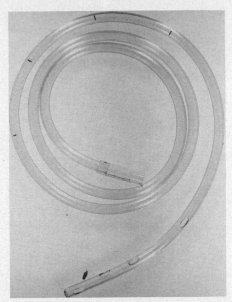

Figure 49–19. Stomach tube for decompression and aspiration in gastric dilation-torsion.

All animals that are successfully decompressed should be examined radiographically to assess the position and degree of filling of the stomach. If the position is normal and the stomach is empty, the animal should not be operated on. If the position is normal and there is only a moderate amount of food or fluid in the stomach, the animal has to be monitored carefully. Metoclopramide* is given intravenously at 0.2 to 0.5 mg/kg to accelerate gastric emptying.[103] Radiography is repeated one hour after the injection. If the degree of filling of the stomach is markedly reduced, the animal should not be operated upon. In all other cases (unsuccessful gastric decompression or evacuation, abnormal position of the stomach) surgery is indicated (Fig. 49–20).

Surgical treatment for gastric dilation-torsion has two objectives: correction of dilation-torsion and prevention of recurrence. In addition, splenectomy may be performed if necessary.

Correction of Dilation-Torsion

The abdominal cavity is entered via a ventral midline incision. After the pylorus and greater curvature have been identified, the surgeon grasps these structures and rotates the stomach back into its normal position. If gastric distension makes this impossible the stomach is punctured with a large-bore needle connected to a suction apparatus. If the stomach is filled with food, suction will not suffice and a gastrotomy may be necessary. In clockwise torsion the stomach has to be punctured or opened through the greater omentum that covers the ventral aspect

of the stomach. The area surrounding the puncture or gastrotomy site should be protected with moist laparotomy sponges to prevent soilage of the abdominal cavity.

Following repositioning of the stomach, all gastric contents should be removed. Gastric lavage, by stomach tube, should be attempted before a gastrotomy is performed. If this method fails the stomach is opened in the middle part of the ventral stomach wall (Fig. 49–21). The area to be incised is grasped with Babcock forceps or stay sutures, brought into the incision, and packed off with moist laparotomy sponges. The incision is made with a scalpel and should be large enough to allow adequate evacuation and inspection of the stomach. Fluid is removed by suction and solid particles with a spoon. It is advisable to use a suction tube with many small holes (Fig. 49–22), as tubes with a single large hole tend to become plugged with mucosa and aggravate preexisting mucosal damage. When all gastric contents have been removed the gastric mucosa and serosa are inspected for signs of devitalization. Gastric necrosis usually begins at the fundus. Necrotic areas may be resected, but if very large parts are affected or if the cardia is involved this is not feasible and euthanasia becomes inevitable.

The incision is closed in two layers: the mucosa with a continuous suture of 4-0 or 3-0 absorbable material and the submucosa, muscularis, and serosa with an interrupted Lembert suture of 3-0 or 2-0 absorbable material. The abdominal incision is closed in a routine manner. Prior to closure the stomach should be intubated with a decompression tube to facilitate treatment of gastric dilation in the immediate postoperative period. Two techniques can be applied to keep the tube in place in the awake animal: pharyngostomy and gastrostomy. Both methods are described in the section on prevention of recurrence.

Prevention of Recurrence

Successful correction of gastric dilation-torsion is likely to be followed by recurrence unless special preventive techniques are applied.[10] Surgical methods currently used can be separated into two groups: methods to prevent gastric retention and methods to prevent dislocation of the stomach. Methods to prevent gastric retention comprise various forms of pyloric surgery and are described in the section on delayed gastric emptying. Delayed gastric emptying may occur after correction of gastric dilation-torsion[25, 46] and can be treated successfully with pyloric surgery.[16] However, in a retrospective study of 25 dogs that underwent pyloric surgery as the sole measure of prevention, five recurrences were noted, indicating that pyloric surgery alone is not completely effective.[145] Methods to prevent dislocation of the stomach include various fixation techniques, such as gastrocolopexy,[19] gastropexy,[11, 83] tube gastrostomy,[109] and circumcostal gastropexy.[41]

Gastrocolopexy is not effective. A retrospective

*Primperan, Delagrange, Paris, France.

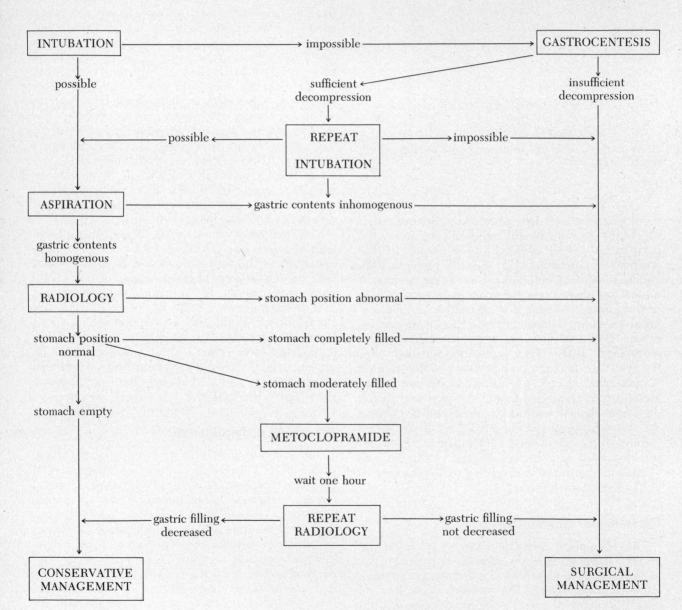

Figure 49–20. Therapeutic approach for gastric dilation-torsion.

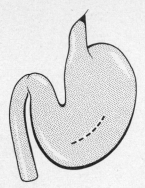

Figure 49–21. Site of incision for gastrotomy.

study of our own patients showed that five of six dogs that underwent gastrocolopexy as the sole method of prevention had a recurrence. During a repeat laparotomy in three of these dogs no permanent adhesions could be found between the greater curvature and the transverse colon, indicating poor fixation.

Gastropexy by simple suturing of the stomach to the body wall is unsuccessful in forming a permanent adhesion,[11, 19, 25] but modified gastropexy techniques in which the peritoneum was incised or scarified yielded a more reliable fixation in experimental animals and prevented recurrence in 44 dogs with gastric dilation-torsion syndrome that have been followed for up to five years.[83]

Tube gastrostomy produces a permanent adhesion of the stomach to the body wall[109] and has the advantage of producing gastric decompression during the immediate postoperative period. Circumcostal gastropexy has only been used in experimental dogs, where it has proved to cause strong adhesions between the stomach and the body wall.[41] Radiographic studies in some of these dogs indicated that gastric emptying time was normal at the fifth postoperative day, suggesting normal antral motility in spite of substantial alterations in the anatomy of the stomach wall. There are, however, no studies on the use of this technique in clinical cases.

In conclusion, two methods have been shown to reduce recurrence rates of gastric dilation-torsion in dogs: gastropexy with scarification or incision of the peritoneum and tube gastrostomy. Tube gastrostomy has the advantage of providing both gastric fixation and decompression in one procedure. In gastropexy, gastric decompression can only be achieved if an additional pharyngostomy is performed to keep the stomach tube in place in the awake animal. Tube gastrostomy is more simple to perform than gastropexy with pharyngostomy but requires more nursing care in the postoperative period. An abdominal bandage is required for at least nine days to keep the dog from disturbing the tube and to prevent excessive skin irritation after the tube is removed. In gastropexy, the pharyngostomy tube may be removed after 48 hours and does not require any specific care thereafter. Both methods are described hereafter.

Gastropexy. After correction of gastric dilation-torsion, the serosa and muscularis on the parietal side of the pyloric antrum are incised parallel to and equidistant from the attachments of the greater and lesser omenta (Fig. 49–23). A second incision is made in the peritoneum and internal fascia of the internal intercostal muscle in the eleventh or twelfth intercostal space (Fig. 49–24). The edges of the abdominal wall incision are sutured to the edges of the incision in the pyloric antrum in a simple continuous pattern with 2-0 monofilament nonabsorbable material (Fig. 49–25). Suturing is best started at the cranial side and completed at the caudal side (Fig. 49–26). Care should be taken to fix the stomach in its normal position with the pylorus located dorsally from the site of fixation.

An 18 French gauge gastrointestinal decompression tube is positioned in the stomach with the tip at the distal part of the corpus. The tube should have a large suction lumen and a smaller venting lumen to prevent plugging when suction is applied (Fig. 49–27). A pharyngostomy is performed to keep the tube in position in the awake animal. An indwelling catheter should not be placed in the external jugular vein at the ipsilateral side to minimize the risk of infecting the venipuncture site.

Tube Gastrostomy. Following correction of gastric dilation-torsion, an 18 to 24 French gauge Foley catheter (Fig. 49–28) is forced through a stab incision in the abdominal wall (Fig. 49–29). The incision is made to the right of the ventral midline approximately 4 cm caudal to the last rib. The stab wound size should not exceed the diameter of the tube and should penetrate all layers of the abdominal wall in a direct manner. Following introduction into the abdominal cavity the tube is allowed to penetrate the greater omentum in close proximity to the pyloric antrum (Fig. 49–30). A purse-string suture of 2-0 absorbable material is placed in the seromuscular layer at the pyloric antrum (see Fig. 49–30). A stab wound is then made in the stomach wall and the tip of the catheter is placed into the stomach. The bulb of the catheter is inflated with 10 to 15 ml of saline and the purse-string suture tied to form a secure seal around the catheter (Fig. 49–31). By applying traction on the catheter, the stomach is drawn to the abdominal wall and fixed with three or four sutures of 2-0 absorbable material (Fig. 49–32). The catheter is firmly secured to the skin to maintain traction on the stomach and the abdominal wall.

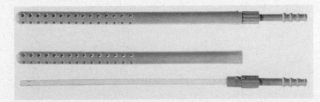

Figure 49–22. Disposable Poole suction tube. Multiple small holes in the detachable outer tube prevent plugging by mucosa or omentum. The flexible inner tube can be used for precise suction.

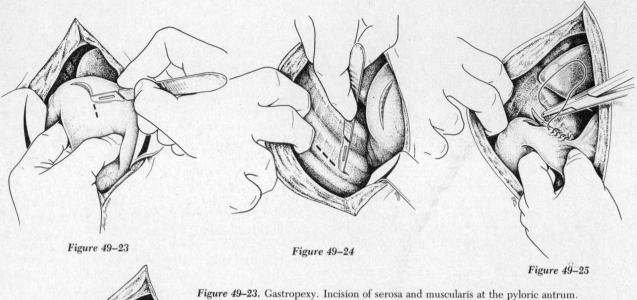

Figure 49–23

Figure 49–24

Figure 49–25

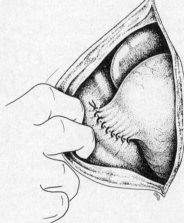

Figure 49–26

Figure 49–23. Gastropexy. Incision of serosa and muscularis at the pyloric antrum.

Figure 49–24. Gastropexy. Incision of peritoneum and internal fascia of the internal intercostal muscle at the right eleventh intercostal space. The incision should be the same length as the incision in the pyloric antrum.

Figure 49–25. Gastropexy. The cranial edge of the incision in the pyloric antrum is sutured to the cranial edge of the incision in the eleventh intercostal space in a simple continuous pattern.

Figure 49–26. Gastropexy. The caudal edge of the incision in the pyloric antrum has been sutured to the caudal edge of the incision in the eleventh intercostal space in a simple continuous pattern.

Figure 49–27. Semipermanent gastrointestinal decompression tube with double lumen. The small tube is continued to the tip as vent lumen to prevent tissue grab during suction.

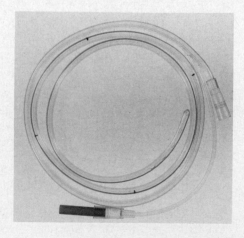

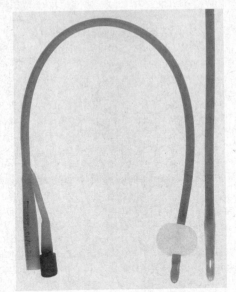

Figure 49–28. Foley catheter with inflated (left) and deflated (right) balloon.

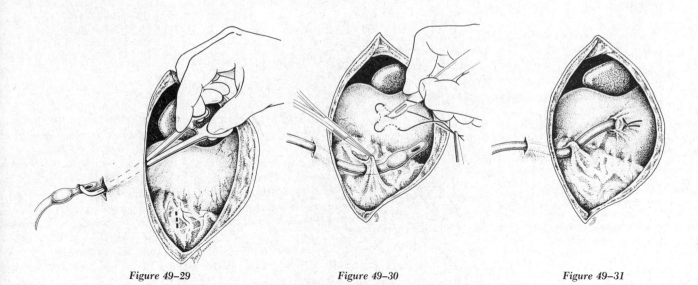

Figure 49–29   Figure 49–30   Figure 49–31

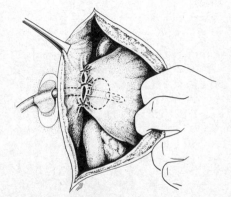

Figure 49–32

Figure 49–29. Tube gastrostomy. Introduction of a Foley catheter through a stab incision in the abdominal wall.

Figure 49–30. Tube gastrostomy. The Foley catheter is forced through the greater omentum and introduced into the stomach through a stab incision in the pyloric antrum. A purse-string suture has been placed at the selected site in the pyloric antrum prior to incision.

Figure 49–31. Tube gastrostomy. The purse-string suture is tied following inflation of the balloon.

Figure 49–32. Tube gastrostomy. The pyloric antrum is sutured to the abdominal wall with simple interrupted stitches. The Foley catheter is secured to the skin so as to maintain traction on the stomach against the abdominal wall.

Splenectomy

Removal of the spleen has been advocated to prevent recurrence of gastric dilation-torsion.[139] A retrospective study of 19 dogs that underwent splenectomy in addition to correction of gastric dilation-torsion indicated only limited preventive value, as five dogs had a recurrence.[144] Removal of the spleen may reduce the blood supply to the fundus of the stomach, because it implies ligation of the short gastric arteries. As the fundus is one of the most severely injured parts of the stomach in gastric dilation-torsion, splenectomy should only be performed if examination of the blood supply indicates damage to the spleen. Following repositioning of the stomach, an opening is made in the ventral leaf of the greater omentum slightly to the left of the midline (Fig. 49–33). This opening facilitates inspection and palpation of the splenic artery and vein, which run adjacent to the left lobe of the pancreas in the dorsal leaf of the greater omentum. If there is evidence of venous thrombosis the spleen should be removed. The opening in the greater omentum does not require suturing.

Prognosis

Surgical correction of gastric dilation has a high mortality and morbidity. In a combined retrospective study of 75 dogs that were operated on for gastric dilation-torsion in three different clinics, mortality was 33.4 per cent.[10] Thirty-six dogs were available for follow-up, 47 per cent of which had a recurrence. In a retrospective study of 70 of our own patients operated on for gastric dilation-torsion, mortality was 63 per cent. Twenty-six dogs were available for follow-up, 62 per cent of which had a recurrence. The higher percentage of recurrences in our own patients may be partially explained by the limited use of surgical methods to prevent recurrence of gastric dilation-torsion as compared with those of the combined study.

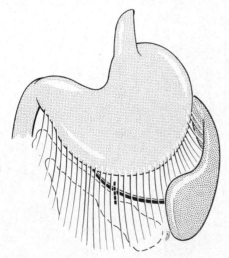

Figure 49–33. Inspection of the splenic artery and vein. Dotted line indicates site of perforation of greater omentum.

Aftercare

During the first 24 hours following surgery the animal should be carefully monitored for cardiac arrhythmias. Fluid, electrolyte, and acid-base imbalances should be corrected during this period by intravenous administration of fluids. No food or drinking water should be given. If a pharyngostomy tube is used it is left in place for 48 hours. As long as the animal is recumbent continuous suction may be applied with a small suction pump and collecting vessel. Following recovery from anesthesia suction can be continued as intermittent aspiration. The amount of aspirated fluid should be measured and replaced intravenously. If it is only minimal and signs of postoperative dilation are lacking, suction may be stopped and the pharyngostomy tube removed after 48 hours. The pharyngostomy heals spontaneously and does not require special care.

Initial aftercare is essentially the same if a tube gastrostomy has been performed, but the tube has to be left in place for seven days to allow the formation of adhesions between the stomach and the abdominal wall. During this period the tube is protected with an abdominal bandage and closed with a cap if no suction is applied. It is pulled out after seven days, creating a gastric fistula. This heals spontaneously but is covered with a protective bandage to prevent excessive skin irritation due to leakage of gastric contents.

Twenty-four hours after surgery small amounts of drinking water may be given. If the animal does not vomit and there are no signs of postoperative gastric dilation, feeding may be started after 48 hours. Small amounts of a bland diet are given every six hours. Drinking water may be offered in small quantities between feeding periods. Oral fluid intake is gradually increased, and intravenous fluid administration is reduced accordingly. Oral food intake is gradually increased until normal levels are reached by the seventh postoperative day. The animal's owner is instructed to continue feeding small quantities two or three times daily and to avoid excessive fluid intake and postprandial exercise.

Complications

The most common complications are cardiac arrhythmias and delayed gastric emptying. Cardiac arrhythmias occur most frequently between 12 and 36 hours after the onset of gastric dilation and are generally ventricular in origin.[97] They may be self-limiting and can be left untreated if pulse quality and capillary refill time are normal and the ECG does not show any paroxysmal ventricular depolarizations. In all other cases antiarrhythmic therapy is indicated as described in the section on preoperative and anesthetic management.

Postoperative delayed gastric emptying indicates disturbed or absent gastric motility, which is also referred to as gastric atony or gastric paresis. It may be caused by ischemic damage or by surgical manipulation and can be aggravated by hypokalemia and the use of opiates as analgesics. In man, delayed gastric emptying has been treated successfully with metoclopramide.*[113] In the dog metoclopramide increases antral motility[65] and accelerates gastric emptying,[103] but its efficacy in clinical cases has not been established. It has few side effects and can be given orally at 0.2 mg/kg three times daily. Coexisting electrolyte imbalances should be corrected and the use of opiates avoided. If delayed gastric emptying persists in spite of this regimen pyloric surgery should be considered.

UPPER GASTROINTESTINAL BLEEDING

Incidence

Upper gastrointestinal bleeding may originate in the esophagus, stomach, or duodenum. It is a relatively rare sign that may occur in dogs and cats of all breeds and ages[131] and is often associated with other diseases such as chronic renal or hepatic disease,[131] mast cell neoplasia,[18, 62, 100, 124] gastrin-producing neoplasia (Zollinger-Ellison syndrome),[56, 69, 129] and gastric neoplasia.[101, 110, 123] It may also be secondary to trauma, shock or sepsis,[95, 148] and disseminated intravascular bleeding[131] or other coagulation disorders.

Pathophysiology

Upper gastrointestinal bleeding indicates mucosal damage in the esophagus, stomach, or duodenum. Esophageal lesions may be caused by gastroesophageal reflux or gastric acid hypersecretion and are discussed in a separate section. Lesions in the stomach and duodenum range from mild inflammation to severe ulceration. The latter can cause serious signs that may require surgical intervention.

This chapter mainly discusses the pathogenesis of gastric and duodenal ulcers. Factors contributing to their development include reduced mucosal blood flow, reflux of bile salts from the duodenum into the stomach, and hypersecretion of gastric hydrochloric acid. Normally the gastric and duodenal mucosa are covered with a layer of mucus that offers protection against the corrosive and digestive effects of gastric acid and pepsin. This mucous layer is composed of sulfated mucins bound to the epithelial cells. When the mucous layer is lost the mucosa comes in direct contact with hydrochloric acid and pepsin, which may result in autodigestion and ulcer development. An important factor in the breakdown of the protective mucous layer is local ischemia due to hemorrhagic shock or sepsis, which may cause a sudden expulsion of apical mucus by a circumscribed population of surface cells.[95] This may partially explain the development of "stress ulcers," which are gastrointestinal ulcers that occur within hours of physical trauma, shock, sepsis, or head injury.[130] Ulceration of gastric neoplasms may also be caused by local ischemia, either by infiltration of neoplastic cells into blood vessels or by dense populations of cells compressing thin-walled vessels.[101]

Another important factor is reflux of duodenal contents into the stomach, which has been proved to cause gastric ulceration in dogs[79] and may play a major role in the development of stress and chronic benign ulcers. Bile salts are more destructive than pancreatic juices[29] because they act as detergents that solubilize lipid cell membranes and can inhibit ion transport systems.[131] As gastric bile concentrations are greatest in the pyloric antrum, most ulcers can be found in this area (sometimes called the ulcer region of the stomach).

A third factor of importance is the presence of gastric hydrochloric acid, without which no ulcers will develop.[95] In fact, gastric acid alone may produce gastrointestinal ulcers if it is secreted in excessive quantities. This hypersecretion may be stimulated by elevated gastrin or histamine production. Excessive gastrin is secreted by gastrinomas, which are non-beta–islet cell tumors of the pancreas that have been proved to cause gastrointestinal ulceration in dogs.[56, 69, 129]

Hypergastrinemia may also occur in uremic patients, as gastrin is removed by the kidney and may accumulate in renal failure.[131] Excess histamine is released from mastocytomas, which have been described in association with gastrointestinal ulceration in dogs[18, 62, 100] and cats.[124] Histamine is also released into the blood stream during endotoxemia and hemorrhagic shock and may play a role in the development of stress ulcers.

Gastric ulcers may also be caused by certain drugs, such as aspirin, phenylbutazone, indomethacine, ibuprofen, and corticosteroids. These drugs decrease the secretion of gastric mucus and alter its biochemical composition, making it less resistant to digestion by proteolytic enzymes.[89] In addition, they reduce the rate of renewal of surface epithelial cells,[87] which may slow down the healing process. The effect of aspirin may be reduced by the administration of enteric-coated preparations that prevent direct absorption of the drug by the gastric mucosa. However, circulating aspirin alone has been proved to cause gastric bleeding in experimental dogs.[89] The ulcerogenic properties of corticosteroids mainly apply to chronic administration. Their use in acute ulceration may even be beneficial, as they may prevent the development of stress ulcers in the restrained rat[71] and in human patients.[66]

Clinical Signs

The most characteristic signs are hematemesis and melena. They may be accompanied by chronic vom-

---

*Primperan, Delagrange, Paris, France.

iting, variable appetite, and weight loss, especially when bleeding is secondary to chronic renal or hepatic disease or to peptic ulceration or gastric neoplasia. Patients with gastrin-producing neoplasms may also have polydipsia[56, 69] and diarrhea.[56] Chronic cases may show acute exacerbations due to hemorrhage or ulcer perforation, which may bring the patient into the emergency room. Characteristic signs in this situation are collapse, abdominal pain, and abdominal distension.[100] Chronically affected patients are usually in poor condition and have pale mucous membranes owing to chronic anemia. There may be icterus if bleeding is secondary to chronic hepatic disease and multiple mucosal erosions in chronic renal disease. The skin should be inspected for multiple tumors that could be mastocytomas. The emergency patient may show signs of shock and sepsis and may indicate pain on abdominal palpation.

Laboratory Findings

In chronically affected patients the most significant finding is microcytic, hypochromic anemia. In acute cases there may be moderate normochromic anemia or no anemia at all if the loss of plasma equals the loss of erythrocytes. Anemia may be nonregenerative if gastrointestinal bleeding is secondary to chronic renal disease. Such patients also have elevated levels of blood urea nitrogen and creatinine and a low specific gravity of urine.

Animals suffering from the Zollinger-Ellison syndrome (recurrent peptic ulcers, hypersecretion of gastric acid, and non-beta–islet cell tumors of the pancreas) may also have low urine specific gravity due to unexplained polydipsia.[56, 69] In chronic hepatic disease serum alkaline phosphatase (SAP), glutamic pyruvate transaminase (SGPT), and glutamic oxaloacetic transaminase (SGOT) activity may be elevated. Plasma albumin may be lowered owing to maldigestion-malabsorption, decreased synthesis due to liver disease, or increased gastrointestinal or renal loss. Chronic vomiting can cause electrolyte and acid-base imbalances. The most commonly found abnormality is metabolic acidosis, but metabolic alkalosis and respiratory acidosis and alkalosis may also occur in vomiting dogs.[22] Metabolic alkalosis may be associated with hypokalemia. The feces of dogs with gastrin-producing tumors may contain large quantities of fat and fatty acids.

Radiographic Findings

Plain abdominal films may aid in the diagnosis of complications such as peritonitis or perforation but are not very helpful in the detection of the site of bleeding. Esophageal, gastric, or duodenal ulcers may be recognized with barium-filling studies and mucosal studies using double contrast radiography. Ulcer craters are detected as outpouchings from the lumen containing contrast material (Fig. 49–34). They

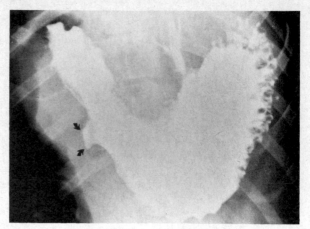

Figure 49–34. Lateral abdominal radiograph of a dog with an ulcerated neoplasm of the pyloric antrum. The ulcer crater is visible as a barium-filled outpouching of the lumen (arrows). (Courtesy of W. Th. C. Wolvekamp.)

are best seen when the radiographic angle is tangential and may be overlooked if positioning is inadequate. Fluoroscopic studies permit variable positioning and may therefore be helpful in the visualization of ulcers.

In spite of good techniques, gastrointestinal ulcers may not be detected radiographically for a variety of reasons: (1) the ulcer may be very shallow; (2) it may be filled with residues of mucus, blood, necrotic tissue, or food; (3) its margins may be so edematous that barium cannot enter the crater; (4) large patient size may preclude good radiologic detail; and (5) small ulcers may be obscured by large rugal folds.[106] Therefore, only positive findings should be considered as diagnostic proof.

Diagnosis

The diagnosis of "upper gastrointestinal bleeding" can be made on the basis of clinical signs alone but is too indefinite for adequate treatment. One should always try to localize the site of bleeding, as this may be helpful in the identification of underlying conditions. In patients with duodenal ulcers, gastric acid hypersecretion due to mastocytomas or gastrinomas should be suspected. Gastrointestinal ulcers can be recognized with radiographic techniques described in the section on radiographic findings. As stated previously, only positive findings should be considered as diagnostic proof. If bleeding is serious and no ulcers can be found other diagnostic methods should be employed, such as endoscopy or exploratory laparotomy. Endoscopy is the method of choice if bleeding is not life-threatening. It is superior to other methods in the detection of superficial erosions and has the advantage of allowing biopsies to be taken. This is of importance, as gastric ulcers may be secondary to gastric neoplasia.[101, 110, 123]

Exploratory laparotomy is indicated if hemorrhage is life-threatening. The technique is described here-

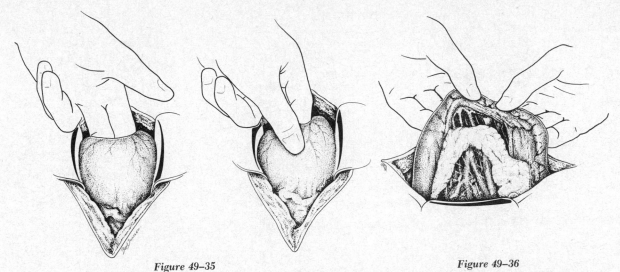

Figure 49–35

Figure 49–36

Figure 49–35. Inspection and palpation of the stomach. The index and middle fingers are brought dorsal to the stomach by blunt perforation of the lesser omentum near the lesser curvature. The stomach is palpated between these fingers and the thumb.

Figure 49–36. Inspection of the right lobe of the pancreas. The pancreas is visualized by lifting the duodenum from the abdominal cavity.

after in the section on surgical methods. Blood should be examined to assess anemia and exclude hepatic and renal disease and bleeding disorders as causative factors. Hypergastrinemia can be diagnosed by radioimmunoassay with antiserum produced against synthetic human gastrin.[77]

Surgical Methods

Surgical treatment of gastrointestinal bleeding is indicated in cases of life-threatening hemorrhage and ulcer perforation. It should also be considered if gastrinomas are suspected or conservative management is unsuccessful.[131]

The abdominal cavity is entered by a cranial midline incision. If necessary, the falciform ligament is amputated to attain better exposure. The lesser omentum is perforated bluntly near the lesser curvature to create an opening of sufficient size to bring the index and middle fingers dorsal to the stomach (Fig. 49–35). With the thumb placed opposite these fingers at the ventral side of the stomach, inspection and palpation are carried out in a systemic way from the fundus up to the pylorus. The presence of ulcers may be indicated by adhesions, serosal scarring, and irregular, thickened areas in the gastric wall. Inspection is continued toward the descending duodenum, which is lifted from the abdominal cavity by its middle part to allow good exposure of the right lobe of the pancreas (Fig. 49–36). This organ should be thoroughly inspected for nodules that might be gastrinomas but must be handled with great care to prevent postoperative pancreatitis.

The left lobe of the pancreas is best approached through the ventral leaf of the greater omentum, which is opened slightly to the left of the midline close to the greater curvature of the stomach (Fig. 49–37). The left lobe of the pancreas lies directly underneath this opening with the splenic artery and vein adjacent to it (Fig. 49–38). If pancreatic nodules are found or ulcer malignancy is suspected, the liver and regional lymph nodes should be inspected for metastasis (Fig. 49–39).

If ulcers cannot be found the stomach has to be opened to allow direct examination of the mucosa. The incision is made in the pyloric antrum, parallel to and equidistant from the greater and lesser curvature. If necessary it is extended toward the duodenum or corpus and fundus. Prior to incision the stomach is walled off with moist laparotomy sponges to avoid spillage of gastrointestinal contents into the abdominal cavity. Small ulcers are removed by elliptical excision. The incision is closed in two layers: the mucosa with a simple continuous suture using 4-0 or 3-0 absorbable material and the submucosa, muscularis, and serosa with an interrupted Lembert suture using 3-0 or 2-0 absorbable material. Multiple or large ulcers in the pyloric part of the stomach are best removed by a Billroth I gastrectomy, which is described in the section on delayed gastric emptying.

Ulcers in the cranial part of the duodenum present a special problem, because they cannot be excised radically without severing the bile and pancreatic ducts. As an alternative procedure the ulcer region may be oversewn with an omental flap after ligation of major bleeding vessels.

Gastrinomas that are confined to one lobe of the pancreas are best removed by en bloc resection of the affected lobe and its regional lymph nodes. Up to 90 per cent of the pancreas can be excised without risk of endocrine or exocrine insufficiency,[31] but if possible the cranial part of the right lobe should be left intact to prevent injury to the pancreatic ducts.

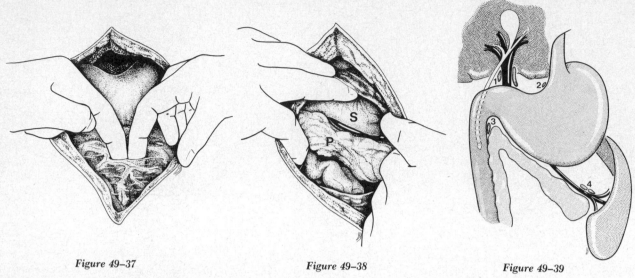

Figure 49–37.   *Figure 49–38.*   *Figure 49–39.*

Figure 49–37. Inspection of the left lobe of the pancreas. The greater omentum is opened slightly to the left of the midline near the greater curvature of the stomach.

Figure 49–38. Inspection of the left lobe of the pancreas. The stomach *(S)* and pancreas *(P)* are visible through the opening in the greater omentum. Adjacent to the cranial side of the pancreas are the splenic artery and vein.

Figure 49–39. Inspection of the regional lymph nodes in upper gastrointestinal disease. *1,* Portal lymph nodes; *2,* omental lymph node; *3,* duodenal lymph node; *4,* splenic lymph nodes.

All resectable metastases should be excised, which may necessitate partial hepatectomy when the liver is involved.

Prognosis

Upper gastrointestinal bleeding due to stress ulcers has a favorable prognosis, provided that the initiating condition can be treated successfully. The prognosis of bleeding due to chronic renal disease, chronic hepatic disease, or blood coagulation disorders depends on the prognosis of the underlying disease but is usually poor. The same applies to ulcers secondary to mastocytomas or gastric neoplasia, which are most commonly diagnosed in an advanced state of the primary disease. Little is known of the prognosis of gastrinomas in small animals, as only two case reports describe their surgical removal in dogs.[56, 129] One dog had liver metastasis at surgery and did not improve following excision of the primary tumor in the pancreas.[129] The other dog had no detectable metastasis and had two small islet cell tumors removed from the pancreas along with the adjacent lymph nodes. The dog improved following surgery but relapsed four and one-half months later and was destroyed. Examination of the removed specimen revealed that the tumors invaded the surrounding tissue and had already spread to the regional lymph node. On autopsy a third tumor was found in the pancreatic remnant, and metastasis were discovered in the liver and regional lymph nodes.[56]

Aftercare

During the first 24 hours following surgery the animal should be carefully monitored for postoperative hemorrhage. Blood transfusions are given to compensate for preoperative and operative losses, if necessary. Fluid and electrolyte balance are maintained by intravenous administration of electrolyte solutions until oral fluid intake is adequate. No food is given during the first 24 hours, but small amounts of drinking water may be offered as soon as the animal has recovered from anesthesia. Feeding is started 24 hours after surgery with small amounts of a high-quality bland diet. The amount of food is gradually increased until normal levels are reached by the fourth postoperative day. If gastric hydrochloric acid hypersecretion or duodenogastric reflux is suspected, cimetidine and metoclopramide may be given as described in the section on GE reflux disease.

Complications

Little is known about complications of partial gastrectomy in small animals. Major complications in man include hemorrhage in the immediate postoperative period due to failure to control bleeding from an ulcer or due to bleeding at the suture line.[133] If serious, they may necessitate reoperation. Late complications of radical gastric resection are discussed hereafter in the section on delayed gastric emptying.

DELAYED GASTRIC EMPTYING

Incidence

The normal gastric emptying time is not a fixed value but varies with the degree of filling of the stomach and the viscosity of its contents. It is best expressed as real half time.[138] Reported mean values for semisolid meals in normal dogs range from 65[138] to 77 min.[132]

Delayed gastric emptying is uncommon in small animals. It can occur in a congenital and an acquired form. The congenital form is caused by pyloric stenosis and occurs almost exclusively in certain breeds. Boxers are most commonly affected,[3, 34, 80, 118, 142] but the disease has also been reported in other brachycephalic breeds, such as the Boston terrier[118] and the bulldog.[76] In cats the most affected breed is the Siamese,[111, 136, 137] but the disease has also been reported in crossbreeds[111, 136] and the Havana.[111] One report mentions a frequent association with esophageal dilation.[111]

Acquired forms of delayed gastric emptying may occur in dogs and cats of all breeds and ages. They may be caused by obstructive diseases such as chronic hypertrophic gastritis,[57] gastric neoplasia,[35] or gastric foreign bodies[131] and by gastric motility disorders.[131]

Pathophysiology

In the normal dog and cat, gastric emptying of liquids differs markedly from that of solids.[72, 85] Liquids are emptied immediately after their ingestion, whereas solids are first subjected to a process of grinding and mixing to break them down into small particles. The duration of this process depends on the size of the fragments, as most solid particles must be less than 1 mm in diameter before they are allowed to pass into the duodenum.[93] Undigestible solids that cannot be broken down to such a small size are retained in the stomach until liquids and digestible solids have been emptied. Undigestible solids are then passed to the duodenum by powerful interdigestive contractions of the pyloric antrum[96] that occur every 100 minutes in the fasting dog.[21]

Gastric emptying of digestible solids is regulated by peristaltic contractions in the distal part of the stomach.[72, 85] These contractions are triggered by action potentials, which in turn are initiated by a pacesetter potential that is generated in an area in the proximal part of the corpus along the greater curvature.[54] The speed of the pacesetter potentials increases in the distal part of the stomach. As a result, the onset of the action potentials throughout the terminal antrum and pylorus occurs nearly simultaneously. Because the diameter of the gastric lumen is smallest at the pylorus, the pyloric contractions obliterate the gastric lumen at the pylorus before the lumen more proximally is closed. The depth of the peristaltic contractions depends on the viscosity of the gastric contents. High viscosity results in a reduction of the depth of the peristaltic wave.[38] As a result of this the central opening of the peristaltic contractions remains wider than the opening of the pylorus. Solid contents are thus retropelled and broken down into smaller particles that become suspended in the liquid phase of the gastric contents.

The emptying of liquids is mainly regulated by the proximal part of the stomach.[72, 85] As a consequence, partial obstruction of the gastric outlet may have little effect on the emptying of liquids. This is especially so in animals with congenital pyloric stenosis, which usually have no symptoms until solid food is given. The nature of the obstruction in this disease has not been fully elucidated. Hypertrophy of the pyloric sphincter is usually seen in the puppy[3, 34, 80, 118, 142] but is consistently absent in the young cat.[111, 136, 137] This finding suggests that disorders of gastric motility might be more important than pure mechanical obstruction, but real evidence for this is lacking. In the acute stage peristalsis may be exaggerated,[106] but in the chronic stages it is usually decreased or completely absent. This may be partially due to the depressive effect of electrolyte imbalances, which frequently accompany delayed gastric emptying.

Surgical intervention may have a profound effect on gastric emptying. In normal dogs, resection of the pylorus and the distal part of the stomach abolishes antral grinding and mixing and accelerates the emptying of solids.[36] The latter effect may be partially obliterated by hypomotility in animals with gastric decompensation, but this does not restore antral grinding and mixing. Resection of the pylorus does not result in duodenogastric reflux because it does not act as a true sphincter. Reflux from the duodenum to the stomach is primarily prevented by the aboral direction and high frequency of duodenal contractions that occur at about 18 cycles/min.[54] This is considerably more often than gastric contractions, which occur about 5 cycles/min.[54]

Clinical Signs

The primary sign is vomiting, which can be projectile. It may occur immediately after eating but can also be delayed for 24 hours or longer. The vomitus may contain undigested food. In congenital pyloric stenosis vomiting usually starts after weaning. Growth may be retarded and the animal may be thin, but otherwise physical examination is unremarkable. Acquired gastric retention usually has a chronic, progressive course. There may be depression, anorexia, weight loss, and signs of dehydration. The stomach can sometimes be palpated as a large fluid-filled bag that may extend beyond the umbilicus. In such cases "water splashing sounds" are frequently heard by the owner.

Laboratory Findings

Chronic vomiting may cause electrolyte and acid-base imbalances. Common findings are hypotonic dehydration and hypokalemic alkalosis, especially in chronic acquired delayed gastric emptying. Dehydration may obscure anemia and hypoproteinemia often present in chronic cases.

Radiographic Findings

Plain films may show various stages of gastric distention (Fig. 49–40). Enlargement of the stomach is characterized by an increased fundic diameter, a markedly convex caudal margin, more caudal than normal location of the fundus and corpus, and increased diameter and length of the lumen of the pyloric portions.[106] Additional information can be obtained from the gas-fluid ratio, which is approximately 5:1 or 6:1 in the normal empty stomach. An alteration of 1:2 or greater indicates retention of gastric and salivary fluids.[106]

Contrast studies are needed to evaluate the gastric mucosa and musculature in the pyloric part of the stomach and to exclude obstruction by radiolucent foreign bodies. Hypertrophic gastritis is characterized by enlargement of the gastric mucosal folds or rugae. Minor or moderate enlargement is difficult to assess, but marked enlargement with rigidity of the rugae can be identified as wide, parallel, radiolucent lines. In gastric neoplasia there may be irregular flattening or ulceration of the mucosa and thickening of the gastric wall.

Radiolucent foreign bodies are best detected with double contrast studies. Fluoroscopy should be used, if available, to evaluate gastric peristalsis and pyloric sphincter action. A barium-impregnated gruel is preferable to more liquid contrast media, as the passage of fluids to the duodenum may be normal in spite of significant delayed gastric emptying. In the early stages of the disease the gastric wall in the terminal pyloric canal and sphincter appears stiff, with exaggerated peristaltic contractions in the pyloric portions.[106] In the chronic stages the length and diameter of the pyloric part increase, whereas peristalsis decreases. In the final stage, which is often referred to as gastric decompensation, the stomach is greatly distended and completely flaccid.[106]

Diagnosis

Delayed gastric emptying and gastric outlet obstruction are diagnosed by radiographic findings. Plain films are taken from the abdomen and the thorax to rule out esophageal dilation and aspiration pneumonia. If these films are not conclusive, a semisolid contrast medium should be administered in sufficient quantity to induce gastric distention. Delayed gastric emptying can be diagnosed by taking serial photographs at predetermined intervals of 30 to 60 minutes. If fluoroscopy is available it should be used to evaluate gastric peristalsis and pyloric sphincter action. Further information can be obtained from contrast studies with liquid contrast media and double contrast or by an exploratory laparotomy. The latter is preferable, because delayed gastric emptying in small animals is usually caused by obstructive diseases of the gastric outlet. This can be assessed and treated in the same surgical procedure. Blood should be examined to check for anemia and hypoproteinemia and to assess electrolyte and acid-base balance. Blood urea nitrogen, creatinine, and urine specific gravity should be determined to rule out concomitant renal failure.

Surgical Methods

Delayed gastric emptying should be treated surgically if it is caused by morphological abnormalities of the gastric wall or functional disorders that are unresponsive to medical management. The surgeon may choose from a great variety of techniqes ranging from simple myotomy to extensive resections such as

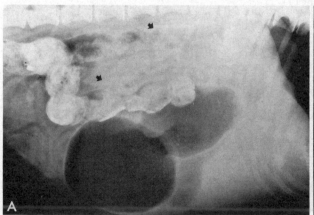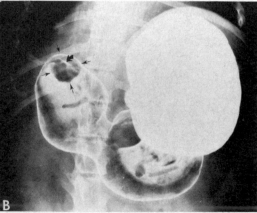

Figure 49–40. Radiographs of a dog with delayed gastric emptying. *A*, On the plain lateral radiograph the stomach is greatly distended and filled with a large amount of fluid (arrows indicate caudal limits of the stomach). *B*, Double contrast radiograph with the dog in dorsal recumbency shows circular filling defect (small arrows) around the pyloric outlet (large arrow), compatible with pyloric mucosal hypertrophy, which was confirmed at surgery. (Courtesy of W. Th. C. Wolvekamp.)

the Billroth I procedure. The method used depends on the nature and the severity of the cause and the personal preference of the surgeon. In general, congenital pyloric stenosis and pure functional disorders can be treated by simple myotomy or Heineke-Mikulicz pyloroplasty. Hypertrophic gastritis may be treated by Finney pyloroplasty or partial gastrectomy. The latter procedure should always be performed if the stomach is seriously enlarged or if gastric neoplasia is suspected.

Following partial gastric resection, continuity can be restored in several ways (Fig. 49–41). The Billroth I gastroduodenostomy is the closest approach to the original anatomy and is the procedure of choice; there is less risk for anastomotic ulcers than with the various gastrojejunostomy procedures. Contraindications for a Billroth I are extensive tension on the anastomosis due to radical gastrectomy and severe scarring of the duodenum due to ulceration. In those cases gastrojejunostomy is a safer procedure. Anastomotic ulcers invariably occur at the jejunal side of the anastomosis. They have been reported as late complications of gastrojejunostomies in man[133] and in a dog[7] and are thought to be principally caused by insufficient neutralization of gastric acid by sodium bicarbonate–rich pancreatic secretions. Hypersecretion of gastric acid due to gastrinomas (Zollinger-Ellison syndrome) or mastocytomas may also be present and should be checked for in any patient presented with an anastomotic ulcer.

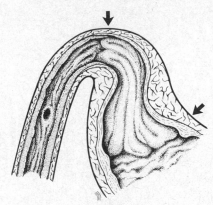

Figure 49–42. Cross section through the canine pylorus. Arrows indicate borders of the pyloric sphincter.

The animal should be carefully prepared for surgery. Electrolyte and acid-base imbalances should be corrected, if possible. The stomach is intubated and aspirated shortly before the induction of anesthesia to prevent aspiration of gastric contents. The stomach tube may be left in place as a pharyngostomy tube until several days after the operation as described in the section on the gastric dilation-torsion syndrome.

Surgical Approach

A cranial midline laparotomy is suitable for all procedures. The falciform ligament should be amputated to attain better access. Blood vessels crossing from the abdominal wall to the falciform ligament are best ligated with transfixation ligatures. Following amputation, the cranial stump is carefully checked for hemorrhage from retracted vessels. A self-retaining abdominal retractor (Balfour) is used in the more extensive procedures. The pylorus is an important landmark in all procedures. It may be several centimeters long with a proximal and a distal sphincter (Fig. 49–42). It can be easily identified on palpation as an area of increased firmness when compared with the remaining part of the stomach and the duodenum.

Pyloromyotomy: the Fredet Ramstedt Procedure

The pylorus is located and grasped between the thumb and index finger of the left hand. A longitudinal incision is made in a relative avascular part of the ventral side of the pylorus (Fig. 49–43). The incision should be carried down to, but not through, the mucosa and should extend 1 to 2 cm on either side of the pylorus. It is easier to carry the incision down to the mucosa over the stomach and then extend it into the duodenum. All fibers of the circular muscle are cut until the mucosa bulges through the incision to the level of the serosa (see Fig. 49–43). Hemorrhage is usually minimal and can be controlled by gentle pressure.

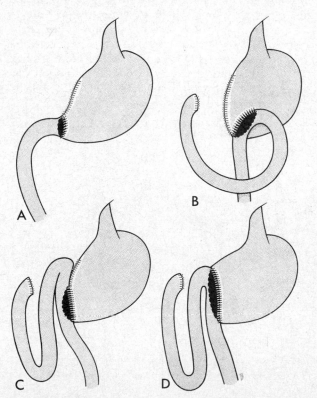

Figure 49–41. Techniques for anastomosis following partial gastric resection. *A*, Billroth I gastroduodenostomy. *B*, Billroth I gastrojejunostomy. *C*, Hofmeister gastrojejunostomy. *D*, Polya gastrojejunostomy.

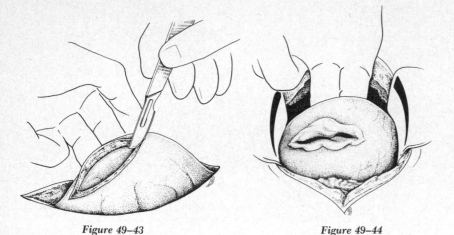

Figure 49–43

Figure 49–44

Figure 49–43. Pyloromyotomy. The pyloric muscle is incised until the mucosa bulges through the incision.

Figure 49–44. Heineke-Mikulicz pyloroplasty. The incision is made through the pyloric muscle and mucosa.

Pyloroplasty: the Heineke-Mikulicz Procedure

The incision is the same as in the Fredet-Ramstedt pyloromyotomy but is made through all layers of the pylorus, including the mucosa (Fig. 49–44). Traction sutures of 3-0 or 2-0 absorbable material are placed approximately 0.5 cm from each side of the incision at its midpoint. When traction is applied the sutures draw the longitudinal incision apart until it becomes first diamond-shaped and then transverse (Fig. 49–45). With traction maintained, the incision is closed transversely in a simple interrupted pattern using 3-0 absorbable suture material. The sutures should be tied loosely and should enclose all layers of the gastric and duodenal wall. The first suture is placed at the ends of the original longitudinal incision to ensure adequate alignment of the wound margins (Fig. 49–46). The rest of the sutures are placed routinely (Fig. 49–47).

Pyloroplasty: the Finney Procedure

The pylorus is located and a traction suture of 3-0 or 2-0 absorbable material is placed at the middle point of the cranial side (Fig. 49–48). A second suture joins a point approximately 5 cm proximal to the pylorus on the greater curvature of the stomach to a point approximately 5 cm from the pylorus on the duodenal wall (see Fig. 49–48). The seromuscular layer of the apposed walls of the stomach and the duodenum are sutured together with a simple continuous suture, using 3-0 absorbable suture material (see Fig. 49–48). This suture should be placed as near the greater curvature margin of the stomach and the inner margin of the duodenum as possible to ensure adequate room for subsequent closure. A V-shaped incision is then made into the stomach from a point just above the caudal suture around through the pylorus and down a similar distance on the duodenal wall adjacent to the suture line (Fig. 49–49).

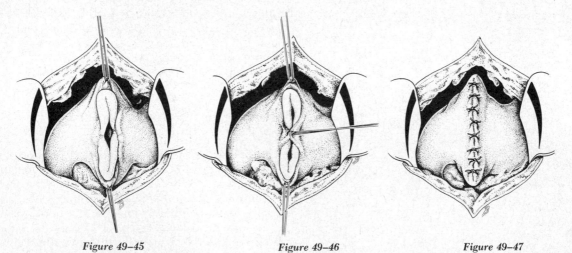

Figure 49–45

Figure 49–46

Figure 49–47

Figure 49–45. Heineke-Mikulicz pyloroplasty. Traction sutures are used to draw the longitudinal incision in a transverse direction.

Figure 49–46. Heineke-Mikulicz pyloroplasty. Closure is started in the middle with a simple interrupted suture through all layers of the stomach wall.

Figure 49–47. Heineke-Mikulicz pyloroplasty. Closure is continued in a simple interrupted pattern.

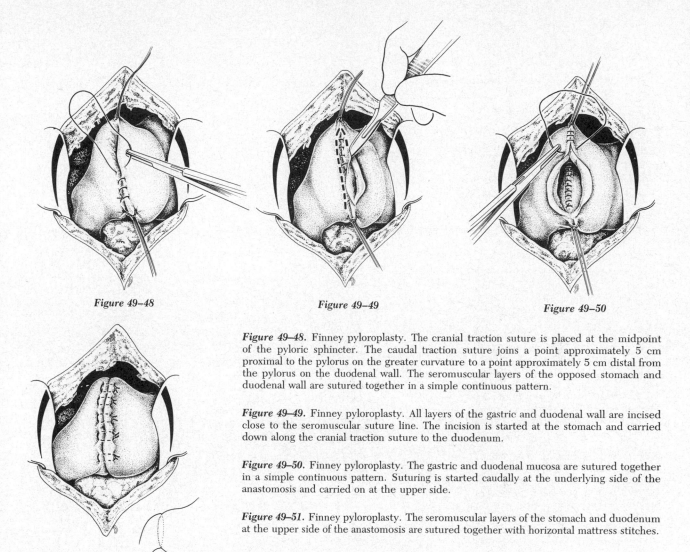

Figure 49–48

Figure 49–49

Figure 49–50

Figure 49–48. Finney pyloroplasty. The cranial traction suture is placed at the midpoint of the pyloric sphincter. The caudal traction suture joins a point approximately 5 cm proximal to the pylorus on the greater curvature to a point approximately 5 cm distal from the pylorus on the duodenal wall. The seromuscular layers of the opposed stomach and duodenal wall are sutured together in a simple continuous pattern.

Figure 49–49. Finney pyloroplasty. All layers of the gastric and duodenal wall are incised close to the seromuscular suture line. The incision is started at the stomach and carried down along the cranial traction suture to the duodenum.

Figure 49–50. Finney pyloroplasty. The gastric and duodenal mucosa are sutured together in a simple continuous pattern. Suturing is started caudally at the underlying side of the anastomosis and carried on at the upper side.

Figure 49–51. Finney pyloroplasty. The seromuscular layers of the stomach and duodenum at the upper side of the anastomosis are sutured together with horizontal mattress stitches.

Figure 49–51

The dorsal side of the incision is closed with a simple continuous suture using 4-0 absorbable suture material (Fig. 49–50). This suture should include all layers of the gastric and duodenal wall and is continued at the ventral side of the incision (see Fig. 49–50). Finally, the seromuscular layers of the stomach and the duodenum at the ventral side of the incision are united with a series of horizontal mattress stitches, using 3-0 suture material (Fig. 49–51). A portion of the greater omentum may be used to cover the anastomosis.

Partial Gastrectomy and Gastroduodenostomy: the Billroth I Procedure

Resection of the stomach is started at the lesser omentum, which is perforated bluntly near the lesser curvature to create an opening of sufficient size to bring the index and middle fingers dorsal from the stomach (see Fig. 49–35). This maneuver allows ad-equate palpation of the distal part of the stomach and facilitates handling during ligation of major vessels at the lesser curvature. Pyloric hypertrophy and neo-plasia of the gastric wall can be readily identified on palpation, but mucosal changes in chronic hyper-trophic gastritis may be subtle and are easily over-looked. If malignancy is suspected the liver and the regional lymph nodes should be inspected for meta-stasis (see Fig. 49–39). The extent of the resection is determined by the location of diseased tissue and by the size of the stomach. The point of resection should always be higher on the lesser curvature than on the greater curvature to obtain a slightly oblique incision (Fig. 49–52). This prevents the formation of a blind sac at the cranial side of the anastomosis.

The lesser curvature is rotated upward to expose the branches of the left gastric artery and vein. These are double ligated with transfixation ligatures and divided at the selected site of resection (Fig. 49–53). An area of at least 2 cm is freed from all fat and omental remnants and marked with a traction suture

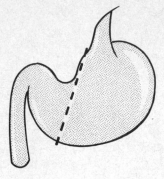

Figure 49–52. Partial gastrectomy. Dotted line indicates a slightly oblique incision to prevent blind sac formation at the lesser curvature.

Figure 49–53. Billroth I gastroduoden-ostomy. Ligation of the branches of the left gastric artery and vein with transfixation ligature. The lesser curvature has been partially freed from fat and omental remnants.

Figure 49–54. Billroth I gastroduoden-osotomy. Ligation of the left gastroepiploic artery and vein. The greater curvature has been partially freed from fat and omental remnants.

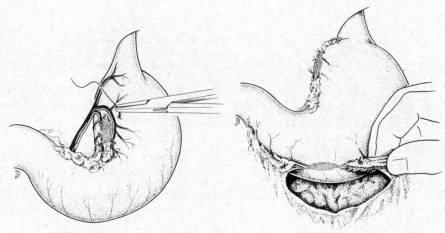

Figure 49–53   ***Figure 49–54***

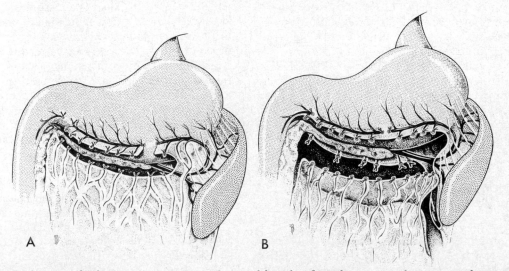

Figure 49–55. Billroth I gastroduodenostomy. *A,* Ligation of omental branches from the gastroepiploic artery and vein in suspected benign disease. *B,* Omental resection in suspected malignant disease. Ligation and division are carried on along the edge of the spleen, the splenic artery and vein, and the left lobe of the pancreas.

of 3-0 or 2-0 absorbable material (see Fig. 49–53). A similar procedure is carried out at the greater curvature, but the ligation of major vessels is slightly different. Instead of using transfixation ligatures, the gastroepiploic vessels are double clamped, divided, and ligated in a routine manner (Fig. 49–54). The omental branches of the gastroepiploic vessels are double ligated and divided close to the greater curvature from the point of division of the gastroepiploic vessels up to the right edge of the greater omentum (Fig. 49–55). If malignancy is suspected, the greater omentum should be included in the resection because it may contain implanted metastasis. In such cases, the dorsal leaf of the omentum is divided close to the left lobe of the pancreas.

The incision is started at the remaining part of the gastroepiploic artery and vein and follows the left gastroepiploic and splenic vessels (see Fig. 49–55). The cranial duodenal flexure is pulled toward the midline and dorsally to expose the common bile duct and the·right gastric artery and vein, which run in the lesser omentum. The right gastric artery and vein are clamped and divided close to the stomach and duodenum to avoid damage to the hepatic and gastroduodenal arteries, which lie in close proximity (Fig. 49–56).

The cranial part of the duodenum is freed from all fat and omental remnants for at least 3 cm distal to the pylorus. The distal part of the stomach is lifted and retracted in a cranial direction to expose the pancreatic angle and duodenal lymph node. The right gastroepiploic artery and vein are hidden in the fat between the pancreas and the stomach and duodenum. They are carefully dissected, clamped, and divided (Fig. 49–57). The area between the pancreatic angle and the right border of the greater omentum is cleared of all fat. The pancreas is carefully

avoided in this procedure. The duodenal lymph node should be removed only if malignancy is suspected. A straight intestinal clamp with atraumatic serrations is applied across the duodenum just proximal to the pancreatic angle. A second clamp is applied distal to the pylorus, leaving a distance of at least 1 cm between the clamps. The duodenum is divided with a knife against the proximal clamp (Fig. 49–58) and the duodenal stump is covered with a moist sponge. Two straight intestinal clamps are applied parallel to each other across the proximal part of the stomach at the site of the traction sutures at the greater and lesser curvature. The clamps are placed approximately 1 cm apart from each other and should be of sufficient length to include all of the stomach.

The stomach is divided with a knife held against the distal clamp (Fig. 49–59), and the distal part of the stomach is removed. Closure of the gastric stump is begun at the lesser curvature and continued up for a distance from the greater curvature to equal the diameter of the transected duodenum. The mucosa is closed with a simple continuous stitch using 4-0 absorbable suture material (Fig. 49–60). The seromuscular layer is closed with an interrupted Lembert suture using 3-0 absorbable suture material (see Fig. 49–60).

The gastric and duodenal stumps are approximated and rotated to expose the seromuscular layers of the underlying side of the anastomosis. These layers are sutured with simple interrupted sutures, using 3-0 absorbable suture material. Suturing is started at the lesser curvature and progresses downward until the greater curvature is reached (Fig. 49–61). Sutures are placed first and tied later. The gastric mucosa is sutured to the duodenal mucosa with a simple continuous suture, using 4-0 absorbable material. Suturing is started at the lesser curvature and progresses

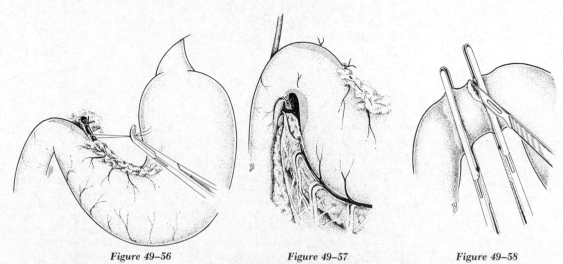

Figure 49–56   *Figure 49–57*   *Figure 49–58*

Figure 49–56. Billroth I gastroduodenostomy. Ligation of the right gastric artery and vein.

Figure 49–57. Billroth I gastroduodenostomy. Ligation and division of the right gastroepiploic artery and vein.

Figure 49–58. Billroth I gastroduodenostomy. Division of the duodenum along the proximal clamp.

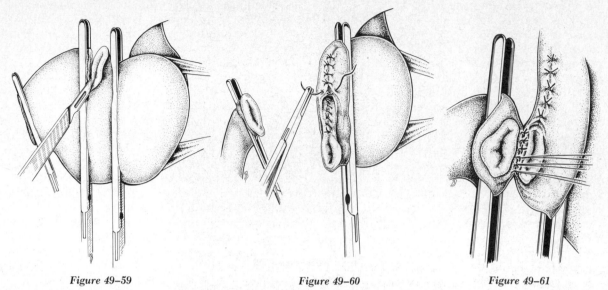

Figure 49–59   Figure 49–60   Figure 49–61

Figure 49–59. Billroth I gastroduodenostomy. Division of the stomach along the distal clamp.

Figure 49–60. Billroth I gastroduodenostomy. Closure of the gastric stump. The mucosa has been closed with a simple continuous suture to leave an opening that equals the size of the transected duodenum. The seromuscular layer is closed with interrupted Lembert sutures.

Figure 49–61. Billroth I gastroduodenostomy. Gastroduodenal anastomosis. The seromuscular layers of the underlying side of the anastomosis are sutured with simple interrupted sutures. Suturing is started at the lesser curvature and progresses downward until the greater curvature is reached.

downward to the greater curvature and continues at the upper side of the anastomosis (Fig. 49–62), where it is tied to the uncut end of the anchoring suture at the duodenal side of the anastomosis.

The anastomosis is completed with a series of interrupted sutures of 3-0 absorbable suture material placed in the seromuscular layers at the upper side of the anastomosis. Suturing is best started at the lesser curvature, which is rotated slightly to facilitate placement of the first sutures (Fig. 49–63). Following removal of the intestinal clamps the anastomosis is inspected for hemorrhage and returned to the abdominal cavity.

Partial Gastrectomy and Gastrojejunostomy: the Billroth II Procedure

The Billroth II procedure allows more radical resections than the Billroth I procedure and may require different techniques of ligation at the proximal side of the anastomosis. If a high resection is planned, ligation of the left gastric artery and vein at some distance from the stomach is easier than ligation of their branches at the gastric wall (Fig. 49–64). Similar ligation of the left gastroepiploic artery and vein leaves the short gastric arteries and veins as the only vessels to nourish the gastric fundus. In man this blood supply is enough for viability.[149]

Following transection of the duodenum as described in the Billroth I procedure, the duodenal stump is closed. The mucosa and submucosa are closed with a simple continuous suture, using 4-0

absorbable suture material. Traction sutures placed at the cranial and caudal margins of the duodenal stump may facilitate handling during suturing (Fig. 49–65). The mucosal suture line is inverted by apply-

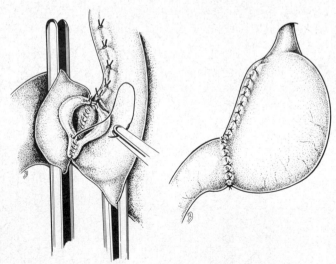

Figure 49–62   Figure 49–63

Figure 49–62. Billroth I gastroduodenostomy. Gastroduodenal asatomosis. The gastric mucosa is sutured to the duodenal mucosa is a simple continuous pattern. The underlying side of the anastomosis is sutured first, starting at the lesser curve. Suturing is carried on at the upper side of the anastomosis.

Figure 49–63. Billroth I gastroduodenostomy. The anastomosis is completed with a row of simple interrupted sutures in the seromuscular layers at the upper side of the anastomosis.

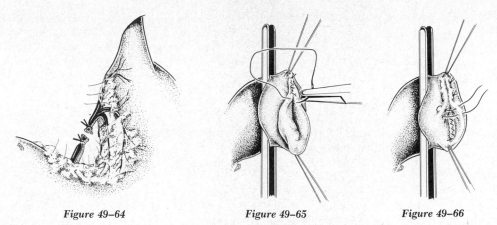

Figure 49–64   Figure 49–65   Figure 49–66

Figure 49–64. Billroth II gastrojejunostomy. Ligation of the left gastric artery and vein near the lesser curvature in radical gastric resection.

Figure 49–65. Billroth II gastrojejunosotomy. Closure of the duodenal stump. The mucosa is sutured in a simple continuous pattern.

Figure 49–66. Billroth II gastrojejunosotomy. Closure of the duodenal stump. The mucosal suture line is inverted by a row of horizontal seromuscular mattress stitches.

ing a row of interrupted mattress sutures of 3-0 absorbable material (Fig. 49–66). The intestinal clamp is removed and the stump is inspected for hemorrhage and returned into the abdomen. The gastric stump is closed in the same manner, but an interrupted Lembert suture may be used instead of mattress sutures to invert the seromuscular layer.

An area at or just cranial from the greater curvature is freed from all fat and omental remnants and clamped with a curved intestinal clamp with atraumatic serrations. A loop of jejunum is brought forward and placed next to the greater curvature of the stomach. The loop should be isoperistaltic and unrestrained but has to be made reasonably short, since longer loops are more prone to subsequent marginal ulceration[149] (see Fig. 49–41). A long intestinal clamp with atraumatic serrations is applied across the jejunal loop, and the seromuscular layers of the stomach and jejunum are approximated with a simple interrupted suture, using 3-0 absorbable suture material (Fig. 49–67). The stomach and jejunum are incised close to this suture line to avoid excessive inversion, which might cause postoperative stenosis (Fig. 49–68). The gastrojejunostomy is completed in the same manner

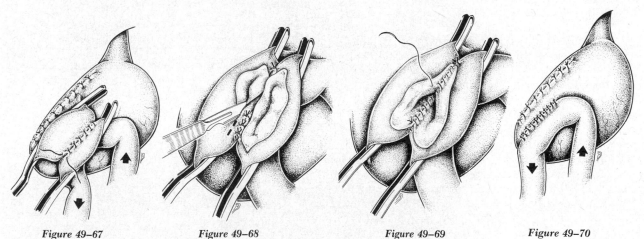

Figure 49–67   Figure 49–68   Figure 49–69   Figure 49–70

Figure 49–67. Billroth II gastrojejunostomy. Gastrojejunal anastomosis. An isoperistaltic jejunal loop is sutured to the stomach with a simple interrupted seromuscular suture.

Figure 49–68. Billroth II gastrojejunosotomy. Gastrojejunal anastomosis. The stomach and jejunum are incised close to the seromuscular suture line.

Figure 49–69. Billroth II gastrojejunostomy. Gastrojejunal anastomosis. The mucosa is closed with a simple continuous suture. Suturing is started at the underlying side of the anastomosis and continued at the upper side.

Figure 49–70. Billroth II gastrojejunosotomy. The anastomosis is completed with a row of simple interrupted sutures in the seromuscular layers at the upper side of the anastomosis.

as the Billroth I gastroduodenostomy (Figs. 49–69 and 49–70).

Gastrojejunostomy: the Polya and Hofmeister Procedures

The Polya and Hofmeister procedures are variations of the Billroth II procedure in which the jejunal loop is anastomosed directly to the gastric stump (see Fig. 49–41). The two methods differ only in the size of the stoma, which is smaller in the Hofmeister method owing to partial closure of the gastric stump. Both methods are less complicated than the Billroth II procedure but offer less freedom in determining the site of anastomosis and the position of the jejunal loop. Since there are no major differences between these procedures and the Billroth I and II, they are not discussed in detail.[84, 125, 149]

Prognosis

Congenital pyloric stenosis has a favorable prognosis if it is not associated with esophageal dilation. The prognosis for acquired delayed gastric emptying depends on the cause of the condition. In our experience chronic hypertrophic gastritis may have a favorable prognosis, even in chronic cases with serious enlargement of the stomach. Gastric neoplasms are usually discovered in an advanced state. If resection is feasible, the prognosis may be favorable in benign neoplasia but is usually poor in malignant tumors.

Aftercare

A gastric decompression tube should be introduced prior to surgery and left in place for at least 48 hours following surgery. This requires a pharyngostomy to keep the tube in place after the animal has recovered from anesthesia. Continuous suction is applied for as long as possible as for gastric dilation-torsion syndrome. The intravenous administration of electrolyte solutions is continued until electrolyte and acid-base imbalances are corrected and oral fluid intake is adequate. Small quantities of drinking water are offered following recovery from anesthesia, but no food should be given during the first 48 hours following surgery. The stomach tube can be removed after 48 hours if the amount of aspirated fluid is only small but may be left in place longer if aspiration yields large amounts of fluid. Following removal of the gastric decompression tube, feeding is started with a liquid food preparation, which is offered in small quantities every eight hours. The amount is gradually increased and replaced by a high-quality bland diet.

If there is gastric atony, metoclopramide* is given subcutaneously in a dose of 0.2 mg/kg every eight

hours 15 to 20 minutes before feeding. This drug is effective in the treatment of delayed gastric emptying in man[113] and accelerates gastric emptying in the dog,[65, 103] but its efficacy in the treatment of delayed gastric emptying in small animals has not been established.

Complications

Aspiration pneumonia is a constant threat to patients with delayed gastric emptying. The risk of aspiration of gastric contents is especially high during the induction of and the recovery from anesthesia, as anesthetics depress the swallowing reflex and may induce vomiting by direct stimulation of the vomiting center. The stomach should, therefore, always be intubated and aspirated before anesthesia is induced.

Few complications are reported following minor surgical procedures such as pyloromyotomy or pyloroplasty. Complications following partial gastrectomy have been reported in man,[133] but little is known about the complications of this surgery in small animal patients. Marginal ulcer following gastrojejunostomy has been reported in a dog.[7] In man, marginal ulcers occur at the intestinal side of the anastomosis and may cause abdominal pain and bleeding. They can be treated medically with antacids and cimetidine, but if medical treatment fails conversion to a Billroth I anastomosis should be undertaken.

GASTRIC FOREIGN BODIES

Incidence

Gastric foreign bodies occur in dogs and cats of all breeds and ages. The incidence is not known but could be quite high, as many small animals consume foreign material.

Clinical Signs

The most characteristic sign is vomiting, which may be intermittent because the vomiting reflex is only triggered when the foreign body is located in the pyloric antrum.[16] Foreign bodies in the corpus and fundus of the stomach usually cause no symptoms. However, if they get stuck in the pyloric portion of the stomach, delayed gastric emptying may develop as discussed in the previous section. Physical examination is usually unremarkable. Gastric foreign bodies cannot be detected on abdominal palpation.

Laboratory Findings

Laboratory findings vary with the severity and duration of vomiting. There may be dehydration and electrolyte and acid-base imbalances. The most com-

---

*Primperan, Delagrange, Paris, France.

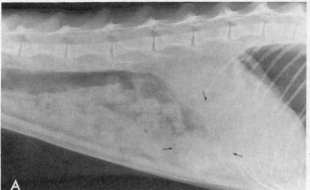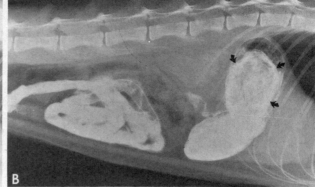

Figure 49–71. Lateral abdominal radiographs of a cat with gastric foreign body. *A,* On the plain radiograph (A) the stomach is filled with fluid-dense material (arrows indicate position of the stomach). *B,* Lateral postevacuation radiograph reveals a large barium-coated foreign body (arrows). (Courtesy of W. Th. C. Wolvekamp.)

mon abnormality in vomiting dogs is metabolic acidosis,[22] but hypokalemic alkalosis may occur in animals with pyloric obstruction.

Radiographic Findings

Plain films are adequate in diagnosing radiopaque foreign bodies, but unfortunately many gastric foreign bodies are radiolucent (Fig. 49–71). Their presence may be indicated by increased width of a localized portion of the stomach.[106] Gas and ingested debris often accumulate around gastric foreign bodies and help to identify them. If contrast studies are necessary, use of air or carbon dioxide as a negative contrast medium is preferable to positive contrast agents, as these tend to mask foreign bodies.[106] The administration of a small amount of barium prior to the introduction of air or carbon dioxide may be helpful, especially if the foreign body absorbs the contrast agent.

Diagnosis

Gastric foreign bodies are diagnosed by radiographic findings. If plain films are inconclusive, positive or double contrast studies should be performed as described previously. Blood should be examined to assess fluid, electrolyte, and acid-base imbalances and to rule out concomitant renal failure.

Surgical Methods

Gastric foreign bodies should be removed when detected because they may cause chronic inflammation of the gastric wall and pyloric or intestinal obstruction. The surgeon may choose from a variety of techniques. The method to use depends on the shape, size, and consistency of the foreign body. Foreign bodies with a rounded shape and a smooth surface can be removed by inducing vomiting 30 minutes after the animal has been fed a regular meal.

In the dog apomorphine can be used at a dose of 1 to 5 mg subcutaneously, but in the cat xylazine* at 1 mg/kg is more effective. If this method fails, the foreign body can be retrieved by endoscopy. A specially designed basket-type grasping forceps (Fig. 49–72) is inserted through the endoscope and manipulated around the foreign body. The basket is closed by sliding it back into the basket tube as far as possible, after which it is withdrawn from the patient together with the endoscope.

Large foreign bodies or foreign bodies with a rough surface that might injure the esophagus when retrieved via the mouth should be removed by gastrotomy. The abdominal cavity is entered by a cranial midline laparotomy. The ventral aspect of the stomach is walled off with moist laparotomy sponges. The incision is made in a relatively avascular area, approximately midway between the lesser and greater curvature and equidistant from the pylorus and cardia[4] (Fig. 49–73). The incision should be large enough to allow the foreign body to pass without tearing. Traction sutures or Babcock tissue forceps should be placed at each end of the incision to elevate the incision and prevent spillage of gastric contents into the abdominal cavity (Fig. 49–74). They will also

---

*Rompun, Bayer, Leverkusen, FRG.

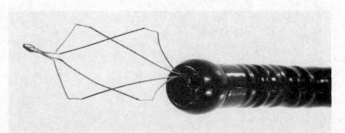

Figure 49–72. Basket-type foreign body grasping forceps protruding from endoscope. The grasping forceps is manipulated around the foreign body and pulled back into the endoscope until it is closed around the foreign body. Endoscope and foreign body are then removed together.

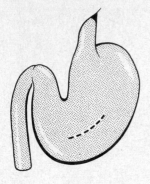

Figure 49–73. Site of incision for gastrotomy.

help to stabilize the incision during suturing. The incision is closed in two layers. The mucosa is closed with a simple continuous suture, using 4-0 absorbable suture material (Fig. 49–75). The seromuscular layer is closed with an interrupted Lembert suture, using 3-0 or 2-0 absorbable suture material (Fig. 49–76). If the abdominal cavity has been contaminated by gastric spillage, it should be thoroughly lavaged with warm saline or lactated Ringer's solution.

Prognosis

Gastrotomy for foreign bodies has a favorable prognosis.

Aftercare

Electrolyte and acid-base imbalances are corrected by intravenous electrolyte solutions. Fluid therapy should be continued until oral fluid intake is adequate. Small amounts of drinking water should be offered as soon as the animal has recovered from anesthesia. If drinking water is retained, feeding can be started 24 hours following surgery with small amounts of a bland diet. The amount of food is gradually increased until normal levels are reached by the fourth postoperative day.

Complications

Gastric foreign bodies may lodge in the pyloric portion and cause delayed gastric emptying, which is discussed in a separate section. Gastrotomy may be complicated by local or generalized peritonitis due to spillage of gastric contents into the abdominal cavity, but this is not a common sequela.

1. Alexander, J. W., Hoffer, R. E., McDonald, J. M., Bolton, G. R., and O'Neil, J. W.: Hiatal hernia in the dog: a case report and review of the literature. J. Am. Anim. Hosp. Assoc. *11*:793, 1975.
2. Andersen, A. C.: Digestive system. *In: The Beagle as an Experimental Dog.* Iowa State University Press, Ames, 1970, Chap. 10.
3. Archibald, J. A., Cawley, A. J., and Reed, J. H.: Surgical technique for correcting pyloric stenosis. Mod. Vet. Pract. *41*:28, 1960.
4. Arnockzy, S. P., and Ryan, W. W.: Gastrotomy and pyloroplasty. Vet. Clin. North Am. 5:343, 1975.
5. Atanassova, E., and Papasova, M.: Gastrointestinal motility. Intern. Rev. Physiol. *12*:35, 1977.
6. Barone, R.: *Anatomie Comparée des Mammifères Domestiques.* Tome 3, Fasc. 1. Splanchnologie. Lab. d'Anatomie, Ecole Nationale Veterinaire, Lyone, 1976.

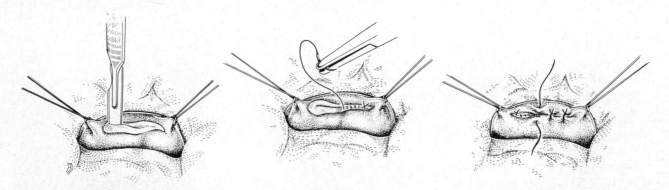

Figure 49–74   **Figure 49–75**   **Figure 49–76**

Figure 49–74. Gastrotomy. Traction sutures are used to stabilize the stomach during incision. The abdominal cavity is walled off with moist laparotomy sponges.

Figure 49–75. Gastrotomy. The mucosa is closed with a simple continuous suture.

Figure 49–76. Gastrotomy. The seromuscular layer is closed with an interrupted Lembert suture.

7. Beaumont, P. R.: Anastomotic jejunal ulcer secondary to gastrojejunostomy in a dog. J. Am. Anim. Hosp. Assoc. 17:233, 1981.

8. Behar, J., Biancani, P., and Sheahan, D. G.: Evaluation of esophageal tests in the diagnosis of reflux esophagitis. Gastroenterology 71:9, 1976.

9. Behar, J., Brand, D. L., Brown, F. C., Castell, D. O., Cohen, S., Crossley, R. J., Pope, C. E. II, and Winans, C. S.: Cimetidine in the treatment of symptomatic gastroesophageal reflux: a double-blind controlled trial. Gastroenterology 74:441, 1978.

10. Betts, C. W., Wingfield, W. E., and Greene, R. W.: A retrospective study of gastric dilatation-torsion in the dog. J. Small Anim. Pract. 15:727, 1974.

11. Betts, C. W., Wingfield, W. E., and Rosin, E.: "Permanent" gastropexy as a prophylactic measure against gastric volvulus. J. Am. Anim. Hosp. Assoc. 12:177, 1976.

12. Blackburn, P. S., and McFarlane, D.: Acute fatal dilatation of the stomach of the dog. Torsion of the stomach. J. Comp. Pathol. 54:189, 1944.

13. Blount, W.-P.: Some normal features of the stomach of the dog. Vet. Red. 10:877, 1930.

14. Bojarb, M. J.: Pathophysiology in Small Animal Surgery. Lea & Febiger, Philadelphia, 1981.

15. Bolton, G. R.: Handbook of Canine Electrocardiography. W. B. Saunders, Philadelphia, 1975.

16. Borison, H. L., and Wang, S. C.: Physiology and pharmacology of vomiting. Pharmacol. Rev. 5:193, 1953.

17. Bourdelle, E., and Bressou, C.: Anatomie Regionale des Animaux Domestiques. IV Carnivores: Chien et Chat. J-B Baillière, Paris, 1953.

18. Carric, C. B., and Seawright, A. A.: Mastocytosis with gastrointestinal ulceration in a dog. Aust. Vet. J. 44:503, 1968.

19. Christie, T. R., and Smith, C. W.: Gastrocolopexy for prevention of recurrent gastric volvulus. J. Am. Anim. Hosp. Assoc. 12:173, 1976.

20. Code, C. F., and Carlson, H. C.: Motor activity of the stomach. In Code, C. F. (ed.): Handbook of Physiology. American Physiological Society, Washington, D.C., 1968, pp. 1903–1916.

21. Code, C. F., and Marlett, J. A.: The interdigestive myoelectric complex of the stomach and small bowel of dogs. J. Physiol. London 246:289, 1975.

22. Cornelius, L. M., and Rawlings, C. A.: Arterial blood gas and acid-base values in dogs with various diseases and signs of diseases. J. Am. Vet. Med. Assoc. 178:992, 1981.

23. Cornelius, L. M., and Wingfield, W. E.: Diseases of the stomach. In Ettinger, S. J. (ed.): Textbook of Veterinary Internal Medicine. W. B. Saunders, Philadelphia, 1975, Chap. 4.

24. Daniel, E. E., and Irwin, J.: Electrical activity of gastric musculature. In Code, C. F. (ed.): Handbook of Physiology. American Physiological Society, Washington, D.C., 1968, pp. 1969–1984.

25. De Hoff, W. D., and Green, R. W.: Gastric dilatation and the gastric torsion complex. Vet. Clin. North Am. 2:141, 1972.

26. Delaney, J. P., and Grim, E.: Canine gastric blood flow and its distribution. Am. J. Physiol. 207:1195, 1964.

27. Delaney, J. P., and Grim, E.: A note on the weight of the dog's stomach. Am. J. Vet. Res. 25:1560, 1964.

28. De Meester, T. R., Wernly, J. A., Bryant, G. H., Little, A. C., and Skinner, D. B.: Clinical and in vitro analysis of determinants of gastroesophageal competence: a study of the principles of antireflux surgery. Am. J. Surg. 137:39, 1979.

29. Den Besten, L., and Hamza, K. N.: Effects of bile salts on ionic permeability of canine gastric mucosa during experimental shock. Gastroenterology 62:417, 1972.

30. De Vries, H. W.: Anesthesia and monitoring of the dog in cardiovascular research. Ph.D. Thesis, Utrecht, The Netherlands, 1976.

31. Dingwall, J. E.: The Pancreas. In Bojrab, M. J. (ed.): Current Techniques in Small Animal Surgery. Lea & Febiger, Philadelphia, 1975.

32. Dodds, W. J.: Instrumentation and methods for intraluminal esophageal manometry. Arch. Intern. Med. 136:515, 1976.

33. Dodds, W. J., Steff, J. J., Arndorfer, R. C., Linehar, J. H., and Hogan, W. J.: Improved infusion system for esophageal manometry. Clin. Res. 22:602, 1974.

34. Douglas, S. W.: Lesions involving the pyloric region of the canine stomach. J. Am. Vet. Rad. Soc. 9:89, 1968.

35. Douglas, S. W., Hall, L. W., and Walker, R. G.: The surgical relief of gastric lesions in the dog: report of seven cases. Vet. Rec. 86:743, 1970.

36. Dozois, R. R., Kelly, K. A., and Code, L. F.: Effect of distal antrectomy on gastric emptying of liquids and solids. Gastroenterology 61:675, 1971.

37. Eastwood, G. L., Castell, D. O., and Higgs, R. H.: Experimental esophagitis in cats impairs lower esophageal sphincter pressure. Gastroenterology 69:146, 1975.

38. Ehrlein, H. J., Pröve, J., and Schweiker, W.: The function of the pyloric sphincter for regulating gastric emptying and preventing reflux in the dog. In Christensen, J. (ed.): Gastrointestinal Motility. Raven Press, New York, 1980.

39. Ettinger, S. J., and Suter, P. F.: Canine Cardiology. W. B. Saunders, Philadelphia, 1970.

40. Evans, H. E., and Christensen, G. C. (eds.): Miller's Anatomy of the Dog, 2nd ed. W. B. Saunders, Philadelphia, 1979.

41. Fallah, A. M., Lumb, W. V., Nelson, A. W., Frandson, R. D., and Withrow, S. J.: Circumcostal gastropexy in the dog—a preliminary study. Vet. Surg. 11:9, 1982.

42. Fink, D. W.: Gastric volvulus: the angiographic appearance. Am. J. Roentgenol. 115:268, 1972.

43. Friedland, G. W., Kohatsu, S., and Lewin, K.: Comparative anatomy of the feline and canine sling fibres. Digest. Dis. 16:495, 1971.

44. Funkquist, B.: Gastric torsion in the dog. Nonsurgical reposition. J. Small Anim. Pract. 10:507, 1969.

45. Funkquist, B.: Gastric torsion in the dog. I. Radiological picture during nonsurgical treatment related to the pathological anatomy and the further clinical course. J. Small Anim. Pract. 20:73, 1979.

46. Funkquist, B., and Garmer, L.: Pathogenetic and therapeutic aspects of torsion of the canine stomach. J. Small Anim. Pract. 8:523, 1967.

47. Gaskell, J. C., Gibbs, C., and Pearson, H.: Sliding hiatus hernia with reflux esophagitis in two dogs. J. Small Anim. Pract. 15:503, 1974.

48. Gaynor, F., Hoffner, R. E., Nichols, M. F., Rosser, E., Moraff, H., Hahn, A. W., and MacCoy, D. M.: Physiologic features of the canine esophagus: effects of tranquilization on esophageal motility. Am. J. Vet. Res. 41:727, 1980.

49. Goldberg, S. L.: Afferent paths of nerves involved in vomiting reflex induced by distension of isolated pyloric pouch. Am. J. Physiol. 99:156, 1931.

50. Grandage, J.: The radiological appearance of stomach gas in the dog. Aust. Vet. J. 50:529, 1974.

51. Grandage, J.: Normal abdominal visceral relationships. Radiol. Proc. 59:241, 1982.

52. Guyton, A. C.: Textbook of Medical Physiology, 6th ed. W. B. Saunders, Philadelphia, 1981.

53. Hall, L. W.: Wrights Veterinary Anesthesia and Analgesia. Baillière Tindall, London, 1971.

54. Happé, R. P.: The gastroduodenal region. In Investigations into disorders of canine gastroduodenal function. Ph.D. Thesis, Utrecht, The Netherlands, 1982.

55. Happé, R. P., and Van der Gaag, I.: Endoscopic examination of the esophagus, stomach and duodenum in the dog. J. Am. Anim. Hosp. Assoc. 19:197, 1983.

56. Happé, R. P., Van der Gaag, I., Lamers, C. B. H. W., Van Toorenburg, J., Larsson, L. I., and Rehfeld, J. F.: Zollinger-Ellison syndrome in three dogs. Vet. Pathol. 17:177, 1980.

57. Happé, R. P., Van der Gaag, I., and Wolvekamp, W. Th. C.: Pyloric stenosis caused by hypertrophic gastritis in three dogs. J. Small Anim. Pract. 22:7, 1981.

58. Henderson, R. D., Mugashe, F., Jeejeebhoy, K. N., Cullen, J., Szczepanski, M., Boszko, A., and Marryat, G.: The role of bile and acid in the production of esophagitis and the motor deficit of esophagitis. Ann. Thorac. Surg. 14:465, 1972.

59. Henschel, E.: Anatomy of the stomach and mechanism of torsion. Proc. Voorjaarsdagen, Netherlands Small Animal Association, 1976.

60. Herr, D. M., Thompson, P. L., and Cunningham, J. H.: What is your diagnosis? J. Am. Vet. Med. Assoc. 162:491, 1973.

61. Hess, W., and Liechti, R.: Gleithernie und Refluxkrankheit. Springer Verlag, Berlin, 1978.

62. Howard, E. B., Sawa, T. R., Nielsen, S. W., and Kenyon, A. J.: Mastocytoma and gastro-duodenal ulceration. Pathol. Vet. 6:146, 1969.

63. Hunt, J. N., and Knox, M. T.: Regulation of gastric emptying. In Code, C. F. (ed.): Handbook of Physiology. American Physiological Society, Washington, D.C., 1968, pp. 1917–1935.

64. Hwang, K., Essez, H. E., and Mann, F. C.: Problems resulting from vagotomy in dogs with special reference to emesis. Am. J. Physiol. 149:429, 1947.

65. Jacoby, H. I., and Brodie, D. A.: Gastrointestinal actions of metoclopramide. An experimental study. Gastroenterology 52:676, 1967.

66. Jama, R. H., Perlman, M. H., and Matsomoto, T.: Incidence of stress ulcer formation associated with steroid therapy in various shock states. Am. J. Surg. 130:328, 1975.

67. Johnson, L. F., and De Meester, T. R.: Twenty four hour pH-monitoring of the distal esophagus: a quantitative measure of gastroesophageal reflux. Am. J. Gastroenterol. 62:325, 1974.

68. Johnson, L. R.: Gastrointestinal hormones and their functions. Ann. Rev. Physiol. 39:135, 1977.

69. Jones, B. R., Nicholls, M. R., and Badman, R.: Peptic ulceration in a dog associated with an islet cell carcinoma of the pancreas and an elevated plasma gastrin level. J. Small Anim. Pract. 17:593, 1976.

70. Kagan, K. G., and Schaer, M.: Gastric dilatation and volvulus in a dog. A case justifying electrolyte and acid-base assessment. J. Am. Vet. Med. Assoc. 182:703, 1983.

71. Kawaruda, Y., Weiss, R., and Matsumoto, T.: Pathophysiology of stress ulcer: Pharmacologic doses of steroid. Am. J. Surg. 129:249, 1975.

72. Kelly, K. A.: Gastric emptying of liquids and solids: roles of proximal and distal stomach. Am. J. Physiol. 239:G71, 1980.

73. Kelly, K. A., and Code, C. F.: Canine gastric pacemaker. Am. J. Physiol. 220:112, 1971.

74. Konturek, S. J.: Gastric secretion. MTP Int. Rev. Sci. 4:227, 1974.

75. Krahwinkel, D. J., Sawyer, D. C., and Evans, A. T.: Neuroleptanalgesia and neuroleptanesthesia. J. Am. Anim. Hosp. Assoc. 8:368, 1972.

76. Lakatos, L., and Ruckstuhl, B.: Hypertrophische Pylorusstenose beim Hund. Schweiz. Arch. Tierheilk. 119:155, 1977.

77. Lamers, C. B. H. W.: Some aspects of the Zollinger Ellison syndrome and serum gastrin. Ph.D. Thesis, Nijmegen, The Netherlands, 1976.

78. Larsen, L. H.: Stomach and small intestine. In Archibald, J. (ed.): Canine Surgery. American Veterinary Publications, Inc., Santa Barbara, 1965, Chap. 20.

79. Lawson, H. H.: Effect of duodenal contents on the gastric mucosa under experimental conditions. Lancet 1:469, 1964.

80. Lawther, W. A.: Pyloric stenosis in a puppy. Aust. Vet. J. 37:317, 1961.

81. Lind, J. R., Duthie, H. L., Schlegel, J. R., and Code, C.

F.: Motility of the gastric fundus. Am. J. Physiol. 201:197, 1961.

82. Lumb, W. V., and Jones, E. W.: Veterinary Anesthesia. Lea & Febiger, Philadelphia, 1973.

83. MacCoy, D. M., Sykes, G. P., Hoffer, R. E., and Harvey, H. J.: A gastropexy technique for permanent fixation of the pyloric antrum. J. Am. Anim. Hosp. Assoc. 18:763, 1982.

84. Maingot, R.: Abdominal Operations. Prentice-Hall Inc., New York, 1974.

85. Malagaleda, J. R.: Physiologic basis and clinical significance of gastric emptying disorders. Digest. Dis. Sci. 24:657, 1979.

86. Malamud, L. S.: GE scintiscanning to detect and quantitate GE reflux. In Second International Symposium on the Esophagus and Gastroesophageal Junction. Biomedical Information Company, New York, 1978.

87. Max, M., and Menguy, R.: Influence of adrenocorticotropin, cortisone, aspirin and phenylbutazone on the rate of exfoliation and the rate of cell renewal of gastric mucosal cells. Gastroenterology 58:329, 1970.

88. McCarthy, L. E., Borison, H. L., Spiegel, P. K., and Friendlander, R. M.: Vomiting: Radiographic and oscillographic correlates in the decerebrate cat. Gastroenterology 67:1126, 1974.

89. Menguy, R.: Gastric mucus and the gastric mucous barrier. Am. J. Surg. 117:806, 1969.

90. Merdan Dhein, C. R., Rawlings, C. A., and Rosin, E.: Esophageal hiatal herniation and eventration of the diaphragm with resultant gastroesophageal reflux. J. Am. Anim. Hosp. Assoc. 16:517, 1980.

91. Merkley, D. F., Howard, D. R., Krehbiel, J. D., Eyster, G. E., Sawyer, D. C., and Krehbiel, J. D.: Experimentally induced acute gastric dilatation in the dog: cardio-pulmonary effects. J. Am. Anim. Hosp. Assoc. 12:143, 1976.

92. Merkley, D. F., Howard, D. R., Krehbiel, J. D., Eyster, G. E., Krahwinkel, D. J., and Sawyer, D. C.: Experimentally induced acute gastric dilatation in the dog: clinicopathologic findings. J. Am. Anim. Hosp. Assoc. 12:149, 1976.

93. Meyer, J. H. S., Mandiola, S., Shadchehr, A., and Cohen, M.: Dispersion of solid food by the canine stomach. Gastroenterology 72:1102, 1977.

94. Miller, M. E. M.: Anatomy of the Dog. W. B. Saunders, Philadelphia, 1964.

95. Moody, F. G., Cheung, L. Y., Simons, M. A., and Zalewsky, C.: Stress and the acute gastric mucosal lesion. Am. J. Dig. Dis. 21:148, 1976.

96. Mroz, C. T., and Kelly, K. A.: The role of the extrinsic antral nerves in the regulating of gastric emptying. Surg. Gynecol. Obstet. 145:369, 1977.

97. Muir, W. W.: Gastric dilatation-volvulus in the dog, with emphasis on cardiac arrhythmias. J. Am. Vet. Med. Assoc. 180:739, 1982.

98. Muir, W. W.: Acid-base and electrolyte disturbances in dogs with gastric dilatation volvulus. J. Am. Vet. Med. Assoc. 181:229, 1982.

99. Muir, W. W., and Lipowitz, A. J.: Cardiac dysrhythmias associated with gastric dilatation-volvulus in the dog. J. Am. Vet. Med. Assoc. 172:683, 1978.

100. Murray, M., McKeating, F. J., and Lauder, I. M.: Peptic ulceration in the dog: a clinicopathological study. Vet. Rec. 91:441, 1972.

101. Murray, M., Robinson, P. B., McKeating, F. J., Baker, G. J., and Lauder, I. M.: Primary gastric neoplasia in the dog: a clinicopathological study. Vet. Rec. 91:474, 1972.

102. Nickel, R., Schummer, A., Sieferle, E., and Sack, W. O.: The Viscera of the Domestic Mammals. Verlag Paul Parey, Berlin, 1973.

103. Nicolai, J. W.: Beschleunigung der Magen-Darm-Passage durch Metoclopramid-dihydrochlorid bei Hunden. Kleinter. Prax. 24:217, 1979.

104. Nissen, R.: Eine einfache Operation zur Beeinflussung der

Refluxoesophagitis. Schweiz. Med. Wochenschr. *86*:590, 1956.

105. Nissen, R., and Rosetti, M.: Die Behandlung von Hiatushernien und Refluxösophagitis mit Gastropexie und Fundoplicatio. Thieme, Stuttgart, 1959.

106. O'Brien, T. R.: *Radiographic Diagnosis of Abdominal Disorders in the Dog and Cat.* W. B. Saunders, Philadelphia, 1978.

107. Okabe, S., Takeuchi, K., Murata, T., and Urushidani, T.: Effects of cimetidine on healing of chronic gastric and duodental ulcers in dogs. Digest. Dis. *23*:166, 1978.

108. Parks, J. L.: Surgical management of gastric torsion. Vet. Clin. North Am. *9*:259, 1979.

109. Parks, J. L., and Green, R. W.: Tube gastrostomy for the treatment of gastric volvulus. J. Am. Anim. Hosp. Assoc. *12*:168, 1976.

110. Pathaik, A. K., Hurvitz, A. I., and Johnson, G. E.: Canine gastrointestinal neoplasms. Vet. Pathol. *14*:547, 1977.

111. Pearson, H., Gaskell, C. J., Gibbs, C., and Waterman, A.: Pyloric and esophageal dysfunction in the cat. J. Small Anim. Pract. *15*:487, 1974.

112. Pearson, H., Darke, P. G. G., and Gibbs, C.: Reflux oesophagitis and stricture formation after anesthesia: a review of seven cases in dogs and cats. J. Small Anim. Pract. *19*:507, 1978.

113. Perkel, M. S., Moore, C., and Hersh, T.: Metoclopramide therapy in patients with delayed gastric emptying. A randomized, double blind study. Digest. Dis. Sci. *24*:662, 1979.

114. Prove, J., and Ehrlein, H. J.: Motor function of gastric antrum and pylorus for evacuation of low and high viscosity meals in dogs. Gut *23*:150, 1982.

115. Punto, L., Mokka, R. E. M., and Kairalvoma, M. I.: Effect of metoclopramide on the lower oesophageal sphincter. An experimental study in dogs. Mcd. Biol. *55*:66, 1977.

116. Rawlings, C. A., Wingfield, W. E., and Betts, C. W.: Shock therapy and anesthetic management in gastric dilatation-volvulus. J. Am. Anim. Hosp. Assoc. *12*:158, 1976.

117. Rees, W. D. W., and Turnberg, L. A.: Mechanisms of gastric mucosal protection: a role for the 'mucus-bicarbonate' barrier. Clin. Sci. *62*:343, 1982.

118. Rhodes, W. H., and Brodey, R. S.: The differential diagnosis of pyloric obstructions in the dog. J. Am. Vet. Radiol. Soc. *6*:65, 1965.

119. Rogers, W. A., and Donovan, E. F.: Peptic esophagitis in a dog. J. Am. Vet. Med. Assoc. *163*:462, 1973.

120. Romanes, G. J. (ed.): *Cunningham's Textbook of Anatomy*, 10th ed. Oxford University Press, London, 1964.

121. Rosin, E., Galphin, S. P., and Bowen, J. M.: Intraluminal esophageal sphincter manometry in dogs immobilized with Xylazin. Am. J. Vet. Res. *40*:873, 1979.

122. Safaie-Shirazie, S., Den Besten, L., and Zike, W. L.: Effects of bile salts on the ionic permeability of the esophageal mucosa and their role in the production of esophagitis. Gastroenterology *68*:728, 1975.

123. Sautter, J. H., and Hanlon, G. F.: Gastric neoplasms in the dog: a report of 20 cases. J. Am. Vet. Med. Assoc. *166*:691, 1975.

124. Seawright, A. A., and Grono, L. R.: Malignant mastcell tumour in a cat with perforating duodenal ulcer. J. Pathol. Bact. *87*:107, 1964.

125. Shackleford, R. T., and Zuidema, G. D.: *Surgery of the Alimentary Tract.* Vol. II, Stomach, Duodenum. Incisions, Sutures. W. B. Saunders, Philadelphia, 1981.

126. Skinner, D. B., and Belsey, R.: Surgical management of esophageal reflux and hiatus hernia. J. Thorac. Cardiovasc. Surg. *53*:33, 1967.

127. Steff, J. J.: Intraluminal esophageal manometry: an analysis of variables affecting recording fidelity of peristaltic pressure. Gastroenterology *67*:221, 1974.

128. Stinson, A. W., and Calhoun, M. L.: Digestive systems. *In* Dellmann, H. D., and Brown, E. M. (eds.): *Textbook of Veterinary Histology.* Lea & Febiger, Philadelphia, 1983.

129. Straus, E., Johnson, G. F., and Yalow, R. S.: Canine Zollinger-Ellison syndrome. Gastroenterology *72*:380, 1977.

130. Stremple, J. F., Mori, H., Lev, R., and Jerzy Glass, G. B.: The stress ulcer syndrome. *In: Current Problems in Surgery.* Year Book Medical Publishers, Inc., Chicago, 1973.

131. Strombeck, D. R.: *Small Animal Gastroenterology.* Stonegate Publishing, Davis, 1979.

132. Theodorakis, M. L.: External scintigraphy in measuring rate of gastric emptying in Beagles. Am. J. Physiol. *239*:G39, 1980.

133. Thompson, J. C.: The stomach and duodenum. *In* Sabiston, D. C., Jr. (ed.): *Textbook of Surgery.* W. B. Saunders, Philadelphia, 1981.

134. Turner, T.: A case of torsion of the stomach in an 11-year old dachshund bitch. Vet. Rec. *76*:243, 1964.

135. Turner, T.: Clinical communication: a case of torsion of the stomach in a five year old cat. J. Small Anim. Pract. *9*:231, 1968.

136. Twaddle, A. A.: Pyloric stenosis in three cats and its correction by pyloroplasty. N. Z. Vet. J. *18*:15, 1970.

137. Twaddle, A. A.: Congenital pyloric stenosis in two kittens corrected by pyloroplasty. N. Z. Vet. J. *19*:26, 1971.

138. Van den Brom, W. E., and Happé, R. P.: Gastric emptying of a radionuclide-labeled test meal in clinical healthy dogs (a new mathematical analysis and reference values). *In* Happé, R. P. (ed.): Investigations into disorders of canine gastroduodenal function. Ph.D. Thesis, Utrecht, The Netherlands, 1982.

139. Vick, K. P., and Dröge, P.: Zum Problem der Magendrehung. Kleinter Prax. *22*:104, 1977.

140. Vitums, A.: Portosystemic communications in the dog. Acta Anat. *39*:271, 1959.

141. Walsh, J. H., and Grossman, M. I.: Gastrin (first of two parts). N. Engl. J. Med. *292*:1324, 1975.

142. While, L. W., and Hose, A. T.: Congenital pyloric stenosis. Vet. Rec. *71*:152, 1959.

143. Wilbur, B. G., Kelly, K. A., and Code, C. F.: Effect of gastric fundectomy on canine gastric electrical and motor activity. Am. J. Physiol. *226*:1445, 1974.

144. Wingfield, W. E., Betts, C. W., and Green, R. W.: Operative techniques and recurrence rates: associated with gastric volvulus in the dog. J. Small Anim. Pract. *16*:427, 1975.

145. Wingfield, W. E., Betts, C. W., and Rawlings, C. A.: Pathophysiology associated with gastric dilatation. J. Am. Anim. Hosp. Assoc. *12*:136, 1976.

146. Winnan, J., Avella, J., Callachan, C., and McCallum, R. W.: Double-blind trial of metoclopramide versus placebo-antacid in symptomatic gastroesophageal reflux. Gastroenterology *78*:1292 (abstr.), 1980.

147. Zeitschmann, O.: The shape and position of the dog's stomach. Vet. Rec. *50*:984, 1938.

148. Zinner, M. J., Turtinen, L., and Gurll, N. J.: The role of acid and ischemia in production of stress ulcers during canine hemorrhagic shock. Surgery *77*:807, 1975.

149. Zollinger, R. M., and Zollinger, R. M., Jr. (eds.): Subtotal gastrectomy. *In Atlas of Surgical Operations.* MacMillan Publishing Co., Inc., New York, 1975.

Chapter 50

The Intestines

Anatomy

John Grandage

The rule of thumb that the carnivore intestine is about five times the length of the trunk applies reasonably well to the dog and cat. The small intestine is about four times the length of the large and measures between 1 and 1.5 meters in the cat and between 2 and 5 meters in the dog.[10, 22]

Being able to distinguish one segment of gut from another avoids unnecessary sifting through loops of intestine at surgery. Only a few features, some subtle or inconstant, can be used to discriminate between segments. Although the small intestine is, on average, slightly narrower than the large, it is not always so because of transient changes in diameter related to physiological activity. The duodenum is best recognized by its relation to the stomach and pancreas and by its position. The jejunum is recognized by its length and emptiness (Latin *jejunum* = empty, hungry) and by the absence of other features. (In many animals the proximal jejunum may be recognized by the simplicity and coarseness of the vascular arcades within its mesentery, in contrast to the distal jejunum, which has more numerous vessels arranged in secondary arcades;[84] in the dog, however, these differences are subtle.[109]) The ileum is recognized by its additional peritoneal membrane, the ileocecal fold that attaches to its antimesenteric border, by the extra blood vessels within this fold, and by the somewhat thicker wall (better-developed circular muscle layer).[11] The cecum, most distinctive of all, is recognized by its blind, short, simple comma shape in the cat and by its longer snail-like coil in the dog. Finally the colon stands out because of its position, its relation to the cecum and rectum, and its often paler color, more prominent longitudinal muscle,[48] and diameter or fecal content. Lymph nodules within the mucous membrane are sometimes visible through the outer coats of the gut wall and appear as extensive aggregates in the small intestine and as solitary nodules in the large (see later).

TOPOGRAPHY AND MESENTERIES

The intestines are the most mobile of the viscera. Mobility is required not only for their own digestive movements but also to allow the abdomen to change shape and capacity, the adjacent viscera to fill and empty, and the spine to flex. Limitless mobility, however, would risk entanglement or vascular occlusion. The mesenteries permit ample mobility while still restricting excessive movement and largely determine intestinal topography; they support, tether,

and convey vital supplies to the intestines and serve as mobile partitions that can be pushed about but not penetrated. The bulk of the mesentery hangs like a full, gathered skirt with the intestines forming the hem. Here the gut can coil and squirm but cannot entangle. Branches of the cranial mesenteric artery radiate through the mesentery and form its principal skeleton. The aortic origin of this artery beneath the first lumbar vertebra is thus a sort of hub to the abdomen and a significant landmark.[47]

As the gut elongates in embryonic life it twists for more than three-fourths of a turn around the cranial mesenteric artery, to resemble two interlocking hooks or question marks, each with ascending, transverse, and descending parts. The transverse colon crosses the abdomen cranial to the artery and the transverse duodenum caudal to it.

Knowledge of the position of the initial and terminal segments of the gut (descending duodenum and descending colon) greatly facilitates exploration of the abdomen. The descending duodenum lies on the right and the descending colon on the left. Their long mesenteries (mesoduodenum and mesocolon) are always the most dorsally located. In the prone position they drape over the rest of the intestines; conversely, in the supine position they cradle the intestines. During a laparotomy one can grasp the descending colon or descending duodenum and draw the whole intestinal mass to one side or the other, exposing the abdominal roof on the left or right (Fig. 50–1).

The ascending parts of the colon and duodenum are held on short mesenteries that tend to fuse with the longer mesenteries overlying them. On the left the ascending duodenum is connected to the descending mesocolon by a short duodenocolic ligament; on the·right the ascending colon is tied to the mesoduodenum. With this basic information, it is possible to find one's way logically to most parts of the gut.

STRUCTURE

In cats and dogs the intestinal wall is thick compared with the size of the lumen,[104] with both mucosal and muscular layers being substantial.[72] The small lumen means the ingesta may be only four per cent of body weight (in ruminants it may reach 25 per cent).

The **mucosa** of the carnivore intestine is without circular folds (plicae circulares), although occasionally

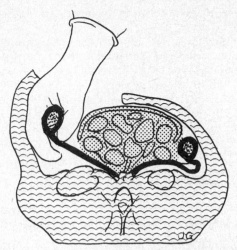

Figure 50–1. Most of the intestinal mass is cradled within the mesoduodenum on the right and mesocolon on the left. The abdominal roof can be exposed by drawing the descending duodenum or descending colon toward the midline.

vestiges of them are seen.[2] The villi are particularly long and slender, most approaching 1 mm in the cat.[111, 112] They are less variable from one segment of the gut to another than in many species[111] and increase the surface area about eight-fold in the dog and up to 15-fold in the cat. The epithelium covering the villi is composed of cells produced in the intestinal crypts; the cells pass up onto the villi and are shed from the apex, with total replacement of the villus epithelium occurring every two to six days. The shed cells add substantially to the protein in the lumen.

About a score of aggregated lymphatic nodules (Peyer's patches), some 2 cm by 1.5 cm, are found roughly opposite the mesenteric attachment in the dog. In this species, but not in many others,[53] they are more numerous in the proximal intestine. The mucosa overlying these aggregations has central craters some 2 to 3 mm deep and 2 to 9 mm wide; when filled with barium during a radiographic examination, these craters resemble ulcers.[85] Such pseudoulcers are particularly common in the descending duodenum.[116] Some claim that six or seven aggregations are also present in the cat,[22, 76, 82] but these are not conspicuous.[111] In the large intestine the lymphoid organs are large solitary nodules. In the dog they have been called lymphoglandular complexes, because large intestinal glands discharge amidst them. They appear as rounded, mucosal elevations, about 3 mm in diameter, which pepper the walls of the large intestine, especially the cecum and rectum in the dog,[3] and exclusively those sites in the cat.[53] The solitary lymphatic nodules are often visible through the serosa of the dog's intestines, and occasionally on radiographs following a barium meal.

The connective tissue of the submucosa is dominated by the left and right spiralling fibers, which provide support while still allowing the intestine to dilate.[6] Earlier opinions that the muscular fibers within the tunica muscularis were spiral too have not been substantiated;[33] instead they consist of the orthodox arrangement of outer longitudinal and inner circular fibers.

VESSELS AND NERVES

Nearly all the intestinal tube is nourished via the cranial mesenteric artery. It anastomoses proximally with a branch of the celiac artery along the descending duodenum, and distally with a branch of the caudal mesenteric along the descending colon. The cranial mesenteric artery itself arises beneath the first lumbar vertebra close to the celiac. Its origin is in the root of the mesentery in association with the mesenteric lymph nodes. It rapidly divides into a leash of about a dozen major branches, only a few of which are named and those only because they supply a part of the digestive tube that is recognizable (e.g., right colic, pancreaticoduodenal). The vessels course in the great mesentery, usually concealed by fat deposits that accumulate around them. They loop and anastomose with their neighbors in a series of arcades that are slightly more complex in the mesentery supplying the more distal parts of the gut. Short vasa recti leave the arcades and run directly to the intestinal wall, where they bifurcate on entry to pass on either side of the tube. They supply two vascular networks, one beneath the serosa, the other in the submucosa.[34, 84, 109]

The caudal mesenteric is a small vessel given off the aorta beneath the fifth lumbar vertebra; it supplies the terminal third of the large intestine.

The veins ultimately drain into the portal vein, which is subject to unique problems associated with the low pressure within it and with its vulnerable location. Most of the tributaries of the portal vein begin as satellites of the arteries, sometimes forming a pair of companion veins. As these vessels ascend in the mesenteries, they depart from the arteries to form three or four major tributaries of the portal vein. The cranial mesenteric vein is the largest of these, receiving blood from the small intestine; the splenic vein is also large and drains not only the spleen but also the stomach and some of the pancreas; the smaller caudal mesenteric vein drains the large intestine and the smallest, the gastroduodenal vein, drains the pylorus, duodenum, and more of the pancreas. The portal vein proper begins after the confluence of the two mesenteric veins. It runs forward in the great mesentery and then further forward it forms the ventral limit to the epiploic foramen as it bridges the short distance to the porta of the liver. It lies well concealed and well secured in the middle of the abdomen, presumably where pressure changes are likely to be least. A number of portosystemic communications (portocaval anastomoses) have been described (see Chapter 79).

Lacteals refers to both the capillary lymphatics

within each villus and the larger grossly visible lymphatics that course through the mesentery. They are conspicuous about an hour or so after a fatty meal, when they may be seen streaming like white linen threads over the mesentery along a course independent of the other vessels. They drain into five or six large mesenteric lymph nodes clustered around the root of the mesentery. A few small nodes may be seen more peripherally, in contact with the gut, and these are named accordingly (duodenal, right colic, left colic, etc.).

The gut has a rich autonomic innervation derived from the cranial and caudal mesenteric plexuses. The autonomic nerves reach the gut in company with the vessels within the mesentery. There are reputedly 5 million myenteric and 15 million submucosal neurons within the cat's small intestine (some 20 times the number of cells in the dorsal root ganglia).[101]

Principles of Intestinal Surgery

Eberhard Rosin

OPERATIVE FLUID THERAPY

Preoperative deficit therapy will blend into, and possibly modify, the fluid therapy given during surgery. A dog presented with intestinal disease may need to be operated on within hours. Hypotension associated with anesthesia and surgery adds to the circulatory disturbance created by fluid loss from vomiting and diarrhea. Unless the fluid deficit is partially corrected before surgery, the animal may not survive the operation. In general, approximately 50 to 75 per cent of the fluid deficit should be corrected before anesthesia is induced.

The management of the animal during surgery is based on the following guidelines: (1) 10 ml/kg body weight/hour of lactated Ringer's solution given for "maintenance" of circulatory volume during procedure; (2) 3 ml of fluid administered for each ml of estimated blood loss; (3) whole blood, approximately 20 ml/kg body weight, administered when the packed cell volume (PCV) falls below 20 and/or the total solids are less than 3.5; and (4) pale mucous membranes, weak pulse, prolonged capillary refill time, or drop of mean arterial blood pressure below 80 torr indicates a need for accelerated rate of administration of lactated Ringer's solution. After the initial deficit is corrected, total fluid volume given over the course of the operation should not exceed 80 ml/kg body weight unless PCV, total solids, and central venous pressure are monitored.

ANTIBIOTIC PROPHYLAXIS

The decision to use an antibiotic for prophylaxis in intestinal surgery, and the choice of the antibiotic to be used, is based on three criteria.[98, 110] First, the patient or operation should carry a risk of infection that exceeds the negative effects associated with the use of an antibiotic. These effects include pain from injection, expense, systemic side effects, and the development of altered microbiological flora. The risk of infection due to contamination from intestinal surgery, particularly from the overgrowth of bacteria in obstructed intestines, warrants the use of antibiotics. Second, the antibiotic should have a microbiological spectrum appropriate to the operation, in this case, the flora responsible for peritonitis. Third, the antibiotic should be administered before wound contamination occurs. Antibiotics must be given within two to three hours of contamination for the antibiotic to be effective against the bacteria introduced into the wound. There is no conclusive evidence to support the use of prophylactic antibiotics beyond six hours after surgery.[16, 113]

The common pathogens responsible for peritonitis following intestinal surgery are *Escherichia coli, Enterococcus,* and coagulase-positive *Staphylococcus aureus.* Selection of antibiotics is also based on knowledge of mean inhibitory concentrations within tissue and peritoneal fluid, when available.[99]

The following two drugs are appropriate choices for antimicrobial prophylaxis for intestinal surgery:[99]

1. Cefazolin, 15 mg/kg intravenously at induction of anesthesia. Second- and third-generation cephalosporins may be equally effective, but insufficient information is available on their use in small animal practice.

2. Trimethoprim-sulfadiazine, 30 ml/kg given subcutaneously two hours before surgery.

A second dose is administered the evening of the operative day, and a third dose is given the following morning. Prophylactic antimicrobial therapy is stopped at that point. If signs of peritonitis develop postoperatively, broad-spectrum antibiotics, selected according to culture and sensitivity data, are given until the animal shows a clinical response to the infection.

If antibiotics have not been given preoperatively or at the time of anesthetic induction and contamination occurs during surgery, antibiotics should be started intravenously during the operative procedure. Aminoglycoside antibiotics cause abnormalities of cardiac muscle function and may induce hypotension and life-threatening arrhythmias.[4]

TIMING OF SURGERY

In general, surgery for mechanical obstruction of the intestines should be performed within 12 hours after the diagnosis is made. The risk of ischemic necrosis caused by vascular disruption at the obstruction increases with time. The consequences of perforation, or even loss of mucosal integrity, and exposure of the systemic circulation to intestinal bacteria are life-threatening. Surgery for penetrating wounds of the abdominal cavity, intestinal perforation, or peritonitis should be scheduled as soon as the diagnosis is made.

ASSESSMENT OF INTESTINAL VIABILITY

Vascular injury to the intestines may occur with venous occlusion (intussusception, torsion, foreign body, strangulated hernia), arterial occlusion (cranial mesenteric artery thrombosis), and arteriovenous injury (traumatic avulsion of mesenteric vessels). These conditions may cause ischemic necrosis of the bowel wall. Assessment of the viability of a segment of intestine may be difficult. Standard clinical criteria are color, arterial pulsations, and peristalsis. However, these factors are often subjective and are not consistently reliable. Clinical judgment of viability is more accurate in cases of venous occlusion, in which the color is blue-black and the bowel is flaccid, than in cases of arterial injury, in which the color may be nearly normal and small vessel thrombosis may be invisible.

Normal appearance does not guarantee that the bowel will heal following resection and anastomosis. If the viability of a segment of bowel is questionable, more should be removed. The risk of short bowel syndrome must be considered if extensive resection is necessary.

A number of techniques have been proposed to increase the accuracy of assessment of intestinal viability, including the use of electromyography, radioactive microspheres, and microtemperature probes.[14, 121] These techniques are technically cumbersome and expensive and are generally not suited for use in clinical veterinary surgery. The use of a Doppler ultrasonic flow probe to detect pulsatile mural blood flow has been reported; however, its accuracy has been challenged by several investigators.[14, 24, 70]

In 1942, Lange and Boyd proposed the assessment of tissue perfusion as indicated by flow of fluorescing solutions as an accurate predictor of tissue viability.[62] This technique has been substantiated in both clinical and laboratory studies.[14, 15, 71] Fluorescein is an organic dye that emits a gold-green fluorescence when exposed to ultraviolet light. After intravenous injection, the fluorescein appears readily in extracellular fluid. The drug reaches its maximum intensity in tissue within minutes; the intensity of staining then diminishes, with total urinary excretion in 24 to 36 hours.

The fluorescein solution is injected intravenously at a dose of 15 mg/kg; side effects are rare. After an equilibration period of two to three minutes, the fluorescent pattern is viewed with a Wood's lamp in a darkened operating room. Six distinct fluorescent patterns have been reported (Table 50–1).[117] Although this technique is a test of vascularity and not specifically of viability, it is a valuable adjunct to clinical judgment in predicting intestinal viability, particularly in arterial injury.[117]

CHOICE OF INSTRUMENTS

The instruments used in intestinal surgery generally are of two types: crushing forceps, used to clamp the ends of the resected segment, and atraumatic (noncrushing) forceps, used to gently occlude the lumen of the segments to be anastomosed. Crushing forceps can be of any pattern that will conveniently fit across the intestine. These forceps, such as Carmalt and Allen, usually have straight blades that hold tissue firmly and often serve as a guide for the scalpel used to transect the intestines.

The choice of noncrushing forceps is more difficult. If an assistant is available, occlusion of the bowel lumen by fingers may be the gentlest means to prevent spillage of chyme.

The open portion of the jaws of Allis forceps can be bolstered as necessary with moist gauze sponges and used to effectively and gently occlude the bowel lumen. The toothed portion of the Allis forceps must be placed with care to avoid mesenteric blood vessels.

The Doyen forceps is a traditional pattern. The shorter pediatric Doyen forceps is more convenient for use in small animal surgery, lessening the risk of lacerating the mesentery by the long tips of the standard Doyen pattern. This injury usually occurs as the bowel is rotated 180 degrees during suturing. Doyen forceps jaws are occasionally covered with rubber tubing. The tubing, particularly after repeated autoclaving, becomes stiff and may cause more dam-

TABLE 50–1. Patterns Seen on Fluorescent Testing of Intestinal Perfusion

Viable intestine	
Normal	Smooth, uniform green-gold
Hyperemic	Brighter than normal color
Fine granular	Finely mottled pattern, not as intense as normal intestine, but no areas of nonfluorescence greater than 3 mm
Nonviable intestine	
Patchy	Blotches of fluorescence with areas of nonfluorescence greater than 3 mm
Perivascular	Staining only in areas adjacent to major arteries
Nonfluorescent	No fluorescence seen

age to bowel wall than the uncovered forceps. The application of rubber shoes over the forceps may also eliminate the flexibility of placing variable tension on the jaws of the Doyen forceps with changes in closing the box lock. This attempt to occlude the intestine with a deforming surface in fact causes additional injury, as the forceps jaws must be closed more forcefully to achieve locking. Rubber covers serve no useful purpose.

The Masters forceps is a slender and more flexible version of the Doyen forceps. Its disadvantage is the long length of the jaws, which makes injury to the mesentery more likely.

Forceps with specially designed replaceable rubber inserts are also available. The Folgerty pattern forceps is an example of this type. The rubber inserts are soft and disposable and reportedly provide atraumatic occlusion of the intestinal wall. Injury to blood vessels is minimized.[40]

Recently, vascular toothed forceps have become increasingly popular. These forceps have rows of short variably patterned teeth that produce minimal trauma to blood vessels. Various patterns of vascular toothed forceps are available, from standard Doyen forceps with vascular teeth to forceps intended primarily for cardiovascular surgery.[74, 83]

CHOICE OF SUTURE MATERIALS

A wide range of suture materials have been used successfully for intestinal anastomosis, including monofilament and multifilament nonabsorbable as well as natural and synthetic absorbable sutures. The surgeon's choice of suture materials is often based on tradition, but with newer materials available and with increased knowledge of their properties and behavior, it is now possible to select sutures that have characteristics more appropriate for use in intestinal surgery.

In contaminated wounds, braided nonabsorbable suture materials increase the likelihood of infection.[29] Braided materials can harbor bacteria and produce a granulomatous inflammation with draining sinus. Multifilament nonabsorbable suture materials, including silk, have been widely used for intestinal surgery without evidence of clinically detectable problems. This clinical experience notwithstanding, there seems little reason to continue the use of multifilament nonabsorbable suture materials for intestinal surgery, because absorbable suture materials that do not have these undesirable side effects are available.

Although surgeons have been satisfied with chromic gut for intestinal surgery, synthetic absorbable suture materials are stronger and more resistant to infection.[63] Differences between gut and the synthetic absorbable sutures include physical properties and method of absorption. Gut is an animal protein manufactured from intestinal serosa or submucosa and is absorbed by enzymatic digestion. The synthetic absorbable materials include polyglycolic acid (Dexon) and polyglactin 910 (Vicryl). These polyester sutures are absorbed primarily by hydrolysis, a process that occurs at the same rate in different tissues and is not affected by changes in tissue environment or bacterial contamination.[63, 96] One disadvantage of these materials compared with chromic gut is their handling characteristics. Polydioxanone (PDS) suture material was developed to overcome the tissue friction and knot security problems associated with Dexon and Vicryl. A monofilament synthetic absorbable suture material, PDS is absorbed by nonenzymatic hydrolysis.[92] This process is independent of inflammation. The inflammatory response to PDS is similar to the response to Dexon and Vicryl.[92] A major advantage of monofilament PDS over Dexon and Vicryl is the lack of tissue drag. PDS has been used successfully in intestinal anastomosis in small animal practice.

PRINCIPLES OF INTESTINAL ANASTOMOSIS

The ideal method for uniting intestinal wounds has probably not been found. Modern surgical techniques for closure of intestinal wounds include various suturing patterns and other techniques such as sutures placed over intestinal stents, mechanical stapling devices, and tissue adhesives. Experimental evaluation of various tissue adhesives has failed to demonstrate an advantage over conventional suture methods for intestinal anastomosis.[73]

Various configurations of intestinal intraluminal stents and approximation plates have been described. Such devices have been constructed of a variety of materials, including metal, bone, wood, potatoes, turnips, and gelatin capsules.[41, 43] No clear advantage of these devices over conventional suturing for anastomosis has been shown.

A variety of stapling instruments have been developed for use in gastrointestinal surgery. These instruments include the LDS (ligating, dividing, and stapling instrument) for double ligation and simultaneous division of vessels; the instruments of the TA (thoracoabdominal) series for closure of incisions and cut ends in the intestinal tract; the GIA (gastrointestinal anastomosis) instrument for anastomosis and for sealed transection of bowel; and the EEA (end-to-end anastomosis) instrument used for end-to-end repair of intestinal resection. Studies show no significant difference in the incidence of anastomotic complications when stapled anastomoses are compared with sutured procedures in the intestinal tract.[21, 54, 91] Stapling instruments are a valuable addition to the surgeon's tool box; however, they are not commonly used in small animal surgery because of the high cost of the instruments and staples.

The surgical literature is replete with studies evaluating and comparing various techniques for intestinal anastomosis. Reconstruction of the intestinal tract following resection can be done by end-to-end,

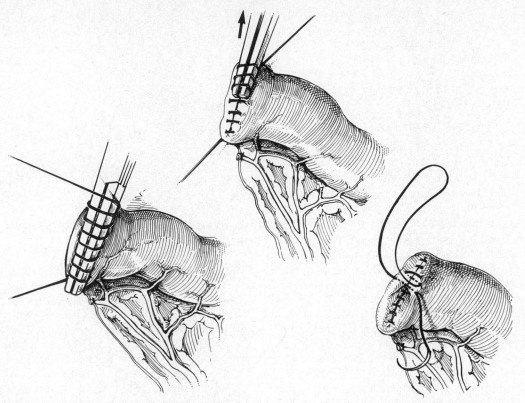

Figure 50–2. Suture patterns used to close the cut ends of the small intestine in preparation for side-to-side anastomosis.

end-to-side, or side-to-side technique. The side-to-side (Figs. 50–2 and 50–3) and end-to-side (Fig. 50–4) techniques are technically more demanding and more time-consuming, involve two to three or more suture lines, and do not reconstruct the intestinal tract in a physiological fashion.[103] There is no reason to select a side-to-side or end-to-side technique in preference to an end-to-end anastomosis for the small intestine. The former techniques are used in alimentary tract surgery, for example, cholecystoenterostomy and gastroenterostomy.

Types of End-to-End Anastomoses

The four main types of sutured end-to-end intestinal anastomosis in the dog and cat are the inverting, everting, invaginating, and approximating suture patterns. Closed intestinal anastomotic techniques, which are an elegant way to minimize contamination while anastomosing the bowel, have not gained popularity in small animal surgery, presumably owing to technical difficulties and the small diameter of dog and cat small intestines.

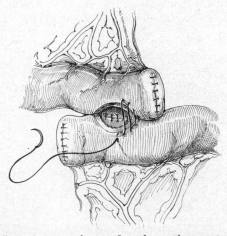

Figure 50–3. Suture technique for side-to-side intestinal anastomosis.

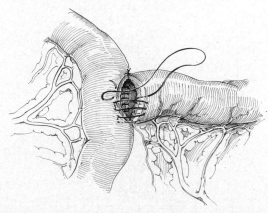

Figure 50–4. Suture technique for end-to-side intestinal anastomosis.

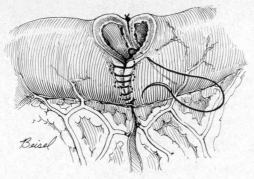

Figure 50–5. Connell suture pattern used as first layer for inverting intestinal anastomosis.

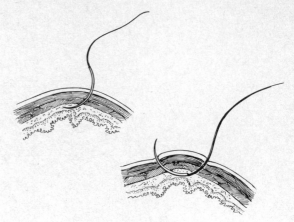

Figure 50–7. Intestinal suture patterns must include the tough submucosa.

The classic technique for intestinal anastomosis is the two-layer inverting technique. This technique is usually performed with a first layer using a Connell suture pattern and a second layer of interrupted sutures in a Lembert pattern inserted to the level of the submucosa (Figs. 50–5 and 50–6). Other suture patterns including the Halsted and Cushing have been described. Lembert in 1826 reported that serosa-to-serosa inverting patterns were necessary for proper intestinal healing.[31] Halsted[50] in 1887 noted that the submucosa is the tough layer of the small intestine and must be penetrated by sutures during anastomosis (Fig. 50–7).[50] The inclusion of the submucosa in an anastomosis for adequate healing has been unchallenged as a basic surgical principle. A single-layer inverting closure using a Connell or Halsted suture pattern has been described.[31, 94]

The everting intestinal anastomosis technique was developed in an attempt to increase the luminal diameter over that achieved with inverting patterns. A horizontal mattress pattern has been described to evert all layers of the intestinal wall (Fig. 50–8).[19, 65] The natural tendency of the cut ends of dog and cat small intestines to evert makes the insertion of horizontal mattress sutures easy to perform.

An invagination technique has also been described. In this technique the mucosa from the distal segment and the muscularis from the proximal segment are removed. The two segments are then telescoped together and held in place by preplaced sutures.[31]

This technique is technically difficult and has not gained popularity in small animal practice.

An end-to-end approximating suture technique has been popular with small animal surgeons. This technique was developed to improve intestinal healing by accurate realignment of cut layers of the intestinal wall and to minimize the possibility of luminal reduction, which may occur with an inverting suture pattern. One of three types of interrupted suture patterns or a continuous pattern can be used. The Gambee pattern is a simple interrupted suture that penetrates the lumen and passes through a small segment of mucosa and submucosa on the same side (Fig. 50–9).[42] The Poth and Gold pattern is a simple interrupted suture that is tied with sufficient tension to cut through the mucosa from beneath and the serosa and muscularis from above and hold just the submucosa in apposition (Fig. 50–10).[89] The appositional technique is a simple interrupted noncrushing suture described by Dehoff (Fig. 50–11).[28]

Intestinal Healing

Inverting Techniques. Inversion of the intestinal wall causes compression of blood vessels and some obstruction of blood flow to the inverted portion. At three days following anastomosis, the mucosa often shows necrosis and edema. At five days, the inverted

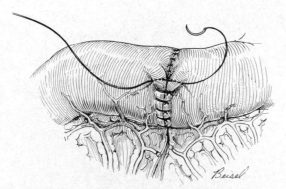

Figure 50–6. Lembert suture pattern used as second layer for inverting intestinal anastomosis.

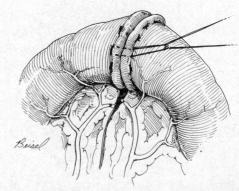

Figure 50–8. Horizontal mattress sutures used for everting intestinal anastomosis.

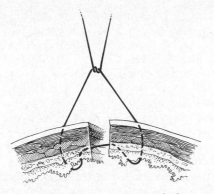

Figure 50–9. The Gambee suture penetrates the lumen and passes though a portion of the mucosa and submucosa to help pull the everted mucosa into apposition.

cuff has usually sloughed, and all strength exists in the submucosa, muscularis, and serosal layers. At 14 days, a scar bridges the suture line, but the individual layers have not reformed.[31, 94]

The single-layer inverting technique produces less necrosis and edema at three days, and the mucosa and submucosa have reestablished continuity at 14 days.[31]

Everting Technique. The everted mucosa trapped between sutures undergoes necrosis. A fibrin seal covers the remainder of the everted mucosa within three hours of completion of the surgery. Carbon particles used to evaluate re-formation of vascular and lymph channels traverse the mucosal and submucosal suture lines more rapidly following everting than inverting repair. Microangiographic evaluation of blood vessel healing, however, showed vessels crossing the incision at one week with inverting pattern but only minimal crossing at three weeks with everting pattern.[1, 31, 90]

The healing process is delayed when compared with that in the inverting anastomosis. At two weeks, histological examination of an inverting anastomosis shows inflammation resolved and healing advanced, whereas examination of the everting anastomosis shows persistence of an inflammatory response and incomplete mucosal healing. The inflammatory response persists longer in the everted pattern, presumably because of the entrapped mucosa. Also, the everted mucosa causes more inflammation at the serosal surface, peritoneal inflammation is enhanced, and adhesions are more likely than with the inverted technique.[31, 90]

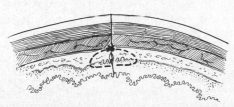

Figure 50–10. The Poth and Gold suture is a "crushing" stitch that passes through the bowel wall and is tied with sufficient tension to cut through mucosa, serosa, and muscularis to hold just the submucosa in apposition.

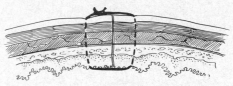

Figure 50–11. Simple interrupted suture used to gently hold the intestine in apposition.

Approximating Technique. The approximating anastomotic technique using a crushing suture pattern produces quicker regeneration of mucosa over the incision, less fibrous connective tissue deposition, and reduced inflammatory response than is seen with either the everting or inverting technique. By the fifth day, mucosal edema is moderate. At 21 days, healing with minimal scar has occurred. The inverting, everting, and crushing patterns of the anastomotic technique have been compared in experimental dogs; the greatest amount of fibrosis was found with the everting technique and the least with the crushing technique.[5, 31]

Tensile Strength

Bursting strength is the intraluminal pressure at which air or water will leak from the anastomotic site. The bursting strength of both inverting and approximating patterns is greater than that of the everting technique during the immediate postoperative period. This difference in bursting strengths disappears as healing progresses.[31, 51]

Breaking strength is determined by traction across the anastomosis until dehiscence occurs. Studies evaluating breaking strength of the three anastomotic patterns have produced conflicting results. Loeb[66] compared the standard two-layer inverting pattern with single-layer inverting, single-layer approximating, and single-layer everting techniques and found the two-layer inverting closure to be slightly stronger than the single-layer inverting and approximating patterns, and significantly stronger than the everting technique immediately postoperatively. Getzen[44] evaluated the strength of a Gambee approximating pattern and found that it was two-thirds as strong as the everted pattern until 21 days after surgery, when the strength is equal. Although Getzen found greater tensile strength with an everted anastomosis than with an inverting pattern, Loeb, McAdams, and Irvin reported opposite results.[31, 66] Hamilton[51] reported that the two-layer inverting technique was the strongest immediately postoperatively, but weaker at 3 to 6 days than either the single-layer inverting or approximating patterns.

Luminal Diameter

Hamilton evaluated luminal diameter after intestinal anastomosis in experimental dogs and reported that the two-layer inverting technique narrowed the luminal diameter an average of 54 per cent, the single-layer inverting technique 39 per cent, the approximating Gambee pattern four per cent, and the everting pattern three per cent.[51] These patterns were all evaluated immediately postoperatively. Bennett[5] studied the luminal diameter of everting, inverting, and crushing suture patterns after healing was complete and reported that the greatest decrease in luminal diameter occurred with the everting pattern and least occurred with the crushing pattern.[5]

Conclusions

The two-layer inverting pattern has the potential for producing a large cuff of inverted tissue and offers greater strength initially but less strength during the early healing period than the single-layer inverting pattern. The available data show little to recommend the everted anastomosis over the approximating pattern for surgery of the intestine. Approximating suture patterns have gained in popularity in small animal surgery in recent years. Approximating patterns offer several advantages over single- or two-layer inverting patterns: ease of application, increased luminal diameter at the anastomotic site, and more rapid mucosal regeneration. Bursting strengths are similar. Approximating patterns also offer some advantages over the everting suture pattern: minimal adhesion formation, more rapid early healing, and better protection against leakage.

Postoperative peritoneal adhesions at the anastomotic site are formed at a rate directly proportional to the amount of mucosa everted. Experimental studies in the dog have shown that inverting suture patterns cause less adhesion than everting patterns in the same dog.[31]

The simple interrupted approximating and simple continuous approximating patterns cause less tissue ischemia at the anastomotic site during the first seven days after surgery than the simple interrupted crushing technique, as evaluated by fluorescein dye and angiographic studies. More tissue necrosis and disruption of blood vessels at the anastomotic site were seen with the crushing technique during the first week postoperatively than with the noncrushing appositional technique. At 21 days there are no significant differences among any of these techniques.[32]

Bursting pressure studies determined that the anastomotic strengths of crushing techniques and simple interrupted noncrushing techniques were similar. Subjective histopathological evaluations of anastomotic sites of both techniques were also similar.[8]

The continuous approximating pattern causes less mucosal eversion and postoperative peritoneal adhesion formation than the interrupted patterns. The continuous pattern also produces more precise submucosal apposition between sutures, with resultant rapid mucosal healing.[32]

All anastomotic patterns, if applied with care and precision, can give good results. Experimental evaluation of healing, strength of anastomosis, compromise of luminal diameter, and adhesion formation indicate an advantage of approximating techniques over inverting or everting techniques. Simple interrupted or simple continuous suture patterns are preferred over a crushing suture pattern for the approximating technique.

Whether a leak develops following anastomosis is determined by a combination of biological factors, particularly vascular supply to the anastomotic site, and is not predictable at the time of surgery. If a leak occurs at the anastomotic site, the site is resected and the same suture pattern can be used to create a new anastomosis. In most instances, a leak from an anastomosis is due not to the choice of suture pattern but rather to some undetermined biological factor of wound healing or to faulty surgical technique.

The Role of the Omentum

The environment of the peritoneal cavity, and particularly the function of the omentum, has considerable impact on the outcome of an intestinal anastomosis. Peacock and Van Winkle suggest that all anastomoses leak to some extent and that a successful anastomosis depends on the natural resistance provided by peritoneal and omental function.[31] An anastomosis isolated from the peritoneal cavity by synthetic wrapping has a greater likelihood of infection, necrosis, and dehiscence. Morrison reported the ability of omentum to plug hernial defects, to seal off infections and perforations, and to impart new blood supply to viscera. He coined the phrase "abdominal policeman."[31]

The first reported use of omentum as a surgical tool was to protect intestinal anastomoses. Mann in 1921 reported that omentum wrapped to form a sleeve around an anastomosis provided significant protection and greatly decreased the incidence of postoperative leakage from the anastomotic site.[100] The value of omental wrapping in enhancing gastrointestinal anastomosis has been proven.[100] The omentum is the most important aid available for the protection of a gastrointestinal anastomosis.

Techniques for Intestinal Anastomosis

Exposure and Examination of Intestines

The intestines are exposed by a ventral midline abdominal incision of sufficient length to permit complete examination of the peritoneal cavity. The falciform ligament is usually not removed. The edges of the incision are protected with moist laparotomy pads, and a Balfour self-retaining abdominal retractor is used to maintain exposure. The Balfour retractor is properly positioned by placing the blades, while the retractor is closed, into the peritoneal cavity. The retractor is spread in stages; each successive spread to the retractor is preceded by a sweeping of the viscera to prevent entrapment between the blades and the abdominal wall.

The entire length of the intestines should be thoroughly and gently examined before a decision about a surgical procedure is made. The duodenum and associated right limb of the pancreas are lifted from the abdominal cavity and examined first. The caudal duodenal flexure can be mobilized by transection of the avascular peritoneal reflexion, which ties the caudal duodenal flexure to the right caudal region of the abdominal cavity. From the caudal flexure, the duodenum runs obliquely forward and is attached to the mesentery of the descending colon by the duodenal colic ligament. The duodenum curves ventrally to form the duodenal jejunal flexure, which may be difficult to see beneath the root of the jejunal mesentery but can be palpated. Traction on the proximal jejunum may bring the duodenal jejunal flexure into view. The jejunum forms several coils. The jejunum is examined by passing the jejunal loops gently through fingers.

The short ileum is identified by the small winding artery located along the antimesenteric border. The ileum joins the cecum and colon at the ileocecal junction.

The intestinal lymph nodes are in the root of the mesentery; they can be seen when the duodenum, jejunum, or ileum is gently lifted to flatten the folds of mesentery. They are examined for size and consistency.

The color of the intestinal serosa is normally glistening pink. Inflammation causes intense hyperemia and fibrin production over the surface of the serosa and mesentery.

If the animal has recently eaten a fatty meal, an extensive branching network of cream-colored channels, the lacteals, is visible on the surface of the intestines and mesentery.

Two types of intestinal contraction may be seen as the normal bowel is examined. A peristaltic wave moves along a short segment of bowel. A segmental contraction causes a tightening of the bowel wall and changes its color from pale pink to white. This contraction usually involves approximately two centimeters of intestine and can last for several minutes.

Particularly in young dogs, small (1-cm) elliptical elevations of the serosa can be seen. These are normal lymphatic Peyer's patches.

Intestinal Resection and Anastomosis

As discussed previously, the procedure of choice is end-to-end appositional anastomosis. In cases of disparity between the luminal diameter of the segments to be anastomosed, one of three techniques can be used: With minor luminal disparity, the spacing between simple interrupted sutures or the spacing between needle passages in a simple continuous pattern is greater on the larger lumen side than on the smaller lumen side, resulting in an end-to-end anastomosis without gap or pucker (Fig. 50–12). With moderate luminal disparity, the bowel with the smaller lumen is transected at an angle rather than perpendicularly across the axis of the bowel, creating

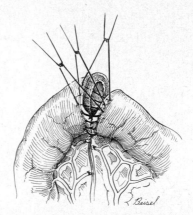

Figure 50–12. With minor luminal disparity between segments to be anastomosed, gaps or puckers are eliminated by spacing each suture further on the larger-lumen side.

a lumen of larger diameter (Fig. 50–13). With marked luminal disparity, the larger lumen is partially closed with a Connell suture pattern oversewed by interrupted Lembert sutures using 3-0 synthetic absorbable suture material (Fig. 50–14). The remaining lumen, now of equal diameter, is anastomosed.

The segment of intestine to be removed is selected after the vascularity of the intestine is assessed.

The jejunal branches of the cranial mesenteric artery, including the terminal arcade, that supply the segment of intestine to be resected are ligated with 3-0 chromic gut with swaged-on taper needle (Fig. 50–15). The vasa recti that leave the terminal arcade and go directly to the intestine to the resected are not individually ligated. The needle is passed carefully through the mesentery and around the jejunal branch(es). Each vessel is doubly ligated with space for transection. With peritonitis, hyperemia and fibrin deposits on the surface of the mesentery may make accurate identification of the jejunal branches difficult. These branches can be more easily seen if the mesentery is transilluminated.

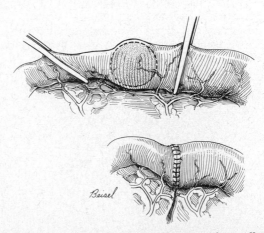

Figure 50–13. With moderate luminal disparity, the smaller segment is transected at an angle, creating a lumen of larger diameter. Anastomosis is done in standard fashion with the segments positioned at approximately 45-degree angle.

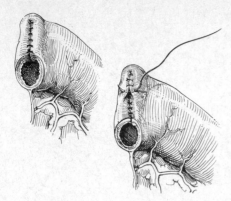

Figure 50–14. With marked luminal disparity, the larger lumen is partially closed by Connell suture pattern oversewn with Lembert suture pattern. The remaining lumen, now of equal diameter, is anastomosed in standard fashion.

The terminal arcade is doubly ligated in similar fashion. The space between these ligatures is the site of transection of the intestine. In obese animals, the mesenteric border may be covered with fat, and the terminal arcade is difficult to see; passing the needle directly adjacent to the bowel wall prevents penetration of the terminal arcade.

The jejunal and ileocolic branches supplying the distal jejunum, ileum, and ileocecal junction may be difficult to identify for ligation, particularly when this area is intussuscepted. Rather than ligating blindly and possibly injuring the blood supply to the transverse colon, my preference is to ligate those branches that can be seen, to transect the mesentery, and to identify the remaining branches as bleeding vessels, which are clamped with hemostatic forceps and individually ligated. This technique results in some blood loss, but there is less risk of damage to branches of the ileocolic artery supplying the ascending and transverse colon.

Crushing clamps are placed across the intestine at the terminal arcade ligature adjacent to the diseased segment. The clamps are placed perpendicular to the axis of the bowel or angled slightly toward the normal segment to ensure adequate blood supply to the antimesenteric border. Noncrushing intestinal forceps are placed approximately two to three centi-

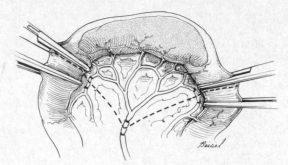

Figure 50–16. After crushing and non-crushing intestinal forceps are placed, the intestine is transected with a scalpel blade using the crushing forceps as a guide. The mesentery and jejunal vessels are transected with scissors.

meters from the crushing clamps (Fig. 50–16). Before these clamps are placed, intestinal contents are milked away from the resection site. The intestine is transected with a scalpel blade, using the crushing clamps as guides. The scalpel blade should pass between the two ligatures on the terminal arcade. The mesentery is transected with scissors, cutting between each pair of ligatures on the jejunal artery branches (see Fig. 50–16).

Intestinal contents adhering to the incised intestinal mucosa are removed with gauze sponges. The cut ends of the intestine often bleed, and the mucosa everts. Arterial bleeding is controlled by ligation. Venous bleeding from the cut surface is controlled by pressure applied with a gauze sponge. The everted mucosa, and inevitably a portion of the submucosa, is trimmed with scissors (Fig. 50–17); the aim is to create a level surface for suturing the bowel wall in an appositional pattern. The circumference is retrimmed immediately prior to suturing if eversion continues.

Anastomosis is done with sutures of 3-0 or 4-0 synthetic absorbable material on a swaged-on taper needle placed in simple interrupted or simple continuous pattern. The suture pattern is started adjacent to the mesenteric border, the mesenteric border is sutured, and the pattern is continued around the circumference of the intestines (Figs. 50–18 and 50–19). The noncrushing intestinal forceps are used

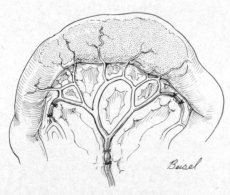

Figure 50–15. The jejunal vessels, including terminal arcade supplying the decreased intestine, are double-ligated.

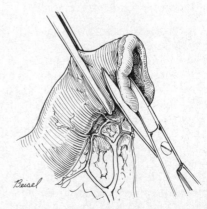

Figure 50–17. The everted mucosa is trimmed with scissors.

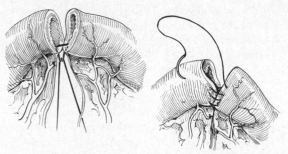

Figure 50–18. The suture pattern is started adjacent to the mesenteric border, the border is sutured, and the pattern is continued toward the antimesenteric side.

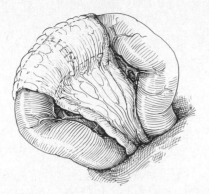

Figure 50–20. The anastomosis is wrapped with omentum. The omentum need not be sutured.

to position and rotate the intestines to facilitate suturing.

Proper spacing between sutures and tension on sutures are determined by clinical judgment, but general guidelines are available. Experimental work evaluating suture placement in intestinal anastomosis in normal dogs has shown that three sutures spaced around the circumference of the anastomosis prevent leakage; leakage of the anastomosis did not occur with a simple continuous pattern in which sutures were spaced 14 millimeters apart.[52] These extremes, however, are not suitable for clinical patients. Sutures should be placed approximately two to three millimeters from the cut surface and three to four millimeters apart. The sutures are passed full-thickness through the bowel wall. They are placed with appositional tension only. Some eversion of intestinal mucosa between sutures is almost inevitable, although the extent of eversion varies considerably. The extent of mucosal eversion can be modified by accurate trimming of the mucosa with scissors, and use of the Gambee suture pattern.

The anastomosis is inspected, and gaps or excess mucosal eversion is corrected by placement of additional sutures in Lembert pattern, though these are usually not required. The defect in the mesentery is sutured with 3-0 absorbable suture material, avoiding the jejunal vessels. The anastomosis is washed with warm, sterile saline and wrapped with omentum (Fig. 50–20). The bowel is replaced in the abdominal caity.

Enterotomy

Intestinal contents are expressed from the region of the enterotomy, and noncrushing intestinal forceps are placed across the bowel to minimize the spillage of chyme. A full-thickness incision is made at the antimesenteric border with a scalpel. The incision may be enlarged as necessary with scissors.

Any everted mucosa is trimmed with scissors before closure is begun. The incision is closed using sutures of 4-0 or 3-0 synthetic absorbable material on a swaged-on taper needle placed in a simple interrupted or continuous pattern. The suture is placed with gentle appositional force. Closure of an enterotomy with a two-layer inverting pattern, the first layer of Connell sutures and the second layer using interrupted Lembert sutures, is the preferred method of closure for biopsy of the intestines in animals with protein-losing enteropathy or when blood supply to the bowel wall may be compromised (Fig. 50–21).

Obstruction of the lumen by a diaphragm of inverted bowel wall, as may occur with a two-layer inverting suture pattern for intestinal anastomosis, should not occur following enterotomy.

The closed enterotomy is washed with a warm, sterile saline solution, covered with omentum, and replaced in the abdominal cavity.

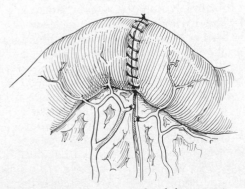

Figure 50–19. The intestine is rotated and the remaining circumference is sutured.

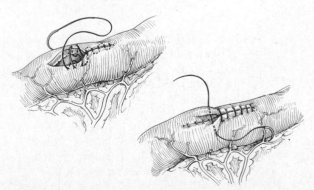

Figure 50–21. Closure of an enterotomy by Connell suture pattern oversewn with Lembert suture pattern. This is the preferred method of closure in cases of possible delayed healing.

ASEPSIS

Every effort should be made to minimize the bacterial contamination of the peritoneal cavity that occurs with intestinal surgery. The segment of intestine prepared for resection and anastomosis or enterotomy is "packed off" from the peritoneal cavity by moist sponges or laparotomy pads. Intestinal contents are displaced from the resection site before the atraumatic forceps are clamped across the intestinal lumen.

Surgical drapes should be impervious to water. Cloth drapes, particularly after a series of washings, lose their barrier properties. Sterile saline solutions used for irrigation will invariably soak fabric drapes and create an environment for bacterial passage. Instruments and equipment used during the intestinal resection and anastomosis or enterotomy are discarded after that procedure is completed, surgical gloves are changed, the peritoneal cavity is thoroughly lavaged, and closure of the incision in the mesentery and closure of the abdominal wall is performed with clean instruments and suture material.

ABDOMINAL LAVAGE AND DRAINAGE

After intestinal surgery is completed, the peritoneal cavity should be thoroughly lavaged with warm, sterile saline solution, 500 ml in a cat, 2 to 4 liters in a large dog. The lavage fluids used must be at body temperature to minimize heat loss.

Although lavage spreads bacterial contamination throughout the peritoneal cavity, its value in the prevention and treatment of peritonitis has been established. Lavage is effective because bacteria, and debris that may compromise phagocytosis of bacteria, are removed. All lavaged fluid must be aspirated. When bacteria are suspended in residual lavage fluid, phagocytosis is impaired.

The efficacy of the addition of povidone-iodine (Betadine) solution to lavage fluid for the prevention or treatment of peritonitis is uncertain at best. The value of adding the solution to lavage fluids has been studied extensively. The results of these studies are difficult to interpret because the data are conflicting; however, the following conclusions can be drawn:[7, 39, 45, 60, 64, 68, 88, 95, 105]

1. The addition of povidone-iodine to lavage fluid can be fatal. Four ml/kg body weight of povidone-iodine instilled into the peritoneal cavity of normal dogs is fatal; 2 ml/kg body weight of povidone-iodine solution instilled into the peritoneal cavity of experimental dogs with peritonitis is fatal.

2. The addition of povidone-iodine solution to the lavage fluid is not as effective as the addition of broad-spectrum antibiotics, for example, kanamycin, for the prevention of experimental peritonitis.

3. Povidone-iodine solution adversely affects phagocytosis and may injure or kill fibroblasts.

In conclusion, the addition of povidone-iodine solution to lavage fluid for the prevention or treatment of peritonitis cannot be recommended.

Experimental studies have shown that the addition of antibiotics to lavage fluid does not improve the survival rate of animals with experimental peritonitis when systemic antibiotics are given concurrently.[61]

The peritoneal cavity cannot be effectively drained by rubber drains or tubes.[49] Drains rapidly become covered with fibrin and omentum, and are no longer effective. Experimental and clinical studies have shown that drainage of the peritoneal cavity by tubes does not increase survival in peritonitis.[49] Additionally, bacteria from the peritoneal cavity may travel along the drains and gain access to the subcutaneous space, causing severe cellulitis.

CLOSURE OF THE ABDOMINAL INCISION

The abdominal wall is closed in standard fashion using synthetic absorbable suture materials. In selected animals with extensive peritoneal contamination and the risk of postoperative infection of the incision, the subcutaneous tissue and skin are left unsutured. The abdominal wall is closed by sutures and the remaining wound is covered with water-soluble antibiotic cream and nonadherent wound dressing, and is protected with an abdominal bandage. The animal is reanesthetized and the incision is closed once inflammation has resolved.

In selected cases with massive peritoneal contamination that cannot be effectively removed, the entire abdominal incision can be left open to drain toxic peritoneal exudate. The open wound is covered by abdominal bandage, which is changed daily. Although this technique has been used to successfully treat severe peritonitis in humans, and has been investigated in an experimental peritonitis model in the dog,[86] its value in treating peritonitis has not been established in clinical practice; my experience suggests that it warrants clinical trial. After completion of the surgery, the incision is not sutured but is protected with a nonadherent dressing and covered with a carefully placed abdominal bandage. The dog is continuously observed, or an aluminum body brace is fitted to prevent self-mutilation. The bandage and wound dressing are changed daily. Fibrous adhesions, which may trap peritoneal exudate, are gently freed. The peritoneal cavity is lavaged with warm sterile fluid as necessary to assure minimal retention of necrotic debris and exudate. If the dog struggles during a bandage change, oxymorphone or meperidine may be given. The bandage change must be done with attention to asepsis to minimize the possibility of additional bacterial infection of the peritoneal cavity or incision. This treatment regimen is continued until the peritoneal inflammation has resolved, usually two to four days. Although granulation tissue will rapidly attempt to cover the incision, a second operation is necessary to close the incision adequately with sutures. Large quantities of fluid are lost into the bandage; fluid balance must be carefully monitored and maintained by administration of intravenous fluids.[86] Hypoproteinemia and hypokalemia may occur; serum electrolytes should be monitored.

POSTOPERATIVE CARE

Three potential problem areas are: fluid and electrolyte balance and nutrition; complications of the abdominal incision; and consequences of intestinal surgery such as peritonitis, adhesions, short bowel syndrome, and adynamic ileus. These problems may be easily solved by offering food and water the day following surgery, or they may require days of intensive care that challenges even the most experienced clinician.

As a general guideline, one should allow a maximum of 72 hours for return of normal bowel function (appetite, no vomiting, and, ideally, normal bowel movement). Surgical exploration is indicated as soon as signs of peritonitis are observed. The early return of oral intake of food and water encourages resumption of intestinal peristalsis and provides the most convenient route for assimilation of water, electrolytes, calories, and protein. The animal is offered a small amount of water the day following surgery. Once initial thirst has been satisfied and no vomiting has occurred, small amounts of bland food are given. If food is refused, a trial feeding of homogenized food can be placed into the cheek pouch or administered by stomach tube. If anorexia persists and no other problems are found, diazepam given intravenously (0.25 to 0.5 mg) or orally (0.2 mg/kg) can be used as an appetite stimulant in the dog. If the animal will not drink water, or vomiting persists, fluid therapy should be given intravenously or subcutaneously while the cause is investigated.

Fluid Therapy

Deficit Therapy. In most cases, dehydration is corrected before surgery. If dehydration is still present after surgery, the replacement volume must be given before maintenance therapy is begun.

Maintenance Therapy. The quantities of water required for maintenance therapy during each 24-hour period are shown in Figure 50–22. For the dog, approximately 40 to 60 ml/kg body weight/24 hours are required. If fluid therapy is required for more than two or three days, electrolyte concentrations, particularly potassium ion, must be monitored. Quantitative laboratory data provide guidelines for the supplementation of potassium to the lactated Ringer's solution used for maintenance therapy (Table 50–2). Potassium may be administered intravenously at a rate not to exceed 0.5 mEq/kg body weight/hour. Solutions containing 35 mEq/liter may be administered subcutaneously.[36] Except when quantitative laboratory data indicate the need for another crystalloid solution, lactated Ringer's is the solution of

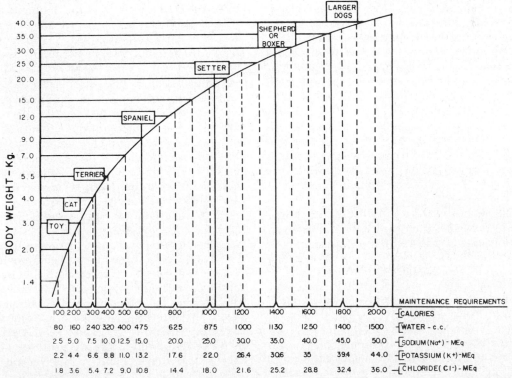

Figure 50–22. Maintenance requirements of calories, water, and electrolytes of caged dogs and cats. (Reprinted with permission from Finco, D. R.: A scheme for fluid therapy in the dog and cat. J.A.A.H.A. 8:178–180, 1972.)

TABLE 50–2. Guidelines for Potassium Ion Supplementation in Maintenance Fluid Therapy

Serum K⁺ (mEq/l)	K⁺ (mEq) Added per 250 ml Lactated Ringer's Solution
3.0–3.5	8
2.5–3.0	12
2.0–2.5	15
<2.0	20

choice for maintenance therapy. This solution is administered intravenously or subcutaneously.

Contemporary Loss. With the animal in the hospital, the clinician can estimate the quantities of fluids lost by vomiting or diarrhea and can increase the quantity of lactated Ringer's administered to replace this loss.

Nutrition

Animals with peritoneal disease may experience a dramatic increase in basal metabolic rate (BMR increases 25 to 50 per cent in severe peritonitis in humans); carbohydrate stores are depleted in 24 hours, and body fats and protein are used as a source of calories. Total body protein metabolism increases, causing a marked negative nitrogen balance, with depletion of the body protein pool and possible impairment of the immune system and of wound healing. In the acute stages, correction of water, electrolyte, and acid-base abnormalities is more important than supplying calories. However, in marked tissue catabolism and weight loss, caloric therapy may be necessary. This is not easy when the animal is not eating. Approximately 60 to 80 calories/kg body weight/24 hours are needed. A 5 per cent glucose solution contains 170 calories/l (4 calories/gm of glucose). Glucose must be administered at a rate of 0.5 to 0.9 gm/kg/hour for efficient use. Because of these limits, total caloric replacement by intravenous glucose may not always be feasible. Fat provides approximate 9 calories/gm and can be used effectively as a source of calories. In the adult dog and cat, 12.5 mg of protein/calorie/day must be synthesized from amino acids for the animal to remain in nitrogen balance.[36]

Nutritional support can be given by either enteric or parenteral routes. Enteral nutrition is defined as supplying nutrients via the gastrointestinal tract using homogenized foods or commercial liquid formula diets. This route avoids the complications and expense associated with parenteral feeding but is contraindicated in vomiting and diarrhea, malabsorption, and adynamic ileus, problems common in animals with surgical intestinal disease. The methods for administration of nutrients by the enteric route include syringe, oral stomach tube, nasogastric tube, pharyngostomy tube, gastrostomy tube, and needle catheter jejunostomy.

Parenteral nutrition is defined as the administration of nutrients through a catheter placed in a central vein. Normal gastrointestinal function is not required; however, this technique is expensive and may cause metabolic abnormalities as well as potential sepsis and thrombosis from the central vein catheter.

Peritonitis

After intestinal surgery, animals must be monitored closely for signs of peritonitis. Both subjective and objective signs may be present. Depression and abdominal pain, of a degree greater than that usually seen in an animal following abdominal surgery, may occur. Although there is considerable variation among animals in response to pain, most animals with peritonitis splint their abdominal walls at the slightest touch. Vomiting, which persists into the first postoperative day, is a prominent sign of peritonitis. Fever and leukocytosis are nonspecific indicators of inflammation and may be present in an animal with peritonitis. Inflammation of the peritoneal cavity causes cessation of normal peristaltic activity and accumulation of fluid and gas. No intestinal sounds are heard. Fluid and gas accumulation may be felt in those animals that tolerate abdominal palpation. Radiographic examination of the abdominal cavity shows fluid and gas accumulation generally throughout the intestinal tract. Free air may be seen within the peritoneal cavity, but it may be the aftermath of the exploratory laparotomy rather than passage of air from a disrupted intestinal anastomosis. Abdominal radiographs also show a lack of intestinal detail and a ground-glass appearance of the abdominal cavity.

These signs are all indicative of, but not pathognomonic for, peritonitis. The single most valuable parameter for diagnosis of peritonitis is cytology of abdominal fluid.

Under sedation, the bladder is expressed, the ventral abdomen is prepared for surgery, and 2 per cent lidocaine is infiltrated into the skin and abdominal wall two centimeters caudal and lateral to the umbilicus. A two-centimeter incision is made through the skin, subcutaneous tissue, and ventral rectus fascia. Blunt dissection is continued through the rectus muscle to the dorsal rectus fascia and peritoneum. After hemorrhage is controlled, the dorsal fascia and peritoneum are elevated with mosquito forceps. A dialysis catheter with the stylet removed is inserted through a stab incision and passed in a dorsal and caudal direction toward the pelvis. If fluid is not obtained, 20 ml/kg of warm lactated Ringer's solution are rapidly infused into the abdominal cavity through the dialysis catheter. The abdomen is massaged gently to distribute the fluid. The fluid bottle is vented with an 18-gauge needle and placed on the floor to collect fluid. The dialysis catheter is withdrawn, and the incisions in the ventral fascia and skin are sutured in routine fashion. A drop of collected lavage fluid is placed on a slide and a smear is

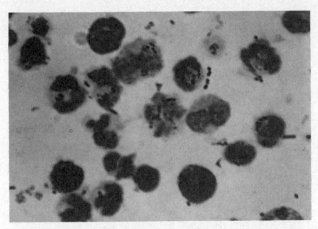

Figure 50–23. Abdominal fluid from a dog with peritonitis. The prominent leukocyte is the degenerating neutrophil showing karyolysis. Bacteria are seen free in the fluid and within neutrophils.

made. The smear is dried and stained by Wright-Giemsa or other rapid stain technique. The slide is examined for bacteria and cell morphology. In animals with peritonitis, the predominant leukocyte is the degenerating neutrophil showing karyolysis; bacteria are seen free in the fluid and possibly within neutrophils (Fig. 50–23). The prominent cell type in peritoneal fluid following uncomplicated intestinal anastomosis of experimental dogs is the nondegenerating neutrophil, and bacteria are consistently absent (Fig. 50–24). Exploratory laparotomy is indicated if an animal shows clinical signs of peritonitis and if degenerative neutrophils and bacteria are seen in fluid obtained by abdominocentesis.[9]

The tenets of treatment of peritonitis are: (1) to stop the source of bacterial contamination; (2) to lavage the peritoneal cavity thoroughly with sterile warm fluids to flush out bacteria and debris; and (3) to administer broad-spectrum antibiotics effective against enteric organisms. Organisms commonly cultured in animals with peritonitis from leakage of intestinal contents include: *Escherichia coli, Entero-*

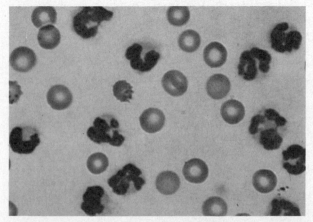

Figure 50–24. Abdominal fluid obtained 24 hours after uncomplicated intestinal anastomosis. The prominent cell type is the nondegenerating neutrophil. No bacteria are seen.

coccus, and coagulase-positive *Staphylococcus aureus.* Selection of antibiotics should be based on sensitivity testing. Antibiotics that may be used until results of laboratory studies are available include trimethoprim-sulfadiazine, 30 mg/kg subcutaneously b.i.d.; chloramphenicol, 50 mg/kg intravenously t.i.d.; and gentamicin, 1 mg/kg subcutaneously b.i.d.[99] Antibiotics are continued as determined by the animal's clinical response. If a favorable response is not noted in seven days, other therapeutic measures should be considered.

Adhesions

Ischemic tissue within the peritoneal cavity is the strongest stimulus to the formation of permanent adhesions. Irritating contaminants that can enter the peritoneal cavity at the time of exploratory laparotomy may cause granulomatous inflammation and the development of fibrous peritoneal adhesions. These substances, which include talc, starch powder, and lint, may act together with other conditions associated with trauma to prevent the reabsorption of fibrinous adhesions.[30]

Injury or inflammation of the peritoneum results in production of serosanguineous exudate. Coagulation of this exudate results in the adhesion of injured peritoneal surfaces within three hours. The majority of early fibrinous adhesions are lysed and absorbed within 72 hours. However, some may persist and become organized by ingrowth of fibroblasts and capillaries to form relatively permanent collagenous adhesions. Fibrinous adhesions are necessary precursors of fibrous adhesions. Mobile intraperitoneal structures will not permanently heal to each other unless they are held in apposition by fibrin until collagen deposition begins on the third postoperative day. The critical factor in the formation of adhesions is whether fibrin is lysed and absorbed or persists and is organized to form fibrous adhesions. Fibrinolytic activity of normal peritoneum is due to activators present in mesothelium and submesothelial blood vessels. These activators convert the enzyme precursor present in blood and fibrinous exudates (plasminogen) to a fibrin-splitting protease (plasmin).[13]

Deperitonealized surfaces that are not otherwise injured heal without permanent adhesions because they retain their ability to lyse fibrinous adhesions before fibroblastic organization can occur. Peritoneum that is made ischemic by tight suturing may lose its ability to lyse fibrin and may actively inhibit fibrinolysis by normal tissues. Other sources of ischemic injury, and contamination with foreign material, may interfere with fibrinolysis, allowing permanent adhesions to develop.[13, 30]

Peritoneal adhesions are best prevented by gentle and precise surgical technique, exacting hemostasis, and deliberate nonsuturing of peritoneal incisions or defects. Fortunately, in contrast to humans and horses, adhesions occur infrequently in small animal surgical patients and rarely cause intestinal obstruction.

Short Bowel Syndrome

Short bowel syndrome is characterized by intractable diarrhea with impaired absorption of fats, vitamins, and other nutrients. Multiple factors may be responsible for short bowel syndrome following intestinal surgery, including: (1) the extent and site of resection; (2) the presence or absence of a functioning ileocecal valve; (3) the function of the remaining digestive organs; and (4) the time allowed for adaptation of the remaining small intestine.

After resection of 80 per cent of small intestine (as measured from the tip of the pancreas to the ileoceal junction), otherwise normal puppies gained weight in normal fashion; resection of 90 per cent of the small intestine produced severe morbidity and significant mortality.[55]

Resection of the ileocecal junction does not produce clinically detectable problems postoperatively. In experimental dogs after resection of the ileocecal junction, an increase was noted in the bacterial flora of the ileum.[43]

Short bowel syndrome can cause maldigestion, malabsorption, bile salt– and fatty acid–mediated diarrhea, bacterial overgrowth, and gastric hypersecretion. Pancreatic enzyme secretion into the intestinal lumen may be reduced in short bowel syndrome, since the stimulating hormones secretin and cholecystokinin, which are normally released from the mucosa of the duodenum and upper jejunum, will be decreased if portions of these bowel sections have been removed. Decreases in digestive enzyme activity in small-intestinal mucosal cell brush border preparations from biopy specimens taken six weeks after a 75 per cent proximal small bowel resection have been reported in the dog. These reductions in enzyme contribute to maldigestion.[18, 23, 38, 118]

Malabsorption probably results from the rapid transit time and reduced small-intestinal mucosal surface area present in short bowel syndrome. Malabsorption of protein, carbohydrate, and fat leads to negative nitrogen balance and tissue catabolism. Unabsorbed sugars may stimulate bacterial overgrowth in the small intestine and may contribute to diarrhea by exerting an osmotic effect to hold water in the intestinal lumen. A chronic deficiency in protein absorption may lead to decreased wound healing and impaired immune system.[18, 23, 38, 118]

Extensive resections of the small intestine can result in bile salt deficiency, since the liver cannot compensate for extensive loss of bile salt in the feces by increased synthesis alone. This bile salt deficiency can contribute to maldigestion of fat with resultant steatorrhea and diarrhea. Steatorrhea is important in the pathogenesis of diarrhea in short bowel syndrome. Experimental studies in the dog have shown that perfusion of the small intestine and colon with fatty acids, as occurs in steatorrhea, reduces absorption of water from the intestinal lumen with resultant diarrhea.

In the absence of an ileocecal valve, bacteria may ascend from the colon into the small intestine. Bacterial overgrowth in the small intestine may contribute to the diarrhea seen in small bowel syndrome. Bacteria hydroxylate fatty acids in the intestinal lumen and thus worsen any fatty acid–mediated diarrhea. Bacteria may also produce toxins that decrease water absorption from the intestinal lumen.[18, 23, 38, 118]

Extensive small bowel resection produces gastric hypersecretion in experimental dogs. Infusion of hydrochloric acid into the stomach and small intestine of experimental dogs produces diarrhea, weight loss, and ulcers in the proximal small intestine.[18, 23, 38, 118]

The small intestine remaining after extensive bowel resection undergoes compensatory changes. The small intestine increases in diameter, the microvilli enlarge, and the number of mucosal cells increases, resulting in increased absorption per unit length. Factors that contribute to this adaptation of the remaining small intestine include: increased concentration of absorbable nutrients in the intestinal lumen; increased blood flow; and increases in concentrations of hormones such as gastrin and cholecystokinin. This adaptation of the remaining small intestine takes several weeks. During this period, parenteral supplementation of fluids, electrolytes, and nutrition may be necessary for survival of the animal.[110, 118, 119]

Long-term medical treatments that may be of value in controlling diarrhea and providing adequate nutrition for dogs with short bowel syndrome have been reported.[118] These treatments include diet modifications such as frequent small meals, low-fat, elemental diet supplements, and medium-chain triglyceride oil; vitamin, mineral, and pancreatic enzyme supplements; and medications including antidiarrheals, oral antibiotics, antacids, and bile salt–binding agents.[118]

A variety of surgical methods to treat short bowel syndrome have been reported, including vagotomy and pyloroplasty, reversal of single and multiple small and large bowel segments, production of artificial sphincters, and construction of intestinal loops. In experimental puppies, transposition of an isoperistaltic colon segment proximal to the small bowel after resection of 90 per cent of the small intestine reduced the morbidity and eliminated the mortality rate; the transposed colon segment was aperistaltic and slowed transit time without causing intestinal obstruction. This procedure resulted in less stool excretion, increased fat absorption, and weight gain of the puppies.[55] These procedures have not been evaluated in clinical trials in small animal practice.

Ileus

Ileus is a form of intestinal obstruction characterized by inadequate peristaltic activity usually involving the entire gastrointestinal tract. Loss of normal gastrointestinal motility may follow any intra-abdominal operation and may also occur with other diseases unrelated to the peritoneal cavity. After the majority of abdominal operations, the reduction in intestinal motility is not of clinical significance. However, following extensive abdominal surgery or in the presence of peritoneal infection, severe ileus may develop. In this condition the intestines are not paralyzed, but effective peristalsis is lost. The intestines rapidly distend with fluid and gas, and absorption is impaired by the increasing intestinal distension. If left untreated, further distension causes greater impairment of absorption.

There is considerable experimental evidence to suggest that ileus is mainly a reflex phenomenon mediated through the sympathetic nervous system. Elimination of sympathetic nerve supply to the intestinal tract reduces or prevents the development of ileus. Whether there is a concomitant reduction in parasympathetic tone in the development of ileus is unknown.[20, 77, 78, 107]

Electrolytes lost into the intestinal lumen include sodium, chloride, and potassium. Loss of potassium has been suggested as a contributory cause of ileus. Normal levels of potassium are essential for proper synthesis of acetylcholine.[20, 77, 78, 107]

Clinical signs of ileus include vomiting, anorexia, and fluid and gas distension of the entire gastrointestinal tract. This fluid and gas can be palpated and can be seen on abdominal radiographs. Characteristically, ileus is not painful. However, peritonitis can be a cause of ileus, and in these cases the clinical signs of peritonitis, including abdominal pain, are superimposed on those of ileus.

Treatment of ileus is difficult. Every effort should be made to prevent this condition by attention to proper surgical techniques. Any coexisting disease, including peritonitis, is treated. Fluid and electrolyte imbalances are corrected, particularly depletion of potassium. Early resumption of oral intake of food and water stimulates gastrointestinal reflexes and may encourage a resumption of normal peristalsis. Treatment of ileus per se has centered on the use of anticholinesterase agents such as neostigmine or the use of cholinergic drugs such as bethanechol chloride. An additional approach to the pharmacological treatment of ileus is the use of pantothenic acid; this substance is an essential component of coenzyme A, which is necessary for the production of acetylcholine. Unfortunately, none of these agents has documented efficacy in the treatment of ileus. In addition, an animal with undiagnosed mechanical intestinal obstruction may be harmed if treated with a parasympathomimetic drug.[81]

Metoclopramide is an effective antiemetic drug that enhances gastrointestinal motility. It stimulates gastric contractions, accelerates gastric emptying, and stimulates smooth muscle contraction in the small intestine, thereby shortening intestinal transit time. Metoclopramide has been used and studied exten-

sively in clinical trials in human patients.[27] Reports of these trials present conflicting evidence; the majority support the value of metoclopramide in reducing postoperative vomiting and nausea in patients following abdominal operations. Though the value of metoclopramide in treating ileus in small animals has not been established, clinical investigation in veterinary surgery is warranted. The dose of metoclopramide is 0.2 to 0.4 mg/kg subcutaneously every six hours, ten to 15 minutes before feeding. It may also be used orally at the same dosage, as necessary.[17]

1. Abramowitz, H. B., and McAlister, W. H.: A comparative study of small bowel anastomoses by angiography and microangiography. Surgery 66:564, 1969.
2. Adam, W. S., Calhoun, M. L., Smith, E. M., and Stinson, A. W.: Microscopic Anatomy of the Dog. Springfield, Charles C Thomas, 1970.
3. Atkins, A. M., and Schofield, G. C.: Lymphoglandular complexes in the large intestine of the dog. J. Anat. 113:169, 1972.
4. Beck, C. C.: Antibiotic-anesthetic interactions. Vet. Med./Sm. Anim. Clin. 70:273–277, 1975.
5. Bennett, R. R., and Zydeck, F. A.: A comparison of single layers suture patterns for intestinal anastomosis. J. Am. Vet. Med. Assoc. 157:2077, 1970.
6. Berry, H. L.: Collagenous fiber patterns in the submucosa of the small intestine of the dog. Anat. Rec. 143:107, 1962.
7. Bolton, J. S., Bornside, G. H., and Cohn, I., Jr.: Intraperitoneal povidone-iodine in experimental canine and murine peritonitis. Am. J. Surg. 137:780, 1979.
8. Bone, D. L., Duckett, K. E., Patton, C. S., and Krahwinkel, D. J.: Evaluation of anastomoses of small intestines in dogs: crushing versus noncrushing suturing techniques. Am. J. Vet. Res. 44:2043, 1983.
9. Botte, R. J., and Rosin, E.: Cytology of peritoneal effusion following intestinal anastomosis and experimental peritonitis. Vet. Surg. 12:20, 1983.
10. Bourdelle, E., and Bressou, C.: Anatomie Régionale des Animaux Domestiques. IV Carnivores: Chien et Chat. Paris, J-B Baillière, 1953.
11. Bradley, O. C., and Graham, T.: Topographical Anatomy of the Dog. 5th ed. Edinburgh, Oliver & Boyd, 1948.
12. Brolin, R. E., and Ravitch, M. M.: Studies in intestinal healing VI. Effect of pharmacologically induced peristalsis on fresh anastomoses in dogs. Arch. Surg. 115:339, 1980.
13. Buckman, R. F., Buckman, P. D., Hufnagel, H. V., and Gervin, A. S.: A physiologic basis for the adhesion-free healing of deperitonealized surfaces. J. Surg. Res. 21:67, 1976.
14. Bulkley, G. B., Wheaton, L. G., Strandberg, J. D., and Zuidema, G. D.: Assessment of small intestinal recovery from ischemic injury after segmental arterial, venous, and arteriovenous occlusion. Surg. Forum 30:210, 1979.
15. Bulkley, G. B., Zuidema, G. D., Hamilton, S. R., et al.: Intraoperative determination of small intestinal viability following ischemic injury. Ann. Surg. 193:628, 1981.
16. Burke, F. J.: The effective period of preventive antibiotic action in experimental incisions and dermal lesions. Surgery 50:161, 1961.
17. Burrows, C. F.: Metoclopramide. Am. Vet. Med. Assoc. 183:1341, 1983.
18. Bury, K. D.: Carbohydrate digestion and absorption after massive resection of the small intestine. Surg. Gynecol. Obstet. 135:177, 1972.
19. Buyers, R. A., and Meier, L. A.: Everting suture of the bowel: experimental and clinical experience in duodenal closure and colorectal anastomosis. Surgery 63:475, 1968.
20. Carmichael, M. J., Weisbrodt, N. W., and Copeland, E. M.: Effect of abdominal surgery on intestinal myoelectric activity in the dog. Am. J. Surg. 133:34, 1977.
21. Chassin, J. L., Rifkind, K. M., Sussman, B. et al.: The

stapled gastrointestinal tract anastomosis: incidence of postoperative complications compared with the sutured anastomosis. Ann. Surg. 5:689, 1978.

22. Chauveau, A.: *The Comparative Anatomy of the Domesticated Animals.* 2nd ed. Translated by G. Fleming. London, Churchill, 1873.
23. Conn, J. H., Chavez, C. M., and Fain, W. R.: The short bowel syndrome. Ann. Surg. 175:803, 1972.
24. Cooperman, M., Martin, E. W., Jr., and Carey, L. C.: Determination of intestinal viability by Doppler ultrasonography in venous infarction. Ann. Surg. 191:57, 1980.
25. Cornelius, L. M.: Fluid therapy in small animal practice. J. Am. Vet. Med. Assoc. 176:110, 1980.
26. Cornelius, L. M., and Rawlings, C. A.: Arterial blood gas and acid-base values in dogs with various diseases and signs of disease. J. Am. Vet. Med. Assoc. 178:992, 1981.
27. Davidson, E. D., Hersh, T., Brinner, R. A., et al.: The effects of metoclopramide on postoperative ileus. Ann. Surg. 190:27, 1979.
28. DeHoff, W. D., Nelson, W., and Lumb, W. V.: Simple interrupted approximating technique for intestinal anastomosis. J. Am. Anim. Hosp. Assoc. 9:483, 1973.
29. Edlich, R. F., Panek, P. H., Rodeheaver, G. T., et al.: Physical and chemical configuration of sutures in the development of surgical infection. Ann. Surg. 177:679, 1973.
30. Ellis, H.: The cause and prevention of postoperative intraperitoneal adhesions. Surg. Gynecol. Obstet. 133:497, 1971.
31. Ellison, G. W.: End-to-end anastomosis in the dog: a comparison of techniques. Comp. Cont. Educ. 3:486, 1981.
32. Ellison, G. W., Jokinen, M. P., and Park, R. D.: End-to-end approximating intestinal anastomosis in the dog: a comparative fluorescein dye, angiographic and histopathologic evaluation. J. Am. Anim. Hosp. Assoc. 18:729, 1982.
33. Elsen, J., and Arey, L. B.: On spirality in the intestinal wall. Am. J. Anat. 118:11, 1966.
34. Evans, H. E., and Christensen, G. C.: *Miller's Anatomy of the Dog.* 2nd ed. Philadelphia, W. B. Saunders, 1979.
35. Finco, D. R.: Fluid therapy—detecting deviations from normal. Am. Anim. Hosp. Assoc. 8:155, 1972.
36. Finco, D. R.: General guidelines for fluid therapy. Am. Anim. Hosp. Assoc. 8:166, 1972.
37. Finco, D. R.: A scheme for fluid therapy in the dog and cat. Am. Anim. Hosp. Assoc. 8:178, 1972.
38. Fletcher, J. T.: Short bowel syndrome. Gastroenterology 77:572, 1979.
39. Flint, L. M., Jr., Beasley, D. J., Richardson, J. D., and Polk, H. C., Jr.: Topical povidone-iodine reduces mortality from bacterial peritonitis. J. Surg. Res. 26:280, 1979.
40. Fogarty, T. J., Raible, D. A., and Krippaehne, W. W.: A new vascular clamp. Am. J. Surg. 112:967, 1966.
41. Fraser, I.: An historical perspective on mechanical aids in intestinal anastomosis. Surg. Gynecol. Obstet. 155:566, 1982.
42. Gambee, L. P.: A single-layer open intestinal anastomosis applicable to the small, as well as the large, intestine. West. J. Surg. Obstet. Gynecol. 59:1, 1951.
43. Gaset, J. C., and Kopp, J.: The surgical significance of the ileocecal junction. Surgery 56:565, 1964.
44. Getzen, L. C., Roe, R. D., and Holloway, C. K.: Comparative study of intestinal anastomotic healing in inverted and everted closures. Surg. Gynecol. Obstet. 123:1219, 1966.
45. Gilmore, O. J. A., Reid, C., Houang, E., and Shaw, E. J.: Intraperitoneal povidone-iodine in peritonitis. J. Surg. Res. 25:471, 1978.
46. Gladen, H. E., and Kelly, K. A.: Electrical pacing for short bowel syndrome. Surg. Gynecol. Obstet. 153:697, 1981.
47. Grandage, J.: Normal abdominal visceral relationships. *In: Radiology. Proceedings.* Vol. 59. Sydney, University of Sydney Postgraduate Committee in Veterinary Science, 1982.
48. Grier, R. L.: The intestines. *In* Bojrab, M. J. (ed.): *Current Techniques in Small Animal Surgery.* Vol. I. Philadelphia, Lea & Febiger, 1975.

49. Haller, J. A., Jr., Shaker, I. J., Donahoo, J. S., et al.: Peritoneal drainage versus non-drainage for generalized peritonitis from ruptured appendicitis in children. Ann. Surg. 177:595, 1973.
50. Halsted, W. S.: Circular suture of the intestine—an experimental study. Am. J. Med. Sci. 94:436, 1887.
51. Hamilton, J. E.: Reappraisal of open intestinal anastomoses. Ann. Surg. 165:917, 1967.
52. Hardy, K. J.: Suture anastomosis: an experimental study using limited suturing of the small bowel in the dog. Arch. Surg. 97:586, 1968.
53. Hebel, V. R.: Untersuchungen uber das Vorkommen von lymphatischen Darmkrypten in der Tunica submucosa des Darmes von Schwein, Rind, Schaf, Hund und Katz. Anat. Anz. 109:7, 1960.
54. Hess, J. L., McCurnin, D. M., Riley, M. G., and Koehler, K. J.: Pilot study for comparison of chromic catgut suture and mechanically applied staples in enteroanastomoses. J. Am. Anim. Hosp. Assoc. 17:409, 1981.
55. Hutcher, N. E., and Salzberg, A. M.: Pre-ileal transposition of colon to prevent the development of short bowel syndrome in puppies with 90 percent small intestinal resection. Surgery 70:189, 1971.
56. Jansen, A., Becker, A. E., Brummelkamp, W. H., et al.: The importance of the apposition of the submucosal intestinal layers for primary wound healing of intestinal anastomosis. Surg. Gynecol. Obstet. 152:51, 1981.
57. Jönsson, K., Jiborn, H., and Zederfeldt, B.: Breaking strength of small intestinal anastomoses. Am. J. Surg. 145:800, 1983.
58. Kratzer, G. L., and Onsanit, T.: Single layer steel wire anastomosis of the intestine. Surg. Gynecol. Obstet. 139:93, 1974.
59. Kratzer, G. L.: Single layer intestinal anastomosis. Surg. Gynecol. Obstet. 153:736, 1981.
60. Lagarde, M. C., Bolton, J. S., and Cohn, I., Jr.: Intraperitoneal povidone-iodine in experimental peritonitis. Ann. Surg. 187:613, 1978.
61. Lally, K. P., Trettin, J. C., and Torma, M. J.: Adjunctive antibiotic lavage in experimental peritonitis. Surg. Gynecol. Obstet. 156:605, 1983.
62. Lange, K., and Boyd, L. J.: The use of fluorescein to determine the adequacy of the circulation. Med. Clin. North Am. 26:943, 1942.
63. Laufman, H., and Rubel, T.: Synthetic absorbable sutures. Surg. Gynecol. Obstet. 145:597, 1977.
64. Lavigne, J. E., Brown, C. S., Machiedo, G. W., et al.: The treatment of experimental peritonitis with intraperitoneal Betadine solution. J. Surg. Res. 16:307, 1974.
65. Leighton, R. L.: Everting end-to-end intestinal anastomosis in the dog. Vet. Med./Small Anim. Clin. 239–248, 1967.
66. Loeb, M. J.: Comparative strength of inverted, everted, and end-on intestinal anastomoses. Surg. Gynecol. Obstet. 125:301, 1967.
67. Lord, M. G., Valies, P., Broughton, A. C.: A morphological study of submucosa of large intestine. Surg. Gynecol. Obstet. 145:55, 1977.
68. Lores, M. E., Ortiz, J. R., and Rossello, P. J.: Peritoneal lavage with povidone-iodine solution in experimentally induced peritonitis. Surg. Gynecol. Obstet. 153:33, 1981.
69. Madden, J. L.: A technique for the performance of an intestinal anastomosis. Surg. Gynecol. Obstet. 136:283, 1973.
70. Mann, A., Fazio, V. W., and Lucas, F. V.: A comparative study of the use of fluorescein and the Doppler device in the determination of intestinal viability. Surg. Gynecol. Obstet. 154:53, 1982.
71. Marfuggi, R. A., and Greenspan, M.: Reliable intraoperative prediction of intestinal viability using a fluorescent indicator. Surg. Gynecol. Obstet. 152:33, 1981.
72. Martin, C. P., and Banks, J.: The amount of mucosal tissue present in the small intestine. J. Anat. 75:135, 1940.

73. Matsumoto, T., Hardaway, R. M., Pani, K. C., et al.: Intestinal anastomosis with *n*-butyl cyanoacrylate tissue adhesive. Surgery *61*:567, 1967.

74. McCaughan, J. J., and Young, J. M.: Intra-arterial occlusion in vascular surgery. Ann. Surg. *171*:695, 1970.

75. Mellish, R. W. D.: Inverting and everting sutures for bowel anastomosis. J. Pediatr. Surg. *1*:260, 1966.

76. Mivart, St. G.: *The Cat: An Introduction to the Study of Backboned Animals*. London, John Murray, 1981.

77. Meshkinpour, H.: Intestinal motility: current concepts. Am. J. Gastroenterol. *71*:101, 1979.

78. Mishra, N. K., Appert, H. E., and Howard, J. M.: Studies of paralytic ileus: effects of intraperitoneal injury on motility of the canine small intestine. Am. J. Surg. *129*:559, 1975.

79. Nahai, F., Lamb, J. M., Havican, R. G., and Stone, H. H.: Factors involved in disruption of intestinal anastomoses. Am. Surgeon *43*:45, 1977.

80. Nance, C. N.: New techniques of gastrointestinal anastomoses with the EEA stapler. Ann. Surg. *189*:587, 1979.

81. Neely, J., and Catchpole, B.: Ileus: the restoration of alimentary-tract motility by pharmacological means. Br. J. Surg. *58*:21, 1971.

82. Nickel, R., Schummer, A., Seiferle, E., and Sack, W. O.: *The Viscera of the Domestic Mammals*. Berlin, Verlag Paul Parey, 1973.

83. Nickell, W. B., Bartley, T. D., and Hartley, C. S.: Arteries and anastomoses—some basic controversies settled. Ann. Thorac. Surg. *7*:221, 1969.

84. Noer, R.: The blood vessels of the jejunum and ileum: a comparative study of man and certain laboratory animals. Am. J. Anat. *73*:293, 1943.

85. O'Brien, T. R., Morgan, J. P., and Lebel, J. L.: Pseudoulcers in the duodenum of the dog. J. Amer. Vet. Med. Assoc. *155*:713, 1969.

86. Orsher, R. J., and Rosin, E.: Open peritoneal drainage in experimental peritonitis. Vet. Surg. 1984 (in press).

87. Ott, B. S., Doyle, M. D., and Greenwald, K. A.: Single layer everted intestinal anastomosis. J. Am. Vet. Med. Assoc. *153*:1742, 1968.

88. Pollock, A. V., Froome, K., and Evans, M.: The bacteriology of primary wound sepsis in potentially contaminated abdominal operations: the effect of irrigation, povidone-iodine and cephaloridine on the sepsis rate assessed in a clinical trial. Br. J. Surg. *65*:76, 1978.

89. Poth, E. J., and Gold, D.: Intestinal anastomosis: a unique technic. Am. J. Surg. *116*:643, 1968.

90. Ravitch, M. M., Canalis, F., Weinshelbaum, A., et al.: Studies in intestinal healing. III: Observations on everting intestinal anastomoses. Ann. Surg. *166*:670, 1967.

91. Ravitch, M. M., and Steichen, F. M.: Technics of staple suturing in the gastrointestinal tract. Ann. Surg. *175*:815, 1972.

92. Ray, J. A., Doddi, N., Regula, D., et al.: Polydioxanone (PDS), a novel monofilament synthetic absorbable suture. Surg. Gynecol. Obstet. *153*:497, 1981.

93. Reiling, R. B., Reiling, W. A., Bernie, W. A., et al.: Prospective controlled study of gastrointestinal stapled anastomoses. Am. J. Surg. *139*:147, 1980.

94. Richardson, D. C.: Intestinal surgery: a review. Comp. Contin. Educ. *3*:259, 1981.

95. Rodeheaver, G., Bellamy, W., Kody, M., et al.: Bactericidal activity and toxicity of iodine-containing solutions in wounds. Arch. Surg. *117*:181, 1982.

96. Rodeheaver, G. T., and Edlich, R. F.:Mechanical performance of polyglycolic acid and polyglactin 910 synthetic absorbable sutures. Surg. Gynecol. Obstet. *153*:835, 1981.

97. Rotering, R. H., Dixon, J. A., Holloway, G. A., and McCloskey, D. W.: A comparison of the He Ne laser and ultrasound Doppler systems in the determination of viability of ischemic canine intestine. Ann. Surg. *196*:705, 1982.

98. Ronald, A. F.: Antimicrobial prophylaxis in surgery. Surgery *93*:172, 1983.

99. Rosin, E.: Gastrointestinal tract (surgical). *In* Johnston, E. D. (ed.): *The Bristol Veterinary Handbook of Antimicrobial Therapy*. Veterinary Learning Systems Co., 1982.

100. Samson, R., and Pasternak, B. M.: Current status of surgery of the omentum. Surg. Gynecol. Obstet. *149*:437, 1979.

101. Sauer, M. E., and Rumble, C. T.: The number of nerve cells in the myenteric and submucous plexuses of the small intestine of the cat. Anat. Record *96*:373, 1946.

102. Schall, W. D.: General principles of fluid therapy. Vet. Clin. North Am. *12*:453, 1982.

103. Schlegel, D. M., and Maglinte, D. T.: The blind pouch syndrome. Surg. Gynecol. Obstet. *155*:541, 1982.

104. Schofield, G. C.: Anatomy of muscular and neural tissues. *In* Code, C. F., and Heidel, W. (eds.): *Handbook of Physiology*, Section 6. Vol. IV: *Motility*. Washington, D.C., American Physiological Society, 1968.

105. Sindelar, W. F., and Mason, G. R.: Intraperitoneal irrigation with povidone-iodine solution for the prevention of intra-abdominal abscesses in the bacterially contaminated abdomen. Surg. Gynecol. Obstet. *148*:409, 1979.

106. Singh, B., and Singh, J.: Evaluation of a single-layer intestinal anastomosis: an experimental study. Aust. N.Z. J. Surg. *45*:102, 1975.

107. Smith, J., Kelly, K. A., and Weinshilboum, R. M.: Pathophysiology of postoperative ileus. Arch. Surg. *112*:203, 1977.

108. Sognen, E., Birkeland, R., and Sohlberg, S.: A gelatine prosthetic aid for intestinal anastomosis. J. Small Anim. Pract. *18*:529, 1977.

109. Thamm, H.: Die arterielle Blutversorgung des Magendarmekanals, seiner Auhangsdrusen (Leber, Pankreas) und der Milz beim Hunde. Morph. Jahrb. *85*:417, 1941.

110. Tilson, M. D., and Wright, H. K.: The effect of resection of the small intestine upon the fine structure of the intestinal epithelium. Surg. Gynecol. Obstet. *134*:992, 1972.

111. Titkemeyer, C. W., and Calhoun, M. L.: A comparative study of the structure of the small intestine of domestic animals. Am. J. Vet. Res. *16*:152, 1955.

112. Trier, J. S.: Morphology of the epithelium of the small intestine. *In* Code, C. F., and Heidel, W. (eds.): *Handbook of Physiology*, Section 6, Vol. III: *Intestinal Absorption*. Washington, D.C., American Physiological Society, 1968.

113. Van Scoy, R. E.: Prophylactic use of antimicrobial agents. May. Clin. Proc. *52*:701, 1977.

114. Vitums, A.: Portal vein in the dog. Zentralbl. Vet. Med. *4*:723, 1959.

115. Vitums, A.: Portosystemic communications in the dog. Acta Anat. *39*:271, 1959.

116. Volini, I. F., Widenhorn, H. L., and De Fio, H.: Pseudoulcers in the duodenum of the normal dog. Arch. Surg. *37*:259, 1938.

117. Wheaton, L. G., Strandberg, J. D., Hamilton, S. R., and Bulkley, G. B.: A comparison of three techniques for intraoperative prediction of small intestinal injury. J. Am. Anim. Hosp. Assoc *19*:897, 1983.

118. Williams, D. A., and Burrows, C. F.: Short bowel syndrome—a case report in a dog and discussion of the pathophysiology of bowel resection. J. Small Anim. Pract. *22*:263, 1981.

119. Wilmore, D. W., Dudrick, S. J., Daly, J. M., and Vars, H. M.: The role of nutrition in the adaptation of the small intestine after massive resection. Surg. Gynecol. Obstet. *132*:673, 1971.

120. Yates, J. L.: An experimental study of the local effects of peritoneal drainage. Surg. Gynecol. Obstet. *1*:473, 1905.

121. Zarins, C. K., Skinner, D. B., Rhides, B. A., and James, A. E.: Prediction of the viability of revascularized intestine with radioactive microspheres. Surg. Gynecol. Obstet. *138*:576, 1974.

51 Small Intestines

Chapter 51

Physiology

Michael A. Pass

DIGESTION AND ABSORPTION OF NUTRIENTS

When food enters the duodenum, it is mixed with secretions from the pancreas, liver, and intestinal mucosa. These secretions contain enzymes and compounds, such as bile salts and colipase, that are essential for digestion and absorption.

The digestive enzymes exert their actions by hydrolyzing dietary components to small molecules that can be readily absorbed (Table 51–1). Salivary, gastric, and pancreatic enzymes act within the gastrointestinal lumen. Enzymes bound to the brush border membranes of the intestinal mucosal cells act when substrates come into close association with the membranes.

Carbohydrates are digested to the monosaccharides glucose, galactose, and fructose, and proteins are hydrolyzed to small peptides and amino acids. Triglyceride digestion is more complex than digestion of other dietary components in that it requres two cofactors, colipase and bile salts. Colipase is a protein secreted by the pancreas that promotes digestion of triglycerides by lipase.[46] The products of digestion of triglycerides are then incorporated into mixed bile salt micelles, a process also promoted by colipase.[46]

Absorption of nutrients in the small intestine occurs by simple diffusion, facilitated diffusion, active transport, or pinocytosis.[16] Glucose and galactose are absorbed by active transport, although at concentrations above the plasma concentration, monosaccharides may be absorbed by diffusion down a concentration gradient.[34] Active transport of monosaccharides is coupled to sodium absorption (Fig. 51–1).[49] Fructose is absorbed by facilitated diffusion.[12]

Amino acids are absorbed by active transport systems coupled to sodium absorption (Fig. 51–1).[49] Dipeptides and tripeptides are also actively absorbed from the small intestine by sodium-coupled carrier systems (Fig. 51–1).[50]

The products of fat digestion, including monoglycerides, free fatty acids, and cholesterol, are incorporated into micelles with bile salts. When the micelles come into close contact with the membrane of an intestinal mucosal cell, the fat digestion products diffuse across the unstirred water layer covering the cell membrane and into the mucosal cells but the bile salts remain in the intestinal lumen.[46] The fatty acids are bound to a fatty acid–binding protein in the cells that may also facilitate transport across the cell membrane.[46] Within the mucosal cell the monogly-

TABLE 51–1. Digestion of Major Nutrients

	Nutrient	Enzyme	Digestion Product(s)	Source(s) of Enzyme
Carbohydrates	Starch	Amylase	Maltose	Pancreas, saliva, stomach
	Maltose	Maltase	Glucose	Brush border
	Lactose	Lactase	Glucose + galactose	Brush border
	Sucrose	Sucrase	Glucose + fructose	Brush border
Proteins	Proteins	Pepsins	Peptides	Stomach
		Trypsin	Peptides	Pancreas
		Chymotrypsin	Peptides	Pancreas
	Peptides	Carboxypeptidase	Amino acids	Pancreas
		Aminopeptidase	Amino acids	Brush border
Lipids	Triglycerides	Lipase	Monoglycerides, free fatty acids + glycerol	Pancreas
	Phospholipids	Phospholipases	Phosphoglycerides + free fatty acids	Pancreas
	Cholesterol esters	Cholesterol hydrase	Cholesterol + free fatty acids	Pancreas
Nucleic acids		Nucleases	Nucleosides + phosphoric acid	Pancreas, brush border

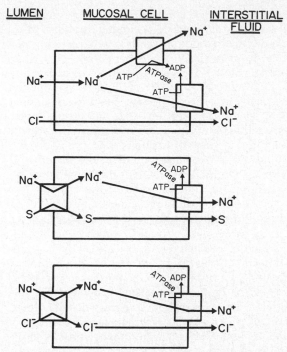

Figure 51–1. Absorption of sodium, chloride, and other substances in the small intestine. There are several transport systems in the small intestine that are driven by the active transport of sodium ions out of the mucosal cells by ATPase-dependent pumps on the lateral and basal plasma membranes. Transport of sodium out of the cells causes sodium to diffuse in from the intestinal lumen, resulting in net absorption of sodium. The uptake of sodium from the intestinal lumen also occurs via carrier molecules, which transport sodium together with either chloride or some other compound (S = D-hexoses, L-amino acids, dipeptides, tripeptides, bile salts, and some water-soluble vitamins). Chloride ions are also absorbed by passive diffusion along an electrochemical gradient established by active absorption of sodium. The movement of chloride and other substances (S) out of the cells occurs by diffusion across the lateral and basal membranes.

cerides and long-chain fatty acids are re-esterified to triglycerides and phospholipids, and cholesterol is re-esterified to cholesterol esters. These compounds are then incorporated into chylomicrons, which are extruded from the cell and removed from the intestine in the lymphatics.[46] The short- and medium-chain fatty acids, which are water-soluble, are not re-esterified to triglycerides but pass out of the cells and are carried away in the portal blood. Although bile salts are essential for maximum absorption of lipids, considerable absorption occurs without them. Conjugated bile salts are reabsorbed in the ileum by active transport.[57] Bile salts that are deconjugated by intestinal bacteria can also be absorbed by diffusion in the jejunum.

The fat-soluble vitamins—A, D, E, and K—are absorbed by diffusion after being incorporated into mixed bile salt micelles. The water-soluble vitamins—ascorbic acid, biotin, choline, folic acid, inositol, nicotinic acid, thiamine and riboflavin—are absorbed by active, sodium-coupled transport systems (see Fig. 51–1).[39] Vitamin B_6 and p-aminobenzoic acid may be absorbed by simple diffusion.[39] Vitamin B_{12}

combines with intrinsic factor, which is secreted by the stomach. In the ileum the vitamin dissociates from intrinsic factor during absorption by pinocytosis.[5]

WATER AND ELECTROLYTE ABSORPTION AND SECRETION

About 2.7 liters of water enter the small intestine of a 20-kg dog each day from ingested fluids and gastrointestinal secretions. (Fig. 51–2).[51] More than 85 per cent of this is absorbed by the small intestine, about 300 ml is absorbed in the colon, and less than 40 ml is passed in the feces (see Fig. 51–2).[51]

Movement of water across the mucosa of the small intestine occurs by passive diffusion along osmotic and hydrostatic pressure gradients. Osmotic gradients across the intestinal mucosa are determined by the osmolality of intestinal contents and by the absorption of sodium and of sodium linked to absorption of chloride or nutrients such as glucose and amino acids (see Fig. 51–1).[41] The hydrostatic pressure in the lumen of the intestine has little effect on absorption of water, but an increase in the hydrostatic pressure in the interstitial fluid of the intestinal mucosa, as occurs in diseases such as lymphangecta-

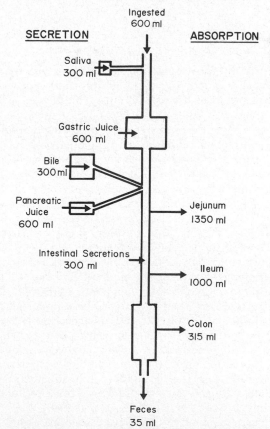

Figure 51–2. Daily secretion and absorption of water across the gastrointestinal tract of a 20-kg dog. (Based on data from Strombeck, D. R.: *Small Animal Gastroenterology.* Davis, CA: Stonegate Publishing, 1979.)

sia, inhibits absorption and may cause movement of water into the intestinal lumen.[12, 24, 53]

Two pathways for diffusion of water across the mucosa have been identified, the transcellular and the paracellular shunt pathways.[9, 53] Diffusion through the transcellular pathway accounts for about 10 per cent of water absorption, and the remainder passes through the alternative pathway through the tight junctions. Water molecules may pass through cell membranes and through pores in the tight junctions.[53] The pores are only a few nanometers in diameter, and in the small intestine they are lined by a negative charge. Thus, only small molecules such as water and urea, and ions can move through them. The negative charge carried on the pores in the small intestine make the pores more permeable to cations than anions, but the reverse may be true in the colon.[53]

Water is secreted by the villous crypt cells of the small intestine in association with active secretion of chloride by the mucosal cells.[36] It is believed that chloride secretion is stimulated by activation of the adenyl cyclase–cyclic AMP mechanism by hormones such as vasoactive intestinal polypeptide and prostaglandins. Acetylcholine and 5-hydroxytryptamine also stimulate secretion by increasing the amount of free calcium in the cell.[36] The cyclic AMP mechanism can also be stimulated by some bacterial toxins such as the heat-labile toxin of *E. coli.*

MOTILITY

Peristaltic and segmental contractions mix the ingesta and propel it along the intestine. Peristaltic contractions consist of a circular contraction of the intestinal wall that progresses along the intestine. As the contraction progresses, the segment in front of the contraction relaxes to accommodate the ingesta being pushed along. Peristaltic contractions usually occur over a few centimeters of the intestine, but occasionally they may traverse its entire length. The vast majority of peristaltic contractions progress distally, but reverse peristalsis occasionally occurs. Peristaltic contractions propel ingesta along the intestine and spread it out over the mucosa.

Segmental contractions consist of a series of circular contractions occurring at intervals of one to two centimeters along a short segment of intestine. The contractions last a few seconds and are then replaced by another series of contractions occurring between the original ones. Alternating contraction and relaxation of adjacent areas continues for several minutes, and this action mixes the food and moves it along the intestine. A series of segmental contractions may remain stationary or may progress a few centimeters distally.

Contractions of the small intestine are associated with electrical discharges in the intestinal muscle. Two types of electrical activity have been recorded, slow wave activity and spike discharges.[2] Slow waves are regular cycles of depolarization and repolarization of the intestinal muscle occurring at about 18 to 20/min in the duodenum and at progressively slower rates distal to the ileum, where they occur at 14 to 15/min.[1] Slow waves originate in a pacemaker located in the longitudinal muscle of the proximal duodenum and are propagated through the intestinal muscle. Slow waves by themselves do not cause intestinal contractions but appear to synchronize intestinal contractions, in that contractions can occur only during the period of depolarization of a slow wave.

Spike potentials occur with intestinal contractions and represent depolarization of the circular muscle layer. They occur in bursts superimposed on the slow waves. Spike potentials have been described as occurring as regular or irregular spiking activity, either of which is associated with contractions.[40]

During fasting the intestine is relatively quiescent. The inactivity of the intestine is interrupted by periods of motility associated with regular spiking activity. The contractions progress distally along the intestine, and the associated electrical activity has been called the migrating myoelectric complex.[59] Contractions that occur during the fasting state serve to clear secretions, cellular debris, and bacteria from the small intestine.[40] Irregular spiking activity occurs after eating and is associated with intense motility, which mixes food with intestinal secretions, exposes ingesta to the mucosa to enhance absorption, and transports ingesta along the intestine.

Generation of slow waves and the migrating myoelectric complex of the fasted state are independent of the extrinsic parasympathetic and sympathetic nerve supply to the small intestine. However, the extrinsic nerves do modulate intestinal motility, with parasympathetic stimulation increasing motility and sympathetic stimulation causing inhibition. The increase in motility after feeding may in part be stimulated by increased vagal activity. Intestinal stasis following trauma and surgery is due to sympathetic stimulation.

The role of gastrointestinal hormones in the control of small-intestinal motility is still unclear. Cholecystokinin and gastrin increase motility and secretin inhibits it.[1] Stimulation of motility by cholecystokinin may be a physiological effect.[21] Gastrin converts the pattern of intestinal motility from the fasted to the fed state; this may be a physiological role of the hormone.[60]

PATHOPHYSIOLOGY OF INTESTINAL OBSTRUCTION

Much of the information on the pathophysiology of intestinal obstruction that is relevant to clinical conditions comes from experimental observations made in the first half of this century, when it was demonstrated that the survival time and the nature of the clinical course of an animal with intestinal obstruction depends on the site of the obstruction, the completeness of the obstruction, and the degree of interference with the intestinal blood flow. In general, proximal obstructions are more acute than distal obstructions, complete obstructions are more acute than partial obstructions, and strangulating obstructions are more acute than simple obstructions. In strangulating obstructions there is interference with blood flow through the affected intestine. Death of animals with intestinal obstruction is caused by a combination of fluid and electrolyte losses, bacterial toxemia, and blood loss. The importance of each of these factors in a particular case depends on the type of obstruction.

It is convenient to classify obstructions as follows: proximal or high simple obstructions of the small intestine, distal or low simple obstructions of the small intestine, strangulating obstructions of the small intestine, partial small-intestinal obstructions, and obstructions of the colon. A condition that has similarities to low intestinal obstruction is adynamic ileus, in which the motility of the intestine is impaired. The pathophysiological consequences of paralytic ileus are similar to those of low intestinal obstruction.

Complete, Simple Obstruction of the Proximal Small Intestine

Experimental obstruction of the pylorus or proximal small intestine in dogs is characterized by persistent vomiting and death in three to four days.[55] If saline is administered parenterally, life is prolonged for three to four weeks; if water is available *ab lib*, animals will survive an average of nine days.[18, 55] In such cases death is due to dehydration and electrolyte losses. The composition of the fluid that is vomited, and the nature of electrolyte losses, depends on the site of the obstruction. In obstructions of the pylorus or duodenum proximal to the entry of the bile and pancreatic ducts, the fluid lost is mainly gastric juice, and the animal develops dehydration with hypochloremia, hypokalemia, and metabolic alkalosis. Obstructions below the entry of the bile and pancreatic ducts cause loss of alkaline fluid in addition to gastric juice, and there is a tendency to develop metabolic acidosis and hypokalemia.[6, 29]

Although death from high intestinal obstruction is due largely to dehydration and electrolyte losses, if the animal survives for a sufficient time, toxemia from bacteria proliferation in the obstructed intestine (see next section) may also contribute to death.[26]

Complete, Simple Obstruction of the Distal Small Intestine

Dogs with experimentally induced intestinal obstruction from the mid-jejunum to the terminal ileum usually survive for about five to seven days.[18, 55] The small intestine becomes greatly distended with fluid and gas. The fluid is composed of secretions from the stomach, intestine, liver, and pancreas.[54] More than 70 per cent of the accumulated gas is swallowed air, and the remainder is from chemical reactions and bacterial fermentation in the intestinal lumen, and from diffusion from the blood.[27]

Failure of the obstructed intestine to absorb secreted fluid is a result of distension caused by accumulation of gas, because the fluid is absorbed if swallowed air is prevented from entering the intestine.[56] Although a considerable amount of fluid becomes sequestered in the intestinal lumen, death in low intestinal obstruction is not due to loss of fluid and electrolytes alone.[18, 55]

Death in low intestinal obstruction has been related to absorption of toxins produced in the intestinal lumen. Evidence for toxemia includes an increase in the survival time of dogs given antibiotics parenterally or into the obstructed loop, and the demonstration that sterilized fluid removed from an obstructed loop of intestine is toxic.[17] The toxins apparently diffuse from the lumen of the intestine into the intestinal wall and peritoneal cavity, where they are removed through the lymphatics and capillaries.

A major factor causing death of animals with low intestinal obstruction is toxemia from proliferation of bacteria in the small intestine. Loss of fluid into the obstructed bowel is also a contributing factor (Fig. 51–3).

Strangulation of the Small Intestine

Strangulation of the intestine refers to conditions in which the flow of blood through the affected area of the intestine is impaired. In these conditions the lumen of the intestine may or may not be obstructed. Strangulating obstructions are generally presented as a more acute clinical picture than simple obstructions. Experimental studies in dogs have shown a difference in the course of the disease, depending on whether the mesenteric arteries or veins have been occluded.[42, 54]

Because of their thinner walls, the mesenteric veins are more susceptible to occlusion than the arteries. In many forms of intestinal strangulation, such as torsion of the mesentery, intussusception, and entrapment of a segment of intestine in a hernia, the veins draining the affected segment are occluded but the arteries are not. Blood flows into the affected intestine and pools in the microcirculation. Hemorrhage into the wall of the intestine and intestinal lumen occurs, and hemorrhagic shock rapidly supervenes. In experimental studies in dogs, ligation of the veins draining a segment of intestine is followed by a severe fall in arterial blood pressure and death in two to 12 hours.[42, 43, 44] Hypotension is a result of loss of blood into the affected intestine.[45] Therefore, death from strangulation of a large segment of intestine occurs because of hemorrhagic shock (Fig. 51–4).

If only a short segment of intestine is affected, the animal may survive for a longer period. Some hem-

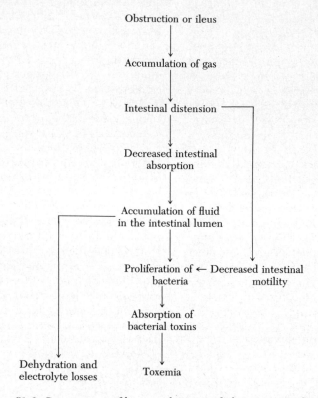

Figure 51–3. Consequences of low, simple intestinal obstruction or adynamic ileus.

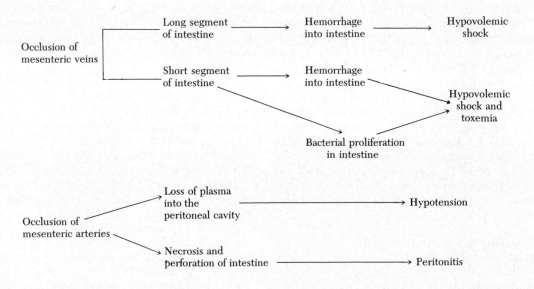

Figure 51–4. Consequences of intestinal strangulation.

orrhage into the intestine occurs, but with time, bacteria proliferate in the affected intestine and the toxins that are produced diffuse into the peritoneal cavity and are absorbed. Death occurs because of a combination of blood loss and toxemia (see Fig. 51–4).[54]

Obstruction to the arterial blood supply, as occurs with mesenteric thrombosis or embolism, has a different course from that of venous obstruction. In experimental studies it was shown that ligation of the mesenteric arteries of dogs causes death of the animal in 16 to 20 hours without a significant fall in arterial blood pressure until just prior to death.[42–44, 54] In many instances the gut wall became perforated and peritonitis occurred.[42, 45] When perforation did not occur, considerable quantities of plasma-like fluid accumulated in the peritoneal cavity.[42] It was concluded that death from occlusion of the mesenteric arteries is due to a combination of loss of plasma into the peritoneal cavity and toxemia (Fig. 51–4).[42, 54]

Obstruction of the Large Intestine

The colon is a very distensible organ that stores feces before they are eliminated. Following obstruction, the ileal effluent accumulates in the colon and water is absorbed. Very large quantities of feces can accumulate in the colon, so the course of the disease is frequently long. Affected animals lose their appetite and die of starvation.[55]

Adynamic Ileus

The motility of the gastrointestinal tract is reduced after anesthesia, surgery, or trauma. In most instances motility returns within a short time and the period of decreased motility is not evident clinically.

Occasionally, however, the period of decreased motility becomes prolonged and progresses to intestinal stasis. The clinical condition associated with intestinal stasis is called adynamic ileus. The cause of adynamic ileus is thought to be increased sympathetic stimulation to the intestine, which inhibits intestinal contractions, or loss of potassium, which decreases the contractility of intestinal muscle.

The pathophysiological effects of intestinal stasis are similar to those of low simple intestinal obstruction (see Fig. 51–3). Stasis is followed by accumulation of gas in the lumen, which distends the intestine. Gas and fluid accumulate, and bacteria proliferate in the intestinal lumen. The final result is toxemia together with fluid and electrolyte losses.

Partial Obstruction of the Small Intestine

Foreign bodies, neoplasms, and intussusceptions can all cause partial obstruction of the small intestine characterized clinically by weight loss and diarrhea. The clinical signs are related to maldigestion and malabsorption of nutrients caused by proliferation of bacteria in the intestine proximal to the partial obstruction. This condition has been called the stagnant or blind loop syndrome.

Normally bacteria are eliminated from the small intestine by contractions of the intestinal wall which continually move bacteria into the large intestine. When the intestine becomes partially obstructed, intestinal contractions are not able to clear ingesta and bacteria from the small intestine effectively. Bacteria proliferate proximal to the obstruction, where ingesta accumulates. Weight loss and diarrhea, which frequently are the most prominent signs of partial intestinal obstructions, are due to the action of bacteria in the intestine (Fig. 51–5). Weight loss is due to bacterially induced carbohydrate, protein,

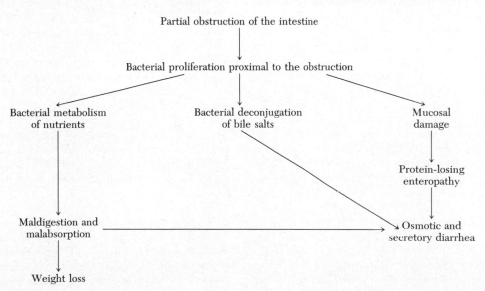

Figure 51–5. Consequences of partial intestinal obstruction.

and vitamin malabsorption, and to bacterial deconjugation of bile salts, which interferes with fat absorption.[14, 15, 22] Mucosal damage caused by bacteria in the stagnant loop may also contribute to malabsorption.[52]

Diarrhea occurs as a result of several mechanisms. Water is retained in the intestine owing to the osmotic effects of unabsorbed nutrients and deconjugated bile salts. Loss of protein across the damaged mucosa of the stagnant loop probably contributes to the development of osmotic diarrhea.[32] Unabsorbed bile salts and fatty acids also stimulate active anion secretion from the intestinal mucosa, causing water to be secreted into the intestinal lumen.[3] Therefore, diarrhea associated with partial intestinal obstruction appears to be due to a combination of osmotic and secretory effects of unabsorbed compounds in the intestinal lumen.

Surgical Disorders

Eberhard Rosin

TRAUMA

Trauma of the small intestine is uncommon. Intestinal and mesenteric injury may occur with bite wounds of the abdomen, when sharp objects or projectiles penetrate the abdominal wall, with self-inflicted injury following evisceration of an abdominal incision, and with blunt trauma from motor vehicle accidents. In a study of 600 cases of motor vehicle accidents in urban dogs, two cases of intestinal injury were reported.[23] Intestinal injuries consisted of contusions of the bowel wall and lacerations of the mesenteric attachment. In both cases, injury to the mesentery deprived a segment of intestine of normal blood supply.[23]

The mechanism of intestinal rupture from blunt abdominal trauma is not established. Experimental findings suggest that injury results primarily from a shearing force. Compression with tearing between two opposing surfaces such as the abdominal wall and spine are apparently the most likely cause of intestinal and mesenteric injury. The site of injury cannot be related directly to intraluminal pressure or to the presence or absence of air and fluid in the intestinal lumen.[61]

Missile, bite, stab, or impalement wounds of the caudal thorax or abdomen may penetrate the peritoneal cavity. The greater the velocity of a missile, the more extensive the damage it can do, although serious injury to the intestines can occur from low-velocity missiles such as air gun pellets. Intra-abdominal injury can occur owing to the concussive effect of a gunshot wound that does not enter the abdomen. Trauma causing multiple perforations of the intestine may appear externally as minor wounds.[4]

Dog bites can cause puncture or severe crushing wounds; the number and location of external bite wounds may not indicate the degree of intestinal damage that has occurred. Stab wounds can cause intestinal injury, but the incidence of associated intra-abdominal injury is low. Self-inflicted injury to the intestines and mesentery is common after evisceration following dehiscence of an abdominal incision.

Clinical Findings

Clinical signs of blunt or penetrating injury to the intestines may be masked by associated injuries such as lacerations, fractures, pneumothorax, or abdominal hemorrhage. The cardinal signs of intestinal injury are: vomiting, abdominal tenderness, bloody stools, or passage of bloody fluid from the rectum. Other signs include depression, anorexia, reluctance to move, and, late in the course of events, shock.[37] In four cases of blunt trauma to the intestines, clinical signs first appeared within 12 hours to three days following injury.[8] Patients with injury to the abdominal cavity often require prolonged observation for development of signs of intestinal disease and peritonitis.

Radiographic Findings

Radiographic examination may allow identification of the projectile, its trajectory, and tissue reaction, which can be seen as an alteration in tissue density. The degree and location of injury may not be apparent on plain radiographs. Accurate diagnosis depends on the recognition of peritonitis. There may be a small amount of or no free gas demonstrable in the abdomen, or gas escaping from ruptured intestines may be trapped, forming gas pockets within adhered loops of intestines. These gas pockets may be identified by their size and lack of conformity to the bowel lumen.[33]

If there is doubt about the need for exploratory celiotomy, a contrast study using oral iodine-containing contrast material can give additional information. Barium should not be used if rupture of the intestines is suspected. Iodine-based contrast material is absorbed by the peritoneum or damaged intestinal mucosa and eliminated by the kidneys. The detection of contrast media in the urinary tract is, therefore, an indication of severe intestinal damage.[30, 31]

Diagnosis

Suspected intestinal injuries are best evaluated by physical examination to detect penetration of the peritoneal cavity, abdominal tenderness, and proctorrhagia. Peritoneal lavage (see Chapter 50) is invaluable; recovered lavage fluid containing bacteria, vegetable fibers, and toxic neutrophils indicates the need for exploratory celiotomy.

In view of the serious consequences of unrecognized and untreated rupture of the intestines, and the low morbidity and mortality associated with exploratory celiotomy, direct examination of the peritoneal cavity should be considered in animals with equivocal signs on physical and radiographic examination.

If intestinal injury is suspected but results of abdominal lavage are equivocal, careful physical examination is repeated twice daily. Radiographic examination and peritoneal lavage are repeated if signs of intestinal injury persist. Exploratory celiotomy should be performed if results of radiographic or lavage examination remain equivocal or are positive for intestinal perforation.

Possible penetration of the peritoneal cavity by a missile requires prompt celiotomy. Stab wounds are not evidence of intestinal injury, and the decision for surgery is based on patient evaluation. Bite wounds are associated with a high incidence of intra-abdominal injury, including intestinal trauma, and in these patients the minimal side effects of a celiotomy with negative results must be weighed against the consequences of delayed or nontreatment of a serious intestinal injury.[4, 13, 48]

Treatment

Treatment of shock and management of cardiovascular and pulmonary injury must precede or occur concurrently with exploratory celiotomy and management of intestinal injury. Broad-spectrum antibiotics are administered preoperatively.

Following incision into the abdomen, the abdominal cavity is thoroughly examined before a decision is made about surgical correction of initially obvious lesions. Adhesions between omentum and intestines or between adjacent intestinal loops are freed to permit inspection of the entire intestinal tract.

Small lacerations or holes in the intestines are debrided and closed with 3–0 synthetic absorbable material placed in simple interrupted or Lembert suture patterns. Larger defects are managed by serosal patching. A segment of healthy intestine, usually jejunum, is sutured in place over the defect(s). One row of simple interrupted sutures is placed circumferentially to secure the healthy serosa over the injury. The sutures should pass through the submucosa of both segments of intestine.[7] More extensive injuries are managed by intestinal resection and anastomosis.

In self-inflicted injury following evisceration, the exposed tissues are gently washed with sterile fluids and the abdomen is explored. Necrotic omentum, mesentery, and intestines are resected. The damage may be so extensive that intestinal resection and anastomosis lead to short bowel syndrome.

Contamination of the peritoneal cavity with intestinal contents is the principal cause of serious complications in intestinal injury. The early use of appropriate broad-spectrum antibiotics such as trimethoprim-sulfadiazine (30 mg/kg subcutaneously b.i.d.), chloramphenicol (50 mg/kg intravenously t.i.d.), or gentamicin (1 mg/kg subcutaneously b.i.d.), thorough irrigation of the peritoneal cavity with warm sterile fluids, aspiration of the lavage fluids, along with delayed closure of the skin and subcutaneous tissues are appropriate measures to treat infection. External drainage in intestinal injury is inadvisable. In rare cases of massive bacterial contamination and infected fibrin deposits that cannot be debrided, the abdominal incision can be left unsutured and the patient treated by open peritoneal drainage.

Postoperatively the animal is supported by fluid, electrolyte, and nutritional therapy and monitored closely for signs of peritonitis. Peritoneal lavage is used as an objective indicator of postoperative peritonitis.

MECHANICAL OBSTRUCTION

Mechanical obstruction is the most common indication for intestinal surgery in small animal practice. Obstruction of the intestinal lumen may occur with foreign bodies, intussusception, neoplasia, and, less commonly, adhesions. The nature and site of the obstruction influence the signs. An object lodged in the proximal small intestines stimulates vomiting with loss of acid secretions from the stomach and alkaline secretions from the gallbladder, pancreas, and duodenum. Dehydration and electrolyte imbalance can be expected. Animals with vomiting may have either normal pH or primary metabolic acidosis. Normal pH following vomiting may result from an equal loss of acid secretions from the stomach and base secretions from the upper intestinal tract. Primary metabolic acidosis is probably due to the relatively greater loss of base fluids from duodenal, pancreatic, and bile secretions than of acid from gastric juice during vomiting. Primary metabolic acidosis may also occur in animals with severe dehydration and inadequate perfusion of splanchnic viscera, skin, and muscle.

Obstruction of the distal jejunum or ileum may not stimulate vomiting, but results in distension of the intestinal lumen by fluid and gas. This gas comes from three sources: (1) swallowed atmospheric air (approximately 70 per cent); (2) decomposition of intestinal contents (10 per cent); and (3) diffusion from blood into the intestinal lumen (20 per cent).[25]

The accumulation of fluid in the obstructed bowel is due to a combination of increased fluid production and decreased fluid absorption. Alterations in blood supply to the intestinal wall and the increase in bacterial population in obstructed bowel contribute to the accumulation of fluid.[10, 19, 28]

Strangulation of the bowel is an infrequent but dangerous and sometimes unsuspected complication of intestinal obstruction. It can be produced by incarceration of the bowel in the neck of a hernial sac or by twisting of the bowel on its mesentery. The mesenteric circulation is blocked, and tissue necrosis follows. The necrotic area allows bacteria and their products to pass through into the peritoneal cavity and into the circulation. The strangulated segment is purple to black, foul-smelling, and friable.

Strangulation of the bowel should be considered in every animal with sudden and severe abdominal pain, a severe systemic reaction, often including shock, that is out of proportion with that seen in intestinal obstruction, and a poor response to supportive treatment. The clinical course of strangulated obstruction depends on the degree and extent of vascular obstruction, the volume of blood lost, and the proliferation and absorption of bacteria and toxins. Strangulated obstruction causes rapid death if not promptly corrected.

Pressure produced by a foreign body or intussusception may cause venous stasis and edema followed by disruption of arterial flow and necrosis of the bowel wall. Once the integrity of the intestinal mucosa is compromised, the alimentary canal is no longer segregated from the systemic circulation. Bacterial products enter the systemic circulation and can produce endotoxic shock.

Foreign Body

A wide variety of foreign objects may be ingested, particularly by young animals. Once the object has passed through the pylorus, the next smallest lumen is the distal duodenum and proximal jejunum, a common site of obstruction (Fig. 51–6).

Clinical Findings

The signs of intestinal foreign body obstruction are variable, depending on the location of the foreign body and the propensity of the foreign body to cause vascular disruption and necrosis of the intestinal wall. Anorexia, depression, abdominal tenderness, and vomiting are commonly seen. Vomiting may be profuse, as with complete obstruction of the proximal small intestine, or sporadic, as with partial obstruction of the distal small intestine. Vomiting may cause dehydration and weakness. Defecation may decrease in frequency and the stools may be blood-tinged.

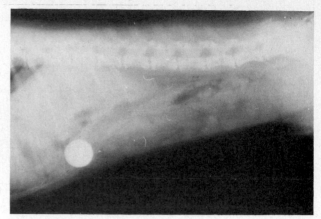

Figure 51–6. Lateral abdominal radiograph of a dog with a marble lodged in the proximal jejunum.

Radiographic Findings

Obstruction of the distal small intestine produces a greater dilation of the bowel with more accumulation of fluid and gas than does obstruction of the proximal small intestine.

A standing lateral projection can be an important addition to the standard recumbent lateral and ventrodorsal projections, as gas-fluid interfaces in dilated loops of obstructed small intestine are more easily seen on this view.

Radiopaque foreign bodies are easily identified. Obstruction by one of the wide variety of radiolucent foreign objects causes enlargement of the diameter of the bowel and retention of gas and fluid, producing the classic radiographic signs of obstruction.

Contrast examination of the small intestine permits confirmation of diagnosis. Intraluminal obstruction often appears as a radiolucent area surrounded by contrast material outlining the foreign body. Radiographic examination six hours after administration of barium suspension permits diagnosis of most proximal small intestine obstructions. Twenty-four hour studies are best in diagnosing most distal small intestine obstructions.

Diagnosis

The diagnosis of foreign body obstruction is based on history, careful abdominal palpation, and abdominal radiographs. The small intestines are "slipped" between the thumb and fingers of one hand in a small dog or cat or between the fingers of both hands in a large dog. If one exerts gradual gentle pressure, only the most nervous or pained dog will resist abdominal palpation. Rapid or rough hand movements cause abdominal splinting, which may be confused with abdominal tenderness associated with disease. Fluid and gas accumulation proximal to the foreign body, and the foreign body itself, can often be palpated.

Intestinal obstruction should be considered in any animal that vomits. Vomiting caused by simple gastritis responds to symptomatic medical treatment. If symptomatic treatment does not improve the animal's condition within 24 hours, further diagnostic evaluation is advisable.

Treatment

The treatment for foreign body obstruction is exploratory celiotomy. The abdomen is exposed by ventral midline abdominal incision of sufficient length to permit adequate inspection of the entire gastrointestinal tract.

If the foreign body has not caused vascular obstruction of the intestinal wall, it is removed through an enterotomy made distal to and slightly over the foreign body. The peritoneal cavity is protected from soilage. The incision is of sufficient length to make removal of the foreign body easy. An incision directly over the foreign body or over the dilated bowel proximal to the obstruction is ill-advised, as some degree of vascular damage to the bowel wall may have occurred that could adversely influence normal healing. The enterotomy incision is closed with a simple interrupted or continuous suture using 3–0 synthetic absorbable material, or a two-layer closure using a Connell suture oversewn with a Lembert suture.

If the foreign body has caused necrosis of the intestinal wall, or if the viability of the bowel wall is in question, a resection and end-to-end anastomosis is indicated. Intravenous injection of fluorescein dye, viewed by Wood's lamp, may aid in the assessment of vascularity of the bowel wall. The abdominal cavity is thoroughly irrigated with warm sterile fluids, and the incision is closed in standard fashion.

Small sharp foreign bodies, such as a sewing needle, are best left alone. The transit of the foreign object through the alimentary canal is monitored by periodic abdominal radiographs, and the animal is monitored for signs of peritonitis. In most cases the needle will pass without complication. Even if it has been localized by abdominal radiographs taken in two projections, the needle can be difficult to find at exploratory celiotomy.

String Foreign Body

String (thread, nylon stocking) can produce a unique form of intestinal obstruction, seen more commonly in cats. The string may extend through much of the intestinal tract and may be visible wrapped around the base of the tongue. The intestine progressively gathers itself in accordion-like pleats along the string. As peristaltic waves continue to attempt to move the irritant along, the string saws through the mesenteric side of the intestine. If the bowel is perforated, signs of peritonitis develop. Occasionally, the inflammation and infection at the sites of laceration are walled off. In these cases, removal of the string is difficult, and the intestines may not resume normal function postoperatively.

Clinical Findings

String foreign bodies cause signs of intestinal obstruction, with variable degrees of vomiting, dehydration, anorexia, and depression. Commonly, obstruction is incomplete and vomiting is not as frequent or severe as with complete obstruction of the proximal intestine. Some intestinal contents may continue to pass through the area of the string obstruction, and blood-tinged feces may be passed.

The string cannot be felt by abdominal palpation; however, abdominal tenderness is usually present, and fluid and gas accumulation and pleating causing irregularity of the small intestine often can be palpated.

Radiographic Findings

Radiographic findings in one study included gathering of bowel loops (50 per cent of affected animals), increased number of intestinal gas bubbles (60 per cent), and peritonitis (40 per cent); contrast examination revealed shortening and eccentric pleating of the small intestine in 43 per cent of affected animals (Fig. 51–7).[38] String foreign body is differentiated from enteritis by the location of the radiographic signs; in enteritis there is symmetrical constriction with centrally located gas bubbles.[33, 38]

String foreign bodies appear as lucent objects within the barium-filled intestinal lumen. After barium passes into the colon, the string may retain barium.

Treatment

The treatment for string foreign body is exploratory celiotomy. For a length of string caught around the

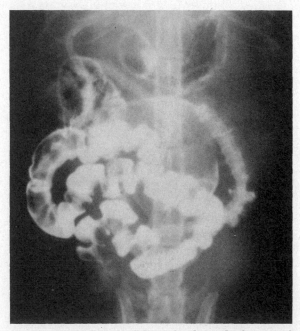

Figure 51–7. Venterodorsal abdominal radiograph of a cat with a string foreign body.

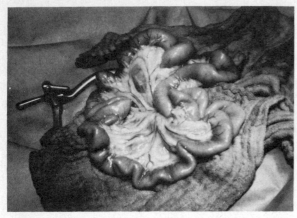

Figure 51–8. A string foreign body in the jejunum of a cat.

tongue, only the most gentle traction on the string in the mouth should be used; if this maneuver fails to deliver the string, it is cut and the remainder is removed from the stomach.

The intestinal tract is exposed by ventral midline abdominal incision, and the entire bowel is gently examined (Fig. 51–8).

An enterotomy incision is made midway along the site of the string obstruction. The string is found along the mesenteric side of the intestinal lumen and pulled from the incision. As much string as possible is delivered by pulling gently and gradually; then the ends are cut (Fig. 51–9). Additional enterotomies are spaced along the intestine to ensure removal of all string while minimizing the risk of lacerating the intestine.

Where localized peritonitis and fibrosis of the mesenteric border of moderate length of intestine are present, a resection and anastomosis should be performed. If the extent of bowel involved is so long

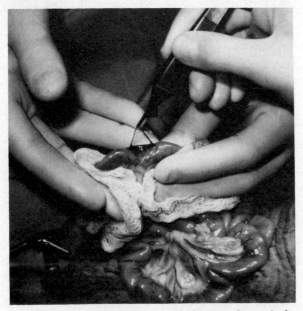

Figure 51–9. Enterotomy for removal of a string foreign body.

that intestinal resection would result in short bowel syndrome, the prognosis for recovery is guarded. The string is hidden within the granulomatous inflammation and may be difficult to find. Even if the string can be extracted successfully, the intestine may not resume normal function postoperatively.

Intussusception

Intussusception is produced by a vigorous contraction that forces the intestine into the lumen of the adjacent relaxed segment. The circumstances that cause the invagination are usually undetermined.

The components of an intussusception include the invaginated section, called the intussusceptum, and the enveloping segment, called the intussuscipiens. The mesentery and blood supply to the intussusceptum are included in the invagination; venous obstruction can progress to arterial occlusion and necrosis. Commonly, fibrin is deposited between the intestinal segments. Double intussusceptions can occur, and triple intussusceptions have been recorded in humans.

An intussusception can progress so that small intestine protrudes from the anus. In this instance an intussusception is differentiated from rectal prolapse by passing a probe between the prolapsed segment and the anus. In intussusception, the probe can be passed without obstruction.

Intussusception occurs most frequently in young animals, at the ileocecal junction. In 45 cases, the age of affected animals ranged from five days to seven years; 37 of the 45 were less than one year old.[62]

Clinical Findings

The cardinal signs of intussusception are vomiting, abdominal pain, passage of bloody mucoid stools, and palpation of a sausage-shaped abdominal mass. These signs are variable and partially depend on the degree of vascular obstruction associated with the intussusception.

Obstruction of the lumen with intussusception can be complete or incomplete. With complete obstruction, extensive accumulation of fluid and gas proximal to the obstruction can be expected. Because the most common site of intussusception is the ileocecal region, this accumulation of fluid and gas may not be emptied by vomiting. If the obstruction is incomplete, feces will pass through the affected region and may accumulate blood and mucus from the diseased mucosa, resulting in the passage of bloody mucoid stools.

Most animals are presented because of bloody diarrhea or vomiting or both, and an elongated mass, usually in the dorsal cranial portion of the abdomen, can be felt on palpation in 67 per cent.[62] Raising the animal's forelimbs while the abdomen is carefully palpated is often helpful. In most instances abdominal pain associated with palpation is minimal.

Intussusception can occur in the dog in an agonal state and should be considered as secondary in these patients. These intussusceptions characteristically have no fibrosis.

Radiographic Findings

The radiographic findings in intussusception are usually those of mechanical obstruction of the intestine. Diagnosis by plain films is difficult. Findings include distension of the intestinal segments proximal to the intussusception with fluid and gas. Because most intussusceptions are ileocolic, the pattern seen on radiographs is usually that of increased tissue density caudal to the stomach with small bowel loops displaced caudally and to the right.

Contrast radiography is usually necessary to differentiate an intussusception from other causes of intestinal obstruction. Since intussusceptions occur most frequently at the ileocecal junction, they are best identified by a barium enema. The intussusception is seen as a compression in the barium column (Fig. 51–10).

Treatment

Reduction of the intussusception by barium enema is possible in approximately 50 per cent of affected infants; this technique has not been reported in small animals. In most instances, the intussusception is

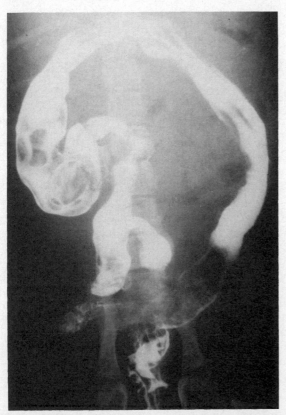

Figure 51–10. Venterodorsal abdominal radiograph of a dog demonstrating barium enema outlining an intussusception.

fixed in position by fibrosis and cannot be manually reduced at surgery.

The treatment of choice is exploratory celiotomy. The abdominal cavity is exposed through a ventral midline abdominal incision, and the entire small and large intestine is carefully examined. Intussusceptions can occur in several locations at the same time, so the entire bowel must be inspected before a decision of resection and anastomosis is made. An attempt is made to manually reduce the intussusception. The intussusception is squeezed while gentle traction is applied to the proximal segment (Figs. 51–11 and 51–12). One of the following scenarios will occur:

1. The intussusception can be successfully reduced (Fig. 51–13). There is no reliable correlation between the duration of signs and the ability to manually reduce the intussusception. The degree of fibrosis and damage to the intussusceptum is related to the degree of vascular obstruction.

2. The intussusception can be reduced; however, in the process, the serosal surface and possibly a portion of the muscular layer of the bowel are split. If superficial, these lacerations can be left alone or can be closed with 3–0 synthetic absorbable suture material placed in simple interrupted pattern.

3. The intussusception cannot be manually reduced, or after reduction, the involved segments of intestine are not viable. Viability is assessed using standard clinical criteria of color, arterial pulsation, and intestinal contraction. The use of intravenous injection of fluorescein dye viewed by Wood's lamp in a darkened operating room helps in evaluating the vascularity of the involved intestine.

If the intussusception cannot be reduced or the intestines are not viable, resection and anastomosis are necessary.

If the intussusception recurs, operative treatment as just described is repeated. Additionally, an attempt should be made to prevent subsequent recurrence. The site of the intussusception can be sutured to the abdominal wall (enteropexy). A method used successfully in children is suturing the small intestine into accordion-like folds by simple interrupted sutures placed to unite adjacent serosal surfaces. The use of these procedures has not been evaluated in reported series of small animals.

Rarely, the recurrence of the intussusception can be seen at surgery as a creeping peristaltic wave (Figs. 51–14 and 51–15). Enteropexy or intestinal plication is performed. The reason for the immediate recurrence of intussusception in these animals is unknown. The prognosis in these cases is guarded.

Adhesions

Adhesions rarely cause intestinal obstruction in small animals, although they frequently develop following traumatic and surgical wounds of the peritoneal cavity. Chronic peritonitis from intra-abdominal

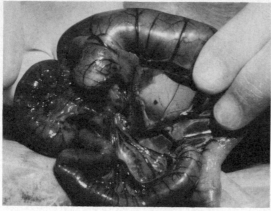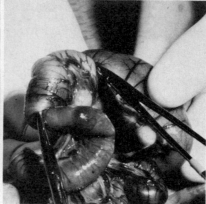

Figure 51–11. Starting manual reduction of an intussusception in a cat.

Figure 51–12. Partial reduction of a double intussusception in the same cat shown in Figure 51–11. Each forceps points to an intussusception.

abscesses and granulomatous inflammation from infected nonabsorbable suture material are exceptions; either may lead to the development of extensive adhesions and interference with normal intestinal peristalsis.

Clinical signs of intestinal obstruction from adhesions cannot be differentiated from intestinal obstruction from other causes. Abdominal palpation may reveal fluid and gas accumulation and an irregular mass of small intestines. Abdominal radiographs may demonstrate altered positions of small intestines and delayed transit time.

Treatment is directed at eliminating the cause of the peritonitis. In rare circumstances in which abdominal trauma has resulted in fibrous bands occluding the intestinal lumen, the bands are resected, and if necessary, involved intestines are resected.

In chronic peritonitis from abscess or granulomatous inflammation associated with foreign bodies, the site of infection is resected. Adhered loops of bowel can occasionally be freed by a combination of blunt

and sharp dissection; however, frequently the plane of dissection is not apparent, and loops of bowel must be resected *en bloc*. With massive adhesions and distortion of normal bowel architecture, the alimentary canal can be difficult to trace, and decisions about appropriate resection and anastomosis can be frustrating. If the site of infection, and the adhered small intestines, can be resected and bowel continuity re-established by anastomosis, prognosis is good. Unfortunately, the infection or granulomatous inflammation may be difficult to control, and extensive intestinal resection may result in short bowel syndrome. The prognosis for return of normal intestinal function is guarded.

Neoplasia

Tumors of the small intestine are uncommon in the dog and cat. Adenocarcinoma and lymphosarcoma are the most common tumor types in the dog. In the cat the most common tumor of the small intestine is lymphosarcoma. Clinical signs of intestinal neoplasia vary with the location of the tumor. Common clinical signs include anorexia, weight loss, and intermittent vomiting or diarrhea. An abdominal mass can usually be palpated.[11, 20]

Abdominal radiographs may demonstrate signs of intestinal obstruction, including accumulation of fluid and gas proximal to the obstruction and delayed intestinal transit time. Mural lesions visible following the administration of contrast material include luminal filling defects, thickening of the bowel wall, mucosal ulceration, and abnormal position of intestinal loops. Constricting annular lesions of the small intestine have also been described.[11, 33]

The definitive diagnosis of small-intestinal neoplasia is made following exploratory celiotomy and histopathological examination of a biopsy specimen.

The location and extent of the tumor determine

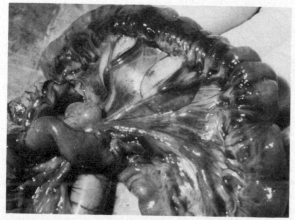

Figure 51–13. Successful reduction of the double intussusception shown in Figure 51–12.

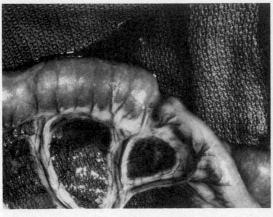 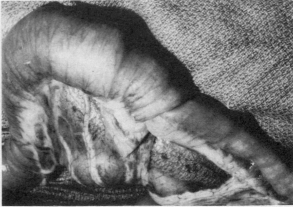

Figure 51–14. An intestinal contraction which will cause the intussusception shown in Fig. 51–15.

Figure 51–15. Operative recurrence of an intussusception in a dog. The cause was not determined.

the possibilities for surgical treatment. Surgery, including resection and intestinal anastomosis, may be combined with chemotherapy. Frequently, the tumor is extensive or metastasis has occurred, and surgical treatment is not possible.

The prognosis for treatment of tumors of the small intestine is guarded. In a report of five cases of tumors of the small intestine, all animals were dead or were euthanized for recurrence of signs within one month after exploratory celiotomy. Two animals died from postoperative complications associated with leakage from intestinal anastomosis.[11]

Mesenteric Torsion

Mesenteric torsion is rare in the dog. The root of the mesentery twists and the anterior mesenteric artery and vein, or branches thereof, are obstructed. The thin-walled veins are occluded more than the mesenteric arteries, and the bowel rapidly turns purple to black and distends with fluid and gas. The integrity of the intestinal mucosa is rapidly compromised. Blood flows into the intestinal lumen, and bacteria and endotoxins enter the peritoneal cavity and systemic circulation.

Clinical Findings

The prominent clinical signs are a distended abdomen and shock. They are sudden in onset and rapidly progressive. Within hours the abdomen becomes markedly distended by gas-filled intestinal loops, and cardiovascular collapse is apparent. The abdomen is tense and tympanitic on percussion. The signs mimic those of gastric dilation-torsion syndrome.

Treatment

Rapid infusion of 80 ml/kg of lactated Ringer's solution is appropriate for replacement of lost blood volume. Exploratory celiotomy is performed imme-

diately. The mesenteric torsion is reduced and the bowel is examined for return of color. Unfortunately the prognosis for resumption of normal circulation is grave. In two reported cases,[35] and in 2 cases seen by the author, circulation did not return. In these cases, the extent of necrosis of the intestine precluded resection and anastomosis. The dogs died or were euthanized.

1. Atanassova, E., and Papaosva, M.: Gastrointestinal motility. Int. Rev. Physiol. *12*:35, 1977.
2. Bass, P.: In vivo electrical activity of the small bowel. *In* Code, C. F. (ed.): *Handbook of Physiology.* Sec, 6, Vol. III. Washington, D. C., American Physiological Society, 1968.
3. Binder, H. J.: Pathophysiology of bile acid– and fatty acid–induced diarrhea. *In* Field, M., Fordtran, J. S., and Schultz, S. G. (eds.): *Secretory Diarrhea.* Bethesda, Md., American Physiological Society, 1980.
4. Bjorling, D. E., Crowe, D. T., Kolata, R. J., and Rawlings, C. A.: Penetrating abdominal wounds in dogs and cats. J. Am. Anim. Hosp. Assoc. *18*:742, 1982.
5. Castle, W. B.: Gastric intrinsic factor and vitamin B_{12} absorption. *In* Code, C. F. (ed.): *Handbook of Physiology.* Sec. 6, Vol. III. Washington, D. C., American Physiological Society, 1968.
6. Cornelius, L. M., and Rawlings, C. A.: Arterial blood gas and acid-base values in dogs with various diseases and signs of disease. J. Am. Vet. Med. Assoc. *178*:992, 1981.
7. Crowe, D. T.: The serosal patch: clinical use in 12 animals. Vet. Surg. *13*:29, 1984.
8. Dorn, Hufford, T. J., and Anderson, N. V.: Four cases of traumatic intestinal injuries in dogs. J. Am. Anim. Hosp. Assoc. *11*:786, 1975.
9. Edmonds, C. J.: Water and ionic transfer pathways of mammalian large intestine. Clin. Sci. *61*:257, 1981.
10. Enochsson, L., Nylander, G., and Öhuman, U.: Effects of intraluminal pressure on regional blood flow in obstructed and unobstructed small intestines in the rat. Am. J. Surg. *144*:558, 1982.
11. Feeney, D. A., Klausner, J. S., and Johnston, G. R.: Chronic bowel obstruction caused by primary intestinal neoplasia: a report of five cases. J. Am. Anim. Hosp. Assoc. *18*:67, 1982.
12. Fordtran, J. S., and Ingelfinger, F. J.: Absorption of water electrolytes and sugars from the human gut. *In* Code, C. F. (ed.): *Handbook of Physiology.* Sec. 6, Vol. III. Washington, D.C., American Physiological Society, 1968.
13. Freeark, R. J.: Penetrating wounds of the abdomen. New Engl. J. Med. *291*:185, 1974.

14. Gracey, M.: The contaminated small bowel syndrome: pathogenesis, diagnosis and treatment. Am. J. Clin. Nutr. 32:234, 1979.

15. Gracey, M., Burke, U., Oshin, A., et al.: Bacteria, bile salts, and intestinal monosaccharide malabsorption. Gut 12:683, 1971.

16. Guyton, A. C.: Textbook of Medical Physiology. 6th ed. Philadelphia, W. B. Saunders Co., 1981.

17. Harper, W. H., and Blain, A., III: The effect of penicillin in experimental intestinal obstruction. Preliminary report on closed loop studies. Bull. Johns Hopkins Hosp. 76:221, 1945.

18. Harper, W. H., and Lemmer, R. A.: Necrosis and ulceration of the intestinal wall in simple intestinal obstruction. Bull. Johns Hopkins Hosp. 179:207, 1946.

19. Heneghan, J. B., Robinson, W. L., Menge, J., and Winistörefer, B.: Intestinal obstruction in germ free dogs. Eur. J. Clin. Invest. 11:285, 1981.

20. Howard, D. R., Schirmer, R. G., Mostosky, U. V., and Michel, R. L.: Adenocarcinoma in the ileum of a young dog: J. Am. Vet. Med. Assoc. 162:956, 1973.

21. Johnson, L. R.: Gastrointestinal hormones and their functions. Ann. Rev. Physiol. 39:135, 1977.

22. Kim, Y. S., and Spritz, N.: Metabolism of hydroxy fatty acids in dogs with steatorrhea secondary to experimentally produced intestinal blind loops. J. Lipid Res. 9:487, 1968.

23. Kolata, R. J., and Johnston, D. E.: Motor vehicle accidents in urban dogs: a study of 600 cases. J. Am. Vet. Med Assoc. 167:938, 1975.

24. Krejs, G. J., and Fordtran, J. S.: Physiology and pathophysiology of ion and water movement in the human intestine. Sleisinger, M. G., and Fordtran, J. S. (eds.): Gastrointestinal Disease: Pathophysiology, Diagnosis and Management. Philadelphia, W. B. Saunders Co., 1977.

25. Lantz, G. C.: The pathophysiology of acute mechanical small bowel obstruction. Comp. Cont. Ed. 3:910, 1981.

26. Markowitz, J., Archibald, J., and Downie, H. G.: Experimental Surgery. 5th ed. Baltimore, The Williams & Wilkins Co., 1964.

27. Miller, L. D., Mackie, J. A., and Rhoads, J. E.: The pathophysiology and management of intestinal obstruction. Surg. Clin. North Am. 41:1285, 1962.

28. Mishra, N. K., Appert, H. E., and Howard, J. N.: The effects of distention and obstruction on the accumulation of fluid in the lumen of small bowel of dogs. Ann. Surg. 5:791, 1974.

29. Nadrowski, L. F.: Pathophysiology and current treatment of intestinal obstruction. Rev. Surg. 31:381, 1974.

30. Nelson, S. W., Christoforidis, A. J., and Roenigk, W. J.: Barium suspensions vs. water-soluble iodine compounds in the study of obstruction of the small bowel. Radiology 80:252, 1963.

31. Nelson, S. W., Christoforidis, A. J., and Roenigk, W. J.: Dangers and fallibilities of iodinated radiopaque media in obstruction of the small bowel. Am. J. Surg. 109:546, 1965.

32. Nygaard, K., and Rootwelt, K.: Intestinal protein loss in rats with blind segments on the small bowel. Gastroenterology 54:52, 1968.

33. O'Brien, T. R.: Radiographic Diagnosis of Abdominal Disorders in the Dog and Cat. Philadelphia, W. B. Saunders Co., 1978.

34. Olsen, W. A., and Ingelfinger, F. J.: The role of sodium in intestinal glucose absorption in man. J. Clin. Invest. 47:1133, 1968.

35. Parker, W. M., and Presnell, K. R.: Mesenteric torsion in the dog: two cases. Can. Vet. J. 13:283, 1972.

36. Powell, D. W., and Field, M.: Pharmacological approaches to treatment of secretory diarrhea. In Field, M., Fordtran, J. S., and Schultz, S. G. (eds.): Secretory Diarrhea. Bethesda, Md., American Physiological Society, 1980.

37. Punzet, G.: Closed traumatic injuries of the small intestine and mesentery in the dog. Wien. Tieraerztl. Monatsschr. 58:339–347, 1971.

38. Root, C. R., and Lord, P. F.: Linear radiolucent gastrointestinal foreign bodies in cats and dogs: their radiographic appearance. J. Am. Vet. Rad. Soc. 12:45, 1971.

39. Rose, R. C.: Transport and metabolism of water-soluble vitamins in intestine. Am. J. Physiol. 240:G97, 1981.

40. Ruckenbusch, Y.: Motor functions of the intestine. Adv. Vet. Sci. Comp. Med. 25:345, 1981.

41. Schultz, S. G.: Cellular models of sodium and chloride absorption by mammalian small and large intestine. In Field, M., Fordtran, J. S., and Schultz, S. G. (eds.): Secretory Diarrhea. Bethesda, Md., American Physiological Society, 1980.

42. Scott, H. G.: Intestinal obstruction; experimental evidence on loss of blood in strangulation. Arch. Surg. 36:816, 1938.

43. Scott, H. G., and Wangensteen, O. H.: Length of life following various types of strangulation obstruction in dogs. Proc. Soc. Exp. Biol. Med. 29:424, 1931.

44. Scott, H. G., and Wangensteen, O. H.: Blood pressure changes correlated with time, length and type of intestinal strangulation in dogs. Proc. Soc. Exp. Biol. Med. 29:428, 1931.

45. Scott, H. G., and Wangensteen, O. H.: Blood losses in experimental intestinal strangulations and their relationship to degree of shock and death. Proc. Soc. Exp. Biol. Med. 29:748, 1931.

46. Shiau, Y. F.: Mechanisms of intestinal fat absorption. Am. J. Physiol. 240:G1, 1981.

47. Shikata, J., Shida, T., Amino, K., and Isioka, K.: Experimental studies on the hemodynamics of the small intestine following increased intraluminal pressure. Surg. Gynecol. Obstet. 156:155, 1983.

48. Shuck, J. M., and Lowe, R. J.: Intestinal disruption due to blunt abdominal trauma. Am. J. Surg. 136:668, 1978.

49. Silk, D. B. A., and Dawson, A. M.: Intestinal absorption of carbohydrate and protein in man. Int. Rev. Physiol. 19:151, 1979.

50. Sleisenger, M. H., and Kim, Y. S.: Protein digestion and absorption. N. Engl. J. Med. 300:659, 1979.

51. Strombeck, D. R.: Small Animal Gastroenterology. Davis, Cal., Stonegate Publishing, 1979.

52. Toskes, P. P., Giannella, R. A., Jervis, H. R., et al.: Small intestinal mucosal injury in the experimental blind loop syndrome. Light- and electron-microscopic and histochemical studies. Gastroenterology 68:1193, 1975.

53. Turnberg, L. A.: Intestinal transport of salt and water. Clin. Sci. Molec. Med. 54:337, 1978.

54. Wangensteen, O. H.: Intestinal Obstructions. 3rd ed. Springfield, Ill., Charles C Thomas, 1955.

55. Wangensteen, O. H., and Leven, N. L.: Correlation of function with cause of death following experimental intestinal obstruction at varying levels. Arch. Surg. 22:658, 1931.

56. Wangensteen, O. H., and Rea, C. E.: The distension factor in simple intestinal obstruction: An experimental study with exclusion of swallowed air by cervical esophagostomy. Surgery 5:327, 1939.

57. Weiner, I. M., and Lack, L.: Bile salt absorption; enterohepatic circulation. In Code C. F. (ed.): Handbook of Physiology. Sec. 6, Vol. III. Washington, D. C., American Physiological Society, 1968.

58. Weipers, W. L., Nagy, L., Pirie, H. M., et al.: A comparison of the toxic effects of intestinal obstruction fluid with those of certain endotoxins. J. Pathol. 110:295, 1973.

59. Weisbrodt, N. W.: Patterns of intestinal motility. Ann. Rev. Physiol. 43:21, 1981.

60. Weisbrodt, N. W., Copeland, E. M., Kearley, R. W., et al.: Effects of pentagastrin on electrical activity of small intestine of the dog. Am. J. Physiol. 227:425, 1974.

61. Williams, R. D., and Sargent, F. T.: The mechanism of intestinal injury in trauma. J. Trauma 3:288, 1963.

62. Wilson, G. P., and Burt, J. K.: Intussusception in the dog and cat: a review of 45 cases. J. Am. Vet. Med. Assoc. 164:515, 1974.

Physiology

Michael A. Pass

The large intestine receives material from the ileum, dehydrates it, and then stores it before it is eliminated from the body. Absorption of water from the fecal material occurs in the proximal colon and cecum, and the dried material is stored in the distal segment of the colon.

Absorption of water by the colon occurs as a result of active absorption of sodium.[24] ATPase-dependent sodium pumps on the basilateral membranes of the mucosal cells transfer sodium ions from the interior of the cells into the interstitial spaces, causing sodium ions to diffuse from the intestinal lumen into the cells. The net movement of sodium from intestinal lumen to interstitial space promotes diffusion of water and chloride ions from the intestinal lumen along osmotic and electrochemical gradients. A similar mechanism occurs in the small intestine.

Potassium is lost in the feces by addition of potassium-rich mucus and cells to the colonic contents and by transport of potassium from the extracellular fluid into the colonic lumen.[24]

Secretion of bicarbonate ions in exchange for absorption of chloride ions occurs in the large intestine.[24] The bicarbonate neutralizes acids produced from bacterial metabolism in the large intestine.

The large intestine contains a variety of bacteria that digest residual food material that cannot be digested by the enzymes of the mammalian alimentary tract. In dogs and cats, this is of little nutritional significance. However, the bacteria of the large intestine are of major importance to surgery, because they are responsible for systemic and wound infections.

The movements of the large intestine are complex. In the cat, ingesta enters the large intestine and is subjected to reverse peristaltic contractions of the proximal colon and cecum.[11, 12] These contractions mix the ingesta. Antiperistaltic contractions occur at a rate of 5 to 6 cycles/min in bursts about every 15 minutes, with each period of activity lasting about 5 minutes. As more ingesta is added to the large intestine, the dehydrated material previously present is displaced distally in the colon, where it is propelled by tonic contractions into the descending colon for storage.[11, 12]

Reverse peristalsis of the pattern seen in cats is not a feature of the large intestine of dogs.[61] Ascending and descending peristaltic contractions and tonic contractions of the colon have been observed in dogs.[33]

The rectum is normally empty, and the anus is kept closed by contraction of the anal sphincter muscles. When contractions of the colon propel feces into the rectum, a reflex is initiated that is conducted through the myenteric plexus. It causes increased motility of the colon and rectum and relaxation of the anal sphincters. This reflex acting alone is not sufficient to cause defecation and is augmented by two spinal reflexes. The first spinal reflex intensifies the contractions in the colon and rectum, and further relaxes the anal sphincters. The second spinal reflex is a respiratory reflex that causes the animal to inhale, close its glottis, and contract its thoracic and abdominal muscles to increase intra-abdominal pressure and force the fecal mass through the anus. Defecation is controlled by several reflexes that can be overcome by voluntary contraction of the external anal sphincter. If this occurs, contractions in the rectum eventually subside, and defecation does not occur until fecal material is again pushed into the rectum.[55]

Surgical Diseases

Michael Aronsohn and Dudley E. Johnston

MEGACOLON

Megacolon is a general term applied to a gross dilation of the large intestine. It is a functional disorder in which accumulated fecal material cannot be evacuated from the colon. Megacolon is congenital or acquired. Congenital megacolon has not been proved to exist in dogs or cats. Acquired megacolon usually results from a lesion that prevents normal defecation over a prolonged period. If no organic lesion can be found, a diagnosis of idiopathic megacolon can be made.

Hirschsprung's Disease

Congenital aganglionic megacolon, or Hirschsprung's disease, has not been satisfactorily documented in the dog or cat but has been extensively studied in humans, in whom the disease is familial

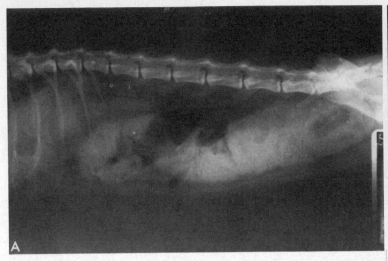

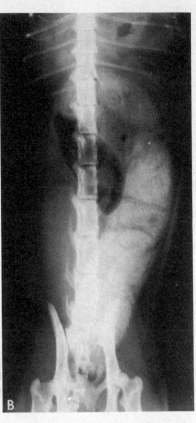

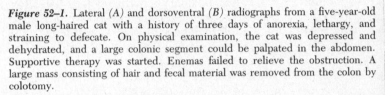

Figure 52–1. Lateral *(A)* and dorsoventral *(B)* radiographs from a five-year-old male long-haired cat with a history of three days of anorexia, lethargy, and straining to defecate. On physical examination, the cat was depressed and dehydrated, and a large colonic segment could be palpated in the abdomen. Supportive therapy was started. Enemas failed to relieve the obstruction. A large mass consisting of hair and fecal material was removed from the colon by colotomy.

and the incidence is one in 5000 live births.[25] The disease is due to congenital absence of intramural ganglion cells in a variable length of large intestine. Typically, the ganglion cells are absent from both Meissner's submucosal plexus and Auerbach's myenteric plexus. The smooth muscle of the affected segment is persistently contracted. The aganglionic segment commonly involves a narrow section of the distal colon or more rarely may extend the entire length of the colon, in which case the small intestine becomes dilated and hypertrophied. The latter condition is called long-segment aganglionosis.[49]

The myenteric ganglia are considered part of the parasympathetic nervous system, and their absence accounts for loss of propulsive peristalsis in the involved colon.[20] The diseased section is normal in

TABLE 52–1. Causes of Constipation

Dietary and environmental	Bones, hair, or foreign material impacted in the colon
	Lack of exercise
	Change of habit or environment
	  No litter box
	  Dirty litter box
	  Hospitalization
		Mechanical obstruction
		continued
			Prostatic hypertrophy
			Pelvic tumor
			Intraluminal
			  Colonic or rectal tumor
			  Perineal hernia

Painful defecation	Anorectal disease
	  Anal sacculitis
	  Anal abscess
	  Perianal fistula
	  Anal stricture
	  Anal spasm
	  Rectal foreign body
	  Pseudocoprostasis
	Trauma
	  Fractured pelvis or limb
	  Dislocated hip
		Neurological disease
		
		"Metabolic" and
		  endocrinological
			Central nervous system dysfunction
			  Paraplegia
			Intrinsic colonic nerve dysfunction
			  Idiopathic megacolon
			Interference with colonic smooth
			  muscle function
			  Hyperparathyroidism
			  Hypothyroidism
			Debility
			  General muscle weakness and
			    dehydration

Mechanical obstruction	Extraluminal
	  Healed fracture of pelvis with
	    narrowing of the pelvic canal
		Drug-induced	Anticholinergics
			Antihistamines
			Barium sulfate
			Diuretics
			Opiates

(Adapted from Burrows, C. F.: Diarrhea and constipation. *In* Ettinger, S. J. (ed.): *Textbook of Veterinary Internal Medicine.* 2nd ed. W. B. Saunders, Philadelphia, 1983.)

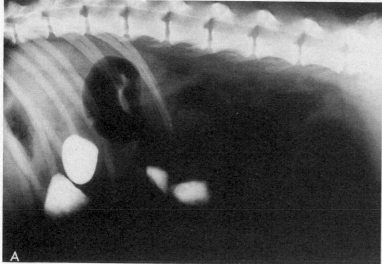

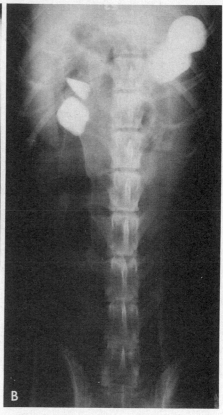

Figure 52–2. Lateral *(A)* and ventrodorsal *(B)* radiographs from a four-year-old female German shepherd with a history of vomiting and anorexia for ten days. The dog was straining to defecate and passing mucus in the feces. Two rocks were present in the stomach and two in the ascending colon. The rocks in the stomach were removed by gastrotomy, and those in the colon were "milked" toward the anus, and removed.

appearance, whereas the dilated section has normal innervation. A definite diagnosis is based on a history of low intestinal obstruction since infancy, contrast radiographic studies of the colon, and histologic demonstration of agangliosis. The disease is usually diagnosed in infancy but occasionally not until adulthood. Definitive surgical treatment is commonly referred to as Swenson's pull-through procedure.[60] Owing to technical difficulties and postoperative complications, various modifications of this technique have been described.[39] The aganglionic segment of colon is removed, and frozen sections are submitted for pathological examination in order to confirm that only normal intestine remains.

Colonic Impaction

Obstipation, or intractable constipation, is an acquired form of megacolon in both dogs and cats. Primary colonic impaction is due to obstruction with foreign material or feces mixed with hair (Fig. 52–1). Secondary colonic impaction is caused by any condition that obstructs the normal passage of feces or causes pain on defecation (Table 52–1; Figs. 52–2 and 52–3).

Clinical Findings

Colonic impaction can occur at any age but is more common in older animals. A history of repeated

Figure 52–3. Lateral radiograph from a ten-year-old male German shepherd with a positive contrast cystogram. The dog had a history of chronic straining to defecate but had deteriorated in the past few days and had pain in the perineal area. Bilateral perineal hernias and enlarged prostate are present along with colonic impaction and retroflexed bladder.

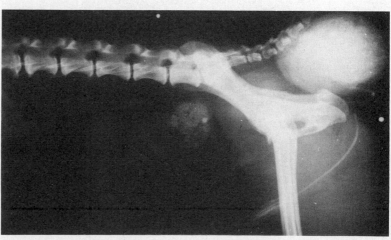

straining to defecate while passing little or no feces is usual. Careful questioning may reveal pertinent information such as feeding of bones or a healed pelvic fracture. Anorexia, vomiting, straining to defecate with passage of small amounts of liquid feces containing blood or mucus, and weight loss may be present. There may be abdominal pain, as evidenced by crying, stiff gait, arched back, and reluctance to move. The patient is usually depressed and may be weak. In acute or partial obstructions, physical findings may be normal. In chronic cases, findings may include severe weight loss, poor hair coat, and dehydration. A large colonic segment can usually be palpated through the abdominal wall. The animal may exhibit pain on abdominal palpation. Plain abdominal radiographs are indicated in all suspected cases of colonic impaction.

Chronic obstipation may be associated with anemia or fluid, electrolyte, and acid-base disturbances. Hypokalemia secondary to vomiting and anorexia is common. A diagnosis of obstipation is usually evident from history and physical examination alone. To classify the underlying cause, radiographic and clinical laboratory data are useful. Proctoscopy and exploratory celiotomy may be indicated for a definitive diagnosis.

Treatment

Therapy is aimed at correction of any fluid, electrolyte, and acid-base disturbances, relief of the obstruction, and management of the underlying cause.

Physical impaction can be removed by a variety of methods, the most conservative being tried first. Oral wetting agents such as dioctyl sodium sulfosuccinate (Colace) and softening and lubricating agents such as mineral oil may relieve acute simple impaction. Enemas and manual decompression are often necessary to relieve a chronic colonic impaction. Sedation or general anesthesia is usually necessary in cats and intractable dogs. Decompression can gen-

erally be accomplished with large-volume soapy water or mineral oil enemas and a sponge forceps to break down and remove the impacted material. It is not recommended that hypertonic sodium phosphate enemas be used in cats, small dogs, or dehydrated and debilitated animals, because large quantities of water may enter the colon while sodium and phosphate are absorbed. Potential damage to the central nervous system can be caused by increased intracellular and extracellular sodium concentrations. Hyperphosphatemia, which will bind and precipitate serum calcium, resulting in hypocalcemia with tetany, may also occur after the administration of hypertonic sodium phosphate enemas.[20, 52] Impacted material can be "milked" caudally toward the anus by gently squeezing the colon through the abdominal wall. It may be necessary to repeat the enemas and manual procedures over a few days to empty the colon completely. It is extremely important that these procedures be done gently to avoid trauma to the colon.

Colotomy may be indicated in extreme cases when other efforts fail or trauma to the colon is likely. Factors such as the animal's ability to undergo general anesthesia and major surgery, and the complications of colotomy, must be weighed against the advisability of continuing with enemas and nonoperative manipulations.

Once the impaction is removed, measures to prevent recurrence are started. With simple bone impaction, bones are eliminated from the diet. Hair ball obstruction in cats can be managed by giving commercial tube laxatives or petrolatum on a regular basis. Constriction of the pelvic canal due to malunion of pelvic fractures may be adequately managed by diet and laxatives. In some cases, pelvic reconstruction is necessary. Techniques for partial hemipelvectomy in animals have been described and used successfully in the treatment of obstipation secondary to malunion of pelvic fractures.[2] Castration and abdominal exploration may be indicated in obstipation sec-

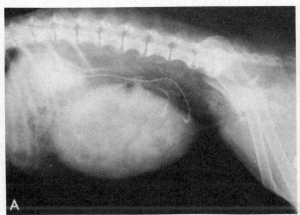 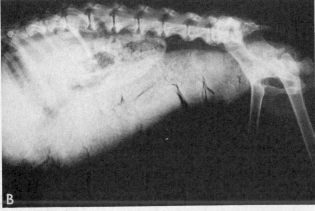

Figure 52–4. *A,* Lateral radiograph from a ten-year-old female beagle that was hit by a car. The dog had flaccid paralysis of the tail and lack of anal and bladder tone. Pelvic radiographs revealed a fracture of the left acetabulum and ilium as well as multiple pelvic floor fractures, but no fractures of the spine or sacrum. *B,* Lateral radiograph taken two years after trauma. Bladder and anal tone had returned, but only partial fecal control was present. The dog was given stool softeners daily and enemas as needed to relieve obstipation.

ondary to prostatic disease. Relief of obstipation associated with perineal hernias usually requires herniorrhaphy.

In recurrent obstipation, long-term medical therapy with dioctyl sodium sulfosuccinate (Colace) or bulk laxatives such as methylcellulose or psyllium hydrophilic mucilloid (Metamucil) along with dietary management such as the use of bran and the occasional use of enemas may be adequate.

The prognosis for colonic impaction depends on the cause. The prognosis for simple bone impaction is excellent, whereas obstruction associated with malunion of a pelvic fracture has a less favorable prognosis. Colonic or extraluminal tumors have a guarded prognosis (Fig. 52–4).

Idiopathic Megacolon

Idiopathic megacolon is an acquired disease for which no clear cause can be determined. It is a well-recognized entity in humans[38, 42] and three cases have been reported in cats.[27, 65]

Clinical Findings

Idiopathic megacolon is seen in adult cats and is characterized by recurrent and possibly progressive episodes of constipation extending over months to years. Treatment with laxatives and enemas along with dietary management usually gives temporary relief, but the problem recurs. Anorexia, vomiting, depression, weight loss, and dehydration have been associated with this condition. Abdominal palpation reveals a distended colon.

Diagnosis can usually be made from the history and physical examination alone, but a complete evaluation, including abdominal radiographs, should be done to rule out a definitive cause of the obstipation.

Treatment

Medical treatment for this condition is unrewarding in both humans and cats, but subtotal colectomy has given good results.[27, 38, 42, 65] Histological examination of the colon in humans has shown that nerve cells are present in the submucosal plexus of Meissner and the myenteric plexus of Auerbach.[38, 42, 54] In one cat, a relative absence of myenteric ganglia in the distal narrowed segment of colon was reported.[65] On the basis of a small number of cats, prognosis following surgical treatment has been excellent, although complications can occur.

TRAUMATIC PERFORATION

Injuries to the colon occur as a result of sharp or blunt trauma to the abdominal wall or from intraluminal trauma. Penetrating abdominal injuries by gunshot wounds, knife wounds, or other sharp objects cause perforation of the colon in the dog.[7] Rarely, bone fragments from a fractured pelvis lacerate the colon. Diagnostic procedures, including protoscopy, colonic biopsy, and positive contrast enemas, can result in perforation of the large intestine, especially when the wall of the colon is diseased. Ingested foreign bodies such as bone and sewing needles can also perforate the colon.

Clinical Findings

Perforation of the colon causes rapidly progressive peritonitis and septic shock. Signs of peritonitis include abdominal tenderness, depression, vomiting, pyrexia, abdominal distension, and ileus. Rapid pulse, pale mucous membranes, and slow capillary refill time are signs of shock. Clinical signs often progress rapidly. An inconsistent sign but a strong indicator of colonic trauma is the passage of bloody feces or mucus. If this is present, there is a high probability of colonic injury. Colonic ischemia or a partial colonic tear may progress to complete perforation after a few days.

Abdominal radiographs show lack of detail and sometimes free air in the abdomen. In perforation of the colon secondary to a positive contrast enema, contrast material is seen free in the abdominal cavity. Positive contrast enemas should not be used when a ruptured colon is suspected.

The diagnosis of colonic perforation is confirmed by microscopic evaluation of fluid recovered by abdominal paracentesis or peritoneal lavage. Peritoneal lavage is a highly accurate method of evaluating abdominal injuries and is significantly more sensitive than needle paracentesis.[19, 35] The presence of a high proportion of degenerate neutrophils and of bacteria within neutrophils and free in the lavage fluid strongly suggests septic peritonitis.[8]

Treatment

An exploratory celiotomy should be performed as soon as possible in suspected or confirmed perforation of the colon. In abdominal trauma, re-evaluation—by observation of the patient's progress, physical examination, and evaluation of peritoneal fluid—is continued until it becomes clear whether exploratory celiotomy is indicated. Fluid replacement and treatment of shock with balanced electrolyte solutions are indicated. Broad-spectrum antibiotics are given as soon as possible. The earlier antibiotics are administered to human patients with penetrating abdominal wounds, the lower the incidence of infectious complications.[28]

A complete exploration is done in all cases because there may be multiple abdominal injuries. Perforations of the large intestine are treated by debridement and primary closure or by resection and anastomosis, depending on the surgical findings.

NONTRAUMATIC PERFORATION

A nontraumatic form of colonic perforation has been seen in dogs after the parenteral administration of dexamethasone following neurosurgical procedures.[5, 34, 63] Seven cases have been reported in dogs that underwent surgery for intervertebral disc herniation and were given dexamethasone during the immediate postoperative period. All dogs died within ten days postoperatively. The combined effect of surgical stress, spinal cord trauma, and corticosteroid therapy has a particularly deleterious effect on the gastrointestinal tract.[63] Experimental studies in dogs indicate that corticosteroids markedly decrease mucous production and alter its histochemical structure, leading to a breakdown of the mucous barrier.[44] In patients with spinal cord injury, colonic motility is usually decreased owing to a number of factors, such as lack of voluntary control of defecation, increased sympathetic tone secondary to distension of the urinary bladder, and lack of normal exercise. Bowel stasis may cause local irritation and ulceration.[63] Corticosteroids interfere with the normal ability of mucosal cells to repair themselves.[44] These small ulcerative lesions may progress to larger ulcers followed by perforation and peritonitis.

The dose of dexamethasone used in dogs following neurosurgery is variable and controversial. We currently use an initial dose of 1 mg/kg intravenously or intramuscularly followed by 0.5 mg/kg every 6 hours, with the dose halved daily and stopped by the fifth postoperative day. The use of cimetidine (Tagamet) along with dexamethasone is advocated by some veterinary surgeons, but its effect in preventing ulceration or perforation of the colon has not been documented.

Colonic perforation has been reported in humans as a complication of steroid therapy but is seen less frequently than perforation of the stomach and duodenum.[21, 64] Colonic perforation in humans is usually caused by long-term steroid therapy in conjunction with some underlying disease of the colon.

Clinical Findings

Anorexia, vomiting, depression, pyrexia, and abdominal pain were observed in the reported cases. A dog may be presented in shock, with death following quickly. The anti-inflammatory effects of steroid therapy may alter the peritoneal and systemic response to perforation and mask the clinical signs. Dogs receiving dexamethasone therapy occasionally develop bloody, mucoid diarrhea. It is best to stop the medication or decrease the dose, because this development may indicate colonic irritation or ulceration that may progress to perforation.

Diagnosis is based on a history of a neurosurgical procedure followed by dexamethasone therapy, physical findings, and results of cytologic examination of peritoneal fluid. Owing to the rapid progression of signs, antemortem diagnosis may not be possible.

Treatment

As with traumatic colonic perforation, immediate treatment of shock, administration of broad-spectrum

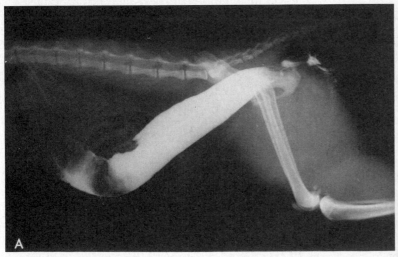
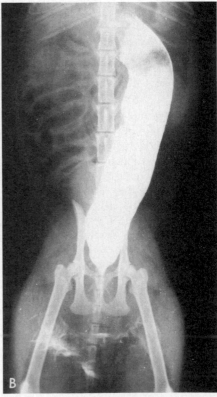

Figure 52–5. Lateral *(A)* and ventrodorsal *(B)* radiographs of a three-month-old male Doberman pinscher given a barium enema, demonstrating inversion of the cecum into the colon. A typhlectomy was performed.

antibiotics, and exploratory celiotomy are essential. The proximal colon is the most common site of perforation. Widespread abdominal contamination may be found because of the anti-inflammatory effects of dexamethasone. Surgical repair, abdominal lavage, abdominal drainage, and postoperative supportive care are the same as for traumatic perforations. Prognosis is grave, since all reported cases have died before or immediately after surgery.

CECAL INVERSION

Inversion of the cecum into the proximal colon of the dog is uncommon.[1, 30, 41, 53] Cecal inversion can cause partial or complete obstruction of the ileocolic junction. The underlying cause of the disorder is unknown.

Clinical Findings

With a partial ileocolic obstruction, a history of chronic intermittent blood-stained feces, occasional vomiting, and slight weight loss may be the only presenting complaints. The history may include multiple negative fecal examination results and no improvement with dietary management. Physical examination is usually nonspecific, although a firm, sometimes painful mass may be palpated in the midventral abdomen.

If complete obstruction of the ileocolic junction has occurred secondary to cecal inversion, clinical signs—vomiting, depression, and dehydration—are acute. A firm, painful abdominal mass can usually be palpated.

Plain abdominal radiographs are usually nonspecific, showing excess amounts of gas in the small intestine. In complete obstruction, gaseous distension of the small intestine is seen. Definitive diagnosis can be made on radiographs taken after oral administration of barium sulfate suspension[30] or barium enema (Fig. 52–5). The inverted cecum appears as a pleated area surrounded by contrast material within the first four to six centimeters of the barium-filled proximal colon.

Treatment

Colotomy and surgical removal of the inverted cecum is curative in most cases. If complete obstruction of the ileocolic junction is present and edema or inflammation of the area is severe, resection is indicated, and the distal ileum is anastomosed to the proximal colon.

CECAL IMPACTION

Impaction of the cecum with inspissated feces or foreign material is rare in dogs.[58] Irritation and typhlitis can occur secondary to the impaction.

Clinical Findings

The presenting history is variable and depends on the size of the impaction, duration of the impaction, and the nature of the material in the cecum. Signs are nonspecific and include vomiting, anorexia, diarrhea, and the passage of feces containing blood or mucus. Pain and a firm mass may be found on abdominal palpation.

Survey radiographs may indicate foreign material in the cecum, the loss of the gas-filled cecal silhouette, or a soft tissue mass in the right craniodorsal abdomen. Delayed emptying time and barium retention in the cecum may be seen after administration of oral barium sulfate suspension.

Treatment

Exploratory celiotomy with typhlectomy is the treatment of choice. If typhlotomy is done, recurrence is possible.

CECAL DILATION

Dilation of the cecum with gas is a rare clinical problem in the dog.[40] History and physical findings are similar to those in cecal impaction. Survey radiographs show a large, dilated cecum filled with gas. Treatment of choice is typhlectomy.

DIAGNOSTIC TECHNIQUES

Endoscopy of the Colon

Endoscopic examination of the colon is a relatively safe procedure that is easy to perform and yields valuable information.

Rigid pediatric human proctoscopes are approximately 2 cm in diameter and 15 cm in length and can be used satisfactorily to examine the distal colon of small dogs and cats. Adult human proctoscopes, approximately 2 cm in diameter and 25 to 30 cm in length, are recommended for large dogs. Such an instrument should be equipped with a high-intensity distal light source, should allow for air insufflation with a hand bulb, and should have a hinged or detachable magnifying window that can maintain a closed system after air has been insufflated. Insufflated air dilates the colon and allows better observation. An obturator with a smooth lubricated tip is used for insertion of the proctoscope. Suction and large cotton swabs should be available to remove blood and debris. Biopsy forceps are passed through the lumen of the instrument, and samples of the mucosa and submucosa are taken.

Flexible fiberoptic tube endoscopes are used to examine the luminal surface of the entire colon of the dog and cat and to obtain biopsy samples of the colonic wall. Flexible endoscopes should be 110 to

150 cm in length and are approximately 1 cm in diameter. They can be adapted for photography. A suction mucosal biopsy capsule, designed for use with flexible endoscopes, is used for obtaining biopsy specimens. Proper preparation of the bowel is essential to ensure good results. A 24-hour fast and a mild enema the evening before the procedure are recommended. Sedation and physical restraint may be all that is necessary, but animals are easier to examine and better results are obtained with general anesthesia.

The patient is placed in right lateral recumbency so that the cecum and colon are less restricted in position and more easily examined. The tip of the endoscope is lubricated and inserted into the anus. Air is insufflated, and the instrument is advanced slowly. The lumen is kept in focus during advance-

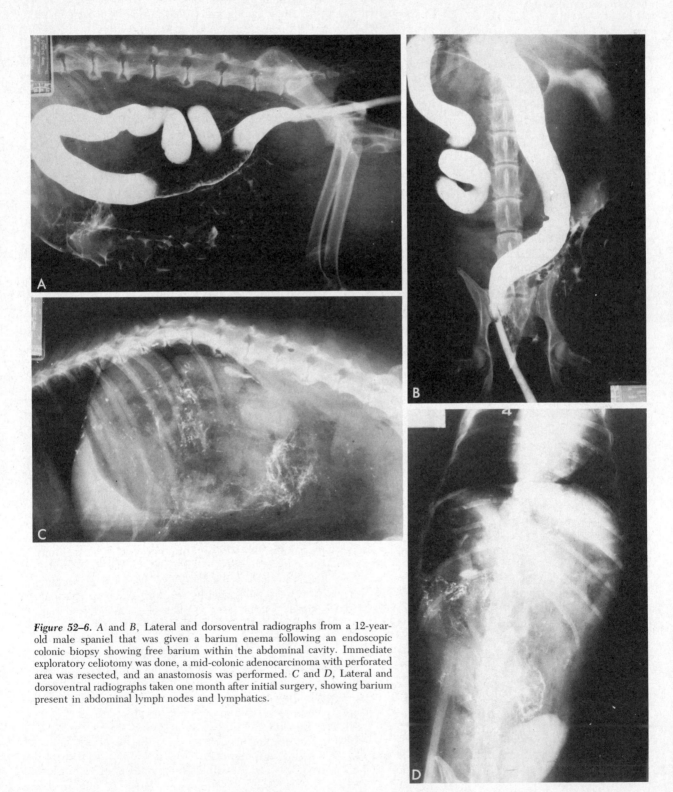

Figure 52–6. A and B, Lateral and dorsoventral radiographs from a 12-year-old male spaniel that was given a barium enema following an endoscopic colonic biopsy showing free barium within the abdominal cavity. Immediate exploratory celiotomy was done, a mid-colonic adenocarcinoma with perforated area was resected, and an anastomosis was performed. C and D, Lateral and dorsoventral radiographs taken one month after initial surgery, showing barium present in abdominal lymph nodes and lymphatics.

ment to prevent entering a diverticulum or perforating the colon.

The entire colon is examined before biopsy specimens are taken. Specimens of mucosa and submucosa are immediately placed in formalin and submitted for histological evaluation. Impression smears can be made for cytological examination. Specimens taken with biopsy forceps may be distorted and difficult for the pathologist to interpret. Mucosal suction biopsy capsules give larger, better-oriented specimens. For optimum results, multiple specimens are submitted for histological evaluation.

An uncommon complication of colonic biopsy is perforation of the colon. Positive contrast radiographic studies should not be performed for two weeks after colonic biopsy in order to avoid perforation of the biopsy site due to increased pressure (Fig. 52–6). Insufflation of air into the colon during proctoscopy creates negative contrast, and radiographs taken at this time may demonstrate lesions beyond the range of a rigid proctoscope.

Radiographic Examination of the Colon

Radiographic evaluation of the colon can aid diagnosis of impaction, perforation, tumor, stricture, and intussusception. Survey radiographs of the colon are difficult to interpret unless the colon is free of fecal material. Food is withheld for 24 hours and a mild enema is given the night before and again one or two hours before radiographic evaluation.

Barium sulfate is used for most positive contrast studies but should not be used if a perforation is suspected. A Foley balloon catheter is inserted into the rectum and inflated. Commercially available barium sulfate, 30 per cent w/w suspension diluted to 10 per cent w/w with water, is infused at 20 to 30 ml/kg for dogs and 10 to 20 ml/kg for cats.[62] Lateral and ventrodorsal radiographs are taken after half of the barium is infused and again when the infusion is complete. The colonic mucosa can be better evaluated with a double-contrast barium enema. Air (22 ml/kg) is insufflated into the colon through a balloon catheter after most of the barium has been allowed to flow out. The remaining barium coats the mucosal surface, contrasting with the insufflated air.

BOWEL PREPARATION FOR COLORECTAL SURGERY

Proper patient preparation for colorectal surgery is important to decrease operative contamination. Mechanical emptying and cleansing of the large intestine and the use of antimicrobial agents significantly reduce the numbers of microorganisms present.

In elective surgery, this process should be started approximately three days prior to surgery. On the third and second days before the procedure, the animal is given a low-residue diet of hamburger and white rice. On the day before food is withheld and

an enema is given. On the day of surgery, abdominal radiographs are taken and examined for feces in the colon. A nonirritating enema such as normal saline is given if feces are present.

Although use of antimicrobial agents continues to be controversial, there seems to be general agreement that antibiotics reduce the risk of infection in large bowel surgery.[15] In humans, infection in colonic surgery can be reduced from 36 to 22 per cent and the mortality rate from 11.2 to 4.5 per cent by the use of antibiotics.[4] The controversy involves the route of administration, how long antibiotics should be given, and what antibiotics should be used.

Nonabsorbable antibiotics can be given orally, or antibiotics can be administered systemically so that blood and tissue concentrations are achieved. Antibiotics can also be administered both orally and systemically. Authors have questioned the value and safety of oral nonabsorbable broad-spectrum antibiotics; if infections develop after their use, the responsible organisms can be highly resistant to antibiotic therapy. Several complications have been reported in humans. These include staphylococcal enterocolitis, pseudomembraneous colitis, and infection caused by opportunistic organisms.[3, 13] Intravenous cephalothin alone is not adequate (infection rate of 39 per cent) compared with oral neomycin and erythromycin or with oral neomycin and erythromycin plus intravenous cephalothin (infection rates of 6 per cent in both groups).[16] On the other hand, intravenous metronidazole may be as effective as orally administered metronidazole;[22] in this case, however, the oral drug is absorbable and systemic levels are obtained from oral administration.

Systemic antibiotics are not beneficial when given in addition to mechanical intestinal cleansing plus oral nonabsorbable and topical antibiotics at surgery.[43] However, one study has shown the incidence of wound infection to be six per cent in patients given systemic cefazolin in addition to oral neomycin and erythromycin, compared with 16 per cent in those given oral neomycin and erythromycin alone.[59]

There is evidence that more than one day of antibiotic prophylaxis is not needed. In one trial of tinidazole and doxycycline in humans,[29] infectious complications occurred in 5.1 per cent of the group receiving one dose of antibiotics, and prolongation of antibiotic administration for five days longer did not reduce the rate of complications.[29] There is strong evidence that prophylactic antibiotics must be administered before bacterial contamination of tissue occurs. In general, antibiotics are started two hours before surgery, and a blood level is maintained for 24 hours after surgery.[9, 29, 59]

Some Common Prophylactic Combinations

Emergency Surgery With No Time for Preoperative Preparation

A cleansing enema should be given if the bowel is not ruptured. At surgery, the surgical site should be regarded as an accidental wound that is heavily contaminated. It should be draped carefully and irrigated repeatedly with saline or an antibiotic solution. A satisfactory antibiotic combination is triple-antibiotic solution containing polymyxin, neomycin, and bacitracin. Systemic antibiotics should be given intravenously before operation, and a blood level should be maintained for 24 hours. The antibiotic should be a broad-spectrum type such as an aminoglycoside. If surgery is delayed so that proliferation of and invasion by bacteria occur, systemic antibiotics should be continued for four to five days.

Elective Surgery When the Large Intestine Cannot Be Emptied

This situation occurs in obstruction caused by constipation or a reduction in size of the lumen. A cleansing enema cannot be given. There is probably no value in preoperative oral administration of antibiotics because they do not pass to the obstructed site. Antibiotic use and wound management are the same as for emergency procedures.

Routine Elective Procedures

There is no doubt about the value of emptying and cleaning the bowel. The three-day regimen described previously is followed, to decrease the total fecal mass with a corresponding, nonselective reduction of colonic and rectal bacteria. There also seems to be no doubt about the value of prophylactic oral antibiotics. A mixture effective against aerobes and anaerobes is needed. Recommended combinations include an aminoglycoside combined with drugs active against anaerobes, such as neomycin plus erythromycin or neomycin plus bacitracin.[14] The combination is given three times on the day prior to surgery. Tetracycline, lincomycin, and metronidazole are also used in combination with an aminoglycoside such as neomycin.[32, 46, 47] Although metronidazole is effective with an aminoglycoside, the marginally increased risk of hepatic toxicity and mutagenesis associated with its administration should be kept in mind.

The significance of systemic antibiotics is not known. The common recommendation for humans is to give a cephalosporin intravenously before surgery and to maintain a blood level for 24 hours. Among human surgeons in the United States, the most common method is the combination of both oral and parenteral antibiotics. The parenteral antibiotic of choice is cephalothin. The oral antibiotics of choice are an oral aminoglycoside (neomycin, kanamycin, or paromomycin) in combination with erythromycin.[16] The surgical wound is irrigated with saline containing antibiotics. Extensive draping is used, and the surgical site is drained, especially if it is retroperitoneal near the rectum.

Minor Procedures in the Rectum and Colon

A minor surgical procedure is required to remove polyps with a small base. The surgical excision does not extend into the submucosa. In these instances, preoperative preparation is minor and includes only emptying and cleaning the large intestine. Antibiotics in any form are probably not justified.

HEALING AND SUTURE METHODS

Many studies have shown that the early phase of healing of colonic and rectal anastomoses is characterized by lysis of mature collagen and loss of tensile strength in the colon or rectum. This finding has influenced methods of suturing and led to concern about the large intestine's ability to withstand stress after surgery.[17, 18, 31]

This concept has been challenged and recent investigations have shown that collagenolysis is not as marked as originally proposed. In a study in 1974, Irvin and Hunt[36] showed that lysis of polymerized tissue collagen does occur during the first three days of healing. However, the actual reduction is variable and of smaller magnitude than previously suggested. In addition, the early phase of healing is not characterized by loss of intestinal strength.[36] More recent work showed that both lysis and synthesis of collagen occur in the entire colon after wounding and that lysis exceeds synthesis for the first three to four days.[37] This is not a surprising finding in light of the inflammation and tissue destruction that occur early in wound healing, followed by fibroblastic activity. Continuous suture patterns appear to lead to a more marked disturbance in the balance between lysis and synthesis and to retarded restoration of collagen concentration.[37] In addition, infection in the wound leads to increased collagenase activity, so that the net amount of collagen in the wound—the resultant amount of residual collagen plus new collagen—can be low for longer than three to four days.

A tight suture can cause increased collagen lysis and delayed collagen production, leading to local ischemia, fewer inflammatory cells, and delayed fibroblastic activity. Collagenolysis occurs because of the presence of collagenase in many large bowel organisms.

In summary, the three most important factors in suturing the colon and rectum are: (1) to avoid continuous suture patterns, (2) to minimize infection, and (3) to ensure adequate blood supply to the healing edge of the incision by avoiding tight sutures.

The selection of the best suture pattern depends on many factors, and there is insufficient evidence to identify the ideal technique. Common patterns in veterinary surgery include inverted patterns such as Connell sutures and interrupted or continuous Lembert sutures.[48] A single-layer anastomosis using interrupted sutures was compared with a two-layer inverting closure.[26] There was no difference in the incidence of wound breakdown cranial to the peritoneal reflection. Caudal to the peritoneum in the rectum, there was a greater incidence of dehiscence with the two-layer closure than with the single-layer closure.[26] These results could be explained by interference with blood supply by the two-layer inverting pattern and difficulty in placing two layers in the pelvic canal. No differences have been found between end-to-end interrupted crushing sutures and interrupted end-to-end inverting sutures in the colon of the dog.[50] Loss of lumen diameter at the anastomotic site with inverting sutures was 63 per cent, compared with 30 per cent with the crushing sutures. However, there did not appear to be any clinical difference between the two groups.

The choice of suture pattern may not be as important as the technique of inserting the sutures, particularly ensuring adequate blood supply to the healing edges. In areas that are difficult to reach, a single interrupted suture through all layers is recommended. Sutures are not tightly placed, and an absorbable material is used. In more accessible areas, and particularly when any tension is present at the suture line, two layers of simple interrupted sutures are recommended. The first sutures are placed through the mucosa and submucosa and the knots are in the lumen. In the second row, the sutures are placed through the serosa (if present), all muscle layers, and, again, the submucosa. Knots are on the outside of the rectal wall. The use of two suture rows is particularly recommended for suturing the end of the rectum to the anus or to the skin when a section of rectum is removed. In this situation there is tension at the anastomotic site. An absorbable material, either chromic surgical gut or a synthetic absorbable material, is used in all situations except for suturing rectal mucosa to skin when monofilament nylon is preferred.

A rubber drain sutured to the site of a colonic anastomosis can prevent the sealing of an anastomotic leak; four of 20 dogs in one study developed diffuse peritonitis due to dehiscence of the suture line.[6] In rats, silicone rubber, PVC, and Teflon do not interfere with healing of a colonic anastomosis; however, latex can lead to significant increase in anastomotic leakage.[56] If the extent of adjacent tissue damage indicates the need for drainage of the area, a Silastic rubber drain should be used; the drain should be placed at least 0.5 cms away from the suture line and should be removed as soon as possible, usually in two to three days.

Although Silastic rubber drains may drain a local anastomotic site adequately, they are not effective for general abdominal drainage. In severe peritoneal contamination in humans, the use of delayed primary closure for general abdominal drainage is beneficial.[23, 51, 57] This technique is currently under investigation by several veterinary surgeons. In humans, the ventral fascia is loosely closed with nonabsorbable suture material such as nylon or polypropylene in a continuous pattern. The subcutaneous tissues and skin are left open and packed with antibiotic ointment and sterile sponges, and the abdomen is wrapped to protect the site. The dressings are changed daily, and the abdomen is closed under general anesthesia

once the infection has been controlled and the patient is stable. Complications associated with this procedure in humans include evisceration, fluid and protein loss, and prolonged hospitalization.[23]

SURGICAL TECHNIQUES

Colotomy

A ventral midline incision is made from umbilicus to pubis. The colon is packed off with saline-soaked laparotomy pads to prevent contamination. Balfour or Gossett self-retaining retractors are used for better exposure. With impaction or foreign body, an incision is made on the antimesenteric border. With biopsy, tumor removal, or perforation, an elliptical incision is made. The colon is closed in one or two layers as previously described. If a large elliptical incision has been made, longitudinal closure may produce narrowing of the lumen. The defect can be closed transversely to preserve normal diameter (Figs. 52–7 and 52–8). The abdomen is lavaged with warm saline or antibiotics. Gloves and instruments are changed prior to routine abdominal closure.

Resection and Anastomosis

The colon is exposed by ventral midline abdominal incision. The branches of the colic artery that supply the diseased colon are ligated and divided. Carmalt forceps are placed across the colon at the transection sites. The colonic contents are "milked" away from the forceps for three to five centimeters, and noncrushing Doyen intestinal forceps are applied. The colon is transected with a scalpel between the crush-

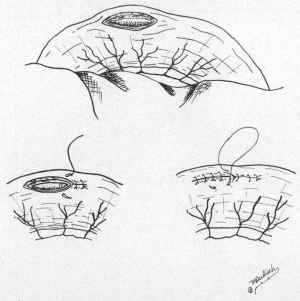

Figure 52–7. Longitudinal closure of the colon using a row of simple interrupted sutures through all layers and a second, reinforcing row of Cushing sutures.

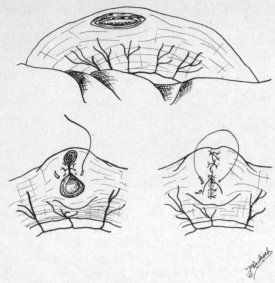

Figure 52–8. When an elliptical segment of colonic wall is removed, a standard longitudinal closure may cause excessive narrowing of the lumen. A transverse closure ensures adequate lumen size.

ing and noncrushing forceps along the edge of the crushing forceps. The resected section of colon with the two crushing forceps is set aside for later examination. If the ileocecocolic junction is removed, the

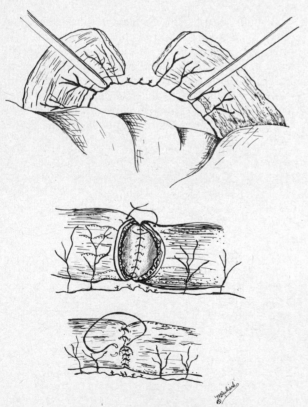

Figure 52–9. Anastomosis of the colon using a row of simple interrupted sutures through all layers and a second, reinforcing row of Cushing sutures. An alternate technique is to place a first layer of simple interrupted sutures through the mucosa and submucosa with the knots tied in the lumen. A second layer of simple interrupted sutures is placed through the serosa, muscularis, and submucosa.

disparity in size between the colon and the small intestine must be considered. It is overcome by cutting the antimesenteric border of the small intestine to the point where the lumens are of equal size. The bulging mucosa is trimmed prior to anastomosis. An alternative method is to cut the small intestine on an angle to expose a larger lumen. A one- or two-layer suture pattern as described for colotomy is used (Fig. 52–9). Suturing is started at the mesenteric border, and the intestine is turned 180 degrees when the antimesenteric border is reached. Suturing is continued from the mesenteric border until the anastomosis is complete. The mesocolon is closed with single interrupted absorbable sutures, blood vessels being avoided. The anastomotic site is examined critically for patency and leaks. The colon and abdomen are lavaged, and the abdomen is closed.

Typhlectomy

The cecum can be removed at its attachment to the colon, or the entire ileocecocolic junction may be removed and the small intestine anastomosed to the colon. The cecocolic opening is located about one centimeter from the ileocolic opening in the dog. The body of the cecum is attached to the terminal ileum by the ileocecal fold consisting of fascia and peritoneum. The cecum gets its blood supply from the ileocecal branch of the ileocecocolic artery. The ileocecal artery passes through the ileocecal fold, sending out ileal and cecal branches, and anastomoses to the last jejunal artery. To remove the cecum, the ileocecal fold is cut and the cecum is dissected from its attachment to the ileum (Fig. 52–10). The ileocecal artery is preserved and the cecal branches are ligated. The small accessory ileocecal fold, extending from the base of the cecum to the proximal colon, is also incised. When the cecum is free of its attachments and blood supply, two Carmalt forceps are placed across its base, and the cecum is amputated by cutting between the two forceps with a scalpel. The remaining forcep is oversewn with 2-0 or 3-0 absorbable suture material in a Parker-Kerr inversion technique. A second layer of continuous Cushing or Lembert sutures is placed.

When the cecum is inverted into the colon, manual reduction may not be possible owing to adhesions. A colotomy is performed, the adhesions are broken down, and the cecum is everted and amputated; if this maneuver is not possible, resection of the ileocecocolic junction may be necessary.

Pull-Through Colonic Resection

A pull-through resection of the colon is indicated in any situation in which an anastomosis has to be made in the pelvic canal, e.g., distal colonic mass lesions, intussusception, and congenital megacolon.

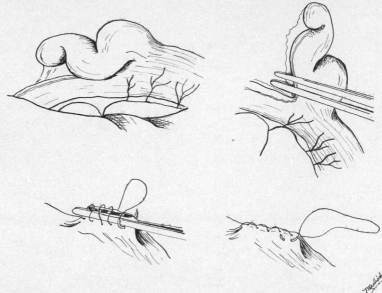

Figure 52–10. To perform a typhlectomy, the cecum is dissected from its attachments to the ilium by blunt incision of the ileocecal fold. The base of the cecum is isolated and double-clamped with intestinal forceps. The cecum is amputated by cutting between the forceps, and a Parker-Kerr inversion is performed.

The patient is placed in dorsal recumbency with the perineal area at the end of the table. The hind legs are fully flexed and pulled cranially in a frog position to allow space to work in the perineal area. The abdominal and perineal areas are draped separately so that two surgeons can work simultaneously—one performing the abdominal phase of the operation and one performing the perineal phase. A separate instrument tray should be used for each phase, and gowns and gloves are changed when indicated.

An abdominal incision is made from the umbilicus to the cranial rim of the pubis. The colon is isolated, and the abdominal viscera are packed off with laparotomy pads. The entire colon and the regional lymph nodes are examined closely; biopsy specimens are taken if indicated. The arteries supplying the section of colon to be resected are identified, ligated, and divided. It may be necessary to ligate and divide the caudal mesenteric artery. The dissection is carried bluntly into the pelvic canal using the fingers to separate the rectal wall from its attachments for 360 degrees circumferentially. The attachments are broken down as close to the rectal wall as possible to prevent damage to parasympathetic nerve fibers. The dissection can be performed to the internal anal sphincter if indicated.

The section of intestine to be removed is isolated, and paired intestinal clamps are placed proximally and distally. The bowel is transected between the paired clamps, and the isolated segment is removed. The proximal and distal cut ends are inverted with 0 or 2-0 silk or nylon in a Parker-Kerr inversion or Lembert pattern, leaving the suture ends five centimeters long. The ends of suture material from the proximal and distal segments are tied together (Fig. 52–11).

At this point, the second surgeon, using another instrument tray, inserts Allis tissue forceps through the anus and into the rectum and grasps the inverted edge of the distal stump. The forceps are withdrawn slowly, everting the rectum through the anus. The everted rectum is transected 180 degrees dorsally at a point two to three centimeters from the anus to expose the suture material attached to the proximal segment. The proximal segment is pulled through the anus to the level of the transected rectum. The surgeon working in the abdomen guides the proximal segment through the anus to ensure that the intestine is not twisted and tension is minimal. If there is tension at the anastomotic site, further dissection of the mesocolon is indicated. Once it is established that the anastomosis can be safely made, the abdomen can be closed by the abdominal surgeon while the perineal surgeon performs the anastomosis.

The anastomosis is begun by suturing the muscular coat of the rectum to the seromuscular coat of the colon. As these sutures are tied, the distal segment is transected further, and suturing is continued until the seromuscular coats are united 360 degrees around the circumference and the distal segment is fully detached. Some sutures can be left long for traction and orientation. The proximal segment is now transected 360 degrees at a distance one to two millimeters distal to the completed seromuscular suture line. The inverted sections of both proximal and distal segments with the connecting suture material are now free and can be laid aside. The mucosa-submucosa layer of the proximal segment is sutured to the mucosa-submucosa layer of the distal segment. The type of suture material used is at the discretion of the surgeon, but it is recommended that a simple interrupted pattern be used in both layers. After suturing is complete and stay sutures are transected, the anastomosis is gently returned to the abdomen through the anal canal. If a mass lesion has been resected, the detached proximal and distal segments should be submitted to a veterinary pathologist.

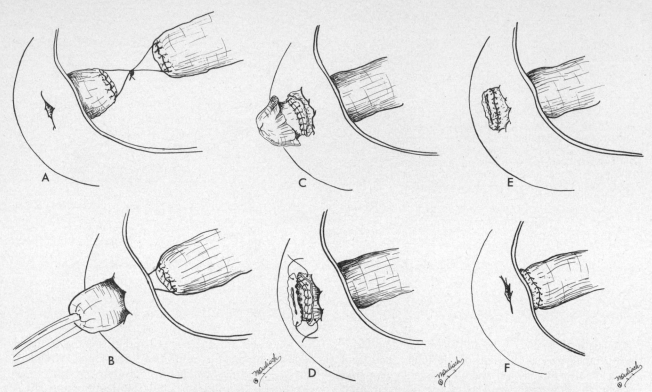

Figure 52–11. A, A Parker-Kerr inversion of the proximal (colonic) and distal (rectal) segments has been completed and the ends of the suture material tied together. B, The distal segment has been inverted with Allis tissue forceps. The proximal segment is drawn through the anus. C, The inverted distal segment to be removed has been detached 360 degrees from the colon, and the seromuscular suture line has been completed. The inverted proximal segment to be removed can now be incised 360 degrees, and both segments, with the attached suture material, can be set aside. D, The mucosa-submucosa layers of both colon and rectum are sutured. E, Suturing is completed. F, The anastomosis has been returned to the abdomen.

POSTOPERATIVE CONSIDERATIONS

The patient is closely observed in the immediate postoperative period. An intravenous catheter is kept in place for the first 24 hours for fluid maintenance. If the animal can hold down water, small amounts of low-residue, easily digestable foods are offered. The patient can be discharged once a normal bowel movement is produced. The most serious complication is peritonitis, which may result from contamination during the surgical procedure or from leakage at the surgical site.

1. Adams, G. B.: Eversion of the cecum of a dog. Southwest Vet. 7:46, 1953.
2. Alexander, J. W., and Carb, A. V.: Subtotal hemipelvectomy in the dog. J. Vet. Orthop. 1:9, 1979.
3. Altemeier, W. A., Hummel, R. P., and Hill, E. O.: The clinical application of antimicrobial treatment in surgery of the colon. In Turrel, R., (ed.): *Diseases of the Colon and Anorectum.* 2nd ed. W. B. Saunders, Philadelphia, 1969.
4. Baum, M. L., Anish, D. S., Chalmers, T. C., et al.: A survey of clinical trials of antibiotic prophylaxis in colon surgery: evidence against further use of no-treatment controls. New Engl. J. Med. 305:795, 1981.
5. Bellah, J. R.: Colonic perforation after corticosteroid and surgical treatment of intervertebral disc disease in a dog. J. Am. Vet. Med. Assoc. 183:1002, 1983.
6. Berliner, S. D., Burson, L. C., and Lear, P. E.: Use and abuse of intraperitoneal drains in colon surgery. Arch. Surg. 89:686, 1964.
7. Bjorling, D. E., Crowe, D. T., Kolata, R. J., and Rawlings, C A.: Penetrating abdominal wounds in dogs and cats. J. Am. Anim. Hosp. Assoc. 18:742, 1982.
8. Botte, R. J., and Rosin, E.: Cytology of peritoneal effusion following intestinal anastomosis and experimental peritonitis. Vet. Surg. 12:20, 1983.
9. Burke, J. F.: The effective period of preventive antibiotic action in experimental incisions and dermal lesions. Surgery 50:161, 1961.
10. Burrows, C. F.: Diarrhea and constipation. In Ettinger, S. J. (ed.): *Textbook of Veterinary Internal Medicine.* 2nd ed. W. B. Saunders, Philadelphia, 1983.
11. Cannon, W. B.: The movements of the intestines studied by means of the roentgen rays. Am. J. Physiol. 6:251, 1902.
12. Christensen, J.: Myoelectric control of the colon. Gastroenterology 68:601, 1975.
13. Clark, C. E., Powis, S. J., Crapp, A. R., et al.: Antibiotic induced pseudomembraneous colitis. Gut 16:824, 1975.
14. Clarke, J. S., Condon, R. E., Bartlett, J. G., et al.: Preoperative oral antibiotics reduce septic complications of colon operations. Ann. Surg. 186:251, 1977.
15. Condon, R. E.: Bowel preparation for colorectal operations. Arch. Surg. 117:265, 1982.
16. Condon, R. E., Bartlett, J. G., Nichols, R. L., et al.: Preoperative prophylactic cephalothin fails to control septic complications of colorectal operations: results of controlled clinical trial. Am. J. Surg. 137:68, 1979.
17. Cronin, K., Jackson, D. S., and Sunphy, J. E.: Changing bursting strength and collagen content of the healing colon. Surg. Gynecol. Obstet. 126:747, 1968.
18. Cronin, K., Jackson, D. S., and Dunphy, J. E.: Specific activity of hydroxyprolinetritium in the healing colon. Surg. Gynecol. Obstet. 126:1061, 1968.
19. Crowe, D. T., and Crane, S W.: Diagnostic abdominal para-

centesis and lavage in the evaluation of abdominal injuries in dogs and cats: clinical and experimental investigations. J. Am. Vet. Med. Assoc. *168*:700, 1976.

20. Davidson, M.: Megacolon in children. *In* Sleisenger, M. H., and Fordtran, J. S. (eds.): *Gastrointestinal Disease.* 2nd ed. W. B. Saunders, Philadelphia, 1978.

21. Diethelm, A. G.: Surgical management of complications of steroid therapy. Ann. Surg. *185*:251, 1977.

22. Dion, Y. M., Richards, G. K., Prentis, J. J., and Hinchey, J. E.: The influence of oral versus parenteral preoperative metronidazole on sepsis following colon surgery. Ann. Surg. *192*:221, 1980.

23. Duff, J. H., and Moffat, J.: Abdominal sepsis managed by leaving abdomen open. Surgery *90*:774, 1981.

24. Edmonds, C. J.: Water and ionic transfer pathways of mammalian large intestine. Clin. Sci. *61*:257, 1981.

25. Ehrenpreis, T.: *Hirschsprung's Disease.* Year Book Medical Publishers, Chicago, 1970.

26. Everett, W. G.: A comparison of one layer and two layer techniques for colorectal anastomosis. Br. J. Surg. *62*:135, 1975.

27. Fellenbaum, S.: Partial colectomy in the treatment of recurrent obstipation/megacolon in the cat. Vet. Med./Small Anim. Clin. *73*:737, 1978.

28. Follen, W. D., Hunt, J., and Altemeier, W. A.: Prophylactic antibiotics in penetrating wounds of the abdomen. J. Trauma *12*:282, 1972.

29. Giercksky, K. E., Danielsen, S., Garberg, O., et al.: A single dose tinidazole and doxycycline prophylaxis in elective surgery of colon and rectum; a prospective controlled clinical multicenter study. Ann. Surg. *195*:227, 1982.

30. Guffy, M. M., Wallace, L., and Anderson, N. V.: Inversion of the cecum into the colon of a dog. J. Am. Vet. Med. Assoc. *156*:183, 1970.

31. Hawley, P. R.: Causes and prevention of colonic anastomotic breakdown. Dis. Colon Rectum *16*:272, 1973.

32. Herter, F. P.: Preparation of the bowel for surgery. Surg. Clin. North Am. 52:859, 1972.

33. Hill, F. W. G., and Hird, J. F. R.: The problem of diarrhoea. *In* Yoxall, A. T., and Hird, J. F. R. (eds.): *Physiological Basis of Small Animal Practice.* Blackwell Scientific Publications, Oxford, 1980.

34. Hoerlein, B. F., and Spano, J. S.: Non-neurological complications following decompressive spinal surgery. Arch. Am. Coll. Vet. Surg. *4*:11, 1975.

35. Hunt, C. A.: Diagnostic peritoneal paracentesis and lavage. Comp. Cont. Ed. *2*:449, 1980.

36. Irvin, T. T., and Hunt, T. K.: Reappraisal of the healing process of anastomosis of the colon. Surg. Gynecol. Obstet. *138*:741, 1974.

37. Jiborn, H., Ahonen, J., and Zederfeldt, B.: Healing of experimental colonic anastomoses. IV: Effect of suture technique on collagen metabolism in the colonic wall. Am. J. Surg. *139*:406, 1980.

38. Lane, R. H. S., and Todd, I. P.: Idiopathic megacolon: a review of 42 cases. Br. J. Surg. *64*:305, 1977.

39. Leape, L. L., and Holder, T. M.: Pediatric surgery. *In* Sabiston, D. C. (ed.): *Davis-Christopher Textbook of Surgery.* 12th ed. W. B. Saunders, Philadelphia, 1981.

40. Le Roux, P. H.: Dilatation of the cecum in dogs. J. S. Afr. Vet. Med. Assoc. *33*:73, 1962.

41. Lorenz, M. D.: Diseases of the large bowel. *In* Ettinger, S. J. (ed.): *Textbook of Veterinary Internal Medicine.* 2nd ed. W. B. Saunders, Philadelphia, 1983.

42. McCready, R. A., and Beart, R. W.: The surgical treatment of incapacitating constipation associated with idiopathic megacolon. Mayo Clin. Proc. *54*:779, 1979.

43. Mehigan, D., Zuidema, G. D., and Cameron, J. L.: The role of systemic antibiotics in operations upon the colon. Surg. Gynecol. Obstet. *153*:573, 1981.

44. Menguy, R., and Masters, Y. F.: Effect of cortisone on mucoprotein secretion by the gastric antrum of dogs: pathogenesis of steroid ulcer. Surgery *54*:19, 1963.

45. Miles, A. A., Miles, E. M., and Burke, J.: The value and duration of defense reactions of the skin to the primary lodgement of bacteria. Br. J. Exp. Pathol. *38*:79, 1957.

46. Nichols, R. L., Broido, P., Condon, R. E., et al.: Effect of preoperative neomycin-erythromycin intestinal preparation on the incidence of infectious complications following colon surgery. Ann. Surg. *178*:453, 1973.

47. Nichols, R. L., and Condon, R. E.: Preoperative preparation of the colon. Surg. Gynecol. Obstet. *132*:323, 1971.

48. Palmenteri, A.: Rectal disease and surgery of dogs. Proc. Am. Anim. Hosp. Assoc. 492–499, 1969.

49. Raffensperger, J. G.: Hirschsprung's disease. *In* Bockus, H. L. (ed.): *Gastroenterology.* 3rd ed. Vol. 2. W. B. Saunders, Philadelphia, 1976.

50. Richardson, D. C., Duckett, K. E., Krahwinkel, D. J., Jr., and Shipman, L. W.: Colonic anastomosis: evaluation of an end-to-end crushing and inverting technique. Am. J. Vet. Res. *43*:436, 1982.

51. Richardson, J. D., and Polk, H. C.: Newer adjunctive treatments for peritonitis (editorial). Surgery *90*:917, 1981.

52. Schaer, M., Cavanagh, P., Hause, W., and Wilkins, R.: Iatrogenic hyperphosphatemia, hypocalcemia and hypernatremia in a cat. J. Am. Anim. Hosp. Assoc. *13*:39, 1977.

53. Schlotthauer, C. F.: Inverted cecum in a dog. J. Am. Vet. Med. Assoc. *125*:123, 1954.

54. Schuster, M. M.: Megacolon in adults. *In* Sleisenger, M. H., and Fordtran, J. S. (eds.): *Gastrointestinal Disease.* 2nd ed. W. B. Saunders, Philadelphia, 1978.

55. Schuster, M. M.: Motor action of rectum and anal sphincters in continence and defecation. *In* Code, C. F., and Heidel, W. (eds.): *Handbook of Physiology.* Sec. 6, Vol. 4. American Physiological Society, Washington, D.C., 1968.

56. Smith, S. R. G., Connolly, J. C., Crane, P. W., and Gilmore, O. J. A.: The effect of surgical drainage materials on colonic healing. Br. J. Surg. *69*:153, 1982.

57. Steinberg, D.: On leaving the peritoneal cavity open in acute generalized suppurative peritonitis. Am. J. Surg. *137*:216, 1979.

58. Stockman, V., and Stockman, J. R.: Cecal impaction in the dog. Vet. Rec. 73:337, 1961.

59. Stone, H. H., Hooper, C. A., Kolb, L. D., et al.: Antibiotic prophylaxis in gastric biliary and colonic surgery. Ann. Surg. *184*:443, 1976.

60. Swenson, O., Sherman, J. O., Fisher, J. H., and Cotten, E.: The treatment and postoperative complications of congenital megacolon: a 25 year follow up. Ann. Surg. *182*:266, 1975.

61. Templeton, R. D., and Lawson, H.: Studies in the motor activity of the large intestine. I: Normal motility in the dog, recorded by the tandem balloon method. Am. J. Physiol. 96:667, 1931.

62. Thrall, D. E.: Gastrointestinal radiology. *In* Anderson, N. V. (ed.): *Veterinary Gastroenterology.* Lea & Febiger, Philadelphia, 1980.

63. Toombs, J. P., Caywood, D. D., Lipowitz, A. J., and Stevens, J. B.: Colonic perforation following neurosurgical procedures and corticosteroid therapy in 4 dogs. J. Am. Vet. Med. Assoc. *177*:68, 1980.

64. Warshaw, A. L., Welch, J. P., and Ottinger, L. W.: Acute perforation of the colon associated with chronic corticosteroid therapy. Am. J. Surg. *131*:442, 1976.

65. Yoder, J. T., Dragstedt, L. R., and Starch, C. J.: Partial colectomy for correction of megacolon in a cat. Vet. Med./Small Anim. Clin. *63*:1049, 1968.

53 Rectum and Anus

Anatomy

John Grandage

Although the rectum and anus are confluent, their differing embryological origins account for substantial differences in structure, innervation, blood supply, and lymphatic drainage.

The rectum is the part of the large intestine that lies within the pelvis. Its origin is often marked by a slight constriction where the circular muscle is thicker and resembles a sphincter.[53] It runs as far as the third caudal vertebra, where it is continuous with the anal canal, a short tube that typically opens beneath the fourth caudal vertebra. The terminal part of the dog's rectum is sometimes slightly dilated to form a rectal ampulla,[44] which is absent in cats. Most of the rectum lies within the peritoneal cavity,[4] although a short segment some two centimeters long continues retroperitoneally before it joins the anal canal.[4] The line of peritoneal reflection is located beneath the second caudal vertebra in the dog and a little further back in the cat; it slopes forward so that much of the ventral surface of the rectum lies retroperitoneally.[8]

STRUCTURE

The rectum is distinguished from the anal canal by the epithelial lining. Columnar epithelium of the rectal mucosa changes to stratified squamous epithelium at the anorectal line. This line marks the site of the cloacal membrane that separated the endoderm from the ectoderm in the embryo; a cloacal membrane of variable thickness is retained in animals with imperforate anus. The rectal mucosa contains large numbers of solitary lymph nodules in both the dog and cat.[15, 24] When the rectum is empty, its mucosa is thrown into a few longitudinal folds that unfold as the organ fills.

The anal canal begins at the anorectal line and is divided into three short segments, a columnar zone, an intermediate zone, and a cutaneous zone (Fig. 53–1). The mucous membrane of the columnar zone is thrown up into about ten short longitudinal folds that do not unfold under modest stretching. These are the anal columns (of Morgagni), which are more conspicuous in the dog than the cat;[62] caudally they loop round to meet each other as the anal valves (of Ball), each loop enclosing a tiny pocket called an anal sinus. The ring of anal valves forms the dentate or pectinate line that marks the caudal limit of this deepest part of the anus. The submucosa of the columnar zone is rich in anal glands (modified tubuloalveolar sweat glands), which may contain tiny, amber-colored beads of lipid secretion.[4, 62] The intermediate zone is a narrow and ill-defined area that lies between the pectinate and anocutaneous lines; it, too, is anointed with anal gland secretion.

The cutaneous zone of the anal canal is distinguished by its keratinized epithelium; it makes up most of the anal region and is further subdivided into an inner, moist zone a few millimeters long that completes the anal canal, and an outer zone that is exposed and relatively hairless, forming the visible disc that advertises the anus. Both zones are rich in glands—true anal glands (i.e., modified sweat glands) present within the inner part and circumanal glands in the outer part. The circumanal glands (perianal, hepatoid glands)[23] are a curious form of sebaceous gland consisting of two distinct parts. A typical se-

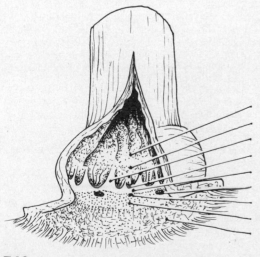

rectum
anorectal line
anal columns
anal sinuses
intermediate zone
opening of anal sac
anocutaneous line
inner cutaneous zone
outer cutaneous zone

Figure 53–1. Some features of the canine anal canal.

baceous part opens through a patent duct into a hair follicle, and a deeper, nonsebaceous part is composed of solid masses of cells filled with proteinaceous material that communicate with the sebaceous portion through solid strands of epithelioid cells.[10] Cells of the nonsebaceous part probably have the potential to transform into true sebaceous cells. Circumanal glands continue to grow throughout life in male dogs,[15] probably accounting for the conspicuous anus of the old dog.

The anal sacs (strictly the paranal sinuses) are paired globular invaginations of the inner cutaneous zone. Their walls are lined with keratinized epithelium and wrapped in a blanket of glandular tissue supported in a connective tissue stroma rich in diffuse lymphoid tissue.[37] The glands of the anal sacs are mostly large, coiled, apocrine, sudoriporous tubules,[15] although in the cat they also include conspicuous spherical sebaceous gland complexes, about three to four millimeters in diameter and partly embedded in the wall.[10, 19, 29] Desquamated epithelial cells plus bacteria and the secretions of these glands are stored in the sacs.[17] The foul-smelling serous or pasty product is discharged at varying stages of defecation in the dog.[4] The anal sacs are located ventrolateral to the anus (at four and eight o'clock); they are typically eight to ten millimeters in diameter and partly collapsed, and they lie sandwiched between the pale internal and the redder external anal sphincters. The single excretory duct for each sac runs a few millimeters and opens at the lateral angle of the anus, usually just out of sight, through an aperture one to two millimeters wide. The apocrine glands within the sac wall liberate most of the proteins and inorganic substances; in addition, there are sebaceous glands within the excretory duct that liberate the lipid (holocrine secretion).[37] The rate of secretion from apocrine and sebaceous glands is surprisingly slow—about 0.1 ml/day or less in dogs.[12]

MUSCLES

The muscle tunics of the rectum are continuous with those of the anal canal. An inner circular layer becomes slightly thickened terminally to form the internal anal sphincter. This lean, smooth muscle sphincter is of questionable significance in fecal continence;[4] it extends slightly more caudally than the external sphincter,[15] from which it is separated by fascia containing fat and the anal sacs. The anus is surrounded by another smooth muscle slip, the anal part of the retractor penis (or retractor clitoridis) muscle; this muscle arises from the first coccygeal vertebra, and most of it terminates at the anal sac.[15] The relatively thick, outer, longitudinal layer of smooth muscle over the rectum fades out at the anal canal. Paired slips detach from the dorsolateral part of this muscle and run to the fifth and sixth tail vertebrae as the rectococcygeus muscles;[4] these muscles probably help evacuate the rectum by drawing

the rectum caudally as the tail is elevated; dogs and cats pump their tails up and down during defecation.

The external anal sphincter is composed of striated muscle and is much larger and thicker than the other components. It is composed of successive rings,[17, 44] which are not particularly easy to differentiate. The caudal or cutaneous part attaches to the skin and on contraction causes the glabrous part of the anal skin to become incorporated into the anal canal. The cranial division is itself partly subdivided into superficial and deep parts that overlie the anal sacs. Most fibers encircle the anus but a few fuse with the bulbospongiosus (or constrictor vulvae) muscle.[17]

RELATIONS

The cranial part of the rectum is suspended by a short mesorectum, about one centimeter long, that is continuous with the mesocolon. The mesorectum allows the limited movement within the restricted space of the pelvis necessary for defecation, whelping, and so on, and is useful during digital exploration. Where the peritoneum reflects back from the rectum over the lateral walls of the pelvis, it creates a pair of pararectal fossae on either side of the rectum. These fossae are only potential spaces that are normally obliterated by fat pushing the pelvic walls medially. The rectum lies above the genital organs. In the male a rectovesical pouch is partly subdivided by a small genital fold carrying the deferent ducts. In the female the genital fold is much larger to accommodate the enclosed uterus and vagina; accordingly, the rectovesical pouch is totally subdivided into a rectogenital pouch above and a vesicogenital pouch below. The prostate and pelvic urethra are normally palpable per rectum in the dog and the cervix and vagina in the bitch. In male cats, the bulbourethral glands are also present and related to the rectum.

The retroperitoneal part of the rectum and the anal canal are supported by fat-laden connective tissue and by the muscles of the pelvic diaphragm. The pelvic diaphragm walls off the pelvic outlet and consists of a pair of muscles on each side, the coccygeus laterally and the levator ani medially. These, above all, are responsible for resisting raised intraabdominal pressure. Should they fail, atrophy, split, or stretch, pelvic and even abdominal viscera are in danger of being squeezed through. Both muscles course obliquely upward and backward from the pelvis to the tail, their principal insertion. Their intimate relation with the pelvic fascia on their deep surfaces and the perineal fascia on their superficial surfaces helps them support the pelvic outlet. The caudal border of the levator ani brushes past the external anal sphincter; it is apparently this site that is most vulnerable to perineal hernia. Frequently, much fat is present, tending to separate the muscles from the rectum.

The ischiorectal fossa is the hollow found above

the pelvis and at the sides of the root of the tail. It lies caudolateral to the pelvic diaphragm and dorsal to the internal obturator muscle that covers that part of the pelvic floor. Except in the leanest of animals this fossa is fat-filled, obliterating much of the fossa itself and tending to obscure the vessels and nerves that lie within it; it is therefore difficult to dissect.

VESSELS

The rectum is supplied mainly by the cranial rectal branch of the caudal mesenteric artery, a vessel that runs within the mesorectum. The retroperitoneal parts of the rectum and anal canal are supplied by a tiny middle artery and a larger caudal rectal artery, both ultimately derived from the internal pudendal artery. The internal pudendal is the largest artery in the ischiorectal fossa, although derivatives of the caudal gluteal artery are also present; numerous small perineal branches further complicate surgery of the region.

Companion veins follow the arteries; significant anastomoses occur between the cranial rectal veins, which drain into the portal system, and the caudal rectal veins, which drain into the caval system.[67]

Lymphatics from the anal skin drain into the superficial inguinal lymph nodes, but the deeper tissues of the anal canal and rectum drain into the large medial iliac lymph node beneath the fifth or sixth lumbar vertebra.[55]

INNERVATION

The rectum is innervated by autonomic nerves from the pelvic plexus. The plexus receives parasympathetic fibers via the pelvic nerves (S1 and S2) and sympathetic fibers via the hypogastrics.

The anus is innervated by the pudendal nerve, a somatic nerve that typically arises from S1, S2, and S3 and runs in the ischiorectal fossa with the internal pudendal vessels. Its caudal rectal branch (mainly from S2 and S3)[16] provides motor fibers to the external anal sphincter, and its perineal branch is sensory to the area.[15] Voluntary control of the external sphincter is lost in animals with spinal or other CNS lesions; such individuals may show fecal incontinence, but constipation is not usually a problem.[46] Apparently, dogs can tolerate unilateral severance of the caudal rectal nerves (as may occur in repair of perineal hernia) without becoming incontinent, but bilateral severence causes incontinence.[15]

The muscles of the pelvic diaphragm are supplied by short branches of sacral nerves (S1, S2, and S3)[16] that enter the dorsomedial borders of these muscles.[4]

Surgical Diseases

Dudley E. Johnston

RECTAL STRICTURES

Rectal strictures are usually associated with anorectal abscess, fistulae, or trauma. In addition, rectal carcinomas tend to involve the rectal wall in a circular manner, leading to severe stricture. Some circular strictures are found two to four centimeters from the anus with no associated perirectal lesion. Such strictures may represent an infection from a penetrating wound of the rectum or may be congenital. Severe stricture of the rectum is seen with perianal fistulae, especially in those dogs with associated proctitis and submucous fistulae in the rectum.

Clinical Signs

Signs are generally obvious, with straining, dyschezia, and constipation. Some animals have severe secondary megacolon with constipation. The stricture can be palpated digitally. Radiography can be used to document the condition but rarely yields more information than finger palpation.

Treatment

Simple circular strictures are treated by repeated bougienage, preferably using one or more lubricated fingers. In this way, the surgeon can feel the band become taut and eventually break, with no tearing of the mucosa. Corticosteroids are given during the healing period of two weeks.

Extensive strictures are excised like sessile rectal polyps. The rectum is incised through 360 degrees approximately one centimeter cranial to the anus. From this point, careful blunt dissection is used to mobilize the rectum until the fibrous ring is reached. The dissected rectum with the stenotic ring is excised. The rectum is sutured to the anus with one buried row of simple interrupted fine absorbable sutures in the submucosa and muscular layer, and one row in the submucosa and mucosa. In some dogs, it is possible to dissect the diseased tissue from the wall of the rectum and then resuture the rectum to the anus without resecting a portion of rectum.[47]

ANAL AND RECTAL PROLAPSE

Several conditions can be associated with prolapse of the anal canal and rectum. These conditions occur most frequently in young, unthrifty, parasitized animals that have diarrhea and tenesmus. The prolapse can occur after administration of parasitides, particularly those agents causing increased gut motility. This occurrence is now rarely seen. Rectal prolapse is commonly seen in association with rectal polyps when severe tenesmus leads to prolapse of the polyp and rectum. After unilateral, or more commonly bilateral, perineal hernia repair, especially when large lateral rectal sacculations are present, prolapse of anus or rectum can be troublesome.

Any prolapse can be a relatively mild condition, leading to local irritation only. In some dogs, the condition is intermittent and is seen for a varying time after defecation. With rectal prolapse, the prolapsed portion becomes increasingly swollen and eventually is traumatized or becomes necrotic.

Clinical Signs

With anal prolapse, a ring of swollen, red, prolapsed mucosa is readily seen. With rectal prolapse, the prolapsed mass is cylindrical and dimpled at the end, and its surface varies from uniform red mucosa to hemorrhagic areas, necrotic areas, and lacerations. The dog may not strain excessively, and the prolapsed mass is relatively insensitive.

Intussusception of the small intestine or colon must be distinguished from rectal prolapse. The prolapsed masses are similar in appearance. However, with an intussusception of colon or small intestine, a finger or long blunt lubricated probe can be passed between the rectal wall and the prolapsed mass. With prolapsed anus, a probe cannot be passed, and with a prolapsed rectum, the probe can be passed only a short distance.

Treatment

The first consideration in rectal prolapse is to determine whether an attempt should be made to reduce the prolapse or whether the prolapsed mass should be removed. The mass is amputated if it is severely lacerated, necrotic, rigid, and unable to be manipulated.

If it is decided to reduce the prolapse, its size is reduced by gentle manipulation and squeezing and is softened by soaking in warm saline solution. Classically, prolapses are treated with cold and hypertonic solutions, powders, or even crystals. Although no satisfactory experimental results are available, theoretical concepts and clinical trials support the use of warm solutions instead of cold ones, and isotonic solutions instead of hypertonic solutions. The mass is edematous and the surface mucosa is abraded. The warmth dilates blood vessels and allows edema to be removed by gentle manipulation. There is no evidence that hypertonic solutions can remove fluids from tissues through intact mucosal surfaces. The use of hypertonic solutions or substances such as alum or sugar can cause mucosal injury, which leads to increased swelling, irritation, and tenesmus.

After reduction of the prolapse, the animal should be given a narcotic agent or tranquilizer, and a purse-string suture can be inserted. Nonabsorbable suture material such as (0 to 2-0) nylon is used, and the suture should not penetrate into the anal sacs. It is possible to make a purse-string suture tight enough that the prolapse does not recur by increasing intra-abdominal pressure but still sufficiently loose to allow passage of soft feces. The animal is given a low-residue diet, such as hamburger and white rice, and Metamucil in the food. The purse-string suture can be removed in four to five days. Application of a topical corticosteroid cream to the anus and rectal mucosa may be helpful in reducing swelling, irritation, and straining. In all cases, the primary cause (parasitism, for example) should be determined and treated.

In mild to moderate rectal prolapse after perineal hernia repair, a purse-string suture should be inserted before the animal is allowed to recover from anesthesia. Some prolapses can occur during the struggling and straining associated with recovery from anesthesia. The loosely tied purse-string suture is left in place for four to five days. In massive rectal prolapse following perineal hernia repair, simple reduction is rarely adequate, and a decision should be made to amputate the prolapsed mass or, alternatively, to reduce the prolapse and prevent recurrence by colopexy (Fig. 53–2). No information is available to support the use of colopexy in this situation, but theoretically, it should be considered. Total amputation of the prolapsed mass has been done on many occasions, with excellent results. Recurrent prolapses after removal of the purse-string suture are treated by re-insertion of the suture, rectal amputation, or colopexy.

Anal prolapse, which is not as serious a condition as rectal prolapse, is often associated only with an unsightly slight protrusion that is more prominent after defecation. The animal licks the area. If treat-

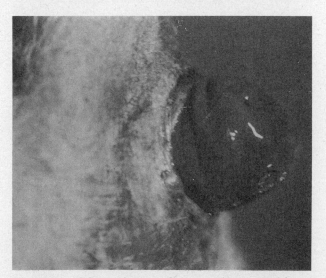

Figure 53–2. Prolapse of anus and rectum after perineal hernia repair. This prolapse did not respond to insertion of a purse-string suture. Amputation or colopexy is indicated.

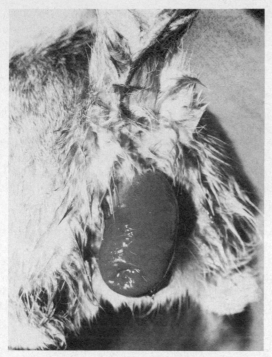

Figure 53–3. Prolapse of the rectum and terminal colon in a cat.

ment is necessary, the prolapsed mucosa can be excised with scissors; suturing is usually not necessary.

Rectal prolapse is a serious disorder in cats (Fig. 53–3). Usually, total prolapse occurs, including part of the colon. There is considerable tenesmus, which can produce catastrophic complications if the pro-

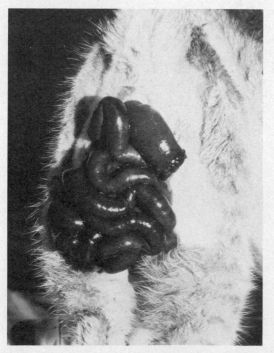

Figure 53–4. Eventration of small intestine through the anastomotic suture line in a cat following resection of prolapsed rectum.

lapsed rectum requires amputation. The continual postoperative straining can lead to passage of abdominal organs, e.g., small intestine, through the pelvis and through the anastomotic suture line in the large intestine (Fig. 53–4). I saw this complication in three cats before amputation of the prolapsed feline rectum was abandoned in favor of abdominal colopexy. The latter procedure gives excellent results.

Amputation of Prolapsed Rectum

This procedure is indicated for treatment of massive prolapses and when the prolapsed portion is necrotic, lacerated, or irreducible.

Submucous resection for rectal prolapse has been described.[60] However, this is a difficult and hemorragic procedure and its efficacy is doubtful. In humans, it has been developed as a salvage procedure for chronic rectal prolapse in sick individuals who cannot tolerate definitive procedures.[65]

Rectal amputation requires general or spinal anesthesia. Preoperative preparation is minimal and includes cleaning the prolapsed portion with nonirritating solutions. In most cases, warm isotonic saline solution is used for the mucosa, and the anus and surrounding skin are cleaned with an antiseptic solution such as povidone-iodine or chlorhexidine. Most reports of rectal amputation describe the use of mattress stay sutures through all layers.[1] However, this method can lead to difficulties in inserting other sutures around the circumference of the rectum. The preferred method is to partly transect the prolapsed mass by a 180-degree transverse incision through the outer and then inner walls of the rectum at the base of the prolapse. A few large vessels are encountered, which should be divided between hemostats and ligated because they may retract and be difficult to find if they are transected without clamping. Then, the two adjacent walls of the rectum are sutured together dorsally. Two rows of sutures are recommended, the first through the submucosa and muscular layer and the second in the submucosa and the mucosa. When suturing is completed in the dorsal 180 degrees of the rectal circumference, further transection and suturing are done until the entire mass is removed. Before the final transection is done ventrally, two long sutures are left to act as stay sutures, to prevent the suture line from disappearing through the anus. Simple interrupted sutures of 2-0 or 3-0 absorbable material are used.

Colopexy

Colopexy is a useful procedure for treatment and prevention of rectal prolapse in cats and dogs. A ventral midline laparotomy is done in the midabdominal region. The descending colon is lifted from the incision and pulled cranially so that a nonsterile assistant with a finger in the rectum may determine that this traction is transmitted to the rectum. The descending colon is sutured to the abdominal wall with the colon in slight cranial traction. The colon is placed against the abdominal wall approximately 2.5 cm away from the linea alba, and simple interrupted absorbable sutures are inserted. The sutures penetrate into the lumen of the colon and are securely fixed to the body wall. The sutures are placed 1.5 to 2 cm apart, and seven or eight are inserted. The colon is then rolled slightly toward the linea alba, and a parallel row of similar sutures is placed between the first row and the linea alba, firmly attaching the colon to the body wall by a double row of sutures.

CONGENITAL ABNORMALITIES OF THE RECTUM AND ANUS

The incidence of these abnormalities in dogs and cats is difficult to determine because many newborn animals with deformities and many unthrifty puppies and kittens are destroyed. The appearance of the various congenital abnormalities can be correlated with the embryological development of the hindgut and the urogenital tract.[2, 50]

There are many classifications of the anatomic varieties of atresia ani. The common classification lists four basic anatomic types.[31] In type I, there is congenital stenosis of the anus. Type II consists of a membranous type of imperforate anus due to persistence of the anal membrane; the rectum ends as a blind pouch immediately cranial to the closed anus. In the type III abnormality, the anus is closed as in type II, but the blind end of the rectum is situated some distance cranial to the anus. In type IV abnormality, the anus and terminal rectum are normal, but the cranial rectum ends as a blind pouch in the pelvic canal.

In these abnormalities, the accessory structures in the anus are usually developed normally. The anal sphincter muscle is present and responds to electrical stimulation. Anal sacs are present and usually open to the exterior. A dimple is seen at the site of the closed anus.

An additional anatomical and functional disability associated with atresia ani is the presence or absence of external or internal fistulae.[18, 21] The incidence of fistulae between the rectum and the urogenital tract is unknown. A common disorder in young females is a fistula between the terminal rectum and the dorsal vaginal wall. The incidence of fistulae between the rectum and urethra in males is unknown.

In addition to congenital abnormalities associated with atresia ani, another group is associated with anogenital clefts in males and females. A cloaca is formed so that feces and urine enter a common cavity and body opening.[68]

Clinical Signs

Clinical signs depend largely upon whether the rectal and anal canal are closed or stenosed and whether the colon and rectum can be decompressed by the presence of a fistula. In general, the fistula allows egress of gas and liquid feces but not normal passage of solid feces.

Animals with stenosis of the anus or rectum are essentially normal until weaning, when various degrees of tenesmus, constipation, and megacolon develop. Diagnosis is confirmed by careful palpation and probing.

Newborn animals with atresia ani and without rectal fistulae are essentially normal clinically for the first two to four weeks of life. Then they show restlessness, abdominal enlargement, and unthriftiness. The diagnosis is easily confirmed by the absence of defecation and of an anal opening. Perineal bulging may be present, depending on the degree of rectal atresia.

The terminal end of the rectum can be immediately cranial to the anus, or can be in any position within the pelvis. Its position can often be determined on radiography, especially if the young animal is radiographed with its anus dorsal so that gas passes upward into the terminal rectum.

An animal with a rectovaginal fistula and atresia ani shows few clinical signs while on a liquid diet. The mother cleans the common opening, and local irritation is minimal. Later, signs of irritation of the vulva, passage of feces via the vulva, and often megacolon are present. The diagnosis is confirmed by local examination and probing (Fig. 53–5). Rarely, radiography is helpful.

No information is available concerning fistulae between the rectum and areas of the urinary tract other than the vagina in dogs and cats. About one-third of

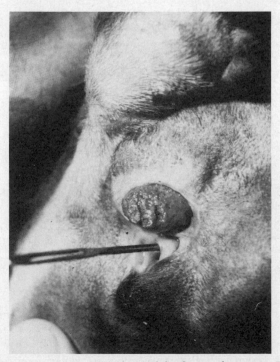

Figure 53–5. Atresia ani with rectal fistula into the vagina. The probe is in the urethra.

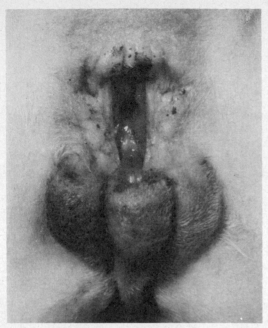

Figure 53–6. Anogenital cleft in a male cat. The anus and urethra have a common opening. The urethra opens on the dorsal aspect of the penis.

human patients with anorectal abnormalities have anomalies in other body areas. This information should be considered and a careful search made for other anomalies in an animal with anorectal fistula. The examination should probably include an evaluation of the urinary tract by excretory urography and cystourethrography. In anogenital clefts in the female, the mucosa of the anus or rectum and the vagina are continuous along the perineal raphe.[68] The anus can be incomplete ventrally, to become the dorsal part of the cleft, or the anus can be atretic, in which case a rectal fistula forms the dorsal part of the cleft. In most cases, feces and urine are passed easily, and the only clinical problems are fecal incontinence, soiling of the perineum with feces and urine, and perineal irritation.

Anogenital clefts are seen in the male. In the example shown in Figure 53–6, the septum dividing the urogenital tract from the hindgut is absent and the urethra is incomplete (hypospadia). The anus and anal sphincter muscle are incomplete ventrally. Defecation and urination take place through a common skin opening. In this cat, there was good control of defecation and urination, but the edges of the skin opening and surrounding hairs were contaminated with feces and urine.

Treatment

Animals with stenosis of the anus or rectum (type I atresia ani) are treated by bougienage, which must be done gently and repeatedly. Satisfactory results are usually obtained. When bougienage is unsuccessful, a surgical procedure such as Z-plasty or total removal of a stenosed portion of rectum is required.

Many serious disorders are encountered in surgical treatment of anomalies associated with atresia ani. The most serious is lack of normal function in the colon and rectum after repair of the anus. This is related either to unknown congenital problems or, more likely, to irreversible damage to the colon and rectum associated with tremendous distension of these organs before the problem is recognized and remedied. These disorders are rarely diagnosed in young animals before several weeks, and most have severe megacolon and abdominal distension by this time.

In type II abnormalities, the anus can be opened easily and the terminal rectal pouch found.[56] A vertical straight incision is made in the skin over the anal dimple, avoiding the anal sacs and openings. The sphincter muscle is identified, and an opening is made through its center. The distal rectal pouch is carefully mobilized, brought out through the sphincter muscle, opened, and sutured to the subcutaneous tissues and skin. One or both ends of the initial skin incision are usually closed by suturing skin to skin. All feces in the colon and rectum are removed, and attempts are made postoperatively to prevent reaccumulation of feces, which unfortunately is likely to happen.

Rectovaginal fistulae are commonly present with type II anal abnormalities. The fistula is carefully dissected through a horizontal straight or curved incision between the anus and the vulva. The fistula is divided, and the openings into the dorsal vagina and ventral rectum are closed, usually by one row of interrupted sutures. Then the anus is opened and the rectum is sutured to the skin as described previously. It is often preferable to transect the rectum cranial to the fistulous opening, remove the segment of the rectum between this point and the anus, and suture the terminal rectum to the anus.

In type III anal and rectal abnormalities, in which the terminal blind end of the rectum is situated in the pelvic canal, successful repair can involve an abdominal approach to mobilize the terminal colon and rectum before the rectum is pulled through the anus and anal sphincter as described for type II abnormalities.[56]

The prognosis for these procedures is guarded. Often, diagnosis is delayed, the colon and rectum are severely distended, and the patient is small and weak. Consequently, surgical mortality is high. In addition, postoperative problems include megacolon and stenosis of the newly formed anal opening. The latter condition should respond to dilation or anoplasty.

Treatment of anogenital cleft in females is generally satisfactory. By an appropriate reconstructive procedure, the anus is opened or re-formed, a rectal fistula is closed if present, and a perineal body is re-formed between the anus and vulva.[68] In the anogenital cleft in the male cat shown in Figure 53–6, excellent functional results were obtained by creating a standard urethrostomy ventrally, removing the testes and scrotum, and re-forming a perineal body.

ANAL SAC DISEASES

The paired anal sacs, which lie on either side of the anal canal between the internal and external anal sphincter muscles, act as reservoirs for secretion from apocrine and sebaceous glands. This dark brown, viscous, malodorous liquid is expressed by action of the external sphincter muscle during defecation.

Disease of the anal sacs is the most common problem in the anal area. It is particularly common in small breeds such as the poodle, although the true incidence in some large breeds, such as the German shepherd, Irish setter, and Labrador retriever, has probably been understated in many surveys.[20, 22, 27]

The cause of anal sac disease is not fully understood in spite of the general statements in most reports of the disorder. Because of the lack of objective investigation, only suggested causes can be offered. For example, anal sac disease seems to be associated with improper diet, soft stools, lack of exercise, lack of adequate external anal sphincter function associated with pudendal nerve disease, perianal fistulae, and scar tissue. It is likely that these possible causes lead to inadequate and irregular emptying of the sac, a process that should take place during defecation if a stool of adequate consistency is forced through a normally functioning anal sphincter.[1] Anal sacs can be emptied purposefully by many dogs and most cats, by voluntary contraction of the external anal sphincter muscle. An association between anal sac disease and systemic disorders such as seborrhea has been suggested but not proven.

Disorders of the anal sacs include impaction, inflammation, and neoplasia. It is likely that impaction and retention of anal sac secretion lead to inflammation and infection. In turn, infection is associated with abscess formation that can lead to rupture of the sac. It is interesting that in small breeds, such as poodles and chihauhaus, rupture occurs in that part of the sac closest to the skin, so that a fistulous tract develops between the sac and the overlying skin. Tissues surrounding the sac are not involved in the inflammatory process. However, in other breeds, notably the German shepherd, the sac is situated much more deeply than in the smaller breeds and lies along the wall of the rectum, rather than projecting out from the rectum under the skin. Rupture of the anal sac in the German shepherd can lead to cellulitis surrounding the sac, spread of the infection along fascial and muscle planes, abscess and granuloma formation, and multiple fistulous tracts opening on the skin surface (see "Perianal Fistulae").[27]

Clinical Signs

Anal sac impaction is invariably associated with licking and biting the area of the anus, tail base, or skin on the side of the perineum. An affected dog characteristically rubs its anus on the ground and may chase its tail.

A sac can be palpated by inserting a finger into the rectum and feeling the sac between this finger and a thumb on the skin over it. No information is available on what constitutes anal sac impaction; however, diagnosis is probably justified if the sac is full, signs of discomfort or pain are present, or the contents of the sac cannot be expressed readily.

Sac contents, in most cases of impaction, are not grossly different from normal, except in quantity. In other cases the contents are inspissated.

Anal sacculitis is associated with increased pain and discomfort and often tenesmus. The contents of the sac are usually thinner than normal, and are purulent or blood-tinged. There may be redness and swelling over the anal sac. Rupture is associated with cellulitis, a discharging fistula or fistulae, and often some relief from the pain in the perianal area. In small breeds, the discharging fistula is usually at four or eight o'clock. In the German shepherd, the area of the anal sac is painful and indurated. The firm swelling can be felt to be spreading around the anus, following the path of the sphincter muscle. Eventually, one or more fistulous tracts develop. Following anal sac rupture, and before fistulous tracts develop, the firm mass in the region of the sac resembles closely a neoplasm of the sac, such as anal sac gland carcinoma.[27] In many cases, differentiation is possible only by excisional, incisional, or needle biopsy.

Treatment

In simple impaction, the sac contents can be readily expressed by pressure between a finger in the rectum and an overlying thumb. Anesthesia or sedation is not usually required. When the contents are inspissated, irrigation with saline may be needed.

Possible contributory factors, such as poor diet, lack of exercise, and diarrhea, should be remedied. It is probably wise to express sac contents again in one to two weeks. Many owners want to perform this procedure, but expression of sac contents can lead to sac irritation and infection if it is done too frequently or with too much pressure.

Surgical removal of impacted anal sacs is indicated if treatment is necessary so often that the dog is becoming apprehensive or if the owner wishes to prevent frequent recurrences. If one sac only is involved, surgical removal of both sacs is advised, to avoid the common involvement of the second sac after a few months.

Anal sacculitis without surrounding cellulitis or fistula can be treated by expression of sac contents every three to four days until the inflammation has subsided. More severe infection requires irrigation of the sac with isotonic saline and instillation of broad-spectrum antibiotics in a cream or solution. Culture and susceptibility testing may be indicated.

The first consideration in treatment of anal sacculitis with surrounding cellulitis is to obtain a diagnosis, and in particular to differentiate between malignant tumor and infection. Some anal sac carcinomas are highly invasive, edematous, and inflamed. Thus they can closely resemble cellulitis. Blood-tinged fluid in the sac can be associated with infection or neoplasia.

When a distinction cannot be made between infection and neoplasia, probably the preferred management is total surgical excision of the mass, including the anal sac and its duct. The wound is left open and heals uneventfully in two to three weeks or is sutured, with a Penrose drain left in place for three to four days. The excised mass should be examined histologically. If the mass appears, at surgery, to be an infected sac, the second sac is removed.

Treatment of ruptured anal sac with a single discharging fistula and no evidence of cellulitis surrounding it is by irrigation of the sac with saline, instillation of antibiotics into the fistula, and use of parenteral antibiotics. The irrigation is repeated at more or less frequent intervals, depending on patient cooperation. If the fistula has not healed in two weeks, the fistula, sac, and duct are excised. The wound is left open or is closed with sutures, with a Penrose drain inserted for three to four days.

Treatment of anal sac rupture with multiple fistulae is discussed under "Perianal Fistulae."

Surgical Excision of the Anal Sac*

Anal Sac Without Infection. Following careful dissection, the resulting cavity is closed and primary healing is obtained. Many techniques are described in the literature for removal of noninfected anal sacs. In my opinion, any technique that transversely incises the anal sphincter causes unnecessary dissection and allows injury to vessels and nerves and is not justified. Numerous cases of incontinence and scarred ani have been seen following anal sac removal (see "Complications of Anal Sac Surgery").

The anal sac is beneath the external sphincter muscle, close to the rectal wall and very close to branches of the caudal rectal artery and vein and branches of the pudendal nerve to the anus. During sac excision, as little muscle is damaged as possible, and blood vessels and nerves must be preserved. Very careful surgical dissection is needed.

The sac can be distended to assist the surgeon in dissection. In large dogs, cotton or umbilical tape can be inserted via the duct. In large and small dogs, a special anal sac gel can be inserted into the sac after being boiled in water for five minutes (Fig. 53–7). This white gel distends the sac, and the heat destroys most of its muscular and fibrous attachments, making dissection easy. No healing problems have been associated with the use of this hot gel.

*Editor's note: Destruction of anal sacs by temporary infusion of solutions containing formalin has been advocated[20] and is said to have a low incidence of complications. In the absence of a large series of cases, the procedure cannot be recommended, because infusion of other substances in the past has resulted in fistulous tracts from residual anal sac wall.

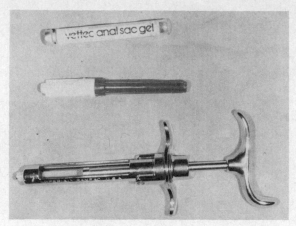

Figure 53–7. Anal sac gel and applicator.

However, in the German shepherd and in any dog with anal sacculitis, rupture of an apparently intact sac has occurred during instillation of the gel, which spreads out into the tissues and can be difficult to remove. Accordingly, the gel must be injected slowly, and the blunt needle should not completely fill the duct.

Anal sac gel is strongly recommended for the inexperienced surgeon. After removing enough anal sacs, the surgeon can readily distinguish the outside of the sac and dissect it free without the gel, the use of which does have complications.

Before surgery, the rectum should be empty. After induction of general anesthesia, the anal area is clipped and prepared for aseptic surgery. The anal sacs are emptied and irrigated with antiseptic solution such as povidone-iodine or chlorhexidine to avoid contamination if the sac is opened accidentally during dissection. A sponge containing antiseptic solution is inserted into the rectum. Anal sac gel may be inserted into the sacs. A vertical incision three to four centimeters long is made over the center of the anal sac. By careful blunt dissection through the sphincter muscle, the sac is reached. Its wall is grasped gently, and the sac is dissected free until it is attached only by its duct. Tuttle forceps are used to grasp the sac atraumatically. Extreme care is necessary at the most cranial aspect of the sac to avoid injury to blood vessels and nerves. No significant bleeding should occur during dissection of the sac.

Two single interrupted sutures of 3-0 or 4-0 absorbable material are inserted into the anal wall immediately cranial and caudal to the anal sac duct. Hemostats are attached to the long ends of these two sutures, which act as marking sutures. The anal sac duct is transected close to the anal wall. The resulting small opening, which tends to be difficult to identify without the two marking sutures, is closed and everted into the anus with two or three interrupted absorbable Lembert sutures. The ends of the two marking sutures are cut short.

The resulting small cavity is irrigated with saline, all bleeding is stopped, and a few fine absorbable sutures are inserted to close dead space. The skin opening is closed with interrupted absorbable sutures in the subcutaneous tissues and interrupted nylon sutures in the skin. If unexpected contamination occurs during surgery, or if cellulitis around the sac is suspected, a 3-mm Penrose drain is inserted into the cavity and removed in one to two days. The second sac is removed in a similar manner. Skin sutures are removed in ten days.

Anal Sac Surrounded by Cellulitis or Ruptured Anal Sac With Fistulae. Removal of an anal sac with surrounding cellulitis or of a ruptured anal sac with one or more discharging fistulae is usually done by inserting the blade of Metzenbaum scissors down the duct into the sac and cutting radially from the anus through the skin, duct wall, and sac wall. The opened sac wall is grasped with five or six hemostats that are clamped together and held as a handle to elevate the sac. The entire sac with duct and anal opening is very carefully dissected free. Fistulae in the skin are excised, and the entire opening is left to heal as an open wound; or if all infected tissue is removed, the cavity is irrigated, a Penrose drain is inserted, the cavity is closed, and the drain is removed in four days.

Complications of Anal Sac Surgery

Anal sac surgery is frequently indicated, and postoperative complications should be few. Unfortunately, when the procedure is done by inexperienced hands, complications are common, and because the anus is involved, severe problems result.

The most common complication is persistent infection with discharging sinuses. It is invariably associated with leaving part of the sac. Because sinuses have been found with the stump of the anal sac duct, simple ligation and transection of the duct is not recommended, because it must leave the part of the duct that is distal to the ligature. Instead, the oversewing technique for total removal of the duct is recommended. Treatment involves finding and removing the cause.

Infection with discharging fistulae has also been encountered. Fistulous tracts generally originate in one of two ways. First, the opening of the duct into the anus is either not closed by suture or ligature or the method of closure fails. The fistula from the anus opens into a lateral abscess cavity, and from this cavity, one or more fistulous tracts open to the skin surface. Treatment is (1) to excise the fistulous tract into the anus and to exteriorize and debride the abscess cavity and leave it open to heal by contraction and epithelialization, or (2) to excise totally the infected tissue, suture the opening, and drain the wound for three to four days. The second manner by which fistulous tracts form is through inadvertent removal of part of the rectal wall. I have seen this situation particularly in German shepherds. In three cases, fistulae developed following anal sac removal; on exploration, the anal sacs were still present, but a section of the rectal wall had been grasped, ele-

vated, and excised. In two other cases, the anal sac had been detached at the duct and probably retracted into the wound, and the wall of the rectum was mistaken for the lost sac and part of it was removed; at exploration, the detached sac and opening into the rectum were discovered.

Failure of the anal sphincter mechanism is another common complication of anal sac surgery. In some cases, there is little or reduced function of the anal sphincter muscle, as determined by its inability to contract and by electromyographic studies. This complication is probably associated with injury to the anal branch of the pudendal nerve. If there is no return of function in three to four months, permanent injury must be suspected, and the dog must be managed by diet and good husbandry procedures or a fascial sling may be used to provide additional continence.[6]

In other dogs, incontinence is present after anal sac surgery but sphincter function appears normal. There is decreased sensation in the anus and anal canal, as judged by applying external stimuli to the area. This development is probably associated with removal of the superficial nerve fibers to the anus by wide and rough dissection during sac removal. Obviously, the main anal nerve to the sphincter muscle is intact. Nerve regeneration takes three to four months. A diet can often be selected by trial to form a relatively dry stool.

Tenesmus and dyschezia can occur following anal sac surgery. Generally, there is some infection following the procedure, and small nodules of scar tissue can be palpated on rectal examination. If active infection is present, exploratory surgery or antibiotics may be necessary. If the surgical site appears inactive, additional healing time should be allowed, with the dog on medical therapy such as a fecal softener (Metamucil). If recovery does not occur, scars should be explored and carefully excised.

PERIANAL FISTULAE

Conditions affecting the anal area in the dog have been reported beginning in 1945.[30] In a report of perianal fistulous tracts in a dog in 1961, Schaffer and Block[52] observed that the condition was seen mainly in male German shepherds and Irish setters and reportedly resulted from infection of the anal sacs complicated by abscess formation. However, these authors stated that the primary cause was the presence of minute fecaliths in the small mucosal pouches or crypts inside the anal opening that caused localized pressure necrosis and infection.

Lewis,[35] in 1968, gave two names to the specific condition that affects mainly German shepherd males over five years of age: "perianal fistulae" and "anal furunculosis." He described the lesions and stated that the origin of infection was the "pouches lying between the columns just inside the anal opening." He commented that the significance of this region seemed to have been overlooked by the clinician. Lewis made several interesting observations. He noted that although he considered that the anal pouches were of prime concern in the cause of the condition, the infection might also arise from impacted anal sacs and other sources. Also, he stressed the significance of the conformation of the German shepherd: long sloping croup, broad loins, long low-slung tail, and broad tail root that is firmly clamped down onto the anal sphincter. This conformation leads to the presence of a thin film of feces in the area, bacterial contamination, and abrasion from the coarser fecal constituents.

Harvey[23] described the age, breed, sex distribution, habitat of the dog, and clinical signs. He discussed the cause of the condition but did not describe a definitive cause. He suggested that the disease resulted from contamination of the anal glands, hair follicles, tubular glands, or sebaceous glands of the perianal skin caused by a fecal film spread over the anal and peripheral area by the broad tail of the German shepherd.

The Lesions of Perianal Fistulae in Dogs

In veterinary literature, there is little discussion of the various types of sinuses or fistulae around the anus, and there has been no general agreement concerning the lesions of perianal fistulae and their cause. Some authors mention the anal sacs in relation to the condition and state that these sacs may or may not be involved.[7, 35, 41] Cases of traumatic rectocutaneous fistulae caused by a dog bite or anal sac surgery have been described.[53] In humans, the situation is much clearer, although in some conditions, the pathogenesis and treatment are vague.[25, 49]

The pathology of the chronic fistulous disease of dogs was described by Levene in 1968,[34] who observed that, "striking though the clinical features are, the histology does not arouse much interest." He described the ulceration and multiple, undermining intercommunicating fistulous tracts. There is a chronic, nonspecific inflammation with fibrosis, granulation tissue, and, in some cases, an epithelial lining of the tracks.[34] The nonspecific nature of the developed lesion is typical of hidradenitis suppurativa in humans.[14, 18] Hidradenitis has been described in canine dermatology, but the name has not been applied to the anal area in the dog.[41]

In an attempt to determine the nature of the sinuses and fistulae in perianal fistulae in dogs, Johnston and Goldschmidt[27] studied 106 cases of perianal fistulae. The primary aim was to describe the actual lesions and to differentiate the various conditions affecting the anus. There were 60 German shepherds, 20 mixed-breed dogs, eight Irish setters, six borzois, four Old English sheepdogs, four springer spaniels, and four retrievers. The age range was two to 12 years, with median age of seven years. There were 69 males and 38 females. Fistulae and sinuses not related to anal inflammation were not included in the survey. The following five distinct lesions were present, singly or in various combinations:

Hidradenitis of the Cutaneous Zone of the Anal Canal

The squamous epithelium and underlying structures were involved. Small skin openings led into subcutaneous cavities. The earliest lesions involved the apocrine sweat glands within the deep portion of the dermis. The glandular lumen contained inflammatory cells with necrosis of the secretory cells and extension through the basement membrane to the periglandular tissue, where occasional giant cells were found. There was subsequent involvement of the periglandular tissue and extension of the inflammation between the lobules of the circumanal (hepatoid) glands. By this stage, the inflammation was both acute and chronic, consisting of neutrophils, macrophages, and lymphoid cells. Eventually, there was involvement of circumanal glands and muscle by the inflammatory process and the formation of sinus tracts. The final lesions consisted of subcutaneous cavities caused by centrifugal spread of the infection from one apocrine gland and one or more skin openings.

These lesions were present in 52 of the 106 dogs. In six of 52 dogs, these lesions were present alone. They occurred in any part of the circumanal area but were particularly severe in the two tail-fold regions. Lesions extended along the ventral surface of the tail (Fig. 53–8).

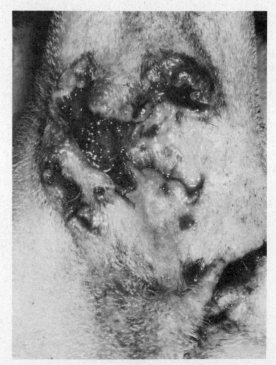

Figure 53–8. Extensive perianal fistulae in a dog. Areas of hidradenitis extend along the tail. There are ruptured anal sacs and fistulae from the anal sinuses (pouches).

In the dog, all structures in the anal area—sebaceous glands and hair follicles—can be involved in addition to apocrine glands. With folliculitis, there is a marked inflammatory reaction secondary to perforation of hair follicles. A pyogranulomatous response is localized around keratin and hair.

The features of these lesions are remarkably similar to those of human hidradenitis.[25, 26, 38, 59, 64] Most important for differential diagnosis is that the lesions are obviously superficial and involve only skin and subcutaneous tissue.

Fistulae of the Anal Sinuses

The anal sinuses are pouches or pockets formed in the columnar zone of the anal canal by the longitudinal ridges that run cranially from the anocutaneous line for about 7 mm.[15] They are the structures referred to previously as small mucosal pouches or crypts.[35, 52] In the study by Johnson and Goldschmidt,[27] fistulae extended from the anal sinuses or pouches at the dentate line either directly to the skin surface or into large perianal subcutaneous abscesses that in turn opened to the skin surface. When fistulae of the anal sinuses were present, they tended to be multiple, usually four to 12 or more.

These anal fistulae were present in 38 dogs. No dogs showed these lesions alone. In six dogs, they were associated with only hidradenitis. Care was needed to distinguish the openings of some of these fistulae from the openings of the anal sacs.

Ruptured Anal Sac

In these cases, skin openings tended to be grouped together: between two and four o'clock or between eight and ten o'clock; however, when hidradenitis was also present, skin openings were randomly located. A probe could be passed into the anal sac from skin openings in most cases or could be passed down the anal sac duct, through the ruptured sac, and out the skin opening. In other cases, it was determined histologically that sacs had ruptured and then healed, leaving a surrounding granulomatous reaction and abscess cavity and fibrosis of the wall of the anal sac. Histologically, there were focal aggregates of neutrophils and epithelioid cells with the formation of granulomas. The remains of apocrine glands of anal sacs were present. In some cases, release of keratinous and pigmented material from the anal sac with phagocytosis by multinucleated giant cells and macrophages was noted. After anal sac rupture, spread of infection was along fascial and muscular planes in the perianal area, producing complex abscess cavities and fistulous tracts.

Ruptured anal sacs were present in 66 dogs, either alone or in association with fistulae of anal sinuses and hidradenitis (Fig. 53–9). Anal sac rupture alone was seen in 24 of the 66 dogs, including 20 German shepherds. Forty of the 66 dogs were German shepherds. In fact, 66 per cent of the German shepherds

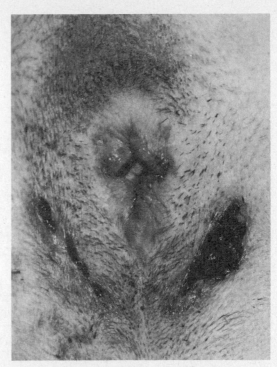

Figure 53–9. Ruptured anal sacs in a German shepherd. Small isolated lesions of hidradenitis are present. The lesions can be treated by excision and suturing of the two main lesions and exteriorization and fulguration of the hidradenitis.

seen had anal sac rupture, and in 50 per cent the only lesions were those caused by anal sac rupture.

Submucous Fistulae and Sinuses of the Rectum

The mucous membrane was severely inflamed, tags of tissue were present, and small (a few millimeters) to long (one to three centimeters) submucous sinuses or fistulae were present in the terminal third of the rectum.[27] These were always associated with severe pain on defecation. Glands resembling circumanal glands were present in the perirectal tissues and showed focal areas of inflammation. Histologically, inflammation followed by local abscess of these glands may lead to formation of the submucous sinuses and fistulae.

These lesions were present in 30 dogs, always in association with other lesions, mainly hidradenitis, fistulae of anal sinuses, and anal sac rupture.

Rectal Fistulae

Rectal fistulae were situated two to six centimeters from the anus and were difficult to find. They explained a failure to heal after surgery. There was usually redness, swelling, and pigmentation of the rectal mucosa at the site of the fistula; however, these features were often obscured by submucous fistulae and perirectal abscesses that eventually burst through the skin. The openings in the rectal wall were small slits in some dogs and were found only after careful search, probing with a tom-cat catheter and injection of fluid. As seen in ruptured anal sacs, the perirectal abscesses were complex. Rectal fistulae with perirectal abscesses were present in six dogs.

The Cause of Perianal Fistulae in Dogs

It is apparent that the cause of perianal fistulae is related to the environment of the area. The low-slung tail and broad-based tail produce the intertriginous lesions peculiar to all skinfold dermatitides. Add to this the moisture from feces, rectal mucus, and anal sac secretion, and an excellent environment for skin maceration followed by inflammation of skin structures is present. This situation closely resembles the experimental situation used by Shelley and Cahn in 1955 to reproduce hidradenitis in animals.[59]

Inflammation of all structures—apocrine and sebaceous glands and hair follicles in the circumanal region, glands in the anal sinuses or pouches, glands in the anal sacs and perirectal glands—is present.

Ruptured anal sacs are seen commonly, although this finding has been reported rarely in previous studies. In some dogs, the ruptured anal sacs are probably overlooked because so much destruction is present that the individual lesions are lost. Sometimes anal sac rupture can be seen histologically, and the sacs are grossly intact, but usually much smaller than normal. Anal sac rupture in German shepherds is common and is clinically different from anal sac rupture in small breeds. In small breeds, there is invariably a single fistulous opening directly over the sac and little, if any, inflammation of tissue surrounding the sac. In German shepherds, rupture of the anal sac occurs deeply in the tissues and is followed by a granulomatous reaction and abscess formation surrounding the sac, infiltration of purulent material along muscle and fascial planes, and production of skin openings that need not be directly over the sac.

The anal sac is situated much more deeply in German shepherds than in small breeds and extends along the rectal wall. Perhaps if an anal sac ruptures on its deep surface in a German shepherd, the inflammation is not restricted by the external anal sphincter as in small breeds, extending instead deep to and outside the external anal sphincter, following fascial and muscular planes. The spread of infection along fascial and muscular planes in the perirectal and perianal area is a critical aspect of the perianal abscesses and fistulae in the dog. This aspect has been studied extensively in humans, and fistulae and abscesses have been designated as intersphincteric, transsphincteric, suprasphincteric, and extrasphincteric. There appears to be no limit to the anatomical paths the fistulae can follow. A similar situation occurs in dogs. Deep subcutaneous abscess cavities are commonly found. Then, in the depths of the abscess cavity, a sinus or fistulous opening can be seen, often with great difficulty. The tract from this opening can pass in many directions but in all cases is controlled by the fascial and muscular planes. In several dogs, abscesses extended as far forward as the coccygeal muscles and spread in a circular path around the rectum. The mechanism of spread can be readily understood by studying the anatomical structures in the anal area.

Treatment

In an early report of the treatment of perianal fistulae, a surgical procedure to obliterate the anal sinuses (crypts or pouches) was described.[52] Lewis[35] in 1968 described two forms of therapy: partial excision and cautery for early cases, and total excision of the anal ring in advanced cases using a technique described in 1961.[11]

Up to 1969, various treatments for the condition were described, including obliteration of the anal sinuses, and partial excision and cautery for early cases. In general, the only treatment for the common advanced case was total excision of the anus with all diseased tissue. Medical therapy was generally regarded as not beneficial. A detailed description of this radical approach to treatment was given by Harvey.[23] The aim of therapy is described in this manner: "Anal sphincter and coccygeal muscle tissue (and tissue of other muscles, when the disease is extensive) should be saved where possible, but not at the risk of leaving diseased tissue in place." The author states that the owners accepted the potential or actual social problems created by this drastic removal of anal structures. Forty-nine per cent of 37 dogs so treated were reported by owners as having flatulence frequently, another 40 per cent occasionally. Twenty-eight per cent of 36 dogs had fecal incontinence frequently, another 4 per cent occasionally.

In 1971, a new approach to the treatment of the condition, cryosurgery, was reported as successful in two dogs.[7] A report followed in 1975 of the use of cryosurgery in 40 cases.[31] In these cases, there was a long healing period, the average time for resolution being 9.8 weeks. The end-results were generally good, and the rates of recurrence and development of complications were considerably less than those following radical excision of the lesions.

A more conservative approach to the management of the anal conditions was reported in 28 dogs in 1973.[51] Differentiation of the cases into degrees of severity was an important consideration in treatment; mild cases were treated by debridement and cauterization, but more severe cases were treated by cryosurgical excision. The objective of treatment was to preserve healthy tissue and stimulate the diseased areas to heal by granulation. In all cases, the anal sacs were removed and then the areas of furunculosis were debrided. The overlying skin and the periphery of the lesions were excised, and any true anal fistulae were opened and debrided. It is important to note that no attempt was made to dissect out and completely resect the diseased tissue. These areas were then cauterized with 75 per cent silver nitrate or 80 per cent liquified phenol. Results were very good: 23 of 24 (96 per cent) animals treated had complete resolution in an average time of 3.5 weeks. Four cases recurred on average eight weeks after the initial resolution. One wonders whether, in fact, these four cases were recurrences or cases of incomplete healing. In two of the four cases, the condition was present for more than a year before cryosurgery was used.

The interesting point in this report is the use of conservative techniques initially to preserve normal structures, and of more drastic excision (by cryosurgery) in nonresponsive cases.

Recommended (Johnston) Surgical Procedure

In the 106 dogs in which the anatomy of the sinus and fistulous tracts was studied, a treatment regimen was devised on the basis of three principles: (1) a knowledge of the likely source and paths of spread of an abscess, sinus, or fistula is necessary, (2) as much normal tissue and anal function as possible must be preserved, and (3) the cause must be removed.[27]

Preparation of the patient for treatment of perianal fistulae is not intensive. Administration of enemas is generally difficult, and prolonged bowel preparation is not warranted. No food is given for 24 hours prior to surgery. The rectum should be emptied, usually after anesthesia is induced. Brief scrubbing of the anus and perianal area and application of a skin disinfectant such as 70 per cent alcohol complete the procedure. An antiseptic-soaked sponge is inserted into the rectum. Antibiotics are not used locally or systemically. Obviously, the wounds are heavily contaminated, but problems with infections have not been encountered. Three basic surgical procedures are used in the treatment of perianal fistulae, depending on the nature and extent of the lesions.

Excision and Closure by Sutures. There is no doubt that rapid healing and excellent function can be achieved by a careful dissection of all diseased tissue with primary closure. This technique is the preferred one, but unfortunately it is not possible in some cases (see hereafter). It is almost always possible when the underlying cause is anal sac rupture and in many cases of abscess from a fistula from an anal sinus. This technique is infrequently appropriate for hidradenitis.

A skin incision is made surrounding fistulous openings in the skin and the opening of the anal sac. The abscess cavity is opened and carefully excised, with all normal tissue spared. Fistulae into anal sinuses can be found and excised. Normal as well as ruptured anal sacs are removed. Rectal fistulae are traced into the rectum, and the opening into the rectum is excised and carefully sutured. The resulting cavity is examined carefully both visually and by palpation to detect any abnormal tissue, which is excised, again with all normal tissue spared. The cavity is irrigated with saline, a Penrose drain is inserted, and the cavity is closed in layers. A few fine absorbable sutures are placed in the middle of the cavity, a row of absorbable sutures is placed in the subcutaneous tissues, and the skin is closed with nylon sutures. The drain is removed in three to four days.

In some cases in which lesions of hidradenitis involving the skin incision are present, the deep tissues, particularly in the cavity from which the anal sac was removed, are closed by sutures as described, but the skin and subcutaneous tissues are not sutured. In these cases, primary healing of the deep cavity is achieved. The hidradenitis, treated as described later, heals by second intention in two to three weeks, compared with four to six weeks if the area is not sutured.

Exteriorization, Saucerization, and Curettage with Open Healing. In hidradenitis and in many advanced cases from other causes, local excision may not be possible because of extensive spread of infection throughout the anal area, and the surgeon has two choices: exteriorization, saucerization, and curettage with open healing, or total ablation of the anus (described later). The former procedure is used if there is any possibility of preserving even some anal function.

The basic technique is exteriorization of the lesion followed by excision of the remaining lesions or electrofulguration (Figs. 53–10 and 53–11).[42, 43] First, skin openings are explored by a probe to determine the extent of the subcutaneous cavities and the pres-

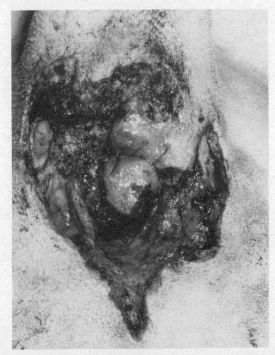

Figure 53–10. Treatment by exteriorization, saucerization, and fulguration of the dog shown in Fig. 53–8. The lesion healed well; however, a decision to excise all lesions and the anus could well have been the correct one.

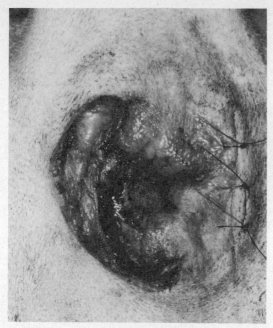

Figure 53–11. Perianal fistulae in a dog. The ruptured anal sac (*right side*) was excised and sutured. The lesions of ruptured anal sac, hidradenitis, and anal fistulae (*left side*) were treated by excision, deep suturing, and superficial fulguration.

ence of fistulae into the anus, rectum, or anal sacs. The skin covering the abscess cavity is removed, leaving no underrun margins of skin. These skin borders are "saucerized." After a cavity is exposed in this manner, the remaining exposed surface or lining of the cavity is examined to determine whether it is a thin granulating membrane over normal tissue or whether scar tissue can be palpated deep to the granulations. If only a thin membrane over normal tissue is present, this membrane is destroyed by electrofulguration. Normal incised tissue at the site of the saucerization is not fulgurated. If scar tissue can be palpated beneath the lining membrane, the membrane and scar tissue are removed by careful excision. This maneuver is necessary because it can expose fistulae that were not previously suspected.

Anal sacs are removed in all cases. When the sac is intact, one blade of a scissors is inserted down the anal sac duct into the sac and the duct and sac are opened in a radial direction from the anus. Skin, subcutaneous tissue, and sac wall are opened. The incised sac wall is picked up with several hemostats and pulled out of the wound. The sac is dissected out with scissors, with all sac and duct removed. Care should be exercised to avoid trauma to the caudal rectal vessels and nerves, which are situated close to the deep portion of the sac. If the artery is cut, it must be carefully ligated, not coagulated, to avoid severe postoperative bleeding. In most cases, the large, clean cavity that is present after anal sac removal is closed with absorbable sutures and a Penrose drain is inserted.

Fistulae into the anus and rectum are excised together with the wall of the anus or rectum caudal to the opening. No attempt is made to close this defect with sutures. Treatment of submucous fistulae is to remove all tags of mucosa in the rectum, to "unroof" and exteriorize (into the rectal lumen) all fistulae, and to fulgurate ulcerated areas.

The important aspects of this technique of exteriorization are to find all sinuses and fistulous tracts and undermined skin, to totally remove or exteriorize these, to "saucerize" the skin edges, and to destroy the lining of the cavity. I previously cauterized this lining with phenol as described by Robins and Lane;[51] however, clinical results have been much better with electrofulguration.

The advantage of fulguration is the control that can be obtained over destruction of the lining membrane. Fulguration is an excellent method for destroying the surface of a lesion. The electrode can be reasonably small; usually, a flat spatula-type electrode approximately three millimeters wide is used. The current setting is kept low so that a vigorous but not violent spark passes from the electrode to the tissues when the gap is approximately two to three millimeters. With fulguration, the tissues are spared severe damage by two mechanisms, unlike with electrocoagulation or electrodessication, in which the electrode is in contact with the surface of the lesion or is inserted beneath the surface of the lesion. Two mechanisms are that the current loses some of its power because of the insulating effect of the two to three millimeters of air and that the eschar that forms on the surface of the lesion following fulguration immediately insulates and spares the underlying tissues. The result is that with electrofulguration, only the surface of a lesion to a depth of no more than one to two millimeters is destroyed. This fine degree of control is not possible with the use of phenol or silver nitrate, or with cryosurgery. Unfortunately, many small modern electrosurgical units have inadequate or no spark-gap current and cannot be used effectively for fulguration. Cryosurgery performed with probes leads to the formation of the typical "ice-ball."[7] All tissues in this frozen ball, normal as well as abnormal, are destroyed and soon slough. The use of a cryosurgical micro-jet, by which liquid nitrogen is sprayed carefully over the surface of the lesion following the exteriorization procedure, could be a suitable alternative to fulguration.

Total Excision of the Anus and Anal Sphincter. In some extremely severe cases, involving sinus and fistulous tracts throughout the entire anus and anal sphincter, and particularly in the presence of painful rectal lesions, total excision of all lesions, including the anus and anal sphincter, is the procedure of choice (Fig. 53–12). A circular incision is made in the skin outside the skin lesions. The incision is extended cranially to the rectal wall so that all lesions are excised, and the rectum is mobilized and withdrawn so that it can be amputated cranial to the rectal lesions.

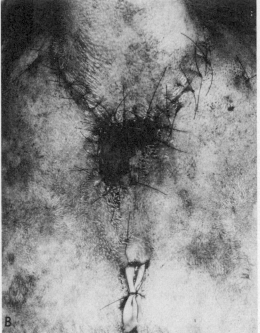

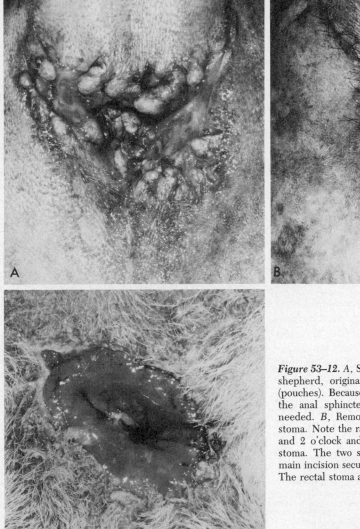

Figure 53–12. A, Several perianal fistulae in a German shepherd, originating in anal sacs and anal sinuses (pouches). Because of destruction and involvement of the anal sphincter, total excision of the anus was needed. *B,* Removal of the anus and formation of a stoma. Note the radiating skin incisions at ten o'clock and 2 o'clock and the Penrose drain ventral to the stoma. The two sutures to the left and right of the main incision secure the top of the Penrose drains. *C,* The rectal stoma after healing.

Generally, the entire external anal sphincter is involved in the inflammatory process and must be removed. In fact, this radical total excision is not used if any normal sphincter exists. A Penrose drain is placed around the rectum in an inverted U shape, with both ends exteriorized via one opening ventral to the stoma. The drain is removed in three to four days. The end of the rectum cranial to the rectal lesions is sutured to the skin opening.

Tension and movement tend to interfere with healing, and the circumference of the rectal opening is considerably less than the skin opening. A suture technique has been devised to avoid these two problems. The rectum is amputated only through the dorsal 180 degrees in the beginning. A row of simple interrupted 2-0 absorbable sutures is placed between the subcutaneous tissues close to the skin edge and the submucosa and muscular layers of the rectum. This row of sutures bears the brunt of all tension and movement in the area. To avoid the disparity between the circumference of the rectum and the skin opening, the sutures are evenly distributed on the rectum and spaced at slightly greater intervals on the skin opening, and large areas of skin openings are avoided entirely. These avoided areas are usually at approximately ten and two o'clock. Occasionally, when the skin opening is not circular because the skin lesions were asymmetrical, other skin areas are omitted from the suture line. After the sutures in the dorsal 180 degrees are completed and traction ends are left on sutures at three and nine o'clock, the remaining rectum is amputated and sutures are placed in the ventral 180 degrees. Skin may need to be avoided at four and eight o'clock. Each avoided skin edge is sutured with subcutaneous absorbable sutures so that the secondary suture line is at 90 degrees to the circumference of the rectum. Finally, rectal mucosa and submucosa are sutured to the skin edge, and skin is sutured to skin in the radiating secondary suture lines with monofilament nylon interrupted sutures.

Postoperative Care

The owner is instructed to wash the sutured anus and open wounds twice daily with warm normal saline. Metamucil is given only if pain on defecation is present. Drains are removed in three to four days and sutures in two weeks. For open wounds, an office visit in four weeks is essential. In the first week after surgery, tissue destroyed by electrofulguration sloughs and the wound does not decrease in size. After this period, healthy granulation tissue is formed, and rapid contraction and epithelization occur. Antibiotics have not been necessary.

Complications During Healing

All dogs that were sutured completely should heal in two weeks. Dogs in which deep cavities are sutured and skin is left open heal in two to three weeks. Most dogs in which wounds are left completely open heal in four to six weeks. One complication during open healing is the development of small superficial ulcers at ten and two o'clock along the tail-folds. At four weeks postoperatively, these ulcers are cauterized with liquid phenol on an out-

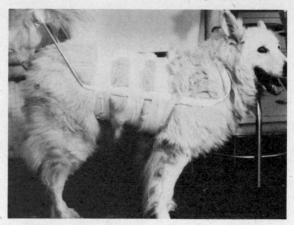

Figure 53–14. Typical tail brace used in dogs to assist healing of wounds in the anal area. Aluminum rod is bent to form a loop around the neck, an arm down each side of the body, and an extension over the back above the tail head.

patient basis and without anesthesia. The twice-daily washing with normal saline is continued, and the animal returns in four weeks (eight weeks postoperatively). At this time, if any areas are not healed, unfavorable prognosis for healing should be given, however, the phenol cauterization is repeated and the animal is seen in four weeks (12 weeks postoperatively). At this time, if any unhealed zones are present, more radical therapy, such as surgical excision of the lesion with primary closure or closure by a reconstructive procedure, is advised. The ulcerated areas are removed by an excision that is either fusiform, square, or triangular. The fusiform wounds can usually be closed in a linear fashion. The square and triangular wounds require a reconstructive procedure, usually undermining and either a sliding flap or a rotational flap (Fig. 53–13). Because these wounds undergo considerable movement and tension during tail movement and defecation, application of

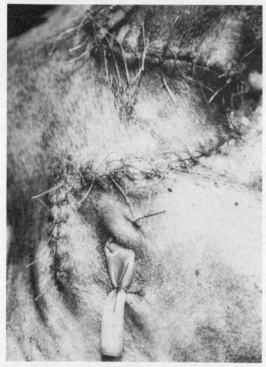

Figure 53–13. Sliding flap procedure to replace an ulcer.

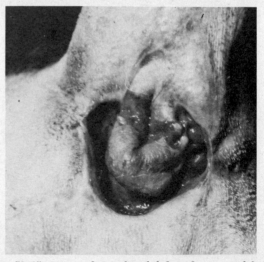

Figure 53–15. A circumferential anal defect after perianal fistulae surgery. This defect requires careful superficial excision of the ulcer area with suturing.

a tail brace is recommended (Fig. 53–14). The use of a tail brace is not consistently successful because many dogs react violently to the brace requiring its removal. When it is tolerated, it is extremely beneficial, especially in preventing movement in sutured wounds and thereby promoting healing. Some dogs will not walk with the brace in place or cannot be trained to tolerate it. In such cases, tail amputation should be considered. The tail must be removed in such a way that no stump or tail-folds remain. This procedure provides excellent results, but it is not acceptable to many owners.

Presence of a sinus or fistulous tract after 12 weeks invariably indicates that a fistula has been overlooked at the initial operation or part of an anal sac remains. A second procedure is needed.

An additional complication is the development of a circumferential defect of 50 per cent or more adjacent to the anus. The granulation tissue in the defect has a smooth, inactive surface, the typical "hygroma" formation in a healing open wound (Fig. 53–15). In these cases, very slow healing is seen, probably because of movement between the skin on one side of the defect and the anal sphincter on the other side. At four and eight weeks, phenol cautery is used, as for radial ulcers; thereafter, the procedures are the same as for radial ulcers. If excision is done, there is careful preservation of normal tissues, especially of as much of the anal sphincter as possible with its nerves and blood supply.

Prognosis and Recurrence Rate

There is no value in stating that a certain percentage of dogs with perianal fistulae have a particular end-result. The end-result depends entirely on the type and extent of the original lesions. All dogs with excised and sutured lesions or superficial hidradenitis should recover and function normally. In other cases, the end-result depends on how much damage has been done to the anus and anal sphincter by the disease process and how much normal tissue must be excised by the surgeon in order to remove all diseased tissue and find and remove all sinuses and fistulae. Equally, there is no value in stating that a given percentage of cases heal in four weeks. These figures are available but are valueless in an understanding of a single case. All dogs with up to moderate involvement should heal in four weeks with normal anal function. With more severe involvement, healing of deep cavities and of superficial ulcers in the tail-folds occurs by eight to 12 weeks. Residual sinuses or fistulae after this time are signs of incomplete removal of the original lesions. Prognosis following total anal resection depends on the dog's house training and the composition of the feces. Excellent primary healing should occur with the techniques described above. The dog that has lost its anal sphincter presents few problems for the owner if the feces are firm and the dog is trained to defecate outside at regular intervals. Uncontrolled passage of gas and liquid feces can be unacceptable to some owners. Unfortunately, German shepherds frequently have soft feces.

When extensive excision of anal lesions is necessary, the scar tissue can lead to anal stenosis. Enlargement of the orifice by Z-plasty is done after healing is complete. Two Z-plasty procedures are done, with the central incision of the Z along the circumference of the anus from ten to eight o'clock and from two to four o'clock. Additional Z-plasty procedures are done, if necessary, from 11 to one o'clock and from five to seven o'clock.

Most cases of recurring perianal fistulae in my experience have represented inadequate surgical excision with incomplete healing, not true recurrences. Careful questioning of an owner often reveals that small nonpainful sinuses or fistulae have been present since the initial procedure. These cases remain dormant for long periods, and usually exacerbation follows; thus, the history of a recurrence. Many anal glands are destroyed or removed in the initial episode, and secretion from anal sacs is not present after sacculectomy. Therefore, the anal area is less moist after successful perianal fistulae treatment. Owners are advised to examine the anal area after healing and to recommence twice-daily washing with warm normal saline if the area is moist and inflamed or if the dog licks it. With the altered anatomy of the area and increased owner awareness of potential problems, true recurrence of perianal fistulae has a very low incidence.

HYPERTROPHY OF THE EXTERNAL ANAL SPHINCTER IN THE DOG

Severe dyschezia is a relatively common clinical problem in dogs, and careful physical examination reveals the cause in most cases. These causes include perianal fistulae in any of their manifestations, anal sac disease, prostatic disease, and rectal tumors and stenosis. Pain can be attributed to scar tissue remaining after healing of anal sac disorders and other anal disorders.

There remains a small but significant group of dogs in which dyschezia is present but no cause can be found for the pain or there is evidence of mild and persistent inflammation of the anus. In addition, in all these dogs, there is a consistent feature, marked hypertrophy of the external anal sphincter muscle. This condition has not been reported previously. No objective studies have been done, but I have seen at least six dogs with this problem.

Clinical Signs

The dog is presented for severe dyschezia. The dog is usually nervous, and external anal examination causes apprehension and resistance. Visually, the external sphincter muscle is markedly hypertrophied. Rectal palpation is done slowly with a lubricated finger, and the hypertrophy and strength of the sphincter muscle are readily apparent. Even when the examining finger is not moved for several seconds to allow the dog to relax, the rhythmic contractions of the muscle continue and are sufficiently strong to produce a numbing sensation in the finger.

Generally, the dog must be sedated or anesthetized to examine the anus and rectum. The only consistent clinical findings are hypertrophy of the anal sphincter and, in some dogs, mild inflammation.

Pathogenesis

There are two possible mechanisms to explain the syndrome, but a common feature is probably a nervous, high-strung dog. All six dogs I have seen had this temperament. In the first mechanism, normal defecation with a large, dry stool could produce sufficient pain or discomfort that the dog contracts the anal sphincter as a defense mechanism. Pushing feces past a contracted anal sphincter causes friction in the anal canal, which in turn causes more pain, more forceful contraction of the sphincter, more irritation, and thus a circle of unrelenting pain and sphincter contraction. An alternative mechanism is that a painful condition such as anal sacculitis could be the precipitating cause of defensive contraction of the anal sphincter.

Treatment

Conservative therapy should be used in the beginning, although results are usually disappointing. Anal sacs are emptied weekly. A local analgesic and anti-inflammatory preparation, used for treating human hemorrhoids, is applied to the anus and into the terminal rectum twice daily. This is not possible in many dogs. A fecal softener such as Metamucil is added to the food. In persistent cases, the anal sacs should be removed surgically.

In four of the six cases I have seen, this therapy was not successful, and the dogs underwent a surgical procedure to temporarily desensitize the anus and to interrupt the cycle of pain and sphincter contraction. The anal branches of the pudendal nerve were isolated and grasped in the jaws of a hemostat, and the hemostats closed completely for a few seconds to crush the nerve bundles but not interrupt their continuity (the nerve injury known as **axonotmesis**). This type of nerve injury is followed by degeneration of the distal axon fragment, then regeneration over a varying period depending on the length of the nerve (at a rate of one to three millimeters a day). These dogs had no anal function after operation and no pain on defecation. Anal function returned in six to eight weeks with no recurrence of dyschezia.

BENIGN AND MALIGNANT TUMORS OF THE RECTUM AND ANUS

Polyps of the Rectum and Anus

Incidence and Pathological Features

Adenomatous polyps of the rectum are not common in dogs. They are raised, sessile, or pedunculated, are commonly multibranched, and can occur in grape-like clusters. Well-differentiated cuboidal or columnar cells cover the surface. The covering epithelial cells show no malignancy, and there is no invasion of the underlying basement membrane or lamina propria.[9]

It is apparent that problems can occur in the identification of rectal polyps, in particular, in distinguishing them from rectal carcinomas and in determining whether so-called premalignant changes exist in a polyp or, alternatively, whether carcinomatous change can occur in benign adenomatous colonic and rectal polyps. There is still insufficient evidence to support or deny these suggestions and to indicate the prognosis following removal of a polyp. Standard pathological terminology is that *malignancy* is an invasion of the basement membrane by tumor cells with extension into the lamina propria. In carcinoma in situ, malignant cells are present in the mucosa, but there is no invasion of underlying layers.

Carcinomatous changes in polyps are apparently rare in animals. One report in 1971 described stromal invasion with atypical cells in the head of a polyp, which was diagnosed as a carcinoma arising in an adenomatous polyp.[61]

Seiler,[57] in 1979, described seventeen cases of colorectal polyps in dogs. The mean age was 6.9 years, and male and female dogs were equally affected. The histopathological classification was hyperplastic polyp, papillary adenoma, tubular adenoma, papillotubular adenoma, and an unclassified type. Severe epithelial atypia, like carcinoma in situ, was apparent in five of the papillotubular adenomas, and these tumors were regarded as more likely to recur or to become malignant.

Polyps are composed of branching lamina propria supporting abnormal epithelium that is contiguous with normal rectal mucosa. Surface ulceration, hemorrhage, and infiltration of inflammatory cells into the stroma are common.

In humans, polyps greater than one centimeter in diameter have a higher potential for malignancy. Five dogs in Seiler's series had polyps greater than one centimeter in diameter, and multiple polyps, marked epithelial atypia, or both developed in these dogs, suggesting a relationship between size of polyps and potential for malignancy.

The cause of colorectal polyps remains unknown.

Polyps vary in number from one to ten or more, and in diameter from a few millimeters to many centimeters in the sessile types. They appear more commonly in the rectum than in the colon, and the most common site is near the anorectal junction.

Clinical Signs

Polyps in the rectum are associated with clinical signs that are typical but not diagnostic. Most dogs have mucus and blood in the feces, and prolonged diarrhea is common. Tenesmus is often present and can lead to prolapse of the polyps or rectum. Some dogs show few signs and the polyp is not detected until it prolapses during defecation.

Diagnosis

Most polyps of the rectum and all polyps of the anal canal can be palpated via the anus and rectum. Bleeding and fragmentation of the polyp occur commonly in the sessile, branched varieties. The pedunculated or sessile mass can be seen early by endoscopy, although emptying and cleaning of the bowel are usually needed. Radiography is generally not helpful in evaluation of polyps of the anus and terminal rectum. Many rectal polyps, however, can be seen on contrast and double-contrast radiography. Usually, little more information is obtained than with palpation and endoscopy.

In all cases, biopsy and histological examination are required for a specific diagnosis. A suitable biopsy specimen can often be obtained by digital palpation when a fragment of the polyp breaks off. In other cases, a wedge-shaped portion of the polyp can be obtained with a suitable retractor or endoscope. Small pedunculated polyps can be removed and then examined.

Removal of Polyps in Dogs

Removal via the anus using electrosurgery is recommended for a pedunculated polyp and for small sessile ones (Fig. 53–16). They must be within the reach of suitable instruments or must occur in the terminal rectum or anus so they can be prolapsed from the anus. All anal and rectal polyps and many polyps in the descending colon can be reached via the anus. A polyp is removed by grasping it and dividing the base with an electrode or tonsil snare acting as an electrode. Overzealous coagulation must be avoided. This procedure requires only evacuation of feces from the colon and rectum as preoperative preparation.

Some surgeons recommend removal of pedunculated or small sessile rectal polyps by ligation or surgical excision and suture.[48] As the polyps do not invade the muscularis mucosa, they can generally be removed in this manner.

Large sessile polyps can be removed by electrocoagulation; however, there is increasing danger of

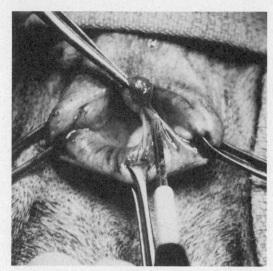

Figure 53–16. This small pedunculated polyp can be removed by electrosurgery.

perforation of the bowel wall or inadequate removal of the polyp with recurrence. The technique can be successful when done by an experienced surgeon. In most cases, however, resection of the affected segment of colon or rectum is recommended (Fig. 53–17A). Antiseptic and antibiotic bowel preparation is needed. The surgical technique is as for removal of rectal carcinomas (Fig. 53–17B).

Prognosis

Survival data after removal of polyps are not available from Seiler's study, but it is noteworthy that in three dogs, polyps recurred between one month and two years after polyp removal.[57] No details of surgical procedure for excision were given. Eight of the 17 dogs lived polyp-free for one to five years, and five of the 17 dogs were not studied after polyp removal.[57] Probably, prognosis is excellent if the polyp can be removed completely. Complete removal is easy in pedunculated polyps and difficult in large sessile ones unless a bowel resection is done. The prognosis following removal of pedunculated or small sessile polyps is excellent.

Rectal Carcinomas

See Chapter 176 for details of tumor biology.

Clinical Signs

Signs can resemble those of polyps but are generally more severe—especially pain. There is straining to defecate, passage of blood and mucus with feces, and painful defecation with passage of ribbon-like feces. Proctoscopic examination may reveal irregular luminal narrowing and ulcerative foci in a bed of firm gray tissue. Some tumors are annular. The mass can be palpated rectally and can be seen on contrast radiography.

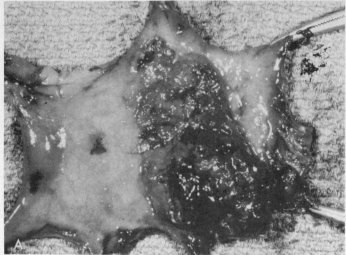

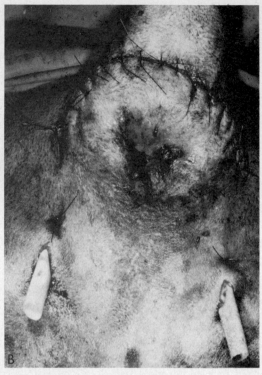

Figure 53–17. *A*, A large sessile bleeding polyp in the mid-rectum. This was removed successfully by total removal of a section of the rectum. *B*, Skin incision and drain placement for removal of the polyp. The Penrose drain is in the shape of a inverted "U" loosely draped over the rectum near the anastomotic site.

Treatment

In removal of rectal masses without prior biopsy, a decision may have to be made, after local excision, to do a more radical excision if the specimen shows malignancy. Excisional biopsy is commonly recommended if a polyp is suspected, although preoperative diagnosis by incisional biopsy is highly recommended if a carcinoma is suspected. The surgeon is able to plan a wider excision and, theoretically, can be more certain of total removal.

Unfortunately, prognosis for long-term survival of dogs with rectal carcinomas is unfavorable.

Anatomical Aspects of Rectal Removal

The pelvic reflection of the peritoneum in the pararectal fossa is at approximately the level of the second coccygeal vertebra. Generally, the peritoneal cavity is not opened when only the caudal half of the rectum is removed. For a short distance cranial to

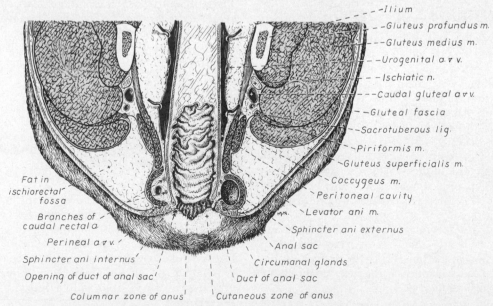

Figure 53–18. Section through anus in horizontal plane, dorsal aspect. (Reprinted with permission from Evans, H. E., and Christensen, G. C. (eds.): *Miller's Anatomy of the Dog.* 2nd ed. W. B. Saunders, Philadelphia, 1979.)

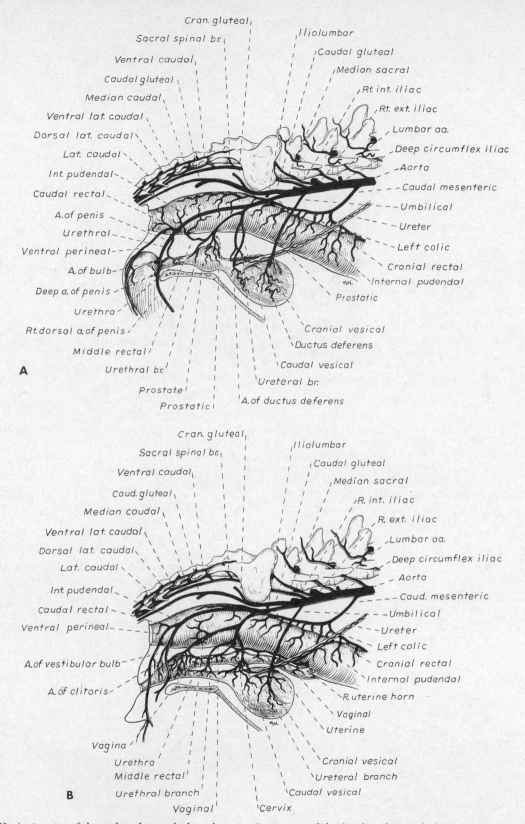

Figure 53–19. *A*, Arteries of the male pelvis, right lateral aspect. *B*, Arteries of the female pelvis, right lateral aspect. (Reprinted with permission from Evans, H. E., and Christensen, G. C. (eds.): *Miller's Anatomy of the Dog.* 2nd ed. W. B. Saunders, Philadelphia, 1967.)

the peritoneal reflection, mobilization of the rectum can be done between the peritoneum and the rectal wall (Fig. 53–18). Opening the peritoneal cavity has not resulted in peritonitis.

Large vessels and nerves pass along or cross the

rectum. They include the internal pudendal artery, which runs parallel to the rectum for about two centimeters before passing lateral to the levator ani muscle (Fig. 53–19). This vessel should not be damaged if mobilization of the rectum is done close to

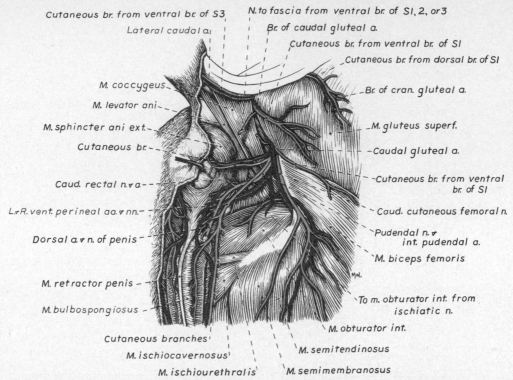

Figure 53–20. Nerves, arteries, and muscles of the male perineum, caudolateral aspect. (Reprinted with permission from Evans, H. E and Christensen, G. C. (eds.): *Miller's Anatomy of the Dog.* 2nd ed. W. B. Saunders, Philadelphia, 1979.)

the rectal wall. In addition, the rectum is crossed laterally by the obturator, ischiatic, pelvic, and anal nerves (Fig. 53–20), which also can be easily separated from the rectum. The coccygeus and levator ani muscles pass around the rectum and are not affected by dissection to mobilize the rectum (Fig. 53–21).

The rectococcygeus muscle is composed of fibers from the external longitudinal musculature of the rectum and passes dorsally and caudally to insert on the fifth and sixth caudal vertebrae. When the tail is

raised during defecation, this muscle shortens the rectum. This muscle is divided at the rectum when more than the terminal rectum is removed (Fig. 53–22).

The retractor penis muscle arises ventrally on each side of the sacrum or the first two caudal vertebrae, passes ventrocaudally across the lateral surface of the rectum, contributes some fibers to the rectal wall, and inserts most of its fibers near the duct of the anal sac and in the external anal sphincter.

When an incision is made between the anus and

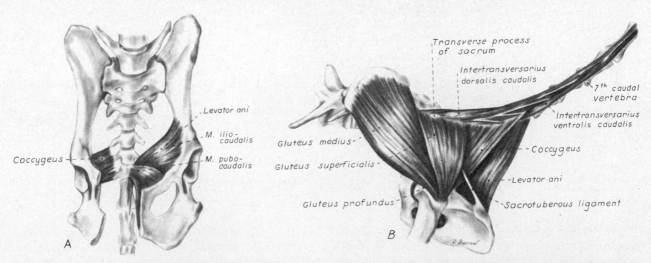

Figure 53–21. Muscles of the pelvis. *A*, Levator ani and coccygeus muscles, ventral aspect. *B*, Caudal and gluteal muscles, lateral aspect. (Reprinted with permission from Evans, H. E., and Christensen, G. C. (eds.): *Miller's Anatomy of the Dog.* 2nd ed. W. B. Saunders, Philadelphia, 1979.)

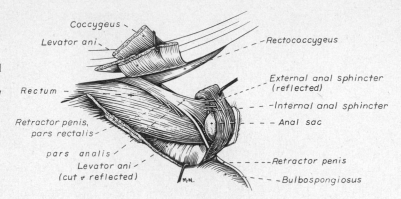

Figure 53–22. Muscles of the anal region, lateral aspect. (Reprinted with permission from Evans, H. E., and Christensen, G. C. (eds.): *Miller's Anatomy of the Dog.* 2nd ed. W. B. Saunders, Philadelphia, 1979.)

tail, the dorsal attachment of the external anal sphincter muscle to the caudal fascia at the level of the third caudal vertebra is divided. Anal sphincter function depends on preservation of anorectal structures and their sensory and motor innervation. In humans, the puborectalis muscle is one of the group of levator ani muscles that form the pelvic diaphragm and is an integral part of the external sphincter apparatus. It contains stretch receptors that signal the arrival of feces in the rectum and initiates reflex contraction of the sphincter. Also, the lower two to three centimeters of anorectal mucosa contain free and specialized nerve endings mediating sensitivity to pain, temperature, light, touch, and pressure. Loss of these receptors results in imperfect continence.[36] Similar information is not available in the dog. However, incontinence occurs too commonly following anal and rectal surgery in dogs, and until objective canine information is available, veterinary surgeons should heed the precautions known to surgeons operating on humans.

A rational plan for management of rectal polyps and carcinomas in the dog must take into account the site and size of the mass and the degree of local invasiveness, as determined crudely by palpation. Few objective facts are available in the dog. In humans, lymphatic spread does not generally occur until the muscularis mucosa is penetrated, and the primary route of spread is upward (cranial). Lateral spread can occur in later stages, but downward (caudal) lymphatic spread occurs only in late cases when proximal lymphatics are obstructed by tumor. Hence, radical resection with sphincter preservation is possible in many cases.[45] Large tumors with evident local invasion probably cannot be removed successfully by any current technique. After biopsy and confirmation of the diagnosis, euthanasia is indicated.

For tumors in the caudal one-third of the rectum that are mobile and show no evidence of metastasis, total local resection can be used. Because these tumors cannot be removed without damage to the anal sphincter, the anus and sphincter should be removed. After patient preparation, a circular incision is made around the anus, and the rectum is gradually mobilized and pulled caudally until it can be transected cranial to the tumor. The rectum is

sutured to the skin opening by two rows of sutures. The first row of 2-0 or 3-0 absorbable simple interrupted sutures is placed in the muscle layers and submucosa of the rectum and the subcutaneous fascia close to the skin edges. The second row of 2-0 or 3-0 interrupted monofilament nylon sutures is placed in the submucosa and mucosa of the rectum and the skin. Penrose drains are placed in the dead space outside the rectum and removed in three days.

Tumors in the terminal colon, or at the colorectal junction, can usually be resected by an abdominal approach with removal of the pubis followed by reattachment of the pubis at the completion of the procedure. A one- or two-layer closure for the anastomosis is done, using simple interrupted absorbable sutures in an appositional pattern without inversion or eversion.

To remove and reattach the pubis, the skin incision is continued caudally as far as the vulva or scrotum. After the abdomen is opened by a midline incision, the incision is continued caudally through the very short aponeurotic attachment between the adductor muscles. These muscles are displaced laterally by blunt dissection as far as the lateral limits of the obturator foramen. With a bone cutter, the pubis is detached by dividing the bone in three places, laterally two to three millimeters medial to the lateral limits of the obturator foramen on both sides (not exactly at the lateral limits of the foramen, to avoid damage to the obturator nerves), and caudally in the midline at the junction with the ischium, the caudal limit of the obturator foramen. The bone is lifted up, completely detached at the two cranial osteotomies, and hinged caudally at the caudal osteotomy. Following surgery in the pelvis, the pubis is reattached cranially by two wire sutures. No caudal suture is needed.

There are two surgical approaches for tumors of the middle third of the rectum that cannot be approached via the abdomen.

1. By means of a U-shaped incision between the anus and the tail, the entire rectum can be mobilized and exteriorized. The affected section is removed and the ends are anastomosed. Two rows of simple interrupted sutures are placed, using 2-0 or 3-0 absorbable material. As the suturing proceeds dorsally, the inner

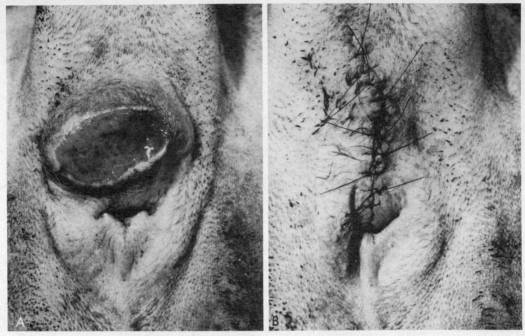

Figure 53–23. *A,* Typical ulcerated perianal adenoma. *B,* Perianal tumors should be excised by a radiating elliptical excision when possible. A sutured incision in this direction interferes with and deforms the anus minimally.

sutures must be inserted first. The knots of the inner layer are placed in the lumen to avoid scar tissue in the rectal wall. The wound is lavaged thoroughly with saline, Penrose drains are inserted, and the subcutaneous tissues and skin are closed. The drains are placed close to, but not touching, the incision line. Drains are removed in three days.

2. A modified "pull-through" procedure can be done. A 360-degree incision is made through the rectal wall approximately one centimeter cranial to the anus. The rectum is pulled caudally while it is mobilized by blunt and sharp dissection, and is then transected cranial to the lesion. A Penrose drain in the shape of an inverted U is draped over the rectum, and both ends are exteriorized below the anus. The cranial cut end of the rectum is anastomosed to the caudal end by two rows of simple interrupted sutures of 3-0 absorbable material as described previously. Drains are removed in three to four days.

In all procedures for removal of rectal tumors, consideration may have to be given to removal of lumbar masses in lymph nodes that can obstruct the pelvic inlet. In these instances, a guarded prognosis must be given.

After extensive rectal surgery, such as resection and anastomosis, the dog is not given food for 24 hours. Then, small amounts of low-residue diet such as hamburger and white rice are given for two to three days. Metamucil is added to the food. The antibiotics that were started preoperatively are continued for 24 hours.

When the anus and anal sphincter have been preserved, excellent results with complete continence can be expected. Stenosis at the anastomotic site has been seen rarely, and removal of all or part

of the rectum does not produce significant changes in defecation.

Perianal Gland Tumors

See Chapter 176 for details of tumor biology.

Treatment

Surgical excision is the preferred treatment and is usually successful (Fig. 53–23). Some perianal gland tumors recur; however, because the tumors occur in old dogs, recurrence may be too late to be significant. The rate of recurrence is greatly reduced by castration.

These tumors appear to be androgen-dependent, and estrogen has been used successfully. However, it cannot be relied upon to do more than cause some reduction in size of the tumor and, in some cases, to relieve ulceration. The oral dose is diethylstilbestrol, 0.5 to 1.0 mg every four days for four to six weeks. No toxic effects have been seen with this low dose.

Perianal gland adenomas respond well to radiation therapy. Because many of them are ovoid, cryosurgical removal can be very successful.

1. Archibald, J., (ed.): *Canine Surgery.* 2nd ed. American Veterinary Publications, Santa Barbara, 1974.
2. Arey, L. B.: *Developmental Anatomy.* 7th ed. W. B. Saunders, Philadelphia, 1965.
3. Arnold, H. L., Jr.: Treatment of hidradenitis suppurativa (letter). J.A.M.A., 223:5, 1973.
4. Ashdown, R. R.: Symposium on canine recto-anal disorders. I: Clinical anatomy. J. Small Anim. Pract. 19:1, 1968.
5. Beahrs, O. H., Theuerkauf, F. J., Jr., and Hill, J. R.:

Procidentia: surgical treatment. Dis. Colon Rectum 15:337, 1972.

6. Bojrab, J. M. (ed.): *Current Techniques in Small Animal Surgery*. Lea & Febiger, Philadelphia, 1983.

7. Borthwick, R.: The treatment of multiple perianal sinuses in the dog by cryosurgery. J. Am. Anim. Hosp. Assoc. 1:45, 1971.

8. Bradley, O. C., and Graham, T.: *Topographical Anatomy of the Dog*. 5th ed. Oliver & Boyd, Edinburgh, 1948.

9. Brodey, R. S.: Canine and feline neoplasia. Adv. Vet. Sci. 14:309, 1970.

10. Calhoun, M. L., and Stinson, A. W.: Integument. In Dellman, H-D., and Brown, E. M. (eds.): *Textbook of Veterinary Histology*. 2nd ed. Lea & Febiger, Philadelphia, 1981.

11. Crighton, G. W.: Surgical removal of the anal ring in the dog. Vet. Rec. 73:416, 1961.

12. Doty, R. L., and Dunbar, I.: Color, odor, consistency and secretion rate of anal sac secretions from male, female and early androyenized female beagles. Am. J. Vet. Res., 35:729, 1974.

13. Dworken, H. H.: *Alimentary Tract: Basic Principles and Case Problems*. W. B. Saunders, Philadelphia, 1974.

14. Ekelund, G., and Lonstrom, C.: Histological analysis of benign polyps in patients with carcinoma of the colon and rectum. Gut, 15:654, 1974.

15. Evans, H. E., and Christensen, G. C.: *Miller's Anatomy of the Dog*. 2nd ed. W. B. Saunders, Philadelphia, 1979.

16. Fletcher, T. F.: Lumbosacral plexus and pelvic limb myotomes of the dog. Am. J. Vet. Res. 31:35, 1970.

17. Fletcher, T. F.: Anatomy of the pelvic viscera. Vet. Clin. North Am. 4:471, 1974.

18. Fox, M. W.: Atresia ani and anus vestibularis in a bitch. Mod. Vet. Pract. 44:53, 1963.

19. Greer, M. B., and Calhoun, M. L.: Anal sacs of the cat (*Felis domesticus*). Am. J. Vet. Res. 27:773, 1966.

20. Halnan, C. R. E.: The frequency of occurrence of anal sacculitis in the dog. J. Small Anim. Pract. 17:537, 1976.

21. Hare, W. D.: Anus vestibularis in a young bitch. Can. J. Comp. Med. Vet. Sci. 23:278, 1959.

22. Harvey, C. E.: Incidence and distribution of anal sac disease in the dog. J. Am. Anim. Hosp. Assoc. 10:573, 1974.

23. Harvey, C. E.: Perianal fistula in the dog. Vet. Rec. 91:25, 1972.

24. Hebel, V. R.: Untersuchungen uber das Vorkommen von lymphatischen Darmkrypten in der Tunica submucosa des Darmes von Schwein, Rind, Schaf, Hund und Katz. Anat. Anz. 109:7, 1960.

25. Hughes, E. S. R.: Inflammations and Infections of the anus. In Turell, R. (ed.): *Diseases of the Colon and Anorectum*. W. B. Saunders, Philadelphia, 1959.

26. Hurley, H. J.: Diseases of the apocrine and eccrine sweat glands. In Moschella, S. L., Pillsbury, D. M., and Hurley, H. J. (eds.): *Dermatology*. Vol. 1. W. B. Saunders, Philadelphia, 1975.

27. Johnston, D. E., and Goldschmidt, M.: The lesions of perianal fistulae in the dog. Comp. Cont. Ed. (in press), 1984.

28. Johnston, D. E.: Treatment of perianal fistulae in the dog. Comp. Cont. Ed. (in press), 1984.

29. Krolling, O.: Entwicklung, Bau und biologische Bedeutung der Analbeuteldrusen bei der Hauskatz. Ztschr. Anat. 82:22, 1926.

30. Lacroix, J. V., and Lacroix, L. J.: Pararectal fistula. N. Am. Vet. 26:39, 1945.

31. Ladd, W. E., and Gross, R. E.: Congenital malformations of the anus and rectum; report of 162 cases. Am. J. Surg. 23:167, 1934.

32. Lane, J. G., and Burch, D. G. S.: The cryosurgical treatment of canine anal furunculosis. J. Small Anim. Pract. 16:387, 1975.

33. Leeds, E. B., and Renegar, W. R.: A modified fascial sling for the treatment of fecal incontinence—surgical technique. J. Am. Anim. Hosp. Assoc. 17:663, 1981.

34. Levene, A.: Symposium on canine recto-anal disorders. II. The surgical pathology of ano-rectal diseases in the dog. J. Small Anim. Pract. 9:323, 1968.

35. Lewis, D. G.: Symposium on canine recto-anal disorders. III: Clinical management. J. Small Anim. Pract. 9:329, 1968.

36. Localio, S. A., and Eng, K.: Sphincter saving operations for cancer of the rectum. N. Engl. J. Med., 300:18, 1979.

37. Montagna, W., and Parks, H. F.: A histochemical study of the glands of the anal sac of the dog. Anat. Rec. 100:297, 1948.

38. Morgan, W. P., and Hughes, L. E.: The distribution size and density of the apocrine glands in hidradenitis suppurativa. Br. J. Surg. 66:853, 1979.

39. Morson, B. C.: The poly-cancer sequence in the large bowel. Proc. Roy. Soc. Med. 67:451, 1974.

40. Moulton, J. E.: *Tumors in Domestic Animals*. University of California Press, Berkeley, 1978.

41. Muller, G. H., Kirk, R. W., and Scott, D. W.: *Small Animal Dermatology*. 3rd ed. W. B. Saunders, Philadelphia, 1983.

42. Mullins, J. F.: Hidradenitis suppurativa. In Conn, H. F. (ed.): *Current Therapy 1972*. W. B. Saunders, Philadelphia, 1972.

43. Newell, G. B., et al.: Treatment of hidradenitis suppurativa. J.A.M.A. 223:5, 1973.

44. Nickel, R., Schummer, A., Sieferle, E., and Sack, W. O.: *The Viscera of the Domestic Mammals*. Verlag Paul Parey, Berlin, 1973.

45. Nicholls, R. R., Ritchie, J. K., Wadsworth, J., and Parks, A. G.: Total excision or restorative resection for carcinoma of the middle third of the rectum. Br. J. Surg. 66:625, 1979.

46. Oliver, J. E., and Selcer, R. R.: Neurogenic disorders of the rectum and anal sphincter. Vet. Clin. North Am. 4:551, 1974.

47. Palminteri, A.: Rectal disease and surgery of dogs. Proc. Am. Anim. Hosp. Assoc. 1969, pp. 492–499.

48. Palminteri, A.: The surgical management of polyps of the rectum and colon of the dog. J. Am. Vet. Med. Assoc. 148:7, 1966.

49. Parks, A. G., Gordon, P. H., and Hardcastle, J. D.: A classification of fistula-in-ano. Br. J. Surg. 63:1, 1976.

50. Rawlings, C. A., and Capps, W. F.: Rectovaginal fistula and imperforate anus in the dog. J. Am. Vet. Med. Assoc., 159:3, 1971.

51. Robins, G. M., and Lane, J. G.: The management of anal furunculosis. J. Small Anim. Pract. 14:333, 1973.

52. Schaffer, A., and Block, I. R.: Pathology and surgical correction of perianal fistulous tracts in a dog. J. Am. Vet. Med. Assoc. 138:22, 1961.

53. Schaller, O.: Gibt es beim Hund einen "Musculus sphincter ani tertius"? Wien. tierarztl. Wschr. 8:614, 1961.

54. Schiller, A. G., Helper, L. C., and Knecht, C. D.: Repair of rectocutaneous fistulas in the dog. J. Am. Vet. Med. Assoc. 150:758, 1967.

55. Schummer, A., Wilkens, H., Vollmerhaus, B., and Habermehl, K-H.: *The Anatomy of the Domestic Animals*. Vol 3: *The Circulatory System, The Skin, and the Cutaneous Organs of the Domestic Mammals*. Verlag Paul Parey, Berlin, 1981.

56. Schwartz, S. I.: *Principles of Surgery*. Vol. 2. McGraw-Hill Book Company, New York, 1979.

57. Seiler, R. J.: Colorectal polyps of the dog—a clinicopathologic study of 17 cases. J. Am. Vet. Med. Assoc. 174:72, 1979.

58. Shaughnessy, D. M., Greminger, R. R., Margolis, I. B., and Davis, W. C.: Hidradenitis suppurativa. J. Am. Vet. Med. Assoc. 222:320, 1972.

59. Shelley, W. B., and Cahn, M. M.: The pathogenesis of hidradenitis suppurativa in man. Arch. Dermatol. 72:563, 1955.

60. Shuttleworth, A. C., and Smythe, R. H.: *Clinical Veterinary Surgery*. Vol. 2. Crosby Lockwood & Son, London, 1960.

61. Silverberg, S. G.: Carcinoma arising in adenomatous polyps of the rectum in a dog. Dis. Colon Rectum 14:3, 1971.

62. Stinson, A. W., and Calhoun, M. L.: Digestive system. In Dellman, H-D., and Brown, E. M. (eds.): *Textbook of Veterinary Histology*. 2nd ed. Lea & Febiger, Philadelphia, 1981.

63. Theuerkauf, F. J., Beahrs, O. H., and Hill, J. R.: Rectal prolapse: causation and surgical treatment. Ann. Surg., 171:6, 1970.

64. Thornton, J. P., and Abcarian, H.: Surgical treatment of perianal and perineal hidradenitis suppurativa. Dis. Colon Rectum, *21*:573, 1978.
65. Uhlig, B. E., and Sullivan, E. S.: The modified Delorme operation; its place in surgical treatment for massive rectal prolapse. Dis. Colon Rectum *22*:513, 1979.
66. Vasseur, P. B.: Perianal fistulae in dogs: a retrospective analysis of surgical techniques. J. Am. Anim. Hosp. Assoc. *17*:177, 1981.
67. Vitums, A.: Portosystemic communications in the dog. Acta Anat. *39*:271, 1959.
68. Wilson, C. F., and Clifford, D. H.: Perineoplasty for ano-vaginal cleft in a dog. J. Am. Vet. Med. Assoc. *159*:871, 1971.

Chapter **54** # Liver and Biliary System

Anatomy

John Grandage

FORM AND LOBATION

A large volume of blood has to percolate at low pressure through the liver. Accordingly, the organ has to be stiff, to resist collapsing on the vessels that run through it; this in turn makes it friable. The vulnerable liver is housed in the most protected part of the abdomen, concealed beneath the ribs, resting on a cushion of falciform fat, molded to the soft dome of the diaphragm, and borne on the springy xiphoid cartilage. Because it fractures if it bends too far, it is fissured to allow it to adapt to the changing form of the diaphragm or the arching of the back (Rouviere's law).[76] The fissures of the carnivore liver are deep, those of the cat especially so, and they allow the lobes to slide over one another like a stack of saucers.[49] Different postures may induce the liver to adopt a different form, so that it can look substantially larger in some radiographic projections than in others.[48]

The seven major lobes or processes are: right and left lobes, each subdivided into lateral and medial parts; the quadrate lobe between them; and the caudate and papillary processes of the caudate lobe. The left lateral lobe is the largest and most mobile. Its peripheral border is irregularly serrated or notched, presumably in association with this mobility. Most of the peripheral borders are sharp (30 degrees or less)[82] but they are less acute in the young, in which the liver is relatively larger, or when the liver swells in hepatomegaly.

FIXATION

The liver is not firmly fixed. Abdominal organs push against its visceral surface and sandwich it against the diaphragm. Its strongest attachment is to the caudal vena cava, which courses through it. It is also bound by the coronary ligament to the diaphragm at the foramen venae cavae. This part of the liver moves least. A few, short, weak peritoneal ligaments radiate from the coronary ligament.[72] The right and left triangular ligaments tether the more central parts of the right and left lobes to the diaphragm; they are sometimes paired.[40] The falciform ligament which runs in the midline is reduced cranially to a delicate membrane or is absent altogether;[102] its caudal part loses direct attachment to the liver but is retained as the fat-laden cushion that forms a useful contrast against the diaphragmatic surface of the liver.

The attachments on the visceral surface are larger but looser. A hepatorenal ligament sweeps from the cranial pole of the right kidney to the depths of the renal fossa of the caudate lobe. The lesser omentum consists of the lace-like and non-supporting hepatogastric ligament, which contains the bile duct, hepatic artery, and the portal vein as well as lymphatics and nerves.[102]

THE BILIARY TREE

Intralobular ducts form within the liver parenchyme from bile canaliculi. These become the tributaries of the lobar ducts, which on emergence from the liver surface are called hepatic ducts. The number and pattern of fusion of the hepatic ducts is highly variable.[40] Five ducts are common, with two to seven being recorded in the dog.[43] Once the hepatic ducts receive the cystic duct from the gallbladder, the single vessel is known as the (common) bile duct. In the dog it runs a fairly straight course for some five centimeters within the lesser omentum from the porta to the duodenum. Its terminal portion runs for some two centimeters within the duodenal wall, finally tapering to a nozzle to open by the side of the pancreatic duct.[22] There is no hepatopancreatic ampulla (of Vater), but instead both ducts open side by side on the major duodenal papilla, a small elevation two to three millimeters high, caudally directed, and located between three and six centimeters from the pylorus in both the cat and the dog.[13, 93] The intramural course within the muscularis of the duodenum may serve as a sphincter.[52] The so-called sphincter of Oddi exists around the papilla despite earlier denials, but its muscle fibers are sparse and scattered, and their precise form is both complex and the subject of conflicting reports.[23, 38, 62] It receives a rich cholinergic innervation.

The cystic duct, short and straight in the dog, longer and more sinuous in the cat,[13, 80] leads into the gallbladder; it does not possess the spiral valve of Heister that is present in the human cystic duct.

The gallbladder is a flattened piriform sac lodged between the quadrate and the right medial lobes of the liver, and of variable shape depending on the degree of distension and the position of the liver. Sometimes it is double.[19] Usually its most dependent part peeps through the parietal surface of the liver to touch the diaphragm. When it is filled with contrast agent, however, radiographs show this contact only when special projections are adopted that take account of the dome-shaped diaphragm; in standard lateral projections the gallbladder is seen a little behind the diaphragm and above the apex of the xiphoid.[36] It is best visualized radiographically when the dog is in an orthograde (upright, bipedal) posture[3] and is always a useful indicator of whether the liver is in the normal position.[1] The delicate wall is lined with a mucus-secreting epithelium and covered with a muscularis that can bring about effective contractions.[18, 35]

BLOOD VESSELS

A dual blood supply to the liver is necessary to serve different needs, sometimes regarded as "private" and "public." The hepatic arteries (vasa privata) may be regarded as the liver's principal maintenance vessels, supplying about 20 per cent of the blood.[69] The portal vessels (vasa publica) supply the remaining 80 per cent of blood, which is delivered straight from the alimentary tract laden with potentially dangerous materials that need to be dealt with rapidly. However, this view should not be taken too literally, for the portal supply is also important for the liver's maintenance. Pancreatic hormones, including insulin and glucagon, within the portal blood have hepatotrophic properties; a depleted portal flow results in liver atrophy and an enhanced flow hypertrophy and hyperplasia.[24, 106]

From two to five proper hepatic arteries arborize in a variety of ways from the parent common hepatic artery.[89, 102] Despite this variability, they ultimately supply the seven obvious lobes in territories superimposable on those of the portal vein and biliary tree.[14, 27, 28]

The portal vein receives its tributaries from most of the gastrointestinal tract (see Chapter 50). Its final course from the root of the mesentery to the porta of the liver is along the short, ventral boundary to the epiploic foramen, where it is vulnerable to pressure and twisting.[124] It breaks up rapidly into seven major radicles that supply the principal lobes and whose pattern is remarkably constant.[26, 27, 102] The embryology of the portal vein is clinically important. It is derived from the vitelline (= omphalomesenteric, cranial mesenteric) vein. In the embryo this vessel is a tributary of the cardinal vein (= azygos vein of later life). The developing liver encroaches upon both the vitelline vein and the left umbilical vein, both of which break up into capillaries to nourish this organ. Umbilical and portal veins thus come into continuity. A large channel, the ductus venosus, remains within the liver to convey oxygenated placental blood rapidly and easily to the caudal vena cava. The ductus venosus normally closes promptly after birth and is left as a ligamentum venosum within the depths of the liver. A persistent ductus venosus, one of the more common portal anomalies in the dog, allows portal blood to bypass the liver sinusoids. Four other congenital portal anomalies have been reported.[112] Two of them involve an anastomosis between the portal and azygos veins (the original venous pathway of the embryo), another between the portal and caval veins directly, and the fourth between the portal vein and a number of smaller mesenteric, splenic, or renal veins (Fig. 54–1).[24, 112] Presumably each of these anomalies represents the retention of some embryonic vascular channel (see also Chapter 79).

Acquired portocaval communications develop as a result of portal hypertension and occur in sites other than those of the congenital anomalies. They appear, predictably, where portal and systemic territories meet: around the terminal esophagus and anus and where mesenteries meet the abdominal wall, either dorsally (and hence into the phrenicoabdominal, renal, gonadal, and circumflex iliac veins) or around the navel (and hence into the various abdominal veins).[117, 118]

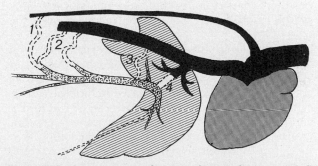

Figure 54–1. Communications between the portal vein (mottled) and systemic veins (black) may persist beyond normal embryonic life as congenital anomalies (white): *1*, portoazygous anastomosis; *2*, peripheral portocaval anastomosis; *3*, central portocaval anastomosis; *4*, patent ductus venosus. Acquired communications may develop at other sites (see text).

Hepatic veins are found exclusively within the substance of the liver where the stiff parenchyme guarantees that they remain patent. They open by many orifices directly into the vena cava as it courses through the dorsal border of the liver.[58] Lymph drains into hepatic and splenic lymph nodes.[40, 41] The liver receives both sympathetic innervation via the celiac plexus and parasympathetic via the vagi.[40]

Physiology

Michael A. Pass

LIVER FUNCTION

The main functions of the liver are to metabolize endogenous and foreign compounds, to secrete bile, and to store blood and some nutrients.

Metabolic Functions of the Liver

The liver metabolizes nutrients, endogenous compounds, and many foreign compounds.[51, 55] Carbohydrates are stored in the liver as glycogen, and galactose and fructose are converted to glucose. The liver also converts amino acids to glucose, and glycogen to glucose, important processes for maintaining the normal blood glucose concentration. Synthesis of lipoproteins, cholesterol, phospholipids, ketone bodies, and bile salts occur in the liver. Carbohydrate and protein in excess of that required for immediate use are converted to triglycerides in the liver and then are transported to adipose tissue for storage. The liver is a major site of protein metabolism and is responsible for synthesizing coagulation factors and most of the plasma proteins; for deaminating amino acids; and for synthesizing amino acids. In the liver, ammonia is converted to urea to be excreted by the kidneys; this is an important process for preventing ammonia toxicity by maintaining a low blood ammonia concentration. The liver stores large quantities of iron and vitamins A, D and B_{12}.[51]

A host of hormones and drugs are metabolized by enzyme systems located in the endoplasmic reticulum and cytosol of the hepatocytes. In general, these reactions convert lipid-soluble compounds into water-soluble metabolites that can be readily excreted in urine or bile.[10, 55, 57] Many hormones and drugs are eliminated from the body after metabolism in the liver, and the activity of the drug-metabolizing enzymes determines the half-life and duration of therapeutic effect of these compounds. In turn the activity of the drug-metabolizing enzymes can be induced or suppressed by a variety of chemicals and environmental factors.[10, 88] Although hepatic metabolism of foreign compounds usually results in the production of nonactive metabolites, in some instances toxic or carcinogenic metabolites are formed that cause diseases in the liver or other tissues.[46, 75, 88]

Metabolism of bilirubin by the liver is of considerable clinical interest not only because unconjugated bilirubin is toxic but because the measurement of bilirubin and its metabolites in body fluids is used in the diagnosis of some liver diseases. Bilirubin is formed from hemoglobin in the cells of the reticuloendothelial system and is transported in the circulation bound to albumen (Fig. 54–2). In the liver it is conjugated to glucuronic acid. The first conjugation occurs in the endoplasmic reticulum to produce bilirubin monoglucuronide, some of which is converted to bilirubin diglucuronide by an enzyme system located on the membrane of the bile canaliculi.[98] Conjugated bilirubin, in both the monoglucuronide and diglucuronide forms, is actively transported into bile and then transported to the intestine. Bilirubin diglucuronide is the major form of bilirubin in bile of dogs and cats. Intestinal bacteria convert bilirubin to urobilinogen, which undergoes further bacterial metabolism to stercobilinogen, which in turn is oxidized to stercobilin and passed in the feces. Some urobilinogen is reabsorbed by the intestine, passes to the liver in the portal blood, and is excreted once again into bile. About five per cent of the reabsorbed urobilinogen is excreted by the kidneys and is oxidlized to urobilin in the urine.

Secretion of Bile

Bile is a yellow or green solution containing electrolytes, bile salts, cholesterol, phospholipids, and bile pigments such as bilirubin. Metabolites of some hormones and many drugs are also secreted into bile.

Bile is formed by secretion of fluid from the hepatocytes and the cells lining the bile ductules.[39] The hepatocytes secrete fluid into the bile canaliculi; the initial process is the active secretion of organic compounds across the canalicular membrane. Water diffuses into the canaliculi along osmotic gradients set up by active transport of organic compounds. This fraction of bile has been called the bile salt–dependent fraction of bile, because bile salts are the major class of organic compound actively secreted into bile.[39] Bile salts such as cholic acid and chenodeoxycholic acid are synthesized in the liver from cholesterol and then conjugated to taurine and glycine before being secreted.[30]

A bile salt–independent fraction of bile, secreted by the canaliculi as a result of active sodium secretion, has been proposed.[39] The existence of this fraction is

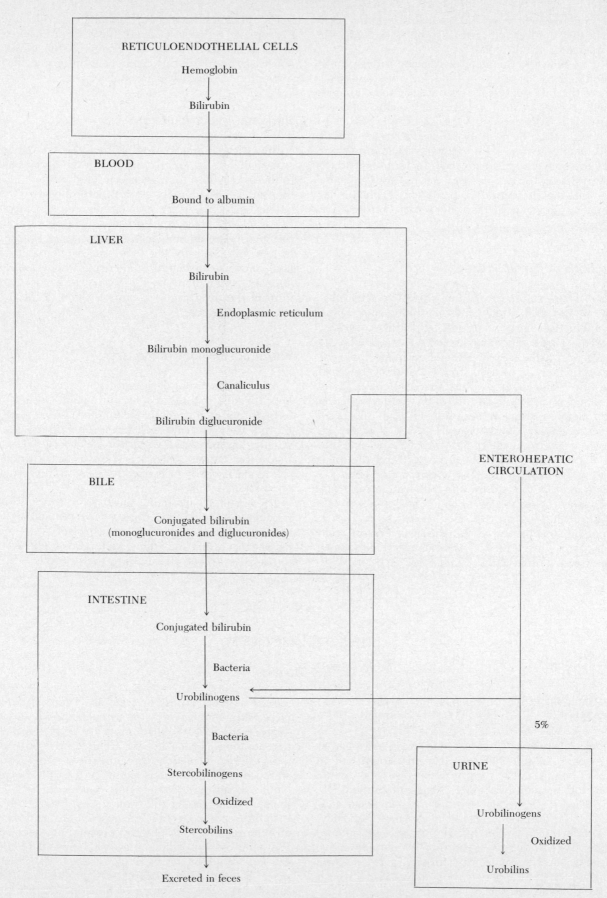

Figure 54–2. Metabolism and excretion of bilirubin.

now somewhat controversial, as it has recently been shown that the fraction could also be associated with the transport of bile salts.[6, 7]

The volume and the electrolyte composition of bile is modified by secretion of fluid from the epithelial cells of the bile ductules. The ductular secretion has a high concentration of bicarbonate ions, and its secretion is stimulated by the gastrointestinal hormone secretin.[39] Secretin is released from the wall of the duodenum when acids enter the small intestine.[92] The bicarbonate neutralizes the acid in the intestine. This mechanism helps protect the intestinal mucosa from the irritant effects of acids and maintains an optimum intestinal pH for the activity of digestive enzymes.

Functions of the Gallbladder

There is a reciprocal relationship between contractions of the gallbladder and the sphincter of Oddi: the sphincter relaxes when the gallbladder contracts, and *vice versa*. The major stimulus to gallbladder contraction is the gastrointestinal hormone cholecystokinin, which is released from the wall of the small intestine when ingesta enters the duodenum.[92] The presence of fats and fat digestion products in the duodenum is a major stimulus for the release of cholecystokinin. Contraction of the gallbladder increases pressure in the biliary tract to expel bile into the duodenum, where the bile salts and phospholipids promote digestion and absorption of fats.

The gallbladder stores bile between meals. The gallbladder concentrates organic compounds in bile by absorbing water and electrolytes.[31, 123] Rise in osmolality of bile and precipitation of organic compounds are prevented by formation of micelles, small aggregates of bile salts, cholesterol, and phospholipids. Micelles have a hydrophobic interior and a hydrophilic exterior, allowing them to be dispersed in solution. The hydrophilic groups in the micelles ionize at the pH of bile, and coalition of micelles is prevented by electrostatic repulsion.

Enterohepatic Circulation

Bile salts are transported to the intestine, actively reabsorbed in the ileum, and pass in the portal blood to the liver where they are re-secreted into bile. The bile salt pool undergoes several enterohepatic circulations each day; during each circulation, small quantities of bile salts escape reabsorption and are lost in the feces. The amount lost is replaced by synthesis of new bile salts by the liver, so that the bile salt pool remains constant.[122] Some drugs undergo enterohepatic circulation. If this occurs with the active form of the drug, the duration of action of the drug may be prolonged.[103]

Vascular Functions of the Liver

About 30 per cent of the cardiac output enters the liver through the portal veins and hepatic artery. Up to eight per cent of the blood volume can be present in the sinusoids and hepatic veins.[51] Sympathetic stimulation associated with exercise, acute stress, or blood loss causes vasoconstriction in the liver, and the blood in the liver is quickly added to the general circulation.

The Kupffer cells lining the hepatic sinusoids are reticuloendothelial cells; they remove particulate material from the blood. They are especially important for phagocytosing and killing bacteria that gain access to the portal blood stream from the intestine.

Surgical Diseases

Richard Walshaw

PORTAL CIRRHOSIS, HYPERTENSION, AND ASCITES

Portal hypertension is a manifestation of a number of diseases of the liver and its circulation and, in human beings, is the complication of hepatic disease that most frequently requires surgical treatment.[84]

In the dog and cat, cirrhosis is seen as an end-stage liver problem, usually of unknown etiology. Viral infections, chronic biliary tract disease, autoimmunity, an ill-defined syndrome of chronic active hepatitis, nutritional factors, toxicity, and long-term drug administration may all be implicated in cirrhosis in the dog and cat.[54]

Cirrhosis is characterized by the presence of widespread hepatic fibrosis or scarring. There is diffuse increase in connective tissue associated with varying degrees of necrosis and attempts at parenchymal cell regeneration. Normal hepatic architecture is lost, and a disordered formation of regenerative nodules separated by fibrous tissue is found. As a result, hepatic blood vessels are compressed and distorted. The hepatic veins, being thin-walled, are affected more than other components of the vasculature, and therefore hepatic venous outflow obstruction develops. Post-sinusoidal obstruction leads to sinusoidal hypertension, which in turn is reflected as an elevation in portal pressure and a decrease in portal blood flow to the liver. As disruption of hepatic integrity progresses, arteriovenous anastomoses develop between

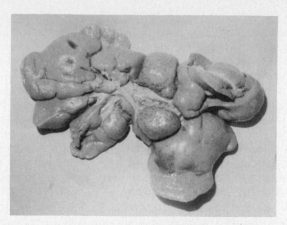

Figure 54–3. Cirrhotic liver from the dog illustrated in Fig. 54–4. The dog died of progressive liver failure and coagulopathy.

branches of the hepatic artery and portal vein, and contribute to the portal hypertension. These anastomoses plus sinusoidal hypertension can result in a reversal of blood flow in the portal vein; diversion of blood away from the hepatic parenchyma compromises nutrition of the liver cells (Fig. 54–3).[54, 84]

To relieve the portal hypertension, portosystemic collateral channels open up. These naturally occurring communicating channels have been well-studied in experimental portal hypertension in the dog and cat. Two major groups of vessels exist, the portoprecaval and portopostcaval systems. Only after portal hypertension develops do these vessels carry any significant blood flow.[54] It is these vessels, in human beings, that lead to the development of varicosities and subsequent hemorrhaging from the esophageal wall, which is associated with a high mortality rate.[84] Despite their large size, the portosystemic anastomoses are unable to accommodate the portal blood flow, and portal hypertension continues to exist. Bleeding esophageal varices do not exist in the dog and cat. The splenomegaly seen in human beings is not reported in the dog and cat either. Collateral omental anastomoses aid splenic venous outflow in these species.[54]

The end-result of progressive postsinusoidal outflow obstruction and continued portal hypertension is ascites. If portal hypertension is present but sinusoidal hypertension is not, ascites rarely develops. Experimentally ascites can be produced by any procedure that obstructs hepatic venous outflow. It does not occur, however, with obstruction of portal venous or arterial inflow. The ascitic fluid leaks from the surface and hilum of the liver, suggesting that it originates from an intrahepatic disturbance. Hepatic sinusoids are lined by discontinuous epithelium, and large gaps exist that permit nearly free passage of plasma proteins into the hepatic interstitium. Any increase in portal pressure results in a massive increase in fluid movement out of the sinusoids and into the hepatic lymphatics. When the carrying capacity of the lymphatics is exceeded, the liver weeps high-protein fluid into the abdominal cavity, producing ascites.[54, 84]

The pathogenesis of ascites is best explained by considering alterations in the Starling forces that operate across the capillary membranes and result from the hydrostatic pressure and oncotic pressure on each side of the membrane. Increased portal pressure is the primary mechanism for the formation of ascitic fluid. However, several other factors are involved, namely, hypoalbuminemia, the sodium ion, and aldosterone. The role that these factors play in the pathogenesis of ascites has only recently been fully evaluated. It is currently thought that increased intrahepatic pressure triggers a series of events that include leakage of fluid, increased secretion of aldosterone, and retention of salt by the kidney, all of which contribute to the formation and persistence of ascites.[54, 84]

Clinical Findings and Diagnosis

Cirrhosis is manifested clinically as impaired liver function, jaundice, portal hypertension, and ascites. It is a chronic insidious problem that slowly becomes clinically noticeable over weeks or months. Weight loss, abdominal enlargement due to ascites, anorexia, polydipsia, polyuria, depression, and lethargy are noted. Rarely, more dramatic signs of hepatic encephalopathy are seen (Fig. 54–4).[54, 110]

Diagnosis of cirrhosis is based on biochemical evidence of impaired liver function, radiographic findings, and liver biopsy results.

If a continuing hepatic inflammatory process is present, serum alanine aminotransferase (ALT) and alkaline phosphatase (AP) concentrations are significantly elevated. However, in advanced cirrhosis, enzyme elevations may be minimal, presumably because few residual hepatocytes remain. An elevation of serum bilirubin concentration is found inconsistently and depends upon the location of the lesion within the liver. Hypoalbuminemia is often found in cirrhotic patients.

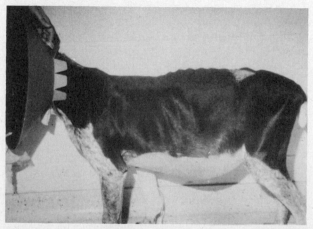

Figure 54–4. Female German shorthaired pointer with emaciation and intractable ascites due to advanced cirrhosis.

Bromsulphalein (BSP) retention is consistently increased in patients with cirrhosis, probably reflecting altered hepatic blood flow. Results of ammonia tolerance tests, however, are usually normal if there are no cerebral signs. If encephalopathy is present, the ammonia tolerance test result is often abnormal.

Radiographs of the abdomen reveal a small liver with an irregular outline, generally reflecting the progressive fibrosis and scar tissue contraction with loss of liver parenchyma.

Histopathological examination of liver biopsy samples confirms the diagnosis of cirrhosis. Biopsy techniques for the liver are described later in this chapter.[54]

Management of Cirrhosis, Portal Hypertension, and Ascites

Because the etiology of cirrhosis is unknown in the dog and cat in practically all cases, it is difficult to devise specific therapy that might slow down or prevent progression of the disease. Cases are frequently presented in an advanced stage, in which loss of liver function is considerable. Therefore, treatment usually involves symptomatic and supportive care.

If hepatic encephalopathy is present, supportive care and dietary adjustments should be instituted as outlined in Chapter 79. No specific drug therapy is effective in preventing progression of the disease. Glucocorticoids have some possible beneficial effect in controlling chronic active hepatitis, if this is still present.[54, 109] However, exact dosage recommendations for treating hepatic failure patients have not been established for animals.[54]

There has been considerable experimental interest in drugs that control or even reverse the fibrosis that occurs in chronic liver disease and cirrhosis. In cirrhosis, it is clear that collagen synthesis is greatly increased in the liver, resulting in severe fibrosis. There appears to be a point at which hepatic fibrosis becomes a self-perpetuating process, even if etiologic agents are removed. Immunological factors may play an important role in this progressive liver destruction. A number of drugs have been investigated in humans and experimental animals as modifiers of the progressive fibrosis. Colchicine, penicillamine, TECA-Medecassol, and L-azetidine-carboxylic acid have shown promise as antifibrosis agents in the liver. However, there are no reports of the clinical use of these agents in the dog and cat.[54]

Generally, a nourishing, well-balanced diet should be fed to dogs and cats with chronic liver failure. The diet should provide adequate quantities of carbohydrates, fats, and proteins. The protein should be fed to increase availability, in order to prevent the breakdown of body protein for energy and the development of hepatic encephalopathy. Extensive descriptions of the dietary management of dogs and cats with hepatic failure are available.[54, 110]

Controlling portal hypertension and ascites can be difficult. In those cases in which treatment of the ascites is considered necessary, therapy is directed at reducing its severity by either pharmacological or mechanical means. It is also essential that measures be taken simultaneously to help improve hepatic function. Different methods of controlling ascites formation and encouraging its elimination include the use of low-sodium diets, diuretics, and paracentesis, and the construction of portocaval or peritoneovenous shunts. Low-sodium diets are used successfully in human beings and, alone, control ascites in a small percentage of cases. Sodium restriction has to be severe and may require the use of home-formulated foods rather than commercially available ones.[54, 110]

If sodium restriction alone is insufficient to control the ascites, distal tubular diuretics, such as spironolactone, that interfere with aldosterone activity may be used. The dose of spironolactone may have to be titrated, as it takes three to four days for this drug to be effective. If these methods are ineffective, powerful "loop" diuretics may be used, such as furosemide and ethacrynic acid. Sodium retention in hepatic ascites occurs at both proximal and distal sites along the nephron, thereby making the loop diuretics very successful at counteracting sodium resorption. Again, diuretic dosage is titrated according to clinical response, and with the loop diuretics, potassium loss is closely followed. Diruetic therapy should result not in dehydration of the patient but in the slow reduction of the amount of ascites present. Serum electrolyte concentrations should be followed closely, and measures taken to correct electrolyte imbalances. If dehydration occurs, it should be promptly corrected and the dose of diuretic suitably adjusted. Although this regimen is successful in the great majority of cases, a small percentage of cases are refractory to salt restriction and diuretics.[54, 110] For these patients, more aggressive, invasive measures should be undertaken.

Paracentesis to remove large quantities of ascitic fluid should be avoided, because the ascitic fluid reforms rapidly. The removal of large volumes of ascitic fluid depletes plasma proteins in a patient that is likely to be hypoproteinemic initially. The synthesis of albumin is severely compromised in these patients and therefore cannot keep up with protein loss. If dyspnea is present or cardiac return is impeded by the intra-abdominal pressure, paracentesis may be indicated. However, it should be limited to as small a volume as possible. Other potential complications include peritonitis, hypovolemia, hepatic coma, and oliguria. Paracentesis can be combined with plasma volume reexpansion, by aseptically collecting the abdominal fluid and infusing it intravenously. This approach, along with diuretic therapy, maximizes the benefits of albumin reinfusion and helps return plasma protein concentrations to normal. This procedure is involved, and complications may follow the repeated collection of abdominal fluid. It can be performed on a continuing basis by an implantable peritoneovenous shunt, as described later.[54, 110]

Because increased hydrostatic pressure within the liver is important in the pathogenesis of ascites, it should be possible to reduce ascites formation by reducing intrahepatic pressure. Decompression of the hepatic vascular bed may be achieved either by reducing the inflow of blood to the liver or by increasing the outflow of blood from it. Improving the outflow of blood from the liver is not possible because of the cirrhosis. Inflow-reducing procedures include hepatic artery ligation and the creation of portacaval shunts. Hepatic artery ligation is no longer used in humans as a means of achieving inflow control, because it is unpredictable and has a high mortality.[84]

Inflow restriction is more easily achieved by portacaval shunts. In humans, the side-to-side portacaval shunt is the most effective in relieving ascites, overcoming intrahepatic hypertension, eliminating the hypersecretion of aldosterone that follows hepatic outflow occlusion, and reducing the markedly increased thoracic duct lymph flow to normal. End-to-side portacaval anastomoses are much less effective. Following shunt creation, human patients have relief of ascites, and a notable improvement in nutritional status and vigor, with gains in lean tissue mass and body fat.[84] This surgical procedure, however, carries significant risk in a patient with hepatic failure; because even more blood is shunted away from the liver, and hepatic encephalopathy may be seen. Therefore intensive and supportive care of these patients during the operative period is required to overcome these significant complications. There is a report[44] but no published series of this procedure in the dog or cat.

A system of continuously removing ascitic fluid from the abdomen and infusing it intravenously in cirrhotic patients has been devised (the LeVeen shunt). It consists of a pressure-sensitive, one-way valve that is implanted in the abdominal wall. Perforated silicone rubber tubing connected to one side of the valve is inserted into the abdomen to drain the ascitic fluid. Silicone rubber tubing from the other side of its valve is tunneled subcutaneously to the cervical region, where it is inserted into the jugular vein and the end is advanced to lie in the anterior vena cava. The valve is designed so that when intra-abdominal pressure is approximately 3 cm H_2O higher than central venous pressure, because of the accumulating ascitic fluid, the valve opens and the fluid flows into the venous system. The valve closes when this pressure gradient is lost and maintains a blood-ascitic fluid interface at the open tip of the venous tubing, preventing entry of blood into the tubing and therefore preventing occlusion due to clot formation (Fig. 54–5).[66, 84]

Recently an extensive review of the use of peritoneovenous shunting for the correction of ascites has

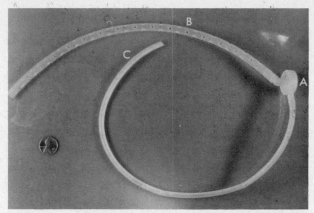

Figure 54–5. The LeVeen peritoneovenous shunt. *A*, pressure-sensitive one-way valve; *B*, perforated abdominal drain; *C*, venous tubing.

been published.[66] The procedure was developed initially in the dog in experimentally created ascites models.[64] Implantation of the peritoneovenous shunt in patients with massive ascites, when combined with vigorous diuretic therapy, often results in the movement of large quantities of fluid from the peritoneal cavity into the circulatory system. Diuresis and natriuresis accompany this fluid movement. In addition, a striking increase in plasma volume, hemodilution, increases in cardiac output and renal plasma flow, and a decrease in plasma renin and aldosterone are noted.[84] There are certain contraindications to shunt placement in ascitic patients, including severe encephalopathy, hepatic coma, jaundice, peritonitis, and serious bleeding diathesis.[37] Significant complications have occurred in humans with the use of peritoneovenous shunts, including local infection, systemic sepsis, coagulopathies, severe electrolyte disorders (hypokalemia), leakage of ascitic fluid, bowel obstruction, congestive heart failure, pulmonary edema, vena cava thrombosis, and air embolism. Also in human beings, esophageal variceal bleeding is seen following shunt placement owing to increased portal venous pressure. Encephalopathy and liver failure also occur.

The techniques for the surgical placement of the shunt in humans and dogs have been well described.[64–66] I have used a LeVeen shunt in one dog with end-stage cirrhosis of the liver to help control intractable ascites (Fig. 54–6). The ascites rapidly resolved, and continued shunt function resulted in no reaccumulation of the fluid (Fig. 54–7). The dog, however, succumbed to progressive liver failure and coagulopathy two months after shunt placement. At this time the shunt was still patent and functioning well. The main problems with the use of peritoneovenous shunting in the dog are the late stage at which cirrhosis is often diagnosed (very little functional liver tissue remains) and the high cost of the LeVeen shunt.

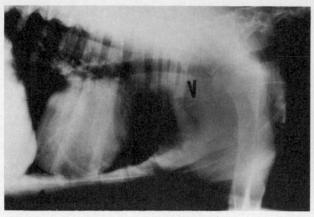
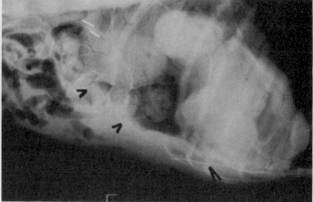

Figure 54–6. Lateral thoracic and abdominal radiographs of dog shown in Fig. 54–4 following placement of LeVeen peritoneovenous shunt. The arrows indicate the path of the shunt from the anterior vena cava to the abdominal cavity.

Prognosis

The prognosis for patients with cirrhosis, portal hypertension, and ascites is poor. Long-term survival is unlikely. However, through institution of aggressive medical management, the problems associated with this syndrome can be minimized and a good quality of life achieved. Surgical intervention, either portacaval shunting or peritoneovenous shunting, should be reserved for those cases resistant to medical management. If surgical intervention is indicated, it should be attempted at an early stage before irreversible liver failure is present. The surgical procedures are associated with significant morbidity and mortality and should not be undertaken lightly.

TRAUMA

Patients with blunt abdominal injuries are often managed in a conservative fashion. Major hemorrhage, due to disruption of solid viscera, or leakage of the contents of a hollow viscus, due to tearing, are indications for surgery.

The liver is the most commonly injured intra-abdominal organ in blunt trauma, such as motor vehicle accidents in which the abdomen is struck laterally. This high incidence of liver injury is probably related to the large size of the organ and its relative friability and immobility.[60, 61]

Blunt abdominal trauma results in acute compression of the liver against the axial skeleton.[4, 5] Transmission of massive pressures to the intra-abdominal viscera causes explosive injuries of the liver. Fracturing and tearing of the parenchyma and capsule are seen, particularly at the relatively more free, caudal aspects of the liver lobes, as compared with the

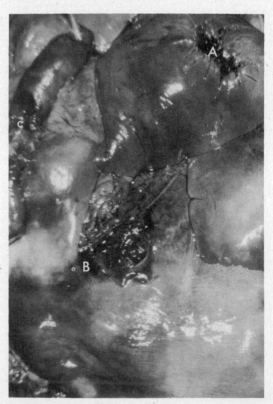

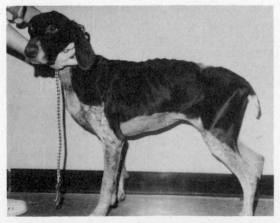

Figure 54–7. Dog shown in Fig. 54–4 a few days following placement of the LeVeen peritoneovenous shunt. There has been complete resolution of the ascites.

Figure 54–8. Necropsy photograph of a dog with multiple abdominal visceral injuries following a gunshot wound. The liver (*A*), stomach (*B*), and small intestine (*C*) have been traumatized.

relatively fixed hilum. These injuries are probably the result of excessive displacement of the free portions. Contusions of the main body of the liver occur as it is compressed on impact. Rarely, fractured or displaced ribs may penetrate and lacerate the liver parenchyma.[60, 68]

Severe blunt abdominal trauma can result in avulsion of hepatic veins or in tearing of the vena cava owing to its relatively fixed position. In these instances fatal hemorrhage usually occurs.[5, 84]

Injury to the extrahepatic biliary system from blunt abdominal trauma is relatively rare.[5, 60, 85] However, as great shearing forces are generated, together with an increase in intraductal pressure due to liver displacement on impact, avulsion of the extrahepatic biliary tree may occur.[60] Avulsion usually occurs close to the duodenum, with resultant bile leakage and the development of peritonitis. The bile leakage that results from liver parenchymal damage is insignificant and self-limiting.

Penetrating abdominal injuries frequently require a more aggressive approach. Multiple viscera are often involved, particularly when the injury is associated with a gunshot wound (Fig. 54–8). Gunshot injuries may result in severe shattering of the liver substance and multiple severe lacerations, particularly when the bullet is of high velocity or large caliber (Fig. 54–9).[68] Frequently the liver is traversed by the bullet as it penetrates other abdominal and possibly thoracic organs. Similarly, the extrahepatic biliary system may be disrupted by penetrating abdominal trauma, possibly resulting in severing of the bile ducts or rupturing of the gallbladder. In human beings, penetrating abdominal trauma makes up the bulk of extrahepatic biliary injuries. Penetrating trauma in this instance includes iatrogenically induced injury due to needle biopsies.[85]

The liver is frequently found in the thoracic cavity in association with a traumatic diaphragmatic hernia. Although the traumatic episode and the diaphragmatic hernia rarely cause any acute hepatic problems, chronic entrapment of the liver in the thorax leads to pleural effusion owing to hepatic congestion. The animal with chronic diaphragmatic hernia is frequently presented because of increasing respiratory problems due to this effusion.

There are two reports of bile pleuritis developing secondary to liver trauma and a small diaphragmatic tear. These two dogs, one injured by a motor vehicle accident and one by a gunshot wound, were presented several days following trauma because of the accumulation of fluid within the thoracic cavity. In both cases the traumatized liver had become adherent to a small hole in the diaphragm and had subsequently leaked bile into the pleural cavity.[9, 94]

It has been reported that following liver trauma, the development of septicemia and toxemia owing to the proliferation of aerobic and anaerobic bacteria (Clostridia) harbored in the dog's liver may be a severe threat to life.[4, 5] It is my opinion that, although it may be possible to demonstrate such problems experimentally, they are not clinically significant.

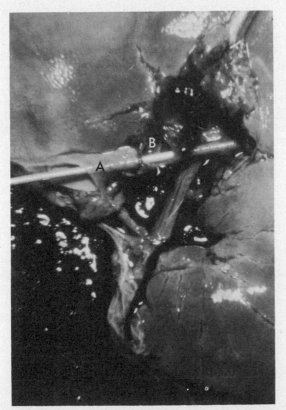

Figure 54–9. Severe liver trauma following a gunshot wound. The vena cava *(A)* and hepatic veins *(B)* have been shattered along with the adjacent hepatic parenchyma.

History

Questions that should be asked include a description of the traumatic episode, if seen, the interval since the injury occurred, the presence or absence of urination prior to or following the accident, whether the animal can walk, whether vomiting has occurred, and whether the animal is demonstrating any difficulty in breathing. Also, it should be determined whether blood was noted in the vomit, feces, or urine.

Few historical signs relate directly to liver injury. However, observation of how the animal was shot or how it was hit by a motor vehicle may make one more suspicious of cranial abdominal injury.[5] Rapid deterioration of the animal's condition after trauma with a noticeably enlarging abdomen may indicate severe intra-abdominal hemorrhage.

Historical findings related to disruption of the biliary system usually take several days or even weeks to become apparent. Generally, affected patients are seen to become progressively more depressed, and to develop anorexia, vomiting, weight loss, and possibly an enlarging abdomen. The owner may notice the development of icterus. If bile pleuritis also occurs, progressive dyspnea will be noted.[9, 11, 94]

Clinical Findings

Clinical examination of any trauma victim should be rapid and thorough. A code for rating the severity of injury sustained by a trauma victim has been established in veterinary medicine, and it is on this basis that trauma patients should be evaluated and treated.[61] Abdominal trauma is in the severe (life-threatening) category and may be fatal within or after 24 hours, depending upon the degree of injury.[61] Liver trauma with signs of hypovolemia due to hemorrhage is life-threatening.

Immediate clinical findings associated with liver injury are related to the amount of blood loss. The majority of animals in which minor lacerations of the hepatic parenchyma are found have no findings directly referable to liver damage. Cranial abdominal pain may be detected, and the animal may assume a tucked-up stance. If a penetrating injury is present, an attempt should be made to assess the direction, depth, and possible extent of the injury.[4, 5] With more extensive liver damage, severe hemorrhage may occur that is detected as an enlarging, fluid-filled abdomen with signs of hypovolemic shock due to blood loss.[4, 5]

Clinical findings related to extrahepatic biliary damage may not become evident for several days or even weeks following the traumatic episode. In these cases, anorexia, depression, icterus, abdominal distension, and the passage of acholic feces indicate the possibility of major biliary leakage. Usually the animal stabilizes following the initial trauma, only to develop these signs at a later date.[4, 5, 11, 94] In other instances biliary system damage is discovered during surgical exploration of the abdomen for more acute problems. Clinical findings are generally related to the developing bile peritonitis and lack of bile entering the gastrointestinal tract. Leakage of bile into the thoracic cavity, due to intrahepatic bile duct rupture plus a diaphragmatic tear, should be considered if a pleural effusion develops.[9]

With cranial abdominal trauma significant enough to cause clinical findings related to liver or extrahepatic biliary system damage, a careful assessment of the thoracic cavity should be made to establish the extent of thoracic organ damage, including a thorough evaluation of diaphragmatic integrity.

Laboratory Evaluation

Hematology

The abnormalities in the hemogram in the acute liver trauma patient reflect blood loss. Early in the clinical course, the hematocrit and hemoglobin values may be normal. If exsanguinating hemorrhage is occurring, there will be no change in the hematocrit. Severe hemorrhage with auto-hemodilution, however, results in a falling hematocrit.[5, 84] The white blood cell count can be elevated, with significant neutrophilia.[84] In chronic cases, with bile peritonitis, an anemia may be present that may or may not be regenerative. A marked neutrophilia is seen, owing to stress and peritonitis.[11, 94]

Serum Biochemistry

Liver function tests rarely provide useful information during the initial 12-hour period, when the clinical diagnosis must be made.[84] However, if liver damage has existed for some time, serum AP and ALT concentrations are increased considerably.[5] If extrahepatic biliary disruption is present, hyperbilirubinemia is found. The conjugated fraction may show the greatest increase, indicating posthepatic biliary leakage, but high concentrations of unconjugated bilirubin may also be seen, possibly owing to reduced hepatic uptake in the presence of high concentrations of conjugated bilirubin resorbed from the peritoneal cavity. Bilirubinuria will also be found.[94]

There may also be other abnormalities related to hypovolemia or the subsequent development of bile peritonitis, such as alterations in BUN, creatinine, and electrolyte concentrations.[11, 94]

Abdominal Paracentesis

The technique of abdominal paracentesis and lavage has been well described.[25, 59] In humans, this technique is one of the most helpful diagnostic procedures for assessing serious intra-abdominal organ damage, having a high degree of accuracy.[84]

When one is considering liver injury, easily obtained free nonclotting blood in the abdominal cavity indicates significant hemorrhage.[84] It is possible to use this test in a quantitative fashion to try to estimate the amount of blood loss into the abdominal cavity.[25] Hemoperitoneum itself is not an indication for surgical exploration, because it can be found in most abdominal trauma patients. However, its presence, together with clinical deterioration following suitable supportive care plus the decline in hematocrit and hemoglobin values may indicate continued excessive intra-abdominal hemorrhage that requires surgical intervention.

If free bile is present in the abdominal cavity, as in extrahepatic biliary disruption, the fluid is typically turbid and green to dark brown and tests highly positive for bilirubin with Ictotest tablets. The fluid has a moderately high white cell count, consisting of mainly mature neutrophils, because it is usually sterile and severe inflammation and suppuration are not present. In microscopic examination of smears from the sediment obtained from the fluid, active mesothelial cells are also seen, these again being associated with sterile inflammation. Many macrophages are found, both of monocytic and mesothelial origin. These cells frequently contain bile pigment.

A yellow-brown granular sediment is seen throughout the smear.[11, 25, 94]

Radiological Findings

Generally, radiographic examination of the abdominal cavity of liver trauma patients provides little information, except for the presence of fluid (blood). Fractures of the caudal ribs, together with clinical findings, may suggest liver damage.[4, 5, 84] If so, a careful radiographic evaluation of the thoracic cavity and diaphragm should be performed to rule out significant thoracic injury or a diaphragmatic hernia. If the diaphragm cannot be clearly identified on plain radiographs, and there is not too much free fluid in the abdominal or thoracic cavities, a celiogram helps determine the integrity of the diaphragm.[109] If significant fluid is present in the thoracic cavity, it is removed to enable assessment of the diaphragm.

In patients with gunshot wounds, the radiographic position of the bullet, together with the position of the entrance wound, may indicate which abdominal organs have been injured. If the bullet has also exited from the body, the assessment of its path through the abdomen together with radiographic findings might aid preoperative evaluation of visceral damage.

In other instances, radiographic findings of other intra-abdominal organ damage may lead to exploratory surgery, at which time liver trauma is diagnosed. Similarly, radiographic examination of the patient with bile peritonitis is likely to result in little confirmatory information, except the presence of fluid in the abdominal cavity.[4, 5, 11, 94]

Diagnosis

In blunt trauma, the diagnosis of liver damage is suspected when historical and clinical evidence of cranial abdominal trauma exists and abdominal paracentesis reveals non-clotting blood. The diagnosis is rarely confirmed in the dog and the cat, because the majority of blunt abdominal injuries do not require exploratory surgery. Liver trauma is confirmed when exploratory surgery is required for other traumatic injuries, e.g., to the urinary or digestive system, or when unrelenting intra-abdominal hemorrhage requires surgical correction.

Penetrating abdominal trauma, in comparison, frequently results in exploratory surgery. Liver damage is identified as the abdominal contents are carefully examined. Trauma to the extrahepatic biliary system, whether due to blunt or penetrating injury, can be more specifically diagnosed prior to exploratory surgery. Historical and clinical findings, together with elevations of serum ALT, AP, and bilirubin levels, should arouse suspicion of such damage. Diagnosis of bile peritonitis is confirmed by abdominal paracentesis with biochemical and microscopic examination of the fluid obtained. In such cases, surgical exploration of the abdomen confirms the diagnosis.

Treatment

Treatment of liver parenchymal trauma depends upon the nature and extent of the injury. The majority of dogs and cats who have suffered liver parenchymal injury require stabilization, supportive care, and treatment of other injuries. Rarely does liver trauma require specific therapy such as emergency surgical intervention.

Management of the trauma patient should be based on a priority system to treat life-threatening injuries first. Therefore attention is first paid to the cardiovascular and respiratory systems.[61] Intra-abdominal hemorrhage, which may be the major cause of the instability of the cardiovascular system, is treated aggressively with the use of intravenous fluid therapy to correct the hypovolemia. Monitoring the patient's packed cell volume and total solids, along with other parameters such as central venous pressure and urine output, allows assessment of the hypovolemia and continued blood loss into the abdomen. Blood transfusions may be required in addition to the crystalloid fluid, if blood loss is considerable as judged by the falling hematocrit and total solids values and inability to correct the hypovolemia.

In the majority of dogs and cats that have suffered liver damage due to either blunt or penetrating trauma, the hemorrhage from the damaged liver surfaces ceases with supportive care. If surgical exploration is undertaken for other reasons once the animal is stable, the liver injuries will not be actively bleeding. Continued intra-abdominal hemorrhage in the face of aggressive supportive care indicates major vascular disruption and the need for surgical intervention. Such injuries include damage to the hilar structures of the liver, hepatic vein avulsion, and major hepatic lobe avulsion.

If surgical exploration is warranted, the patient should be stabilized as rapidly and completely as possible prior to the induction of anesthesia. Broad-spectrum prophylactic antibiotic therapy is provided because the extent of injury is unknown preoperatively, particularly in penetrating abdominal trauma, in which multiple visceral injuries may exist.

Once the abdomen has been opened, the blood removed, and the liver exposed, an attempt is made to identify the source of the hemorrhage and achieve rapid, if only temporary, control of it. A tear of the vena cava can be temporarily controlled by occluding the vena cava cranial and caudal to the liver or by partially occluding it with a suitable vascular clamp. In addition, temporary occlusion of hepatic vascular inflow reduces the hemorrhage. The vena cava can only be occluded for short intervals (less than 15 minutes) without causing severe hypotension. Therefore, either partial or intermittent occlusion should be used. Repair of the vena cava should be undertaken as rapidly as possible if it is feasible.[4, 5, 84]

Hepatic vein avulsion should be recognized promptly. Besides leading to exsanguination, this injury and vena caval tearing can lead to air embolism.[84] Vena cava occlusion and hepatic vascular inflow occlusion are used to identify and repair the vascular damage. Occlusion of the hepatic artery and portal vein is helpful in controlling hemorrhage while repairing massive liver injuries.[4, 5, 17, 84] Vascular occlusion is tolerated for 20 minutes at normal body temperatures in humans. This period can be extended by using hypothermia and also by using intermittent occlusion.[84] Repair of the avulsed hepatic veins can be undertaken in a controlled manner.

Hemorrhage from severely traumatized liver lobes is temporarily stopped by direct pressure until hemorrhage is controlled. Temporary occlusion of the portal vein and main hepatic artery may be necessary in order to identify the site of damage.[17, 84] Arterial hemorrhage should be controlled before venous hemorrhage. Arterial hemorrhage can be controlled by direct ligation of damaged vessels within the traumatized lobe or by ligation of the main hepatic artery supplying that lobe. If adequate portal blood flow and normovolemia are maintained and the patient is well-oxygenated, ligation of major branches of the hepatic artery is a safe procedure that does not result in extensive hepatic necrosis. Venous hemorrhage is similarly controlled.

If hemorrhage continues or it is impossible to perform the foregoing procedures, lobectomy is indicated to control the hemorrhage and remove the injured tissue.[4, 5, 17, 84]

Liver parenchymal damage should be carefully examined, once the major hemorrhage has been controlled. Devitalized tissue is removed to prevent delayed necrosis, possible infection, and late hemorrhage. Many lacerations or penetrating wounds of the parenchyma do not require debriding or suturing providing that they are not actively bleeding.[4, 5, 17, 45]

There is considerable controversy regarding the advisability or necessity of closing larger defects of the liver parenchyma.[4, 5, 17, 45] It is difficult to approximate the edges of such defects with sutures, owing to the lack of significant capsule in the liver of the dog and cat and to the friability of the parenchyma. In addition, closure of such defects can lead to continued intrahepatic bleeding and therefore hematoma formation, with subsequent necrosis and abscess formation. It is better to leave such defects open. The hepatic area can be drained if continued hemorrhage or bile leakage occurs from the traumatized parenchyma. There is even controversy about the need for routine use of such drainage techniques. The use of indwelling sponges or gauze packing of defects is to be avoided because of the potential for complications such as abscess.[17, 45, 85]

If parenchymal damage is significant, with possible involvement of major ducts or vessels, partial or total lobectomy is the treatment of choice. Tube drainage of the extrahepatic biliary system to provide biliary decompression, and thus to reduce bile leakage from the damaged parenchyma, cannot be recommended. Tube drainage does not decrease intrahepatic biliary pressure or reduce bile leakage. Such procedures are associated with considerable morbidity in humans.[84]

A thorough exploration of the abdomen should be performed, once hemorrhage has been brought under control, particularly with penetrating injuries, in which multiple organs may have been damaged. The integrity of the diaphragm should also be assessed. The abdominal cavity should be thoroughly lavaged with copious volumes of warm saline to remove all debris and blood clots prior to closure.

Treatment of extrahepatic biliary disruption requires either surgical repair of or diversion proximal to the area of trauma and bile leakage. As there is probably significant bile peritonitis by the time this problem is diagnosed, preoperative patient stabilization is usually necessary to alleviate the poor condition of the patient. Electrolyte imbalances and dehydration are corrected with appropriate intravenous electrolyte solutions. Significant anemia, possibly nonregenerative, and hypoproteinemia may be present, requiring either blood or plasma transfusions. In patients with bile peritonitis, bile salts cause hemolysis and may be fibrinolytic. Hemorrhage may be a complicating factor during treatment and again may require the use of fresh blood transfusions.[11, 94]

Although uncomplicated bile peritonitis is usually sterile, prophylactic broad-spectrum antibiotic therapy should be instituted. There are anaerobic bacteria (Clostridia) present in the liver of the dog that could possibly contaminate the peritoneal cavity via the leaking bile, but such a possibility has not been demonstrated clinically.[11, 94] Tissue damage caused by peritonitis and other traumatic lesions warrants antibiotic coverage.

When the abdomen is opened, the abdominal fluid is removed. Careful retraction of the duodenum and stomach caudally and the liver cranially exposes the extrahepatic biliary system. An assessment should be made of its integrity and the site of leakage should be identified. Bile duct disruption usually occurs close to its entrance into the duodenum. Small tears in the gallbladder can usually be repaired by primary suturing. However, larger disruptions are better treated by cholecystectomy.[5, 17, 85]

Many methods have been described for repair of tears or transections of the common bile duct in humans, although there are few reports of such techniques in veterinary surgery. Procedures used for repair of common bile duct injuries include primary suturing and anastomosis, T-tube or Y-tube repair, cholecystoenterostomy, reimplantation of the bile duct, seromuscular patch grafting, and the use of indwelling polyethylene catheters. Many of these procedures are technically difficult to perform because of the small diameter of the common duct in the dog or cat.[11, 94] The one technique that can be universally applied, because the diameter of the common duct is not a problem, is cholecystoenterostomy, usually cholecystoduodenostomy. This procedure, when performed correctly, is successful in the dog.[113] Reports in humans describe serious ascending infections and cholangitis with this technique.[104] These complications do not occur when cholecystoenterostomy is used in the dog.[113]

Following repair of the traumatized bile duct, the abdomen should be thoroughly lavaged with warm saline to remove debris, bile, and blood. Bile salts are soluble in saline. Copious quantities of saline are required to clean the abdomen.[11] As bile peritonitis is usually sterile, its resolution following repair should be uncomplicated. Cultures may be taken from the abdominal cavity at surgery. Drainage of the area of the gallbladder and bile duct is not indicated unless necessitated by other injuries.

Treatment of peritonitis is discussed in Chapter 44. In bile peritonitis, open peritoneal drainage may be used for up to 72 hours postoperatively to treat severe peritonitis following operative lavage.[113]

Following intra-abdominal operative procedures, a loose simple continuous suture of a monofilament nonabsorbable material, such as polypropylene, is placed in the body wall. The edges of the body wall incision are allowed to gape approximately two to three centimeters. No attempt is made to close the subcutaneous tissue or skin. A sterile, nonadherent dressing, such as sterile petroleum jelly gauze, is placed over the incision, followed by sterile absorbent dressings. A pad of cotton is placed over the ventral abdominal area. The dressings are held in place by routine bandage materials. The bandage is changed as frequently as necessary depending upon the amount of drainage. By about 48 to 72 hours postoperatively, drainage is minimal and is a clear serosanguineous fluid. At this time, providing that the patient is stable, the animal can be returned to the operating room and the abdomen closed.

During open peritoneal drainage, the animal should be monitored closely for hypovolemia, hypoproteinemia, and electrolyte disturbances.

Postoperative Care and Recovery

Recovery is rapid in the majority of cases. Blunt trauma to the liver parenchyma in the dog and cat rarely leads to complications during the recovery phase.

Additional supportive care should consist of continuation of postoperative antibiotic therapy, until the patient is stable and perihepatic drains have been removed. Oral feeding is begun as soon as possible. If drains were placed around liver parenchymal damage, these should be removed once drainage becomes minimal and is bile-free (usually in three to four days). While in place, the drains should be protected by sterile dressings, and postoperative antibiotic therapy should be continued. The drains can usually be removed in three to four days. Rarely are T-tubes or

Y-tubes used in veterinary surgery. However, if they have been used in bile duct repair, they should also be protected with sterile dressings. These tubes are usually removed in ten to 14 days.[11, 56] With extrahepatic biliary system disruption and subsequent bile peritonitis, extensive postoperative care is usually required. Uncomplicated bile peritonitis usually resolves without complication.

Hematological and serum biochemistry evaluations are performed during the postoperative period. Regeneration of the anemia and a return to normal of the hypoproteinemia should occur as the bile peritonitis resolves. Electrolyte imbalances should return to normal with appropriate intravenous fluid and electrolyte therapy. Bilirubin concentrations return to normal levels as bile flow is re-established. Similarly the bilirubinuria should resolve. Serum concentrations of AP and ALT take a few weeks to return to normal, but a decline should be noted during the postoperative period, indicating a resolution of hepatic damage.[11, 94]

Intravenous fluid and electrolyte therapy is continued until the animal is able to maintain itself orally. If hypokalemia is present during the postoperative period, additional intravenous supplementation is required.

Prognosis

The prognosis for complete recovery following trauma to the liver is excellent. The determinants for complete recovery are rarely associated with the liver trauma itself unless massive injury such as hepatic vein avulsion has occurred. It is more likely that other injuries will determine whether successful recovery is possible. Liver failure as a direct result of uncomplicated hepatic trauma is extremely rare.[84]

With extrahepatic biliary trauma, complete recovery depends on early recognition of the problem, good supportive care of the patient, and technically accurate and successful surgical repair of the problem. Surgical failure, due to bile duct strictures or leaking suture lines, for example, is probably the most common complication. However, in extrahepatic biliary disruption with uncomplicated bile peritonitis, a successful outcome should be anticipated, providing that other injuries do not result in morbidity or mortality.

CHOLELITHIASIS

Cholelithiasis is rare in the dog; less than 30 cases have been reported.[12, 22, 34, 53, 71, 74, 77, 79, 87, 95–97, 99, 116, 119] It is even rarer in the cat.[83] The majority of reported cases in the dog were asymptomatic, and cholelithiasis was noted at necropsy or when the dogs were used for experimental surgical procedures (12 out of 9,600 dogs).[77] Symptomatic cases were associated with either choledocholithiasis or peritonitis secondary to erosion and perforation of the gallbladder due to chronic cholecystolithiasis. Only 25 per cent of recorded cases of cholelithiasis in the dog were symptomatic.[77]

An extensive review of the pathogenesis of human gallstones is available.[100] The pathogenesis of cholelithiasis in the dog and cat is not understood. Choleliths in the dog and cat contain many substances found in human gallstones, namely cholesterol, bilirubin, biliverdin, calcium, phosphate, oxalate, magnesium, iron, fibrin and bacteria.[77] The majority are not composed primarily of cholesterol, but accurate quantitative analysis of these stones is lacking. It is unlikely that choleliths in the dog contain as much cholesterol as do choleliths in human beings, because canine bile is much less saturated with cholesterol than is human bile.[78] In cholelithiasis reported in the veterinary literature, no attempt has been made to analyze the bile of these animals to determine the concentrations of cholesterol, bile salts, and lecithin. A number of the choleliths appeared to be pigment stones.[77] In one canine case, a negative bile culture was obtained, whereas bacteria were seen on examination of a cross-section of a cholelith from another dog.[12, 99] Experimentally in several laboratory animal species including the dog, dietary alterations have resulted in cholelithiasis. However, the diet that produces cholelithiasis in one species bears little resemblance to the diet that is effective in another.[99]

It is unlikely that a primary hepatic disorder resulting in the production of bile supersaturated with cholesterol (as in human cholesterol cholelithiasis) is a significant cause in the dog and cat. Whether problems resulting in bile stasis, recurrent inflammatory disease, or infection are involved in the etiology is uncertain.

The actual incidence of the disease in the dog and cat is also unknown. It is possible that many dogs and cats may have choleliths but are asymptomatic. Such is the case in human beings, and a significant number of the cases reported in animals were also asymptomatic. However, necropsy series reveal an extremely low incidence of this disease in the dog and cat and probably accurately reflect the true incidence.[77, 111]

History

Cholecystolithiasis may cause no symptoms.[34, 71, 79, 97, 116] If recurrent cholecystitis occurs or choledocholithiasis develops secondary to cholecystolithiasis, signs referable to obstructive disease of the biliary system are seen.[53, 83, 95, 97, 99]

Typical signs in symptomatic cases are depression, anorexia, vomiting, and diarrhea. The owner may notice icterus. Weight loss may also be seen with chronic or recurrent disease. Frequently, the patient has recurrent episodes of illness before the diagnosis of cholelithiasis is made, presumably related to recurrent obstruction of the biliary system and associated inflammatory disease.

Two cases have been reported in dogs in which the biliary system had perforated with cholelithiasis. These dogs were more severely depressed and had a more rapid clinical deterioration owing to developing peritonitis.[77, 95]

Clinical Findings

Although rare, cholelithiasis must be ruled out when clinical findings suggest obstructive icterus.

In symptomatic cases of cholelithiasis, clinical findings generally support the history. The patient may be depressed and dehydrated. The animal may be pyrexic at examination if active inflammatory disease or associated infection is present. Severely depressed animals may be hypothermic, and the mucous membranes and sclera are icteric. Cranial abdominal pain, and possibly liver enlargement, may be detected.[77, 83, 95, 99]

Laboratory Evaluations

Hematology

Probably the most significant abnormality in the hemogram is an elevated while blood cell count, associated with neutrophilia. It reflects the inflammatory disease and possible infection that is present. Anemia can also be seen in these cases.[53, 77, 83, 95, 99]

Serum Biochemistry

The most significant biochemical abnormalities are associated with abnormal hepatic function. Hyperbilirubinemia is present with a predominance of conjugated bilirubin. Elevation of serum AP concentrations sometimes occurs prior to the elevation of serum bilirubin concentrations and is associated with increased production of AP, hepatic necrosis, and lack of biliary secretion. Serum ALT concentrations are also elevated but often not as much as serum AP concentrations. The ratio of serum albumin to globulin may be altered because of abnormal liver function. Other abnormalities in the serum biochemistry evaluations may indicate dehydration, debilitation or other organ disease.[53, 77, 83, 95, 99] If icterus is marked, bilirubinuria may be found, with decreased levels of urobilinogen in the urine.

Radiological Findings

The preoperative diagnosis of cholelithiasis depends heavily upon radiological studies. Pure cholesterol stones are radiolucent, and pigment stones and mixed stones are variably radiopaque. In humans, only 20 to 30 per cent of choleliths are sufficiently

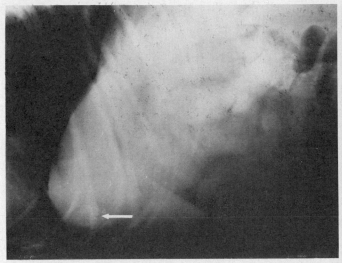

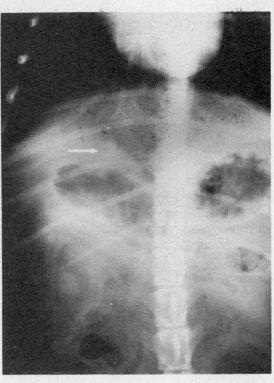

Figure 54–10. Lateral and ventrodorsal abdominal radiographs of a dog with asymptomatic cholecystolithiasis *(arrow).*

calcified to be apparent on plain radiographs.[99] Therefore plain radiography is not a highly successful method for diagnosis. Plain radiography has been diagnostic in both the dog and the cat in some cases.[77, 83, 95, 99] This difference may reflect the very low incidence of choleliths, with a high cholesterol content, and the greater incidence of mixed or pigment stones in the dog and cat. In these cases a radiodense mass was visible in the right cranial abdomen, adjacent to the liver and pylorus (Figs. 54–10 and 54–11).

Cholecystography and cholangiography using oral and intravenous contrast administration in the dog and cat have been reviewed.[2, 3, 19, 20, 81] Oral cholecystography produces radiographic opacification of the gallbladder by administration of an organic iodide-containing compound. The substance is absorbed from the intestine, excreted by the liver in the bile, and concentrated in the gallbladder (Fig. 54–12). Several factors may result in failure of the contrast material to be excreted in the bile: liver dysfunction or bile duct obstruction, failure of contrast material to enter the gallbladder due to cystic duct obstruction, and failure of the gallbladder to concentrate the

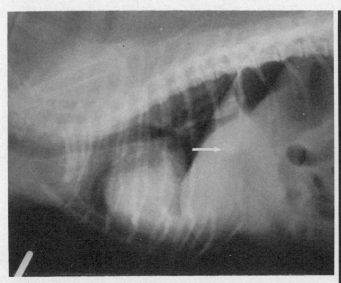

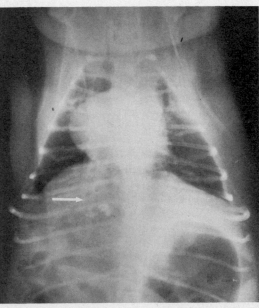

Figure 54–11. Lateral and ventrodorsal abdominal radiographs of a dog with asymptomatic choledocholithiasis *(arrow),* confirmed at necropsy.

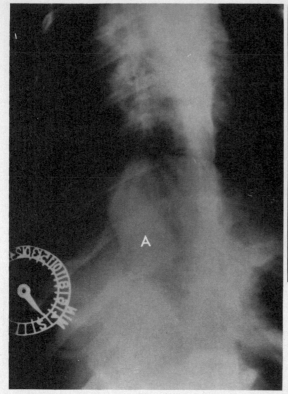

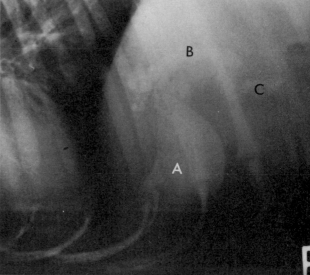

Figure 54–12. Lateral and ventrodorsal abdominal radiographs of a dog demonstrating oral cholecystography. The gallbladder *(A)* and common bile duct *(B)* are outlined. Dye can also be seen entering the duodenum *(C)*.

media due to cholecystitis. Visualization of the gallbladder rarely occurs using this technique if the serum bilirubin concentration is greater than 3 mg/dl. The contrast medium and bilirubin compete for the same excretion pathway in the liver.[77, 85]

There are two important diagnostic findings with oral cholecystography. First, radiolucent shadows in the opaque dye are usually choleliths. Second, failure to visualize the gallbladder may indicate bile duct obstruction or other disease. Caution should be used when interpreting this finding, and the procedure should be repeated.[85]

Intravenous cholecystography with cholangiography involves the use of dyes such as sodium iodipamide that do not require gallbladder concentration to visualize the biliary system. Primarily designed to visualize the extrahepatic bile ducts, this procedure also allows gallbladder visualization. It is indicated in patients who cannot take the oral dye or who have already had a cholecystectomy and when detailed visualization of the extrahepatic bile ducts is required. Dilation or stricture of the bile ducts, choledocholithiasis, choledochal cysts, and cystic duct remnants can be demonstrated. If acute cholecystitis is present, the gallbladder will not be visualized; conversely, gallbladder visualization rules out this diagnosis.[85] When its results are positive, intravenous cholangiography has a high degree of accuracy, but a negative result does not rule out disease.

Because of these problems and the generally low diagnostic rate achieved, oral and intravenous cholecystography and cholangiography, as preoperative diagnostic procedures, have fallen from vogue in human medicine and are considered obsolete.[56] Studies now receiving considerable interest in human medicine are ultrasonography, computerized axial tomography, endoscopic retrograde cholangiopancreatography, and percutaneous transhepatic cholangiography.

Both ultrasonography and computerized axial tomography (CAT scanning) are attractive in that they are noninvasive techniques that carry no risks and can be used in patients with elevated serum bilirubin concentrations. Ultrasonography has the added advantage of being relatively inexpensive. CAT scanning overall appears to offer little advantage over ultrasonography in the diagnosis of cholelithiasis and therefore is not widely used.[56, 85]

Ultrasonography is increasingly used in the diagnosis of obstructive jaundice. Bile duct dilation, both intrahepatic and extrahepatic, and choleliths can be detected. Ultrasonography is more accurate than cholecystography and in humans is recommended as the initial diagnostic procedure in patients suspected of having gallstones.[56, 85] The use of ultrasonography in the diagnosis of liver disease, including cholelithiasis, has been reported in dogs and cats.[21]

Diagnosis

The diagnosis of cholelithiasis in symptomatic patients should be suspected when signs of obstructive icterus are found. The problem is often recurrent, with periods of complete remission, and may be associated with cranial abdominal pain and fever.

Obstructing lesions of the biliary system, such as neoplasms, produce progressive obstruction with unrelenting icterus. Findings associated with cholelithiasis include anorexia, vomiting, diarrhea, depression, and dehydration. Serum biochemical evaluations reveal elevated bilirubin, AP, and ALT concentrations owing to the biliary obstruction and associated liver damage. Plain radiographic studies of the abdomen may reveal radiopaque masses near the gallbladder. Special radiological studies, as previously described, may confirm the diagnosis of cholelithiasis. A definitive diagnosis of cholelithiasis as a primary disease entity will be made at operation.

Treatment

The treatment of choice for symptomatic cholelithiasis is surgical removal of the stones. This usually involves cholecystectomy and possibly also common duct exploration, if choledocholithiasis is present or suspected. Surgery constitutes, at present, the only effective, safe, and practical method of therapy for cholelithiasis, as there is no form of medical therapy available for this problem in the dog and cat.

The preoperative preparation of a dog or cat with cholelithiasis should include correction of fluid deficits and electrolyte imbalances by intravenous fluid therapy. Perioperative prophylactic antibiotic therapy is probably indicated, especially if evidence of acute inflammatory disease or sepsis is detected during patient evaluation. In humans, a significant reduction in wound infection and sepsis was found when prophylactic antibiotics were administered to patients with choledocholithiasis and active disease.[56]

Exploration of the gallbladder and extrahepatic biliary system should be approached via cranioventral midline abdominal incision, which can be extended into a right paracostal incision if exposure is insufficient. Retracting the stomach and duodenum caudally and the mass of the liver cranially with moistened laparotomy sponges allows identification of the gallbladder and common bile duct.

The entire extrahepatic biliary system should be observed and gently palpated to help determine the presence of cholelithiasis. Gallbladder distension and common bile duct dilation will strongly support the presence of an obstructing lesion. An attempt is made to gently express the gallbladder contents, providing that marked pathological changes are not present, as a crude estimate of the patency of the cystic and common bile ducts. The finding of cholecystolithiasis, together with a dilated common bile duct and evidence of obstructive icterus, indicates that the patient also has choledocholithiasis.

Other possible causes of extrahepatic biliary obstruction, such as neoplasia, should be ruled out at this time. Sclerosing cholangitis, may be the cause of the obstruction in the cat.[37]

If cholecystolithiasis is confirmed, a cholecystectomy is usually performed. Concern has been expressed in the veterinary literature as to the consistent significant choledochal dilation that occurs in the dog follwing cholecystectomy. The long-term consequences of the dilation are not known. The dilation may occur because of the significant increase in intraductal pressure that is required to open the sphincter of the bile duct into the duodenum.[17, 95, 121] Therefore cholecystotomy with stone removal may be considered preferable.[95]

Whether exploration of the common bile duct will be required depends upon whether choledocholithiasis is present or not. In humans, certain findings are considered absolute evidence of choledocholithiasis and indicate common duct exploration. These are palpable stones in the ducts, obstructive icterus with cholangitis, the demonstration of stones by cholangiography, and significant common duct dilation. Relative indications for duct exploration include recurrent icterus, small stones in the gallbladder (or sludge), biliary-enteric fistula, and pancreatitis.[56, 85] The more of these factors that are present, the greater the chance of finding choledocholithiasis.

Prior to duct exploration, the true position of the duct should be identified by fine-needle aspiration, so that a vessel such as the portal vein is not opened. The bile aspirated can be used for microbiological culture and analysis. If the facilities are available, a pre-exploratory cholangiogram should be obtained at this time. A catheter can be inserted into the common duct through the stump of the cystic duct if a cholecystectomy has been performed, or through a cholecystotomy incision.[56, 85]

If common duct exploration is to be performed, an incision should be made into the duct distal to the entrance of the cystic duct. The incision should be in the most dilated portion so that the possibility of stricture formation is minimal. The duct should be gently massaged from both proximal and distal ends to the incision to allow removal of the stones. Specific probes, scoops, and stone forceps are designed for further exploration in human surgery. It is important to determine that the bile duct entrance into the duodenum is patent. A suitable probe is inserted distally in the duct into the duodenum to ascertain patency. The duct system is thoroughly irrigated with saline using either soft or metal catheters to remove as much debris as possible. It is suggested that dilation of the sphincter is appropriate to allow residual debris or small stones to pass easily into the duodenum.[56, 85]

A piece of equipment widely used in human surgery to aid in the removal of biliary calculi is the Fogerty balloon-tipped catheter. After the catheter is passed beyond the stone and the balloon is carefully inflated, the catheter can be slowly withdrawn, bringing the stone with it. This technique is reported to be particularly useful for removing stones in the intrahepatic bile ducts.[56, 85]

If it is determined that the bile duct is obstructed at the sphincter and it cannot be relieved by the methods described above, a duodenotomy may be performed to expose and catheterize the duct in a retrograde manner. Narrowing of the duct opening may require surgical correction by sphincteroplasty or choledochoduodenostomy.[17, 77, 85]

Although primary closure of the duct is possible following common duct exploration in human surgery, significant complications can be prevented by external T-tube drainage.[56, 85] Because experience is limited in veterinary medicine, no strict rules can be given for the use of T-tubes in the dog and cat. The size of the patient may preclude their use in some cases. One author has questioned the routine use of such tubes because of the possible stimulation of scar tissue formation.[17] T-tube placement is performed to provide drainage of the common bile duct and to prevent the development of abscess and fistula formation. In addition, post-exploratory and postoperative cholangiography can be performed through the T-tube to evaluate the completeness of stone removal and the flow of contrast material into the duodenum.

If the small size of the patient prohibits the use of a T-tube, biliary drainage can be achieved by placing a catheter in the common duct and directing it into the duodenum. The catheter is buried in the duodenal wall for approximately 1 cm and exteriorized through the abdominal wall in association with a duodenopexy.[33]

Following completion of the surgical procedures, the operative area is thoroughly lavaged with warm saline to remove debris and bile. A Penrose drain may be placed in the area of the choledochotomy wound, and another adjacent to the bed of the gallbladder, if a cholecystectomy was performed. The abdominal incision can then be closed routinely.

Surgical treatment of cholelithiasis in the dog and cat has consisted of cholecystectomy, cholecystotomy with flushing of the ducts, T-tube drainage, choledochotomy, and attempted transduodenal approach to the common bile duct.[12, 22, 53, 77, 79, 95, 99]

Postoperative Care and Recovery

Postoperative care consists of a continuation of intravenous fluid therapy until the patient has returned to full oral feeding. Antibiotics should probably be continued until the Penrose drain has been removed. Whether antibiotics need to be continued until the T-tube is removed is debatable. The Penrose drain can usually be removed on about the third postoperative day, when drainage is minimal. A sterile dressing should be placed over the abdomen to protect the abdominal drains and tubes. Serum AP, ALT, and bilirubin concentrations are followed postoperatively. A return of these values to normal indicates adequate biliary drainage and repair of liver damage.

If a T-tube has been used initially, it should be left unclamped to provide biliary drainage. Prior to clamping, a cholangiogram can be performed through the T-tube to ensure adequate flow of bile into the

duodenum prior to tube removal. In human surgery this is performed on the fifth to seventh postoperative day, and the cholangiogram is used to confirm that the biliary system is free of choleliths. At this point the T-tube can be periodically clamped, increasing the amount of time the T-tube is closed each day. If progress is satisfactory, the tube can be left clamped all the time, to prevent bile loss. The T-tube is usually removed 14 days postoperatively; at this time a well-established tract has formed, and bile peritonitis following removal is unlikely.[56, 85]

Prognosis

The prognosis for dogs and cats with cholelithiasis is difficult to predict because of the small number of reported cases. There are few reported long-term follow-ups on these cases to indicate whether the problem recurred.[99] Whether factors such as cholecystectomy, dietary alterations, and long-term medical therapy affect recurrence in dogs or cats is unknown.

SURGICAL PROCEDURES FOR THE LIVER AND BILIARY SYSTEM

Liver Biopsy

Many types of liver disease in the dog and cat result in similar clinical findings and similar abnormalities in laboratory studies of liver function. Without a definitive diagnosis, it is often hard to institute specific treatment and to give an accurate prognosis. Liver biopsy is frequently the only method of providing such diagnostic information. Many different methods of liver biopsy are available to the clinician, each having its advantages, disadvantages, indications, and associated possible complications.[86]

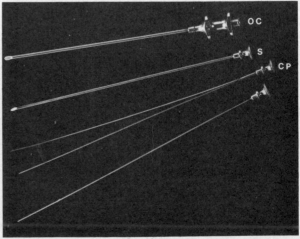

Figure 54–13. Franklin-modified Silverman biopsy needle. *OC*, outer cannula; *S*, stylet; *CP*, cutting prongs. The tips on the cutting prongs are sealed so as to retain the biopsy sample.

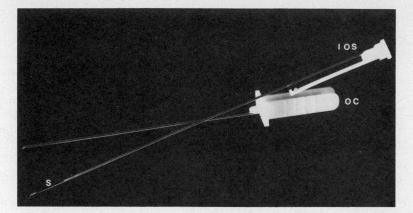

Figure 54–14. Tru-Cut disposable biopsy needle. *OC*, outer cannula; *IOS*, inner obturator–specimen rod; *S*, specimen notch in inner obturator–specimen rod.

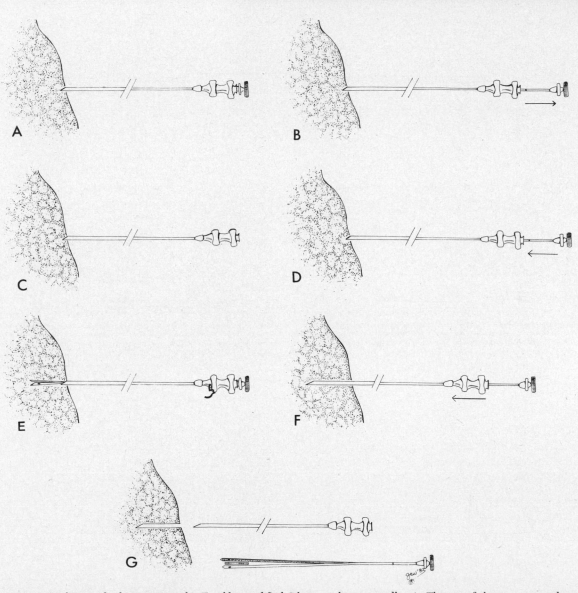

Figure 54–15. Technique for biopsy using the Franklin-modified Silverman biopsy needle. *A*, The tip of the outer cannula, with the stylet inside, is in contact with the liver surface. *B, C,* and *D,* The stylet is removed and then replaced with the cutting prongs. *E,* The cutting prongs have been thrust into the liver. The resistance imparted by the liver parenchyma has forced the blades of the cutting prongs apart. *F,* The outer cannula is advanced over the cutting prongs, forcing them into apposition. The outer cannula is advanced sufficiently to ensure complete coverage of the cutting prongs. *G,* The outer cannula and cutting prongs, containing the biopsy specimen, are removed together from the liver *(upper).* The biopsy specimen is shown after the cutting prongs have been removed from the outer cannula *(lower).*

Liver biopsy techniques range from closed to semi-open procedures. Generally the closed techniques are more suited to diffuse liver disease in which there is a high degree of probability of obtaining a representative sample of liver tissue. Conversely, in focal liver disease, for example metastatic neoplasia, closed techniques have a low probability of being successful. In these cases, an invasive technique may be chosen. The closed techniques are generally less stressful to the patient and do not usually require general anesthesia. The semi-open and open techniques usually require general anesthesia, and although the accuracy of the procedure is greatly increased, the added stress of general anesthesia in a patient with altered liver function may significantly increase the morbidity.[86]

The general indications for liver biopsy are: differential diagnosis of increased or decreased liver size, abnormal laboratory test results, and jaundice; diagnosis of primary liver neoplasia; evaluation of the liver as a site of metastatic neoplasia; assessment of progression or regression of liver disease compared with previous biopsy results; and evaluation of treatment regimens for liver disease.[42, 86]

Certain contraindications to liver biopsy are rec-

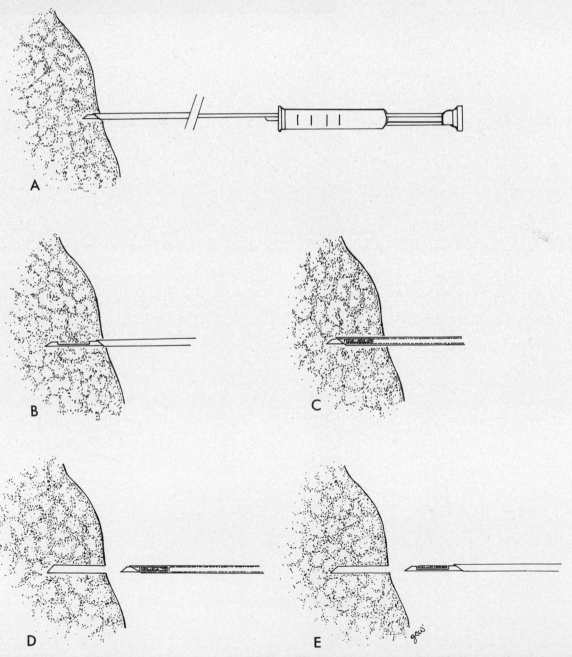

Figure 54–16. Technique for biopsy using the Tru-Cut biopsy needle. *A*, The tip of the outer cannula, with the inner obturator–specimen rod inside, is in contact with the liver surface. *B*, The inner obturator–specimen rod has been thrust into the liver. *C*, The outer cannula has been rapidly advanced over the specimen notch in the stationary inner obturator–specimen rod. *D*, The biopsy needle, containing the specimen, has been removed from the liver. *E*, The outer cannula has been pulled back to expose the specimen notch containing the biopsy sample.

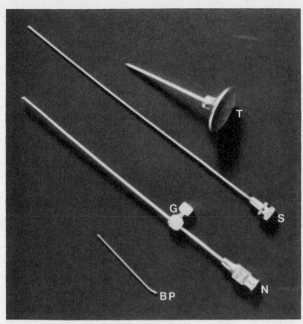

Figure 54–17. Menghini biopsy needle. *T*, trochar; *S*, stylet; *N*, needle; *G*, guard; *BP*, blocking pin.

ognized. They apply primarily to closed techniques, in which correction of problems should they arise is difficult. With open techniques there are no real contraindications. Bleeding disorders, whether congenital or acquired, are a potential problem, particularly with the closed techniques. An evaluation of the patient's coagulation systems should be performed prior to biopsy. General screening tests that can be employed include measurements of activated clotting time, bleeding time, and a platelet count. If abnormalities are detected by these tests, more specific tests should be performed, such as measurements of prothrombin time, partial thromboplastin time, fibrinogen concentration, and fibrin degradation products.[86]

Percutaneous Needle Biopsy

Percutaneous needle biopsy is performed using either a Franklin-modified Silverman biopsy needle, a Tru-cut disposable biopsy needle, or a Menghini needle. The Menghini needle is a coring and aspirating biopsy needle that is designed to aspirate a plug of tissue from soft parenchymal organs such as the liver.

The Franklin-modified Silverman needle and the Tru-cut needle are shown in Figs. 54–13 and 54–14. The operation of the two needles is basically the same, except that using the modified Silverman needle is a two-person procedure, whereas the Tru-cut needle can be operated single-handed. When the cutting prongs, or inner cannula, are advanced into the tissue, a small cylindrical specimen is obtained that is cut from the surrounding tissue by advancing the outer cannula over the inner one. The technique

for the two needles is illustrated in Figs. 54–15 and 54–16.[86]

The Menghini needle is available in different lengths and diameters. The 7-cm, 1.2-mm diameter needle is recommended for most dogs and cats.[86] It has a number of special features, including an extremely thin wall, a convex cutting edge that has been sharpened around its entire circumference, and a small blocking pin that is narrower than the internal diameter of the needle. The blocking pin is designed so that it will not fall through the needle or be aspirated into the syringe. Because of its design, the needle cuts a small core specimen from the liver while causing little damage to the surrounding tissue. The blocking pin prevents aspiration and fragmentation of the biopsy specimen in the syringe barrel and helps control negative pressure in the syringe (Fig. 54–17).[86]

The Menghini needle can be operated by either one or two people. Prior to biopsy a 10- to 12-ml syringe containing approximately 5 ml of saline is attached to the needle. If this is a two-person procedure, a length of tubing can be placed between the syringe and needle. The needle is advanced to the liver surface and its lumen cleared prior to biopsy by flushing with 1 to 2 ml of saline from the syringe. A negative pressure is created in the syringe by withdrawing the plunger and is maintained throughout the biopsy procedure. The needle is advanced rapidly into and out of the liver to a predetermined depth in one continuous motion lasting only a fraction of a second. Following removal of the needle from the patient, the specimen is flushed from the needle using the remainder of the saline in the syringe (Fig. 54–18).[86] Alternatively, the needle can be used with a stylet and without the blocking pin. In this instance, the needle is advanced to the liver surface with the blunt stylet in place. This feature is particularly useful in the transthoracic approach, as damage to the lungs is minimized. Once the liver has been contacted, the stylet is quickly removed and the syringe attached. As the biopsy specimen is cut from the liver, the negative pressure causes the specimen to be drawn into the saline in the syringe, from which it can be retrieved.[42]

The Menghini needle has a high failure rate when used on fibrotic or cirrhotic liver, because the negative pressure is inadequate to remove the specimen intact from the liver.[86]

Prior to needle biopsy of the liver the patient should be fasted for 12 hours to prevent inadvertent puncture of a distended stomach. One half to one hour prior to biopsy, a small quantity of fat or oil is given to stimulate contraction of the gallbladder. Radiographs of the abdomen should be obtained to confirm the size and position of the liver relative to other organs, as these factors may influence the approach used. If ascitic fluid is present, it should be removed by paracentesis. The fluid should be examined cytologically, for possible additional diagnostic information.[42, 86]

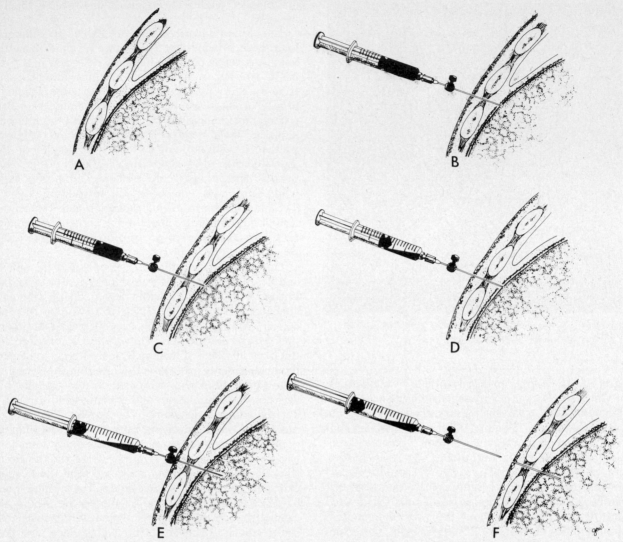

Figure 54–18. Technique for biopsy using the Menghini biopsy needle. *A*, Cross-section of body wall illustrating close association of ribs, pleural space, diaphragm, and liver. *B*, The needle, with syringe containing saline attached, is inserted to the level of the diaphragm. *C*, One to 2 ml of saline is injected through the needle to clear it of any tissue that may have occluded the lumen. *D*, A negative pressure is then created in the needle by withdrawing the syringe plunger. This pressure is maintained throughout the rest of the biopsy procedure. The guard is set on the needle at this time so as to allow approximately 10 to 15 mm of liver penetration by the needle. *E* and *F*, The needle is rapidly and smoothly moved into and out of the liver in one continuous motion. The needle is then quickly withdrawn from the body, ensuring that the biopsy specimen is sucked up into the needle.

In the majority of dogs and cats sedation and local anesthesia are adequate for needle liver biopsy. If general anesthetic agents have to be used, agents that depend on the liver for metabolism and excretion should be avoided. Therefore, reversible narcotic agents or inhalant anesthetics can be used relatively safely.[42, 86]

Transthoracic Percutaneous Liver Biopsy. This approach is the most widely accepted technique for liver biopsy in humans. Success depends on accurate location of the liver and having the patient control respiration in forced expiration, thereby approximating the diaphragm as closely as possible to the thoracic wall. The right side is chosen, as there is a significantly greater liver mass on this side.[86]

A right-sided approach is also used in the dog and cat, although the right side of the liver is smaller than the left, because a greater portion of the right hepatic lobes face the right thoracic wall. The close association of the stomach and diaphragm make the left-sided approach unsuitable. In the conscious dog and cat, voluntary respiratory control cannot be achieved. Therefore, this technique tends to be more difficult to perform in the dog and cat than in humans.[42, 86]

To obtain a liver biopsy specimen by the transthoracic approach, the animal can be placed in left lateral[42] or dorsal or sternal recumbency.[86] The right thoracic wall over the fourth to ninth intercostal spaces is clipped and aseptically prepared in a routine manner. The exact site for biopsy should be determined by evaluating two radiographic views of the thorax and abdomen. It is usually about the right seventh intercostal space, dorsal to the costochondral junctions (Fig. 54–19). The incision is infiltrated with two per cent lidocaine down to the parietal pleura

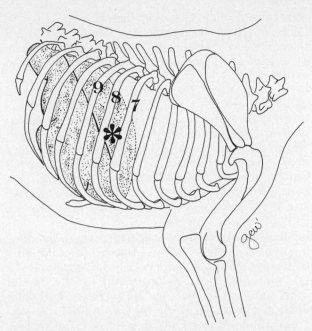

Figure 54–19. Illustration of the site for insertion of the biopsy needle through the thoracic wall for transthoracic percutaneous liver biopsy.

and is draped, and a small skin incision is made to allow entrance of the needle. On entering the thoracic cavity, the needle is directed caudally until the diaphragm is reached. The biopsy procedure is completed as rapidly as possible, the actual technique depending upon the type of needle being used, as soon as the animal has fully exhaled. The needle is completely removed and handed to an assistant for processing of the specimen. A suture may be used to close the stab incision. After a sterile sponge is placed over the incision, the animal is immediately placed in right lateral recumbency for approximately five minutes, thereby allowing compression of the biopsy site in the liver against the body wall to help control hemorrhage.[42, 86]

Transabdominal Percutaneous Liver Biopsy. The transabdominal approach, used as a blind biopsy technique, can be difficult in the dog and cat because of the variable position of the liver and its movement with respiration. If the liver is small, the degree of difficulty is increased.[86]

The procedure can be performed with the animal in either dorsal or left lateral recumbency. In dorsal recumbency the liver falls toward the vertebrae and away from the ventral body wall. In left lateral recumbency it is hard to determine the position of the gallbladder. Therefore both positions have disadvantages. However, dorsal recumbency is usually preferred.

The cranial ventral abdominal midline is clipped and prepared. A small skin incision is made between the left lateral border of the xiphoid process and the left costal arch. The biopsy needle is inserted through this incision into the abdominal cavity and directed in a craniodorsal direction at an approximate angle of 20 to 30 degrees left of the midsagittal plane (Fig.

54–20). Once the liver is encountered, the biopsy procedure is completed, the actual technique depending on the type of needle being used. The needle should not be advanced into the liver any farther than absolutely necessary to avoid damaging the deeper-lying major vessels.[86]

The accuracy of the transabdominal approach can be greatly increased by combining it with a "keyhole" technique. In this instance, a small cranial ventral midline incision is made into the abdominal cavity such that one or two fingers can be inserted. This allows palpation of the liver surface, and some attempt can be made at directing the needle to representative portions of the liver. Also, the gallbladder and other structures can be avoided.[86]

Once the selected site for biopsy has been chosen, that portion of the liver is supported by the operator's fingers. It can be immobilized against other portions of the liver, diaphragm, body wall, or other abdominal structures. The biopsy needle is inserted through a separate stab incision, into the portion of the liver to be biopsied. Multiple specimens can be obtained by this technique from different areas and depths of the liver, and diagnosis of focal hepatic disease is significantly increased. Hemorrhage from the biopsy site can be controlled by direct pressure with a finger or sponge.[86]

The major complications associated with blind needle biopsy of the liver, via either a transthoracic or transabdominal route, are gallbladder puncture, biopsy of adjacent organs, hemoperitoneum, and the transfer of ascites into the thorax.[54] Gallbladder puncture may require surgical correction or it may seal itself following needle drainage.[54, 86] Pneumothorax may also be associated with the transthoracic approach.

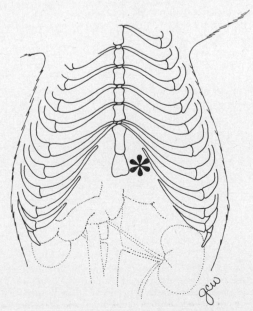

Figure 54–20. Illustration of the site for insertion of the biopsy needle for transabdominal percutaneous liver biopsy.

Laparoscopy

The liver of the dog and cat is easily examined by laparoscopy, thereby allowing guided biopsies of both generalized and focal liver disease.[29, 45, 86] The probability of obtaining diagnostic representative samples of hepatic tissue is greatly increased over that in either blind or "keyhole" percutaneous needle biopsies.

Laparoscopy for examination of the liver can be performed from either a ventral midline, left paralumbar, or right paralumbar approach. Which approach is chosen depends upon prior examination of the patient, evaluation of abdominal radiographs, and what other abdominal organs the clinician wishes to examine. Examination of the liver is enhanced during this procedure by tilting the patient in approximately a 30-degree head-up position, thereby allowing the gastrointestinal tract to fall caudally away from the liver. Biopsy cup forceps that can be introduced either through the scope or through a second puncture site provide tissue for histological evaluation. Guided biopsies can therefore be made anywhere across the liver surface using these forceps. If a deeper biopsy sample is required, the laparoscope can be used to guide a biopsy needle, which has been introduced into the abdomen through a separate stab incision, to a specific area of the liver that the clinican wishes to biopsy.

The author routinely uses laparoscopy for liver biopsy in the dog and cat because of its significantly increased rate of obtaining diagnostic samples. It is a safe procedure that, if performed correctly, carries little risk for the patient. Laparoscopy has some disadvantages. Usually the procedure has to be performed under general anesthesia, but it can be performed under sedation and a local anesthetic. Careful selection of the anesthetic agents used, for example, inhalant anesthetics and reversible narcotics, involves minimal risk to the animal with compromised liver function. Massive ascites, which can be associated with certain forms of liver disease, should be drained prior to laparoscopy; otherwise poor observation results. If significant congenital or acquired bleeding disorders are present, fresh whole blood transfusion may be required prior to laparoscopy and liver biopsy to minimize hemorrhage.

Possible complications that can arise from laparoscopic liver biopsy include hemorrhage, perforation of an abdominal viscus, pneumothorax, subcutaneous emphysema, and air embolism.

While laparoscopy is being performed, the rest of the abdominal contents should be examined, for possible additional diagnostic information. Also, laparoscopy may demonstrate to the clinician that an exploratory laparotomy should be performed. Surgically treatable lesions may be found or biopsy of other organs that cannot be reached through the scope may need to be done.

Surgical Biopsy Procedures

A number of different methods of surgical biopsy of the liver during abdominal exploration in the dog have been described.[4, 17, 33, 90]

Because the liver in the dog and cat has multiple lobes, liver biopsy in the dog and cat can be performed by simple ligation of a tapering edge of a lobe. The tip of one of the lobes is grasped gently with a moist sponge. A ligature of absorbable suture material is tightened around this portion of the liver as far back as necessary to obtain the required size sample. The ligature fractures the parenchyma and occludes the blood vessels and bile ducts. The biopsy sample is amputated with a scalpel. Large amounts

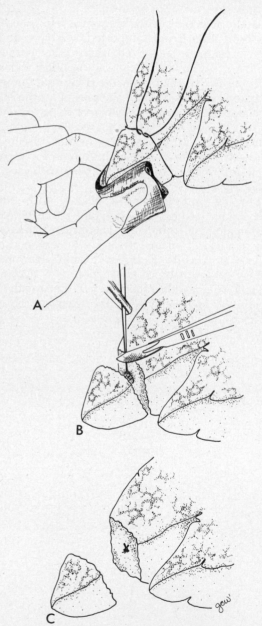

Figure 54–21. Surgical biopsy of the liver by ligature fracture. *A,* Tip of liver lobe is gently grasped with a moist sponge. A ligature has been placed around the lobe tip at a suitable point. *B,* The ligature is tightened so as to cut through the liver parenchyma and also to occlude major blood vessels and bile ducts. *C,* The biopsy sample is amputated with a scalpel.

of liver tissue can be obtained by this technique (Fig. 54–21).[17, 90]

Liver biopsy can also be performed by wedge resection.[4, 33] Two rows of horizontal mattress sutures of absorbable suture material are placed through the liver tissue along the margins of the tissue wedge to be excised. The sutures should overlap each other slightly. The two suture lines meet proximally to form a V. The sutures are tied so that they gently compress the liver tissue, to minimize hemorrhage after resection. The wedge of tissue between the suture lines is sharply excised with a scalpel so that an undamaged biopsy specimen is obtained. After excision, the edges of the wedge can be drawn together by absorbable sutures that encircle the two suture lines (Fig. 54–22). Problems encountered with this technique include hemorrhage and the tendency for the sutures to pull out of the hepatic parenchyma.

It has been suggested that it is inappropriate to bury significant quantities of such material in the hepatic parenchyma as described, and that approximating cut edges of hepatic tissue could result in intrahepatic hematoma formation due to continued bleeding. Therefore a technique similar to partial hepatectomy is considered more appropriate.[17]

The disadvantages of the surgical techniques just described are that they allow biopsy of only the edges of the liver lobes and, with the wedge resection technique, are very time-consuming. Because of these disadvantages, I prefer to use a Keyes cutaneous punch. With this technique any portion of the liver parenchyma can be sampled, possibly providing more representative examples of liver lesions, particularly when focal disease is present. This technique is also rapidly performed. A suitable punch is chosen considering the side of the liver and focal lesions to be sampled. The Keyes punch is used much like a cookie cutter to cut out a cylinder of tissue. Once the punch has been drilled into the hepatic parenchyma to the required depth, it is gently twisted so that the base of the specimen is cut off. The biopsy punch containing the sample is removed. Hemorrhage from the hole in the liver parenchyma is controlled by inserting a rolled piece of absorbable gelatin sponge (Gelfoam). Pressure, with a gauze sponge, should be gently applied for a couple of minutes. Specimens should be taken from the convex cranioventral surface of the liver and should not penetrate more than halfway through the lobe to avoid the larger vessels that lie closer to the concave surface (Figs. 54–23 and 54–24).

Biopsy needles, such as previously described, can also be used at the time of abdominal exploration to obtain samples from different areas of the liver.[86] The

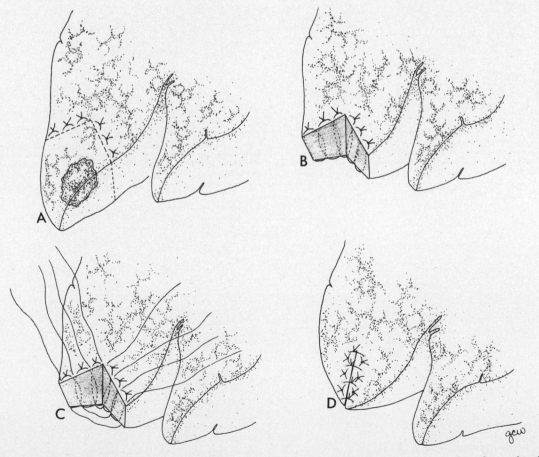

Figure 54–22. Surgical biopsy of the liver by wedge resection. *A*, Two rows of horizontal mattress sutures have been placed along the margins of the wedge to be excised. *B*, The liver wedge has been sharply excised with a scalpel. *C*, Sutures are placed so as to encircle the two lines of mattress sutures. *D*, The incised edges of the wedge are drawn together by the encircling sutures.

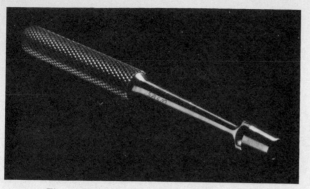

Figure 54–23. Keyes cutaneous biopsy punch.

advantage of needle biopsy is that focal areas can be sampled. The disadvantage is that only small, possibly inadequate samples are obtained.

Partial Hepatectomy

Severe trauma, neoplasia, focal abscess, and other localized hepatic diseases may require partial or total amputation of a liver lobe. The most commonly described method for performing a partial hepatic lobectomy in the dog and cat is the "finger fracture" technique.[4, 17, 32, 33, 45] The advantages of this tech-

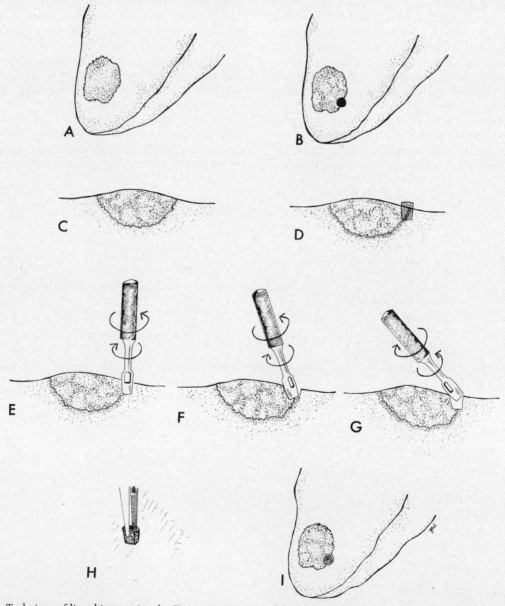

Figure 54–24. Technique of liver biopsy using the Keyes cutaneous punch. *A* and *B*, Surface view of liver lobe indicating lesion and site of biopsy. *C* and *D*, Cross-section views of liver lobe indicating lesion and site of biopsy. *E*, The punch is drilled into the hepatic parenchyma to the required depth. *F* and *G*, The punch is gently twisted so that the base of the specimen is cut off. The biopsy punch containing the sample is removed. *H*, A piece of absorbable gelatin sponge is rolled up to form a cylinder slightly bigger than the size of the Keyes punch used. *I*, The rolled piece of absorbable gelatin sponge is inserted into the biopsy hole in the liver to control hemorrhage.

nique are that hemorrhage and bile leakage from inadvertently severed vessels and bile ducts are avoided.[4] However, an accurate dissection line is not always achieved, and capsular or parenchymal fissures may be created in the surrounding normal tissue. A scalpel handle instead of fingers may be used to overcome this problem.[45] Similarly, in small patients a tissue forceps instead of fingers can be used for parenchymal dissection. By placing the closed narrow jaws of the forceps into the tissue, and opening them, one divides the parenchyma without trauma to the blood vessels or bile ducts.[17]

The liver is approached through cranioventral (midline) abdominal incision. If exposure is inadequate, the incision can be extended into a right or left paracostal incision. Also the incision can be extended cranially into a median sternotomy if greater exposure of the diaphragmatic surface of the liver is required or if exposure of the vena cava is necessary to aid in control of hemorrhage.

The portion of the liver lobe to be resected is supported with moist sponges and is retracted caudally. The liver capsule is scored along the proposed line of resection with a blunt instrument such as a scalpel handle to provide a clean line of dissection. The thumb and forefinger of the surgeon's hand are inserted along the line of dissection and worked through the parenchyma with a rubbing motion, thereby "fracturing" the parenchyma. The main ducts and vessels are identified by their difference in resistance. The hepatic tissue is carefully removed from the ducts and vessels, which are then ligated and divided. Hemoclips can be used instead of suture ligatures. The dissection is continued until that portion of the liver lobe has been completely removed (Fig. 54–25).[17, 32, 33, 45]

Hemorrhage from the exposed parenchymal sur-

face is minimal. Some authors have recommended suturing omentum or falciform ligament over this surface.[63, 64] Others, however, make no attempt to cover the raw surface of the liver.[33] Similarly, the need for drainage is controversial.[33, 63]

For distal partial lobectomies where the liver lobe is relatively thin, electrosurgical resection has also been used successfully.[45] This is a simple, quick technique. Small vessels and ducts can be transected by a combination of coagulation and cutting current. Larger structures are identified and ligated prior to transection. Oozing of blood from the cut surface is negligible.

If total, or near-total, amputation of a liver lobe is to be attempted, it may be necessary to control blood flow to the liver to avoid major hemorrhage. The hepatic artery and portal vein can be occluded by cross-clamping the hepatoduodenal ligament. Warm ischemia times of more than 10 minutes should be avoided. If longer control of the blood inflow is required, intermittent occlusion is used. Similarly, umbilical tape tourniquets can be used to temporarily occlude the prehepatic and posthepatic caudal vena cava. The vena cava should be occluded only if uncontrollable hemorrhage occurs.[17, 33, 45] The vessels and ducts at the base of the lobe to be resected are carefully identified, ligated, and divided prior to lobe removal. The liver lobes closely associated with the vena cava require careful dissection to identify the hepatic veins and to avoid tearing the veins or the vena cava.[17]

Following partial hepatectomy, the animal should be monitored carefully for evidence of postoperative intra-abdominal hemorrhage. Prophylactic antibiotic therapy is indicated. Intravenous fluid and electrolyte therapy should be continued until oral feeding can be instituted.

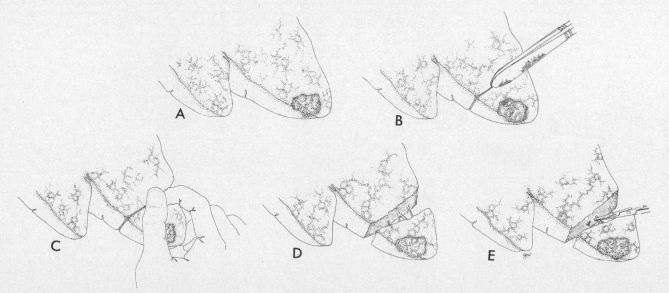

Figure 54–25. Partial hepatic lobectomy using the "finger-fracture" technique. *A,* The portion of the liver to be resected is packed off with moist sponges and retracted caudally. *B,* The liver capsule is scored along the proposed line of resection with a blunt instrument such as a scalpel handle. *C,* The thumb and fingers are used to "fracture" the liver parenchyma along the line of resection. *D,* The major blood vessels and bile ducts are left intact and are therefore easily identified. *E,* The vessels and ducts are then ligated and divided.

Cholecystectomy

The potential indications for cholecystectomy in the dog and cat are neoplasms of the gallbladder, irreparable trauma to the gallbladder, cholecystitis, and cholelithiasis.[4, 17, 33]

The gallbladder is approached via cranioventral midline abdominal incision. An extension of the incision into a right paracostal incision may be required in certain animals, such as a deep-chested dog, to gain adequate exposure. The gallbladder can be removed either by starting the dissection at the fundus and working proximally toward the cystic duct or by identifying the cystic duct and cystic artery with the initial dissection and working distally toward the fundus. In either technique atraumatic forceps, such as Babcock forceps, or stay sutures can be applied to the fundus of the gallbladder to provide traction during the dissection. The gallbladder may be decompressed prior to dissection. The suggested advantages of initial decompression are that the gallbladder is smaller and there is less danger of bile spillage during dissection. The main disadvantage to initial decompression is that the dissection plane between the gallbladder and its bed is less distinct.[17]

When working from the fundus, gentle traction on the gallbladder helps identify the plane of dissection between it and the liver parenchyma. The visceral peritoneum is incised and the gallbladder is gently freed from the liver by blunt dissection. The dissec-

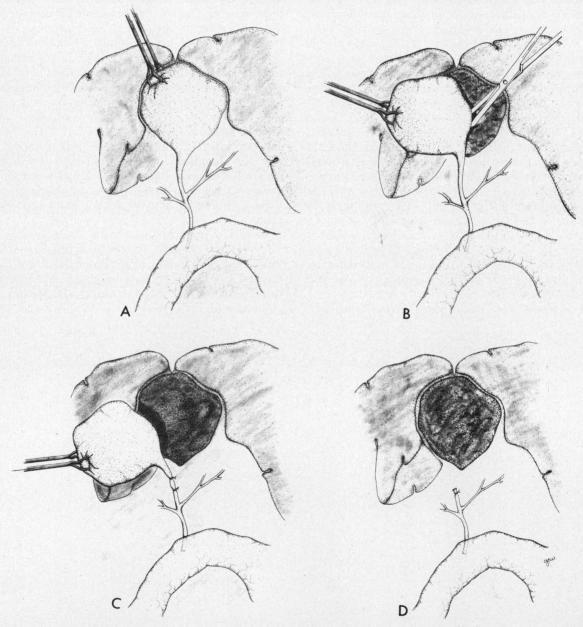

Figure 54–26. The technique of cholecystectomy proceeding from the fundus. *A,* The fundus of the gallbladder is supported with Babcock forceps. Initial decompression of the gallbladder may be indicated. *B,* With gentle traction on the gallbladder, the visceral peritoneum is incised and the gallbladder is gently freed from the liver by blunt dissection. *C* and *D,* The cystic duct and artery are identified, ligated, and divided.

tion is continued until the cystic duct and cystic artery are identified. The duct and artery are clamped, transected, and double-ligated (Fig. 54–26).[4, 33] Care should be taken to properly identify and isolate the cystic duct prior to transection and ligation in order to avoid damage to the adjacent hepatic ducts and common bile duct. Hepatic ducts or the common duct can be inadvertently included in clamps and ligatures, causing biliary strictures or acute occlusion.[84]

If the structures at the liver hilus can be clearly identified, cholecystectomy can proceed from the cystic duct. The cystic artery and cystic duct should be dissected so that they can be individually clamped, transected, and double-ligated. By application of traction to the proximal end of the gallbladder, the dissection can continue between the gallbladder and

the liver. Any additional vessels between the gallbladder and the liver should be carefully identified and individually ligated. The dissection is continued distally until the gallbladder is freed from its bed in the liver (Fig. 54–27).[17]

Following cholecystectomy, hemorrhage from the exposed liver surface is controlled by pressure. No attempt is made to appose the serosal edges of the gallbladder bed.[4, 17] Once hemorrhage has ceased, the area is flushed with warm saline to remove any bile and debris, and the abdomen is closed in a routine manner. Drainage is not required.

Prophylactic antibiotic therapy is indicated in patients undergoing cholecystectomy, because the biliary system is being invaded and often a significant inflammatory or infectious process is present. Postoperative care consists of intravenous fluid and elec-

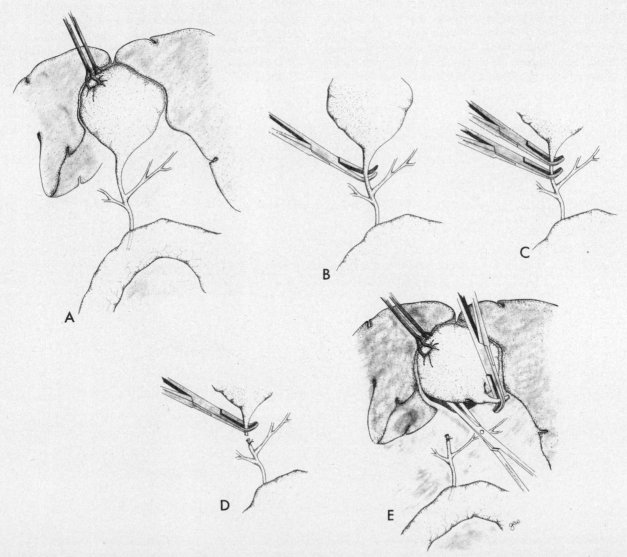

Figure 54–27. The technique of cholecystectomy proceeding from the cystic duct. *A,* The fundus of the gallbladder is supported with Babcock forceps. Initial decompression of the gallbladder may be indicated. *B,* The cystic duct, and associated cystic artery, should be dissected free from the surrounding structures. *C* and *D,* The cystic duct and artery are individually clamped and divided. The proximal ends of these structures are subsequently ligated. *E,* Traction is applied to the proximal end of the gallbladder to allow dissection to continue between the gallbladder and the liver in a distal direction.

trolyte therapy until oral feeding can be instituted. The patient should be evaluated for signs of newly appearing or unresolving obstructive jaundice, which indicates either pathological or iatrogenic bile duct obstruction.

Cholecystoenterostomy

If trauma, inflammation, or neoplasia has obstructed or disrupted the common bile duct, a surgical procedure is required to redirect the flow of bile into the intestinal tract. A choledochoenterostomy is a technically difficult procedure to perform in the dog and cat and has limited assurance of long-term successful results, owing to the small size of the bile ducts.[17, 113]

The procedure of choice for biliary redirection in the dog and cat, when feasible, is a cholecystoenterostomy, in particular either a cholecystoduodenostomy or a cholecystojejunostomy. Either procedure produces a direct communication between the gallbladder and the intestinal tract and obviates the need for the common bile duct. Cholecystoenterostomy is a controversial procedure, because it was believed that reflux of intestinal contents into the anastomosed gallbladder would always result in chronic cholangitis and an infected biliary system. Recently it has been shown that reflux of intestinal contents causes little change in the bile ducts and gallbladder, providing that the refluxed material can freely drain back into the intestine. Free drainage is ensured by an accurately performed procedure that creates a large (approximately 2.5 cm) permanent opening between the gallbladder and the intestinal tract.[113, 114]

The cholecystoenterostomy procedure commonly described in the veterinary literature is the "suture cutting" technique.[4, 33] It is inadequate in the dog because it results in a stenotic opening between the gallbladder and the intestinal tract and has a significant rate of postoperative complications. A small opening contributes to the pathogenesis of cholangitis.[113] This procedure cannot be recommended.

A mucosal approximating technique has been described in dogs that yields a large permanent opening between the gallbladder and intestine.[17, 113, 114] The technique gives excellent long-term functional results with no progressive cholangitis or chronic infection.[113]

Depending upon the degree of mobility of the gallbladder, it may require dissection from its fossa

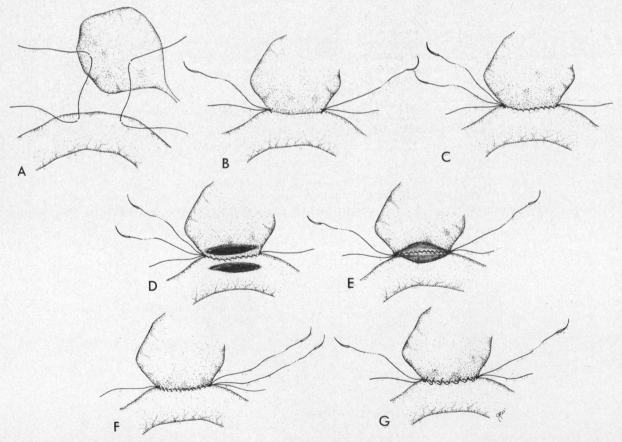

Figure 54–28. The technique of cholecystoenterostomy—mucosal approximating technique. *A* and *B*, The fundus of the gallbladder and the antimesenteric border of the intestine are approximated with two fine sutures. These should be placed approximately 3 cm apart. *C*, The serosal surfaces of the gallbladder and intestine are approximated with a simple continuous pattern. *D*, 2.5-cm incisions are made in both the gallbladder and intestine. The contents of each are carefully aspirated. *E*, The posterior mucosal edges are approximated with a continuous suture pattern. *F*, The anterior mucosal edges are approximated with a continuous suture pattern. Care should be taken to ensure complete sealing of the anastomosis at each end. *G*, The near serosal surfaces are approximated with a similar suture pattern to complete the anastomosis.

to allow a tension-free anastomosis with the intestinal tract. Two sutures of five (4-0) synthetic absorbable suture material are used to approximate the fundus of the gallbladder to the antimesenteric border of the intestine. These should be placed so that eventually a 2.5-cm incision can be made in the adjoining walls of the two structures. A two-layer anastomosis is then performed. The serosal surfaces of the gallbladder and intestine are approximated between the two stay sutures using a simple continuous suture pattern of 4-0 synthetic absorbable material. A stab incision is made into the gallbladder and the bile is aspirated. The incision is enlarged to 2.5 cm, between the two original stay sutures. A similar 2.5-cm incision is made in the antimesenteric border of the intestine. If a cholecystojejunostomy is being performed, it is suggested that the intestine is occluded proximal and distal to the anastomosis site to minimize intestinal spillage. The width of the opening can be increased by excising a two- to three-millimeter-wide strip of tissue from the edge of the incised wall of each organ. The near and far sides of the gallbladder-to-intestine anastomosis are completed using a simple continuous suture pattern to achieve mucosal approximation. The near side serosal layers are then approximated using a similar suture pattern. Omentum should be draped over the anastomosis site (Fig. 54–28). [17, 113]

Following completion of the anastomosis, the surgical site is thoroughly lavaged with warm saline, and the abdomen is closed in a routine manner. Drainage is not required. Prophylactic antibiotic therapy is indicated because of the invasion of both the biliary and intestinal tracts.

Postoperative care consists of intravenous fluid and electrolyte therapy. Anorexia, nausea, and vomiting can be seen postoperatively owing to surgical trauma to the pancreas, duodenum, and gallbladder. Fluid therapy is continued until oral feeding can be instituted when vomiting ceases. Function of the cholecystoenterostomy can be assessed by measuring serum concentrations of bilirubin, AP, and ALT. Cholecystography can be performed postoperatively to evaluate gallbladder function and the size of the anastomotic opening. An upper gastrointestinal barium radiographic study can be used to evaluate reflux into the gallbladder. Failure to demonstrate reflux of barium into the gallbladder or prolonged retention of barium in the biliary system indicates progressive stenosis of the opening, thereby indicating future obstruction and cholangitis. [113]

1. Allan, G. S.: Use of contrast radiography of the gall bladder in the diagnosis of diaphragmatic hernia. N.S.W. Vet. Proc. 10:51, 1974.
2. Allan, G. S., and Dixon, R. T.: Cholecystography in the dog: the choice of contrast media and optimum dose rates. J. Am. Vet. Radiol. Soc. 16:98, 1975.
3. Allan, G. S., and Dixon, R. T.: Cholecystography in the dog: assessment of radiographic positioning and the use of double contrast examination by visual and densitometric methods. J. Am. Vet. Radiol. Soc. 18:177, 1977.

4. Archibald, J., and Hofmeyer, C. F. B.: Liver and biliary system. Archibald, J. (ed.): In Canine Surgery II. American Veterinary Publications Inc., Santa Barbara, 1974.
5. Archibald, J., Holt, J. C., Sokolovsky, V., and Catcott, E. J. (ed.): Management of Trauma in Dogs and Cats. American Veterinary Publications, Inc., Santa Barbara, 1981.
6. Baker, A. L., Wood, R. A. B., Moossa, A. R., and Boyer, J. L.: Sodium taurocholate modifies the bile acid–independent fraction of canalicular bile flow in the Rhesus monkey. J. Clin. Invest. 64:312, 1979.
7. Balabaud, C., Kron, K. A., and Gumucio, J. J.: The assessment of the bile salt–nondependent fraction of canalicular bile water in the rat. J. Lab. Clin. Med. 89:393, 1977.
8. Barrett, R. E., et al.: Four cases of congenital portacaval shunt in the dog. J. Small Anim. Pract. 17:71, 1976.
9. Bellenger, C. R., Trim, C., and Sumner-Smith, G.: Bile pleuritis in a dog. J. Small Anim. Pract. 16:575, 1975.
10. Bend, J. R., and Hook, G. E. R.: Hepatic and extrahepatic mixed-function oxidases. In Lee, D. J. K. (ed.): Handbook of Physiology. Vol. 9. American Physiological Society, Bethesda, Md., 1977.
11. Berzon, J. L.: Surgical repair of traumatic injuries of the biliary system: Case report and discussion. J. Am. Anim. Hosp. Assoc. 17:421, 1981.
12. Binns, R. M.: Cholelithiasis causing obstructive jaundice in a boxer dog. Vet. Rec. 76:239, 1964.
13. Bourdelle, E., and Bressou, C.: Anatomie régionale des animaux domestiques. IV. Carnivores: Chien et Chat. J-B Bailliere, Paris, 1953.
14. Bressou, C., and Vladutiu, O.: Les artères, les veins, et les canaux biliares intra-hépatiques chez le chat. Rec. Med. Vet. 120:161, 1944.
15. Breznock, E. M.: Surgical manipulation of portosystemic shunts in dogs. J. Am. Vet. Med. Assoc. 174:819, 1979.
16. Breznock, E. M., et al.: Surgical manipulation of intrahepatic portocaval shunts in dogs. J. Am. Vet. Med. Assoc. 182:798, 1983.
17. Breznock, E. M.: Surgery of the liver and biliary system. In Bojrab, M. J. (ed.): Current Techniques in Small Animal Surgery II. Lea & Febiger, Philadelphia, 1983.
18. Burgener, F. A., and Fischer, H. W.: Contraction of the canine gall bladder in different regions of common bile duct obstruction. Radiology 116:49, 1975.
19. Carlisle, C. H.: Radiographic anatomy of the cat gallbladder. J. Am. Vet. Radiol. Soc. 18:170, 1977.
20. Carlisle, C. H.: A comparison of techniques for cholecystography in the cat. J. Am. Vet. Radiol. Soc. 18:173, 1977.
21. Cartee, R. E.: Diagnostic real time ultrasonography of the liver of the dog and cat. J. Am. Anim. Hosp. Assoc. 17:731, 1981.
22. Cartmell, W. B., Edwards, H. G., and Hammonds, P.: Cholelithiasis in a dachshund bitch and its surgical treatment. Vet. Rec. 76:1323, 1964.
23. Casas, A. P.: Contribution à l'étude du sphincter d'Oddi chez Canis familiaris. Acta Anat. 34:130, 1958.
24. Cornelius, I. M., Thrall, D. E., Halliwell, W. H., et al.: Anomalous portosystemic anastomoses associated with chronic hepatic insufficiency in six young dogs. J. Am. Vet. Med. Assoc. 167:220, 1975.
25. Crowe, D. T., and Crane, S. W.: Diagnostic abdominal paracentesis and lavage in the evaluation of abdominal injuries in dogs and cats: clinical and experimental investigations. J. Am. Vet. Med. Assoc. 168:700, 1976.
26. Cuo, P.: La segmentation hépatique des carnivores. Rec. Med. Vet. 141:233, 1965.
27. Cuo, P., Blin, P.-C., and Berenger, A.: Topographie de la veine porte intra-hépatique du chien. Rec. Med. Vet. 141:5, 1965.
28. Cuo, P., Blin, P.-C., and Berenger, A.: Topographie artérielle du foie du chien. Rec. Med. Vet. 141:123, 1965.
29. Dalton, J. R. F., and Hill, F. W. G.: A procedure for examination of the liver and pancreas in dogs. J. Small Anim. Pract. 13:527, 1972.
30. Danielsson, H.: Mechanisms of bile acid biosynthesis. In

Nair, P. P., Kritchevsky, D. (eds.): *The Bile Acids: Chemistry, Physiology and Metabolism.* Plenum Press, New York, 1973.

31. Diamond, J. M.: Transport mechanisms in the gallbladder. *In* Code, C. F., (ed.): *Handbook of Physiology.* Sec. 6, Vol. 5. American Physiological Society, Washington, D. C., 1968.

32. Dingwall, J. S., et al.: A new technique for liver resection in the dog. J. Small Anim. Pract. 7:429, 1970.

33. Dingwall, J. S.: The liver and biliary system. *In* Bojrab, M. J. (ed.): *Current Techniques in Small Animal Surgery I.* Lea & Febiger, Philadelphia, 1975.

34. Doster-Virtue, M. E., and Virtue, R. W.: Gallstones in a dog. J. Am. Vet. Med. Assoc. 101:197, 1942.

35. Dubois, F. S., and Hunt, E. A.: A comparative study of the emptying of the gall bladder in the opossum and the cat, together with notes on the anatomy of the biliary tract of the opossum. Anat. Rec. 54:289, 1932.

36. Dyce, K. M.: An experimental study of the biliary tract of the dog. Zentralbl. Vet. Med. 3:717, 1956.

37. Edwards, D. F., McCracken, M. D., and Richardson, D. C.: Sclerosing cholangitis in a cat. J. Am. Vet. Med. Assoc. 182:710, 1983.

38. Eichorn, E. P., Jr., and Boyden, E. A.: The choledocho-duodenal junction in the dog—a restudy of Oddi's sphincter. Am. J. Anat. 97:431, 1955.

39. Erlinger, S., and Dhumeaux, D.: Mechanisms and control of secretion of bile water and electrolytes. Gastroenterology. 66:281, 1974.

40. Evans, H. E., and Christensen, G. C. (eds.): *Miller's Anatomy of the Dog.* 2nd ed. W. B. Saunders, Philadelphia, 1979.

41. Ewing, G. O., Suter, P. F., and Bailey, C. S.: Hepatic insufficiency associated with congenital anomalies of the portal vein in dogs. J. Am. Anim. Hosp. Assoc. 10:463, 1979.

42. Feldman, E. C., and Edwards, D. F.: Percutaneous liver biopsy in the dog. *In* Bojrab, M. J. (ed.): *Current Techniques in Small Animal Surgery II.* Lea & Febiger, Philadelphia, 1983.

43. Florentin, P., Cuo, P., and Leroy, G.: Topographie des voies biliares du chien. Bull. Assoc. Anatomistes. 48th Reunion, Toulouse, 1962, p. 605.

44. Furneaux, R. W.: End-to-end portacaval anastomosis for the correction of ascites in a terrier dog. J. Am. Anim. Hosp. Assoc. 19:562, 1973.

45. Furneaux, R. W.: Surgical techniques for the liver and spleen. Vet. Clin. North Am. 5:363, 1975.

46. Gillette, J. R.: Formation of reactive metabolites of foreign compounds and their covalent binding to cellular constituents. *In* Lee, D. H. K. (ed.): *Handbook of Physiology.* Sec. 9. American Physiological Society, Bethesda, Md., 1977.

47. Grafton, N.: Surgical ligation of congenital portosystemic venous shunts in the dog: a report of three cases. J. Am. Anim. Hosp. Assoc. 14:728, 1978.

48. Grandage, J.: The radiology of the dog's diaphragm. J. Small Anim. Pract. 15:1, 1974.

49. Grandage, J.: Normal abdominal visceral relationships. *In* Radiology Proc. (University of Sydney Postgraduate Committee in Veterinary Science) 59:241, 1982.

50. Griffiths, G. L., Lumsden, J. H., and Valli, V. E. O.: Hematologic and biochemical changes in dogs with portosystemic shunts. J. Am. Vet. Med. Assoc. 17:705, 1981.

51. Guyton, A. C.: Textbook of Medical Physiology. 6th ed., W. B. Saunders, Philadelphia, 1981.

52. Halpert, B.: The choledocho-duodenal junction—a morphological study in the dog. Anat. Rec. 53:83, 1932.

53. Harari, J., Ettinger, S., and Lippincott, C. L.: Extrahepatic bile duct obstruction due to cholecystitis and choledocholithiasis: Case Report. J. Am. Anim. Hosp. Assoc. 18:347, 1982.

54. Hardy, R. M.: Diseases of the liver. *In* Ettinger, S. J. (ed.): *Textbook of Veterinary Internal Medicine II.* W. B. Saunders, Philadelphia, 1983.

55. Holligworth, R. M.: Biochemistry and significance of transferase reactions in the metabolism of foreign chemicals. *In* Lee, D. H. K. (ed.): *Handbook of Physiology.* Sec. 9. American Physiological Society, Bethesda, Md., 1977.

56. Jordan, G. L.: Choledocholithiasis. Curr. Prob. Surg. 14:12, 1982.

57. Kappas, A., and Alvares, A. P.: How the liver metabolizes foreign substances. Sci. Am. 232:22–31, 1975.

58. Kershner, D., Hooten, T. C., and Shearer, E. M.: Production of experimental portal hypertension in the dog: anatomy of the hepatic veins in the dog. Arch. Surg. 53:425, 1946.

59. Kolata, R. J.: Diagnostic abdominal paracentesis and lavage: experimental and clinical evaluations in the dog. J. Am. Vet. Med. Assoc. 168:697, 1976.

60. Kolata, R. J., and Johnston, D. E.: Motor vehicle accidents in urban dogs: a study of 600 cases. J. Am. Vet. Med. Assoc. 167:938, 1975.

61. Kolata, R. J., Kraut, N. H., and Johnston, D. E.: Patterns of trauma in urban dogs and cats: a study of 1,000 cases. J. Am. Vet. Med. Assoc. 164:499, 1974.

62. Kyosola, K., and Reichart, L.: The anatomy and innervation of the sphincter of Oddi in the dog and cat. Am. J. Anat. 140:497, 1974.

63. LeVeen, H. H., et al.: Peritoneovenous shunting for ascites. Ann. Surg. 180:580, 1974.

64. LeVeen, H. H., and Wapnick, S.: Operative details of continuous peritoneovenous shunt for ascites. Bull. Soc. Int. Chir. 6:579, 1975.

65. LeVeen, H. H., et al.: Further experience with peritoneovenous shunt for ascites. Ann. Surg. 184:574, 1976.

66. LeVeen, H. H., et al.: Ascites: its correction by peritoneovenous shunting. Curr. Prob. Surg. 16:2, 1979.

67. Levesque, D. C., et al.: Congenital portacaval shunts in two cats: diagnosis and surgical correction. J. Am. Vet. Med. Assoc. 181:143, 1982.

68. Litwin, M. S.: Trauma: management of the acutely injured patient. *In* Sabiston, D. C. (ed.): *Davis-Christopher Textbook of Surgery XII.* W. B. Saunders, Philadelphia, 1981.

69. Markowitz, J., Rappaport, A., and Scott, A. C.: The function of the hepatic artery in the dog. Am. J. Digest. Dis. 16:344, 1949.

70. Marretta, S. M., et al.: Urinary calculi associated with portosystemic shunts in six dogs. J. Am. Vet. Med. Assoc. 178:133, 1981.

71. Martensson, K.: Studies on the etiology of gallstones: a subtilis-like bacilli-group as an etiologic factor. Acta Chir. Scand. Suppl. 62:1, 1941.

72. Martin, E., Poey, V., Saffadi, L., et al.: Triangular ligaments of the canine liver and their role in holding the liver in place. Gaceta Veterinaria 42:198, 1980.

73. Meyer, D. J., et al.: Ammonia tolerance test in clinically normal dogs and dogs with portosystemic shunts. J. Am. Vet. Med. Assoc. 173:377, 1978.

74. Millar, J. A. S., and Hubbard, D. W.: Gallstones in a dog. J. Am. Vet. Med. Assoc. 108:160, 1946.

75. Mitchell, J. R., Nelson, S. D., Thorgeirsson, S. S., et al.: Metabolic activation: biochemical basis for many drug-induced liver injuries. Prog. Liver Dis. 5:259, 1976.

76. Monro, A.: A treatise on comparative anatomy. *In A System of Anatomy and Physiology.* Vol. III. Elliot, Edinburgh, 1787.

77. Mullowney, P. C., and Tennant, B. C.: Choledocholithiasis in the dog: a review and a report of a case with rupture of the common bile duct. J. Small Anim. Pract. 23:631, 1982.

78. Nakayama, F.: Composition of gallstone and bile: species differences. J. Lab. Clin. Med. 73:623, 1969.

79. Nelson, C. N., Piker, J. F., and Welsch, R. A.: Cholelithiasis in a dog. J. Am. Vet. Med. Assoc. 152:47, 1968.

80. Nickel, R., Schummer, A., Seiferle, E., and Sack, W. O.: *The Viscera of the Domestic Mammals.* Verlag Paul Parey, Berlin, 1973.

81. O'Brien, T.: Cholecystography. *In: Radiographic Diagnosis of Abdominal Disorders in the Dog and Cat.* W. B. Saunders, Philadelphia, 1978.

82. O'Brien, T. R.: *Radiographic Diagnosis of Abdominal Disorders in the Dog and Cat*. W. B. Saunders, Philadelphia, 1978.

83. O'Brien, T. R., and Mitchum, G. D.: Cholelithiasis in a Cat. J. Am. Vet. Med. Assoc. *156*:1015, 1970.

84. Orloff, M. J.: The liver. *In* Sabiston, D. C. (ed.): *Davis-Christopher Textbook of Surgery XII*. W. B. Saunders, Philadelphia, 1981.

85. Orloff, M. J.: The biliary system. *In* Sabiston, D. C. (ed.): *Davis-Christopher Textbook of Surgery XII*. W. B. Saunders, Philadelphia, 1981.

86. Osborne, C. A., et al.: Liver biopsy. Vet. Clin. North Am. *4*:333, 1974.

87. Parascandolo, C.: Obstruction des Ductus choledochus durch Gallensteine beim Hunde-Operation und Heilung. Arch. Wissensch. u. Prakt. Thierh. *28*:484, 1902.

88. Pass, M. A.: The relationship of hepatic drug metabolism to hepatotoxicity with some examples in sheep. Vet. Ann. *22*:129, 1982.

89. Payer, V. J., Riedel, J., Minar, J., and Moravec, R.: Der extra hepatale Abschnitt der Leberarterie des Hundes vom Gesichtspunkt der chirurgischen Anatomie. Anat. Anz. *103*:246, 1956.

90. Putnam, C. W., and Starzl, T. E.: Simplified biopsy of the liver in dogs. Surg. Gynecol. Obstet. *144*:759, 1977.

91. Rawlings, C. A.: Presentation at the Annual Surgical Forum, Am. Coll. Vet. Surg., Chicago, 1981.

92. Rayford, P. L., Miller, T. A., and Thompson, J. C.: Secretin, cholecystokinin and newer gastrointestinal hormones. New Engl. J. Med. *294*:1093, 1976.

93. Revell, D. G.: The pancreatic ducts in the dog. Am. J. Anat. *1*:443, 1902.

94. Robins, G., Thornton, J., and Mills, J.: Bile peritonitis and pleuritis in a dog. J. Am. Anim. Hosp. Assoc. *13*:55, 1977.

95. Schall, W. D., et al.: Cholelithiasis in dogs. J. Am. Vet. Med. Assoc. *163*:469, 1973.

96. Schlotthauer, C. F.: Gallstones in dogs: reports of two cases. North Am. Vet. *26*:349, 1945.

97. Schlotthauer, C. F., and Stalker, L. K.: Cholelithiasis in dogs: report of two cases. J. Am. Vet. Med. Assoc. *88*:758, 1936.

98. Schmid, R.: Bilirubin metabolism: state of the art. Gastroenterology *74*:1307, 1978.

99. Scott, D. W., et al.: Cholelithiasis in a dog. J. Am. Vet. Med. Assoc. *163*:254, 1973.

100. Shaffer, E. A., and Small, D. M.: Gallstone disease: pathogenesis and management. Curr. Prob. Surg. *13*:7, 1976.

101. Simpson, S. T., and Hribernik, T. N.: Porto-systemic shunt in the dog: two case reports. J. Small Anim. Pract. *17*:163, 1976.

102. Sleight, D. R., and Thomford, N. R.: Gross anatomy of the blood supply and biliary drainage of the canine liver. Anat. Rec. *166*:153, 1970.

103. Smith, R. L.: *The Excretory Function of Bile: The Elimination of Drugs and Toxic Substances in Bile*. Chapman and Hall, London, 1973.

104. Starzl, T. E., and Koep, L.: Liver homotransplantation. *In* Sabiston, D. C. (ed.): *Davis-Christopher Textbook of Surgery XII*. W. B. Saunders, Philadelphia, 1981.

105. Starzl, T. E., and Teiblanche, J.: Hepatotrophic substances. *In* Popper, M., and Schaffner, F. (eds.): *Progress in Liver Disease VI*. Grune & Stratton, New York, 1979.

106. Starzyl, T. E., Francavilla, A., Halgrimson, C. G., et al.: The origin, hormonal nature and action of hepatotrophic substances in portal venous blood. Surg. Gynecol. Obstet. *137*:179, 1973.

107. Starzl, T. E., Porter, K. A., and Putnam, C. W.: Intraportal insulin protects from the liver injury of portacaval shunt in dogs. Lancet *2*:1741, 1975.

108. Steinberg, D.: On leaving the peritoneal cavity open in acute generalized suppurative peritonitis. Am. J. Surg. *137*:216, 1979.

109. Stichle, R.: Personal communication. Michigan State University, 1983.

110. Strombeck, D. R.: Portosystemic vascular anastomoses. *In*: *Small Animal Gastroenterology*. Stonegate Publishing, Davis, Ca., 1979.

111. Strombeck, D. R.: Diseases of the gallbladder. *In*: *Small Animal Gastroenterology*. Stonegate Publishers, Davis, Ca., 1979.

112. Suter, P. F.: Portal vein anomalies in the dog: their angiographic diagnosis. J. Am. Vet. Radiol. Soc. *16*:84, 1975.

113. Tanger, C. H.: A comparison of two methods of cholecystoduodenostomy. Masters Thesis, Texas A&M University, 1982.

114. Tanger, C. H., Turrel, J. M., and Hobson, H. P.: Complications associated with proximal duodenal resection and cholecystoduodenostomy in two cats. Vet. Surg. *11*:60, 1982.

115. Tennant, B. C., and Hornbuckle, W. E.: Diseases of the liver. *In* Anderson, N. V. (ed.): *Veterinary Gastroenterology*. Lea & Febiger, Philadelphia, 1980.

116. Verine, H. J., et al.: Cholelithiasis in a bitch. Vet. Rec. *84*:75, 1969.

117. Vitums, A.: Portosystemic communications in the dog. Acta Anat. *39*:271, 1959.

118. Vitums, A.: Portosystemic communications in animals with hepatic cirrhosis and malignant lymphoma. J. Am. Vet. Med. Assoc. *138*:31, 1961.

119. Volkmar, F.: Cholelithiasis in dogs. Vet. Med. *33*:31, 1938.

120. Vulgamott, J. C., et al.: Congenital portacaval anomalies in the cat: two case reports. J. Am. Anim. Hosp. Assoc. *16*:915, 1980.

121. Wakim, K. G., and Mahour, G. H.: Pathophysiological consequences of cholecystectomy. Surg. Gynecol. Obstet. *133*:113, 1971.

122. Weiner, I. M., and Lack, L.: Bile salt absorption; enterohepatic circulation. *In* Code, C. F. (ed.): *Handbook of Physiology*. Sec. 6, Vol. 3. American Physiological Society, Washington, D.C., 1968.

123. Wheeler, H. O.: Concentrating function of the gallbladder. Am. J. Med. *51*:588, 1971.

124. Wingfield, W. E., Betts, C. W., and Rawlings, C. A.: Pathophysiology associated with gastric dilation-volvulus in the dog. J. Am. Anim. Hosp. Assoc. *12*:136, 1976.

Anatomy

John Grandage

LOCATION

The pancreas develops from the first parts of the duodenum, to which it retains a close association. The organ is ensheathed by adjacent mesenteries, and in the dog and cat it is long and slender. In most species the pancreas is one of the most fixed of the abdominal viscera,[2] but in carnivores it is more mobile, with a lobulated form that allows it to bend within the mesentery. It adopts a V or L shape with the angle located against the cranial part of the duodenum. Its weight may vary by as much as threefold,[25, 31] although such differences are not striking at either surgery or autopsy.

The larger segment (the right lobe, duodenal limb) is also the longer. It runs beside the descending duodenum either against the right flank or as high as the abdominal roof. It is located in the mesoduodenum, sandwiched betweeen the duodenum (ventrolaterally) and the ascending colon (dorsomedially). As the middle part of the descending duodenum is the most mobile, so too is the adjacent part of the pancreas.

The smaller, shorter, thicker, segment (left lobe, gastric limb, tail) lies in the deep leaf of the greater omentum and runs obliquely caudally, dorsally, and to the left. It is not intimately related to a specific segment of gut and is found high in the abdomen, lodged between the left kidney, stomach, and transvese colon.[24] It lies beneath the great vessels, including the portal vein. Left and right limbs meet at the apex of a V (the body of the pancreas, pancreatic angle), which is the only part that closely embraces the cranial part of the duodenum. It may, with care, be parted from the duodenum by blunt dissection or by "rubbing away."[13]

The pancreas is invisible radiographically, and its position must be inferred from its relation to the pylorus or duodenum. These adjacent organs can provide important clues about pancreatic status.[19, 27]

It is worthwhile to conjure a simple picture of its normal location (Fig. 55–1).

DUCTS

Pancreatic ducts are totally concealed within the substance of the gland. Large interlobular ducts run longitudinally in the middle of the gland and terminate in the duodenum without ever becoming visible. Unlike the bile duct, the pancreatic ducts course straight through the gut wall at right angles to it. The ducts are sometimes palpable, are tough, and can be exposed by blunt dissection.

Because the pancreas arises from both dorsal and ventral primordia, it usually has two ducts, a pancreatic duct and an accessory pancreatic duct, although an additional one has been recorded in about eight per cent of dogs.[26] Many variations in form and development of the ducts are recorded, and their unpredictability may present problems for the surgeon. In nearly all cases the ducts communicate with each other within the substance of the gland,[26, 31] usually uniting in the body of the gland where the two limbs meet.[6] Surgically it is not possible to determine the precise duct pattern except by blunt dissection. The one, two, or three ducts all open within about four centimeters of each other. A sphincter has been described for each.[15] The *pancreatic duct* (of Wirsung) arises from the ventral primordium and usually opens with the bile duct on the major duodenal papilla five centimeters or so from the pylorus. It is always present and is the principal and usually the only duct in the cat. It is small in the dog and drains only the left lobe. Sometimes it may open directly into the bile duct, and at other times independently of the bile duct.[6] The *accessory pancreatic duct* (of Santorini) arises from the dorsal primordium. It is present in only about 20 per cent of cats but is the larger duct in the dog. It opens onto the minor duodenal papilla, some two centimeters distal to the major papilla.

Nodular accessory pancreases may be found in the wall of the stomach, gut, or gallbladder and may be dislocations of primordia. Occasionally a so-called pancreatic bladder is seen, particularly in the cat; this is a dilated pancreatic duct and should be regarded as an insignificant pathological variant.[4]

VESSELS AND NERVES

The pancreas is supplied by several small-caliber arteries.[2, 7] Precise patterns vary, but the following

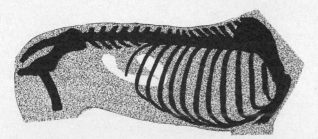

Figure 55–1. The typical location of the pancreas. The part of the right limb shown beneath the last rib is the most mobile; the body and the adjacent part of the left limb are the least mobile.

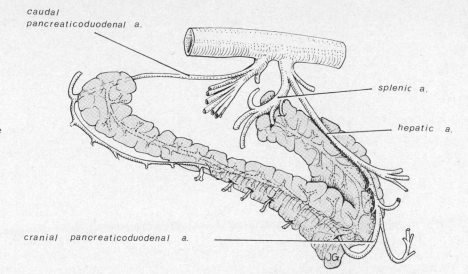

Figure 55–2. Blood supply to the canine pancreas viewed from the right side.

scheme generally applies (Fig. 55–2). The celiac artery supplies most of the gland, with the cranial mesenteric artery supplying only the caudal part of the right limb. Two of the three branches of the celiac artery contribute radicles to the pancreas: branches of the splenic artery enter the end of the left limb, and branches from a distal segment of the hepatic (gastroduodenal) artery supply the body of the pancreas; the terminal branch of the hepatic artery becomes the cranial pancreaticoduodenal artery, which plunges into the body of the gland and supplies the cranial half of the right limb. Duodenal branches are given off from this vessel and course through the pancreatic tissue to supply the gut itself. The remaining portion of the pancreas is supplied by the caudal pancreaticoduodenal branch of the cranial mesenteric artery. Anastomoses between these various vessels occur within the substance of the gland.[16] Several portal tributaries drain the various parts.

A few autonomic nerves reach the pancreas, which is curiously populated with Vater-Pacini corpuscles.[24, 37] The corpuscles are especially numerous in both the cat and dog. Lymphatics are abundant[2] and drain into the duodenal lymph node, if present, or into the mesenteric lymph nodes.

Physiology

Michael A. Pass

PANCREATIC EXOCRINE FUNCTION

Pancreatic juice is secreted into the duodenum by the exocrine portion of the pancreas. It contains several important digestive enzymes or their precursors, including trypsinogen, chymotrypsinogen, procarboxypeptidase, prophospholipase A, proelastase, lipase, amylase, cholesterol hydrase, and nucleases (Fig. 55–3). Pancreatic juice has a high content of bicarbonate ions, which help to neutralize gastric acid in the intestine, and also contains colipase, which is important for the digestion of triglycerides.

The pancreatic enzymes are secreted by acinar cells. The electrolyte concentrations of the acinar secretion are similar to extracellular fluid, but the electrolyte concentrations of pancreatic juice are modified by secretion from the pancreatic ducts. The ductular secretion has a high concentration of bicarbonate ions, so the secretion that enters the duodenum is alkaline.

The enzymes trypsin, chymotrypsin, carboxypeptidase, phospholipase A, and elastase are secreted as inactive forms. Trypsinogen is activated to trypsin in the lumen of the intestine by the enzyme enterokinase, which is secreted by the small intestine in response to chyme in the intestinal lumen. Trypsin then activates the other enzymes (see Fig. 55–3).

Pancreatic secretion is stimulated by the vagus nerves and the gastrointestinal hormones cholecystokinin and secretin.[29, 35] The sight, smell, or taste of food and distention of the stomach increase secretion of pancreatic enzymes by vagal stimulation. Enzyme secretion is also stimulated by the gastrointestinal hormone cholecystokinin, which is released from the small intestine in response to chyme in the intestinal lumen (see Fig. 55–3). Food in the small intestine also causes release of the gastrointestinal hormone secretin, which is the major stimulant to secretion of the bicarbonate-rich fluid from the pancreatic ductules.

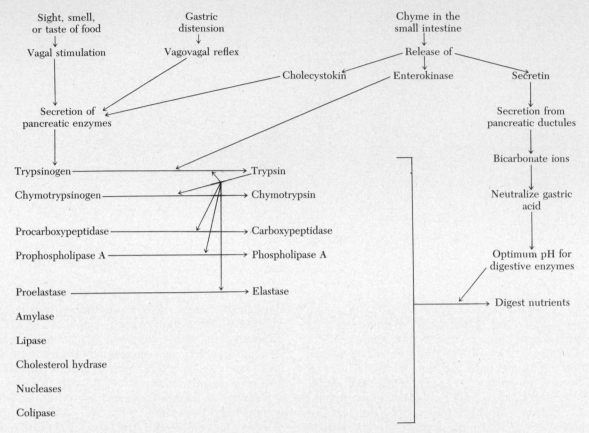

Figure 55–3. Scheme for control of pancreatic secretion and activation of pancreatic enzymes.

Surgical Diseases of the Exocrine Pancreas

Richard Walshaw

PANCREATITIS

In the dog and cat, pancreatitis is either acute edematous or necrotizing, hemorrhagic) or chronic (relapsing). In the chronic form, repeated bouts of acute pancreatitis can lead to an anatomic and functional destruction of both the endocrine and exocrine portions of the pancreas. Results of this destructive pancreas include end-stage pancreatic insufficiency, diabetes mellitus, and gastrointestinal and bile duct obstruction.[17, 23]

Pancreatitis is relatively common in dogs but it is rare in cats, possibly owing to the fact that cats experience a more chronic, frequently subclinical, low-grade interstitial pancreatitis.[14, 33, 38]

Middle-aged, obese, sedentary dogs are affected, and there is a higher incidence in females. Pancreatitis is rare in healthy, physically active dogs.[17, 33] A typical profile for cats with pancreatitis is unavailable because of the low incidence of the disease, except for trauma-induced pancreatitis in cats with the "high-rise syndrome."[1, 14, 33]

Etiology

The etiology of pancreatitis in the dog and cat is obscure; suggestions are based on inference from what is known in humans and from experimental acute pancreatitis in dogs.[18, 34, 39] Table 55–1 lists the known causes in humans and experimental animals. In the dog, most cases of pancreatitis are diagnosed as idiopathic.

Pathophysiology

Injury to the pancreatic acinar cells and obstruction of the pancreatic ducts are important factors in the development of pancreatitis.[11] The pancreas is normally protected from autodigestion by storing its digestive enzymes in zymogen granules, by synthesizing some enzymes in an inactive precursor form, and by the presence of trypsin inhibitors in the cells.[17, 22] Injury to the acinar cells results in the release of digestive enzymes and the premature ac-

TABLE 55–1. Causes of Pancreatitis in Dogs and Cats

Suggested Etiology	Comments
Bile reflux	No evidence to support this as being a clinical problem in the dog and cat.
Occlusion of the pancreatic ducts—without impairment to bile flow and with continued stimulation of pancreatic secretion	Experimentally, produces pancreatitis in the dog. Severity increased if vascular supply compromised.
Reflux of duodenal contents into pancreatic ducts	Experimentally, produces severe pancreatitis, but no conclusive evidence to show that this happens naturally.
Nutrition	High-fat diets for extended periods.
Bacteria	Of unknown importance.
Viruses	Have been associated with pancreatitis in humans; pancreatitis possibly occurs with parvovirus in puppies.
Autoimmune or allergic mechanisms	—
Trauma	Real, post-surgical (iatrogenic)
Drug-induced pancreatitis	An increasingly recognized problem in humans and animals. Many drugs are known to cause this but glucocorticoids and ACTH have the highest incrimination rate.
Hereditary pancreatitis	Known to occur in humans.
Metabolic disorder resulting in hyperlipidemia, uremia, hypercalcemia, increased incidence with these problems	—

tivation of proenzymes with subsequent pancreatic autodigestion and necrosis. Damage can be variable, from a localized edematous pancreatitis to severe autodigestion with spillage of proteolytic and lipolytic enzymes into the abdominal cavity. Severe peripancreatic fat necrosis and abscess formation and spreading peritonitis may develop. Owing to the acute inflammatory changes in the peritoneal cavity, large quantities of fluid may be sequestered here and in the paralyzed gastrointestinal tract.[17, 33, 34, 38]

Fluid sequestration in the peritoneal cavity, the gastrointestinal tract, the pancreas itself, and the splanchnic circulation, together with the systemic effects of released vasoactive agents and toxic factors including myocardial depressant factor and endotoxins from the destroyed pancreas, can lead to a progressive hypovolemic and toxic shock in severe cases.[17, 33, 34, 38]

Other systemic effects have been noted in pancreatitis patients.[17, 33, 38] The released digestive enzymes can activate the clotting mechanism, resulting in both local and disseminated intravascular coagulation.

The pulmonary edema seen in these patients may result from injury to pulmonary capillaries and digestion of surfactant by circulating pancreatic enzymes. This vascular damage allows plasma to leak into the interstitial spaces of the lung and into alveoli.

Hepatitis and hepatic necrosis and nephrosis have also been reported and are probably the result of circulating pancreatic enzymes and toxins. Cardiomyopathy and arrhythmias may be caused by toxic factors released by the pancreas or may be the result of a direct effect of pancreatic enzymes on the heart muscle itself.

Electrolyte alterations can occur from fluid loss and sequestration and tissue destruction. In particular, hypocalcemia is seen, probably owing to a combination of factors such as the precipitation of calcium in the soaps that form in the necrotic fat, low plasma protein levels with reduced calcium carrying capacities, and a reduced parathomone response.

Hyperglycemia is also commonly seen because of exocrine glucagon release or inadequate insulin release. Diabetes mellitus produced during acute pancreatitis is usually transient, but if the islet cell population is reduced by previous or recurring attacks, diabetes become permanent.

Acute Pancreatitis

History[17, 33, 38]

The history includes: vomiting (occasional to many times per hour), depression, anorexia, and nausea (as expressed by ptyalism, repeated swallowing, restlessness, and pacing). Diarrhea may be present if portions of the intestinal tract surrounding the pancreas are involved in the disease process.

Abdominal pain is one of the most consistent symptoms. It is signified by a stiff gait, arched back, reluctance to move, lying down on cool surfaces, lying in an abnormal position in an attempt to relieve the pain, and obvious discomfort when handled. The degree of abdominal pain exhibited varies considerably from animal to animal.

Clinical Findings[17, 33, 38]

Pancreatitis is variable in its clinical presentation, there being no consistent pathognomonic signs. The clinical picture can vary from one of an apparent mild gastric problem to that of a peracute abdomen. Abdominal pain, particularly localized to the right cranial portion of the abdomen, when associated with vomiting is highly suggestive of pancreatitis. The absence of pain, however, does not rule out this diagnosis.

A mild elevation of body temperature is often noted but the temperature may become subnormal with progressive shock in severely affected cases. Varying degrees of dehydration are present owing to fluid loss from vomiting, diarrhea, and fluid sequestration within the abdominal cavity. There may be overt signs of hypovolemic or endotoxic shock.

Abdominal distension due to fluid accumulation, paralytic ileus, and aerophagia may be detected. Diarrhea is inconsistent.

The potential list of "rule-outs," based on these historical and clinical findings and their variability, is large. A number of diagnostic studies are required to complete the minimum data base for these patients.

Laboratory Evaluations

Serum Amylase and Lipase Determinations.[17, 33, 38] Increased serum levels of amylase and lipase in a patient with the previously described clinical presentation are generally diagnostic of pancreatic acinar cell injury.

Serum amylase levels, however, can be elevated in a number of different disease processes. This finding by itself is not diagnostic of pancreatitis. Some controversy exists as to the diagnostic usefulness of elevated serum amylase levels in cats. Increased serum lipase levels are a generally consistent and diagnostic finding in pancreatitis in the dog, there being no other known disease process causing elevation of these levels. Generally, a three to four-fold increase in serum lipase levels is diagnostic. How-

ever, normal plasma lipase activity does not completely obviate a diagnosis of pancreatitis. Increased serum lipase levels have not been found consistently in cats with confirmed pancreatitis. Levels of both enzymes should be measured and followed to increase diagnostic accuracy. Changes in amylase and lipase levels generally follow each other closely. These levels should be monitored daily during the course of the disease to assess progress and effectiveness of the therapy. Monitoring following recovery may help identify chronic relapsing, but asymptomatic, cases.

Abdominal Paracentesis.[17, 33, 38] In the evaluation of an animal with acute abdomen, abdominal paracentesis with fluid analysis can be one of the most useful diagnostic procedures available to the clinician. The finding of serosanguineous fluid with extremely high amylase levels (1,000 S.U./ml) supports the diagnosis of pancreatitis.[9]

Other acute abdominal problems also result in abdominal fluid with a reasonably high amylase level, but generally, in pancreatitis, this level is extremely high. If simple paracentesis fails to yield fluid for analysis, abdominal lavage can be performed, and the fluid obtained can be used for amylase determinations.[9]

Other Blood Evaluations.[17, 33, 38] The hemogram usually reflects a stress response, showing neutrophilia. In peracute conditions, however, with extreme pancreatic destruction and peritonitis, a degenerative left shift is present. Hemoconcentration is also evident.

Blood glucose levels may be elevated owing to transient diabetes caused by the inflammatory process. A controlled diabetic patient may be deregulated

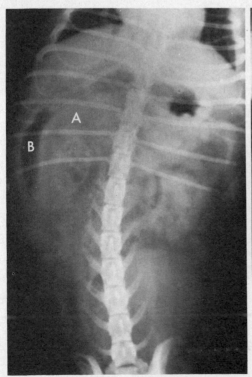

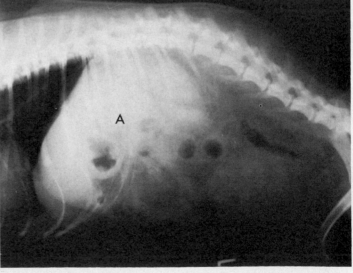

Figure 55–4. Acute pancreatitis in a dog. Plain radiographs demonstrate an increase in radiographic density and loss of detail in the area of the pancreas (A) and a dilated, gas-filled duodenum (B).

because of an attack of pancreatitis, in which case marked hyperglycemia, glucosuria, ketonuria, and ketoacidosis occur.

Liver enzyme elevation, due to hepatic damage that occurs during acute pancreatitis, is usually noted. Underlying liver disease needs to be differentiated from liver disease caused by the acute episode.

Prerenal uremia due to the hypovolemic state may also be noted.

Radiography.[17-19, 33, 38] Radiographic findings in acute pancreatitis may include the following (Fig. 55–4):

1. Evidence of localized peritonitis near the pancreas, suggested by an increase in radiographic density and a loss of detail.

2. A poorly defined "mass" in the area of the pancreas.

3. A dilated, gas-filled duodenum pushed against the right body wall.

4. Ileus of adjacent loops of bowel.

5. Evidence of peritoneal fluid.

The absence of other radiographic findings may help eliminate other causes of the clinical signs. An upper gastrointestinal contrast series outlines the swollen pancreas, further demonstrates disease and fixed position of the duodenum, and excludes other causes of acute vomiting and abdominal pain (Fig. 55–5).

Diagnosis

A diagnosis of acute pancreatitis is based on a summation of historical and clinical findings, elevated serum amylase and lipase levels, plus additional information provided by hemograms, other blood chemistry studies, and radiography.

Treatment

Correct medical therapy cures the majority of cases of acute pancreatitis. The main aim of this therapy is to reduce the synthesis and secretion of pancreatic enzymes to a minimum, while supporting the patient until the acute inflammatory process has subsided. Patient care consists of (1) recognition of shock and correction of fluid, electrolyte, and acid-base abnormalities, (2) inhibition of pancreatic enzyme secretion, (3) control of pain, (4) correctly timed surgical intervention in appropriate cases, and (5) a carefully monitored recovery and convalescence.[17] Even with correctly instituted therapy, patient mortality cannot always be predicted, and careful monitoring is required.

Medical Therapy

Fluid and Electrolyte Thearapy.[17, 33, 38] Vigorous volume replacement therapy is essential, because death usually results from hypovolemic or endotoxic shock. Hypovolemia is marked; experimentally, plasma losses of 30 to 40 per cent may occur. Owing to the acute inflammatory reaction and peritonitis that exist, large quantities of plasma protein are also lost.[17]

Because large volumes of fluid, and possibly plasma, are rapidly administered to these patients, careful patient monitoring is required. An indwelling central venous catheter is necessary. In severe cases it may be necessary to monitor central venous pressure and place an indwelling urinary catheter to monitor urinary output, thereby assessing fluid therapy and renal function. An isotonic multiple electrolyte replacement solution is the fluid of choice for correcting the hypovolemia. Deficits should be corrected as quickly as possible, using packed cell vol-

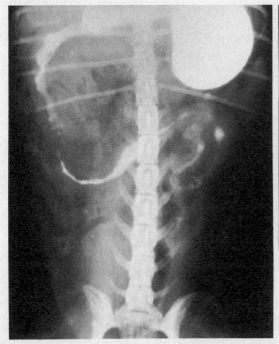

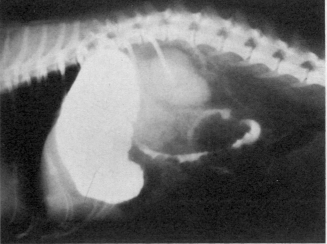

Figure 55–5. An upper gastrointestinal contrast series of the dog with acute pancreatitis shown in Fig. 55–4. Note the laterally displaced, fixed position of the duodenum as it surrounds the swollen pancreas. There is marked irregularity in the duodenal pattern owing to the adjacent severe inflammatory process.

ume, total solids, and, in severe cases, central venous pressure and urinary output to judge the adequacy of therapy.

The patient should be closely monitored for the development of pulmonary edema. Extravasation of fluid into the extravascular space due to a generalized increase in capillary permeability can be seen with acute pancreatitis. Extreme care is required when plasma is used as a replacement fluid to correct hypoproteinemia, because it could exacerbate pulmonary edema.[38]

Low-molecular-weight dextran has been used in humans and experimentally in dogs with pancreatitis. This agent increases pancreatic microcirculation and supports overall blood volume and flow. Occasional bleeding problems have been noted in humans with this plasma expander; therefore careful monitoring is required.[17]

Hypokalemia may be present owing to losses through vomiting and anorexia. Supplementation with potassium chloride, in addition to the potassium already present in the multiple-electrolyte solution, may be required. The acid-base status of the patient is often unpredictable. The severe vomiting may induce metabolic alkalosis. However, in the face of marked hypovolemia and possible endotoxemia, metabolic acidosis can be seen. The patient with acute pancreatitis may well be eubasic owing to these conflicting mechanisms. Acid-base problems are usually corrected by vigorous fluid therapy and the return of renal function. If the equipment is available, acid-base determinations should be made.

Improvement of local pancreatic blood flow is necessary to help prevent the progression of severe hemorrhagic pancreatitis. Certainly, correct fluid therapy will help, but specific therapy aimed at preventing microthrombus formation, lysing newly formed clots, and restoring reduced pancreatic blood flow to normal may be indicated; heparin, fibrinolysin, and vasopressin therapy, respectively, have been shown experimentally to be useful adjuncts in maintaining adequate perfusion of the pancreatic microcirculation. Their use in clinical acute pancreatitis in the dog has not been investigated.

Suppression of Pancreatic Enzyme Secretion. Suppression of pancreatic enzyme secretion is one of the most important parts of therapy. All oral intake is prevented, stopping the physiological chain of events that results in pancreatic enzyme release. Oral feeding should stop until vomiting has ceased for at least 48 to 72 hours.[17, 33, 38]

Anticholinergic drugs, such as atropine, are not beneficial in treating acute pancreatitis. There is no evidence to suggest that they inhibit pancreatic secretion in the unstimulated pancreas. In addition, secretion ceases in acute pancreatitis. Anticholinergic drugs also have marked side effects, including a further reduction of gastrointestinal motility, which is already impaired because of the adjacent acute inflammatory process. The resultant ileus will not help in restoring normal gastrointestinal function.

Anticholinergic agents, such as atropine, cannot be recommended.[33, 38]

Glucagon has been shown experimentally to reduce pancreatic exocrine secretion and also to increase splanchnic blood flow. These properties have yet to be demonstrated to be of clinical use in the dog and cat.[17, 33, 38]

The routine use of corticosteroids to help decrease pancreatic inflammation is contraindicated. Glucocorticoids are known to cause acute pancreatitis in the dog. They result in sludging of the pancreatic secretions and a narrowing of the duct system due to ductular epithelial proliferation, thus impairing drainage of the acinar tissue. Steroid therapy should be reserved for use only in the treatment of endotoxic shock, a situation in which it is definitely indicated.[17, 33, 38]

Analgesia. Meperidine hydrochloride is the drug of choice if the pharmacological control of pain is indicated. Morphine is contraindicated because of its side effects of pancreatic duct sphincter spasm, increasing intraductal pressure, and elevating serum amylase levels. These side effects occur also with meperidine, but to an insignificant degree. Analgesic therapy, if indicated, is required for only one to two days.[17, 38]

Antibiotic Therapy. Prophylactic antibiotic therapy does not improve recovery rates from acute pancreatitis. Antibiotics should be reserved for those patients in which sepsis can be documented and for prophylaxis in surgical exploration. The antibiotic should be determined by Gram stain and culture and sensitivity testing whenever possible.[5, 17, 33]

Surgical Therapy. Very few cases of acute pancreatitis in the dog require surgical intervention. Indications for surgical intervention in acute pancreatitis in dogs are: (1) deterioration in spite of intensive medical therapy; in humans, 48 hours is suggested an appropriate time before surgery is considered;[5, 30] (2) where suspicion of pancreatic abscess or significant peritonitis requiring operative drainage and lavage; (3) where inability to make a definitive diagnosis; and (4) persistence or development of bile duct obstruction after the initial acute inflammatory response has subsided.

The treatment of complications arising from the acute episode are the most likely reason for surgical exploration. Pancreatic abscess formation in humans is associated with mortality rates of close to 100 per cent without surgical intervention and 30 to 50 per cent with drainage.[5] In patients who are progressively deteriorating in spite of aggressive medical therapy, surgical intervention is a controversial issue. Although mortality rates are very high following surgery, it is claimed that operative peritoneal lavage and drainage yield better results than no treatment. Generally, once surgery is considered part of treatment for a patient with acute pancreatitis, the patient has an extremely guarded prognosis.[5, 30]

Following appropriate patient stabilization, the abdomen is explored through cranioventral midline incision. As soon as the abdomen is opened, culture specimens are taken from any fluid and the rest of the fluid is removed with suction to allow easy exploration. It is likely that multiple loose adhesions have formed between the omentum and loops of small intestine covering the duodenum and the inflamed area of the pancreas. These should be carefully broken down, and any abscess pockets should be sampled for culture and evacuated.

Retracting the greater omentum and stomach cranially and using the colon to retract the small intestine caudally completely exposes the duodenum and both limbs of the pancreas. The dorsal leaf of the greater omentum is opened to expose the ventral surface of the left pancreatic limb. Great care should be taken when handling the structures surrounding the pancreas. At this point, the diagnosis of acute pancreatitis should be obvious.

An assessment needs to be made of the viability of the various portions of the pancreas, the extent of damage to the adjacent wall of the duodenum, whether abscesses have developed in and adjacent to the pancreas, and the presence of obstruction of either the bile duct or gastrointestinal tract. The pancreas is greatly lavaged with warm saline to remove debris. Necrotic, ischemic portions of the pancreas, particularly distal portions of the limbs, can be resected providing that the main draining duct system is not damaged. Total pancreatectomy may be indicated if the pancreas is completely destroyed by the disease process. Large abscesses within the substance of the pancreas should be opened, sampled for culture, flushed, and drained.

Duodenal and bile duct involvement in the inflammatory process should be assessed. Extensive inflammatory disease of the duodenal wall and also of the pylorus could lead to partial or complete obstruction of the gastrointestinal tract and biliary system as a long-term complication. These problems may need surgical correction at a later date if clinical signs of gastrointestinal or bile duct obstruction become apparent.

Following surgical correction of pancreatic disease, a complete and thorough abdominal lavage is indicated to rid the peritoneal cavity of contamination. Warm saline solution is used, and the procedure is repeated until the fluid is clear and free of debris.

Prior to abdominal closure, if extreme pancreatic damage is present, the pancreas should be drained. A Penrose drain of suitable size should be placed along each side of the right limb of the pancreas and brought out through an incision in the right abdominal wall. The left limb should be similarly drained through the left body wall. The drains are removed when drainage ceases. If peritonitis is significant, it may be considered appropriate to delay the closure of the abdomen for two to three days. Nonoperative and postoperative peritoneal lavage may be beneficial in severe acute pancreatitis in both humans and dogs.[5, 28, 30, 31] However, in man, no significant overall reduction in mortality rate has been achieved by this technique.[5, 30, 31] The one report of this procedure in the dog did not establish any value for lavage, because no controls were included.[28] Also, significant complications such as anemia, electrolyte disturbances, hypoproteinemia, and infection are associated with these techniques.[5, 30]

Postoperative care consists of continued intravenous fluid and electrolyte therapy, broad-spectrum antibiotic therapy, and no oral feeding. A sterile dressing is placed over the drains to assess drainage and prevent contamination and is changed as often as required until drain removal.

Recovery and Convalescence[17, 38]

Serum amylase and lipase levels should be monitored closely during the recovery or postoperative phase. Return of these levels to normal helps determine when oral feeding can be started. Other blood parameters, such as the white blood cell count, and levels of liver enzymes, serum bilirubin, glucose, and bood urea nitrogen, should be followed to determine resolution.

Intravenous fluid and electrolyte therapy is continued until vomiting has ceased and the patient is able to maintain itself orally. During intravenous fluid therapy, hypokalemia may develop owing to zero intake and continued losses. Multiple electrolyte replacement fluids may have to be supplemented with additional potassium chloride.

If pancreatic drains have been placed during abdominal exploration, they are left in place until the acute inflammatory process has subsided and drainage is minimal. Once the patient has returned to normal feeding, the drains can be removed.

When the patient resumes eating, foods should be used that are least stimulatory to pancreatic secretion. High-carbohydrate diets are used initially. Proteins are gradually introduced, especially those of high biological value. Because diets high in fat contribute to pancreatitis in the dog, they must be avoided. If there is an extended recovery period before oral intake can be resumed, total parenteral nutrition, which does not stimulate the exocrine pancreas, may have to be instituted to support the patient. Ideally, a low-fat diet should be initiated as a long-term measure. If necessary, low-fat prescription diets or fat-free diets, to which medium-chain triglycerides are added, may be used.[38]

Amylase and lipase levels are monitored during convalescence. Pesistently high levels may indicate a chronic, relapsing problem with potentially serious sequelae.

Prognosis[17, 38]

The prognosis of canine or feline pancreatitis depends on establishing an early diagosis, instituting effective and aggressive therapy, and controlling potential complications. Providing that these criteria are met, the majority of animals with acute pancrea-

titis recover uneventfully. Delay in establishing the
diagnosis and instituting effective therapy, however,
can result in significant morbidity and mortality. If
extensive destruction of the pancreas has occurred
because of acute disease, diabetes mellitus and pancreatic exocrine insufficiency may result. Recurrent
pancreatitis may be a major cause of diabetes mellitus
in the dog.

Chronic Pancreatitis

Repeated attacks of acute pancreatitis result in
progressive destruction of the pancreatic glandular
tissue with increasing amounts of fibrous connective
tissue as wound healing continues. Potential sequelae
are diabetes mellitus, exocrine pancreatic insufficiency, and obstruction of the gastrointestinal tract
and biliary tree by scar tissue and adhesions.[17, 33, 38]
This discussion is limited to the obstructive problems
associated with chronic pancreatitis.

History

The animal may be presented for a repeat attack
of acute pancreatitis. The history associated with such
a case may include previous episodes of acute pancreatitis (see previous discussion).

Generally, a patient with obstructive problems
secondary to chronic pancreatitis shows a progressively more frequent vomiting over several weeks to
months. The vomiting may be associated with eating,
and an increased intolerance of solid foods is noted.
Weight loss is seen, and there may be vague indications of abdominal discomfort. Increasing icterus may

be observed. Repeated episodes of acute pancreatitis
may be reported as having occurred months or years
previously. In some cases, however, no such prior
history is given, this presentation being the first
symptomatic episode that the animal has experienced. In others, a definitive diagnosis of acute
pancreatitis may never have been made prior to
presentation, previous bouts of illness being attributed to "gastritis."

Clinical Findings

On physical examination, icterus and weight loss
may be noted. Abdominal palpation may reveal some
discomfort with an ill-defined mass in the right cranial
portion of the abdomen. Dehydration may be present
owing to vomiting and progressive anorexia. If the
patient is experiencing a repeat attack of acute pancreatitis, findings previously described are detected.

The clinical findings are not likely to be diagnostic,
and a number of "rule-outs" can be entertained in a
differential diagnosis. As with acute pancreatitis, additional studies are required to reach a definitive
diagnosis.

Laboratory Evaluations

Serum Amylase and Lipase Determinations.
These values will be abnormal only if the patient is
experiencing acute pancreatitis. With quiescent
chronic pancreatitis, they are normal or even subnormal, a reflection of the severity of glandular
destruction that has occurred previously.[17, 33]

Other Blood Evaluations. The hemogram is likely
to be normal unless an active inflammatory process

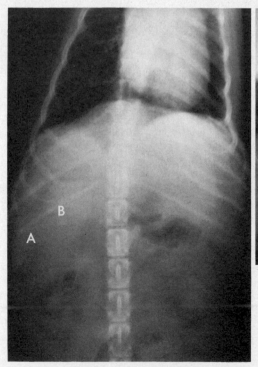
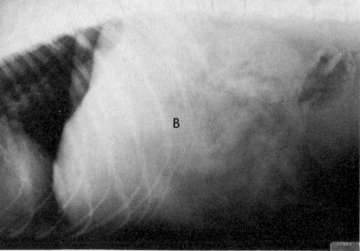

Figure 55–6. Chronic pancreatitis in a dog, resulting in gastrointestinal and
bile duct obstruction. On the ventrodorsal radiograph the duodenum is
pushed laterally owing to an ill-defined mass in the area of the pancreas (A).
An increase in radiographic density and loss of detail are present in the area
of the pancreas (B).

is in progress. Hyperglycemia may be present because of progressive loss of islet cells. Whether the patient is overtly diabetic depends on the extent of this loss.[33] Liver enzyme levels in the blood will probably be elevated, owing to long-standing hepatic damage from the recurrent bouts of acute pancreatitis. Also, extrahepatic bile duct obstruction, if present, is reflected by increases in these enzymes and in serum conjugated bilirubin.

Radiography. Survey abdominal radiographs may reveal an ill-defined mass in the right cranial abdomen. The duodenum, if gas-filled, is seen to be pushed laterally and to have an irregular outline. Gallbladder distention, due to bile duct obstruction, may be detected (Fig. 55–6). An upper gastrointestinal contrast series reveals varying degrees of pyloric or duodenal obstruction. Owing to the encroaching scar tissue and adhesions, an irregular shape and pattern of the pyloric antrum and descending duodenum is seen (Fig. 55–7). These findings, however, are not diagnostic for chronic pancreatitis, even though highly suggestive; neoplasia, for example, cannot be ruled out (Fig. 55–8).

Diagnosis

A diagnosis of obstructive disease due to chronic pancreatitis is suggested by the history, clinical findings, and laboratory evaluations, but definitive diagnosis cannot be made without exploratory surgery and biopsy. Signs and symptoms of other diseases, particularly exocrine pancreatic adenocarcinoma, may mimic these findings.

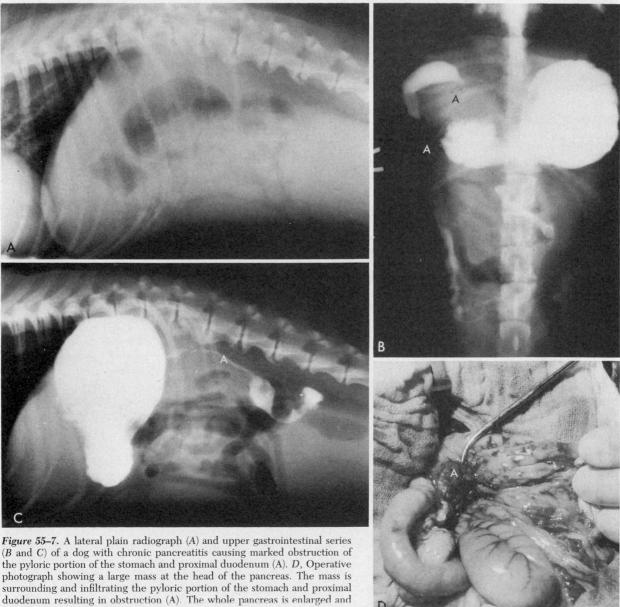

Figure 55–7. A lateral plain radiograph (A) and upper gastrointestinal series (B and C) of a dog with chronic pancreatitis causing marked obstruction of the pyloric portion of the stomach and proximal duodenum (A). D, Operative photograph showing a large mass at the head of the pancreas. The mass is surrounding and infiltrating the pyloric portion of the stomach and proximal duodenum resulting in obstruction (A). The whole pancreas is enlarged and fibrotic.

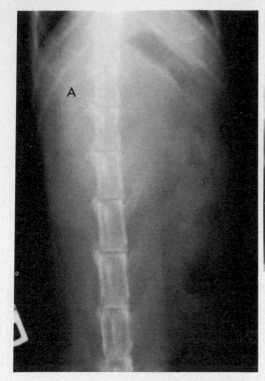

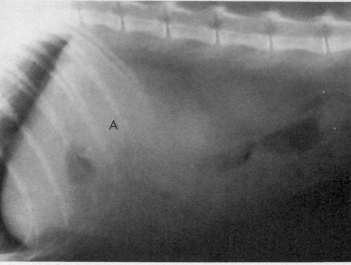

Figure 55–8. Pancreatic adenocarcinoma in a cat. Note the similarity between these radiographs and those shown in Fig. 55–6. An increase in radiographic density and loss of detail in the area of the pancreas (A) in a dog or cat with gastroduodenal or bile duct obstruction is seen with both pancreatic adenocarcinoma and chronic pancreatitis.

Treatment

The patient diagnosed as having chronic relapsing pancreatitis and experiencing an acute episode at the time of presentation should be treated as described in the section on acute pancreatitis.

In chronic pancreatitis with biliary or gastrointestinal obstruction, surgical exploration of the abdomen is indicated. Fluid and electrolyte imbalances should be corrected prior to surgery, and the patient started on broad-spectrum prophylactic antibiotics.

Chronic, persistent pain, a significant problem in humans with chronic pancreatitis due to chronic ductal distension, is not reported in the dog and cat. Also, primary biliary disease is not a cause of pancreatitis as it is in humans, so surgical intervention for this reason is not indicated.[5, 8]

Exploration of the abdominal cavity is performed through a cranioventral midline incision. Many adhesions may be present near the pancreas. These are carefully broken down to identify both limbs of the pancreas, the pylorus and duodenum, and the biliary tree.

An attempt is made at this time to differentiate chronic pancreatitis from pancreatic exocrine adenocarcinoma. These two diseases, unless obvious metastasis to the liver is present, may look grossly similar. Therefore suitable biopsy specimens should be taken and examined. Either frozen sections for histopathological evaluation or impression smears for cytological evaluation are made to provide a tentative diagnosis at surgery. Establishing a diagnosis at this stage may significantly alter treatment. Biopsy samples should be placed in a suitable fixative so that permanent sections can also be made.

The extent of the disease should be assessed at this time to determine what surgical correction is necessary. Generally, it is preferable to avoid extensive resections of the pancreas and duodenum, as such procedures are technically difficult and associated with a high morbidity and mortality. The animal may already be borderline exocrine- or endocrine-deficient. Extensive pancreatectomy may simply aggravate the problems; palliative procedures should be performed to re-establish bile drainage and gastrointestinal continuity. The duodenum should be left intact to drain the remaining pancreatic secretions. Pancreatic resections should be limited to easily accessible, acutely diseased areas, where there is little risk of devascularizing the duodenum. Pancreatic or peripancreatic abscesses should be sampled for culture and evacuated; prior to closure, Penrose drains should be placed in and around them and brought to the outside.

When bile duct obstruction has been caused by the encroaching chronic inflammatory reaction, drainage is most easily re-established by performing a cholecystojejunostomy. This is a functional and well-tolerated procedure if performed correctly in the dog and the cat and will provide adequate biliary tree drainage above the site of obstruction (see Chapter 54).

The invading inflammatory reaction, and subsequent scar tissue formation, can create a functional partial obstruction of the pylorus and descending duodenum. There is rarely complete obstruction of this portion of the gastrointestinal tract. To bypass this poorly functioning portion of the tract, a gastrojejunostomy can be performed to provide good outflow to the stomach. It is not necessary, and owing to the massive inflammatory reaction, it is unadvisable to disconnect the stomach from the duodenum, thereby creating a blind duodenal loop. Gastrojejunostomy is a well-tolerated, functional procedure with few reported problems in the dog and cat (see Chapter 49). Rarely, peptic ulceration of the jejunum at the anastomotic site can occur, but generally, excellent gastrointestinal function is achieved. Pancreatic duct obstruction is not a cause of acute pancreatitis in the dog and cat. Therefore leaving the duodenum intact continues to provide a drainage route for pancreatic secretions.

If extensive disease is present, subtotal pancreatectomy may be necessary. This procedure may well involve removal of portions of the duodenum as well, owing to its intimate involvement in the disease process. Total or subtotal pancreatectomy can be performed. A total pancreatectomy may be technically easier to perform but postoperative patient management may be difficult.

Following completion of the necessary surgical procedures, the abdominal cavity is thoroughly lavaged with warm saline. Penrose drains should be placed around the pancreas, if either severe active inflammation or abscesses are present, and brought to the outside through separate incisions.

Recovery and Convalescence

As with acute pancreatitis, it may be appropriate to monitor serum amylase and lipase levels during the postoperative period, particularly if active disease is present at operation.[17, 38] Iatrogenic pancreatitis may be caused by surgical manipulation and may be detected by serum enzyme monitoring. If bilirubin and liver enzyme levels were elevated preoperatively owing to bile duct occlusion, a decrease in these values indicates successful biliary drainage.

Intravenous fluid and electrolyte therapy is continued until normal gastrointestinal function has returned. The creation of a gastrojejunostomy should allow early return to oral feeding, because the inflamed, irritated portion of the gastrointestinal tract has been bypassed.

If prophylactic antibiotics were used preoperatively, surgical contamination was minimal, and there is no evidence of continued infection, antibiotics can be stopped within 12 to 24 hours postoperatively. However, if Penrose drains were placed, pancreatic abscess was present, and there is evidence of continued infection, a therapeutic regimen of antibiotics should be instituted. Abdominal Penrose drains should be removed when the drainage is minimal and there is no evidence of a continuing pancreatic problem. Diet during the recovery and convalescence phase is as described for acute pancreaputis.[38]

Both exocrine and endocrine pancreatic insufficiency may occur in the dog or cat with chronic relapsing pancreatitis and will be compounded if extensive pancreatic resection has been undertaken.[17, 33, 38]

Prognosis

The prognosis for the animal with chronic relapsing pancreatitis remains guarded, because there may be recurrent episodes, particularly in the cat, in which chronic pancreatitis is usually persistent, producing smoldering inflammation and vague signs of illness.[33] In the dog, complete resolution may occur, particularly if contributing factors are avoided.

With regard to the surgical correction of biliary and gastrointestinal obstruction, providing that technically correct procedures have been performed, prognosis should be favorable for continued normal function. There has been one report in the veterinary literature regarding anastomotic ulceration at the site of a gastrojejunostomy. Appropriate medical therapy should resolve this problem.

Correction and long-term control of both exocrine and endocrine pancreatic deficiencies may prove limiting factors in the management of chronic pancreatitis.

PANCREATIC INJURY

Pancreatic trauma is extremely rare in the dog and cat. In one survey of motor vehicle accidents in 600 dogs, pancreatic injury was not detected.[30] Traumatic pancreatitis due to blunt abdominal trauma occurs in the cat as part of the "high-rise" syndrome.[1, 33, 39]

Pancreatic injury is more likely to result iatrogenically or from penetrating injuries than from blunt abdominal trauma. Penetrating injuries include stab, gunshot, and bite wounds. They also include foreign bodies penetrating outward from the duodenum.[1]

Iatrogenic injury during surgery can be caused by improper handling of the pancreas while adjacent organs are being operated on or by improper techniques of pancreatic surgery, which may result in pancreatic ischemia and necrosis.

History

Signs similar to those previously described for acute pancreatitis become evident following trauma, usually within 12 to 24 hours. Acute and persistent vomiting, evidence of abdominal pain, anorexia, and depression are noted.[1]

If other abdominal organs are also damaged as the result of the injury, signs related to pancreatic injury may be masked by those associated with more acute problems, such as hemoperitoneum.

A history of a previous traumatic episode such as those described in the introduction may be available. With ingestion of a linear or sharp foreign body, intermittent vomiting and a decreased appetite or anorexia may have been observed before the acute episode.

Clinical Findings

As with acute pancreatitis, cranial abdominal pain is present in an acutely depressed, vomiting patient. The patient should be carefully examined for external signs of trauma, such as entrance wounds for bullets or sharp objects or multiple bite wounds, particularly over the right lateral thorax and abdomen.

If the history suggests foreign body ingestion, the oral cavity, particularly the frenulum, should be thoroughly examined for a linear foreign body. Cats suffering from the "high-rise" syndrome often have mandibular or maxillary fractures and thoracic trauma, such as pulmonary contusions. Occasionally, a diaphragmatic hernia may also be present. The clinical signs of traumatic pancreatitis may be masked by these more immediate problems.[39]

Because the injury to the pancreas causes progressive damage, clinical signs of hypovolemic or endotoxic shock may become evident. Fluid may be detected in the abdominal cavity, and generalized abdominal pain may become apparent as peritonitis develops.[1]

Laboratory Evaluation

The detection of elevated serum amylase and lipase levels in a patient presented as outlined previously indicates pancreatic glandular damage.[40] Depending upon which other organ systems have also been injured, abnormalities in other blood values may be noted. Liver enzyme and bilirubin levels are of particular interest. Elevation may indicate associated bile duct or liver damage. Also, the white blood cell count and the differential give some indication of the seriousness of intra-abdominal injury. For example, a degenerative left shift indicates extensive tissue destruction and peritonitis.

Frequently abdominal radiography is initially unrevealing in pancreatic trauma without additional injury. As hemorrhagic pancreatitis progresses, characteristic radiographic changes are detected. An increasing diffuse density in the right cranial abdomen becomes apparent, usually by about the third day after trauma. Dorsal displacement of the duodenum with ileus and corrugation and spasticity of its wall are seen. As the inflammatory process spreads, it involves the entire ventral portion of the abdomen. These radiographic findings have been described in cats with the "high-rise" syndrome. Associated abdominal injuries, including the presence of blood or other fluid in the cavity, tend to obscure the specific radiographic findings. When penetrating abdominal wounds or duodenal perforation is the possible cause of pancreatic injury, free gas may be detected on abdominal radiographs. Localization of gas to the duodenum and pancreas may aid in the diagnosis of pancreatic damage.[39]

Diagnosis

Pancreatic injury is suspected on the basis of history and clinical findings, elevated serum amylase and lipase levels, and characteristic findings on abdominal radiographs. Abdominal paracentesis and lavage are useful in diagnosing pancreatic injury and in assessing the abdominal trauma patient in general. With extensive pancreatic glandular damage, amylase levels in the abdominal fluid are greatly increased (over 1,000 S.U./ml). These levels also increase with intestinal injury and ischemia, but they do not reach such high values. When intestines are damaged, microscopic examination of the abdominal fluid reveals septic peritonitis and possibly intestinal contents.[5]

In either penetrating abdominal trauma or bowel perforation, surgical exploration of the abdomen confirms the diagnosis of pancreatic injury. Generally, all cases of penetrating abdominal injury should be surgically explored, as the chance of significant intra-abdominal organ damage is high.

Treatment

If blunt abdominal trauma has induced acute pancreatitis, the disorder is treated medically: supportive fluid and electrolyte therapy, no oral feeding until vomiting has ceased, and possibly, in the case of trauma, antibiotic therapy. Serum amylase and lipase levels can be used to monitor resolution of the process. With the same criteria as described in the section on acute pancreatitis, surgical exploration of the abdomen may be indicated if the disease process is progressing in spite of intensive medical therapy.[5]

Cats that develop traumatic pancreatitis associated with "high-rise" syndrome develop a severe form of the disease, with extensive pancreatic damage and peritonitis, that is associated with a high mortality. Surgical intervention may have to be considered early in the clinical course.[31]

Penetrating abdominal trauma almost uniformly results in intra-abdominal organ damage that requires surgical correction. In these cases exploratory laparotomy is indicated, in addition to intensive medical therapy, to correct such problems. Certain surgical procedures are useful in the management of different types of pancreatic injury.[1, 5, 12, 21]

When contusion or laceration of the pancreas has occurred without disruption of the major duct system, external drainage after careful debridement and operative lavage is often the treatment of choice. Debridement of contused or necrotic tissue should be performed cautiously to avoid damage to the major ducts. Thorough intraoperative abdominal lavage is performed to remove all debris from the cavity. Penrose drains are placed adjacent to the injured portions of the pancreas and are brought to the outside through separate incisions. Complications that can occur following such treatment include fistula formation and the development of pseudocysts due to leakage of secretions from small duct ruptures.[1, 5, 12]

If damage is severe, particularly in the more distal portions of the right limb and the whole left limb, partial pancreatic resection is probably better than external drainage. It may be safer to perform a partial pancreatectomy than to leave damaged, leaking portions of the pancreas in the abdomen.[1, 5, 12]

Severe trauma to the body of the pancreas, with major duct disruption and duodenal damage, may require a total pancreatectomy and possibly resection of portions of the duodenum.[5, 12, 21] If so, cholecystojejunostomy and gastrojejunostomy may be required to reconstruct the gastrointestinal tract and provide an avenue for biliary drainage. If the duodenum and its blood supply are intact, a total pancreatectomy can be performed, with preservation of these structures.

The patient can maintain normal exocrine and endocrine function with at least 80 per cent of the pancreas resected, providing that the major duct systems are intact and the duodenum is viable.[1, 5, 12]

Recovery and Convalescence

Postoperative care is the same as for acute and chronic pancreatitis. If a pancreatic fistula develops owing to external drainage, the patient should be carefully monitored for potential problems associated with the loss of large volumes of pancreatic fluid, which is rich in bicarbonate. Hyponatremia, acidosis, and hypovolemia may occur. Small fistulas usually close spontaneously following drain removal, particularly if pancreatic secretion can be minimized.[5, 12] Large fistulas may require reoperation with resection and duct ligation. Cyst formation in the dog and cat is rare. Cysts are not usually associated with any clinical signs and may not require removal.[11] In humans, cyst removal or drainage is usually recommended because the results of nonoperative prolonged observation are poor.[5]

Prognosis

The prognosis for animals with traumatic pancreatitis depends on pancreatic damage, associated injuries and early recognition and diagnosis. In one report of traumatic pancreatitis in cats due to the "high-rise" syndrome, the mortality rate was extremely high and probably reflected an inability to recognize the problem and to institute appropriate aggressive therapy early enough.[39]

SURGICAL PROCEDURES

Pancreatic Biopsy

Pancreatic biopsy can be performed either as a surgical procedure at the time of abdominal exploration or via laparoscopy. In humans, needle aspiration biopsy has been successfully performed.[17, 38]

Laparoscopy allows good observation of the right limb of the pancreas, the duodenum, and adjacent structures.[10] The left limb, however, cannot be seen via this technique. Laparoscopy can be performed either from a ventral midline position or from the right paralumbar area. Biopsy cup forceps provide suitable pieces of tissue for histological evaluation. Laparoscopy with biopsy may be an important step in differentiating pancreatic adenocarcinoma from the obstructive sequelae of chronic pancreatitis without subjecting the patient to surgery. The extensive adhesions that are often present may obscure the pancreas. During a laparoscopic examination of the abdomen in suspected pancreatic carcinoma, the liver is thoroughly examined for metastases. These may be the only lesions easily visible, and biopsy samples should be taken. Also, seeding of pancreatic adenocarcinoma through the omentum and mesentery may be present and, biopsy of suspicious lesions should be performed.

Pancreatic biopsy should be performed at the time of surgical exploration of the abdomen if other procedures have failed to provide a definitive diagnosis. When obstruction of the biliary tree and gastrointestinal tract is present and is thought to be due either to chronic relapsing pancreatitis or to pancreatic exocrine adenocarcinoma, a thorough exploration of the whole cranial abdomen is performed. Enlarged lymph nodes or suspicious liver lesions are sampled and may provide a definitive diagnosis. Similarly, in patients with islet cell carcinoma, the draining lymph nodes and the liver are carefully examined and sampled.

Surgical biopsy of the pancreas for diffuse disease should be performed at the distal extremity of the limbs to avoid damage to major ducts and blood vessels. For lesions restricted to the main body of the pancreas, as pancreatic carcinoma frequently is, great care is taken when obtaining the specimen to avoid penetrating deeply into the tissue and thereby disturbing major duct systems and blood vessels.

Biopsy specimens are taken from the extremities of the limbs by gently separating adjacent pancreatic lobules using blunt dissection until a pedicle is created. The major pancreatic ducts are preserved by this method. The pedicle, which consists of the smaller ducts to those lobules, can be safely ligated and the biopsy specimen removed. The pancreas should be handled with extreme care during this procedure to avoid iatrogenic pancreatitis. Using blunt dissection minimizes hemorrhage and leakage of pancreatic secretions from adjacent lobules (Fig. 55–9).

Biopsy of more solid lesions, such as exocrine adenocarcinoma, can be obtained either by wedge incisional biopsy or use of a 4-mm Keyes biopsy punch. When the specimens are obtained, impression smears are made by cytological evaluation. Examining these immediately may make it possible to obtain a diagnosis that may significantly alter the course of treatment. The remaining specimens are placed in fixative for permanent sectioning. Hemorrhage from the biopsy site is best controlled with pressure or electrocautery.

Islet cell carcinomas are sampled by complete

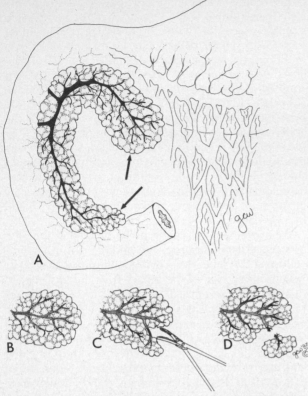

Figure 55–9. Pancreatic biopsy. *A, Arrows* indicate the extremity of the two pancreatic limbs where surgical biopsy specimens can be safely taken without disruption of major ducts, in cases of diffuse disease. *B* and *C,* The portion of the pancreas to be sampled is identified. The adjacent pancreatic lobules are gently separated using blunt dissection. The duct structures will be identified. *D,* The ducts have been ligated and divided and the biopsy specimen has been removed.

excision. These lesions are usually solitary in the pancreas, although metastasis to regional lymph nodes and liver may have occurred. If the lesion is in the left limb or the distal portion of the right limb, it is most easily removed by partial pancreatectomy. However, if the lesion is well circumscribed, as is most often the case, and is in the right limb adjacent to the duodenum, it must be carefully freed by blunt dissection from the rest of the pancreas without disturbing the blood supply to the duodenum and the pancreas or the major ducts. The surgical site is lavaged with saline to remove released pancreatic enzymes prior to closure of the abdomen.

Operative Pancreatic Lavage and Drainage

Lavage of the peritoneal cavity in acute pancreatitis in the dog is believed to increase survival rate as a result of removal of destructive pancreatic enzymes from the abdominal cavity.[18, 39] Although this procedure is of some immediate clinical benefit in humans[5, 30, 31] there are no controlled clinical studies in the dog to demonstrate it. One study in which peritoneal lavage was reported for the treatment of pancreatitis in the dog did not establish any definite value for the procedure, owing to the small number of patients and lack of control dogs.[30]

However, operative lavage of the pancreas and peritoneal cavity (as previously described for acute pancreatitis) may be of potential benefit in patients who are deteriorating in spite of aggressive medical therapy. Following debridement of areas of pancreatic necrosis and drainage of abscess cavities, the pancreas should be thoroughtly lavaged with copious amounts of warm saline. The whole abdominal cavity is similarly lavaged until the return fluid is clear and free of debris. With the use of copious volumes of warm saline, debris, pancreatic enzymes and bacteria can be diluted out and removed.

Following completion of this procedure, the pancreas can be drained. Penrose drains of suitable size are placed along each side of right limb of the pancreas and brought out through an incision in the right abdominal wall. The left limb can be similarly drained through the left body wall (Fig. 55–10).

If peritonitis is severe, closure of the abdomen can be delayed. This technique has been well described for the treatment of acute generalized suppurative peritonitis in humans and has been used successfully to treat peritonitis associated with acute pancreatitis.[36] I have used open peritoneal drainage successfully to treat acute peritonitis or various etiologies in the dog. Postoperative peritoneal lavage cannot be recommended, because it is not effective and it possesses a number of potentially serious complications.[28] The drains are left in place until drainage ceases, the patient has returned to oral feeding, and the acute inflammatory process has subsided.

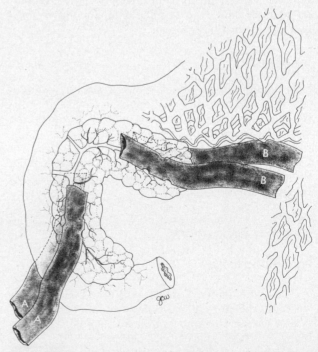

Figure 55–10. Operative pancreatic drainage. *A,* Penrose drains placed along each side of the right limb of the pancreas and exiting through the right abdominal wall. *B,* Penrose drains placed along each side of the left limb of the pancreas and exiting through the left abdominal wall.

Partial Pancreatectomy

Partial pancreatectomy is indicated when extensive necrosis has occurred to a portion of the pancreas as part of the disease process of pancreatitis. Animals with cysts or abscesses secondary to pancreatitis may require partial pancreatectomy. The other main indication is in the surgical treatment of islet cell neoplasia in which the tumors are large and invasive and are situated in either the distal portion of the right or any portion of the left limb of the pancreas.

The pancreas is surgically exposed by making a cranial ventral midline abdominal incision. Self-retaining retractors are required for the body wall. The omentum can be mobilized cranially and retracted from the abdomen. Careful packing-off of the omentum with saline-moistened laparotomy sponges and similar packing-off and caudal retraction of the colon expose the left limb of the pancreas. To examine the ventral surface of this limb, the omental sac is opened adjacent to the pancreas. In neoplastic disease, the draining lymph node chains running along the splenic vessels and the portal vein are carefully examined.

The right limb of the pancreas is exposed by mobilizing the duodenum and packing off the small bowel and colon medially and caudally with saline-moistened laparotomy sponges. The lymph nodes at the head of the pancreas and the hilus of the liver can be examined at this time. Performing these maneuvers exposes the whole pancreas. The blood supply to the two limbs of the pancreas should also be carefully examined to determine the position of the cranial and caudal pancreaticoduodenal vessels and the splenic vessel branches that supply the left limb of the pancreas. The position of these vessels may well determine the extent of the pancreatic resection.

During a partial pancreatectomy, care should be taken to avoid iatrogenic damage to the remaining pancreas. This organ should be handled as little as possible during the surgical procedure.

Working from the distal end of the limb to be

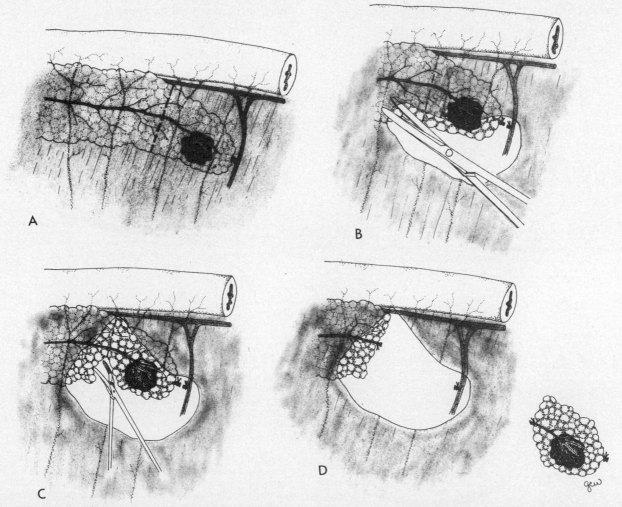

Figure 55–11. Partial pancreatectomy—removal of the distal portion of the right limb. *A*, The duodenum is carefully elevated to expose the right limb of the pancreas containing the lesion. The area is packed off from the rest of the abdomen with moist laparotomy sponges. *B*, The mesentery is incised, and appropriate blood vessels are ligated and divided to free the limb up to the intended point of resection. *C*, The mesentery covering the pancreas is carefully incised to expose the pancreatic lobules, which are then carefully separated using blunt dissection until the major duct is identified. *D*, The duct is then ligated and divided, and the distal portion of the limb is removed. The mesenteric defect should be closed to prevent herniation.

resected, the mesentery is incised and the appropriate blood vessels are ligated and divided to free the limb to the intended point of resection (Fig. 55–11). At the point of resection, the mesentery covering the pancreas is carefully incised to expose the pancreatic lobules. The pancreatic lobules are separated using blunt dissection with forceps or mosquito hemostats from both sides of the limb until the major duct is identified. When the duct is suitably exposed, it can be ligated. Gut suture is not used because of possible rapid enzyme digestion. The duct is transected and the portion of the pancreas removed.[13] The operative area is lavaged with warm saline to remove any debris and dilute and to remove pancreatic sections. Whether the area of resection should be drained depends on the reason the partial pancreatectomy was performed, the extent of the disease, and degree of iatrogenic damage to the pancreas during the procedure. In resection for islet cell carcinoma, there is little indication to drain the operative site, providing that good surgical technique has resulted in minimal trauma to the remaining pancreas. When resection is performed for pancreatic necrosis or

abscess formation, the pancreas should be drained as described previously.

Partial pancreatectomy of the right limb extending into the doudenal segment can be performed, providing that the blood supply to the duodenum is left intact and the location and possible variation of the pancreatic ducts are taken into consideration. Only a small percentage of dogs have a single duct draining into the duodenum, but it is virtually impossible to visualize the duct system at the surgery.[13] Partial pancreatectomy extending onto the duodenal segment is best avoided.

Following partial pancreatic resection, the patient is managed as if acute pancreatitis were present. Intravenous fluid and electrolyte therapy is used until nausea and vomiting cease and oral feeding can be safely reinstituted. Measurement of serum amylase and lipase levels helps monitor the patient's progress. For uncomplicated partial pancreatic resections, as for islet cell carcinoma removal, perioperative antibiotic therapy is not indicated. However, in severe necrotizing pancreatitis, antibiotics are necessary because of the potential for sepsis.

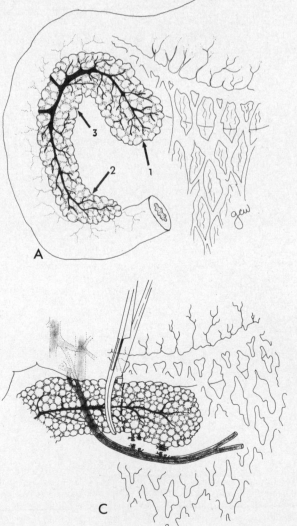

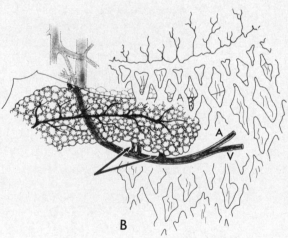

Figure 55–12. Total pancreatectomy without duodenectomy—removal of the left pancreatic limb. *A,* The sequence for removing the different portions of the pancreas when performing a total pancreatectomy. *1,* left limb; *2,* distal portion of right limb; *3,* remainder of right limb and body. *B,* The mesentery is incised around the limb to free the lobe and expose the blood supply (*arrows*) entering the dorsal edge of the pancreas. The blood vessels, which are branches from the splenic artery (*A*) and vein (*V*) should be carefully identified. *C,* The blood supply to the pancreas is carefully ligated and divided, with damage to the main splenic vessels being avoided. A clamp is then placed across the limb at the angle of the pancreas, and the left limb is removed.

If drains have been placed during surgery, they are protected postoperatively with sterile dressings. The drains can be removed once normal pncreatic function has returned and drainage has ceased.

Total Pancreatectomy

Total pancreatectomy, by itself, is rarely performed in the dog and cat. Experimentally, however, it is a successful way of producing diabetes mellitus. Total pancreatectomy is rarely indicated for exocrine pancreatic carcinoma, because usually by the time of surgical exploration the neoplasm involves the duodenum and metastases are present; if a massive resection is to be undertaken, the duodenum has to be removed as well. In humans, pancreaticoduodenectomy is the only surgical therapy with proven efficacy for the control of neoplasia of the head of the pancreas.[5]

Total Pancreatectomy Without Duodenectomy

The surgical approach is as for partial pancreatectomy. The left limb should be exposed and removed first. The mesentery surrounding the left lobe is incised to free the lobe and to allow exposure of the blood supply. The blood supply, branches from the splenic artery and vein, enters the dorsal edge of the pancreas. Care should be taken in identifying, ligating, and dividing these vessels. There are several sets of vessels along the length of the left limb, and during ligation and division of them damage to the main splenic vessel must be avoided. Once the limb has been dissected free to the angle of the pancreas, a clamp can be placed across the pancreas at this point and the left limb can be removed (Fig. 55-12).

The distal portion of the right limb can be removed next. There is great variation in the position of the caudal pancreaticoduodenal vessels. They should be clearly identified and preserved during resection. The branches supplying the distal portion of the right limb are carefully dissected free, ligated, and divided. The mesentery surrounding the distal right limb is incised up to the duodenum. At this point, a clamp can be placed across the pancreas and the distal portion can be removed (Fig. 55-13).

Removal of the remaining portion of the pancreas is difficult, and care has to be taken to avoid destroying the blood supply to the descending duodenum. Methods of "rubbing" the pancreas away from the duodenum and its vessels have been described,[13] but they are often unsatisfactory. Considerable hemorrhage is encountered because of the tearing of the many branches of the pancreaticoduodenal vessels that supply this portion of the pancreas, making further dissection very difficult. Also, the pancreas does not easily "rub off" the duodenum as described.

The most satisfactory way to remove this portion of the pancreas is to use a combination of blunt dissection with mosquito hemostats and electrocau-

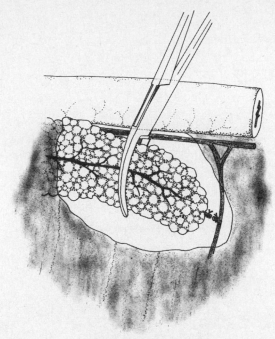

Figure 55–13. Total pancreatectomy without duodenectomy—removal of the distal portion of the right limb. The mesoduodenum surrounding this portion of the pancreas is incised. The blood supply, from the caudal pancreaticoduodenal vessels, is identified, ligated, and divided. A clamp is placed across the pancreas, close to the duodenum, and the distal portion of the pancreas is removed.

tery. The mesoduodenum is incised to the head of the pancreas. Mosquito hemostats are used to bluntly undermine the mesentery covering the junction between the pancreas and the duodenum. Electrocautery is used to incise this mesentery. Dissection is started on the lateral side of the pancreas and duodenum, beginning at the caudal end. If one slowly works along the pancreas-duodenal junction, each vessel branching from the pancreaticoduodenal vessels can be identified, cauterized, and divided. Using this technique, one can maintain excellent hemostasis, making dissection much easier. Once the division between the duodenum and the pancreas has been established, the main pancreaticoduodenal vessels are visible for the entire length of the pancreas. Dissection continues as previously described until the pancreas has been completely dissected free from the major vessels on the lateral side.

Dissection is continued in the same manner on the medial side of the duodenum. In the majority of dogs, the dorsal pancreatic duct is encountered close to the caudal end of this portion of the pancreas. The duct is easily identified and can be sectioned without ligation. Working cranially along the medial side of the duodenum, one continues blunt dissection and vessel identification using mosquito hemostats and electrocauterization of vessels. As the head of the pancreas is approached, the pancreaticoduodenal vessels (one or two major arterial branches) that enter the head of the pancreas are exposed. These may have to be clamped and ligated rather than cauterized, owing to their size. The bile duct is not en-

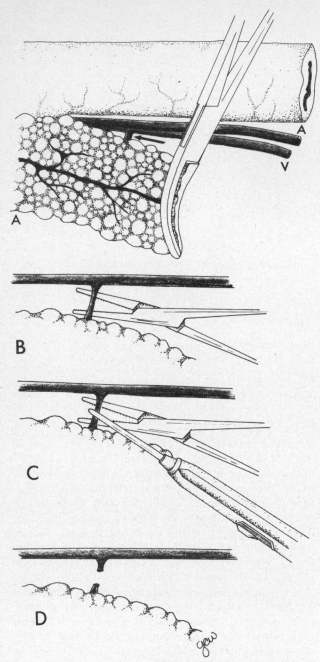

Figure 55–14. Total pancreatectomy without duodenectomy—removal of the body of the pancreas. *A,* Following incision of the mesoduodenum to the head of the pancreas, dissection starts at the distal end of the remainder of the right limb. Care must be taken to avoid damaging the pancreaticoduodenal vessels (*A* and *V*). A major branch of these vessels into the pancreas will need to be ligated and divided at this point (*arrow*). *B* and *D,* Each vessel branching from the pancreaticoduodenal vessel is identified and undermined with mosquito hemostats. The branches are cauterized and divided using electrocautery, as illustrated. Excellent hemostasis can therefore be maintained, making dissection much easier.

countered during this dissection, and the ventral pancreatic duct, being much smaller than the dorsal duct, is rarely identified as a significant structure. Once the head of the pancreas is dissected free, the rest of the pancreas is removed from the abdomen. The area should be inspected for any significant

hemorrhage, which should be stopped. The tear in the mesoduodenum is closed to prevent internal herniation of the bowel. A simple continuous suture pattern of fine absorbable suture material reattaches the mesoduodenum to the duodenum. Care must be taken to avoid suturing through the pancreaticoduodenal vessels or strangulating them in the suture pattern. The abdomen is flushed with warm saline and closed. If a total pancreatectomy has been performed, there is no indication for drainage of this area (Fig. 55–14).

Postoperative care consists of supportive fluid and electrolyte therapy. Because of the prolonged handling of the duodenum that occurs during this operation, nausea and vomiting are commonly encountered. Therefore, intravenous fluid therapy is continued and oral feeding is withheld. Owing to the extensiveness of this surgical procedure, prophylactic antibiotics are indicated.

The greatest postoperative problem encountered is the immediate diabetic state. Also, exocrine pancreatic insufficiency is present and requires replacement therapy.

Total Pancreatectomy With Duodenectomy

This procedure involves resection of the distal portion of the stomach, including the pylorus, the duodenum, and the entire pancreas. In exocrine adenocarcinoma, total pancreatectomy has the advantage of preventing local recurrence in the pancreatic remnant. Postoperatively, both exocrine and endocrine replacement therapy is required. For these reasons, in human surgery, some surgeons will preserve the unaffected tail of the pancreas.[5] This preservation, however, has not been described clinically in the dog or cat.

The surgical exposure of the pancreas and duodenum has been described in the previous sections. The left limb of the pancreas is mobilized and removed as previously described. The common bile duct is identified distal to the junction of the cystic duct. At this point the duct is ligated and divided. The stomach is transected in its distal third so that most of the pyloric antrum and pylorus are removed. The proximal end is oversewn in preparation for gastrojejunostomy.

Starting cranially, the pyloric portion of the stomach, proximal portion of the duodenum and the head of the pancreas are dissected free from the surrounding structures. Great care must be taken to avoid damaging the major branches of the celiac artery, namely the hepatic arteries and splenic and left gastric arteries, during this dissection. Also, the portal vein and its branches should be identified as they run adjacent to the head of the pancreas and bile duct towards the hilus of the liver. The dissection is continued caudally so that the duodenum and the remaining portions of the pancreas can be removed. The duodenum is transected distal to the area of involvement in the disease process, and the end is

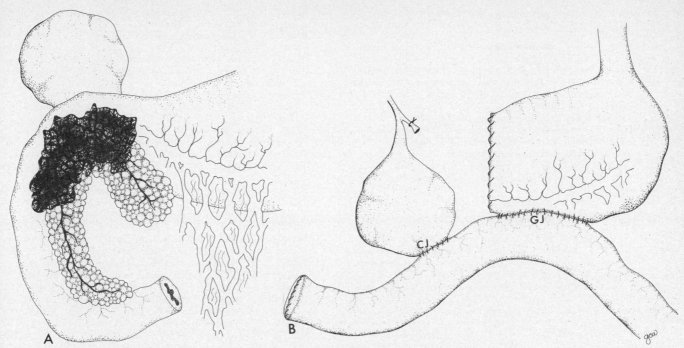

Figure 55–15. Total pancreatectomy with duodenectomy. *A,* Extensive lesion involving the head of the pancreas, duodenum, and surrounding structures. *B,* Following pancreatectomy with duodenectomy, the gastrointestinal and biliary systems are reconstructed by creation of a gastrojejunostomy (*GJ*) and a cholecystojejunostomy (*CJ*).

oversewn. At this point the distal stomach, duodenum, and pancreas can be completely removed.

A cholecystojejunostomy is performed to reestablish biliary drainage. Distal to it, a side-to-side gastrojejunostomy is performed to provide continuity to the gastrointestinal tract (see Chapters 49 and 54). Following completion of the anastomoses, the abdomen is thoroughly lavaged with warm saline and closed (Fig. 55–15).

Prophylactic antibiotic therapy is indicated in this procedure because of the extent of the disease process and the surgical procedure and because both the biliary system and gastrointestinal tract have been invaded during the surgery. Postoperatively, supportive intravenous fluid and electrolyte therapy is required until oral feeding can be instituted. The adequacy of biliary drainage should be monitored via serum bilirubin and liver enzyme levels. Gastrointestinal function can be monitored by observing the effects of feeding.

1. Archibald, J., Holt, J. C., Sokolovsky, V., and Catcott, E. J.: Abdominal injuries. In: *Management of Trauma in Dogs and Cats.* American Veterinary Publications, Inc., Santa Barbara, 1981.
2. Barone, R.: *Anatomie Comparée des mammiféres domestiques.* Tome 3, Fasc. 1: Splanchnologie. Lyons Lab. d'Anatomie, Ecole Nationale Veterinaire, 1976.
3. Beaumont, P. R.: Anastomotic jejunal ulcer secondary to gastrojejunostomy in a dog. J. Am. Anim. Hosp. Assoc. *17*:233, 1981.
4. Boyden, E. A.: The problem of the pancreatic bladder. Am. J. Anat. *36*:151, 1925.
5. Bradley, E. L., III, and Zeppa, R.: The pancreas. *In* Sabiston, D. C. (ed.): *Davis-Christopher Textbook of Surgery XII.* Philadelphia, W.B. Saunders, 1981.
6. Bradley, O. C., and Graham, T.: *Topographical Anatomy of the Dog.* 5th ed. Edinburgh, Oliver & Boyd, 1948.
7. Cadete, L. A.: The arteries of the pancreas of the dog. An injection corrosion and microangiographic study. Am. J. Anat. *137*:151, 1973.
8. Cooperman, A. M.: Chronic pancreatitis. Surg. Clin. North Am. *61*:71, 1981.
9. Crowe, D. T., and Crane, S. W.: Diagnostic abdominal paracentesis and lavage in the evaluation of abdominal injuries in dogs and cats: clinical and experimental investigations. J. Am. Vet. Med. Assoc. *168*:700, 1976.
10. Dalton, J. R. F., and Hill, F. W. G.: A procedure for the examination of the liver and pancreas in dogs. J. Small Anim. Pract. *13*:527, 1976.
11. DeHoff, W., and Archibald, J.: Pancreas. *In* Archibald, J. (ed.): *Canine Surgery II.* Santa Barbara American Veterinary Publications, 1974.
12. Dickerman, R. M., and Dunn, E. L.: Splenic, pancreatic and hepatic injuries. Surg. Clin. North Am. *61*:3, 1981.
13. Dingwall, J. S.: The pancreas. *In* Bojrab, M. J. (ed.): Current Techniques in Small Animal Surgery. Philadelphia, Lea & Febiger, 1975.
14. Duffell, S. J.: Some aspects of pancreatic disease in the cat. J. Small Anim. Pract. *16*:365, 1976.
15. Eichhorn, E. P., and Boyden, E. A.: The choledochoduodenal junction in the dog—a restudy of Oddi's sphincter. Am. J. Anat. *97*:431, 1955.
16. Evans, H. E., and Christensen, G. C.: *Miller's Anatomy of the Dog.* 2nd ed. W. B. Saunders, Philadelphia, 1979.
17. Hardy, R. M.: Inflammatory pancreatic disease. *In* Anderson, N. V. (ed.): *Veterinary Gastroenterology.* Lea & Febiger, Philadelphia, 1980.
18. Kleine, L. J.: Clinical and radiographic aspects of acute pancreatitis in the dog. Comp. Cont. Ed. *2*:295, 1980.
19. Kleine, L. J., and Hornbuckle, W. E.: Acute pancreatitis: the radiographic findings in 182 dogs. J. Am. Vet. Radiol. Soc. *14*:102, 1978.

20. Kolata, R. J., and Johnston, D. E.: Motor vehicle accidents in urban dogs: a study of 600 cases. J. Am. Vet. Med. Assoc. *167*:938, 1975.

21. Litwin, M. S.: Trauma: management of the acutely injured patient. *In* Sabiston, D. C. (ed.): *Davis-Christopher Textbook of Surgery XII.* W.B.Saunders, Philadelphia, 1981.

22. Longnecker, D. S.: Pathology and pathogenesis of diseases of the pancreas. Am. J. Pathol. *107*:103, 1982.

23. Mallory, A., and Kern, F., Jr.: Drug-induced pancreatitis: a critical review. Gastroenterology *78*:813, 1980.

24. Martin, E., Poey, V., Saffadi, L., et al.: Triangular ligaments of the canine liver and their role in holding the liver in place. Gaceta Veterinaria *42*:198, 1980.

25. Nickel, R., Schummer, A., Seiferle, E., and Sack, W. O.: *The Viscera of the Domestic Mammals.* Verlag Paul Parey, Berlin, 1973.

26. Nielsen, S. W., and Bishop, E. J.: The duct system of the canine pancreas. Am. J. Vet. Res. *15*:266, 1954.

27. O'Brien, T. R.: Radiographic diagnosis of abdominal disorders in the dog and cat. W.B. Saunders, Philadelphia, 1978.

28. Park, J. L., Gahring, D., and Greene, R. W.: Peritoneal lavage for peritonitis and pancreatitis in twenty-two dogs. J. Am. Anim. Hosp. Assoc. *9*:442, 1973.

29. Preshaw, R. M.: Pancreatic exocrine secretion. MTP Int. Rev. Sci. *4*:265, 1974.

30. Ranson, J. H. C.: Acute pancreatitis. Curr. Prob. Surg. *16*:1, 1979.

31. Ranson, J. H. C.: Acute pancreatitis—Where are we? Surg. Clin. North Am. *61*:55, 1981.

32. Revell, D. G.: The pancreatic ducts in the dog. Am. J. Anat. *1*:443, 1902.

33. Rogers, W. A.: Diseases of the exocrine pancreas. *In* Ettinger, S. J. (ed.): *Veterinary Internal Medicine II.* W.B. Saunders, Philadelphia, 1983.

34. Schaer, M.: The pancreas. *In* Bojrab, M. J. (ed.): *Pathophysiology in Small Animal Surgery.* Lea & Febiger, Philadelphia, 1981.

35. Singh, M., and Webster, P. D.: Neurohormonal control of pancreatic secretion. Gastroenterology *74*:294, 1978.

36. Steinberg, D.: On leaving the peritoneal cavity open in acute generalized suppurative peritonitis. Am. J. Surg. *137*:216, 1979.

37. Stinson, A. W., and Calhoun, M. L.: Digestive system. *In* Dellman, H. D., and Brown, E. M. (ed.): *Textbook of Veterinary Histology.* 2nd ed. Lea & Febiger, Philadelphia, 1981.

38. Strombeck, D. R.: The Pancreas. *In: Small Animal Gastroenterology.* Stonegate Publishing, Davis, 1979.

39. Suter, P. F., and Olsson, S.-E.: Traumatic hemorrhagic pancreatitis in the cat: A report with emphasis on the radiological diagnosis. J. Am. Vet. Radiol. Soc. *10*:4, 1969.

40. Warren, K. W., and Hoffman, V.: Changing patterns in surgery of the pancreas. Surg. Clin. North Am. *56*:615, 1976.

Section VII

Hernias

Christopher R. Bellenger
Section Editor

56 Hernias

Christopher R. Bellenger

A hernia is defined as the protrusion of an organ or part through a defect in the wall of the anatomical cavity in which it lies or into a subsidiary compartment of that cavity. The majority of hernias involve protrusions of abdominal contents through part of the abdominal wall, diaphragm, or perineum. Herniation may occur elsewhere in the body, for example, tentorial herniation, but such lesions have not been included here.

CLASSIFICATION

Anatomical Site

There are a number of ways in which hernias may be classified, the most common being the anatomical *site* of the hernia. In Section VII, four chapters deal with the four principal anatomical areas that are involved: the cranial abdominal, caudal abdominal, diaphragmatic, and perineal areas. There are further subdivisions within each area (Table 56–1).

Congenital versus Acquired Hernias

A *congenital* hernia is due to a defect already present at birth, although the herniation itself may not develop until later. *Acquired* hernias in which the abdominal wall defect occurs after birth are caused principally by external blunt trauma, especially from motor vehicle accidents or as a result of poor closure or partial disruption of an abdominal incision. In the case of perineal hernia, however, neither trauma nor incision is usually involved; the acquired perineal hernia probably represents a combination of degenerative changes in the structures of the pelvic diaphragm.

Reducible Versus Incarcerated Hernias

In addition to the classifications listed in Table 56–1, which take into consideration only the defect in the restraining wall, hernias may also be classified according to the state of their contents. If the contents of the hernia can be returned to the abdomen by manipulation, a hernia is *reducible*, whereas the hernia whose contents are fixed in the abnormal location is *incarcerated*, or irreducible. Surgical correction of a reducible hernia is generally easier than that of an incarcerated hernia, and the risk of strangulation is less. In a *strangulated* hernia the blood vessels supplying the herniated tissues are constricted, usually at the edge of the defect in the abdominal wall. Strangulation eventually results in

tissue necrosis and is a most serious development, especially when intestinal loops are involved.

Type of Herniated Tissue

Finally, hernias can be classified according to their contents, such as intestine or omentum.

PARTS OF A HERNIA

The parts of a hernia include the hernial *ring* or neck, the *sac*, and the *contents*. The neck or ring is the actual defect in the limiting wall, e.g., tear in the diaphragm. The size may vary from a few millimeters to several centimeters. It may become indurated as a result of inadequate spontaneous repair processes, and collagen maturation and scar contraction may induce strangulation. The sac comprises the tissues that cover the herniated contents. In congenital umbilical hernia this includes a peritoneal lining, subcutaneous tissue, and skin. If large, this hernia assumes a flasklike shape.

In traumatic hernias the sac, at least initially, does not have a peritoneal lining, although peritonealization may occur even in perineal hernia. In indirect scrotal hernias the normal peritoneal lining of the vaginal process lines the sac. In traumatic diaphragmatic hernias the function of the sac is assumed by the thoracic walls. The *contents* of a hernia includes the organs or tissues that have moved to the pathological location. The contents of a hernia are fairly predictable at most anatomical sites of herniation, although some variation is possible.

EPIDEMIOLOGY

The only hernias commonly apparent at birth are umbilical hernias and, to a lesser extent, congenital inguinal and peritoneopericardial hernias. Table 56–2 summarizes the incidence of congenital hernias per

TABLE 56–1. Sites and Types of Hernias

Anatomical Area	Types of Hernia
Cranial abdominal (ventral and lateral)	Umbilical
	Traumatic
	Incisional
Caudal abdominal	Inguinal
	Scrotal
	Femoral
Diaphragmatic	Peritoneopericardial
	Hiatal
	Traumatic
Perineal	Perineal

TABLE 56–2. Prevalence of Congenital Hernias in Dogs and Cats Per 1000 Hospital Patients

	Dog		Cat	
	A	B	A	B
Diaphragmatic	0.49	—	0.66	—
Umbilical	1.71	2.35	1.43	1.66
Inguinal	0.40	0.54	0.25	0.20

Notes: Data in column A are from Priester, W. A., Glass, A. G., and Waggoner, N. S.: Congenital defects in domesticated animals: General considerations. Am. J. Vet. Res. *31*:1871, 1970. Data in column B are from Hayes, H. M.: Congenital umbilical and inguinal hernias in cattle, horses, swine, dogs, and cats: Risk by breed and sex among hospital patients. Am. J. Vet. Res. 35:839, 1974.

1000 hospital patients.[6,16] Traumatic hernias are seen most commonly in young to middle-aged animals. Perineal hernias are seen in middle-aged to old dogs.

Perineal hernia in dogs occurs almost exclusively in the male. Inguinal herniation occurred more frequently in the bitch than the stud at the University of Sydney Veterinary Hospital (USVH) (ratio 1.75:1) although not in a large United States series.[6] Pregnancy may result in the extra-abdominal development of fetuses in the herniated uterine horn. Umbilical hernias are found more frequently in females than in males.[6]

Some striking differences are observed between man and the dog in the common sites of herniation. In man hernia is almost synonymous with a groin hernia in the male, as direct and indirect inguinal hernias represent about 75 per cent of the total number of hernias.[11,14] Another common area includes incisional and ventral hernias. Rates of herniation after ventral abdominal closure in humans range from 1 to 2 per cent in primarily healed wounds to 10 per cent after infection and 30 per cent after dehiscence and closure.[7] In the dog, diaphragmatic, perineal, and umbilical hernias are most frequently observed. At the USVH, the number of hernias seen in 13,529 canine and 4,573 feline accessions from 1974 to 1982 included (feline numbers in parentheses) perineal 63(0), umbilical 42(11), diaphragmatic 15(21), inguinal-scrotal 33(2), incisional 1(4), and traumatic abdominal 1(2), giving a hernia rate per 1000 hospital cases of 11.5(8.8). These figures may reflect the referral nature of the practice.

Breed differences in incidence have been observed with most hernias, and these are referred to in subsequent chapters. The increased prevalence of congenital hernias among certain dog breeds indicates a pattern of familial inheritance. The variation in prevalence seen between males and females in some hernias suggests that such genetic factors may be sex linked. However, it should not be assumed that all congenital hernias are heritable defects.

Both vitamin A deficiency[12] and the estrus-suppressing drug methallibure[20] induce diaphragmatic hernias in pigs. Methylmercuric chloride is teratogenic for umbilical hernia in cats.[9] Most congenital diaphragmatic hernias in dogs are not considered to be inherited.[4] Blanket recommendations for the neutering of all animals with congenital hernias need to be reviewed in the light of an increasing understanding of the interplay between genetics and the environment. Also, the presence of a possibly inherited condition needs to be weighed against the value of the other inherited characteristics of the breed.

SIGNS OF HERNIATION

The most easily elicited clinical sign of herniation is swelling, resulting from the separation of muscle layers and the intrusion of the abdominal contents. This sign is not seen in diaphragmatic hernia; respiratory signs predominate owing principally to the thoracic space occupied by abdominal organs. The skin over the swelling may be inflamed if recent trauma has occurred or if the contents have become strangulated, but otherwise inflammation is generally not observed. Pain is usually not manifest on palpation, and the sac takes on the consistency of the contents. Additional signs depend mainly on the nature and state of the contents of the hernia, e.g., reducible hernias compared with strangulated intestinal hernias.

DIAGNOSIS

It is difficult to generalize about the diagnosis of herniation.

A history of access to highways and a recent absence from the home coupled with dyspnea is suggestive of diaphragmatic hernia or other thoracic trauma. A history of recent surgery may also be of significance if wound swelling is apparent. Observation and palpation are important in most cases. Swelling due to herniation needs to be differentiated from swelling caused by neoplasia, abscess, lymphadenopathy, or hematoma. Plain and contrast radiography may be required to positively identify intestinal loops or other viscera in the sac. Centesis is rarely indicated except in bladder herniation.

PRINCIPLES OF HERNIORRHAPHY

The first record of an operation (in man) for hernia relief is said to have been made by Celsus[21] in the first century A.D. Since that time, herniorrhaphy has attracted considerable attention.[17]

There are four main aims of hernia repair:

1. Return of viable contents to their normal anatomical location within the abdomen;
2. Secure closure of the neck of the hernia, thus preventing recurrence;
3. Obliteration of any redundant tissue in the sac; and
4. Use of the patient's own tissues whenever possible.

Surgical access is usually obtained by incision either directly over or around the hernial sac, although in some cases of bilateral inguinal hernia in the bitch a midline incision may be used and the hernias reduced by traction from within the abdomen. In diaphragmatic hernia, an indirect approach via celiotomy or thoracotomy is required. Herniated tissues may have reduced viability and increased friability, requiring careful handling. If devitalized, excision is required. Adhesions in incarcerated hernias may require separation by blunt and sharp dissection, and the neck of the hernia may need to be enlarged to facilitate return of the tissues engorged by venous and lymphatic obstruction or normal physiological processes such as pregnancy. The returned tissues should be placed in their normal location in the abdomen.

The basic principle of hernia repair is to close normal tissue to normal tissue without undue tension.[7] Closure of the neck of the hernia is most commonly and preferably performed by direct suture approximation of local tissues. Specifics for suture types are given in the following section. It is essential to recognize the specific anatomical structures that have sufficient holding power to resist disruption and incorporate them in the closure. Thus, an accurate knowledge of the anatomy of the area is fundamental to repair. In the majority of cases local tissues can be readily approximated, although some initial dissection may be required to allow them to stretch over the defect.

When direct approximation of local tissue is not possible, local muscle and fascial tissue flaps that retain an adequate blood supply are the best alternatives, such as superficial gluteal or obturator muscle flaps in perineal herniorrhaphy or reflection of flaps of the external lamina of the rectus abdominis muscle sheath to cover midline defects. Failing this, free flaps of autogenous tissue such as fascia lata or skin[13,22] or prostheses have been used.

Prosthetic Implants in Hernia Repair

Implants are of greatest value when a large defect makes the approximation of normal tissue impossible without undue tension.[18] Although wire meshes of tantalum and stainless steel have been used,[10,15] constant flexion of the area tends to produce fragmentation.[15,18]

Nonporous synthetic cloth materials are inferior to meshes both in the rate of increase of tensile strength and in tolerance by the host.[2]

Synthetic meshes woven of a single or multiple filament fiber have flexibility, are less damaging than wire if displaced, and are well incorporated by fibrous connective tissue. The most commonly used is a monofilament plastic knitted mesh made from polyethylene or polypropylene.[3,8,14] This material is well tolerated in wounds, does not disintegrate with age, and can stretch in two directions to distribute the load more evenly.[5] Granulation tissue and capillaries grow through the mesh, building a strong layer of connective tissue in four to six weeks.[19] The disadvantages include the possibility of rejection and irritation of adjoining tissue. Polypropylene mesh can be implanted into moderately infected wounds as long as drainage is adequate.[5]

Numerous techniques have been described for inserting prosthetic mesh including the use of one to three layers of mesh.[14] For best results the mesh should extend 1.5 to 3.0 cm beyond the margins of the defect. It should be anchored to strong supporting structures with interrupted sutures of synthetic monofilament nonabsorbable material placed at intervals of 4 to 6 mm. The sutures should extend to the outer edge of the mesh. The mesh should be implanted as deeply into the abdominal wall as is reasonable for the particular hernia.[1,14] Once the contents are returned and the neck is closed, the stretched and redundant subcutaneous tissue and skin of some hernias often remain. If skin closure without tension can still be achieved, this redundant tissue may be removed to provide a more aesthetic closure and to aid in obliteration of dead space.

Recurrence of a hernia results from failure of the repair process and, as with wound breakdown in general, indicates infection, extreme tension, or inadequate nutrition of the apposed tissues or obvious technical failures such as the use of incorrect suture material or inappropriate tissue layers. In man, "whether a herniorrhaphy is successful or not is determined by the time the last suture has been placed. Although all surgeons must be prepared to admit that recurrences will occur, the only proper attitude to take is that any recurrence is the fault of the surgeon."[17]

1. Adler, R. H., Mendez, M., and Darby, C.: Effects of implanted mesh on the strength of healing wounds. Surgery 52:898, 1962.
2. Arnaud, J. P., Eloy, R., Adloff, M., and Grenier, J. F.: *In vivo* exploration of the tensile strength of the abdominal wall after repair with different prosthetic materials. Eur. Surg. Res. 11:1, 1979.
3. Cady, B., and Brooke-Cowden, G. L.: Repair of massive abdominal wall defects—combined use of pneumoperitoneum and Marlex mesh. Surg. Clin. North Am. 56:559, 1976.
4. Foley, C. W., Lasley, J. F., and Osweiler, G. D.: *Abnormalities of Companion Animals: Analysis of Heritability.* Iowa State University Press, Ames, 1979.
5. Goris, J. A.: Ogilvie's method applied to infected wound disruption. Arch. Surg. 115:1103, 1980.

6. Hayes, H. M.: Congenital umbilical and inguinal hernias in cattle, horses, swine, dogs and cats: Risk by breed and sex among hospital patients. Am. J. Vet. Res. 35:839, 1974.

7. Hunt, T. K.: Disorders of repair and their management. In Hunt, T. K., and Dunphy, J. E. (eds.): Fundamentals of Wound Management. Appleton-Century-Crofts, New York, 1979, pp. 68–168.

8. Kaufman, M., and Weissberg, D.: Marlex mesh in giant ventral hernia repair. Isr. J. Med. Sci. 16:739, 1980.

9. Khera, K. S.: Teratogenic effects of methylmercury in the cat: Note on the use of this species as a model for teratogenicity studies. Teratology 8:293, 1973.

10. Koontz, A. R.: On the need for prostheses in hernia repair. Am. Surg. 28:342, 1962.

11. Nyhus, L. M., and Bombeck, C. T.: Hernias. In Sabiston, D. C. (ed.): Textbook of Surgery, 12th ed. W. B. Saunders, Philadelphia, 1981, pp. 1328–50.

12. Palludan, B.: The teratogenic effect of vitamin A deficiency in pigs. Acta Vet. Scand. 2:32, 1961.

13. Peacock, E. E.: Subcutaneous extraperitoneal repair of ventral hernias: A biological basis for fascial transplantation. Ann. Surg. 181:722, 1975.

14. Ponka, J. L.: Hernias of the abdominal wall. W. B. Saunders, Philadelphia, 1980.

15. Preston, D. J., and Richards, C. F.: Use of wire mesh prostheses in the treatment of hernia. Surg. Clin. North Am. 53:549, 1973.

16. Priester, W. A., Glass, A. G., and Waggoner, N. S.: Congenital defects in domesticated animals: General considerations. Am. J. Vet. Res. 31:1871, 1970.

17. Ravitch, M. M.: Repair of Hernias. Year Book Medical Publishers, Chicago, 1969.

18. Stock, F. E.: Repair of large herniae with nylon mesh. Lancet 1:395, 1954.

19. Usher, F. C., and Ochsner, J. L.: Marlex mesh: a new polyethylene mesh for replacing tissue defects. Surg. Forum 10:319, 1960.

20. Vente, J. P., Wrathall, A. E., Hebert, N., and Hoskin, B. D.: Quantitative anatomical study of methallibure-induced malformations in piglets. Res. Vet. Sci. 13:169, 1972.

21. Warwick, B. L.: A study of hernia in swine. Res. Bull. 69, Univ. Wisconsin Agric. Expt. Station, 1926.

22. Zimmerman, L. M.: The use of prosthetic materials in the repair of hernia. Surg. Clin. North Am. 48:143, 1968.

Chapter 57 Cranial Abdominal Hernias

Richard Read

The hernias discussed in this chapter include all those involving the abdominal wall, except for inguinal, scrotal, and femoral hernias (see Chapter 58) and are listed according to their etiology: congenital, traumatic, and incisional. Although hernias have been separated into umbilical and ventral in the past, the term *ventral hernia* is inappropriate to small animal surgery, as many hernias occur in the flank region.

CONGENITAL HERNIAS

Umbilical Hernia

Pathological Anatomy

The abdominal wall is formed in the embryo by the migration of the cephalic, caudal, and two lateral folds. These four folds meet at the umbilicus, where the yolk sac is continuous with the developing midgut. During its elongation, the midgut enters the umbilical cord but returns to the abdominal cavity well before parturition.[21]

The umbilical aperture in the fetus allows passage of the umbilical blood vessels, the vitelline duct, and the stalk of the allantois. After these structures are disrupted at birth, this opening normally closes rapidly.[24] If closure does not occur, a defect remains in the ventral midline, forming the umbilical hernial ring. Depending on the size of the ring, the hernia

may contain falciform ligament, omentum, or small intestine.

Etiology

There is evidence for a genetic basis for umbilical hernia.[18, 32] Although the incidence is low, the Airedale, basenji, Pekingese, pointer, and Weimaraner breeds are more at risk than others. Females have a higher incidence than males.[18] One family of Cornish Rex cats showed a high incidence of umbilical hernia.[32] The genetic defect has been described as a polygenic threshold character, possibly involving a major gene whose expression is mediated by the genetic background of the breed.[32] A high incidence of umbilical hernia has been noted in dogs with other congenital abnormalities, particularly cryptorchidism.[30]

Improper transection of the umbilical cord at birth may result in failure of the umbilical ring to close normally.[3] However, it is unlikely that this mechanism is involved in the majority of cases.

Clinical Signs

Most umbilical hernias are small, soft, reducible masses found at the site of the umbilical scar and are of little clinical importance. The size of the hernial ring is noted and the contents of the sac determined by palpation. In most cases where the hernial ring is less than 2 to 3 cm in diameter, the contents consist of falciform fat and occasionally omentum.

The presence of adhesions between the contents and the edge of the hernial ring and the presence of intestine are determined by palpation. Occasionally, large umbilical hernias are seen and the contents may include liver, spleen, and small intestine.

Most umbilical hernias do not inconvenience the animal. If the contents become incarcerated or their blood supply becomes occluded, local signs of pain and swelling develop rapidly. If intestine is involved, intestinal obstruction may occur.

Diagnosis

The diagnosis of umbilical hernias is usually simple. In incarcerated and strangulated hernias, it can be difficult to determine the precise nature of the contents. Radiography may help to differentiate intestine and omentum by the presence of gas-filled loops on a plain lateral film. If the contents are reducible, the hernial ring can usually be palpated, confirming the diagnosis.

An incarcerated hernia may be difficult to differentiate from an abscess by palpation alone. The site of the lesion and an accurate history usually remove any doubt. If radiography fails to provide the answer, paracentesis of the mass may be used, but this is rarely necessary.

Treatment

Since the majority of umbilical hernias are small and cause no clinical signs, the question inevitably arises as to whether treatment is warranted. Umbilical hernias are rarely treated surgically in children because spontaneous closure occurs in most cases by two years of age.[27] Many mature dogs with persistent umbilical hernias are encountered in veterinary practice. Spontaneous closure has been recorded in pups up to six months of age.[3]

Many small umbilical hernias are repaired surgically; in females this is most easily performed during ovariohysterectomy. The midventral incision is extended through the hernial sac and the sac is dissected free, making sure any adhesions to hernial contents are carefully resected. Closure is usually effected with simple interrupted sutures of an absorbable suture material, resulting in apposition of the edges of the hernial ring. An alternative that may provide a more secure closure is an overlapping, or "pants-over-vest" closure (Fig. 57–1). However, the recurrence rate following simple repair of umbilical hernias is low as long as proper surgical principles are followed.

In a large umbilical hernia, simple closure may result in excessive tension on the wound edges, with a greatly increased risk of recurrence of the hernia. In these cases, the hernial sac can be preserved by releasing it from the external lamina of the rectus sheath on one side only. After initial closure, the

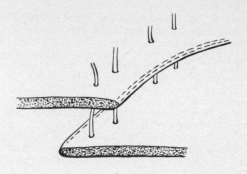

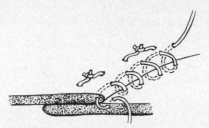

Figure 57–1. The overlapping, or "pants-over-vest," technique.

excess fascia is flapped over the suture line and sutured to the opposite side, providing a second layer of support.[3] Alternatively, prosthetic materials can be used to help bridge the gap. The most commonly used material is polypropylene mesh, which can be applied in a number of different ways and sutured to the abdominal wall with nonabsorbable sutures of a similar material (see Incisional Hernias). Excessive loose skin associated with a large umbilical hernia should be excised prior to closure.

Small hernias are more prone to incarceration and subsequent strangulation of intestine than large hernias, and adequate supportive treatment for the shock and toxemia associated with strangulating intestinal obstruction is of paramount importance. The viability of the affected loops of intestine must be accurately assessed and resection and anastomosis performed if necessary. The hernia is repaired as previously mentioned.

Because of the genetic predisposition to umbilical hernia in dogs and cats, desexing should also be considered when discussing treatment of this condition, particularly in breeds with a higher than average incidence of umbilical hernia.

Other Developmental Abnormalities

If the midgut fails to return to the abdominal cavity, the condition is described as cord hernia.[21] This is a slight variation on an umbilical hernia, but treatment must be instituted immediately owing to fluid loss from the exposed intestine. Failure of any of the folds to properly migrate results in an omphalocele, in which a large defect is present around the umbilicus and the viscera are covered only with a layer of amnion and chorion. In children, this condition is frequently associated with other congenital abnormalities, resulting in a poor prognosis.[21] Omphalocele has been reported in an entire litter of kittens.[20] The true incidence of these conditions is hard to determine, as many animals probably die or are destroyed without veterinary attention being sought.

Umbilical hernia has been reported with other defects in dogs. In one case, the rectus abdominis muscles were apparently hypoplastic,[31] and in another, a large umbilical hernia was accompanied by a deformed penis and failure of the preputial tissues to meet in the midline.[33] This latter case also had a defect in the diaphragm, as did two other dogs with large umbilical hernias.[26, 35] These differed from true omphaloceles in that the skin was largely intact over the hernia and abdomen. However, their occurrence emphasizes the fact that developmental abnormalities of the abdominal wall do occur in small animals and may complicate an outwardly simple surgical repair for umbilical hernia. The use of prosthetic materials may be indicated in repair of these defects.

TRAUMATIC HERNIAS

Etiology, Pathogenesis, and Anatomical Considerations

Hernias caused by trauma usually lack a peritoneal covering to the hernial contents and hence have been called false hernias.[3] The most common site for traumatic hernias is the flank; this is probably due to less elasticity of the tissues in this area compared with the costal attachments, linea alba, and prepubic tendon.[3, 28] In addition, the muscles of the abdominal wall may be contracted in fear at the time of impact, particularly in cases of automobile trauma.[3] Sharp and blunt trauma can result in hernia formation. The most common form of blunt trauma is the motor vehicle accident,[22] whereas gunshot and dog bite wounds are generally a combination of sharp and blunt trauma.

With blunt trauma, penetrating wounds are often not present or, if they are, do not reflect the extent of the underlying damage. Hernias can develop weeks after the original trauma, particularly in dog bite wounds, because of injury to deeper structures.[3]

A sudden increase in intra-abdominal pressure can cause a traumatic hernia, but this is unlikely unless a pre-existing weakness of the abdominal wall is present, e.g., in hyperadrenocorticism and diabetes mellitus.[3, 29] Ventral abdominal hernia has been reported in sheep owing to violent straining during parturition.[8]

Traumatic herniation of the urinary bladder ventrally through a separated pubic symphysis has been reported.[9] This condition also occurs occasionally in man, and it has been suggested that the supporting ligaments to the bladder must also be damaged for

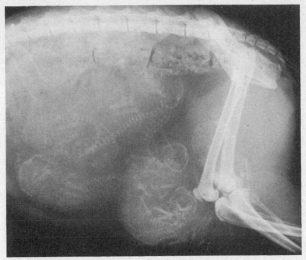

Figure 57–2. Lateral radiograph of a ten-month-old cat with a ventral hernia and ruptured uterus, with fetuses in the hernia.

this to occur because surgical resection of the pubis does not result in herniation of the bladder.[12, 13]

The extent of damage to underlying structures must always be accurately assessed, particularly when penetrating wounds have occurred. The site of the hernia determines which organs are most likely to be injured. Damage to parenchymatous organs such as spleen and liver is likely to result in abdominal hemorrhage, which may lead to hypovolemic shock. Penetrating and crushing intestinal injuries can lead to leakage of intestinal contents, peritonitis, and toxemia. Other hollow organs, such as urinary bladder, stomach, and uterus, that are distended at the time of trauma are prone to rupture (Fig. 57–2).

Extensive damage to the abdominal wall and subcutaneous tissues is common when cats are mauled by large dogs. Aside from herniation and trauma to abdominal viscera, signs of toxemia can develop owing to extensive necrosis of muscle and subcutaneous tissues. Because they lack a peritoneal covering, the hernial contents in these cases are in direct contact with the traumatized abdominal wall. This predisposes to incarceration and strangulation because of adhesion formation and the possibility of constriction of blood supply by wound contraction as healing progresses.[28]

Clinical Signs

Signs directly referable to the hernia are asymmetry and swelling at the site of injury. The size of the swelling may reflect the extent of the herniation, particularly in ventral hernias. However, paracostal and lumbar hernias may show little external swelling, because the hernial contents fall back into the abdominal cavity. Paracostal hernias may be associated with diaphragmatic rupture, and the abdominal contents may fall forward into the thorax rather than prolapsing into the subcutaneous tissues.

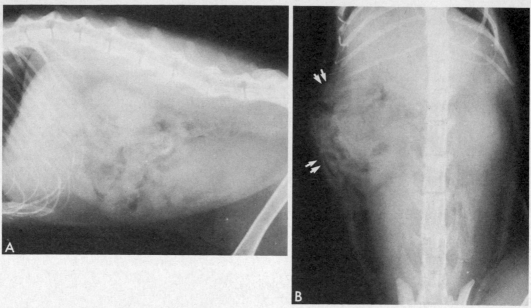

Figure 57–3. Lateral (*A*) and ventrodorsal (*B*) radiographs of a cat with a hernia in the right flank after a dog bite. Note that the hernia is not visible on the lateral film but that a fracture/dislocation is present at the L5–6 vertebral junction. The arrows mark the limits of the hernia on the ventrodorsal film.

The signs of herniation are often masked by the effects of trauma to skin, subcutaneous tissue, and muscle. Severe bruising and swelling of these tissues is common with and without actual herniation. In penetrating wounds, the hernia may be some distance from the wound site. Entry and exit points should be sought with gunshot wounds to determine the path of the missile. Other clinical signs depend on the involvement of other structures and the extent of damage to them. In the early stages, hypovolemic shock may be present owing to blood loss, and peritonitis and toxemia may develop later on owing to damage to the gastrointestinal tract. Incarceration or strangulation of intestine in the hernia may cause signs of intestinal obstruction. Jaundice and other signs of liver failure may develop where massive soft tissue necrosis is occurring. Involvement of the urinary bladder in a hernia may cause urinary obstruction.

Diagnosis and Differential Diagnosis

Careful palpation of the trauma site may reveal an abdominal wall defect. The point of largest swelling may not be the site of the hernia because intestine can migrate in the subcutaneous space.[3] In some cases the outer muscle layer remains intact, making diagnosis more difficult. Occasionally, thorough palpation must be delayed because of patient discomfort until anesthesia can be safely induced. Gentle palpation is essential, as the tissues are prone to further damage.

Diagnosis of a hernia by palpation alone can be difficult owing to other signs of trauma. Radiography is particularly useful in these cases.[3, 34] The shape and size of the abdomen are examined first, and

closer attention is then paid to any area of focal swelling (Figs. 57–3 and 57–4). All abdominal viscera, particularly those adjacent to an area of swelling, should be sought and identified. The absence of a structure from its normal position is suggestive of a hernia.[34] In addition, subcutaneous emphysema may be present if the skin or intestine has been penetrated. The diagnosis of trauma to viscera can be aided by abdominal paracentesis. Cytology and biochemistry of abdominal fluid may indicate involvement of the gastrointestinal or urinary tract. Peritoneal lavage is more accurate in determining trauma than simple paracentesis.[7]

In chronic traumatic hernia, the outward signs of

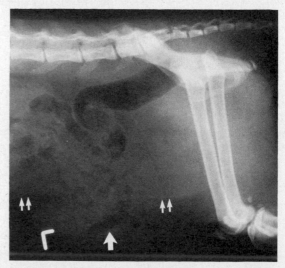

Figure 57–4. Lateral radiograph of a cat with a ventral abdominal hernia following automobile trauma. Note the ventral abdominal wall (*double arrows*) and the herniated, gas-filled intestinal loops (*single arrow*).

trauma may have subsided. If penetrating wounds were involved, subcutaneous infection and abscessation may mask the hernia.

Treatment and Patient Management

Many cases of traumatic abdominal herniation are emergency situations. Life-threatening problems must obviously be dealt with first. These may include extensive abdominal hemorrhage, ruptured intestine, and consequences of thoracic trauma such as pneumothorax, hemothorax, pulmonary contusion, and diaphragmatic hernia.

The timing of repair of a traumatic hernia is important. The first consideration is the animal's general condition. One or more days of resuscitation may be necessary before the patient is fit to undergo definitive repair. The exception to this rule is when radiography or abdominal paracentesis suggests a serious intra-abdominal problem, in which case immediate surgery may be indicated, accompanied by the appropriate supportive therapy. In some cases, a delay of up to five days can be beneficial. Recently traumatized tissues hold sutures poorly, and a delay to allow acute inflammation to subside and hematomata to resolve is advised.[10, 36] However, too long a delay results in retraction of the wound edges and an increased chance of adhesion formation and strangulation of hernial contents.[36]

An extensive area of skin should be prepared for surgery because the extent of the injuries to the muscle wall is frequently not known and the surgeon must be prepared to extend the initial incision. Sufficient exposure must be obtained to adequately explore the abdominal contents for signs of damage. Individual muscle layers should be identified and areas of suspect viability debrided. Once all necrotic tissue has been removed, the muscle layers can be individually reapposed. In the lumbar area, all three layers should be sutured separately.

Sutures may have to be anchored around the last rib in paracostal hernias. Synthetic absorbable suture material on an atraumatic needle is the material of choice, even when contamination is present. There is evidence to suggest that breakdown products of polyglycolic acid may be bacteriostatic.[11]

As in the repair of umbilical and incisional hernias, excessive tension on suture lines must be avoided. Where extensive tissue loss has occurred, prosthetic materials may be required to close the deficit (see Incisional Hernias). Adequate drainage of the abdominal cavity, abdominal wall, and subcutaneous tissues must be provided in all cases of traumatic abdominal hernia repair. Penrose rubber drains are adequate in most instances and should be removed within four to five days. When severe contamination and infection have occurred, the skin wound may need to be left open to granulate. The wound should be covered with moist dressings, which require regular changing.

In chronic traumatic hernias, the individual muscle layers may become fibrosed together, making identification of layers difficult.[3] The extensive debridement required to separate the layers adequately for suturing may not be warranted. As an implant is more likely to be necessary in these cases, the fibrosed combined muscle layer can be sutured as one unit to the prosthesis.

Aftercare and Prognosis

In addition to supportive measures for visceral trauma, the patient must be kept confined for at least five days. Drains are not removed, and it is important to restrict movement to a minimum. Paracostal hernia repairs in particular are under increased load because of the continual movement associated with respiration, and this may delay wound healing.[3]

Extensive injury to the abdominal wall and subcutaneous tissues should be monitored carefully for further tissue necrosis and subsequent reherniation or toxemia.

INCISIONAL HERNIAS

Etiology, Pathogenesis, and Anatomical Considerations

Incisional hernia is a serious postoperative complication of abdominal surgery. It can develop following any laparotomy, but is most commonly associated with midline laparotomies, which carry the highest chance of complete wound disruption and subsequent evisceration. The weight of the abdominal contents exerts a distracting force on the edges of a sutured midline laparotomy incision. Any factor that either increases that pressure or weakens the suture line predisposes to incisional hernia. In contrast, when a flank laparotomy is performed through a muscle-splitting grid incision, the wound edges are drawn together by the weight of the abdominal contents, particularly when the animal is standing. This is perhaps the greatest advantage of the flank incision for laparotomy. However, the disadvantage of limited exposure generally restricts its use to specific procedures such as renal biopsy.

Increased intra-abdominal pressure can predispose to incisional hernia. Prolonged postoperative vomiting or coughing or, in dogs, excited barking, greatly increases the distracting force on the suture line. Severe obesity in human patients is associated with a higher rate of incisional hernia.[17] During the first five days of healing, an incised wound has no strength of its own, the edges being held in apposition by the sutures and a thin layer of fibrin.[29] Wound strength increases rapidly from days 6 to 15 as collagen is laid down, but experiments in rabbits show that recovery of the initial wound strength may be as low as 45 per cent up to two to four months later.[1] The choice of suture material must be made in light of knowledge of wound healing and wound strength. These figures suggest that nonabsorbable sutures should always be used to close a laparotomy, but clinical results with

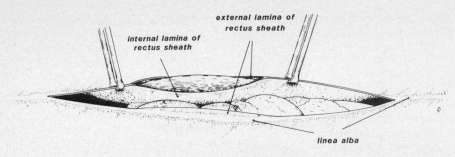

Figure 57–5. The internal rectus sheath and peritoneum retract from the wound edge, leaving the rectus muscle belly exposed.

absorbable sutures are satisfactory. This indicates that the physical and chemical properties of suture materials are generally of minor importance to wound stability.[2]

If wound healing is less than optimal, the choice of suture material can become important. If the rate of gain of tensile strength in the wound is slower than normal, a critical point may be reached when an absorbable suture material is failing and wound strength is insufficient to prevent disruption. This applies particularly to surgical gut in the first ten days after surgery. Two important factors affecting the rate of gain of tensile strength in the wound are wound nutrition and oxygenation and wound infection. In severely debilitated patients or when heavy wound contamination is suspected, nonabsorbable suture material should be used, and a monofilament plastic material such as polypropylene is preferred. Many other factors can influence the rate of wound healing, and the possibility of the presence of any of these factors must be examined in any case of incisional hernia. For example, prolonged systemic corticosteroid therapy can substantially delay the increase in tensile strength of a surgical wound.[29]

Although the previously mentioned factors can be involved in incisional hernia, technical failure on the part of the surgeon is far more significant. Incorrect tying of knots, damaging and therefore weakening suture material (particularly surgical gut), and cutting suture ends too short can result in suture failure. A simple interrupted pattern is recommended for routine closure of all midline laparotomy incisions. Failure of one knot or suture loop in the case of a continuous suture pattern is far more likely to result in evisceration than a similar failure when a simple interrupted pattern is used.

The veterinarian's control over the postoperative activity of his patients is often minimal, and many dogs feel well enough to resume normal activity within one to three days following a routine procedure such as ovariohysterectomy. The advantages of a continuous closure include the saving of time and a more even distribution of tension along the wound. If a continuous suture pattern is used to close a midline laparotomy incision, a nonabsorbable, inert suture material is essential and extra care must be taken with suture placement and knot stability.

Failure to place sutures correctly is another cause of incisional hernias. If the incision through the linea alba deviates from the midline, the internal lamina of the rectus sheath and attached peritoneum retract away from the incision (Fig. 57–5). This exposes the belly of the rectus abdominis muscle, which has poor holding power for sutures. The strong fascia of both

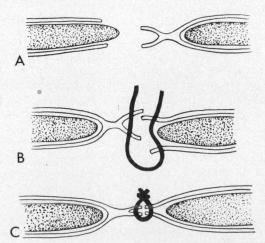

Figure 57–6. Correct method for suturing a midline laparotomy incision when the rectus muscle is exposed.

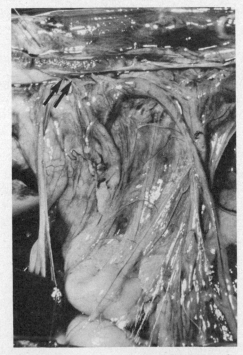

Figure 57–7. Autopsy showing extensive adhesions to the ventral midline. The arrows point to the line of adhesions between the omentum and the peritoneal surface of the wound.

the internal and external laminae of the rectus sheaths must be included in the sutures to achieve adequate wound strength. Primary healing of the muscle sheaths requires their apposition by the sutures. Sutures must therefore be placed by picking up the external and internal muscle sheaths separately on each side, avoiding the belly of the rectus muscle, and thus reconstructing the linea alba (Fig. 57–6). In addition, failure to reappose the internal rectus sheaths leaves an area of muscle belly exposed to the abdominal contents and extensive adhesions of omentum or other organs may occur (Fig. 57–7). All sutures should be placed 3 to 5 mm from the wound edge to ensure adequate anchorage. In male dogs, the preputial fascia must not be confused with the laminae of the rectus sheaths. Both layers must be sutured separately.

Clinical Signs

Most incisional hernias develop in the first two weeks after surgery, most frequently in days 3 to 5. The presence of a small hernia may be an incidental finding when the animal is presented for suture removal because the hernia often causes no outward signs of discomfort (Fig. 57–8). Unless infection is present, the swelling is usually soft and painless, but adhesions to the hernial ring frequently make complete reduction of the contents difficult. A serosanguineous discharge is often present and is noteworthy.

Larger hernias that tend toward eventration may show pallor or cyanosis of the overlying skin. These signs may be masked by discharge if the wound breakdown has been aided by infection or inadequate hemostasis.

When eventration has already occurred, damage to the protruding intestine and omentum rapidly ensues and the animal is frequently presented in severe shock. Dogs and cats often mutilate protruding viscera, and it is not uncommon to find loops of intestine completely devoid of any mesenteric attachment and lacking blood supply. Apart from self-trauma, damage from contact with the ground exacerbates the problem.

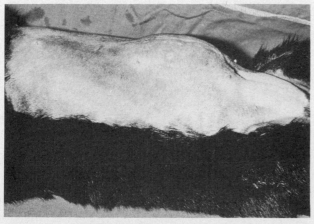

Figure 57–8. Incisional hernia in a cat.

Diagnosis and Differential Diagnosis

Any swelling of the suture line should be examined closely and carefully palpated for texture and pain or heat. Since wound infection may be associated with incisional hernia, it can be difficult to confirm the presence of a small hernia. A hernial ring is the definitive sign, but palpation of the contents may confirm the presence of omentum or loops of intestine. If a hernia is suspected, an attempt to gently reduce the contents may permit palpation of the hernial ring and confirmation of the diagnosis.

Some cats develop a firm swelling in the skin and subcutaneous tissues five to ten days after midline laparotomy. Some discomfort is evident on palpation, and the swelling is generally adherent to the underlying abdominal wall. These cases require careful examination to rule out incisional hernia. A needle aspirate usually reveals a small amount of serosanguineous fluid, and bacteriological culture is often negative. These cases seem to be distinct from wound infections and may be a reaction to suture material or excessive trauma to subcutaneous tissues. I have encountered this with both chromic gut and synthetic absorbable suture materials, and the inexperience of the surgeon and the duration of surgery cannot always be implicated in the etiology. These cats are generally given antibiotics as a precaution against infection, but this is probably unnecessary as the swelling subsides after two to three weeks, leaving little or no evidence of its occurrence. Many young cats have minimal subcutaneous fat in the ventral abdominal area, and it is debatable whether subcutaneous sutures are required. A subcuticular skin closure using fine synthetic absorbable suture material is possibly the best compromise and gives excellent cosmetic results.

Treatment

Simple Acute Hernias

Incisional hernias are treated without delay, particularly those encountered immediately after midline laparotomy. Although small hernias may stabilize and cause no clinical problem, there is a danger that further breakdown of the wound may occur, predisposing to eventration. Alternatively, as wound healing progresses and wound contraction takes place, incarceration of the contents may result.

Treatment involves reopening the skin and subcutaneous wounds through the original incision and carefully freeing any adhesions to the abdominal wall. These adhesions are usually poorly organized and can be freed with little difficulty. Despite the presence of the hernia, the wound edges will be actively involved in the healing process, requiring minimal debridement. Because the substrate phase of wound healing has already occurred, healing of these wounds occurs more rapidly than in a primary wound.

The edges are reapposed with simple interrupted sutures of a synthetic absorbable material, making certain the sutures are securely anchored, correctly placed, and tied. Prior to closure of the final 3 to 4 cm of the abdominal wound, the remainder of the sutured incision should be checked for weak points by inserting a finger into the peritoneal cavity and palpating the incision from the inside, checking for loose sutures, excessive gaps between sutures, and areas where the internal lamina of the rectus sheath has been omitted from the suture.

It is important to determine the cause of the herniation: knots coming undone, suture material breaking (particularly at the knot), or sutures pulling through the tissues. If there is any doubt concerning the security of the remaining, nonherniated part of the original wound, it is resutured. If it is suspected that the herniation was associated with wound infection, bacteriological cultures are taken from the wound and appropriate antibiotic treatment begun. Chromic gut should not be used in a contaminated wound as the proteolytic enzymes produced by inflammatory cells attack the suture material and cause rapid loss of tensile strength.[29] If there is any likelihood that wound healing will be less than optimal, a nonabsorbable suture material such as polypropylene, nylon, or stainless steel should be used.

Chronic Incisional Hernias

This type of hernia is far more common in humans than in small animals. In some cases, multiple attempts at closure have already been made. Retraction of the edges of the abdominal wound occurs over a period of time, resulting in excessive tension on the sutures when the wound edges are apposed. This is often the cause of repeated failure of attempts to close the defect. Aside from the detrimental effect on wound healing, excessive tension in the abdominal wall puts pressure on the viscera, with subsequent cardiorespiratory embarrassment due to pressure on the diaphragm and great veins. As in all hernia repairs, adhesions to the edges of the hernial ring must be carefully broken down prior to closure, taking care not to damage any associated abdominal viscera.

Primary closure of the edges may not be possible. Chronic iatrogenically induced pneumoperitoneum has been used in human patients to stretch the abdominal wall prior to surgery and facilitate primary closure.[5, 17] However, technical problems and poor patient acceptance may preclude its use in small animals. Various special closure techniques have been described using the hernial sac or rectus sheaths to close the defect.[6, 23] These involve incising the external lamina of the rectus sheath laterally and releasing it from the surface of the rectus muscle on each side of the hernial ring. These flaps are inverted and overlapped, sutures being placed between the two sheaths and in some cases incorporating flaps made from the hernial sac. Others have described suture patterns designed to counteract the distracting force,[4, 25] such as a double loop closure where the inner loop is tightened by the distracting force of abdominal wall contraction.

Direct contact between the aponeurotic sheaths is

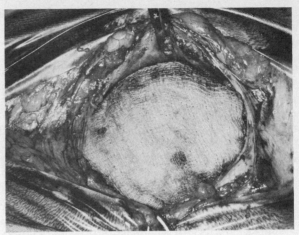

Figure 57–9. The hernial contents of the cat in Figure 57–8 have been returned to the abdomen, revealing the deficit in the abdominal wall. The viscera are covered with a gauze sponge.

the preferred form of treatment because a stronger repair results.[5] However, there are some circumstances in which prosthetic closure is required (Fig. 57–9). The most commonly used material is polypropylene mesh (Marlex).

Single-, double-, and triple-layer techniques have all been described for inserting prosthetic mesh.[5, 14, 15, 19] In some cases the sharp edges are turned under to minimize irritation.[5] The mesh is sutured to the surrounding abdominal wall with sutures of a similar material. The subcutaneous tissues and skin are closed over the top. For a more detailed discussion of the use of prosthetic materials in hernia repair, see Chapter 56.

Herniation with Evisceration

Immediate therapy for shock is indicated, even if outward signs are minimal. Intravenous fluid therapy plus administration of broad spectrum antibiotics should be established as soon as practicable. All exposed viscera must be protected with clean abdominal sponges and washed with large volumes of

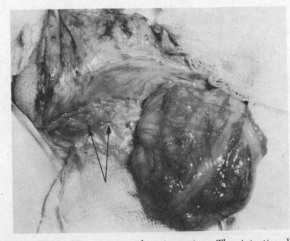

Figure 57–10. Herniation with evisceration. The intestine has remained within the omental sac and the hernial contents have been surrounded by gauze sponges prior to surgical correction. Note the remaining gut sutures of the original wound closure (*arrows*).

warmed balanced electrolyte solution (Fig. 57–10). Once the animal's condition has been sufficiently stabilized, anesthesia is carefully induced, the animal is placed in dorsal recumbency, and the area is prepared for surgery, taking care to avoid contact between the exposed viscera and potentially cytotoxic skin disinfectants. The wound is extended to allow full examination of all the abdominal viscera, particularly the omentum, small and large intestines, and mesentery. All damaged areas are exposed and checked for irreversible damage. Particular attention is paid to areas where the mesentery has been damaged. If self-mutilation has occurred, resection of nonviable intestine and anastomosis of remaining segments is frequently required. Extensive resection of small intestine may be necessary. The likelihood of long-term gastrointestinal problems occurring depends on the amount of intestine remaining. As long as the ileocecal valve remains intact, up to 80 per cent of the small intestine can be resected with little likelihood of problems developing.[16] However, if the ileocecal valve is resected, this figure drops to 50 per cent.[16]

Once all nonviable tissue has been removed, the abdomen is thoroughly lavaged with warmed balanced electrolyte solution. An antibiotic such as crystalline penicillin can be added to the final lavage solution, but the dilution of bacterial numbers and mechanical removal of debris by the solution itself are more important than local antibiotic therapy. The abdominal wound is closed with nonabsorbable suture material if heavy contamination is present.

Aftercare and Prognosis

Minimal postoperative care is indicated in simple, acute herniation, aside from restriction of exercise and removal of underlying causes that predispose to herniation such as wound infection and persistent vomiting. The prognosis is generally good.

Strict postoperative confinement is indicated in chronic incisional hernia, particularly when some tension was required to close the deficit or a prosthetic material was implanted. The prognosis is always guarded in recurrent incisional hernia, particularly if no underlying cause can be found.

When evisceration has occurred, treatment includes strict confinement, close monitoring for signs of peritonitis or ileus, continued therapy for shock, and other nursing care applicable to intestinal surgery. The prognosis is favorable as long as peritonitis does not develop and sufficient viable intestine remains.

Prevention

Incisional hernia is a largely preventable condition. It is the surgeon's duty to observe the principles of aseptic surgery and proper wound closure to minimize its occurrence.

1. Adamson, R. J., and Kahan, S. A.: The rate of healing of incised wounds of different tissues in rabbits. Surg. Gynecol. Obstet. *130*:837, 1970.
2. Andersen, J. R., Burcharth, F., Larsen, H. W., Roder, O., and Andersen, B.: Polyglycolic acid, silk and topical ampicillin. Arch. Surg. *115*:293, 1980.
3. Archibald, J., and Sumner-Smith, G.: *Canine Surgery*, 2nd ed. American Veterinary Publications, Inc., Santa Barbara, 1974, pp. 511–514, 535–538.
4. Burleson, R. L.: Double loop mass closure technique for abdominal incisions. Surg. Gynecol. Obstet. *147*:414, 1978.
5. Cady, B., and Brooke-Cowden, G. L.: Repair of massive abdominal wall defects—combined use of pneumoperitoneum and marlex mesh. Surg. Clin. North Am. *56*:559, 1976.
6. Chaimoff, C., and Dintsman, M.: Repair of huge midline hernias in scar tissue. Am. J. Surg. *125*:767, 1973.
7. Crane, S. W.: Evaluation and management of abdominal trauma in the dog and cat. Vet. Clin. North Am. *10*:655, 1980.
8. O'Connor, J. J. (ed.): *Dollar's Veterinary Surgery*. 4th ed. Bailliere, Tindall and Cox, London, 1950, p. 676.
9. Dorn, A. S., and Olmstead, M. L.: Herniation of the urinary bladder through the pubic symphysis in a dog. J. Am. Vet. Med. Assoc. *168*:688, 1976.
10. Dubois, P. M., and Freeman, J. B.: Traumatic abdominal wall hernia. J. Trauma *21*:72, 1981.
11. Edlich, R. F., Panek, P. H., and Rodeheaver, G. T.: Physical and chemical configuration of sutures in the development of surgical infection. Ann. Surg. *177*:679, 1973.
12. Foster, E. J., Murray, D. G., and Gregg, R. O.: Chronic bladder herniation associated with pubic diastasis. J. Trauma *21*:80, 1981.
13. Fuhs, S. F., Herndon, J. H., and Gould, F. R.: Herniation of the bladder—an unusual complication of traumatic diastasis of the pubis. J. Bone Joint Surg. *60A*:704, 1978.
14. Furneaux, R. W.: Abdominal wall reconstruction in a cat. Feline Pract. *4*:28, 1974.
15. Goris, J. A.: Ogilvie's method applied to infected wound disruption. Arch. Surg. *115*:1103, 1980.
16. Grier, R. L.: Techniques for intestinal anastomosis. *In* Bojrab, M. J. (ed.): *Current Techniques in Small Animal Surgery*. Lea & Febiger, Philadelphia, 1975, p. 121.
17. Hamer, D. B., and Duthie, H. L.: Pneumoperitoneum in the management of abdominal incisional hernia. Br. J. Surg. *59*:372, 1972.
18. Hayes, H. M.: Congenital umbilical and inguinal hernias in cattle, horses, swine, dogs and cats—risk by breed and sex among hospital patients. Am. J. Vet. Res. *35*:839, 1974.
19. Hilbert, B. J., Slatter, D. H., and McDermott, J. D.: Repair of a massive abdominal hernia in a horse using polypropylene mesh. Aust. Vet. J. *54*:588, 1978.
20. Howard, D. R.: Omphalocele in a litter of kittens. Vet. Med./Small Anim. Clin. *68*:879, 1973.
21. Klein, M. D., and Hertzler, J. H.: Congenital defects of the abdominal wall. Surg. Gynecol. Obstet. *152*:805, 1981.
22. Kolata, R. J., Krant, N. H., and Johnston, D. E.: Pattern of trauma in urban dogs and cats: a study of 1,000 cases. J. Am. Vet. Med. Assoc. *164*:499, 1974.
23. Lazaro da Silva, A.: Surgical correction of longitudinal median or paramedian incisional hernia. Surg. Gynecol. Obstet. *148*:579, 1979.
24. Miller, M. E., Christensen, G. C., and Evans, H. E.: *Anatomy of the Dog*. W. B. Saunders, Philadelphia, 1968, p. 670.
25. Moss, G.: Technique for repair of ventral hernia. Surg. Gynecol. Obstet. *141*:607, 1975.
26. Nicholson, C.: Defective diaphragm associated with umbilical hernia (letter). Vet. Rec. *98*:433, 1976.
27. Nyhus, L. M., and Bombeck, C. T.: Hernias. *In* Sabiston, D. C. (ed.): *Davis-Christopher Textbook of Surgery*. 11th ed. W. B. Saunders, Philadelphia, 1977, pp. 1141–1165.
28. Parks, J.: Herniation. *In* Bojrab, M. J. (ed.): *Pathophysiology in Small Animal Surgery*. Lea & Febiger, Philadelphia, 1981, pp. 420–424.

29. Peacock, E. E., and Van Winkle, W.: *Wound Repair*, 2nd ed. W. B. Saunders, Philadelphia, 1976, p. 218.
30. Pendergass, T. W., and Hayes, H. M.: Cryptorchidism and related defects in dogs—epidemiological comparisons with man. Teratology *12*:51, 1975.
31. Ripley, W. A., and McCarnan, H. R.: Umbilical hernia repair with mersilene mesh. Can. Vet. J. *15*:357, 1974.
32. Robinson, R.: Genetic aspects of umbilical hernia incidence in cats and dogs. Vet. Rec. *100*:9, 1977.

33. Sawyer, S. L.: Defective diaphragm associated with umbilical hernia (letter). Vet. Rec. *98*:490, 1976.
34. Silverman, S., and Ackerman, N.: Radiographical evaluation of abdominal hernias. Mod. Vet. Pract. *58*:781, 1977.
35. Swift, B. J.: Defective diaphragm associated with umbilical hernia (letter). Vet. Rec. *98*:511, 1976.
36. Tirgari, M.: Ventral hernia in the sheep. Vet. Rec. *106*:7, 1980.

Chapter 58 Caudal Abdominal Hernias

D. D. Smeak

The caudal abdominal hernias include inguinal, scrotal, and femoral hernias. Most published information regarding caudal abdominal hernias consists of isolated case reports and anecdotal citings.

Two general categories have been developed to describe hernias in the inguinal region. *Indirect* hernias involve the abdominal viscera entering the cavity of the vaginal process, which forms a hernial sac (Fig. 58–1A). This is the most common type of inguinal hernia found in small animals[8] and man.[30] *Direct* hernias pass through the inguinal rings adjacent to the normal evagination of the vaginal process (Fig. 58–1B). Except in traumatic cases, the contents are covered by a separate outpocketing of peritoneum.

INGUINAL HERNIAS

An inguinal hernia results from a defect in the inguinal ring through which the abdominal contents protrude.[3,20,30] The term *inguinal hernia* generally denotes direct and indirect hernias in the female and direct hernias in the male. Indirect hernias in the male are considered separately as scrotal hernias.

Congenital inguinal hernias in the dog and cat are rare.[25] The Basenji, Pekingese, and West Highland white terrier appear to have a greater risk of developing this condition. Congenital umbilical and inguinal hernias often exist in the same animal.[9] Males are more susceptible than females to developing congenital inguinal hernias.[7] This may be due to delayed inguinal ring narrowing because of late testicular descent in dogs.[12]

Acquired inguinal hernias are common in the dog and most often involve the middle-aged intact bitch.[3,19,20,27] No breed predilection has been documented,[29] although toy breed dogs may be clinically over-represented. Sporadic cases of acquired inguinal hernias in the cat have been described with equal occurrence among the sexes and breeds examined.[9]

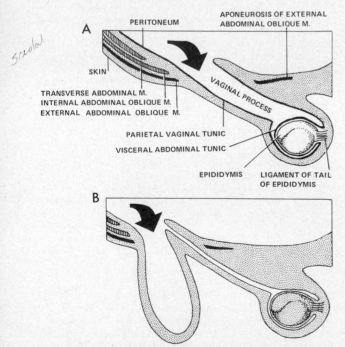

Anatomy[6] (Fig. 58–2)

The passageway for the vaginal process with the spermatic cord in the male or the round ligament in the female, through the opening in the caudoventral abdominal wall, is called the inguinal canal. In both sexes, the genital branch of the genitofemoral nerve, artery, and vein and the external pudendal vessels pass through the caudomedial aspect of these canals. The inguinal canal is a sagittal slit between the

Figure 58–1. Sagittal section of the inguinal canal and vaginal process in the male dog. Arrows indicate route of herniation in indirect (*A*) and direct (*B*) inguinal hernias.

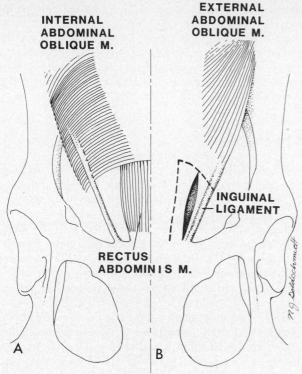

INTERNAL
ABDOMINAL
OBLIQUE M.

EXTERNAL
ABDOMINAL
OBLIQUE M.

INGUINAL
LIGAMENT

RECTUS
ABDOMINIS M.

A   B

Figure 58–2. Schematic diagram of the inguinal ring anatomy in the dog. *A*, Internal inguinal ring. *B*, External inguinal ring. Dotted line illustrates the superimposition of the inguinal rings.

abdominal muscles connected by the external and internal inguinal rings. The internal inguinal ring is bounded medially by the rectus abdominis muscle, cranially by the caudal edge of the internal abdominal oblique muscle, and both laterally and caudally by the aponeurosis of the external abdominal oblique muscle and inguinal ligament. The external inguinal ring is a slit in the aponeurosis of the external abdominal oblique muscle. The close superimposition of the external and internal inguinal rings in small animals does not form a canal, as its name implies, but a potential gap where hernial disruption may occur.

Pathogenesis

Numerous unconfirmed explanations have been presented regarding the pathogenesis of inguinal hernias. Few studies have definitively shown a significant heritable influence. Heritable inguinal hernias, however, have been documented in the golden retriever,[15] cocker spaniel, and young dachshund. Inheritance in the latter two breeds is thought to be polygenic.[27] It has been recommended that small animals with inguinal hernias be neutered until conclusive evidence is demonstrated regarding the heritable nature of this disease process.[7] Factors possibly involved in inguinal hernias can be grouped in three major areas: anatomical, hormonal, and metabolic.

An anatomical defect in the inguinal area is considered the most important factor in the etiology of inguinal hernias.[9,30] Specifically, enlargement of the vaginal orifice, which, unlike that in man, remains open, is the most important cause of inguinal hernias in domestic animals.[9] A congenital persistent vaginal orifice, however, is essential in the development of indirect inguinal hernias in man.[4,24] The internal abdominal oblique muscle in man acts as a shutter to prevent herniation of abdominal contents with abdominal contraction.[30] Prevention of inguinal hernias in small animals may depend on a similar neuromuscular reflex in addition to a normal anatomical barrier at the inguinal rings.[17] Bitches may be predisposed because the inguinal canal is both shorter and of larger diameter for passage of the round ligament.[2] Congenital inguinal hernias may disappear spontaneously at 12 weeks of age owing to a decrease in the relative size of the inguinal rings.[7] The occurrence of traumatic inguinal hernias in the dog may be due to a pre-existing anatomical weakness in the area.[19]

There is evidence that sex hormones play a role in the etiology of inguinal hernias. The majority of inguinal hernias appear in the estral or pregnant bitch. Acquired inguinal hernias have not been reported in the neutered female. Therefore, estrogen production may have a close relationship in their development.[27] Sex hormones may change the strength and character of the connective tissue, which may weaken or enlarge the inguinal rings.[21] Experimentally, sex hormone imbalance has been directly linked to inguinal hernia formation in male and female mice.[11]

Weakening of the abdominal wall may be due to altered nutritional or metabolic status of the animal.[20] Obesity may predispose the animal to inguinal herniation because of increased abdominal pressure forc-

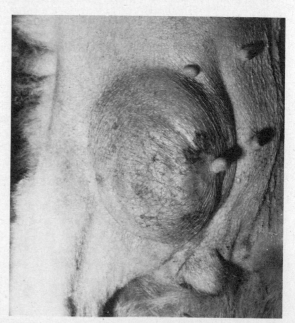

Figure 58–3. An inguinal hernia containing jejunum in a mature Pomeranian bitch.

ing abdominal fat through the inguinal canals.[19] Hernia in obese bitches is also associated with the accumulation of fat around the round ligament dilating the vaginal process and inguinal canal.[4]

Clinical Signs

Affected animals are most commonly presented with a painless,[13,19,28] unilateral[8] or bilateral mass with a soft doughy consistency,[8,19] although the appearance may vary depending on the amount of vascular occlusion and the contents of the hernia. Inguinal hernias may be undetectably small or very large, containing, for example, a gravid uterus or bladder (Fig. 58–3). Large inguinal hernias in the bitch may extend caudally following the round ligament to the vulva, thus resembling a perineal hernia.[7,19] Direct inguinal hernias in the male dog may resemble scrotal hernias because of swelling and edema of the testicle and spermatic cord from venous or lymphatic obstruction at the inguinal ring.

Diagnosis

Careful history taking and palpation are all that may be required to diagnose inguinal herniation. Vomiting, abdominal pain, and depression should suggest the possibility of obstructed intestine. Prior breeding or vaginal discharge associated with an inguinal mass may indicate uterine involvement. A history of stranguria may be elicited with bladder herniation. The history often will not reveal any clues to herniation when protrusion of omentum or prostatic fat occurs through the inguinal canals.

Diagnosis is confirmed by reduction of the hernia and palpation of the inguinal rings. Reduction is facilitated by elevating the hind quarters while the animal is in dorsal recumbency to reduce caudal intra-abdominal pressure.[3] Careful palpation of *both* inguinal rings is recommended, since inguinal hernias can be small and can remain undetected.

Incarcerated hernias present more of a diagnostic challenge, since palpation may not yield a definitive diagnosis. All inguinal masses, including mammary tumors and cysts, lipomas, enlarged lymph nodes, abscesses, and hematomas, must be considered as differential diagnoses. Although immediate surgical exploration facilitates diagnosis of an inguinal mass or hernia, surgical correction of such disorders proceeds with greater precision if the anatomical aspects are delineated first. Plain and contrast radiographs can be used to confirm the nature of the hernial contents. Reported contents of inguinal hernias include omentum, prostatic fat, uterus, intestine, colon, bladder,[5] and spleen.[1] A herniated gravid uterus is easily detected on plain radiographs by the appearance of the fetal skeleton after 43 days gestation or as a lobulated fluid density before skeletal ossification.[5] Catheterization of the bladder followed by

withdrawal of urine and possibly pneumocystography may be used to detect any involvement of the bladder. Fine-needle aspiration to help diagnose an inguinal mass or hernia should proceed with caution, especially if a loop of intestine or pyometra is suspected, because of the potential for leakage and the resultant sepsis.

Surgical Repair

Inguinal hernias are best repaired at the time of diagnosis, since delay may result in more difficulty in performing the operation and may increase the risk of complication. Successful surgical repair of inguinal hernias depends on knowledge of the anatomy of the area and good surgical technique consisting of apposition of strong tissues without tension and high hernial sac ligation. Adequate preoperative evaluation and stabilization of the patient are necessary.

The conventional approach to inguinal hernias[13,14,19,28] begins with an incision over the medial aspect of the swelling, parallel to the flank fold. The hernial sac is exposed through blunt dissection, and reduction is performed by milking the contents back or grasping the sac and twisting to force the contents through the canal. If the hernia cannot be reduced, the hernial sac is opened and the canal is enlarged by incising through the abdominal wall in a craniomedial direction. Excision of diseased hernial contents may be performed through this approach. The neck of the hernial sac is ligated as close to the internal inguinal ring as possible, and the sac is amputated. The incisions in the abdominal wall and enlarged external inguinal ring are closed with a synthetic absorbable material in a simple interrupted fashion. In traumatic inguinal hernias or when the external inguinal ring is weak, sutures can be placed between the inguinal ligament, rectus abdominis muscle, and internal abdominal oblique muscle to aid in hernia closure. The subcutaneous tissues and skin layers are then closed.

The midline approach[19,22,23] (Fig. 58–4) may be preferred over the conventional approach in several instances. The midline approach avoids incising through mammary tissue in the lactating animal. If bilateral hernias are suspected, repair through this approach can be carried out through one skin incision. Some surgeons routinely explore both inguinal rings, since small hernias are frequently missed on palpation.[19,22,29] In complicated hernias, entrance into the abdomen through the midline approach is more familiar to most surgeons.

The simplest option for treating a herniated gravid uterus in a domestic pet is ovariohysterectomy. If a valuable litter is expected in a breeding bitch, successful repair of the hernia and replacement of the incarcerated uterus have been accomplished up to the seventh week of gestation. Past seven weeks an ovariohysterectomy or hysterotomy is recommended

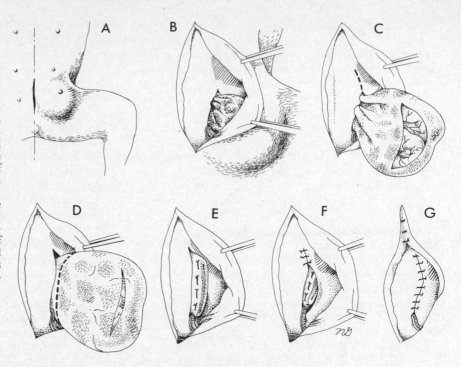

Figure 58–4. Midline approach to inguinal hernia repair. *A,* Proposed skin incision. *B,* Approaching the hernial sac by dissecting along the external lamina of the rectus sheath. *C,* The hernial sac is isolated and opened to expose the hernial contents. The dotted line indicates the direction of the abdominal wall incision if canal enlargement will facilitate reduction or resection of the hernial contents. *D,* Reduction of the hernial contents. The sac is severed at its base (dotted line). *E,* Hernial sac ligation with horizontal mattress sutures. *F,* Reduction in the size of the hernial ring with simple interrupted sutures. *G,* Wound closure. Subcutaneous tissue is tacked down to the external lamina of the rectus sheath.

depending on the health and value of the bitch as a breeding animal.[27]

In most cases inguinal hernias can be repaired with the patient's own tissues without resorting to prosthetic materials. Occasionally patients with large defects due to trauma or recurrent inguinal hernias require reinforcement of the primary hernia repair. The use of Marlex mesh as an onlay graft has not been reported but might be considered in selected cases for repairing inguinal hernias.

Complications

The most common complication is hematoma formation from inadequate hemostasis during herniorrhaphy. Swelling and tenderness in the inguinal area may be associated with incorporation of the nerves and vessels in the repair of the hernia or ensuing infection. If suppuration occurs, the skin and subcutaneous layers are opened and the usual local measures taken for treatment.

Recurrence of inguinal hernias after surgery is uncommon.

Postoperative Management

No antibiotics or bandages are generally used. If excessive dead space is anticipated, dressings with or without Penrose drain placement may help prevent seroma formation. Exercise is limited until suture removal. Controlled walking soon after surgery is encouraged to decrease postoperative edema and pain. The incision is monitored for swelling or discharge, and skin sutures are removed in seven to ten days.

SCROTAL HERNIAS

Scrotal hernias result from a defect in the vaginal orifice that allows the abdominal contents to protrude into the vaginal process beside the spermatic cord down to the level of the testicle. Indirect inguinal hernias (scrotal hernias) in the male dog and cat are rare.[6,16,18] The majority of case reports from England and the United States involve young, chondrodystrophic breeds of dogs.[8,13,16,23] No surveys of age or breed prevalence are available.

Pathogenesis

The literature regarding the pathogenesis of scrotal hernias is limited. Unlike the situation in man, the heritability of this disorder in dogs and cats remains unknown.[3] There may be a congenital anatomical defect or weakness in the vaginal orifice in those dogs with scrotal hernias.[29] Trauma may be related to scrotal hernia formation.

Anatomy

The anatomical boundaries of the inguinal rings have been previously described. The relative size of the inguinal canal and the structures found within the inguinal rings differ between the sexes. The cremaster muscle in the male is a continuation of the free caudal border of the internal abdominal oblique muscle. The spermatic cord passes through the inguinal rings within the vaginal process. In scrotal hernias, the abdominal contents herniate within the vaginal process alongside the spermatic cord (Fig. 58–1A).[6]

Clinical Signs

The presenting signs of scrotal herniation result from the protrusion of abdominal contents through the vaginal process into the scrotum.[3] This hernia is predominantly unilateral.[3] One bilateral case has been reported.[8] In man, 15 per cent of patients presented with unilateral scrotal hernia eventually develop this disease on the other side.[26]

The external appearance of this hernia depends on the contents and amount of venous obstruction present at the hernial ring. The swelling is generally cordlike, extending from the inguinal ring to the caudal aspect of the scrotum[16] (Fig. 58–5). Since the inguinal canal is smaller in the male, strangulation is more frequently seen than in the female with indirect hernias.[27] Strangulated hernias may show a dark discoloration of the tissues within the hernia, which is often visible externally. In addition, sharp pain is commonly elicited on palpation of these hernias.

Diagnosis

The diagnosis of a scrotal hernia can be confirmed by reducing the contents of the hernia and palpating the hernial ring. Reduction is facilitated by the same procedure as that described for inguinal hernias. Careful palpation of a cordlike structure travelling from the external inguinal ring to the scrotum generally rules out severe scrotal inflammation, orchitis, and tumors of the testes or scrotum. Distinguishing scrotal hernia from hydrocele[26] or torsion of spermatic cord is reportedly difficult in man.[30]

The diagnostic aids utilized for inguinal hernia may also be employed for scrotal hernias. The contents of scrotal hernias have been reported to consist of prostatic fat, omentum, and intestine.[8,13]

Surgical Repair

Repair of scrotal hernias should be considered as soon as a definitive diagnosis has been made and the patient is stabilized. Rapid diagnosis and repair are especially important in scrotal hernias, since strangulation of the hernial contents frequently occurs.

The surgical approach to scrotal herniation begins by incising the skin over the inguinal rings parallel to the flank fold. Care is taken when dissecting around the sac or inguinal rings to avoid disrupting the hernial contents.

Reducible and incarcerated scrotal hernias are repaired in a manner similar to that employed for inguinal hernias. The hernial sac is exposed, opened if necessary, and the abdominal contents replaced or resected. If the testicle is to be preserved (Fig. 58–

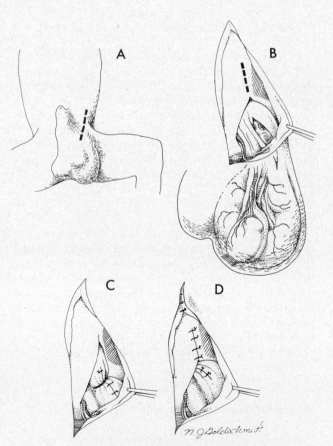

Figure 58–6. Repair of scrotal hernia (noncastration). *A,* Proposed skin incision. *B,* Approach to the inguinal canal by blunt dissection. Evaluation of the hernial contents is made through an incision in the parietal vaginal tunic (hernial sac). Dotted line indicates the direction of the abdominal wall incision if canal enlargement will facilitate reduction or resection of the hernial contents. *C,* Following reduction, a transfixing ligature closes the enlarged vaginal orifice. *D,* Simple interrupted suture closure of the abdominal wall, cranial part of external inguinal ring, parietal vaginal tunic, and subcutaneous tissues.

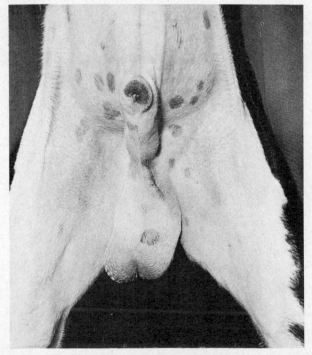

Figure 58–5. Left-sided scrotal hernia in a one-year-old Great Dane.

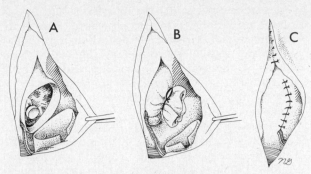

Figure 58–7. Repair of scrotal hernia (castration). *A*, The skin incision, approach, and reduction of the hernial contents are performed as in Figure 58–4*A*, *B*, and *C*. The hernial sac is severed and the spermatic cord is ligated. *B*, The testicle is removed and the hernial sac is closed with a transfixing ligature. *C*, Closure of the hernial ring and subcutaneous tissue.

6), the enlarged neck of the hernial sac (parietal vaginal tunic) is reduced in size by a transfixing ligature or several horizontal mattress sutures. These sutures are placed as close to the internal inguinal ring as possible. The external inguinal ring is partly closed with simple interrupted sutures without obstructing the spermatic cord, external pudendal vessels or genital artery, vein, and nerve branches.

When castration is intended (Fig. 58–7), the hernial sac is opened, and the spermatic cord is transfixed separately from the hernial sac. The testicle is removed following disruption of the ligament of the tail of the epididymis. The hernial sac is ligated at the level of the internal inguinal ring. The external inguinal ring is closed, leaving ample room for the genital artery, vein, and nerve branches and external pudendal vessels. There is usually no need to remove the parietal vaginal tunic distal to the ligation, since this can lead to further surgical trauma and hemorrhage.[26] Scrotal ablation is indicated if the scrotum is redundant.

Bilateral castration is currently recommended in conjunction with scrotal hernia repair. Recurrence of scrotal hernia is common if castration is not performed.[3] An increased incidence of testicular tumors in dogs has been associated with scrotal hernias.[10]

Complications

Scrotal dermatitis and scrotal hematomas are the most common sequelae of surgery. Scrotal dermatitis is commonly caused by rough clipping or scrubbing and is perpetuated by licking of the inflamed skin. Scrotal hematoma occurs from inadequate hemostasis following castration. Attempts to aspirate the hematoma are generally fruitless. In man, mild cases of scrotal hematoma may benefit from external support.[26] Scrotal hematoma is generally self-limiting and rarely requires surgical exploration.

If castration is not performed as a part of the herniorrhaphy, swelling in the scrotal area following surgery may result from occlusion of the lymphatic or venous drainage of the testicle. This complication may be prevented by palpating the involved testicle shortly after closure of the inguinal rings. Any change in consistency of the involved testicle compared with the opposite testicle necessitates re-evaluation of the inguinal ring closure.

Postoperative Management

In most instances no antibiotics or bandages are used. Suture removal and exercise restrictions are similar to those following inguinal herniorrhaphy. Scrotal dermatitis is controlled by preventing irritation caused by licking and using topically applied anti-inflammatory ointments.

FEMORAL HERNIAS

Femoral hernias are characterized by protrusion of fat or abdominal contents through a defect in the femoral canal. The occurrence of femoral hernias in small animals is very rare.[3]

Anatomy (Fig. 58–8)

The femoral opening in the caudal abdominal wall is composed of two separate areas contained within the limits of the inguinal ligament and pelvis caudolateral to the inguinal canal. The muscular lacuna contains the femoral nerve within the substance of the iliopsoas muscle. The vascular lacuna lies craniomedial to the muscular lacuna and contains the femoral artery and vein and the saphenous nerve. Each lacuna is separated by the iliopectineal arch composed of iliac and transversalis fascia. The transversalis fascia also surrounds the femoral vessels, forming the funnel-shaped femoral sheath. Hernia-

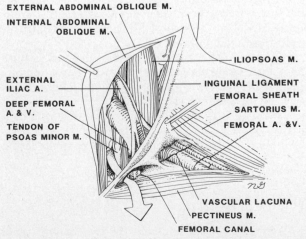

EXTERNAL ABDOMINAL OBLIQUE M.
INTERNAL ABDOMINAL OBLIQUE M.
ILIOPSOAS M.
EXTERNAL ILIAC A.
DEEP FEMORAL A. & V.
TENDON OF PSOAS MINOR M.
INGUINAL LIGAMENT
FEMORAL SHEATH
SARTORIUS M.
FEMORAL A. & V.
VASCULAR LACUNA
PECTINEUS M.
FEMORAL CANAL

Figure 58–8. Anatomy of the femoral region. Arrow indicates the path of femoral herniation. (Inguinal canal is cranial and medial to the inguinal ligament.)

tion most likely occurs in a potential space caudomedial to the femoral vessels known as the femoral canal.[6]

Pathogenesis

Femoral hernias in man are primarily due to an anatomical weakness in the borders of the femoral canal.[24] The same may be true in the dog and cat. Hormonal, metabolic, or hereditary causes may also play a role in the development of femoral hernias, as in inguinal hernias.[24] Iatrogenic femoral hernias may be created by transecting the origin of the pectineus muscle in subtotal pectineal myectomy or a ventral approach to the coxofemoral joint. A part of the transversalis fascia of the femoral sheath is removed with the origin of the pectineus muscle, creating a weakness in the caudolateral femoral canal. This complication is prevented by transecting the pectineus muscle well away from its origin on the pubis.

Clinical Signs

Animals with femoral hernias may appear clinically similar to animals with inguinal hernias. The hernial enlargement is generally on the medial aspect of the thigh but may also extend into the inguinal area. The size and consistency of the swelling are variable depending on the hernial contents and the amount of vascular obstruction of the contents at the hernial ring.

Diagnosis

Femoral herniation may be diagnosed by careful palpation of the femoral ring after reduction of the hernial contents into the abdomen. If reduction is not possible, differentiation from inguinal hernias can be difficult. With the animal standing on its hind limbs, inguinal hernias are palpated medial and cranial to the pelvic brim. In femoral hernias the swelling is caudal to the inguinal ligament and ventrolateral to the pelvic brim.[3]

The same diagnostic aids used in inguinal hernias may be used for femoral hernias. Differentiation of a femoral hernia from an enlarged lymph node or mass may not be obvious. Historically, the sudden onset of a swelling is more likely suggestive of hernia than of lymphadenitis or lipoma.[26] Prostatic fat and cysts have been reported as femoral hernia contents in the dog.[20]

Surgical Repair

Knowledge of the anatomy of the femoral canal and surrounding structures is essential for successful surgical repair of femoral hernias. Even though this surgical procedure is rarely performed, familiarity with the region is recommended. Femoral hernias may be incorrectly diagnosed as inguinal hernias because of their similar appearance and relatively rare occurrence. Therefore, the surgeon should be ready to repair either hernia when the definitive diagnosis is uncertain.

In approaching uncomplicated femoral hernias, the skin is incised parallel to the inguinal ligament. The hernial sac is exposed and the contents are reduced into the abdomen. Ligation of the hernial sac should be as high in the femoral canal as possible. The femoral canal is closed by placing sutures between the inguinal ligament and pectineal fascia (Bassini procedure in man).[24] The canal may also be closed by placing sutures between the inguinal ligament and the tendinous portion of the psoas minor muscle. Because of the important structures in the area, extreme care in placing the sutures is advised. Closure of the subcutaneous tissue and skin is routine.

If strangulation or incarceration is suspected, the abdominal midline approach may be used. Closure of the hernial sac is performed intra-abdominally by inverting and ligating the hernial sac. If needed, reconstruction of the femoral canal can be performed as previously stated.

Complications

Seromas and infections are the most common complications of femoral herniorrhaphy in man.[24] Scrotal swelling may appear if damage or occlusion of the spermatic cord occurs during closure of the hernia.

1. Alvarenga, J.: Unusual inguinal hernia in a bitch. Mod. Vet. Pract. 56:35, 1975.
2. Archibald, J., and Ellett, E. A.: Hernia. In Archibald, J. (ed.): Canine Surgery, 1st ed. American Veterinary Publications, Santa Barbara, CA, 1965.
3. Archibald, J., and Sumner-Smith, G.: Abdomen. In Archibald, J. (ed.): Canine Surgery, 2nd ed. American Veterinary Publications, Santa Barbara, CA, 1974, pp. 515–554.
4. Ashdown, R. R.: The anatomy of the inguinal canal in the domestic mammals. Vet. Rec. 75:1345, 1963.
5. Bartels, J. E.: How to delineate canine and feline hernias radiographically. Mod. Vet. Pract. 53:27, 1972.
6. Evans, H. E., and Christenson, G. C.: Miller's Anatomy of the Dog, 2nd ed. W. B. Saunders, Philadelphia, 1979.
7. Fox, M. W.: Inherited inguinal hernia and midline defects in the dog. J. Am. Vet. Med. Assoc. 143:602, 1963.
8. Grier, R. L., Hoskins, J. D., and Wahlstrom, J. D.: Inguinal hernia and Richter's hernia. J. Am. Vet. Med. Assoc. 159:181, 1971.
9. Hayes, H. M.: Congenital umbilical and inguinal hernias in cattle, horses, swine, dogs, and cats: risk by breed and sex among hospital patients. Am. J. Vet. Res. 35:839, 1974.
10. Hayes, H. M., and Pendergrass, T. W.: Canine testicular tumors: epidemiologic features of 410 dogs. Int. J. Cancer. 18:482, 1976.
11. Hazary, S., and Gardner, W. V.: The influence of sex hormones on abdominal musculature and the formation of inguinal and scrotal hernias in mice. Anat. Rec. 136:437, 1960.

12. Hobday, F. T. G.: *Castration (Including Cryptorchidism and Caponing) and Ovariotomy*, 2nd ed. Johnston, London, 1914.
13. Iverson, W. O.: Strangulated inguinal hernia in a basset hound. Vet. Med./Sm. Anim. Pract. 72:408, 1977.
14. Kipnis, R. M., and Hill, R. B.: An ectopic pregnancy within an inguinal hernia. Canine Pract. 5:45, 1978.
15. Larson, R. E., Dias, E., Flores, G., and Selden, J. R.: Breeding studies reveal segregation of a canine robertsonian translocation along mendelian proportions. Cytogenet. Cell Genet. 24:95, 1979.
16. Leighton, R. L., Cordell, J. T., and Ewald, B. H.: Scrotal hernia in a dog. J. Am. Vet. Med. Assoc. 139:1098, 1961.
17. Lunn, H. F.: Observations on the mammalian inguinal region. Proc. Zool. Soc. London 118:345, 1948.
18. Marwah, K., and Kulkarni, P. E.: Inguinal hernia in a male dog—a case report. Indian Vet. J. 54:571–572, 1977.
19. North, A. F.: A new surgical approach to inguinal hernias in the dog. Cornell Vet. 49:379, 1959.
20. Parks, J.: Herniation. *In* Bojrab, M. J. (ed.): *Pathophysiology in Small Animal Surgery*. Lea & Febiger, Philadelphia, 1981, pp. 420–424.
21. Peacock, E. E., and VanWinkle, W.: *Surgery and Biology of Wound Repair*. W. B. Saunders, Philadelphia, 1976.
22. Peddle, J. F.: Inguinal hernia repair in the dog. Mod. Vet. Pract. 61:859, 1980.
23. Pennock, P. W.: Strangulated inguinal hernia in a male dog. Mod. Vet. Pract. 43:88, 1962.
24. Ponka, J. K.: *Herniation of the Abdominal Wall*. W. B. Saunders, Philadelphia, 1980.
25. Priester, W. A., Glass, A. G., and Waggoner, S. S.: Congenital defects in domestic animals: general considerations. Am. J. Vet. Res. 31:1872, 1970.
26. Ravitch, R. M.: *Repair of Hernia*. Year Book Medical Publications, Chicago, 1969.
27. Roberts, S. J.: *Veterinary Obstetrics and Genital Diseases (Theriogenology)*, 2nd ed. Edward Brothers, Ann Arbor, MI, 1971.
28. Snow, R.: Inguinal metrocele (gravid) in a bitch. J. Am. Vet. Med. Assoc. 129:359, 1956.
29. Wright, J. G.: The surgery of the inguinal canal in animals. Vet. Rec. 75:1352, 1963.
30. Zimmerman, L. M.: *Anatomy and Surgery of Hernia*. Williams & Wilkins, Baltimore, 1967.

Chapter **59** # Diaphragmatic Hernias

Peter I. Punch and Douglas H. Slatter

A diaphragmatic hernia is a protrusion of the abdominal viscera through the diaphragm into the thoracic cavity.[5, 6, 23] In the majority, the viscera are not trapped within the thorax and may return through the diaphragmatic defect to the abdominal cavity.[2, 3, 39, 40, 49, 64, 78] Clinical signs may therefore be intermittent, and because many patients show few signs, the diagnosis of diaphragmatic hernia may be difficult.

ETIOLOGY

Diaphragmatic hernias may be congenital[9, 23, 33, 35, 46] or acquired.[4, 13, 19, 23, 32, 39, 46, 55, 66, 76, 78] This classification has its limitations, because the two are not distinct. For example, congenital defects such as a poorly developed central tendon of the diaphragm may predispose to an acquired diaphragmatic hernia in later life.[4, 47]

Virtually all acquired diaphragmatic hernias result from trauma.[5, 6, 23, 49, 78] Congenital defects develop *in utero* when the diaphragm's embryonic segments fail to fuse.[5, 9, 23, 33, 34, 35] They can range in size from a small defect to complete absence of the diaphragm.[6]

Traumatic Diaphragmatic Hernias

Traumatic pleuroperitoneal hernias are the most common. In one survey, 116 dogs and cats with diaphragmatic hernias, 76.8 per cent were of traumatic origin, 9.5 per cent were congenital, 16 (13.8 per cent) were of unknown etiology, and a hiatal hernia was iatrogenic.[78] The trauma is generally caused by a motor vehicle, but a kick or blow to the abdomen, a fall or sudden twist, and a penetrating wound may result in herniation.[4, 13, 45, 76, 78] When an animal experiences a sudden powerful blow against the abdominal wall, there is an abrupt increase in intra-abdominal pressure. The flexible diaphragm is pushed violently cranially, and if the glottis is open the lungs deflate, resulting in a large pleuroperitoneal pressure gradient. The diaphragm disrupts at its weakest point(s), allowing abdominal contents to enter the thorax.[4, 13, 49, 73]

Congenital Pleuroperitoneal Hernias

In children, congenital pleuroperitoneal hernia generally occurs as an acute respiratory emergency during or shortly after birth and has a mortality rate of 12 to 30 per cent.[61] In dogs and cats this condition is rare. Congenital pleuroperitoneal hernias occurred in four out of 17 pups in two consecutive litters from a Labrador bitch bred to an American foxhound.[36] Three of the affected pups, two males and one female, died at birth. The fourth pup, a female, died four days after birth. Autopsy revealed major defects in the diaphragm. The central tendon and crural attachments were absent, and only traces of the lateral attachments of the diaphragm were present. The 1:3 ratio of affected to normal pups suggested autosomal recessive transmission. The condition was unlikely to be sex-linked because equal numbers of male and female pups were affected.[36]

A cat with a congenital pleuoperitoneal hernia of the left diaphragm suffered constant dyspnea but lived a comparatively normal life.[45]

Congenital Peritoneopericardial Hernias

The most commonly described congenital hernia in dogs, and more rarely in cats, is the peritoneopericardial hernia. It is congenital rather than acquired, because in the dog and cat there is no direct communication between the pericardial and peritoneal cavities after birth.[29] The diaphragmatic defect, sometimes triangular, is located in the ventral midline of the diaphragm (Fig. 59–1).[23, 49] A number of theories have been suggested for the embryogenesis of these lesions,[29] but the hypothesis that is most widely accepted is that the hernia arises because of faulty development or prenatal injury of the septum transversum (see Fig. 59–1), permitting peritoneal and pericardial communication.[9, 15, 23, 28, 37] An unknown teratogen resulted in congenital peritoneopericardial hernias and cardiac abnormalities in four collie pups.[35] Cardiac abnormalities, sternebra malformations, and umbilical hernias may occur concurrently in peritoneopericardial hernias.[33, 35] Weimaraners are predisposed to umbilical herniation,[42] and a number have had both umbilical and diaphragmatic hernias.[33, 63] Concurrent congenital peritoneopericardial and umbilical hernias have been reported in a German shepherd, a Labrador retriever, and a crossbred dog.[21, 34] The umbilical defect that occurred in one of the Weimaraners was a triangular area covered by a serous membrane.[63] This condition (omphalocele; see Chapter 57) also occurs in children with peritoneopericardial hernias.[53]

An attempt was made to determine whether peritoneopericardial hernias are heritable in cats, but this issue was not substantiated.[46]

Hiatal Hernias

A hiatal hernia is defined as the protrusion or herniation of any structure through the esophageal hiatus of the diaphragm into the thorax.[61] In humans, at least four types of hiatal hernia have been described.[61] These hernias may be congenital or acquired, and the cause of the latter is often unknown.[61]

Sliding hiatal hernias, in which the diaphragm can move up and down the esophagus, resulting in temporary or permanent displacement of a portion of the stomach through the esophageal hiatus, have been described in the dog and cat (see Fig. 59–9).[2, 29, 40, 65] The majority of these have been in young animals and are probably congenital. Rolling or paraesophageal hernias, in which the esophagus remains in the normal position but a portion of the stomach herniates into the mediastinum adjacent to the thoracic esophagus, may occur in dogs.[23]

ANATOMY

Diaphragm

The diaphragm develops from six embryonic segments. The largest section is the transverse septum (Fig. 59–2), which migrates from the cervical region.[7] During migration the transverse septum is innervated by branches of the fourth to seventh cervical nerves, which combine to form the phrenic nerves.[33, 68] Bilateral phrenicotomy does not compromise respiration in the dog.[33]

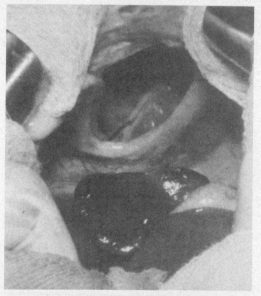

Figure 59–1. Peritoneopericardial hernia in a dog. Note the ventral midline position and triangular shape of the diaphragmatic defect. (Reprinted with permission from Archibald, J., and Harvey, C. E.: Thorax. *In* Archibald, J. (ed.): *Canine Surgery.* 2nd ed. American Veterinary Publishers, Santa Barbara, 1974.)

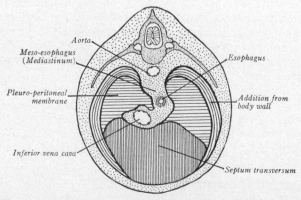

Figure 59–2. Embryonic components of the mammalian diaphragm. (Reprinted with permission from Arey, L. B.: *Developmental Anatomy.* 5th ed. W. B. Saunders Co., Philadelphia, 1946.)

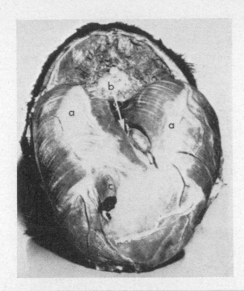

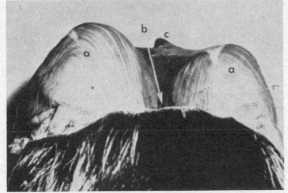

Figure 59–3. The diaphragm of an embalmed dog. Upper: cranial view. Lower: dorsal view. Note the size and position of the crura (a), the deep intercrural cleft (b) and the posterior vena cava (c). (Reprinted with permission from Grandage, J.: The radiology of the dog's diaphragm. J. Small Anim. Pract. *15*:1, 1974.)

The dome-shaped adult diaphragm projects into the thorax and consists of two single-layered muscle masses separated by a central collagenous tendon.[27, 34] The central tendon is relatively small and is strengthened by the two-layered disposition of the tendon fibers.[33] The diaphragm is separated from the pleural and peritoneal cavities by the endothoracic fascia and transversalis fascia, respectively.[33] It is attached to the lumbar vertebrae, the ribs, and the sternum. The diaphragm is not a single dome but consists of three partially molded lobes arranged in the form of a Y (Fig. 59–3).[41] The arms of the Y are the left and right crura, which are separated by the deep intercrural cleft. The right crus is readily distinguished radiographically from the left because the vena cava passes through it.[41] The stem of the Y is the cupula, which lies ventral to the intercrural cleft.[41] The crura remain relatively immobile during respiration, but the cupula is the most mobile section of the diaphragm.[41] An intact diaphragm is not essential for respiration, because other abdominal and thoracic muscles can assume its role, generally resulting in increased abdominal and thoracic movement during respiration.[13, 49]

There are three places where viscera pass through the diaphragm.[33, 41] The vena caval hiatus has been briefly mentioned. The aortic hiatus, through which pass the aorta, azygos vein, and thoracic lymphatic duct, is ventral to the lumbar vertebral bodies between the left and right diaphragmatic crura (see Fig. 59–3).[34] The esophagus and the vagal nerves pass through the diaphragm at the esophageal hiatus, which is supported by the right crus. The configuration of the right crus enables the muscle to play an important role in normal distal esophageal function during swallowing and vomiting.[30, 51] Herniation may occur at any of the diaphragmatic hiatuses.[78]

Pleural Cavity

Pleura is the mesothelial lining of the lungs, thoracic walls, and the structures of the mediastinum. It forms two complete sacs referred to as the pleural cavities.[22, 33, 60] In the normal dog each pleural sac contains 3.5 ml of fluid for lubrication, and the pleural cavity is only a potential space.[22, 33] The pleural fluid flows from the parietal pleura into the pleura cavity, and through the pulmonary pleura into the lung capillaries and lymphatics.[47] This fluid flow pattern results from differences in the colloidal osmotic, hydrostatic, and transpulmonary pressures in the respective tissues.[59]

An increase in the pleural fluid drainage rate can be accommodated to a limited extent, but if excess fluid or fluid containing plasma proteins accumulates in the pleural cavities, the normal hydrostatic and osmotic colloidal pressure gradients are counteracted, and further fluid accumulates.[57] Owing to the flimsiness of the caudal ventral mediastinum, pleural effusions that accumulate in one side soon enter the other pleural cavity.[61] The pleural and peritoneal cavities communicate by lymphatics and micropores in the diaphragm.[60]

PATHOPHYSIOLOGY

The pathophysiology of diaphragmatic hernias is variable and depends on a number of interdependent factors, including the etiology and chronicity of the hernia, the size of the defect and its location, organs which herniate, the viability of the herniated organs, and the presence or absence of adhesions, pleural effusion, and pulmonary edema.[23, 34, 39, 49, 70]

Traumatic Diaphragmatic Hernias

The location of the diaphragmatic tear depends on the position of the animal at the time of impact and the location of the viscera. The area of the diaphragm least protected by the viscera at the time of impact ruptures.[23] Trauma may result in the herniation of the diaphragm at more than one site.[78] Some workers have reported the incidence of left-sided hernias to

TABLE 59–1. Incidence of Traumatic Diaphragmatic Hernia Sites

Species	Total Number*	Incidence (%)				Reference
		Left Side	*Right Side*	*Both Sides*	*Other Sites*	
Dog	26	61.5	23.1	11.5	3.8	4
Dog and cat	61	50.8	49.2	—	—	19
Dog	25	24.0	64.0	12.0	—	39
Cat	15	40.0	20.0	—	—	
Dog	18	33.3	66.6	—	—	76
Cat	14	35.7	28.6	—	35.7†	

*Number of animals in study for which information was available.
†Radial tears.

be twice that of right-sided hernias,[4] whereas others have reported the reverse.[79] Overall there appears to be little difference in the incidence of left- and right-sided hernias (Table 59–1), and some animals suffer bilateral tears. The muscular sections of the diaphragm are more susceptible to rupture than the central tendon,[39, 46, 49, 76, 78] and the tear may be circumferential, radial, or a combination (Fig. 59–4) (Table 59–2).[39]

The location and size of the diaphragmatic tear to a large extent determine which organs herniate from the abdomen to the thorax. For example, in a right-sided tear, the liver generally herniates, whereas in a left-sided tear, the stomach herniates.[76] The liver herniates most frequently, followed by small intestines, stomach, and spleen.[39, 78] Virtually any of the abdominal viscera, including the omentum, pancreas, colon, gallbladder, cecum, kidney, falciform ligament, and even a gravid uterus, may herniate into the pleural cavities.[4, 39, 46, 78]

Herniation of the liver may result in hydrothorax and ascites if the hepatic venous drainage is compromised. Hydrothorax and ascites can be caused by a rise of 5 to 10 mm Hg in intrahepatic pressure, which results in exudation of large quantities of fluid through the capsule of Glisson and serosa.[15, 71] In one study 26 (22.4 per cent) of 116 dogs and cats with diaphragmatic hernias had hydrothorax. Of those 26 animals, 24 had herniated livers, but 67 other animals had herniated livers without pleural effusion.[71] Hemothorax and chylothorax are other forms of pleural effusion that may result from the traumatic insult that produces diaphragmatic hernias.[22, 24, 39, 55, 60, 66, 78]

The major effect of organ herniation from the abdomen into the thorax and pleural effusion is

pulmonary atelectasis, which may result in a significant loss of functional lung capacity. The great veins may also be compressed, causing decreased venous return and reduced cardiac output.[23, 49] However, dogs and cats at rest can tolerate severe hypoxia,[56] and many animals with diaphragmatic hernias show few clinical signs.[78] Concurrent interstitial pulmonary edema arising from traumatic thoracic injury may further decrease oxygen uptake and result in hypoxemia and acidosis.[23, 73] Affected patients may be precariously close to respiratory decompensation and fatal shock. Extreme care must be exercised in their handling.[39, 73]

Diaphragmatic herniation of the stomach may result in gastric tympany. The accumulation of gas within the stomach severely compromises cardiovascular function by compressing the vena cava and dramatically reduces lung capacity. Failure to alleviate this condition results in death.[39, 49, 76]

A number of other pathological disorders may arise following traumatic diaphragmatic herniation. Intestinal obstruction or strangulation may occur because of the formation of adhesions, constriction of the hernia, or volvulus,[23, 49] and jaundice may develop owing to biliary obstruction.[49] In a more chronic hernia the pressure of viscera against the edge of the hernia may result in ulceration or hemorrhage. If the blood supply is severely compromised, ischemic necrosis, intestinal perforation, and abscess formation may occur.[23]

Congenital Hernias

The rare congenital pleuroperitoneal hernias are similar in pathophysiology to acquired pleuroperito-

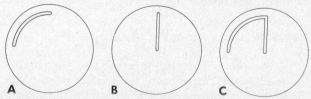

Figure 59–4. Types of diaphragmatic tear: *A*, circumferential; *B*, radial; *C*, both. (Reprinted with permission from Garson, J. L., Dodman, N. H., and Baker, G. J.: Diaphragmatic hernia. Analysis of fifty-six cases in dogs and cats. J. Small Anim. Pract. *21*:469, 1980.)

TABLE 59–2. Type of Traumatic Diaphragmatic Tear*

Species	No. of Cases	Incidence (%)			Reference
		Circumferential	*Radial*	*Both*	
Dog	25	40.0	40.0	20.0	39
Cat	17	58.8	17.6	23.5	
Dog	18	100.0	—	—	76
Cat	14	64.3	35.7	—	

*See Fig. 59–4.

neal hernias and generally result in death.[36] In the more common peritoneopericardial hernias there is frequently little pathological change because the mediastinum is intact and the lungs can function reasonably normally.[15, 49] However, if a substantial amount of the abdominal viscera herniates into the thorax, cardiovascular and pulmonary disorders develop from compression. Cardiac murmurs and changes in the ECG may result from compression and distortion of the atrioventricular valves, pulmonic stenosis, or displacement of the heart.[15, 28, 33, 37, 49] More than 40 cases of peritoneopericardial hernias have been reported (see Table 59–3). Weimaraners and German shepherds have been more commonly reported as having hernias than other breeds.

The organs most commonly herniated are the liver and gallbladder, followed by the small intestine, spleen, stomach, and, occasionally, omentum or falciform ligament.[34] Incarceration or strangulation of the liver, stomach, or small intestines in the hernia may result in vomiting, diarrhea, ascites, or intestinal obstruction or rupture.[33, 37, 63] In one case hepatic ischemic cirrhosis developed because of reduced liver perfusion, producing hepatoencephalopathy.[33] In a cat with severe right-sided congestive heart failure, the heart and liver were found to be fused at autopsy.[38]

Hiatal hernias generally cause no pulmonary or cardiovascular problems, and the clinical signs are referable to the gastrointestinal system. Esophagitis and inhalation pneumonia may develop owing to the frequent reflux of gastric contents.[40, 65] In addition, hiatal hernias may predispose the animal to gastroesophageal intussusception. The diaphragm may rupture at the time of intussusception, and in most cases the condition is fatal.[67]

DIAGNOSIS

Clinical Signs

The clinical signs of diaphragmatic hernias are not pathognomonic. The etiology and type of hernia, the severity of pulmonary and cardiac compression, which organs herniate, the degree of luminal and vascular obstruction, and the chronicity of the condition influence the presenting signs.[4, 6, 13, 23, 34, 49, 76, 78] Clinical signs may be intermittent because the herniated organs return to the abdomen, and some animals may have a diaphragmatic hernia for years without showing clinical signs.[78]

Traumatic Diaphragmatic Hernias

There is no breed, age, or sex predisposition to traumatic diaphragmatic hernia.[4, 39, 78] A history of trauma may be known, and the time between the traumatic insult and presentation can vary from none to more than six years.[78] In a recent report more than 80 per cent of traumatic hernias were diagnosed less than 4 weeks after injury.[39] Animals with acute traumatic hernias are frequently presented in shock with the accompanying signs of pale or cyanotic mucous membranes, tachypnea, tachycardia, decreased peripheral circulation, slight fever, and oliguria. Injuries to the skeleton, particularly the pelvis and hind legs, and to abdominal viscera, lungs, and central nervous system may overshadow signs of diaphragmatic hernia.[4, 23, 49, 76, 78] Shock is life-threatening and must be treated before one considers surgical correction of a diaphragmatic hernia.[6, 23, 44, 58]

Dyspnea, sometimes accompanied by hyperpnea and cyanosis resulting in fatigue and lethargy, is observed in the majority of dogs and cats with traumatic diaphragmatic hernias and is the most common clinical sign.[6, 13, 19, 23, 39, 76, 78] Animals may prefer a sitting or standing position, sometimes with abducted elbows or extended neck, and may object to lying down.[23, 39, 49, 58] Orthopnea may be due either to sternal pain or to the abdominal organ pressure on thoracic structures.[23] An animal exhibiting orthopnea should not be restrained in lateral recumbency. Neither should the hindquarters of an animal with suspected diaphragmatic hernia be elevated to see if dyspnea is increased, because of the serious risk of pulmonary decompensation, which may result in collapse and death.[5, 49] Generally the more abdominal viscera displaced into the thorax, the greater the interference with respiration and circulation.[6] In animals with chronic hernias there is some ability to compensate for reduced lung capacity, but exercise intolerance or chronic respiratory disease may be seen.[6, 78] Gastric tympany may add to respiratory distress.[6, 39, 76]

In some animals, enteric signs due to a compromised gastrointestinal system may be observed, with or without respiratory signs.[39] Enteric signs may include dysphagia, emesis, anorexia, and diarrhea or constipation.[19, 39, 58, 78]

Congenital Peritoneopericardial Hernias

The clinical signs of approximately 40 animals with congenital peritoneopericardial hernias are listed in Table 59–3. This condition may be diagnosed after a pup or kitten is weaned and is being fed solid food. Dyspnea, vomiting, abdominal pain, and diarrhea may be seen following ingestion of food.[6, 12, 28] Occasionally, this condition is diagnosed in unthrifty kittens or pups.[39, 63] However, many animals show few clinical signs, and the hernia is frequently an incidental finding during investigation of some other problem.[21, 39]

Clinical signs may occur at any age (see Table 59–3) and may have an acute onset. Gastrointestinal signs of vomiting, anorexia or polyphagia, diarrhea, and weight loss are common, as are respiratory signs of dyspnea, coughing or wheezing, and poor exercise tolerance. In two cases, one in the dog and the other in a cat, there were neurological signs of head pressing, blindness, and convulsions, probably owing to hepatoencephalopathy.[39] Owing to compromised venous return and pressure by the abdominal visceral

TABLE 59–3. Clinical Reports of Congenital Peritoneopericardial Hernias in Dogs and Cats

Species and Breed	Age*	Sex†	Presenting Signs	Herniated Organs‡	Reference
Dogs					
Weimaraner	4 mo	M	Poor growth	Liver and gallbladder	34
	2.5 yr	M	Vomiting, pawing, and head pressing	Mesentery, small intestine	34
	2.5 yr	M	Hit by car, incidental finding	Small intestine, liver, and gallbladder	34
	3 yr	M	Acute onset of vomiting	NA	34
	2.5 yr	F	Abnormal abdominal swelling	Liver, spleen, pancreas, omentum, small intestine	52
	4 mo	M	Poor growth, omphalocele, vomiting, distress after eating	None, organs slipped back to abdomen	63
	15 yr	FS	Anorexia, vomiting,- lethargy	Omentum, duodenum, liver and gallbladder	75
German Shepherd	4 yr	M	Vomiting	Omentum, jejunum	9
	7 wk	M	No clinical signs, muffled heart sounds	Small intestine	15
	6 mo	M	Anorexia, reduced exercise, polydipsia, dark feces	Omentum, liver, small intestine	63
	1.5 yr	M	Lethargy, abdominal distension	Liver	77
Great Dane	3.5 yr	F	Underweight, polyphagia	Liver, spleen, and gallbladder	34
	4 mo	NR	Dyspnea	Small intestine	43
	1 yr	M	Failure to thrive	Small intestine and liver	50
English Setter	5 wk	M	Vomiting, diarrhea	Small intestine, omentum, mesenteric lymph nodes	28
	14 wk	M	Heart murmur, incidental finding	NA	34
	4 yr	M	Nasal discharge, cough	Omentum, falciform ligament	34
Golden Retriever	2 yr	M	Low exercise tolerance, listless, anorexia	Omentum, mesentery, falciform ligament	34
	11 mo	F	Vomiting	Spleen, duodenum, pyloric antrum, pancreas	72
Pekingese	2.5 yr	F	Lethargy, wheezing	Liver and omentum	34
	6 yr	F	Cough, gag, wheezing	Liver	34

on the heart, signs of congestive heart failure may be present.[37, 38]

Hiatal Hernias

Hiatal hernias in dogs and cats are rare, and most are congenital.[29, 40] Clinical signs may be observed first when the animal is weaned onto solid food and are generally seen within the first 12 months of life.[2, 4, 29, 62, 65] The most consistent clinical signs are regurgitation or vomiting and excessive salivation.[2, 29, 40, 62, 65] Regurgitation is passive, and there is no consistent time lapse between ingestion and regurgitation.[2, 40, 62] Dyspnea and exercise intolerance may be seen in severe cases.[2]

Physical Examination

Traumatic Diaphragmatic Hernia

The results of physical examination, as with the clinical signs, depend on the severity and location of the hernia. On auscultation, the heart beat is generally muffled, but the intensity of cardiac sounds may be increased if the heart is displaced toward one side.[6, 49, 73] Percussion of the chest generally reveals decreased resonance, and sometimes a fluid line can be located. If the stomach becomes tympanic, resonance is increased on the left side.[5, 6, 49, 73] Borborygmi due to the presence of intestines in the thoracic cavity are heard infrequently and should not be relied

TABLE 59–3. Clinical Reports of Congenital Peritoneopericardial Hernias in Dogs and Cats *Continued*

Species and Breed	Age*	Sex†	Presenting Signs	Herniated Organs‡	Reference
Dogs Continued·					
Collie (4 pups)	4 mo	3F, IM	Heart murmurs	NA	35
Dachshund	4 wk	M	Dyspnea	Small intestine	12
Doberman	1.5 yr	F	Anorexia, weight loss	Part of stomach, liver, spleen	34
Gordon Setter	2 yr	M	Dyspnea, emaciation	Small intestine	54
Labrador	8 mo	M	Umbilical hernia, incidental finding	NA	21
Manchester Terrier	2 yr	F	Diarrhea, anorexia, CHF	Liver, fat, small intestine	37
Miniature Poodle	2 yr	M	Vomiting, diarrhea	Small intestine	24
Mixed breed	6 mo	F	Incidental finding at surgery for umbilical hernia and spay	Liver and gallbladder, fat	34
	2 yr	M	Salivation, dyspnea	NA	34
Viszla	2 yr	M	Vomiting, anorexia, lethargy	Small and large intestine	11
Cats					
Persian	4 mo	F	Anorexia, vomiting	Spleen, liver, pyloric antrum, duodenum, omentum	10
	8 yr	FS	Seizures	NA	34
	10 yr	F	Vomiting	NA	34
Domestic Short-Hair	7 yr	FS	Occasional vomiting, dyspnea	Omentum, small intestine, liver	8
	2 mo	F	Marked dyspnea	NA	34
	10 yr	F	Vaginal discharge, incidental finding	Pylorus, spleen, liver and gallbladder	34
Siamese	2 yr	MC	Weight loss, vomiting	Small intestine and liver	14
Siamese X	5 mo	M	Ascites, CHF	Liver, heart and liver fused	38

*Age at time of diagnosis.
†M = male; MC = male castrated; F = female; FS = female spayed; NR = not recorded.
‡Na = not available, either not recorded or no surgery or autopsy performed.

on for the diagnosis of diaphragmatic hernia.[39, 76, 78] Similarly the "wasp waist," "tucked-up," or "empty" appearance of the abdomen due to displacement of abdominal viscera into the thoracic is observed infrequently.[39, 78]

Congenital Hernias

Congenital pleuroperitoneal hernias have findings similar to those of acquired hernias. Physical findings in animals with congenital peritoneopericardial hernias also depend on the severity of herniation. Pleural effusion is generally not present because the mediastinum is intact, but ascites is occasionally present. The heart beat may be muffled, and a murmur may be heard owing to displacement of the heart by visceral organs or pulmonic stenosis.[9, 15, 34] Skeletal and ventral abdominal wall abnormalities, including pectus excavatum, fusion, absence or malformation of stenebrae, omphalocele, and umbilical hernias, may occur concurrently.[21, 34, 63] In one dog the umbilical and diaphragmatic hernias were so large that the heart could be palpated through the abdominal wall.[21] Borborygmi are occasionally heard in the thorax.[6, 33]

Physical examination of animals with hiatal hernias is often unrewarding. The animals may be cachectic, and dehydration and depression due to repeated vomiting may be observed.[40, 65] Areas of lung consolidation due to inhalation pneumonia may be located by auscultation and percussion.[40, 65]

Differential Diagnosis of Diaphragmatic Hernias

The differential diagnosis of traumatic and congenital pleuroperitoneal diaphragmatic hernias varies according to the presenting clinical signs and physical findings, and includes all forms of pleural effusion (hydrothorax, chylothorax, pyothorax, and hemothorax),[22, 25, 60] pneumonia, acute gastric dilation or torsion, congestive heart failure, and intestinal accidents.[6, 13, 76]

Differential diagnosis of congenital peritoneopericardial defects includes traumatic and congenital pleuroperitoneal hernias, respiratory diseases, congestive heart failure, congenital heart diseases, gastric dilation or torsion, intestinal obstruction, and congenital gastrointestinal and esophageal disorders.

The differential diagnosis of hiatal hernias includes all causes of persistent vomiting: cricopharyngeal or esophageal achalasia, foreign body obstruction, vascular ring stricture of the esophagus, esophageal diverticulum, peritoneopericardial hernias, and pyloric stenosis.[62]

Radiography

Pleuroperitoneal and Peritoneopericardial Hernias

A tentative diagnosis of diaphragmatic hernia may be made on the basis of the history, clinical signs, and physical examination, but radiography is essential for definitive diagnosis.[9, 23, 34, 39, 49, 78] Familiarity with the normal radiographic appearance of the diaphragm is essential to avoid misdiagnosis. More than 50,000 variations in the radiographic outline of the diaphragm due to breed, positioning of the animal and x-ray source, obesity, respiration, age, and posture are possible in the normal dog.[42] Despite the low prevalence of traumatic diaphragmatic hernias, any animal that has suffered severe trauma should be routinely radiographed to check the diaphragm.[44, 58]

If possible, both lateral and ventrodorsal radiographs should be obtained. Animals with a suspected diaphragmatic hernia should be handled carefully with minimal restraint, and if they continue to struggle, anesthesia should be used. Owing to reduced respiratory and cardiac function, care must be exercised when anesthesia is induced—a considerable number of the animals that succumb to diaphragmatic hernias die because of poor anesthetic technique.[39, 78] The radiographic signs of traumatic pleuroperitoneal and congenital peritoneopericardial hernias are listed in Table 59–4. Not all signs are present in one animal, and repeat radiographic examinations may be necessary for diagnosis because viscera may return to the abdomen.[23, 49, 78]

Pleural effusions, which are common in pleuroperitoneal hernias but usually do not occur with peritoneopericardial hernias, are observed more easily on

TABLE 59–4. Radiographic Signs of Diaphragmatic Hernias

Type of Hernia	Radiographic Signs
Traumatic diaphragmatic*	Loss of diaphragmatic line
	Loss of cardiac silhouette
	Pleural effusion
	Dorsal or lateral displacement of lung fields
	Presence of gas- or barium-filled intestine in the thoracic cavity
	Presence of air or contrast medium in thorax from a peritoneogram
Congenital peritoneopericardial‡	Enlarged cardiac silhouette†
	Dorsal displacement of trachea
	Overlap of the diaphragmatic and caudal heart borders
	Discontinuity of diaphragmatic silhouette
	Presence of gas- or barium-filled small intestine or stomach in the pericardium
	Presence of air or contrast medium in the pericardium from a peritoneogram
	Concurrent sternal abnormalities

*Compiled from references 39, 49, and 64.

†Cardiac silhouette is defined as the radiographic density including the heart, pericardium, and any abnormal pericardial sac contents.[34]

‡Compiled from references 9, 12, 15, 24, and 34.

a ventrodorsal than on a dorsoventral view.[22] Because an animal that has severely compromised respiratory function may develop respiratory failure if placed in a ventrodorsal position, a dorsoventral view may be safer.[22] Small quantities of pleural fluid may not be detected,[60] but large amounts of fluid are readily seen on recumbent or standing lateral views.[22] Radiographic signs of pleural fluid include interlobar pulmonary fissure lines, rounding of the lung margin at the costophrenic angles, masking of the cardiac and diaphragmatic silhouettes, and separation of the lung margins from the thoracic wall.[22, 60] If herniated abdominal viscera can be seen, no further radiographs are required, but if large amounts of fluid are present, thoracocentesis may be necessary for diagnostic radiographs.

Thoracocentesis should be done with the animal awake and standing.[22] Skin over the seventh or eighth intercostal space on both sides is routinely prepared, and local anesthesia of the skin and underlying muscle is induced.[22, 60] A 16- or 18-gauge needle is attached via a three-way valve to a 20-ml syringe. The skin is displaced from the site of thoracocentesis, in order to ensure occlusion of the puncture following removal of the needle, and the needle is inserted in the middle of the intercostal space to avoid the intercostal artery, which lies at the caudal border of the rib.[60] The bevel of the needle should be directed toward the chest wall as it is introduced, and gentle suction should be applied to the syringe so that fluid is seen

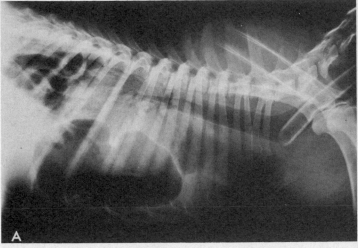
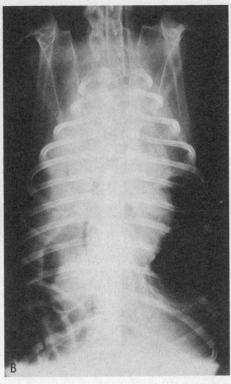

Figure 59–5. Lateral (*A*) and ventrodorsal (*B*) views of a dog with a bilateral circumferential traumatic diaphragmatic hernia (etiology: motor vehicle accident 12 months previously). *A*, Note the gas-distended stomach superimposed over the cardiac shadow, the presence of some pleural fluid, gas-filled intestine in the thorax, and the loss of the ventral diaphragmatic silhouette. *B*, Note the severe compression of the lungs, the loss of diaphragmatic outline, and the presence of gas-filled intestine and stomach.

as soon as the pleural cavity is entered.[22, 60] Large amounts of fluid may be withdrawn from the pleural cavity via the three-way valve. A sample is kept for later analysis, and the volume of fluid is measured. Both pleural cavities may require drainage before diagnostic radiographs can be obtained.[60] Care must be taken not to induce a pneumothorax during thoracocentesis.[60] There is less danger of iatrogenic lung injury if a short plastic intravenous catheter is used instead of a hypodermic needle. For the removal of large volumes of fluid or when pleural effusion continues, an indwelling chest drain is better than a needle (see "Treatment").

A definitive diagnosis of pleuroperitoneal (Figs. 59–5 and 59–6) or peritoneopericardial hernias (Fig. 59–7) can generally be made using plain films (see Table 59–4). The site of a pleuroperitoneal hernia

may be determined according to which organs herniated. For example, the stomach may herniate through a left-sided tear, and the liver generally herniates in a right-sided tear.[6, 76] However, a recent study showed that right-sided diaphragmatic hernias are underdiagnosed and left-sided hernias overdiagnosed on the basis of radiographic findings.[39] Frequently the site of traumatic hernias cannot be located radiographically.[6, 76, 78]

Contrast radiographic studies are undertaken only if a definitive diagnosis cannot be made using plain films.[6, 39, 64, 76, 78] The most commonly used techniques have been barium swallows and pneumoperitoneograms.[23, 34, 39, 76, 78] Owing to partial gastrointestinal obstruction, there may be a considerable delay in the time it takes the contrast medium to appear in the small intestine.[76] The presence of gas- or barium-

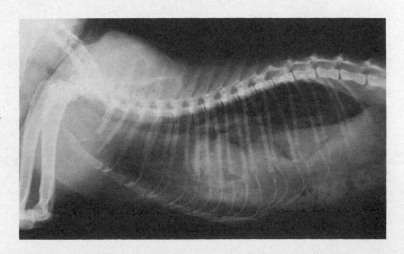

Figure 59–6. A cat with a traumatic diaphragmatic hernia. Note dorsal displacement of the lungs, loss of diaphragmatic lobe, obscuring of the cardiac silhouette, and the presence of large intestine containing fecal material.

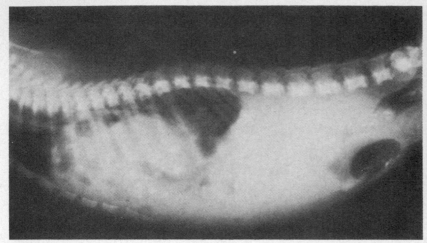
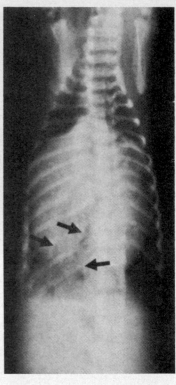

Figure 59–7. Congenital peritoneopericardial diaphragmatic hernia in a two-month old domestic short-hair cat. *A*, Lateral radiograph of the thorax and abdomen. The cardiac silhouette is enlarged, and the trachea is displaced dorsally. Gas-filled intestine can be seen within the cardiac silhouette, and the ventral diaphragmatic silhouette cannot be seen. *B*, The ventrodorsal view shows a greatly enlarged cardiac silhouette and gas-filled loops of bowel in the pericardium (*arrows*). The central section of the diaphragm is obliterated. (Reprinted with permission from Evans, S. M. and Biery, D.: Congenital peritoneopericardial diaphragmatic hernia in the dog and cat: A literature review and 17 additional case histories. Vet. Radiol. *21*:108, 1980.)

filled stomach or intestine in the thorax is diagnostic for diaphragmatic hernia (see Table 59–4). The location of the gastrointestinal tract in either the pleural cavity or the pericardium is useful for distinguishing pleuroperitoneal and peritoneopericardial hernias, respectively (Fig. 59–8).

A pneumoperitoneogram is performed by injecting 20 to 30 ml of air or gas into the abdominal cavity and holding the animal upright for approximately five minutes.[49] A standing lateral radiograph shows a pneumothorax within the dorsal pleural space in animals with a pleuroperitoneal hernia and air in the pericardium of animals with a peritoneopericardial hernia.[4, 77] A false-positive result occurs if air is accidentally injected through the diaphragm. A pleuroperitoneogram in a normal animal outlines the intact diaphragm cranial to the liver.[4] Positive-contrast peritoneography using a water-soluble, iodinated organic

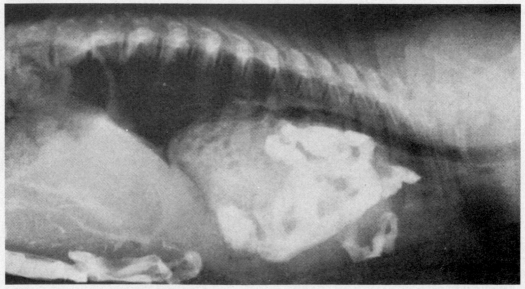

Figure 59–8. Congenital peritoneopericardial hernia in a seven-week-old German shepherd pup. The pup was given a barium meal 2 hours prior to the taking of the radiograph. Note that the intestines are confined within the pericardial sac. (Reprinted with permission from Bolton, G. R., Ettinger, S., and Roush, J. C.: Congenital peritoneopericardial diaphragmatic hernia in a dog. J. Am. Vet. Med. Assoc. *155*:723, 1969.)

contrast medium injected intra-abdominally, at 1 to 2 ml/kg, is a safer technique than pneumoperitoneography.[64] If pleural effusion is present, the fluid is removed before the contrast medium is injected. Barium sulfate is not used for peritoneography.[64] In animals with a diaphragmatic hernia, contrast medium in the thorax is easily observed and is diagnostic. False-negative results may occur if the hernia is obstructed by viscera or if the medium is diluted by a pleural effusate and can no longer be visualized on radiographs. False-positive results may be due to paracostal hernias, accidental injection of medium into the thorax, or an intercostal tear that permits medium to enter the pleural cavity without passing through the diaphragm.[64]

Radiographic diagnosis of the herniation of solid viscera, e.g., liver and spleen, may be more difficult than that of herniation of the gastrointestinal tract. Intravenous hepatography was suggested but required slow intravenous infusion over two hours.[26] Angiography of the celiac or cranial mesenteric arteries permits the visualization of the blood supply to the liver, spleen, stomach, small intestines, and omentum and determination of an abnormal position of these viscera.[48] The catheter must be precisely positioned using fluoroscopy.[48] Cholecystography may be used for the diagnosis of herniated gallbladder.[3] Intravenous iodamide allows rapid visualization of the gallbladder but is contraindicated in animals with suspected diaphragmatic hernias because of the high incidence of vomiting and the accompanying risk of respiratory decompensation. Oral media are well absorbed, but it takes 10 to 12 hours for sufficient amounts to accumulate in the gallbladder for diagnostic radiographs.[3]

Hiatal Hernias

The least common of the diaphragmatic hernias can be the most difficult to diagnose with routine radiographic techniques. Plain films sometimes reveal a soft tissue mass in the dorsal caudal thorax (Fig. 59–9A)[29] and barium meals may outline the stomach if it is entrapped within the thorax. Plain films and contrast radiography may not reveal any abnormality in animals with sliding hiatal hernias, however, because the stomach can return to the abdominal cavity (Fig. 59–9B).

Fluoroscopy, using barium sulfate as a contrast medium, may be essential for the diagnosis of sliding hiatal hernias.[40, 65] Esophageal peristalsis may be normal. Repeated reflux of barium sulfate from the stomach into the esophagus is frequently accompanied by herniation of the stomach, which is intermittent and diagnostic.[40, 65]

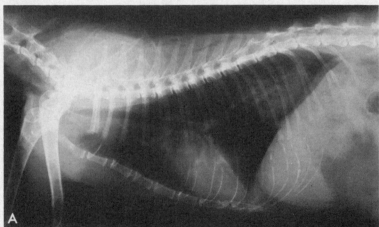

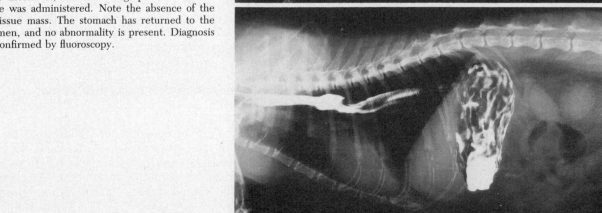

Figure 59–9. Sliding hiatal hernia in a cat. *A*, Lateral plain film. Note the soft tissue mass in the caudal dorsal thorax. *B*, Lateral radiograph after barium sulfate was administered. Note the absence of the soft tissue mass. The stomach has returned to the abdomen, and no abnormality is present. Diagnosis was confirmed by fluoroscopy.

Laboratory Findings

Blood and serum for complete blood count and biochemical evaluation of liver enzymes (serum glutamic oxaloacetic transminase and alkaline phosphatase) and blood urea nitrogen are collected to check for anemia, dehydration, infection, nephritis or hepatitis.[4, 39, 49]

If a pleural or peritoneal effusion is present, a sample is submitted for cytological analysis and bacterial culture.[22, 60, 66] The fluids most commonly recovered are transudates and modified transudates[22, 39, 66, 69] from a herniated liver or, occasionally, small intestine.[78] Hemothorax due to a ruptured liver, spleen, or fractured ribs[39] and chylothorax[55] have also been associated with traumatic diaphragmatic hernias.

In one dog, fibrinolysis resulting in clotting abnormalities occurred when the liver was traumatically herniated into the thorax.[32] Blood coagulation was normal but the clot was lysed in three to five minutes instead of more than 24 hours.

Miscellaneous Tests

An ECG can confirm cardiac displacement and concurrent congenital cardiac abnormalities or cardiac contusion.[1, 15, 34, 35] Cardiac arrhythmias, resulting from myocardial injury, significantly increase the danger of anesthesia.[1]

Aids to the diagnosis of hiatal hernia include gastroscopy, esophageal manometry, and measurement of esophageal pH.[18, 40, 63] A consistently acid pH in the esophagous is a indication of gastric reflux,[18] and gastroscopy may reveal peptic esophageal ulceration.[40, 65]

TREATMENT

Surgical correction of diaphragmatic hernia is not an emergency procedure, unless respiration is severely compromised, and may be postponed until the animal's condition has stabilized.[23, 39, 49, 78] Shock following trauma is treated as the first priority. Animals with myocardial injuries are allowed to recover before being anesthetized.[1, 23, 78] Some elderly animals with long-standing hernias and few clinical signs are left untreated and may continue to lead reasonably normal lives.[39] Whether other injuries, such as fractures, sustained at the time of traumatic herniation should be treated before or after the correction of the hernia remains controversial, and a decision must be made on an individual basis.[39, 78]

Left-sided hernias may allow the stomach to enter the thorax and dilate, severely reducing respiration. An emergency thoracocentesis is performed to deflate the stomach, and surgical correction is carried out as soon as possible.[39, 49, 76] A stomach tube should not be used to relieve gastric tympany, because the esophagus frequently undergoes torsion and an attempt to pass the tube may provoke struggling that can result in death.[76] In general, surgery should be carried out as soon as practical after the diagnosis of diaphragmatic hernia.[23, 49]

Surgical Approaches

Three surgical approaches have been recommended for the repair of traumatic diaphragmatic hernias: (1) lateral thoracic approach,[6, 19] (2) midline laparotomy, which may be extended by a median sternotomy,[4, 5, 6, 13, 23, 39, 49, 76, 78] and (3) transthoracic approach.[12, 20]

A lateral thoracotomy is simple and provides good exposure of the herniated viscera.[6, 19] The major reason for using a lateral thoracotomy is that adhesions are readily accessible and easily broken.[19] However, adhesions are extremely uncommon,[4, 6, 39, 76, 78] and the side on which the hernia is located must be known prior to performing surgery.[5, 6] If the location of the hernia is unknown, is misdiagnosed, or extends bilaterally, the surgeon may be obliged to extend the incision to a transthoracic approach through the sternum or, alternatively, to perform a thoracotomy on the other side.[6, 39, 78]

A midline laparotomy is simple, causes less postoperative pain than a thoracotomy, and has the advantage of providing exposure and access to the diaphragmatic hernia regardless of the site.[6, 23, 39, 49, 76] In addition, an abdominal approach permits examination of all abdominal viscera for injury.[76] Disadvantages of a midline laparotomy are that the diaphragm is approached from its concave surface and is slightly less accessible and that when intrathoracic adhesions occur they may be more difficult to reduce.[6]

The midline laparotomy, with a median sternotomy for better exposure if necessary, is the most commonly used technique for the correction of diaphragmatic hernia.[4, 5, 6, 23, 34, 39, 49, 76, 78] A thoracotomy is contraindicated in animals with a congenital peritoneopericardial hernia because of poor access to the herniated organs, the need to disrupt the mediastinum to gain access to the hernia, and the production of pneumothorax, which does not normally occur in a midline laparotomy because the mediastinum and pericardium are intact.[34]

Peritoneopericardial and Pleuroperitoneal Hernias

Positive-pressure ventilation is required for animals with pleuroperitoneal hernias and for some animals with peritoneopericardial hernias. An intravenous catheter should be inserted for fluid replacement. The ventral abdomen and thorax are prepared routinely for surgery.[23, 39, 49] The fluids should be warmed and the animal kept on a heated pad to prevent hypothermia.[39]

The initial incision is started in the midline at the xiphoid cartilage and extended caudally along the linea alba as far as necessary for good exposure. Generally, extension just caudal to the umbilicus is sufficient.[6, 13, 49, 76] Artificial respiration is started immediately after the abdomen is opened in animals with pleuroperitoneal hernias. A self-retaining retractor should be positioned and the faliciform ligament either removed or split.[49] Excess pleural or ascitic fluid is removed. When this fluid is removed, significant body protein loss occurs, and the remaining body fluid is redistributed, perhaps predisposing the animal to pulmonary edema due to reduced plasma oncotic pressure.[70] Pulmonary edema, a frequent complication of re-expansion of chronically collapsed lungs after correction of a diaphragmatic hernia, may have fatal consequences.[69] Careful attention to the artificial respiration to avoid over-expansion of the lungs will reduce this danger.[39]

Congenital peritoneopericardial hernias are located in the ventral midline of the diaphragm and are readily identifiable (see Fig. 59–2).[15, 33, 63] Traumatic pleuroperitoneal hernias are commonly located in the ventral diaphragm and are easily seen, but hernias in the more dorsal diaphragm may not be visible and are located by palpation.[4, 6, 39, 49, 78] More than one hernia may occur, and the entire diaphragm should be carefully examined for defects.[78] In most cases, the herniated organs can be returned to the abdominal cavity by gentle traction. Great care must be taken when handling the liver and spleen, because these organs are frequently severely congested and highly susceptible to rupture.[6, 49] If the abdominal organs are incarcerated within the thorax, or the liver is severely swollen, the hernia is enlarged by incising the diaphragm.[4, 23]

When adhesions have formed and cannot be reduced from the abdomen, or the diaphragmatic hernia cannot be seen, the abdominal incision is extended cranially and a median sternotomy is performed.[4–6, 39, 40] A sternotomy should not be performed unless necessary, because it causes much postoperative pain.[5] The posterior half of the sternum is split in the midline. Lateral deviation may result in laceration of the internal thoracic arteries with subsequent hemorrhage.[5] The sternum may be split with a scalpel blade,[5] but if necessary, bone-cutting scissors, an osteotome, or an oscillating bone saw can be used.[49] To obtain adequate exposure the diaphragm can be incised down to the hernial defect, with care taken to avoid the phrenic nerves and posterior vena cava.[5, 49]

Adhesions between the thoracic and abdominal viscera must be broken down carefully by blunt or sharp dissection.[23, 49] If adhesions to the lung have developed, care must be taken not to damage the surface of the lung, or a fatal pneumothorax may develop postoperatively.[19] After reduction of the hernia the abdominal contents are packed caudally to permit greater access to the diaphragm.[5, 23, 49] The edges of chronic and congenital hernias should be debrided.[21, 23, 34, 49, 63, 76] Prior to closure, a chest drain can be inserted in animals with a pleuroperitoneal hernia, but in most cases a drain should not be necessary in animals with a congenital peritoneopericardial hernia.[39, 49] The air trapped in the pericardium is slowly absorbed over the next week.[63, 77]

To close the diaphragmatic defect, the surgeon grasps the edges of the hernia with Allis tissue forceps and approximates them for suturing,[4–6] starting at the deepest end of the tear and using sterile nonabsorbable suture material.[23, 39, 49] A simple continuous or continuous-lock suture pattern is generally recommended for the closure of the defect.[4, 23, 49, 78] If the defect is large, it is good practice to interrupt the pattern in two or three places. In larger animals a second layer of sutures should be inserted.[49] Considerable care is required when suturing around the vena cava, because constriction of this vessel may result in ascites due to an increase in intrahepatic pressure.[4, 16, 71] Ideally, an attempt should be made to return the diaphragm to its original anatomic structure and position, but if costal detachment of the diaphragm has occurred this may not be possible. The diaphragm can be anchored to the costal arch or abdominal wall, and despite the inaccurate repair, tidal volume soon returns to normal after surgery.[76] If a median sternotomy was performed the sternum is closed by placing two to four stainless wire sutures through the cut sternebrae rather than encircling them, in order to avoid the risk of injury to the thoracic organs if a wire breaks.[5, 49]

In dogs and cats with pleuroperitoneal hernias, the pneumothorax that was induced when the abdomen was opened can be reduced by inflating the lungs to maximum capacity prior to tying the last suture.[4, 6, 39, 76] Alternatively, the diaphragm can be closed, the lungs inflated, and the pneumothorax reduced via a chest drain previously inserted or via thoracocentesis.[39, 49] A combination of the two methods may be used. The use of a chest drain may reduce the incidence of pulmonary edema from over-expansion of the lungs.[39] After closure of the diaphragm, sufficient warm saline to cover the defect can be poured into the anterior abdomen, and the lungs can be reinflated to check for major leaks. Any major defects are closed with interrupted sutures, but small openings seal rapidly.[23]

The edges of the hernia can usually be joined together, but occasionally the defect is sufficiently large to require the use of an autogenous, homologous, or synthetic graft.[4, 17, 23, 63, 74] Teflon mesh,[23, 63] Silastic sheeting,[74] tensor fasciae latae from the thigh,[5, 63] a sliding graft from the lateral abdominal wall,[23] and, recently, an omental pedicle flap[17] have been used to close diaphragmatic defects. The use of the omentum was stated to have the advantages of being readily available, producing minimal donor defect, and having no rejection problems because of its autogenous source.[17] Left and right omental pedicles can be obtained by ligating and severing the right and left gastroepiploic arteries, respectively,

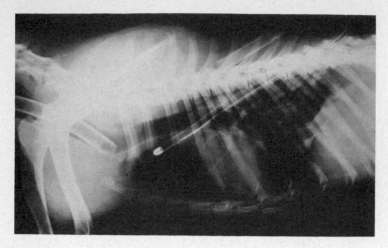

Figure 59–10. Postoperative radiograph of the dog with traumatic diaphragmatic hernia shown in Figure 59–5. Note the presence of small amounts of pleural effusion and the poor positioning of the indwelling chest drain.

then ligating and severing the small gastric branches along the greater curvature of the stomach.[17] The technique appears tedious, and as yet no clinical report on its use in dogs and cats has been published.

Prior to the abdominal closure, the viscera should be carefully inspected for signs of trauma or lack of viability.[76] In most cases and despite congestion, removal of organs is unneccessary.[39, 49, 78] Abdominal closure is routine, and sutures are removed ten days after surgery.

A postoperative radiograph is taken to check for pleural effusion, pneumothorax, and collapsed lung lobes and to ensure that no defects were missed (Fig. 59–10). This film is also useful for comparison with later radiographs that may be taken to monitor the patient's progress.

Sliding Hiatal Hernias

Owing to the rarity of sliding hiatal hernias in domestic animals and even greater rarity of surgical repair of this condition, it is difficult to generalize about which technique is the most useful. The aim of surgical correction of sliding hiatal hernias is to restore gastroesophageal competence and thereby control the esophagitis.[18, 61] In human medicine, the three most commonly used procedures are Nissen fundoplication (Fig. 59–11), the Besley procedure (Fig. 59–12), and the Hill procedure.[18, 31, 61] The Nissen fundoplication, performed by a midline laparotomy, has been performed on at least three dogs.[29, 40] Surgery was successful on a 8-week-old male Irish setter pup,[40] but was unsuccessful in another Irish setter[40] and in a Shetland sheepdog.[29] The second Irish setter died because of gastric prolapse one month after surgery.[40] A lateral thoracotomy at the ninth intercostal space on the left side was performed and the Besley procedure was used on the Shetland sheepdog.[29] Gastric reflux initially was prevented but subsequently restarted. The dog died of gastric wall necrosis two weeks after gastric antacids were withdrawn. A cause-and-effect relationship was not established.[29]

Postoperative Care

Broad-spectrum systemic antibiotics are administered for five days postoperatively. All patients, particularly animals that had pleuroperitoneal hernias, are carefully monitored for the first 24 hours postoperatively. Mucous membrane color and capillary

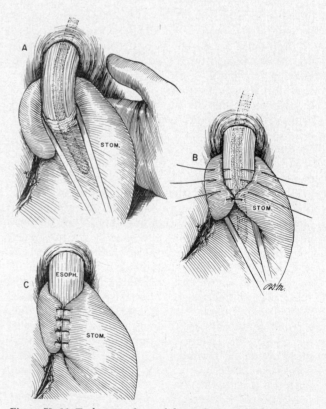

Figure 59–11. Technique of transabdominal Nissen fundoplication. Above: Abdominal exposure and mobilization of the distal esophagus and upper stomach in preparation for carrying out a fundoplication. *A*, Mobilized fundus is displaced behind the esophagus by the surgeon's right hand. *B*, Placement of sutures so as to encircle the distal esophagus with a generous portion of fundus. Note indwelling #40 F gastric tube. *C*, Completed procedure. (Reprinted with permission from Ellis, F. H., Jr.: Gastroesophageal reflux: Indications for fundoplication. Surg. Clin. North Am. 51:575, 1971.)

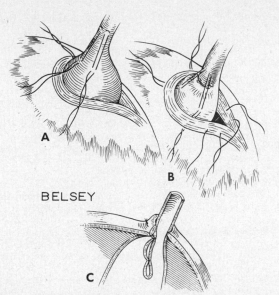

BELSEY

Figure 59–12. Belsey Mark IV transthoracic repair of sliding esophageal hiatal hernia. Exposure is gained through a left thoracotomy incision. After complete mobilization of the cardia, the lower 4 cm of esophagus is cleared of connective tissue. *A,* Mattress sutures are placed between gastric fundus and muscular layers of esophagus 1 to 2 cm above and below the esophagogastric junction. *B,* After these mattress sutures are tied, a second row of mattress sutures is placed to imbricate additional fundus onto the lower esophagus. Note that these sutures pass through the hiatus and out through the tendinous portion of the diaphragm. Before these sutures are tied, crural sutures are placed to narrow the esophageal hiatus. *C,* Completed repair after reduction of hernia and tying of sutures to maintain reconstruction. Previously placed crural sutures have been tied behind the esophagus to narrow the hiatus. (Reprinted with permission from Payne, W. S., and Ellis, F. I.: Esophagus and diaphragmatic hernias. *In* Swartz, S. I. (ed.): *Principles of Surgery.* 2nd ed. Vol. 2. McGraw-Hill, New York, 1974.)

refill, respiratory rate and pattern, temperature, and fluid balance are regularly checked. Oxygen support may be necessary in some cases, and if a chest drain has been inserted the animal must be constantly supervised. Analgesics may be necessary to relieve pain, but respiratory depressants (e.g., narcotics) must not be used. Fluid support should be administered until the animal's appetite returns, but care must be taken to prevent fluid overload.[6, 23, 29, 39, 49] Animals with surgically corrected hiatal hernia should remain on oral antacid therapy indefinitely.[29]

PROGNOSIS

The prognosis for animals with traumatic diaphragmatic hernias is guarded, and there is no correlation between the severity of clinical signs, the chronicity of the hernia, and survival.[39] The survival rate of animals with traumatic diaphragmatic hernias is listed in Table 59–5; Walker and Hall[76] reported a much higher survival rate than the other studies; this difference may be due to their failure to include operative deaths. An average survival rate of 50 to 60 per cent should be expected in both dogs and cats with traumatic hernias.

Causes of preoperative death have included multiple organ failure and shock due to the initial trauma, compromised respiration due to gastric tympany or the presence of abdominal viscera in the thorax, and shock following thoracocentesis.[39, 78] Animals have also died when being restrained for radiographs or following a pneumoperitoneogram.[78] The majority of animals that die during operation do so at induction of anesthesia or, less frequently, owing to poor maintenance of anesthesia and artificial respiration.[39, 78] Approximately 50 per cent of deaths following operation occur within the first hour,[39] and if the animal survives 24 hours it has a good prognosis.[39, 78] The most common causes of death within the first 24 hours postoperatively are hemothorax, pneumothorax, pulmonary edema, shock following abdominocentesis, and the initial trauma.[39, 76, 78] Death that occurs a considerable time after operation is generally due to gastrointestinal problems, including gastric

TABLE 59–5. Survival Rates in Dogs and Cats with Traumatic Diaphragmatic Hernias

No. Cases	Species	Deaths Before Operation		Deaths During or After Operation							Survivals		Reference
				Surgery and Anesthesia		< 24 Hours Postoperatively		> 24 Hours Postoperatively					
		No.	%	No.	%	No.	%	No.	%		No.	%	
62	Dogs	15	21.4	Operative deaths 23 (32.9%)*							32	45.7	19
8	Cats												
35	Dogs	3	8.6	2	5.7	8	22.9	3	8.6		19	54.3	39
23	Cats	0			17.4	6	26.1	1	4.3		12	54.3	
18	Dogs	0	0	0	0	0	0	3†	9.4		29	90.6	76
14	Cats												
94	Dogs	19	16.4	9	7.8	12	10.3	2	1.7		74	63.8	78
22	Cats												

*Time and cause of deaths not specified.
†All were dogs

torsion, ruptured ileum, intestinal stenosis, necrotic enteritis, and intestinal infarction.[39, 78]

The results of surgery for congenital peritoneopericardial hernias are much better. Of the animals listed in Table 59–3, 35 dogs and cats were operated on. Four animals (11.4 per cent) died during operation; one of these had perforated intestines,[11] and the other 3 were collie pups with congenital cardiac abnormalities.[35] Three animals were euthanized postoperatively, one because of peritonitis,[9] one because of continued vomiting,[34] and one because of hepatoencephalopathy.[34]

The results of surgical correction of sliding hiatal hernia in dogs have already been discussed. Owing to a lack of data it is not possible to give statistically signifcant success rates for surgery. Therefore, at this stage the prognosis must be considered "guarded."

DIAPHRAGMATIC EVENTRATION

Eventration of the diaphragm is a unilateral elevation of the intact diaphragm into the thoracic cavity.[29, 61] This condition is not a diaphragmatic hernia, but a brief summary is included. In humans, the condition may be congenital or acquired. It results from developmental or acquired defects of the diaphragm or its innervation.[61] Surgical correction involves reducing the eventration by excising the defect, inserting a prosthesis, or plication.[61] An esophageal hiatal hernia with eventration of the diaphragm was reported in an 18-month-old male Shetland sheepdog.[29] The animal was presented with the clinical signs of a hiatal hernia. Both defects were due to a congenitally weak central tendon of the diaphragm. The weak area was plicated, and correction of the hiatal hernia was attempted via a combination of Nisson fundoplication and the Besley procedure.[29]

1. Alexander, J. W., Bolton, G. R., and Koslow, G. L.: Electrocardiographic changes in nonpenetrating trauma to the chest. J. Am. Anim. Hosp. Assoc. *11*:160, 1975.
2. Alexander, J. W., Hoffer, R. E., MacDonald, J. M., et al.: Hiatal hernia in the dog: a case report and review of the literature. J. Am. Anim. Hosp. Assoc. *11*:793, 1975.
3. Allan, G. S.: Cholecystography—an aid in the diagnosis of diaphragmatic hernias in the dog and cat. Aust. Vet. Pract. *3*:7, 1973.
4. Al-Nakeeb, S. M.: Canine and feline traumatic diaphragmatic hernias. J. Am. Vet. Med. Association *159*::1422, 1971.
5. Archibald, J., and Harvey, C. E.: Thorax. *In* Archibald, J. (ed.): *Canine Surgery*, 2nd ed. American Veterinary Publishers, Santa Barbara, 1974.
6. Archibald, J. A., Reed, J. H., Cawley, A. J.: Surgical techniques for correcting diaphragmatic hernia in the dog. Mod. Vet. Pract. *41*:28, 1960.
7. Arey, L. B.: *Developmental Anatomy*. 7th ed. W. B. Saunders, Philadelphia, 1966.
8. Atkins, E.: Suspected congenital peritoneopericardial diaphragmatic hernia in an adult cat. J. Am. Vet. Med. Assoc. *165*:175, 1974.
9. Baker, G. J., and Williams, S. C. F.: Diaphragmatic pericardial hernia in the dog. Vet. Rec. *78*:578, 1966.
10. Barrett, R. B., and Kittrell, J. E.: Congenital peritoneoperi-

11. Bistner, S. and Butler, W. B.: What is your diagnosis? J. Am. Vet. Med. Assoc. *151*:763, 1967.
12. Björck, G. R., and Tigershiöld, A.: Peritoneopericardial diaphragmatic hernia in a dog. J. Small Anim. Pract. *11*:585, 1970.
13. Blakely, C. L., and Munson, T. O.: Rupture of the diaphragm. J. Am. Vet. Med. Assoc. *107*:292, 1945.
14. Bolland, E., Goverts, J. T., and Osinga, E. C.: What is your diagnosis? Tijdochr. Diergeneesk *103*:1076, 1978.
15. Bolton, G. R., Ettinger, S., and Roush, J. C.: Congenital peritoneopericardial diaphragmatic hernia in a dog. J. Am. Vet. Med. Assoc. *155*:723, 1969.
16. Brauer, R. W., Holloway, R. J., and Leong, G. F.: Changes in liver function and structure due to experimental passive congestion under controlled hepatic vein pressure. Am. J. Physiol. *197*:681, 1959.
17. Bright, R. M., and Thacker, H. L.: The formation of an omental pedicle flap and its experimental use in the repair of a diaphragmatic rent in the dog. J. Am. Anim. Hosp. Assoc. *18*:283, 1982.
18. Brindley, G. V., and Hightower, N. C.: Surgical treatment of gastroesophageal reflux. Surg. Clin. North Am. *59*:841, 1979.
19. Brodey, R. S., and Sauer, R. M.: Clinico-pathologic conference. J. Am. Vet. Med. Assoc. *145*:1213, 1964.
20. Butler, H. C.: Transthoracic approach for diaphragmatic hernia repair in cats and dogs. J. Am. Vet. Med. Assoc. *131*:167, 1957.
21. Butler, H. C.: Congenital diaphragmatic hernia and umbilical hernia in a dog. J. Am. Vet. Med. Assoc. *136*:559, 1960.
22. Cantwell, H. D., Rebar, A. H., and Allen, A. R.: Pleural effusion in the dog: principles for diagnosis. J. Am. Anim. Hosp. Assoc. *19*:227, 1983.
23. Carb, A.: Diaphragmatic hernia in the dog and cat. Vet. Clin. North Am. *5*:477, 1975.
24. Clinton, J. M.: A case of congenital pericardio-peritoneal communication in a dog. J. Am. Vet. Radiol. Soc. *8*:57, 1967.
25. Creighton, S. R., and Wilkins, R. J.: Thoracic effusion in the cat. Etiology and diagnostic features. J. Am. Anim. Hosp. Assoc. *11*:66, 1975.
26. Dalgard, D. W., Adamson, R. H., and Verness, M.: Diaphragmatic herniation of the liver in macaques demonstrated by intravenous hepatograph. Lab. Anim. Sci. *25*:753, 1975.
27. DeTroyer, A., Sampson, M., Sigrist, S., and Macklem, P. I.: The diaphragm: two muscles. Science *213*:237, 1981.
28. Detweiler, D. K., Brodey, R. S. and Flickinger, G. L.: Diaphragmatic hernia. J. Am. Vet. Med. Assoc. *137*:177, 1960.
29. Dhein, C. R. M., Rawlings, C. A., Rosin, E., et al.: Esophageal hiatal and eventration of the diaphragm with resultant gastroesophageal reflux. J. Am. Anim. Hosp. Assoc. *16*:519, 1980.
30. Duron, M. B., Jung-Caillol, M-C., and Marlot, D.: Effets des distensions etagées de l'oesphage thoracique sur l'activité spontanée du diaphragm chez le chat et le lapin. C. R. Seances Acad. Sci. (Paris) *281*(Serie D):183, 1975.
31. Ellis, F. H.: Gastroesophageal reflux. Indications for fundoplication. Surg. Clin. North Am. *51*:575, 1971.
32. Engen, M. H., Weirich, W. E., Lung, and J. E.: Fibrinolysis in a dog with diaphragmatic hernia. J. Am. Vet. Med. Assoc. *164*:152, 1974.
33. Evans, H. E., and Christensen, G. C. (eds.): *Miller's Anatomy of the Dog.*, 2nd ed., W. B. Saunders, Philadelphia, 1979.
34. Evans, S. M., and Biery, D.: Congenital peritoneopericardial diaphragmatic hernia in the dog and cat: a literature review and 17 additional case histories. Vet. Radiol. *21*:108, 1980.
35. Eyster, G. E., Evans, A. T., Blanchard, G. L., et al.: Congenital pericardial diaphragmatic hernia and multiple cardiac defects in a litter of collies. J. Am. Vet. Med. Assoc. *170*:516, 1977.
36. Feldman, D. B., Bree, M. M., and Cohen, B. J.: Congenital

diaphragmatic hernia in neonatal dogs. J. Am. Vet. Med. Assoc. *153*:942, 1968.

37. Finn, J. P., and Martin, C. L.: Diaphragmatic pericardial hernia. J. Small Anim. Prac. *10*:295, 1969.

38. Frye, F. L., and Taylor, D. O. N.: Pericardial and diaphragmatic defects in a cat. J. Am. Vet. Med. Assoc. *152*:1507, 1978.

39. Garson, H. H., Dodman, N. H., and Baker, G. J.: Diaphragmatic hernia. Analysis of fifty-six cases in dogs and cats. J. Small Anim. Pract. *21*:469, 1980.

40. Gaskell, C. J., Gibbs, C., and Pearson, H.: Sliding hiatus hernia with reflux oesophagitis in two dogs. J. Small Anim. Pract. *15*:503, 1974.

41. Grandage, J.: The radiology of the dog's diaphragm. J. Small Anim. Pract. *15*:1, 1974.

42. Hayes, H. M.: Congenital umbilical and inguinal hernias in cattle, horses, swine, dogs and cats: risk by breed and sex among hospital patients. Am. J. Vet. Res. *35*:839, 1974.

43. Hobson, H. P., and Knauer, C. W.: Congenital pericardial diaphragmatic hernia; the surgical correction of a clinical case. Southwest. Vet. *27*:25, 1974.

44. Kagan, K. G.: Thoracic trauma. Vet. Clin. North Am. *10*:641, 1980.

45. Keep, J. M.: Congenital diaphragmatic hernia in a cat. Aust. Vet. J. *26*:193, 1950.

46. Kent, G. C.: Feline diaphragmatic hernia. J. Am. Vet. Med. Assoc. *116*:348, 1950.

47. Kinasewitz, G. T., Groome, L. J., Marshall, R. J., and Diana, J. N.: Permeability of the canine visceral pleura. J. Appl. Physiol. *55*:121, 1983.

48. Koper, S., Mucha, M., Silmanowicz, P., et al.: Selective abdominal angiography as a diagnostic method for diaphragmatic hernia in the dog: an experimental study. Vet. Radiol. *23*:50, 1982.

49. Krahwinkel, D. J.: Lower respiratory tract trauma. *In* Kirk, R. W. (ed.): *Current Veterinary Therapy VI.* W. B. Saunders, Philadelphia, 1977.

50. Leighton, R. L.: Peritoneopericardial hernia in a dog. Vet. Med. Small Anim. Clin. *l72*:1843, 1977.

51. McCarthy, L. E., Bonson, I. L., Spiegel, P. K., and Friedlander, R. M.: Vomiting: radiographic and oscillographic correlates in the decerebrate cat. Gastroenterology *67*:1126, 1974.

52. McClellan, J. E., Olson, R. E., and McClelland, J. E.: What is your diagnosis? J. Am. Vet. Med. Assoc. *170*:549, 1977.

53. McCrory, W. W., and Bunch, R. F.: Omphalocele with diaphragmatic defect and herniation of the heart into the pericardial cavity. J. Pediatrics *31*:45, 1947.

54. Magy, A. Z., and Schecter, R.: What is your diagnosis? J. Am. Vet. Med. Assoc. *171*:1115, 1977.

55. Meinche, J. E., Hobbie, W. V., and Barto, L. R.: Traumatic chylothorax with associated diaphragmatic hernias in the cat. J. Am. Vet. Med. Assoc. *155*:15, 1969.

56. Miller, R. A., Heagan, B. S., and Taylor, C. B.: The oxygen content of arterial blood in dogs breathing air at low barometric pressure. Am. J. Physiol. *150*:1, 1947.

57. Misercocchi, G., Negrini, D., Mariane, E., and Passafro, M.: Reabsorption of of a saline or plasma-induced hydrothorax. J. Appl. Physiol. *54*:157, 1983.

58. Morgan, R. V.: Respiratory emergencies. Part II. Comp. Cont. Ed. *5*:305, 1983.

59. Murray, J. F.: *The Normal Lung.* W. B. Saunders, Philadelphia, 1972.

60. Osborne, C. A., and Perman, V.: Pleural effusion. *In* Kirk, R. W. (ed.): *Current Veterinary Therapy V.* W. B. Saunders, Philadelphia, 1974.

61. Payne, W. S., and Ellis, F. H.: Esophagous and diaphragmatic hernias. *In* Swartz, S. I. (ed.): *Principles of Surgery.* 2nd ed., Vol. 2. McGraw-Hill, New York, 1974.

62. Pearson, H.: The differential diagnosis of persistent vomiting in the young dog. J. Small. Anim. Pract. *11*:403, 1970.

63. Reed, J. H., and Pennock, P. W.: Concurrent ventral and pericardial diaphragmatic hernias in 2 dogs. Mod. Vet. Pract. *52*:47, 1971.

64. Rendano, V. T.: Positive contrast peritoneography: an aid in the radiographic diagnosis of diaphragmatic hernia. J. Am. Vet. Radiol. Soc. *20*:67, 1979.

65. Rogers, W. A., and Donovan, E. F.: Peptic esophagitis in a dog. J. Am. Vet. Med. Assoc. *163*:462, 1973.

66. Roudebush, P., and Burns, J.: Pleural effusion a sequela to traumatic diaphragmatic hernias: a review of four cases. J. Am. Anim. Hosp. Assoc. *15*:699, 1979.

67. Rowland, M. G. and Robinson, M.: Gastro-oesophageal intussusception in an adult dog. J. Small Anim. Pract. *19*:121, 1978.

68. Sant'Ambrogio, G., Frazier, D. T., Wilson, M. F., and Agostoni, E.: Motor innervation and pattern of activity of cat diaphragm. J. Appl. Physiol. *18*:43, 1963

69. Staub, N. C.: Alveolar flooding and clearance. Am. Rev. Respir. Dis. *127*:544, 1983.

70. Staub, N. C., Nagano, H., and Pearce, M. L.: Pulmonary edema in dogs, especially the sequence of fluid accumulation in the lungs. J. Appl. Physiol. *22*:227, 1967.

71. Szabo, G., Jakab, R., and Sugar, I.: The effect of occlusion of liver lymphatics on hepatic blood flow. Res. Exp. Med. (Berlin) *169*:1, 1976.

72. Teague, H. D., Cook, M., Brunell, W. K., and Erikson, J.: Surgical repair of a diaphragmatic hernia in a dog. Canine Pract. *5*:63, 1978.

73. Ticer, J. W. and Brown, S. G.: Thoracic trauma. *In* Ettinger, S. J. (ed.): *Textbook of Veterinary Internal Medicine.* Vol 1. W. B. Saunders, Philadelphia, 1975.

74. Touloukian, R. J.: A "new" diaphragm following prosthetic repair of experimental hemidiaphragmatic defects in the pup. Ann. Surg. *187*:47, 1978.

75. Tucker, E. W.: What is your diagnosis? J. Am. Vet. Med. Assoc. *151*:1101, 1967.

76. Walker, R. G., and Hall, L. W.: Rupture of the diaphragm: report of 32 cases in dogs and cats. Vet. Rec. 77:830, 1965.

77. Weitz, J., Tilley, L. P., and Moldoff, D.: Pericardiodiaphragmatic hernia in a dog. J. Am. Vet. Med. Assoc. *173*:1336, 1978.

78. Wilson, G. P., Newton, C. D., and Burt, J. K.: A review of 116 diaphragmatic hernias in dogs and cats. J. Am. Vet. Med. Assoc. *159*:1142, 1971.

79. Wilson, G. P.: Unpublished data (1984).

60 Perineal Hernia

Chapter

Rhondda B. Canfield
and Christopher R. Bellenger

Perineal hernia results from failure of the pelvic diaphragm to support the rectal wall. Stretching and deviation occur in the course of the rectum. In advanced cases, pelvic and occasionally abdominal contents protrude between the pelvic diaphragm and the rectum. A subcutaneous swelling occurs ventrolateral to the anus, and in bilateral cases, caudal projection of the anus is also seen.

SURGICAL ANATOMY

The perineum is the part of the body wall that covers the caudal pelvic aperture and surrounds the anal and urogenital canals.[42] The skeletal boundaries of the caudal pelvic aperture, or pelvic outlet, are the first caudal vertebra dorsally and the right and left ischiatic tuberosities and ischiatic arch ventrally. The lateral borders are formed by the sacrotuberous ligament, which extends from the lateral angle of the ischiatic tuberosity to the transverse process of the first caudal vertebra, and the caudal end of the sacrum.[25] Unlike that in other domestic mammals, this aperture in carnivores is similar in size or larger than the cranial pelvic aperture or inlet.[61]

The principal structure of the perineum is the pelvic diaphragm. It consists of the coccygeus and levator ani muscles, together with their external and internal fascial coverings.[42] These muscles are anchored to the pelvis and caudal vertebrae.

The perineal fascia consists of superficial and deep layers. The superficial layer is continuous with the fascia of the tail, rump, and thigh regions and converges toward the anus. The deep layer covers the dorsal surface of the internal obturator muscle, attaches to the ischiatic tuberosities and adjacent sacrotuberous ligament, and extends cranially between the rectum and the urogenital canal. In the median plane, fibers of the deep perineal fascia "directly unite the complex musculature between the anal canal and the vagina or the bulb of the penis," forming a fibromuscular node called the perineal body.[25]

A topographical feature of the area is the ischiorectal fossa. The walls of this wedge-shaped depression are formed by the external anal sphincter, the coccygeus and levator ani muscles medially, the internal obturator muscle ventrally, and the caudal part of the superficial gluteal muscle laterally. A varying amount of fatty tissue, which is incorporated in the superficial perineal fascia, occupies this space.

The perineal region is the surface area bounded by the base of the tail dorsally and the skin covering the caudal border of the superficial gluteal muscle and the lateral angle of the ischiatic tuberosity bilaterally. The ventral boundary is formed by the caudodorsal aspect of the scrotum in the male and the dorsal margin of the vulval lips in the female.

Structures of Surgical Importance for Herniorrhaphy (Figs. 60–1 through 60–3)

Coccygeus Muscle

Origin. Medial aspect of the ischiatic spine.

Insertion. Transverse processes of the second to the fourth or fifth caudal vertebra.

Vascular Supply. Branches derived from the caudal gluteal artery penetrate the dorsolateral and ventrolateral surfaces. The medial circumflex femoral artery supplies a branch that ascends through the obturator foramen.

Innervation. Fibers that leave the ventral branch of the second and/or third sacral nerve pass caudally between the ventrolateral sacrocaudalis and pirifor-

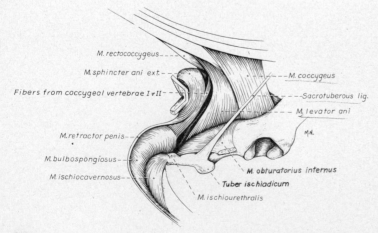

Figure 60–1. Superficial perineal muscles of the male dog (lateral view). (Reprinted and modified with permission from Evans, H. E., and Christensen, G. C.: *Miller's Anatomy of the Dog*, 2nd ed. W. B. Saunders, Philadelphia, 1979.)

M. rectococcygeus

M. sphincter ani ext.

Fibers from coccygeal vertebrae I v II

M. retractor penis

M. bulbospongiosus

M. ischiocavernosus

M. coccygeus

Sacrotuberous lig.

M. levator ani

M.N.

M. obturatorius internus

Tuber ischiadicum

M. ischiourethralis

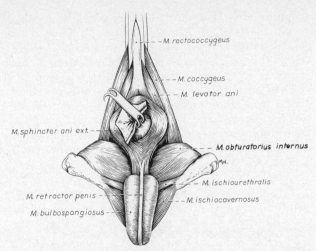

Figure 60–2. Superficial perineal muscles of the male dog (caudal view). (Reprinted and modified with permission from Evans, H. E., and Christensen, G. C.: *Miller's Anatomy of the Dog*, 2nd ed. W. B. Saunders, Philadelphia, 1979.)

mis muscles and penetrate the middle of the medial surface of the coccygeus muscle.

Relationships. The medial surface is related to the levator ani muscle and the lateral surface to the superficial gluteal muscle cranially and the fat of the ischiorectal fossa caudally.

Action. Bilateral: to draw the proximal part of the tail against the anus. Unilateral: lateral flexion of the tail.[25]

M. Levator Ani

The levator ani muscle is divided into two parts, the iliocaudal muscle cranially and the pubocaudal muscle caudally. This division may be visible throughout the course of the muscle.

Origin. Iliocaudalis muscle: medial surface of the body of the ilium. Pubocaudalis muscle: dorsal surface of the pubis cranial to the obturator foramen and the pelvic symphysis.

Insertion. Iliocaudalis muscle: the fibers converge caudodorsally to a long thin tendon that passes caudally, flattening out over the ventral surface of the tail muscles. The tendon inserts onto the hemal arches, which articulate with the cranial ends of the fifth and sixth caudal vertebrae. It may extend as far as the seventh caudal vertebra. In those breeds in which the tail has been docked, the tendon disappears into the fascia covering the tail stump.[15] Pubocaudalis muscle: the fibers pass dorsally, with the majority having a strong fascial attachment to the ventral surface of approximately the fourth caudal vertebra. Some fibers may insert on the tendon of the iliocaudal muscle.

Vascular Supply. Vessels from a branch of the medial circumflex femoral artery penetrate the lateral surface of the muscle. A small branch from the deep femoral artery also passes into this muscle.

Innervation. A nerve derived from fibers of the third and occasionally second sacral nerve penetrates the dorsal border of the iliocaudalis muscle. Another nerve, of similar origin, traverses the medial surface of the iliocaudalis muscle and supplies the pubocaudalis muscle.

Relationships. The medial surface of the iliocaudalis muscle is related to a varying amount of retroperitoneal fat, which may separate the dorsal part of the muscle from the peritoneum that lines the lateral wall of the pararectal fossa. This fossa, divided dorsally from that of the other side by the mesorectum, is formed when the peritoneum lining the dorsolateral wall of the pelvic cavity reflects onto the wall of the rectum. Ventrally the muscle is separated from the prostate gland by retroperitoneal fat. The medial surface of the pubocaudalis muscle has a firm fascial attachment to the lateral rectal wall. The dorsal border of the iliocaudal muscle converges toward the ventral border of the ventrolateral sacrocaudalis muscle, and the caudal border of the pubocaudalis muscle is firmly bound to the external anal sphincter by fascia. At the level of the ventral wall of the rectum, a few muscle fibers from the caudomedial part of the pubocaudalis muscle radiate into the perineal body and the deep part of the external anal sphincter.[15, 62]

Action. As for the coccygeus muscle.[25] This muscle also compresses the lateral rectal wall during defecation. Distension receptors for this reflex may be

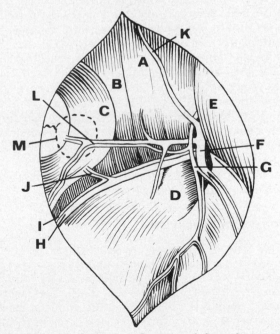

Figure 60–3. Blood vessels and nerves of the male perineum (caudolateral view, right-hand side). *A,* Coccygeus muscle; *B,* levator ani muscle; *C,* external anal sphincter; *D,* internal obturator muscle; *E,* superficial gluteal muscle; *F,* caudal gluteal artery; *G,* caudal cutaneous femoral nerve; *H,* internal pudendal artery; *I,* pudendal nerve; *J,* caudal rectal artery and nerve; *K,* lateral caudal artery; *L,* dorsal perineal artery and perineal nerve; *M,* position of the anal sac. (Redrawn and modified from Greiner, T. P., Johnson, R. G., and Betts, C. W.: Diseases of the rectum and anus. *In* Ettinger, S. J. (ed.): *Textbook of Veterinary Internal Medicine,* 2nd ed. W. B. Saunders, Philadelphia, 1983.)

present in the muscular layer of the rectal wall or in the levator ani muscle.[12]

M. Internal Obturator

Origin. Ischiatic table and the cranial and medial borders of the obturator foramen.

Insertion. The fibers converge laterally and pass over the lesser ischiatic notch to a strong, flat tendon embedded in the gemelli muscles. This tendon inserts in the trochanteric fossa.

Vascular Supply. The medial circumflex femoral artery sends branches that penetrate the ventral surface of the muscle covering the obturator foramen. Branches of the caudal gluteal artery provide a collateral supply.

Innervation. As the ischiatic nerve passes over the greater ischiatic notch it sends a branch caudally toward that part of the muscle covering the lesser ischiatic notch. This nerve divides and penetrates the dorsal surface of the muscle adjacent to the sacrotuberous ligament.

Action. In conjunction with other muscles, outward rotation of the femur.[25]

Superficial Gluteal Muscle

Origin. The gluteal fascia cranially, the lateral part of the sacrum, the first caudal vertebra, and the cranial half of the sacrotuberous ligament.

Insertion. A broad, flat tendon passes over the lateral surface of the greater trochanter to insert on the third trochanter.

Vascular Supply. Branches of the caudal gluteal artery, which passes ventral and parallel to the sacrotuberous ligament, penetrate the dorsomedial surface of the muscle.

Innervation. The caudal gluteal nerve, which may arise from either the ischiatic nerve or the first and second sacral nerves,[25] penetrates the medial surface of the dorsocaudal part of the muscle.

Action. In combination with other gluteal muscles, extension of the hip joint.[25]

External Anal Sphincter

This striated, voluntary muscle, which surrounds the anal canal, may be divided into three parts. The cutaneous part lies directly underneath the skin in the subcutaneous tissue; the superficial fibers, which directly or indirectly attach to the third or fourth caudal vertebra, pass over the lateral surface of the anal canal and anal sacs, and attach to the bulbospongiosus muscle (male) or constrictor vulvae muscle (female); the deep fibers surround the anal canal, passing medial to the anal sacs. Superficial fibers may cross ventral to the anus or interchange with deep fibers.

Innervations. Via a branch of the caudal gluteal artery.

Innervation. The sole nerve supply is the caudal rectal nerve, which leaves the pudendal nerve at the caudal border of the levator ani muscle and penetrates the caudolateral part of the external anal sphincter in the ventral ischiorectal fossa region.[25]

Relationships. The rectococcygeus muscle, which arises from the longitudinal muscle layer of the rectum, passes caudally through an arch formed by the external anal sphincter dorsal to the anal canal. It inserts on the ventral surface of the fourth or fifth caudal vertebra, anchoring the rectum to the axial skeleton.[25]

The small retractor penis muscle arises on the sacrum or first two caudal vertebrae and passes caudoventrally medial to the levator ani muscle. Some fibers (pars rectalis) insert on the rectum, others (pars analis) end between the fibers of the external anal sphincter near the anal sac duct, and the remainder course distally in the median plane, inserting ventrally on the penis. The deep surface of the external anal sphincter is related to the internal anal sphincter, which is composed of circular muscle fibers of the anal canal.

Pudendal Nerve

The pudendal nerve and internal pudendal artery and vein pass into the ischiorectal fossa on the ventrolateral surface of the coccygeus muscle. They are bound together by connective tissue and continue caudomedially across the dorsal surface of the internal obturator muscle. A short branch, the caudal rectal nerve, leaves the pudendal nerve to supply the external anal sphincter. Other branches, the perineal nerves, supply the skin of the anal and scrotal (labial) regions and the mucous membrane of the anus. The terminal branch of the pudendal nerve is the sensory, dorsal nerve of the penis. Entering the ischiorectal fossa adjacent to the pudendal nerve is the caudal cutaneous femoral nerve, which branches and passes through the fat in the fossa, accompanied by branches of the caudal gluteal artery. The pudendal nerve and accompanying vessels are generally related to the ventral part of the perineal hernial sac.

Anatomical Variation

The levator ani muscle in the bitch is more powerful, being broader as well as thicker, and more adherent to the rectal wall over a longer distance, than the same muscle in the male dog.[58] In a study of 39 mixed breed dogs, the ratios of the weight of the levator ani muscle to body weight and the length of the levator ani muscle to pelvic and vertebral column lengths were significantly greater in the female than the male.[19] The results were similar when the ratios of the sacrotuberous ligament weight to body weight were compared. It has been stated that "the pelvic diaphragm is more powerful in the female to bear the load of parturition" and that "this offers a plausible explanation of the fact that perineal hernia is almost never seen in females."[19]

Preliminary analysis of data recorded from the dissection of 24 normal dogs in another anatomical study[15] indicates that the problem is more complex than is suggested by previous authors.[19, 58] Within each of three breeds studied (boxer, corgi, and greyhound) there were no significant differences between male and female dogs when the percentage of the weight of the levator ani and coccygeus muscles (individually and combined) was compared with either the body weight or the total dissected thigh muscle weight. However, significant anatomical differences exist between the breeds considered in this study. Those breeds susceptible to perineal herniation (boxer and corgi) had significantly, relatively heavier combined levator ani and coccygeus muscles than the nonsusceptible breed (greyhound) when comparisons were made on a percentage basis with both body weight and total dissected thigh muscle weight.

ETIOLOGY

Predisposition

The following data and discussion are confined to the dog unless otherwise specified.

Species

Perineal hernia has been documented in the human and the dog and rarely in the cat,[3, 43, 50] cow, and ewe.[22]

Human. Perineal hernia is the rarest hernia except sciatic hernia, with most cases occurring between the ages of 40 and 60 years.[47] Herniation anterior to the superficial transverse muscle of the perineum appears to be confined to women[16, 47] and results in a swelling in the major labium of the vulva.[75] Herniation posterior to the superficial transverse muscle of the perineum occurs in both men and women[47, 60] and results in a swelling in the buttock between the rectum and ischiatic tuberosity.[56] Both types of perineal hernia occur either between the fibers of the levator ani muscle or between this muscle and the

coccygeus muscle.[16, 47, 80, 90] Rectal sacculation or dilation is not generally seen, possibly because in the human, the levator ani muscle not only inserts on the coccyx and perineal body but also has fibers (puborectal muscle) that blend with the longitudinal muscle layer of the rectum.[53, 85] In contrast, in the dog and cat, there is no rectal insertion. Conditions that increase intra-abdominal pressure and, in some cases, a congenital predisposition are regarded as important factors in the etiology of perineal hernia.[47, 56]

Dog. The prevalence of perineal hernia in the dog is low. In the United States a review of 800,000 medical extracts found 771 cases (0.1 per cent incidence),[37] whereas in Australia the prevalence was 0.4 per cent.[5]

Cat. Perineal hernia is rare in the cat. Five cases have been documented.[3, 43, 50]

Age

Perineal hernia is most common in dogs from seven to nine years of age.[37] When cases were grouped according to breed, a variation was found: The estimated relative risk of herniation was greatest between 7 and 9 years of age in Boston terriers, boxers, and Pekingese and between 10 and 14 years in collies and mongrels.

Sex

Perineal hernia occurs commonly in the male and rarely in the female.[37, 68, 71]

Breed

Reports on perineal hernia cases taken from veterinary hospital records have shown an over-representation of certain breeds, including the Boston terrier,[13, 37] boxer,[5, 13, 37] collie,[13, 37, 88] corgi,[5, 13, 88] kelpie and kelpie crosses,[5] and Pekingese.[37, 88] Both sexes of the Pekingese are also predisposed to herniation at other sites.[36]

Right versus Left Side

It may be anticipated that unilateral herniation would occur with equal frequency on either side of

TABLE 60–1. Incidence of Unilateral and Bilateral Perineal Hernia

Reference	No.	Unilateral Right	Left	Bilateral No.
Bellenger[5]	24	13	11	11
Burrows and Harvey[13]	43	36	7	28
Harvey[34]	13	11	2	1
Holmes[39]	5	4	1	0
Martin[54]	12	4	8	3
Pettit[69]	20	16	4	19
Weaver and Omamegbe[88]	65	35	30	36
Totals	182	119 (65%)	63 (35%)	98

the anus, although this is not the case in most reports (Table 60–1).

On the basis of published figures, there is a clear predisposition for the right side, although authors have been unable to explain this occurrence. In 32 clinically normal dogs of various breeds, it was found that the weight of the levator ani and coccygeus muscles varied between the right and left sides randomly and within ± 17 per cent.[15]

Although herniation occurs unilaterally, the contralateral side is frequently weak.[13, 21] The decision to classify a case as either unilateral or bilateral is subjective and depends on the criteria used. The side on which herniation occurs may be related to the rate and extent of tissue deterioration on that side of the pelvic diaphragm rather than to causes affecting one side or the other preferentially.

Pathogenesis

Events preceding the appearance of a perineal swelling, which is indicative of herniation, have not been determined. Perineal herniation commonly occurs between the external anal sphincter and the levator ani muscle and occasionally between the levator ani and coccygeus muscles. In the only reported canine case of sciatic hernia, herniation occurred between the coccygeus muscle and the sacrotuberous ligament.[23]

Herniation depends on the deterioration of the supporting function of the pelvic diaphragm.[20, 29, 37, 51, 54] Whereas one author[58] stated that there was a partial or total rupture of the levator ani muscle, others[7, 49] referred to a fascial weakening followed by the separation of the external anal sphincter from the pelvic diaphragm muscles. Masses of pelvic fat may push between these muscles "along the classic route of perineal hernia," and the natural fissures in the levator ani muscle for the passage of the obturator nerve and between the iliocaudal and pubocaudal muscles can be widened.[2] Deterioration of the levator ani muscle results in the reduction of rectal wall support. In hernias involving retroperitoneal fat and rectal sacculation, frequently only the cranial remnants of the levator ani muscle can be found lying medial to the coccygeus muscle. In larger hernias it may be absent, and the coccygeus and internal obturator muscles may be reduced in size.

The cause of this muscular deterioration could be one or a combination of the following pathological processes.

Atrophy. This is a progressive shrinkage of muscle fibers resulting predominantly in a reduction in fiber diameter.[59]

Neurogenic atrophy is the result of partial or total interruption of the nerve supply to a muscle. Affected muscle fibers are reduced in size yet retain normal structure. "It is not until late in these diseases that structural changes in the atrophied fibers and interstitial tissue occur."[70] Biopsy specimens of the levator

ani muscle taken during herniorrhaphy have shown atrophy of groups of muscle fibers indicative of neurogenic atrophy. The inconsistent changes found may have been "the result of stretching of the motor nerves due to straining at defecation."[34] The relationship between herniation and abdominal straining has not been determined. Tenesmus may precede[21, 76] or may occur subsequent to perineal swelling.[14, 86] In some cases tenesmus may not be a significant part of the clinical picture,[34] or it may be present over a long interval without herniation.[14] More information correlating histopathological changes and clinical signs is required to determine the importance of neurogenic atrophy in the etiology of perineal herniation.

Senile atrophy is a general morphological expression of aging.[59] Decrease of the levator ani muscle tone would result in a weakening of rectal wall support. This may be a minor contributing cause of herniation.

Because the levator ani and coccygeus muscles function in tail movement, their relative size and strength may be reduced (*disuse atrophy*) in short-tailed dogs.[20] This could be a contributing factor for the predisposition of the Boston terrier, boxer, and corgi breeds.

Myopathies. These are primary degenerative conditions that are noninflammatory and nondystrophic and are not caused by denervation. The microscopic appearance of the tissue is nonspecific. In the majority of cases, scattered degenerative changes of the muscle fibers are present.[70] Conditions secondary to or at least associated with endocrine disorders are included. Male predisposition to perineal herniation may suggest that sex hormones are involved in the maintenance of muscle strength or tone of the pelvic diaphragm.[37]

Estrogen secretion by the aging testis,[73] testicular and prostatic tumors, and clinical signs of endocrine imbalance[20] may be associated with perineal hernia. In biopsy specimens of testes in some hernial cases, no lesions were found that could be related to the condition; however, it was stressed that histological appearance is not indicative of endocrine activity.[69] Nevertheless, perineal hernias have been found concomitant with testicular neoplasms in other dogs, the proportion varying with the tumor type. Herniation was present in one of 46 cases (2 per cent) of Sertoli cell tumor, 10 of 67 cases (15 per cent) of interstitial cell tumor, nine of 47 cases (19 per cent) of seminoma, and four of 38 cases (11 per cent) of mixed-type tumors.[52] Clinical changes associated with interstitial cell tumors and seminomas were similar in frequency.[52] Sertoli cell tumors were associated with feminization owing to their estrogen secretion[44] and with the lowest level of herniation. Therefore, if perineal hernias are associated with a hormonal imbalance, either absolute or relative androgen, rather than estrogen, levels appear to be involved.

The effect of androgen levels on the pelvic diaphragm has not been established. In the rat, there is a decrease in the weight of the combined bulbocavernous, ischiocavernous, and levator ani muscles, penis, and bulb following castration.[84] Testosterone and 5α-dihydrotestosterone are bound to receptor protein in the "bulbocavernous/levator ani" muscle.[45] However, it has been suggested that this muscle is part of the male reproductive system and not homologous to the levator ani muscle in man, dog, and cat.[38] In a preliminary study of the effect of testosterone on the status of the levator ani muscle in six male dogs there was no correlation between testosterone levels, muscle fiber size, and fiber type 1 and 2 distribution.[19]

Prostatic Involvement

Hypotheses linking perineal hernia to prostatic hypertrophy are inevitable, as both occur predominantly in middle-aged to old male dogs. A direct causal relationship is not favored, but most authors consider prostatic enlargement to be a contributing factor.

Benign hyperplasia is the most common prostatic condition in the dog. Although the majority of dogs with benign hyperplasia have no initial signs, this, together with other pathological conditions resulting in prostatic enlargement, generally results in tenesmus associated with defecation or urination.[14, 30, 40, 87]

Prostatitis, which may occur in association with hyperplasia,[44] can be acute or chronic. Although the gland is not palpably enlarged, the animal may experience tenesmus related to defecation. In chronic cases, the gland can become fibrous, shrinking in size and obstructing the urethra.[8]

When abdominal pressure is increased in association with voiding, the freely movable prostate can be forced into the pelvic region, creating tension on the weakened pelvic tissues.[28, 72, 76] The result may be a gradual breakdown of the pelvic diaphragm with a passage produced between the pelvic cavity and perineal subcutaneous tissue, allowing herniation.

The relationship between the prostate gland and perineal hernia may not be fully understood until there is adequate documentation of the size and histopathological status of the gland in hernia cases. Radiographic measurement[78] and biopsy are both required in preference to subjective assessment by rectal and abdominal palpation.

Perineal Hernia in the Cat

Five cases of perineal hernia in the cat have been documented.[3, 43, 50] Two were castrated males aged six and ten years; two were spayed, aging females; and one was an entire 15-month-old male. Bilateral herniation was diagnosed in all cats, with the right side being more extensively involved in two.[3, 50] Two cats had no clinical signs prior to the perineal swelling. Two males had undergone a perineal urethrostomy one to two months before developing intermittent constipation; perineal herniation was diagnosed

one and five years postoperatively. One female had a three-year history of intermittent constipation prior to presentation with a tail base abscess; one month later a bilateral perineal swelling was observed. All cases involved rectal wall dilation, and in one, fatty vascular tissue was present in the hernia.[50]

The etiology of the herniation was apparent only in the perineal urethrostomy cases, in which surgical separation of the pelvic urethra from the surrounding tissue resulted in chronic obstipation/constipation secondary to perineal hernia.[43] At surgery, it was found that there had been a separation of the external anal sphincter and the levator ani muscle; in one case the levator ani muscle was indistinct and fibrous. In two of the remaining cases there was no apparent cause, and in the other, the role that the abscess played in the development of the hernia was debatable. From these cases, it cannot be determined whether atrophy of the levator ani muscle or merely separation of connective tissue between the external anal sphincter and the levator ani muscle results in the loss of rectal wall support in the cat. The anatomy of the pelvic diaphragm is similar in the dog and cat with one exception: The cat has no sacrotuberous ligament.[55]

CLINICAL SIGNS

The majority of animals are presented with a reducible perineal swelling and one or more of the following signs: constipation (difficult defecation or defecation at prolonged intervals), obstipation (intractable constipation), tenesmus (straining to defecate or urinate without evacuation of feces or urine),

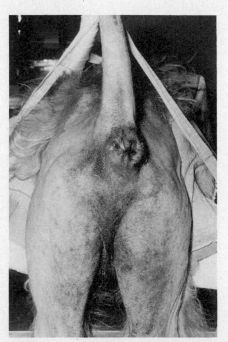

Figure 60–4. Afghan with left sided perineal hernia, positioned on the operating table. Note the swelling ventrolateral to the anus on the left.

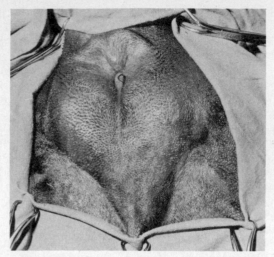

Figure 60–5. German short-haired pointer with bilateral perineal hernia. Note the more ventral swelling and caudal projection of the anus. A purse-string suture has been placed in the anus.

and dyschezia (painful defecation).[67] The swelling is usually ventrolateral to the anus (Fig. 60–4), although in some bilateral cases ventral swelling with caudal projection of the anus becomes evident (Fig. 60–5). This swelling may not be obvious in all cases.[13] In one survey[13] diarrhea occurred, at least occasionally, in over 50 per cent of cases. Stranguria (painful urination, with urine being voided drop by drop)[67] may occur in association with prostatic disease or retroflexion of the bladder and prostate (Fig. 60–6). Other symptoms occurring occasionally are ulceration of the skin overlying the swelling, fecal incontinence,[13] and altered tail carriage.[5]

The contents of the hernia most commonly include rectal sacculation, prostate gland, fluid, connective tissue, and retroperitoneal fat. The last two may

resemble omentum and may contain small, firm nodules and areas of necrosis. Some authors have used the terms rectal sacculation, dilation, flexure, deviation, and diverticulation synonymously. *Rectal sacculation* occurs when unilateral loss of support for the rectal wall enables it to expand to one side; *dilation* of the rectal lumen results from a bilateral loss of wall support; and rectal *flexure* or *deviation* occurs when the rectum herniates, resulting in a bend in the course of the rectum. Some consider rectal flexure to be a separate entity from perineal hernia and a diagnosis of rectal sacculation and diverticulum to be erroneus; in one survey, approximately 50 per cent of swellings examined radiographically were due to rectal flexure.[77] An acquired *diverticulum,* defined as representing a herniation of the mucous membrane through the muscular wall of an organ,[67] may not be considered synonymous with sacculation. A rectal diverticulum may exist alone or with perineal herniation;[51] it is generally related to trauma and may be difficult to palpate.[31]

Occasionally, fatty tissue and fluid alone form the hernial contents.[13] Bladder, jejunum, prostatic cyst,[5] or colon[57, 79] may be present in the sac. The bladder is often present in perineal hernia in the bitch, and the consequent swelling tends to be ventral.

External hernias generally consist of a sac formed as a pouch of parietal peritoneum; however, only a few authors refer to this mesothelial membrane in perineal hernia.[7, 39, 58, 65, 77, 88] One view was that peritoneal involvement in herniation varied with the location of the levator ani muscle rupture; either the membrane ruptured with the muscle,[7, 58] or, in areas involving retroperitoneal fat and rectal ectasia (dilation), it was not affected.[58] Others considered a peritoneal sac to be associated only with a hernia and not with a rectal flexure.[77] Cytological examinations of hernial sacs indicate that mesothelial cells are present in sheet form. Whether this mesothelium is associated with an outpocketing of peritoneum or mesothelial proliferation subsequent to membrane rupture has not been established.

CONSERVATIVE THERAPY

Medical and Dietary Treatment

This form of treatment may be indicated as an adjunct to surgical procedures or when straining to defecate is infrequent. Information on the success of medication and dietary management as the only form of treatment is scanty. Seven of ten dogs treated with stool softeners and fecal removal when required subsequently underwent surgery or were euthanized.[34] Only in the two cases in which straining had not been part of the presenting clinical picture were the dogs functioning normally approximately 15 months after the initial examination.

The following diet and medication regimens should be adjusted to obtain soft feces and regular defecation.

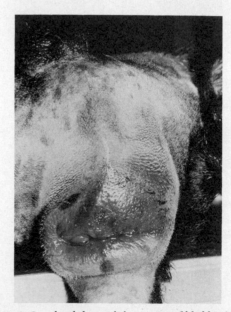

Figure 60–6. Crossbred dog with herniation of bladder and retroperitoneal adipose tissue. The anus and perineum are swollen and inflamed.

Diet. A diet high in fiber (bran) and moisture content should be given.

Bulk-Forming Laxatives. These include methylcellulose (a semisynthetic cellulose derivative) and psyllium preparations (e.g., psyllium mucilloid powder). Via their hydrophilic or osmotic properties, they retain water and electrolytes in the intestinal lumen and soften and increase fecal bulk. The latent period before effect is one to three days.[27, 81]

Docusates. These may be distinguished from the previous group by their action on the intestines, reducing net absorption of electrolytes and increasing the permeability of the mucosa.[27] Dioctyl sodium sulfosuccinate and dioctyl calcium sulfosuccinate are commercially available. They are used to keep feces soft and to avoid straining. The latent period before effect is one to three days. They may be used routinely, together with the diet previously described. Dioctyl sodium sulfosuccinate in solution is also avilable as an enema.

Hormone Therapy. Castration is the treatment of choice for prostatic hyperplasia. Clinical signs may be alleviated initially by low-dosage estrogen therapy;[8, 87] however, squamous metaplasia with a further increase in gland size and bone marrow depression with neutropenia, nonregenerative anemia and thrombocytopenia can result from excessive estrogen levels.[6] Prior to treatment plain radiographs and a pneumocystograph should be taken, and a sterile urine and prostatic wash sample submittted for cytology and culture. If bacterial growth is present, the appropriate antibiotics are administered.

Chlormadinone acetate, a progestin with antiandrogenic activity, has reduced prostatic size in cases of hyperplasia.[10, 74] In contrast to the toxic side effects associated with estrogen therapy, chlormadinone acetate was well-tolerated, even after long-term administration.[10] Another highly potent antiandrogen, cyproterone acetate, was successful experimentally in reducing enlarged prostate glands in dogs.[9]

Supportive Apparatus

There have been two reports of the use of external devices to support the perineum.[82, 83]

SURGICAL THERAPY

Preoperative Procedures

Normal preoperative examinations for geriatric patients are undertaken.[11]

Catheterization. A small percentage of perineal hernia cases are presented with retroflexion of the bladder and partial or total urethral obstruction. Urethral catheterization should be attempted, but if it is unsuccessful, the urine may be aspirated through a hypodermic needle placed aseptically in the perineal swelling. With the bladder evacuated, it may be possible to reduce the hernia manually by pressure

on the perineal region. A catheter may be used to maintain urethral patency. Fluid, electrolyte, and acid-base imbalances are corrected and the patient is stabilized before surgical treatment is attempted.

Enema. A warm water enema to which a stool softener may be added should be given to all constipated animals approximately 18 hours prior to surgery. This interval is required to allow total evacuation of fluid from the large intestine and avoid surgical site contamination.

Radiographs. Radiographs that delineate anatomical structures present at the hernial site provide information that enables the surgeon to anticipate possible problems and determine the best surgical procedure for repair of the defect.[4] The position of the bladder can be demonstrated by positive or negative contrast cystography. Pneumoperitoneography, which involves the introduction of a negative contrast medium such as CO_2 or N_2O into the peritoneal cavity, may be useful in silhouetting the pelvic viscera.[64] This technique is not commonly used.

To illustrate any deviation in the passage of the rectum, a barium meal is preferable to a barium enema.[77] Ideally, the gastrointestinal tract should be empty for this procedure. The contrast medium should be present in the large intestine within three to five hours following administration; however, the transit rate is variable.[64] If the animal is constipated, radiography may be delayed until the following day to allow time for the barium sulfate to mix with the feces in the rectum. Rectal sacculation and flexure are best observed from a dorsoventral projection; displacement due to an enlarged prostate gland is best seen from a lateral projection.

Restrictions. Food should be withheld 24 hours prior to surgery. Intravenous fluid therapy may be required during this period if the animal is dehydrated or has been uremic.

Surgical Procedures

After induction of general anesthesia, intravenous electrolyte infusion is commenced; the flow rate varies with the state of hydration of the animal, cardiovascular parameters, and the extent of hemorrhage during surgery. The surgical area, including the scrotal and prescrotal regions, is clipped (Fig. 60–7). A rectal examination allows assessment of the laxity in rectal wall support (Fig. 60–8) and prostatic size. Feces, if present, are removed, and a pursestring suture is placed around the anus after insertion of a plug of absorbent cotton. The skin is scrubbed with povidone-iodine scrub solution and the animal transferred to the operating theater.

Standard Herniorrhaphy. The patient is positioned in sternal recumbency. The cranial thigh region is cushioned against the table to avoid placing unnecessary pressure on the femoral nerve. The tail is secured cranially over the body, and skin disinfection is completed (see Fig. 60–4). Drapes are placed

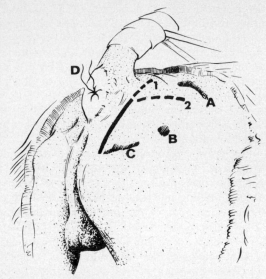

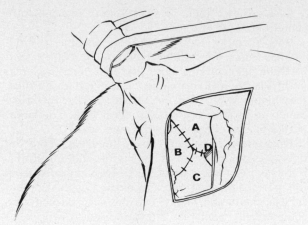

Figure 60–9. Suture placement in standard herniorrhaphy (caudolateral view). *A,* Coccygeus muscle; *B,* external anal sphincter; *C,* internal obturator muscle; *D,* pudendal nerve, internal pudendal artery and vein.

Figure 60–7. Surgical preparation of the perineal area. Incision 1: standard perineal herniorrhaphy. Incision 2: superficial gluteal transposition. *A,* Iliac crest; *B,* greater trochanter of the femur; *C,* ischiatic tuberosity; *D,* purse-string suture in the anus.

around the surgical site and tail (see Fig. 60–5). The exposed skin is covered with a sterile adhesive plastic drape. An incision, curving ventromedially, is made from a point lateral to the tail base to the medial angle of the ischiatic tuberosity (Fig. 60–7). Skin edge drapes are attached. Hemorrhage is controlled by ligation or electrocautery. The hernial sac is opened with blunt dissection, avoiding damage to any organ present. Fat in the hernial sac is usually left but may be ligated and excised. Pelvic and abdominal contents are identified and returned to their original location. A moistened sponge attached to a clamp may be used to keep these organs repelled. The internal pudendal artery and vein, which may be markedly dilated, and the pudendal nerve are located in the ventral region of the sac. Care must be exercised to avoid damaging the pudendal nerve or its branch, the caudal rectal nerve. An intact motor supply to the external anal sphincter is essential for normal defecation.[12]

The external anal sphincter, rectum, and coccygeus and internal obturator muscles are exposed. The levator ani muscle, if identifiable, may be located medial to the coccygeus muscle. The sacrotuberous ligament is palpated. Single interrupted surgical gut or synthetic absorbable sutures (size 1 USP) are inserted but not tied. Approximately four sutures are placed between the coccygeus muscle and the cranial portion of the external anal sphincter. One or two sutures are each placed from the internal obturator muscle to the external anal sphincter and from the internal obturator to the coccygeus muscle. The rectal wall and anal sacs are not incorporated in the closure. The sponge is removed, and progressing in either a dorsal or ventral direction, the sutures are tied, with care being taken to avoid placing pressure on the internal pudendal blood vessels. Unless the hernia is bilateral or muscles other than the levator ani muscle have atrophied, this closure provides adequate reconstruction of the pelvic diaphragm with minimal tension on individual sutures (Fig. 60–9). The subcutaneous tissue is approximated with absorbable sutures and the skin with polypropylene.

In bilateral herniation, both combined[5, 13] and staged procedures with an interval of three to four weeks[88] have been advocated. This decision should depend on individual case assesment. The purse-string suture is removed. Palpation of the internal rectal wall confirms that support has been re-established and that no sutures have penetrated the rectal lumen. The dog is placed in dorsal recumbency and a prescrotal castration performed.

Additional Procedures
Elevation of the Internal Obturator Muscle.[24] In the ventrolateral region of the caudal pelvic outlet there may be considerable tension placed on the sutures apposing the internal obturator muscle to the external anal sphincter or coccygeus muscle. This point is emphasized by the finding that the ventral repair area was more likely to be weaker and permit hernial recurrence than the dorsal and lateral areas.[13]

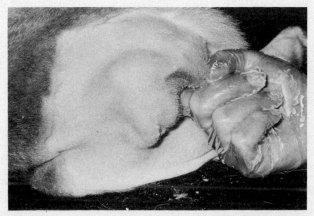

Figure 60–8. Corgi with perineal hernia. The tip of the examining finger is in the rectal sacculation and can be seen elevating the skin over the pararectal fossa.

This problem may be avoided by elevating the internal obturator muscle from the ischium.[24] An incision is made along the ischiatic tuberosity and a periosteal elevator used to raise the muscle and the periosteum as far cranially as the caudal limit of the obturator foramen. Damage to the muscular nerve supply must be avoided. The tendon of insertion may be severed to further free this muscle. Sutures are placed as previously described.

Incorporation of the Sacrotuberous Ligament in Sutures Dorsolateral to the External Anal Sphincter.[7, 13, 69] When the coccygeus muscle, together with the levator ani muscle, appears weakened, the sacrotuberous ligament may be included in the dorsolateral sutures to strengthen the closure of the pelvic diaphragm. The sciatic nerve, which passes cranioventral to the ligament, must be avoided. The caudal gluteal blood vessels, running between the ligament and the sciatic nerve, may be encountered.

Subcutaneous Perineal Fascia Reconstruction. A flap of fascia is dissected from the deep lateral side of the incision and sutured to the external anal sphincter, thus covering the deeper muscular sutures. Although it has been claimed that this procedure alone provided adequate closure of the pelvic defect,[7] the claim is not adequately substantiated by the results of postsurgical follow-up examinations.

Transposition of the Superficial Gluteal Muscle.[77] This procedure may be used (1) routinely, (2) as an alternative to the incorporation of the sacrotuberous ligament in a standard herniorrhaphy when coccygeus muscle is deficient, or (3) to provide additional support over the standard closure.

The skin is prepared farther cranially than was indicated for the previous procedure, and the dog is placed in lateral recumbency. The skin incision extends over the superficial gluteal muscle (see Fig. 60–7). The hernial sac is opened and its contents are reduced. The external anal sphincter, coccygeus and

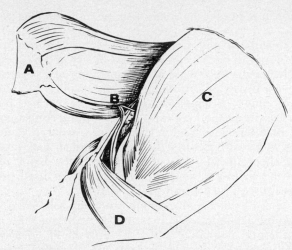

Figure 60–11. Surgical reflection of the superficial gluteal muscle (lateral view, right-hand side.) *A*, Tendon of insertion of the superficial gluteal muscle; *B*, vascular and nervous supply to the superficial gluteal muscle; *C*, middle gluteal muscle; *D*, biceps femoris muscle.

internal obturator muscles, internal pudendal vessels, and pudendal nerve are identified. Fascia overlying the superficial gluteal muscle is reflected (Fig. 60–10). The cranial border of the muscle is located and under-run in a caudoventral direction. The insertion of this muscle on the third trochanter of the femur and a section of the caudal part of the fascia lata tensor muscle are transected. The ventral border of this flap must allow broad apposition with the cranial border of the external anal sphincter. The remainder of the superficial gluteal muscle is under-run until the vascular and nervous supply is located entering the medial surface. This muscular flap is reflected toward the external anal sphincter (Fig. 60–11). To gain apposition without tension, it is frequently necessary to sever the cranial border of the superficial gluteal muscle from the gluteal fascia and occasionally necessary to incise part of the muscular attachment to the sacrum. The flap is now sutured to the external anal sphincter caudally and to the underlying tissue dorsally and ventrally. The subcutaneous tissue is apposed and the wound is closed.

A modification of this procedure is transposition of the superficial gluteal muscle flap through a 45-degree angle. The tendon of insertion is sutured to the ischial fascia and the internal obturator muscle. The caudal border of the muscle is sutured to the external anal sphincter and the cranial border to the sacrotuberous ligament.[88]

Placement of Prosthetic Implants. There are only a few reports of the use of synthetic materials in perineal hernias in the dog. Implants have been placed in position via both perineal[46, 48] and abdominal[17] approaches. Critical assessments of the long-term effectiveness of any of the techniques employed have been minimal. Four of five cases in which polyester mesh was used were successfully treated, with recurrence of herniation in one case after 19 months.[63] Information on the use of

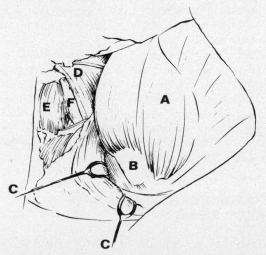

Figure 60–10. Surgical exposure of the superficial gluteal muscle (lateral view, right-hand side). *A*, Superficial gluteal muscle; *B*, greater trochanter of the femur; *C*, retraction of biceps femoris muscle, *D*, coccygeus muscle; *E*, external sphincter ani; *F*, rectal wall (exposed by atrophy of the levator ani muscle).

prostheses in hernia repair may be found in Chapter 56.

Cystopexy and Colopexy. These procedures, together with partial closure of the defect in the caudal pelvic wall, were used in the treatment of a perineal hernia involving retroflexion of the bladder.[26] Cystopexy alone, although temporarily effective, was not successful in the long term in preventing recurrence of bladder herniation.[33] Cystostomy, using a Foley catheter exiting through the abdominal wall, may enhance adhesion formation, the catheter being removed in five to seven days. Colopexy is used primarily with recurring rectal prolapse.

The bladder and rectum are approached via a midline laparotomy and sutured to opposing sides of the lateral abdominal wall. The ventral wall, adjacent to the incision, should be avoided, as another operator at a later date may incise the linea alba and inadvertently the bladder or rectum. Sutures must not penetrate the mucosa of either structure.

Anal Splitting.[35, 89] Although the results have not been entirely satisfactory, this technique has been advocated in hernial cases that have recurred following standard perineal herniorrhaphy.[35] The major complications are fecal incontinence and anal soiling. Development of techniques such as transposition of the superficial gluteal muscle and elevation of the internal obturator muscle make anal splitting an operation of last resort.

A dorsolateral incision is made through the skin, rectal wall, and intervening tissue (which includes the external anal sphincter) from the anal ring to the full depth of the rectal sacculation. The anal sacs and the caudal rectal nerve are avoided. The wound, beginning at its craniolateral extent, is closed by suturing the rectal wall to the skin.

Postoperative Management

Contamination of the healing wound must be avoided. Antibiotics are not used unless there is evidence of infection. An Elizabethan collar prevents the patient from irritating the wound or removing the sutures. Conditions leading to abdominal straining should be avoided. Diet regulation and medication, as discussed previously, assist in achieving this aim. Skin sutures may be removed ten to 14 days postoperatively.

Surgical Complications

Wound Infection. The incidence of infection or wound breakdown following standard herniorrhaphy has been recorded as 13,[88] 20,[5] and 26 per cent.[13] Following superficial gluteal muscle transposition, 58 per cent experienced wound breakdown, which was primarily superficial.[88] *E. coli* was the most commonly isolated organism in one study, with *Proteus, Staph-*

ylococcus, Klebsiella, and *Bacteroides* species occurring occasionally.[5] Routine use of antibiotics has little effect on the postoperative development of infection.

Fecal Incontinence. Fecal incontinence following standard perineal herniorrhaphy has been recorded in less than ten per cent of cases.[5, 13, 34] Damage to the pudendal or caudal rectal nerves may result in decrease or loss of external anal sphincter function. The degree of neurological injury may be reflected in the speed of functional recovery. With permanent damage to the nerve on the operative side, several weeks may be required for reinnervation of the sphincter from the contralateral side.[66] Permanent fecal incontinence generally results from bilateral nerve damage.

Urinary Tract Malfunction. Fifteen per cent of animals suffered postsurgically from "acute urinary problems" that "were mainly attributable to anuria following retroflexion of the bladder."[13] Neurological injury may result in anuria or urinary incontinence. Signs are generally transient, with recovery of normal bladder function within one week.[5, 13] Postoperative dysuria followed by spontaneous recovery has also been recorded.[66]

Tenesmus. This postoperative complication occurs in a varying percentage of cases, from less than 10 per cent[5, 13] to 25 per cent.[34] Signs frequently resolve with time. If this problem is due to sutures inadvertently placed through the rectal wall, they should be removed.[41]

Rectal Prolapse. This may be a transient problem.[5, 13] Prolapse may necessitate resection[34] and, if persistent, colopexy.

Sciatic Nerve Paralysis. Damage to this nerve during standard perineal herniorrhaphy can result in temporary or permanent lameness.[13, 66] In cases with sciatic paralysis, the hind limb can support weight; however, "the tarsus is overflexed and sinks close to the ground, and the paw is dragged on its dorsum and placed with the dorsum on the ground surface. Hip flexion and stifle extension are normal."[18] Superficial gluteal muscle transposition does not interfere with locomotion.[88]

Other Complications. Other complications occasionally encountered have included prolonged postoperative hemorrhage and pain[13] and rectal constriction subsequent to combined rectal diverticulectomy and herniorrhaphy.[5] Anal splitting may result in permanent anal and perianal soiling, which is "probably due to inability to control and direct the bowel movement during defecation."[35]

RECURRENCE OF HERNIATION AFTER SURGICAL REPAIR

Factors to be considered when evaluating documented recurrence rates are as follows.

Follow-up Time. The overall recurrence rate, in surveys involving detailed postoperative follow-up

TABLE 60–2. The Effect of Castration on Recurrence of Herniation Following Perineal Herniorrhaphy

Reference	Castrated		Not Castrated	
	Total No. Dogs	No. Recurrences	Total No. Dogs	No. Recurrences
Bellenger[5]	24	2	8	2
Burrows and Harvey[13]	14	6	22	10
Harvey[34]	14	5	26	10
Hayes, Wilson, and Tarone[37]	81	18	46	22
Totals	133	31	102	44
Per cent recurrence		23		43

investigations, ranges between 31[37] and 45 per cent.[13] Within six to 12 months of surgery, herniation recurred in 11 per cent (one in nine)[13] and 18 per cent (seven in 36)[37] of cases. More than one year postoperatively, 25 per cent (11 in 44) and 50 per cent (12 in 24)[13] of cases experienced repeated herniation. The recurrence, when the follow-up time was greater than one year, is possibly associated with the continued deterioration of the perineal tissue rather than surgical technical factors, which are likely to influence the high percentage of recurrence[37] in the immediate postoperative period.

Variation in Surgical Competence. A comparative study of the effect of surgical skill on the recurrence of herniation revealed that the recurrence rate was significantly higher when standard herniorrhaphy was performed by less experienced surgeons.[13] This finding has not been confirmed by other investigators.[88]

Effect of Castration. Many authors have suspected that the prostate gland or testicular hormonal imbalance plays a role in the pathogenesis of perineal hernia.

A comparison was made between dogs castrated in association with perineal herniorrhaphy and those left entire.[37] Variations in the time interval between surgery and the acquisition of follow-up information were taken into consideration when the data were analyzed. The authors found that the recurrence risk among noncastrated animals was 2.7 times greater than among castrated males (p < 0.01). Analysis of pooled data (Table 60–2) indicates that castration significantly reduces the recurrence of herniation subsequent to perineal herniorrhaphy. In unilateral perineal hernia cases undergoing surgery, it was found that castration had no effect on the rate of herniation on the contralateral side.[13]

Type of Suture Material Used in Repair. Recurrence was reported in 14 out of 26 (54 per cent) cases in which nonabsorbable sutures were used and in three out of 11 (27 per cent) in which surgical gut was used.[13] Although this difference was not statistically significant, the high rate of wound infection suggests that absorbable sutures are preferable.

Number of Times Herniorrhaphy Has Been Performed. The risk of recurrence in animals having repeated herniorrhaphy is higher than in animals undergoing initial hernia repair.[13]

1. Amand, W. B.: Nonneurogenic disorders of the anus and rectum. Vet. Clin. North Am. 4:535, 1974.
2. Ashdown, R. B.: Symposium on canine recto-anal disorders—I: Clinical anatomy. J. Small Anim. Pract. 9:315, 1968.
3. Ashton, D. G.: Perineal hernia in the cat—a description of two cases. J. Small Anim. Pract. 17:473, 1976.
4. Bartels, J. E.: How to delineate canine and feline hernias radiographically. Mod. Vet. Pract. 53:27, 1972.
5. Bellenger, C. R.: Perineal hernia in dogs. Aust. Vet. J. 56:434, 1980.
6. Betts, C. W., and Finco, D. R.: Diseases of the canine prostate gland. In Kirk, R. W. (ed.): Current Veterinary Therapy V. W. B. Saunders, Philadelphia, 1974, pp. 938–941.
7. Blakely, C. L.: Perineal hernia. In Mayer, K., Lacroix, J. V., and Hoskins, H. P. (eds.): Canine Surgery, 4th ed. American Veterinary Publications, Inc., Santa Barbara, 1957, pp. 458–468.
8. Borthwick, R., and MacKenzie, C. P.: The signs and results of treatment of prostatic disease in dogs. Vet. Rec. 89:374, 1971.
9. Bovee, K. C.: Canine prostatic diseases. In Proc. Univ. of Sydney Post-Grad. Comm. in Vet. Sc.: Nephrology, Urology and Diseases of the Urinary Tract. 61, 1982, pp. 355–360.
10. Brass, W., Ficus, H. J., and Jöchle, W.: Antiandrogen-Behandlung der Prostatavergrösserung beim Hund. Kleintierpraxis, 16:95, 1971.
11. Brunson, D. B., and Short, C. E.: Anaesthesia for small animal geriatric patient. Cornell Vet. 68(Suppl. 7):15, 1978.
12. Burrows, C. F.: Diseases of the colon, rectum and anus in the dog and cat. In Anderson, N. V. (ed.): Veterinary Gastroenterology. Lea & Febiger, Philadelphia, 1980, pp. 553–592.
13. Burrows, C. F., and Harvey, C. E.: Perineal hernia in the dog. J. Small Anim. Pract. 14:315, 1973.
14. Campbell, J. R., and Lawson, D. D.: The signs of prostatic disease in the dog. Vet. Rec. 75:4, 1963.
15. Canfield, R. B.: Anatomical aspects of perineal hernia in the dog. Master's thesis, University of Sydney.
16. Chase, H. C.: Levator hernia (pudendal hernia). Surg. Gynecol. Obstet. 35:717, 1922.
17. Clarke, R. E.: A new method to repair a perineal hernia in the dog caused by a haemangiosarcoma in a retained testicle. Aust. Vet. Pract. 9:71, 1979.
18. de Lahunta, A.: Veterinary Neuroanatomy and Clinical Neurology. W. B. Saunders, Philadelphia, 1977.
19. Desai, R.: An anatomical study of the canine male and female pelvic diaphragm and the effect of testosterone on the status of levator ani of male dogs. J. Am. Anim. Hosp. Assoc. 18:195, 1982.
20. DeVita, J.: Factors responsible for perineal hernia in male dogs. In Mayer, K., Lacroix, J. V., and Hoskins, H. P. (eds.): Canine Surgery, 4th ed. American Veterinary Publications, Inc., Santa Barbara, 1957, pp. 456–457.
21. Dieterich, H. F.: Perineal hernia repair in the canine. Vet. Clin. North Am. 5:383, 1975.

22. Dollar, J. A. W.: Perineal hernia. *In Regional Veterinary Surgery and Operative Technique.* Gay and Hancock Ltd., London, 1912, pp. 558–559.

23. Dorn, A. S., Cartee, R. E., and Richardson, D. C.: A preliminary comparison of perineal hernia in the dog and man. J. Am. Anim. Hosp. Assoc. *18:*624, 1982.

24. Earley, T. D.: Personal communication, 1983.

25. Evans, H. E., and Christensen, G. C.: *Miller's Anatomy of the Dog,* 2nd ed. W. B. Saunders, Philadelphia, 1979.

26. Eyestone, H.: A successful operation for perineal hernia. Vet. Med. *36:*531, 1941.

27. Fingl, E.: Laxatives and cathartics. *In* Gilman, A. G., Goodman, L. S., and Gilman, A. (eds.): *The Pharmacological Basis of Therapeutics,* 6th ed. Macmillan Publishing Co., New York, 1980, pp. 1002–1012.

28. Gadd, J. D.: Hypertrophy of the prostate gland. J. Am. Vet. Med. Assoc. *104:*15, 1944.

29. Genevois, J. P.: Pathologie ano-rectale et périnéale. III. Hernie périnéale. Rev. Med. Vet. *132:*575, 1981.

30. Greiner, T. P., and Johnson, R. G.: Diseases of the prostate gland. *In* Ettinger, S. J. (ed.): *Textbook of Veterinary Internal Medicine,* 2nd ed. W. B. Saunders, Philadelphia, 1983, pp. 1459–1493.

31. Greiner, T. P., Johnson, R. G., and Betts, C. W.: Diseases of the rectum and anus. *In* Ettinger, S. J. (ed.): *Textbook of Veterinary Internal Medicine,* 2nd ed. W. B. Saunders, Philadelphia, 1983, pp. 1493–1521.

32. Gordon, N.: The position of the canine prostate gland. Am. J. Vet. Res. *22:*142, 1961.

33. Harvey, C. E.: Anal and perineal diseases of the dog. *In* Grunsell, C. S. G., and Hill, F. W. G.: *The Veterinary Annual,* 17th ed. Year Book Medical Publishers, Chicago, 1977, pp. 150–155.

34. Harvey, C. E.: Treatment of perineal hernia in the dog—a reassessment. J. Small Anim. Pract. *18:*505, 1977.

35. Harvey, C. E.: Anal splitting in dogs with perineal hernia: technique and results. J. Am. Anim. Hosp. Assoc. *14:*243, 1978.

36. Hayes, H. M., Jr.: Congenital umbilical and inguinal hernias in cattle, horses, swine, dogs and cats: risk by breed and sex among hospital patients. Am. J. Vet. Res. *35:*839, 1974.

37. Hayes, H. M., Jr., Wilson, G. P., and Tarone, R. E.: The epidemiologic features of perineal hernia in 771 dogs. J. Am. Anim. Hosp. Assoc. *14:*703, 1978.

38. Hayes, K. J.: The so-called "levator ani" of the rat. Acta Endocrinol. *48:*337, 1965.

39. Holmes, J. R.: Perineal hernia in the dog. Vet. Rec. *76:*1250, 1964.

40. Hornbuckle, W. E., MacCoy, D. M., Allan, G. S., and Gunther, R.: Prostatic disease in the dog. Cornell Vet. *68*(Suppl. 7):284, 1978.

41. Houlton, J. E. F.: Surgical treatment of perineal hernia in dogs. Vet. Ann. *23:*208, 1983.

42. International Committee on Veterinary Anatomical Nomenclature: *Nomina Anatomica Veterinaria,* 2nd ed. Adolf Holzhausen's Successors, Vienna, 1973.

43. Johnson, M. S., and Gourley, I. M.: Perineal hernia in a cat: a possible complication of perineal urethrostomy. Vet. Med./Small Anim. Clin. *75:*241, 1980.

44. Jubb, K. V. F., Kennedy, P. C., and McEntee, K.: The male genital system. *In* Jubb, K. V. F., and Kennedy, P. C. (eds.): *Pathology of Domestic Animals,* Vol. 1, 2nd ed. Academic Press, New York, 1970, pp. 443–485.

45. Krieg, M., Szalay, R., and Voigt, K. D.: Binding and metabolism of testosterone and of 5α-dihydrotestosterone in bulbocavernosus/L.A. (BCLA) of male rats: in vivo and in vitro studies. J. Steroid Biochem. *5:*453, 1974.

46. Koger, R. B.: Polyethylene sponge in perineal herniorrhaphy. Vet. Med. *49:*451, 1954.

47. Koontz, A. R.: *Hernia.* Appleton-Century-Crofts, New York, 1963.

48. Larsen, J. S.: Perineal herniorrhaphy in dogs. J. Am. Vet. Med. Assoc. *149:*277, 1966.

49. Leighton, R. L.: Surgical procedures for the routine small animal practice. Perineal herniorrhaphy. Vet. Med. *55:*33, 1960.

50. Leighton, R. L.: Perineal hernia in a cat. Feline Pract. *9:*44, 1979.

51. Lewis, D. G.: Symposium on canine recto-anal disorders—III: Clinical management. J. Small Anim. Pract. *9:*329, 1968.

52. Lipowitz, A. J., Schwartz, A., Wilson, G. P., and Ebert, J. W.: Testicular neoplasms and concomitant clinical changes in the dog. J. Am. Vet. Med. Assoc. *163:*1364, 1973.

53. Magnus, R. V.: The comparative anatomy of the levator ani and ano-rectal muscles. Victorian Vet. Proc. 41, 1967–1968.

54. Martin, M.: La hernie périnéale modification de la herniopexie classique. Rec. Méd. Vét. *158:*441, 1982.

55. Martin, W. D., Fletcher, T. F., and Bradley, W. E.: Perineal musculature in the cat. Anat. Rec. *180:*3, 1974.

56. Maull, K. I., and Fleishman, H. A.: Hedrocele: report of a case and review of the literature. Dis. Colon Rectum *21:*107, 1978.

57. Mitchell, J. M.: Successful perineal hernia operation. Vet. Rec. *60:*685, 1948.

58. Moltzen-Nielsen, H.: Perineal hernia. Proc. XVth Int. Vet. Congr. *1:*971, 1953.

59. Montgomery, C. A.: Muscle disease. *In* Benirschke, K., Garner, F. M., and Jones, T. C.: *Pathology of Laboratory Animals.* Springer-Verlag, New York, 1978, pp. 821–879.

60. Moschcowitz, A. V.: Perineal hernia. Surg. Gynecol. Obstet. *26:*514, 1918.

61. Nickel, R., Schummer, A., and Seiferle, E.: *The Viscera of the Domestic Mammals,* 2nd ed. Verlag Paul Parey, Berlin, 1973.

62. Nitschke, T.: Diaphragma pelvis, Clitoris und Vestibulum vaginae der Hündin. Anat. Anz. *127:*76, 1970.

63. Nommensen, C.: Versuche zur Behandlung von Dammbrüchen beim Hund mit Hilfe eines Polyesternetzes. Tieraerztl. Umsch. *29:*79, 1974.

64. O'Brien, T. R.: *Radiographic Diagnosis of Abdominal Disorders in the Dog: Radiographic Interpretation, Clinical Signs, Pathophysiology.* W. B. Saunders, Philadelphia, 1978.

65. O'Connor, J. J. (ed.): Perineal hernia. *In Dollar's Veterinary Surgery,* 4th ed. Bailliere, Tindall and Cox, London, 1965, pp. 679–680.

66. Omamegbe, J. O.: A study of external hernias in domestic animals, with particular reference to canine perineal hernia. Thesis, University of Glasgow, 1979.

67. Osol, A. (ed.): *Blakiston's Gould Medical Dictionary,* 3rd ed. McGraw-Hill Book Co., New York, 1956.

68. Pettit, G. D.: Perineal hernia in a bitch. Can. Vet. J. *1:*504, 1960.

69. Pettit, G. D.: Perineal hernia in the dog. Cornell Vet. *52:*261, 1962.

70. Rosai, J. (ed.): Skeletal muscle. *In Ackerman's Surgical Pathology,* Vol. 2, 6th ed. C. V. Mosby, St. Louis, 1981, pp. 1629–1636.

71. Sandwith, D. J.: Perineal hernia in the bitch. Vet. Rec. *99:*18, 1976.

72. Schlotthauer, C. F.: The prostate gland in the dog. Proc. Am. Vet. Med. Assoc. 234, 1955.

73. Schnelle, G. B.: Perineal hernia. Proc. XVth Int. Vet. Congr. *2:*377, 1953.

74. Schörner, Von G.: Konservative Behandlung der Prostatahypertrophie beim Rüden mit Δ1-Chlormadinonazetat (Tardak). Wien. Tieraerztl. Monatsschr. *64:*231, 1977.

75. Skandalakis, J. E., Gray, S. W., and Akin, J. T., Jr.: The surgical anatomy of hernial rings. Surg. Clin. North Am. *54:*1227, 1974.

76. Sparks, E. R.: Prostatectomy in the reduction of perineal hernias in the dog. Vet. Med. *28:*508, 1933.

77. Spreull, J. S. A., and Frankland, A. L.: Transplanting the superficial gluteal muscle in the treatment of perineal hernia and flexure of the rectum in the dog. J. Small Anim. Pract. *21:*265, 1980.

78. Stone, E. A., Thrall, D. E., and Barber, D. L.: Radiographic interpretation of prostatic disease in the dog. J. Am. Anim. Hosp. Assoc. *14*:115, 1978.

79. Thayer, C. B.: Surgical correction of a perineal hernia. Vet. Med. *43*:35, 1948.

80. Thomford, N. R., and Sherman, N. J.: Primary perineal hernia. Dis. Colon Rectum *12*:441, 1969.

81. Upson, D. W.: Pharmacologic principles of gastrointestinal therapy. Vet. Clin. North Am. *2*:49, 1972.

82. Vendrig, A. A. A.: Use of a truss in canine perineal hernia. Tijdschr. Diergeneeskd. *107*:325, 1982.

83. Vinson, F.: "Leatherpants" for perineal hernia. Vet. Med. *32*:83, 1937.

84. Wainman, P., and Shipounoff, G. C.: The effects of castration and testosterone on the striated perineal musculature in the rat. J. Endocrinol. 29:975, 1941.

85. Warwick, R., and Williams, P. L. (eds.): *Gray's Anatomy*, 35th ed. Longman Group Ltd., Edinburgh, 1973.

86. Weaver, A. D.: Differential diagnosis of tenesmus in the dog. J. Small Anim. Pract. *15*:609, 1974.

87. Weaver, A. D.: Prostatic disease in the dog. Vet. Ann. *20*:82, 1980.

88. Weaver, A. D., and Omamegbe, J. O.: Surgical treatment of perineal hernia in the dog. J. Small Anim. Pract. *22*:749, 1981.

89. Whittlestone, J. F.: Perineal hernia. J. Small Anim. Pract. *14*:828, 1973.

90. Zimmerman, L. M., and Anson, B. J.: *Anatomy and Surgery of Hernia*. Williams & Wilkins, Baltimore, 1953.

Section VIII

Respiratory System

A. Wendell Nelson
Section Editor

61 Functional Anatomy

John Grandage and Ken Richardson

The organs of the respiratory system consist of the passageways that conduct, control, modify, and exploit air as it passes from the nose to the pulmonary alveoli. They have only a few features in common, such as their serial arrangement, the stiffness of their walls, and the continuity of their mucous membranes.

UPPER RESPIRATORY TRACT

The respiratory tract is arbitrarily divided at the cricotracheal junction into upper and lower parts. The upper part includes the nose, nostrils, nasal chambers and their contents, paranasal sinuses, pharynx, and larynx.

Nose and Nasal Chambers

Nasal Plate

The hairless part of the nose of the dog and cat, the *nasal plate* or planum nasale, is covered with thick keratinized epidermis.[21] In the cat, its surface is made up of fine tubercles,[56] but in the dog it is arranged in polygonal plaques (areae) delineated by sulci, which provide patterns unique to each individual. Noseprints are used for identification.[42]

The canine nasal plate is often wet yet is free from local glands.[74] The wetness is caused primarily by secretions of the remote lacrimal and lateral nasal glands, which convey their secretions to the nasal vestibule by long ducts. The opening of the nasolacrimal duct is easily identified on the floor of the nasal vestibule just inside the nostril. Frequently, an accessory opening is present caudal to the nasal vestibule in the middle meatus level with the canine tooth.[11] The duct of the lateral nasal gland opens more dorsally, at the rostral end of the dorsal nasal concha.[28] The duct is only about 0.5 mm in diameter and can be difficult to identify even in dissected dogs. In live animals experimentally subjected to heat stress, the nasal gland discharges copious serous fluid.[15] The secretion is one of the principal sources of fluid for evaporative cooling.[53, 68] Although cooling may be its principal function, the fluid also contains a high proportion of IgA.[1] A few much smaller medial nasal glands are found on the rostral part of the septum. They open at the caudal limit of the vestibule and contribute marginally to the wetness of the nose. Whereas a healthy animal usually has a wet nose and occasionally a dry one, a febrile animal nearly always has a dry nose unless rhinitis is present.

In cats, the lateral nasal gland and its duct are

visible only microscopically, and their secretion is mucous instead of serous.[17]

Pigmentation of the nasal plate varies according to breed, although the plate is commonly black in the dog and rose in the cat. Some nonpigmented or weakly pigmented, flesh-colored noses ("Dudley noses")[70] or the butterfly (spotted) noses of harlequin varieties are predisposed to photosensitivity reactions and melanomata. The junction between the hairless skin and hairy skin is particularly vulnerable to solar dermatitis (Collie nose).[60]

Nostrils and Nasal Vestibule

The *nostrils* (nares) and the associated structures immediately inside the nasal vestibule impede the flow of air into the nasal chambers. Minor variations in form can be physiologically or clinically significant. In the dog, each nostril is typically comma-shaped when viewed from the front. The tail of the comma curves to the side of the nose as a short slot that leads into a caudally directed, tapered alar groove a few millimeters long beneath the *wing of the nose* (ala nasi). The function of this groove has not been determined, but its location suggests that it aids directional scenting.

The nostrils are bordered medially by a vertical pillar (the *columella*), which forms the rostral end of the nasal septum (Fig. 61–1). In both cat and dog, it is furrowed in the midline by the philtrum, a groove that continues over the upper lip. The roof of the nostril is supported by a curved canopy of dorsolateral nasal cartilage[29, 67] that has been called the alar cartilage.[11] It arches laterally to support the wing of the nose. The floor of the nostril *(sill)* is stiffened by a flimsy rod of cartilage *(accessory nasal cartilage)*. Laterally, the nostril is breached by the *alar groove*, which separates the wing of the nose from the sill and upper lip (Fig. 61–1).

The *nasal vestibule* is not empty (as in the human nose) but is occupied by the swollen end of the ventral nasal concha, called the alar fold or swell body. This bulbous, fleshy fold of mucous membrane lies in the depths of each nostril like a loose-fitting plug, attached and supported by a ventrolateral nasal cartilage. It bulges medially from the wing of the nose and limits the air inlet to a falciform crevice. Its removal greatly enlarges the airway. In the rat or rabbit, the diameter of this fold can change according to vascular engorgement and cyclically promotes or discourages the flow of air through each nasal chamber.[18] It may regulate a similar nasal cycle in the dog, justifying its alternative name "swell body." Recent work suggests that the vascular architecture may be inappropriate for such a function.[2] It is this fold or its attachment to the wing of the nose that is typically

The authors acknowledge the valuable assistance of Richard Krumins in the preparation of the section on the larynx.

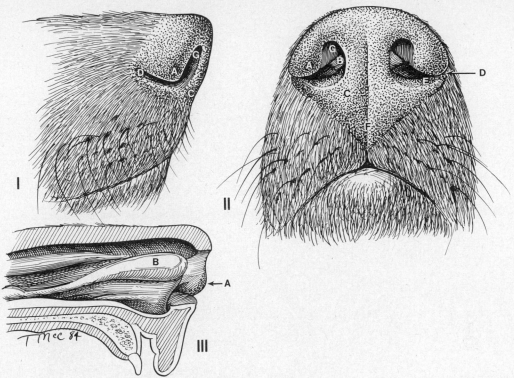

Figure 61–1. Nose and nasal vestibule. *I* and *II*, Lateral and rostral views of mesaticephalic canine nose. *III*, Left nasal vestibule viewed from the right side with the septum removed. Important structures are identified: *A*, wing of the nostril; *B*, alar fold; *C*, columella; *D*, alar groove; *E*, nasal sill; *F*, philtrum; *G*, nostril.

excised in the treatment of stenotic nares.[37] Such removal leads to greater exposure of the deepest part of the vestibule, known as the *atrium*, a small chamber that leads mainly into the middle nasal meatus. The blood supply to these portions of the nasal plate and alar fold is via numerous small branches of the infraorbital arteries.[22]

The embryological development of the nose is important because of its association with those anomalies usually referred to as harelip or cleft lip (or, more comprehensively, "cleft of the primary palate").[35] These anomalies are often associated with various forms of cleft palate ("cleft of the secondary palate"), yet the two groups of anomalies are embryologically and etiologically distinct.[54]

In the dog embryo of about 25 days, a pair of olfactory pits are separated from each other by a broad column of tissue that is the anlage for the end of the nasal septum, medial portions of the upper lip, and associated portions of the incisive bones. This median process, which separates the nostrils, is destined to fuse on each side with a finger-like maxillary process that grows inwards, beneath the nostrils. A plate of epithelial cells, the "nasal fin,"[33] which normally exists only transiently, can remain and prohibit the fusion of the median and maxillary processes. The result is a cleft of the primary palate, which can involve all or part of one lip, the sill of the nostril, the alveolar process of the incisive bone, or all of the incisive bone.

Development of the secondary palate succeeds that of the primary palate and involves the inward growth of a pair of mesenchymal shelves called lateral max-

illary processes. These meet and fuse to each other at the midline, to the primary palate in front, and to the nasal septum above. These events occur at about 33 days gestation in the dog.[29] They bring about separation of nasal chambers from the oral cavity and allow digestive and respiratory activities to proceed independently. Failure of the lateral processes to meet results in cleft of the secondary palate. The more caudal parts of the palate remain unossified and become the fleshy soft palate.

The major palatine arteries supply the oral mucosa of the hard palate, the periosteum, and the bone that forms the alveoli (Fig. 61–2A). These paired arteries branch frequently as they travel rostrally to the back of the incisor teeth, where they anastomose with each other and send branches through the incisive foramina to anastomose with the lateral nasal arteries.[29]

The sphenopalatine artery arises from a common trunk with the major palatine artery (Fig. 61–2B). It supplies the mucoperiosteum of the side and floor of the nasal fossa, adjacent nasal septum, and ventral nasal conchae.

Nasal Cavity

The nasal cavity is probably the dog's most variable feature, yet it is remarkably uniform in the cat. The *nasal septum,* which divides the cavity into two, is mostly cartilaginous but does have an osseous periphery. In the dog, a middle section is membranous and allows the end of the nose to move, in turn enabling the dog to nip the surface of a flat object with its incisors while its nose is pushed dorsally out of the

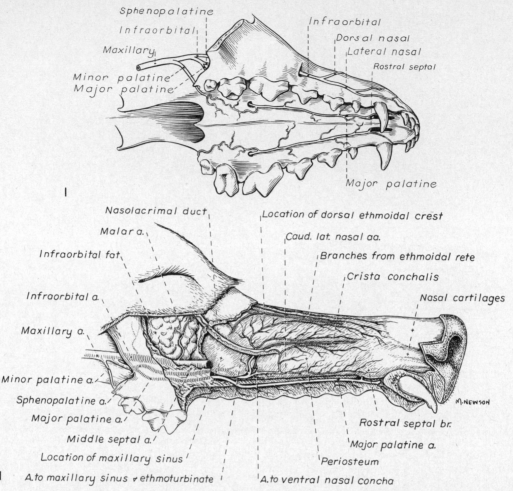

Sphenopalatine
Infraorbital
Maxillary
Minor palatine
Major palatine

Infraorbital
Dorsal nasal
Lateral nasal
Rostral septal

Major palatine

I

Nasolacrimal duct
Malar a.
Infraorbital fat
Infraorbital a.
Maxillary a.

Minor palatine a.
Sphenopalatine a.
Major palatine a.
Middle septal a.
Location of maxillary sinus

Location of dorsal ethmoidal crest
Caud. lat. nasal aa.
Branches from ethmoidal rete
Crista conchalis
Nasal cartilages

Rostral septal br.
Major palatine a.
Periosteum

M. NEWSON

II   A. to maxillary sinus v ethmoturbinate   A. to ventral nasal concha

Figure 61–2. Ventrolateral (I) and lateral (II) views of the distribution of the arterial supply to the hard palate. (Reprinted with permission from Evans, H. E., and Christensen, G. C. (eds.): *Miller's Anatomy of the Dog.* 2nd ed. W. B. Saunders, Philadelphia, 1979.)

way. The cat's nose is not mobile, and its cartilages resemble shortened canine nasal cartilages.[61]

The bulk of the muzzle is made up of two nasal fossae, irregular passageways between the nostrils and the openings into the nasopharynx (*choanae*). The fossae are almost filled with conchae (Fig. 61–3), scrolls of bone or cartilage that project medially from the sides and roof and are covered with a vascular and glandular mucous membrane. In the dog the ventral nasal concha is easily distinguished from the others. It occupies the rostral and ventral quarter of the nasal fossa and consists of a caudal lamellar part connected to the alar fold of the vestibule by an isthmus. It is supported by a thin basal lamella (conchal crest), which arises from the maxilla and whose lineal shadow is one of the more distinctive radiographic features of the conchae. The basal lamella is continuous with a spiral lamella, which supports thirty or more secondary lamellae. Even slight inflammation of the mucous membrane over these lamellae can lead to total airway obstruction.[23] All other conchae are ethmoturbinates, a series of folds of varying complexity, the longest and most dorsal of which is known as the dorsal nasal concha. In the cat, the ventral nasal concha is smaller and

there is compensatory development of lamellae in the adjacent conchae.

The air passages are restricted by the conchae to narrow meatuses. A thin, vertical, common meatus is found on either side of the septum; it unites and is coextensive with the dorsal, middle, and ventral meatuses, which occupy the spaces between the conchae. The ventral meatus is the largest and leads into the choana via an unobstructed bony tube, the nasopharyngeal meatus. Even the ventral meatus is narrow, however, as it passes beneath the lamellar part of the ventral nasal concha. Which route forms the principal airway to the pharynx is a matter of contention; some claim it to be via the ventral meatus,[13] and others via the dorsal meatus.[24]

The rostral quarter of the nasal cavity is lined with stratified squamous epithelium, and the remainder with pseudostratified ciliated columnar respiratory epithelium.[2] Much of the nonolfactory mucous membrane may be likened to erectile tissue. Thirty per cent or more of this membrane is made up of large thin-walled veins, which serve as both heat exchangers and capacitance vessels. The heat exchangers are so efficient that dogs can exhale air 16.5° C below body temperature, saving 75 per cent of the water

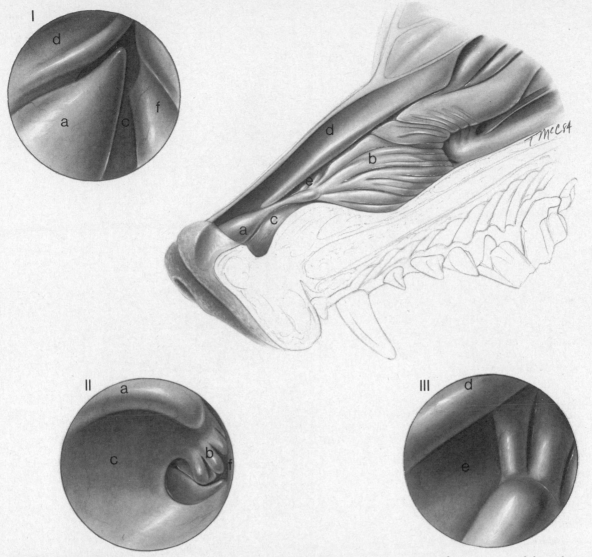

Figure 61–3. Medial view of the canine nasal conchae and nasal passages. Three common endoscopic views of the right nasal passages are presented for spatial orientation. *I*, The endoscope is positioned at the mid medial side of the alar fold *(a)* and just caudal to the wing of the nostril, with the ventral *(c)* and dorsal *(d)* meatuses and nasal septum *(f)* noted. *II*, The endoscope is positioned just cranial to the junction of the alar fold *(a)* and the ventral nasal conchae *(b)*, viewing the ventral meatus *(c)*, and nasal septum *(f)*. *III*, The endoscope is positioned as in *II* but viewing the ventral nasal concha, the dorsal nasal concha *(d)*, and medial nasal meatus *(e)*.

and 80 per cent of the heat in dry air at 0° C.[32] The degree of filling of capacitance vessels determines the degree of congestion, or conversely, the degree of nasal patency.[2] The mucous membrane of the rostral half of the nasal cavity carries a rich complement of tubuloacinar nasal glands. Stimulation of this portion induces a vigorous sneeze reflex,[23] so that rhinoscopy may even require a local as well as a general anesthetic.

Macrosmatic (smelling) species such as the dog have an extensive olfactory mucous membrane. It is found in the caudodorsal part of the nose, where in German shepherds, for example, it is reputed to cover an area of 150 cm² and support over 200 million receptors.[27] The appearance of the olfactory membrane differs little from that of the remainder of the mucous membrane, although it may be marginally thicker and grayer.[74]

Paranasal Sinuses

The cat and dog possess frontal sinuses and maxillary recesses. The maxillary recess is not a true sinus, because it does not lie between two plates of a cranial bone but is instead bound laterally by the maxilla and medially by the ethmoid.[56]

The *frontal sinus* is the biggest and occupies the brow ridge and supraorbital process of the frontal bone. The size of this sinus is not only absolutely but also relatively bigger in large dogs. Boxers, Great Danes, and mastiffs have huge frontal sinuses, whereas toy breeds, especially brachycephalic toy breeds, have tiny or nonexistent ones. The sinuses of carnivores grow until the animal is mature.

Right and left frontal sinuses are separated by a median septum (Fig. 61–4). In the dog, but not the cat, each is composed of three separate cavities,

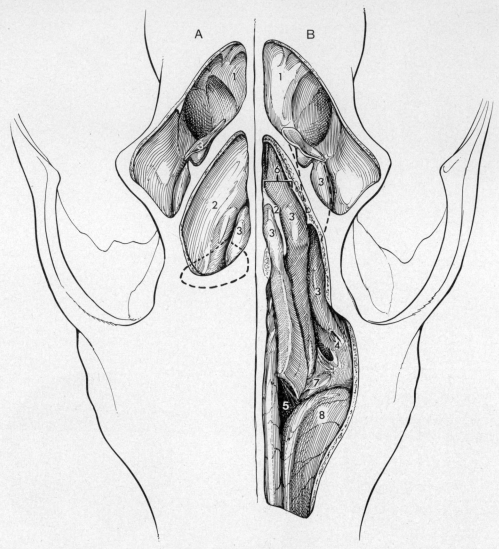

Figure 61–4. Frontal sinus of the dog. *A*, The dorsal view of the right frontal sinus is presented to show the lateral (*1*) and rostral (*2*) compartments with the sinus portion of ectoturbinates (*3*) projecting into these compartments of the sinus through the nasofrontal opening (*dotted line*) in the rostral sinus septum. *B*, The floor of the rostral compartment of the left frontal sinus has been removed to expose the medial compartment (*6*). This compartment is located rostral to the lateral compartment (*1*) and ventral to the rostral compartment (*2*). The lateral compartment drains into the nasal passages just medial to the orbit (*4*) and caudal to the ventral nasal conchae (*8*). The rostral compartment drains more medial just lateral to the dorsal nasal cochae (*5*) together with the medial compartment. The drainage of the lateral compartment (*4*) is lateral and slightly ventral to the drainage of the medial compartment (*7*).

lateral, medial, and rostral, which communicate separately via nasofrontal openings with the nasal fossa.[29] The lateral compartment is much larger and may be partially subdivided by incomplete septa. It usually contains one of the ethmoturbinates that just enter the rostral part of its floor. The smaller medial compartment and the smallest rostral compartment are filled with ethmoturbinates and are therefore less easy to identify on radiographs. The scrolls of bone within them are covered with the yellowish-gray olfactory mucous membrane.

The maxillary recess is found at a level of the carnassial tooth between the orbit and infraorbital canal. It communicates with the middle meatus by a roomy nasomaxillary opening, which is flanked by the nasal conchae. The recess houses the broad, flat,

lateral nasal gland on its lateral wall; the gland appears grossly like thickened mucous membrane and cytologically like a serous salivary gland.[53] The medial wall bears small compound alveolar glands; because the wall also contains many nerve endings it may serve a sensory function.[12] A small sphenoid sinus is present in the cat, and a similar cavity is found in the dog but is filled with ethmoturbinates.

Many functions have been proposed for mammalian sinuses, such as imparting resonance to the voice, humidifying the inspired air, increasing olfactory surface area, shock absorbing, mucous secreting, thermally insulating, growth modifying, skull lightening, and atavistic remnant,[14] yet the number of proposals is itself indicative that the function of the sinuses remains largely unknown.

Nasopharynx

The respiratory tract develops mostly from the floor of the digestive tube, where it is in constant danger of being flooded with ingesta. The pharyngeal chiasma is an ingenious crossroads that has evolved to cope with this design flaw. The two roads are the nasopharynx and larynx in one direction, and the oropharynx and esophagus in the other.

The nasopharyngeal conduit is a relatively large tubular space extending from the choanae to the intrapharyngeal ostium. Only its floor is extensively mobile. The rest of the nasopharynx moves little and remains permanently patent. The choanae are fixed apertures in its roof on either side of the vomer. The walls of the nasopharynx are relatively featureless except for a small mucosal cushion that lies just behind the slit-like opening of each auditory tube. These openings are located high on the lateral walls of the nasopharynx and are about ten and four millimeters long in the dog and cat, respectively.[56] Tubal tonsils are absent but a flat pharyngeal tonsil is present in the roof. Digital pressure in this area is said to stimulate respiration.[23]

Soft Palate

The soft palate forms the floor of the nasopharynx and the roof of the oropharynx. It is a mobile, valve-like partition that can be elevated to close off the proximal airway during swallowing or depressed to close off the oral cavity during nose-breathing. During swallowing it works with the epiglottis, which closes off the distal airway, to allow a bolus of ingesta to cross the respiratory tract. A soft palate that is resected too radically may be unable to close off the nasopharynx during swallowing, thereby permitting aspiration of food.[38]

The free edge of the soft palate curves laterally to form two palatopharyngeal arches; these pass caudally and merge with the walls of the pharynx, leaving a large caudoventrally directed central hole—the intrapharyngeal ostium. The three parts of the pharynx (nasal, oral, and laryngeal) meet at this ostium; a pair of palatopharyngeal muscles serves as its sphincter. The epiglottis frequently pokes through the ostium so that its apex rests on the dorsal surface of the palate. In these circumstances air always passes through the nose; when the epiglottis lies ventral to the soft palate, air may pass through the nose or the mouth, depending on the relation of the soft palate. At rest, air is usually both inhaled and exhaled through the nose. During panting, the nasal heat exchanger is circumvented, and air is usually inhaled through the nose but exhaled through the mouth. During severe heat stress, air is inhaled and exhaled through both nose and mouth.[32] The oscillating tongue, so obvious in the panting dog, signals the complex movements of larynx, hyoid, and soft palate that occur at this time.

The soft palate is usually conspicuous on lateral radiographs because of the contrast afforded by air above and below it. It is long in both brachycephalic and dolichocephalic breeds.[29] Radiographs of brachycephalic breeds usually reveal it to be thickened, suggesting that these animals need to sustain contractions of the longitudinal muscles in their palates in order to maintain a patent airway. The pharynx is rarely seen clearly on radiographs of brachycephalic breeds, presumably because of the restricted air space.

Tensor and levator muscles of the palate run over the sides of the nasopharynx to a common aponeurosis on the midline that provides structural support for the soft palate (Fig. 61–5). The tendinous insertion of the tensor veli palatini muscle passes over the ventral edge of the hamulus of the pterygoid bone to insert rostrally in the soft palate.[29] This arrangement creates caudolateral tension on the soft palate. The tendinous portion is transected at the pterygoid bone in patients with cleft soft palate in order to reduce tension on the suture closure. The mucous membrane is of the respiratory type on the dorsal surface of the

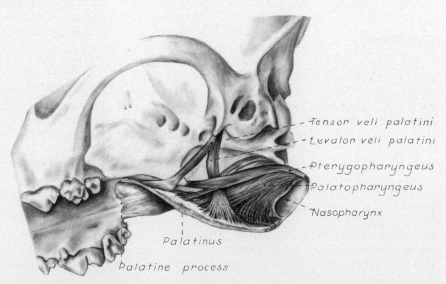

Figure 61–5. Muscles of the pharynx and soft palate. (Reprinted with permission from Evans, H. E., and Christensen, G. C. (eds.): *Miller's Anatomy of the Dog.* 2nd ed. W. B. Saunders, Philadelphia, 1979.)

Tensor veli palatini

Levator veli palatini

Pterygopharyngeus

Palatopharyngeus

Nasopharynx

Palatinus

Palatine process

soft palate and of the digestive type on the ventral surface. The oral surface is richly endowed with glands and lymphoid tissue, although such features are relatively sparse on the nasal side.[56] The minor palatine artery supplies most of the soft palate. This slender vessel arises from the maxillary artery at the level of the last cheek tooth and runs longitudinally close to the midline.[29] Nerves from the pharyngeal plexus (derived from cranial nerves IX and X) supply the soft palate.

Larynx

The larynx supports two sets of ingenious valvular mechanisms, the epiglottis and the glottis. The epiglottis acts mostly passively as a hinged lid that can be pushed over the entrance to the larynx (the aditus laryngis) and thereby protect the lower airway against aspiration of liquids and solids during swallowing. It also acts as a vane that can deflect air into or select air from the nose or mouth according to need (for temperature regulation, olfaction, vocalization).

The glottis is a more refined, active valve made up of a pair of vocal folds and associated cartilages that encroach on the airway. Normally, it widens slightly during inspiration and narrows during expiration. Acting as double doors, the vocal folds are the last defense against inhalation of noxious material, and efficient neural mechanisms prompt their rapid closure. As seals, they can close off the lower airway (when thoracic or abdominal pressure is raised during parturition, coughing, etc). They can close off the upper airway (when thoracic pressure is lowered during early vomition, windsucking, etc.). As elastic membranes, they vibrate for phonation, either slowly (for low pitch) or rapidly (for higher pitch), at different lengths (for different harmonics), and at different amplitudes (for different volumes). As slowly oscillating shutters, they generate the purr of the cat (frequency 20 to 30 Hz) by a mechanism involving the muscles of both the larynx and diaphragm, which are activated simultaneously but out of phase.[63]

Cartilages

The larynx is basically a fibroelastic membranous tube in which stiff hyaline cartilages are embedded to maintain a patent airway and to provide support for the moving parts. The cricoid and thyroid mineralize early in life, especially in the giant dog, making them even stiffer and, incidentally, more conspicuous on radiographs.[30, 57] The ring-shaped cricoid, the most rigid, forms a chassis supporting the thyroid and paired arytenoid cartilages, which articulate with it.

Right and left arytenoid cartilages covered with mucous membrane intrude into the lumen of the larynx, with the gap between them forming the dorsal part of the glottal cleft (Fig. 61–6). A vocal ligament arises from the most ventral portion of both arytenoids (the vocal process). They stretch side-by-side

and meet at the internal ventral midline of the thyroid. They form the core of the vocal folds and the ventral part of the glottal cleft. The glottal cleft is thus a rhomboidal space of which a ventral intermembranous part lies between the vocal folds and a dorsal intercartilaginous part lies between the arytenoids. Rotation of the arytenoids in a ventromedial direction adducts the vocal folds and changes the shape of the cleft from a broad diamond to a narrower one, until it is totally obliterated. Rotation in the opposite direction restores the original aperture.

Similar but smaller and less intrusive vestibular folds lie parallel and rostral to the vocal folds. They bound a vestibular cleft that is broader than the glottal cleft. The thyroid cartilage swings like a visor from the cricoid to assist in lengthening or shortening the vocal and vestibular folds.

The remaining cartilages are wholly or partly elastic. They are found in those rostral parts of the larynx that project into the pharyngeal lumen and encircle the aditus (see Fig. 61–6). Elastic cartilages tolerate buffeting by food during swallowing. The principal element, the epiglottis, is pointed and V-shaped in the dog and cat. It is quite exposed and, according to circumstances, can rest on the caudal part of the soft palate or on the root of the tongue or can fold back into the laryngopharynx to form a cap over the aditus. The seal to the epiglottic lid is completed by the aryepiglottic fold, a fold of mucous membrane running from epiglottis to arytenoid. In the dog, the corniculate and cuneiform tubercles project like pairs of small horns on each side of the aditus. These tubercles are independent cartilages in some species, but in the dog they are processes of the arytenoid cartilage.[19] The cuneiform process is elongated, and its ventral part gives rise to the vestibular fold (or false vocal cord). Both the corniculate and cuneiform processes are absent from cats.[36]

The aditus laryngis is the irregularly shaped entrance to the larynx that lies between the aryepiglottic folds and their enclosed cartilages. Its widest part is found ventrally, abutting onto the rim of the epiglottis and the cuneiform processes. Its caudodorsal part is narrower, almost cleft-like, and lies between the cuneiform and corniculate tubercles (see Fig. 61–6).

Laryngeal Lumen

The larynx projects into the pharynx, and its entrance is held away from the pharyngeal wall. Fluids are unable to flow directly into the laryngeal lumen but are directed by the epiglottis into the surrounding gutter-like recesses made up of the paired valleculae beneath the epiglottis and the piriform recesses on each side. These recesses fill with contrast agent during a barium swallow.

The cavity of the larynx extends from the aditus to the first tracheal ring. It is divided by the glottal cleft into a short, rostral, irregularly cup-shaped part—the laryngeal vestibule—and a larger, caudal, cylindrical part—the infraglottic cavity. The glottal cleft is the

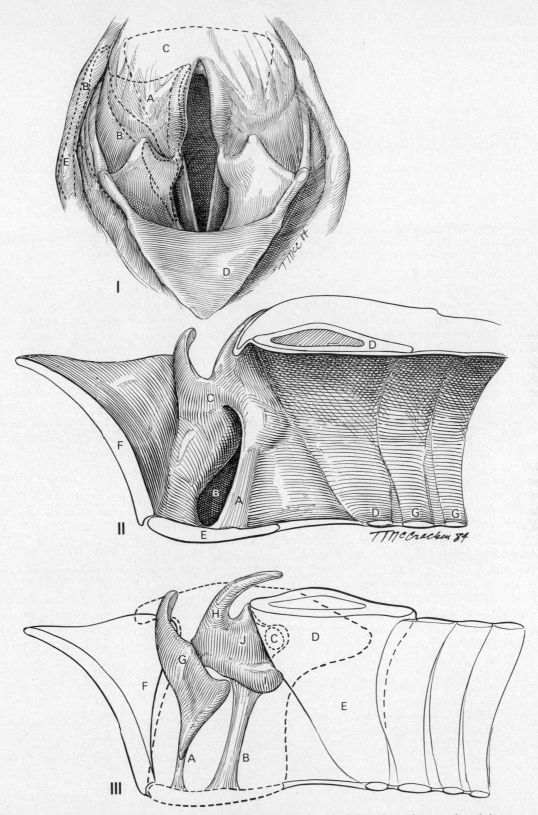

Figure 61–6. Larynx and laryngeal cartilages. *I,* Rostral surface of the larynx viewed from the oral approach with locations of arytenoid *(A),* thyroid *(B),* cricoid *(C),* and epiglottic *(D)* cartilages, and thyrohyoid articulation *(E)* identified. *II,* Medial surface of the right side of the larynx showing vocal fold *(A),* entrance to the ventricle *(B),* and mucosal surface over the arytenoid cartilage *(C).* The normal topography of the laryngeal mucosa is presented. Cut surfaces of the cricoid *(D),* thyroid *(E),* epiglottic *(F),* and tracheal ring *(G)* cartilages are identified. *III,* The medial view of the right side of the larynx is illustrated, with the vestibular ligament *(A),* vocal ligament *(B),* and articulation between the arytenoid and cricoid cartilages *(C)* labeled. The thyroid cartilage *(D; dotted line),* cricoid cartilage *(E; solid line),* and epiglottis *(F; solid line)* are indicated. Arytenoid cartilage is indicated by shaded detail—cuneiform process *(G),* corniculate process *(H),* vocal process *(I),* and body *(J).*

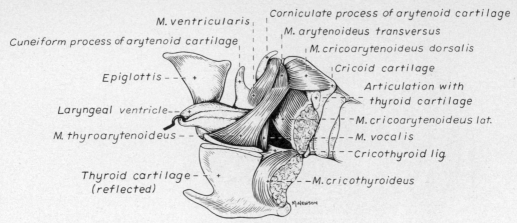

Figure 61–7. Laryngeal muscles, lateral aspect. (Thyroid cartilage is cut left of midline and reflected.) (Reprinted with permission from Evans, H. E., and Christensen, G. C. (eds.): *Miller's Anatomy of the Dog.* 2nd ed. W. B. Saunders, Philadelphia, 1979.)

narrowest part of the airway. Any inflammatory swelling at this site may reduce its diameter, with the risk of asphyxia. The risk of edema is reduced by modifications to the mucous membrane. The membrane has a thin submucosa over the vocal folds that is devoid of glands (hence less chance of edema). The epithelial lining is stratified squamous in the vestibule and reverts to the normal respiratory type only in the infraglottic cavity.[56]

The dog, but not the cat, possesses large laryngeal ventricles. Each is composed of two parts, a depression lying lateral to the vocal fold and a saccule lying lateral to the vestibular fold (see Fig. 61–6). The ventricular depression is a deep vertical trough that opens into the larynx by a broad fissure between the vocal and vestibular folds. At its base, a small oval fissure about three millimeters long leads anteriorly into a larger saccule about the size and shape of an almond ($22 \times 12 \times 6$ mm). This sac is lodged mainly between the mucosa of the vestibular fold and the end of the lamina of the thyroid cartilage. Glands within it are thought to bathe the vocal and vestibular folds with secretions that prevent desiccation. The ventricular depressions form a space lateral to the vocal folds and probably provide room for the folds

to vibrate during barking. Support for this concept of vocal function is provided by the Basenji breed, which apparently never barks and in which ventricles are reduced or absent.[7] Ventriculocordectomy (debarking) by partial or total resection of the vocal fold may quieten a dog but will not make it totally mute.[8]

The rapid flow of air over the ventricular orifices probably reduces the intraluminal pressure and contributes to their pathological eversion in brachycephalic breeds. Correction of this disorder necessitates radical excision of the ventricular mucosa.[39, 49]

Muscles

Extrinsic muscles of the larynx work in harmony with the muscles of the hyoid to elevate, depress, protract, or retract. Intrinsic muscles are striated and mostly concerned with movement of the vocal folds, especially their adduction (Fig. 61–7). Sustained adduction of the vocal folds (laryngospasm), commonly induced in the cat, is caused by spasm of the cricoarytenoid, thyroarytenoid (adductors), and cricothyroid (tensor) muscles.[64, 65] It is uncommon in the dog.[34] The dorsal cricoarytenoid is the only abductor of the vocal folds. Laryngeal hemiplegia following distur-

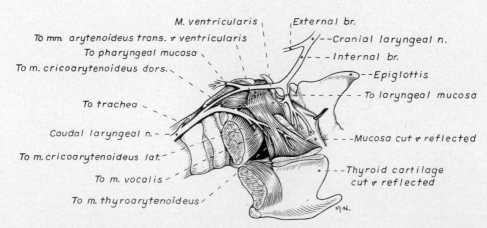

Figure 61–8. Distribution of laryngeal muscles and nerves, lateral aspect. (Reprinted with permission from Evans, H.E., and Christensen, G. C.: *Miller's Anatomy of the Dog.* 2nd ed. W. B. Saunders, Philadelphia, 1979.)

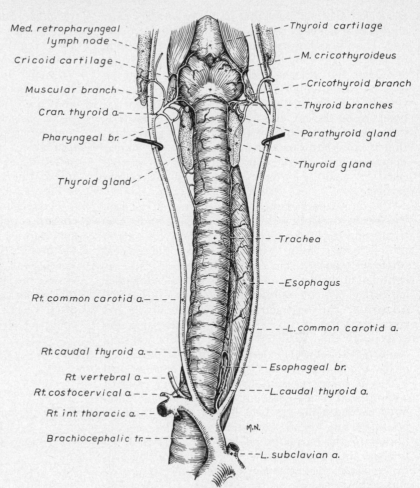

Med. retropharyngeal lymph node
Cricoid cartilage
Muscular branch
Cran. thyroid a.
Pharyngeal br.
Thyroid gland

Thyroid cartilage
M. cricothyroideus
Cricothyroid branch
Thyroid branches
Parathyroid gland
Thyroid gland

Trachea
Esophagus

Rt. common carotid a.

L. common carotid a.

Rt. caudal thyroid a.

Esophageal br.

Rt. vertebral a.

L. caudal thyroid a.

Rt. costocervical a.

Rt. int. thoracic a.

M.N.

Brachiocephalic tr.

L. subclavian a.

Figure 61–9. Distribution of major arterial supply to the larynx and trachea, ventral aspect. (Reprinted with permission from Evans, H. E., and Christensen, G. C. (eds.): *Miller's Anatomy of the Dog.* 2nd ed. W. B. Saunders, Philadelphia, 1979.)

bance to this muscle or its nerve is rare in the dog.[49] Bilateral laryngeal paralysis resulting from recurrent laryngeal nerve degeneration (neuropathy or myopathy) occurs frequently enough in middle-aged dogs to be considered a major differential diagnosis in laryngeal stridor.[40] The larynx is partly concealed by the pharyngeal constrictors (hyo-, thyro-, and cricopharyngeals), which originate on both sides of the larynx and join on the midline dorsal to the pharynx (Section VI).

Nerves and Vessels

The recurrent laryngeal branch of the vagus nerve supplies all the intrinsic muscles of the larynx except the cricothyroid (Fig. 61–8). It reaches the larynx by passing along the dorsolateral surface of the trachea and continues over the lateral surface of the dorsal cricoarytenoid muscle before plunging deep to the thyroid lamina. The external branch of the cranial laryngeal nerve supplies the cricothyroid. The internal branch of the cranial laryngeal is a sensory nerve to the laryngeal mucosa. It gains access to the interior by passing between the junction of the thyrohyoid and the pharyngeal constrictors, then through the rostral thyroid notch.

The cranial laryngeal artery provides the principal blood supply. It originates from the external carotid and courses with the cranial laryngeal nerve through the rostral thyroid notch. Its companion cranial laryngeal vein empties via the hyoid venous arch into the external maxillary vein. Each caudal thyroid vein drains into the internal jugular.

Lymphatics drain into the medial retropharyngeal lymph node.[69]

Palpation and Topography

Parts of the hyoid and larynx can be palpated immediately caudal to the angle of the mandible in the midline. The transversely running basihyoid is the most rostral component. It is flanked by the paired keratohyoid bones, which project forward, and the paired thyrohyoids, which run obliquely caudally. Two further prominences are easily identifiable in the midline, namely, the thyroid prominence and, just caudal to it, the cricoid cartilage. Sternohyoid, geniohyoid, and sternothyroid muscles interfere with but do not totally prevent palpation of the laryngeal region.

LOWER RESPIRATORY TRACT

Trachea

C-shaped cartilages stiffen the elastic tubular trachea and help keep it patent. They alternate with elastic annular ligaments that unite the cartilages and allow the trachea to stretch and bend without buckling. The amount of stretching required by an arching neck or an extending head can be substantial.[51] There are about 40 cartilages in the cat and 35 to 45 in the dog, but the number varies among breeds and individuals.[11] Each cartilage is thickest ventrally and tapers along the curved arms to terminate dorsally as thin, flexible overlapping blades. The first tracheal ring is complete dorsally in the dog, has a similar shape to that of the caudal edge of the cricoid cartilage, and is partially covered by the cricoid cartilage.

The dorsal part of the trachea is free of cartilage and is composed of a wide band of mucosa, connective tissue, and tracheal muscle. In carnivores this smooth muscle inserts on the external surface of the tracheal cartilages some distance lateral to their tips. Its contraction draws the ends of the cartilages together and even past one another so that they overlap like a keyring. This contraction narrows the airway and reduces the dead space,[55] in turn increasing the velocity of the ventilated air and perhaps assisting the expulsion of mucus during coughing. Contraction of the tracheal muscle also stiffens the trachea[58] and makes it more resistant to collapse from external compression. It may prevent sucking of the membranous part into the tracheal lumen, which tends to occur during forced expiration (dynamic collapse) because of the Bernouilli effect.[45, 46] Relaxation of the tracheal muscle allows the tips of the cartilages to spring apart, increases the diameter of the airway, and reduces airway resistance. Excessive spreading of the cartilages is the main feature of collapsed trachea syndrome.

The diameter of the tracheal lumen also varies because of breed characteristics. On the basis of radiographic appearance, bulldogs and brachycephalic breeds have narrow tracheas[41] whereas dachshunds and basset hounds have wide ones.

The mucous membrane of the trachea bears pseudostratified ciliated epithelium kept moist by secretions of goblet cells and mucus-secreting tracheal glands found mainly in the submucosa.[16, 56] The cilia sweep a continuous layer of mucus towards the larynx.[20] Thus, a tight-fitting tracheotomy or endotracheal tube is likely to obstruct its flow and become plugged.

The pleated mucosa of the membranous portion allows tracheal expansion with muscle relaxation.[71, 72] It is the only part of the trachea to be completely ciliated in newborn puppies, with the rest remaining inconsistently ciliated for several days.[77]

The trachea is loosely enclosed in a sleeve of fascia.[29] The deeper leaf forms part of the prevertebral fascia that separates the trachea from the longus colli muscle. It also contributes to the carotid sheath, a tube of fascia that encloses vagus and sympathetic nerves (or vagosympathetic trunk), carotid artery, internal jugular vein, and, sometimes, tracheal lymph trunk. The carotid sheath is found dorsolateral to the trachea, with the recurrent laryngeal nerve running

a similar but independent course. The esophagus runs mostly dorsal to the trachea, drooping to the left at the thoracic inlet. Sternothyroid, sternohyoid, and sternocephalic muscles lie ventral to the trachea.

Cranial and caudal thyroid arteries are slender vessels that supply most of the trachea (Fig. 61–9). They are of variable origin, run in the loose tracheal fascia,[29] and frequently are associated with the recurrent laryngeal nerves. The small branches of the thyroid and bronchial arteries that supply the trachea penetrate between the tracheal rings on each lateral side of the trachea. They arborize in the submucosa to form an interconnecting network of vessels.

The terminal trachea, carina, and pulmonary bronchi are supplied with blood via the bronchoesophageal arteries.[29] The bronchial branches arborize over the bronchi from a dorsal approach and traverse the airway walls proximally and distally. The proximal vessels anastomose with the branches of the caudal thyroid arteries on the distal tracheal wall, and the distal vessels follow the bronchi into the lung parenchyma. Bronchial arteries supply the tissue of the

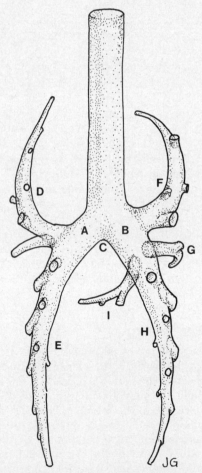

Figure 61–10. The canine bronchial tree, dorsal aspect. The left (A) and right (B) segmental bronchi are the first branches of the trachea and form the carina (C). The left segmental bronchus divides into the left cranial bronchus (D), supplying the left cranial and middle lobes, and the left caudal bronchus (E), supplying the left caudal lobe. The right segmental bronchus divides into the right cranial (F), middle (G), caudal (H), and accessory (I) lobar branches.

lung (they are the *vasa privata*, in contrast to the pulmonary vessels, the *vasa publica*).

Transection of a bronchus near its origin interrupts its bronchial vessels and results in a poor blood supply to the distal segment of the bronchus that is extrapulmonary. This situation is sufficient to prolong healing time if the bronchus is anastomosed without resection of most of the distal extrapulmonary segment of the bronchus.

The tracheal mucosa and its smooth muscle are innervated by the recurrent laryngeal nerve. In general, the receptors for vagal afferents are concentrated in the larger airways, including the trachea. Subepithelial receptors are responsible for initiating the cough reflex.[16]

Bronchial Tree

At its termination the trachea divides into two short principal bronchi, which subdivide successively into lobar, segmental, and several smaller generations of bronchi. The number of generations depends on the size of the animal and is proportional to the cube root of the body weight,[43] (i.e., between nine and ten generations in Labrador retrievers).[44]

Each of the six lobar bronchi is recognizable on a lateral radiograph. The origins of the two cranial lobar bronchi show as black overlapping discs near the tracheal bifurcation. The disc of the right cranial lobar bronchus is more cranial than the disc of the left. The caudal limit of these bronchi is super-

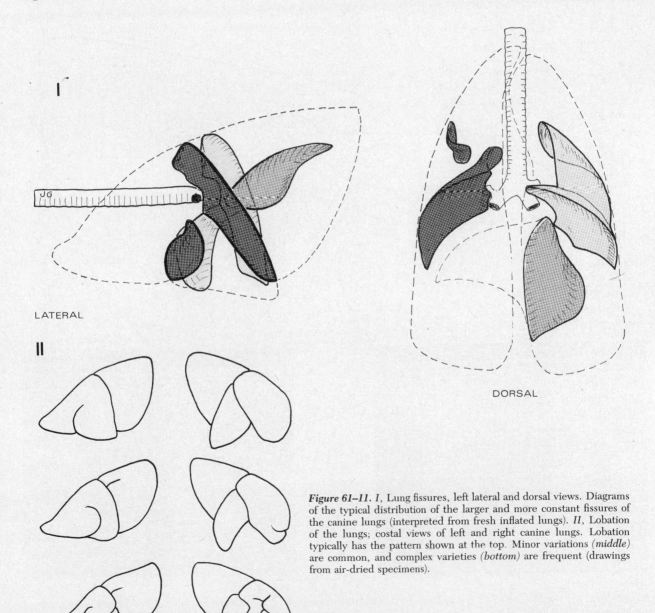

Figure 61–11. I, Lung fissures, left lateral and dorsal views. Diagrams of the typical distribution of the larger and more constant fissures of the canine lungs (interpreted from fresh inflated lungs). *II,* Lobation of the lungs; costal views of left and right canine lungs. Lobation typically has the pattern shown at the top. Minor variations *(middle)* are common, and complex varieties *(bottom)* are frequent (drawings from air-dried specimens).

imposed over the carina—the median crest of the tracheal bifurcation (Fig. 61–10).

The two lungs can be subdivided into about 30 bronchopulmonary segments, each a territory of lung supplied by a segmental bronchus. Each segment is independent, although some gaseous communication between adjacent segments can occur through the interalveolar pores of Kohn.[5] The precise definition of a segmental bronchus is somewhat arbitrary, because authors differ as to basis of nomenclature.[3, 9, 10, 75] It is possible to isolate one bronchopulmonary segment from its neighbors, but such isolation is rarely practical or necessary except in partial lobectomy for metastatic disease.

The tracheal cartilage rings gradually give way to variously shaped cartilaginous plates that surround the bronchi distal to the carina. The plates are oak leaf-shaped, overlapping in distribution, and attached distally to the submucosa. Bronchial transection leaves pieces of loosely attached cartilage along the incision.

Bronchioles are usually less than one millimeter in diameter, have no cartilaginous support, and usually have no glands in their walls.[56] In the cat, however, glands are present.[25] The terminal bronchioles give rise to respiratory bronchioles whose walls bear some alveoli. These in turn lead into alveolar ductules that end in alveolar saccules. The precise form of the terminal part of the airway is debatable, some authors claiming that the form in the dog is unique.[59] Most

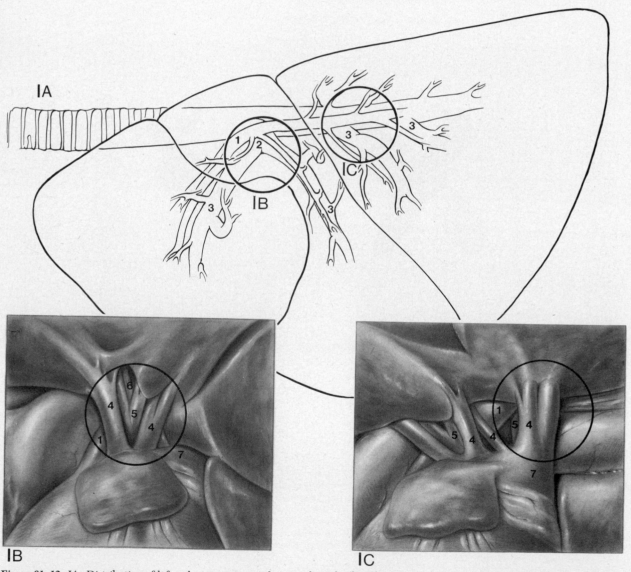

Figure 61–12. *IA*, Distribution of left pulmonary artery relative to bronchi *(line drawing)*. The left pulmonary artery *(1)* passes dorsal to the left segmental bronchus *(2)*, giving rise to lobar branches that are spatially related to the craniodorsal side of the lobar bronchi *(3)*. The detailed *inserts* illustrate the surgeon's view of the ventromedial aspect of the hilar region with the cranial and middle *(IB)* and caudal *(IC)* lobes of the left lung reflected dorsally. The locations of the left lobar veins *(4)*, bronchi *(5)*, and arteries *(6)*, and left atrium *(7)* are noted.

Illustration continued on opposite page

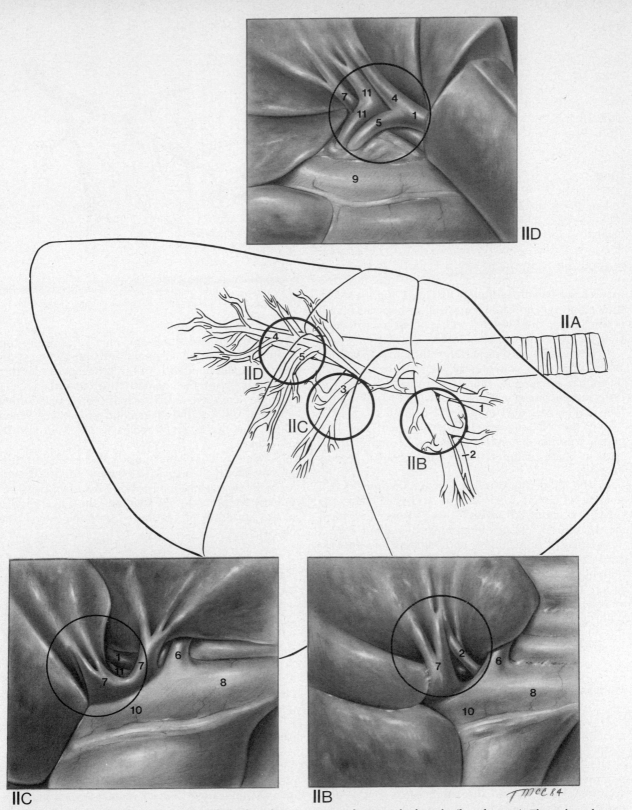

Figure 61–12 *Continued. IIA,* Distribution of the right pulmonary artery relative to the bronchi *(line drawing).* The right pulmonary artery *(1)* passes ventral to the carina to emerge at the hilus between the right cranial and middle lung lobes and courses dorsally to the bronchus of the middle lung lobe. The right cranial lobar artery *(2)* is located at the cranioventral edge of the bronchus, while the middle *(3)* and caudal *(4)* arteries are craniolateral to the respective bronchi. The artery of the accessory lobe *(5)* is ventral to its bronchus. The detailed *inserts* illustrate the surgeon's view of the ventral medial aspect of the hilar region with the cranial *(IIB),* middle *(IIC),* and caudal and accessory *(IID)* lobes of the right lung reflected dorsally. The locations of the azygous vein *(6),* lobar veins *(7),* cranial vena cava *(8),* caudal vena cava *(9),* and right atrium *(10)* are labeled. *IIB,* The cranial right lobar artery *(2)* crosses dorsal to the lobar veins *(7)* obscuring the lobar bronchus. *IIC,* The right pulmonary artery *(1)* is seen between and dorsal to the lobar veins *(7),* which cover most of the lobar bronchus *(11). IID,* Dorsal to the caudal vena cava *(9),* the terminal branching of the right pulmonary artery *(1)* gives rise to the caudal *(4)* and accessory *(5)* lobar branches coursing along their respective bronchi *(11).* Lobar vein *(7)* is passing ventral toward the left atrium.

cells lining the alveoli are squamous type I pneumocytes. Scattered among them are the cuboidal type II pneumocytes that secrete pulmonary surfactant.[25] Surfactant reduces the surface tension as alveoli shrink (by ten-fold when cat lungs deflate from 70 to 40 per cent capacity).

Lung

The lungs of the dog and cat are deeply fissured into distinct lobes. Fissuring allows the lungs to change shape with movements of the diaphragm or bending of the spine (Rouviere's law).[26, 66] Lobation is surgically convenient because it allows segments of lung to be isolated and excised. Because the fissures are usually obliquely disposed (Fig. 61–11A), they stand out on radiographs only when the pleura is thickened, fluid resides within them, or the adjacent parenchyme is consolidated.

Lobation follows typical rather than strict patterns. Both lungs are consistently divided by a caudal interlobar fissure into cranial and caudal lobes. The right lung is larger and further divided into a middle lobe and an accessory lobe (Fig. 61–11B). The cranial lobe of the left lung is usually partly subdivided into cranial and caudal parts. Resection of one of these parts is made simpler if the whole cranial lobe is excised.

In the moderately inflated state, the lung has a density of about 0.25. In the collapsed state, its density is about 0.5 owing to its content of residual air. In the fetal stage, lung density is about 1.06.[11] The density, functioning, and radiographic appearance are greatly influenced by gravity because the dependent parts are hypostatically congested and the upper parts are better inflated.[31] In human lungs, ventilation of air and perfusion of blood are not uniformly distributed, whereas recent work in standing dogs suggests that during tidal breathing, ventilation and perfusion are uniform.[4]

Pulmonary Vessels

The differences between pulmonary arteries and pulmonary veins are less striking than between their systemic counterparts because of the lower pressure of the pulmonary circuit.[50] Nevertheless, the large pulmonary trunk still has the creamy appearance of a systemic artery, and the subdivisions of the pulmonary arteries are typically of the elastic type. Elastic arteries accompany bronchi to form bronchovascular bundles; the vessels taper until about one millimeter in diameter, at which point they change to muscular vessels that continue to accompany the smaller airways. Radiographically, the pulmonary arteries run conspicuously lateral and adjacent to most of the airways (Fig. 61–12).

The pulmonary veins lie medial to the lobar bronchi. Their terminal portions may be seen subpleurally

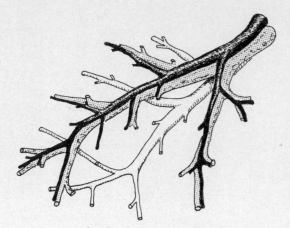

Figure 61–13. Peripheral pulmonary vessels. Pulmonary arteries *(black)* retain a close, segmental relation with the smaller bronchi *(gray)*, and veins *(white)* become intersegmental peripherally.

on the mediastinal surface of some lobes before they empty into the left atrium. More peripherally, the veins run independently of the bronchovascular bundles, usually intersegmentally (Fig. 61–13).

Some deoxygenated bronchial venous blood drains into and dilutes the oxygenated pulmonary venous blood, but the larger bronchial veins drain into the azygos vein.[56]

Pulmonary lymphatics mostly drain into the three groups of tracheobronchial lymph nodes located around the tracheal bifurcation. In a few dogs pulmonary lymph nodes are found on the dorsal surfaces of the lobar bronchi at the edge of the lung parenchyma.[29]

Pleura

The mesothelium of the carnivore is supported on an unusually thin connective tissue layer. The caudal mediastinal pleura is so thin that it is transparent and ruptures easily. It is not normally fenestrated,[29] although some authors claim that it often is.[73] After the mediastinum is perforated, air and fluids in one pleural sac can move into the other to give bilateral pneumothorax or hydrothorax. The pulmonary pleura is particularly thin in carnivores,[47, 48, 74] whereas the parietal pleura is of more variable thickness.

The lungs, covered with their own pulmonary pleura, are vacuum-packed in large sacs of parietal pleura that are collapsed around them. Consequently, folds exist where parietal pleura is in contact with more parietal pleura. The potential spaces between the two layers are known as pleural recesses; they can open to receive the expanding lung during inspiration or fill with air or fluid in pathological states. The costodiaphragmatic and costomediastinal recesses are perhaps the most important surgically, because they mark sites where the pleural cavities can be entered without danger of penetrating the lung. The costodiaphragmatic recess is about four centimeters wide in the dog and runs roughly parallel and cranial to the costal arch. The diaphragm is pushed hard against the costal wall for the length of this recess, with only a thin film of fluid separating the two layers of parietal pleura.

Elsewhere, the parietal pleura is in contact with visceral (pulmonary) pleura except for the thin film of lubricating fluid. The pressure within the pleural cavity and hence within the liquid is negative. The liquid pressure declines even more within the interlobar fissures where two layers of visceral pleura are in contact with each other.[52] When the chest cavity is opened, air rushes in, so that the lungs collapse and the thoracic cavity expands as the ribs spring apart. The pleural sacs extend a short distance cranial to the first rib as the pleural cupolae; puncture at this site can cause pneumothorax.

The mediastinal pleura encloses most of the thoracic viscera other than the lungs. Air that leaks along the sides of the bronchial tree can track to the hilus of the lungs and then around the trachea and other mediastinal structures to create a pneumomediastinum. The caudal lobe of the lung is tethered to the mediastinum by a slender web of pleura (pulmonary ligament) that runs for several centimeters caudal to the hilus. The accessory lobe of the lung is housed in a special compartment between the mediastinum on the left and the plica venae cavae on the right.

The parietal pleura is supplied by spinal nerves and is sensitive to tactile or thermal stimuli. The visceral pleura conveys afferents via autonomic nerves that only mediate pain.[76] Analgesic requirements relate to the chest wall rather than to the lung itself.

1. Adams, D. R., Deyong, D. W., and Griffith, R.: The lateral nasal gland of the dog: its structure and secretory content. J. Anat. 132:29, 1981.
2. Adams, D. R., and Hotchkiss, D. K.: The canine nasal mucosa. Anat. Histol. Embryol. 12:109, 1983.
3. Adrian, R. W.: Segmental anatomy of the cat's lung. Am. J. Vet. Res. 25:1724, 1964.
4. Amis, T. C., Jones, H. A., Rhodes, C. G., et al.: Regional distribution of pulmonary ventilation and perfusion in the conscious dog. Am. J. Vet. Res. 43:1972, 1982.
5. Angulo, A. W., Kownacki, V. P., and Hessert, E. C.: Additional evidence of collateral ventilation between adjacent bronchopulmonary segments. Anat. Rec. 130:207, 1958.
6. Arnoczky, S. P., and O'Neil, J. A.: Lung lobectomy. Vet. Clin. North Am. 9:219, 1979.
7. Ashdown, R. R., and Lea, T.: The larynx of the Basenji dog. J. Small Anim. Pract. 20:675, 1979.
8. Baker, G. J.: Surgery of the canine pharynx and larynx. J. Small Anim. Pract. 13:505, 1972.
9. Barone, R.: Arbre bronchique et vaisseaux pulmonaires chez le chien. Compt. Rend. de l'assoc. Anat XLIV Reunion, 1972, pp. 132–144.
10. Barone, R: Les images radiologiques normales des poumons et de leur arbre broncho-vasculaire chez le chien. Rev. Med. Vet. de Toulouse 121:1, 1970.
11. Barone, R.: Anatomie Comparée des mammifères domestiques. Tome 3, Fasc. 1: Splanchnologie. Lab. d'Anatomie, École Nationale Vétérinaire, Lyon, 1976.
12. Bast, T. H.: The maxillary sinus of the dog, with special reference to certain new structures probably sensory in nature. Am. J. Anat. 33:449, 1924.
13. Becker, R. F., and King, J. E.: Delineation of the nasal air streams in the living dog. Arch. Otolaryngol. 65:428, 1957.
14. Blanton, P. L., and Biggs, N. L.: The paranasal sinuses: 400 years of controversy. Am. J. Anat. 124:135, 1969.
15. Blatt, C. M., Taylor, C. R., and Habal, M. B.: Thermal panting in dogs: the lateral nasal gland, a source of water for evaporative cooling. Science 177:804, 1972.
16. Bojrab, M. J., and Nafe, L. L.: Tracheal reconstructive surgery. J. Am. Anim. Hosp. Assoc. 12:622, 1976.
17. Bojsen-Moller, F.: Topography of the nasal glands in rats and some other mammals. Anat. Rec. 150:11, 1964.
18. Bojsen-Moller, F., and Fahrenkrug, J.: Nasal swell bodies and cyclic changes in the air passage of the rat and rabbit nose. J. Anat. 110:25, 1971.
19. Bradley, O. C., and Graham, T.: Topographical Anatomy of the Dog. 5th ed. Oliver & Boyd, Edinburgh, 1948.
20. Bridger, G. P.: Mucociliary function in dog's larynx and trachea. Laryngoscope 82:218, 1972.
21. Calhoun, M. L., and Stinson, A. W.: Integument. In Dellman, H-D., and Brown, E. M. (eds.): Textbook of Veterinary Histology, 2nd ed. Lea & Febiger, Philadelphia, 1981.
22. Christensen, G. C., and Toussaint, S.: Vasculature of external nares and related areas in the dog. J. Am. Vet. Med. Assoc. 131:504, 1957.
23. Cook, W. R.: Observations on the upper respiratory tract of the dog and cat. J. Small Anim. Pract. 5:309, 1964.
24. Dawes, J. D. K.: The course of the nasal airstreams. J. Laryngol. Otol. 66:583, 1952.
25. Dellman, H-D.: Respiratory system. In Dellman, H-D., and Brown, E. M. (eds.): Textbook of Veterinary Histology. 2nd ed. Lea & Febiger, Philadephia, 1981.
26. Diaconescu, N., and Veleanu, C.: Die Rolle der Brustwirbelsaulendynamik bei der Lobierung des Lungenparenchyms. Anat. Anz. 117:96, 1965.
27. Droscher, V. B.: The Magic of the Senses. W. H. Allen, London, 1969.
28. Evans, H. E.: The lateral nasal gland and its duct in the dog. Anat. Rec. 187:574, 1977.
29. Evans, H. E., and Christensen, G. C.: Miller's Anatomy of the Dog. 2nd ed. W. B. Saunders, Philadelphia, 1979.
30. Gaskell, C. J.: The radiographic anatomy of the pharynx and larynx of the dog. J. Small Anim. Pract. 15:89, 1974.
31. Glazier, J. B., Hughes, J. M. B., Maloney, J. E., et al.: Vertical gradient of alveolar size in lungs of dogs frozen intact. J. Appl. Physiol. 23:694, 1967.
32. Goldberg, M. B., Langman, V. A., Taylor, C. R.: Panting in dogs: paths of air flow in response to heat and exercise. Resp. Physiol. 43:327, 1980.
33. Haines, R. W., and Mohiuddin, A.: Handbook of Human Embryology. 5th ed. Churchill Livingstone, Edinburgh, 1972.
34. Hall, L. W., and Clarke, K. W.: Veterinary Anaesthesia. 8th ed. Bailliere Tindall, London, 1983.
35. Hammer, D. L., and Sacks, M.: The palate. In Bojrab, M. J. (ed.): Current Techniques in Small Animal Surgery. Lea & Febiger, Philadelphia, 1975.
36. Hare, W. C. D.: Carnivore respiratory system. In Getty, R. (ed.): Sisson and Grossman's The Anatomy of the Domestic Animals. 5th ed. W. B. Saunders, Philadelphia, 1975.
37. Harvey, C. E.: Stenotic nares surgery in brachycephalic dogs. J. Am. Anim. Hosp. Assoc. 18:535, 1982.
38. Harvey, C. E.: Soft palate resection in brachycephalic dogs. J. Am. Anim. Hosp. Assoc. 18:538, 1982.
39. Harvey, C. E.: Everted laryngeal saccule surgery in brachycephalic dogs. J. Am. Anim. Hosp. Assoc. 18:545, 1982.
40. Harvey, C. E.: Partial laryngectomy in brachycephalic dogs. J. Am. Anim. Hos. Assoc. 18:548, 1982.
41. Harvey, C. E., and Fink, E. A.: Tracheal diameter: analysis of radiographic measurements in brachycephalic and non-brachycephalic dogs. J. Am. Anim. Hosp. Assoc. 18:570, 1982.
42. Horning, J. G., McKee, A. J., Keller, H. E., and Smith, K. K.: Nose printing your cat and dog patients. Vet. Med. 21:432, 1926. (Cited by Evans and Christensen[29].)
43. Horsfeld, K.: Postnatal growth of the dog's bronchial tree. Resp. Physiol. 29:185, 1977.

44. Horsfeld, K., and Cumming, G.: Morphology of the bronchial tree in the dog. Resp. Physiol. 26:173, 1976.

45. Knudson, R. J., and Knudson, D. E.: Pressure-flow relationships in isolated canine trachea. J. Appl. Physiol. 35:804, 1973.

46. Knudson, R. J., and Knudson, D. E.: Effect of muscle contraction of flow limiting collapse of isolated canine trachea. J. Appl. Physiol. 38:125, 1975.

47. McLaughlin, R. F., Tyler, W. S., and Canada, R. O.: Subgross pulmonary anatomy in various mammals and man. J.A.M.A. 175:694, 1961.

48. McLaughlin, R. F., Tyler, W. S., and Canada, R. C.: A study of the subgross pulmonary anatomy in various mammals. Am. J. Anat. 108:149, 1965.

49. Leighton, R. L.: The larynx. In Archibald, J. (ed.): Canine Surgery. American Veterinary Publishers, Santa Barbara, 1974.

50. Michel, R. P.: Arteries and veins of the normal dog lung: qualitative and quantitative structural differences. Am. J. Anat. 164:227, 1982.

51. Miserocchi, G., and Agostini, E.: Longitudinal forces acting on the trachea. Resp. Physiol. 17:62, 1973.

52. Miserocchi, G., Nakamura, T., Mariani, E., and Negrini, D.: Pleural liquid pressure over the interlobar mediastinal and diaphragmatic surfaces of the lung. Resp. Physiol. 46:61, 1981.

53. Moe, H., and Bojsen-Moller, F.: The fine structure of the lateral nasal gland (Steno's gland) of the rat. J. Ultrastructure Res. 36:127, 1971.

54. Moore, K. L.: Before We Are Born: Basic Embryology and Birth Defects. 2nd ed. W. B. Saunders, Philadelphia, 1983.

55. Mortola, J. P., and Fisher, J. T.: Comparative morphology of the trachea in newborn animals. Resp. Physiol. 39:297, 1980.

56. Nickel, R., Schummer, A., Seiferle, E., and Sack, W. O.: The Viscera of the Domestic Mammals. Verlag Paul Parey, Berlin, 1973.

57. O'Brien, J. A., Harvey, C. E., and Tucker, J. A.: The larynx of the dog: its normal radiographic anatomy. J. Am. Vet. Radiol. Soc. 10:38, 1969.

58. Palombini, B., and Coburn, R. E.: Control of the compressibility of the canine trachea. Resp. Physiol. 15:365, 1972.

59. Park, J. F., Clarke, W. J., and Bair, W. J.: The respiratory system. In Anderson, A. C. (ed.): The Beagle as an Experimental Dog. Iowa State University Press, Ames, 1970.

60. Patterson, J. M.: Nasal solar dermatitis in the dog—a method of tattooing. J. Am. Anim. Hosp. Assoc. 14:370, 1978.

61. Popovic, S.: Eine Darstellung der morphologischen Eigentumlichkeiten des knorpeligen Nasengerustes bei Haussaugetieren. Anat. Anz. 114:379, 1964.

62. Reeves, J. T.: Microradiography of intrapulmonary bronchial veins of the dog. Anat. Rec. 159:255, 1967.

63. Remmers, J. E., and Gautier, H.: Neural mechanisms of feline purring. Resp. Physiol. 16:351, 1972.

64. Rex, M. A. E.: A review of the structural and functional basis of laryngospasm and a discussion of the nerve pathways involved in the reflex and its clinical significance in man and animals. Brit. J. Anaesth. 42:891, 1970.

65. Rex, M. A. E.: Laryngospasm and respiratory changes in the cat produced by mechanical stimulation of the pharynx and respiratory tract: problems of intubation in the cat. Br. J. Anaesth. 45:54, 1971.

66. Rouviere, H., and Cordier, G.: La raison d'être des fissures. Loi de fissuration. C.R. Ass. Anat. 29th réunion, Lisbonne, 1933, pp. 578–585.

67. Schaller, O., Habel, R. E., and Frewein, J.: Nomina Anatomica Veterinaria. International Committee for Veterinary Anatomical Nomenclature, Vienna, 1973.

68. Schmidt-Nielsen, K., Bretz, W. L., and Taylor, C. R.: Panting in dogs: unidirectional air flow over evaporative surfaces. Science 169:1102, 1970.

69. Schummer, A., Wilkens, H., Vollmerhaus, B., and Habermehl, K. H.: The Circulatory System, the Skin and Cutaneous Organs of the Domestic Mammals. Paul Parey, Berlin, 1981.

70. Spira, H. R.: Canine Terminology. Harper & Row, Sydney, 1982.

71. Tandler, B., Sherman, J. M., and Boat, T. F.: Surface architecture of the mucosal epithelium of the cat trachea. I: Cartilaginous portion. Am. J. Anat. 168:119, 1983.

72. Tandler, B., Sherman, J. M., and Boat, T. F.: Surface architecture of the mucosal epithelium of the cat trachea. II: Structure and dynamics of the membranous portion. Am. J. Anat. 168:133, 1983.

73. Ticer, J. W., and Brown, S. G.: Thoracic trauma. In Ettinger, S. J. (ed.): Textbook of Veterinary Internal Medicine. W. B. Saunders, Philadelphia, 1975.

74. Trautmann, A., and Febiger, J.: Fundamentals of the Histology of Domestic Animals. Habel, R. E., and Biberstein, E. L., transl. Comstock Publishing Associates, Ithaca, 1957.

75. Tucker, J. L., and Krementz, E. T.: Anatomical corrosion specimens. II: Bronchopulmonary anatomy in the dog. Anat. Rec. 127:667, 1957.

76. Warwick, R., and Williams, P. L. (eds.): Gray's Anatomy. 35th ed. Longman, London, 1973.

77. Wright, N. G., and Brown, R. M. H., McCandlish, I. A. P., et al.: Patterns of cilia formation in the lower respiratory tract of the dog: a scanning electron microscope study. Res. Vet. Sci. 34:340, 1983.

62 Pathophysiology of Surgically Correctable Diseases of the Respiratory System

Alan Tucker

The purpose of this chapter is to provide a sound physiological base for surgeons diagnosing and treating diseases and injuries of the respiratory system. Emphasis is placed on determining the specific causes of respiratory dysfunction and determining potential consequences of respiratory dysfunction on gas exchange.

PHYSIOLOGY OF THE NORMAL LUNG

The primary function of mammalian lungs is to exchange gas between atmospheric air and venous blood returning from metabolizing cells. Secondary functions include warming and humidifying inspired air, vocalization, and temperature regulation. The lung circulation has other nonrespiratory functions, such as serving as a filter to remove embolic material from the blood and activation and metabolism of vasoactive substances in blood.[3, 23, 64] To ensure adequate gas exchange, the following processes must be maintained: (1) alveolar ventilation; (2) even distribution of inspired gas; (3) even perfusion of pulmonary capillaries; (4) diffusion of gases across the alveolar-capillary membrane; (5) matching of ventilation and perfusion; and (6) gas transport in blood. A working knowledge of these processes of gas exchange is essential to understand the pathophysiology of respiratory dysfunctions. The mechanisms of respiratory control and lung defense mechanisms are also discussed, completing this review of lung function.

Functions of the Airways

The olfactory sense is highly developed in both the dog and cat. The ethmoturbinates provide the primary olfactory mucous membrane, whereas the maxilloturbinates serve as accessory regions of olfaction and primary regions of humidification of inspired air. The maxilloturbinates branch extensively and occupy much of the space in the nasal chamber, resulting in high resistance to airflow. Inflammation or edema of the mucous membranes in this region further increases resistance to airflow, causing dyspnea and labored breathing. The branching maxilloturbinates also participate in lung defense by trapping inspired particles and foreign bodies. Most foreign bodies lodge in the anterior third of the nasal chamber, where they can be seen and removed.[19] The two lateral nasal glands, located in each maxillary sinus, supply a large part of the water for evaporative cooling during panting in dogs.[7]

The pharynx, a relatively large structure, is a frequent site of foreign body penetration. The soft palate is a thick, fleshy structure in the dog. Prolongation of the soft palate can give rise to a variety of clinical problems and signs. The canine larynx possesses deep, laryngeal saccules and prominent vocal cords, performs the usual functions of respiration and phonation, as in other animals, and regulates temperature.[67] Panting in the dog puts extra stress on the larynx, particularly in brachycephalic dogs, in which the airway is already restricted. The feline larynx has a highly sensitive mucous membrane. Stimulation of this mucous membrane can precipitate violent coughing and laryngospasm. The epiglottis is well developed in dogs and cats and functions to close the larynx during deglutition. Flaccidity of the epiglottis often causes laryngeal obstruction and increased resistance to airflow.

The trachea is the major airway leading to the bronchial tree, which, despite incomplete cartilage rings, can be compressed or collapsed or can become stenotic.[38, 40]

Ventilation—Mechanics of Respiration

Normal resting ventilation is accomplished primarily by contraction of the diaphragm.[12, 44] During inspiration, the diaphragm moves caudad and pulls the caudal surfaces of the lung with it. During expiration, which is normally passive, the diaphragm relaxes and the elastic recoil of the lungs and chest wall returns the lung to its pre-inspiratory position. When ventilatory demands are increased, other muscles are used.[51] The external intercostals, sternocleidomastoids, ventral serrati, and scaleni aid inspiration by moving the ribs in a rostral direction, thus pulling the lung surfaces outward. Contraction of the internal intercostals and abdominal recti aids in forceful expiration and during periods of labored breathing. These changes in chest cavity volume and the subsequent changes in lung volume produced by respiratory skeletal muscle contraction initiate the movement of air through the airways and down to the alveoli.

Respiratory Pressures

Air moves into and out of the lungs by moving along pressure gradients generated by changes in the volume of the chest cavity. Pressure within the alveoli becomes subatmospheric during inspiration, returning to atmospheric pressure at the end of inspiration (Fig. 62–1). This small pressure gradient is sufficient to move air through the airways to the alveoli. As air moves into the lungs, the alveolar pressure returns toward atmospheric pressure so that at end-inspiration there is no pressure gradient and thus no air flow. A positive alveolar pressure is produced during expiration as the chest wall and lungs recoil (see Fig. 62–1), producing a pressure gradient that pushes air out of the lungs. Again, at end-expiration there is no pressure gradient and no air flow.

The magnitude of the alveolar pressure change is dependent on the movement of the diaphragm and chest wall and on intrapleural pressure.[12] This pressure, to which the lung surface is exposed, is negative relative to atmospheric pressure. The negative intrapleural pressure is due, in part, to the continuous absorption of pleural fluid and air by the visceral pleural capillaries and to the elastic recoil of the lungs, which tends to pull the lung surfaces away from the parietal pleura of the chest wall.[31] Direct measurements of intrapleural pressure are difficult to make; however, estimates can be obtained by measuring esophageal pressure with a balloon catheter. During the breathing cycle, intrapleural pressure changes as shown in Figure 62–1. As the diaphragm and chest wall move away from the lung surfaces during inspiration, intrapleural pressure becomes more negative. At end-inspiration, intrapleural pressure is lowest because the diaphragm and chest wall are farthest from their resting positions. During expiration, intrapleural pressure returns to its pre-inspiratory value (see Fig. 62–1). Intrapleural pressures remain subatmospheric throughout the respiratory cycle during quiet resting breathing but can become positive during a forced active expiration.

Forces to Be Overcome During Ventilation

The change in intrapleural pressure during quiet breathing is approximately 3 cm H_2O, but the change in alveolar pressure during the same cycle is only 1 cm H_2O. This pressure change of 1 cm H_2O is the energy used to move air into the lungs. The remaining 2 cm H_2O change is used to overcome several forces opposing expansion of the lung.[47] These include elastic structures that have to be stretched, airways that offer resistance to airflow, tissue that offers resistance to distortion, and surface tension in the alveoli that limits alveolar expansion.

Compliance. Energy is required to stretch the elastic components of the lung and chest wall during inspiration. The energy requirements can be estimated by a pressure-volume curve (Fig. 62–2). This curve describes the relationship between lung volume changes (ΔV) produced by changes in pressure (ΔP) throughout the range of lung volumes.[57] The slope of the pressure-volume curve ($\Delta V/\Delta P$) at any particular point is the pulmonary compliance at that lung volume; the steeper the slope, the greater the compliance. Thus, the greatest pulmonary compli-

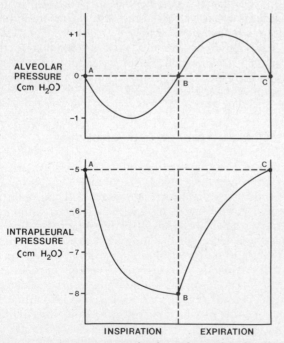

Figure 62–1. Changes in intra-alveolar and intrapleural pressure during one breathing cycle. Point A is pre-inspiration, point B is at end-inspiration, and point C is at end-expiration. (Redrawn from West, J. B.: *Respiratory Physiology—The Essentials*, 2nd ed. Williams & Wilkins, Baltimore, 1979, p. 103.)

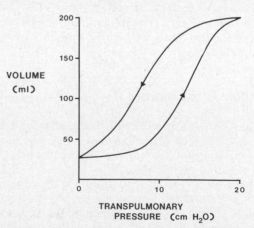

Figure 62–2. Pressure-volume curve in isolated dog lungs. Note the phenomenon of hysteresis during inspiration and expiration. (Redrawn from Bruderman, I., Somers, K., Hamilton, W. K., Tooley, W. H., and Butler, J.: Effect of surface tension on circulation in the excised lungs of dogs. J. Appl. Physiol. *19*:707, 1964.)

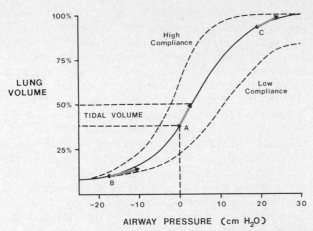

Figure 62–3. Pressure-volume curves in artificially ventilated lungs. Point A represents the high compliance normally seen during the tidal volume breathing, point B represents low compliance at low lung volumes, and point C represents low lung compliance at high lung volumes. The left-shifted curve demonstrates a pressure-volume curve in highly compliant lungs, such as exhibited in early emphysema. The right-shifted curve demonstrates a pressure-volume curve in low compliant lungs, such as exhibited with lung fibrosis.

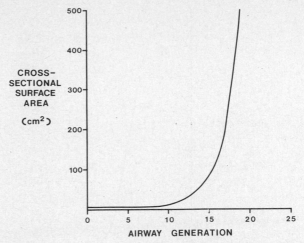

Figure 62–4. The rapid increase in the total cross-sectional surface area of the airways seen with increasing airway generation. (Redrawn from West, J. B.: *Respiratory Physiology—The Essentials,* 2nd ed. Williams & Wilkins, Baltimore, 1979, p. 7.)

ance is usually measured in the tidal volume range (Fig. 62–3). At both high and low lung volumes, compliance of the normal respiratory system is reduced, indicating that more energy is required to expand the lungs by the same volume. Normal values for pulmonary compliance in dogs and cats are shown in Table 62–1. Lung compliance can be reduced by lung fibrosis or pulmonary edema. In these less expansible lungs, more energy is required to expand the lungs during inspiration (see Fig. 62–3). The energy used to stretch the elastic structures of the lung and chest wall is energy that is stored, not dissipated. During subsequent expiration this energy (*lung elastic recoil*) is used to move air back through the airways. The lower the pulmonary compliance, the greater the elastic recoil. Thus, some of the energy used in the inspiratory effort is regained during expiration, even when compliance is markedly reduced. If lung compliance is increased, as in normal aged dogs, a loss of lung recoil is apparent.[60]

Airway Resistance. The branching pattern of the airways offers resistance to airflow. At branch points, each proximal airway divides into two smaller distal airways, each of which has a higher resistance than the proximal airway. However, the two distal airways together offer less resistance to airflow than does the single proximal airway. This airway branching pattern results in an exponential increase in the cross-sectional area of the airways (Fig. 62–4). Since resistance to airflow depends on the total number of airways, airway resistance decreases as the air moves more distally into the lung (Fig. 62–5). The external nares, nasal cavity, pharynx, larynx, and trachea offer the greatest resistance to airflow, whereas the respiratory and terminal bronchioles offer the least resistance. Total airway resistance has been partitioned for the dog lung.[24, 45, 52] During quiet respiration, inspiratory resistance was estimated as 79 per cent nasal, 6 per cent laryngeal, and 15 per cent small airway. Expiratory resistance was estimated as 74 per cent nasal, 3 per cent laryngeal, and 23 per cent small airway.[52] Measurements of total airway resistance (pressure gradient along the airways/airflow) reflect airway resistance of the upper airways and are not greatly affected by changes in lower airway diameter. It is for this reason that small airway disease is difficult to diagnose until the disease has progressed to the stage at which small airway resistance is markedly increased. Normal values for total airway resistance in dogs and cats are shown in Table 62–1. Because of the shape of their head, brachycephalic dogs (e.g., English bulldogs, Boston terriers, pugs, Shih Tzu, Pekingese, and boxers) have increased nasopharyn-

TABLE 62–1.   Pulmonary Compliance and Airway Resistance in Normal Dogs and Cats*

Species	Body Weight (kg)	Lung Weight (g)	Pulmonary Compliance (ml/cm H$_2$O)	Lung Compliance (ml/cm H$_2$O)	Respiratory Resistance (cm H$_2$O/ml/sec)	Upper Airway Resistance (cm H$_2$O/ml/sec)
Dog (large)	26.0	294	48.1	65.3	0.008	—
Dog (small)	13.6	112	16.6	20.1	0.008	0.0042
Cat	3.0	24	10.1	14.5	0.020	0.0407

*Data obtained from Bennett, F. M., and Tenney, S. M.: Comparative mechanics of mammalian respiratory system. Resp. Physiol. *49*:131, 1982.

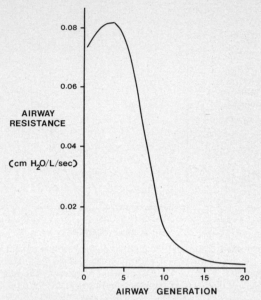

Figure 62–5. Changes in airway resistance seen with increasing airway generation. Note the very high resistance in the large airways. (Redrawn from Pedley, T. S., Schrater, R. C., and Sudlow, M. F.: The prediction of pressure drop and variation of resistance within the human bronchial airways. Resp. Physiol. 9:387, 1970.)

geal resistance[38] and may be severely compromised without additional insult to the respiratory system.

Airway resistance has to be overcome during both inspiration and expiration. The energy (pressure gradient) used during inspiration is supplied by respiratory muscle contraction. During expiration, the energy used to overcome airway resistance is normally derived from the energy stored as elastic lung recoil. When airway resistance is increased, more energy must be generated to move air through the narrowed airways. Airway diameters can be altered by either mechanical, neural, or chemical actions. Airway obstructions (mucus, edema, inflammatory exudate, neoplasms, or foreign bodies) block the airways, reduce the diameter, and increase airway resistance.

Another mechanical effect on airway resistance is produced by changes in lung volume during the process of ventilation itself.[9] As lung volume increases during inspiration, airway resistance decreases because airways are pulled open by the expanding parenchyma. During expiration, lung volume decreases and the tension on the airways is removed. The airways return to smaller diameters with higher resistance. Small airway closure can also occur at low lung volumes, trapping air distal to the site of closure.[75]

Neural control mechanisms play an important role in regulating airway caliber and tone.[59] Parasympathetic stimulation, with the release of acetylcholine, causes bronchoconstriction and increased airway resistance. Sympathetic stimulation, on the other hand, causes bronchodilatation due to the action of norepinephrine on beta-adrenergic receptors. Vasoactive

agents also modify bronchomotor tone.[65] Both histamine, by acting on histamine H_1 receptors,[33] and 5-hydroxytryptamine (serotonin)[13] induce bronchial smooth muscle contraction. Prostaglandins and leukotrienes can also exert marked bronchoconstrictor actions. Reduction in the P_{CO_2} in the air flowing through the airways also causes bronchoconstriction.

Surface Tension. Energy is used to overcome the tension at the surface of the alveoli.[15] When two dissimilar substances come into contact at a common surface, a surface tension develops. An air-liquid interface generates a high surface tension that resists deformation. Since the alveolar surfaces are air-liquid interfaces, surface tension should be high. However, measurements of surface tension indicate that the liquid lining the alveoli has a low surface tension (Fig. 62–6). This is due to the surface-active phospholipid—surfactant—synthesized by alveolar type II cells and secreted onto the alveolar surfaces.[37] In addition to reducing surface tension, surfactant also varies surface tension, depending on the size of the individual alveoli. Laplace's law, describing the pressure and surface tension of bubbles

$$P = \frac{2\,T}{r}$$

where P is the pressure inside the bubble,
T is the surface tension, and
r is the radius of the bubble,

indicates that as the area of the bubble changes at constant surface tension, the pressure within the bubble changes accordingly. Thus, a small bubble has high pressure. If alveoli followed the same physical principle, large alveoli would have relatively low pressures, whereas small alveoli would have relatively high pressures. Since alveoli are interconnected, small alveoli should collapse into large alveoli, resulting in areas of lung with overexpanded alveoli and areas of lung with collapsed alveoli (atelectasis). In the lung, however, surfactant serves to

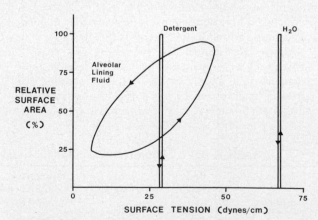

Figure 62–6. Plots of surface tension and area for water, detergent, and washings of alveolar lining fluid. Note that the alveolar lining fluid exhibits a low surface tension with a small area and a higher surface tension with a larger area. (Redrawn from West, J. B.: *Respiratory Physiology—The Essentials,* 2nd ed. Williams & Wilkins, Baltimore, 1979, p. 94.)

vary the surface tension as the size of an alveolus changes. The ability of surfactant to reduce surface tension depends on its relative concentration on the alveolar surfaces. In small alveoli, surfactant reduces surface tension to the extent that the ratio of surface tension to radius remains constant; thus, intra-alveolar pressure does not change. In large alveoli, surfactant is spread thinly on the surface and reduces surface tension to a lesser extent, so the surface tension increases as the radius increases. This concentration dependence of surfactant allows alveoli of different sizes to coexist and lessens the development of atelectasis. The alveolar surface tension also contributes to lung recoil. Some of the energy used to expand the alveoli is stored as increased surface tension and is used during the following expiration to return alveoli to pre-inspiratory volumes.

Surfactant serves the following functions: (1) it indirectly increases lung compliance by lowering surface tension; (2) it promotes alveolar stability and minimizes atelectasis; and (3) it greatly reduces the amount of work needed to expand the lungs. Surfactant deficiency causes respiratory distress in the neonate. These patients are affected by "stiff" lungs, areas of atelectasis, pulmonary edema, and labored breathing. Since the surfactant system is one of the last to mature during gestation, premature birth can result in respiratory distress.

Work of Breathing

Energy is used throughout the respiratory cycle to move air into and out of the lungs. During normal quiet breathing this energy is produced by contraction of the inspiratory muscles. The intrapleural pressure change, generated primarily by diaphragmatic contraction,[62] is the energy used to overcome the elastic, resistive, and surface tension forces in the lung (Fig. 62–7). If diaphragmatic function is reduced (e.g., phrenic nerve compression or trauma or bilateral phrenic nerve resection), the intercostal and accessory muscles become the primary muscles of respiration. Expiration is normally passive, with the energy used to overcome airway resistance derived from the energy stored in elastic structures and as increased surface tension. When lung function is depressed, expiration becomes active as additional energy is supplied by contraction of expiratory muscles, greatly increasing the energy requirements for ventilation.[63]

Alveolar Ventilation

Expired ventilation can be measured by determining respiratory frequency and the tidal volume of each breath. For diagnostic purposes, it is not the total volume of air moved that is important but, rather, whether the ventilation is adequate to meet metabolic needs. Therefore, measurements of alveolar ventilation are necessary. Expired ventilation can be subdivided into alveolar ventilation and dead space ventilation. Alveolar ventilation includes all gases participating in gas exchange. Dead space ventilation includes air in the conducting airways (anatomical dead space) and air in alveoli that are not perfused and are not participating in gas exchange. The total dead space volume can be calculated as follows:

$$V_D = \frac{Pa_{CO_2} - PE_{CO_2}}{Pa_{CO_2}} \times V_T$$

where Pa_{CO_2} is the partial pressure of CO_2 in arterial blood,

PE_{CO_2} is the partial pressure of CO_2 in mixed expired air,

V_T is tidal volume.

Note: PA_{CO_2} (partial pressure of CO_2 in alveolar gas) can be substituted for Pa_{CO_2}.

Then, alveolar ventilation can be calculated as follows:

$$\dot{V}_A = f(V_E - V_D) \text{ or } \dot{V}_A = \dot{V}_E - \dot{V}_D$$

where f is the respiratory frequency,

V_E is the expired volume,

$\dot{V}_E$ is the expired ventilation, and

$\dot{V}_D$ is the dead space ventilation.

Alveolar ventilation is indirectly related to arterial levels of carbon dioxide:

$$Pa_{CO_2} = \frac{\dot{V}_{CO_2} \times 0.863}{\dot{V}_A}$$

where $\dot{V}_{CO_2}$ = CO_2 production by metabolizing cells.

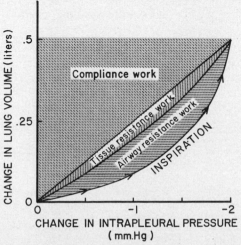

Figure 62–7. Graphical representation of three types of work accomplished during inspiration: (1) compliance work; (2) tissue resistance work; and (3) airway resistance work. (Reprinted with permission from Guyton, A. C.: *Textbook of Medical Physiology,* 6th ed. W. B. Saunders, Philadelphia, 1981, p. 479.)

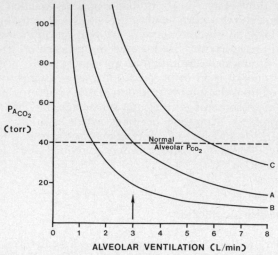

Figure 62–8. Effect of changes in alveolar ventilation on alveolar P_{CO_2} in a dog at three levels of CO_2 production: *A*, 140 ml CO_2/min; *B*, 70 ml CO_2/min; and *C*, 280 ml CO_2/min.

Small changes in alveolar ventilation can markedly affect carbon dioxide levels (Fig. 62–8) and, subsequently, acid-base balance. This intimate relationship between alveolar ventilation and carbon dioxide is considered again in the discussion of control of ventilation.

The maintenance of constant alveolar ventilation is essential during artificial respiration of an anesthetized patient or one in which respiratory function is depressed. Inappropriate settings on the respirator can lead either to hypoventilation, with consequent hypoxemia, hypercapnia, and acidosis, or to hyperventilation, with consequent hypocapnia and alkalosis. In addition, intermittent positive pressure ventilation can have significant cardiovascular effects. When air is forced into the lung under positive pressure, blood flow into the chest from the peripheral veins is impeded. Thus, venous return falls and cardiac output is reduced during periods of increased pressure. Exposure of the lung to airway pressures of greater than 20 torr may cause overinflation of lung units and in diseased lungs may cause alveolar rupture and pneumothorax. Positive end-expiratory pressure (PEEP) can also alter cardiorespiratory dynamics. In particular, PEEP has been shown to reduce cardiac output[56] and impair gas exchange.[20]

Blood Flow—Perfusion of Pulmonary Capillaries

Another important component of gas exchange is maintenance of even perfusion of pulmonary capillaries with hypoxemic, hypercapnic blood. This function is performed by the pulmonary circulation. In addition to gas exchange, the pulmonary circulation serves as a reservoir of blood for left ventricular ejection and a filter to remove embolic material and

TABLE 62–2. Pulmonary and Systemic Hemodynamics in an Awake Dog

	Pulmonary	Systemic
Mean arterial pressure (torr)	15	100
Mean capillary pressure (torr)	10	20
Mean atrial pressure (torr)	5 (left)	1 (right)
Cardiac output (L/min)	3.0	3.0
Vascular resistance (torr/L/min)	3.3	33.0

is important in the synthesis, activation, and metabolism of several vasoactive agents.

The pulmonary circulation differs from the systemic circulation in several respects. The pulmonary circulation is a low-pressure, low-resistance vascular bed (Table 62–2). Pulmonary arterial pressure is approximately one-seventh and pulmonary vascular resistance (PVR) approximately one-tenth those of comparable systemic values.[27] The vascular resistance is distributed evenly between the arterial, capillary, and venular beds. Several passive hemodynamic and respiratory factors can influence PVR. Increases in pulmonary arterial pressure and/or pulmonary blood flow (cardiac output) result in reductions in PVR[75] (Fig. 62–9A). This paradoxical effect is caused by the

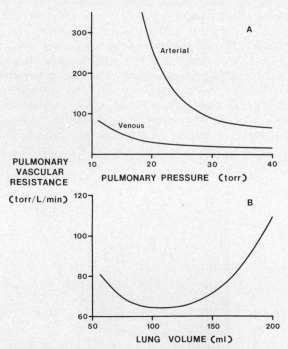

Figure 62–9. Changes in pulmonary vascular resistance in isolated dog lungs. *A*, Changes caused by changes in pulmonary arterial or venous pressure. (Redrawn from West, J. B., and Dollery, C. T.: Distribution of blood flow and the pressure-flow relations of the whole lung. J. Appl. Physiol. *20*:175, 1965.) *B*, Changes caused by changes in lung volume at constant capillary transmural pressure. (Redrawn from West, J. B.: *Respiratory Physiology—The Essentials*, 2nd ed. Williams & Wilkins, Baltimore, 1979, pp. 37 and 39.)

recruitment of previously closed capillaries and the distention of previously open capillaries. The increased cross-sectional surface area of the capillary bed decreases vascular resistance. Obstruction of pulmonary vessels by embolic material (e.g., thromboemboli, heartworms) increases vascular resistance. This increased PVR can cause pulmonary hypertension and right ventricular hypertrophy. Changes in lung volume also influence the caliber of vessels within the lung[54, 75] (Fig. 62–9B). At low lung volumes, the expanding forces exerted on the lungs are reduced and the large vessels tend to collapse, increasing their vascular resistance. At high lung volumes, the greater expanding forces tend to pull open the larger vessels, simultaneously compressing the small vessels within the alveolar walls by the tension applied to elastic structures within the walls. This effect predominates, and vascular resistance increases at high lung volumes.

Several active mechanisms also alter PVR. Stimulation of the sympathetic nervous system generally causes a slight increase in PVR and a decrease in vascular compliance.[35] Parasympathetic stimulation has little effect, although acetylcholine is a pulmonary vasodilator. Vasoactive agents that alter systemic vascular tone have similar actions on the pulmonary vascular bed, with a few exceptions.[5, 69] Angiotensin II and several of the prostanoids (PGF$_{2\alpha}$, PGH$_2$, thromboxane A$_2$, leukotrienes) are vasoconstrictors, whereas bradykinin and other prostanoids (PGE$_1$, prostacyclin) are vasodilators. Histamine can be either a vasoconstrictor or vasodilator, depending on which receptors are activated (H$_1$ and H$_2$ receptors, respectively).[72] 5-Hydroxytryptamine (serotonin) is usually a pulmonary vasoconstrictor.[69] However, none of these neurohumoral agents is as important in regulating pulmonary vascular tone as is a reduction in partial pressure of alveolar oxygen. Local alveolar hypoxia causes smooth muscle contraction in vessels supplying the hypoxic region of lung. This "hypoxic pulmonary vasoconstriction" is effective in directing blood flow away from hypoxic (poorly ventilated) areas of the lung to better ventilated areas of the lung.[22] This mechanism functions remarkably well in local regulation of vascular tone and in balancing ventilation and blood flow in the lung.

What happens when the entire lung becomes hypoxic? All of the lung units "sense" a local hypoxia, resulting in vasoconstriction throughout the lung and the development of pulmonary hypertension, which persists and may lead to right ventricular hypertrophy and failure if hypoxia is continued.

Diffusion

Once ventilation brings air into the alveoli and perfusion brings blood into the pulmonary capillaries, oxygen and carbon dioxide are transferred across the tissue barrier separating air and blood. The gases move across the alveolar-capillary membrane by simple diffusion.[29, 32] Oxygen and carbon dioxide diffuse along their concentration, or partial pressure, gradients. In addition, several other factors are important in determining the rates of diffusion, and Fick's law describes this relationship:

$$\dot{V}_{gas} = \frac{A}{T}D(P_1 - P_2)$$

where A is the surface area available for diffusion,
    T is the thickness of the alveolar-capillary membrane,
    D is the diffusion constant for a specific gas
    $(D\alpha \sqrt{solubility/molecular\ weight})$,
    $(P_1 - P_2)$ is the partial pressure gradient across the alveolar-capillary membrane.

The physical characteristics of the alveolar-capillary membrane are important in determining diffusion across the membrane (Fig. 62–10). Reductions in membrane surface area (caused by emphysema or lung removal) or increased membrane thickness (caused by fibrosis or pulmonary edema) markedly decrease gas diffusion. Likewise, a decrease in the pressure gradient across the alveolar-capillary membrane reduces diffusion.

The pressure gradient favors the transfer of oxygen ($\Delta P = 60$ torr for O$_2$, whereas $\Delta P = 6$ torr for CO$_2$), but the solubility favors CO$_2$ transfer (20 times greater

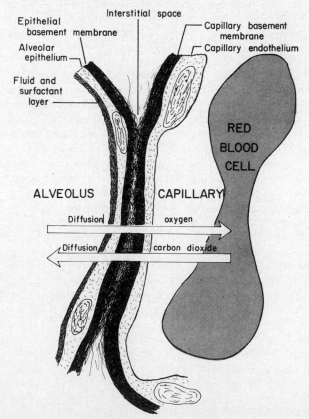

Figure 62–10. Structure of the alveolar-capillary membrane. (Reprinted with permission from Guyton, A. C.: *Textbook of Medical Physiology*, 6th ed. W. B. Saunders, Philadelphia, 1981, p. 498.)

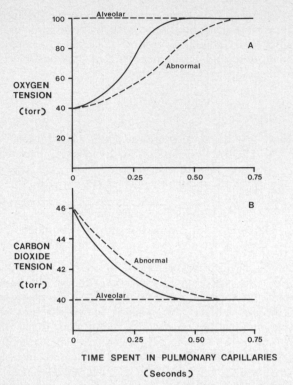

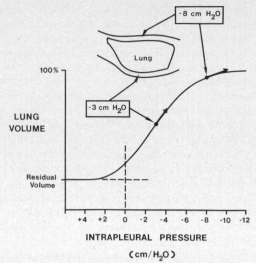

Figure 62–12. Primary cause of the regional differences in ventilation across the thorax. The intrapleural pressure is less negative at the ventral portion of the lung because of the effect of gravity on the lung. Similarly, the intrapleural pressure is more negative at the dorsal portion of the lung. As a consequence, lung compliance and ventilation are greater in the ventral alveoli and lower in the dorsal alveoli. (Redrawn from West, J. B.: *Ventilation/Blood Flow and Gas Exchange*, 3rd ed. Blackwell Scientific Publications, Oxford, 1977, p. 28.)

Figure 62–11. *A,* Uptake of O_2 from alveolar gas into blood during passage through the pulmonary capillaries in normal and abnormal (e.g., lung fibrosis) lungs. *B,* Release of CO_2 from blood into alveolar gas during passage of blood through the pulmonary capillaries in normal and abnormal lungs. (Redrawn from Wagner, P. D., and West, J. B.: Effects of diffusion impairment on O_2 and CO_2 time courses in pulmonary capillaries. J. Appl. Physiol. 33:62, 1972.)

of the lung are equally perfused and ventilated and that ventilation and blood flow are evenly distributed to all alveoli and capillaries. However, these conditions rarely, if ever, occur in normal or diseased lungs. The result of nonuniform distribution of ventilation and perfusion is the development of gas exchange abnormalities.

The distribution of ventilation is markedly affected by gravity.[36, 50] In the standing animal, gravitational forces, acting on the lung suspended in the thoracic cavity, pull the lungs toward the sternum. The intrapleural space is compressed at the ventral surfaces and expanded along the dorsal aspects of the lung. Accordingly, intrapleural pressure is higher at the

than O_2 solubility in water or tissue). Since the surface area and membrane thickness are the same for the two gases at any particular time, CO_2 diffusion or transfer should be ten times greater than O_2 diffusion or transfer. The greater solubility of CO_2 is the reason that diffusion impairment rarely causes significant CO_2 retention when O_2 transfer has been markedly reduced. Oxygen transfer across the alveolar-capillary membrane has been estimated as a function of time spent by red blood cells in the pulmonary capillaries (Fig. 62–11A). Pulmonary capillary P_{O_2} increases rapidly and reaches the alveolar P_{O_2} well within the normal time spent by erythrocytes in the capillaries. Complete oxygen transfer still occurs within the available time in lungs with abnormally thickened alveolar walls, although impairment of diffusion occurs during exertion, when less time for diffusion is available. Carbon dioxide transfer follows a similar pattern (Fig. 62–11B), except that CO_2 moves from capillary blood to alveolar air and is less susceptible to impairment of diffusion.

Ventilation-Perfusion Relationships

The previous discussion of normal lung physiology has been based on the assumption that all portions

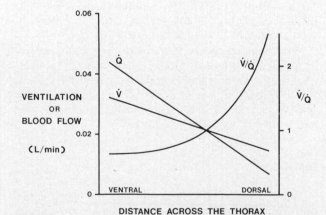

Figure 62–13. Distribution of ventilation, blood flow, and ventilation-perfusion ratios across the thorax of a dog. (Redrawn from West, J. B.: *Ventilation/Blood Flow and Gas Exchange*, 3rd ed. Blackwell Scientific Publications, Oxford, 1977, p. 30.)

bottom of the lung and lower at the top of the lung (Fig. 62–12). Since intrapleural pressure is an expanding pressure, dorsal alveoli are exposed to a greater expanding pressure and therefore have a greater volume.[25] Conversely, ventral alveoli exposed to a lower expanding pressure have smaller volumes. These differences in alveolar volumes have considerable effects on alveolar compliance (see Fig. 62–12) and, subsequently, on ventilation. Thus, dorsal alveoli have high expanding pressures, large volumes, low compliance, and low ventilation, whereas ventral alveoli have low expanding pressures, small volumes, high compliance, and greater ventilation (Fig. 62–13). The magnitude of the gravitational effect is dependent on the size of the animal. Larger animals with larger lungs exhibit a more nonuniform distribution of ventilation.

In addition to gravitational effects, collateral pathways for airflow contribute to nonuniform distribution of ventilation.[46, 71] Interalveolar pores and communications between bronchioles can be used for distributing air to areas of lung with poor ventilation. These air channels have high airway resistance and therefore play a minor role in the normal lung but may become very important with lung disease.[43] There is also a tremendous species difference in the existence and magnitude of collateral ventilation.[61, 78] Cows and pigs have little or no functional collateral ventilation, whereas collateral ventilation is extensive in dogs and sheep. Robinson and Sorenson[61] have speculated that differences in collateral ventilation account for the susceptibility of different species to lung diseases. The dog, with its extensive collateral ventilation, suffers from few chronic pulmonary diseases that result in impaired gas exchange.

A third modifier of ventilatory distribution is uneven compliance and airway resistance. Highly compliant areas of the lung are better ventilated. Also, variable compliance results in different time constants for expansion and deflation of lung units. Thus, it is possible for some lung units to be deflating while other lung units are still expanding. Poor mixture of alveolar gas results and alveolar P_{O_2} may be reduced in the lung units with slow time constants. In a similar manner, uneven airway resistance can affect the distribution of ventilation, resulting in poorly and well-ventilated areas of the lung.

The distribution of blood flow is markedly affected by gravity.[21, 36, 76] In the standing animal, dorsal portions of the lung are above heart level, whereas the ventral portions are below the heart, indicating that dorsal vessels are poorly perfused and ventral vessels are well perfused (Fig. 62–13). Again, this gravitational effect is more pronounced in larger animals with large lung volumes. The development of shunts, where blood bypasses the gas exchange area, also leads to a poor distribution of perfusion and consequent gas exchange abnormalities.

A description of potential maldistributions of ventilation or perfusion is actually not sufficient to predict gas exchange disorders; the balance between venti-

TABLE 62–3. Regional Alveolar Gas Composition in a Standing Dog*

	$\dot{V}_A$ (ml/min)	$\dot{Q}$ (ml/min)	$\dot{V}/\dot{Q}$	$P_{A_{O_2}}$ (torr)	$P_{A_{CO_2}}$ (torr)
Dorsal	180	100	1.8	120	30
Ventral	450	550	0.8	92	42

*Data adapted from West, J. B.: *Ventilation/Blood Flow and Gas Exchange,* 3rd ed. Blackwell Scientific Publications, Oxford, 1977.

lation and blood flow in each individual alveolus or gas exchange unit is required. This parameter is the ventilation-perfusion ratio ($\dot{V}/\dot{Q}$). A perfect match of ventilation and perfusion would be a $\dot{V}/\dot{Q}$ of 1.0. However, as can be seen in Figure 62–13, very little of the lung has a $\dot{V}/\dot{Q}$ of 1.0. The dorsal portions of the lung have a $\dot{V}/\dot{Q}$ in excess of 2.0, whereas the ventral portions have a $\dot{V}/\dot{Q}$ of approximately 0.8. The indicates that dorsal alveoli are relatively overventilated (or underperfused) and ventral alveoli are relatively underventilated (or overperfused). Figure 62–13 illustrates the $\dot{V}/\dot{Q}$ relationships of the normal lung. In the diseased lung this normal nonlinear distribution can be altered even more, resulting in further mismatching of ventilation and blood flow.[78]

The significance of $\dot{V}/\dot{Q}$ relationships can best be expressed by determining regional alveolar gas composition (Table 62–3). Alveoli with a $\dot{V}/\dot{Q}$ greater than 1 have alveolar O_2 partial pressures ($P_{A_{O_2}}$) greater than 100 torr and alveolar CO_2 partial pressures ($P_{A_{CO_2}}$) less than 40 torr. Alveoli with $\dot{V}/\dot{Q}$ less than 1 have $P_{A_{O_2}}$ less than 100 torr and $P_{A_{CO_2}}$ greater than 40 torr. In normal lungs, blood leaving the capillaries has an oxygen tension equal to the corresponding $P_{A_{O_2}}$. Owing to the nonlinear characteristics of oxygen transport (discussed later), alveoli with high $P_{A_{O_2}}$ cannot compensate for alveoli with low $P_{A_{O_2}}$. Therefore, $\dot{V}/\dot{Q}$ maldistribution leads to a fall in arterial O_2 partial pressure (Pa_{O_2}). Thus, an O_2 gradient develops between alveolar gas and arterial blood [$(A-a)D_{O_2}$], which is caused by $\dot{V}/\dot{Q}$ imbalance. The greater the maldistribution of $\dot{V}/\dot{Q}$, the greater the $(A-a)D_{O_2}$ and the more severe the arterial hypoxemia. Ventilation-perfusion mismatching is probably the most common cause of arterial hypoxemia.

Gas Transport in Blood

Once oxygen diffuses across the alveolar-capillary membrane, it is transported in the blood to the sites of metabolism. Oxygen can be carried in blood via two mechanisms. First, oxygen can be dissolved in plasma. The amount dissolved depends on the solubility and partial pressure of O_2. Despite a P_{O_2} of almost 100 torr, the low solubility of O_2 results in only about 3 per cent of the O_2 being carried in the dissolved state. The second method of transport is in combination with hemoglobin. The O_2 content of

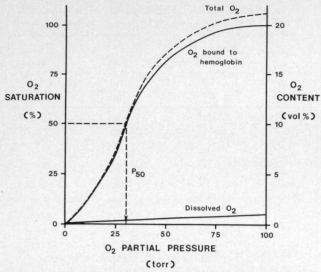

Figure 62–14. O_2-hemoglobin dissociation curve (solid line) obtained under conditions of pH 7.4, P_{CO_2} 40 torr, and 37°C. The total O_2 content is also shown. The P_{50} of dog blood (as shown) is approximately 29 torr, whereas the P_{50} of cat blood is about 36 torr. (Redrawn from West, J. B.: *Respiratory Physiology—The Essentials,* 2nd ed. Williams & Wilkins, Baltimore, 1979, p. 71.)

blood is the actual amount of O_2 combined with hemoglobin. The percentage of hemoglobin combined with oxygen (per cent saturation) is calculated by deriving the O_2 content/O_2 carrying capacity ratio.

The interactions between O_2 and the heme moieties of hemoglobin are described by the O_2-hemoglobin dissociation curve (Fig. 62–14). There are several aspects of this dissociation curve that emphasize the O_2-hemoglobin binding characteristics. The sigmoid-shaped curve is caused by the different binding affinities of the four heme moieties of hemoglobin. The first and fourth heme groups bind O_2 more avidly, resulting in the relatively flat portions of the curve. The second and third heme groups have a lower affinity for O_2, resulting in the relatively steep portion of the curve. In the P_{O_2} range corresponding

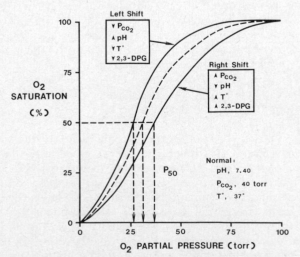

Figure 62–15. Shifts in curve position and P_{50} caused by changes in P_{CO_2}, pH, T°, and 2,3-DPG concentration.

to the steep portion of the O_2-hemoglobin dissociation curve, O_2 unloading is facilitated at the tissue level. At a P_{O_2} of 80 torr or more only a small increase in O_2 saturation is observed. This relationship increases O_2 uptake into blood in the pulmonary capillaries. Furthermore, the O_2-hemoglobin relationship is affected by other factors that can alter the affinity of hemoglobin for oxygen.[68] For example, an increase in P_{CO_2} (Bohr effect), a decrease in pH (increase in H^+ concentration), an increase in temperature, and an increase in 2,3-diphosphoglycerate (2,3-DPG) concentration decrease the O_2-hemoglobin affinity, shifting the O_2-hemoglobin curve to the right (Fig. 62–15) and indicating that oxygen delivery to the tissues is enhanced. Changes in the opposite direction (e.g., a decrease in P_{CO_2}) increase the O_2-hemoglobin affinity, shifting the curve to the left (see Fig. 62–15) and indicating that oxygen uptake at the pulmonary capillaries is enhanced.

Carbon dioxide transport in blood from metabolizing tissues to the lungs occurs by three mechanisms. Dissolved CO_2 accounts for about 7 per cent of transported CO_2, and the amount dissolved depends on the solubility and partial pressure of CO_2. Carbon dioxide is also transported by chemical combination with blood proteins as carbamino compounds. Hemoglobin is the primary protein that binds CO_2, and this transport mechanism accounts for approximately 20 per cent of excreted CO_2. CO_2 is primarily transported in the form of bicarbonate. In plasma, the hydration of CO_2 is a slow process that yields carbonic acid, which dissociates into a bicarbonate ion and a proton (Fig. 62–16). However, within red blood cells, an intracellular enzyme (carbonic anhydrase) catalyzes this reaction,[46] yielding bicarbonate ions, which diffuse out of the red blood cells (see Fig. 62–16). Chloride ions and water move into the cells to maintain electrical and osmotic balance. In the tissues, CO_2 moves into blood, increasing the P_{CO_2} and HCO_3^- concentration. In the lungs, ventilation removes CO_2, lowering P_{CO_2} and reversing the hydration of CO_2. The degree of O_2-hemoglobin saturation affects the magnitude of CO_2 transport. Upon oxygenation of hemoglobin, a hydrogen ion is released. This ion increases the hydrogen ion concentration, forcing the CO_2 hydration reaction back toward free CO_2. Therefore, when de-oxygenated blood in the pulmonary capillaries becomes oxygenated, a greater number of CO_2 molecules are simultaneously released. This enhancement of CO_2 transport by the O_2-hemoglobin interaction is known as the Haldane effect.

Control of Ventilation

Alveolar ventilation is precisely matched to metabolic needs so that arterial P_{O_2} and P_{CO_2} vary little with physical activity. From the extremes of sleep to intense running, ventilation is adjusted to maintain adequate oxygen uptake and carbon dioxide elimi-

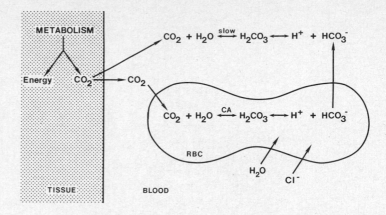

Figure 62–16. Schema showing how CO_2, produced by the tissues, is taken up in blood and converted to HCO_3^-. The hydration of CO_2 is slow in plasma but increased in the presence of the intracellular enzyme carbonic anhydrase (CA). The chloride (Cl^-) shift is also demonstrated.

nation. This precise control of ventilation is accomplished by the integration of three different components. A central controller, or "respiratory center," generates the breathing rhythm[17] and adjusts the tidal volume of each breath, and chemical and neural reflexes adjust ventilation to the needs of the animal.

The respiratory center is located in the medulla and is made up of two relatively distinct groups of neurons (Fig. 62–17). The dorsal respiratory group is primarily composed of inspiratory neurons that discharge during inspiration. The ventral respiratory group is composed of both inspiratory and expiratory neurons. The dorsal respiratory group appears to drive the ventral respiratory group and is probably the origin of the respiratory rhythm. Pontine activity also influences the respiratory pattern. The apneustic center facilitates inspiration, whereas the pneumotaxic center inhibits inspiration. These pontine centers support the medullary center by fine-tuning the respiratory pattern. The signals generated by the respiratory center are sent along descending pathways to the spinal cord. Along these pathways all respiratory inputs are integrated to achieve the appropriate respiratory output for the muscles of respiration.

Chemoreceptor reflexes are the most important regulators of ventilation. Changes in arterial P_{CO_2}, P_{O_2}, and pH are capable of altering ventilation by stimulating central and peripheral chemoreceptors. Of these chemical factors, the respiratory system is most sensitive to carbon dioxide. During normal physical activity, arterial P_{CO_2} varies less than 3 torr. A small increase in P_{CO_2} causes a substantial increase in ventilation (Fig. 62–18), which then returns P_{CO_2} to its original value. In contrast, a reduction in P_{CO_2} leads to a decrease in ventilation, thus allowing P_{CO_2} to return to the baseline value. This action of carbon dioxide is due primarily to activation of the central chemoreceptor,[42] located on the ventral surface of the medulla (Fig. 62–19). The blood brain barrier is relatively impermeable to HCO_3^- and H^+, so the action of carbon dioxide is due to the diffusion of free CO_2 through the barrier. Once CO_2 is dissolved in the medullary extracellular fluid, it is hydrated to

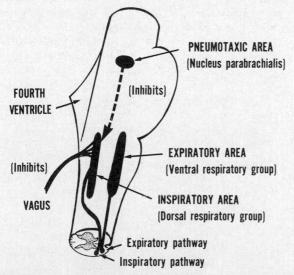

Figure 62–17. Organization of the mammalian respiratory center. (Reprinted with permission from Guyton, A. C.: *Textbook of Medical Physiology*, 6th ed. W. B. Saunders, Philadelphia, 1981, p. 516.)

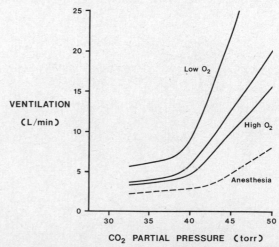

Figure 62–18. Ventilatory response to CO_2 under normal, low, and high O_2 conditions. The dotted line represents the effects of anesthesia on hypercapnic ventilatory drive. (Redrawn from Nielsen, M., and Smith, H.: Studies on regulation of respiration in acute hypoxia. Acta Physiol. Scand. 24:293, 1951.)

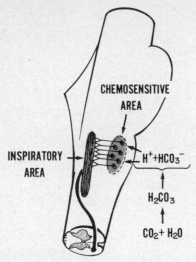

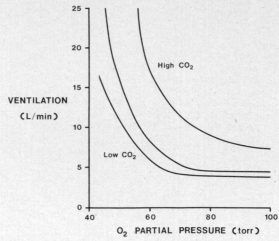

Figure 62–19. Drawing of the central chemoreceptor (chemosensitive area) located bilaterally in the medulla. This area is sensitive primarily to changes in blood P_{CO_2}, but H^+ ions are the final stimulators of ventilation. (Reprinted with permission from Guyton, A. C.: *Textbook of Medical Physiology*, 6th ed. W. B. Saunders, Philadelphia, 1981, p. 518.)

Figure 62–21. Ventilatory response to low O_2 under normal, low, and high CO_2 conditions. (Redrawn from Loeschke, H. H., and Gertz, K. H.: Effect of oxygen pressure in inspired air on respiratory activity of the human, tested under the constant behavior of alveolar carbon dioxide pressure. Pfluegers Arch. 267:460, 1958.)

HCO_3^- and H^+. These H^+ ions stimulate chemoreceptors to elicit the ventilatory response to carbon dioxide. The extreme sensitivity to carbon dioxide is due to two factors. First, in extracellular fluid pH is lower than that of arterial blood. Second, there is little protein in extracellular fluid; therefore, a low buffering capacity exists. Small changes in CO_2 result in greater changes in H^+ concentration in extracellular fluid than in blood, which is buffered by plasma proteins and hemoglobin.

Carbon dioxide can also stimulate the peripheral chemoreceptors located in the carotid and aortic bodies (Fig. 62–20). The resulting ventilatory response is usually rapid, of smaller magnitude, and shorter than the ventilatory responses observed with central chemoreceptor stimulation. Since H^+ ions cannot easily permeate the blood brain barrier, ventilatory responses to acute changes in pH are due to stimulation of peripheral chemoreceptors. However, sustained pH imbalance can lead to stimulation of central chemoreceptors as an equilibrium is reached across the blood brain barrier.

The ventilatory control system is less sensitive to changes in arterial P_{O_2} than to changes in arterial P_{CO_2} (Fig. 62–21). No change in ventilation is observed in the normal range of oxygen levels, even with changes in Pa_{O_2} of 15 torr, indicating that oxygen levels are not involved in the normal breath to breath adjustments of ventilation. However, if Pa_{O_2} falls below 60 to 70 torr, a vigorous ventilatory response is initiated. This hypoxic ventilatory drive may be essential for the maintenance of ventilation under a number of circumstances, particularly if CO_2 responsiveness has been altered by lung disease and acid-base disturbance. The response to reductions in Pa_{O_2} is due to stimulation of the peripheral chemoreceptors (see Fig. 62–20). Stimulation of the carotid bodies[6] increases nerve impulse activity in the glossopharyngeal nerves, which are integrated with the

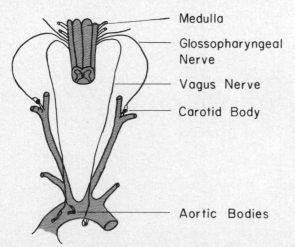

Medulla

Glossopharyngeal Nerve

Vagus Nerve

Carotid Body

Aortic Bodies

Figure 62–20. Location of the carotid and aortic bodies. (Reprinted with permission from Guyton, A. C.: *Textbook of Medical Physiology*, 6th ed. W. B. Saunders, Philadelphia, 1981, p. 520.)

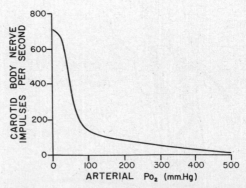

Figure 62–22. Effect of arterial P_{O_2} on nerve impulse rate from the carotid body of a cat. (Reprinted with permission from Guyton, A. C.: *Textbook of Medical Physiology*, 6th ed. W. B. Saunders, Philadelphia, 1981, p. 520.)

central ventilatory drive (Fig. 62–22). Stimulation of the aortic bodies increases nerve impulse activity in the vagi.

The neural respiratory reflexes[71] are less important in the control of normal ventilation but may play an important role when lung function is altered. The inflation stretch reflex (Hering-Breuer reflex) causes termination of inspiration as the lungs are inflated. Stretch receptors in the airways are stimulated as the lung expands, and inspiration is terminated before the lung is overexpanded. This vagal negative feedback system may be involved in the frequency–tidal volume selection related to changes in the work of breathing. Chest wall reflexes, such as the muscle spindle reflex, also seem to stabilize ventilation in the face of changes in lung mechanics. Upper airway reflexes, such as the irritant reflex, cause coughing and bronchoconstriction when foreign gases or particles are inhaled. This reflex protects the lung, particularly the alveolar surfaces, from the inhaled particles and gases.

Anesthetics may adversely affect the control of respiration (see Fig. 62–18). Barbiturates are central respiratory depressants that cause alveolar hypoventilation and subsequent hypoxemia, hypercapnia, and acidosis. Narcotic analgesics and general anesthetics also depress breathing. These agents reduce hypoxic and hypercapnic ventilatory drives. In addition, anesthetics inhibit contraction of the intercostal muscles, so that inspiration depends entirely on diaphragmatic contraction.

Lung Defense Mechanisms

The respiratory system is particularly susceptible to particles and toxic agents, since there is direct contact between atmospheric air and the functional elements of the lungs. Lung tissue can be easily damaged when exposed to toxic materials, leading to abnormalities in gas exchange and respiratory dysfunction. Fortunately, the lungs have a series of structures and processes that either prevent or reduce the potential damage from inhaled material.[11, 16]

The first line of defense is the filtration of particulate matter in the upper airways. During nasal breathing, the majority of large particles (5 to 30 μm) contact the mucous membranes of the nares and nasopharynx. The mucosal folds and sinus cavities create turbulent airflow, facilitating contact of inhaled particles. Smaller particles (1 to 5 μm) may pass through these upper airways but usually settle in the bronchioles and adhere to the mucous lining the airways. Very small particles (<1 μm) may move by bulk flow to the respiratory bronchioles and diffuse into alveoli, where they reside until removed by alveolar macrophages.

Particles that touch or settle on the mucous lining of the airways are removed by the mucociliary cells. The cilia of epithelial cells beat in a layer of mucus, pushing the mucus and impacted particles toward

the nasopharynx.[8, 28] The cilia beat approximately 15 to 20 beats/sec, but this rate may be markedly reduced by drugs (such as barbiturates) or airway disease.[70] Particles in alveoli may be moved, by physical forces caused by respiration, up to the terminal bronchioles, where they can be removed by ciliary action. These particles may also be phagocytized by alveolar macrophages, which then migrate to the cilia or lymphatics.

Lung reflexes also play an important part in the lung defense mechanisms.[2, 66] Stimulation of receptors in the upper airways by noxious agents can cause apnea, preventing further inhalation of the agents. Laryngeal reflexes appear to be well organized, particularly in the cat, in which laryngospasm can become a surgical problem. Mechanical stimulation of the larynx, soft palate, pharynx, and trachea of the cat can cause dramatic, intense laryngospasm.[58] Endotracheal intubation is a frequent cause of mechanically induced laryngospasm. Initiation of the irritant reflex induces sneezing, coughing, and bronchoconstriction, causing forceful expulsion of the noxious agents. These reflexes, in combination with the alveolar macrophages and cilia, are essential for maintaining a viable gas exchange surface. Any disruption of defense mechanisms increases the susceptibility of the lung to infection and injury.

DYSFUNCTION OF THE RESPIRATORY SYSTEM

Maintenance of normal arterial levels of oxygen and carbon dioxide and normal pH requires the proper functioning of all of the processes of gas exchange. Even a slight structural or functional dysfunction can cause respiratory failure, leading to hypoxemia, hypercapnia, and acidosis (Fig. 62–23). Hypoxemia and its attendant gas exchange abnormalities may have one or more causes: (1) alveolar hypoventilation, (2) impairment of diffusion, (3) pulmonary shunting, (4) ventilation-perfusion imbalance, (5) decreased inspired P_{O_2}, or (6) altered blood gas transport (Fig. 62–24).

Terminology and Definitions

Hypoxemia below normal content of oxygen in arterial blood

Hypercapnia above normal partial pressure if carbon dioxide in arterial blood

Respiratory acidosis decreased arterial pH caused by carbon dioxide retention (e.g., alveolar hypoventilation)

Respiratory alkalosis increased arterial pH caused by excessive carbon dioxide elimination (e.g., hyperventilation)

Hypoventilation reduced alveolar ventilation in relation to metabolism, such that arterial carbon dioxide partial pressure rises

Hyperventilation increased alveolar ventilation in

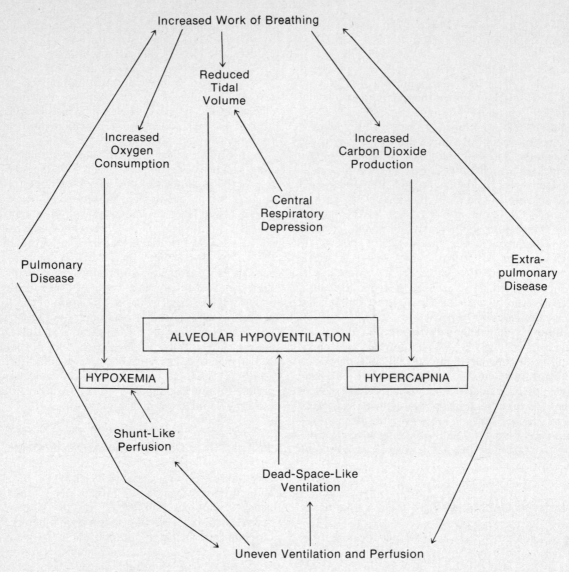

Figure 62–23. Schematic representation of the mechanisms producing alveolar hypoventilation and subsequent hypoxemia and hypercapnia. (Reprinted with permission from Ettinger, S. J.: *Textbook of Veterinary Internal Medicine*, Vol. 1. W. B. Saunders, Philadelphia, 1975, p. 562.)

relation to metabolism, such that arterial carbon dioxide partial pressure falls

Dyspnea   subjective difficulty or distress in breathing

Hyperpnea   increased ventilation in conjunction with increased metabolism

Apnea   absence of breathing

Cyanosis   a dark bluish or purplish coloration of mucous membranes and skin due to oxygen deficiency

Hypoxia   relative deficiency of oxygen

Causes and Effects of Respiratory System Dysfunction

Nasopharyngeal obstruction or compression is usually caused by stenotic nares, granulation tissue, polyps and tumors, palate deformations, foreign bodies, scarring secondary to trauma, or inflammatory disorders. In dogs, stenotic nares, nasal tumors, and foreign bodies are most common, whereas rhinitis and sinusitis are more common in cats. Congenital or acquired stenotic nares, usually due to occlusion of the external nares by the dorsal parietal cartilage, causes inspiratory distress with open-mouth breathing. The primary pathophysiological changes with nasal obstruction are increased airway resistance and decreased pulmonary compliance.[53] Examples of changes in respiratory parameters with experimental nasal obstruction in dogs are shown in Table 62–4. Episodic or continuous respiratory distress may progress to cyanosis or collapse. The greatly increased nasal resistance necessitates a change to mouth breathing to avoid a greatly increased energy usage in breathing.[52] However, in the process, normal olfactory function and the warming, humidification, and filtration of inspired air are impaired.

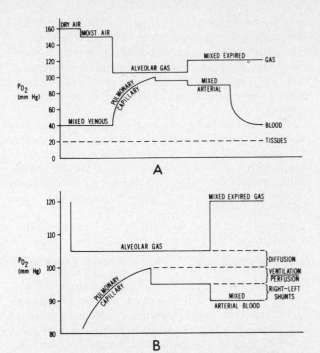

Figure 62–24. Oxygen tensions in blood and gas phases. *A,* Oxygen partial pressure (P_{O_2}, mm Hg) in blood and gas phases of the respiratory system. *B,* Blood and gas oxygen tensions within the lung showing factors comprising the alveolar-arterial oxygen difference. (Reprinted with permission from Ettinger, S. J.: *Textbook of Veterinary Internal Medicine,* Vol. 1. W. B. Saunders, Philadelphia, 1975, p. 538.)

As air is inspired through the nares, it is warmed and humidified. Also, large particles are trapped in either the external nares or the turbinates. These particles will remain lodged unless the sneeze reflex is initiated by irritation of the nasal passages. Sneezing can continue for some time if the foreign body is not cleared; however, the intensity abates with time. Foreign bodies in the nasal passages increase airway resistance and the work of breathing if the animal continues nose breathing.

Tumors arising in the nasal cavities also obstruct air flow. If nasal breathing continues, air movement distal to the site of obstruction may be impaired. The increased upper airway resistance may cause alveolar hypoventilation and subsequent hypoxemia and hypercapnia. In addition, the affected animal may try to overcome the increased airway resistance by making vigorous inspiratory efforts, with resultant signs of dyspnea. Since the obstruction is in the upper airways, markedly increased stress and strain on distal lung components result from the greater changes in intrapleural pressure and increased negative inspiratory pressure.[53] Eversion of laryngeal saccules may occur because of the greater changes in airway pressure,[39] thus complicating the airway obstruction. If the animal switches to mouth breathing to bypass the obstruction site, none of these complications will result. Dogs and cats resist mouth breathing even with very high nasopharyngeal resistance.

Inflammation in the turbinates results in necrosis and ulceration of the nasal mucosa, and hypersecretion of mucus causes nasal obstruction and increased airway resistance. The pathophysiological responses and respiratory adjustments to chronic rhinitis-sinusitis are similar to those described for nasal tumors.

The larynx and trachea must perform several functions in the maintenance of normal respiration; they must be (1) relatively rigid to prevent collapse, (2) flexible to accommodate changes in air volume, (3) able to trap and remove particles suspended in the inspired air, and (4) flexible enough to allow movements of the head and neck. Laryngeal obstruction or compression can be caused by trauma (crushing or laceration), everted laryngeal saccules, laryngospasm, obstructive laryngeal webbing, tumors and foreign bodies, laryngeal paralysis and swelling, and proliferative or granulomatous laryngitis. Another laryngeal complication is aspiration, which is often categorized as chronic bronchopneumonia or aspiration pneumonia. Obstruction or compression of the trachea can be caused by tracheal collapse or stenosis, trauma, neoplasms, and foreign bodies. Tracheal collapse or stenosis is usually associated with a long history of chronic coughing that may be accentuated by exertion or excitement. The cough is initiated by stimulation of nerve endings in the trachea.

Obstruction of airflow in these large airways produces pathophysiological changes similar to those observed in nasopharyngeal obstruction. Airflow is impaired, and the animal hypoventilates, resulting in respiratory acidosis unless the increased resistance is overcome by vigorous respiratory efforts. Increased inspiratory efforts result in markedly subatmospheric intrapleural and airway pressures distal to the site of

**TABLE 62–4. Per Cent Changes in Respiratory Parameters in Dogs
After Four Months of Nasal Obstruction***

	Unilateral Obstruction	Partial Bilateral Obstruction	Bilateral Obstruction
Compliance	−3.8	−4.3	+27.1
Resistance (lower airway)	−7.3	+154.6	−50.0
Functional residual capacity	+5.9	+24.0	+12.4
Intrapleural pressure	−4.6	−30.2	−75.0
Body weight	+5.0	−9.4	+73.0

*Data obtained from Ohnishi, T., Ogura, J. H., and Nelson, J. R.: Effects of nasal obstruction upon the mechanics of the lung in the dog. Laryngoscope *81*:712, 1971.

obstruction. Laryngeal and pharyngeal edema may result, accompanied in some animals by the medial movement of the aryepiglottic folds and arytenoid cartilages and eversion of the laryngeal saccules. Active expiration may be caused by airway obstruction, and additional complications, such as distal airway closure, may occur. All of these changes exacerbate the existing obstructive disorder and compound the respiratory dysfunction. The large swings in intrapleural and airway pressures may also cause poor distribution of ventilation and perfusion, leading to arterial hypoxemia. The dyspnea resulting from laryngeal or tracheal obstruction may be either inspiratory or expiratory, but it is usually more severe during expiration. Chronic laryngeal or tracheal obstruction can also cause secondary pulmonary hypertension and right heart failure. The respiratory adjustments to this type of airway obstruction probably include a change in the frequency–tidal volume selection to slow deep respirations. Open-mouth breathing would have little benefit, since the obstruction is distal to the nasopharynx.

Small airway obstruction or compression can result in several different types of pathophysiological changes. Abscesses and neoplasms, excessive bronchoconstriction, edema and excessive mucus production, bronchiolitis, emphysema, and foreign bodies can all cause small airway complications. The primary effect is an increase in airway resistance in the affected airways. This, in turn, produces a maldistribution of ventilation, with hypoventilation of the lung distal to the small airway obstruction. Alveolar P_{O_2} falls in these lung units; thus, blood leaving these lung units carries less oxygen. The ventilation-perfusion imbalance that occurs produces arterial hypoxemia, the severity depending on the extent of small airway dysfunction. Alveolar ventilation may be adequate to maintain relatively normal levels of carbon dioxide, but arterial P_{O_2} cannot be maintained in the face of a ventilation-perfusion imbalance. The hypoxemia may be severe enough to produce cyanosis.

If a number of small airways are affected, the increased airway resistance may result in increased work of breathing. However, the dyspnea noted with upper airway obstruction is not evident unless the majority of small airways are affected. Regional differences in airway pressure can also occur, leading to atelectasis in lung units distal to small airway obstructions and causing alveolar overdistension in lung units unaffected by airway obstruction.

In response to small airway obstruction, several respiratory adjustments may be invoked.[10, 49] First, an increase in ventilation may be evident, particularly if sufficient arterial hypoxemia develops to stimulate the peripheral chemoreceptors. Second, in the hypoventilating lung units, alveolar P_{O_2} falls and hypoxia stimulates vasoconstriction of the vessels supplying blood to these areas. The net result is a redistribution of perfusion to match the maldistribution of ventilation. In this manner, a potentially marked ventilation-perfusion imbalance can be avoided and severe arterial hypoxemia can be prevented. The signs of small airway obstruction are evident only if a large proportion of the airways is involved. If this occurs, labored breathing, dyspnea, and cyanosis may be present. However, involvement of a small proportion of small airways can cause minimal signs of respiratory dysfunction.

Interstitial and alveolar lung complications are less amenable to surgical correction but produce a variety of pathophysiological changes. Lung fibrosis, lung compression due to space-occupying lesions, pneumonia, pulmonary edema, pulmonary contusion and "shock lung," and constrictive pleuritis can cause interstitial-alveolar respiratory dysfunction.

A decrease in lung compliance is the primary defect in restrictive lung disorders;[14] more energy is required to expand the lung to the same extent, and the work of breathing is markedly increased. A reduction in lung reserve is usually noted. Restrictive conditions impair full expansion of the lungs most during exertion. As the ventilatory demands increase with physical activity and if the animal cannot meet these demands, exertional dyspnea develops. The level of physical activity may be reduced concurrently with signs of respiratory dysfunction. Another important consequence of restrictive lung disorders may be diffusion impairment.[26] If the alveolar-capillary membrane is thickened, whether by interstitial cellular proliferation, fluid accumulation, or inflammation, oxygen transfer is impaired, whereas carbon dioxide transfer is virtually unaffected. This results in arterial hypoxemia without concurrent hypercapnia. Diffusing capacity is decreased under these conditions.

A change in the frequency–tidal volume selection would probably be the most obvious change in respiration with restrictive lung disorders. Since lung compliance is reduced whereas airway resistance is unaffected, the work of breathing is minimized with shallow rapid respirations. If the alveolar-capillary membrane is only slightly thickened, the resting animal exhibits no signs of respiratory dysfunction. A further thickening of the membrane may still not impair oxygen transfer at rest; however, on exertion a diffusion impairment may develop, producing hyperventilation and possibly dyspnea.

Abnormalities of the chest wall and diaphragm can alter the mechanics of ventilation sufficiently to cause respiratory system dysfunction.[4] Chest wall pain and trauma, pneumothorax, diaphragm deformation and paralysis, diaphragmatic herniation, neoplasms, pleural effusion, and pleuritis can restrict movement of the chest wall or diaphragm, causing impaired ventilation.

Restriction of chest wall expansion and/or diaphragmatic contraction causes varying degrees of alveolar hypoventilation. Decreased chest wall compliance and altered intercostal muscle function can affect ventilation, particularly during physical activity. Diaphragmatic dysfunction decreases ventilation both at rest and during exertion. If the restriction of chest wall expansion is limited to specific areas, regional disparities in intrapleural pressure may develop, leading to ventilation-perfusion imbalance (see "Ventilation-Perfusion Relationships"). Arterial hypoxemia occurs, depending on the severity of the chest wall dysfunction and the magnitude of the ventilation-perfusion imbalance.

Multiple rib fractures result in a number of pathophysiological responses. Pain is aggravated by chest motion and initiates voluntary restricted intercostal respiratory activity. In multiple rib fractures the chest wall may lose its stability and traumatic "flail chest" may develop. The unstable portion of the chest wall on the injured side moves paradoxically, being sucked in by the negative intrapleural pressure during inspiration and pushed out during expiration. The distribution of ventilation is markedly impaired, even with relatively shallow motion of the flail segment, respiratory dead space increases, and cyanosis frequently develops.

When air enters the pleural space a pneumothorax develops. Air can enter the pleural space either from outside the chest wall (thoracic cage injury) or from the lung itself (tear in the main bronchus or lung parenchyma). The severity of the pneumothorax depends on the amount of air that enters. As the lung collapses, effective lung volume is lost and alveolar hypoventilation may occur. If only a small amount of air enters, lung mechanics are affected in that region, and maldistribution of ventilation can occur. The mediastinum in dogs provides an effective barrier between the pleural cavities and prevents leakage of air or fluids from one cavity into the other.[73] Thus, a bilateral pneumothorax rarely develops when only one pleural cavity is traumatized. A tension pneumothorax, in the presence of which air can enter the intrapleural space during inspiration but cannot escape during expiration, can compromise the contralateral ventilating lung and thus further impair gas exchange.

When fluid enters the pleural space a pleural effusion develops. Fluid displaces functional lung, as does air and abdominal viscera, and causes alveolar hypoventilation, ventilation-perfusion imbalance, hypoxemia, hypercapnia, and acidosis. Large accumulations of fluid produce severe respiratory distress and dyspnea as well as chronic wasting disease.

The respiratory adjustments associated with chest wall and diaphragmatic abnormalities usually involve the recruitment of accessory respiratory muscles. If alveolar hypoventilation develops, muscles of the shoulder girdle and abdominal muscles may be recruited to aid in changing the size of the thoracic cavity to permit adequate ventilation. Tachypnea is often observed in these compromised animals. Labored breathing is often accompanied by evidence of abdominal respiratory effort and mouth breathing.

Respiratory dysfunction can also be caused by vascular obstruction or vasoconstriction, although these disorders are not as amenable to surgical correction as other lung disorders. Pulmonary embolism (particularly from heartworms, *Dirofilaria immitis*), pulmonary vasoconstriction, pulmonary arteritis and vascular muscularization, pulmonary congestion, and pulmonary edema are examples of major vascular disorders that can cause respiratory dysfunction. The majority of these conditions are secondary to other lung diseases or abnormalities. The primary consequence of these vascular disorders is the development of pulmonary hypertension. The distribution of blood flow may be altered under these conditions, leading to ventilation-perfusion imbalance and arterial hypoxemia. Patent ductus arteriosus can also cause pulmonary hypertension[34, 55] and capillary congestion, which can elicit neural reflexes that increase ventilation, but may also cause dyspnea. In addition, if arterial hypoxemia results from the vascular disorders, hypoxia-stimulated hyperventilation may be observed.

Pre- or postsurgical pulmonary edema can present several problems. Surgical procedures on edematous lung are particularly difficult, and postsurgical recovery can be impaired by fluid accumulation within the lungs. Pulmonary edema is particularly debilitating because of the multiple pathophysiological consequences. Maldistribution of pulmonary blood flow,[41] changes in lung mechanics,[18] maldistribution of ventilation,[30] and impaired gas diffusion[75] have all been reported with progressive pulmonary edema.

1. Agostini, E.: Mechanics of the pleural space. Physiol. Rev. 52:57, 1976.
2. Angell-James, J. E., and Daly, M. B.: Some aspects of upper respiratory tract reflexes. Acta Otolaryngol. 79:242, 1975.
3. Bakhle, Y. S., and Vane, J. R.: Pharmacokinetic function of the pulmonary circulation. Physiol. Rev. 54:1007, 1974.
4. Bergofsky, E. H.: Respiratory failure in disorders of the thoracic cage. Am. Rev. Resp. Dis. 119:643, 1979.
5. Bergofsky, E. H.: Active control of the normal pulmonary circulation. *In* Moser, K. M. (ed.): *Pulmonary Vascular Diseases.* (Lung Biology in Health & Disease Ser.: Vol. 14.) Marcell Dekker, New York, 1979, p. 233.
6. Biscoe, T. J.: Carotid body: Structure and function. Physiol. Rev. 51:427, 1971.
7. Blatt, C. M., Taylor, C. R., and Habal, M. B.: Thermal panting in dogs: The lateral nasal gland, a source of water for evaporative cooling. Science 117:804, 1972.
8. Bridger, G., and Proctor, D.: Mucociliary function in the dog's larynx and trachea. Laryngoscope 82:218, 1972.
9. Briscoe, W. A., and Dubois, A. B.: The relationship between airway resistance, airway conductance and lung volume in subjects of different age and body size. J. Clin. Invest. 37:1279, 1958.
10. Brown, R., Woolcock, A. J., Vincent, N. J., Macklem, P. T.: Physiological effects of experimental airway obstruction with beads. J. Appl. Physiol. 27:328, 1969.
11. Camner, P.: Alveolar clearance. Europ. J. Resp. Dis. 61(Suppl. 107):59, 1980.
12. Campbell, E. J. M., Agostoni, E., and Davis, J. N.: *The Respiratory Muscles: Mechanics and Neural Control.* W. B. Saunders, Philadelphia, 1970.
13. Chand, N.: Reactivity of isolated trachea, bronchus and lung strip of cats to carbachol, 5-hydroxytryptamine and histamine: Evidence for the existence of methysergide-sensitive receptors. Br. J. Pharmacol. 73:853, 1981.
14. Cherniack, R. M., Cherniack, L., and Naimark, A.: *Respiration in Health and Disease,* 2nd ed. W. B. Saunders, Philadelphia, 1972.
15. Clements, J. A., Brown, E. S., and Johnson, R. P.: Pulmonary

surface tension and the mucous lining of the lung: some theoretical considerations. J. Appl. Physiol. 12:262, 1958.

16. Cohen, A. B., and Gold, W. M.: Defense mechanisms of the lung. Ann. Rev. Physiol. 37:325, 1975.

17. Cohen, M. I.: Neurogenesis of respiratory rhythm in the mammal. Physiol. Rev. 59:1105, 1979.

18. Cook, C. D., Mead, J., Schreiner, G. L., Frank, N. R., and Craig, J. M.: Pulmonary mechanics during induced pulmonary edema in anesthetized dogs. J. Appl. Physiol. 14:177, 1959.

19. Cook, W. R.: Observations on the upper respiratory tract of the dog and cat. J. Small Anim. Pract. 5:309, 1964.

20. Dueck, R., Wagner, P. D., and West, J. B.: Effects of positive end-expiratory pressure on gas exchange in dogs with normal and edematous lungs. Anesthesiology 47:359, 1977.

21. Edmunds, L. H., Gold, W. M., and Heymann, M. A.: Lobar distribution of pulmonary arterial blood flow in awake standing dogs. Am. J. Physiol. 219:1779, 1970.

22. Fishman, A. P.: Hypoxia on the pulmonary circulation. How and where it acts. Circ. Res. 38:221, 1976.

23. Fishman, A. P.: Nonrespiratory functions of the lungs. Chest 72:84, 1977.

24. Frank, N. R., and Speizer, F. E.: SO_2 effects on the respiratory system in dogs. Arch. Environ. Health 11:624, 1965.

25. Glazier, J. B., Hughes, J. M. B., Maloney, J. E., and West, J. B.: Vertical gradient of alveolar size in lungs of dogs frozen intact. J. Appl. Physiol. 23:694, 1967.

26. Gracey, D. R., Divertie, M. B., and Brown, A. L., Jr.: Alveolar-capillary membrane in idiopathic interstitial pulmonary fibrosis. Electron microscopic study of 14 cases. Am. Rev. Resp. Dis. 98:16, 1968.

27. Haddy, F. J., Campbell, G. S., Adams, W. L., and Visscher, M. B.: A study of pulmonary venous and arterial pressures and other variables in the anesthetized dog by flexible catheter techniques. Am. J. Physiol. 158:89, 1949.

28. Hilding, A. C.: Ciliary streaming through the larynx and trachea. J. Thorac. Surg. 37:108, 1959.

29. Hlastala, M. P.: Diffusion in lung gas and across alveolar membrane in mammalian lungs. Fed. Proc. 41:2122, 1982.

30. Hogg, J. C., Agarawal, J. B., Gardiner, A. J. S., Palmer, W. H., and Macklem, P. T.: Distribution of airway resistance with developing pulmonary edema in dogs. J. Appl. Physiol. 32:20, 1972.

31. Hoppin, G. G., Jr.: Distribution of pleural surface pressures in dogs. J. Appl. Physiol. 27:863, 1969.

32. Horsfield, K.: Gaseous diffusion in the lungs. Br. J. Dis. Chest 74:99, 1980.

33. Irvin, C. G., and Dempsey, J. A.: Role of H_1 and H_2 receptors in increased small airways resistance in the dog. Resp. Physiol. 35:161, 1978.

34. Jeraij, K., Ogburn, P., Lord, P. F., and Wilson, J. W.: Patent ductus arteriosus with pulmonary hypertension in a cat. J. Am. Vet. Med. Assoc. 172:1432, 1978.

35. Kadowitz, P. J., and Hyman, A. L.: Effect of sympathetic nerve stimulation on pulmonary vascular resistance in the dog. Circ. Res. 32:221, 1973.

36. Kaneko, K., Milic-Emili, J., Dolovich, M. B., Dawson, A., and Bates, D. V.: Regional distribution of ventilation and perfusion as a function of body position. J. Appl. Physiol. 21:767, 1966.

37. King, R. J.: The surfactant system of the lung. Fed. Proc. 33:2238, 1974.

38. Knecht, C. D.: Upper airway obstruction in brachycephalic dogs. Comp. Cont. Ed. 1:25, 1979.

39. Leonard, H. C.: Eversion of the lateral ventricles of the larynx of the dog—five cases. J. Am. Vet. Med. Assoc. 131:83, 1957.

40. Leonard, H. C.: Collapse of the larynx and adjacent structures in the dog. J. Am. Vet. Med. Assoc. 137:360, 1960.

41. Levine, O. R.: Extravascular lung water and distribution of pulmonary blood flow in the dog. J. Appl. Physiol. 28:166, 1970.

42. Loeschcke, H. H.: Respiratory chemosensitivity in the medulla oblongata. Acta Neurobiol. Exp. 33:97, 1973.

43. Macklem, P. T.: Airway obstruction and collateral ventilation. Physiol. Rev. 51:368, 1971.

44. Macklem, P. T.: Respiratory muscles: The vital pump. Chest 78:753, 1980.

45. Macklem, P. T., Woolcock, A. J., Hogg, J. C., Nadel, J. A., and Wilson, N. J.: Partitioning of pulmonary resistance in the dog. J. Appl. Physiol. 26:798, 1969.

46. Maren, T. H.: Carbonic anhydrase: Chemistry, physiology, and inhibition. Physiol. Rev. 47:595, 1967.

47. Mead, J.: Mechanical properties of lungs. Physiol. Rev. 41:281, 1961.

48. Menkes, H., Lindsay, D., Gansu, G., Wood, L., Muir, A., and Macklem, P. T.: Measurement of sublobar lung volume and collateral flow resistance in dogs. J. Appl. Physiol. 35:917, 1973.

49. Metcalf, J. F., Wagner, P. D., and West, J. B.: Effect of local bronchial obstruction on gas exchange in the dog. Am. Rev. Resp. Dis. 117:85, 1978.

50. Milic-Emili, J., Henderson, J. A. M., Dolovich, M. B., Trop, D., and Kaneko, K.: Regional distribution of inspired gas in the lung. J. Appl. Physiol. 21:749, 1966.

51. Ogawa, T., Jefferson, N. C., Toman, J. E., Chiles, T., Zambetoglou, A., and Necheles, H.: Action potentials of accessory respiratory muscles in dogs. Am. J. Physiol. 199:569, 1960.

52. Ohnishi, T., and Ogura, J. H.: Partitioning of pulmonary resistance in the dog. Laryngoscope 79:1847, 1969.

53. Ohnishi, T., Ogura, J. H., and Nelson, J. R.: Effects of nasal obstruction upon the mechanics of the lung in the dog. Laryngoscope 81:712, 1971.

54. Permutt, S.: Effect of lung inflation on static pressure-volume characteristics of pulmonary vessels. J. Appl. Physiol. 16:64, 1961.

55. Pyle, R. L., Park, R. D., Alexander, A. F., and Hill, B. L.: Patent ductus arteriosus with pulmonary hypertension in the dog. J. Am. Vet. Med. Assoc. 178:565, 1981.

56. Qvist, J., Pontoppidan, H., Wilson, R. S., Lowenstein, E., and Laver, M. B.: Hemodynamic responses to mechanical ventilation with PEEP. Anesthesiology 42:45, 1975.

57. Rahn, H. A., Otis, A. B., Chadwick, L. E., and Fenn, W. O.: The pressure-volume diagram of the thorax and lung. Am. J. Physiol. 146:161, 1946.

58. Rex, M. A.: Laryngospasm and respiratory changes in the cat produced by mechanical stimulation of the pharynx and respiratory tract: Problems of intubation in the cat. Br. J. Anaesth. 43:54, 1971.

59. Richardson, J. B.: Nerve supply to the lungs. Am. Rev. Resp. Dis. 119:785, 1979.

60. Robinson, N. E., and Gillespie, J. R.: Lung volumes in aging beagle dogs. J. Appl. Physiol. 35:317, 1973.

61. Robinson, N. E., and Sorenson, P. R.: Collateral flow resistance and time constants in dog and horse lungs. J. Appl. Physiol. 44:63, 1978.

62. Rochester, D. F., and Bettini, G.: Diaphragmatic blood flow and energy expenditure in the dog. J. Clin. Invest. 57:661, 1976.

63. Roussos, C. H.: The failing ventilatory pump. Lung 160:59, 1982.

64. Said, S. I.: Metabolic functions of the pulmonary circulation. Circ. Res. 50:325, 1982.

65. Said, S. I., Kitamura, S., Yoshida, T., Preskitt, J., and Holden, L. D.: Humoral control of airways. Ann. N.Y. Acad. Sci. 221:103, 1974.

66. Sasaki, C. T., and Suzuki, M.: Laryngeal reflexes in cat, dog, and man. Arch. Otolaryngol. 102:400, 1976.

67. Schmidt-Nielsen, K., Bretz, W. L., and Taylor, C. R.: Panting in dogs: Unidirectional airflow over evaporative surfaces. Science 169:1102, 1970.

68. Shappel, S. D., and Lenfant, C. J. M.: Adaptive, genetic and iatrogenic alterations of the oxyhemoglobin dissociation curve. Anesthesiology 37:127, 1972.

69. Su, C., and Bevan, J. A.: Pharmacology of pulmonary blood vessels. Pharmacol. Ther. [B] 2:275, 1976.

70. Toremalm, N.-G.: Factors influencing the mucociliary activity

in the respiratory tract. Europ. J. Resp. Dis. *61*(Suppl. 107):41, 1980.

71. Traystman, R. J., Batra, G. K., and Menkes, H. A.: Local regulation of collateral ventilation by oxygen and carbon dioxide. J. Appl. Physiol. *40*:819, 1976.

72. Tucker, A., Weir, E. K., Reeves, J. T., and Grover, R. F.: Histamine H$_1$- and H$_2$-receptors in pulmonary and systemic vasculature of the dog. Am. J. Physiol. *229*:1008, 1975.

73. von Recum, A. F.: The mediastinum and hemothorax, pyothorax, and pneumothorax in the dog. J. Am. Vet. Med. Assoc. *171*:531, 1977.

74. Wagner, P. D., Laravuso, R. B., Goldzimmer, E., Naumann, P. F., and West, J. B.: Distribution of ventilation-perfusion ratios in dogs with normal and abnormal lungs. J. Appl. Physiol. *38*:1099, 1975.

75. West, J. B.: *Ventilation/Blood Flow and Gas Exchange*, 3rd ed. Blackwell Scientific Publications, Oxford, 1977.

76. West, J. B., Dollery, C. T., and Naimark, A.: Distribution of blood flow in isolated lung: relation to vascular and alveolar pressures. J. Appl. Physiol. *19*:713, 1964.

77. Widdicombe, J. B.: Respiratory reflexes in man and other mammalian species. Clin. Sci. *21*:163, 1961.

78. Woolcock, A. J., and Macklem, P. T.: Mechanical factors influencing collateral ventilation in human, dog, and pig lungs. J. Appl. Physiol. *30*:99, 1971.

Chapter 63

Preoperative Assessment and Care of the Respiratory Patient

A. Wendell Nelson and Richard D. Park

Injury to or dysfunction of the respiratory system can rapidly lead to death. Even chronic respiratory disease can change into a life-threatening condition with only a small increase in the severity of the disease. Therefore, patients having signs of respiratory disease should be examined with care, and items needed for respiratory support should be readily available.

A patient with respiratory signs may be responding to changes in other than the respiratory system or to a combination of problems. A patient in respiratory distress may tolerate only a limited initial examination to assess vital body functions (i.e., respiratory, cardiovascular, and central nervous systems) before or during supportive therapy.[22] Thus, when examining the critical patient the clinician must obtain a pertinent history, rapidly assess vital functions, and provide supportive care simultaneously. As the patient becomes stable, a complete history is obtained from the owner and a complete physical examination is done.

The complete physical examination and history are augmented by laboratory support.[1] The thoroughness and accuracy of the diagnosis and prognosis depend on the capability of the diagnostician and the availability of equipment and laboratory support. Pertinent information can be obtained from radiological (plain film and contrast), visual (fiberoptic), hematological (hemogram, blood gases), and cytological/bacteriological (tracheal wash, thoracentesis, biopsy) studies.

The primary aims of examination, diagnosis, and care of the distressed respiratory patient are: (1) maintaining vital body functions through supportive care (i.e., ventilation, circulation, cerebration); (2) minimizing or preventing secondary problems from augmenting the progression of the disease (e.g., hypoxia, inhalation pneumonia, tension pneumothorax); (3) reduction of pain or anxiety to improve patient comfort yet retain patient awareness of its injuries (sedation, local anesthesia, high-oxygen atmosphere); and (4) elimination of the cause of respiratory dysfunction.[22]

CRITICAL CARE PATIENT

Physical Examination

The patient in respiratory distress is quickly but carefully evaluated for ability to ventilate (air movement and mucous membrane color), character of respiratory movements, and level of respiratory system involved (nares, larynx, trachea, or lungs).[10, 13] Immediate administration of oxygen via a nose cone or oxygen cage and thoracentesis may be necessary to overcome hypoxia and accompanying anxiety, allowing a more accurate examination. The excitement of a strange environment may be enough to decompensate some borderline dyspneic patients.

Ventilation

Adequate ventilation depends on an unobstructed airway, an intact respiratory mechanism, and exchange of gases at the alveolus.[22] The entire system must be assessed rapidly, and measures to prevent or correct hypoxemia or hypercapnia must be taken immediately. The mouth and the oropharynx are cleared of any solid or liquid foreign material that may be obstructing the airway. If signs of hypoxia or impaired ventilation persist, the larynx and cervical trachea are auscultated for obstruction. Stridorous respiratory sounds, loudest and clearest in this region, indicate a stenosis, and intubation should be considered. An obstructing foreign body located in this region could be driven deep into the trachea by intubation; the existence of a foreign body should be determined from the history of possible inhalation, palpation, and visual inspection prior to passing the tube.

Endotracheal Intubation

Because intubation is usually not possible in conscious animals, chemical restraint is needed. Intravenous oxymorphone (0.012 to 0.05 mg/kg) or meperidine hydrochloride (0.1 to 0.5 mg/kg) is frequently adequate for intubation.[22] These narcotic agents are reversed with naloxone hydrochloride (Narcan) when sedation is no longer desired. Phenathiazine tranquilizers are useful but are avoided if hypotension is a potential problem. Succinylcholine, used intravenously at the rate of 0.1 to 0.3 mg/kg body weight, is effective for simple restraint, but the animal loses all ability to ventilate spontaneously, and mechanical ventilation is needed. Thiobarbiturate (Pentothal) given as an intravenous bolus (0.5 to 1.0 mg/kg body weight) provides good short-term restraint for intubation.

In patients with possible laryngeal or tracheal mucosal lacerations or airway discontinuity, the endotracheal tube is carefully inserted with a laryngoscope and digital palpation. This practice reduces the chance of leaving the lumen of the airway or obstructing the tube and airway by elevating mucosal flaps.

A clear plastic endotracheal tube with a high-volume, low-pressure cuff is the tube of choice. Such a tube allows observation of accumulated fluid or exudate, and the low-pressure cuff reduces pressure necrosis when inflated for extended periods.

Tracheostomy

Unless a life-threatening upper cervical airway obstruction is present and long-term endotracheal tube intubation is impractical, tracheostomy is avoided. Although emergency tracheotomy can be done under adverse conditions, tracheostomy should be done in the operating room under aseptic conditions and preferably with an endotracheal tube in place to allow control of ventilation during insertion (see Chapter 65).

Continued poor ventilation with a clear upper airway indicates oxygen therapy and examination for the source of the problem (e.g., chest injury, air or fluid in the pleural space, lung injury, blood-alveolar gas exchange, pulmonary thrombosis, diaphragmatic hernia).[1, 3, 4, 10, 12, 17]

Oxygen Therapy

Oxygen therapy is indicated when ventilation with room air is not adequate to oxygenate the blood. Hyperpnea, cyanotic mucous membranes, and low arterial P_{O2} and oxygen saturation are signs of inadequate oxygenation.[20]

Oxygen delivery systems should be simple and effective.[10, 13] A nose cone on a non-rebreathing system is the easiest and safest method. Most conscious animals tolerate the system if they are slowly introduced to it and the nose cone is large enough to allow open-mouth breathing. This system conveniently supplies oxygen while a physical examination and other procedures are done.

A transtracheal catheter is a convenient method for delivering oxygen. A long (20 to 30 cm) catheter is placed through a needle introduced percutaneously into the midcervical trachea.[13] The catheter is connected to a metered oxygen source for continuous delivery. The addition of nebulized water and mucokinetic drugs can aid in the breakup and expulsion of thick mucus. Water alone, as steam or aerosol, is as efficacious as acetylcysteine, proteolytic enzymes, sodium bicarbonate, or ethyl alcohol.[30]

An oxygen cage is convenient and effective for providing an oxygen rich atmosphere to a conscious animal over a long period. Most cages waste considerable oxygen and rarely supply a continuous oxygen concentration of greater than 50 per cent with practical oxygen flows. Oxygen should be cool and well-humidified if it is to be used for long periods. Systems for temperature and humidity control and CO_2 removal are necessary.

Efficient closed systems using endotracheal or tracheostomy tubes for oxygen delivery can maintain a 100 per cent oxygen atmosphere. High-volume, low-pressure cuffs should always be used on the endotracheal tubes to reduce injury to the tracheal mucosa. The oxygen supplied in this system should be humidified.

A 100 per cent oxygen atmosphere can usually be tolerated for up to 24 hours before oxygen toxicity occurs. Occasionally, even a 100 per cent O_2 atmosphere will not properly oxygenate the blood.[10]

Chest Wounds

Open chest wounds result in the loss of negative intrapleural pressure and pneumothorax (see Chapter 41). This type of wound must be covered quickly with any reasonable material that forms an airtight seal. The pneumothorax is drained immediately to allow more complete lung expansion. Definitive wound care is given after the patient is stable and more serious problems have been corrected.

Pneumothorax

Pneumothorax, or free air in the pleural space, occurs primarily as a sequel to trauma.[12, 13, 22] It results from an open chest wound, as described previously, or from air entering the pleural space through an injury to the trachea, bronchus, or lung. A tension pneumothorax develops as pleural space pressure approaches atmospheric pressure. The diagnosis of tension pneumothorax is based on a hyperexpanded thorax, a reduced movement of air during ventilation, increased pulmonary resonance, and decreased heart sounds. Tension pneumothorax must be treated immediately by thoracentesis (see "Chest Drainage").

Hemothorax

Hemothorax is found primarily in trauma patients and is characterized by pale mucous membranes, dyspnea, reduced or muffled chest sounds on auscultation, dullness on percussion, and the presence of blood on thoracentesis. Dyspnea and hypoxemia are the major problems. Hemothorax is an emergency more because of blood loss than because of lung compression, although lung contusion, edema, and compression are additive problems. A chest drain is placed to evacuate the chest, monitor the volume of blood loss, and document continued hemorrhage. Continued hemorrhage (more than 2 ml/kg/hr) that cannot be compensated for by transfusion and fluid therapy is an absolute indication for surgical exploration of the thorax.

Flail Chest

A section of the chest wall will become unstable when four or more ribs are fractured, each in at least two places.[10, 12, 13] This condition results in paradoxical movements of the chest wall during ventilation. Treatment consists of outward traction of the unstable segment so that it cannot collapse inward. In addition, segment motion can be reduced and efficiency of ventilation enhanced by a light pressure wrap on the chest (see Chapter 41).[13]

Diaphragmatic Hernias

Diaphragmatic hernia may be symptomatic in the acute phase.[12] It is usually characterized by dyspnea, tendency to assume a sitting position to reduce abdominal pressure on the diaphragm, and muffled heart and respiratory sounds (usually on one side). Chronic lung compression by abdominal viscera or from fluid accumulation secondary to a liver lobe incarcerated by a diaphragmatic laceration can cause subtle respiratory signs. In comparison, the patient can become hypoxic and die rapidly if the stomach becomes trapped in the chest and dilates. Therefore, surgical correction of a diaphragmatic hernia is indicated (see Chapter 59).

Impaired Alveolar Gas Exchange

Hypoxia in the presence of a patent airway and intact ventilatory mechanism originates from inadequate exchange of gases between the alveoli and blood (see Chapters 62 and 188). Gas exchange is altered by pulmonary contusion or edema, aspiration of fluid, intra-alveolar hemorrhage, and severe pneumonia. Alveolar gas exchange should be evaluated by arterial blood gases and by the color of mucous membranes. Assisted ventilation or supplemented oxygen should be started immediately if gas exchange is inadequate to support the patient. Inflation pressure is limited to that needed for adequate gas exchange, since excessive pressure can result in reopening of lung and bronchial lacerations, rupture of bullae, and parenchymal lung damage.

Radiographic Examination of the Stable Dyspneic Animal

Information obtained from the radiographic examination consists of the anatomical structures involved, the severity of the condition, and, with proper observance of radiographic signs, a specific diagnosis. This information is valuable in establishing, changing, or maintaining therapy and helps in arriving at an accurate prognosis. However, two questions should be asked before the dyspneic but stable animal is radiographed: Is information needed, for diagnostic or therapeutic reasons, that will justify and be obtained from a radiographic examination at this time? Can the animal withstand the physical stress needed for a radiographic examination without endangering its life?

With patience and care, a dyspneic animal can be radiographed with minimal stress. Oxygen and equipment for ventilation must be available, and the animal continuously observed for signs of respiratory difficulty. A complete radiographic examination is performed if possible, i.e., all views are taken. A minimal examination (lateral view) is performed if the animal is extremely debilitated or dyspneic. The immediate safety of the dyspneic animal should take precedence over obtaining additional radiographic views.

STABILIZED RESPIRATORY PATIENT

It is important to reevaluate the patient constantly for the progression of the disease as therapy is instituted. All systems are examined and therapy altered to meet changing signs. After the patient has been stabilized, a thorough evaluation is carried out.

History

The owner is questioned carefully concerning signs of disease, and current problems are categorized as to those preexisting and those that are new.[25] The owner is asked to describe signs rather than to identify them by name. The owner's idea of a cough, for example, may be different from that of the diagnostician. Objective and subjective observations are examined to determine the true magnitude of the current disease state. The chronological sequence and changing characteristics of each of the presented signs are evaluated to assist in the diagnosis and prognosis of the disease.

Age and Breed. The age and breed incidences of certain disease categories may help to streamline diagnosis.

Young patients are more likely to have infections and congenital diseases, whereas older patients are more likely to have neoplastic disease. Vaccination status is important in these patients to rule out certain diseases.

Certain breeds have genetic or conformational predispositions to specific respiratory disorders. Brachycephalic breeds frequently have upper respiratory tract stenosis, (e.g., stenotic nares, elongated soft palate, everted saccules, laryngeal collapse).[18]

Residence. The geographic residence may aid diagnosis of chronic infectious diseases (e.g., coccidioidomycosis, histoplasmosis).[24] The present residence (urban, rural) and personal habits (indoor, outdoor—confined or free) may indicate exposure to trauma, infectious disease, or inhaled foreign bodies.

Previous Diseases. A thorough record of past illness, medication used, and outcome of treatment is important when considering the current problem. Current disease may be directly or indirectly related to previously diagnosed problems, such as cardiac failure, elongated soft palate, and malignant neoplastic disease. A recurring process may warrant a change in medication or reevaluation for a missed diagnosis. Past trauma may have resulted in undiagnosed damage (chylothorax, diaphragmatic hernia) with delayed onset of respiratory signs.

Current Problem. A detailed chronological account of the current problem is obtained. Time of onset, initial signs, progress of disease, and new signs that have developed recently are important.[25] The owner should describe sounds and activities rather than assigning them names (e.g., cough, gag, retch). Appetite, excretory habits, and interest in spontaneous exercise are noted. The owner should also be asked whether signs of disease are enhanced by eating, drinking, exercise, excitement, periods of inactivity, or sleep. If this is a chronic disease, whether it has responded to any medication given and in what way should also be ascertained.

Physical Examination

The physical examination of the patient with respiratory signs should not be limited to the respiratory system.[17, 25] The extent of the initial examination depends on the condition of the patient and its response to handling.

Initial observation should be made of the freely moving patient.[25] Character of respiratory movements, mental acuity, general body condition, and ability to walk are noted. Dyspnea, open-mouth breathing, and signs of hypoxia are assessed quickly and the patient is stabilized prior to continuing the physical examination. Obvious wheezing (stridor) indicates partial airway obstruction. The volume of air movement should be noted. The amount of the air coming from both and each nostril and the difference in air movement with an opened or closed mouth are subjectively estimated, in order to differentiate nasal and lower airway obstruction.

Hydration

Hydration can be assessed using skin elasticity, sunken eyes, total serum protein, and serum osmolality. Dehydration, in addition to other systemic effects, causes increased viscosity of bronchial secretions, which leads to accumulation of exudates and formation of mucous plugs and bronchial obstruction. Reduction in circulating blood volume in the dehydrated patient can be severe enough to cause physiological shunting (ventilation-perfusion mismatch).

Rehydration should be done carefully in the patient with cardiac and respiratory tract lesions.[20] Compensated heart failure, myocardial and lung contusions, sepsis, and hypoalbuminemia complicate the process of rehydration by increasing the chance of pulmonary edema, especially in cats. Rehydration is done with intravenous Ringer's solution while the patient is monitored for increases in central venous pressure and for moist respiratory sounds. Considerable rehydration takes place in patients in a controlled atmosphere into which water or saline is being nebulized.[28] Overhydration can occur in this situation.

Palpation

The entire body should be palpated for abnormal conditions—dehydration, wounds, pain, swelling or mass, subcutaneous emphysema, rib, skull or long bone fractures, collapsed soft trachea, and weak or irregular peripheral pulse.[1, 17] The examination should start at the nose and end at the tip of the tail, with a systematic coverage of the entire body. Specific abnormalities are reexamined in detail after the initial examination is complete.

The larynx and trachea are examined for swelling or displacement caused by trauma, infection, or neoplasia.[1] Light compression of the larynx and trachea will incite a cough when inflammation, partial obstruction, or collapse is present. Abnormal flattening of the cervical trachea can be palpated.

Subcutaneous emphysema is usually related to lacerations of the esophagus, larynx, trachea, or mainstem bronchi and can cause pneumomediastinum and pneumothorax. Lung laceration usually results in pneumothorax without subcutaneous emphysema. Skin lacerations in the axillary or inguinal regions frequently cause "sucking" type wounds as the patient walks, leading to subcutaneous emphysema.

Enlargement of lymph nodes, spleen, liver, or other tissues can indicate neoplastic disease. Advanced metastatic lung disease causes respiratory insufficiency as a result of decreased functional lung. Fluid accumulation in the thorax or abdomen directly interferes with lung expansion and frequently is coincident with neoplastic and cardiovascular disease.

Lacerations, hernias, and fractures indicate trauma and possible central nervous system, lung, and myocardial contusions. Such contusions can progress significantly, especially if they remain undetected and the patient is anesthetized. Usually, lung contusions resolve in three to seven days without specific treatment. When diagnosed, lung contusions serve as a warning to be cautious (1) with positive-pressure ventilation in order to reduce the chance of reopening lung lacerations and (2) with fluid therapy in order to decrease the risk of pulmonary edema.

Peripheral pulse is palpated and mucous membranes are observed to differentiate hypoxemia of cardiovascular and pulmonary origin. A full pulse with moist mucous membranes and a rapid capillary refill usually indicates adequate circulation and a probable respiratory origin for coexisting hyperpnea and hypoxemia. Anemia has to be ruled out as a cause of hypoxemia. The lack of proper hemoglobin oxygenation with adequate cardiac output is related to decreased oxygen delivery to the perfused pulmonary capillaries (see Chapter 62). Respiratory tract obstruction (usually larynx to bronchi), severe lung disease (edema, pneumonia), pulmonary shunting and inability to expand lungs (flail chest, pleural effusion, pneumothorax, atelectasis, diaphragmatic hernia, neoplasia) are common causes of poor oxygen delivery.

Auscultation

Auscultation of the entire respiratory system in a quiet room helps localize stenosis, fluid accumulation, and nonaerated portions of the lung. The sounds generated by air movement are related to changes in its velocity and of laminar flow to turbulent flow.[1] The addition of fluid modifies these sounds.

A comparison of sounds heard at the thoracic wall, cervical trachea, larynx, and nose helps determine where sounds originate. Sounds are usually loudest and clearest when the stethoscope is placed nearest to their origin. Each sound is evaluated as to its type (crackle, wheeze, friction rub, or miscellaneous).

The *crackle* (rale) is a discontinuous, nonmusical, discrete explosive noise that has no recognizable tone.[24] High-pitched or *fine crackles* (dry rales) generally are associated with interstitial pulmonary edema, chronic interstitial pneumonia, and chronic pulmonary fibrosis. They are heard during the latter part of inspiration and may be the result of equilization of pressure between upper and lower sections of small bronchial airways, with explosive opening of collapsed or obstructed regions.

Coarse crackles (moist rales) are lower in pitch and have a bubbling or gurgling type of sound.[24] They are associated with the early part of inspiration and inflammation and fluid in the large airways. Coarse crackles are heard in the late states of pulmonary edema and bronchial pneumonia, when intraluminal fluid accumulation occurs.

Wheezing is a continuous musical sound of one or more notes resulting from air passing through a narrowed airway.[24] They are high-pitched (sibilant) or low-pitched (sonorous) and associated with inspiration or expiration. The pitch is associated with the mass and elasticity of the oscillating structure and with the linear velocity of air passing through the stenosis. *Stridor* is a term frequently used for an intense inspiratory wheeze originating in the larynx or trachea during severe stenosis.

Wheezes are associated with functional (bronchospasm or laryngospasm) or physical (laryngeal collapse, foreign body, mucous plugs, tumors) narrowing of the airway. Lower-pitched wheezes are associated with secretions in the airway and coarse crackles. A cough usually changes these sounds.

Friction rub is a combination of loud, coarse sounds of both a continuous and discontinuous nature. It is generated from the parietal and visceral pleural surfaces, which have been roughened by fibrin deposition and inflammation, as they slide over each other during respiration. These sounds are similar to crackles, only more focal, louder, and lower-pitched.

Areas of silence in the lung field indicate lack of air movement (complete bronchial obstruction or parenchymal consolidation) or lack of lung contact with the thoracic wall (effusion, pneumothorax, diaphragmatic hernia). Normal cats may have inaudible respiratory sounds while they are at rest.

A cough indicates irritation or fluid accumulation in the lower respiratory tract.[1, 8, 18] Aspiration of liquid or particulate material initiates the cough reflex. If this occurs frequently during eating or drinking, laryngeal dysfunction or cleft palate is suspected. A moist cough is frequently related to alveolar pulmonary fluid accumulation (e.g., bronchiectasis, pneumonia, pulmonary edema). Airway inflammation (without exudation), neoplasia, emphysema, and physical deformities of the trachea result in a dry cough.

Heart sounds are evaluated at the same time for

determination of loudness, abnormal sounds (murmurs), presence of normal sounds, and synchrony with the peripheral pulse.

Percussion

Percussion of the thorax is useful in determining areas of decreased or increased resonance.[17, 19] Areas of dullness (decreased resonance) on the thoracic wall indicate solid tissue (consolidated lung lobe, abdominal organs) or fluid within the chest adjacent to the area percussed. Increased resonance indicates pneumothorax.

Blood Analysis

Cytological examination of blood provides preoperative baseline data and an indication of a systemic reaction to respiratory problems. Blood gas studies can identify abnormal O_2, CO_2, and pH levels and assist in differentiating hypoxia, hypercapnea, and acid-base balance or the cause of abnormal respiratory signs. Knott's test is a screening test for heartworm infestation. A basic automated chemistry panel (measuring glucose, BUN, creatinine, albumin, globulin, electrolytes, and tissue enzymes) and a standard urinalysis are used to complement a thorough physical examination and assist in assessing nonrespiratory disease that may be concurrent with the respiratory problem.

Thoracentesis

Complete drainage of pleural fluid should be done early in the diagnostic process. A smear of the fluid should be examined for cellular content (including microorganisms) and an aliquot should be taken for culture and antibiotic sensitivity testing. The pleural space is completely drained, if possible, to determine the amount of fluid that is present, to improve lung expansion, and to allow radiographs to be taken that are not obscured by the fluid density.

Rate of fluid accumulation is recorded, as well as any change in its character, by periodic drainage through an indwelling chest tube. Persistent or recurring hemothorax not treatable by transfusion and drainage or pneumothorax not treatable by drainage is grounds for exploratory thoracotomy.

Aspiration and Diagnostic Lavage

Secretions and exudates of the airway from the nostrils to the mainstem bronchi are evaluated to assist in diagnosis. Deep swabs, brushing, and lavage of the nasal passages require sedation or anesthesia in most cases to prevent sneezing and damage to tissue due to patient movement. Sterile culture swabs and brushes are usually sufficient to obtain exudate and soft tissue samples from the nose. More dense tissue is removed with a biopsy needle or forceps, curette, or trephine.

Nasal lavage technique is described in the section on rhinoscopy. A Foley catheter is used to obstruct the caudal nasal passage, and debris is flushed out of the nostrils by a stream of saline solution introduced through the catheter. Both swab and lavage techniques can be used to help distinguish between infection and neoplasia.

Transtracheal Lavage

Diagnostic transtracheal lavage and aspiration are done before endoscopy to prevent translocation of upper respiratory organisms to the tracheobronchial area. The skin over the cricothyroid membrane or proximal trachea is clipped and prepared. Local anesthesia is used, and some sedation may be needed in the anxious patient. A needle (16-gauge in dogs, 18- or 20-gauge in cats) is inserted through the skin and cricothyroid membrane or between tracheal rings.[22, 23] A plastic catheter* is passed through the needle and advanced into the distal trachea or mainstem bronchus. A small amount of sterile saline (2 to 5 ml) is flushed into the airway in 0.5-ml increments and immediately aspirated. The fluid is cultured, and centrifuged sediment is smeared for cytological examination.[19, 23]

Radiographic Examination of the Stable Respiratory Patient

Radiographic examination of the stable respiratory patient is supplemental to the physical examination, used in conjunction with other clinical data to arrive at a diagnosis or confirm other findings. The information obtained can change the diagnosis or therapeutic approach; for example, neoplastic pulmonary metastasis can be found in a patient with a previously identified, surgically resectable primary neoplasm.

A radiographic examination is an excellent means to assess both the approximate extent and the character of disease processes in the respiratory system. The determination as to whether the disease involves respiratory or adjacent structures can usually be made radiographically. The radiographic findings often serve as an important pivotal point in determining appropriate therapy or diagnostic tests.

Plain Film Studies

Films of good technical quality and proper patient positioning are necessary for accurate radiographic evaluation of the respiratory system. An underexposed film made on expiration can create the appear-

---

*Intracath, Abbott Laboratories, North Chicago, IL.

ance of diffuse lung disease, and actual focal lung lesions may not be seen.

The plain film examination is the "cornerstone" of the radiographic examination. Other examination techniques, such as fluoroscopy, special positioning, and contrast studies, should be performed if additional information is needed.

It is important to do a complete radiographic study of the part being examined. Radiographic views that best demonstrate each region or disease are necessary. Metastatic lesions or other small focal lesions in the lung may be missed with only one view of the thorax. Thoracic masses surrounded by pleural fluid may be missed unless positional films are made to gravitate the fluid away from the suspected masses. The end-result of an incomplete radiographic examination may be a misdiagnosis, erroneous therapy, or an inaccurate surgical approach. Areas in the respiratory tract that can be satisfactorily examined radiographically are the nasal cavity, paranasal sinuses, pharynx and larynx, trachea, and lungs.[8, 14, 26]

Nasal Cavity and Paranasal Sinuses. Accurate radiographic examination of the nasal cavity and paranasal sinuses requires general anesthesia. The open-mouth ventrodorsal view and the dorsoventral view of the nasal cavity with the film positioned in the mouth are the most valuable views to evaluate nasal cavity disease. One or both of these views should always be included in a nasal cavity study (Fig. 63–1A). Non-screen film (film in cardboard holders or dental occlusal film) can be used for the intraoral, dorsoventral nasal cavity study to obtain fine film detail not possible with intensifying screens. Comparisons between right and left sides are made when interpreting films of the nasal cavity to assist in finding subtle changes.

The frontal sinuses can be evaluated best with oblique and rostrocaudal views (Fig. 63–1B). Frontal sinuses of small dogs and cats may not always be seen on the rostrocaudal view.

Pharynx and Larynx. Lateral views of the pharynx and larynx usually provide the most information. A view made on inspiration is usually most satisfactory, because gas volume in the pharynx and larynx is increased during inspiration and provides better contrast for pharyneal and laryngeal structures.

Trachea. Lateral views of the trachea are most informative. In small dogs and cats, the entire trachea may be included on one lateral view. In large dogs, a separate view over the thoracic inlet is usually necessary to compensate for the increased soft tissue thickness. Depending on the position of the head, the trachea may have a slight normal dorsal deviation in the cranial mediastinal area. This deviation appears when the head and neck are flexed and usually disappears when they are extended.

Several views and techniques may be used to evaluate the trachea for collapse. Lateral radiographs are made on inspiration and expiration (Fig. 63–2). The head is hyperextended to demonstrate and accentuate cervical and thoracic inlet tracheal collapse (Fig. 63–2A), and a tangential view of the trachea is used to demonstrate thoracic inlet tracheal collapse (Fig. 63–2B) or a pendulous dorsal tracheal muscle.

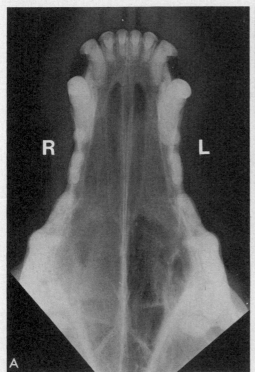

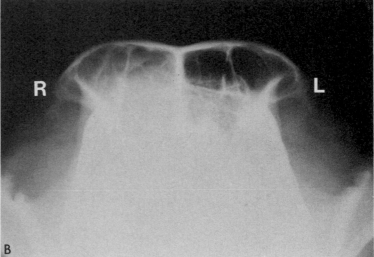

Figure 63–1. A, An oral ventrodorsal radiograph. This view provides unobstructed visualization of the nasal cavity. There is increased soft tissue density in the caudal right nasal cavity compared with the normal left nasal cavity. The small nasal turbinates have been destroyed or are not visible in the caudal right nasal cavity but are distinctly seen on the left. This animal had a nasal adenocarcinoma in the caudal right nasal cavity, but the radiographic signs are nonspecific and compatible with neoplasia or rhinitis. *B,* A rostrocaudal radiograph of the frontal sinuses in the same animal. This view provides an unobstructed view of the frontal sinuses with side-to-side comparison and is important for frontal sinus evaluation. An increased soft tissue density can be seen in the right frontal sinus. This appearance is compatible with inflammatory fluid, hemorrhage, or neoplastic infiltration. The fluid was secondary to the adenocarcinoma in the right nasal cavity.

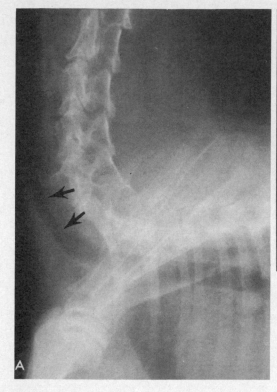

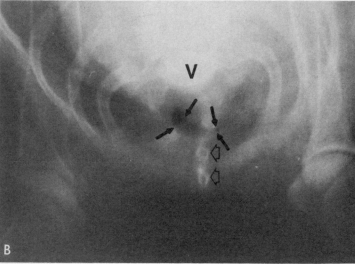

Figure 63–2. *A,* A lateral radiographic view of the trachea with the neck hyperextended. This view is sometimes helpful to demonstrate cervical and thoracic inlet tracheal collapse. A mild to moderate cervical tracheal collapse is present *(arrows)*. *B,* Tangential craniocaudal radiographic view of the trachea at the thoracic inlet. This view provides an end-on projection of the trachea to evaluate size and shape. The superimposed end-on caudal cervical vertebrae (V) are dorsal and the sternebrae *(open arrows)* are ventral to the trachea. The trachea *(solid arrows)* has a dorsal ventral collapse.

If fluoroscopy is available, tracheal movements with inspiration and expiration can be observed. Cervical, thoracic inlet, and thoracic tracheal collapse can all be readily observed with fluoroscopy. Bronchial collapse is observed best on expiratory films and with endoscopy.

Lungs. Routine radiographs of the thorax should be made on inspiration with exposure times of 1/20 second or less. The entire thorax should be included on the film. A lateral view and a dorsoventral or ventrodorsal view constitute a complete study in most cases. When one is checking for small focal lesions, two lateral views (a left-to-right and a right-to-left) should be obtained. Many focal lesions can be missed

if the second lateral view is not added because the denser dependent lung or pleural fluid can reduce the tissue contrast needed to outline the lesion (Fig. 63–3). When pleural fluid is present and mass lesions are suspected in the lungs or other thoracic structures, various body positions can be used to gravitate fluid away from the suspected mass(es) while films with a horizontal beam projection are made to more clearly demonstrate the lesion(s).

Contrast Studies

Bronchography. Bronchography is a technique used to outline the mucosal surfaces of the trachea

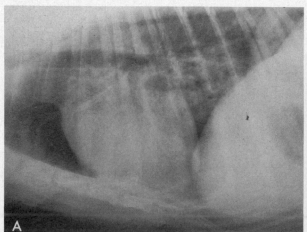

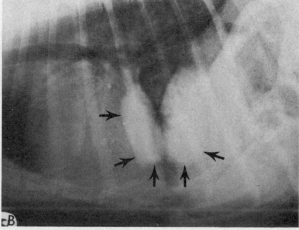

Figure 63–3. Recumbent lateral thoracic radiographs. *A,* Left recumbent lateral thoracic radiograph. There is an apparent ill-defined increased interstitial lung density present between the heart and diaphragm. *B,* Right recumbent lateral thoracic radiograph. A lung mass is present with well-defined borders *(arrows)*. The mass is in the left caudal lung lobe and is seen most distinctly on the right recumbent lateral view because the air-tissue contrast is enhanced by increased inflation of the (upper) left lung.

and bronchi with radiopaque contrast material. It has not been widely used in veterinary medicine.[2, 5-7, 15, 16] The indications for its use are few, and because it compromises respiratory function, bronchography is used with caution.

Indications. The most common indication for bronchography is to demonstrate bronchiectasis in an animal with chronic, nonresponsive cough. Not all cases of bronchiectasis are recognizable on plain radiographs. Bronchiectasis is usually generalized in the dog, but segmental bronchiectasis does occur and would be surgically correctable if diagnosed.[5, 15]

Other, less common indications are to demonstrate tracheal or bronchial foreign bodies, stenoses and tears, lung lobe displacement, and *Filarioides* lesions within the trachea, and to differentiate primary lung neoplasia and infection. Bronchoscopy-assisted biopsy is better than bronchography for differentiating neoplasia, infection, and parasitic granulomas.[9]

Contraindications. Acute tracheobronchial inflammation and any condition that is a contraindication for general anesthesia are contraindications for bronchography.

Contrast Material. Recommended contrast material for bronchography include aqueous propyliodone,* barium-carboxymethylcellulose, and tantalum oxide powder.† These contrast agents produce minimal side effects and have physical properties that produce good bronchial opacification. Because tantalum oxide powder must be atomized for distribution to the bronchi, it must be administered with bronchial catheterization techniques.

Technique. Bronchography can be performed under general anesthesia with tracheal intubation and bronchial catheterization or by percutaneous, transtracheal injection. The patient is premedicated with atropine to reduce the amount of bronchial secretion.

Intubation Technique. A small rubber or polyethylene catheter is placed through the tracheal tube to the desired location in a bronchus. Contrast material is slowly injected, under fluoroscopy, until the desired filling is achieved. If the procedure is performed without fluoroscopy, 0.25 to 0.5 ml/kg body weight of contrast material is injected into the distal trachea with the animal positioned in lateral recumbency. This amount usually fills the dependent lung.

Transtracheal Injection Technique. Injections are made into the ventral proximal trachea with the patient in lateral recumbency. First, 2 to 3 ml or 4 per cent lidocaine hydrochloride (Xylocaine) are injected for topical anesthesia. Liquid contrast material, 0.25 to 0.5 ml/kg body weight, is injected next, and the animal is positioned to gravitate contrast material into the dependent lung. Severe respiratory dysfunction is minimized by placing contrast medium in one lung at a time. Twenty-four or 48 hours later, the other lung is examined if desired.

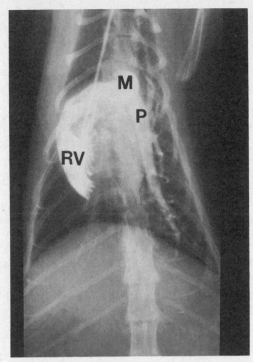

Figure 63–4. A ventrodorsal thoracic radiograph of an angiocardiogram with opacification of only the left pulmonary arteries. The injection of contrast material was made in the ventricle *(RV)*. The contrast material reached the main pulmonary artery segment *(M)* and the left pulmonary arteries *(P)*. Because there was congenital absence of the right pulmonary vessels, no opacification was seen on the angiogram.

Pulmonary Angiography. Pulmonary angiography is a technique of injecting contrast material to opacify pulmonary arteries and veins.

Indications. Indications for pulmonary angiography include detection of congenital pulmonary vascular abnormalities (Fig. 63–4), diagnosis of pulmonary

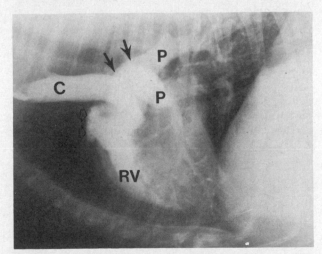

Figure 63–5. A lateral thoracic radiograph of a nonselective angiocardiogram in a case of pulmonary thromboembolism. The cranial vena cava *(C)*, right auricle *(open arrows)*, right ventricle *(RV)*, main pulmonary artery segment *(solid arrows)*, and pulmonary arteries to the caudal lung lobes *(P)* are opacified by contrast material. The main pulmonary artery segment is enlarged. The caudal lung lobe pulmonary arteries are large and tortuous and do not fill peripherally. The changes are compatible with pulmonary thromboembolism and pulmonary hypertension.

---

*Dionosil, Glaxo Operations Ltd., Greenford, England.

†Tantalum oxide powder, Fansteel Metallurgical Corp., North Chicago, IL.

thromboembolism[3] (Fig. 63–5), and demonstration of hypertensive changes in pulmonary vessels. Hypertensive-appearing vessels can be present with reversed cardiac shunts and heartworm disease. Selective angiography demonstrates mild hypertensive changes in secondary and tertiary pulmonary artery branches with mild or occult heartworm disease when such changes are not apparent in primary pulmonary artery branches.

Technique. Depending on the condition of the animal and the suspected disease process, either nonselective or selective pulmonary angiography can be performed. A nonselective study can be performed by injecting contrast material into a jugular or cephalic vein. A bolus of approximately 10 to 25 ml of contrast material, depending on the animal's size, should be injected as rapidly as possible. Films then should be made to record the pulmonary vascular phase of the angiogram, which may vary from five to 30 seconds, depending on the degree of vasculature obstruction.

A selective angiogram may be performed by positioning a catheter in the main pulmonary artery or one of its branches. This technique is superior to the nonselective technique for demonstrating mild peripheral lesions, but it cannot easily be performed in debilitated animals or without fluoroscopy.

ENDOSCOPY OF THE RESPIRATORY SYSTEM

Endoscopy of the respiratory system is convenient for localizing the inciting cause of unexplained coughing, sneezing, hemoptysis, wheezing, stridor, stertor, and discharge.[17]

Anesthesia

General anesthesia should be used for all endoscopy procedures in animals because of the inability to control the awake patient and its reflexes, and in order to prevent damage to the animal and equipment. Deep general anesthesia is needed to examine the upper respiratory system, especially the nasal passages.[22] A lighter plane of anesthesia can be used if it is augmented by a topical anesthetic—lidocaine hydrochloride, one to two per cent solution; tetracaine hydrochloride, 0.5 per cent solution (dogs only); or mepivacaine hydrochloride, two per cent solution. Care must be exercised not to exceed the toxic limits of any of these agents. The total safe dose of the agent should be calculated, drawn into a syringe, and administered in fractionated doses. The anesthetic is administered through the endoscope as various levels of the respiratory tract are explored.

Atropine sulfate is used sparingly or not at all in the patient undergoing endoscopic examination of the respiratory system. This agent decreases secretions of the mucous membranes, allowing the surfaces to dry, thereby increasing friction between the endoscope and mucosa and causing more damage to the mucous membrane. If copious amounts of secretion are encountered during the examination and become a problem to the endoscopist, atropine sulfate can be given intramuscularly (1 mg/kg) or by nebulization (0.1 mg/kg) to control the secretions.[29]

Either gas or intravenous general anesthetics are used for endoscopy. Gas anesthesia is less risky for the patient and can be administered through special adaptors attached to the endotracheal tube or endoscope (see Chapter 28). These adaptors allow maintenance of anesthetic gas levels in the patient while protecting the examiner from exposure.

Position of the Patient

The patient is placed in either dorsal or lateral recumbency for examination of the respiratory system. Dorsal recumbency is generally more comfortable and less confusing for the examiner.

Passage of the rigid bronchoscope through the larynx and down the trachea is facilitated by keeping the head of the patient at the edge of the examination table. The patient's head is easily extended and the endoscopist is not restricted by the close proximity of the table surface.

Upper Respiratory System

Rhinoscopy

Rhinoscopy is useful in exploring lesions observed on radiographs or as a primary method of examining the nasal passages for the detection of foreign bodies, granulomas, tumors, infectious processes, or parasites. The major problems encountered in small animal rhinoscopy are the small nasal passages, large volume of fragile turbinates, and the delicate mucous membrane. The endoscopist must have a detailed knowledge of the anatomy of the turbinates to understand the structures being observed. Significant hemorrhage during physical examination is highly probable. Extreme care and small instruments are necessary.

The otoscope can be used to examine the region immediately inside the external nares, the alar cartilage, and the rostral ventral turbinates.

The instrument most commonly used for extensive exploration of the nasal passages is the small rigid arthroscope (see Chapter 28). The outside diameter of the examining piece is approximately 2.5 mm. This instrument gives a reasonable field of view to examine the turbinates and nasal passages in small dogs (five to seven kilograms) and some cats.[22] Larger arthroscopes and flexible bronchoscopes can be used in large dogs.

The rigid fiberoptic system provides a good view

of the rostral end of the nasal meatus, ventral turbinates, and alar cartilage. The ventral nasal passage can be viewed for most of its length, although the ethmoid turbinates and caudal aspect of the ventral turbinates are rarely seen. Relatively deep anesthesia is important because the sneeze reflex is initiated even under general anesthesia.

A primary requirement for good rhinoscopy is initial preparation of the field of examination. The nasal passages are irrigated well through a Foley catheter passed into the caudal nasal passageway via the oral pharynx. A No. 12 Fr Foley catheter with a 5-ml cuff is used in small dogs and large cats, and a No. 20 to 22 Fr Foley catheter with a 30-ml cuff in giant dogs. The tip of the catheter is amputated about one centimeter from the balloon cuff so that there is a single end-port. A small amount of air is placed in the cuff to aid in manually placing the catheter tip in the caudal nasal passage. The soft palate is pulled rostrally as the catheter tip is placed dorsal to the palate and passed dorsorostrally. More air is added to the cuff so that it can be palpated dorsal to the soft palate. The balloon is milked rostrally to the pterygoid bones by palpation through the soft palate. The balloon is filled until it completely occludes the nasal passageway (Fig. 63–6).

Dorsal recumbency places the nose in an elevated relationship to the nasopharynx. This arrangement produces a fountain-like function of the nasal irrigation system, eliminating the majority of the bubble formation that may occur along the nasal turbinates. It is a convenient position for examining the nasal passages on both sides of the septum. The endotracheal tube cuff must be tested to make sure it is functional in order to prevent aspiration of flushing solution.

Cool saline or Ringer's solution is irrigated through the nasal passageways via the Foley catheter to clear the majority of mucus and exudate. Also the constant flush of cool electrolyte solution causes blood vessels to contract, decreases congestion, and carries blood away from the area if the mucous membrane is lacerated. It also provides a better examination of the mucous membrane, because mucous strands, proliferative tissue, and exudates are lifted from the surface. Neosynephrine (1 per cent) added to the fluid aids blood vessel constriction.[21] It is desirable to irrigate the nasal passageways well before attempting a visual examination. Perfusion of the nasal passages is continued during the entire examination.

The endoscope is introduced into the external nares and passed dorsal to the alar fold. The arthroscope is slowly and gently passed into the dorsal meatus while the operator observes the passageway through the scope. In this way one can avoid impacting the end of the scope against the dorsal nasal concha or surrounding mucous membrane. The extent of the dorsal meatus to the ethmoid turbination

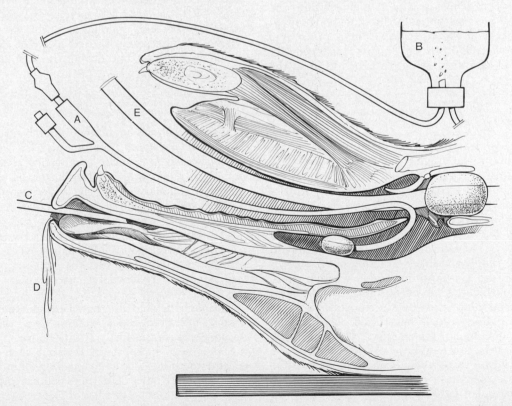

Figure 63–6. Nasal flushing system. A drawing of a dog's skull demonstrates the position of a Foley catheter (A) with the balloon end in the caudal nasal passage. The pressurized fluid reservoir (B) is used as a source of cold flushing solution. The tip of the rigid fiberoptic unit (C) is shown in the ventral meatus, and flush solution (D) is flowing from the nostrils. A cuffed endotracheal tube (E) is in position to prevent inhalation of flush solution.

is examined, after which the tip of the scope is withdrawn slightly and depressed ventrad along the nasal septum into the middle meatus. The ethmoidal conchae and the dorsal aspect of the ventral nasal concha can be examined as the scope is withdrawn to the alar fold. The scope is passed into the ventral nasal meatus as the rostral cartilaginous nose is bent dorsally to assist in passage of the endoscope. The endoscope is guided caudally under the view of the operator, and the nasal passageway is examined to the level of the balloon on the Foley catheter. The Foley catheter is removed. The endoscope is advanced into the caudal nasal passageway for further examination of this area.

Obstruction of the caudal nasal passage eliminates this route for a constant flush system. Each nostril can be flushed independently using a soft rubber feeding tube, or the solution can be flushed in one nostril and out the other. The flush technique is not essential to, but is helpful for, rhinoscopy.

The laryngoscope is used to examine the complete oral cavity, oral pharynx, and glottic region. The addition of an angled dental mirror to the laryngoscope can allow the examiner to explore the caudal aspect of the nasopharynx.[22] Exploration is facilitated by catching the free edge of the soft palate with a traction suture or retractor (snook hook) and retracting it rostrally.

The flexible fiberoptic bronchoscope or gastroscope can be used to examine the caudal nasal passage from the oral cavity.[22] The instrument is passed into the oral cavity of the anesthetized patient and retroflexed so that the tip of the fiberoptic unit is protruding into the caudal nasal pharynx.[17] This maneuver provides a good view of the entire area rostral to the hard palate.

Laryngoscopy

Flexible or rigid fiberoptic laparoscopes can be used to examine the epiglottis and structures of the glottic opening (aryepiglottic fold, mucous membrane covered arytenoid cartilages, vocal folds, and ventricular openings). The rigid fiberoptic laparoscope gives a larger field of view.

The epiglottis and entire glottic rim are examined for pathological conditions. The examiner should spend some time watching the motion of the various structures of the glottis to determine whether there are any abnormalities. A fairly light plane of anesthesia is needed to evaluate the function of these structures, because deep anesthesia abolishes the majority of movement in the larynx.[26] The vocal folds, true vocal cords, and openings of the ventricles are examined as the bronchoscope is advanced into the larynx. Areas of tissue irritation or proliferation are noted and sampled for biopsy.

The flexible fiberoptic unit is convenient for observation of the epiglottis, ventricular opening, ventricular fold, and vocal folds from various angles by its inherent capability to look around corners.

Lower Respiratory System

Trachea and Bronchi

As the bronchoscope is advanced into the trachea, motion of the tracheal rings and dorsal tracheal membrane is observed. Narrowing of the airway is noted as to type and location.

The bronchoscope is passed into the intrathoracic segment of the trachea, and again the walls are observed for abnormal motion.[27] The normal tracheobronchial wall dilates on inspiration and constricts with expiration. Coughing results in approximately a 50 per cent decrease in tracheal diameter.[17] A collapsing trachea is made obvious by the redundant dorsal membrane and flattening of the tracheal rings as the examiner views the trachea during the various phases of respiration. The carina and mainstem bronchi are observed for the character of the mucous membrane lining and any exudates.[17, 23] Foreign bodies may be observed in this region or deeper in the various branchings of the bronchial tree. The depths of this tree are best reached with the flexible pediatric bronchoscope, which can be advanced easily to the tertiary bronchi in most dogs.

Trachea and bronchi are examined for tumors located in the wall. Neoplasia may emanate from the lung parenchymal tissue and erode into the bronchial lumen.

Foreign bodies deep within the bronchial tree usually cannot be retrieved and incite a local infection. With the aid of a bronchoscope, purulent material may be seen draining from the affected bronchus. This information is used to direct the surgeon to the appropriate lobe during the ensuing exploratory thoracotomy.

Thoroscopy

Direct examination of the pleural space can be done with fiberoptic equipment.[11, 17, 18] This technique is used to evaluate penetrating chest trauma, persistent pneumothorax of undiagnosed origin, suspected pulmonary neoplasia with negative biopsy results, and the pleural space in high-risk surgical patients.

Thoroscopy is a relatively low-risk procedure and provides considerable information when done by experienced thoroscopists. The number of thoracotomies can be reduced by initial examination with this technique.

Although flexible fiberoptic equipment has been used, rigid thoroscopes, arthroscopes, and laparoscopes work satisfactorily. Units with a biopsy port are the most appropriate. Without such a port, a second incision is used to insert a blunt probe to displace lung lobes and mediastinum or a biopsy instrument to obtain samples of pleura, mediastinum, or lung. An electric-tipped cautery probe can be inserted to seal small areas of hemorrhage or air leakage secondary to biopsy, trauma, or ruptured blebs.

Thoroscopy requires general anesthesia or heavy sedation and local anesthesia. The patient is placed in dorsal or lateral recumbency and a mild pneumothorax is created. The pleural space can be entered through an intercostal space, although a cranial or caudal substernal approach provides a better view of the hemithorax. The cranial approach is used for caudal lesions, and the caudal approach for cranial lesions.

At the completion of the study, the pneumothorax is reversed by suction through the thoroscope, and the skin incisions are closed with one or two sutures.

ANESTHESIA FOR RESPIRATORY DISEASE PATIENTS

Patients with respiratory disease are prime candidates for respiratory and cardiac failure during induction of anesthesia (see Chapter 188). Care is taken not to excite the patient during the preanesthetic period. Oxygen therapy may be needed during this period and is administered through a nose cone or, for small dogs and cats, in an anesthesia box.

Anesthesia is inducted as rapidly as possible so that the anesthetist can gain control of the airway to ensure adequate ventilation. Intubation must be done quickly and accurately, and assisted ventilation must be used until the patient is stable. In a patient with laryngeal or proximal tracheal stenosis, a tube tracheostomy must be performed under sedation and local anesthesia prior to induction with a general anesthetic, to ensure an adequate airway throughout the periods of anesthesia and postoperative recovery (see Chapter 65).

Monitoring of the Anesthetized Patient

Monitoring of the patient during surgery is discussed in detail in Chapter 29. In the patient with depressed lung function, arterial blood gases and pH are monitored during operation and recovery from general anesthesia. In addition, all atelectatic areas of lung are observed for inflation with normal ventilatory pressures before the chest is closed.

Hypothermia

The anesthetized small dog or cat loses body temperature rapidly during extended diagnostic procedures, during preparation for thoracic surgery, and while the thorax is open. An external heat source as well as insulation against cold surfaces should be provided for these patients.

Radiant heat (heat lamp), heated water bed, and padded electric heating pad are common methods of applying external heat. The water bed is the safest method. Frequently, however, a water bed is not sufficient to maintain body temperature, especially if large areas have been clipped free of hair and the skin is wet from water and alcohol solutions. A heat lamp is a convenient heat source during skin preparation and prior to draping. The eyes are protected from drying by conjunctival ointments and shade.

A heavy pad is placed between the table and a water bed or heating pad to reduce heat loss into the table. A heavy towel is placed between the patient and the water bed or heating pad to absorb fluid and distribute the heat more evenly over the contact surface of the patient.

The heated skin surface is evaluated frequently for areas of excessive heat to prevent local burns. Core body temperature is monitored continuously in all anesthetized animals, especially small dogs and cats, so that hypothermia can be prevented.

1. Bauer, T., and Thomas, W. P.: Pulmonary diagnostic techniques. Vet. Clin. North Am. Small Anim. Pract. *13*:273, 1983.
2. Bishop, E. J., Medway, W., and Archibald, J.: Radiographic methods of investigating the thorax of small animals including a technique for bronchography. N. Am. Vet. *36*:477, 1955.
3. Burns, M. G., Kelly, A. B., Hornof, W. J., and Howerth, E. W.: Pulmonary artery thrombosis in three dogs with hyperadrenocorticism. J. Am. Vet. Med. Assoc. *178*:388, 1981.
4. Chambers, J. N., and Rawlings, C. A.: Ventilation-perfusion mismatching precipitating hypoxemia in two dogs. J. Am. Anim. Hosp. Assoc. *13*:335, 1977.
5. Douglas, S. W.: The interpretation of canine bronchograms. J. Am. Vet. Radiol. Soc. *15*:18, 1974.
6. Douglas, S. W., and Hall, L. W.: Bronchography in the dog. Vet. Rec. *71*:901, 1959.
7. Dyce, K. M.: Experimental bronchography of the dog. Br. Vet. J. *111*:323, 1955.
8. Ettinger, S. J.: Differential diagnosis of coughing. *In* Ettinger, S. J. (ed.): *Textbook of Veterinary Internal Medicine.* 2nd ed. W. B. Saunders, Philadelphia, 1983.
9. Fraser, R. G., and Paré, J. A. P.: *Diagnosis of Diseases of the Chest.* W. B. Saunders, Philadelphia, 1977.
10. Harvey, C. E., and O'Brien, J. A.: Management of respiratory emergencies in small animals. Vet. Clin. North Am. *2*:243, 1972.
11. Jackson, A. M., and Ferreira, A. A.: Fluoroscopy as an aid to the diagnosis of diaphragmatic injury in penetrating wounds of the lower left chest: a preliminary report. Injury *7*:213, 1975.
12. Kagan, K. G.: Thoracic trauma. Vet. Clin. North Am.: Small Anim. Pract. *10*:641, 1980.
13. Kolata, R. J.: Management of thoracic trauma. Vet. Clin. North Am.: Small Anim. Pract. *11*:103, 1981.
14. Morgan, J. P., and Silverman, S.: *Techniques of Veterinary Radiography.* 3rd ed. Veterinary Radiological Associates, Davis, 1982.
15. Myer, W., and Burt, J. K.: Bronchiectasis in the dog: its radiographic appearance. J. Am. Vet. Radiol. Soc. *14*:3, 1973.
16. Nelson, S. W., Christoforidis, A. J., and Pratt, P. C.: Bronchography. *In* Felson, B. (ed.): *Roentgen Techniques and Laboratory Animals.* W. B. Saunders, Philadelphia, 1968.
17. O'Brien, J. A.: A diagnostic approach to respiratory disease. Curr. Vet. Ther. *7*:203, 1980.
18. Ogburn, P., and Bistner, S. I.: Examination of the respiratory system. Vet. Clin. North Am.: Small Anim. Pract. *11*:623, 1981.
19. Pecora, D. V.: Bacteriologic cultural examination of the lower respiratory tract of laboratory dogs. Am. J. Vet. Res. *37*:1511, 1976.
20. Peters, R. M., and Hogan, J. S.: Fluid overload and the post-

traumatic respiratory distress syndrome. J. Trauma *18*:83, 1978.

21. Rebar, A. H., DeNicola, D. B., and Muggenburg, B. A.: Bronchopulmonary lavage cytology in the dog: normal findings. Vet. Pathol. *17*:294, 1980.

22. Rodkey, W. G.: Initial assessment, resuscitation, and management of the critically traumatized small animal patient. Vet. Clin. North Am.: Small Anim. Pract. *10*:563, 1980.

23. Roudebush, P.: Diagnostics for respiratory diseases. *In* Kirk, R. W. (ed.): *Current Veterinary Therapy. VIII. Small Animal Practice.* W. B. Saunders, Philadelphia, 1983.

24. Roudebush, P.: Lung sounds. J. Am. Vet. Med. Assoc. *181*:122, 1982.

25. Schaer, M., and Ackerman, H.: Diagnostic approach to the patient with respiratory disease. *In* Ettinger, S. J. (ed.): *Veterinary Internal Medicine.* 2nd ed. W. B. Saunders, Philadelphia, 1983.

26. Ticer, J. W.: *Radiographic Techniques in Veterinary Practice.* 2nd ed. W. B. Saunders, Philadelphia, 1984.

27. Venker-vanHaagen, A. J.: Bronchoscopy of the normal and abnormal canine. J. Am. Anim. Hosp. Assoc. *15*:397, 1979.

28. Venker-vanHaagen, A. J., Hartman, W., and Goedegebuure, S. A.: Spontaneous laryngeal paralysis in young Bouviers. J. Am. Anim. Hosp. Assoc. *14*:714, 1978.

29. Zavalla, D. C., Godsey, K., and Badell, G. N.: Response to atropine sulfate given by aerosol and intramuscular routes to patients undergoing fiberoptic bronchoscopy. Chest 79:512, 1981.

30. Zenoble, R. D.: Respiratory pharmacology and therapeutics. Comp. Cont. Ed. 2:586, 1980.

Chapter **64**

Upper Respiratory System

A. Wendell Nelson and Peggy M. Wykes

CONGENITAL ANOMALIES

Stenotic Nares

Stenotic nares are frequently found in brachycephalic dogs and occur with other conditions causing resistance to air flow (i.e., elongated soft palate, collapsed larynx, everted laryngeal saccules, paralyzed vocal cords (Fig. 64–1).[48, 59, 67] Interference with inspiration by the obstructed nares can lead to secondary airway changes (i.e., everted saccules, laryngeal collapse, tracheal collapse), but the reverse does not occur.

Stenotic nares are frequently diagnosed in younger, brachycephalic dogs (less than two years) with overlong soft palate and have a good prognosis after surgical treatment.[42] In older brachycephalic dogs (more than 2 years), stenotic nares are associated with additional airway obstruction, and these patients have a guarded prognosis even with treatment.[41]

Stenotic or obstructed nares affect the mechanics of the lungs.[20, 85] The greatest changes are observed in dogs with partial bilateral nasal obstruction and high nasal resistance. Increases in end-expiratory intrapleural negative pressure, functional residual capacity, and pulmonary resistance occur. Increased tone of respiratory muscles and bronchial smooth muscle may be the cause of these changes.

Clinical Signs

The principal sign of stenotic nares is inspiratory dyspnea, which is relieved by open mouth breathing.[67] The wing of the nostril fills the majority of the external nares, is sucked inward on inspiration, and occludes the nostril airway. Additional signs such as coughing, gagging, and stridorous respiration are commonly related to extension of the long soft palate into the larynx.[42, 67]

Surgical Plan

The patient should be hyperoxygenated, the anesthesic should be given rapidly, and intubation of the trachea should be quickly accomplished. Struggling on induction can result in acute hypoxia and respiratory acidosis.

The stenosing wings of the nostrils are resected so there is adequate cross-sectional area of the nostril to allow unobstructed inspiration. The patient is then temporarily extubated, and the soft palate and larynx are examined for additional obstructive lesions. If the soft palate is determined to be interfering with air passage into the larynx, it should be shortened at this time (see "Overlong Soft Palate"). Everted laryngeal saccules, if found, can be resected at this time.

Surgical Approach

The wing of the nostril is examined to determine the amount of tissue to be removed for optimal air flow. The wing is continuous with the alar fold as it tapers caudally to the alar cartilage. Part of this fold may need to be excised to open the airway. This tissue is highly vascular and bleeds profusely when incised. Pressure against the first incision of the wedge with a suction tip controls the hemorrhage and removes most of the blood as a second incision is made. Electrosurgery should not be used because it destroys too much tissue. Epinephrine-soaked, cotton-tipped swabs are helpful in reducing the hemorrhage as the edges are sutured together.

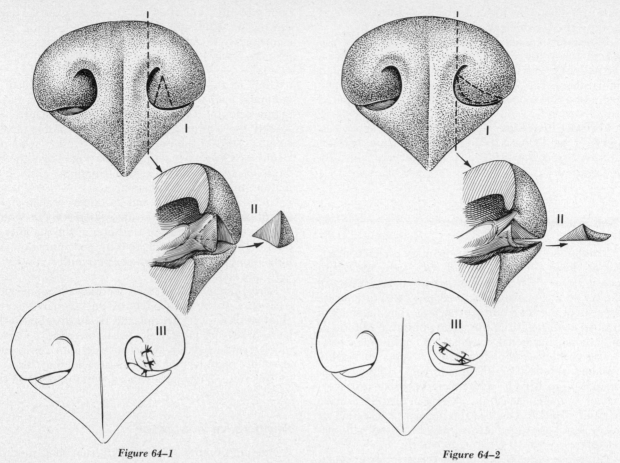

Figure 64–1

Figure 64–2

Figure 64–1. Repair of stenotic nares using vertical wedge. *I*, Vertical wedge incisions on the wing of the nostril. The vertical dotted line indicates the plane of the cutaway view (see II). *II*, The incisions to remove the vertical wedge from the wing of the nostril. The depth of the wedge is indicated by the dotted lines going to the alar cartilage. *III*, Line drawing illustrating the placement of sutures to close the wedge defect.

Figure 64–2. Repair of stenotic nares using horizontal wedge. *I*, Dotted lines on the mucosa of the wing of the nostril indicates the mucosal incision. The vertical dotted line indicates the plane for the cutaway diagram (see II). *II*, A cutaway diagram of the external nares and proximal nasal passages. The depth of the horizontal wedge is indicated by dotted lines going to the alar cartilage. *III*, The line drawn indicates the closure of the incision with interrupted sutures.

Vertical Wedge Resection. The technique of removing a vertical wedge from the wing of a nostril and extending the incision caudally to include part of the alar cartilage has been useful in eliminating stenosis. The incision is made with a No. 11 Bard Parker or No. 65 Beaver blade. The tip of the blade is introduced at the apex of the wedge and directed caudally with the cutting edge directed medially to the free edge of the wing of the nostril. The apex of the wedge is the pivot point of the flap created to allow the edges of the incision to come together evenly and without tension. The blade is again introduced at the apex of the wedge and the cutting edge is directed ventrolaterally as the tip is pushed caudally to end at the same point the first incision did. The wedge is removed and the edges are sutured with 5-0 or 6-0 fine absorbable suture using a small half-circle cutting needle (Fig. 64–1). Three or four interrupted sutures are needed to close the wound, one being placed at the mucocutaneous junction.

Horizontal Wedge Resection. A second method removes a wedge of the nostril in a medial to lateral direction.[42, 59] The incision is started near the medial edge of the wing and continued along the ventral edge to the lateral border. This incision is deepened dorsocaudally to the alar fold (Fig. 64–2*I*). A second incision is made horizontally across the rostral surface of the wing of the nostril, dividing it into dorsal and ventral segments (2/3 and 1/3, respectively). The horizontal incision is deepened caudally to meet the first incision at the alar fold, and the wedge of tissue is removed (Fig. 64–2*II*), Leaving a flap of mucosa from the ventral surface of the wing of the nostril. The flap is elevated dorsally to close the defect. Absorbable 5-0 to 6-0 suture material is used to close the defect.

Lateral Wedge Resection. A third method for enlarging stenotic nares is the resection of a portion of the caudolateral border of the wing or the nostril and a wedge of skin adjacent to it.[57] A triangular lesion is created with the apex directed caudolaterally and the base perpendicular to the ventral edge of the wing. All points of the triangle converge caudally toward the alar cartilage and the pyramid of tissue is cut free. The free portion of the wing is pulled laterally as a rotational flap and sutured to the skin.

Fine monofilament nonabsorbable sutures are used to close the skin defect.

Comment. In all three methods the sutures are placed to simply appose tissue. Tight sutures cause the patient to rub the surgical site, resulting in wound dehiscence. The long-term results of the first two techniques have been good. The third has had limited use.

Postoperative Care. The surgical site is kept clean and protected from rubbing (self-mutilation) with an Elizabethan collar. Additional medical care is usually not needed.

Cleft Palate

Congenital diseases of the primary and secondary palate have been reported in both dogs and cats.[25, 36, 55, 56, 58, 93, 110] The primary palate consists of the tip and premaxilla, whereas the secondary palate consists of the hard and soft palates. The incomplete closure of these structures is attributed to inherited, nutritional, hormonal, mechanical, and toxic factors.

The incidence of cleft palate is higher in brachycephalic breeds (i.e., Boston terrier, Pekingese) although other breeds (schnauzer, Labrador retriever, cocker spaniel, dachshund, German shepherd) have been involved.[58] A cleft of the primary and secondary palate has been reported in cats,[93, 110] especially Siamese.

Clefts are inherited as either recessive or irregular dominant traits.[27, 39, 58, 65] All types of clefts, from partial unilateral to complete bilateral, have been produced in dogs in mating trials.[58] Mating phenotypically cleft parents produced offspring with a 41.7 per cent cleft occurrence rate, and the severity of the cleft in the parents did not influence the severity of the cleft in the puppies. Unilateral clefts are more common on the left side.

Nutritional, hormonal, and mechanical factors enhance the formation of clefts in genetically predisposed fetuses.[39, 58, 106] Rate of growth of the palatine plates must compete successfully with the growth of the skull width to achieve midline closure of the palatine plates.[37, 65] Broad-headed fetuses have a greater tendency to develop a cleft palate and to be affected by nutritional, hormonal (steroid), and toxic (including viral infections) factors. Toxic agents and intrauterine viral infections can produce animals with clefts if the insult occurs at a specific time in fetal development (25th to 28th day in the dog).[58]

Clinical Diagnosis

Primary cleft palate (harelip) is obvious at birth as an abnormal division in the upper lip. The affected animal should be examined for coexisting clefts of the secondary palate (hard and soft palate). Clefts of the secondary palate are more common and frequently go unnoticed until the neonate demonstrates signs of poor growth; drainage of milk from the external nares during or after nursing; coughing, gagging, and sneezing while eating; and respiratory tract infection (rhinitis, laryngotracheitis, and inhalation pneumonia).

Cleft of the distal one-half of the soft palate is generally well tolerated, because inhalation pneumonia seldom develops. The animal is usually presented for slower growth, chronic rhinitis, and a cough. Clefts of the entire soft palate allow food and liquid easy access to the nasal passage, resulting in nasal discharge, sneezing and coughing, and, ultimately, inhalation pneumonia.

Clefts of the primary and secondary palate cause conditions similar to those described for the secondary cleft palate, with the addition of the inability to nurse. The neonate is affected by poor nutrition and inhalation pneumonia, which frequently results in early postnatal death.

Early diagnosis and tube feeding allows surgical treatment to be delayed until the animal is six to eight weeks of age. During this delay the cleft in the hard palate frequently decreases in width, making more tissue available for reconstruction. The tissues are more mature and have better holding strength by this time, and there is more working room in the small oral cavity.

Preoperative Preparation

Nursing puppies are not taken from their mothers until just prior to surgery. Older patients are not fed in the morning and are brought to surgery as early in the day as practical. Patients with signs of pneumonia should be appropriately treated and tube fed until they are good surgical risks.

Inhalation anesthesia is induced with the patient in an anesthesia box. A close-fitting (preferably cuffed) endotracheal tube is passed *per os* and taped to the lower jaw.

Surgical Technique

Meticulous care of tissue is needed at all stages of cleft reconstruction. Crushing and drying of tissue should not be tolerated. The injection of epinephrine solution and the use of electrosurgical equipment are avoided. Retraction is done with traction sutures and fine skin hooks.[56] All sutures (4-0 to 6-0) should have swaged-on needles.

The patient is placed in ventral recumbency during repair of clefts of the primary palate and in dorsal recumbency for those of the secondary palate. No hair clipping is necessary. The oral and nasal cavities are flushed clear of debris with saline and then four to six times with a tissue-compatible antiseptic.

The animal's chin is placed on folded towels and the surgeon is seated to obtain good working position for a cleft of the primary palate. Movement of the head and muscle should not be restricted by tape or heavy draping material, because soft tissue symmetry

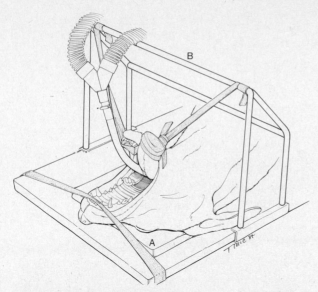

Figure 64–3. Head restraint for palate surgery. The line drawing demonstrates the head placed on a pad *(A)* and the upper jaw taped to the surgical table. The lower jaw is taped to the anesthesia screen *(B)* with one-inch adhesive tape. The tongue is dried and taped to the tape holding the lower jaw. The anesthesia tubes are draped over the corner of the anesthesia screen and held in place with tape.

and open mouth positions are important. The dorsally recumbent patient needs a skull pad, and the mouth is taped in an open position for exposure of the secondary palate. The tongue and endotracheal tube are taped to an anesthesia screen to provide better exposure of the surgical field (Fig. 64–3).

Clefts of the Primary Palate

The main objective in repairing primary cleft palate is closure of the nasal floor. Without adequate closure of the nasal mucosa over the cleft, realignment of the remaining tissue is meaningless, as dehiscence with secondary repair requires taking down of the lip closure.

Cleft Lip (Harelip). The objective of cleft lip closure is to align the natural adjoining edge of the cleft so that distance from the ventral nostril to the free ventral edge of the lip is the same on the cleft and unaffected sides.[33, 37, 39] The ventral rim of the nostril and the floor of the rostral nasal passage must make a smooth, sealed junction. The alveolabial sulcus is established to provide mucosal continuity of the oral side of the cleft.

The normal side of the nose is measured for width of the lip in the same area as that of the cleft. This dimension is compared with the two edges of the cleft. The edge of the lip is shortened by resection of a wedge of tissue and is lengthened by making an incision perpendicular to the cleft edge, which is sutured open.

The columella and philtrum are examined carefully (preferably with the aid of enlarged photographs) to identify the proper location of incisions and to allow accurate reconstruction of the lip. Frequently the medial edge of the philtrum of the cleft side lies

nasally along the edge of the columella (Fig. 64–4). The epithelial surface of the columella and adjacent tissue (pore size, pigmentation, surface pattern, and presence of hair) is compared with that of the normal side to determine the proper final location of each portion of tissue. The same is done for the cleft side of the lip (Fig. 64–4).

Although a single case is used here as an example for simplicity, the basic principles described hold true for most clefts of the lip.

In Figure 64–4, the ventral medial edge of the nostril-columella junction (*b–d*) is fused ventrally with the ventral medial ridge of the philtrum. This fusion plane is incised (*a–b*), and the incision is extended along the edge of the nasal mucosa (*b–c*) to produce a flap of tissue that forms the ventromedial rim of the nostril. The incision (*a–b*) is deepened and continued along the ventral mucosal border of the lip (*b–d–e*) to produce two layers of tissue that when sutured together will form the philtrum. A narrow rim of mucosa is left attached to the flap to form the normal midline crease in the philtrum.

In the normal nostril, the ventral edge, as it extends from lateral to medial, is progressively more elevated above the floor of the rostral nasal passage. This is taken into consideration in constructing the ventral rim of the nostril. The lateral edge of the cleft is brought to its normal location at the columella and philtrum, and the natural folding point (*f′*) of the buccal mucosa is noted (Fig. 64–4II). This point is used as the lateral end of the nasal mucosa pedicle flap raised from the rostral extent of the floor of the nares. The incision is extended medially from point *f′* to the alveolabial sulcus of the columella (*b*). The ventral edge of this incision (*b–f′*) will be the location of the alveolabial sulcus. The mucosal pedicle flap of the nasal floor is completed with a short incision (*f–g*) along the junction of the labial mucosa with the gingival mucosa. The nasal floor mucosal flap is undermined and is used later to cover the denuded surface of the nasal side of the ventral rim of the nostril.

Prior to alignment of the ventral edge of the nostril, the buccal mucosa is dissected off the lateral edge of the cleft by lateral extension of the mucosal incision along the alveolabial sulcus (*f–f′*) and the ventro-lateral edge of the nasal floor (*g–h*) toward the lateral commissure of the nostril (Fig. 64–4III). This incision is extended to the mucocutaneous junction of the nostril rim (*n–i–l*) and ventrally along the mucocutaneous junction of the lateral edge of the cleft (*i–j*). The mucosal flap (*f–j*) is undermined and tailored to construct the alveolabial sulcus and fill mucosal deficits on the oral side of the lip.

An incision is made in the mucocutaneous junction of the medial extent of the ventral rim of the nostril (*k–i–l*). The mucocutaneous tissue outlined by this incision is undermined, producing a flap (2) of tissue, which is used to replace part of the deficit in the columella left by the nasal rim flap (3) and philtrum (4) (Fig. 64–4IV).

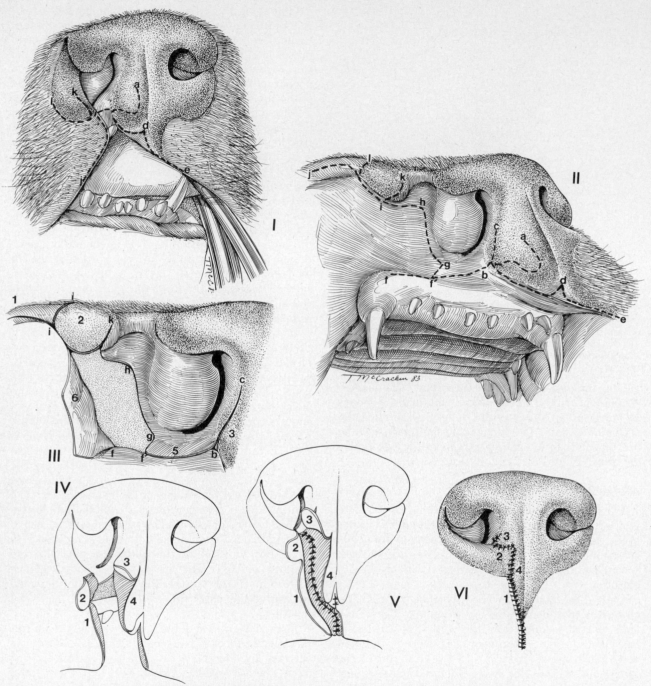

Figure 64–4. Surgical correction of cleft lip (harelip). *I,* The rostral view of the cleft lip is illustrated with the lips in a natural position. The incisions are noted with dotted lines. The *a–d* incision is made to create the right side of the philtrum when aligned with the *d–e* incision. The junction points of the ventral edge of the lip are at *j* and *e. II,* The *c–b–f'–j* incision outlines the flap of mucosa raised from the floor of the nostril to provide a bed for the lip at the alveolar labial sulcus and is used to cover the caudal side of the ventral rim of the nostril. The *f–f'–g–h–i* incision outlines a flap of mucosa that is used to rebuild the alveolar labial sulcus by suturing its free edge to the *f–f'–b–e* line. The *k–i–l* and *a–b–c* flaps are raised to allow the medial edge of the ventral rim of the nostril to be sutured to the lateral side of the columella. *III,* The incisions are made, and the flaps are given numbers (1–6). *IV,* The flaps are lifted and the lip is rotated into position. The *a–b–d* flap (4) is rotated ventrally to align the philtrum. The mucosal incisions *h–g* and *h–i* are aligned and sutured as the ventral rim of the nostril is rotated into position. *V,* The sutures unite the fibromuscular layer of the lip and the mucosa at the philtrum. Flap 2 *(k–i–l)* is used to fill the mucosal deficit left by flaps 3 and 4. Flap 3 *(a–b–c)* is rotated slightly caudally to complete the mucosal cover on the dorsal edge of the ventral rim of the nostril. *VI,* The completed mucosal and skin suture lines with the final placement of flaps 2 and 3 are shown.

The edges of the cleft are aligned (points *k* and *a* are in apposition). The *a–b–c* flap (3) is rotated nasally to reconstruct the medial ventral edge of the nostril (Fig. 64–4V). Some trimming of flaps may be necessary to provide good closure.

The incised edges *g–h* and *h–k* are sutured together to provide mucosal continuity in the lateral nasal floor. The nasal floor mucosal flap (5) provides mucosa to cover remaining mucosal defects on the nasal side of the ventral rim of the nostril (Fig. 64–4V). Fine absorbable, simple interrupted sutures (4–0 to 6–0) close these incisions in the mucosa. Sutures are placed in the fibromuscular tissue of the junction of the medial and lateral components of the cleft (Fig. 64–4V). This suture layer and the layers of the mucosa and of the skin provide a three-layer closure. Interrupted sutures are used in all layers.

The philtrum is sutured by closing the incision *b–d* and *d–e* on the midline with fine absorbable suture. The mucosal edge left on the philtrum is sutured in the midline crease with the knots buried in the submucosa.

The skin is examined to identify ventral junction points (*e* and *j*) of the cleft. Frequently, full thickness lip incision (*i–l*) under the ventral rim of the nostril at the haired-nonhaired junction is needed. When stretched open, this incision increases the length of the lateral edge of the cleft. The length of this incision is half of the desired increase in the length of the edge of the cleft (see Fig. 64–4III). The skin covering the lip near the cleft is undermined liberally (*flaps 1* and *2* in Fig. 64–4V) so that it can be aligned smoothly as it is sutured closed.

Alignment of the skin at the cleft midline is made by matching like tissues (and hair) opposite each other. Simple interrupted monofilament sutures are used to accurately appose the skin edges.

The buccal mucosal flap (*flap 6* in Fig. 64–4III) is used to close the alveolabial sulcus and cover the denuded surface of the oral side of the lip. Undermining and rotation of the mucosa from under the columella may be necessary to cover this area without causing tension bands on the lip. Soft, braided, absorbable suture material is used to close the mucosal incisions in this area.

Rotation of the dorsolateral cartilage (wing of the nostril) into its normal position may place excessive tension on the primary suture lines. A padded tension suture is used to hold the cartilage in its normal position during healing.[37]

A butterfly tape or padded tension suture is applied across the cleft to take tension off the suture lines and to protect the sutures from licking by the patient or littermates. Oral feeding should begin as soon as recovery from anesthesia is complete.[56] A slurry of canned food and water is used for two to three days, then gradually replaced by canned food by the seventh day. Skin sutures are removed in 14 days.

Complete Primary Cleft Palate. Complete cleft of the lip is repaired as described whether it occurs alone or in conjunction with a cleft of the premaxilla.[33, 39] The cleft in the premaxilla is closed first with two mucoperiosteal flaps raised from the nasal floor (Fig. 64–5). The incisions (*f–f'* and *b–b'*) at the junction of nasal and gingival mucosa are continued caudally along the edge of the cleft in the premaxilla to the caudal extent of the cleft (Fig. 64–5II and III). These mucosal edges are undermined to create two long narrow flaps, one nasal and one oral, along each side of the cleft premaxilla. The two nasal flaps are sutured together, closing the nasal floor over the cleft

(Fig. 65–5IV). Simple interrupted absorbable sutures (4-0 to 6-0) are preplaced and tied sequentially from caudal to rostral with knots buried in the submucosa. The rostral nasal floor is closed by suturing of the rostral edge of these flaps to the ventral rim of the nostril (see Fig. 64–4). The remaining hard palate and gingival cleft are closed through the use of similar flaps raised along the ventral edge of the cleft in the premaxilla (Fig. 64–5IV). These flaps are sutured on the oral midline by similar sutures, which are not preplaced. Closure of the lip is the same as described for cleft lip.

Complete Bilateral Clefts of the Primary Palate. This condition is rarely presented for treatment owing to the severe problems in postnatal feeding, which lead to early death from dehydration and inhalation pneumonia.

The basic approach is the same for unilateral complete cleft of the primary palate. An additional problem arises from the close adherence of the philtrum to the incisive gingiva and a deficiency of tissue in the lip that prevents the closure of the mucosal defect behind the philtrum that is needed to create the alveolabial sulcus.

Mucous membrane on the caudal surface of the philtrum is raised as a flap based ventrally on the gingiva and is used to extend the alveolar mucosa dorsally. The denuded caudal surface of the philtrum is covered by single pedicle flaps of mucosa raised from the lateral edges of the cleft lip, which are sutured together on the midline behind the philtrum.[37] The nasal floor is closed as previously described. The skin edges of the cleft are sutured to the columella, philtrum, and each other to close the midline defect using the same principles as described for a unilateral cleft. The rostrally protruding premaxilla repositions itself gradually after the lip cleft has been closed and lip pressure has been established.

Clefts of the Secondary Palate

Cleft hard palate may occur as a sole entity or may be part of a primary or soft palate cleft. Major clefts of the hard palate usually involve the soft palate.

Closure of the palate defects in the neonate is fraught with problems, such as sutures placed too tightly and suture line tension (secondary to incomplete tissue mobilization, growth stresses, lack of available tissue, movement of tissues from tongue motion, and respiratory pressures) leading to dehiscence. Healing of areas left open by shifted palate mucoperiosteal flaps cause palate growth abnormalities as a result of contraction of the collagen in the granulation tissue next to the dental arcade.[64] Both narrowing and shortening of the maxilla have been demonstrated.[63, 68] This problem can be reduced by covering the defect left by the mucoperiosteal flap with a pedicled buccal mucosal graft.[64] Multiple operations may be needed to close palate defects, especially in the young, rapidly growing patient.[109, 110]

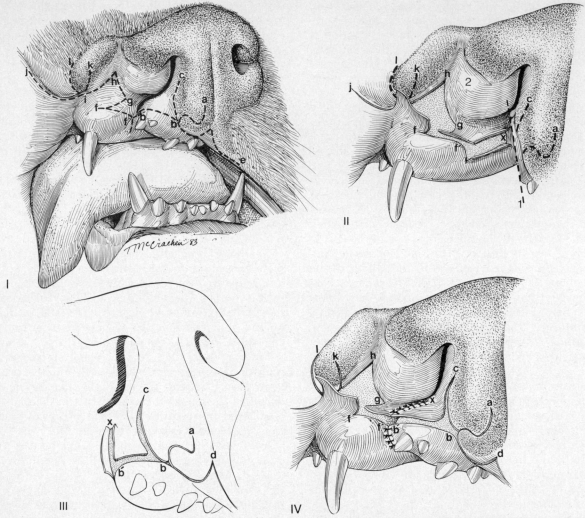

Figure 64–5. Repair of the cleft primary palate. *I,* The cleft primary palate with the lip held laterally to expose the cleft in the incisor bone. Similar flap incisions *(dotted lines)* are indicated as shown in the harelip illustration (Fig. 64–4). *II* and *III,* Three-quarter views of the incisive cleft to illustrate the mucosal flaps *(f′–x* and *b′–x)* raised from the opposite edges of the cleft in the incisive bone. *IV,* The two flaps *c–b–b′–x* and *g–f–f′–x* are sutured together at the cleft to form a single flap used to close the cleft in the floor of the nostril (incisive bone) and cover the caudal aspect of the ventral rim of the nostril (see Fig. 64–4*II*). The oral side of the cleft on the incisive bone is closed with two flaps *(f′–x* and *b′–x).* (See Fig. 64–4 for lip alignment and closure.)

Cleft Hard and Soft Palate

Midline clefts of the hard and soft palates have been closed by several methods. The techniques described satisfy the basic criteria of multilayer closure, off-setting suture lines, and low tension closure necessary for success.

Technical Considerations

Hard Palate. Hard palate clefts are closed with two tissue layers and off-setting suture lines. Palate mucosal deficits secondary to flap production and movement should be covered with buccal mucosal flaps.

Soft Palate. The musculature of the nasopharynx is oriented to elevate its floor (soft palate), to constrict the orifice of the nasopharynx, and to pull the laryngeal pharynx rostrally and constrict it (see Chapter 61).[76] The tensor and levator veli palatini and palatopharyngeus muscles place lateral tension on the soft palate, which would cause tension on the suture lines closing a cleft. The palatinus muscle is paired and lies on each side of the midline in the soft palate. It pulls the soft palate rostrally and can place a shearing force on the palate sutures, especially near the free edge of the soft palate.

In most cases, maintaining soft palate muscular function is not seriously considered during cleft reconstruction in dogs and cats because voice modulation is not important. However, failure to consider the tensing effects of these muscles on the cleft suture lines can lead to postoperative dehiscence.

Tension from the tensor veli palatini muscle is nullified by its transection during the placement of relaxing incisions along the lateral border of the soft palate. The remaining muscle tension on sutures in the mucosa is relieved by suturing the muscular layer separate from the nasal and oral mucosae (a three-layer closure). This is difficult, at best, to do in puppies, and frequently the nasal mucosa is closed with the muscle layer. Muscular tension leading to dehiscence is more significant in partial or complete clefts with a tissue deficit and little room for a relaxing incision (see "Lateral Cleft of the Soft Palate"). Oral mucosal flaps can be used to repair this defect, but the repair does not reconstruct the balance of muscular function around the nasal pharynx.[36] The mucosal flap does close the defect and produces a marked reduction in postoperative signs of the cleft.

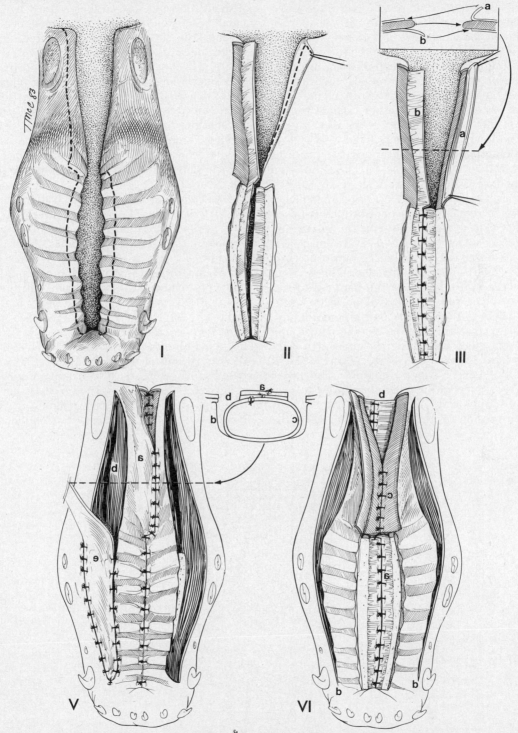

Figure 64–6. Closure of the complete cleft for the secondary palate. *I*, Incisions (*dotted line*) in the mucoperiosteum of the hard palate and the mucosa of the soft palate. *II*, Flaps are raised along the cleft and hinged at the edge of the cleft to provide nasal mucosa. The flap incision (*dotted line*) in the nasal surface of the soft palate will be used to replace oral mucosa. *III*, Rostral nasal mucosa continuity is completed (sutures) with hard palate mucosa. Oral (*a*) and nasal (*b*) flaps are raised on the soft palate. Tissue alignment for the soft palate is indicated. *Inset*, A cross-section through the soft palate. *IV*, Nasal mucosa (*a* and *b*) is sutured. The first few sutures (*c*) are shown closing the muscular portion of the soft palate. Lateral mucosal relaxing incisions (*d*) are made along both sides of the hard and soft palate. *V*, Oral mucosa at the cleft is sutured (*a*), and the relaxing incision (*b*) is deepened between the nasal mucosa (*c*) and the pterygoid bones (*d*) or the soft tissue in its plane (see *inset*). The buccal mucosal flap (*e*) is shown sutured into the defect left after undermining and moving the hard palate mucoperiosteal flap.

Surgical Repair

Hard Palate. A two- or three-layer closure with off-setting suture lines provides the most reliable cleft seal.[55] The width of the bone defect is measured digitally and by hypodermic needle palpation of the osseous plate. Bilateral pedicle flaps of mucoperiosteum, based on the nasal sides of the cleft, are raised along the length of the hard palate cleft (Fig. 64–6*I* and *II*). A scalpel and a periosteal elevator are used to free the soft tissue from the medial edges of the cleft in the bone.[37, 99] The total width of the hard palate flaps, when sutured together, should exceed the width of the hard palate defect by 10 to 20 per cent. The midline closure is completed to the hard-soft palate junction with simple interrupted sutures of fine gut (5-0 to 6-0) with the knots on the nasal side. Redundant tissue at closure is gently pushed toward the nasal passage as the oral closure is made. Another flap of remaining mucoperiosteum is raised from the left side to the palate with the rostral and caudal pedicles intact (Fig. 64–6*IV*). An incision is made just medial to the dental arcade (alveolar ridge) to form the lateral edge of this flap. The incision extends for the entire length of the hard palate and that portion of the soft palate involved in the cleft. The hard palate portion of the flap is undermined, moved over to cover the midline osseous defect, and sutured to the mucosa covering the remaining right side of the hard palate (Fig. 64–6*V*). This is a modification of the vomer flap technique.[55] The major palatine artery is carefully avoided in order to preserve blood supply to the flap.

Excessive tension on the oral mucosa suture line or a wide bony defect requires a second mucoperiosteal flap raised from the opposite side of the hard palate (Fig. 64–6*IV* and *V*). The second flap should allow adequate tension release and defect coverage without allowing the midline suture line (oral and nasal) to be superimposed. Movement of air or fluids through the suture lines is eliminated by the technique, because each suture line is backed by viable tissue.

A single- or double-pedicle flap of buccal mucosa is constructed, rotated into the deficit in the hard palate mucosa next to the dental arcade, and sutured to adjacent mucosa. Rapid coverage of this area reduces granulation tissue production and dental arcade deformity.[63, 64] The base of the buccal mucosa pedicle(s) is transected in two weeks, and incisions are sutured.

Soft Palate. Repair of a soft palate cleft, with (see Fig. 64–6) or without (see Fig. 64–7) a co-existing hard palate cleft, is done with either overlapping flap technique or midline appositional two- or three-layer closure.

The *overlapping flap* technique produces two flaps, one based on the nasal side and the other on the oral side of the palate (see Fig. 64–6*III*). The right side of the soft palate is tensed orally and laterally to expose the nasal side. An incision is made in the nasal mucosa from the hard palate junction to the caudal end of the cleft. The width of this orally based mucosal flap is 5 to 6 mm. A second flap of comparable size is developed with a nasal base on the opposite side of the soft palate cleft. The orally based mucosal flap is sutured into the mucosal defect

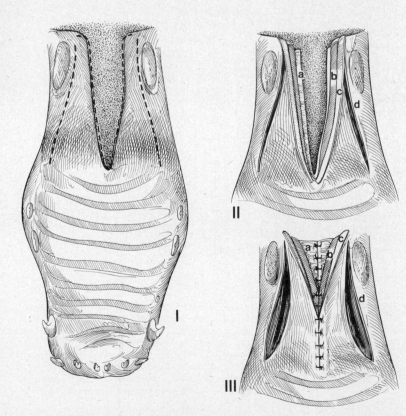

Figure 64–7. Appositional repair of cleft soft palate. *I*, The lateral relaxing and cleft incisions (*dotted lines*) are indicated. The mucosal incision is made along the entire free edge of the cleft. *II*, The free edge of the cleft is dissected to create three layers: nasal mucosa (*a*), muscular layer (*b*), and oral mucosa (*c*). The tension-reducing incisions (*d*) are also shown. *III*, The cleft is partially sutured showing three layers: nasal mucosa (*a*), muscular layer (*b*), and oral mucosa (*c*). The tension-reducing incisions have been deepened.

left by elevation of the nasally based flap. An interrupted pattern of 5-0 absorbable suture is used, with the knots placed on the nasal side. The palatine muscles are sutured along the midline with 5-0 absorbable suture in the same pattern. The right mucosal flap is stretched into the defect on the left side using 5-0 monofilament, nonabsorbable suture in a simple interrupted pattern (see Fig. 64–6V).

Relaxation of the soft palate tissues is obtained by lateral mucosal incisions extending from the medial side of the last molar to the caudal edge of the soft palate at its lateral junction with the oral pharynx (see Figs. 64–6V and Fig. 64–7). The incision passes just dorsal to the palatine tonsil. The mucosal incision is deepened by blunt dissection. The tensor veli palatini muscle is transected as it crosses the annulus of the pterygoid bone (Fig. 64–6V, *inset*). Blunt dissection is continued submucosally between the pterygoid annulus and the nasal mucosa lining the lateral wall of the nasal pharynx. This plane is carried caudally between the levator veli palatini and palatopharyngeous muscles to the caudal edge of the nasal pharynx. The incision is left open to heal by second intention. In patients with combined midline clefts of the hard and soft palates, this incision is a direct continuation of the relaxing incision in the oral mucoperiosteal tissue of the hard palate, which extends along the medial aspect of the alveolar ridge.

The *appositional repair* of a soft palate cleft uses two- or three-layer closure and bilateral relaxing incisions (Fig. 64–7). A stay suture is placed at each junction of the cleft with the caudal free border of the soft palate. A long needleholder or similar forceps are used to grasp the stay suture close to the knot and tense that edge of the cleft caudally. The initial incision is made along the edge of the cleft from the rostral to the caudal end using a No. 65 Beaver or No. 11 Bard Parker blade. Care is taken to complete the incision at the rostral junction of the cleft. A No. 15 Bard Parker blade is used to dissect the oral mucosa away from the palate musculature as the incised edge of the oral mucosa is gently held with fine vascular forceps. The oral mucosa is reflected laterally for half the width of the palate (4 to 5 mm) on each side of the cleft. The procedure is repeated for the nasal mucosa by holding the palate muscular layer with thumb forceps and dissecting it away from the nasal mucosa for a distance of 1 to 2 mm. After both edges of the cleft have been dissected, a two- or three-layer closure of the cleft is made.

The nasal mucosa, if strong enough, is sutured with fine (5-0 or 6-0) gut in a simple interrupted or continuous pattern, with the caudal sutures placed first and the knots on the nasal side. The muscular layer (nasal mucosa may be included if not previously sutured) is sutured with interrupted horizontal mattress sutures of 4-0 to 5-0 absorbable suture beginning at the caudal end of the incision. The oral mucosa is sutured with 5-0 nonabsorbable monofilament suture without including deeper tissues and with the knots on the oral side. Each suture should be placed only

tight enough to appose tissue surfaces, because postoperative swelling will increase tissue pressure. Sutures placed too tightly will cut through the tissue, resulting in dehiscence within two to four days.

Suturing of the palatine muscles as a separate layer reduces the effect of tension and shearing forces generated by the palatine muscles on the oral mucosa during healing. Nonabsorbable sutures may be used in the muscular layer if it is being sutured separately from the mucosal layers.

Lateral Cleft of the Soft Palate. A unilateral or bilateral cleft can be located lateral to the palatine muscles. The tensor and levator veli palatini muscles or palatopharyngeus muscle pull the free edge of the cleft laterally, opposing cleft reconstruction. In bilateral clefts, a central strip of palate containing the palatine muscles covered by mucosa can be seen and may be shorter than normal.

Mucosal Flap Closure. A technique has been described in which the lateral soft palate cleft is closed with a nasal pharyngeal mucosal flap.[36] The mucosa dorsolateral to the cleft is harvested with the flap based just dorsal to the palatine tonsil and the free edge originating from the dorsolateral wall of the nasopharynx, including the vestige of the lateral portion of the palate (Fig. 64–8). The length and width of the flap are established by measuring the size of the defect in the palate and adding 2 mm to the width.

The medial edge of the cleft is incised along its

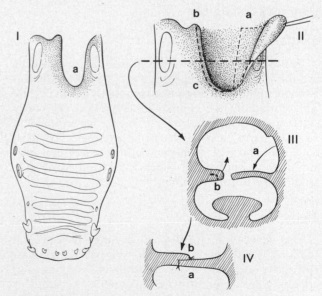

Figure 64–8. Repair of a unilateral cleft of the soft palate. *I,* The palate of the dog with a unilateral cleft (*a*) of the soft palate. *II,* The lateral edge of the cleft is retracted with a suture and the incision (*a, dotted line*) in the lateral nasopharynx is indicated. The incisions on the oral surface near the medial edge (*b*) and at the rostral edge of the clefts (*c*) are indicated (*dotted lines*). *III,* A cross-section through the cleft illustrates the lateral nasal pharyngeal flap (*a*), the medial palate mucosal flap (*b*), and the tongue (*c*). *IV,* This cross-section of the palate closure illustrates the junction of the pharyngeal (*a*) and the palate (*b*) flaps and the location of the suture lines.

entire length to form two layers of tissue. The incision is deepened 1 to 2 mm and separated to receive the free edge of the nasal pharyngeal mucosa flap. Interrupted penetrating sutures of fine (4-0 to 5-0) gut hold the flap between the two edges of the palate. This procedure closes the palate defect but does not provide muscular function to this area, and the nasal surface is left to granulate and epithelialize.

Postoperative Care of Cleft Palate Patients

Postoperative care of cleft palate patients is related to maintaining adequate alimentation without placing tension on the suture lines. A wide cleft with a tenuous closure should be bypassed with a pharyngostomy tube so that the patient can be fed without disturbing the incisions.[109] Patients with a supple palate after two- or three-layer closure can be fed a gruel in 24 to 48 hours and soft food in 72 hours.[55] Dry food is not introduced into the diet for six weeks. Edema or infection is rarely a problem. Dehiscence is the result of motion, tight sutures, or tension. Oral sutures are not removed because they gradually work their way out.

Long-Term Dehiscence. The reconstructed neonatal palate grows rapidly, causing stretching and thinning of some of the hard palate closures.[109] This process results in various-sized oronasal fistulae, which are repaired after the patient is eight to ten months old.[99]

Overlong Soft Palate

Incidence

Approximately 80 per cent of overlong soft palates are found in brachycephalic dogs, with English and French bulldogs being most frequently involved.[43, 95] This condition is accompanied by other respiratory tract anomalies including, in decreasing frequency, stenotic nares, laryngeal saccule eversion, laryngeal collapse, tracheal stenosis, and tracheal collapse. Edematous pharyngeal mucosa and enlarged, protruding tonsils are common.

Signs

The severity of inspiratory dyspnea depends on the length and congestion of the soft palate and other restrictive or obstructive conditions. Gagging and coughing are frequently accompanied by a rattling or snoring noise during ventilation, especially inspiration.

The free border of the overlong soft palate extends beyond the tip of the epiglottis to interfere with laryngeal function. This border may lie on the epiglottis or may be sucked into the glottis during inspiration, causing injury to the palate and larynx and leading to inflammatory edema.

Surgical Procedures

The intention of palate resection is to shorten the soft palate so that its free border lies slightly rostral to or just covers the tip of the epiglottis.[42]

The dog is intubated with a cuffed endotracheal tube and general anesthesia is maintained. The mouth is held open with a mouth gag, and the tongue is extended to provide adequate exposure of the oral pharynx. A pair of malleable ribbon retractors are helpful in moving soft tissues while the resection level is being determined.

The point at which the tip of the epiglottis touches the soft palate is noted and marked with a traction suture or a sterile felt-tipped marking pen. The free border of the palate is grasped with forceps, and both sides of the palate as well as the oral cavity are swabbed with antiseptic. Injection of the resection site with diluted epinephrine is *not* desirable, because hemorrhage is not a problem and edema occurs more frequently with its use.

Crush Technique. The palate is clamped with large curved hemostats or similar crushing forceps to form an arch at the reference mark or traction suture. The forceps are left in place while the palate is transected along their distal side with a scalpel, scissors, or electroscalpel. The forceps are left in place for four to five minutes. Some hemorrhage and postoperative edema should be expected.

Non-Crush Technique. The palate is prepared as described for the crush technique, and the traction suture is placed at the level of the tip of the epiglottis (Fig. 64–9). The free edge of the palate is retracted rostrally with forceps. A fine (4-0 to 5-0) absorbable suture is tied at the lateral edge of the traction suture. The palate is incised half of its width with a scalpel or scissors while light tension is applied on the forceps. The incised edge is sutured with a simple continuous pattern, with stitches placed through both the nasal and oral mucosa 1 mm from the cut edge and 2 mm apart. The "cut and sew" technique is continued until the palate transection and incision closure is completed.

The closely placed sutures provide a smooth hemostatic closure and should not shorten the width of the soft palate. Postoperative hemorrhage or edema is minimal.

Postoperative Care. Steroids are useful in decreasing edema. Dexamethasone (0.5 to 1.0 mg/kg) is given just prior to surgery and every eight hours for three doses.[43] Antibiotics are not needed.

Rathke's Cleft Cyst

Persistent remnants of Rathke's cleft may become cystic in the dog and should be considered as part of the differential diagnosis of nasal pharyngeal obstruction.[100] The patient is presented for signs of hypopituitarism accompanied by progressive obstruction of

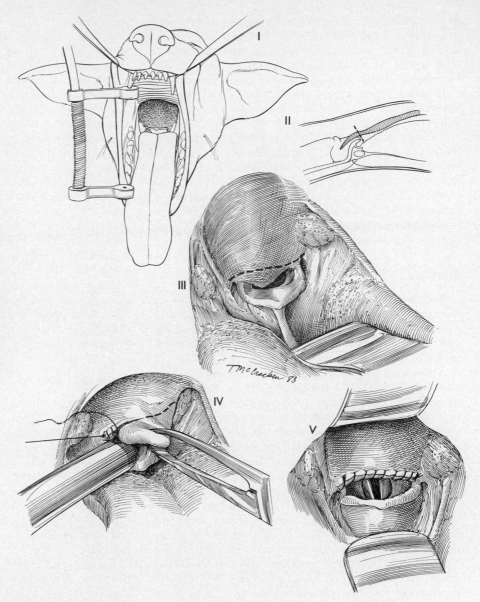

Figure 64–9. Resection of the over-long soft palate—non-crushing technique. *I,* Standard head restraint used during soft palate resection (also used for partial laryngectomy and vocal fold resection). The upper jaw is suspended by tape from an anesthesia screen (see Fig. 64–3) and jaws are held open with a standard mouth gag. *II,* Excision (*dotted line*) of the soft palate is shown. *Inset,* A cross-section of the larynx indicates the relation of excision to the tip of the epiglottis. *III,* The free end of the palate is grasped with forceps, and the edge of the palate at the beginning of the suture line is tensed with a suture. The incision is started, and the first sutures are placed. *IV,* The completed suture line is illustrated.

the nasal pharynx. A cyst-like, hard mass compressing the dorsal nasopharynx can be palpated through the soft palate. It is evident on radiographs as a soft tissue mass with some bone in the wall.

Surgical Approach. Inhalation anesthesia is used, and the oral cavity and pharynx are lavaged with iodophor antiseptic. A mandibular symphysiotomy exposes the soft palate and nasopharynx.

An incision is made on the midline of the soft palate between the palatine muscles and penetrating into the nasopharynx. The mucosa is incised over the mass, the ventral wall is broken down, and the contents removed. The remaining bony wall is removed with rongeurs until the pituitary fossa and gland are visible. The mucosa over the cyst is not sutured. The soft palate incision is closed in two layers (nasal and oral mucosa) with 4-0 to 5-0 gut suture using an interrupted pattern. The mandibular incision is closed routinely.

Postoperative Care. The patient can be offered food and water as soon as it has recovered from

anesthesia. Antibiotics are continued for 5 to 7 days postoperatively. Good recovery can be expected.

TRAUMA TO THE UPPER RESPIRATORY TRACT

External Nares (Nostrils)

Trauma to the external nares may lead to stenosis or obstruction. The loss of one of the nares does not impede normal resting ventilation. Chronic bilateral stenosis or obstruction may cause secondary lung changes (see Chapter 61) and weight loss. Weight loss may be due to the difficulty in eating and mouth-breathing, whereas lack of appetite may be due to the inability to smell.

Lacerations

Patients with lacerations of the nose, nostrils, and proximal nasal passage should be evaluated as soon as possible to prevent additional tissue loss as a result of drying or infection. Adequate but not unnecessary debridement, to remove foreign material and nonviable tissue, is followed by copious flushing of the remaining tissue with saline and tissue-compatible antiseptic. This area has an abundant blood supply, and relatively long, narrow pieces of tissue are viable and should be retained.

Careful identification of the remaining tissue is necessary to establish proper alignment. Mucous membrane and mucocutaneous continuity must be preserved to maintain patency of the airway.[21] Mucosal lacerations are repaired with simple interrupted sutures of 4-0 to 6-0 absorbable material. Large flaps of mucosa are sutured at their edge and held into their bed by soft stents (see "Soft Stents for Nostrils").

Stenosis

Acquired stenosis is difficult to repair, because an adequate opening and mucosal membrane continuity must be attained. The wing of the nostril is usually scarred to the nasal septum just caudal to the columella.

A rhinotomy is made at the caudolateral commissure of the nostril, proceeding in a dorsocaudal direction. The junction between the wing of the nostril and the alar cartilage may need to be incised and the wing elevated to obtain the necessary exposure. The junction of normal tissue and scar is incised, and the scar is removed en bloc, leaving any normal mucosa behind. The remaining mucosa is sutured over the defect to establish mucosal continuity with 5-0 or 6-0 absorbable suture. If small mucosal defects remain, a soft conforming stent is left in the nasal passage, extending caudal to the lesion and just protruding from the nostril (see "Soft Stents for Nostrils"). The stent is removed after mucosal coverage is complete (ten days to two months). Gentle rhinoscopy with the patient anesthetized is used to evaluate mucosal healing.

Oral mucosa taken as a free, full-thickness graft from the buccal surface of the lip is used to line a large defect.[21] The mucosa is excised, leaving only a thin sheet of fascia closely adherent to it. Four to six sutures of fine, absorbable suture are used to align the graft in its bed. A soft stent is laid in the nostril to hold the graft against the wall of the nostril. The lateral nostril wall is sutured into normal position. If the lesion extends to the mucocutaneous junction, nonabsorbable 5-0 to 6-0 in an interrupted pattern can be used to sew the graft to the skin. Careful suturing is needed to obtain accurate tissue alignment and proper suture tension.

Soft Stents for Nostrils

These are used to hold the flaps and grafts of the mucosa against the nasal walls and to provide gentle counterpressure against a denuded surface in order to retard granulation tissue growth while the mucosa regenerates. A loose, longitudinal roll of soft rubber sheeting, loosely packed Vaseline-impregnated gauze, or a very soft, thin-walled silicone rubber tubing are used for the stents.

Pressure of the stent against the graft should be sufficient to barely hold the graft against its bed.[79] The stent must slide easily against the mucosa, must conform to the shape of the nostril and passageway, and should fill but not distend the nostril to obtain mucosal growth without pressure points. Rubber or plastic tubing that resists collapse should not be used as a stent. The nasal passage is not round, and a piece of tubing of sufficient size to act as a stent to most of the nasal surface would dilate or stretch some areas, causing pressure points. The tissue at these points would become necrotic and slough. The granulation tissue response in this area can be enough to cause stenosis.

Bone and superficial tissue repair is completed after the mucosal repair. The initial repair is allowed to heal completely for two to four months before a secondary reconstruction for airway stenosis is attempted.

Traumatic Split Palate (see Chapter 162)

The cat is prone to a midline fracture of the maxilla with laceration of the soft tissue of the hard palate in falls from heights ("high-rise syndrome") and occasionally in vehicle accidents.[30, 83] Concurrent injuries to the mandibular symphysis and soft tissue, nasal turbinates, and teeth occur frequently. Respiratory distress may accompany these injuries because of nasal obstruction, soft tissue swelling, and chest trauma. Repair of these structures should occur after stabilization of the patient and repair of more critical injuries.

Several techniques are used to repair midline fractures of a hard palate. The simplest procedure entails placing Kirschner wires through the palate from the one side to the opposite side, leaving the pin exposed 1 to 2 mm beyond the gingiva on each side. Figure-of-eight wires are placed across the oral surface of the hard palate and looped around the exposed ends of the pins. As these wires are tightened, the midline fracture is stabilized.

The soft tissues are sutured with interrupted sutures of monofilament, nonabsorbable suture when the palate is unstable. Most patients with such injuries heal without surgical repair of the palate. Healing occurs readily because blood supply is abundant. The wires and pins are removed within four to five weeks.

Oronasal Fistula

Oronasal fistula occurs secondary to tooth extraction, resection or irradiation of nasal and maxillary neoplasia, and penetrating injury of the palate or maxilla. Presence of infection, necrotic tissue, or food in the nasal passage leads to chronic rhinitis and nasal discharge.

Surgical closure of an oronasal fistula depends on well-supported mucosal advancement or rotation flap(s) that, when sutured in place provides an air-tight seal. A relatively thin flap moves according to intranasal air pressure during closed-mouth ventilation, resulting in a gradual dehiscence. A flap of mucoperiosteum from the hard palate or a double-flap closure providing a mucosal surface for both the nasal and oral sides usually resists motion and dehiscence. The flap covering the oral side of the fistula should be larger than the bony defect, so that the suture lines occur over a stable surface with a good blood supply.

Oronasal fistulas are either healed (mucosal continuity between oral and nasal cavities) or nonhealed. Healed fistulas provide surgical alternatives, because one or more of the flaps can be based at the edge of the fistula, obtaining their blood supply from the nasal vessels.

Preoperative Preparation. The nasal and oral cavities are flushed liberally with saline to remove debris. Flushing is repeated with an antiseptic. Positioning and draping are as described for cleft secondary palate.

Single-Flap Closure. A single flap is used to close a *nonhealed* fistula of relatively small (less than 1.5 cm) diameter. Gingival mucosa and adjacent periosteum or buccal mucosa and submucosa are used as a single pedicle advancement flap to close the smaller of the fistulas in this group.[79] Any raised bony edge of the fistula is reduced to the level of adjacent bone to provide an even graft bed. The flap is made larger than the fistula, and a bed of sufficient size is made for it. The flap edges are sutured to the surrounding mucosa with 4-0 or 5-0 nonabsorbable suture in an interrupted pattern.

A thicker flap can be raised from the buccal mucosa and submucosal tissues or the oral mucoperiosteum of the hard palate than can be obtained from the gingiva. Thicker flaps are used to cover the larger fistula in this group to appose flap movement.

Double-Flap Closure. Double-flap methods are used for healed and nonhealed fistulas. A graft of mucosa and submucosal tissue is prepared to provide a mucosal surface for the nasal passage and a vascularized support for the oral graft. In both cases, the oral surface is covered by a hard palate mucoperiosteal flap.

Healed Fistula Repair. The healed fistula allows a gingival or hard palate mucosal flap to be based at the edge of the fistula and to close the nasal mucosal deficit. Two small flaps are better than one large one, because they have a better blood supply and the suture line uniting them on the midline is easily placed and off-set from suture lines of the oral flap (Fig. 64–10II). The width of each flap is half the diameter of the fistula. The flap width is measured from the nasal edge onto the nasal mucosa in four to five locations, each point being marked. An incision is made in the oral mucosa, connecting each of the points and the mucosa is dissected free from the oral edge of the fistula, leaving its nasal attachment in place. Rostral and caudal incisions are made in the rim of mucosa, creating two flaps (Fig. 64–10II). The edges of the flaps are trimmed free of excess mucosa until they fit together to form a relatively smooth nasal mucosal layer when sutured with 5-0 to 6-0 absorbable sutures in an interrupted pattern.

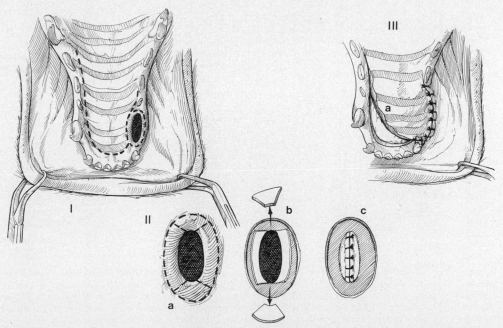

Figure 64–10. Repair of the healed oronasal fistula. *I*, The incision lines are located (*dotted lines*) for the tissue used to close the nasal and oral sides. *IIa*, The incisions to produce mucosal flaws are indicated by *dotted lines*. *b*, Pieces of mucosa are resected to produce two flaps, which are sutured together (*c*) to provide nasal mucosa continuity. *III*, The oral side of the fistula is covered with a hard palate mucoperiosteal flap (*a*).

In patients with either healed or nonhealed fistula, the oral side is covered with a single pedicle flap of mucoperiosteum elevated from the hard palate (Fig. 64–10*III*). Interrupted 4-0 to 5-0, nonabsorbable, monofilament suture is used to secure the palate flap in its new bed.

Lyophilized cartilage plates have been used in dogs to cover a palate bone defect; the oral mucosa is closed over such a plate.[61] The denuded nasal surface is rapidly covered by granulation tissue and epithelium. The cartilage is slowly resorbed and replaced by bone.

Nonhealed Fistula Repair. A nonhealed fistula requires the nasal graft to be based away from the edge of the fistula. The nasal graft is a pedicled island graft that is harvested from the buccal or oral mucosa with a broad submucosal pedicle to ensure a good blood supply (Fig. 64–11*II*). This procedure provides a free mucosal border that may be sutured to nasal mucosa, turbinates, or bony rim of the fistula. A single- or double-pedicled buccal mucosal flap can be used instead, but a second operation is needed to incise the pedicle(s) and suture the free edge(s) to the nasal mucosa. The oral side is covered with a mucoperiosteal flap from the hard palate (see Fig. 64–11*IV*).

The nasal passages are gently lavaged clear of blood clots and debris with warm saline solution through a Foley catheter placed in the external nares or nasopharynx. The catheter should not be advanced into the surgical site, because the sutures in the nasal mucosa or turbinates have little holding strength and may be torn out.

Postoperative Care. The patient is allowed to eat and drink 24 hours after surgery. Only soft food is allowed for six weeks, and bones are permanently

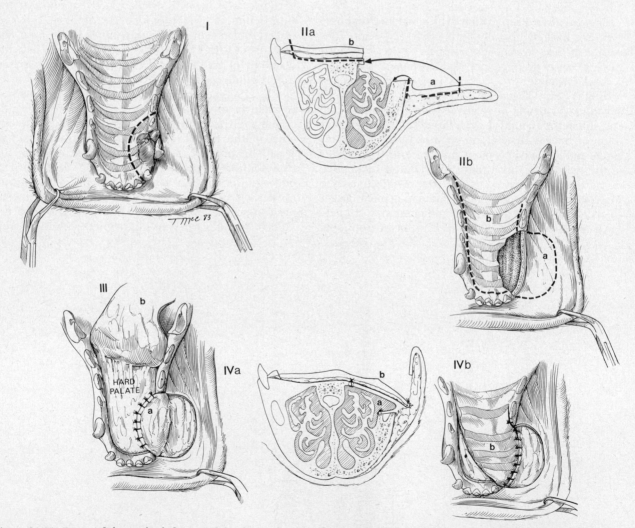

Figure 64–11. Repair of the nonhealed oronasal fistula. *I,* The area of excision or fistula (*dotted line*). *IIa,* Dotted lines indicate the position of the incisions to create the buccal mucosa (*a*) and hard palate mucoperiosteal (*b*) flaps. *IIb,* Cross-section of the oronasal fistula shows the position of the buccal mucosa (*a*) and hard palate mucoperiosteal (*b*) flaps, indicated by *dotted lines. Arrow* indicates the direction of rotation of the buccal mucosal flap to its final resting place to provide mucosal coverage for the nasal passage. *III,* The buccal mucosal flap (*a*) is sutured in place to the palate bone and nasal mucosa and the hard palate mucoperiosteal flap (*b*) is elevated, exposing the palatine bone. *IVa,* The oronasal fistula has been closed on the oral side with the mucoperiosteal flap (*b*) sutured into place to the subcutaneous tissue of the lip. *IVb,* A cross-section through the completed repair of the oronasal fistula, indicating the buccal mucosal flap (*a*) in position with sutures in the surrounding bone and nasal mucosa and the mucoperiosteal hard palate flap (*b*) in place providing oral coverage with sutures holding it to the submucosal tissues of the lip.

removed from the diet. A pharyngostomy tube may be used in patients with a tenuous closure of a large defect. Gruel feedings are given through this tube until the fistula is healed, usually three to four weeks.

Nasal Trauma

Crush Injury

Crush injury to the nasal passages should be explored early to remove fractured turbinates, bone fragments, and devitalized soft tissue. This practice provides an open airway in a shorter time, eliminates the prolonged fetid discharge, and reduces the chance for airway stenosis by scarring of malaligned tissue.

Penetrating injuries of the nose and nasal passages frequently disrupt mucosal membrane, cartilage, and bone. However, the excellent blood supply of these tissues and the warm, moist environment leads to rapid tissue proliferation. Granulation tissue and bony callus occlude the nasal passage if mucosal discontinuity is large compared with the airway cross-sectional area.

Obstruction of one nasal passage is usually tolerated well, because the other compensates for resting air flow needs.[20, 85] Bilateral obstruction is not tolerated well, however, since dogs and cats still try desperately to breathe through their noses and change to mouth-breathing only during hypoxia. Severe damage to both nasal passages should be aggressively treated.

Endoscopic Debridement. Endoscopic exploration via the external nares and endoscopic surgery of the nasal passages are limited to medium and large dogs, in which there is adequate room for a small arthroscope and fine alligator forceps. Blood clots, mucus, and other debris are teased away and flushed out with saline (see Chapter 63). Severely fractured turbinates are removed with alligator forceps until the airways are clear. Mucosal flaps are teased back into normal alignment as the last part of the procedure after the flush has been stopped.

Hemorrhage is controlled or decreased with cold saline and occasional use of epinephrine. The flow of saline carries the blood cloud away, leaving a rivulet of blood hugging the mucosal surface and a clear view of the surrounding tissue. Instruments are moved slowly to avoid disturbing the laminar flow pattern, because turbulence produces another blood cloud.

Surgical Approach to Nasal Passages. Dorsal and lateral depressed fractures of nasal bones and maxilla can be elevated from the external approach. Small pins and wires are used to maintain alignment.

The rostral passages can be exposed from the dorsal or ventral sides, but the region caudal to the ethmoid turbinates is approached from the palate side only. The dorsal approach is the traditional entrance to the nasal passages and sinuses.[53] The ventral approaches can be used to explore ventral regions of the passages without injury to uninvolved major turbinates.[79, 84] The general conformation of the nasal passages and frontal sinuses varies in dolichocephalic and brachycephalic dogs and cats (see Chapter 61).[53]

Dorsal Nasal Approach. The standard approach to the nasal passage is via a dorsal midline incision caudal to the *nasal plane* to the level of the medial canthi (Fig. 64–12).[53] The incision is extended caudal to the dorsal orbital rims if the frontal sinuses are to be explored at the same time.

The skin, subcutaneous tissue, and periosteum are incised. The periosteum is elevated and reflected laterally with its covering of skin. One or both sides of the nose can be entered.

The nasal bone and dorsolateral aspect of the incisive, maxillary, and frontal bones are exposed. Either a single-bone flap covering both nasal passages or two bone flaps (one for each side) can be raised. If the septum has been or will be destroyed, a single flap should be raised to reduce the tendency for central collapse. When the single flap is cut, a thin osteotome is driven centrally under the bone flap along its length to cut the septal attachments.

The limits of the bone flap(s) are cut with either a bone saw or osteotome. The lateral limits should remain medial to the lacrimal duct and infraorbital canal. The bone sections are hinged rostrally on periosteum or are removed and kept moist by wrapping in moist sponges.

After the bone flaps are removed, the passages are washed gently to remove loose blood clots and debris. Damaged tissue and hematomas are removed gently, leaving healthy tissue intact. With thorough knowledge of turbinate anatomy and careful orientation, nasal reconstruction frequently can be accomplished without destruction of all turbinate architecture.

Iced saline or saline slush, epinephrine (1:100,000) packs, and careful use of cautery will help control hemorrhage. Major hemorrhage is controlled with transfixing sutures. Blood for transfusion should be obtained prior to surgery for critical patients requiring major turbinate resection or dissection.

Temporary ligation of both carotid arteries can be used to reduce the hemorrhage during intranasal surgery.[51] The carotid artery on each side of the neck is approached caudal to the cranial thyroid artery and is removed from the carotid sheath to avoid injury to the vagosympathetic trunk. The artery is occluded with noncrushing vascular clamps or umbilical tapes. Carotid flow is reestablished as soon as the intranasal operation is complete.

The nasal passage is flushed clear of blood clots during the operation and again at completion of the palate closure, in order to reduce airway obstruction, decrease subsequent nasal discharge, and provide a cleaner environment for healing in the postoperative period.

The nasal passages are packed with moist or Vaseline-impregnated cotton gauze if continued hemor-

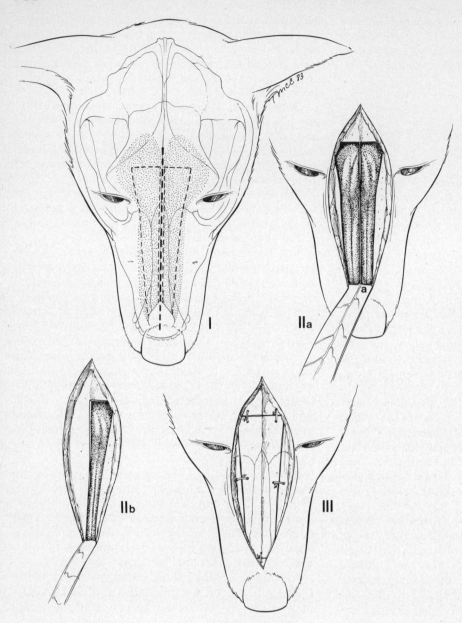

Figure 64–12. Dorsal approach to the nasal passage. *I,* Location of the frontal sinuses and nasal passages (*dotted areas*) and the incisions in the skin and bones (*dashed lines*). *IIa,* The skin incision is shown, with the nasal and frontal bones elevated to bilaterally expose the nasal passage and entrance into the frontal sinus. The bones are hinged on the cartilaginous junction (*a*) at the rostral end of the nasal bones. *IIb,* A similar approach to one nasal passage. *III,* The bone flaps are replaced and held in position with sutures. Suture holes are made with a bone drill or Steinmann pin.

rhage is a problem or mucous membrane flaps or grafts need to be held in place. The packing should be placed with an accordian fold, beginning at the caudal end of the surgical field and working rostrally with the ends of the packing left protruding out one or both nostrils. The packing should be removed during the second to fourth postoperative day—a little at a time.

The excised bone segments are sutured into place with 3-0 or 4-0 wire placed through predrilled holes in the segments and adjacent bone.[53] The periosteum and subcutaneous tissues are closed with 3-0 absorbable suture in a simple continuous pattern. The skin is closed and a tie-on bandage is placed to prevent subcutaneous emphysema.

The oropharynx and nasopharynx are cleared of all fluid and debris before the patient is extubated. The head is kept slightly lower than the thoracic inlet during recovery to prevent aspiration of any remaining fluid or debris. Antibiotics are not used unless infection existed prior to surgery. The antibiotic selection should be based on bacterial culture and sensitivity data.

Ventral Approach to Rostral Nasal Passages. The ventral rostral approach to the nasal passage requires entrance through the hard palate, rostral to the foramina of the major palatine neurovascular bundle (Fig. 64–13).[79, 88] A mucoperiosteal incision is made along the entire lingual edge of the alveolar ridge. The palate periosteum is undermined with a periosteal elevator, and the mucoperiosteal flap is reflected caudoventrally attached at its caudal edge. Hemorrhage is controlled with cold saline packs, dilute epinephrine (1:100,000), and ligation of large vessels. Electrocautery of flap vessels is avoided.

A section of palatine bone smaller than the mucoperiosteal flap is removed with a bone saw, cutting burr, or osteotome.[79] If the palatine bone is to be

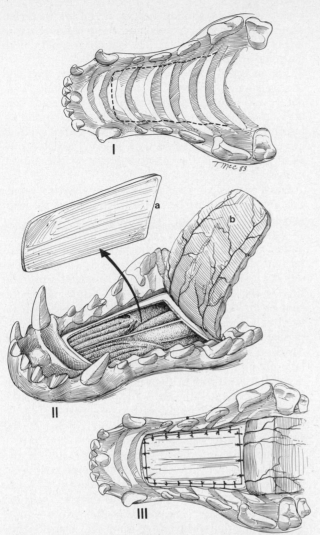

graft is made larger than the bone defect, and the mucosa is removed from one side. The denuded surface is faced toward the oral cavity and is covered by the oral mucoperiosteal flap, which is returned to its normal location and held in place with simple interrupted sutures of 3-0 to 5-0 nonabsorbable suture.

Ventral Approach to Caudal Nasal Passages. The caudal nasal passages are approached via midline incisions in the hard or soft palate (Fig. 64–14).[79] The mucoperiosteum of the hard palate is elevated lateral to the alveolar ridge, with the palatine neurovascular bundles spared (as they emerge from the major palatine foramen). The mucoperiosteum and soft palate attachments to the caudal edge of the palatine bone are incised, and the midline incision is extended into the soft palate as far as necessary. The soft palate is incised through its full thickness.

The incision edge is retracted with tension sutures. The palatine bone is removed as needed for exposure. Full-width sections should be left intact and replaced,

Figure 64–13. Ventral approach to the nasal passage. *I,* The surface of the hard palate with a mucoperiosteal incision (*dotted lines*). *II,* The mucoperiosteal flap (*b*) is raised and the bone plate (*a*) is resected as one piece. The bone plate is slightly smaller than the mucoperiosteal flap to provide a firm base for the soft tissue suture line. *III,* The bone plate is held in place with sutures passed through predrilled holes.

saved and replaced, the vomer-septum junction is cut in a rostral to caudal direction with a thin osteotome. The remaining septum supplies a central support for the palatine bone when it is replaced. This approach can cause injury to the vomer bone, which results in muzzle shortening in growing dogs.[108] This does not occur in the cat.[28] The remaining surgical manipulations and nasal packing are conducted as outlined above (see "Dorsal Nasal Approach").

Closure requires replacement of the large segments of palate (palatine and maxilla) that were removed. This bone provides a stable backing for the mucoperiosteal flap when it is repositioned. Palatine-maxilla wires (interfragment wiring) or two to three transpalatine Kirschner wires are used to stabilize the palatine bone (see "Traumatic Split Palate").

A cartilage plate harvested from the nasal septum can be used to cover a palatine bone defect.[62] The

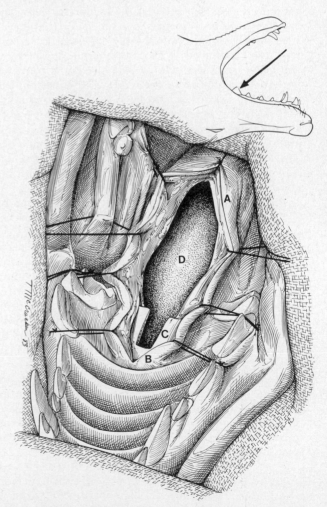

Figure 64–14. Ventral approach to the caudal nasal passage. The drawing indicates the incision through soft (*a*) and hard (*b*) palates. The incision is held open with stay sutures. The palate bone (*c*) is resected as necessary to gain exposure to the nasal passage (*d*). *Inset,* The head position needed for this approach (see Fig. 64–3).

but partial-width sections can be discarded. The palatine vascular pedicle is kept intact to maintain adequate blood supply to the soft tissues of the palate.

Dissection of the turbinates, callus, or granulation tissue requires hemorrhage control, removal of clots, and packing as described for the dorsal nasal approach. Replacement of the bony palate by wire fixation has been described previously. The soft tissues of the palate are sutured with simple interrupted or continuous patterns. The nasal mucosa of the soft palate is closed with absorbable material, and the oral mucosa of the hard and soft palate is closed with monofilament nonabsorbable suture. The bone defect left in the palate will fill in with fibrous connective tissue, not bone.[69]

The caudal edge of the soft palate is retracted rostrally and the nasopharynx, oropharynx, and laryngopharynx are cleaned of fluid, clots, and debris. The patient is recovered in a moderate head-down position until the swallowing reflex is effective.

Ventral Approach to the Nasopharynx. A midline incision in the soft palate is used to approach the nasopharynx. The incision can extend through the caudal edge of the soft palate, but if this extension can be avoided, closure is technically simpler. A mandibular symphysiotomy may be necessary to obtain good exposure of the nasopharynx through the soft palate incision. The palate incision is retracted with sutures placed in the edges of the incision and held with forceps or sutured into the oropharynx ventral to the tonsillar crypt.

The palate incision is closed in two layers, nasal and oral, with simple interrupted or continuous sutures of absorbable 3-0 to 5-0 material in the nasal mucosa and nonabsorbable material in the oral mucosa.

Postoperative Care. Antibiotics are maintained for a minimum of five days after soft palate approaches and ten days after hard palate approaches when large pieces of hard palate bone are resected and replaced. The surgical site should be examined at five days for possible dehiscence and at 14 days for completeness of healing. Only soft food is fed during the first ten days and is slowly converted to canned food by three weeks. Tenuous closures should be bypassed by placing a pharyngostomy tube and feeding a gruel for ten days. Hard food should not be fed for four to six months, especially after a hard palate approach.

Intranasal Repair. The dorsal and ventral approaches to the nasal passage provide adequate exposure of the injured area. Local debridement of injured turbinates and nasal passages is done to provide an airway and prevent occlusion of the passage by granulation tissue and scarring.

Frequently, a ragged, bleeding bed of tissue and exposed bone and cartilage remain after debridement and should be lavaged clean with cold saline to remove debris and stop hemorrhage. In these patients, a two-stage procedure is done to allow a healthy granulation bed to develop. The area should be loosely but completely packed with Vaseline-soaked gauze or similar soft, nonirritating material. The bone flaps are replaced and the remaining tissue layers closed as described. The patient is treated with systemic antibiotics.

The incision is reopened in three to four days and the packing is removed gently. Mucus, blood, exudates, and any devitalized tissue are removed. The area is lavaged liberally with a dilute (1:10) iodophor antiseptic to reduce the bacterial flora. Large surfaces of granulation are grafted with free or pedicled mucosal grafts from the nasal septum or the buccal mucosa.[21, 79]

Nasal septum or septal mucosa is used to repair the granulating surface of the rostral nasal passage. Loss of turbinates or nasal wall from trauma or resection can result in large area(s) devoid of mucosa and occasionally in full-thickness bone loss. The septal mucosa and cartilage can be used to repair these defects.[79] The septal mucosa is removed from the side of the septum and held in a saline-moistened sponge for use as a free graft. The cartilage can be used as a free composite (mucosa or cartilage) or a pedicled graft hinged on its mucosa on one side. The cartilage-mucosa graft is swung on its pedicle dorsolaterally into position or is excised and used as a free graft. It is sutured to the remaining nasal tissue or bone predrilled with holes by means of horizontal mattress sutures. The excised nasal septal mucosa or buccal mucosa is used as a free graft to cover the remaining nasal mucosal defects.[21, 79]

If the mucosal defect includes the site of the surgical approach, the area is not covered with graft until the nasal passage has been packed with Vaseline-soaked gauze. The caudal-to-rostral accordion packing technique is used, with the rostral end of the material left protruding from the nostril. After packing is complete, the remaining portion of the graft is sutured into place using 5-0 to 6-0 absorbable suture (over the packing), completely lining the nasal passageway. The packing should gently hold the grafts in place during the healing process. Excessive pressure results in necrosis of the grafts.

Postoperative Care. Antibiotics are continued as long as the packing is in place. The external nares are kept clear of dried exudate by gentle washing with saline. The packing is removed in ten to 14 days with the patient heavily sedated and its head under solid restraint while gentle traction is placed on the packing. Part (a third to half) of the packing is removed at each of two or three sessions. The nasal passage should be examined endoscopically in three to four weeks if there are signs of nasal obstruction. A similar second procedure may be needed, or a local area of granulation tissue can be excised under endoscopic guidance.

Nasopharynx Trauma

Injury to the nasopharynx is rare. Objects such as sticks and porcupine quills may penetrate the soft palate and injure the mucosa of the nasopharynx. Surgical sites in the caudal nasopharynx that leave large mucosal defects should be closed.

Surgical exposure of the area is accomplished through a midline incision in the soft palate. Mucosal defects caused by tissue debridement or resection of neoplastic tissue can be covered by advancement flaps from the dorsal or dorsolateral aspects of the laryngeal pharynx. Sharp dissection is necessary to undermine these flaps for a sufficient distance to allow adequate stretching to cover the defect. If this mucosa is not sufficient to cover the entire defect, a free mucosal graft may be obtained from the buccal mucosa. The edges of such grafts should be sutured so that mucosal continuity is attained.

Packing of this area is usually not necessary unless there is difficulty in maintaining contact between the graft and the host bed. If packing is needed, a procedure similar to that described for the nasal approach can be used.

Nasal Foreign Bodies

Most small foreign bodies that gain access to the nasal passages are filtered from the air by the rostral turbinate system[13] and are expelled by sneezing. Occasionally, they become embedded in mucosa and cause a severe inflammatory response.[111, 115]

Signs

Epistaxis is seen in both acute and chronic stages of inflammation and infection caused by a foreign body. Mucosal erosion or paroxysms of sneezing can cause hemorrhage.

As the barbs of the plant material begin to disintegrate, the foreign body can be dislodged and expelled. The inflammation and infection initiated by the foreign body can persist as a chronic rhinitis.[13] A unilateral mucopurulent discharge accompanies the foreign body.

Diagnosis

An otoscope can be used to examine the rostral nasal passage, and occasionally the foreign body is seen and removed with small alligator forceps. A small flexible fiberoptic bronchoscope or ridged arthroscope allows a better view (see Chapter 63). The constant flush system described in Chapter 63 for rhinoscopy aids in removing mucopurulent exudate from the passages to provide a clearer view.

Radiographic examination is useful in determining the presence of radiopaque foreign bodies. For outlining of radiolucent bodies, contrast media may have to be injected into the passages, although small foreign bodies are difficult to find this or any other way. Instillation of 30 per cent barium sulfate (1 ml/ 5 kg body weight) through a preplaced catheter as

the catheter is withdrawn is adequate to outline the passage and foreign body surfaces.[31] Filling defects on the dorsoventral and lateral radiographs indicate the probable location of a foreign body or other radiolucent mass. After 24 hours the barium is usually gone from the area, and if needed, the study is repeated on the opposite side.

Removal of Foreign Body

A rostrally located foreign body can be removed with forceps. A foreign body located deep in the nasal passage may be seen with an endoscope but generally is not accessible from the nares. Occasionally, in large dogs, a pair of fine alligator forceps can be used along with the endoscope to remove the foreign material.

Foreign bodies found in the caudal nasal passage and nasopharynx were grasped orally and either were partially swallowed and retched into the area or penetrated the soft palate. They may be embedded in the mucosa (or deeper) or free in the nasal passage.

A visual exploration of the nasopharynx can be done through the nose of small dogs and cats with a small arthroscope or through the oral cavity with a flexible fiberoptic system or hand-held rotating laryngoscope.[19] Rostral traction on the free edge of the soft palate facilitates examination with the rotating laryngoscope. The nasal passages in larger dogs can be explored with a flexible fiberoptic system (bronchoscope). The foreign body may be dislodged by the endoscope and pushed into the oropharynx, where it is easily retrieved. Generally, the embedded foreign body is located and surgical approach is made through the soft palate (see discussion of ventral approaches to the nasal passages).

Surgical Approach. Inaccessible foreign bodies should be surgically removed through a dorsal or ventral approach to the nasal passage, as previously described.[111, 115] The foreign body is located and removed, and the incision is explored for other debris.[111] Hemorrhage is controlled with cold saline and epinephrine (1:100,000).

Abnormal tissue should be debrided until only healthy tissue remains. The area is lavaged. Closure of the mucous membrane is usually not needed if the defect is relatively small (<1.0 cm). Larger defects should be covered with mucosal grafts (see "Nasal Trauma"). The palate is closed and postoperative care given as previously described (see "Nasal Trauma").

NEOPLASTIC DISEASE OF THE NASAL PASSAGES

Patients with neoplastic disease of the nasal passages are presented with nasal passage obstruction, purulent or hemorrhagic nasal discharge, facial swelling, or the presence of a mass on the palate or gingiva.[11, 13] Sneezing, epistaxis, and stridorous nasal sounds are common. Malignant neoplasms are very invasive and can destroy large segments of the turbinates, nasal bones, and palate (see Section 19).

Benign tumors and polyps are found in the nasal passages and growing out of the eustachian tube into the nasal pharynx. These are obstructive, are accompanied by a mucoid exudate, and may recur after excision.

Surgical Approach

Dorsal and ventral approaches to the nasal passages are used in neoplastic disease. Considerable hemorrhage accompanies this type of surgery, and packing of the area with iced saline and dilute solutions of epinephrine helps control hemorrhage. Temporary occlusion of the carotid arteries by atraumatic clamps or ligatures is also helpful.[51] Larger vessels should be ligated or cauterized.

Wide excision of malignant neoplasms (1 to 2 cm margins) is necessary, and resections involving the maxilla and palatine bones frequently result in large oronasal fistulas. Radiation therapy causes bone necrosis and results in a similar condition or may worsen an existing fistula. Reconstruction of these defects has already been described (see "Oronasal Fistula").

CHRONIC SINUSITIS

Chronic sinusitis in cats occurs as the result of mucosal damage secondary to feline viral rhinotracheitis or calicivirus.[13] Severe mucosal ulceration and turbinate resorption allows secondary bacterial infection (streptococci, staphylococci, pasteurella, or coliforms).[82] Normal drainage of the frontal sinus fails because of thickening of the mucosa and submucosa in and around the sinus osteum. Chronic infection occurs with or without mucocele formation.

Surgical Approach

Medical therapy alone is generally not satisfactory. Surgical drainage of the sinus is needed. The sinus is trephined with an intramedullary pin to allow irrigation and drainage.

Sinus Flushing. Placement of the trephine hole varies with the age of the cat (Fig. 64–15).[114] In kittens three to four months old, the hole is placed just lateral to the midline, halfway between a line connecting the rostral margins of the supraorbital processes and a line connecting the medial canthi. In mature cats the hole is placed just lateral to the midline on the line connecting the rostral margins of the supraorbital processes. A small skin incision is made, and the hole is drilled into the sinus.

Curette biopsy and swab specimens should be obtained as soon as the sinuses are opened. Direct smears are helpful in directing initial therapy. Histological examination and bacterial culture and sen-

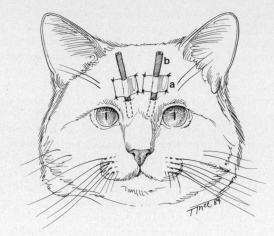

Figure 64–15. Placement of plastic tubes into the frontal sinuses for irrigation. Small pieces of adhesive tape (*a*) are placed around the tubes (*b*) and are sutured to the skin to prevent tube displacement.

sitivity testing of the biopsy specimens are needed for definitive diagnosis.

Small-diameter tubing (IV tubing) is placed through the hole and into the sinus (Fig. 64–15).[114] Adhesive tape tabs (double-eared) are placed on the tubing and their other ends are sutured to the skin between the eyes and the forehead. A second method to secure the tubing is to place a suture in the skin, tie the knot, and pass the two ends of the suture completely around the tubing in opposite directions. The suture is tightened until the tube wall is slightly constricted and then tied. These techniques will hold the tube in place while medication is infused to flush the sinuses.

The sinuses are flushed two to three times a day with a trypsin solution (one part trypsin powder to two parts water), 0.5 to 1.5 ml/sinus,[114] to aid in dissolving the heavy mucus.

Sinus Drainage. A more radical approach is needed if the sinonasal opening remains occluded after flushing. A midline incision is made and the skin is undermined over the sinus. The periosteum is elevated. The superficial bone plate over the sinus is removed with a burr or rongeurs. Turbinates extending into the sinus are removed (Fig. 64–16).

In unilateral involvement in which one aperture into the frontal sinus is occluded, the wall separating the two sinuses is completely removed to provide drainage into the normal sinus and osteum. This procedure plus medical therapy is usually successful.

Maxillary sinusitis is commonly secondary to periapical dental abscess of the carnassial tooth. Extraction of the affected tooth allows ventral drainage, which combined with appropriate antibiotic therapy is usually curative.[13]

Sinus Obliteration. Bilateral sinus involvement has been treated in the cat by obliterating the sinuses.[2, 14, 75, 109] The occluded apertures into the frontal sinuses are enlarged with a bone burr, mucosal lining and a layer of superficial bone being removed.

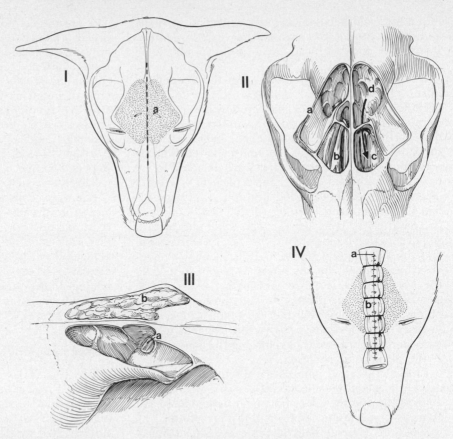

Figure 64–16. Obliteration of the frontal sinus in the dog. *I*, Outline of the frontal sinuses (*shaded area*), aperture into the frontal sinus (*a*), and skin incision (*dotted line*). *II*, The bone plate (*a*) has been removed over the frontal sinus and caudal nasal passage, exposing the ethmoturbinates (*b*) as they enter the frontal sinuses from the nasal passage (*c*). The opposite sinus (*d*) has had the compartment divisions and mucosal lining of the sinus and the aperture into the frontal sinus (*arrow*) removed with a pneumatic bone burr. *III*, The aperture into the frontal sinus (*a*) has been covered by a free fascial graft, and the left sinus has been filled with a fat graft (*b*). *IV*, The primary incision (*a*), shown through the bandage, is covered by a tie over the bandage (*b*) to prevent subcutaneous emphysema.

The mucosa and underlying cortical bone are removed from the remaining sinus(es) with a bone burr. A fascial patch (harvested locally) is placed over each aperture, the area is flushed with antibiotics, and the cavities are filled with fat, bone chips, plaster of Paris, or polyester sponge.[1, 2, 7, 14, 24, 78, 97, 98, 103] Polyester sponge is soaked in antibiotic prior to implantation.

The periosteum is sutured in place and subcutaneous tissue and skin are closed routinely. The si-

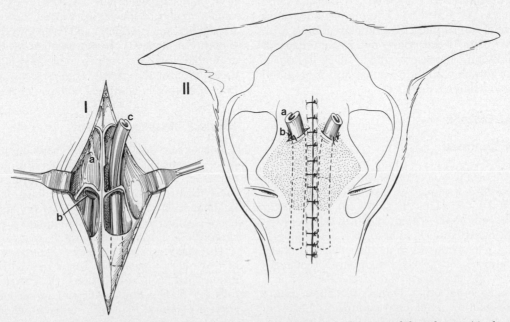

Figure 64–17. Re-establishing normal drainage from the frontal sinus in the dog. *I*, In the exposed frontal sinus (*a*), the compartment divisions have been removed and the aperture diameter (*b*) has been increased with a bone burr without removing excess sinus mucosa. A loose roll of silicone rubber sheeting (*c*) is placed through the aperture into the nasal passage. *II*, The rolls of sheeting are brought through incisions (*a*) in the periosteum and skin near the caudodorsal aspect of the sinuses. The rolls are held in place by sutures (*b*) placed through the sheeting and skin.

nuses heal and become occluded with fibrous tissue and bone during the ensuing six to 12 months.[2] Recurrent mucocele can be a problem unless all mucosa is removed.[2, 75, 78, 96]

Reconstruction of Apertures into the Frontal Sinuses. Bilateral frontal sinusitis in the dog with occluded apertures has been treated by reestablishing normal intranasal drainage.[81] A similar approach is used in the cat, with removal of the bone plate over the sinus. The bone over the sinuses is removed by osteotome or saw. The apertures are enlarged to 1.0 to 1.5 cm with a bone burr, and a piece of 0.125-mm silicone rubber sheet rolled into four thicknesses is laid loosely in each opening so that it extends into the nasal cavity (Fig. 64–17). The other end of each roll of sheeting is brought out through the periosteum and the skin, lateral to the midline incision. A nonabsorbable monofilament suture is placed to include the sheeting as it passes through the skin. The sheeting is left in place for two months while the mucosa regenerates. Wiring the bone plate(s) back in place provides only a slight improvement in cosmetic appearance over not replacing the bone as long as the periosteum is closed.

Rubber tubing (9 mm o.d. × 6 mm i.d.) has been used in place of the silicone rubber sheeting, but the edge of the aperture does not cover with mucosa and stenosis or occlusion recurs within four months.[81] A roll of soft gauze is held in place over the surgical site by tie-over sutures. This reduces postoperative swelling and subcutaneous emphysema. The bandage is removed by the fourth to sixth postoperative day.

Postoperative Care. Systemic antibiotics are desirable. The exposed rubber sheeting is cleaned daily at the skin interface, and a nonirritating ointment (antiseptic or antibiotic) is applied. Irrigation around the sheeting is not effective. The openings left after the removal of the rubber sheeting close rapidly with granulation tissue if they have not reepithelialized. If new epithelium has grown down along the tract, resection of the new epithelium and scar is required to obtain good skin closure.

LARYNGEAL DISEASE

Laryngeal Collapse

Laryngeal collapse occurs as the result of either cartilage fracture (trauma) or loss of the supporting function of the cartilages (Fig. 64–18).[70] The latter condition is commonly recognized in brachycephalic breeds (Pekingese, pug, Boston terrier, and bulldogs) and is sometimes referred to as the "brachycephalic airway syndrome."[42–45, 83] The sequence of changes that occur in the larynx are thought to develop as a secondary effect of other forms of upper airway stenosis pre-existing in affected patients.[49, 50] Most of these dogs have varying degrees of respiratory obstruction due to stenotic nares or elongated soft palate. These two conditions amplify the respiratory malfunction already present because of the head and pharyngeal conformation of these "pug-nosed" breeds. Selective breeding has caused the upper airways, especially the nasal and pharyngeal passages, to be shortened and dorsoventrally compressed, resulting in greater resistance to breathing and increased upper airway noise. Collectively, these obstructive conditions predispose the dog to abnormal stresses within the larynx that lead to progressive distortion and ultimate collapse of the arytenoid cartilages (stages 1 to 3).[50, 70] Respiration is further impeded in the dog with coexistent hypoplastic or collapsing trachea or cardiovascular disease.

Laryngeal collapse, as seen in the brachycephalic airway syndrome, is a progressive disease in which the prognosis deteriorates with time.[50, 70] If the predisposing causes for laryngeal collapse (stenotic nares, elongated soft palate) are treated early, the laryngeal cartilage changes can be transient. However, the folding of the cuneiform and corniculate tubercles can be irreversible and finally suffocating in chronic, untreated cases.

Pathophysiology

The first stage in the pathogenesis of laryngeal collapse involves eversion of the laryngeal saccules into the cavity of the glottis (see Fig. 64–18).[70, 82] This is caused by an abnormally elevated negative pressure created at the glottis during inspiration. The vacuum that develops in the glottis results from increased inspiratory effort necessary to ventilate through the stenotic nares or elongated soft palate. Inflammation and edema of the mucosa usually accompany saccule eversion and contribute to the dyspnea. During stage 2 the cuneiform process at each arytenoid cartilage, which normally extends to the caudal region of the larynx during inspiration, loses its rigidity and gradually collapses into the laryngeal lumen. In stage 3, the corniculate process of each arytenoid cartilage, which normally maintains the dorsal arch of the glottis, collapses toward the midline, resulting in complete collapse of the larynx.

Surgical Treatment

Laryngeal surgery in brachycephalic breeds is tedious because of the limited working area, the redundancy of pharyngeal tissue, and the tendency of these tissues to become rapidly edematous with minimal handling.[45] Thus, a temporary tracheostomy may be necessary to ensure an adequate airway during surgery and during postoperative recovery.

The dog with stenotic nares, elongated soft palate, or everted laryngeal saccules is treated for this condition first (see discussions of individual procedures).[45, 48] The dog is allowed to recover, and the clinical response is used to indicate whether further tissue resection is necessary.

Dogs with persistent stage 2 disease, even after resection of the soft palate and nares, may require partial arytenochordectomy to enlarge the laryngeal

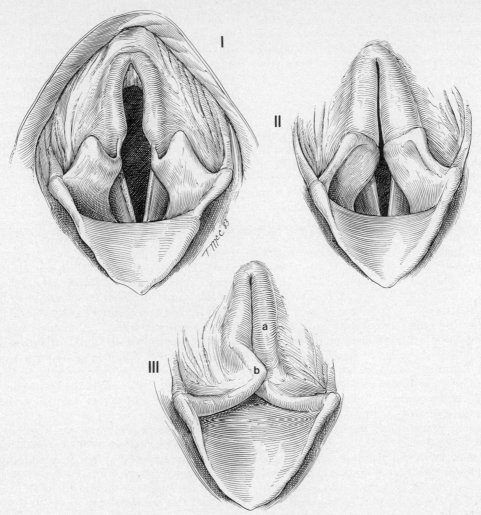

Figure 64–18. Comparative positioning of the arytenoid cartilage in laryngeal paralysis and collapse. *I*, A normal larynx with the arytenoid cartilages in a resting position. *II*, The paralyzed larynx allows the arytenoid cartilages to rotate medially until there is only a slight opening between them. The corniculate processes of the arytenoid cartilages are shown in almost complete apposition. *III*, In the collapsed larynx, the arytenoid cartilage corniculate (*a*) and cuneiform (*b*) processes are touching each other; they tend to overlap with more extensive change.

opening (see discussion of partial laryngectomy). Brachycephalic dogs and small breed dogs with stage 3 laryngeal collapse do not show significant improvement when treated with partial laryngectomy.[45] An alternative treatment for dogs with severe laryngeal collapse that do not improve after resection of the elongated soft palate, stenotic nares, or laryngeal saccules is a permanent tracheostomy (see Chapter 65).[48]

Laryngeal Paralysis

Laryngeal paralysis in the dog and cat usually occurs from an interruption of the innervation to the intrinsic muscles of the larynx.[38, 83, 84, 89, 106] Disruption of the normal nerve transmission of the vagus or recurrent laryngeal nerves may be either congenital or acquired (idiopathic, traumatic, iatrogenic).[106, 107] The result is a failure of the arytenoid cartilages and

vocal folds to abduct, leading to mechanical airway obstruction (see Fig. 64–18).

A congenital predisposition has been suggested in dogs less than one year of age that show signs of laryngeal paralysis.[46] The breeds affected by the congenital form vary with the geographical area: Siberian huskies in the United States, Bouvier de Flanders in the Netherlands, and bulldogs in Britain.[89, 107] In one review, a close genetic relationship between some of the Bouviers developing spontaneous laryngeal paralysis was found, suggesting a hereditary factor.[107] A similar relationship occurs in humans.[34]

Idiopathic acquired laryngeal paralysis, the most common form, is usually seen in large dogs (St. Bernard, Labrador retriever, golden retriever, Siberian husky) more than nine years old.[46]

Severe damage or severance of the laryngeal nerves subsequent to cervical surgery or trauma also results in laryngoplegia. Space-occupying masses in the neck or cranial mediastinum (i.e., cervical abscesses, thyroid carcinomas, heart base tumors, lymphosarcoma) can compress or infiltrate laryngeal nerves, disrupting innervation to the larynx.[94] Viral infection may have similar results.[72]

History

The presenting signs are similar in the two age groups.[45] Early signs include change in voice followed by gagging and coughing, especially during eating or drinking. Endurance decreases and laryngeal stridor (especially inspiratory) increases as the airway occlusion worsens. Episodes of severe dyspnea, cyanosis, or syncope are seen in the severely affected patient. The progression of signs is often slow; it may be months to years before the animal develops severe respiratory distress.[83]

Diagnosis

Examination of the entire respiratory tract is necessary to localize the obstructed area and determine whether other diseases (e.g., collapsing trachea, congestive heart failure) coexist. A high-pitched noise in the laryngeal region on auscultation suggests laryngeal stenosis. Radiography is helpful only to rule out the causes of respiratory compromise.[82] The diagnosis is ultimately made on laryngoscopy when the dog is under light anesthesia.

The animal with laryngeal paralysis is unable to abduct the arytenoid cartilages and vocal folds during inspiration. The arytenoid processes rest in a more midline position, creating a smaller lumen, and their movement is out of phase with respiration. Inflammation of the tonsils, pharynx, and larynx is often associated with the condition.

The majority of animals presented with clinical laryngeal airway obstruction have bilateral dysfunction of the dorsal cricothyroid muscles. Unilateral laryngeal paralysis (hemiplegia) in the dog and cat is recognized but usually causes minimal respiratory distress. Consequently, laryngeal hemiplegia is rarely diagnosed clinically except in very athletic animals.

The cause of both congenital and idiopathic laryngeal paralysis is postulated as neurogenic atrophy of the intrinsic laryngeal muscles.[84, 106] Examination of the laryngeal nerves demonstrate varying degrees of nerve degeneration. Bilateral recurrent laryngeal nerve lesions are most common, although concurrent vagal and central nervous system lesions have been identified.[84]

Medical Treatment

Most animals in a cyanotic crisis precipitated by an upper airway obstruction recover initially with medical therapy. Oxygen is administered by mask, oxygen cage, or endotracheal tube to alleviate the hypoxia. Hyperventilating hyperthermic animals (temperature greater than 105°F [40.5°C]) must be cooled with an alcohol or iced water bath. Corticosteroids (intravenous dexamethasone, 0.2–1.0 mg/kg three times a day) reduce laryngeal inflammation and edema. Fluids should be administered, but with caution, because some animals with severe upper respiratory obstruction develop pulmonary edema; diuretics are indicated in these patients. An emergency tracheostomy is needed for severely dyspneic animals.

Surgical Treatment

Laryngeal surgery is directed at removing or repositioning laryngeal cartilages that obstruct the rima glottidis. The three currently recognized surgical procedures used to correct laryngeal paralysis are: (1) unilateral or bilateral arytenoid cartilage lateralization; (2) ventricular chordectomy or partial arytenoidectomy via the oral or ventral laryngotomy approach; and (3) permanent tracheostomy.[40, 41, 46, 92] More recently described in the veterinary literature is a technique using castellated laryngofissure to increase the glottic and subglottic diameter in laryngeal paralysis.[32] Sufficient long-term results are not available to evaluate this procedure. The technique selected is determined by the size of the animal, the severity of the obstruction, and the preference of the surgeon.

A prophylactic temporary tracheostomy (see Chapter 65) is suggested as the first step in major elective laryngeal surgery.[5, 46, 50] The tracheostomy has several advantages: (1) air can bypass the obstructed region, (2) gas anesthesia is administered at a constant level through the tracheostomy tube, (3) the surgeon has more oral space in which to work, and (4) aspiration of blood is reduced. Also, the tracheostomy minimizes air flow through the surgical site, decreasing the chance of postoperative laryngeal edema. The major disadvantage of the tracheostomy tube is the tedious postoperative care necessary to keep it patent (see Chapter 65).

Arytenoid Cartilage Lateralization. This procedure has been used successfully to treat laryngeal paralysis in medium-sized and large dogs.[92] The technique can be performed unilaterally or bilaterally, depending on the relative increase in glottic diameter needed to produce an airway of adequate size yet prevent aspiration.[41]

The animal is positioned in dorsal recumbency and a paramedian skin incision is made over the larynx. The sternohyoideus muscles are separated to expose the ventral aspect of the thyroid and cricoid cartilages. The larynx is rotated to expose the thyropharyngeal muscle for transection at the dorsal caudal edge of the thyroid cartilage. The recurrent laryngeal and vagus nerves and cranial thyroid and carotid arteries are located and identified to avoid injury. The wing of the thyroid cartilage is retracted laterally, the cricothyroid junction is incised, and the cricothyroid muscle is transected to allow disarticulation of the cricothyroid junction (Fig. 64–19). Separation of

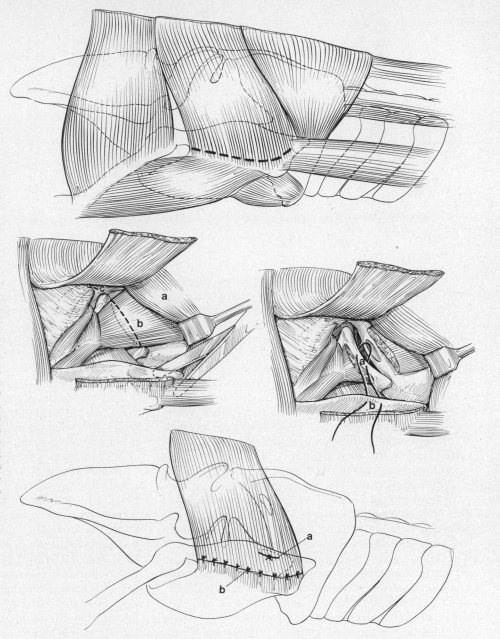

Figure 64–19. Lateralization of the arytenoid cartilage. *I*, The larynx and some of the adjacent musculature. The thyropharyngeus muscle is transected near its attachment to the thyroid cartilage (*dotted line*). *II*, The cricopharyngeal muscle (*a*) is retracted caudally, exposing the cricothyroid articulation, which is transected with scissors to allow retraction of the thyroid cartilage. The cricoarytenoideus dorsalis muscle (*b*) is transected (*dotted line*) over the cricoarytenoid articulation. The junction between the corniculate processes (*c*) is severed (*dotted line*) without incising the mucosa beneath. *III*, The cricoarytenoid articulation has been incised and a suture placed through the dorsal portion of the arytenoid (articular surface) (*a*) and thyroid cartilages (*b*). *IV*, The suture (*a*) between the arytenoid and the thyroid cartilages has been tied, pulling the arytenoid cartilage laterally as the thyroid cartilage is allowed to return to its normal position. The thyropharyngeus muscle (*b*) is sutured in place.

the arytenoid cartilages is completed after division of the cricoarytenoideus dorsalis muscle and the sesamoid band connecting the arytenoid cartilages dorsally. Invasion through the laryngeal mucosa is avoided. Heavy (0-0, 1-0, or 2-0), nonabsorbable suture is placed in an interrupted pattern from the muscular process of the arytenoid cartilage to the dorsal caudal edge of the thyroid cartilage and tightened to abduct the arytenoid cartilages. An assistant should be available to observe *per os* the size of the laryngeal opening achieved to ensure that adequate abduction of the laryngeal cartilages has been obtained.[92] The wound is closed by suturing the thyropharyngeus muscle and routinely closing the subcutaneous tissue and skin.

Partial Laryngectomy *per os.* Partial laryngectomy for the treatment of laryngeal paralysis involves re-

moval of one or both vocal folds and unilateral resection of the corniculate and vocal processes of the arytenoid cartilage.[40, 41, 46, 50] The procedure is relatively easy to perform, essentially noninvasive, and effective in medium-sized to large dogs. Partial laryngectomy for the treatment of severe laryngeal cartilage collapse has met with poor results in brachycephalic dogs and is no longer recommended as a primary form of treatment in these breeds.

A prophylactic tracheostomy is performed just prior to positioning of the animal for partial laryngectomy. With the animal in sternal recumbency, the head is suspended by the maxilla, and the mandible is held open with a mouth gag. The rima glottidis is observed while the soft palate is elevated and the base of the tongue is depressed with malleable retractors (see Fig. 64–9). If the laryngeal saccules are

I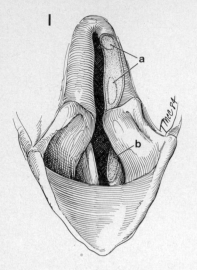

II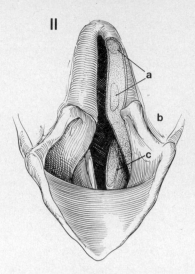

Figure 64–20. Partial resection of the larynx. *I*, The larynx is illustrated from the oral approach. The corniculate process (*a*) of the arytenoid cartilage has been removed, beginning slightly ventral to the dorsal commissure. The vocal fold (*b*) has been removed on the same side, leaving the ventral commissure intact. *II*, A more radical partial laryngectomy with resection of the corniculate process (*a*), the majority of the cuneiform process (*b*), false vocal fold, and the true vocal fold (*c*). The ventral commissure of the vocal folds is left in place.

everted, they are grasped with forceps and resected with long scissors (see "Everted Laryngeal Saccules").

The surgical procedure for laryngeal paralysis and laryngeal cartilage collapse is initially limited to one side of the larynx.[46] Unilateral resection of the vocal fold and a portion of the arytenoid cartilage usually provides an adequate airway opening, minimizes scar tissue webbing across the glottis, and reduces aspiration (Fig. 64–20). The other side is resected at a later date only if the unilateral procedure proves inadequate. We prefer to perform a bilateral ventricular chordectomy along with unilateral partial arytenoidectomy as the first procedure. It is rarely necessary to operate on the opposite side.

Long-handled muscle biopsy or laryngeal cup forceps are used to remove first the vocal fold and then the corniculate and vocal processes of the most affected arytenoid cartilage. Bites of tissue and cartilage are removed until the desired opening is obtained. The aryepiglottic fold and cuneiform process of the arytenoid cartilage are avoided. The dorsal and ventral commissures of the glottis, where the vocal folds meet ventrally and the arytenoid cartilages join dorsally, are also preserved to minimize scar tissue webbing across the rima glottidis (Fig. 64–20).[46]

The objective is to resect enough tissue to provide a functional airway without significantly compromising laryngeal function. The size of the airway created may be equivalent to maximal abduction of the vocal folds and arytenoid cartilages in the normal dog under light anesthesia.[46, 50] Resection of too much tissue results in a laryngeal closure defect and aspiration problems. If unilateral arytenoid chordectomy fails to relieve airway obstruction due to laryngeal paralysis, other forms of airway disease must be reconsidered.

In our experience, St. Bernards do not experience the same degree of improvement as other breeds after partial laryngectomy.

The use of electrocautery for the resection of the laryngeal structures and to control hemorrhage should be avoided in order to reduce postoperative swelling and formation of granulation tissue. Any

bleeding can easily be controlled by direct pressure with gauze sponges. The mucosal edges are trimmed free of ragged tissue tags. Mucosal suturing is not necessary.

Partial Laryngectomy via Ventral Laryngotomy Approach. The indications for this approach are similar to those for oral laryngectomy. It is particularly useful in patients weighing less than 7 kg.

The animal is positioned in dorsal recumbency, and the head is extended and secured to the operating table. A tracheostomy is performed and the patient is ventilated through the tracheostomy tube. The ventral midline skin incision is made over the larynx. The underlying sternohyoideus muscles are separated. The cricothyroid membrane and thyroid cartilage are incised on the midline and the edges are retracted to expose the arytenoid cartilages and vocal folds. The mucosa is incised over the corniculate and vocal processes of the arytenoid cartilage to facilitate their removal as well as that of the entire vocal fold. Any redundant mucosa is excised, and the mucosal defect is sutured or allowed to heal by second intention. The thyroid cartilage incision is sutured with interrupted absorbable sutures that do not penetrate the laryngeal lumen. The subcutaneous tissue and skin are routinely closed.

This approach offers better exposure of the endolaryngeal structures and more operative space than the oral approach. The size of the functional airway created is more difficult to appreciate unless the airway is observed *per os*. Varying degrees of scar tissue form across the glottic floor with this approach. The granulation tissue can be reduced at the ventral glottic commissure if the mucosa is sutured. Scar tissue formation in this area is minimal and usually not a problem.

Postoperative Management. A broad-spectrum antibiotic is administered at surgery and continued for three to five days postoperatively. Corticosteroids (prednisolone, 0.5–1.0 mg/kg) are used in an effort to minimize laryngeal edema and inflammation during the first one to three postoperative days.[46] Feeding is begun 12 to 24 hours after surgery. Abrasive or sloppy food is avoided for the first month after surgery to reduce aspiration. The patient, when fed canned dog food, will swallow discrete boluses of food, reducing the changes of aspiration. Water can be provided initially in the form of ice cubes. All dogs will experience some coughing and gagging associated with eating for varying periods.[48]

Strenuous exercise and barking should be discouraged for at least six weeks. Such laryngeal stress will provoke mucosal edema and increased granulation tissue formation. Tranquilizers should be given to the excitable patient.

Complications of Partial Laryngectomy. Several potential surgical complications are associated with a partial laryngectomy procedure.[40, 46] Coughing, gagging, and periodic retching caused by edema and inflammation are common after surgery. These signs persist when excessive removal of the aryepiglottic fold or cuneiform process has resulted in incomplete epiglottic closure during swallowing. Fatal aspiration pneumonia may occur. Associated neuromuscular disease involving both the pharyngeal and laryngeal regions may also alter swallowing function.[49] Partial laryngectomy, in itself, does not interfere with swallowing.[40]

Laryngeal stenosis can develop after partial laryngectomy, especially if the dorsal and ventral glottic commissures are removed and mucosal continuity is not restored with proper suturing (see "Laryngeal Stenosis"). It is best to avoid these commissures, if possible, to eliminate suturing.

Persistent airway aspiration secondary to swallowing dysfunction can be prevented by total laryngectomy or laryngeal diversion in conjunction with a permanent tracheostomy. Laryngeal diversion entails anastomosing the proximal trachea to the esophagus.[71] The trachea, at approximately the fourth or fifth ring, is anastomosed to the esophagus in an end-to-side manner. A longitudinal incision is made in the esophagus, and the end of the proximal trachea is sutured to the submucosa and muscular tissue of the esophagus. Nylon 3-0 suture is used in an interrupted pattern without penetrating into the lumen of either. The proximal end of the remaining trachea is anastomosed to the skin to form a permanent tracheostomy (see Chapter 65).

Everted Laryngeal Saccules

Everted laryngeal saccules are most frequently seen in brachycephalic breeds, either as a single entity or in association with other respiratory obstructive conditions (elongated soft palate, stenotic nares).[44, 70] Laryngeal saccule eversion is uncommon in other breeds even when other causes of severe laryngeal obstruction exist. The saccules (ventricles) evert in response to the decrease in pressure that is created within the larynx during inspiration (Fig. 64–21). The everted tissue rapidly becomes edematous and partially occludes the ventral rima glottidis.

Surgical Resection

The patient is placed in sternal recumbency with the mouth held open, as described for partial laryngectomy. The saccule is grasped with Allis forceps, and rostral traction is supplied (Fig. 64–21). The saccule is amputated at its base with scissors or a long-handled scalpel. Hemorrhage is minor and can be controlled by pressure. Inflammation is reduced by avoiding the electroscalpel.

Reverse Sneeze

An intermittent problem in many toy breed dogs that is frequently manifest as an upper respiratory

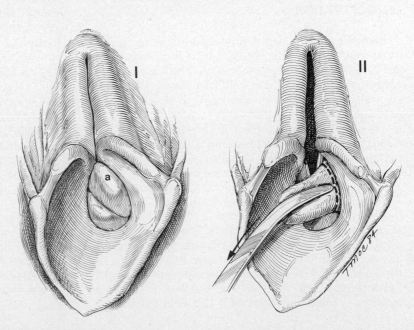

Figure 64–21. Surgical removal of everted saccules. *I,* A collapsed larynx with everted saccules (*a*). *II,* The saccule is grasped with long forceps, retracted, and incised (*dotted line*). The process is repeated for the other saccule.

spasm is termed the reverse sneeze. This condition is usually observed during excitement. It can be classified as a nuisance or may develop into a spastic condition resulting in cyanosis and syncope. It is associated with retention of the epiglottis over the rima glottidis with entrapment by the soft palate. Nasopharyngeal spasm may also be associated with the condition.

Surgical Approach

Surgical removal of approximately 1 to 2 mm of the free margin of the epiglottis offers partial to total relief. The incised area heals with the production of a small amount of granulation tissue, which upon maturing causes an eversion of the edge of the epiglottis. This distortion of conformation probably decreases the chance that a suction seal will be produced.

Inflammation of the Larynx

Inflammation of the laryngeal tissue causing dyspnea must be differentiated from surgically correctable laryngeal obstruction. Few primary inflammatory diseases occur in the larynx of the dog or cat. Epitheliotropic viral infections (i.e., distemper) are the most common diseases producing a true laryngitis.[5, 66] Erythema and edema of the laryngeal mucosa and tonsillar enlargement are common signs.

Laryngeal edema and spasm can be induced in very obese or brachycephalic dogs by excessive panting from overheating or prolonged excitement. Local laryngeal irritation causes severe laryngospasm in the cat. These situations can lead to an acute airway obstruction and death if not recognized and treated early.

DEVOCALIZATION

Phonation in the dog is produced by the forcing of air through the larynx, which causes the vibration of structures within. The lips, tongue, and fauces aid in phonation, but the true and false vocal folds and ventral processes of the arytenoid cartilages are the principal sources of sound.

The aim of devocalization is to remove all of the laryngeal tissue that can emit sound. It is not possible to totally silence a dog without performing a total laryngectomy.[5] In general, the more tissue that is excised, the greater is the reduction in phonation.[66]

Several surgical procedures have been described to eliminate the function of the laryngeal structures associated with sound production. The use of a biopsy punch, scissors, or cautery to remove the vocal folds has been described in the literature.[5, 52] Resection of the true vocal folds alone may provide only transient devocalization and result in a muted bark.[116] Bilateral resection of the true vocal folds and ventricular folds

(true and false vocal folds, respectively) has also been used. More radical laryngeal excision involves additional removal of portions of the arytenoid cartilages.[5, 50, 116] The removal of structures associated with phonation is approached either orally or through a ventral laryngotomy incision.[52, 116]

Vocal Chordectomy *per os*. A short-acting barbiturate usually provides adequate anesthesia and ample time to perform the procedure. The animal is placed in ventral recumbency with the head suspended by the maxilla and the mouth held open with a mouth gag. The vocal folds are exposed by elevation of the soft palate and depression and extension of the tongue with malleable retractors. Simple excision of the vocal folds requires securing the cord with tissue forceps and resection with long, curved scissors. Care should be taken to avoid disruption of the ventral commissure of the vocal fold attachment, as it would enhance bridging by granulation tissue and subsequent ventral glottic stenosis.

Of one thousand experimental dogs "debarked" by this technique, 90 per cent were muted or aphonic three to four months after operation. Eventually, 60 per cent of these dogs developed scar tissue at the surgical site that allowed them to have a muted bark.[52]

A more extensive resection for "debarking" *per os* involves the removal of not only the true and false vocal folds but also the ventral cuneiform and vocal processes of each arytenoid cartilage.[115] Long-handled biopsy cup forceps are used to remove these structures. Each part to be removed is stabilized with tissue forceps, then completely excised via a series of bites with the biopsy instrument. The ventral commissure is spared. Hemorrhage is usually unremarkable and can be controlled by direct pressure with gauze sponges.

Vocal Chordectomy via Ventral Laryngotomy (Laryngofissure). This approach was originally suggested to provide better surgical exposure for more accurate vocal fold dissection in an effort to provide better long-term results than those obtained by cord excision *per os*.[116] It has become the recommended approach when devocalization is essential.

The animal is placed in dorsal recumbency, the neck is extended, and the head is secured. A 6- to 7-cm ventral midline skin incision is made from the hyoid apparatus to the second or third tracheal ring. The larynx is seen after the subcutaneous tissue and sternohyoideus muscles are separated. The borders of the thyroid and cricoid cartilages are identified prior to incision of the cricothyroid ligament. The ventral midline incision is extended cranially through the body of the thyroid cartilage. Self-retaining retractors are used to separate the edges of the thyroid cartilage. The vocal folds (including the vocalis muscle) and ventral arytenoid projections (vocal processes) are moved in one piece with scissors. The mucosal edges may be sutured.

If the vestibular folds (false vocal folds) and the lateral wall of the ventricle are removed along with the aforementioned structures, the wound cannot be sutured. This technique leaves a large denuded area that has a greater tendency for webbed stenosis. The cricothyroid membrane is closed with absorbable suture, and the thyroid cartilage edges are apposed with simple interrupted, nonpenetrating sutures. Occasionally, small dogs (less than 18 kg) require a tracheostomy tube for the first 24 hours after surgery. A similar laryngotomy procedure can be used in cats.[116] The closely associated ventricular and vocal folds are removed, resulting in a significant decrease in the amplitude of vocalization and loss of the "purr."

Postoperative Care. It is essential that the dogs have limited exercise and be discouraged from barking for four to six weeks after surgery. Excitement with associated high air flow through the larynx can cause significant inflammation and granulation tissue production. This will result in the return of some degree of phonation. Corticosteroids can be used for two to three days postoperatively to reduce edema and inflammation of the surgical site. Additional medical therapy is generally not needed.

LARYNGEAL TRAUMA

Laryngeal trauma can be induced either intrinsically or extrinsically. The most common cause of intrinsic laryngeal damage is rough intubation for anesthesia or bronchoscopic examination. Repeated trauma to the arytenoid processes and vocal folds causes varying degrees of hyperemia and edema of laryngeal mucosa as well as occasional ulceration. The resultant airway obstruction may not become apparent until the animal is extubated. To reduce these complications, the appropriate size tube or endoscope should be selected and adequately lubricated prior to insertion.

Foreign bodies more typically lodge in the pharyngeal region and esophagus rather than the larynx, but sticks, needles, plant material, and bones have been extracted from the larynx of dogs and cats. Minor injury results in simple mucosal regeneration, whereas full-thickness mucosal injury induces granulation tissue formation and webbing between vocal folds and arytenoid cartilages, respectively. Diaphragm-like or broad-based circumferential stenosis occurs after loss of a large segment of the laryngeal mucosa.

Extrinsic laryngeal trauma from vehicle accidents is not commonly seen in dogs because the larynx is anatomically well protected. Choke chain, dog bite, and gunshot injuries account for most laryngeal trauma.[73] Guard or show dogs controlled by choke chains can fracture laryngeal cartilages or hyoid bones during training periods. The same type of "strangulation injury" is observed in dogs that are suddenly stopped by a long tether line. Laryngeal and perilaryngeal edema and hematoma can rapidly cause dyspnea and even suffocation, especially if laryngeal cartilage fracture and collapse occur. Local emphysema

secondary to laryngeal laceration may extend into the mediastinum and break into the pleural space, causing a pneumothorax. The healing of malaligned cartilage fragments can lead to delayed airway obstruction due to subsequent granulation tissue formation; this is accentuated by scar tissue contracture, causing further cartilage collapse and laryngeal stenosis later in the healing process.

Penetrating injuries of the neck inflicted by animal bites or bullets frequently cause extensive damage to multiple cervical structures. Damage to deep structures include laryngeal and tracheal perforation, esophageal laceration, nerve and vascular injury, as well as soft tissue disruption. Hematomas and tissue edema may mask some of the signs associated with these injuries. Local infection with subsequent abscess or fistula formation, mediastinal emphysema, infection, pneumothorax or pyothorax, or laryngeal paralysis can occur. The chance to stabilize and align cartilage fractures and repair mucosal lacerations, without significant loss of tissue, may be forfeited if the clinician procrastinates for 24 hours. Early exploration, debridement, alignment of tissue, and drainage along with medical therapy is necessary whenever laryngeal, tracheal, or esophageal injury is suspected. Prevention of airway stenosis is of primary concern.

Diagnosis

Thorough evaluation of the entire patient as well as local examination of tissue damage is critical to establish short- and long-term therapy. Affected animals can tolerate only minimal stress if respiratory compromise is severe. A respiratory crisis can be prevented if a temporary tracheostomy is performed early.

Palpation of the laryngeal region is helpful, but soft tissue swelling usually prevents evaluation of deep cervical structures. Auscultation of the upper airway usually helps localize stenosis. Radiographic examination of the larynx is most helpful in adult animals, which have calcified laryngeal cartilage whereby laryngeal and hyoid structures can be evaluated.[28, 82]

Laryngoscopy and esophagoscopy are important methods of examining every patient showing signs of injury to the airway or esophagus or in which injury is likely to have occurred. These examinations require general anesthesia.

Patients should be preoxygenated to have maximum time for laryngeal and tracheal examination before intubation is required. Oxygen is given through the endoscope during the airway examination. Intubation is done after laryngeal damage is assessed and, when possible, under the guidance of endoscopic view to decrease the chance of additional damage to laryngeal tissues. The esophagus is examined after airway control has been achieved.

Submucosal hemorrhage, mucosal laceration, and luminal obstruction due to cartilage malalignment or hematoma are indications of laryngeal damage. Lack of motion of the arytenoid processes (when the animal is examined under light anesthesia) suggests laryngeal paralysis. Direct injury to the intrinsic muscles of the larynx may cause similar loss of function.

Criteria for exploration of laryngeal injuries are airway obstruction sufficient to require a tracheostomy, emphysema involving the fascial planes of the neck, exposed cartilage in lumen of larynx, and fractured cricoid cartilage.[12]

Treatment

Surgical exploration of the site of injury through a ventral midline incision is indicated.[12] Vessel laceration and thrombosis are treated by thrombus removal and vessel ligation next to the nearest functional branch. Vessel debridement and anastomosis should be considered in bilateral injuries of major vessels.

The laryngeal lumen is approached by a ventral midline thyrotomy or through the fractured cartilage.[12] Simple lacerations of the mucosa are trimmed free of devitalized tissue and sutured with fine absorbable interrupted suture. Malaligned flaps of mucosa without cartilaginous damage are debrided and sutured with preplaced sutures, the mucosa being tacked to the cartilage with penetrating absorbable 4-0 to 6-0 sutures.

Advancement flaps of mucosa from the pyriform area are used for cartilage surfaces that cannot be covered with mucosa by careful suturing of lacerations.[12]

Alignment of the mucosa and cartilage edges can be done simultaneously if the lacerations coincide. Fractured cartilages are debrided, trimmed for accurate alignment of fragments, and closed with preplaced interrupted absorbable or nonabsorbable 3-0 to 5-0 monofilament sutures.[12] With calcified cartilage, suture holes must be predrilled before suture closure is attempted. Small defects in cartilage continuity may be patched with local pedicle muscle flaps (see "Laryngeal Stenosis"). The ventral laryngotomy is closed with interrupted sutures splitting the cartilage thickness to prevent overriding of the apposed edges.

Small (1-cm wide) resection or loss of the ventral cricoid cartilage can be left to heal by second intention[91] without resulting in significant stenosis.

If the arytenoid cartilage is avulsed from its attachment to the cricoid cartilage, it is better to remove the arytenoid than to attempt to reposition it.[12] Partial disruption of an arytenoid cartilage is repaired with absorbable horizontal mattress sutures between the arytenoid and cricoid cartilages. Torn mucosa is meticulously closed.

Mucosal flaps and cartilage fragments are held in position with laryngeal luminal stents or Montgomery T tubes (see discussion of laryngeal and tracheal stents).[12] These are surgically implanted via laryngotomy or tracheotomy incisions. Final location of the repositioned flap is verified by endoscopic examination.

Postoperative Care. General postoperative care is followed (see Chapter 66). Antibiotics are used routinely and are initiated after the contaminated tissues have been sampled for culture. They are continued for three to five weeks.[17, 60] Corticosteroids (prednisone, 1.0 mg/kg/24 hours) are given at surgery and are continued for 48 to 72 hours postoperatively to reduce edema.[17]

Stents for Laryngeal and Tracheal Repair

After resection or realignment of obstructing tissue, it is difficult to prevent transverse adhesion of the dorsal (arytenoid) or ventral (vocal fold) commissures, collapse of damaged cartilage secondary to granulation tissue contracture, and excessive granulation tissue production during healing of large defects in the mucosa. Stents are generally used to maintain normal tissue contour, separate adjacent healing surfaces, retard the proliferation of granulation tissue toward the airway lumen, and hold a mucosal graft adjacent to the airway wall while it heals into its new bed.

The "keel" type of stent is used to separate adjacent healing surfaces of the vocal folds and arytenoid cartilages to prevent web formation.[79] Stenosing webs can be seen after laryngeal injury, complete vocal chordectomy, and bilateral partial arytenoidectomy, which leave denuded surfaces on both sides of the commissure. Silicone rubber or Teflon keels are commonly used in humans and have been used in dogs.[77, 79] The silicone keel* is the most versatile (Fig. 64–22). The soft but resistant consistency of the keels allows laryngeal motion without damaging tissue and resists granulation tissue webbing during epithelialization of the surface.

The umbrella-shaped keel is placed through a ventral incision in the thyroid cartilage (Fig. 64–22I). The keel is trimmed to length so that it does not traumatize the dorsal interarytenoid commissure. Two figure-of-eight, 3-0 monofilament nonabsorbable sutures hold the keel in place against the thyroid cartilage (Fig. 64–22II). The keel is removed through a small ventral cervical skin incision after healing of adjacent tissues is complete (two to three weeks). The result is regeneration of a sharp commissure.

Laryngeal lumen stents* cast from soft silicone rubber are available in human but not dog sizes.[79, 96] Similar stents can be constructed from a finger cot and a properly trimmed piece of foam rubber so the lumen of the larynx is just filled (Fig. 64–22III).[101] The stent is trimmed for the length, and the open end is tied off with suture. A similar stent is made from 0.05-mm Silastic sheet loosely rolled to fit into the lumen.[100] The stents are soft and flexible and hold the mucosa or graft against the laryngeal wall without causing pressure necrosis. The stent is held in place with penetrating sutures tied over buttons on the skin surface on each side of the neck (Fig. 64–22).

---

*E. Hood Benson & Co., Duxbury, MA 02332.

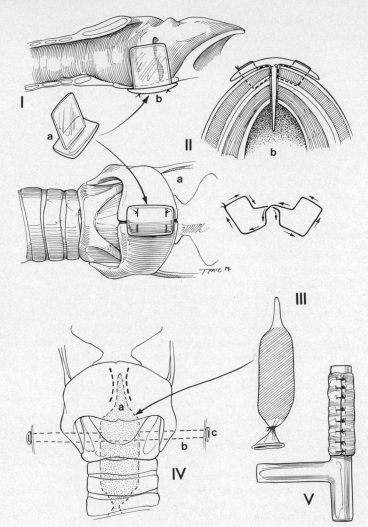

Figure 64–22. Internal stents for laryngeal stenosis. *I,* Silicone rubber "keel" stent (*a*) in place between the vocal folds (*b*). *II,* The figure-of-eight suture pattern used to hold the "keel" in place and the cartilage in alignment is shown from the ventral view (*a*) and the cross-sectional view (*b*). *III,* A full luminal stent made from a finger cot and soft foam rubber. This partially filled cot leaves a thin (unfilled) end that will act as a "keel" stent when placed between the vocal folds, while the remaining portion fills the laryngeal lumen. *IV,* The full-lumen stent (*a*) held in place with a 4-0 wire suture (*b*) placed from skin surface to skin surface and tied through buttons (*c*). *V,* The Montgomery "T" tube is shown with a free mucosal graft mounted on it. The Montgomery tube is placed via the tracheostomy, provides an airway, and holds the mucosal graft gently against the denuded air wall while it heals in place.

The sutures are placed under direct vision while the laryngeal incision is still open. Because this type of stent obstructs the airway, a tracheostomy tube is needed.

The stent is removed through a ventral thyrotomy in six to eight weeks, depending on the severity of the injury. A keel is placed after the lumen stent is removed to provide a sharp ventral commissure. The keel is removed in two weeks.[96]

A Montgomery T tube is used in caudal laryngeal (subglottic) and tracheal injuries to provide both a luminal stent and an airway.[77, 79] This very soft, flexible tube should be accurately sized to just fill the airway lumen and still move easily. Montgomery T tubes are used as supportive stents for injuries and as carriers for mucosal grafts (Fig. 64–22*III*). The tube is placed through a tracheotomy (see Chapter 65). These tubes are tolerated well in humans and dogs and have been kept in place for months with good results.[77, 79]

Most materials are not suited for use as stents because they are not soft enough or are improperly sized. Pressure points, sharp edges, and inflexibility are not tolerated by the delicate tissues of either larynx or trachea.

STENOSIS

Laryngeal Stenosis

Obstruction of the larynx by granulation tissue and cartilage degeneration and collapse results in progressive reduction in airway diameter. These lesions vary from partial diaphragm or web stenoses to broad-based scar tissue covered by mucosa. Focal and circumferential involvement can occur. Laryngeal stenosis is a complication of laryngeal surgery.

Glottic Stenosis

Etiology

Various types of trauma lead to primary or secondary glottic stenosis (see "Laryngeal Trauma"). Transluminal webs of mucosa-covered granulation tissue occur after injury to both arytenoids or both vocal folds (i.e., arytenoidectomy, vocal chordectomy). Prolonged intubation is a major cause of laryngotracheal injury leading to long segmental stenoses in humans.[77] Such stenosis has been noted in the dog and will become more common in animals as prolonged respiratory support of salvage patients occurs.

Diagnosis

Laryngeal stenosis secondary to granulation tissue manifests as a progressive dyspnea after a traumatic incident or prolonged intubation. A patient with early signs of dyspnea can have as much as a 60 per cent reduction in luminal size and remain clinically unchanged for weeks. Inflammatory edema or mucous accumulation further reduces the lumen size, and the patient can become acutely dyspneic and may die if not treated immediately.[10] Chronic minor dyspnea alone is sufficient reason to perform a thorough airway examination.

Direct examination of the entire system from the nasopharynx to the treachea with endoscopic equipment is the best method to assess lesions (see Chapters 23 and 63). The condition of the supraglottic tissue, pyriform fossa, and esophagus must also be noted in case major reconstruction of the larynx using these structures is required.

Tomography may assist in the evaluation of the lesion, especially if the area is too small to allow passage of the bronchoscope. Contrast laryngography may be disastrous in the presence of inflamed mucosa, because the airway may close immediately.

Treatment

A plan must be developed to reduce the stenosis.[77] The best treatment is to prevent stenosis in surgical patients by accurate tissue apposition and in acutely injured patients by surgical exploration and reconstruction within 24 hours of injury.[10] Local tissue swelling is not a reason to delay surgical correction. Accurate anatomic alignment and stabilization of cartilage fragments and mucosa are necessary (see "Laryngeal Trauma").

Corticosteroid and antibiotic therapy reduces the severity of stenosis in acute injuries by reducing infection and granulation tissue production. Dilation, surgical repair, and laser vaporization have been used to reduce the stenosis, with reasonable success in selected cases.

Mechanical Dilation. Dilation is best suited for thin web lesions less than four weeks old, and it is not effective for the broad-based lesions.[18] Stenosis from external trauma is not responsive to dilation. Dilation by rigid bronchoscope stretching will increase the lumen size. It is done under general anesthesia, usually six times in an eight-week period.[10] Intralesional or systemic corticosteroids are used in conjunction with this treatment. Internal stenting is not necessary.[10]

Surgical Repair. Fusion of the dorsal and ventral commissures of the glottis frequently occurs after bilateral arytenoidectomy and ventricular chordectomy, respectively. Many narrow-based (rostrocaudal) adhesions heal with an adequate glottic opening after simple sharp excision of the web via the oral or ventral routes.[77, 79, 96]

Broad-based adhesions must be sharply resected to normal tissue in order to reestablish the glottic airway. High recurrence rates of this lesion are reduced by stenting (see discussion of laryngeal and tracheal stents).[96] Recurrence can be prevented by placing a piece of silicone rubber sheeting or "keel" in the airway between the granulating surfaces and keeping it in place with sutures.

A tracheotomy is made three to four rings below the larynx, and a tracheostomy tube is placed (see Chapter 65). It is maintained during surgery and postoperatively until the stent is removed.

Full luminal laryngeal stents are used in circumferential mucosal loss. They are used to retard granulation tissue production by contact and to hold mucosal grafts against the laryngeal wall (see discussion of laryngeal stents).[10, 79] Stents are left in place for two weeks to two months, with periodic removal of granulating foci until epithelial coverage is complete.[96]

Subglottic Stenosis

Surgical Repair

Thick-based stenoses involve a large area of laryngeal wall and may cause the collapse of damaged cartilage by contraction of maturing collagen. Loss of cartilage due to infection, trauma, and resection predisposes to this problem. Reconstructive techniques for severe stenosis include laryngorrhaphy with stenting or grafting, cricolaryngotomy with splinting, hemilaryngectomy, and segmental resection and anastomosis.

Surgical Approach. A standard ventral midline, upper cervical approach is made for each of the procedures. A tracheostomy tube should be placed for the operation and maintained for 24 to 72 hours postoperatively to provide an unobstructed view during the procedure and patient airway protection during recovery.

Laryngorrhaphy. This procedure requires the presence of at least a small laryngeal lumen.[16] Obliteration of the lumen secondary to post-traumatic scarring is not helped by this technique. Lateral and ventral approaches through the laryngeal wall have been used.[111] Lateral (bilateral) incisions involving all layers of the laryngeal wall are made over the length of the stenosis, the more dorsally located laryngeal nerves being avoided. Ventral incision of the thyroid and cricoid cartilages and the first tracheal ring provides adequate exposure of the lumen (Fig. 64–23). The incision is spread to produce a fusiform opening through the wall and scar, and into the lumen. This opening is covered with a patch graft of costal cartilage (perichondrium on the luminal side), nasal septum (with mucosa toward the lumen), sternohyoideus muscle (as a pedicle graft), or 1- to 2-mm-thick silicone rubber sheeting, which acts as a

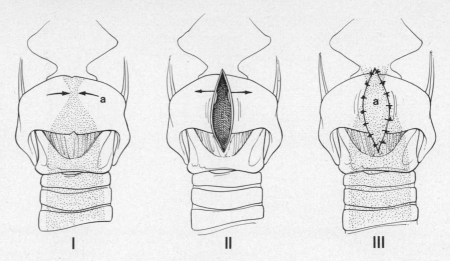

Figure 64–23. Laryngorrhaphy. *I,* The airway is narrowed (*a*) in the region of the vocal folds. The airway lumen is indicated by shading. *II,* The thyroid cartilage is excised, and the incision is expanded to increase the cross-sectional area of the airway. *III,* The incision is patched with a cartilage implant (*a*), which is sutured in place. The expanded airway is indicated by shading.

stent to hold the incision edges apart and seal the opening created.[8, 10, 16, 23, 90, 103, 104, 112]

Cartilage and mucosal grafts are trimmed to fit into the defect, and muscle and silicone are used as external overlay (Fig. 64–23).[16] Granulation tissue covers the surface of the cartilage, muscle, or silicone rubber, after which epithelium will grow over the granulation tissue. Granulation tissue may become extensive if epithelium does not cover it within three to four weeks. Nasal septal cartilage provides less long-term stenting than costal cartilage because it partially collapses with contraction of the scar and is partially resorbed.[102, 103]

Buccal mucosa grafts are used as free grafts to cover the luminal side of large, full-thickness defects in an effort to limit the granulation tissue growth and to provide epithelial surface immediately for the larynx.[90] The external side of the mucosal graft is supported with a muscle flap or cartilage graft. Internal stenting provides support for the cartilage grafts during healing and keeps the mucosal graft in contact with the host bed (see Fig. 64–22).[96]

Cricolaryngotomy with Splinting. The basihyoid bone, as a free graft or attached to a sternohyoideus muscle pedicle, has been effectively used as an implant in subglottic stenosis.[3, 22, 26] The middle three-fourths of the basihyoid bone is dissected free of all its soft tissue attachments except the insertion of one of the sternohyoideus muscles, which provides a blood supply to the bone. The airway is not entered. Small bone cutters are used to transect the basihyoid near its articulation with the remaining hyoid apparatus. Close attachments of bone and muscle to the surrounding tissue are incised, and the bone segment and its muscle pedicle are moved caudally to the cricoid cartilage (Fig. 64–24).

The laryngorrhaphy incision is made on the midline from the cricoid cartilage to the first tracheal ring. Submucosal scar is removed where possible, leaving the mucosal lining intact. The cricoid ring is distracted laterally and connective tissue constraints are freed until the basihyoid bone will fit between its cut ends. Stainless steel wire suture is used to suture the cricoid cartilage to the hyoid bone after holes are drilled in the bone or through its central cavity. A fine cutting needle with 4-0 or 5-0 steel is used, because the cricoid cartilage is narrow and tends to split when the needle is pushed through it. Additional sutures are placed in the surrounding muscle and connective tissue to strengthen the fixation of the basihyoid implant.

The remaining sternohyoideus muscle is sutured to the geniohyoideus and mylohyoideus muscles at their insertions to reestablish the continuity lost by removal of the basihyoid bone. The remaining soft tissue is closed.

A free basihyoid segment has been used in the same technique to spread the cricoid cartilage. This procedure has been successful in the long-term maintenance of laryngeal dilation in humans and dogs, although some bone resorption has occurred.[29] Allografts are rejected.

Hemithyroidectomy and Total Laryngectomy. These procedures are used more frequently in patients with proliferative laryngeal disease of septic or neoplastic origin, but they can be adapted for treatment of laryngeal stenosis (see "Neoplasia of the Larynx").

Caudal Segmental Laryngeal Resection. Patients with glottic stenosis involving the cricoid cartilage or neoplasia of the ventral airway in this area respond well to partial cricoid resection and reconstruction using the proximal trachea.[35] The procedure replaces the resected ventral aspect of the cricoid cartilage with the ventral one-half to two-thirds of two tracheal rings.

The sternohyoideus muscles are separated on the midline, exposing the thyroid and cricoid cartilages. Transection of one of the sternohyoideus muscles at its insertion provides better exposure and more working room. Cricothyroideus muscles are transected close to the cricoid cartilage and are preserved. The cricoid cartilage is resected ventral to the articulation with the thyroid cartilage to avoid injuring the recur-

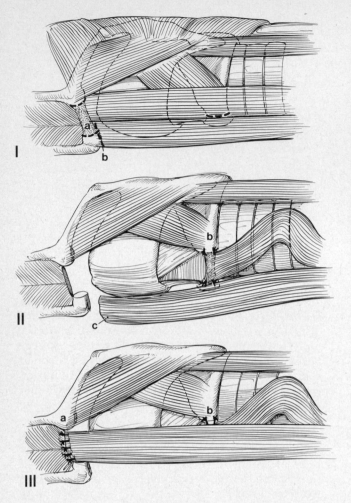

Figure 64–24. Cricolaryngotomy with splintage. *I*, The incisions in the basihyoid bone (*a*), sternohyoideus muscle (*b*), and cricoid cartilage (*c*) are indicated (*dotted lines*). *II*, The basihyoid bone has been resected on its sternohyoideus muscle pedicle and implanted (*b*) between the ends of the transected cricoid cartilage. The free end of the other sternohyoideus muscle (*c*) is shown. *III*, The free end of the sternohyoideus muscle is sutured to the myohyoideus muscle (*a*) and covers the basihyoid implant site (*b*).

rent nerves, which are buried in the connective tissue dorsal to the articulation. The first and second tracheal rings, if involved, are resected (Fig. 64–25).

The remaining larynx is examined, and any additional stenosing scar is removed. Mucosal defects of the dorsal and lateral surfaces can be covered with free buccal mucosal grafts or pedicle mucosal grafts from the interhyoid region or pyriform fossa. Mucosal loss from the remaining cricoid is covered by the mucosa-lined dorsal tracheal membrane, which is

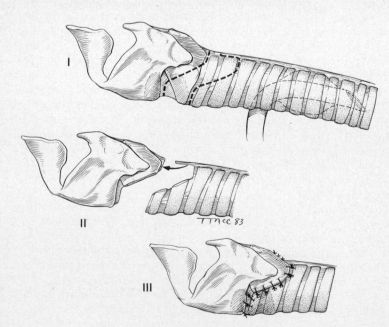

Figure 64–25. Caudal segmental laryngeal resection. *I*, The segment of cricoid cartilage and trachea to be resected is outlined (*dotted line*) and the cricoid muscle (*shaded area*) is left attached to the thyroid cartilage. The tracheostomy route for the endotracheal tube is used. *II*, The segment is resected, leaving the dorsal tracheal membrane with its mucosa intact to line the dorsal cricoid region. The mucosa of the remaining cricoid cartilage may have to be removed if it is involved in the disease process. *III*, The completed anastomosis with the cricoid cartilage arch reconstructed. The cricothyroid muscle is sutured to the trachea (*shaded area*).

spared during shaping of the rostral trachea for anastomosis to the larynx (see Fig. 64–25II). A traction suture is placed on the ventral midline around the third tracheal ring caudal to the resection. The trachea is pulled rostrally and shaped to fit into the defect in the cricoid. The lateral portions of the first two remaining tracheal rings are resected so that the remaining ventral segments adequately replace the resected cricoid cartilage.

The first sutures align the mucosa of the remaining cricoid cartilage with the dorsal tracheal membrane. Knots are placed on the extraluminal side. Simple interrupted, nonabsorbable 3-0 to 4-0 sutures are preplaced, with careful alignment of cartilage and mucosal interfaces. Partial-thickness sutures may be needed in the cricoid and thyroid cartilages to obtain good alignment with the trachea. A small hand drill or hand chuck and K-wire are needed to make suture holes in mineralized cartilage.

After all sutures are preplaced, the larynx and trachea are pulled together and their alignment is examined. When the alignment is perfect, the sutures are tied. The cricothyroideus muscles are sutured to the trachea with interrupted sutures to aid in making the anastomosis air-tight, to provide tissue with a good blood supply adjacent to the anastomosis for optimal healing, and to strengthen the anastomosis. The remaining tissues are sutured into normal anatomic alignment.

Postoperative Care. Airway maintenance is a primary concern in all laryngeal patients (see Chapter 66). Preoperative antibiotics are continued for five days and steroids are continued for 72 hours if excessive tissue edema is expected.

Laser Excision. Vaporization of glottic and subglottic stenoses with CO_2 laser has met with varied success in the dog and humans.[4, 61, 74, 101, 105] The CO_2 laser is used in conjunction with an operating microscope and a micromanipulator. It generates a beam of less than 2 mm diameter, operates at 10.6-μ wave length with power of 70 ma and 20 watts. Exposures of 0.1 to 1 second are used. Tissue necrosis occurs 2 mm beyond the edge of the vaporized lesion.

Adjacent tissues are protected from injury by saline-soaked gauze sponges. The endotracheal tube is wrapped with aluminum foil to prevent burning, and the oxygen concentration should be 30 per cent or less in inspired gas to prevent a flash fire. Smoke and vapors are carried away from the site by suction.

Tissue reaction is minimal for three weeks, and little edema or granulation tissue develops during this time.[74, 105] Epithelialization is progressive during this period, and small lesions heal completely. Large, denuded areas follow the same pattern, but if they are not healed in three weeks, granulation tissue production becomes rapid and stenosis recurs. After laser excision of large lesions, early surface coverage with a suitable mucosal graft may prevent re-stenosis (see Chapter 65). Stents (keel, rolled silicone sheet) reduce the chances of re-stenosis (see discussion of laryngeal stents),[100] by holding mucosal grafts in place

and reducing adhesions between adjacent denuded surfaces.

Postoperative Care. Antibiotics and steroids are started postoperatively and continued. Methylprednisolone is given intralesionally, 10 to 15 mg (80 mg/ml) as a single dose.[61]

Cryosurgery. Cryosurgical techniques have been used to freeze laryngeal tissue.[54, 80] A closed probe with circulating liquid nitrogen is used *per os* or via a thyrotomy to freeze the tissue. Surrounding tissues are insulated from the probe with rigid polystyrene foam wafers or urethane sponge. A two-minute freeze after the probe reaches $-196°C$ will cause a 2-mm-deep lesion. A second freeze is used after a slow thaw.

Tissue edema develops in the first 48 hours, soft tissue sloughs in three to seven days, and cartilage sloughs in five to 20 days. Healing occurs by 35 days.[80] Cartilage heals with a fibrous plate.

A second technique using a fine spray of liquid nitrogen has been used in dogs and humans to remove small lesions on the mucosa from the vocal folds.[54] Two 30-second freezes result in mucosal sloughs and healing in seven days. A temperature of $-30°C$ is reached in the submucosa. Two one-minute freezes result in necrosis and scarring of the vocal fold, with considerable loss of phonation as a sequel.

PROLIFERATIVE DISEASE OF THE LARYNX

Granulomatous Laryngitis

Granulomatous laryngitis is a chronic, proliferative inflammatory disease seen in dogs.[47, 82] It must be differentiated from ulcerating forms of laryngeal neoplasia by biopsy. The proliferating lesions tend to be found around the arytenoid processes and cause laryngeal stenosis. Regression of the lesion usually occurs with debulking of the mass and steroid therapy. Prednisolone (0.2 to 1 mg/kg) is administered daily for two to four weeks, then intermittently as needed to reduce granulation tissue.[47]

Neoplasia of the Larynx

See also Chapter 185.

Primary neoplasia of the larynx is rare in the dog and cat.[113] Various laryngeal tumors have been reported, including squamous cell carcinoma, mast cell tumor, oncocytoma, and mixed cell tumor.[6, 47, 49, 113] Of these, squamous cell carcinoma is the most common primary laryngeal neoplastic lesion seen in small animals. Other tumors, such as lymphosarcoma, plasma cell tumor, and thyroid neoplasia, have been found to metastasize to the laryngeal region. Inflammatory polyps and laryngeal cysts are seen occasionally in the laryngeal region and must be differentiated from neoplasia.[15, 47]

Voice alteration is an early sign with masses in the

larynx (particularly the vocal cords). Progressive encroachment on the airway results in partial obstruction and respiratory noise or distress. Acute dyspnea and hypoxia develop when inflammatory edema and excessive tracheal secretion compound the obstruction. Inflammation and ulceration (pain) can initiate laryngeal spasm in cats (less easily in dogs), resulting in acute hypoxia and cyanosis.

A temporary tracheostomy is needed in some patients to provide an airway during diagnostic evaluation (see Chapter 65). The tracheostomy should be placed well below the larynx, between tracheal rings four and eight, so that sufficient trachea will be available for laryngeal reconstruction.

Surgical resection of benign tumors and cysts in small animals is curative; surgical treatment for malignant disease is usually only palliative. The clinical application of these techniques is feasible in selected cases. Partial, hemi- and total laryngectomy can be used in animals because speaking ability is not critical.

Identification of the tumor type, size, and location is needed to develop a surgical plan. Adequate surgical margins should be taken but all remaining tissues should be spared to rebuild the larynx. A tracheotomy is made in all cases to facilitate anesthesia and postoperative airway maintenance. Chemotherapy or radiation treatment has been used in conjunction with palliative surgery in dogs, but the response has been poor.[113]

Partial Segmental Laryngectomy. Small tumors involving mucosa of the vocal cord and adjacent superficial tissues can be excised via partial laryngectomy.[8, 79, 86, 87, 89] A midline ventral approach is made to the larynx and extended into the lumen via a midline thyrotomy. The tissues are examined, tumor margins are established, and outlining incisions are made in the mucosa. Similar incisions are made in the overlying thyroid cartilage, and the full-thickness laryngeal segment is removed (Fig. 64–26II and III). Mucosal and cartilage defects are repaired by suturing or by replacing large tissue defects with implants to reestablish normal tissue continuity.

The tissue implants—i.e., nasal septum, rib carti-

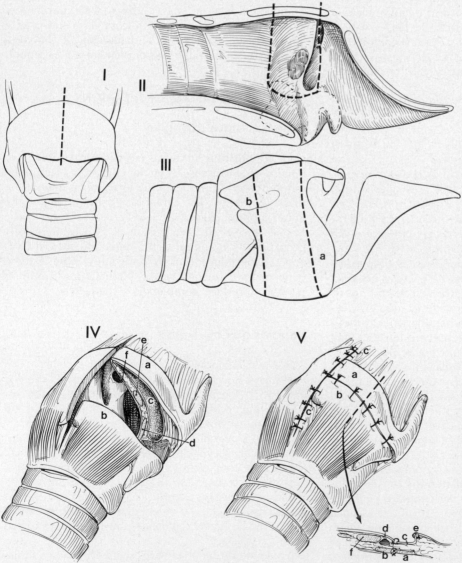

Figure 64–26. Partial segmental laryngectomy. *I,* Ventral incision is made in the thyroid cartilage (also the cricoid cartilage if needed) to expose the vocal fold and surrounding structures. *II,* The incision in the mucosa, arytenoid cartilage, and muscles (*dotted line*) is deepened to the level of the thyroid cartilage. *III,* The incision through the lateral side of the thyroid cartilage is indicated (*dotted line*) leaving cranial (*a*) and caudal (*b*) segments to be sutured. *IV,* The segment of tissue is removed, leaving the cranial (*a*) and caudal (*b*) portions of the thyroid cartilage, the rostral part of the saccule mucosa (*c*), the cut surfaces of the vocal process (*d*), ventral portion of the cuneiform process of the arytenoid cartilage (*e*), and the edge of laryngeal mucosa (*f*). *V,* The thyroid cartilage segments (*a* and *b*) are aligned and sutured. The midline sutures (*c*) join the thyroid cartilage and soft tissue to close the unequal cartilage edges. *Inset,* a cross-section through the resection site, showing the various suture lines. The thyroid cartilage segments (*a* and *b*) are sutured. The mucosa of the saccule (*c*) is sutured to the cricoid cartilage (*f*). The mucosa of the saccule (*e*) and remaining false vocal fold are sutured to close this defect.

lage, buccal mucosa, thyroideus muscle or combinations of these (see "Laryngeal Stenosis")—are used only when most of the thyroid cartilage is resected. The thyroid cartilage is sutured to the implant with 3-0 or 4-0 absorbable suture on a cutting needle. In dogs with mineralized cartilages holes may have to be drilled in the cartilage edge through which sutures are passed. The exterior of the implant is supported by remaining laryngeal muscle, strap muscles, and subcutaneous tissue.

Implants that are not covered with a mucosal surface may require periodic resection of granulation tissue while epithelial tissue grows in from the surrounding mucosa. Excision of excessive granulation tissue is done *per os* with biopsy forceps, shielded electrocautery, or CO_2 laser with vision of the area through a bronchoscope.[86]

The more common repair involves anastomosis of the remaining tissue. The ventral lateral thyroid cartilage resection is continued dorsally to include its full width (see Fig. 64–26*IV*), to allow the cranial segment of the thyroid cartilage to be moved caudally and sutured to the remaining caudal segment. The mucosa is tailored to provide a smooth alignment as the thyroid cartilage is sutured. Closure of the ventral thyrotomy has minor complications due to the mismatched cartilage width at the cranial end. The mismatch is adjusted for by careful soft tissue and soft tissue–cartilage closure (Fig. 64–26*V*).

Mucosal involvement over the cricoid cartilage is treated by full-thickness wall resection. The trachea is used to reconstruct the resected cricoid cartilage and mucosa (see "Caudal Segmental Laryngeal Resection").

Postoperative Care. Care of the respiratory patient is routine (see Chapter 66). The tracheostomy is maintained through the postoperative period (two to ten days). Antibiotics are given postoperatively for five days. Pharyngostomy tube feeding is used for ten to 14 days to reduce tissue motion Mucosa dehiscence is a complication.

Total Laryngectomy. Tumors involving both sides of the larynx are treated by total laryngectomy.[79] A ventral midline approach is made to the larynx and trachea. Traction sutures are placed around the fourth tracheal ring, and the trachea is transected caudal to the cricoid cartilage. A sterile endotracheal tube is placed into the distal trachea to maintain anesthesia (Fig. 64–27).

The thyropharyngeus, cricopharyngeus, sternothyroideus, and thyrohyoideus muscles are transected at their laryngeal attachments. The sternohyoideus muscle is left undisturbed. The caudal aspect of the larynx is grasped, elevated, and dissected free from remaining attachments. The mucosa is incised at the rostral edge of the larynx, and the entire larynx, including the epiglottis, is removed. The pharyngeal mucosa is closed with a simple, continuous pattern

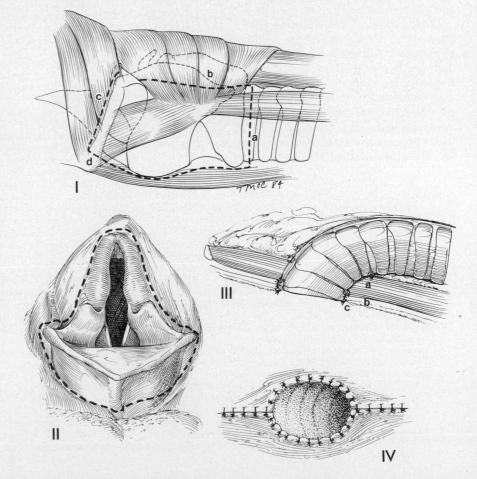

Figure 64–27. Total laryngectomy with permanent tracheostomy. *I,* Dotted lines indicate the location of incisions to transect the trachea (*a*), the cricopharyngeus and thyropharyngeus muscles (*b*), hyopharyngeus muscle (*c*), and thyrohyoid bone and ventral soft tissue (*d*). *II, Dotted line* indicates incision in the pharyngeal mucosa area which is made from the caudal (submucosal) approach as the larynx is removed. *III,* The trachea is positioned for a permanent tracheostomy. Sutures are placed between the sternohyoideus muscle (*a*) and the trachea to hold it in position. Additional sutures are placed between the trachea and the subcutaneous tissue (*b*) and skin (*c*). *IV,* Good alignment of the skin and mucous membrane must be obtained. Fine nonabsorbable sutures correctly align the tissues.

using 3-0 absorbable suture. The thyropharyngeus and cricopharyngeus muscles, which were transected at the thyroid cartilage, are sutured together ventral to the esophagus.

The resulting dead space is closed with adjacent soft tissue, and a Penrose drain is placed to prevent seroma formation. The proximal end of the trachea is brought ventrally between the sternohyoideus muscles with a slight bend to bring the orifice nearly parallel with the skin surface. The tracheal orifice is trimmed to provide an even contour relative to the skin. The sternohyoideus is sutured to the trachea with interrupted sutures to hold it in the ventral position (see Fig. 64–27). Excess skin and subcutaneous tissue are removed to eliminate folds of skin around the permanent tracheostomy. A round piece of skin is resected to provide an opening equal to or slightly larger than the trachea. Subcutaneous tissue is sutured to the tracheal wall, and skin is sutured to the tracheal mucosa with 3-0 or 4-0 absorbable suture in an interrupted pattern.

A temporary tracheotomy is made caudal to the permanent tracheostomy, and the endotracheal tube is removed. A tracheostomy tube is placed in the caudal tracheotomy to maintain an airway while the permanent tracheostomy site heals. This procedure decreases tissue irritation and stenosis at the permanent tracheostomy. The remaining cervical incision is closed, and a sterile Vaseline-soaked gauze pad and an absorbent bandage are placed over the drain and permanent tracheostomy.

Postoperative Care. Routine care of the tracheostomy tube is important to maintain an adequate airway (see Chapter 65). The bandage is changed daily for five to six days, and the drain is removed as soon as it is relatively nonproductive (24 to 72 hours). The bandage is removed permanently as soon as the postoperative inflammation subsides at the permanent tracheostomy site and healing is progressing well. The tracheostomy tube is removed at this time, and the site is debrided and sutured.

1. Abramson, A. L., and Eason, R. L.: Experimental results of cancellous autografts and frozen allografts transplanted into the canine frontal sinus. Laryngoscope 87:1312, 1977.
2. Abramson, A. L., and Eason, R. L.: Experimental frontal sinus obliteration: long term results following removal of mucous membrane lining. Laryngoscope 87:1066, 1977.
3. Alonso, W. A.: Hyoid arch transposition. Otolaryngol. Clin. North Am. 12:903, 1979.
4. Andrews, A. H., Goldenberg, R. A., Moss, H. W., and Shaker, M. H.: Carbon dioxide laser for laryngeal surgery. Surgery Ann. 6:459, 1974.
5. Baker, G. J.: Surgery of the canine pharynx and larynx. J. Small Anim. Pract. 13:503, 1972.
6. Beaumont, P. R.: Mast cell sarcoma in the larynx of a dog: a case report. J. Small Anim. Pract. 20:19, 1979.
7. Beeson, W. H.: Plaster of Paris as an alloplastic implant in the frontal sinus. Arch. Otolaryngol. 107:664, 1981.
8. Biller, H. F., and Lucente, F. E.: Reconstruction of the larynx following vertical partial laryngectomy. Otolaryngol. Clin. North Am. 12:761, 1979.
9. Blaugrund, S. M., and Kurland, S. R.: Replacement of the arytenoid following vertical hemilaryngectomy. Laryngoscope 85:935, 1975.
10. Bone, R. C.: Subglottic stenosis. Otolaryngol. Clin. North Am. 12:869, 1979.
11. Bradley, P. A., and Harvey, C. E.: Intranasal tumors in the dog: an evaluation of the prognosis. J. Small Anim. Pract. 14:459, 1973.
12. Brandenburg, J. H.: Management of acute blunt laryngeal injuries. Otolaryngol. Clin. North Am. 12:741, 1979.
13. Bright, R. M.: Nasal foreign bodies, tumors and rhinitis/sinusitis. In Bojrab, M. J. (ed.): Pathophysiology in Small Animal Surgery. Lea & Febiger, Philadelphia, 1981.
14. Bright, R. M., Thacker, H. L., and Brunner, R. D.: Fate of autogenous fat implants in the frontal sinuses of cats. Am. J. Vet. Res. 44:22, 1983.
15. Caywood, D., Wallace, L. J., Alsaker, R. D., and Lord, P. F.: A laryngeal cyst in the dog: a case report. J. Am. Anim. Hosp. Assoc. 13:87, 1977.
16. Cotton, R. T.: Laryngotracheal reconstruction in children. Five year follow-up. Ann. Otol. Rhinol. Laryngol. 90:516, 1981.
17. Croft, C. B., Zub, K., and Borowiecki, B.: Therapy of iatrogenic subglottic stenosis: a steroid/antibiotic regime. Laryngoscope 89:482, 1979.
18. Crysdale, W. S.: Laryngeal and tracheal stenosis in children. Otolaryngol. Clin. North Am. 12:817, 1979.
19. Curley, B. M., Nelson, A. W., and Kainer, R. A.: Mandibular symphysiotomy in the dog and cat: a surgical approach to the nasopharynx. J. Am. Vet. Med. Assoc. 160:981, 1972.
20. Cvetnic, V., Cvetnic, S., and Grbac, I.: Comparison of gas quantities in the blood of patients with nasal packing for epistaxis, after nasal surgery and experimentally. Rhinology 17:257, 1979.
21. Denecke, H. J., and Meyer, R.: Plastic Surgery of the Head and Neck. Vol. 1: Corrective and Reconstructive Rhinoplasty. Springer-Verlag, New York, 1967.
22. Druck, N. S., Alonso, W. A., and Ogura, J. H.: Hyoid arch transposition. Trans. Am. Acad. Ophthalmol. Otolaryngol. 82:175, 1976.
23. Duncavage, J. A., Toohill, R. J., and Isert, D. R.: Composite nasal septal graft reconstruction of the partial laryngectomized canine. Otolaryngology 86:ORL285, 1978.
24. Eason, R. L., Abramson, A. L., and Pryor, W. H.: Experimental results of autogenous cancellous bone chips transplanted into the infected canine frontal sinus cavity. Trans. Am. Acad. Ophthalmol. Otolaryngol. 82:148, 1976.
25. Edmonds, L., Stewart, R. W., and Selby, L.: Cleft lip and palate in Boston terrier pups. Vet. Med. Small Anim. Clin. 67:1219, 1972.
26. Finnegan, D. A., Wong, M. L., and Kashima, H. K.: Hyoid autograft repair of chronic subglottic stenosis. Ann. Rhinol. Laryngol. 85:643, 1975.
27. Fogh-Andersen, P.: Inheritance of hare lip and cleft palate. Ejnar Munksgaard, Copenhagen, 1943.
28. Freng, A.: Mid-facial saggital growth following resection of the nasal septum-vomer: a roentgencephalometric study in the domestic cat. Acta Otolaryngol. (Stock.) 92:363, 1981.
29. Gaskell, C. J.: The radiographic anatomy of the pharynx and larynx of the dog. J. Small Anim. Pract. 14:89, 1974.
30. Geffen, L. R.: Traumatic cleft palate in a cat. Vet. Rec. 72:572, 1960.
31. Gorling, R. L., and Ticer, J. W.: Contrast rhinography: a radiographic technique for evaluating diseases of the nasal cavity and paranasal sinuses in the dog. Presented at Am. Coll. Vet. Surg. Ann. Mtg., Feb., 1982.
32. Gourley, I. M., Paul, H., and Gregory, C.: Castellated laryngofissure and vocal fold resection for the treatment of larnygeal paralysis in the dog. J. Am. Vet. Med. Assoc. 182:1084, 1983.
33. Graham, W. P.: The plastic surgery of clefts. In Cooper, H. K., Harding, R. L., Krogman, W. M., et al. (eds.): Cleft Palate and Cleft Lip. W. B. Saunders, Philadelphia, 1979.
34. Gracek, R. R.: Hereditary adductor vocal cord paralysis. Ann. Otolaryngol. 85:90, 1976.
35. Grillo, H. C.: Primary reconstruction of airway after resection of subglottic laryngeal and upper tracheal stenosis. Ann. Thorac. Surg. 33:3, 1982.

36. Hammer, D. L., and Sacks, M.: Surgical closure of cleft soft palate in a dog. J. Am. Vet. Med. Assoc. *158*:342, 1971.

37. Hammer, D. L., and Sacks, M.: The palate. *In* Bojrab, M. J. (ed.): *Current Techniques in Small Animal Surgery*. Lea & Febiger, Philadelphia, 1979.

38. Hardie, E. M.: Laryngeal paralysis in three cats. J. Am. Vet. Med. Assoc. *179*:879, 1981.

39. Harding, R. L.: Surgery. *In* Cooper, H. K., Harding, R. L., Krogman, W. M., et al. (eds.): *Cleft Palate and Cleft Lip*. W. B. Saunders, Philadelphia, 1979.

40. Harvey, C. E.: Partial laryngectomy in the dog. I: Healing and swallowing function following surgery (submitted for publication).

41. Harvey, C. E.: Partial laryngectomy in the dog. II: Assessment of the intermediate increase in glottic area obtained and compared with other laryngeal surgical procedures (submitted for publication).

42. Harvey, C. E.: Upper airway obstruction surgery. 1: Stenotic nares surgery in brachycephalic dogs. J. Am. Anim. Hosp. Assoc. *4*:535, 1982.

43. Harvey, C. E.: Upper airway obstruction surgery. 2: Soft palate resection in brachycephalic dogs. J. Am. Anim. Hosp. Assoc. *18*:538, 1982.

44. Harvey, C. E.: Upper airway obstruction surgery. 3: Everted laryngeal saccule surgery in brachycephalic dogs. J. Am. Anim. Hosp. Assoc. *18*:547, 1982.

45. Harvey, C. E.: Upper airway obstruction surgery. 4: Partial laryngectomy in brachycephalic dogs. J. Am. Anim. Hosp. Assoc. *18*:548, 1982.

46. Harvey, C. E. and O'Brien, J. A.: Upper airway obstruction surgery. 5: Treatment of laryngeal paralysis in dogs by partial laryngectomy. J. Am. Anim. Hosp. Assoc. *18*:551, 1982.

47. Harvey, C. E., and O'Brien, J. A.: Upper airway obstruction surgery. 6: Surgical treatment of miscellaneous laryngeal conditions in dogs and cats. J. Am. Anim. Hosp. Assoc. *18*:557, 1982.

48. Harvey, C. E.: Upper airway obstruction surgery. Overview of results. J. Am. Anim. Hosp. Assoc. *18*:567, 1982.

49. Harvey, C. E.: The larynx. *In* Bojrab, M. J. (ed.): *Pathophysiology in Small Animal Surgery*. Lea & Febiger, Philadelphia, 1981.

50. Harvey, C. E., and Venker-van Haagan, A.: Surgical management of pharyngeal and laryngeal airway obstruction in the dog. Vet. Clin. North Am. *5*:515, 1975.

51. Hedlund, C. S., Tangner, C. H., Elkins, A. D., and Hobson, H. P.: Temporary bilateral carotid artery occlusion during surgical exploration of the nasal cavity of the dog. Vet. Surg. *12*:83, 1983.

52. Henrikson, D. M.: Technique of devocalizing dogs. J. Am. Vet. Med. Assoc. *155*:21, 1969.

53. Hoerlein, B. F.: The nasal cavity. *In* Bojrab, M. J. (ed.): *Pathophysiology in Small Animal Surgery*. Lea & Febiger, Philadelphia, 1981.

54. Hong, S. W., Silverstein, H., and Sadeghee, S.: The effect of cryosurgery on the canine and human larynx. Laryngoscope *87*:1079, 1977.

55. Howard, D. R.: Mucoperiosteal flap technique for a cleft palate repair in dogs. J. Am. Vet. Med. Assoc. *165*:352, 1974.

56. Howard, D. R., Merkley, D. F., Lammerding, J. J., et al.: Primary cleft palate (hare lip) and closure repair in puppies. J. Am. Anim. Hosp. Assoc. *12*:636, 1976.

57. Jeddicke, K.: Surgical treatment of nasal stenosis of the dog. Prakt. Tier. Arzt. *59*:420, 1978.

58. Jurkiewicz, M. J., Bryant, D. L.: Cleft lip palate in dogs: a progress report. Cleft Palate J. *5*:30, 1968.

59. Knecht, C. D.: Upper airway obstruction in brachycephalic dogs. Comp. Cont. Ed. *1*:25, 1979.

60. Koopman, C. F., Jr., Feld, R., and Coulthard, S. W.: Effects of antibiotics and injury of cricoid cartilage in cricothyrotomy. Surg. Forum *30*:507, 1979.

61. Koufman, J. A., Thompson, J. N., and Kohut, R. I.: Endoscopic management of subglottic stenosis with CO_2 surgical laser. Otolaryngol. Head Neck Surg. *89*:215, 1981.

62. Krajnik, J., Gawronski, M., Knapik, S., et al.: Healing of bone defect in nasal cavity following application of cartilaginous plate. Acta Chir. Plast. (Praha.) *20*:1, 1978.

63. Kremenak, C. R., Huffman, W. C., and Olin, W. H.: Growth of maxilla in dogs after palatal sugery. I. Cleft Palate J. *4*:6, 1967.

64. Kremenak, C. R., and Searls, J. C.: Experimental manipulation of midfacial growth: a synthesis of five years of research. J. Dent. Res. *50*:1488, 1971.

65. Krogman, W. M.: Craniofacial growth: prenatal and postnatal. *In* Cooper, H. K., Harding, R. L., Krogman, W. N., et al. (eds.): *Cleft Palate and Cleft Lip*. W. B. Saunders, Philadelphia, 1979.

66. Lane, J. G.: Canine laryngeal surgery. Vet. Ann. *18*:239, 1978.

67. Lamberding, J. J., and Howard, D. R.: Stenotic nares. *In* Bojrab, M. J. (ed.): *Pathophysiology in Small Animal Surgery*. Lea & Febiger, Philadelphia, 1981.

68. Latham, R. A., Deaton, T. G., and Calabrese, C. T.: A question of the role of the vomer in the growth of the premaxillary segment. Cleft Palate J. *12*:351, 1975.

69. Lee, D. A., and Wright, W. K.: Regeneration of nasal skeletal structures after subperiosteal and subpericondrial resection. Arch. Otolaryngol. *103*:281, 1977.

70. Leonard, H. C.: Collapse of the larynx and adjacent structures in the dog. J. Am. Vet. Med. Assoc. *137*:360, 1960.

71. Lindeman, R. C.: Diverting the paralyzed larynx: a reversible procedure for intractable aspiration. Laryngoscope *85*:157, 1975.

72. Magnussen, C. R.: Herpes simplex virus and recurrent laryngeal nerve paralysis. Arch. Intern. Med. *139*:1423, 1979.

73. Manus, A. G.: Canine epihyoid fractures. J. Am. Vet. Med. Assoc. *147*:129, 1965.

74. McGee, K. C., Nagle, J. W., and Toohill, R. J.: CO_2 laser repair of subglottic and upper tracheal stenosis. Otolaryngol. Head Neck Surg. *89*:92, 1981.

75. McNeil, R. A.: Surgical obstruction of the maxillary sinus: a clinical and experimental study. Laryngoscope *77*:202, 1967.

76. Miller, M. E., Christensen, G. C., and Evans, H. E.: *Anatomy of the Dog*. Philadelphia, W. B. Saunders, 1964.

77. Montgomery, W. W.: Management of glottic stenosis. Otolaryngol. Clin. North Am. *12*:841, 1979.

78. Montgomery, W. W.: The fate of adipose implants in a bony cavity. Laryngoscope *74*:816, 1964.

79. Montgomery, W. W.: *Surgery of the Upper Respiratory System*. Vol. 2. Lea & Febiger, Philadelphia, 1983.

80. Mulvaney, T. J., and Miller, D.: Endolaryngeal cryosurgery. An improved technique. Arch. Otolaryngol. *102*:226, 1976.

81. Neel, H. B., Whicker, J. H., and Lake, C. F.: Thin rubber sheeting in frontal sinus surgery: animal and clinical studies. Laryngoscope *86*:524, 1976.

82. O'Brien, J. A.: The larynx of the dog: Its normal radiographic anatomy. J. Am. Vet. Radiol. Soc. *10*:38, 1969.

83. O'Brien, J. A., and Harvey, C. E.: Diseases of the upper airway. *In* Ettinger, S. J. (ed.): *Veterinary Internal Medicine*. W. B. Saunders, Philadelphia, 1982.

84. O'Brien, J. A., Harvey, C. E., Kelly, A. M., and Tucker, J. A.: Neurogenic atrophy of the laryngeal muscles in the dog. J. Small Anim. Pract. *14*:521, 1973.

85. Ohnishi, T.: Effects of nasal obstruction upon mechanics of the lung in the dog. Laryngoscope *81*:712, 1971.

86. Park, N. H., Major, J. W., and Sauers, P. L.: Hemilaryngectomy and vocal cord reconstruction with gastric tendon graft. Surg. Gynecol. Obstet. *155*:253, 1982.

87. Pleet, L., Ward, P. H., DeJager, H. J., and Berci, G.: Partial laryngectomy with imbrication reconstruction. Trans. Am. Acad. Ophthalmol. Otolaryngol. *85*:ORL882, 1977.

88. Ranger, D.: Transpalatal approach to the postnasal space. *In* Ballantyne, J. (ed.): *Operative Surgery—Fundamental International Techniques—Nose and Throat*. 3rd ed. Butterworths, London, 1976.

89. Reinke, J. D., and Suter, P. F.: Laryngeal paralysis in a dog. J. Am. Vet. Med. Assoc. 172:714, 1978.

90. Rice, D. H., and Coulthard, S. W.: The growth of cartilage from a free perichondral graft in the larynx. Laryngoscope 88:517, 1978.

91. Romita, M. C., Colvin, S. B., and Boyd, A. D.: Cricothyrotomy—its healing and complications. Surg. Forum 28:174, 1977.

92. Rosin, E., and Greenwood, K.: Bilateral arytenoid cartilage lateralization for laryngeal paralysis in the dog. J. Am. Vet. Med. Assoc. 180:515, 1982.

93. Saperstein, G., Harris, S., and Leipold, H. W.: Congenital defects in domestic cats. Feline Pract. 6:18, 1976.

94. Schaer, M., Zaki, F. A., and Harvey, H. J.: Laryngeal hemiplegia due to neoplasia of the vagus nerve in the cat. J. Am. Vet. Med. Assoc. 174:513, 1979.

95. Schafer, B.: Shortening of the vellum palatinum—evaluation of surgical results (in dog). Klein. Tier Praxis 22:323, 1977.

96. Schenck, N. L.: Frontal sinus disease. III: Experimental and clinical factors in failure of the frontal osteoplastic operation. Laryngoscope 85:76, 1975.

97. Schenck, N. L., Tomlinson, M. J.: Frontal sinus trauma: experimental reconstruction with Proplast. Laryngoscope 87:398, 1977.

98. Schenck, N. L., Tomlinson, M. J., and Ridgley, C. D.: Experimental evaluation of a new implant material in frontal sinus obliteration: a preliminary report. Arch. Otolaryngol. 102:524, 1976.

99. Sinibaldi, K. R.: Cleft palate. Vet. Clin. North Am.—Small Anim. Pract. 9:245, 1979.

100. Slatter, D. H., Schirmer, R. G., and Krehbiel, J. D.: Surgical correction of cystic Rathke's cleft in a dog. J. Am. Anim. Hosp. Assoc. 12:641, 1976.

101. Strong, M. S., Healy, G., Vaughan, C. W., et al.: Endoscopic management of laryngeal stenosis. Otolaryngol. Clin. North Am. 12:897, 1979.

102. Thomas, G. K., and Marsden, J.: Subglottic enlargement using cartilage-mucosa autograft, a preliminary experimental study. Arch. Otolaryngol. 101:689, 1975.

103. Tomlinson, M. J., and Schenck, N. L.: Autogenous fat

104. Toothill, R. J., Martinalli, D. L., and Janowak, M. C.: Repair of laryngeal stenosis with nasal septal grafts. Ann. Otol. Rhinol. Laryngol. 85:600, 1976.

105. Vaughan, C. N.: Transoral laryngeal surgery using the CO_2 laser: laboratory experiments and clinical experience. Laryngoscope 88:1399, 1978.

106. Venker-van Haagan A. J.: The source of normal motor unit potentials in supposedly deinnervated laryngeal muscles of dogs. Zentralbl. fur Vet. 25A:751, 1978.

107. Venker- van Haagan, A. J., Hartman, W., Goedege, B., and Uure, S. A.: Spontaneous laryngeal paralysis in young bouviers. J. Am. Anim. Hosp. Assoc. 14:714, 1978.

108. Wada, T., Kremanek, C. R., and Miyazaki, T.: Midfacial growth effects of surgical trauma to the area of the vomer in beagles. J. Osaka Univ. Dent. Sch. 20:241, 1980.

109. Wallace, L. J.: An alternative procedure for repair of cleft hard palate and soft palate in the dog. In Bojrab, M. J. (ed.): Current Techniques in Small Animal Surgery. Lea & Febiger, Philadelphia, 1981.

110. Wardrip, S. J.: Cleft palate repair in a kitten. Vet. Med. Small Anim. Pract. 77:227, 1982.

111. Weerda, H.: Treatment of long rigid tracheal stenoses: an experimental study on animals. Otorhinolaryngology 140:181, 1978.

112. Wells, M. J., Coyne, J. A., and Prince, J. L.: What is your diagnosis? Foreign body in the nasal pharynx. J. Am. Vet. Med. Assoc. 180:83, 1982.

113. Wheeldon, K. B., Suter, P. F., and Jenkins, T.: Neoplasia of the larynx in the dog. J. Am. Vet. Med. Assoc. 180:642, 1982.

114. Winstanley, E. W.: Trephining frontal sinuses in the treatment of rhinitis and sinusitis in the cat. Vet. Rec. 95:289, 1974.

115. Wright, W. D.: Removal of a hairpin from the nasal cavity of a dog. Vet. Med. Small Anim. Clin. 77:388, 1982.

116. Yoder, J. T., and Starch, C. J.: Devocalization of dogs by laryngofissure and dissection of thyroarytenoid folds. J. Am. Vet. Med. Assoc. 145:325, 1964.

Chapter **65** Lower Respiratory System

A. Wendell Nelson

ANATOMY OF THE TRACHEA AND BRONCHI

Anatomic features of the canine and feline trachea have been discussed (see Chapter 61). The trachea has 34 to 44 C-shaped cartilaginous rings connected by elastic tissue, allowing considerable movement during respiration and swallowing.[11, 28] The tracheal rings are incomplete distal to the carina and form overlapping oakleaf-shaped plates of cartilage on the main bronchi. These plates are based distally and slide over each other during respiration, allowing the bronchi to expand and lengthen. During inhalation, the tracheal rings recoil (open) and the dorsal tracheal membrane widens and moves toward or away from the lumen as relative pressure affects it. These movements are normal unless the cross-sectional area is

greatly decreased. The length of the trachea decreases with cranial displacement of the carina during lung inflation. Movement of the carina relative to the placement of the endotracheal tube is important, since insertion into the carina allows the mucosa of the carina to be injured by the tube during inspiration.

Vessels supplying the tracheal wall enter from both the cranial and caudal thyroid and bronchial arteries.[23] They provide a major intercommunicating network of small vessels that connect both the left and right main vascular supplies.[112] This longitudinal vascular network supplies segmental branches that penetrate the annular ligament between each ring and arborize in the submucosa.[35]

On the right side the cranial and caudal thyroid

arteries are held to the external surface of the trachea by short segmental branches. The left cranial and caudal thyroid arteries are in close proximity to the esophagus and send relatively long segmental branches to the trachea at each annular ligament.

Tracheal mucosa supplies mucus and water to the lumen, replacing its cell population every few days and moving the mucous layer orally via beating cilia. The mucosal cells are replaced every three to five days.[26] Disruption of mucosal continuity incites the rapid production of granulation and epithelial tissues.[40, 79] This aggressive response of granulation tissue frequently leads to lumen stenosis.[79]

Recurrent laryngeal nerves are intimately associated with the dorsolateral edges of the trachea cranial to the heart, and the vagus nerves assume a similar position caudal to the aortic arch.

CONGENITAL DISEASE OF THE TRACHEA AND BRONCHI

History

Pathological conditions affecting the trachea and bronchi are associated with a cough, reverse sneeze, retch, gag, wheeze, or whistle. The nature and frequency of these signs and a history of conditions that incite them may assist in a definitive diagnosis.[28, 83]

Stridorous sounds and dyspnea are present in some cases with a narrowed airway. Coughs related to inflamed mucous membranes are usually incited by ingestion of food or water, excitement, or light tracheal pressure. Coughing after eating is incited by esophageal abnormalities.[28] Fluid in the trachea and bronchi is sufficient to incite a cough without additional stimuli. These patients have periods of coughing during or after rest.

Physical Examination

Close attention to respiratory sounds assists in diagnosing tracheal disease.[28, 83] Relatively quiet to mildly resonant respiratory sounds indicate a non-fluid-producing inflammatory condition. Palpation of the trachea initiates a resonant, harsh cough, which may be associated with nonproductive retching or gagging. Moist, rattling respiratory sounds are associated with a more productive and mainly mucoid tracheal fluid. Palpation causes some gagging with the production of a white, mucoid to frothy, possibly blood-tinged fluid. Tracheal collapse or cardiac problems may produce this reaction. Tracheal collapse causes a "honking" type of cough.

Palpation of the trachea may reveal abnormalities in anatomical conformation. Heavy sedation or anesthesia may be needed to provide sufficient relaxation so that the entire cervical trachea can be palpated without distressing the patient. Examination for ab-

normal texture of the tracheal wall (i.e., soft, rigid), angulation or flattening of the curvature to the tracheal rings, intraluminal masses that appose digital collapse of the trachea, and abnormally small circumference of the trachea is important.[28, 112] The thyroid gland as well as lymph nodes in the area should be palpated for possible enlargement causing tracheal compression.

Intrathoracic portions of the trachea and bronchial tree must be studied by other methods. Conformation of these structures may be outlined by radiographic techniques, whereas internal characteristics are examined with a bronchoscope (see Chapter 63).

Special Diagnostic Techniques

Radiography

Lateral and dorsoventral radiographs of the trachea and bronchi provide information on their size, shape, and location. Small changes in the diameter of adjacent segments of the normal trachea can be found. A transverse projection of the trachea may be obtained at the thoracic inlet. It is important that these be examined during both inspiration and expiration.

The normal diameter of the trachea should be approximately three times the diameter of the proximal third of the third rib or equal to the diameter of the cricoid cartilage lumen. A more reliable method of determining relative tracheal diameter is comparison with the thoracic inlet. A ratio of the internal diameter of the trachea to the distance between the ventral edge of the first thoracic vertebra and the dorsal edge of the manubrium is made. A ratio of 0.16 or greater indicates a normal diameter.[46] A hypoplastic trachea is abnormally small, the cartilage rings are closed dorsally, and the tracheal lumen does not change in diameter during the respiratory cycle. A collapsing trachea varies greatly in diameter during the respiratory cycle. Intraluminal obstruction or extraluminal compression is noted as nonchanging local reduction in the tracheal air shadow. If an obstruction is found, the entire respiratory tract should be examined for additional areas of obstruction prior to surgical exploration. Radiodense foreign bodies are seen on plain radiographs. Radiolucent foreign bodies should be considered if there is obstruction of a distal bronchus, causing secondary lobar atelectasis. Positive contrast tracheobronchograms are needed to outline these foreign bodies.

Overlapping of the airway with the forelimbs interfers with radiographic studies. The head and neck should be kept in a normal position unless exaggerated flexion or extension of the occipitoatlantal articulation is used to stress the trachea. This maneuver exaggerates abnormalities, especially tracheal collapse. The forelimbs may be pulled caudally or cranially to obtain detailed films of the trachea over its entire length. The overlying shadow of the esophagus may obscure the true tracheal shadow and confuse film interpretation, especially if there is significant gas within the esophagus. Sufficient exposure eliminates this overlying shadow and allows the tracheal lumen to be traced.[28]

Positive contrast study of the trachea and bronchi requires general anesthesia. This study should be combined with tracheal culture, endoscopic examination, and definitive surgical intervention to decrease the number of anesthetic periods.

Positive contrast studies of the trachea and bronchi outline disruptions in the tracheal wall, radiolucent foreign bodies, abnormalities of the tracheal conformation, and intraluminal masses (see Chapter 63). Contrast material may cause mucosal inflammation, especially in patients with acute pulmonary infection. Hypersensitivity to the contrast material should be determined prior to its use. Atropine sulfate should not be used, as it interferes with mucociliary action, which is needed to remove the contrast material.[28]

An endotracheal tube is passed to provide a patent airway and a pathway through which the contrast media is introduced. The contrast material of choice is a 50 to 60% weight/volume suspension of barium sulfate in carboxymethylcellulose base. Dilution is made with sterile saline, and 1 cc/5 kg body weight is injected through the endotracheal tube into the cervical trachea. The patient is allowed to respire normally for approximately one minute before standard radiographs are taken. Additional contrast medium is used if there is not sufficient outline of the bronchial tree. Motion studies via a fluoroscope with image intensification provide the best evaluation of tracheal function as well as the necessary examination of the tracheal lumen. Studies during inspiration, expiration, and induced cough aid in examination of the trachea and bronchial tree.

Culture

The trachea should be cultured before it is examined endoscopically or has contrast material instilled into it. After heavy sedation or induction of anesthesia, the trachea is cultured via the oral cavity with a sterile swab. The epiglottis is depressed as the swab is carefully introduced between the vocal cords and a deep sample is obtained. In large dogs, a uterine swab (large animal type) can be used for this purpose. Tracheal wash and aspiration of the deep bronchial tree are done at this time (see Chapter 63).

Endoscopy

A complete endoscopic evaluation of the trachea and bronchial tree should be done before the mucous membrane's color and typical exudate have been obscured by the contrast material (see Chapter 63).

COLLAPSING TRACHEA

Incidence

The majority of the 133 cases of collapsing trachea reviewed in the literature between 1967 and 1979 were found in miniature or toy breeds.[2, 7, 24, 25, 111] Pomeranian (30), miniature and toy poodle (26), Yorkshire terrier (26), Chihuahua (17), and pug (5) were the most common breeds affected. In a review of 2,780 dogs of all breeds seen for the first time between 1971 and 1973, 15 cases (0.5 per cent) had a collapsing trachea.[2] Of the 521 toy dogs in this review, 14 cases (2.7 per cent) of collapsing trachea were recorded, whereas 4 cases were seen out of 136 miniature or toy poodles (2.9 per cent) and 4 cases were seen out of 43 Pomeranians (9.3 per cent).

History

The condition is seen in dogs of all ages, with the average age of diagnosis being seven years.[23–25] Signs of respiratory distress have usually been evident for an average of two years.[22, 23] There is no sex predilection. The early signs are a mild productive cough and mild exercise intolerance in a normally active patient. This progresses into a more severe exercise intolerance (to cyanosis) and the development of a honking cough. Harsh rales may be present. Dyspnea is noted during inhalation (cervical trachea) or exhalation (thoracic trachea) with an abdominal lift or both. Obesity is a frequent but not consistent finding. A history of medical therapy with only transitory benefit is common.[28]

Pathophysiology

The dorsal tracheal membrane or cartilaginous rings or both may be involved (Fig. 65–1). If the tracheal rings are reasonably normal and the dorsal membrane is redundant or weak (Grade 1 or 2), the

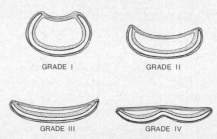

GRADE I   GRADE II

GRADE III   GRADE IV

Figure 65–1. Classification of collapsed trachea. Grade I. The trachea is nearly normal. The tracheal membrane (trachealis muscle) is slightly pendulous, and the tracheal cartilages maintain a normal "C" shape. The tracheal lumen is reduced by approximately 25 per cent. Grade II. Tracheal membrane is widened and pendulous. The tracheal cartilages are partially flattened, and the tracheal lumen is reduced by approximately 50 per cent. Grade III. Tracheal membrane is almost in contact with the dorsal surface of the tracheal cartilages. The tracheal cartilages are nearly flat, and the tracheal lumen is reduced by approximately 75 per cent. Grade IV. Tracheal membrane is lying on the dorsal surface of the tracheal cartilages. The tracheal cartilages are flattened and may invert dorsally (retroflex). The cartilage lumen is essentially obliterated. (Redrawn from Tanger, C. H., and Dobson, H. P.: A retrospective study of 20 surgically managed cases of collapsed trachea. Vet. Surg. *11*:146, 1982.

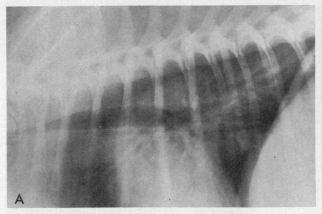

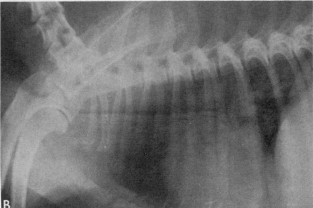

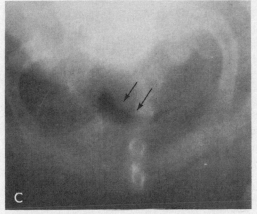

Figure 65–2. Radiographs of a collapsing trachea. *A,* During inspiration, the distal thoracic trachea is normal. *B,* During expiration, the thoracic trachea is nearly collapsed. *C,* The cross section of the trachea at the thoracic inlet demonstrates the flattened rings and redundant tracheal membrane (*arrows*). (From Dr. R. D. Park, Colorado State University, Fort Collins, CO.)

membrane is drawn into the cervical tracheal lumen during inspiration and forced into the intrathoracic trachea and mainstem bronchial lumen during expiration, causing a functional stenosis.[112] If the cartilaginous rings are hypoplastic or fibrodystrophic, they lack the ability to maintain their "C" configuration. These rings are shorter in length and collapse laterally to form either a flattened oval or a slitlike lumen (Grade 3 or 4).[7, 25, 115] In the latter case, the tracheal rings are nearly straight and may be retroflexed at the thoracic inlet. This results in an extremely small cross-sectional area of functional tracheal lumen and high airway resistance. Abnormal rings in the cervical region collapse on inspiration, whereas those in the thoracic portion collapse on expiration (Fig. 65–2). Tissues forming the tracheal wall, although flattened, are adequate to provide an airway if maintained in the expanded state.

Diagnosis

The severe dyspnea of some patients makes diagnostic tests difficult and dangerous. Simple digital palpation of the trachea incites severe coughing spasms and hypoxia. Palpation of the cervical trachea reveals a dorsoventral flattened trachea with narrow borders. Hyperextension of the occipitoatlantal joint may increase the severity of the dyspnea owing to dorsoventral tracheal flattening.[23, 25]

Radiographs of the lateral cervical and thoracic trachea taken in the unanesthetized patient during inspiration and expiration are usually diagnostic for this condition. Severely affected patients are radiographed in the standing lateral position with a horizontal beam if they resist being held in lateral recumbency. Preoxygenation of the patient reduces respiratory distress.

Endoscopy is the best technique to evaluate the trachea and bronchi prior to surgery and should be done in conjunction with anesthesia for surgery. Oxygen should be infused through the bronchoscope during the examination. Endotracheal tubes for miniature dogs are usually too small to pass an endoscope through and cannot be used (see Chapter 23). The effects of respiration and head and neck extension on the trachea and bronchial lumen should be noted. The degree of dorsal tracheal membrane laxity, the shape of tracheal rings, and the flattening of the trachea and bronchi should be closely observed to aid in developing the surgical plan. Reconstruction of one segment of the system may be followed in a few days by signs of collapse of another segment.

The surgical correction of collapsing trachea should not be undertaken unless the remainder of the respiratory system is free of disease. Upper respiratory obstruction, stenotic nares, overlong soft palate, laryngeal paralysis or collapse, and everted ventricles should be relieved prior to correction of lesions involving the trachea or bronchi. Correction of these may relieve the dysplasia sufficiently to eliminate the need for surgical correction of the collasping trachea and bronchi.

Methods of Repair

Four basic methods have been devised to support an airway that lacks sufficient rigidity to withstand the pressure changes of ventilation and remain patent. These methods have provided relief in clinical cases for varying postoperative periods.

Dorsal Tracheal Membrane Plication

This technique is used with reasonable success, especially in patients that have firm, C-shaped tracheal rings (near normal length) and a stretched or lax tracheal membrane (Grades 1 and 2).[115] A patent resting trachea is occluded during inspiration (cervical trachea) and expiration (thoracic trachea) by the internal negative pressure and external positive pressure, respectively.

Preoperative Preparation. Preoperative antibiotics are given and continued for 24 hours. Oxygen is given as required during all phases of animal preparation. Atropine is not used unless excess secretions are encountered. Viscous tracheal secretions, caused by atropine, are difficult to remove and can lead to tracheal stenosis during recovery from anesthesia.

Surgical Approach. A midline cervical incision exposes the trachea and is continued as a sternotomy incision if the thoracic trachea is involved (see hereafter). A right lateral dissection is made to expose the dorsal aspect of the trachea. The width of the lax tracheal membrane is reduced by plication with 3–0 or 4–0 monofilament nonabsorbable interrupted horizontal mattress sutures (Fig. 65–3).[10, 102] This prevents the redundant membrane from sagging into the tracheal lumen and obstructing air flow.

In severe tracheal collapse, the cartilaginous rings are flattened (dorsoventrally) and comprise only one-half of the tracheal circumference (Grades 3 and 4).[115] The plication technique used in these cases causes severe narrowing of the trachea as the tips of the rings are drawn toward each other to assume a "C" shape. When the width of the dorsal membrane equals one-half of the tracheal circumference (i.e., complete dorsoventral flattening), approximately 25 per cent of the existing circumference is lost in the plication technique. This results in approximately a 44 per cent decrease in the potential cross-sectional area of the collasped trachea. Only minor additional reduction in lumen area due to mucous plugs or inflammation and edema of the mucosa will cause clinical signs of stenosis. Therefore, plication should be reserved for those patients with reasonable cartilage development and tracheal stenosis caused by dorsal tracheal membrane laxity (Grade 1 or 2).[115]

Internal Stents

Long-term internal support of the weak trachea in the dog with a straight tubular stent has not been successful, since it has a tendency to be dislodged, become obstructive, or be coughed out.[66]

Internal tracheal support as an emergency method for maintaining an airway can be achieved with an endotracheal tube placed through a tracheotomy site and passed distally into the thoracic trachea to a point that relieves respiratory distress (see Tracheostomy). The tracheotomy approach allows the tube to be cleaned and replaced as necessary with little discomfort to the patient. Suctioning of the distal trachea and bronchial tree is done through this tube.

A Montgomery "T" tube* (see Laryngeal Stents, Chapter 64) of soft Silastic has been used successfully to support the larynx and trachea during the postsurgical healing period. Its conformation provides good stability at the tracheotomy and proximal and distal to this site. This is a noncuffed tube used with a tracheotomy that allows air and fluid to pass through and around it (Fig. 65–4). The tube is slightly smaller than the internal diameter of the trachea, and mucosal damage is prevented by a good fit, soft consistency, light weight, and good stability. The tube is seldom changed and is easily cleaned while in place.

Tracheal Ring Transection

Satisfactory improvement in the cross-sectional area of the trachea has been obtained by transecting alternate tracheal rings at the ventral midline.[65] Lat-

---

*E. Bensen Hood Laboratories, Inc., Duxbury, MA.

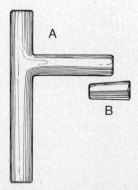

Figure 65–4. A, Montgomery "T" tube made from soft Silastic rubber. Available in sizes from 4.5 to 18 mm OD tubing and 22 to 161 mm overall length. B, The tube is furnished with a plug with a side arm.

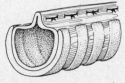

Figure 65–3. Grade II collapsing trachea with the dorsal membrane plicated with interrupted horizontal mattress sutures.

eral tracheal collapse occurs when every tracheal ring is transected. Transection of alternate rings allows the dorsal tracheal membrane to shorten and pull the ends of the tracheal rings toward the midline, whereas the intact rings prevent lateral collapse of the trachea.

The trachea is approached from the ventral midline while the neck is held in dorsiflexion. Alternate rings are transected on the ventral midline beginning with the first ring. This is done without cutting the tracheal mucosa.

Some of the cranial throacic trachea can be reached by traction on the cervical trachea. If a significant portion of the thoracic trachea is involved, a combined cervicothoracic incision must be used (see hereafter).

Postoperative Care. The patient is confined to a cage for five to ten days. Other therapy is not needed unless there is pre-existing pulmonary or cardiac disease.

External Support

An external structure to prevent flattening of the trachea and mainstem bronchi without interfering with segmental motion or vascular supply is most suitable for prolonged tracheal support. Several attempts have been made to use relatively long pieces of material to support the trachea.[12] However, these are not as functional as individual split rings and interfere more with tracheal motion.

Plastic split rings have been made to partially encircle the trachea or mainstem bronchus (Fig. 65–5). When sutured to the ring, the airway wall is held in an expanded form.[106, 115] The split rings are placed one to three tracheal rings apart to provide the flexibility needed for tracheal movement.[115] These rings are implanted without interfering with the vascular and nerve supply of the larynx, trachea, or bronchi.

Polypropylene syringe cases and Teflon tubing have been the source of tubular material sectioned to construct support rings of varying ring widths (4.8

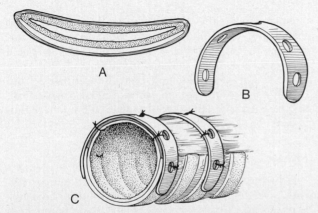

Figure 65–5. Use of plastic rings to support a collapsing trachea. Grade III collapsing trachea (A) is tented on a fenestrated plastic partial ring (B). C, The plastic ring is sutured to the tracheal ring and the dorsal membrane.

to 9.5 mm wide).[106, 115] The internal diameters are selected according to the size of the trachea around which they are to be implanted. Currently used rings and materials have been adequate for the trachea, but they are too coarse for the mainstem bronchus. Other material, such as high-density porous polyethylene, is needed for these small airways.

Broad spectrum antibiotics and corticosteroids are given preoperatively. These are used to decrease the potential of infection in a contaminated area and reduce postoperative swelling of the tracheal mucosa.

Surgical Approach. A cervicothoracic incision is required to approach the cervical and cranial thoracic trachea. A cervical approach is used if the intrathoracic lesion is confined to the thoracic inlet. The ventrocervical area is prepared from the larynx to the second sternabra. If the lesion extends into the thoracic trachea and mainstem bronchi, the ventrocervical as well as the ventral and right sides of the thorax are prepared.

The cervical trachea is exposed through a midline ventral incision made from the larynx to the thoracic inlet. A combination of sharp and blunt dissection separates the midline musculature to the trachea. The cranial 3 to 4 cm of thoracic trachea is reached from the thoracic inlet by blunt dissection of the surrounding loose areolar tissue of the mediastinum and traction of the cervical trachea. If the thoracic trachea is involved, the cervical skin incision is extended to the fifth intercostal space and continued dorsally along the interspace. The right intercostal incision is completed into the thorax and the ventral midline incision is deepened, exposing and splitting the sternum on the midline from the manubrium through the fifth sternabra.

The azygous vein is superficial to the carina, and the mainstem bronchi and must be ligated and transected before these structures are approached. As the trachea is exposed, neurovascular structures along the dorsolateral border are left intact (see Chapter 61).

Tracheal support rings are placed without interrupting or compressing the neurovascular supply of the trachea.[114] A tunnel is made between the trachea and the recurrent laryngeal nerves and right thyroid artery at each ring implant site so that each ring can be passed around the dorsal aspect of the trachea. Although separation of the entire trachea from surrounding tissue does not interfere with healing of the tracheal resection and anastomosis,[19] it may result in avascular necrosis of the trachea when plastic rings are placed. The pressure of these rings compromises blood flow in the nutrient vessels lying on the external surface of the trachea. If the split ring is slightly small for the trachea, the ring should be retroflexed or straightened, after which it will retain a larger arc and will not exert excessive pressure.

The open end of each ring should lie along the ventral border of the trachea. Approximately two-thirds to three-quarters of the trachea is encircled by each split ring.

Each ring is passed through the tunnel with the aid of right-angle forceps and is held in place by suturing it to the adjacent tracheal cartilage or soft tissue. The wide (5 to 9 mm) Teflon and polypropylene rings have holes drilled in them so that the suture can pass through and granulation tissue can grow and anchor the ring.[111, 115] Approximately five sutures are placed on each ring: one near each ring end, two in the tracheal membrane, and one on each lateral side of the trachea. The sutures completely encircle the cartilaginous tracheal ring and penetrate or encircle the plastic ring. Suturing the tracheal membrane to the dorsal aspect of each split ring prevents the tracheal membrane from collapsing into the lumen of the trachea. Fine, monofilament nonabsorbable suture is used for its strength, long life, and tissue compatibility. Simple interrupted sutures hold the ring in place until connective tissue binds the trachea to it.

Postoperative Care. This includes antibiotics for five to ten days and corticosteroids for at least three days postoperatively. The dog frequently has a persistent cough during the healing phase.[115] This is related to tracheal inflammation and edema from the endotracheal tube as well as the penetrating sutures holding the trachea to the plastic rings. A persistent cough while continuing administration of bronchial dilators,[66] anti-inflammatory agents, and cough suppressants should be cause for examination. The persistent cough may be related to a collapsing mainstem bronchus or myocardial disease. Bronchoscopy is used to evaluate the internal structure of the trachea and bronchi during the postoperative period. If myocardial problems have not been previously diagnosed, the cardiovascular system should be re-examined.

HYPOPLASIA OF THE TRACHEA

Dorsally closed tracheal rings are a congenital condition resulting in a narrow trachea and are characterized by chronic cough, wheezing, recurrent respiratory infection, and dyspnea (both inspiratory and expiratory).[46, 113] The puppy has a slow growth rate and exercise intolerance. The small, firm trachea is found by palpation and confirmed by radiography. Positive contrast bronchography outlines the narrowed trachea.

This condition should be differentiated from other tracheal stenoses, since there is no surgical cure for this anomaly. Segmental stenoses are repaired by resection and anastomosis or by implanted prosthesis (see Tracheal Stenosis).

INTERNAL INJURY TO THE TRACHEA

Injury During Intubation

Injury of the tracheal mucosa by prolonged use of cuffed endotracheal tubes is directly related to the pressure exerted by the inflated cuff and the tip of the tube on the tracheal wall.[21, 87, 89, 106] The normal trachea is not a true circle, and cuff expansion causes uneven contact with the wall. High pressures (one to three times systemic blood pressure) are attained at initial contact points as the cuff has expanded to occlude the trachea.[21] Even "just seal" pressure often exceeds 160 mm Hg pressure.[21] Blood flow studies in the canine tracheal mucosa noted that minimal surface pressure (20 mm Hg) were needed to obstruct capillaries.[21, 106] After four hours of this pressure, the canine mucosa was damaged sufficiently so that it lost its cilia and became mildly inflamed within the next 24 hours.[106] The cilia returned in 7 to 14 days.[89, 106] Twenty mm Hg of pressure in a tracheal tube cuff is extremely low compared with that attained in high pressure cuffs (130 to 370 mm Hg).[89] These high pressures cause local collapse of mucosal vessels and nutrient vessels of the cartilage rings. The result is ischemic necrosis of mucosa and, possibly, the entire thickness of the tracheal wall.[21] Granulation tissue filling the defect encroaches upon the lumen and, by proliferation and contraction, results in stenosis. The initial squamous epithelium eventually converts to a partial or fully ciliated surface.[87]

Similar lesions can be caused by pressure of the endotracheal tube tip.[21, 79] Curvature of the tube should match that of the trachea so that pressure points are held to a minimum. Tracheostomy tubes are more likely to cause damage with the cuff and tip owing to their prolonged use. The weight of anesthesic or ventilation tubes attached to the tracheostomy tube may rotate the tube against the tracheal wall and accentuate the pressure points developed by the tube itself (see Tracheostomy).

Endotracheal tubes sterilized with ethylene oxide cause mucosal irritation or necrosis unless they are properly degassed.[120] Large sections of mucosa are sloughed in severe cases. Stenosis may result.

Tracheal Stenosis

Narrowing of the tracheal lumen due to scar tissue may result from endotracheal tube pressure, blunt or penetrating trauma, tracheostomy, or tracheal anastomosis with or without irritation.[19, 39, 41, 59, 72, 79, 98, 115, 122] This condition must be differentiated from extraluminal compression, intraluminal obstruction, and tracheal hypoplasia and collapse. Similar pathological changes of the larynx must be ruled out.

History

A history of trauma, inhalation anesthesia, or tracheal anastomosis under tension is common. Dyspnea is observed during inspiration and expiration and is progressive.[28, 59, 79] An active or athletic patient has signs of dyspnea with less reduction of lumen diameter (40 to 50 per cent) than sedentary dogs (60 to 70 per cent).[69] As the stenosis limits luminal size to 10 to 15 per cent of normal, resting dyspnea is obvious with cyanosis upon exercise. At this point, a small reduction in the stenotic lumen (e.g., mucous plugs, edema, or external pressure) can produce very high resistance to ventilation and cause asphyxia.

Preoperative Examination

The stenotic patient is examined in the awake state while oxygen is provided (see Chapter 63). Auscultation of air movement in the trachea generally locates the stenosis by relatively high-pitched local sounds.[28, 86] Radiographic examination confirms the presence of luminal stenosis and assists in characterization of the obstruction. Flat film imaging can be combined with positive contrast studies to outline the surface of the airway lumen.

Tracheoscopy provides visual identification of changes in lumen shape and lining tissue. A ventilating bronchoscope should be used to provide an adequate airway during this examination. A visual examination and biopsy of the stenosing tissue should be done to obtain a proper diagnosis and prognosis, especially if the site is not going to be resected.

Nonsurgical Approach

Tracheal bougienage has been used in man as primary therapy for stenosis with reasonable success.[73] Dilation of the stenosis is produced by passing progressively larger rigid bronchscopes and must be done with care so that the trachea is not lacerated. This has been combined with steroid therapy and stenting (i.e., Montgomery "T" tube).[41, 73] Triamcinolone acetonide (40 mg/ml, 0.1 to 0.2 ml) injected intralesionally followed by high doses of prednisone systemically for six weeks has been used successfully.[72] Repeated treatments may be needed with stenting for up to three years.

A modification of the Montgomery "T" tube was made to stent a long section of the thoracic trachea including the carina.[124] The distal limb of the "T" tube had a Y piece added that fit into the carina. The whole assembly was placed via tracheotomy. The implant was not removed until the trachea was lined with mucosa and the tracheal wall was strong enough not to collapse during respiration.

Small web stenoses have been removed from the trachea with CO_2 laser equipment.[73] Similar techniques are used as described under Laryngeal Stenosis (see Chapter 64).

Surgical Approach

The specific location and estimated size of the mass and length of trachea involved must be determined before surgery is attempted. Resection of long tracheal segments may require special techniques to allow successful anastomosis (see Tracheal Anastomosis and Reconstruction). A history of prior tracheal resection and the length of the segment resected must be considered in the preoperative planning for reconstruction, since these factors limit the length of a second resection.[19, 72]

The stenotic section is carefully examined and initially transected near its distal end.[79, 100] The distal segment is intubated with a sterile endotracheal tube to maintain anesthesia if the orally placed tube cannot be passed into the distal segment while the stenotic segment is excised. Serial transections are made proximally until normal tracheal lumen and mucosa are found.[100] The ends of the trachea are anastomosed. The surgical technique for tracheal resection is described elsewhere (see Tracheal Resection and Reconstruction).

Foreign Bodies of Trachea and Bronchi

Tracheal and bronchial foreign bodies (e.g., rocks, safety pins, and plant materials) have been reported in the dog and cat.[27, 29, 45, 93, 98] Small light objects may be inhaled deep within the bronchial tree or coughed up and removed. Chronic pneumonia, abscesses, and fistulous tracts may develop from the presence of these foreign bodies.[28]

History

The history of an acute onset of coughing and possibly dyspnea is common. High-frequency rales may be heard in the vicinity of the foreign body if it is partially obstructing air flow. The initial signs of coughing and dyspnea generally recede only to reappear as the surrounding airway becomes inflamed. Chronic infection may occur and may temporarily improve with medical therapy.

Diagnosis

Radiopaque foreign bodies are confirmed with flat film radiographs. Radiolucent foreign bodies can be demonstrated by positive contrast bronchography and bronchoscopy.[28, 130] Exudate emanating from the bronchus may be seen even if the foreign body is not. This indicates the location of the foreign body and should correlate with radiographic evidence of lung inflammation or consolidation.

Therapy for Retrievable Foreign Bodies

Foreign bodies lying in the trachea or mainstem bronchus are removed from most patients with a rigid hollow bronchoscope and appropriate grasping equipment (see Chapter 23).

The bronchoscope is advanced close to the foreign body and the appropriate wire basket or grasping forcep is passed through the bronchoscope to the object. A firm grip is obtained on the object, and it is drawn snugly against the bronchoscope and withdrawn. As the larynx is approached, the foreign body is positioned so that it will cause the least damage as it is pulled between the vocal cords and through the glottis.

Foreign bodies that are difficult to grasp are retrieved with the aid of a Fogarty catheter.[61] The catheter tip is passed through a rigid bronchoscope and advanced past the foreign body, and the balloon cuff is inflated. The foreign body is pulled toward the bronchoscope with the aid of the balloon, held against the bronchoscope tip, and withdrawn.

Therapy for Nonretrievable Foreign Bodies

Bronchial foreign bodies are frequently not retrievable and require a surgical approach.[27, 45, 93] Broad-spectrum antibiotic therapy is initiated prior to surgery. A lateral thoracotomy at the appropriate interspace is used to approach the affected lung, and tissue is inspected for consolidation and palpated for location of the foreign body. A decision must be made whether to do a bronchotomy or a lobectomy to remove the foreign body.

The presence of significant chronic inflammation and consolidation dictates a lobectomy (see hereafter). If the lobe is relatively normal except for atelectasis, the involved bronchus is incised and the foreign body removed.

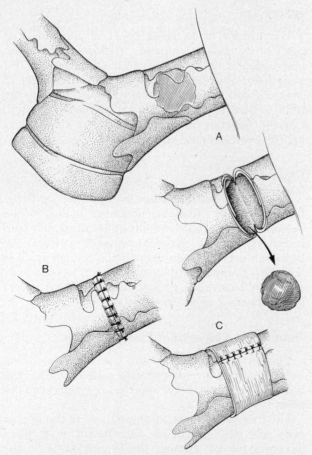

Figure 65–6. Bronchial foreign body retrieved by bronchotomy. *A,* Accurate mucosal alignment is achieved with simple interrupted sutures. *B,* Incomplete cartilage plates are aligned where possible. *C,* A pleural patch is sutured over the primary suture line.

Left lung lobes are approached from the caudodorsal direction, whereas right lung lobes are approached from the craniodorsal direction to avoid the pulmonary vessels. The bronchus is dissected free of surrounding soft tissues, and a noncrushing clamp is placed proximal to the foreign body prior to the bronchial incision. This is not possible if the foreign body is too close to the orifice of the mainstem bronchus, in which case the mainstem bronchus is clamped. The bronchial wall is incised through normal-appearing tissue rostral to the foreign body. If this is not possible, the incision is made directly over the foreign body. An incision is made extending more than half way around the bronchus and the foreign body is removed (Fig. 65–6).

If the deeper, supporting tissue and mucosa are necrotic for more than one-third of the circumference of the bronchus, the entire section (360°) is excised so that healthy ends can be anastomosed. Lobectomy is considered when most of the visible bronchus is severely damaged or the lung lobe consolidated. Mucosal loss with submucosal damage exceeding one-third the circumference of the bronchus usually leads to airway stenosis.[41]

Smaller areas of mucosal damage can be debrided and the bronchotomy incision closed. Simple interrupted absorbable sutures (3–0 to 5–0) are preplaced through cartilage and mucosa for closure of the bronchotomy or bronchial anastomosis. Mucosal alignment is most important, as cartilage closure is variable owing to incomplete rings. The suture line is examined for air leaks and covered with a vascular pedicle flap of pleura, pericardium, or omentum (see Fig. 65–6). This prevents rubbing of the suture knots on adjacent blood vessels, which can cause a bronchiovascular fistula or major local hemorrhage.[41] The tissue flap aids in sealing the bronchial incision (see Bronchial Anastomosis).

EXTERNAL INJURY TO THE TRACHEA AND BRONCHI

Direct injury to the trachea and bronchi can be caused by either blunt or penetrating trauma to a cervical or thoracic area.[52, 114, 122] Persistent peritracheal, subcutaneous, and/or mediastinal emphysema indicates the need for a careful examination for trachea or bronchial damage.

The incidence of airway injury is low considering the number of blunt trauma cases in small animals. Since the majority of blunt injuries occur from the lateral side in animals, the trachea is not crushed against the spine and can move laterally with the impact.

Cervical Trachea

Cervical trachea laceration due to nonpenetrating injury is uncommon but occurs in choke chain and dog bite wounds. Small lesions are commonly self-limiting and are undiagnosed. Lacerations of the trachea may be severe enough to produce significant subcutaneous and mediastinal emphysema.[11, 28, 114]

Extensive tissue damage frequently accompanies penetrating bite and gunshot wounds.[11, 28, 52, 114] Tracheal transection with soft tissue interposition, hematoma obstruction, and injury to major vessels frequently results in early death of the patient.[78, 114] The severely injured animal must have a cervical airway established quickly or be lucky enough to breathe through the skin laceration to survive for definitive treatment.

Emergency Care

Intubation per os or through the laceration is done quickly to gain control of the airway. Intubation via the laceration is selected in cases of large defects that distort the path of the trachea. The distal tracheal segment is hooked by suture or forceps introduced through the laceration, and the lumen is cleared of debris and intubated. In distal third cervical tracheal transections, the distal segment may retract into the thoracic inlet. It must be retrieved and traction sutures placed before intubation.[52]

Initial wound clean-up is completed, the cervical area is prepared for surgery, and the wound is explored. The extent of damage is determined and appropriate care is given to damaged nonairway structures.[114]

Surgical Approach

Cartilage and mucosa of the trachea are debrided, aligned, and sutured in position with fine monofilament nonabsorbable material (see Tracheal Anastomosis).[41, 79] Excessive numbers of sutures are not desirable. General alignment of cartilage and mucosa can be aided by an intraluminal stent placed through a tracheotomy incision (e.g., Montgomery "T" tube or tracheostomy tube) (see Fig. 65–4).[22, 41, 79] These stents should be small enough to fit easily yet large enough to almost fill the tracheal lumen. The tube provides an airway during postoperative recovery and aids in maintaining alignment as granulation tissue fills in gaps and epithelialization takes place. Correct-fitting "T" tubes are well tolerated for months.[22, 41]

Postoperative Care

Drainage from the peritracheal area is required until the infection is under control. Broad spectrum bactericidal antibiotic therapy is started prior to exploration and continued for ten days postoperatively (see Chapter 66). Small areas of granulation tissue can be removed through a bronchoscope at periodic examinations during the healing period. Permanent removal of the tube is governed by reduction of inflammatory tissue and a smoothly healed or nearly healed mucosal surface.[41]

Intrathoracic Trachea and Bronchus

Penetrating injury or inward collapse of the chest wall during impact causes significant damage to the trachea and mainstem bronchi. Minor punctures or lacerations supported by healthy peritracheal tissue are self-limiting. Unsupported lacerations, especially involving the distal trachea and bronchi, may cause extensive pneumomediastinum and tension pneumothorax.[78, 114]

Intrathoracic lacerations of the trachea or bronchi are commonly caused by vehicular and occasionally by "big dog–little dog" injuries. These are due to crushing of the trachea between the collapsing thoracic walls or laceration by a penetrating tooth or fractured rib. The majority are self-limiting as long as pneumothorax is controlled by suction drainage. Mediastinal and subcutaneous emphysema can be reduced by placing a tracheostomy tube, which decreases airway resistance. A persistent nonresolving pneumothorax after three to four days of conservative therapy or an inability to control the pneumothorax by suction drainage is a criterion for exploratory thoracotomy.

Preoperative Assessment

Preoperative location of the involved airway is desirable if not mandatory. Positive contrast bronchography and endoscopic examination of the trachea, bronchi, and pleural cavity normally locate the involved area (see Chapter 63). If the precise location of the disrupted airway is not determined, an approach should be made on the side with the most trauma (i.e., contusions, fractured ribs, and so on). However, the laceration may not be in this area.

Surgical Approach

These procedures require general anesthesia. Hyperoxygenation, rapid induction, and complete control of ventilation are important for satisfactory production of a stable anesthetized patient.

A lateral thoracotomy (see Chapter 41) approach is made in the intercostal space caudal to the fractured rib or over the known laceration site. The approach is made with adequate preparation so that the incision can be extended to the opposite side (transverse thoracotomy). Flooding of the pleural space with saline aids location of the air leak.

Closure of the debrided laceration depends on the defect (see Tracheal and Bronchial Reconstruction, Lung Laceration). Subsequent lavage of the pleural space cleans the area and aids in identification of other existing air leaks. The space is flooded and air pockets eliminated before identifying bubbles as air leaks. The lungs are inflated several times before the system is declared sealed. A chest drain is placed and a standard incision closure is done.

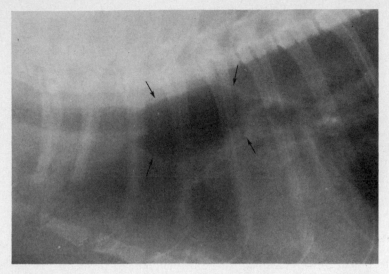

Figure 65–7. Radiograph of a traumatic transection of the distal trachea in a cat. The distal pseudotrachea (*arrows*) is present connecting the distracted ends of the trachea. (From Dr. R. D. Park, Colorado State University, Fort Collins, CO.)

Postoperative Care

Standard monitoring of the thoracic patient is done (see Chapter 66).

Tracheal Transection

In cats, this condition occurs near the carina and may be due to violent stretching (i.e., secondary to hyperextension of the head and neck), injury induced by a large dog, or other trauma.[31, 57, 103] The carina and lungs are a fixed point that is stronger than the tracheal wall. As the trachea is stretched against this point, it ruptures just proximal to the carina.[78] This injury is compromising but not lethal if the peritracheal tissues maintain continuity and provide an airway. The initial dyspnea may persist or resolve until subsequent stenosis or displacement of the trachea causes its return. Diverticula may form in this pseudotrachea.[57]

History

The patient is presented with a history of trauma and dyspnea. The respiratory distress can be intermittent, continuous, or progressive. The constant work of respiration needed just to stay alive may interfere with the eating habits and debilitate the cat. Sibilant wheezing is heard in the hilar region, and any struggling precipitates severe dyspnea.

Diagnosis

Radiographs of the trachea show the discontinuity of the trachea (Fig. 65–7). The air density shadow is continuous, but the wall is less dense and may balloon on inspiration and flatten on expiration.[57, 103] The distal trachea and bronchial tree are normal.

Anesthesia

Care is required during induction of anesthesia. The cat is placed comfortably in an induction (cat) box and oxygenated well before the anesthetic is added. Atropine should not be used, as thick secretions may cause tracheal obstruction or impair passage of the endotracheal tube. The head and neck are extended so that the distal trachea is slightly stretched at the avulsion site to keep the airway open.

The anesthetist should not try to pass the endotracheal tube past the lesion at this time. The endotracheal tube length should be sufficient to intubate the trachea beyond the lesion (see Fig. 65–7). The tube is advanced during surgery under the surgeon's guidance. The cat is allowed to breathe on its own, as positive pressure respiration may rupture the airway.

Surgical Approach

A right lateral thoracotomy is made at the fourth interspace. The cranial lung lobe is packed caudally with a moist gauze sponge, and the azygous vein is ligated and transected. The carina is located by gentle palpation and the vagus nerve located and freed from the carina. The carina is secured with a single traction suture (3–0), the remaining tissues are incised over the pseudo airway, and the endotracheal tube is passed distally into the left main bronchus.

The distracted ends of the trachea are isolated by gentle dissection, preserving local vessels and nerves. In longstanding lesions, considerable scar tissue may be encountered at the transection site. As the tissue is dissected from the trachea, care must be used to leave vessels and nerves intact. These structures are best freed by sharp dissection, originating in normal tissue and working slowly into the scar tissue. Abnormal trachea is removed and a standard anastomosis made using six or seven preplaced 4–0 monofilament nonabsorbable interrupted sutures (see Tracheal Anastomosis).

The endotracheal tube is withdrawn proximal to the anastomosis. An airtight seal in the trachea is verified by submersion of the anastomosis in saline as the ventilation pressure is elevated to 20 to 30 cm H_2O. A pleural patch is harvested and sutured around the trachea to support the anastomotic site.

NEOPLASIA OF THE TRACHEA AND BRONCHI*

Diagnosis

Tracheal obstruction due to intra- and extraluminal neoplastic disease is not common in dogs and rare in cats (see Section 19).[4, 5, 8, 17, 18, 49, 53, 80, 120, 128] The tumor type is academic, since it is the obstruction that is the immediate life-threatening problem. The primary concern is mass resection and maintenance of an unobstructed airway. The diagnosis of tracheal obstruction has been previously discussed (see Tracheal Stenosis). The progressive development of dyspnea without a history of tracheal trauma, intubation, or surgery should place neoplasia high on the differential diagnosis list.[8, 18, 28] Conformation of luminal neoplasia is made with radiographic and endoscopic examination and tissue biopsy. Presurgical biopsy is desirable for planning the pre- and postsurgical workup, therapy, and prognosis discussions with the client.

Surgical Resection

Benign Tumors

Resection in the neoplastic mass does not always include airway wall resection. Benign lesions have been removed without recurrence of local stenosis.[53, 120] Animals are rarely examined early enough in the disease process to permit excision of these masses with bronchoscopic equipment. A tracheotomy incision between two rings or through the dorsal tracheal membrane is adequate to approach these lesions.[8, 53] Care must be taken to preserve the recurrent nerves and main tracheal vessels as the approach and tracheal incisions are made.[42] Sharp dissection of the benign neoplastic mass along a normal tissue plane is adequate to remove the tumor and prevent recurrence.[8, 53] The remaining mucosa and tissue lining the resection bed should be healthy and nontraumatized. Regrowth of epithelium should be complete and without significant luminal stenosis unless the mass is large.

Malignant Tumors

Deep penetration of neoplastic tissue, either benign or malignant, into the tracheal wall necessitates full thickness tracheal resection and reconstruction.[41, 42] Occasionally only a window of full thickness wall need be resected and the tracheal wall patched with synthetics or autogenous tissue (see Tracheal Reconstruction). Although partial wall resection with anastomosis has been reported, it has no advantage over complete resection of the involved segment and anastomosis.[41]

The surgeon should not allow the amount of resection required to be modified by complexity of the repair needed. After adequate resection has been attained, a reasonable repair can be made with a combination of autogenous tissues and synthetic materials.

If the neoplastic mass involves peritracheal tissues, it may be difficult to determine whether the recurrent laryngeal nerves are involved. These nerves are isolated in normal tissue above or below the lesion and their dissection continued into the neoplastic tissue. If the nerve cannot be salvaged, especially if both nerves are involved, stabilization of the arytenoid cartilages must be done to maintain an adequate airway after surgery (see Laryngeal Paralysis).

The bronchus supplying an involved lung lobe may contain neoplastic tissue. If this extends to the junction with the mainstem bronchus, a portion of the mainstem bronchus is removed with the lobe during lobectomy. This necessitates anastomosis of the mainstem bronchus or resection of the distal lung lobes (see Bronchial Resection and Anastomosis).

After tracheal and bronchial resection, irradiation of the anastomosis can produce severe stenosis. Tracheal anastomoses irradiated three weeks postsurgery with over 4000 RAD developed moderate to severe ring stenosis.[121]

Cryosurgery

Freezing of the intra- and extraluminal tracheal neoplasms by surface and transmural techniques has been well tolerated by dogs and man.[20, 40, 82, 117] Solid-tipped probes are directed via a bronchoscope to obtain accurate placement.

Two- to four-minute freezes produce ice balls with temperatures of $-60°C$ at the probe and $-30°C$ 1 cm from the probe. Necrosis is complete by 14 days, and the lesion is fibrotic by 21 days. Airways remain intact, and ciliated epithelium returns in 180 days. Stenosis does not occur.[117]

Hemorrhage and pneumothorax may occur occasionally during tissue necrosis.[40] Mucosal laceration results if the probe is dislodged before thawing is complete.[20]

TRACHEAL AND BRONCHIAL RESECTION AND RECONSTRUCTION

Preoperative Evaluation and Preparation

Resection of the trachea is not undertaken until the lesion and the proposed segment for resection are evaluated in relation to the reparative procedure. Preparations must be made for maintenance of ventilation during all phases of the procedure. The patient should be under full control at all times so that unanticipated or hurried procedures do not occur.

A longstanding stenotic lesion in the trachea may cause secondary degenerative changes in the distal trachea, bronchial tree, and lungs (see Chapter 62). The respiratory system distal to the stenosis should

---

*See also Chapter 185.

be thoroughly evaluated along with pulmonary function. Radiographic examination during inspiration and expiration and blood gas analysis assist in identification of coexisting problems.

Preoperative x-rays should be available at the time of surgery. These should have adequately localized the lesion for resection and identified any other possible lesions in the respiratory system. Positive contrast radiography assists in outlining questionable lesions (see Chapter 63).

Endoscopic evaluation of the mass and biopsy of the lesion should have been done prior to initiation of definitive procedures. Endoscopic evaluation of the obstructing mass assists in determining the cross-sectional patency of the airway. Significantly reduced airway (less than 15 per cent patency) causes CO_2 retention during the preresection period of the operation.

The trachea is not a sterile environment, nor can it be sterilized prior to surgical intervention. Culture and antibiotic sensitivity testing of the prominent bacteria causing airway sepsis should be conducted and the appropriate antibiotics identified prior to surgery. The antibiotics can be given orally or intramuscularly within 12 hours or intravenously 2 to 3 hours prior to the surgical procedure to have adequate blood and tissue levels at surgery.

Endotracheal tube length should be selected so that the cuffed portion of the tube reaches into the distal portion of the trachea beyond the anastomosis.

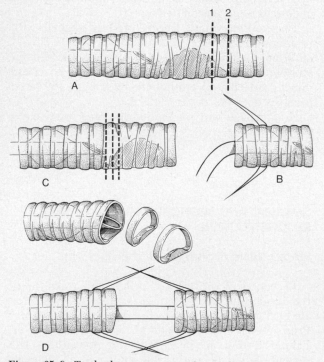

Figure 65–8. Tracheal resection. *A*, The trachea is transected through the obstruction (1) and again at the distal edge of the obstruction (2) under direct observation. *B*, A sterile endotracheal tube is placed into the distal segment. *C*, The trachea is segmentally sectioned to the proximal extent of the lesion. *D*, Traction sutures are used to approximate and align the proximal and distal tracheal segments while the distal endotracheal tube is removed and the proximal tube is advanced into the distal trachea.

If an impassable obstruction exists, care should be taken not to push the tube into the mass. The tube end should be left just proximal to the obstruction until mass resection allows advancement of the tube into the distal segment (Fig. 65–8).

A sterile endotracheal tube and "Y" piece extension should be available for distal segment intubation during the surgical procedure.[41] This allows greater flexibility for distal dissections by being able to move the intubated segment independently from the upper trachea. In procedures involving the carina, two additional sterile systems are needed; one for the left lung and one for the right, including two complete gas machines. An endotracheal tube is placed into each mainstem bronchus, and each lung is ventilated separately. This allows a very complicated resection to take place without cardiopulmonary bypass.[41]

Limitations of Tracheal Resection

Dogs undergoing tracheal resection and anastomosis respond to increasing longitudinal tension on the trachea with an increased potential for tracheal stenosis.[9, 19, 63, 72, 85] Evidence of cartilage necrosis and a decrease in cartilage ring growth can be seen in puppies at the anastomotic site sutured under excessive tension (more than 1000 gm).[72, 77] The amount of trachea that can be removed varies with age.[19, 72] Young patients have more elasticity in the tracheal tissues, allowing a long resection and anastomosis to be accomplished. However, the tissues contain less collagen and more water and lack the tensile strength of adult tissues. Thus, puppies cannot withstand the same increase in tension at the anastomotic site that adults can. As the tension at the anastomotic site in puppies increases to 250 gm, separation of the anastomosis begins in the lateral segments of the tracheal wall.[72] This results in a 2- to 3-mm separation involving approximately 25 per cent of the suture line and a 10 per cent stenosis in 50 per cent of cases. The separation is filled with granulation tissue, which causes stenosis.

As the tension increases toward 1000 gm, the separation increases and also involves the ventral segment of the tracheal wall. Tension exceeds the strength of the cartilaginous tissue, and the surfaces begin to cut through.[77] A six- to seven-ring resection in puppies results in 500 to 750 gm of tension at the surgical site, whereas increasing this to eight or nine rings brings the tension to 1000 gm or more. Tensions in excess of 1,250 gm resulted in complete disruption of the anastomosis and approximately 50 per cent death rate due to tracheal stenosis.

Similar dehiscence occurs in the adult dog as the tension increases above 1,700 gm, approximately a 50 per cent resection of the tracheal length.[19] This is similar to the lesion in puppies that develops after approximately 25 per cent of the tracheal length (eight to nine rings) has been resected.

Anastomosis under tension (greater than 250 gm)

in puppies causes a retardation in growth of the tracheal rings adjacent to the anastomosis in addition to dehiscence.[72] This tension is more of a problem in puppies than in adult dogs. Thus, a 20 to 25 per cent resection of the trachea in the puppy and a 50 per cent resection in the adult dog is tolerated.[19, 72] This may be applied to the cat; however, sufficient research has not been conducted to provide that information.

As tension is applied at the surgical site, the annular ligaments begin to stretch in the adjacent intertracheal ring spaces. As the tracheal ends are brought under more tension, sequential stretching of the annular ligaments takes place, radiating from the surgical site. Tethering at the points of blood vessel penetration and fascia attachment opposes this stretch. Thus, freeing of the trachea cranially and caudally from the resection site allows the ends of the trachea to be brought together under less tension.

Considering the tension factors and the sequence by which the anastomosis undergoes dehiscence with excessive tension, the application of supplemental support becomes important in long resections. The lateral walls of the anastomosis are the first to dehisce, and this progresses to the ventral wall as more tension is applied.[72] These stress points can be reduced by the application of tension sutures in the tracheal wall and the maintenance of cervical flexion during a one- to two-week period of healing (see Figs. 65–8 and 65–10).[9, 63, 72, 79]

Cervical Trachea

Surgical Approach

The surgical approach to the cervical trachea is via the ventral midline. The patient is placed in dorsal recumbency with the front legs tied toward the rear of the animal. The skin incision is deepened to the level of the sternohyoid muscles, which are separated on the midline. The trachea is approached through the paratracheal fascial planes until the ventral aspect of the rings is exposed. Lateral dissection of the trachea is done cautiously so that the vascular supply to the trachea and the position of the recurrent laryngeal nerves can be identified. Cranial and caudal circumferential dissection should be restricted to the segment to be resected and the adjacent 1 to 2 cm of trachea. This minimal dissection is aimed at protecting the segmental blood supply entering the tracheal wall. Circumferential tracheal dissection from the level of the cranial thyroid artery caudally to the origin of the left and right caudal thyroid arteries does not interfere with healing of a tracheal resection and anastomosis in adult dogs.[19] This may not be true in all tracheal surgery, and the blood supply should be protected.[41, 115]

Traction sutures are placed in the trachea proximal and distal to the resected segment, preventing the trachea from retracting after it is transected.[41] After resection and distal tracheal intubation, anastomosing

sutures are preplaced (see Fig. 65–8). The ends of the trachea are held in apposition with traction sutures while the preplaced sutures are tied.

Suturing Techniques

Two suture patterns have been used commonly in tracheal anastomosis. In man and other animals, the simple interrupted suture pattern penetrating the cartilaginous rings adjacent to the incision is the best method to obtain good tissue alignment (Fig. 65–9).[41, 72, 77] Interrupted sutures of monofilament nonabsorbable or braided absorbable (4–0 to 5–0) suture are placed with the knots on the external surface of the trachea. Braided nonabsorbable suture causes a higher incidence of granuloma formation and should not be used.[37] Tracheal rings of young animals are quite friable and have a tendency to tear when penetrated by a needle. Very fine suture material (5–0) with a fine cutting needle reduces this problem.

Tracheal ring encircling sutures can be used in place of penetrating sutures.[9, 39, 63, 79, 122] Frequently, these sutures cause the two rings to override unless a segment of trachea has been removed. In one report the distal tracheal segment was invaginated into the proximal segment and sutured.[128] This did not significantly inhibit mucous flow within the trachea, nor did it cause significant stenosis at the surgical site. Slight tension applied to the mucosa actually increases the rate of mucous flow over the ciliated mucosal surface.[38]

Accurate mucosal alignment is strived for at the anastomosis, as defects in mucosal continuity may lead to granulation tissue growth, scarring, and possible stenosis.[41, 79]

Two methods of applying tension sutures have been described (see Fig. 65–9). The first method is encircling of a tracheal ring with nonabsorbable sutures (3–0 or 4–0 monofilament) two to three rings from the anastomosis in the proximal and distal segments.[9, 10] These sutures are tied together on the outside of the trachea at the tension that relaxes the primary suture line. Three of these sutures are equally spaced on the circumference of the tracheal

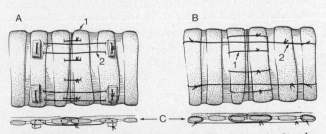

Figure 65–9. Two methods of tracheal anastomosis. *A*, Simple interrupted sutures are penetrating the cartilage rings (1) adjacent to the incision while padded partially penetrating mattress sutures (2) reduce anastomosis tension. *B*, Simple interrupted sutures are shown encircling the cartilage rings (1) adjacent to the incision while the cartilage ring–encircling sutures are tied and their long ends are tied together to act as tension sutures (2). *C*, Longitudinal section of tracheal wall demonstrates the suture positioning.

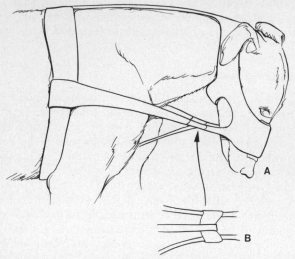

Figure 65–10. A dog with a tape neck splint in place to hold the neck in a flexed position to reduce tension on the trachea postoperatively. *B*, Ventral side of tie down for nose.

rings, carefully avoiding nutrient vessels and recurrent nerves.

A second method utilizes a technique to keep suture material from entering the lumen of the trachea. This entails the placement of steel suture (5–0) through the tracheal rings in a horizontal mattress fashion after penetrating a small Teflon pad.[63] The Teflon pad prevents the suture from pulling through the cartilaginous ring. The addition of tension sutures significantly reduces incisional separation and granulation tissue production in anastomoses with excessive tension on the primary suture line.

After the anastomosis is lavaged with saline and antiseptic, the surrounding soft tissue is sutured over the anastomosis to eliminate dead space and assist in sealing the tracheal incision. The strap muscles are sutured at the midline and the skin incision is closed. The anastomotic site is drained if significant contamination occurred.

Tension at the surgical site can be decreased by cervical flexion, which pushes that proximal trachea toward the chest.[42, 79] The head of the patient is held in a flexed position by placing heavy suture material through the intermandibular skin and attaching it to the skin at the sternum. The sutures are tightened until the head and neck are in a flexed position, relaxing the surgical site. A similar result can be attained by placing the neck in a tape splint, holding it in a flexed position (Fig. 65–10).[41]

Cranial Thoracic Trachea

Surgical Approach

The cranial thoracic trachea is approached through the right third or fourth intercostal space. The trachea lying within the thoracic inlet is approached by adding a partial sternotomy to the lateral fourth intercostal thoracotomy (see Chapter 41). The midline sternotomy from the fourth interspace is continued cranially as a midline cervical incision. The forequarter on the right side can be retracted craniodorsally, exposing the mediastinal area and giving access to the entire trachea from larynx to carina.

The pleura is incised over the trachea, and the azygous vein is isolated, double ligated, and transected. The vagus, phrenic, and recurrent laryngeal nerves are identified and retracted with traction sutures (3-mm umbilical tape). Soft tissue around the trachea is dissected away, and the caudal blood supply to the trachea and esophagus is identified and preserved.

Considerable scar tissue may be encountered if tracheal injury was chronic (see Tracheal Avulsion). The scar is not dissected until tissue planes have been established in the uninjured tissue and vital structures located. The dissection is carried toward the scar along established tissue planes.

Suturing Techniques

Traction sutures are placed in the trachea proximal and distal to the lesion (2-0 silk) to control tracheal movement. The location of the endotracheal tube is reviewed at this point and sterile endotracheal tubes and extension anesthesia lines are prepared if their need is anticipated. The orally placed endotracheal tube is manipulated past the lesion with the aid of the anesthetist if it is not already present in the distal segment. If this is not possible owing to obstruction, the distal extent of the lesion is located, the trachea is incised at this point, and a sterile endotracheal tube is placed into the distal segment (see Fig. 65–9). One must verify adequate gas flow and lung inflation through the new tube before proceeding..

Resection of the lesion is completed while preserving blood supply to the trachea and esophagus. Ventral and lateral dissection (blunt) is carried cranially to gain tracheal laxity.[41, 42] This is augmented by neck flexion to obtain sufficient length of trachea to allow anastomosis of the incised ends. Monofilament nonabsorbable or absorbable sutures (3-0 or 4-0) are preplaced as described for the cervical trachea. After this is completed the sterile endotracheal tube is removed, the ends of the trachea are approximated, the oral endotracheal tube is passed into the distal segment, and the cuff is inflated. Adequate ventilation is verified. Sutures are tied and tension sutures added as needed. Endotracheal tube and cuff are relocated proximal to the anastomosis.

The anastomosis site is lavaged with warm saline and examined for air leaks while 25 to 30 cm of water pressure is applied by the anesthetist. Additional sutures are placed to close any leaks.

A pleural or pericardial patch is harvested and placed around the trachea to reinforce the anastomosis. Suture knots are situated away from adjacent blood vessels to prevent vessel erosion by rubbing on the knots.[41, 42]

Distal Thoracic Trachea and Carina

Surgical Approach

A fifth intercostal lateral thoracotomy is made. The visceral pleural incision is extended caudally to the carina and over the right main bronchus. All vital structures mentioned in dissection of the cranial thoracic trachea (nerves and vessels) plus the pulmonary arteries must be identified and preserved. The azygous vein is ligated and transected.

Salvageable main bronchi are identified and appropriately sized sterile endotracheal tubes are selected to intubate them (Fig. 65–11). The right and left main bronchi are isolated by reflecting the soft tissue including the vagus nerve, trunks of the bronchial arteries, and esophagus dorsally. Traction sutures are placed in the wall of each bronchus distal to the point of transection. The main bronchi are transected as close to the carina as possible, the distal segments intubated with sterile tubes, and the lungs ventilated.[71]

The carina is dissected free from surrounding soft tissue, avoiding the main trunks of the bronchoesophageal arteries and the vagus nerves. The distal trachea is dissected as necessary to provide a 1- to 2-cm length proximal to the lesion. Traction suture is placed and the trachea transected at the proximal edge of the lesion.

Both lungs are ventilated while the right bronchus sutures to the trachea are preplaced (see Fig. 65–11). The discrepancy between the size of these two structures requires careful suturing to produce an airtight seal. The rings are sutured first, and the major mismatch in size is adjusted in suturing the tracheal membrane. After all sutures are preplaced, the right bronchus is extubated, the orally placed tracheal tube is advanced into the right bronchus, the cuff is inflated, the lung is ventilated, and the sutures are tied.

The anastomotic site for the left bronchus on the trachea is located by placing the left bronchus in a comfortable position next to the trachea and the size of the stoma established. The left lung is ventilated while a stoma is cut in the trachea for the left bronchus, and the sutures are preplaced in the left bronchus and tracheal stoma (see Fig. 65–11). The bronchus is extubated and the sutures tied while the right lung is ventilated.

Incomplete cartilage rings in this region complicate bronchial anastomosis. Sutures must be placed to provide accurate mucosal alignment at the anastomosis. Cartilage is included, as it can provide stability, yet it should not interfere with mucosal alignment. The endotracheal tube is withdrawn proximal to the anastomosis, both lungs are inflated, and the suture lines are checked for leaks.

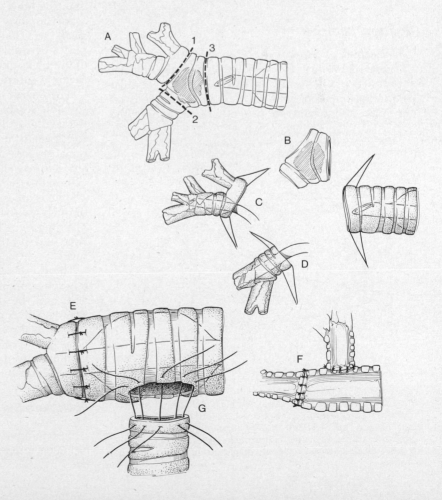

Figure 65–11. Resection of the carina. *A*, The incision sequence for resecting the carina (*B*), is left bronchus (*1*), right bronchus (*2*), and trachea (*3*). *C* and *D*, sterile endotracheal tubes are placed in the mainstem bronchi as they are transected to support ventilation while anastomosing sutures are preplaced. *E*, The right mainstem bronchus is anastomosed to the distal trachea. *F*, The size mismatch is compensated for when anastomosing the dorsal tracheal membrane. *G*, The left mainstem bronchus is anastomosed to an os created in the wall of the trachea.

Pleural pedicle flaps can be raised and the anastomosis is wrapped to strengthen the closure and protect adjacent vessels from erosion due to rubbing on the suture knots.[41–43]

Anastomosis of bronchi can sufficiently interfere with the blood supply to the distal segment to slow healing and cause dehiscence.[60] Bronchial arteries should be preserved to offset this. In addition, an omental pedicle flap is brought through the diaphragm and wrapped around the anastomosis.[68] This provides the same protection as the pleural patch, revascularizes the surgical site, and improves healing. All lung lobes should be checked for inflation and proper positioning. The chest is lavaged clean, a drain placed, and the incision closed (see Chapter 41).

Caudal Displacement of Trachea

If more trachea is needed than can be advanced by general mobilization procedures to obtain approximation of the ends of the divided thoracic trachea, the proximal cervical trachea is transected and its distal end drawn down into the thorax.[41, 79, 110] This is an extreme procedure but can be done when additional trachea is needed. The cervical tracheal defect must be reconstructed or a permanent tracheostomy made (see Tracheal Reconstruction).

Tracheal Stretch

A method of extending the length of the trachea without increasing the tension at the anastomosis above acceptable limits is incision of the annular ligaments between each ring.[79] Lateral incisions on one side above and on the other side below the

anastomosis allow the rings to stretch apart with only the mucous membrane remaining intact. This allows the blood supply to remain intact on one side of the trachea above and on the other side below the anastomosis. This provides a relatively weak structure; however, it does provide an adequate airway. Care must be used that the mucosa is left intact in making these incisions; otherwise, significant air leakage occurs and granulation tissue forms. Any mucosal defects should be sutured with fine absorbable material.

Bronchial Resection and Anastomosis

Severe injuries to or neoplastic involvement of the bronchial junction requires resection of the junction and the associated lung lobe.[71] The resulting disruption of mainstem bronchial continuity requires anastomosis of the bronchus or a loss of the remaining lung lobes supplied by the distal segment.

Surgical Approach

A standard intercostal incision is used and the bronchus is approached as described previously. The mainstem bronchus is dissected free from the adjacent structures, crossclamped above and below the resection site with noncrushing clamps, and resected with the lung lobe.

Anastomosis of bronchi is difficult because of their small size and incomplete cartilage rings. Small pieces of disjointed cartilage are left around the edge of the transected bronchus, tending to interfere with accurate suture placement (Fig. 65–12).

A primary suture line of simple interrupted absorbable stitches is placed with mucosal alignment as the goal. Cartilage plates may be incorporated in the sutures only if they allow mucosal alignment. Additional stitches of 4-0 to 6-0 monofilament nonabsorbable suture may be placed through the cartilage rings external to the mucosa to obtain better wall stability. The anastomosis is wrapped with omentum brought through the diaphragm with its blood supply intact.[13] This improves the blood supply to the healing bronchus and protects the pulmonary vessels from sutures.[68]

The chest is lavaged and suctioned clean, the lung lobes are inflated and their proper positioning verified, and the chest drain is placed. Standard chest wall closure is done (see Thoracotomy).

Bronchial wall instability (collapse) and lumen stenosis are potential postoperative complications.[68] Gradual onset of a cough, harsh localized lung sounds, and retention of secretion occur.

Postoperative Care

Preoperative antibiotics are continued for 24 hours or longer in patients with existing infections (Chapter 66).

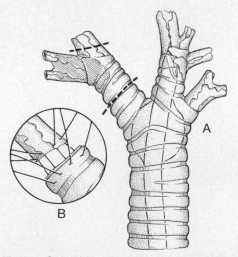

Figure 65–12. Lobectomy involving the mainstem bronchus. *A,* The endotracheal tube is advanced into the other mainstem bronchus while the inflated cuff obstructs the orifice of the involved bronchus. *B,* The transected bronchus is anastomosed after lobectomy with preplaced simple interrupted sutures. Cartilage plates in the wall of the distal segment complicate the accuracy of the anastomosis.

Replacement of Tracheal Wall

Partial Replacement

Partial circumferential tacheal defects have been patched with dermis, fascia, dura mater, periosteum, cartilage, polypropylene mesh, and silicone rubber with good success.[33, 58, 104, 109, 123]

The patching material is sewn to the trachea to provide a good seal, and adjacent muscle and connective tissue are sutured to the graft area to add strength and a good blood supply. A layer of granulation tissue forms on the lumen surface and becomes covered with tracheal epithelium.

Vascular pedicle grafts of the diaphragm and stomach will have been used to patch tracheal wall with good success.[88, 125] External support for these implants is not necessary if they are narrow (i.e., less than 35 per cent of circumference of trachea) and do not exceed four or five tracheal rings in length or are relatively thick or firm.[58, 109]

Segmental Replacement

Replacement of 1- to 4-cm circumferential segments of the tracheal wall can be accomplished using autogenous tissues. Rib periosteum or perichondrium has been used as a free graft.[64, 86, 118] Sufficiently long segments of tissue are harvested to completely surround the trachea. A standard rib resection is done, and the periosteum and perichondrium are resected as a single strip. These tissues are sutured directly to the tracheal rings to bridge the defect. These tissues have been transplanted with vascular pedicles, which are anastomosed to vessels in the neck.[64] This does not seem to be necessary to obtain tissue survival but may be needed to produce bone or cartilage in the graft. The graft is sutured to overlying neck muscles to provide good stability and increase the success of the procedure. Varying degrees of tracheal stenosis occur as collagen contracts in the healed implant, and external support (i.e., plastic rings) should be used to maintain an adequate airway.[118]

Cartilage has been harvested from the pinna of the ear and nasal septum to use as a free tracheal graft. The cartilage is resorbed and replaced by granulation tissue with varying degrees of stenosis.[32, 94, 118] Buccal mucosa grafted to the pinna of the ear, with the mucosa and cartilage subsequently harvested as a compound graft, has been used to replace the tracheal wall.[30] Two to four rings have been replaced successfully with this implant.

Synthetic Replacement

Various combinations of synthetic materials in the form of mesh grafts and porous materials have been used for partial and complete circumferential tracheal reconstruction.[62, 91, 127] However, most of these failed owing to infection and stenosis. Mesh with a loose weave and some stiffness to resist collagen contraction

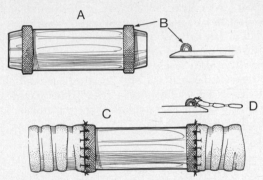

Figure 65–13. *A,* A silicone rubber (Silastic) tracheal prosthesis with tapered ends and sewing ring *(B). C,* The prosthesis is anastomosed to the trachea with a longitudinal section of the wall *(D)* at the anastomosis.

has allowed granulation tissue encapsulation and epithelialization without serious stenosis.[91]

Nonporous Silastic tubing has been used to repair segmental defects in the trachea.[83, 84, 109] Tubes to replace the straight trachea and carina have been used in dogs and man with relatively good results (five-year follow-ups).[83] The silicone rubber tubes require a sewing ring on the outside, which is covered with a fabric (Fig. 65–13). The tapered ends of the graft, which extend beyond the sewing ring, are telescoped into the trachea for a few millimeters, and the ends of the remaining trachea are sutured to the fabric-covered rings. The ends of the trachea and implant are covered with adjacent soft tissue to provide a seal and blood supply to the area.[82, 84] The external surface of these grafts is completely covered with fibrous connective tissue, preventing infection and air leakage into the surrounding tissue. The inner surface is nonwettable and is not covered by an epithelial surface.[58, 83, 84] Small granulomas develop at the distal ends of the prosthesis where it is attached to the trachea. These have been controlled by removal via the bronchoscope using biopsy and instruments. There appears to be little problem with the movement of mucus from the distal to the proximal end of these protheses in both dog and man.[82, 84]

Tracheal Allografts

Allografts of tracheal segments have been used without long-term success. These tissues are rejected or replaced with collagen, resulting in severe stenosis and complete obstruction.[32]

TRACHEOSTOMY

Indications

Tracheostomy is indicated for either life-threatening upper respiratory obstruction or the anticipation of its development. A tracheostomy provides access to the trachea for ventilatory assistance, removal of heavy secretions and aspirated material, and inhalation anesthesia for an upper respiratory or intraoral surgical procedure.[13, 48, 55, 79] It is the best if not the only method to maintain prolonged ventilatory support for the critical but conscious surgical patient during the postoperative recovery period.

Tracheotomy does not affect the growth of the trachea significantly, yet it can result in a subclinical stenosis at the tracheostomy site.[76] This occurs more frequently when the trachal rings are transected or partially resected.[47, 76, 79]

Temporary Tracheostomy

Transverse Tracheostomy

No tissue is removed from the tracheal wall, since the incision is made between the tracheal rings and through the annular ligament and mucosa (Fig. 65–14).[47, 76] The ventral two-thirds of the circumference of the trachea is incised to provide a large enough opening to admit the tracheostomy tube. The presence of a tube in this opening results in pressure against the surrounding tissues and can cause pressure necrosis of the adjacent cartilage rings and mucosa with prolonged use. Aseptic conditions are desirable whenever a tracheotomy is performed. However, emergency situations require that it be conducted under less than aseptic situations, and the resulting tissue contamination must be treated. If tolerated by the patient, tracheotomy can be done under local anesthesia. A roll of towels or cotton may

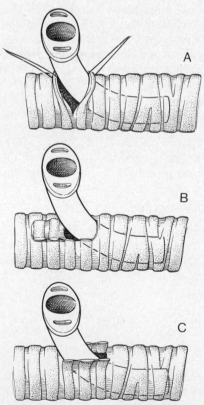

Figure 65–14. Three methods of creating a temporary tracheostomy: *A*, transverse tracheotomy; *B*, tracheal flap; *C*, vertical tracheotomy.

be placed under the neck to cause a dorsal flexion in the cervical region, which assists in keeping the trachea near the skin surface and the site open. The surgical site is prepared and a midline skin incision is made from approximately the first to the eighth tracheal ring. The interspace between the fourth and fifth tracheal rings is incised through the annular ligament and mucosa (Fig. 65–14). The edge of the fifth tracheal ring is gripped with a tissue hook, spay hook, or suture so that it can be elevated relative to the fourth tracheal ring. Scissors are used to extend the incision around the ventral aspect of the trachea, incising approximately 65 per cent of the tracheal circumference. As the scissors are advanced dorsally, the recurrent laryngeal nerve must be avoided. A suture is left in the fifth ring so that the ring can be manipulated during intubation or re-intubation at a later time if the tube becomes dislodged.

The trachea is suctioned clean of blood, mucus, and other debris as soon as the tracheotomy is completed and prior to intubation. The skin incision is loosely sutured, an antiseptic ointment is applied to the skin incision and the tube is tied in place with tapes placed around the neck.

As soon as the upper airway has been re-established and the tracheotomy is no longer needed, the tube may be removed and the trachea suctioned clear of fluid and debris. The surgical site is allowed to granulate or is sutured with four or five interrupted absorbable sutures placed through the tracheal rings. Good tissue approximation decreases granulation tissue formation at the surgical site.[47] Primary closure of the temporary tracheostomy does not lead to stenosis unless significant pressure has been borne by the adjacent tracheal tissues from the tracheostomy tube to cause tissue necrosis.[47] Air leaking from the trachea dictates that skin and other soft tissue be left open for 48 to 72 hours under an antibiotic ointment pack while granulation tissue seals the leaks, after which the skin is sutured. If air leakage occurs with the skin closed, significant subcutaneous and mediastinal emphysema will develop.

Vertical Tracheostomy

A vertical incision is made through the ventral midline of three tracheal rings. These rings must be retracted laterally with stay sutures, and the endotracheal tube is placed (see Fig. 65–14). There is a tendency toward transverse narrowing during healing after extubation owing to medial collapse of the cut rings.[76, 79]

Tracheal Flap

A third technique has been suggested to eliminate excessive granulation tissue that frequently occurs with the excision of the ventral portion of two or three tracheal rings. A U-shaped incision based at the second tracheal ring and extending two rings distally is made in the ventral aspect of the trachea (see Fig. 65–14).[13, 56] The flap is raised as a door so that the endotracheal tube or tracheostomy tube can be placed. This provides a tracheotomy incision that eliminates excessive pressure from the tracheostomy tube on the surrounding tissue. The flap technique is best suited for long-term intubation (weeks to months). After extubation, the tracheostomy site is debrided free of granulation tissue and the flap mobilized and sutured into its original bed. Interrupted sutures of fine absorbable material are used to approximate each tracheal ring to obtain accurate tissue alignment. The area heals with limited granulation tissue production.

Tube Placement

Proper sizing and tube alignment within the trachea allow prolonged use without damage to the mucosa and cartilage. A too deep or twisted insertion of the curved tracheostomy tube causes excessive pressure by the arch of the tube on the dorsal wall of the trachea and the tip of the tube on the ventral wall of the trachea (Fig. 65–15). Prolonged improper positioning can lead to serious mucosal erosion and cartilage injury with formation of granulation tissue and airway stenosis.[79] Pneumatic cuff inflation to high pressure causes similar lesions (see Intubation Injury to the Trachea). After the tube is placed, the skin is loosely sutured, the tube secured with neck ties, and a light sterile bandage placed around the neck.

Postoperative Care

Antibiotic therapy is maintained for approximately seven days to control infection. Corticosteroids are also valuable in decreasing inflammation in the immediate postoperative period (72 hours).

Humidification

Humidification of inspired air is more important in patients with tracheostomy tubes in place.[13, 48, 79]

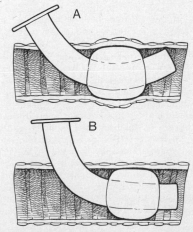

Figure 65–15. A, The improper placement of a tracheostomy tube with the cuff overinflated and the end of the tube pressing against the ventral wall. B, The proper placement of a tracheostomy tube.

Moisture can be added to the inspired air in the patient's cage by a nebulizer. Saline solution (0.5 to 1.0 ml) is injected through the tracheostomy tube every two hours to aid in humidifying the trachea and loosening the mucus.[56, 79] A mucolytic agent (acetylcysteine) may be added to the saline to assist in breaking down thick mucous secretions; however, this is irritating to the trachea in dogs.[48]

Cleaning of the Tracheostomy

This is extremely important and probably the major factor in the success of a tracheostomy.[13, 56, 79] Patients with an irritated trachea produce large amounts of mucus, which obstructs a tracheostomy tube or site rapidly. Tracheostomy tubes in these patients need to be cleaned every 10 to 15 minutes in extreme cases and every four to six hours in nonreactive cases. It is of the utmost importance that the tracheostomy tubes be closely examined frequently so that the build-up of dry mucus on the inside of the tube is discovered before it interferes with adequate ventilation. Tracheostomy tubes with liners aid in the ease of cleaning. The inner liner is removed and cleaned without dislodging the entire system. This type of tube is usually made out of metal and does not have an inflatable cuff.

Plastic cuffed and uncuffed tracheostomy tubes are single units that require removal for thorough cleaning. Flexible swabs and suction can be used to clean these tubes while they are in place. The curve prevents thorough examination to determine if cleaning is complete.

Airway suctioning in the awake animal may meet with significant resistance. The instillation of local anesthetics decreases the sensitivity of the tracheal mucosa. It is best to avoid suctioning the trachea immediately after eating, since this may cause vomition. Suctioning may cause respiratory distress and vagal stimulation.

Care must be taken to suction the proximal end of the respiratory system whenever the tube is removed. The animal should not be in a standing position when these tubes are removed, since fluids or debris in the proximal respiratory system gravitates into the lungs.

Removal of Tracheostomy Tube

The tracheostomy tube is removed as soon as a normal airway is established. In the majority of small animal patients that undergo upper respiratory surgery, the tracheostomy tube is removed in 24 to 48 hours. In patients with considerable airway damage, prolonged intubation may be needed for days or even weeks. These patients are more prone to damage the tracheal mucosa at the tracheostomy site and at the tube cuff.

The tracheostomy tube is removed and replaced with a smaller one if possible. The patient is observed for the next ten minutes to evaluate ventilation through the upper airway and around the tube. If the respiration is not labored, the orifice of the tube is covered. If the patient is dyspneic with this maneuver, the smaller tube should be left in place for another 24 hours and the procedure repeated. When adequate ventilation occurs with the small tube obstructed, the tube is removed and the tracheostomy site occluded. If ventilation is still adequate, the tracheostomy is surgically repaired. This procedure allows extubation as soon as possible.

Patients with significant upper and lower respiratory pathology should be observed for prolonged periods before determining whether adequate ventilation has taken place. The 10 to 15-minute observation period should be extended to one to two hours at each stage before final evaluation is made.

High tracheostomies with or without a tracheostomy tube in place may interfere with swallowing. The trachea is tethered in position and does not slide during swallowing. The animal usually adjusts to this within a relatively short period of time. More distally placed tracheostomy sites are better tolerated.

Permanent Tracheostomy

Two similar techniques for permanent tracheostomy have been used successfully in dogs. The surgical site is centered over the sixth tracheal ring and a midline approach to the trachea is made. The sternohyoideus muscles are separated, and the ventral aspect of the trachea is exposed. The dissection is carried along the lateral walls of the trachea so that it can be elevated to the skin. Approximately 3 cm of the dorsal aspect of the trachea is freed from surrounding soft tissue. Nonabsorbable monofilament suture (3-0) is used to suture the medial edges of the

sternohyoideus muscle bellies together dorsal to the trachea (Fig. 65–16). Usually two or three horizontal mattress sutures are placed through these muscles and drawn into position dorsal to the trachea. The proximal and distal ends are left attached in their normal positions. If this places the trachea in an extreme ventral position, these muscles can be sutured to the lateral tracheal fascia instead. This decreases tension on the skin–mucosa anastomosis and reduces the tendency for dehiscence. The ventral aspect of two to four tracheal rings is removed, leaving the mucosa intact. The section of tracheal wall removed in this manner should be approximately 50 per cent larger than the desired size of the tracheostomy. Excessive skin or subcutaneous fat in the region acts as a flap, which may close over the tracheostomy. This must be excised so that there is a smooth comformation to the ventral aspect of the neck and an even transition between the skin surface and the tracheal mucosa at the anastomosis. After the tracheal rings have been removed, an incision is made in the tracheal mucosa.

In the first technique the incision is linear and in the midline extending approximately three-quarters of the distance between the proximal and distal rings.[50] An oval piece of skin the size of the tracheostomy is excised and the subcutaneous tissues are sutured to the lateral tracheal fascia near the edge of the incised tracheal rings (simple interrupted 3-0 absorbable suture). The skin is anastomosed directly to the tracheal mucosa using simple interrupted sutures of 4-0 fine absorbable material. This technique produces stress points at the two ends of the incision, frequently resulting in minor dehiscence of the area and granulation tissue formation.

A second method of closing the skin–mucous membrane incision is to produce skin flaps and mucosal

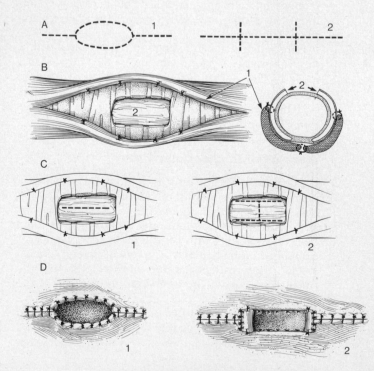

Figure 65–16. Two methods of making a permanent tracheostomy. First method: An oval piece of skin (A-1) is resected at the tracheostomy site, and the trachea is stabilized in a ventral position by suturing the sternohyoideus muscle to its lateral and dorsal wall (B-1). The ventral sections of three tracheal rings are removed (B-2), leaving the mucosa intact. The mucosa is incised on the midline (C-1) and the skin sutured to the mucosa (D-1). Second method: Two incisions are made perpendicular to the midline skin incision (A-2) to create two skin flaps. The trachea is stabilized (B-1) and the ventral tracheal rings are resected (B-2) as in the first method. An H-shaped mucosal incision is made (C-2), creating two mucosal flaps oriented perpendicular to the skin flaps. The mucosal flaps are externally reflected and sutured to the skin edge left by the internally reflected skin flaps (D-2). The free edges of the skin flaps are sutured to the incised mucosa at the level of the tracheal lumen.

flaps at 90° angles to each other (see Fig. 65–16). The incision in the mucosa is an H shape but is placed so that two flaps are formed at the cranial and caudal ends of the incision. These flaps are raised to suture to the skin and seal the tracheostomy site at the cranial and caudal borders. At the same time, a pair of skin flaps equal in width to the length of the mucosal incision at the tracheostomy site are raised from the midline incision. These are depressed toward the tracheal lumen to be anastomosed to the incision in the mucosa along the lateral edge of the tracheostomy. This eliminates the high tension points and provides complete mucocutaneous anastomosis around the entire tracheostomy. Hair from the skin flaps grows into the tracheostomy site, which can be kept clear by judicious trimming.

Normal ciliated epithelium returns to the region of the permanent tracheostomy within 16 weeks.[50] Adequate function of the ciliated epithelium seems to be maintained in adjacent areas during this period, and no loss of movement of tracheal mucus is noted.

It is important to be precise in the anastomosis of the mucous membrane to the skin with both methods. When defects are left in this suture line, granulation tissue forms and significantly adds to stenosis. Since these tracheostomies are designed for lifetime use, it is desirable to have a clean, nonirritated, well-healed site.

Postoperative Care

The long-term care of a permanent tracheostomy site entails cleaning of the opening, removal of hair or debris, and application of ointments such as boric acid or povidone iodine to the mucocutaneous junction. This helps to decrease drying and cracking of the mucosa during the adjustment period. Ointments also assist in the removal of mucus that dries on the surface of the tracheostomy site, requiring frequent removal. The majority of patients with permanent tracheostomies do not need altered atmospheric humidity.[50] The tracheal mucosa adjacent to the permanent tracheostomy usually adapts to the lower humidity over a period of time by undergoing squamous metaplasia in the immediate area of the tracheostomy site.[50]

Care must be used in handling the patient so that foreign bodies are not inhaled into the respiratory system. This is a problem during the warm weather months when the patient has access to weeds or grasses and may inhale pieces of plant material into the trachea. The patient must be kept away from the water so that he does not attempt to swim.

LUNG

Congenital and acquired diseases of the lung that require surgical intervention are intimately associated with and similarly presented as medical problems. The overlapping signs and conditions require careful evaluation and diagnosis. An inappropriate preoperative work-up that prolongs anesthesia and increases surgical trauma cannot be tolerated by the thoracic patient.

Lung and chest sounds or their absence assists in characterizing basic fluid, inflammatory, and air flow changes. Microscopic analysis of aspirates, radiographic shadow patterns, and endoscopic visual surveys are intensively used in the diagnosis of thoracic pathology. Ultrasound is adding another dimension to diagnosis (see Chapter 63).

Congenital Lung Disease

Congenital disease of the lung is usually completely compatible or incompatible with life.[55] The severe anomalies of agenesis or hypoplasia cause death shortly after birth. Hypoplasia of one lung or lung lobe is rarely diagnosed unless chest radiographs are taken or a necropsy is performed.[55, 107] Congenital tracheoesophageal or bronchoesophageal fistulae have not been reported in the dog and cat (see Acquired Tracheoesophageal Fistula).

Cysts

Pulmonary cystic disease can be congenital or acquired.[36, 55, 75, 129] Thin-walled congenital pulmonary cysts are lined with bronchial epithelium and can be small or lung lobe in size. They contain air or fluid, or both in their lumens. Large cysts are referred to as pneumatoceles. Infected cysts may lead to abscess formation with scarring and loss of epithelial lining. These cysts cannot be differentiated from infected bullae or lung abscesses.

Bullae

Lung bullae and blebs are similar to cysts; they may be congenital or acquired and have no epithelial lining.[6, 55, 75, 129] Bullae are large air spaces that develop within the lung parenchyma, whereas blebs are small accumulations of air between the visceral pleura and the lung parenchyma.[6] These cavities develop from traumatic rupture and coalescence of alveoli and are frequently secondary to obstructive lung disease. (Fig. 65–17). Bullae and cysts show similar complications of infection, abscessation, rupture causing pneumothorax, and local compression of lung tissue leading to dyspnea, exercise intolerance, and abdominal respiration.[6, 75, 129] Auscultation may reveal decreased ventilation sounds on the affected side and increased heart sounds on the contralateral side (displaced heart due to space-occupying cyst).

Spontaneous idiopathic pneumothorax warrants close examination of radiographs detailing lung profile and parenchyma for bleb, bulla, or cyst formation. Atelectasis of the lobe containing the ruptured cavity occurs and may obscure underlying cysts. Thoroscopy

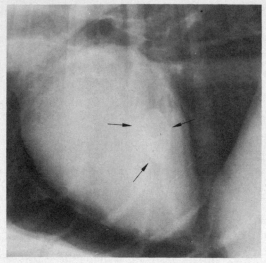

Figure 65–17. Radiograph of a traumatic bulla partially filled with blood in a lung lobe *(arrows)*. (From Dr. R. D. Park, Colorado State University, Fort Collins, CO.)

assists in evaluating visceral surfaces for additional cysts and locating the ruptured cavity. A combination of rigid and flexible fiberoptics may be necessary to provide a thorough examination of the lung surface (see Chapter 63).

Conservative control of pneumothorax by continuous chest drainage should be tried for two to three days before partial or complete lobectomy is done.[6] Many cases respond to this therapy, but the recurrence rate is high.[129] Pleurectomy or pleural abrasion with dry gauze sponges to cause complete pleural adhesion has been used in recurring pneumothorax. Successful production of a complete adhesion or control of the disease is uncommon.[129]

Acquired Lung Disease

Abscess

Lung abscess and associated pyothorax are more common in cats than in dogs, although they are relatively uncommon in both. Abscess formation is secondary to foreign body obstruction or migration, chronic lung infection (i.e., bacterial bronchopneumonia, bronchiectasis, penetrating wounds, or vascular obstruction and infarction by emboli, especially bacterial, fungal, or parasitic) and neoplastic tissue.[75]

History. This condition is manifested as a chronic debilitating disease with varying degrees of respiratory distress, persistent low grade fever, and severe leukocytosis with a degenerative left shift. Anemia of a chronic disorder may be present. The abscess may involve part or all of the lobe, may be thick- or thin-walled, or may rupture into the airway or pleural space but rarely erodes a blood vessel.[75] Ventilatory sounds range from moist rales and friction rub to no sounds over the mass and muffled sounds (including cardiac) from pleural effusion. Chest drainage to

relieve the respiratory distress may be necessary before the patient will tolerate detailed examination.

Chest radiographs aid in locating the involved region. The pleural space may have to be lavaged and drained before a definite radiographic diagnosis can be made. An abscess has a water density unless it has ruptured and drained (Fig. 65–18). In the latter case, air contrast may be seen in the abscessed cavity if it connects with the respiratory system.

Medical Approach. Medical management should be exhausted before surgical intervention is begun. Appropriate antibiotics are given, and bilateral chest drainage and lavage should be actively pursued. Insignificant improvement in lung expansion, loculation of fluid, and an unresolving lung density are indications for exploratory thoractomy.

Surgical Approach. An aggressive approach to surgical exploration is frequently beneficial since it decreases recovery time by removing the initiating cause. The patient should be prepared so that exposure of both hemithoraces is possible. A lateral thoracotomy with the option of extending this to a transverse thoracotomy has been my choice. The incision into the thorax is made with great care, since adhesions of lung lobes to the lateral wall are common. These can be dissected free by careful digital pressure and sharp dissection without significant lung damage (except in organized lesions).

The involved lung lobe is located and a partial or complete lobectomy is done. Occasionally two lobes are involved. The remaining interlobar fissures are explored and adhesions between lung lobes freed until all lobes are moveable and loculated areas of exudate are cleared. Sheets of fibrin covering lung surfaces are undesirable and should be removed (see Restrictive Pleuritis). Chest drains are placed and the thoracic cavity closed. Postoperative care is discussed hereafter.

Restrictive Pleuritis

Trauma, inflammation, and septic injury to the pleura may result in heavy deposition of fibrin on the pleural surface. Pulmonary compression (i.e., hemic and inflammatory pleural effusion) allows the collapsed lung to become entrapped in an organized fibrin jacket that opposes reinflation even after adequate chest drainage. This sequela should be considered in patients whose respiratory distress or exercise intolerance continues after adequate chest drainage. Patients should be monitored for evidence of noninflating lungs by serial inspiratory radiographs one to two days apart. Static or decreasing inflation of the lungs is indicative of restrictive pleuritis. Exploratory thoracotomy is considered in the stabilized patient as soon as restrictive pleuritis is diagnosed. In septic pleuritis, appropriate antibiotics are identified and administered for at least 24 hours prior to thoracotomy to decrease the chance of infection of the incision.

The stages of restrictive pleuritis were reviewed

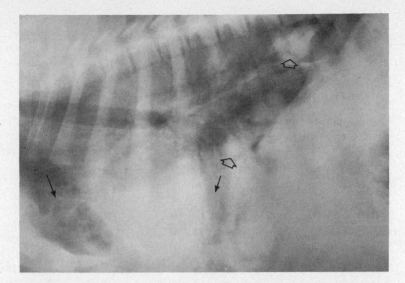

Figure 65–18. Radiograph of a lung abscess *(open arrows)* and pleural effusion *(solid arrows)*. (From Dr. R. D. Park, Colorado State University, Fort Collins, CO.)

recently.[97] Fibroblastic and angioblastic infiltration into the fibrin layer deposited on the pleural surface may occur as early as seven days after injury. Collagen fibers are laid parallel to the pleural surface, whereas capillary ingrowth is perpendicular to the pleura and emanates from it. Mature collagen formation in the outer portion of the fibrin "peel" may be seen at four weeks post injury. This reaction continues to mature in ensuing weeks until a mature fibrous encasement develops with fibrovascular tufts penetrating and anchoring it to the lung parenchyma.

Considering the histological documentation of this condition, it is obvious that early resection of the fibrinous and fibrous envelope is simpler and less traumatic to pulmonary tissue. Within two to three weeks of its onset, the cleavage plane at the pleural surface can still be identified with relative ease. Every effort is made to follow this plane and remove large sheets of tissue one at a time. Gentle traction and blunt dissection with occasional transection of fibrovascular adhesions are adequate. The dissection is continued until adequate expansion of the lung occurs during inflation with normal respiratory pressures.

Attempts at decortication of the lung entrapped in a mature fibrous tissue have not been very beneficial. Significant damage to the pleural and parenchymal lung tissue occurs, and recurrence should be expected.

Postoperative Care. Standard postoperative monitoring of the chest patient is performed (see Chapter 66). Drainage is established, and, after decortication, the thorax is lavaged two to four times a day until the effusion begins to clear. Each lavage consists of evacuation of existing fluid followed by two or three flushes of Ringer's electrolyte solution, two or three flushes of antiseptic (iodophor) electrolyte solution, and one or two rinsing flushes of electrolyte solution. Appropriate antibiotics can be replaced in the chest after the last flush. The frequency of lavaging is reduced as the pleura heals and the effusion clears. Thoracic lavage is needed from two to ten days, depending on the severity of the condition. Without lavage, postoperative inflammatory effusion from the original condition and the surgical trauma can cause return of restrictive pleuritis. Cytology of the effusion should demonstrate more normal leukocytes and decreasing total cell count as the pleura heals. Radiographic examination of the lung fields should indicate lung expansion being maintained or improving toward near normal limits.

Blood electrolytes and protein levels are monitored. Significant leaching of electrolytes (especially if saline lavage is used) and protein can occur.

Bronchiectasis

Chronic respiratory disease can result in or be caused by saccular or cylindric dilations of bronchi or bronchioles or both.[55, 75] Bronchiectasis in young animals can be assumed to be congenital. The acquired condition is the result of infection combined with bronchial obstruction by copious tenacious exudates. Collateral ventilation is interfered with by these exudates, resulting in peripheral atelectasis. The inflamed bronchial walls lose collagen and elastin, and a granulomatous reaction develops. Dilated and sacculated bronchi develop and retain secretions, resulting in recurring infections.[75]

Recurrent infections perpetuate the lesion and increase the number of affected bronchi. The cranial and middle lobes tend to be affected more frequently, although multiple lobe involvement is common in dogs.[75] Recurrent fever with signs of respiratory infection, anorexia, and debilitation with exercise intolerance are present in these patients. A "crackling" type of respiratory sound is heard in advanced disease.

Thoracic radiographs show signs of atelectasis, consolidation, and fibrosis. Contrast bronchography is needed to outline the bronchi for positive diagnosis. Dye is placed in only one lung, since the dye causes an inflammatory reaction and can lead to respiratory collapse. Tracheal wash with culture will identify the bacteria involved. Bacterial sensitivity studies should be done to identify the appropriate antibiotics.

Lobectomy of the affected lobes has been the definitive treatment in those patients with one or two involved lobes (see Lobectomy). Removal of affected lobes eliminates the initiating foci for recurrent infection. Continuous monitoring of remaining lobes and intense medical management of respiratory infection is mandatory to prevent recurrence of this condition. Patients with more than two lobes involved are treated medically with good nutrition, antibiotics, and frequent examination for respiratory disease.[75]

Foreign Body (see Tracheal and Bronchial Foreign Bodies)

Barbed seeds or hulls (grass awns) and other small bodies inhaled into the bronchi resist dislodgment by coughing and work their way along the small air passages.[75] A plant awn frequently breaks into parenchymal tissue and causes a septic focus that develops into an abscess. Distant migration may occur, leaving lung abscess, pyothorax, and draining tracts in its wake. Occasionally as the barbs begin to disintegrate, the remaining plant material may be dislodged and expelled by coughing. Small oval rocks, nuts, or other dense objects that enter the bronchial tree may obstruct or act as a one-way valve at a small bronchus.[75, 94] Usually part of the involved lobe becomes atelectic and secondarily septic, especially if the foreign body is irritating or toxic to the adjacent tissue.

History. Vague and intermittent signs of respiratory disease may be seen. Initial inhalation of the foreign body causes severe dry coughing. This is followed by periods without clinical signs and periods of low-grade respiratory infection with a moist cough and fever. A temporary response to antibiotic therapy is common.

Diagnosis. Radiographic examination may show an area of increased lung density compatible with local atelectasis, bronchopneumonia, abscess, or granuloma. Radiopaque bodies are easily seen, whereas radiolucent bodies are difficult to outline when located deep in the bronchial system.

Exudate from a single main bronchus during bronchoscopy is supportive of a diagnosis of local infection, with a high index of suspicion for a foreign body.

Surgical Approach. Partial or complete lobectomy is the method of choice for removing deep-seated foreign bodies. A lung abscess and pyothorax may accompany the foreign body (see Lung Abscess).

Lung Laceration

Lung lacerations are usually small and resolve on their own or with the aid of chest drainage to control the accumulation of air and blood in the chest. Rupture of the pleural pulmonary surface induced by blunt trauma is commonly associated with rib fractures. Fractured rib ends lacerate the parenchyma and bronchi as they are depressed medially by the impact and can impale a lung on rib splinters, causing deep lacerations. Lung lacerations not anatomically near fractures have been noted.[36, 49] Lateral compression of the chest wall with a closed glottis causing a rapid increase in intra-airway pressure has been suggested as a cause of explosive rupture. The rapid decrease in these pressures immediately following chest compression may result in additional shearing tears.[44]

Penetrating wounds of the chest causing lung lacerations are frequently lethal unless only the peripheral lung is involved.[44] Crushing chest injuries of small dogs and cats caused by large dogs may tear the intercostal muscles and lung without penetrating the skin. Gunshot wounds of the lung are highly fatal unless the projectile is of low velocity or affects only the peripheral lung tissue. High-velocity bullet wounds cause blebs, bullae, and secondary ruptures in lung parenchyma adjacent to the bullet path (see Gunshot Wounds).

Radiographic evidence of fractured ribs, increased lung density (contusion, edema), and free air and fluid in the thorax aid in identifying lung lobe lacerations.[75, 95] Air and fluid are quickly dispersed to both sides of the thorax in most trauma cases.

Prior to surgical intervention, a serious effort is made to locate the laceration. Bronchoscopy is used to locate lacerations of the trachea or main bronchi, with hemorrhage from a main bronchus probably identifying an involved lobe. Thoroscopy has been used to locate lacerations and cauterize bleeding points with good success (see Chapter 63). The combination of thoroscopy and bipolar electrocautery in the treatment of bleeding lacerations has significantly reduced the number of exploratory thoracotomies in human trauma patients.[44]

All penetrating wounds of the chest should be explored as soon as the patient is stabilized. Life-threatening hemorrhage into the bronchial tree, hemorrhage into the chest greater than 2 cc/kg/hr, and unresolving or uncontrollable pneumothorax with chest drainage are reasons for exploratory thoracotomy.[41, 44]

Surgical Approach. The lateral intercostal approach is used through the intercostal space closest to the laceration (see Thoracotomy). Without an accurate location, the intercostal incision is made over the lung lobe most damaged as noted on radiographs.

Superficial lacerations usually seal on their own but may be reopened with positive pressure respiration. These are closed with a simple, continuous, inverting mattress suture (Lembert type) of fine absorbable suture (4–0 or 5–0) (Fig. 65–19). Contused or edematous lung is friable and tends to tear when sutured. In these cases large horizontal mattress sutures of similar material are placed across the laceration and tightened gently until the air leak

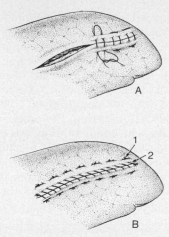

Figure 65–19. A, Superficial lung laceration closed with an interrupted Lembert mattress suture pattern. B, Deep lung laceration sutured with hemostatic mattress sutures (1) and closed with a simple continuous suture pattern (2).

stops. Deep lacerations into the lung parenchyma may involve vessels and airways that leak profusely. Two approaches can be taken.

In the first, the base of the involved lobe is gently crossclamped (noncrushing vascular forceps) to reduce or stop air and blood flow. The wound is explored for lacerated bronchioles and vessels, and these are individually ligated with fixation ligatures. Pedicle compression is released periodically to allow tissue perfusion and evaluate the ligatures. The edges of the laceration are apposed by the loose Lembert or simple continuous suture technique to realign the pleural surface.

The second approach is rapid placement of deep penetrating hemostatic sutures along the edge of the laceration (see Fig. 65–19). These should collapse the bleeding tissue and provide an adequate seal of small vessels and bronchioles. Torn larger bronchi should be located and individually ligated, since hemostatic sutures will probably not occlude them. The laceration is closed with a simple continuous suture pattern.

With both techniques, the lobe is evaluated for ventilation and perfusion after the leaks are controlled. If either appears to be compromised, a partial or complete lobectomy is done. The remaining visceral pleura is examined for lacerations. Flooding the chest with saline during positive pressure ventilation will locate any air leaks. The thorax is closed with a suction drain in place (see Thoracotomy and Chapter 66).

Lung Lobe Torsion

Lung lobe torsion is an uncommon condition that has been reported in at least 19 dogs and 5 cats.[1, 15, 70, 81, 96] Dogs with deep, narrow chests have a higher incidence of lung torsion, and the right cranial and middle lobes are more frequently affected.[1, 15, 70, 81, 96] Most torsions cause venous and

bronchus obstruction while a portion of the arterial blood flow remains. The lobe becomes severely congested and consolidated as fluid moves into the interstitial tissue and airways. The condition is associated with chronic respiratory disease, chylothorax, trauma, thoracic surgery, and neoplasia.[70]

Clinical Signs. Although nonspecific, these are related to local and systemic effects of the consolidated or necrotic lung lobe and accumulation of fluid in the pleural space. Patients are depressed and have a cough and varying degrees of respiratory distress. Anorexia with weight loss and occasional vomition occur in longstanding cases (one to three weeks). Moist rales are heard with muffled respiratory and cardiac sounds due to accumulation of pleural fluid.

Diagnosis. Thoracocentesis produces large amounts of a serosanguineous or chylous fluid. Cytology of this fluid reveals significant numbers of red blood cells and leukocytes but rare evidence of sepsis.

Radiographs show evidence of pleural effusion and lung consolidation. Pleural fluid may have to be drained before the consolidated lung lobe can be seen. Fluid may remain trapped around the affected lobe after chest drainage. Early in the process, radiographs of the lobe indicate air bronchograms, but this air is absorbed and replaced by fluid within two to three days. The lobe may reach an inflated size but will be consolidated.

The obstructed orifice of the main bronchus supplying the affected lobe can be demonstrated by positive contrast bronchography and bronchoscopy. The orifice may have ridges of wrinkled musoca and appear narrow when observed through the bronchoscope.[81] Oily radiopaque dye deposited in the area fails to drain into the suspected bronchus, and this can be demonstrated by radiographs.

Medical Therapy. Initial therapy is symptomatic and aimed at stabilization. Respiratory distress is relieved with chest drainage, elevated oxygen atmosphere, and medical care of associated respiratory disease. Intravenous fluid therapy is indicated if dehydration is present and is given prior to surgery in all cases to provide a good circulating blood volume. Antibiotics are given before surgery.

Surgical Approach. Total lobectomy of the involved lung lobe is the treatment of choice. Most twisted lung lobes are congested and friable, may be necrotic, and should not be salvaged even if they "reinflate" with untwisting. The pedicle of the lung should be clamped with noncrushing forceps before it is untwisted.[70, 116]

The remaining lung lobes are examined for physical condition and normal positioning and the thorax lavaged. Resistance to full lung inflation due to restrictive pleuritis should be noted and the interfering fibrin dissected from the visceral pleura (see Restrictive Pleuritis).

Postoperative Care. Presurgical antibiotics are continued for at least five days (see Chapter 66).

NEOPLASTIC DISEASE OF LUNG (see Chapter 185)

Primary and metastatic neoplasia of the lung is not surgically approached unless it appears as a solitary nodule, diagnostic biopsy is desired, or a salvage procedure is feasible. Solitary nodules should be differentiated from fluid-filled cysts, bullae, and abscesses. Clinical signs, history, radiographic examination, and biopsy should be used in each diagnosis. Neoplasia is more common in animals over seven years of age. Thoracic masses of this type may cause hypertrophic osteoarthropathy.

Lung Biopsy

Needle Biopsy

Percutaneous fine needle aspiration with the aid of bipolar fluoroscopy or thoroscopic direction yields good results in experienced hands.[54, 101, 126] Pneumothorax and hemothorax are real complications and occasionally require chest drainage. Deaths have occurred. Cutting or high-speed-drill-driven trephine needles provide better tissue samples.[101] A higher complication rate from hemorrhage and pneumothorax occurs with this technique, which provides little advantage over other closed techniques.

Endoscopy can be used effectively to obtain lung biopsies. The tracheobronchial route is used for intraluminal masses, and, when peripheral guidance is adequate, biopsies can be obtained by penetrating the bronchial wall. Obtaining tissue from a divisional septum at a bronchial branch point can result in severe hemorrhage, and this technique should be avoided. Biopsies obtained are small, crushed, and frequently nondiagnostic (37 per cent positive).[34]

Rigid and flexible endoscopes can be used for thoroscopy and surface lesions approached under visual control. Hemo- and pneumothorax may result but may be controlled by cauterizing the site with shielded bipolar cautery probes passed through the scope. Similar small biopsy specimens are obtained.

Open chest lung biopsy is the preferred technique in diffuse disease.[34] A small lateral thoracotomy is made and the edge of a lung lobe is allowed to herniate. It is grasped by noncrushing forceps, and a partial lobectomy is performed. More solitary or deeper lesions are approached through a lateral thoracotomy, and a partial or complete lobectomy is performed.[34] An adequate tissue sample, an accurate diagnosis and prognosis, and possibly a cure can be obtained with a single procedure while the complications of pneumothorax and hemothorax are essentially eliminated. Open chest lung biopsy is rapid with the aid of stapling equipment (see Lobectomy).

Cryosurgery (see Chapter 173)

Cryosurgical techniques have been adapted for use through rigid, hollow bronchoscopes.[20, 40] The probes can be introduced into the tracheal bronchial tree by the oral or tracheostomy route. The same technique can be utilized during thoroscopy exams to approach surface lesions. Full thickness freezing of trachea, bronchi, and lung parenchyma has been well tolerated and heals without stenosis.[40] Three freezes per site are used with temperatures of $-60°C$ at probe site and $-30°C$ 10 mm from the probe.[20, 40]

Hemorrhage and pneumothorax can occur in 5 to 15 days during tissue dissolution. Significant hemorrhage has occurred when the cryoprobe has moved before the tissue had thawed.[19] Uninvolved tissues should be shielded by insulation of the inflow and outflow tubing of the solid probe tip. Local necrosis and resolution occur in 21 days in most cases.

LOBECTOMY

Partial Lobectomy

Excision of a portion of a lung lobe for isolated disease or diagnostic biopsy is relatively safe and rapidly performed. Lesions involving the distal two-thirds or less of a lung lobe can be excised using partial lobectomy. Nonresponsive lung abscesses, cysts or bullae, small tumors, and severe lacerations are treated by this technique. Of all biopsy techniques, direct observation of the tissue being removed provides the pathologist with the best tissue selection.[34]

The affected lobe is approached through a lateral thoracotomy. If the affected area is near the apex of a lung lobe, a simple wedge or distal lobe amputation is done. The area of the lung lobe to be removed is identified, and a pair of crushing forceps is placed across the lobe proximal to it (Fig. 65–20). If a wedge is taken out, two pairs of forceps are used to outline the wedge, and a continuous horizontal mattress suture (3–0 or 4–0 absorbable suture) is placed on the proximal side of the forceps. The suture is tied so that a piece (8 to 10 cm long) is left to control the lung at each side of the lobe. The lung lobe is incised on the proximal side of the forceps leaving a narrow

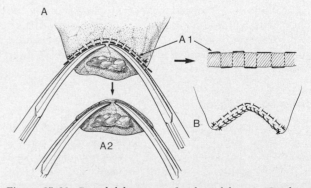

Figure 65–20. Partial lobectomy of a lung lobe. *A,* Crushing forceps are placed proximal to the lesion. *A1,* A hemostatic continuous horizontal mattress suture is placed 2 mm proximal to the forceps. *A2,* The segment is excised. *B,* A simple continuous pattern is used to oversew the incision in the lung.

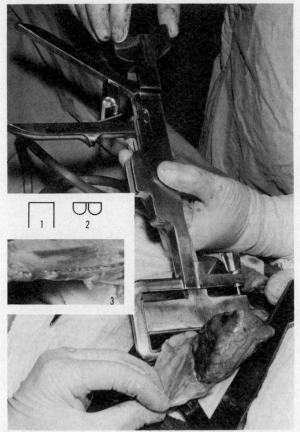

Figure 65–21. Partial lobectomy using stapling equipment. Stapler is placed across the lung lobe proximal to the lesion, and two rows of staples are simultaneously placed to seal the lung edge. The lung lobe distal to the stapler is excised and the stapler removed. *Inset,* Staple before *(1)* and after *(2)* closure and stapled lung lobe *(3)*.

strip of uninjured lung distal to the suture. The edge of the lung incision is oversewn with a very closely spaced simple continuous suture pattern of absorbable suture (4–0 or 5–0). The lobe is allowed to drop back into the thoracic cavity, the chest is filled with saline until the incision is covered, and the lungs are inflated so that the suture line can be checked for air leaks. Leaks are closed with simple interrupted or cruciate sutures of similar suture material.

Partial lobectomy in the proximal third of the lobe will encounter relatively large bronchi and blood vessels. These are ligated individually with suture ligatures (fixation ligatures) to reduce the chance of hemorrhage or air leak, and the lung edge is sutured as described.

Mechanical stapling equipment can be used in lieu of suture techniques.[51] The stapler is placed across the lobe proximal to the lesion and a double row of fine staples is placed (Fig. 65–21). The lobe distal to the staples is clamped to prevent leakage and excised. Occasionally there will be small air leaks and hemorrhage along the stapled surface since the physical construction of the staples in a "B" configuration allows small vessels and bronchi to remain patent. These leaks are controlled by a few interrupted sutures. This is a very rapid technique and is warranted in critical patients. Stapling equipment is too large to use in the thorax of small patients.

The chest is evacuated of all fluid and other debris and a chest drain placed (see Chest Drain Placement). The intercostal incision is closed routinely (see Chapter 41). If there is no accumulation of fluid or air in the chest cavity within the first 24 hours, the chest drain is removed. Postoperative care is discussed in Chapter 66.

Complete Lobectomy

The excision of one or two lung lobes is necessary when extensive disease or injury occurs. The surgical approach is through a standard lateral thoracotomy over the affected lung area and its hilus. It is better to be one interspace caudal rather than cranial if there is any question as to the specific location of the diseased lobe (the ribs are retracted cranially more easily). The remaining lung lobes are packed out of the way with moist laparotomy sponges, and the visceral pleura is incised to expose the pulmonary vessels.[4]

The arterial supply to the lobe is approached first to control blood flow to the lobe, preventing congestion and reducing the chance of severe arterial hemorrhages as the hilar dissection is made. There is little chance of "seeding" the vascular system from the lobe manipulation with an intact venous outflow. The drastic reduction in intravenous hydrostatic pressure and collapse of the microvasculature after arterial ligation prohibit significant venous outflow. Venous backflow from the pulmonary vein can occur if the vein is incised and is more of a nuisance than a problem.

The pulmonary artery supplying the affected lung lobe is dorsal to the left bronchi and ventrolateral to the right bronchi (see Chapter 61). The pulmonary artery is exposed by sharp and blunt dissection until its circumference is clear of pleura and perivascular tissue (Fig. 65–22). Right-angle forceps assist in dissection of the blind side. A piece of 3-mm moistened umbilical tape is passed around the artery for traction, facilitating movement of the vessel while ligatures are placed and acting as an emergency ligature in case the vessel is torn. A simple ligature of 2–0 or 3–0 suture material (nonabsorbable) is tied at the proximal end of the artery near its branch point, taking care not to encroach on the lumen of the parent vessel. A similar suture is placed distal to the point at which the artery will be transected. A transfixing suture is tied 1 mm distal to the proximal suture to prevent migration (see Fig. 65–22). The artery is transected between the two distal sutures.

The lobe is retracted dorsally and the pulmonary vein is approached on the ventral side of the bronchus (see Chapter 61). Care should be taken as the dissection is extended around the pulmonary vein to prevent laceration of this delicate vessel. Sharp dissec-

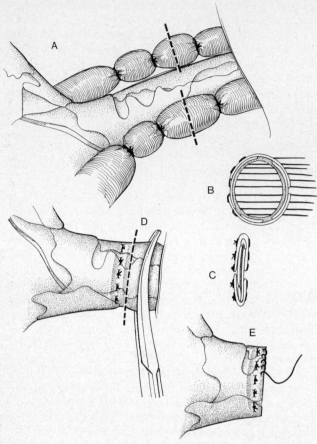

Figure 65–22. Lung lobectomy. *A*, The artery and vein supplying the lung lobe are each triple ligated with the central ligatures as fixations. The vessels are transected *(dashed line)*. *B*, The clamped bronchus has preplaced interrupted horizontal mattress sutures, which when tied collapse the bronchus *(C)*. *D*, The bronchus is transected. *E*, The end is oversewn with a simple continuous suture pattern.

tion (scissors) combined with gentle blunt dissection with forceps or Q-tips is needed to isolate the vein. The vein is ligated as for the artery. The venous drainage from other lung lobes in the area should not be interfered with by incorporating an adjacent vein in the ligatures.

The main bronchus supplying the lobe is dissected free of remaining tissue. The bronchus is cross-clamped with two crushing forceps proximal and distal to a convenient point for transection close to the lung lobe (see Fig. 65–22). The bronchus is transected between the forceps and the lung is removed.[3] Thus, more room is provided in the chest to complete the operation. The bronchus, near its origin proximal to the remaining clamp, is sutured with preplaced interrupted horizontal mattress sutures (2–0 to 3–0 nonabsorbable monofilament suture). These sutures collapse the bronchus as they are tied. The bronchus is transected just distal to these sutures, leaving minimal noncrushed bronchus remaining distal to the mattress sutures. A simple continuous suture pattern is used to oversew the mucosa and cartilage on the distal end of the bronchus (3–0 or 4–0 absorbable suture). The bronchial suture

line is tested for air leaks by flooding the thorax with warm saline and producing 25 to 30 cm of water pressure in the ventilation system. Additional sutures may be placed to close major leaks. Suture hole leaks are closed by suturing surrounding pleura and sub-pleural tissue over the end of the bronchus and vessel stumps. Complete coverage of the raw tissues exposed during surgery aids in decreasing adhesions, reduces postoperative air leaks, and aids in healing of exposed stumps.

An alternative technique is mechanical suturing with automatic stapling equipment. Stapling the entire pedicle in situ has met with few problems.[51, 90, 110] The equipment is difficult to handle in a small thorax, exclusion of adjacent tissue is troublesome, and leakage of air and blood through the B-shaped staples is an occasional problem. Sutures are used to stop minor leaks. When this technique is used, it decreases surgery time.

Necrotic Lobes

Resection of a twisted lung lobe occasionally means handling friable tissue and vessels containing large loose clots and autolyzed blood. Such lobes should be retracted gently and not untwisted until the pedicle is clamped.[70, 116]

The bronchus and vascular pedicle are superficially dissected in the rotated position until grossly separate from the adjacent tissues. The pedicle is cross-clamped with two pair of forceps near the lung lobe and severed between them. The lobe is removed from the thorax, leaving more working room at the hilus.

The remaining pedicle is dissected free of pleura and superficial adipose and loose connective tissue. The pedicle is clamped with noncrushing forceps close to its root. The distal forcep is removed and the vessels and bronchus flushed to remove clots and debris. The structures are each clamped separately with a pair of hemostats, the noncrushing clamp is removed, and their trunks are dissected free of surrounding tissue. The vessels are double ligated and the bronchus oversewn as described (see Lobectomy). Excess vessel and bronchial tissue is amputated and the stumps are checked for hemorrhage and air leaks. The same technique can be used for lobes containing large abscesses or neoplasms that obstruct the surgeon's view of the hilus.

The remaining part of the operation is identical to a standard lobectomy. The pleural space is flushed liberally with antiseptic solution followed by saline or Ringer's solution. All lung lobes are examined for proper positioning, a chest drain is placed, and the incision is closed.

Postoperative Care

Preoperative antibiotics are continued and standard postoperative monitoring of the chest patient is done (see Chapter 66).

PNEUMONECTOMY

Excision of an entire lung is tolerated if the remaining lung is reasonably healthy. Transient respiratory acidosis has been noted in dogs undergoing pneumonectomy.[16] Healthy dogs undergoing staged lobectomies over a six-month period can survive on the equivalent of one and one-half healthy caudal lung lobes. Restriction of over 60 per cent of the pulmonary artery is fatal in dogs, which correlates well with dogs surviving a 50 per cent total lung loss and dying with a 75 per cent loss.[16] Some lung regeneration can be anticipated in a subtotal lobectomy, especially if two other lobes are simultaneously removed. This may account for gradual improvement in exercise tolerance in these patients.[16]

Pneumonectomy is indicated for lesions already described that have extended to all lobes of one lung while sparing the contralateral lung. The same surgical conditions exist as those described for lobectomy (i.e., neoplasia, abscess, trauma), and the same sequence of vessel and bronchial ligation is followed. Lobes that are large and consolidated undergo pedicle clamping and lobe excision prior to pedicle dissection and vessel ligation. This provides improved working room in the thorax in small dogs and cats.

Control of the main pulmonary artery (lobar) branch early in the procedure reduces the chance of major hemorrhage during hilar dissection. A 25-cm piece of 3-mm moistened umbilical tape is passed around the lobar artery close to the branch of the main pulmonary artery and the two ends passed through a 3- to 5-cm piece of rubber tubing. This noose can be tightened to stop flow in the lobar artery or it can be used for traction. The artery is ligated or transected and oversewn. Prior to oversewing the lobar artery, a noncrushing vascular clamp is placed on the artery just distal to the umbilical tape noose, a crushing clamp is placed more distal, and the artery is transected. The cut edge of the proximal segment of the lobar artery is oversewn with a double layer of simple continuous monofilament nonabsorbable suture (4–0 to 5–0) (Fig. 65–23). In small dogs and cats, the lobar artery is ligated twice (1 cm apart) and a fixation ligature juxtapositioned distal to the proximal ligature. The vessel is transected between the two distal sutures. The veins are ligated using the same method in all dogs and cats.

The bronchus is transected using the cut-and-sew technique, and the endotracheal tube is advanced into the contralateral bronchus. Monofilament nonabsorbable suture is anchored in the tracheal wall immediately adjacent to the bronchus and used for traction. The bronchus is clamped distal to the amputation site. The incision is started approximately 1 cm distal to the carina and advanced about one-third of the bronchial diameter. Simple interrupted sutures are placed through the bronchial rings close to the orifice (3–0 or 4–0 monofilament nonabsorbable suture). The incision is advanced and sutured closed until the bronchus has been transected. The ends of

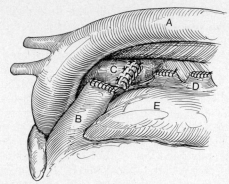

Figure 65–23. Pneumonectomy. The removal of the lung is complete. The left pulmonary artery (A) and pulmonary veins (B) are oversewn with a simple continuous suture close to their base to prevent cul-de-sacs where thrombi could form. The left mainstem bronchus is oversewn (C), producing a smooth contour to the tracheal wall.

the incision may have to be tapered to obtain a smooth closure and good seal. The resection and closure should not reduce the size of the other bronchus.

All ligatures are checked for security and the endotracheal tube is withdrawn proximal to the carina. The tracheal incision is submerged in saline and examined for air leaks while the intratracheal pressure is raised to 25 to 30 cm H_2O. Extra sutures are used as needed to stop air leaks.

Pleura is sutured over the hilar area. The thorax is lavaged, suction cleaned, and closed as previously described. Adequate chest drains are placed and monitored for fluid and air accumulation for at least 24 hours (see Chapter 66).

Lung Reimplantation

Lung reimplantation is used in research models to study the deinnervated lung responses to various pharmacological and toxic conditions.[99] Studies of the technical and physiological problems related to lung reimplantation are the basis for lung transplantation in man.[99, 105] A detailed publication concerning the technical aspect of autogenous lung reimplantation was recently published.[99]

All dogs are screened for existing respiratory and pulmonary vascular disease. Thoracic radiographs, blood analysis, Knott's test, and pulmonary vascular pressures are examined for abnormalities. The patient is prepared for lateral thoracotomy at the fifth interspace, anesthetized with gas anesthesia, and ventilated with oxygen. Intravenous Ringer's solution is given during surgery (2.0 to 2.5 ml/kg/hr).

Surgical Procedure

A complete hilus dissection is made, isolating the main pulmonary lobar artery–left atrial junction with the pulmonary veins and the mainstem bronchus. A piece of umbilical tape is placed around the bronchus to retract this structure while the final dissection is made and vascular clamps are placed on the artery and atrium.

Two noncrushing vascular clamps are used to occlude the bronchus while the lung is held inflated in 20 cm H_2O. The first clamp is placed near the carina where the vagus nerve crosses the bronchus, and the second clamp is placed near the junction of the bronchus to the cranial lobe and the mainstem bronchus. The bronchus is transected, leaving a proximal segment adequate for suturing. Two noncrushing vascular clamps are placed across the lobar artery with the proximal clamp located next to but not occluding the main pulmonary artery. The other clamp is placed parallel to the first clamp and perpendicular to the branching of the cranial lobe artery. The latter is used as a landmark for proper alignment for reclamping the distal segment of the lobar artery prior to anastomosis. The artery is transected with sharp scissors, leaving approximately 1 cm of vessel beyond the proximal clamp.

The atrial dissection is completed, exposing the atrium and the pulmonary veins. A noncrushing vascular clamp is placed across the atrium so that there is sufficient atrial wall included to allow anastomosis without interfering with the ostia of the pulmonary veins. Care is taken not to interfere with the veins draining the opposite lung. The atrium is transected with scissors, leaving 4 to 5 mm of wall beyond the clamp.

The excised lung is placed in cold lactated Ringer's solution and perfused with 60 cm H_2O pressure via the artery with cold lactated Ringer's solution containing 1000 units of heparin. Air is excluded from the artery by keeping the lung submerged during the perfusion. The artery is reclamped perpendicular to the cranial lobe branch while still submerged.

The bronchus clamp is removed and the bronchial wall trimmed to leave 4 to 5 mm of wall beyond the beyond the lobar orifices. This leaves minimal bronchial wall that is perfused by vessels from lung parenchyma and reduces delayed healing and dehiscence.[60] This problem can be eliminated by wrapping the bronchial anastomosis with an omental pedicle flap.[14, 68]

Reimplantation is begun with the anastomosis of the atrium. The corners of the atrial cuffs contained in the clamps are united by 5–0 monofilament nonabsorbable suture. These sutures are continued in a simple continuous pattern, closing the dorsal and then the ventral wall of the anastomosis. Intima-to-intima apposition is important. The distal venous clamp is removed prior to tightening the last suture to allow blood to flush the air out of the anastomotic site. The last suture is tied and leaks are repaired.

The artery is anastomosed next using the biangulation technique and 5–0 monofilament nonabsorbable suture in a simple continuous pattern (see Vascular Anastomosis). Care is taken to assure proper alignment of the artery prior to suturing. Before tightening the last suture, the remaining atrial and distal arterial clamps are removed and air is flushed from the arterial anastomosis. Sutures are tied and the anastomosis leaks are repaired if significant. The proximal arterial clamp is removed, establishing blood flow to the lung.

Bronchial anastomosis is made with 4–0 monofilament nonabsorbable suture using a simple continuous pattern. Braided or twisted nonabsorbable suture causes a higher incidence of inflammation, infection, and fistula formation.[108] The ventral wall is sutured first, working from within the lumen. Then the dorsal wall is sutured to complete the anastomosis. Suture placement is designed to obtain perfect alignment of the mucosa. This may be difficult, since the loss of complete tracheal rings and the appearance of irregular cartilage plates near the lobar bronchi result in small pieces of cartilage along the suture line, which tend to interfere with accurate mucosal alignment.

The thorax is lavaged and suctioned free of fluid and debris. All suture lines are checked for leaks and repaired if necessary. A chest drain is placed and the thorax closed after the lung is fully inflated.

Postoperative Care

Standard chest patient care is followed (see Chapter 66). The patient is kept in an oxygen cage with a 60 per cent O_2 environment. Preoperative antibiotics are continued for five days, and lung changes are monitored by radiographs every 48 hours. Reinnervation is complete in 8 to 11 months.[92]

1. Alexander, J. W., Hoffer, R. E., and Boltona, G. R.: Torsion of the diaphragmatic lobe of the lung following surgical correction of a patent ductus arteriosis. Vet. Med./Small Anim. Clin. 69:595, 1974.
2. Amis, T. C.: Tracheal collapse in the dog. Aust. Vet. J. 50:285, 1974.
3. Arnoczky, S. B.: Lung lobectomy. Vet. Clin. North Am. 9:219, 1979.
4. Aron, D. N., DeVries, R., and Short, C. E.: Primary tracheal chondrosarcoma in a dog: a case report with description of surgical and anesthetic techniques. J. Am. Anim. Hosp. Assoc. 16:31, 1980.
5. Beaumont, P. R.: Intratracheal neoplasia in two cats. J. Small Anim. Pract. 23:29, 1982.
6. Berzon, J. L., Rendano, V. T., and Hoffer, R. E.: Recurrent pneumothorax secondary to ruptured pulmonary blebs: a case report. J. Am. Anim. Hosp. Assoc. 15:707, 1979.
7. Binnington, A. G., and Kreplin, C. M. A.: An unusual lateral tracheal collapse in a dog. Can. Vet. J. 18:190, 1977.
8. Black, A. P., Liu, S., and Randolph, J. F.: Primary tracheal leiomyoma in a dog. J. Am. Vet. Med. Assoc. 179:905, 1981.
9. Bojrab, M. J., and Dallman, M. J.: Tracheal resection and anastomosis. Canine Pract. 7:69, 1980.
10. Bojrab, M. J., and Nafe, L. L.: Tracheal reconstructive surgery. J. Am. Anim. Hosp. Assoc. 12:622, 1976.
11. Bojrab, M. J., and Renegar, W. R.: The trachea. In Bojrab, M. J. (ed.): Pathophysiology in Small Animal Surgery. Lea & Febiger, Philadelphia, 1981.
12. Boyd, C. L., and Hanselka, D. V.: Prosthesis for correction of collapsed trachea. J. Am. Anim. Hosp. Assoc. 12:829, 1976.
13. Brant, L. R., Spencer, F. C., Boyd, A. D., and Daly, J. F.: Tracheostomy and assisted ventilation. In Sabiston, D. C.,

and Spencer, F. C. (eds.): *Gibbon's Surgery of the Chest.* W. B. Saunders, Philadelphia, 1976.

14. Bright, R. M., and Thacker, H. L.: The formation of an omental pedicle flap and its experimental use in the repair of a diaphragmatic rent in the dog. J. Am. Anim. Hosp. Assoc. *18*:283, 1982.

15. Brown, N. O., and Zontine, W. J.: Lung lobe torsion in the cat. Am. Vet. Rad. Soc. *17*:219, 1976.

16. Brugarolas, A., and Takita, H.: Regeneration of the lung in the dog. J. Thorac. Cardiovasc. Surg. *65*:187, 1973.

17. Bryan, R. D., Frame, R. W., and Kier, A. B.: Tracheal leiomyoma in a dog. J. Am. Vet. Med. Assoc. *178*:1069, 1981.

18. Cain, G. R.: Tracheal adenocarcinoma in a cat. J. Am. Vet. Med. Assoc. *182*:614, 1983.

19. Cantrell, J. R., and Folse, J. R.: The repair of circumferential defects of the trachea by direct anastomosis: experimental evaluation. J. Thorac. Cardiovasc. Surg. *42*:589, 1961.

20. Carpenter, R. J., Neel, H. B., and Sanderson, D. R.: Cryosurgery of bronchiopulmonary structures: our approach to lesions inaccessible to the rigid bronchoscope. Chest *72*:279, 1977.

21. Cooper, J. D., and Grillo, H. C.: The evolution of tracheal injury due to ventilatory assistance through cuffed tubes: a pathologic study. Ann. Surg. *169*:334, 1969.

22. Cooper, J. D., Todd, T. R. J., Ilves, R., and Pearson, F. G.: Use of the silicone treated T-tube for the management of complex tracheal injuries. J. Thorac. Cardiovasc. Surg. *82*:559, 1981.

23. Done, S. H.: Canine tracheal collapse: etiology, pathology, diagnosis and treatment. Vet. Ann. *18*:255, 1978.

24. Done, S. H., Clayton-Jones, D. G., and Price, E. K.: Tracheal collapse in the dog: a review of the literature and report of two new cases. J. Small Anim. Pract. *11*:743, 1970.

25. Done, S. H., and Drew, R. A.: Observations on the pathology of tracheal collapse in dogs. J. Small Anim. Pract. *17*:783, 1976.

26. Donnelly, G. M., Haack, D. G., and Heird, C. S.: Tracheal epithelium: cell kinetics and differentiation in normal rat tissue. Cell Tissue Kinet. *15*:119, 1982.

27. Eyster, G. E., Evans, A. T., O'Handley, P., and Steffers, J.: Surgical removal of a foreign body from the tracheal bifurcation of a cat. J. Am. Anim. Hosp. Assoc. *12*:481, 1976.

28. Ettinger, S. J., and Ticer, J. W.: Diseases of the trachea. *In* Ettinger, S. J. (ed.): *Veterinary Internal Medicine*, 2nd ed. W. B. Saunders, Philadelphia, 1982.

29. Evans, H. E., and Christensen, G. C. (eds.): *Miller's Anatomy of the Dog.* 2nd ed. W. B. Saunders, Philadelphia, 1979.

30. Farmer, A. F., Gain, G., and Farkas, L. G.: Composite grafts for tracheal defects. Mod. Vet. Pract. *52*:37, 1971.

31. Feeney, D. A., Malnati, G., and Mahaffey, M. B.: What is your diagnosis? Ruptured trachea. J. Am. Vet. Med. Assoc. *175*:303, 1979.

32. Flemming, I., and Hommerich, K. W.: Surgery of the tracheal and laryngotracheal stenosis: tracheal stenosis, development and latest state of experimental surgery. J. Fr. Otorhinolaryngol. *23*:387, 1974.

33. Furneaux, R. W.: Tracheal reconstruction with knitted polypropylene mesh in a dachshund dog. J. Small Anim. Pract. *15*:619, 1973.

34. Gaensler, E. A., and Carrington, C. B.: Open biopsy for chronic, diffuse, infiltrative lung disease: clinical, roentgenographic and physiological correlations in 502 patients. Ann. Thorac. Surg. *30*:411, 1980.

35. Galoob, N. D., Norris, C. W., and Toledo, P. S.: In vivo observation of tracheal microcirculation in dogs. Ann. Otol. Rhinol. Laryngol. *86*:204, 1977.

36. Ganske, J. G., Dennis, D. L., and VanderVeer, J. B.: Traumatic lung cyst: case report and literature review. J. Trauma *21*:493, 1981.

37. Gibbons, J. A., Peniston, R. L., Raflo, C. P., Diamond, S. S., and Arron, B. L.: A comparison of synthetic absorbable suture with synthetic nonabsorbable suture for construction of tracheal anastomosis. Chest *79*:340, 1979.

38. Giordano, A., and Holsclaw, D. S.: Tracheal resection and microciliary clearance. Ann. Otol. Rhinol. Laryngol. *85*:631, 1976.

39. Gordon, W.: Surgical correction of tracheal stenosis in a dog. J. Am. Vet. Med. Assoc. *162*:479, 1973.

40. Goerenstein, A., Neel, H. B., and Sanderson, D. R.: Transbronchoscopic cryosurgery of respiratory structures: experimental and clinical studies. Ann. Otol. Rhinol. Laryngol. *85*:670, 1976.

41. Grillo, H. C.: Congenital lesions, neoplasms and injuries of the trachea. *In* Sabiston, D. C., and Spencer, F. C. (eds.): *Gibbon's Surgery of the Chest*, 3rd ed. W. B. Saunders, Philadelphia, 1976.

42. Grillo, H. C.: Reconstruction of the trachea after resection for neoplasm. Otolaryngol. Head Neck Surg. *4*:2, 1981.

43. Grillo, H. C.: Primary reconstruction of airway after resection of subglottic laryngeal and upper tracheal stenosis. Ann. Thorac. Surg. *33*:3, 1982.

44. Hankins, J. R., McAslan, T. O., Shin, B., Ayella, R., Cowley, R. A., and McLaughlin, S.: Extensive pulmonary laceration caused by blunt trauma. J. Thorac. Cardiovasc. Surg. *74*:519, 1977.

45. Harris, L. T.: Tracheal foreign body in a cat. Vet. Med./Small Anim. Clin. *77*:1088, 1982.

46. Harvey, C. E., and Fink, E. A.: Tracheal diameter: analysis of radiographic measurements in brachiocephalic and non-brachiocephalic dogs. J. Am. Anim. Hosp. Assoc. *18*:570, 1982.

47. Harvey, C. E., and Goldschmidt, M. H.: Healing following short duration transverse incision tracheotomy in the dog. Vet. Surg. *11*:77, 1982.

48. Harvey, C. E., and O'Brien, J. A.: Tracheotomy in the dog and cat: Analysis of 89 episodes in 79 animals. J. Am. Anim. Hosp. Assoc. *18*:563, 1982.

49. Harvey, H. J., and Sykes, G.: Tracheal mast cell tumor in the dog. J. Am. Vet. Med. Assoc. *180*:1097, 1982.

50. Hedlund, C. S., Tangner, C. H., Montgomery, D. L., and Hobson, H. P.: A procedure for permanent tracheostomy and its effects on tracheal mucosa. Vet. Surg. *11*:13, 1982.

51. Hess, J. L., DeYoung, D. W., and Grier, R. L.: Use of mechanical staples in veterinary thoracic surgery. J. Am. Anim. Hosp. Assoc. *15*:569, 1979.

52. Hill, F. W. G.: Repair of traumatic rupture of the trachea of a dog. Vet. Rec. *95*:265, 1974.

53. Hough, J. D., Krahwinkle, D. J., Evans, A. T., Carrig, C. B., Tvedten, H. W., and Schirmer, R. G.: Tracheal osteochondroma in a dog. J. Am. Vet. Med. Assoc. *170*:1416, 1977.

54. Jamplis, R. W., Stevens, M. G., and Lillington, G. A.: Percutaneous needle aspiration biopsy of the lung. Am. J. Surg. *116*:243, 1968.

55. Jubb, K. V. F., and Kennedy, P. C.: Respiratory system. *In* Jubb, K. V. K., and Kennedy, P. C. (eds.): *Pathology of Domestic Animals*, 2nd ed. Academic Press, New York, 1970.

56. Kenan, P. D.: Complications associated with tracheostomy: prevention and treatment. Otolaryngol. Clin. North Am. *12*:807, 1979.

57. Kennedy, R. K.: Traumatic tracheal separation with diverticuli in a cat. Vet. Med./Small Anim. Clin. *71*:1384, 1976.

58. Klopper, P. J.: Experimental reconstruction of the trachea with silicone rubber. Arch. Chir. Neerl. *21*:293, 1969.

59. Knecht, C. D., Schall, W. D., and Barrett, R.: Iatrogenic tracheal stenosis in a dog. J. Am. Vet. Med. Assoc. *160*:1427, 1972.

60. Koerner, S., Pinisker, K., Torres, M., Colon, I., Hagstrom, J., Crane, R., and Veith, F. J.: Lobar bronchial anastomosis to improve bronchial healing in lung transplantation. Surg. Forum *27*:195, 1976.

61. Kosloske, A. M.: The Fogarty balloon technique for removal of foreign bodies from the tracheobronchial tree. Surg. Gynecol. Obstet. *55*:72, 1982.

62. Kosoy, J., Homsy, C. A., Greenberg, S. D., and Prewitt, J.

M.: Proplast tracheal prosthesis: a preliminary report. Ann. Otol. Rhinol. Laryngol. 86:392, 1977.

63. Kotake, Y., and Grillo, H. C.: Reduction of tension at the anastomosis following tracheal resection in puppies. J. Thorac. Cardiovasc. Surg. 71:600, 1976.

64. Krespi, Y. P., Baek, S. M., Marovitz, W. F., and Biller, H. F.: Revascularized free pleuroperiosteal flap to correct full thickness tracheal defects. Bull. N.Y. Acad. Med. 55:939, 1979.

65. Leonard, H. C.: Surgical correction of collapsed trachea in dog. J. Am. Vet. Med. Assoc. 158:598, 1971.

66. Leonard, H. C., and Wright, J. J.: An intraluminal prosthetic dilator for tracheal collapse in the dog. J. Am. Anim. Hosp. Assoc. 14:464, 1978.

67. Lett, A. R., and Munoz, N. M.: Interrelationship between alpha- and beta-adrenergic antagonists and histamine in canine airways. J. Allergy Clin. Immunol. 64:300, 1981.

68. Lima, O., Goldberg, M., Peters, W. J., Ayabe, H., Townsend, E., and Cooper, J. D.: Bronchial omentopexy in canine lung transplantation. J. Thorac. Cardiovasc. Surg. 83:418, 1982.

69. Lindholm, C. E.: Prolonged endotracheal intubation. Acta Anaesthesiol. Scand. 33:1, 1969.

70. Lord, P. F., Greiner, T. P., Greene, R. W., and DeHoff, W. D.: Lung lobe torsion in the dog. J. Am. Anim. Hosp. Assoc. 9:473, 1973.

71. Lowe, J. E., Bridgman, A. H., and Sabiston, D. C.: The role of bronchioplastic procedures in the surgical management of benign and malignant pulmonary lesions. J. Thorac. Cardiovasc. Surg. 83:227, 1982.

72. Maeda, M., and Grillo, H. C.: Effect of tension on tracheal growth after resection and anastomosis in puppies. J. Thorac. Cardiovasc. Surg. 65:658, 1973.

73. Maniglia, A. J.: Tracheal stenosis: conservative surgery as a primary mode of management. Otolaryngol. Clin. North Am. 12:877, 1979.

74. McGee, K. C., Nagle, J. W., and Toohill, R. J.: CO$_2$ laser repair of subglottic and upper tracheal stenosis. Otolaryngol. Head Neck Surg. 89:92, 1981.

75. McKiernan, B. C.: Lower respiratory tract diseases. In Ettinger, S. J. (ed.): Veterinary Internal Medicine, 2nd ed. W. B. Saunders, Philadelphia, 1982.

76. Mendez-Picon, G., Ehrlich, F. E., and Salzberg, A. M.: The effect of tracheostomy incisions on tracheal growth. J. Pediatr. Surg. 11:681, 1976.

77. Mendez-Picon, G., Hutcher, N. E., Neifeld, J., and Salzberg, A. M.: Long-term study of tracheal growth after segmental resection in puppies. J. Pediatr. Surg. 9:615, 1974.

78. Mills, S. A., Johnston, F. R., Hudspeth, A. S., Breyer, R. H., Myers, R. T., and Cordell, A. R.: Clinical spectrum of blunt tracheobronchial disruption illustration in seven cases. J. Thorac. Cardiovasc. Surg. 84:49, 1982.

79. Montgomery, W. W.: Surgery of the Upper Respiratory System, Vol. 2. Lea & Febiger, Philadelphia, 1973.

80. Morrison, R. R.: Surgical removal of an intratracheal nodule of ectopic bone and cartilage. Can. Vet. J. 21:290, 1980.

81. Moses, B. L.: Fiberoptic bronchoscopy for diagnosis of lung lobe torsion in a dog. J. Am. Vet. Med. Assoc. 76:44, 1980.

82. Neel, H. B., Farrell, K. H., and DeSanto, L. W.: Cryosurgery of respiratory structures: 1. cryonecrosis of trachea and bronchus. Laryngoscope 83:1062, 1973.

83. Neville, W. E.: Prosthetic reconstruction of the trachea and carina. Nippon Kyobu Geka Gakkai Zasshi 27:405, 1979.

84. Neville, W. E., Balanowski, P. J. P., and Soltanzadeh, H.: Prosthetic replacement of the trachea and carina. J. Thorac. Cardiovasc. Surg. 72:525, 1976.

85. O'Brien, J. A.: A diagnostic approach to respiratory disease. In Kirk, R. (ed.): Current Veterinary Therapy VII. W. B. Saunders, Philadelphia, 1980.

86. Ohlsen, L., and Nordin, U.: Tracheal reconstruction with perichondrial grafts. Scand. J. Plast. Reconstr. Surg. 10:135, 1976.

87. Paegle, R. D., Ayres, S. M., and Davis, S.: Rapid tracheal

88. Papachristou, D., and Fortner, J. G.: Experimental use of a gastric flap on an omental pedicle to close defects in the trachea, pharynx or cervical esophagus. Plast. Reconstr. Surg. 59:382, 1977.

89. Pedersoli, W. M., and Krista, L. M.: Alterations in tracheal epithelium in dogs due to endotracheal intubation. Vet. Anesth. 4:34, 1979.

90. Petrova, N. P., Rabinovich, J. J., Kapitanov, N. N., and Bogomolova, O. R.: Employment of two new stapling devices (models SV-2 and US-18) in experimental combined resections of the bronchus and pulmonary artery. Ann. Thorac. Surg. 19:67, 1975.

91. Pizzoferrato, A., Leake, D., Michieli, S., Haubold, A., and Freeman, S.: Preliminary histologic evaluation of a biocompatible mesh for tracheal reconstruction. Biomater. Med. Devices Artif. Organs 7:321, 1979.

92. Planche, C., Weiss, M., and Verriest, C.: Two-stage bilateral lung reimplantation in the dog. J. Thorac. Cardiovasc. Surg. 74:238, 1977.

93. Pritchard, D. L.: What is your diagnosis—bronchial foreign bodies. J. Am. Vet. Med. Assoc. 176:1385, 1980.

94. Quisling, R. W.: Experimental tracheal reconstruction with external ear cartilage autografts. Arch. Otolaryngol. 104:311, 1978.

95. Rawlings, C. A.: The lungs. In Bojrab, M. J. (ed.): Pathophysiology in Small Animal Surgery. Lea & Febiger, Philadelphia, 1981.

96. Rawlings, C. A., Lebel, J. L., and Mitchum, G.: Torsion of the left apical and cardiac pulmonary lobes in a dog. Am. Vet. Med. Assoc. 156:726, 1970.

97. Read, R. A.: Successful treatment of organizing hemothorax by decortication in a dog: a case report. J. Am. Anim. Hosp. Assoc. 17:167, 1981.

98. Richards, C. D., and Kallenbach, W. W.: Resection and anastomosis of the trachea for removal of an intraluminal foreign body. Vet. Med./Small Anim. Clin. 74:1275, 1979.

99. Rosin, E., and Galphin, S.: Surgical technique of left lung reimplantation in the dog. Vet. Surg. 7:18, 1978.

100. Ross, J. A. T.: Techniques in surgical repair of tracheal stenosis. Otolaryngol. Clin. North Am. 12:893, 1979.

101. Roudebush, P., Green, R. A., and Digilio, K. M.: Percutaneous fine-needle aspiration biopsy of the lung in disseminated pulmonary disease. J. Am. Anim. Hosp. Assoc. 17:109, 1981.

102. Rubin, G. J., Neal, T. M., and Bojrab, M. J.: Surgical reconstruction for collapsed tracheal rings. J. Small Anim. Pract. 14:607, 1973.

103. Ryan, C. O., and Smith, R. A.: Separation of tracheal rings in a cat (What is your diagnosis?). J. Am. Vet. Med. Assoc. 161:1151, 1972.

104. Sabas, A. A., Uez, J. B., Rojas, O., Inones, A., and Aranguren, J. A.: Replacement of the trachea with dura mater: experimental work. J. Thorac. Cardiovasc. Surg. 74:761, 1977.

105. Salem, G., Schlick, W., Keiler, A., Moschl, P., Glockler, M., Radaszkiewicz, T., and Kreuzer, W.: Allotransplantation of the lung in dogs with experimental lung damage. World J. Surg. 3:511, 1979.

106. Sanada, Y., Kojima, Y., and Fonkalsrud, E. W.: Injury of cilia by tracheal tube cuffs. Surg. Gynecol. Obstet. 154:648, 1982.

107. Saperstein, G., Harris, S., and Leipold, H. W.: Congenital defects in domestic cats. Feline Pract. 6:18, 1976.

108. Sawasaki, H., et al.: Postoperative bronchopleural fistula: clinical and experimental study. Chest 76:702, 1975.

109. Schneider, K. M., Smolansky, S. J., Weinberg, G., Morecki, R., and Ruben, R. J.: An external "barrel stave" prosthesis in laryngotracheal reconstruction. Trans. Am. Acad. Ophthalmol. Otolaryngol. 85:ORL866, 1977.

110. Scott, R. N., Faraci, R. P., Hough, A., and Chretien, T. B.: Bronchiol stump closure techniques following pneumonectomy: a serial comparative study. Ann. Surg. 18:205, 1976.

111. Slatter, D. H., and Pettit, G. D.: Surgical method of

correction of collapsed trachea in a dog. Aust. Vet. J. 50:41, 1974.

112. Sobin, S. S., Frasher, W. G., Herta, M., Tremer, H. M., and Hadley, G. G.: Microcirculation of the tracheal mucosa. Angiology 14:165, 1963.

113. Suter, P. F., Colgrove, D. J., and Ewing, G. O.: Congenital hypoplasia of the canine trachea. J. Am. Anim. Hosp. Assoc. 8:120, 1972.

114. Symbas, P. N.: Bullet wounds of the trachea. J. Thorac. Cardiovasc. Surg. 83:235, 1982.

115. Tangner, C. H., and Hobson, H. P.: A retrospective study of 20 surgically managed cases of collapsed trachea. Vet. Surg. 11:146, 1982.

116. Teunissen, G. H., Wolverkamp, W. T., and Goedegebuure, S. A.: Necrosis of a pulmonary lobe in a dog. Tijdschr. Diergeneeskd. 101:1129, 1976.

117. Thomford, N. R., Wilson, W. H., and Blackburn, E. D.: Morphological changes in canine trachea after freezing. Cryobiology 7:19, 1970.

118. Toohill, R. J.: Autogenous graft reconstruction of the larynx and upper trachea. Otolaryngol. Clin. North Am. 12:909, 1979.

119. Trim, C. M., and Simpson, S. T.: Complication following ethylene oxide sterilization: a case report. J. Am. Anim. Hosp. Assoc. 18:507, 1982.

120. Troy, G. C.: Surgical removal of a tracheal osteochondroma. Canine Pract. 5:47, 1978.

121. Tsubota, N., Simpson, W. J., VanNostrand, A. W., and Pearson, F. G.: The effects of preoperative radiation of primary tracheal anastomosis. Ann. Thorac. Surg. 20:152, 1975.

122. Vasseur, P.: Surgery of the trachea. Vet. Clin. North Am. Small Anim. Pract. 9:231, 1979.

123. Weerda, H.: Treatment of long, rigid tracheal stenoses: an experimental study of animals. J. Otol. Rhinol. Laryngol. 40:181, 1978.

124. Westaby, S., Jackson, J. W., and Pearson, G. F.: A bifurcated rubber stent for relief of tracheobronchial obstruction. J. Thorac. Cardiovasc. Surg. 83:414, 1982.

125. Westaby, S., Shepard, M. P., and Nohl-Oser, H. C.: The use of diaphragmatic pedicle grafts for reconstructive procedures in the esophagus and tracheobronchial tree. Ann. Thorac. Surg. 33:486, 1982.

126. Westcott, J. L.: Direct percutaneous needle aspiration of localized pulmonary lesions: results in 422 patients. Radiology 137:31, 1980.

127. White, R. A., White, E. W., and Nelson, R. J.: Uniform microporous biomaterials prepared by Relamineform technique. Biomater. Med. Devices Artif. Organs 7:127, 1979.

128. Withrow, S. J., Holmberg, D. L., Doige, C. E., and Rosychuk, R. A. W.: Treatment of a tracheal osteochondroma with an overlapping end-to-end tracheal anastomosis. J. Am. Anim. Hosp. Assoc. 14:469, 1978.

129. Yoshioka, M. M.: Management of spontaneous pneumothorax in 12 dogs. J. Am. Anim. Hosp. Assoc. 18:57, 1982.

130. Zavala, D. C., and Rodes, M. L.: Foriegn body removal: a new role for the fiberoptic bronchoscope. Ann. Otol. Rhinol. Laryngol. 84:650, 1975.

Chapter **66** # Postoperative Care of Respiratory Patients

A. Wendell Nelson

During the final stages of a surgical procedure, problems likely to occur in recovery from anesthesia and surgery are anticipated and eliminated, circumvented, or prepared for. Of primary concern are a patent airway, adequate ventilation and gas exchange, strong cardiovascular system, and normal body temperature.

PATENT AIRWAY

The obvious causes of airway obstruction (e.g., blood, mucus, fluids) are suctioned and drained via the trachea, pharynx, and caudal nasal passage. The "head-down" position is used in the immediate postoperative period to drain minor hemorrhage or fluid pockets from the nasal and pharyngeal regions.[8, 13] Care is used in placing the patient in a head-down position so that the trachea and neck vessels are not compressed by the edge of the table and the weight of the abdominal viscera on the diaphragm does not interfere with ventilation.

Depressed patients are kept intubated until conscious with a strong swallowing reflex. This practice is also used in patients that are likely to have partial occlusion of the respiratory system (e.g., edematous tissue, laryngeal paralysis, collapsing trachea). The tube is secured to the upper jaw with gauze to keep the tube in place without interfering with swallowing or vomiting. The cuff on the tube should remain inflated until it is removed. For the patient in which the cervical trachea or larynx has been the surgical site and significant postoperative congestion and edema are anticipated, steroid and antibiotic therapy is initiated and a tracheostomy tube is placed.

Relatively large doses of corticosteroids are given to patients with inflammatory or granulating lesions. Initial doses of dexamethasone (1.0 to 2.0 mg/kg) or prednisolone (5.0 to 10.0 mg/kg) are given systemically and tapered during a five- to ten-day postoperative period.[24] Prednisolone (1.0 to 2.0 mg/kg) has been used daily until the mucosa is healed.[5] These are most effective in suppressing the acute inflammatory response to injury (surgery) and decreasing granulation tissue production (stenosis).[5] Corticosteroids potentiate beta-2 stimulators, which improve ciliary clearance and decrease production of mucus.[24]

A single intralesional injection of triamcinolone (40

mg divided in 5 to 10 sites) into the granulation tissue causing airway stenosis is effective in reducing the final volume of tissue produced.[1, 13]

Bactericidal and broad-spectrum antibiotics are used to protect against infection when immunosuppressive levels of corticosteroids are used. These should be continued until after the effects of the steroid have dissipated. Antibiotics are not effective in altering the growth of granulation tissue in airway injury and the ultimate development of stenosis.[12] Methods of tracheostomy tube placement are discussed in Chapter 64.

Care of the Tracheostomy

The most critical aspect of providing an airway with a tracheostomy tube is maintaining it correctly.[16] Keeping the local area clean and the tube completely clear are the primary aims of aftercare. The surgical site is cleaned with a tissue-compatible antiseptic each time the tube is changed.[13] Between changes the exposed subcutaneous tissue and surrounding skin are protected by antibacterial ointment to decrease the chances of infection and tissue dehydration.

The frequency of cleaning depends on the amount of serum and mucus that is expelled from the trachea and varies considerably between patients.[13] Small accumulations of mucus can be removed with a sterile cotton swab moistened with sterile saline while the tube remains in place. Patients with irritated respiratory tracts and other conditions that produce significant mucus in the trachea frequently require cleaning of the tracheostomy tube. Cleaning may be carried out by suctioning the tube lumen and distal respiratory tree every 15 minutes to one hour during the initial phase. In addition, the tracheostomy tube lumen must be frequently inspected for the build-up of dried or inspissated mucus coating the walls. Rapid occlusion of the tube can occur from coughing a blood clot or mucous plug into the tube. This occurrence must be treated immediately to prevent asphyxiation. It is unwise to place a tracheostomy tube in an animal that is not constantly supervised.

The tube can be slowly occluded by small amounts of mucus, serum, blood, or exudate continuously gaining access to the tube and then being dried by the air moving through the tube. This process produces many layers of dry material that reduce the lumen diameter. A tube with a liner sleeve is cleaned by removing the sleeve and replacing it with a clean, sterile sleeve. A sleeveless tube is removed for cleaning and immediately replaced with a clean tube. The lumen of the removed sleeve or tube is cleaned by vigorous brushing with a test tube brush and detergent solution.[16] A piece of gauze bandage threaded through the lumen of the tube can also be used. The tube is held under running water while the gauze is pulled back and forth through it until all of the debris is removed. The cleaned tube or sleeve is held in an antiseptic solution until it is needed, at which time it is rinsed with saline and reused.

A cuffed tracheostomy tube is used whenever there is a chance of aspiration of food, liquid, or exudate from the pharynx or proximal airway or when the tube is used for anesthesia or positive-pressure ventilation. A high-volume, low-pressure (less than 25 cm H_2O) cuff is used to decrease damage to the tracheal mucosa and cartilage. The cuff is deflated whenever it is not needed.

Care must be taken to clean the proximal end of the respiratory system whenever the tube is removed. The animal should not be in a sitting position when the tube are removed, so that fluids or debris in the proximal trachea will not gravitate to the lungs.

Patient activity is restricted so that foreign bodies are not inhaled. Inhalation is particularly a problem during warm weather months, when the patient has access to weeds or grasses and can inhale pieces of plant material. The patient must be kept away from water so that it does not attempt to swim.

Airway Suctioning

Airway suctioning in the awake animal can meet with significant patient resistance. The instillation of local anesthetics decreases the sensitivity of the tracheal mucosa. It is best to avoid suctioning the trachea immediately after eating because it can cause vomiting. Suctioning may also cause respiratory distress and vagal stimulation.

Tracheobronchial suction in the conscious patient requires a tracheostomy and strict sterile technique.[15] A nasotracheal tube can be used in some dogs, but patience is required on the part of the animal and the nurse. A smooth-tipped, side-hole catheter is used to prevent mucosal damage.

The patient is oxygenated, and a sterile catheter is inserted through the nose or a trachesotomy tube into the trachea. It is advanced to the mainstem bronchi, and suction is applied as the catheter is rotated and withdrawn. Maximum suction time is limited to ten seconds, after which the patient is re-oxygenated and the procedure repeated.[15] Small amounts of sterile saline are flushed into the airway to help liquefy thick mucus. Airway suctioning can cause hypoxia, lung collapse, cardiac arrhythmias, hypotension, and vomiting. Although the patient is at risk, excessive airway fluid is dangerous and cannot be ignored.

Removal of the Tracheostomy Tube

The tracheostomy tube is removed as soon as a normal airway is established so that comfortable respiration can ensue. In the majority of the small animal patients undergoing upper respiratory surgery, the tracheostomy tube can be removed in 24 to 48 hours. When considerable airway damage has occurred, prolonged intubation may be needed, for days or even weeks, and the patient is more prone to secondary damage to the tracheal mucosa with stenosis at the tracheostomy site and at the level of the balloon pressure on the trachea.

After the tracheostomy tube has been removed, the patient should be observed closely for the next 30 minutes to evaluate its ability to ventilate through the upper airway. If ventilation is normal after 30 minutes, the patient is monitored every two to four hours for 24 hours. If the patient becomes distressed, the original tube is replaced for another 24 to 72 hours and the procedure is repeated.

The airway may be open but narrow with ventilation slightly deficient, or the tube may have been supporting a weak airway wall that slowly collapses after extubation. These problems are difficult to detect initially and are manifested by a slowly developing respiratory insufficiency over hours or days. If this occurs, the airway is re-evaluated endoscopically and a plan for surgical repair or long-term support (e.g., Montgomery T tube) is determined.

A Montgomery T tube is used in patients with laryngeal or tracheal damage that has a high probability of leading to stenosis[16] (see Fig. 65–4, page 994). The soft silicone rubber tube just fits into the lumen of the trachea. The tube has no cuff and serves more as a support (stent) than as an airway. The side-arm of the tube extends out of the tracheostomy and stabilizes the tube in place. The side-arm is plugged, when possible, to prevent drying of the mucosa and to reduce mucus production.[13] Maintenance of the tube is similar to a regular tracheostomy tube. The tube is cleaned *in situ* with suction equipment, or the tube is flexible enough to be removed through the tracheostomy and replaced after cleaning.

After extubation is complete and the airway is adequate, the tracheostomy either is allowed to granulate closed or is surgically repaired. Surgical repair is selected in patients that did not undergo tracheal ring excision (see Chapter 65) or that can tolerate tracheal resection and anastomosis, in order to reduce the chance of local stenosis.

Local infection is always a concern, since many of these patients are being treated with corticosteroids to reduce inflammation and granulation tissue. Thus, broad-spectrum antibiotics are used with the steroids until all skin and mucosal surfaces have healed.[13]

RESPIRATORY SUPPORT

Volume of air movement during ventilation is an important factor in the postoperative patient. Reasonable air movement without excessive work is desired and subjectively evaluated in the extubated patient. In the intubated patient, a pneumotachometer can be attached to the endotracheal tube to measure tidal volume. This is a critical evaluation in the postoperative patient and a difficult one to assess correctly in the pharmacologically depressed patient. Shallow breaths can reflect CNS depression, incision pain, or lung compression.

Hypoventilation of central nervous system origin can be diagnosed by evaluating other responses (e.g., conscious sensory responses and reflexes) to assess CNS depression. Narcotics, anesthetics, anesthetic accidents, and incision pain should be considered as causes of hypoventilation and should be appropriately treated.

The work of ventilation accomplished by the muscles of the chest, diaphragm, and abdomen increases considerably in dyspneic and hyperpneic patients.[20] An increase in cardiac output needed by the muscles of ventilation can be as much as five to seven times above that at rest. Thus, the heavy workload of strenuous respiration can deprive the rest of the body of needed energy. The ventilating muscles may in turn be deprived of adequate energy to maintain ventilation in low cardiac output states and may eventually fail.[23] This process can also occur during rapid and sustained contractions of muscle, which interfere with its blood supply. Thus, a more normal energy balance and blood flow distribution between tissues is attained in patients in respiratory distress by mechanically assisting ventilation and providing an oxygen-rich atmosphere.[19]

Respiratory support may be required only during the immediate postoperative period or for several days. It may entail an elevated oxygen atmosphere, assisted ventilation, complete positive ventilation, or positive end-expiratory pressure (PEEP) (see Chapter 188). Most postoperative patients are safely and rapidly removed from oxygen therapy, with or without assisted or controlled positive-pressure ventilation.

Hypercarbia and acidemia are overlooked in oxygen therapy and are frequently the cause of respiratory distress after oxygen therapy is started. They are related to inadequate ventilation and respond to assisted ventilation with air or oxygen. Hypoxemia requires the addition of oxygen to the ventilating gas. Failure of the patient to respond to this treatment requires careful evaluation of the arterial and venous blood gas and pH levels, volume of air (gas) moved, and cardiovascular function. Continued hypoventilation, hypoxemia, and hypocarbia require prolonged respiratory support. The system used is dictated by the type of ventilatory assistance and the gas atmosphere needed.

Prolonged breathing of a high-oxygen atmosphere can depress pulmonary surfactant activity, predisposing to alveolar collapse. Oxygen concentrations of 30 to 50 per cent are usually satisfactory to correct hypoxemia caused by most respiratory disease.[15] The effectiveness of oxygen therapy is determined by monitoring the physical response of the patient and changes in arterial and venous blood gas levels. High oxygen tension in inspired gas as well as infection and inflammation inhibit ciliary function[11, 24] and dehydrate mucus in the airway. Thick mucus may obstruct small airways and trap oxygen-rich gas in the lung segments. The oxygen is rapidly absorbed and the region becomes atelectatic. Collapse is enhanced, and re-expansion is more difficult if the surfactant level is low. The chance that this disorder will develop can be reduced by humidifying the oxygen delivered, keeping the oxygen concentration as low as possible while still adequately oxygenating the patient, and using oxygen therapy only as long as it is absolutely needed. Humidification is used to prevent drying of the mucous membranes and to decrease the viscosity of mucus produced in the airway. If additional moisture is needed to reduce mucus viscosity, a nebulizer is used in place of a humidifier (see "Airway Hydration").

Bronchial dilators are used with humidification to aid movement of water into and mucus out of the small airways. Isoetharine hydrochloride (.25 to .5 ml of 0.5% solution) can be nebulized in saline and aminophylline (10 mg/kg) can be given intravenously four to six times per day.[6]

Oxygen Delivery

A face mask is a simple method of supplying an oxygen-rich atmosphere to the patient, although the awake patient tends to resist its application. Considerable oxygen is lost in flushing expired gases out of the mask and leakage around the mask. In addition, attempts to provide ventilatory support through a face mask may result in gastric distension and pressure on the diaphragm.

A more effective delivery system of oxygen is via an intranasal or transtracheal tube.[14] A measured oxygen flow is delivered through a well-lubricated soft rubber tube placed through the nostril and advanced into the nasopharynx so that the tip lies dorsal to the soft palate. The tube is taped to the nose or head and neck to allow more freedom of head movement.

The transtracheal method uses a technique similar to that for a transtracheal wash.[11, 14] A small flexible catheter (14- or 16-gauge) is passed into the trachea through a needle pushed through the skin and cricothyroid membrane. The needle is withdrawn, and the catheter is passed into the distal cervical trachea. The external catheter is taped in place to allow head and neck movement without dislodging of the catheter.

Both the nasal and transtracheal techniques require less oxygen (two to four liters) than the face mask and a system to deliver humidified oxygen.[14] The patient has greater freedom of movement, an assistant is not needed to hold the face mask in place, and the patient can be examined (especially in the head region) and treated more conveniently.

An oxygen cage with heat and humidity control provides a convenient oxygen-rich moist atmosphere for long-term oxygen therapy. The conscious animal tolerates the system well as long as the noise level of the cooling unit's compressor is low. The oxygen level seldom can be maintained above 60 per cent in oxygen cages, and the oxygen-rich atmosphere is lost each time the door is opened to examine or treat the patient.[14]

Assisted or controlled positive-pressure respiration is needed to treat hypoventilation and improve oxygen transport.[15, 19] It provides the energy needed to expand the collapsing (atelectatic) lungs and to increase tidal volume. The trachea must be intubated with a tube (endotracheal or tracheostomy) fitted with a large-volume, low-pressure cuff.[15] Either a rebreathing or a nonrebreathing system can be used; the former uses less oxygen. The tracheostomy tube is tolerated by most conscious patients and is the method of choice for long-term ventilatory assistance. Moist oxygen or room air is needed for long-term therapy. The lowest oxygen concentration that provides adequate oxygenation is used, in order to decrease the chance of oxygen toxicity.

Ventilation assistance can be augmented by positive end-expiratory pressure (PEEP) therapy. PEEP opposes the development of atelectasis and pulmonary edema by maintaining a minimum positive pressure (5 to 10 cm H_2O) within the distal airways at all times.[15] It should be used only in the patient with a closed chest, because an open chest allows overexpansion of the lungs and the development of emphysema.

PEEP and positive-pressure respiration elevate intrathoracic pressure in the closed chest and decrease venous return to the heart, thereby decreasing cardiac output and tissue perfusion.[15] These techniques should be limited to patients requiring this type of therapy in practices with equipment capable of safely providing the therapy and trained personnel for constant monitoring.

The conscious patient in respiratory distress becomes less anxious, lies down and rests, and has a more normal respiratory rate when therapy is adequate. The response of the unconscious patient is monitored by a return toward normal respiratory rate, tidal volume, heart rate, ECG, blood gas levels, and mucous membrane color. If the patient doesn't respond to therapy, at least to some degree, within five to fifteen minutes, the treatment must be re-evaluated.

Body Position

The patient that was in lateral recumbency should not be turned to its opposite side during recovery from anesthesia. The "down" lung during anesthesia is overperfused and underventilated and can be partially atelectatic. If the "down" lung is positioned on top during recovery, its weight may interfere with ventilation of the other lung, particularly if the lungs were packed off during chest surgery and pneumothorax or atelectasis is still present.

After the patient is sufficiently awake, it is placed in sternal recumbency to allow both lungs to be expanded and congestion to dissipate.

Lung Expansion

Pneumothorax is the most common postoperative complication leading to lung compression. The thorax remains partially distended during expiration. Chest percussion and auscultation are the quickest methods to evaluate the presence of air in the pleural space. Extreme care should be used to prevent iatrogenic lung laceration during needle aspiration of the chest (see Chapter 41).

Atelectasis and shallow respiration are common in patients that have undergone thoracic surgery. Adequate chest drainage, positive-pressure respiration (especially with 5 to 10 cm H_2O positive end-expiratory pressure), and intercostal local anesthesia aid significantly in attaining lung expansion. Chest drainage is discussed in Chapter 41.

Local anesthesia of the chest incision is attained by placing bupivacaine (0.5 per cent) or mepivacaine (2 per cent) hydrochloride around the intercostal nerves supplying the surgical region. This procedure gives four to eight hours of analgesia. The patient breathes more deeply and relaxes during recovery without being sedated.[15] Maximum doses of local anesthetics should not be exceeded.

Airway Hydration

Ultrasonic nebulization is used to provide a moisture-rich atmosphere to assist in reducing the viscosity of mucus in the airways and protect the airway mucosa from the drying action of a high-oxygen atmosphere.[8] It is a poor method to deliver drugs to the small bronchi and alveoli. Overhydration of small (less than 5 kg) patients, overheating (dogs and cats are unable to cool themselves in 100 per cent humidity), and contamination (nebulized bacteria, viruses) are problems to be avoided.[14]

Nebulizing equipment provides much more water than humidifiers and thus hydrates the airway rapidly. Intermittent therapy (30 to 40 minutes three to four times per day) is done in a closed cage to hydrate and loosen mucus and exudates. Each period of therapy is followed by mild exercise, chest coupage and vibration, and cough induction to assist removal of secretions.[14]

Causes of Inadequate Ventilation

If inadequate ventilation is still apparent (high Pa_{CO_2}) after the aforementioned treatments are given, some of the following causes should be considered: a tight chest bandage, distended stomach, depression, paralysis of the respiratory muscles, persistent atelectasis and pneumothorax, lung lobe torsion, inhalation pneumonia, pulmonary contusion, and pulmonary edema, as well as hypothermia, anemia, and hypoperfusion.

Tight Body Bandage

A tight padded bandage to protect the chest incision or chest drain can inadvertently interfere with expansion of the chest, especially in the anesthetized patient with shallow respiratory movements and less muscle tone. A chest bandage should be checked after it is in place, preferably with the patient in sternal recumbency or standing. One or two fingers should be placed under the bandage and held there for two or three respirations, in each of several locations around the chest. The bandage should be tight only at the end of inspiration.

Inhalation Pneumonia

Aspiration of low-pH gastric contents during recovery from anesthesia can be fatal, especially with existing airway disease. Rapid treatment (alveolar lavage, corticosteroids, and positive-pressure respiration) is critical to reduce pulmonary tissue damage.[3, 4, 9] Injury to alveolar epithelium and endothelium predisposes to pulmonary edema, especially in patients that require large volumes of fluid.[17, 18] Involvement of more than one lung lobe has a high mortality (90 per cent).[3]

Alveolar lavage of the affected lobes with small amounts (4 to 5 ml) of 7.5 per cent sodium bicarbonate solution is aimed at neutralizing the acid and removing particles of material to reduce the severity of the damage.[9] A larger volume of this solution might lead to foaming. Lavage must be done immediately, because delays of 15 to 20 minutes allow significant damage to occur. Lavage is the most important treatment.

Corticosteroids are given to reduce the extent of injury and subsequent inflammation, although they do not change the morbidity or mortality rates under experimental conditions.[17] Positive-pressure ventilation reduces the magnitude of intrapulmonary shunting and the tendency to develop thrombosis of small pulmonary arteries.[4]

Phrenic Nerve Injury

Paralysis of the diaphragm occurs after bilateral phrenic nerve transection during surgery or as part of bilateral brachial plexus avulsion. Such paralysis may interfere with ventilation, especially when combined with depressed skeletal muscle function or other disease processes that reduce lung capacity (e.g., general anesthesia, lung lobe torsion, pleural fluid, lobectomy, pneumonia).

Occasionally a segment of each nerve is removed

with a mediastinal mass, and nothing less than nerve grafting and anastomosis would be reasonable therapy. However, such measures would not change the inefficient ventilation during the recovery from anesthesia, during which time respiratory support could be needed.

Unsuspected bilateral phrenic nerve damage is signalled by excessive abdominal muscle activity during respiration, paradoxical respiration (abdominal collapse during inspiration), and little change in the shadow of the diaphragm during fluoroscopy. Unilateral phrenic nerve paralysis is usually asymptomatic.

Atelectasis

Atelectasis (pulmonary collapse) is caused by complete airway obstruction (blood clots, mucus plug, foreign body, lung lobe torsion), external lung compression (pleural effusion, pneumothorax, "packing off" during surgery) and hypoventilation during inhalation anesthesia. Atelectasis is prolonged or exacerbated by decreased mucus clearance, shallow respiration, depressed cough reflex, and continued lateral recumbency.[14] Thus, the postoperative patient is a prime candidate for atelectasis, which is usually manifested by prolonged recovery from anesthesia, polypnea, cyanosis, and reduced arterial oxygen pressure. The reduction in ventilation-perfusion ratio is the primary cause of hypoxemia.[14] Prevention in the surgical patient is attained by light terminal anesthesia, adequate lung inflations during anesthesia, reduction of the time of lung compression from surgical packing to 30 minutes, positive-pressure ventilation to inflate atelectatic lung caused by surgical packing, adequate chest drainage to remove residual pneumothorax and pleural fluid, and use of local anesthesia of the chest wall incision at the end of the operation.

Postoperative treatment of suspected atelectasis is aimed at adequate lung inflation, sufficient oxygen concentration to reverse hypoxemia, and removal of bronchial secretions. If this meets with only limited success, positive-pressure respiration and positive end-expiratory pressure are needed to reverse the atelectasis. Room air is used, after adequate lung inflation is established and hypoxemia has been eliminated, to reduce the alveolar oxygen concentration and rapid absorption collapse of alveoli (see "Oxygen Delivery"). Thoracic radiographs are taken to rule out other problems. Failure to correct the atelectasis predisposes the patient to pneumonia.

Lung Lobe Torsion

Lung lobe torsion can occur during thoracic surgery as a result of accidental displacement or improper replacement of one or more of the lobes. Thus, prevention is the best approach, and careful inspection of lung lobe orientation at the end of a thoracic procedure and chest drain placement is very important. The diagnosis, pathogenesis, and treatment of lung lobe torsion are discussed in Chapter 65.

Pulmonary Edema

Most cases of pulmonary edema in postoperative patients result from increased pulmonary capillary permeability.[22] Edema, congestion, and hemorrhage in lung tissue reduce the capacity both to ventilate and to transfer gases across the alveolar wall. Increased crackles and areas of no lung sounds indicate possible fluid accumulation in lung tissue and can be accompanied by dyspnea, polypnea, and cyanosis.

Aggressive treatment is necessary in patients that do not respond to high oxygen tension environment. Sedation with small doses of morphine (0.05 to 0.1 mg/kg every two to three minutes) intravenously is done to control the effect of the drug.[7, 21] The endpoint is relief of the anxiety and dyspnea. Intravenous fluids are stopped, sternal (rather than lateral) recumbency is encouraged, and cough reflex is stimulated by a tracheal or laryngeal squeeze and chest slap.[15] If there is considerable airway fluid, oxygen therapy is of marginal benefit without additional treatment.

Reduction of pulmonary fluid is accomplished by reducing total body fluid (diuretics), inflammation (corticosteroids), and airway fluid (suction and reducing surface tension of existing fluid).[21] The diuretic of choice for acute pulmonary edema secondary to fluid overload or excessive pulmonary hydrostatic pressure is furosemide (1.0 to 2.0 mg/kg) given intravenously and repeated in two hours if needed.[21]

Corticosteroids are given in relatively high initial doses and rapidly decreased.[7] Dexamethasone (0.5 to 1.0 mg/kg body weight) given intravenously or subcutaneously every eight hours is effective. Prednisolone (5 to 10 mg/kg) is also used.

Nebulization of 20 to 30 per cent ethyl alcohol in saline solution in a cool oxygen cage (maximum 65°F [18°C]) helps break down frothy bronchial fluid.[8, 13] Similar therapy can be combined with positive-pressure ventilation through a tracheostomy tube to provide good lung expansion and PEEP to reduce fluid accumulation. This therapy requires nursing staff to maintain constant monitoring. Frequent changes in patient status require alteration of therapy. Tracheal suction is used in conjunction with alcohol nebulization to remove major pockets of fluid (see "Airway Suctioning").

Alcohol nebulization is stopped when the airway fluid loses its frothy nature. The nebulized saline also provides a water source that hydrates (or overhydrates) the patient and needs close monitoring.[14, 15] The patient should be removed from the ventilator as soon as its unassisted ventilation is able to maintain adequate blood gas and pH values. The patient is monitored for recurrence of pulmonary edema.

Pulmonary edema as a result of left heart failure or low plasma protein is treated with rapid digitalization or plasma infusion, respectively.[7]

CARDIOVASCULAR SUPPORT

The maintenance of adequate blood pressure, cardiac output, and tissue perfusion is essential in the postoperative care and evaluation of the respiratory system (see also Section IX). Poor tissue perfusion has the same signs as respiratory failure (e.g., acidosis, hyperpnea, tachycardia) and interferes with interpretation of diagnostic signs. Peripheral pulse (rate and character), mucous membranes (refill and color intensity), heart sounds, and ECG are standard parameters for postoperative monitoring of the cardiovascular system. Maintenance of circulating blood volume with a balanced electrolyte solution, plasma, and whole blood is of primary importance. The packed cell volume should be maintained between 20 and 30 per cent to ensure good oxygen-carrying capacity, and the total serum protein level at 2.5 gm/100 ml to provide adequate oncotic pressure and viscosity of the circulating blood.[10, 11] Maintenance and monitoring of cardiac function, cardiac output, and tissue perfusion are discussed in detail in Chapter 29.

Fluid therapy is commonly used during surgery and is continued into the recovery phase to maintain patient hydration and to provide a ready avenue for drug administration. The length of time and volume of treatment depend on the fluid requirements of the patient. Sufficient fluid intake is needed at least to provide normal urine production, maintain circulating blood volume, and achieve adequate tissue hydration. Postoperative fluid therapy should be monitored carefully so that these needs are met but not exceeded. The patient with damaged lung tissue, septicemia, toxemia, or left heart failure has a greater tendency to develop pulmonary congestion and edema, which can be aggravated by fluid therapy.[18]

An isotonic, crystalloid solution similar in electrolyte concentrations to serum is used as a basis for most replacement therapy in respiratory patients. Plasma is added to combat hypoproteinemia (less than 2.5 gm/100 ml total serum protein) in high-volume therapy, although other oncotic agents (e.g., dextran, hydrolyzed starch) can be used. Whole blood is used only when the packed cell volume is less than 20 per cent in the acutely anemic patient.[11]

Any patient that has been fasted or is anorectic for more than 24 hours is or can potentially be hypoglycemic and should be given dextrose in the maintenance fluid. Low sugar reserves allow hypoglycemia to develop within 24 hours after surgery, during which time most patients have not been fed. Hypoglycemia could prolong recovery time, cause generalized weakness, and precipitate seizures, which can allow inhalation of gastric contents or damage surgical repairs.

HYPOTHERMIA

Hypothermia is a problem in the patient exposed to long periods of anesthesia or large incisions, especially with an open body cavity. It is common for the respiratory patient to have radiographic and endoscopic examinations in addition to a major surgical procedure. Hypothermia is likely to be more profound in the smaller patient with a larger ratio of body surface area to mass.

Prevention or reduction of the degree of hypothermia is important to aid in a rapid recovery from anesthesia and a return of normal metabolic function. Methods of keeping the preoperative patient warm are described in Chapter 63; similar techniques are used in the postoperative patient. It is important to provide a safe rewarming procedure and to monitor its effectiveness.

The aim of surface rewarming is to provide a continuous source of heat that produces a constant skin temperature of 10° C (18° F) above core body temperature but not exceeding 42° C (108° F). The hair and skin are dried to prevent heat loss from evaporation, and the body should be insulated from surrounding surfaces to prevent heat loss by conduction.

Moving warm air is used as the heating system in oxygen cages and can actually cool the patient with a damp or wet body surface. Therefore, if this system is used, the patient must be dry, and the air temperature well above body temperature (40 to 44° C [105 to 111° F]).

If the heat source is placed under the anesthetized or depressed patient, a relatively thick pad is placed between the patient and the heat source to prevent heat concentration at pressure points, to distribute the heat more evenly, and to reduce the chance of skin burns. When a heat lamp is used, the patient is covered by a light cloth to even out the heat distribution, to prevent "sunburn" of the clipped surface, and to shade the eyes and exposed mucous membranes.

The skin–heat source interface is monitored frequently "by feel" to evaluate temperature conditions. The skin should be warm but not hot to palpation. Core body temperature should be monitored continuously in critical cases to ensure a continued rise. A digital electronic thermometer that reads the temperature to the nearest .01° and uses a flexible probe is the most desirable system. The .01° sensitivity provides data that are constantly changing and indicate immediately the progress of rewarming. The core body temperature should increase at a relatively steady rate and should not "plateau" at a hypothermic level. Cessation of rewarming or increasing hypothermia requires evaluation and calibration of the monitoring equipment and heating system. Changing or combining heating systems can be required to attain the desired results.

Continous body temperature monitoring is also important to avoid *hyperthermia*. The patient is removed from the exogenous heat source but remains insulated from surrounding surfaces when the core body temperature reaches 38° C (100° F).

During the period of recovery from anesthesia, the patient responds to hypothermia by shivering. This intense muscular activity increases caloric and oxygen consumption. It becomes a significant problem in patients with other high oxygen demands (tissue trauma), low tissue and blood sugar (anorexia, hypoglycemia), and limited cardiopulmonary reserve. Adequate oxygen and caloric therapy are needed in these patients, whereas more normal patients are able to compensate with their own body reserves.

CHEST DRAINAGE

Chest drainage is an important component of the postoperative care of the patient after thoracic surgery. The details of rationale for use, technical considerations, and systems used are covered in Chapter 42. Specific items are worth stressing here, however. The security of the entire system is extremely important and requires close attention to details. The drain is sutured to the skin of the patient, and each junction of tubing is secured sufficiently to prevent leaks and resist disconnection by strenuous traction. The portion of the drain near the patient is protected by a body bandage and an elizabethan collar. The system should be rechecked periodically to assess patency and security.

The collection system and all connecting tubing to the patient are sterile to begin with and the tube lumen is kept in this state during all handling procedures. The one-way drainage system must be sized for the patient and the volume of drainage expected.[10] The Heimlich valve should be used only in medium to large dogs, since small dogs and cats usually do not develop sufficient expiratory pressure for effective drainage.[2, 10]

COUGH

Cough suppression after surgical manipulation of the respiratory system is generally undesirable.[15] A good cough reflex is helpful in a patient that needs to remove mucus, blood, and exudate from the distal airway or that has a tendency to inhale material from the upper respiratory system or during eating and drinking.

Chronic cough in patients with minor tracheitis secondary to sutures is treated with systemic corticosteroids (dexamethasone, prednisolone) and centrally active antitussives (hydrocodone, butorphanol).[6] Thus, the cough reflex is not blocked but is reduced so that the patient can have some rest. Nonnarcotic agents can usually provide this degree of relief.[24]

1. Bone, R. C.: Subglottic stenosis. Otolaryngol. Clin. North Am. 12:869, 1979.
2. Butler, W. B.: Use of a flutter valve in treatment of pneumothorax in dogs and cats. J. Am. Vet. Med. Assoc. 166:473, 1975.
3. Cameron, J. L., Mitchell, W. H., and Zuidema, G. D.: Aspiration pneumonia. Arch. Surg. 106:49, 1973.
4. Cameron, J. L., Caldina, P., Thoung, J. K., and Zuidema, G. D.: Aspiration pneumonia: physiologic data following experimental aspiration. Surgery 72:238, 1972.
5. Croft, C. B., Zub, K., and Borowiecki, B.: Therapy of iatrogenic subglottic stenosis: a steroid/antibiotic regimen. Laryngoscope 89:482, 1979.
6. Davis, L. E.: Antitussive therapy in small companion animals. J. Am. Vet. Med. Assoc., 108:1105, 1982.
7. Davis, L. E.: Management of acute pulmonary edema. J. Am. Vet. Med. Assoc. 175:97, 1979.
8. Harvey, C. E., and O'Brien, J. A.: Management of respiratory emergencies in small animals. Vet. Clin. North Am. 2:243, 1972.
9. Head, J. R., Suter, P. F., and Ettinger, S. J.: Lower respiratory tract diseases. In Ettinger, S. J. (ed.): Textbook of Veterinary Internal Medicine. W. B. Saunders, Philadelphia, 1975.
10. Kagan, K. G.: Thoracic trauma. Vet. Clin. North Am.: Small Anim. Pract. 10:641, 1980.
11. Kolata, R. J.: Management of thoracic trauma. Vet. Clin. North Am. 11:103, 1981.
12. Koopmann, C. F., Jr., Feld, R., and Coulthard, S. W.: Effects of antibiotics and injury of cricoid cartilage in cricothyroidotomy. Surg. Forum 30:507, 1979.
13. Manigila, A. J.: Tracheal stenosis: conservative surgery as a primary mode of management. Otolaryngol. Clin. North Am. 12:877, 1979.
14. McKiernan, B. C.: Lower respiratory tract diseases. In Ettinger, S. J. (ed.): Textbook of Veterinary Internal Medicine. 2nd ed. W. B. Saunders, Philadelphia, 1983.
15. McKiernan, B. C.: Principles of respiratory therapy. In Kirk, R. W. (ed.): Current Veterinary Therapy VIII: Small Animal Practice. W. B. Saunders, Philadelphia, 1983.
16. Montgomery, W. W.: Tracheal stenosis. In Surgery of the Upper Respiratory System. Lea & Febiger, Philadelphia, 1973.
17. Peitzman, A. B., Shires, G. T., III, Illner, H., and Shires, G. T.: The effect of intravenous steroids on alveolar-capillary membrane permeability in pulmonary acid injury. J. Trauma 22:347, 1982.
18. Peters, R. M., and Hogan, J. S.: Fluid overload and post-traumatic respiratory distress syndrome. J. Trauma 18:83, 1978.
19. Pinilla, J. C.: Acute respiratory failure and severe blunt chest trauma. J. Trauma 22:221, 1982.
20. Roussos, C., and Macklem, P. T.: The respiratory muscles. N. Engl. J. Med. 307:786, 1982.
21. Suter, P. F., and Ettinger, S. J.: Pulmonary edema. In Ettinger, S. J. (ed.): Textbook of Internal Medicine. 2nd ed. W. B. Saunders, Philadelphia, 1983.
22. Tranbaugh, R. F., and Lewis, F. R.: Mechanisms and etiologic factors of pulmonary edema. Surg. Gynecol. Obstet. 158:193, 1984.
23. Viires, N., Sillye, G., Rassidakis, A., et al.: Effect of mechanical ventilation on respiratory muscle blood flow during shock. Physiologist 23:1, 1980.
24. Zenoble, R. D.: Respiratory pharmacology and therapeutics. Comp. Cont. Ed. 2:586, 1980.

Section IX

Cardiovascular System

George Eyster
Section Editor

The anatomy of the cardiovascular system must be considered with respect to the thoracic cavity and the relationship between tissues of surgical interest and the surrounding external structures. The two most commonly used surgical approaches to the thoracic cavity are the lateral thoracotomy and the median sternotomy. Selection of one of these approaches will, to a large extent, be dictated by the anatomic exposure of surgically important tissues that can be obtained by the technique.

The left lateral thoracotomy through the fourth rib space is a suitable approach for several commonly performed procedures (Fig. 67–1). This approach provides adequate exposure of and access to the right ventricular outflow tract, main pulmonary artery, and ductus arteriosus. The brachiocephalic artery and left subclavian artery can be dissected and isolated as

they leave the ascending aorta cranial to the heart. The cranial and caudal venae cavae may be approached from the left, but because they lie to the right of the mediastinum, isolation requires deep dissection. The descending aorta and left auricle are also adequately exposed at the posterior aspect of the incision.

The left vagus nerve passes across the base of the heart, and the left phrenic nerve crosses slightly more ventrally. Fibers that make up the left recurrent laryngeal nerve leave the vagus at the aortic arch and loop around the arch caudal to the ligamentum arteriosum. The left ventricle can be seen through the fourth rib space, but adequate exposure for surgical manipulation usually requires an incision at the fifth or sixth rib space.

The ribs displace cranially more readily than cau-

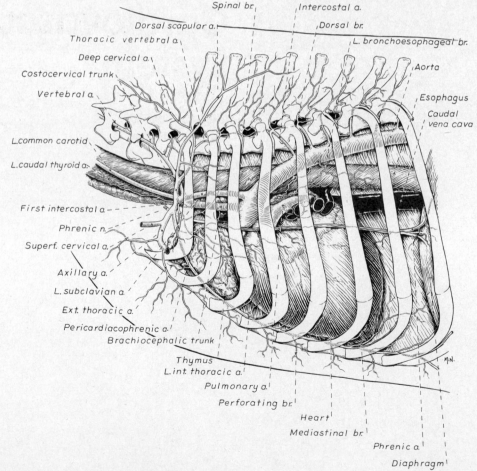

Figure 67–1. Arteries of the left thorax. (Reprinted with permission from Evans, H. E., and deLahunta, A.: *Miller's Guide to the Dissection of the Dog.* 2nd ed. W. B. Saunders, Philadelphia, 1980.)

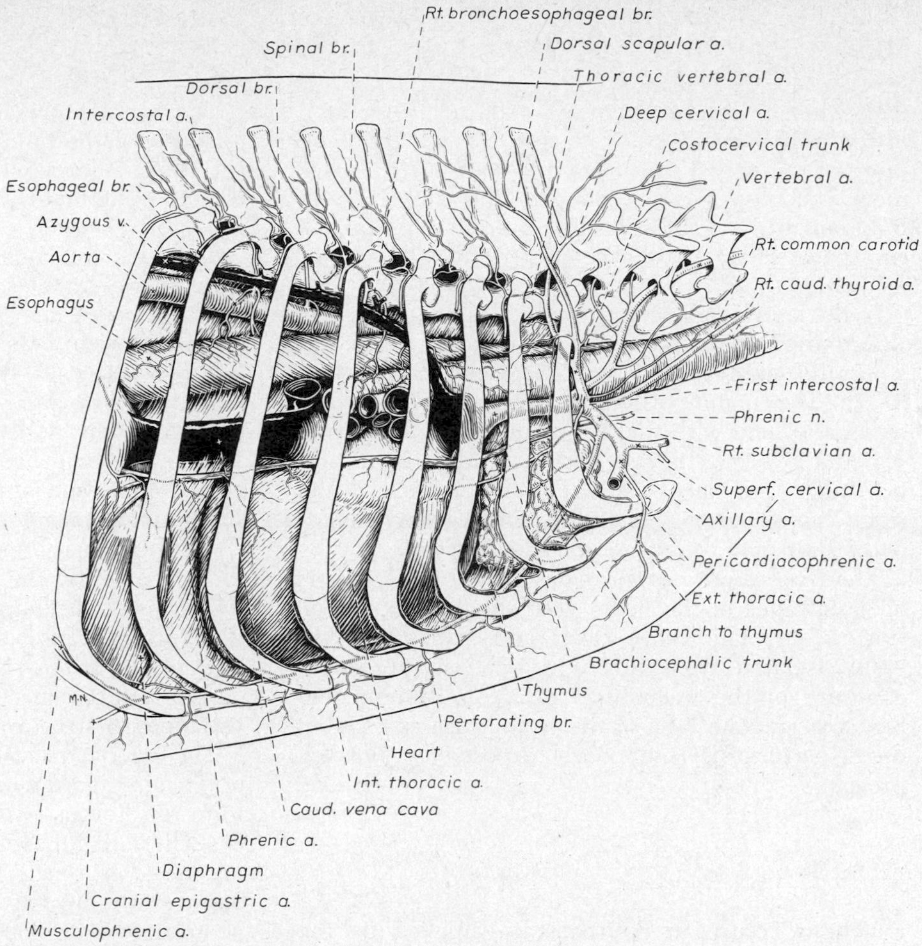

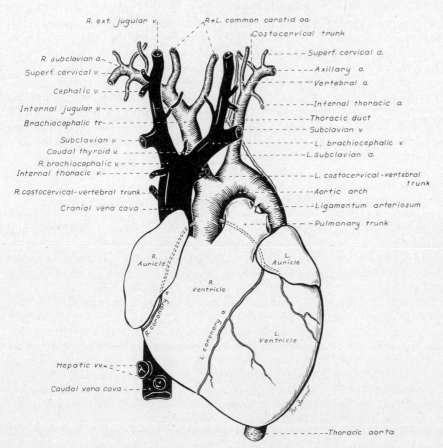

Figure 67–2. Arteries of the left thorax. (Reprinted with permission from Evans, H. E., and deLahunta, A.: *Miller's Guide to the Dissection of the Dog.* 2nd ed. W. B. Saunders, Philadelphia, 1980.)

Rt. bronchoesophageal br.

Spinal br.

Dorsal scapular a.

Dorsal br.

Thoracic vertebral a.

Intercostal a.

Deep cervical a.

Costocervical trunk

Esophageal br.

Vertebral a.

Azygous v.

Aorta

Rt. common carotid

Esophagus

Rt. caud. thyroid a.

First intercostal a.

Phrenic n.

Rt. subclavian a.

Superf. cervical a.

Axillary a.

Pericardiacophrenic a.

Ext. thoracic a.

Branch to thymus

Brachiocephalic trunk

Thymus

Perforating br.

Heart

Int. thoracic a.

Caud. vena cava

Phrenic a.

Diaphragm

Cranial epigastric a.

Musculophrenic a.

R. ext. jugular v.

R.+L. common carotid aa.

Costocervical trunk

Superf. cervical a.

R. subclavian a.

Axillary a.

Superf. cervical v.

Vertebral a.

Cephalic v.

Internal thoracic a.

Internal jugular v.

Thoracic duct

Brachiocephalic tr.

Subclavian v.

Subclavian v.

L. brachiocephalic v.

Caudal thyroid v.

L. subclavian a.

R. brachiocephalic v.

Internal thoracic v.

L. costocervical-vertebral trunk

R. costocervical-vertebral trunk

Aortic arch

Cranial vena cava

Ligamentum arteriosum

Pulmonary trunk

R. Auricle

L. Auricle

R. Ventricle

R. coronary a.

L. coronary a.

L. Ventricle

Hepatic vv.

Caudal vena cava

Thoracic aorta

Figure 67–3. Diagram of heart and great vessels, ventral view. (Reprinted with permission from Evans, H. E., and deLahunta, A.: *Miller's Guide to the Dissection of the Dog.* 2nd ed. W. B. Saunders, Philadelphia, 1980.)

dally when a rib space is opened, so structures located in the caudal third of the rib space may be exposed more completely if the incision is made one rib space more caudally. For the same reason, structures in the cranial thorax may often be suitably exposed one rib space caudal to that expected by radiographic evaluation.

Right lateral thoracotomy provides surgical exposure to the cranial and caudal venae cavae, the azygos vein, the right auricle, and the right atrium (Fig. 67–2). The main portion of the right ventricle is accessible, and with slight rotation the right ventricular outflow tract is also. The ascending aorta may be isolated, if necessary, from this approach. The right vagus nerve and right phrenic nerve follow paths similar to those seen on the left side.

Median sternotomy provides access to chambers on both sides of the heart with slight manipulation (Fig. 67–3). The venae cavae and azygos vein are easily isolated from this approach, and excellent exposure of the ascending aorta can be obtained. Structures at the base of the heart, such as a patent ductus arteriosus, are poorly exposed by this approach.

VESSELS

Venous return to the heart is supplied by the cranial and caudal venae cavae. Both vessels lie to the right of the mediastinal tissue and enter the right atrium. The azygos vein is the last branch to enter the cranial vena cava. The azygos vein originates dorsally in the abdomen and collects the dorsal intercostal veins on each side. The venous return supplied by the azygos vein is an important consideration during inflow occlusion and cardiopulmonary bypass.

The presence of a persistent left cranial vena cava has been reported by several authors.[2, 8, 9] Patterson[5] reported 13 cases among 290 dogs with congenital heart disease. This anomaly may occur alone or in conjunction with other congenital defects. Buchanan described the vessel as following the coronary groove until joining the coronary sinus and entering the right atrium near the opening of the caudal vena cava.[2] Because occasionally the right cranial vena cava is absent, the left cranial vena cava should not be ligated unless adequate alternative venous drainage is present. Although a persistent left cranial vena cava does not produce any clinical abnormalities, it may cause confusion during diagnostic angiography or surgical procedures.

The pulmonary trunk and its branches carry unoxygenated blood to the lungs. The trunk arises from the pulmonary fibrous ring and divides into the right and left pulmonary arteries. The pulmonary trunk contacts the aorta along its medial surface as the vessels spiral and cross each other. For this reason, isolation of either the pulmonary artery or aorta requires careful dissection to separate the desired vessel from the remaining one.

The ligamentum arteriosum arises before the bifurcation of the pulmonary trunk and passes to the aorta. Anatomical closure of this vessel does not usually occur until puppies are six to eight days of age.[6]

The right pulmonary artery leaves the pulmonary trunk at right angles and lies across the base of the heart between the venae cavae. The first branch enters the right cranial lobe and branches to supply the remainder of the right lung lobes. The left pulmonary artery is slightly smaller in diameter than the right artery. It divides into two or more branches. The smaller branches enter the cranial portion of the cranial lobe and the larger branch subdivides to supply the remainder of the left lobe of the lung.

The pulmonary veins return oxygenated blood to the left atrium. The pulmonary veins from each of the lobes of the lungs usually retain their separate structure all the way to the heart. Occasionally, fusion of veins from the right caudal and accessary lobes occurs before entrance to the left atrium. Other variations in structure also commonly occur.

The arterial blood supply to the systemic organs originates from the aorta. The ascending aorta arises from the fibrous base of the heart and turns dorsocaudally and to the left as the aortic arch and descending aorta. Normally the aortic arch arises embryologically from the left fourth arch; however, numerous anomalies of development resulting in abnormal development of the systemic arteries have been reported. The first large branch to leave the aortic arch is the brachiocephalic trunk, which terminates in the common carotid arteries and the right subclavian artery. The second major branch off the aortic arch is the left subclavian artery. This vessel has a rather extended course before it branches, allowing mobilization of the left subclavian artery for anastomosis in palliative surgical procedures for some congenital defects. The remainder of the aortic arch continues as the descending aorta until it terminates in the iliac branches.

NERVES AND INNERVATION

The autonomic nervous system, sympathetic and parasympathetic branches, provide the innervation to the heart. The effects of the autonomic nervous system include control of heart rate, rate of impulse transmission, and force of contraction.[5]

Parasympathetic innervation is provided by the vagus nerve. The right vagus nerve supplies fibers primarily to the sinoatrial node and the left vagus nerve to the atrioventricular node. The atria receive parasympathetic fibers as well, but parasympathetic innervation to the ventricles is minimal. Parasympathetic effects are mediated by acetylcholine and result in decreased heart rates and slower impulse conduction.[5]

Sympathetic fibers are distributed to both the atria and ventricles. These fibers originate in the thoracic spinal cord. Sympathetic effects are mediated by norepinephrine and produce increases in heart rate, impulse transmission, and strength of contraction.[5]

PERICARDIUM

The pericardium is divided into an outer fibrous part and an inner serous part. The fibrous pericardium is a thin sac that contains the heart and is continued on the arteries and veins associated with the heart. The apex is continued to the ventral part of the diaphragm, where it becomes the sternopericardiac ligament.

The serous pericardium has parietal and visceral layers. The parietal layer is fused to the fibrous pericardium. The visceral layer is attached firmly to the heart muscle. The pericardial cavity lies between these two layers. Normally this cavity contains a small amount of clear fluid but is a potential space that can expand and contain large amounts of fluid in pathological conditions.

HEART

The heart lies obliquely in the thorax with the base directed craniodorsally and the apex directed caudoventrally. A small area located on the caudodorsal surface adjacent to the apex is closely associated with the diaphragm. The remainder of the heart predominantly faces the sternum and ribs.

The heart usually extends from the third rib to the sixth rib, but variation is seen among different breeds. This fact is important in selecting the rib space for a surgical incision, especially in chondrodystrophic breeds. Normally the lungs cover most of the heart's surface, but the cardiac notch on the right side does allow direct access to the right ventricle. This anatomic relationship is useful during diagnostic and therapeutic procedures.

Internally, the heart is divided into four chambers which can be identified by superficial external landmarks. The coronary groove, which contains the major coronary vessels, demarcates the atria and ventricles. The interventricular grooves separate the right and left ventricles. The paraconal interventricular groove crosses the cranioventral surface of the heart, and the subsinosal interventricular groove divides the caudodorsal surface (Figs. 67–4 and 67–5).

CORONARY VESSELS

Blood supply to the heart muscle is provided by the right and left coronary arteries. They arise from the aortic bulb beyond the aortic valve. The left coronary artery is a very short trunk that divides into the circumflex, paraconal interventricular, and occasionally septal branches. The circumflex branch lies in the coronary groove and passes to the left and across the caudodorsal surface of the heart and turns toward the apex of the heart. Here it becomes the subsinosal interventricular branch (caudal descending coronary artery) (Fig. 67–4). Branches of the circumflex artery supply both the atria and ventricles.

The paraconal interventricular branch (cranial descending coronary artery) winds distally across the heart in the paraconal interventricular groove, reaching the apex of the heart (see Fig. 67–4). Branches supply both the right and left ventricles, the left ventricular branches usually being more numerous. The septal branch usually arises from the paraconal interventricular branch but may arise as a terminal branch of the left coronary artery. It supplies blood to most of the septum.

The right coronary artery curves to the right in the coronary groove. It is initially bordered by the pulmonary artery and conus arteriosus. The right auricle covers it dorsally. The major branch to the ventricle is the right marginal branch supplying the middle of

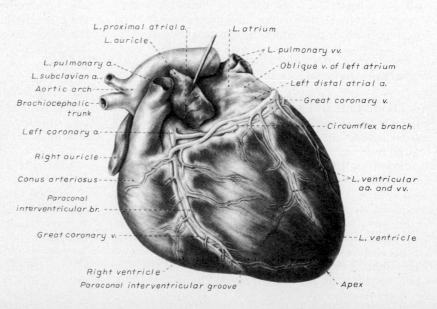

Figure 67–4. The heart, left lateral aspect. (Reprinted with permission from Evans, H. E., and Christensen, G. C.: *Miller's Anatomy of the Dog.* 2nd ed. W. B. Saunders, Philadelphia, 1979.)

L. proximal atrial a.
L. auricle
L. pulmonary a.
L. subclavian a.
Aortic arch
Brachiocephalic trunk
Left coronary a.
Right auricle
Conus arteriosus
Paraconal interventricular br.
Great coronary v.
Right ventricle
Paraconal interventricular groove
L. atrium
L. pulmonary vv.
Oblique v. of left atrium
Left distal atrial a.
Great coronary v.
Circumflex branch
L. ventricular aa. and vv.
L. ventricle
Apex

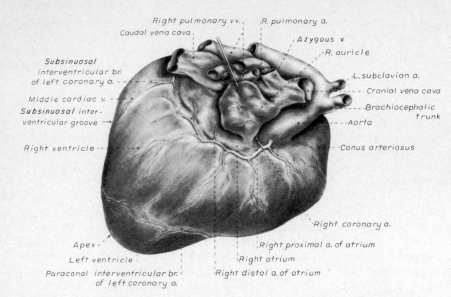

Figure **67–5.** The heart, right lateral aspect. (Reprinted with permission from Evans, H. E., and Christensen, G. C.: *Miller's Anatomy of the Dog.* 2nd ed. W. B. Saunders, Philadelphia, 1979.)

the right ventricular wall. An atrial branch that is larger than the other atrial branches supplies the sinoatrial node (see Fig. 67–5).

Venous return to the heart is primarily through the coronary sinus to the right atrium. The coronary sinus is the termination of the great coronary vein, which lies in the dorsodextral part of the coronary groove. It opens into the right atrium ventral to the caudal vena cava.

The great coronary vein originates near the apex of the heart and courses dorsally in the paraconal interventricular groove. It collects numerous veins from the ventricles and atria and completes its course in the coronary groove. At the level of the coronary sinus, the dorsal vein of the left ventricle enters the great coronary vein. The middle cardiac vein ascends the subsinosal interventricular groove and empties into the coronary sinus (see Figs. 67–4 and 67–5).

The right cardiac veins return blood from the right ventricle and enter the small cardiac veins or right atrium directly. The small cardiac veins are microscopic channels that enter all heart chambers but predominate in the right ventricle and right atrium.

FIBROUS SKELETON

The fibrous skeleton of the heart is composed of fibrous tissue and some cartilage. It forms the structural scaffolding of the heart and also separates the atrial and ventricular muscle masses. Electrical communication between the atria and ventricles is therefore limited to the specialized conducting pathways. The fibrous base consists of a narrow ring surrounding each of the atrioventricular valves and a scalloped ring surrounding each of the great arteries that leave the heart. The area between the two atrioventricular rings and the aortic ring is well developed and called the right fibrous trigone. To the left of this area lies the smaller left fibrous trigone.[4] The relationships

within the fibrous skeleton are important in understanding and characterizing congenital cardiac defects.

ATRIA

The right atrium receives venous blood from the systemic circulation and venous return from the coronary vessels. Systemic blood enters through the cranial or caudal vena cava, whereas coronary blood is returned through the coronary sinus, which enters the atrium from the left.

The intervenous tubercle, a transverse ridge on the dorsal wall of the right atrium between the vena caval openings, directs venous return into the right ventricle. Caudal to this structure is the fossa ovalis, a slit-like depression in the atrial septum. This is the site of the foramen ovale, which allows communication between the right and left atrium in the fetus. The opening functionally closes at birth because an oblique membranous flap does not permit flow from the higher-pressure left atrium to the right atrium. Anatomic closure occurs during the first few weeks of life.

The right auricle is a blind appendage that leaves the cranial surface of the right atrium and extends ventrally. The walls of this structure contain branching, interwoven muscle bands that originate from a semilunar crest or crista terminalis. This ridge separates the atrioventricular annulus from the cranial vena cava and also the main atrial chamber from the right auricle.

The left atrium consists of a main chamber and a left auricle. The left auricle lies caudal to the pulmonary trunk and overlies the proximal portion of the paraconal interventricular groove. The two atria are separated by the atrial septum. The dorsal aspect of the left atrium is the site of the pulmonary veins opening into the chamber. The right lung lobes drain

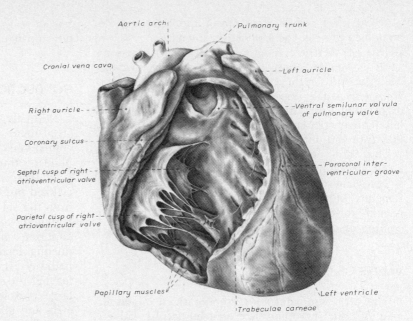

Figure 67–6. A dissection showing the interior of the right ventricle, ventral aspect. (Reprinted with permission from Evans, H. E., and Christensen, G. C.: *Miller's Anatomy of the Dog.* 2nd ed. W. B. Saunders, Philadelphia, 1979.)

craniodorsally and the left lung lobes caudodorsally. The membranous flap of the foramen ovale can be seen from this side.

VENTRICLES

The right ventricle, which is crescent-shaped in cross-section, lies cranial and ventral to the left ventricle in the thoracic cavity (Fig. 67–6). Because it functions in a lower-pressure system, the right ventricular wall is thinner than the left. The entrance to the right ventricle is controlled by the right atrioventricular valve. Blood leaving the right ventricle passes through the pulmonic valve.

Within the right ventricle the supraventricular crest separates the conus arteriosus and the right atrioventricular valve. Muscular projections, papillary muscles, give rise to the chordae tendinae. Although variation is common, there are usually three main papillary muscles in the right ventricle. The chordae tendinae arise from the apices of the papillary muscles and attach to the atrioventricular valve cusps. They prevent eversion of the valve leaflets; tear or rupture of the chordae tendinae may be associated with exaggerated valve motion.

The right ventricle has multiple trabecular ridges that run from base to apex and give the right ventricle a distinctive angiographic appearance. A muscular strand crosses the lumen from septal wall to peripheral wall. It is called the trabecula septomarginalis, previously known as the moderator band. This struc-

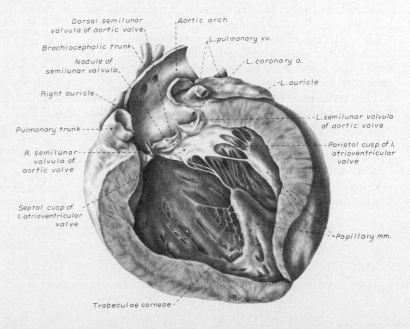

Figure 67–7. A dissection showing the interior of the left ventricle, left lateral aspect. (Reprinted with permission from Evans, H. E., and Christensen, G. C.: *Miller's Anatomy of the Dog.* 2nd ed. W. B. Saunders, Philadelphia, 1979.)

ture carries Purkinje fibers from the right bundle branch to the right ventricular free wall.

The left ventricle is conical and, since it functions as the systemic pump, has a thicker more muscular wall than the right ventricle (Fig. 67–7). The left ventricle usually has two large papillary muscles originating from the left ventricular free wall. The left atrioventricular valve and the aortic valve control flow into and out of the left ventricular chamber.

The interventricular septum is composed of a small, dorsal membranous portion and a more extensive ventral muscular portion. The membranous portion lies under the septal cusp of the right atrioventricular valve. Congenital defects in the septum most commonly occur in this area.[3]

VALVES OF THE HEART

The atria and ventricles are separated on either side by the right and left atrioventricular valves. They attach peripherally to the fibrous skeleton and are stabilized by multiple chordae tendinae. Innervation to the valve leaflets arises from the atrial subendocardium.

The right atrioventricular valve (tricuspid valve) has two cusps, the septal cusp and the parietal cusp (see Fig. 67–6). These cusps merge at their extremities and may form subsidiary cusps. The left atrioventricular valve, the mitral valve, is also a bicuspid valve (see Fig. 67–7). The valve is anatomically suited to the higher-pressure system in which it functions, because the chordae tendinae and papillary muscles are larger. The leaflets are also known as the septal and parietal leaflets. Common usage in humans identifies the septal leaflet as the anterior leaflet and the parietal leaflet as the posterior leaflet. These terms are also found in some veterinary literature.

The semilunar valves normally consist of three leaflets attached peripherally to the aortic or pulmonic fibrous ring. The free border of each cusp has a nodule in the middle that helps to complete the valve closure during diastole. Beyond the valve cusps lies a dilated area associated with each cusp. This forms the aortic bulb on the left side and a similar structure in the pulmonary artery on the right.

The pulmonic valve consists of right, left, and intermediate cusps. The aortic valve consists of right, left, and septal cusps. These cusps are more developed than on the right side because of the greater pressures in the left ventricle and aorta. The coronary vessels arise from the right and left aortic sinuses. It is important to appreciate the close relationship between the aortic and mitral valves at their common border so that surgical manipulations of one valve do not impair the function of the other.

CONDUCTION SYSTEM

Normally, cardiac impulses originate at the sinoatrial node, which is located at the junction of the cranial vena cava and right atrium. Nutrition is supplied by the sinus node artery. The sinoatrial node is composed of dense fibrous stroma containing specialized muscle cells.[1] Conduction across the atrium from the sinoatrial node to the atrioventricular node is thought to occur via the three internodal pathways (anterior, middle, and posterior). The major conducting load is carried by the anterior internodal pathway. It joins Bachmann's bundle shortly after leaving the sinoatrial node. Bachmann's bundle is a large muscle bundle connecting the right and left atria and allowing rapid distribution of impulses to the left atrium.[1, 7]

The atrioventricular node begins in the septal wall of the right atrium. It lies dorsal to the septal leaflet of the tricuspid valve and anterior to the ostium of the coronary sinus. The atriventricular bundle (of His) emerges from the atrioventricular node and continues ventrally through the fibrous base of the heart. The bundle divides into the right and left bundle branches. The right bundle branch traverses the septum as a single structure that branches near the right ventricular apex. The left bundle branch is broader and fans over a more diffuse area. The bundle branches terminate in the endocardium as Purkinje fibers.

1. Bigger, J. T.: Mechanisms and diagnosis of arrhythmias. *In* Braunwald, E. W. (ed.): *Heart Disease.* W. B. Saunders, Philadelphia, 1980, pp. 630–634.
2. Buchanan, J. W.: Persistent left cranial vena cava in dogs: angiocardiography, significance and coexisting anomalies. J. Am. Vet. Radiol. Soc. *4*:1, 1963.
3. Buchanan, J. W., and Patterson, D. F.: Selective angiography and angiocardiography in dogs with congenital cardiovascular disease. J. Am. Vet. Radiol. Soc. *6*:21, 1965.
4. Evans, H. E., and Christensen, G. C.: *Miller's Anatomy of the Dog.* W. B. Saunders, Philadelphia, 1979, pp. 632–654.
5. Guyton, A. C.: *Textbook of Medical Physiology*, 6th ed. W. B. Saunders, Philadelphia, 1976, pp. 183–184.
6. House, E. W., and Ederstrom, H. E.: Anatomical changes with age in the heart and ductus arteriosus in the dog after birth. Anat. Rec. *160*:289, 1968.
7. Netter, F. H.: *The Ciba Collection of Medical Illustrations.* Vol. 5: *Heart.* CIBA, Summit, NJ, 1969, pp. 13–15.
8. Patterson, D. F.: Epidemiologic and genetic studies of congenital heart disease in the dog. Circ. Res. *23*:171, 1968.
9. Stoland, O. O., and Latimer, H. B.: A persistent left superior vena cava in the dog. Trans. Kansas Acad. Sci. *50*:84, 1947.

Chapter 68

Cardiovascular Physiology and Pathophysiology

Mark D. Kittleson

INTRODUCTION

Heart failure is a common pathophysiological state. An understanding of cardiovascular physiology and pathophysiology is essential to recognize and treat heart failure.

Heart failure is the consequence of various diseases. Its treatment depends on the type of underlying disease and its stage. There is no simple definition of heart failure. Acute heart failure is a pathophysiological state in which a cardiac lesion or insult has resulted in a sudden decrease in cardiac output severe enough to create clinical signs of poor tissue perfusion; e.g., an anesthetic overdose. In chronic heart failure cardiac output has gradually decreased so that reserve mechanisms in the body are stimulated to retain salt and water, to increase heart rate, and to increase contractility, if possible, to compensate for the inadequate tissue blood flow. Chronic heart failure is characterized by a progression of cardiovascular abnormalities that usually starts with ventricular dilation secondary to increased salt and water retention within the vascular space. This progresses to increased ventricular diastolic blood pressures and edema with additional fluid retention and, finally, low cardiac output when the compensatory mechanisms are overwhelmed. In acute heart failure, dilation may not be present, ventricular diastolic pressure may be normal, and cardiac output may be low because of inadequate time for fluid retention.

CARDIOVASCULAR PHYSIOLOGY AND PATHOPHYSIOLOGY

The cardiovascular system has three essential functions: to maintain (1) systemic arterial blood pressure, (2) adequate tissue perfusion, i.e., cardiac output, and (3) venous blood pressures. The cardiovascular system works within a framework of priorities. As cardiovascular function fails, the lower priority functions are lost sequentially. The first priority is to maintain systemic arterial blood pressure within a normal range so that blood flow to essential organs is maintained. The next is to maintain adequate cardiac output to provide blood flow to all tissues, and the last is to maintain reasonable venous pressures.

A critical systemic arterial blood pressure is essential for the immediate survival of a patient. Flow to all tissues depends on the system having a certain driving force per unit area (pressure) within the circulatory system. The brain, heart, and kidneys need higher pressures (60 to 70 mm Hg) to maintain adequate flow than other organs because the resistance to flow through their vascular beds is greater than that of other tissues. The cardiovascular system maintains a blood pressure reserve such that mean pressure in the systemic arteries is 100 to 110 mm Hg. Without adequate cerebral blood flow mammals die immediately, so the cardiovascular system maintains a high cerebal perfusion pressure. For example, when an acute cardiovascular disease interferes with the heart's pumping ability, the sudden decrease in cardiac output (flow) results in a decrease in blood pressure (pressure = flow × resistance). The immediate response of the cardiovascular system to the decrease in cardiac output is to increase peripheral vascular resistance and return pressure to normal. This is done at the expense of blood flow, since the increase in resistance decreases cardiac output even further. This maintains flow to the essential organs but diminishes flow to less vital organs.

The next priority of the cardiovascular system is to maintain cardiac output. Without adequate oxygen delivery to all organs and muscles, anaerobic metabolism begins, resulting in cellular acidosis and cell death, followed by patient death within hours to days. The cardiovascular system uses reserve mechanisms to return cardiac output, and therefore oxygen delivery, to normal after cardiovascular injury. To accomplish this, the body increases catecholamine stimulation of the heart, which increases heart rate and contractility. In addition, the amount of fluid in the vascular space increases, resulting in increased diastolic blood volume in the affected ventricular chamber. The increased blood volume (volume overload) increases the stretch on myocardial fibers, which increases the force of their contraction (Frank-Starling mechanism). The increased diastolic blood volume also gives the ventricle a mechanical advantage in that it can expel a small percentage of its contents while achieving the same stroke volume. In this situation the myocardial fibers shorten less to achieve the same stroke volume.

As an example, a normal left ventricle with an end-diastolic volume of 80 ml and an end-systolic volume of 30 ml has a stroke volume of 50 ml and an ejection fraction of 62.5 per cent. If the contractility of this ventricle decreased and the ejection fraction decreased to 25 per cent, the end-systolic volume would increase to 60 ml and stroke volume would decrease to 20 ml. With fluid retention the end-diastolic volume could increase to 110 ml, which would bring the stroke volume back to normal while the ejection fraction (45 per cent) would still be markedly reduced from normal.

The increase in blood volume has a distinct disadvantage, however, in that it may result in increased venous pressure. In the normal dog there are low-pressure receptors in the cardiovascular system that monitor intracardiac diastolic and venous blood pressures. When these pressures rise above normal they activate changes that result in fluid loss from the vascular space. Venous pressures return to normal. These receptors are located in the left atrium, the ventricles, and the pulmonary arteries. In chronic heart failure these low-pressure receptors become desensitized to diastolic pressure increases, and diastolic pressures within the vascular space are allowed to remain elevated.[12, 39]

Systolic Function

The heart's ability to pump an adequate amount of blood to peripheral tissues is determined by four factors: preload, afterload, contractility, and heart rate. Cardiac output can be increased by a decrease in afterload or an increase in contractility, preload, or heart rate.

Preload

Preload is the amount of stretch placed on a myocardial sarcomere at the end of diastole.[29] Starling's law of the heart states that increased sarcomere stretch results in a more forceful contraction. The amount of stretch placed on this basic myocardial contractile structure is determined by the pressure in the ventricular chamber at end-diastole, the size of the chamber at end-diastole, the compliance of that chamber, the orientation of the sarcomere to the forces acting upon it, and the number of sarcomeres in series within the cell. Clinically, either end-diastolic pressure or end-diastolic volume is used to measure preload. Neither equate exactly with the degree of sarcomere stretch, since other factors play a role in its determination. However, they are readily measurable and important clinically. In chronic heart failure Starling's law helps increase cardiac output. Renal retention of salt and water and stimulation of thirst result in increased intravascular volume, specifically ventricular volume. Systemic venoconstriction occurs concurrently, shifting blood from systemic veins into the ventricles. This increase in end-diastolic volume dilates the affected ventricle, increases the diastolic stress on the ventricular walls, and effectively increases end-diastolic sarcomere stretch.

Renal retention of salt and water is extremely important in heart failure. It helps the heart compensate for its decreased cardiac output by increasing preload, but it produces many of the clinical signs usually seen in chronic heart failure.[15]

The renin-angiotensin-aldosterone system (RAAS) is probably the best explained system for salt and water retention in heart failure. Renin release by the juxtaglomerular apparatus is stimulated by many different mechanisms. This region is innervated by sympathetic nervous fibers, and beta receptor stimulation causes the release of renin. Stretch receptors also apparently lie in the media of the afferent renal arterioles. They detect decreases in afferent arteriolar blood pressure and stimulate renin release. The macula densa is a region of specialized tissue in the distal tubule that is closely associated with the juxtaglomerular apparatus. It plays a role in the modulation of renin secretion, but the mechanism is poorly understood. Some studies suggest that a decreased sodium load at the macula densa stimulates renin release,[36] whereas others show that increased sodium concentrations act similarly.[34] In addition, a number of humoral factors (sodium and potassium concentrations, circulating angiotensin II and vasopressin concentrations) also affect renin release.

Renin is an enzyme that converts angiotensinogen, a protein formed in the liver, to angiotensin I. This, in turn, is converted to angiotensin II by a converting enzyme found predominantly in endothelial cells of the lung. Angiotensin II is a potent vasoconstrictor[7] that also stimulates thirst[9] and aldosterone secretion.

Aldosterone secretion is controlled by angiotensin II, plasma potassium concentration, and, to a lesser degree ACTH. It is the final mediator in the RAAS system, and its major action is to promote sodium reabsorption and potassium excretion in the distal tubules of the kidney. Plasma aldosterone concentrations are elevated in dogs[21] and humans with heart failure.[8] The elevations in plasma aldosterone concentration are higher in dogs when the clinical signs of heart failure are more severe. Similarly in man, aldosterone concentrations are highest when patients are in severe heart failure and are clinically unstable. Therefore, aldosterone concentrations correlate well with clinical signs. Neither aldosterone concentrations nor clinical signs correlate well with hemodynamic parameters.

Along with the altered RAAS, changes in renal blood flow distribution, proximal tubular fluid reabsorption, circulating vasopressin concentrations, and possibly plasma concentrations of a natriuretic hormone aid in the retention of salt and water in heart failure. When cardiac output decreases, renal blood flow distribution changes so that an increased percentage of the renal blood flow goes to the juxtamedullary nephrons, away from the cortical nephrons.[33] Since the juxtamedullary nephrons travel deeper into the renal medulla, they are able to conserve larger quantities of sodium.

When cardiac output decreases, renal blood flow decreases. This decrease is probably disproportionately high compared with other organs because of afferent renal vasoconstriction, which occurs secondary to sympathetic stimulation.[6] To maintain normal filtration, the efferent arteriole of the glomerulus constricts secondary to angiotensin II stimulation. The afferent arteriole, although constricted, remains relatively dilated compared with the efferent arteriole. This increases the pressure within the glomerular capillaries, which increase the percentage of serum filtered from the blood (filtration fraction). This increase maintains a normal glomerular filtration rate, whereas total renal blood flow is reduced, until renal blood flow is severely compromised. The increase in filtration fraction results in the blood within the efferent arteriole and peritubular capillaries being relatively dehydrated or hyperosmolar as compared with normal. The plasma protein concentration (oncotic pressure) within these vessels is increased, and the hydrostatic pressure is decreased. As blood traverses the peritubular capillaries, a greater percentage of fluid is resorbed into the vascular space from the proximal tubules.

Plasma vasopressin (ADH) concentrations are elevated in congestive heart failure patients.[3, 11] Vasopressin aids in water retention and in severe, terminal heart failure. It can be present in concentrations high enough to cause hyponatremia. Vasopressin also stimulates thirst in heart failure patients, which helps increase intravascular volume.

For many years a hormone that promotes renal sodium loss (nutriuretic hormone) has been postulated to be present in normal animals. This hormone may be decreased in heart failure. To date its presence or absence has not been proved.[6]

In summary, with chronic heart failure, renal retention of salt and water, increased thirst, and systemic venoconstriction cause increases in intracardiac diastolic volumes. This increase in volume increases the stretch on the myocardium (preload), which enables it to contract more forcefully. The increased volume also gives the ventricle a geometric advantage so that the sarcomeres do not have to shorten as far to achieve the same ejected volume. On the other hand, this fluid retention is also harmful. If severe, it results in edema behind the affected ventricle by increasing intraventricular diastolic pressures. It also increases the size of the ventricular cavity, which, as will be seen in the following section, increases myocardial oxygen consumption by altering afterload.

Afterload

Afterload is systolic myocardial wall stress.[28] It is the force that opposes muscle shortening. If the myocardium was arranged as a linear strip of muscle with a weight attached to one end and the other end fixed, afterload would be the mass of the weight. In the heart, the weight, or force, that the muscle has to overcome to shorten and eject blood is approximated by systolic wall stress. Systolic intraventricular pressure is not synonymous with afterload because of the geometric considerations of muscle stretched around the ventricular chamber. The calculation of wall stress can be approximated by the formula ventricular wall stress = intraventricular pressure × chamber radius/ventricular wall thickness.[28] This formula should not be used for a thick-walled chamber,[38]

but it can aid in explaining the relationships that determine afterload. Based on the formula, afterload is increased whenever intraventricular pressure is increased, chamber volume (radius) is increased, or ventricular wall thickness is decreased during systole. In chronic myocardial failure, e.g., congestive cardiomyopathy, fluid retention generally causes the ventricle to dilate. This increases the chamber radius and causes the wall to thin. The net result is a large increase in afterload because of the increase in systolic chamber radius and the decrease in the wall thickness. The ventricle compensates for this by adding new sarcomeres to help lift the load and the wall thickens (hypertrophies), effectively reducing afterload. In pressure overloads, as seen in aortic or pulmonic stenosis, intraventricular pressure is increased but chamber size is normal. Again, afterload is increased, so the wall hypertrophies to decrease wall stress. This is concentric hypertrophy (a thick wall around a normal size chamber) as opposed to eccentric hypertrophy (normal to slightly thickened wall around a dilated chamber) in the case of a volume overload as in the previous example.

Afterload almost always increases when cardiac problems exist. The heart has only one way to compensate for it, i.e., to hypertrophy. If the heart cannot compensate, the sarcomeres are under a chronically increased load, which generally means that they cannot shorten as far, i.e., lift the weight as far. This means that the entire chamber does not eject its contents sufficiently and stroke volume decreases. An increase in contractility can offset this adverse condition but usually at a terrible price—myocardial hypoxia.

The amount of oxygen extracted from each unit volume of blood by the myocardium is much higher than in any other organ in the body. This means that myocardial blood flow is not as optimal as flow is for other organs. Subsequently, there is very little reserve for myocardial oxygen delivery. Therefore, myocardial oxygen consumption must stay within a relatively narrow range or myocardial hypoxia occurs. Myocardial oxygen consumption is governed primarily by heart rate, contractility, and afterload.[31] When any of these factors increases, myocardial oxygen consumption increases. These factors are usually kept within narrow limits in the normal animal so that myocardial hypoxia and resultant myocardial failure are prevented.

Afterload is highly dependent on systolic intraventricular pressure. The pressure that a ventricle generates during systole is determined by aortic input impedance, stroke volume, and velocity of flow. Aortic input impedance is another factor that increases in heart failure.[27]

Impedance is the force opposing forward flow in a system, e.g., cardiovascular system, where pulsed or cyclic flow is present.[26] *Resistance* is the term applied to the similar opposing force in a steady flow system. Impedance is a frequency-dependent characteristic. In a system of tapered elastic tubes, e.g., the mammalian arterial system, input impedence refers to the pressure-flow relationships at a specific frequency (heart rate) of operation. In the same system the term *characterisitc impedance* is used to refer to the arithmetic average input impedance over a range of frequencies, i.e., DC to the 10th harmonic of the basic frequency.

Aortic input impedance and characteristic impedance change with alterations in muscular tone in the arterial system, particularly at the level of the arterioles. Arterial compliance changes also affect characteristic impedance. Heart failure stimulates the constriction of these arterioles by increasing sympathetic tone and increasing circulating levels of angiotensin II. This action on arterioles causes an increase in input and characteristic impedance in the arterial system, yielding a greater opposing force for the ventricle to overcome while ejecting blood, i.e., a need for a relatively increased intraventricular pressure.

Aortic input impedance is determined by systemic vascular resistance, arterial compliance, and the inertance of the blood. An increase in resistance or a decrease in arterial compliance increases input impedance.

Contractility

The third determinant of cardiac output is contractility. Contractility is an inherent myocardial cellular property that can be changed by extracellular influences. Contractility, preload, and afterload influence the force and velocity with which the sarcomere contracts. One way to define contractility is to say that it is myocardial performance (force and velocity of contraction) independent of load. However, this does not provide any clearcut understanding of the principle of contractility.

The myocardial cell is made up of the usual metabolic and reproductive elements along with contractile proteins and proteins involved with calcium transport. The contractile proteins are actin and myosin, which make up the sarcomere. Myosin acts as an ATPase, which is stimulated by Ca^{++} and inhibited by Mg^{++}. When myosin combines with actin, the ATPase is activated, resulting in contraction. Two regulatory proteins are associated with the actin-myosin complex: troponin and tropomyosin. Tropomyosin is a rod like protein that intertwines through the center of the actin filament. Troponin is associated with tropomyosin but is a complex sitting by itself every 365 Å along the tropomyosin molecule. Tropomyosin prevents actin and myosin from interacting. Troponin regulates tropomyosin's position. Troponin is deactivated by Ca^{++}, resulting in tropomyosin moving so that actin and myosin touch each other and active contraction occurs.

Calcium ions are stored in the cell primarily on the sarcoplasmic reticulum. This protein structure actively binds Ca^{++} during diastole, keeping intracellular Ca^{++} concentrations around 10^{-7} M. During systole, the entrance of Ca^{++} into the cell during phase 2 of the action potential stimulates the release of calcium from the intracellular binding sites. This increases the intracellular Ca^{++} concentration to approximately 10^{-5} M[14]. Calcium binds to troponin and contraction occurs. The maximal force generated by a contraction depends on the number of troponin molecules that receive calcium. The rate of tension rise (dP/dT) reflects the rate at which Ca^{++} is bound to troponin,[17, 18] and maximal shortening velocity (Vmax) is determined by the rage of actin-myosin interaction.

Increasing contractility increases the amount of calcium released from the sarcoplasmic reticulum and the rate at which it is released. The increased systolic calcium release is caused by positive inotropic agents increasing the amount of Ca^{++} bound to the sarcoplasmic reticulum during diastole. Catecholamines with beta adrenergic activity increase the amount of intracellular cyclic AMP by stimulating adenyl cyclase. Cyclic AMP in turn stimulates a protein kinase system that phosphorylates a protein on the sarcoplasmic reticulum called phospholamben.[17] This phosphorylation allows the sarcoplasmic reticulum to bind more calcium during diastole and subsequently release more Ca^{++} during systole. Apparently beta adrenergic stimulation also increases the rate at which Ca^{++} is bound and released.

Preload (the amount of sarcomere stretch) also changes force development chracteristics of the myocardium, probably through changes in intracellular Ca^{++} kinetics. In skeletal muscles, an increase in muscle length results in an increased sensitivity of troponin for Ca^{++}. This may also occur in cardiac muscle.[18]

Heart Rate

Heart rate is normally controlled by the rate of diastolic depolarization in the sinus node. The rate of diastolic depolarization is altered by a variety of influences such as temperature, metabolic rate, sympathetic tone, and parasympathetic tone. Diverse influences such as fever, thyrotoxicosis, excitement, and exercise cause an increase in heart rate. Each situation that results in heart rate elevation does so because the body is demanding an increased cardiac output. The increase in heart rate is generally beneficial but may be detrimental to the heart because of the rise in myocardial oxygen consumption. Tachydysrhythmias that result in heart rates greater than 200 beats/min may also be detrimental because of inadequate ventricular filling time.

The integration of the three factors that determine stroke volume (preload, contractility, and afterload) is best explained with stress-volume loops (Fig. 68–1). Myocardial wall stress is represented on the abscissa and intraventricular volume on the ordinate. One cardiac cycle is completed with each loop. In this discussion the loop starts at point A, which is end-diastole. At this point the ventricle has a certain

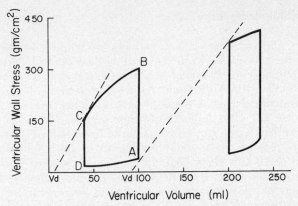

Figure 68–1. Stress-volume loops from a normal dog and a dog with severe myocardial failure. The loop on the left is from a normal 30-kg dog. Point A is end-diastole, point B is onset of ejection, point C is end-systole, and point D is onset of ventricular filling. The dashed line is Emax (contractility). Dead volume is labelled Vd. The loop on the right is from a patient with congestive cardiomyopathy and no secondary mitral regurgitation. End-diastolic volume is markedly increased. Contractility is markedly depressed and systolic wall stress (afterload) is increased because of the large increase in chamber diameter (chamber dilation).

end-diastolic volume, which can be determined by drawing a line perpendicular from the x axis to point A. This volume generates a certain ventricular wall stress (end-diastolic wall stress), which can be determined by drawing a perpendicular line from the y axis to point A. Point A represents ventricular preload. At point A active contraction also begins, so the mitral valve closes. Isovolumic contraction takes place between points A and B. As can be seen on the loop, wall stress rises, whereas volume remains constant (isovolumic). The wall stress increases because only intraventricular pressure increases during this phase of the cardiac cycle. The pressure rises because the ventricle is contracting against closed aortic and mitral valves. At point B the aortic valve opens. Between points B and C the ventricle ejects its contents against an afterload. Afterload (systolic wall stress) decreases throughout ejection. As can be seen in Figure 68–1, peak wall stress occurs at the onset of ejection. After that time intraventricular pressure increases mildly and then decreases while the ventricular radius decreases in size and the ventricular wall thickens, resulting in a reduction in wall stress or afterload. The volume change from point B to point C is stroke volume. Point C is the end-systolic stress-volume point where the aortic valve closes. The change from point C to D is isovolumic relaxation. At point D the mitral valve opens. From D to A the ventricle fills.

Contractility cannot be determined by analyzing one stress-volume loop. Contractility can be determined if afterload is changed acutely by altering systemic blood pressure. When afterload is increased by giving an alpha receptor agonist such as methoxamine, the end-systolic stress-volume point changes. End-systolic wall stress increases because of the increase in pressure. End-systolic volume increases because the myocardial fibers cannot shorten as far when the force that inhibits their contraction (after-

load) is increased and contractility is held constant. If several stress-volume loops are generated, each at different afterloads, a line can be drawn through the end-systolic stress-volume points. The slope of this straight line is called Emax. The intercept or the x axis is called dead volume (Vd). Emax and Vd define contractility. When contractility decreases, Emax decreases and Vd increases. A decreased Emax translates into a larger end-systolic volume for a given wall stress. As contractility decreases end-systolic volume increases, resulting in a decreased stroke volume if end-diastolic volume remains constant. The hemodynamic abnormalities in each type of heart failure presented in this chapter are explained with stress-volume loops. For purposes of illustration, a specific normal value has arbitrarily been chosen for each parameter. End-diastolic volume is 100 ml; end-systolic volume is 40 ml; stroke volume is 60 ml; wall stress at the onset of ejection is 300 gm/cm^2; and wall stress at end-systole is 150 gm/cm^2. Diastolic wall thickness is 1.0 cm and end-systolic wall thickness is 1.5 cm. End-diastolic pressure is 10 mm Hg.

Diastolic Function

To this point the discussion has been limited to systolic function of the heart. Diastolic function also influences cardiac function and can cause signs of heart failure. Diastolic function is the ability of the heart to fill during diastole. Diastolic ventricular compliance, ventricular relaxation rate, and filling time are the major factors determining the amount of blood that can fill a chamber and the diastolic pressure that results. Filling time is influenced only by heart rate. Compliance is the amount of pressure change generated for a given change in volume ($\Delta P/\Delta V$).[22] It is the reciprocal of stiffness. The stiffer a chamber is the greater the diastolic pressure in that chamber for any given volume of blood. Compliance decreases in myocardial failure,[23] and pressure overload and may increase in volume overload.[23-25] If a heart has a very stiff or incompliant chamber the patient may show signs of edema behind that chamber even though the chamber size is normal and systolic pumping ability is normal. The classic examples of this are hypertrophic and restrictive cardiomyopathies. Diseases that result in increased intracellular diastolic calcium concentrations, e.g., myocardial failure, may produce poor cardiac relaxation because of residual calcium on the contractile proteins. This results in the affected chamber needing more time to fill and higher filling pressures.

HEART FAILURE

There is a myriad of diseases and lesions that result in clinical signs of heart failure. Instead of discussing each disease or lesion as a separate entity, they will be divided into groups based on chronicity (acute versus chronic), clinical signs (forward versus backward failure), clinical severity (mild to severe) and type of failure (myocardial failure, volume-overloaded failure, pressure-overloaded failure). This organization allows clinicians to make more logical decisions when planning therapeutic interventions.

Forward versus Backward Failure

Heart failure may be forward or backward failure. Signs of forward failure are referable to low forward flow or cardiac output and occur because vascular beds are underperfused and poorly oxygenated. Clinical signs consist of weakness, lethargy, and decreased exercise tolerance. Laboratory signs include decreased cardiac output, widened arteriovenous oxygen difference, decreased mixed venous oxygen tension, and, when severe, azotemia and metabolic acidosis. Backward failure refers to high diastolic intracardiac pressures that result in edema in the tissues behind the affected chamber. The high pressures result from increased intravascular volumes or incompliant chambers. Clinical signs depend on which side of the heart is affected. Left-sided backward failure causes pulmonary edema and right-sided backward failure causes hepatomegaly, ascites, hydrothorax, or peripheral edema. Clinical signs depend on the location of the edema. Laboratory confirmation depends on pressure measurements of the appropriate venous or capillary bed. In right heart failure central venous pressure measurement confirms the diagnosis. In left heart failure pulmonary artery diastolic or pulmonary capillary wedge pressures are most commonly measured. However, the severity of the pulmonary edema on a chest radiograph probably correlates well with the pulmonary capillary pressures, so pressure measurements generally are not measured in veterinary medicine. They may be crucial, however, in selected patients to differentiate cardiac from noncardiac pulmonary edema.

Acute versus Chronic Failure

Heart failure is also classified as acute or chronic. Acute heart failure can be caused by anesthetic or other drug overdoses, dysrhythmias, acute myocardial trauma, or acute valvular lesions such as ruptured chordae tendinae and so on. It most commonly occurs as forward failure. These patients may be hypotensive because of poor cardiac output and may be in cardiogenic shock because of poor tissue perfusion. However, as in the case of ruptured chordae tendinae, backward failure can predominate. In chronic heart failure, signs of backward failure (pulmonary edema, ascites) usually predominate and are most apparent. Forward failure is usually present in a milder form in chronic heart failure in that cardiac output is adequate at rest but becomes inadequate when the patient is exercised. Signs of forward failure do become apparent at rest, however, when chronic heart failure becomes severe.

Clinical Severity

Chronic heart failure patients are commonly classified according to the severity of their clinical signs. Humans are classified according to a system devised by the New York Heart Association (NYHA). NYHA functional class I patients have evidence of cardiac disease, e.g., a heart murmur and an identifiable cardiac lesion but no evidence of heart failure. Class II patients have slight limitations of their physical activity and show signs of fatigue or dyspnea upon exercise. Class III patients exhibit clinical signs with any physical activity or are dyspneic when recumbent (orthopnea), and class IV patients have evidence of failure at rest.

Acute heart failure patients are generally recognized when their signs are severe and so are generally in class IV at the time of therapy. These patients should be classified according to Forrester's system, which separates patients according to presence or absence of backward and forward failure.[10] Subset I includes those patients with no evidence of backward or forward failure who have been mistakenly diagnosed as having heart failure or who have minimal heart failure. Subset II patients have backward failure only (pulmonary edema, high pulmonary capillary wedge pressure). Subset III patients have evidence of only forward failure (low cardiac output, low mixed venous oxygen tension), and subset IV patients have evidence of both. This classification system is useful when planning therapy for either acute or chronic heart failure patients. In general, subset II patients are treated with diuretics or venodilators or both, whereas subset III patients are treated with positive inotropic agents (if myocardial failure is present) or anteriolar dilators or both. Subset IV patients are treated with combinations of these.

Heart Failure Secondary to Myocardial Failure

Myocardial failure is defined as a loss of myocardial contractility. It can be primary or secondary. In Syrian hamsters, an inherited primary defect has been identified in the sarcoplasmic reticulum (SR).[24] This defect results in poor calcium binding by the SR during diastole and, subsequently, poor systolic release of calcium (poor contractility). A similar primary defect may exist in dogs, cats, and humans with congestive cardiomyopathy. Myocardial failure may also develop secondary to chronic pressure and volume overloads (aortic stenosis, mitral regurgitation). A similar SR defect develops in this situation that decreases contractility. Troponin also decreases its affinity for calcium, reducing the ability of the heart to respond to an increased preload.[32] In addition to the decrease in contractility, when the SR stops binding an appropriate amount of calcium, diastolic calcium concentrations increase. This is harmful to the cell in several ways. First, it results in poor removal of calcium ions from troponin and poor relaxation of the sarcomeres. Second, it causes cellular electrical instability.[35] The instability is usually manifested as increasing voltage fluctuations after cellular repolarization called late afterdepolarizations. If these voltage fluctuations reach electrical threshold, they result in cellular depolarization. On a surface electrocardiogram they occur as premature depolarizations. Third, the high diastolic calcium concentrations result in mitochondrial damage. When the SR can no longer bind all of the intracellular calcium, other intracellular structures increase their binding. The mitochondria bind up to 20 times their usual amount of calcium. This helps intracellular calcium kinetics but the calcium poisons the mitochondria, resulting in less efficient energy production.[16] This probably decreases contractility further.

The decreased contractility in myocardial failure initially results in a decreased stroke volume and a poor cardiac output. If the contractility defect occurs acutely and is severe, the patient shows clinical signs of poor tissue perfusion (poor mucous membrane color, prolonged capillary refill time). If the defect is very severe, hypotension ensues, which, if left untreated, causes death from cardiogenic shock. If the myocardial failure is chronic, the decreased cardiac output stimulates compensatory mechanisms. Intraventricular blood volume and heart rate are increased by the mechanisms explained previously. Catecholamine stimulation increases contractility in the remaining viable cells to compensate for the dead and dying cells. If the myocardial failure is not severe, the patient may only show signs of cough and dyspnea when exercised vigorously. If the failure is very severe, patients show signs of forward and backward failure at rest. The backward failure is due to the increased vascular volume and poor ventricular compliance. The poor compliance may be related to myocardial fibrosis secondary to cell necrosis and high diastolic intracellular calcium concentrations.

To illustrate the changes seen in myocardial failure an acute cardiac insult is postulated that results in a sudden decrease in left ventricular contractility. The decrease in myocardial contractility results in a decreased Emax (slope of the line joining dead volume and the end-systolic stress-volume point). This results in decreased myocardial fiber shortening, assuming that afterload and preload are constant. The decreased myocardial fiber shortening results in a larger end-systolic volume (the chamber does not eject as much of its contents) and a decreased ejection fraction and stroke volume. This results in an initial decrease in systemic arterial blood pressure and systolic intraventricular pressure and, subsequently, an initial decrease in afterload. Arteriolar constriction occurs and increases aortic input impedance. This returns blood pressure back to normal. The subsequent increase in afterload results in a further increase in end-systolic volume and a further decrease in stroke volume. Catecholamine release increases heart rate, which helps increase cardiac output and blood pressure, as well as stimulates renin release. The renin release, along with the other mechanisms for increasing circulating blood volume, results in an increased blood volume and cardiac dilation. Therefore the end-diastolic volume increases as the myocardial failure moves into the subacute and chronic phases. The increased end-diastolic volume results in an increase in stroke volume, an increase in end-diastolic wall stress, and an increase in afterload because of the increase in ventricular volume throughout systole. When the ventricular chamber initially dilates, the ventricular wall thins as it has the same mass stretched around a larger chamber. The thin wall also contributes to an increased afterload. With time the ventricular wall thickens as new sarcomeres are added into the wall. The wall eventually attains a slightly increased thickness, if it is able to respond normally, which reduces the afterload. Hearts with myocardial failure, however, are often unable to generate as much hypertrophy as hearts with valvular lesions and similar volume overloads (increased end-diastolic volumes).

As an example, a patient with severe chronic myocardial failure is illustrated in Figure 68–1. The patient has an end-systolic volume of 200 ml, an end-diastolic volume of 230 ml, a stroke volume of 30 ml, a wall stress at the onset of ejection of 420 gm/cm^2, and a wall stress at end-systole of 380 gm/m^2. The diastolic wall thickness is 1.0 cm and end-systolic wall thickness is 1.1 cm. The end-systolic volume has increased primarily because of a decrease in cardiac contractility. However, the increase in end-systolic wall stress has also helped increase the end-systolic volume by impeding systolic contraction. The end-diastolic volume is increased because of renal salt and water retention. There has been partial compensation for the decrease in contractility and the increase in afterload so that stroke volume is still reasonable but the dog is in forward failure because of the poor stroke volume. The increase in diastolic volume coupled with a decrease in left ventricular compliance has resulted in an elevated end-diastolic pressure. Subsequently the patient has pulmonary edema (backward failure). The large increase in systolic wall stress in this patient results in an elevated myocardial oxygen consumption. If coronary flow cannot compensate for this, myocardial hypoxia and a continuous deterioration in cardiac function will occur.

Myocardial failure is a disease that has been treated pharmacologically. The signs of backward failure are treated with diuretics, low-salt diets, and venodilators, all given to reduce ventricular diastolic volumes and thus reduce diastolic pressures and edema. Both backward and forward failures are treated with positive inotropic agents such as the digitalis glycosides, milrinone, and dobutamine. Unfortunately not all patients respond to the initial administration of these drugs,[20] and almost all patients lose their responsiveness to these drugs over time. The increase in contractility produced by these agents results in an increased cardiac output, which in turn results in less renal salt and water retention. Forward failure is also treated with arteriolar dilators in those patients refractory to positive inotropic drugs. The medical therapy of choice for this disease is some form of long-term positive inotrope since, this is the only therapy that prolongs survival time in the dog.[20]

Surgical therapy now appears to be an alternative therapy in man. Cardiac transplantation prolongs life significantly in those patients that do not reject their transplant. Artificial heart replacements may also become feasible means of prolonging life in the near future. Unfortunately they will probably be cost-prohibitive for animals.

Heart Failure Secondary to Severe Left-to-Right Shunts

A left-to-right shunt occurs when there is an abnormal communication between the systemic and the pulmonary circulations, resulting in increased pulmonary blood flow. They may be isolated lesions or parts of or in conjunction with more complex malformations. The effects that they have on the circulation and the type of heart failure that they produce depend on the location of the shunt (see Chapter 71). Regardless of location, left-to-right shunts produce a volume overload of the chambers or vessels involved. For example, a ventricular septal defect (VSD) results in shunting of blood from the left ventricle to the right ventricle. To compensate for the loss of left ventricular stroke volume, the body retains and takes in more salt and water to increase blood volume. A large part of this increase in volume (volume overload) is shifted into the left ventricle. A portion of this volume is ejected into the aorta to keep the forward cardiac output adequate, and the rest of it contributes to the abnormal flow through the VSD. Because of the increased diastolic volume in the left ventricle it becomes dilated. Larger lesions result in larger flows with a greater loss of forward stroke volume. As a result, the body must increase its blood volume more so larger lesions result in greater left ventricular volume overload and dilation. If the lesion is severe, massive salt and water retention results in elevated left ventricular diastolic pressures when the compliance of the left ventricular myocardium is overwhelmed, creating pulmonary edema.

In addition to the left ventricular volume overload, the structures into which the shunted blood flows are volume overloaded and dilated. These include the right ventricle, pulmonary vasculature, and left atrium in a VSD. If the VSD is in the inflow portion of the left ventricular septum, all of the right ventricle will be volume overloaded (dilated), whereas if it is high in the septum, only the right ventricular outflow tract may be overloaded. As such, right ventricular enlargement is variable in VSDs.

A patent ductus arteriosus (PDA) is similar, except the shunt is beyond the level of the right ventricle so it is not involved. An atrial septal defect (ASD) or anomalous pulmonary venous return creates a volume overload of the left atrium, the right atrium and ventricle, and the pulmonary vasculature. The left ventricle is not involved.

The size of the left-to-right shunt is determined by the resistance to flow across the defect, the pressure gradient across the defect, and the effects of streaming. The resistance to flow is generally determined by the size of the defect. The larger the defect, the less resistance it presents to flow. The pressure gradient is usually determined by the site of the lesion. As an example, a VSD has a high systolic pressure differential from the high-pressure left ventricle to the lower-pressure right ventricle. An ASD, on the other hand, has a very small difference in pressure across it. Large shunt flow can still be produced by an ASD because blood flow is preferentially shunted in a stream toward the defect.

Patent ductus arteriosus (PDA) is the most common congenital defect in the dog and by far the most common surgical procedure performed by the veterinary cardiovascular surgeon. It is an example of a severe volume overload causing signs of heart failure in which the myocardium is usually normal. In PDA a portion of the left ventricular stroke volume is shunted away from the aorta and peripheral tissues into the pulmonary artery. To compensate for the lost cardiac output, total blood volume is increased by all of the mechanisms discussed previously and systemic venoconstriction takes place. The net result is an increased left ventricular end-diastolic volume. Since end-systolic volume is normal and end-diastolic volume is increased, total left ventricular stroke volume is increased in compensation for the stroke volume lost through the PDA. If the PDA is small, this compensation results in relatively normal hemodynamics. However, if the PDA is large there must be a large increase in the left ventricular end-diastolic volume to compensate for the decreased effective stroke volume. This results in elevated left ventricular diastolic pressures and pulmonary edema. It is theoretically possible that a PDA could be so large that complete compensation for the decreased effective stroke volume could not occur; however, this rarely happens clinically. Therefore, most young dogs with PDA have heart failure with signs of left ventricular backward failure (pulmonary edema) and not forward failure.

Older dogs that have had a smaller PDA for many years are occasionally presented in heart failure. Often they are in atrial fibrillation. Usually these dogs mave myocardial failure along with their shunt. The myocardial failure occurs in these dogs secondary to the prolonged increase in cardiac preload, afterload, and myocardial oxygen consumption.

Left-to-right shunts that have resulted in heart failure have been treated as if myocardial failure was always present. This concept may be changing now that patients are being studied more rigorously by noninvasive techniques.[4, 37]

The evidence that dogs with PDA do not have myocardial failure is circumstantial. Young dogs presented with pulmonary edema secondary to PDA are surgically corrected and live a normal life. It is extremely unlikely that a dog with any degree of myocardial failure would live 12 to 16 years after ductus correction. In children with PDA, indices of myocardial contractility are normal when studied 24 hours after surgical ligation. When studied preoperatively, children with PDA have volume-overloaded left ventricles and left atria, increased shortening fractions, and normal end-systolic diameters.[1] This suggests a volume-overloaded state with normal contractility. Indices of ventricular function were not improved when digoxin was administered.[1] Therefore, positive inotropic therapy is not recommended for the treatment of young dogs with heart failure secondary to PDA. Instead, diuretic therapy is recommended to abolish the pulmonary edema prior to anesthesia. Surgical correction is the therapy of choice once the patient has stabilized.

The older patient presented with PDA, atrial fibrillation, and heart failure should be treated with a positive inotrope (digitalis glycosides, milrinone), diuretics, and so on, and surgical correction should be performed.

Other left-to-right shunts (ventricular septal defects, atrial septal defects, endocardial cushion defects, and so on) presumably follow a similar course. In early cases that have heart failure, the failure is probably secondary to a large volume overload associated with a large defect. As time progresses, myocardial failure probably becomes a contributing factor. Unfortunately the development of myocardial failure is variable and the only way to judge the severity of the decrease in myocardial contractility in a patient is to measure hemodynamic parameters.

One study has evaluated ventricular function in children with VSDs before and after digoxin therapy.[4] This study examined 21 patients with an average pulmonary to systemic flow ratio of 2.6 ± 1.1 (SD). Six had evidence of myocardial failure, whereas 15 did not. The group of six with myocardial failure responded clinically and hemodynamically to digoxin. None of the 15 without myocardial failure responded hemodynamically to digoxin, but 6 responded clinically. In eight of the patients that responded clinically, including three that did not respond hemodynamically, tissue oxygen consumption decreased. This suggests that the digitalis glycosides may improve the balance between tissue oxygen delivery and tissue oxygen consumption either by improving cardiac output, and therefore tissue oxygen delivery, or by decreasing tissue oxygen consumption. This latter possible benefit needs additional study before it can be used as a rationale for using the digitalis glycosides in heart failure patients without myocardial failure.

Accepted surgical therapy of VSD includes repair of the defect and pulmonary artery banding to increase the impedance to pulmonary flood flow. The latter decreases the left-to-right shunt. Accepted medical therapy includes diuretic administration to decrease the left ventricular volume overload and so reduce the amount of pulmonary edema and vasodilator administration. Arteriolar dilators reduce aortic input impedance, which reduces the magnitude of the left-to-right shunt. In one study in seven infants with a large VSD, hydralazine reduced the systemic to pulmonary flow ratio from 3.4 to 2.3 and decreased shunt flow from 10.8 to 8.2 L/min/m² by decreasing systemic vascular resistance index (one component of aortic input impedance) from 13.9 to 9.5 mmHg/L/min/m².[2]

Heart Failure Secondary to Severe Regurgitation

The pathophysiology of mitral regurgitation is very similar to that of ventricular septal defect. In each case the left ventricle ejects a percentage of its stroke volume into a low-pressure chamber. Each lesion creates a left ventricular volume overload that compensates for a less effective forward stroke volume. The degree of left ventricular volume overload (left ventricular dilation) is related to the magnitude of the regurgitation and the degree of myocardial failure.

Mitral regurgitation in the dog can be a primary or a secondary lesion. Primary lesions produce pathology of the mitral valve apparatus itself. Examples include endocardiosis of the valve, ruptured chordae tendinae, and bacterial endocarditis of the valve. Secondary lesions are the consequence of other disease processes. The most common example is mitral regurgitation secondary to congestive cardiomyopathy, in which the mitral valve and chordae tendinae are normal but the mitral valve annulus is dilated secondary to the left ventricular dilation. The annular dilation results in loss of normal valvular coaptation and subsequent regurgitation.[5]

The pathophysiology of mitral regurgitation in the dog depends on the type of lesion present. Mitral regurgitation secondary to congestive cardiomyopathy always has myocardial failure associated with it, and the mitral regurgitation is essentially a complicating factor. Mitral regurgitation due to mitral valve endocardiosis is very different, however. This disease of small dogs is associated with destruction of the valve, and myocardial failure is usually mild or absent. The signs of heart failure in this situation are created mostly by massive regurgitation and not myocardial failure.

Small dogs with primary mitral regurgitation due to endocardiosis and severe heart failure (class IV) have been studied to determine the pathophysiology of this disease. Early in the course of class IV failure (clinical signs of severe failure present for less than one month) myocardial failure is not present. After this time myocardial failure may be present but the tendency is for mild myocardial failure to develop. Those dogs with failure refractory to diuretic therapy generally have massive regurgitant fractions (89 ± 5 per cent) and variable degrees of myocardial failure.[19]

The primary reason for the signs of heart failure in this population of dogs is massive mitral regurgitation. Signs of backward failure are caused by the enormous quantity of blood ejected into the left atrium during systole coupled with the increased blood volume that occurs with renal salt and water retention. The left atrium dilates to accommodate this increase in blood volume, but at some point its compliance is overwhelmed. When this occurs left atrial pressures increase. Pulmonary capillary pressures reflect the left atrial pressures. When the hydrostatic pressures increase to a point that other Starling forces in the pulmonary capillaries are overwhelmed, transudation of fluid into the pulmonary interstitial spaces occurs. The transudate is initially removed via the pulmonary lymphatics. When this system is overwhelmed, edema fluid accumulates, first in the interstitial space and then in the alveolar space.

As long as the regurgitant lesion is not overwhelming, compensation for the loss in left ventricular stroke volume with fluid retention and an increase in heart rate occurs. Therefore cardiac output is generally normal or adequate at rest in most patients until the late stages of heart failure. Cardiac output may not be adequate for exercise. When regurgitation becomes overwhelming or moderate to severe myocardial failure appears, even the massive volume overload cannot compensate for the lost stroke volume and resting cardiac output becomes inadequate. This results in forward failure.

The stress-volume loop in Figure 68–2 depicts a

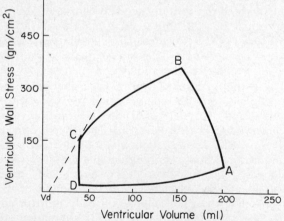

Figure 68–2. A stress-volume loop from a patient with severe mitral regurgitation due to endocardiosis and normal myocardial contractility. The end-diastolic volume is markedly increased, which increases end-diastolic wall stress and contributes to increasing systolic wall stress. There is no isovolumic systole because of the incompetent mitral valve, so volume decreases between points A and B. Since contractility and end-systolic wall stress is normal, end-systolic volume is normal. Total left ventricular stroke volume is markedly increased (160 ml), but in this patient 80 per cent is ejected into the left atrium.

patient with mitral regurgitation due to endocardiosis of the mitral valve. This patient has normal myocardial contractility. Therefore Emax and Vd are normal, which means that the end-systolic volume is normal (40 ml). End-systolic volume, pressure, and wall thickness are all normal, so end-systolic wall stress is normal (50×10^3 dynes/cm²). The wall stress at the onset of ejection is mildly increased (360×10^3 dynes/cm²), which means that total afterload (wall stress throughout systole) is increased slightly. There is no isovolumic systole in this disease because the mitral valve is incompetent, so there is blood leaking into the left atrium throughout systole. Total stroke volume of the left ventricle is the volume at point A minus the volume at point D. Total stroke volume of this ventricle is markedly increased to 160 ml because end-diastolic volume is increased to 200 ml and end-systolic volume is normal. In this patient most of the blood leaks back into the left atrium rather than being ejected into the aorta. The regurgitant fraction is 80 per cent, not depicted in the figure. As a result, for each heart beat 128 ml of blood is ejected into the left atrium while 32 ml is ejected into the aorta. The ejection fraction is increased to 80 per cent. The geometric advantage of having a dilated ventricle is of paramount importance, since it allows the ventricle to increase its stroke volume to a point where there is compensation for the loss of the regurgitant flow. The Frank-Starling mechanism is also important since it allows the ventricle to increase the force of contraction so that it can expel the additional volume without any increase in contractility.

The diastolic properties of the ventricle depicted in Figure 68–2 are relatively normal. Compliance is only mildly decreased, but the large increase in diastolic volume has overwhelmed even this relatively normal compliance so that end-diastolic pressure and wall stress have increased. The increased intraventricular diastolic pressure will cause pulmonary edema.

Since myocardial failure is not a prominent feature of mitral regurgitation in most small patients in class IV, surgical replacement of the valve is the ideal method for treating this disease. However, since surgery requires open heart techniques and since cardiac bypass cannot be readily performed on small dogs, this is not presently a viable alternative. Medical therapy is used to treat this disease. Diuretics are used in all cases that have evidence of pulmonary congestion or edema. Low-salt diets are used whenever possible. These two methods are used to control the signs of backward failure until the patient becomes refractory to their use or until signs of forward failure become evident. At that time hydralazine administration is indicated.

Hydralazine is an arteriolar dilator. It relaxes the smooth muscles of systemic arterioles, reducing aortic input impedance and systolic left ventricular pressure. The reduction in intraventricular pressure reduces the systolic pressure gradient across the mitral valve, which decreases regurgitant flow. In addition, decreasing aortic input impedance allows the ventricle to eject more blood into the systemic circuit. The combination of increased forward flow and decreased backward flow results in the left ventricular chamber becoming smaller. As a result, the mitral annulus decreases in size and effectively reduces the regurgitant fraction further.

If the patient becomes refractory to hydralazine or develops a supraventricular tachydysrhythmia (sinus tachycardia, atrial premature depolarizations, atrial tachycardia, flutter, or fibrillation, and so on), a digitalis glycoside (digitoxin or digoxin) is added to the therapeutic plan.

Heart Failure Secondary to Pressure Overloads

Stenotic lesions cause a pressure overload of the affected ventricle. That is, they increase the systolic intraventricular pressure. This increased pressure translates into an increased afterload. The myocardium compensates for this increased load with myocardial hypertrophy, which reduces the wall stress. As long as this compensation is adequate ventricular function is relatively normal, at least at rest.[30] Myocardial function, however, is altered. The alteration consists mostly of a decreased velocity of shortening, although tension development may also be affected. This has been interpreted as a decrease in contractility in the past, but recent evidence suggests that it may instead be a compensatory change by the contractile proteins. In chronic pressure overloads the myosin ATPase changes to a "slower" form, resulting in a decreased rate of ejection but allowing the muscle to increase mechanical efficiency when contracting with elevated wall stresses.

Along with systolic dysfunction, patients with stenotic lesions and concentric myocardial hypertrophy also commonly have diastolic dysfunction. The thicker muscle of concentric hypertrophy is stiffer than a normally thick muscle. Therefore, it is common for these patients to exhibit signs of backward failure since relatively small compensatory increases in ventricular diastolic volumes can increase diastolic pressures.

Severe or critical stenoses of the aortic or pulmonic valves can cause signs of heart failure by themselves; however, this is unusual. More commonly, stenotic lesions cause myocardial failure. Myocardial failure, in conjunction with the increased aortic input impedance, results in heart failure.

To understand the cardiovascular changes associated with a severe pressure overload, aortic banding is used as an example. In one study, a constricting band was placed around the proximal aorta.[30] This increased aortic input impedance enough to increase peak systolic intraventricular pressure from its normal value of 140 to 220 mm Hg. This increased peak systolic wall stress from 300 to 434 gm/cm². The acute increase in afterload decreased per cent diameter

shortening (a correlate of ejection fraction) from 30.0 to 22.4 per cent, which resulted in an increased end-systolic volume and a decreased stroke volume. The decrease in ejected volume coupled with a normal blood volume resulted in a slightly increased end-diastolic diameter (46.0 to 47.2 mm) and an increased end-diastolic pressure (11.0 to 17.0 mm Hg).

One week following the aortic banding the heart compensated for the decreased stroke volume by increasing left ventricular volume further. The end-diastolic diameter increased further to 48.8 mm and the end-diastolic pressure increased to 22 mm Hg, both indicative of an increased diastolic volume in the left ventricle. End-diastolic wall thickness gradually increased from 11.8 to 12.5 mm, which decreased peak systolic wall stress to 418 gm/cm². Per cent diameter shortening increased to 25.1 per cent because of the decrease in afterload. However, these dogs remained in backward failure (left ventricular end-diastolic pressure = 22 mm Hg) and systolic wall stress remained elevated during the study, so afterload was chronically increased and myocardial oxygen consumption would have been elevated. These changes are illustrated in Figure 68–3. More myocardial hypertrophy should have occurred with time, which would have reduced afterload.

When myocardial failure occurs in association with a pressure overload, ventricular function deteriorates markedly. Myocardial failure results in a decreased cardiac output, which stimulates fluid retention, producing a volume overload in addition to the pressure overload. Hypertrophy usually compensates for the increased pressure. The newly increased ventricular diameter, however, increases systolic wall stress and the ventricle appears to be unable to generate further hypertrophy to offset this increase in afterload.[13] In this case, ventricular function deteriorates because of the decreased contractility and the increased wall stress. The net result can be a rapidly deteriorating clinical course.

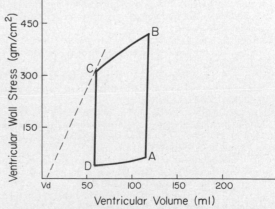

Figure 68–3. A stress-volume loop from a dog with induced aortic stenosis from aortic banding one week after banding. Systolic wall stress is elevated because of the increase in intraventricular pressure. End-diastolic wall stress is elevated because of an increase in end-diastolic pressure. An appropriate increase in left ventricular wall thickness (left ventricular concentric hypertrophy) should reduce both stresses.

The preferred therapy for severe stenotic lesions is surgical relief of the stenosis, preferably before massive hypertrophy has taken place. Medical therapy may be beneficial when myocardial failure develops but is of little benefit before that time.

1. Baylen, B., Meyer, R. A., Korfhagen, J., Benzing, G. III, Bubb, M. E., and Kaplan, S.: Left ventricular performance in the critically ill premature infant with patent ductus arteriosus and pulmonary disease. Circulation 55:182, 1977.
2. Beekman, R. H., Rocchini, A. P., and Rosenthal, A.: Hemodynamic effects of hydralazine in infants with a large ventricular septal defect. Circulation 65:523, 1982.
3. Belleau, L., Mion, H., Granger, P., Bertranou, E., Nowaczynski, W., Boucher, R., and Genest, J.: Studies on the Mechanism of Experimental Heart Failure in Dogs. Canad. J. Physiol. Pharmacol. 48:450, 1970.
4. Berman, W., Jr., Yabek, S. M., Dillon, T., Niland, C., Corlew, S., and Christensen, D.: Effects of digoxin in infants with a congested circulatory state due to a ventricular septal defect. N. Engl. J. Med. 308:363, 1983.
5. Boltwood, C. M., Tei, C., Trim, P., Wong, M., and Shah, P. M.: The mechanism of mitral regurgitation in nonischemic dilated cardiomyopathy. Circulation 66:II, 1982.
6. Cannon, P. J.: The kidney in heart failure. N. Engl. J. Med. 296:26, 1977.
7. Curtiss, C., Cohn, J. N., Vrobel, T., and Franciosa, J. A.: Role of the renin-angiotensin system in the systemic vasoconstriction of chronic congestive heart failure. Circulation 58:763, 1978.
8. Dzau, V. U., Colucci, W. S., Hollenberg, N. K., and Williams, G. H.: Relation of the renin-angiotensin-aldosterone system to the clinical state in congestive heart failure. Circulation 63:645, 1981.
9. Fitzsimmons, J. T., and Simons, B. J.: The effect on drinking in the rat of intravenous infusion of angiotensin given alone or in combination with other simuli of thirst. J. Physiol. 203:45, 1969.
10. Forrester, J. S., Diamond, G., Chatterjee, K., and Swan, H. J. C.: Medical therapy of acute myocardial infarction by application of hemodynamic subsets. N. Engl. J. Med. 295:1356, 1976.
11. Goldsmith, S. R., Francis, G. S., Cowley, A. W., Levine, T. B., and Cohn, J. N.: Increased plasma vasopressin in patients with congestive heart failure. Circulation 66:II, 1982.
12. Greenberg, T. T., Richmond, W. H., Stocking, R. A., Gupta, P. D., Meehan, J. P., and Henry, J. P.: Impaired atrial receptor responses in dogs with heart failure due to tricuspid insufficiency and pulmonary artery stenosis. Circ. Res. 32:424, 1973.
13. Gunther, S., and Grossman, W.: Determinants of ventricular function in pressure-overload hypertrophy in man. Circulation 59:679, 1979.
14. Harigaya, S., and Schwartz, A.: Rate of calcium binding and uptake in normal animal and failing human cardiac muscle. Circ. Res. 25:781, 1969.
15. Humes, H. D., Gottlieb, M. N., and Brenner, B. M.: The kidney in congestive heart failure. In Brenner, B. M., and Stein, J. H. (eds.): Sodium and Water Homeostasis. Churchill Livingstone, New York, 1978, p. 51.
16. Ito, Y., and Chidsey, C. A.: Intracellular calcium and myocardial contractility. IV. Distribution of calcium in the failing heart. J. Mole. Cell Cardiol. 4:507, 1972.
17. Katz, A. M.: Mechanical and biochemical correlates of cardiac contraction. Mod. Con. Cardiovasc. Dis. 40:45, 1971.
18. Katz, A. M.: Congestive heart failure: Role of altered cellular control. N. Engl. J. Med. 293:1184, 1975.

19. Kittleson, M. D., Eyster, G. E., Anderson, L. K., Knowlen, G. G., and Olivier, N. B.: Myocardial function in dogs with chronic mitral regurgitation and severe congestive heart failure. Scientific Proc. Am. Coll. Vet. Intern. Med., 1982.
20. Kittleson, M. D., Eyster, G. E., Knowlen, G. G., Oliver, N. B., Anderson, L. K., and Crawford, M. A.: The effect of digitalis glycosides on peripheral tissue oxygen delivery and myocardial function in dogs with congestive cardiomyopathy. Scientific Proc. Am. Coll. Vet. Intern. Med., 1982.
21. Knowlen, G. G., Kittleson, M. D., Nachreiner, R., and Eyster, G. E.: Comparison of plasma aldosterone concentration to the clinical status of dogs with chronic heart failure. Scientific Proc. Am. Coll. Vet. Intern. Med., 1983.
22. Levine, H. J., and Gaasch, W. H.: Diastolic compliance of the left ventricle. Mod. Con. Cardiovasc. Dis. 47:95, 1978.
23. Lord, P. F.: Left ventricular diastolic stiffness in dogs with congestive cardiomyopathy and volume overload. Am. J. Vet. Res. 37:953, 1976.
24. McCollum, W. B., Crow, C., Harigaya, S., Bajusz, E., and Schwartz, A.: Calcium binding by cardiac relaxing system isolated from myopathic Syrian hamsters (strains 14.6, 82.62, and 40.54). J. Molec. Cell Cardiol. 1:445, 1970.
25. McCullagh, W. H., Covell, J. W., and Ross, J., Jr.: Left ventricular dilatation and diastolic compliance changes during chronic volume overloading. Circulation 45:943, 1972.
26. Milnor, W. R.: Arterial impedance as ventricular afterload. Circ. Res. 36:565, 1975.
27. Pepine, C. J., Nichols, W. W., and Conti, C. R.: Aortic input impedance in heart failure. Circulation 58:460, 1978.
28. Quinones, M. A., Mokotoff, D. M., Nouri, S., Winters, W. L., Jr., and Miller, R. R.: Noninvasive quantification of left ventricular wall stress: Validation of method and application to assessment of chronic pressure overload. Am. J. Cardiol. 45:782, 1980.
29. Ross, J., Jr.: Afterload mismatch and preload reserve: A conceptual framework for the analysis of ventricular function. Prog. Card. Dis. 18:255, 1976.
30. Sasayama, S., Ross, J., Jr., Franklin, D., Bloor, C. M., Bishop, S., and Dilley, R. B.: Adaptations of the left ventricle to chronic pressure overload. Circ. Res. 38:172, 1976.
31. Sonnenblick, E. H., and Skeleton, C. L.: Oxygen consumption of the heart: Physiologic principles and clinical implications. Mod. Conc. Cardiovasc. Dis. 40:9, 1971.
32. Sordahl, L. A., McCollum, W. B., Wood, W. G., and Schwartz, A.: Mitochondria and sarcoplasmic reticulum function in cardiac hypertrophy and failure. Am. J. Physiol. 224:497, 1973.
33. Sparks, H. V., Kopald, H. H., Carriere, S., Chimoskey, J. E., Kinoshita, M., and Barger, A. C.: Intrarenal distribution of blood flow with chronic congestive failure. Am. J. Physiol. 223:840, 1972.
34. Thurau, K., Schnermann, J., Nagel, W., Horster, M., and Wohl, M.: Composition of tubular fluid in the macula densa segment as a factor regulating the function of the juxtaglomerular apparatus. Circ. Res. 21 (Suppl. 11):79, 1967.
35. Tsien, R. W., and Carpenter, D. O.: Ionic mechanisms of pacemaker activity in cardiac Purkinje fibers. Fed. Proc. 37:2127, 1978.
36. Vander, A. J., and Miller, R.: Control of renin secretion in the anesthetized dog. Am. J. Physiol. 207:537, 1964.
37. White, R. D., and Lietman, P. S.: Commentary: A reappraisal of digitalis for infants with left-to-right shunts and "heart failure." J. Pediatr. 92:867, 1978.
38. Yin, F. C. P.: Ventricular wall stress. Circ. Res. 49:829, 1981.
39. Zucker, I. H., Earle, A. M., and Gilmore, J. P.: The mechanism of adaptation of left atrial stretch in dogs with chronic congestive heart failure. J. Clin. Inv. 60:323, 1977.

69 Pathophysiology of Arteriovenous Fistulae

N. Bari Olivier

INTRODUCTION

Since their initial recognition in the 18th century, abnormal communications between the arteries and veins (arteriovenous fistulae) have been studied in man and animal with great interest. This interest in an otherwise simple anatomical lesion is due mainly to its ability to produce profound local and systemic cardiovascular abnormalities. These changes can be severe enough to endanger the viability of the local tissue or the circulatory system. Although arteriovenous fistulae are relatively uncommon in animals, their potential morbidity necessitates a basic understanding of the pathophysiology to develop a rational therapeutic approach.

Arteriovenous fistulae can be classified as either congenital or acquired based on their onset of development. Embryologically, primitive vessels serve both arterial and venous functions. As they differentiate, small communications transiently persist that join the new artery and vein. Normally, these small communicating vessels degenerate and are permanently closed. The persistence of these communicating vessels provides the basis for congenital fistulae.[1, 2] Congenital fistulae are identified by the same clinical features as acquired fistulae; in fact, their pathophysiology is identical except for magnitude. Although congenital forms can be multiple, they are generally small with mild local and systemic effects. The other form of arteriovenous fistula is the acquired fistula. Vascular trauma is probably the most common cause of acquired fistula formation and may be in the form of blunt trauma, penetrating trauma including surgery, venipuncture, and aneurysmal rupture. Other inciting causes include neovascularization, either with neoplasia or as collateral circulation develops in ischemic tissue. In recent years, iatrogenic fistulae have been surgically created in animals to aid hemodialysis.

Clinical findings of arteriovenous fistula vary but include dilation of involved arteries and veins with venous pulsation and a continuous murmur often accompanied by a palpable thrill. Varying degrees of edema and ischemia may be present in the tissue normally served by the affected vessels. Hyperthermia may be noted at and above the fistula and hypothermia distal to the lesion. Heart rate is generally normal at the time of recognition but may be elevated in a fistula of short duration or if cardiac decompensation has occurred. With larger fistulae, occlusion of fistula flow causes an abrupt fall in heart rate (Branham's sign). With a compensated fistula, systolic arterial pressure is usually normal but may be slightly increased because of a large left ventricular stroke volume. A more prominent decrease in both diastolic and mean arterial pressure occurs. This reduction is due mainly to a decrease in peripheral vascular resistance and rapid diastolic runoff into the capacitant venous circulation.[6] The result is a pulse pressure that is widened with the systolic pressure rising rapidly and the diastolic pressure falling rapidly (water-hammer pulse). Cardiac output is elevated, sometimes by as much as two to three times normal.[3] Large fistulae, especially of longer duration, show cardiac enlargement with pulmonary overcirculation. Venous oxygen saturations are elevated in large shunts owing to the functional peripheral left-to-right shunt.

Although many cases are recognized by the local effects of the fistula, some cases are presented for signs of congestive circulatory failure. This systemic effect, usually seen with large distensible fistulae, is generally the most serious threat to the patient. The triad of congestive circulatory failure, elevated cardiac output, and high venous oxygen saturation suggests an arteriovenous fistula.

PATHOPHYSIOLOGY

Local Effects

With the development of an arteriovenous fistula, a new circulatory circuit is established through which blood flows preferentially. The fistula joins the arterial system of high resistance, pressure, and oxygen saturation to the venous system of low resistance, pressure, and oxygen saturation and high capacitance. Blood flow follows the path of least resistance no matter how circuitous. The arterial flow thus leaks into the capacitant venous system. Two circulatory pathways are now established: the normal arterial-capillary-venous system and a new system that acts as a short cut and robs the normal pathway of its flow (Fig. 69–1).

The initial effects of this new pathway include a decrease in total peripheral vascular resistance causing arterial hypotension, a decrease in the circulation to the tissues normally served by the affected artery, and varying degrees of venous hypertension with increased venous return to the heart. The rapid flow, turbulence, and vascular vibrations through the fistula and receiving veins are the source of the continuous murmur and thrill common in arteriovenous fistulae. The physiological response to the opening of a fistula is similar to that of acute hemorrhage, with an autonomic increase in heart rate and force of contraction to increase cardiac output and peripheral

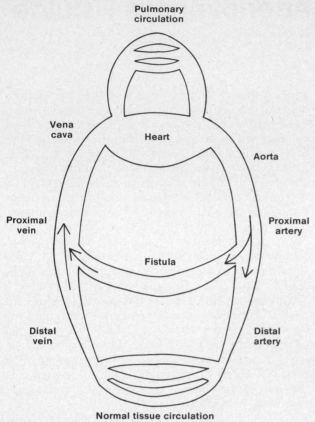

Pulmonary
circulation

Vena
cava

Heart

Aorta

Proximal
vein

Proximal
artery

Fistula

Distal
vein

Distal
artery

Normal tissue circulation

Figure 69–1. The new flow circuit established by an arteriovenous fistula that circumvents the normal circulation. The entire fistulous circuit includes the fistula itself, proximal vein and vena cava, heart and pulmonary circulation, aorta, and proximal artery.

vasoconstriction to restore arterial blood pressure.[6] The diastolic and mean arterial blood pressures usually remain low owing to the continued shunting of blood through the low-resistance shunt. Renal and other mechanisms of fluid conservation eventually increase the blood volume sufficiently to replace these initial autonomic changes.[1, 3] The magnitude of these changes is dependent primarily on the amount of shunt flow through the fistula, which depends on several factors. The size of the original artery involved and its inherent velocity of flow initially influence the amount of blood available for fistula flow. Subsequent collateral circulation may increase the available supply, which can shunt through the fistula and exacerbate systemic clinical signs. The size of the fistula influences not only the magnitude of the fall in vascular resistance, which attracts or favors shunt flow, but also the *maximal* amount of blood that may traverse it in a given time (flow). Thus, the maximum potential for shunt flow is determined by fistula size, whereas the degree to which this potential is reached is determined by the available arterial blood flow supplied by the original artery and any subsequent collaterals.

The progression, or fate, of a newly formed fistula is determined largely by its elasticity or distensibility.

If the fistula is initially small and nonexpansile, it may remain small with negligible effects or may even spontaneously close owing to increasing connective tissue formation. If the fistula is distensible, regardless of initial size, it favors an ever increasing flow and with time is likely to cause significant local and systemic effects.

Distal tissues served by the affected vessels may undergo several changes. Arterial flow to this tissue may be compromised owing to competition with the fistula for the arterial supply and venous hypertension in the distal vein, which, in some cases, may further retard flow through the capillary beds. Ischemia, edema, and organ dysfunction may develop as a result. In contrast, with most fistulae the flow to distal tissue is normal owing to an effective compensatory increase in cardiac output and the development of collateral circulation.[4] The establishment of collateral circulation following the opening of a fistula can be quite extensive, even exaggerated. This collateral circulation primarily represents the dilation of pre-existing unused arterial communications. These unused channels are progressively opened as blood is shunted through the fistula and away from deprived distal tissue.

The degree of collateral development seems to be influenced by at least three factors.[3] The first is the size of the fistula and its total shunt flow. The second factor is the duration of the fistula, since in many cases collateral development is a continuous process. The third factor involves the ability of the proximal arterial blood flow to supply the fistula. For example, equal-sized fistulae in the femoral and iliac arteries might be associated with different degrees of collateral development. The smaller femoral artery, with a lower inherent blood flow, even with progressive dilation, may not provide enough blood to attain maximal shunt flow; hence, collateral development is extensive as it too follows the path of least resistance and contributes to shunt flow. In contrast, the iliac artery, with its greater blood flow, can more adequately supply the same fistula as well as distal tissue and thus develop less collaterals. It is interesting to note that iliac fistulae of even moderate size can be rapidly fatal in the dog because of the immense shunt flow and rapid cardiac volume overload. Thus, for a given fistula size and elasticity, morbidity is greater with fistulae located more centrally involving larger vessels with greater inherent flow rates.

Blood flow through a large fistula can be so intense as to cause retrograde flow from the distal artery into the fistula.[3, 4] This phenomenon can be seen immediately upon opening a large fistula. Distal arterial blood flow becomes retrograde and is supplied by pre-existing distal arterial collaterals.

Arteriovenous fistulae are often remarkably dilated. The amount of dilation depends on the distensibility of the fistula and time. Classically the entire fistulous circuit dilates owing to an increasing blood volume, which it must accommodate (see Fig. 69–1).

Accompanying this gross dilation are histological changes in the affected vessels. Arteries begin to look more like veins and veins like arteries, processes called venification and arterialization, respectively.

Various other local effects may develop in relation to the specific location of the fistula. Appendicular growth may be exaggerated with a large fistula in an extremity owing, in part, to increased blood volume in the fistulous circuit of the affected extremity.

Pulmonary arteriovenous fistulae deserve special mention. The basic principles of pathophysiology apply, yet this vascular bed does not normally have a high resistance across the capillaries so the attraction of blood flow through a fistula and vascular pressure changes do not occur with the same magnitude as with a similar systemic fistula.[5, 6] The other obvious difference is the establishment of a functional right-to-left shunt resulting in varying degrees of arterial hypoxemia. Such fistulae are often congenital and may be single or multiple. There is usually a continuous murmur with systolic intensification that may be louder on inspiration. Changes in heart rate with opening and closing of the fistula are either absent or minimal owing to negligible changes in systemic arterial pressure. Blood volume may increase, but again in less magnitude than with a comparable systemic fistula.

Systemic Effects

Some of the systemic effects of an arteriovenous fistula have already been mentioned. The majority of the effects involve alterations in the cardiac system (Fig. 69–2). As previously stated, the opening of an arteriovenous fistula establishes a circulatory pathway that bypasses the normal capillary resistance bed. As a result of this arterial "hemorrhage" into the capacitant venous circulation, a significant drop in peripheral resistance and systemic arterial blood pressure occurs (systolic, mean, and diastolic). In contrast, venous pressure and flow increase. An increase in heart rate, cardiac output, and peripheral vasoconstriction develops rapidly to restore arterial pressure to normal, although mean and diastolic pressures may remain low.

If the fistula is initially large or expansile, an increase in blood volume gradually takes place as the renal conservation of water is stimulated. It is not unusual for blood volume to expand to 30 per cent or more above the prefistula value.[3] The magnitude of this increase is directly related to total fistula flow. Heart rate and peripheral vasoconstriction diminish as the blood volume increases, yet cardiac output remains elevated. The long-term increase in cardiac output is due to increased venous return (increased

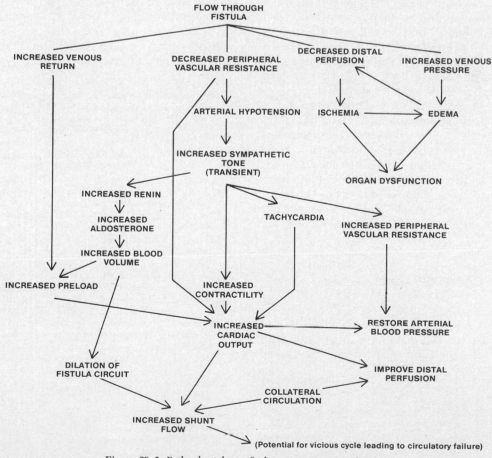

Figure 69–2. Pathophysiology of a large arteriovenous fistula.

preload) through the Frank-Starling mechanism as well as decreased peripheral vascular resistance (decreased afterload). The elevation in cardiac output is both a necessary compensatory mechanism and an obligatory event driven by these changes in preload and afterload. Occlusion of such fistula flow by external digital pressure or surgical ligation reverses these changes with an initial rise in arterial pressure above normal. This is followed by vagal slowing of the heart rate, restoring the blood pressure and cardiac output toward normal. A renal water diuresis ensues, restoring the blood volume toward normal.

Although the changes in blood volume and cardiac output are important in compensation following fistula formation, they also contribute to the morbidity of the disease. As cardiac output and blood volume increase, the entire fistulous circuit expands, favoring an even greater flow. This results in an even greater increase in blood volume and cardiac output, thereby establishing a vicious cycle. This phenomenon may take months or even years to develop but can be ultimately expected with any fistula capable of continued expansion.

A characteristic finding with arteriovenous fistulae is a variable increase in oxygen saturation in the venous circulation proximal to the fistula. This systemic effect is not deleterious to the patient.

Congestive circulatory failure remains the most serious potential systemic effect of most arteriovenous fistulae. The load of increasing venous return to the heart and pulmonary circuit may eventually exceed the capabilities of the central circulation. This results in elevated venous pressures and, ultimately, edema (congestive heart failure). If heart failure develops, it may be due to the severe volume overload by itself or in combination with valvular incompetence secondary to severe cardiac dilation or myocardial failure or any combination of these factors. In any case, signs of congestive failure develop. These changes are dramatically reversible with permanent closure of the fistula if myocardial failure has not occurred. If myocardial failure is too extensive or if pulmonary vascular changes secondary to pulmonary hypertension have progressed too far, cardiopulmonary decompensation may continue despite closure of the fistula.

THERAPEUTIC CONSIDERATIONS

Some of the earliest attempts at surgical repair of an arteriovenous fistula in man involved ligation of the proximal artery. These attempts usually met with disastrous results, primarily gangrenous necrosis of the distal tissue. These unfortunate results stressed the importance of the collateral circulation in the ultimate survival of the distal tissue.[3] With ligation of only the proximal artery, the distal collaterals began diverting their effective distal tissue blood flow to the fistula (retrograde flow). Ligation of the proximal vein or proximal vein and artery was usually unsuccessful as well, since collateral venous drainage developed rapidly and re-established the fistula flow. The desired approach seems to be either quadruple ligation (ligation of proximal and distal artery and vein) and resection of the fistula and affected proximal and distal vessels or closure of the fistula itself and surgical repair of the affected vessels. The latter technique is often advocated in man to circumvent insufficient distal collateral circulation.[1] This is not as critical in small animals with their well-developed natural collateral circulation. Thus, in all but the major vessels, quadruple ligation and resection is adequate. Intravenous balloon embolization has also been used successfully to occlude fistulae in areas inaccessible to surgical ligation.[7, 8]

The systemic effects of local repair must also be considered. By closing the fistula, an abrupt rise in peripheral vascular resistance (increased afterload) occurs, which, in conjunction with the increased blood volume, might be an excessive acute strain on a failing or near failing central circulatory system. Cautious venesection or diuretic administration before or even during surgical repair might prevent or minimize these risks.

Attention to these and other principles of the pathophysiology involved is important to the successful repair of any arteriovenous fistula.

1. Gomes, M., and Bernatz, P.: Arteriovenous fistulas: A review and ten year experience at the Mayo Clinic. Mayo Clin. Proc. 45:81, 1970.
2. Holman, E.: Abnormal arteriovenous communications. Circ. 32:1001, 1965.
3. Holman, E.: *Abnormal Arteriovenous Communications*, 2nd ed. Charles C Thomas, Springfield, 1968.
4. Lough, F., Giordano, J., and Hobson, R.: Regional hemodynamics of large and small femoral arteriovenous fistulas in dogs. Surgery 79:346, 1976.
5. Moyer, J., Glantz, G., and Brest, A.: Pulmonary arteriovenous fistulas. Am. J. Med. 32:417, 1962.
6. Nakano, J., and DeSchryuer, C.: Effects of arteriovenous fistula on systemic and pulmonary circulations. Am. J. Physiol. 207:1319, 1964.
7. Terry, P. B., Barth, K. H., Kaufman, S. L., and White, R. I.: Balloon embolization for treatment of pulmonary arteriovenous fistulas. N. Engl. J. Med. 302:1189, 1980.
8. Terry, P. B., White, R. I., Barth, K. H., Kaufman, S. L., and Mitchell, S. E.: Pulmonary arteriovenous malformations: Physiologic observations and results of therapeutic balloon embolization. N. Engl. J. Med. 308:1197, 1983.

Chapter 70

Diagnostic Methods

Lorel K. Anderson

Diagnostic procedures involving the cardiovascular system are directed toward an accurate diagnosis, evaluation of the severity of the disorder, development of possible therapeutic plans, and an assessment of prognosis. This information is essential in deciding whether surgical intervention is appropriate, in selecting the surgical procedure to be used, and in evaluating the probable outcome of surgery.

ANAMNESIS

Despite the development of new diagnostic techniques and equipment, it is important to remember the significance of information obtained through a complete history and physical examination. Many of the decisions about diagnostic tests and therapy are based on knowledge gained during these procedures. Astute observations and questions at this stage may streamline the entire process of evaluation, diagnosis, and therapy.

The breed of dog or cat may be an aid to diagnosis, since certain cardiac diseases, both congenital and acquired, have breed predispositions. The poodle has an incidence of patent ductus arteriosus exceeding that of the general population, and English bulldogs have a disproportionately high incidence of pulmonic stenosis.[31] Patient age is significant, because young dogs are more likely to have congenital defects and older dogs more frequently have acquired disorders. The patient's sex is less significant in disease distribution, although patent ductus arteriosus is more common in females and cardiomyopathy is more frequent in male cats.[27,33] It is important to recognize existing trends and to maintain an open mind in evaluating diagnostic data.

The history includes identification of the chief complaint, a chronologic history of the current problem, pertinent past disorders, and environmental and vaccination details. Since several cardiac diseases are hereditary and others are possibly genetically transmitted, a complete family history is valuable. Comparative data concerning growth and activity of littermates may also be helpful.

The animal's environment and level of activity are useful in assigning it to one of the four classes of heart failure described by the New York Heart Association; this assessment can be used as a guide in selecting appropriate therapy:

Class I animals have cardiac disease, but no evidence of clinical signs even with exercise.

Class II patients develop clinical signs with exercise.

Class III patients exhibit clinical signs with normal activity or demonstrate orthopnea.

Class IV animals have clinical signs even at rest.

Information about the animal's diet is also important, because weight control and limited sodium intake may be part of the therapeutic plan. Dietary changes resulting in increased sodium intake may precipitate sudden progression of clinical signs in a previously well-controlled animal.

The owner's desired use for the pet should be considered in selecting a therapeutic program and in evaluating the prognosis. A dog with congenital heart disease may be inappropriate to use in a breeding program but suitable as a pet. Moderate exercise intolerance may be acceptable in a house pet but unsatisfactory in a field trial dog. These factors can influence the extent of work-up requested and the type of therapy recommended.

An important aspect of the history lies in assessing whether clinical signs are referable to the cardiovascular system. Many of the signs commonly seen with cardiac disease can also be seen with other disorders. In a coughing dog, for example, the clinician must decide whether the cough is related to cardiac disease or to a primary respiratory problem. Similar decisions must be made concerning signs like ascites, dyspnea, collapsing episodes, and tissue edema.

Frequently, cardiac disease arises secondary to other disease processes or may result in disorders involving other organ systems. It is important, in obtaining a history, to pursue questions that assess not only the cardiovascular system but all other systems as well. In evaluating and treating a patient, the clinician must remember that he is not treating pulmonic stenosis but an animal with pulmonic stenosis.

PHYSICAL EXAMINATION

Like the history, the physical examination is directed at evaluating the entire animal and identifying all abnormalities. A history of cardiovascular problems may focus additional attention on the cardiac and pulmonary systems.

Observation of the animal in the waiting room and as it enters the examination room allows assessment of gait, attitude, general appearance, and response to limited activity. This is an ideal time to identify lameness, abdominal distension, tissue edema, and respiratory distress. Positional dyspnea, open-mouth breathing, tachypnea, and obstructive dyspnea can all be seen.

Examination of the cardiac and pulmonary systems includes evaluation of other body areas frequently altered by cardiovascular disease. The capillary perfusion time is determined and the color of mucous membranes is evaluated. Prolonged perfusion time is consistent with decreased cardiac output. Pale membranes may indicate poor cardiac perfusion as well as anemia. Cyanotic membranes are associated

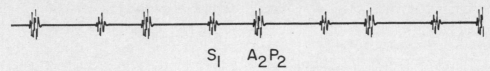

$$S_1 \qquad A_2 P_2$$

Figure 70–1. Split second heart sound. Closure of the pulmonic valve is delayed. S_1, first heart sound; A_2, aortic valve closure; P_2, pulmonic valve closure.

with decreased oxygen saturation. Mucous membranes of the oral cavity, vulva, prepuce, or conjunctiva are suitable for evaluation. Multiple areas should be examined to identify differential cyanosis, which may be seen in right-to-left–shunting patent ductus arteriosus.

The neck is examined for jugular distension or a jugular pulse, and the arterial pulse is also evaluated. The rate should be identical to the heart rate. A pulse deficit may accompany some dysrhythmias. The intensity of the pulse is also important, because it may change with certain diseases. Weak pulses can reflect poor cardiac output, whereas run-off or "water hammer" pulses accompany patent ductus arteriosus and aortic regurgitation.

Palpation of the thorax is useful in identifying traumatic lesions, structural anomalies, and masses. The point of maximal intensity (PMI) of the cardiac thrust can usually be palpated at the left fifth rib space at the costochondral junction. This point may shift with cardiac enlargement, masses in the thorax, and pulmonary disorders. Very loud cardiac murmurs may also be palpable on the chest wall, producing a "thrill."

Percussion may be used to localize the heart or other solid tissue masses, that give off a dull sound. Air-filled lungs are recognized by a resonant sound. Air-fluid lines may also be evaluated similarly, with a dull sound below the line and greater resonance above.

AUSCULTATION

Auscultation is an important step in evaluation of the patient with cardiac disease. A good stethoscope, a quiet room, a cooperative patient, patience, and concentration are required for this part of the examination.

Auscultation is best performed with the animal in a standing position, to allow the heart and lungs to assume their normal anatomic positions. All areas of the heart and lung field are ausculted in an orderly manner. The heart is evaluated over the pulmonic, aortic, mitral, and tricuspid areas. In addition, the

remainder of the chest, thoracic inlet, neck, and head are evaluated for radiation of murmurs. The diaphragm and the bell of the stethoscope should be used to identify both high-frequency and low-frequency murmurs. The lung fields are auscultated over multiple sites on both sides of the chest.

Vibrations of the heart muscle and vessel walls secondary to changes in blood flow produce normal and abnormal sounds that can be heard on auscultation. In the dog and cat, a first heart sound (S_1) associated with atrioventricular valve closure and a second heart sound (S_2) at the time of semilunar valve closure are normally heard. S_1 is low-pitched and is heard best over the apex of the heart. S_2 is higher-pitched than S_1 and the other heart sounds and is quite distinctive; it is heard best over the base of the heart.

Closures of the aortic and pulmonic valves are asynchronous but separated by such a short interval that normally it can't be recognized on auscultation. Splitting of S_2 may be heard when pulmonic valve closure is delayed by pulmonary hypertension, right bundle branch block, left ventricular premature beats, pulmonic stenosis, and some left-to-right shunts (Fig. 70–1). Paradoxical splitting of S_2, with the aortic valve closing after the pulmonic valve, may occur with systemic hypertension, left bundle branch block, right ventricular premature beats, and aortic stenosis.[2,17]

The third heart sound (S_3) occurs during diastole and the period of rapid ventricular filling. In the dog and cat it is usually associated with heart failure and ventricular dilation. The fourth heart sound (S_4) is heard just prior to S_1 and is associated with atrial contraction (Fig. 70–2). The presence of S_4 indicates heart failure or a disorder altering left ventricular distensibility.[18] The presence of S_3 or S_4 or both is described as a diastolic gallop rhythm.

Systolic clicks are high-pitched additional sounds occurring between S_1 and S_2. These may be ejection sounds associated with aortic or pulmonic valvular disease. A murmur often follows the ejection sounds. Systolic clicks may also be associated with mitral valve prolapse, producing billowing of the mitral valve leaflets into the left atrium during systole.[20,26,30]

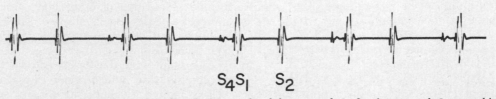

$$S_4 S_1 \qquad S_2$$

Figure 70–2. Fourth heart sound. Presystolic gallop rhythm. S_4, fourth heart sound; S_1, first heart sound; S_2, second heart sound.

Cardiac Murmurs

Turbulent flow through the heart and vessels can produce auscultable murmurs. These may be (1) innocent flow murmurs, which are heard most frequently in young dogs or cats, (2) murmurs arising from physiological changes such as anemia with a PCV less than 15 per cent, or (3) murmurs due to cardiac disease. Evaluation of a murmur includes identification of the time of occurrence, duration, type, intensity, location in the thoracic cavity, and radiation.

Systolic murmurs occur during ventricular contraction, between S_1 and S_2, and are the most commonly identified murmurs. They may be produced by atrioventricular valvular insufficiency, semilunar valvular stenosis, or ventricular septal defects. Diastolic murmurs are less common, and in the dog and cat they are usually associated with aortic or pulmonic regurgitation. Continuous murmurs are heard most commonly with patent ductus arteriosus but can accompany any arteriovenous fistula.

The duration of the murmur within systole or diastole may vary. Holosystolic murmurs occupy the entire systolic period, whereas crescendo-decrescendo (ejection) murmurs occur only during ventricular emptying. The murmurs of mitral regurgitation, tricuspid regurgitation, and ventricular septal defect are, therefore, of longer duration than the murmurs of aortic or pulmonic stenosis.

Several different grading systems are used to identify the intensity of a murmur. The most commonly used system is a I through VI rating. A *grade I* murmur is the softest murmur that can be heard and its recognition usually requires considerable time and experience. A *grade VI* murmur is the loudest murmur and can be heard even when the stethoscope is no longer in contact with the chest wall. The other grades of murmurs fall in between these extremes, allowing a semiquantitative assessment of the murmur and a means of reporting changes in the murmur's intensity.

The type of the murmur reflects those factors influencing modulation of intensity. Plateau murmurs are the same intensity throughout. Variable-intensity murmurs may be crescendo, decrescendo, or crescendo-decrescendo in nature. Aortic and pulmonic stenosis have a diamond-shaped, crescendo-decrescendo pattern (Fig. 70–3).

In describing a murmur, one also must note the area of maximal intensity on the thoracic cavity. This position varies, depending on why and from where the murmur arises. Radiation of the murmur is also important diagnostically, since some murmurs are quite localized but others, such as the murmur of aortic stenosis, may radiate to the thoracic inlet and up the carotid arteries.

When all of these factors are taken into consideration during the evaluation of a murmur, auscultation can be a very discriminating diagnostic procedure. A high level of discrimination at this stage of patient evaluation increases efficiency in the selection and application of additional diagnostic procedures.

PHONOCARDIOGRAPHY

The phonocardiogram provides a graphic display of those heart sounds identified on auscultation. A crystal microphone applied to the skin is the source of the signal, which is filtered to allow selective passage of sounds and then amplified for display. The phonocardiogram is simultaneously recorded with an electrocardiogram, to allow assessment of the shape and frequency of murmurs as well as confirmation of their position during the cardiac cycle. The phonocardiogram also allows accurate timing and sequencing of heart sounds, thereby permitting definitive identification of third and fourth heart sounds, split second heart sounds, and systolic ejection sounds and clicks (see Figs. 70–1 to 70–3).

ELECTROCARDIOGRAPHY

The electrocardiogram is a recording of electrical activity in the heart as reflected by electrodes on the surface of the body. The signal arises from the inherent automaticity of the cardiac tissues and the sequential transmission of electrical impulses through the conduction system. The electrocardiogram provides a means of recognizing some alterations in electrical activity. Changes in the electrocardiogram may be associated with cardiac enlargement, myocardial disease, conduction disorders, and dysrhythmias. Application of this information in the surgical patient is useful in diagnosis, prognosis, anesthetic management, and postoperative care.

Several different lead systems have been used in small animal electrocardiography. A combination of these systems gives the most complete information. The hexaxial lead system is composed of three bipolar leads (I, II, III) and three augmented unipolar leads (AVR, AVL, AVF). All six leads compare electrical

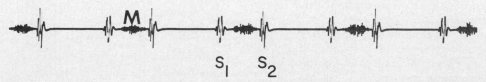

Figure 70–3. Crescendo-decrescendo murmur of pulmonic stenosis. The murmur begins after S_1 and ends before S_2. The intensity varies, producing a diamond shape. *M*, murmur; S_1, first heart sound; S_2, second heart sound.

TABLE 70–1. Normal Values for Canine and Feline Electrocardiograms

Measurement (Units)	Dog	Cat
Heart rate (beats/minute)	70–180	160–240
P wave width (seconds)	Maximum 0.04	Maximum 0.04
P wave amplitude (millivolts)	Maximum 0.4	Maximum 0.2
QRS complex width (seconds)	Maximum 0.05 small breeds, 0.06 large breeds	Maximum 0.04
R wave amplitude (millivolts)	Maximum 2.5 small breeds, 3.0 large breeds	Maximum 0.9
T wave amplitude (millivolts)	Less than ¼ R wave	Maximum 0.3
P-R interval (seconds)	0.06–0.13	0.05–0.09
Q-T interval (seconds)	0.15–0.25	0.12–0.18
S-T segment depression (millivolts)	Less than 0.2	No numerical value
S-T segment elevation (millivolts)	Less than 0.15	No numerical value
Mean electrical axis of QRS complex-frontal plane (degrees)	+40–+100	0–+160

(Data from Tilley, L. P.: *Essentials of Canine and Feline Electrocardiography.* C. V. Mosby, St. Louis, 1979.)

voltage in the right arm, left arm, and left leg in various combinations. The hexaxial system is useful in determining the mean electrical axis in the frontal plane.

Another view of the heart is obtained from the unipolar precordial leads (CV_5RL, CV_6LL, CV_6LU, V_{10}). The orthogonal lead system used in vectorcardiography (Leads X, Y, and Z, respectively) is approximately equal to Lead I, Lead AVF, and Lead V_{10}. Additional data are available from esophageal and invasive leads.

The electrocardiogram is recorded with the patient in right lateral recumbency, limbs perpendicular to the body, and electrodes attached at the olecranon and stifle. This is the reference position for recording tracings and must be used for comparisons with normal values.[6,47] Different positioning of cats produces less variation than of dogs. Although sternal positioning in the cat does not produce marked differences in amplitude or conformation, right lateral recumbency is still the accepted standard.[12,22,47] Positioning is not critical in the evaluation of dysrhythmias.

Normal values for the feline and canine electrocardiogram are listed in Table 70–1.

Cardiac Enlargement

Changes in the duration and amplitude of the P wave may occur with atrial enlargement. The right atrium depolarizes first and inscribes the initial part of the P wave. Left atrial depolarization occurs slightly later, producing the remainder of the P wave. When the right atrium enlarges, portions of the right and left atrial depolarization overlap; this superimposition results in increased P wave amplitude. In left atrial enlargement, the second half of the P wave is prolonged, resulting in an increased P wave duration. Biatrial enlargement produces a combination of the two changes. These changes may occur in diseases that potentially increase atrial pressure or atrial blood volume, such as pulmonic stenosis and mitral regurgitation.

Left ventricular enlargement is often associated with increased amplitude of the R waves in leads facing the left ventricle. Other changes seen in animals with enlarged left ventricles include prolongation of the QRS complex, S-T segment slurring, and increased T wave amplitude. Deviation of the mean electrical axis to the left is not always associated with left ventricular enlargement. A mean electrical axis of greater than +100° in the dog is a useful indicator of right ventricular enlargement (Fig. 70–4). Other criteria include S waves in Leads I, II, III; deep Q waves in Leads I, II, III, except in deep-chested

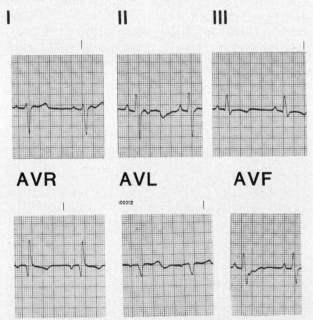

Figure 70–4. Electrocardiogram from a 5-month-old male beagle with severe pulmonic stenosis. Right ventricular enlargement is indicated by $S_1S_2S_3$ pattern and right axis deviation. (50 mm/sec, 1 cm = 1 mv.)

dogs; and positive T waves in lead V_{10}. Biventricular enlargement produces a combination of alterations such as tall R waves in Leads II, III, AVF plus right axis deviation.

Myocardial Damage

The electrocardiogram can be used to recognize some types and degrees of myocardial damage. The identification of these patterns is useful in assessing severity of disease, establishing a prognosis, and in managing anesthesia. Myocardial impairment may occur as a sequel to primary cardiac disease or, frequently, as the result of trauma to the thoracic cavity, e.g., in an automobile accident.

Myocardial changes are most dependably recognized when one is evaluating serial electrocardiograms. If a normal pattern has been established, sudden changes are more easily identified and more likely to be associated with disease than with normal patient variation. Alterations that might be expected include the development of deep Q waves,[40,47] particularly in transmural myocardial damage. Deep Q waves may occur normally in thin, deep-chested dogs and also in right ventricular enlargement, so assessment should be made with these facts in mind.

Elevation or depression of the ST segment is a rapidly developing response to myocardial hypoxia or injury. The ST segment is elevated in leads oriented toward the injured surface and depressed in leads directed away from the injured surface. The mechanism responsible for ST segment change is still controversial. One theory describes a diastolic current of injury at rest due to altered resting potential in injured myocardial tissue, and resulting in an apparent ST segment alteration. In addition, a systolic current of injury resulting in impaired depolarization or early repolarization produces true ST segment alteration. The combination of these two currents of injury results in the ST segment changes recognized clinically.[23,40] Resolution of ST segment changes indicates myocardial recovery.

Finally, changes in repolarization of injured myocardial tissue may produce T wave alterations. The T wave may initially become more peaked and symmetrical and later become inverted. Inversion is probably due to a reversal in the direction of repolarization.[23,40] Resolution of T wave changes again indicates recovery. The wide variability of T waves in dogs and cats emphasizes the importance of serial electrocardiograms.

Conduction Disorders

Conduction disorders may involve any level of the normal conduction pathway. The abnormalities may range from alterations in impulse generation to delay or complete obstruction of conduction. These disorders are important to the surgeon, because they may accompany some operable cardiovascular diseases, influence anesthetic protocols or management procedures, or require surgical implantation of a cardiac pacemaker.

Alterations in sinoatrial conduction can be inferred from long pauses without P waves on the surface electrocardiogram. Recordings from the sinoatrial node are required for definitive identification of sinoatrial arrest or varying degrees of sinoatrial block. Excessive vagal tone may produce sinoatrial conduction disorders, but in many patients, particularly in older animals, the abnormalities are due to progressive fibrous replacement of the sinoatrial node. Frequently, the electrocardiographic changes are intermittent, so ambulatory monitoring of the electrocardiogram for varying intervals is beneficial in diagnosis. Clinical signs and electrocardiographic findings can be related with this technique.

Conduction disorders at the atrioventricular (AV) node may also vary in severity. The different degrees of atrioventricular nodal block can be identified by surface electrocardiograms. First-degree AV block is characterized by delayed conduction and a prolonged PR interval. Second-degree AV block is associated with intermittent obstruction of conduction, resulting in P waves that are not followed by QRS complexes. Although frequent in diseased hearts, first-degree and, occasionally, second-degree AV block may occur in otherwise normal dogs. This alteration may be responsive to atropine.[11] Third-degree or complete AV block produces atrioventricular dissociation, since no atrial impulses are conducted to the ventricle and ventricular depolarization is the result of an escape rhythm arising below the atrium. This condition is often unresponsive to medical therapy and if not reversible may require a pacemaker.[8]

A better understanding of the location and mechanism of AV node conduction disorders can be gained through intracavitary electrograms. The His bundle electrogram is recorded from a bipolar electrode catheter passed down the jugular vein to the AV node. It allows the examiner to localize the conduction problem to the area between the atrium and bundle of His or the area between the bundle of His and the ventricle.[5,46] This information is useful therapeutically and in assessing prognosis.

Intraventricular conduction defects can accompany congenital abnormalities, cardiomyopathies, neoplasia, and other cardiac conditions.[16,32,49] Right bundle branch block may be seen as an incidental finding in otherwise normal dogs.[32] Because the right bundle branch is more discrete, disruptions of conduction to the right ventricle are more common than abnormalities of the left bundle branch. Delayed or obstructed conduction in either system destroys the normal synchrony of ventricular depolarization. The asynchrony is reflected in the electrocardiogram by a prolonged and distorted QRS complex.

Although complete left bundle branch block is uncommon, obstruction of either the left anterior or the left posterior fascicle may occur with greater

LEAD II 50mm/sec

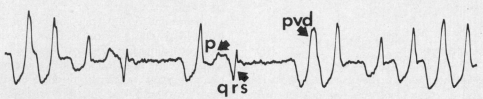

Figure 70–5. Paroxysmal ventricular tachycardia in a dog with aortic stenosis. *p*, atrial systole; *grs*, normal ventricular systole; *pvd*, premature ventricular depolarization. (50 mm/sec, 1 cm = 1 mv.)

frequency. The left anterior fascicle is most likely to be involved, because it is longer, narrower, less vascular, and lies nearer the left ventricular outflow tract. The electrocardiogram in a patient with left anterior fascicular block demonstrates slight prolongation of the QRS complex and severe left axis deviation.

An important consideration in conduction disturbances is the possibility that surgical intervention in a susceptible area may produce one or more of these disorders. The surgeon should be familiar with pertinent anatomy and able to recognize the electrocardiographic changes accompanying conduction defects.

Dysrhythmias

Abnormalities in rate and rhythm other than those previously discussed are also important considerations before, during, and after cardiovascular surgery. Both bradyarrhythmias and tachyarrhythmias may be seen. Abnormalities in rhythm may be precipitated by changes in the supraventricular tissues (sinoatrial node, atrium, and atrioventricular node) or in the ventricular tissues. This is an important distinction, because the precipitating disorders, clinical signs, and therapies may be significantly different.

Many of the supraventricular dysrhythmias develop in animals with unilateral or bilateral atrial enlargement. Atrial enlargement predisposes to myocardial changes that may alter automaticity and also favors re-entry pathways that can perpetuate abnormal rhythms. Paroxysmal supraventricular dysrhythmias may also occur in hypertrophic cardiomyopathy as a result of ventricular pre-excitation and in the tachycardia-bradycardia episodes associated with sick sinus syndrome.[4,47,48]

Premature atrial depolarizations are identified by the early appearance of P waves with abnormal conformation. These P waves are usually followed by normal QRS complexes. The ectopic beats may occur singly, in pairs, or in runs producing paroxysmal atrial tachycardia. Atrioventricular nodal or junctional premature depolarizations are also usually followed by normal QRS complex. The P wave, if visible, is inverted owing to retrograde conduction to the atria.

Paroxysmal atrioventricular junctional tachycardia may be difficult to distinguish from atrial tachycardia, because the P waves may be superimposed on the QRS complexes or T waves, thus impairing assessment of atrial activity from the surface electrocardiogram. *Paroxysmal supraventricular tachycardia* describes those dysrhythmias in which atrial activity cannot be evaluated.

Atrial fibrillation may occur with congenital or acquired disorders. It may manifest, for example, as a preoperative complication in patent ductus arteriosus with severe mitral regurgitation and left atrial enlargement.[1,47] The electrocardiogram is characterized by the absence of discernible P waves, an irregular ventricular rate, variable second-degree atrioventricular block, and usually a rapid ventricular rate. Atrial fibrillation as a complication of progressive disease has a poor long-term prognosis. If the underlying disorder can be corrected, such as in patent ductus arteriosus, the dysrhythmia may be manageable medically for a longer period.

Ventricular dysrhythmias may range from periodic ventricular premature depolarizations to ventricular tachycardia with only occasional capture or fusion beats (Fig. 70–5). The QRS complexes are usually bizarre and prolonged. They occur early in the cardiac cycle, prior to normal ventricular depolarization, and are disassociated from the P waves of sinoatrial node–generated atrial depolarization. Ventricular dysrhythmias are particularly likely to occur in disorders that negatively alter the relationship between cardiac muscle mass and coronary perfusion, such as aortic stenosis.[37] Frequent premature depolarizations, multifocal premature depolarizations, R-on-T phenomenon, and activity-induced or activity-aggravated premature depolarizations may all be associated with a more severe prognosis and should be treated aggressively.

RADIOLOGY

Radiographs, like electrocardiograms, are rapidly available, noninvasive sources of diagnostic information. A radiograph can be used to visually assess cardiac size and shape, vascular conformation, pulmonary pattern, and other noncardiopulmonary thoracic structures. It rarely gives direct evidence of the kind of cardiac disease present, but rather demonstrates changes in the thoracic structures that occur in response to cardiac disease. The examiner must then integrate radiographic findings, history, and other clinical data to determine the diagnosis. A systematic approach is essential to avoid missing important changes and to insure completeness.

The position of the heart in the thorax may vary. Normally, the apex of the heart lies in the left hemithorax, but primary dextrocardia may occur with situs inversus or severe cardiac malformation.[15] Secondary dextroposition may occur in response to diseases that produce extracardiac thoracic changes or to cardiac disease and cardiomegaly. The apex may shift to the left in response to right ventricular enlargement. These changes can influence radiographic evaluation.

Cardiac size is an important indicator of heart disease. Cardiomegaly occurs as a result of cardiac dilation, eccentric hypertrophy, pericardial effusion, or peritoneopericardial hernia. Microcardia is most frequently related to hypovolemia. Cardiac size may be assessed by direct measurement or may be subjectively evaluated. Measurement, although reasonably consistent, is slow and tedious.[45] Most evaluators subjectively assess cardiac size on the basis of previous films or past experience with radiographs of normal animals. It is important in subjective evaluation to consider the dog's breed and conformation. Deep-chested dogs may have narrower, more vertical hearts, whereas wide-chested breeds have a more dorsoventrally compressed thorax and greater sternal contact. The cardiac silhouette is more elongated in the cat than in the dog, so evaluation of feline cardiac size requires experience with normal cat thoracic radiographs and slightly different criteria. Significant cardiac disease can occur with no evidence of cardiac enlargement on the radiographs, particularly with concentric hypertrophy, which may accompany hypertrophic cardiomyopathy and similar disorders.

Evaluation of cardiac shape helps to localize cardiac enlargement to the right, left, or both sides. Changes in the contour of the heart in both the dorsoventral and lateral views can coincide with enlargement of one or more of the cardiac chambers (Fig. 70–6). Distension or distortion of major cardiac vessels provides additional information. The aortic arch and main pulmonary artery areas—one o'clock and two o'clock, respectively, in the dorsoventral film—dilate in response to increased or turbulent flow (see Fig. 70–6). Although some disorders may accentuate chambers and vessels, the loss of the normal cardiac shape and the absence of typical silhouette structures suggests pericardial effusion or peritoneopericardial hernia. The cranial waist may be filled by the aortic arch or main pulmonary artery. In aortic stenosis, post-stenotic dilation of the aorta produces a distinctive radiographic pattern (Fig. 70–7).

Examination of the vascular pattern is helpful in assessing blood supply to and from both sides of the

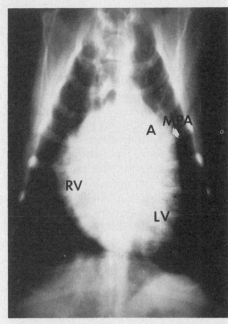

Figure 70–6. Dorsoventral thoracic radiograph of a 1½-year-old female mixed-breed dog with patent ductus arteriosus. Biventricular enlargement is present, and the aorta and main pulmonary artery are dilated and prominent. *LV*, left ventricle; *RV*, right ventricle; *A*, aorta; *MPA*, main pulmonary artery.

heart. The overall vascularity of the lung field should be evaluated, in particular the size of the artery and vein to the right cranial lung lobe. Many diseases retain normal pulmonary vascularity, but separating other disorders according to whether the lungs are undercirculated or overcirculated is helpful diagnostically. Marked decrease in pulmonary vascularity is expected in tetralogy of Fallot, whereas left-to-right shunting, as in patent ductus arteriosus, produces pulmonary overcirculation. Passive pulmonary congestion can also be signified by dilation of the pulmonary veins.

Pulmonary pattern is routinely assessed because many cardiovascular diseases affect the respiratory tract. The inverse relationship is also true. Three

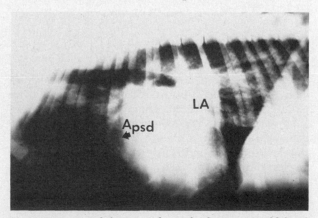

Figure 70–7. Lateral thoracic radiograph of a two-year-old female German shepherd with aortic stenosis. The anterior waist is filled by the post-stenotic dilatation of the aorta, and the left atrium is enlarged. *Apsd*, post-stenotic dilatation of the aorta; *LA*, left atrium.

major radiographic pulmonary patterns have been described—alveolar, interstitial, and bronchovascular.[44] Some diseases produce a combination of changes seen in more than one pattern. Of particular interest to the cardiologist are the vascular patterns seen with heartworms and left-to-right shunts, the bronchial patterns seen with chronic bronchitis producing cor pulmonale, and the interstitial and alveolar patterns of pulmonary edema.

Dirofilariasis is often associated with predominantly pulmonary signs, and these changes must be addressed during therapy. Recognition of and medical attention to the pulmonary overcirculation found in left-to-right shunts can facilitate anesthesia and surgery. Right-sided failure is frequently secondary to cor pulmonale in older dogs with chronic obstructive airway disease. Changes in the bronchovascular markings may help to identify this cause of right heart failure. Finally, left heart failure can produce progressive degrees of pulmonary congestion, ranging from venous engorgement to interstitial edema and, most significantly, alveolar edema. Edema is often greatest in the perihilar area initially, with progressive peripheral involvement as severity increases.[43] Recognition of these changes is important diagnostically and also prognostically, in evaluating response to therapy.

Evaluation of other thoracic and nonthoracic tissues and structures is important in integrating the lesions and pathogenesis. Pleural effusion, ascites, and hepatomegaly are all sequelae to right heart failure that are radiographically recognizable. Abnormal masses in the thorax impair circulation by obstructing venous return or forward cardiac output.

Space-occupying lesions or effusions in the thorax may interfere with evaluation of the heart. Sometimes it is not possible to distinguish soft tissue structures from compartmentalized fluid or free fluid. Positional radiographs can be obtained by changing the position of the animal, the beam, or both. Fluid can be redistributed to improve cardiac visibility or to discriminate between fluid and nonmoveable, radiodense masses.

Contrast Radiography

Although general assessments can be made from plain radiographs, contrast radiography allows evaluation of wall thickness, chamber and vessel size, and flow patterns. This information is essential in the diagnosis and development of therapeutic plans for some cardiovascular disorders. Contrast techniques may employ intravascular or extravascular administration of radiopaque agents.

Because pericardial effusion may occur secondary to space-occupying lesions involving the base of the heart or atria, contrast studies may be used as part of the diagnostic plan in animals with pericardial disease. Gastrointestinal contrast studies may help to outline displaced bowel loops in peritoneopericardial

hernias. Intravascular studies can help to identify pericardial effusion and related cardiac abnormalities, such as atrial masses and, occasionally, heart base tumors.[13] In some cases, a pneumopericardium may be performed. Effusion is removed via pericardiocentesis, and carbon dioxide is reinfused as a contrast medium. Carbon dioxide rather than room air is employed in order to decrease the risk of embolization. Caution should be used, since this procedure can induce hemodynamic changes similar to those seen in pericardial effusion.[28,39]

Intravascular angiography may be accomplished nonselectively, through percutaneous catheterization of the jugular or cephalic vein, or selectively, following direct catheterization of right- or left-sided structures through the jugular vein, carotid artery, or femoral vessels. The contrast agent used should be of low toxicity, high opacity, and low viscosity; this combination allows use of small volumes of contrast to be easily injected at low risk. Diatrizoate meglumine, diatrizoate sodium, iothalamate meglumine, and iothalamate sodium have all been used as contrast agents. Each compound has strengths and weaknesses, and as yet the ideal contrast medium has not been found.

Nonselective venous angiography is less precise but more easily and rapidly accomplished. Chemical restraint of some type is usually required, but the depth and duration are shorter than for selective catheterization. The technique can be adapted to private practice; although a rapid film changer is helpful, manual techniques are adequate. This procedure is most applicable in small dogs and cats, because the volumes of contrast required in large breeds are difficult to inject rapidly by hand and dilution of contrast may impair evaluation. Pressure data and blood gas information cannot be obtained with this technique, but an anatomic diagnosis and subjective assessment of severity are usually possible.

Although different methods can be used, we prefer left lateral recumbency with placement of an 18- to 20-gauge catheter in the right jugular vein. Approx-

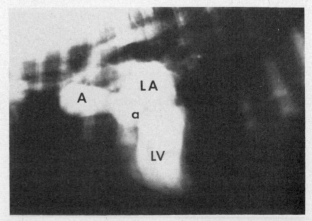

Figure 70–8. Nonselective venous angiogram from a three-month-old female German shepherd with aortic stenosis. The post-stenotic dilatation of the aorta is demonstrated. *LA*, left atrium; *LV*, left ventricle; *a*, aortic valve; *A*, aorta.

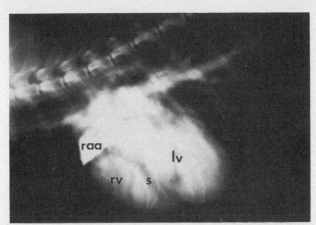

Figure 70–9. Nonselective venous angiogram from a one-year-old female mixed-breed cat with a ventricular septal defect. The film demonstrates reopacification of the right ventricle through the ventricular septal defect after contrast media had been cleared from the right ventricle. *raa*, right atrial appendage; *lv*, left ventricle; *rv*, right ventricle; *s*, septum.

imately 1 ml/kg of iothalamate meglumine is injected as rapidly as possible. The first film is taken just prior to completion of the injection and at intervals of 0.5 to 1.0 second thereafter, depending on the tentative diagnosis. If a manual technique is used to change films, the films can be taken as quickly as feasible. A film taken at 6 to 8 seconds after injection provides a left ventricular study without right-sided superimposition in most animals. Adjustments in timing must be made in animals with prolonged circulation times.

This technique can be used to distinguish between hypertrophic and congestive cardiomyopathy in cats. Aortic thromboemboli can also be identified and evaluated. A lateral radiograph centered over the abdomen and taken 10 to 15 seconds after injection usually provides adequate aortic contrast to localize vascular obstruction.[29] Obstructive defects such as pulmonic stenosis and aortic stenosis are usually well demonstrated. Post-stenotic dilations and secondary ventricular changes are outlined by the contrast medium (Fig. 70–8).

Right-to-left shunts can be readily recognized, but left-to-right shunts are much more difficult to diagnose (Fig. 70–9). Disorders such as tetralogy of Fallot produce simultaneous opacification of the right and left sides with immediate presence of contrast in the aorta. Although left-to-right shunts are difficult to identify, if large enough, they can be signified by the reopacification of the right side when contrast medium reaches the left side.

Some complicated disorders may be evaluated more completely if dorsoventral films are taken as well as the lateral films, allowing relationships of structures that might be obscured on the lateral view to be visible. Because of dye dilution during circulation, small defects may not be visible in a nonselective study.

Nonselective techniques may be ineffective for diagnosis of some cardiac disorders. Mitral and tri-cuspid regurgitation, for example, cannot be directly identified using this procedure, but their secondary effects can be seen.

CARDIAC CATHETERIZATION AND SELECTIVE ANGIOGRAPHY

Selective angiography is usually performed in conjunction with cardiac catheterization. This latter procedure is more invasive and requires greater anesthetic management, more time, and additional special equipment. Cardiac catheterization is used to confirm a tentative diagnosis, to identify additional abnormalities, and to determine the exact nature of and severity of a particular lesion.

In addition to angiography, cardiac catheterization provides assessment of pressures, oxygen tensions, cardiac output, and shunt quantitation. All of this information may not be necessary in every case, and a protocol for the most complete and efficient evaluation should be prepared for each patient. To obtain this type of data, the following additional equipment is required: a monitor with electrocardiograph and pressure channels, a recorder to use in conjunction with the monitor, fluoroscopic capabilities, a pressure transducer, and appropriate catheters. Recording of angiograms requires a rapid film changer, a videotape recorder, or cineangiographic equipment. An image intensification system helps to reduce radiation exposure for both patient and operator.[3] Cardiac output determination and evaluation of oxygen tensions require some type of indicator dilution cardiac output technique and oximetry. Because of the significant equipment needs, cardiac catheterization is usually limited to large institutions.

Cardiac catheterization is a surgical technique, and the risks of the anesthesia and procedure should always be weighed against the value of the information obtained. Potential complications include vascular damage during catheter placement, cardiac perforation, emboli, adverse reaction to contrast media, dysrhythmias, sepsis at the surgical site, and trauma to the vagosympathetic trunk.[3] Because catheter-induced dysrhythmias may arise, appropriate antidysrhythmic drugs and a defibrillator should be immediately available.

Surgical Approach

The surgical approach for cardiac catheterization is via the carotid artery and external jugular vein or the femoral vessels. Use of the right carotid artery and jugular vein avoids angiographic confusion and difficulty with catheter manipulation, which may occur in those animals with persistent left cranial vena cava. These vessels are usually sacrificed at the conclusion of the procedure, although they can be repaired if necessary. The jugular vein provides the easiest access to the pulmonary outflow tract, since the path through the right atrium, right ventricle, and pulmonary outflow tract requires only one bend in the catheter and then follows the natural curve of the catheter. The left ventricle can be entered easily from the cranial or caudal position, although catheterization of the left atrium requires a sharp turn in the catheter's pathway.

Catheter Selection

Catheter selection is important and varies depending on the information desired and the area under study. Most catheters are constructed of woven Dacron, polyethylene, polyurethane, or Teflon. These materials influence the shape, stiffness, and coefficient of friction for each catheter. Reinforcement is added to increase the stiffness of some catheters, to aid in passing them within the vessel. Guide-wires can be used to increase the stiffness of soft catheters. Although greater stiffness aids in catheter manipulation, it also increases the risk of cardiac trauma. Preformed catheters with a particular curve or shape are used to catheterize specific structures where little additional manipulation is required. Non-preformed catheters are softer and more malleable. An important characteristic of these catheters is memory, or the ability to retain the shape that has been produced during passage through cardiac structures.

End-hole catheters are suitable for recording of pressures, particularly pulmonary artery wedge pressures. Because of catheter recoil, they are not suitable for power contrast injections.[3,21] Other catheters are excellent for contrast studies but less suitable for pressure recording. The clinician has the alternative of using different catheters for various aspects of the study, which is time-consuming, or using a catheter that is suitable, if not ideal, for multiple purposes. We frequently use a ventriculography catheter because it is adaptable to pressure recording and angiography. In addition, the tapered end facilitates passage through obstructed pulmonary or aortic outflow tracts.

Catheter size and length are also important. French (Fr) units express outside diameters of catheters. Each French unit is 0.33 mm. Most dogs require 5 to 8 Fr catheters, and cats require smaller sizes. The catheter must be compatible with all ancillary equipment, such as needles, guide-wires, and sheaths. The largest-diameter catheter that can be safely used should be selected. Shorter catheters produce less pressure damping and better recordings so the minimum functional catheter length is recommended.

Catheters may be modified for special applications. Balloon catheters, such as the Swan-Ganz, allow flow-directed placement and recording of wedge pressures. Multiple-lumen catheters permit simultaneous sampling of multiple areas from several ports at different levels. Thermistors can be added to permit thermodilution cardiac output determinations. Catheter electrodes permit simultaneous pressure and electrocardiographic recordings.

Technique

Although in some instances only right-heart catheterization is performed, in most cases in which cardiac catheterization is performed to confirm or establish a diagnosis, both sides should be evaluated. Frequently, multiple defects may be present, and some of these may not be suspected, so complete catheterization helps to avoid errors of omission. Anesthesia should be monitored carefully during catheterization, and the patient kept in as light an anesthesia plane as possible so that pressures and cardiac outputs are reasonable reflections of these values in the awake animal.

Pressure Recordings

Pressure tracings should be recorded from all chambers and vessels entered. Normal values are listed in Table 70–2. The right atrial pressure tracing is characterized by two positive deflections, the a wave and the v wave. The a wave reflects pressure during atrial systole, and the v wave represents pressure during atrial filling. Both waves are recorded, and a mean pressure is calculated electronically.

Right ventricular pressures are recorded during systole and diastole. Right ventricular end-diastolic pressure is recorded immediately after atrial systole and prior to ventricular contracture. Systolic, dia-

TABLE 70–2. Normal Pressure and Oxygen Saturations for Canine Heart Chambers

Chamber	Pressure (mm Hg)		O₂ Saturation (%)
Vena cava	5/−1	mean 3	75
Right atrium	5/−1	mean 3	75
Right ventricle	20/0	end-diastolic 3	75
Pulmonary artery	20/10	mean 15	75
Pulmonary artery wedge	12/6	mean 8	98
Left atrium	14/5	mean 8	98
Left ventricle	120/0	end-diastolic 6	98
Aorta	120/80	mean 100	98

stolic, and mean pulmonary artery pressures are recorded. A slight (≤ 5 mm Hg) pressure gradient may exist between the right ventricle and pulmonary artery in normal dogs.

Left atrial pressure is usually evaluated indirectly via the pulmonary artery wedge pressure, because the left atrium is difficult to catheterize. This technique also allows evaluation of left atrial pressure using only a right-sided catheter. The wave form is somewhat damped, but a and v waves are still present. These should be recorded along with the mean pressure. To assure proper wedge position the mean pulmonary artery pressure should exceed the mean pulmonary artery wedge pressure, and a blood sample from this area should be arterialized.[3]

Pressure tracings of the left ventricle are similar to those of the right ventricle, but the pressure levels reflect the greater thickness of the left ventricular wall. The same measurements are recorded on the left side as on the right side. Aortic pressure tracings demonstrate a systolic peak followed by the incisura, denoting aortic valve closure, and a gradual drop in pressure as blood flows peripherally. Systolic, diastolic, and mean pressures are also recorded.

Abnormalities in pressure recordings may be diagnostic of various conditions. Aortic and pulmonic stenosis both produce pressure gradients between the ventricular chamber and related great vessels. This information is obtained by recording pressures as the catheter is pulled from the pulmonary artery to right ventricle or from the left ventricle to the aorta. The nature and location of the pressure change can help localize the lesion to the subvalvular, valvular, or supravalvular area. In addition, the rise in aortic pressure with aortic stenosis is slow and delayed compared with the left ventricular pressure development.

Aortic regurgitation produces wide aortic pulse pressures and marked increase in left ventricular end-diastolic pressure. Pulmonary hypertension is reflected in elevated pulmonary artery pressure. Mitral and tricuspid stenosis produce diastolic gradients between the atria and ventricles. Mitral regurgitation results in elevated pulmonary artery wedge pressures and exaggerated v waves.

Cardiac Output Measurement

Cardiac output determinations are accomplished via some indicator dilution technique. In the Fick method, oxygen is the indicator. Indocyanine green is the most commonly used dye indicator. More recently, thermodilution techniques using cold or room-temperature saline have become widely used. The major advantage of the thermodilution technique is that it can be repeated numerous times without indicator build-up and interference. Indicator dilution techniques can also be used to recognize shunts. Right-to-left shunts produce an early appearance of indicator on the left side, and left-to-right shunts

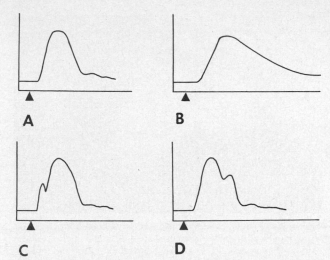

Figure 70–10. Cardiac output curves typical of various cardiac conditions (injections made in the right atrium and sampled from the aorta). *Triangles* represent the injection. *A*, Normal dilution curve. The appearance time is 4–6 sec. There are recirculation "bumps," depending on the indicator used. *B*, Dilution curve seen with AV valve regurgitation. The appearance time may be slightly delayed. The curve is long and low, representing the to-and-fro flow at the lesion. *C*, Dilution curve of right-to-left shunt. The early appearance at 1–2 sec is due to the right-to-left shunted indicator. *D*, Dilation curve of left-to-right shunt. The large "bump" on the down slope of the curve is due to the indicator that has quickly recirculated back through the lungs to be observed in the aorta again.

produce an early recirculation "bump" on the output curve (Fig. 70–10).

Oximetry

Oximetry is useful in the diagnosis and quantitation of shunts. Normal blood saturations are listed in Table 70-2. Left-to-right shunts are signified by increased right side oxygen saturation. Multiple samples should be checked to insure repeatability of the data. This information can also be used to quantitate the amount of blood being shunted across a defect (see Chapter 71). Unidirectional shunts can be calculated simply by comparing pulmonary flow to systemic flow. In bidirectional shunts, more complex mathematical manipulation are required to assess the amount of shunting. This is an important determination, since small shunts may be well tolerated and may require no surgical intervention.

Selective Angiography

Selective angiography is accomplished by direct catheterization of the desired vessel or chamber. Since the catheter can be placed at the desired injection site, less contrast medium is required, and better demonstration of the lesion obtained. Figures 70–11 and 70–12 demonstrate selective angiograms in aortic stenosis and pulmonic stenosis, respectively. Location of the obstruction, wall thickness, and cham-

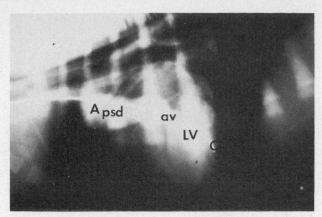

Figure 70–11. Selective left ventricular angiogram from the same three-month-old female German shepherd as in Fig. 70–8. Post-stenotic dilatation of the aorta is demonstrated. A pressure gradient of 40 mm Hg existed between the left ventricle and aorta. *C,* catheter in the left ventricle; *LV,* left ventricle; *av,* aortic valve; *Apsd,* post-stenotic dilatation of the aorta.

ber size can all be assessed from selective angiograms. In addition, selective catheter placement allows evaluation of valvular regurgitation, septal defects, and other shunts. If all data obtained by catheterization is integrated, the clinician can determine systolic and diastolic chamber size, valve orifice area, vascular resistance, and regurgitant flow.

Therapeutic Uses

Although infrequently accomplished in veterinary medicine, cardiac catheterization can be used as a therapeutic technique. Balloon atrial septostomy is a standard procedure to improve systemic and pulmonary mixing in transposition of the great vessels.[38] Catheterization techniques have also been used to obstruct shunts, remove emboli or catheter fragments, and produce embolization.[3] This area has great potential for expansion in veterinary surgery.

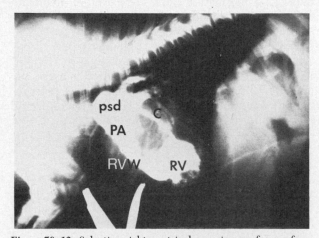

Figure 70–12. Selective right ventricular angiogram from a four-month-old male Scottish terrier with severe pulmonic stenosis. Marked right ventricular hypertrophy and post-stenotic dilatation of the main pulmonary artery are present. *C,* catheter in the right ventricle; *RV,* right ventricle; *RVW,* right ventricular wall; *PA,* main pulmonary artery; *psd,* post-stenotic dilatation.

ECHOCARDIOGRAPHY

In recent years, echocardiography has become a useful noninvasive diagnostic technique in animals. Most of the veterinary literature deals with applications of M-mode echocardiography, but the increasing availability of two-dimensional equipment should result in a proliferation of reports of use and applications.

Echocardiography uses the imaging capabilities of ultrasound to identify and evaluate various cardiac structures. The ultrasound transducer acts as a transmitter and receiver. It generates high-frequency sound waves, which reflect or echo from cardiac structures, and then collects these reflected waves so they can be integrated and displayed on an oscilloscope. M-mode, or motion, echocardiography is produced when the transducer is placed in a fixed position and the changes in position of cardiac structures during the cardiac cycle are recorded. The echocardiogram that results shows time on the horizontal axis and distance from the transducer on the vertical axis. An electrocardiogram is used as a reference for the phases of the cardiac cycle.

Although different transducer positions have been used, in small animals the recording is usually made with the patient in left lateral recumbency and the transducer placed at the ventral right hemithorax. Palpation of the right chest wall helps to locate the area of maximal cardiac intensity and the proper transducer position. Selection of a transducer is influenced primarily by the size of the patient and is usually a compromise, permitting adequate penetration but retaining sufficient resolution and detail. Use of ultrasonic coupling gel is essential to eliminate the air space between transducer and chest wall. Transducer placement is adjusted slightly to record tracings from all desired positions.

Echocardiograms in animals are generally comparable qualitatively to those recorded in man. Human references are therefore helpful in recognizing normal patterns and alterations that accompany disease. Beginning with transducer artifact, the structures on the echocardiogram appear in the following order: right ventricular wall, right ventricular chamber, ventricular septum, left ventricular chamber, mitral valve, left ventricular wall, and pericardium (Fig. 70–13). If the transducer is rotated ventrally, the left ventricle can be seen below the mitral valve. Craniodorsal rotation produces a view of the aortic root and left atrium. The mitral valve has a distinctive appearance. The anterior leaflet inscribes an M and the posterior leaflet a W. These are helpful landmarks when one is trying to establish correct transducer position. The aortic root has parallel walls that both move toward the transducer in systole and away from the transducer during diastole, in contrast to the left ventricle, in which the septum and left ventricular wall move toward each other in systole and away from each other in diastole.

Because M-mode echocardiography produces an

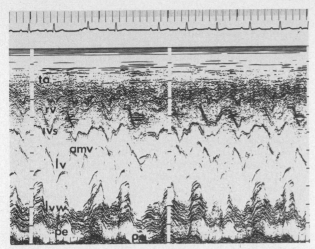

Figure 70–13. Echocardiogram from a two-year-old male Old English sheepdog with idiopathic pericardial effusion. The transducer beam passes through the left ventricle at the level of the mitral valve. *ta*, transducer artifact; *rv*, right ventricle; *ivs*, interventricular septum; *amv*, anterior leaflet of the mitral valve; *lv*, left ventricle; *lvw*, left ventricular wall; *pe*, echo-free space behind the left ventricle, representing pericardial effusion; *p*, pericardium.

"icepick" view of the heart, many cardiac defects cannot be seen, but secondary changes are often readily evaluated. Measurement of intracardiac dimensions, ventricular wall thickness, valve position, and valve motion is a useful means of assessing chamber enlargement and muscular hypertrophy. For comparison, it is best to index these values to body surface area or weight.

Left ventricular function can be evaluated by determination of end-systolic and end-diastolic diameters, per cent shortening fraction, left ventricular ejection time, pre-ejection period, and the ratio of pre-ejection period to ejection time. The systolic intervals are heart rate–dependent and must be corrected for variation in cardiac rate.[19,34,36] Systolic and diastolic left ventricular volumes may be calculated if some assumptions are made concerning ventricular shape. These assumptions may be reasonably accurate for the normal heart, but cardiac chamber shape frequently changes in the small or very dilated heart.[19]

Contrast echocardiography can be used to identify shunts and valve regurgitation. Contrast can be produced by rapid injection of isotonic saline, the patient's blood, indocyanine green dye, or a combination of these agents. Rapid injection creates microcavitation, producing echo-dense targets in the otherwise echo-free chamber. The targets can be followed through the circulation to demonstrate right-to-left shunts, left-to-right shunts, and mitral valve regurgitation.[9] Right-to-left shunts can be identified by venous injection of contrast, whereas studies of the left side require selective left ventricular catheterization.

Few congenital defects can be seen directly with M-mode echocardiography. However, right ventricular hypertrophy accompanying pulmonic stenosis, left atrial and ventricular dilation secondary to patent ductus arteriosus, and right ventricular volume overload and paradoxical septal motion seen with atrial or ventricular septal defects are all examples of compensatory changes identified on echocardiography. In some patients with tetralogy of Fallot, the presence of an overriding aorta may be signified on the echocardiogram by loss of the normal continuity between the ventricular septum and aortic root. Aortic stenosis in the dog is usually subvalvular, and the subvalvular fibrous obstruction can be seen as a slight narrowing in the left ventricular outflow tract below the aortic valve. Post-stenotic dilation of the aorta may also be seen.

Acquired cardiac defects also produce echocardiographic changes. The echocardiogram is an excellent way to diagnose pericardial effusion. Because both the pericardium and epicardium can be visualized, it is more definitive than radiographs alone. Pericardial effusion is seen as an echo-free space, which is usually of greatest degree at the cardiac apex between the epicardium and pericardium (Fig. 70–13). Pleural effusion can be distinguished from pericardial effusion on the basis of location and radiographic findings.

The cardiomyopathies are usually indicated by the respective changes in ventricular diameters, left atrial dimensions, wall thickness, septal thickness, and ventricular function. Echocardiography is an alternative to angiography in distinguishing hypertrophic from congestive cardiomyopathy, particularly in cats.

Although subtle changes in the valves may accompany endocardiosis, changes in chamber dimensions are much more pronounced in disorders such as mitral regurgitation.[35] In combination with other diagnostic procedures, echocardiography can support a diagnosis of valvular regurgitation and provide some information on the severity of the lesion. Vegetative lesions of bacterial endocarditis are much more easily seen on M-mode echocardiograms. They produce thickened, irregular echo-dense masses associated with the affected valves.[7,10,41] The mitral and aortic valves are most frequently involved in small animals. Small vegetative lesions may not be discerned on the echocardiogram, so absence of lesions on the echocardiogram does not preclude their presence in the patient.

MISCELLANEOUS DIAGNOSTIC PROCEDURES

Additional diagnostic procedures may be indicated, depending on the underlying problem and presenting clinical signs. Complete blood counts are important in disorders produced by infectious agents, such as bacterial endocarditis and dirofilariasis. Laboratory evaluations are indicated to assess organ dysfunction occurring secondary to or concomitantly with cardiac disorders. Suspected dirofilariosis may require microfilaria evaluation or occult heartworm assessment using fluorescent antibody techniques.

Thoracocentesis or pericardiocentesis is indicated as both a diagnostic and a therapeutic technique in patients with thoracic or pericardial fluid (see Chapter

74). Evaluation of the fluid allows characterization of the type of effusion. The etiology may be identified from the results of fluid evaluation, but frequently the findings are inconclusive.[14,42]

Blood gas values provide important information in assessing the nature and severity of alterations in cardiopulmonary function. Venous partial pressure of oxygen is a useful indirect indicator of cardiac output.[24] It is particularly helpful to evaluate progression of disease or response to therapy according to the changes in venous partial pressure of oxygen.

Evaluation of central venous pressure is a useful means of assessing backward failure on the right side. Although a transducer can be used, a simple manometer is a quick, effective way to monitor changes in pressure in response to therapy. Monitoring arterial pressure is not performed as frequently in animals because of inadequate technology and expensive equipment requirements. This information, however, is important in assessing disorders that produce hypertension or hypotension, in evaluating effectiveness of supportive therapy, and in monitoring response to various drugs that act as vasodilators or vasopressors.

Arterial pressure can be measured by direct catheterization of a superficial artery, frequently the femoral artery, or by indirect ultrasonographic or oscillometric techniques.[25] Problems can arise with any technique and these problems include restraint, patient size, vessel size, accuracy, and repeatability. As technology improves, indirect techniques are becoming increasingly more accurate and available. The ability to monitor arterial pressure routinely provides an important source of patient information.

Additional pulmonary diagnostic procedures may be indicated in patients with interrelated cardiac and pulmonary diseases. As with other diagnostic techniques, those procedures that provide significant information with justifiable risk should be considered.

Cardiac disease occurs rarely as an isolated syndrome but more often as part of a continuum that is affected by other systems and in turn produces changes in those systems. Diagnostic procedures should, therefore, be directed toward overall patient evaluation and should include not only those tests that will yield a diagnosis of the disorder but also those that assess the disorder's effect on the patient.

1. Ackerman, N., Bunk, R., Hahn, A. W., and Hayes, H. M.: Patent ductus arteriosus in the dog: A retrospective study of radiographic, epidemiologic, and clinical findings. Am. J. Vet. Res. 39:1805, 1978.
2. Adolph, R. J.: Second heart sound: the role of altered electromechanical events. In Leon, D. F., and Shaver, J. A. (eds.): Physiologic Principles of Heart Sounds and Murmurs. American Heart Association, Inc., New York, 1975.
3. Barry, W. H., and Grossman, W.: Cardiac catheterization. In Braunwald, E. (ed.): Heart Disease: A Textbook of Cardiovascular Medicine. W. B. Saunders, Philadelphia, 1980.
4. Beckett, S. D., Branch, C. E., and Robertson, B. T.: Syncopal attacks and sudden death in dogs: mechanisms and etiologies. J. Am. Anim. Hosp. Assoc. 14:378, 1978.
5. Bigger, J. T.: Mechanisms and diagnosis of arrhythmias. In Braunwald, E. (ed.): Heart Disease: A Textbook of Cardiovascular Medicine. W. B. Saunders, Philadelphia, 1980.
6. Bolton, G. R.: Handbook of Canine Electrocardiography. W. B. Saunders, Philadelphia, 1975.
7. Bonagura, J. D.: M-mode echocardiography: basic principles. Vet. Clin. North Am. 13:299, 1983.
8. Bonagura, J. D., Helphney, M. L., and Muir, W. W.: Complications associated with permanent pacemaker implantation in the dog. J. Am. Vet. Med. Assoc. 182:149, 1983.
9. Bonagura, J. D., and Pipers, F. S.: Diagnosis of cardiac lesions by contrast echocardiography. J. Am. Vet. Med. Assoc. 182:396, 1983.
10. Bonagura, J. D., and Pipers, F. S.: Echocardiographic features of aortic valve endocarditis in a dog, a cow and a horse. J. Am. Vet. Med. Assoc. 182:595, 1983.
11. Branch, C. E., Robertson, B. T., and Williams, J. C.: Frequency of second-degree atrioventricular heart block in dogs. Am. J. Vet. Res. 36:925, 1975.
12. Calvert, C. A., and Coulter, D. B.: Electrocardiographic values for anesthetized cats in lateral and sternal recumbencies. Am. J. Vet. Res. 42:1453, 1981.
13. Cantwell, H. D., Blevins, W. E., and Weirich, W. E.: Angiographic diagnosis of heart base tumor in the dog. J. Am. Anim. Hosp. Assoc. 18:83, 1982.
14. Cantwell, H. D., Rebar, A. H., and Allen, A. R.: Pleural effusion in the dog: principles for diagnosis. J. Am. Anim. Hosp. Assoc. 19:227, 1983.
15. Carrig, C. B., Suter, P. F., Ewing, G. O., and Dungworth, D. L.: Primary dextrocardia with situs inversus, associated with sinusitis and bronchitis in a dog. J. Am. Vet. Med. Assoc. 164:1127, 1974.
16. Chastain, C. B., Reidesel, D. H., and Graham, D. L.: Ventricular septal hemangiosarcoma associated with right bundle branch block in a dog. J. Am. Vet. Med. Assoc. 165:177, 1974.
17. Craige, E.: Heart sounds. In Braunwald, E. (ed.): Heart Disease: A Textbook of Cardiovascular Medicine. W. B. Saunders, Philadelphia, 1980.
18. Craige, E.: The fourth heart sound. In Leon, D. F., and Shaver, J. A. (eds.): Physiologic Principles of Heart Sounds and Murmurs. American Heart Association, Inc., New York, 1975.
19. Crawford, M. H.: Value and limitations of echocardiography for determining left ventricular size and performance. Coun. Clin. Card. Am. Heart Assoc. Nwsltr. 6:1, 1981.
20. Fontana, M., Kissel, G., and Criley, J. M.: Functional anatomy of mitral valve prolapse. In Leon, D. F., and Shaver, J. A. (eds.): Physiologic Principles of Heart Sounds and Murmurs. American Heart Association, Inc., New York, 1975.
21. Fox, P. R., and Bond, B. R.: Nonselective and selective angiocardiography. Vet. Clin. North Am. 13:259, 1983.
22. Gompf, R. E., and Tilley, L. P.: Comparison of lateral and sternal recumbent positions for electrocardiography of the cat. Am. J. Vet. Res. 40:1483, 1979.
23. Horan, L. G., and Flowers, N. C.: Electrocardiography and vectorcardiography. In Braunwald, E. (ed.): Heart Disease: A Textbook of Cardiovascular Medicine. W. B. Saunders, Philadelphia, 1980.
24. Kittleson, M. D.: Concepts and therapeutic strategies in the management of heart failure. In Kirk, R. W. (ed.): Current Veterinary Therapy VIII: Small Animal Practice. W. B. Saunders, Philadelphia, 1983.
25. Kittleson, M. D., and Olivier, N. B.: Measurement of systemic arterial blood pressure. Vet. Clin. North Am. 13:321, 1983.
26. Leatham, A.: Right ventricular outflow obstruction. In Leon, D. F., and Shaver, J. A. (eds.): Physiologic Principles of Heart Sounds and Murmurs. American Heart Association, Inc., New York, 1975.
27. Liu, S.: Pathology of feline heart diseases. Vet. Clin. North Am. 7:323, 1977.
28. Lombard, C. W.: Pericardial disease. Vet. Clin. North Am. 13:337, 1983.
29. Owens, J. M., and Twedt, D. C.: Nonselective Angiocardiography in the cat. Vet. Clin. North Am. 7:309, 1977.
30. Paley, H. W.: Left ventricular outflow tract obstruction. In

Leon, D. F., and Shaver, J. A. (eds.): *Physiologic Principles of Heart Sounds and Murmurs.* Am. Heart Association, Inc., New York, 1977.

31. Patterson, D. F.: Epidemiologic and genetic studies of congenital heart disease in the dog. Circ. Res. 23:171, 1968.

32. Patterson, D. V., Detweiler, D. K., Hubben, K., and Botts, R. P.: Spontaneous abnormal cardiac arrhythmias and conduction disturbances in the dog. Am. J. Vet. Res. 22:355, 1961.

33. Patterson, D. V., and Pyle, R. L.: Genetic aspects of congenital heart disease in the dog. Gaines Vet. Symp., Ames, Iowa, 1971.

34. Pipers, F. S., Andrysco, R. M., and Hamlin, R. L.: A totally noninvasive method for obtaining systolic time intervals in the dog. Am. J. Vet. Res. 39:1822, 1978.

35. Pipers, F. S., Bonagura, J. D., Hamlin, R. L., and Kittleson, M.: Echocardiographic abnormalities of the mitral valve associated with left-sided heart diseases in the dog. J. Am. Vet. Med. Assoc. 179:580, 1981.

36. Pipers, F. S., Reef, V., and Hamlin, R. L.: Echocardiography in the domestic cat. Am. J. Vet. Res. 40:882, 1979.

37. Pyle, R. L.: Congenital heart disease. *In* Ettinger, S. J. (ed.): *Textbook of Veterinary Internal Medicine.* W. B. Saunders, Philadelphia, 1983.

38. Rashkind, W. J., and Miller, W. W.: Creation of an atrial septal defect without thoracotomy: a palliative approach to complete transposition of the great vessels. J.A.M.A. 196:991, 1966.

39. Reed, J. R., and Thomas, W. P.: Hemodynamics of progressive pneumopericardium in the dog. Am. J. Vet. Res. 45:301, 1984.

40. Schamroth, L.: *An Introduction to Electrocardiography.* Blackwell Scientific, Oxford, 1976.

41. Sisson, D., and Thomas, W. P.: Endocarditis of the aortic valve in the dog. J. Am. Vet. Med. Assoc. 184:570, 1984.

42. Sisson, D., Thomas, W. P., Ruehl, W. W., and Zinkel, J. G.: Diagnostic value of pericardial fluid analysis in the dog. J. Am. Vet. Med. Assoc. 184:51, 1984.

43. Suter, P. F.: The radiographic diagnosis of canine and feline heart disease. Comp. Cont. Ed. Prac. Vet. 3:441, 1981.

44. Suter, P. F., and Chan, K. F.: Disseminated pulmonary diseases in small animals: a radiographic approach to diagnosis. J. Am. Vet. Radiol. Soc. 9:67, 1968.

45. Suter, P. F., and Lord, P. F.: A critical evaluation of the radiographic findings in canine cardiovascular diseases. J. Am. Vet. Med. Assoc. 158:358, 1971.

46. Tilley, L. P.: Advanced electrocardiographic techniques. Vet. Clin. North Am. 13:365, 1983.

47. Tilley, L. P.: *Essentials of Canine and Feline Electrocardiography.* C. V. Mosby, St. Louis, 1979.

48. Tilley, L. P., and Gompf, R. E.: Feline electrocardiography. Vet. Clin. North Am. 7:257, 1977.

49. Troy, G. C., and Turnwald, G. H.: Atrial fibrillation and abnormal ventricular conduction presented as right bundle branch block in a dog with an atrial septum primum defect. J. Am. Anim. Hosp. Assoc. 15:417, 1979.

Chapter **71**

Cardiac Disorders

George E. Eyster and Bonnie DeYoung

The major cardiac disorders in the dog and cat can be divided into two categories: the congenital, often hereditary conditions and the acquired disorders. Acquired cardiovascular disease in animals is usually not amenable to surgical intervention. Fortunately, many of the common congenital cardiac diseases can be treated surgically. The most common congenital disorders are also the most easily repaired or palliated by surgery, and many of these procedures can be performed in the fully equipped surgical practice. Details of correction of specific disorders can be found in Chapter 73. In this chapter, the more common cardiac disorders the pathophysiology and diagnosis of diseases of surgical relevance are reviewed.

CONGENITAL CARDIAC DISORDERS

A summary of known breed dispositions for congenital heart diseases in dogs is seen in Table 71–1.

Development

In the developing fetus, the heart forms from a single tube and, through a series of bends and separations, eventually becomes a four-chambered structure. In the developing heart, partially oxygenated placental blood is diverted away from the lungs, which develop later. In the fetus, the right side of the heart and pulmonary circulation is a high-pressure, high-resistance circuit, which persists until the lungs inflate immediately after birth. As a result, the right side of the developing fetal heart is the high-pressure system, whereas in the postnatal animal, the left side is the high-pressure system.

During fetal development, connections between the two parallel circuits, the developing right side of the heart and the developing left, will as a result of the high resistance to pulmonary flow shunt from right to left. The fetal circulation consists of partially oxygenated placental blood that reaches the right atrium and divides to flow to the right ventricle or left atrium via the foramen ovale. Blood reaching the right ventricle is diverted through the ventricular foramen to the left ventricle or into the pulmonary artery. Blood reaching the pulmonary artery is diverted through the ductus arteriosus to the aorta, with a small amount continuing to supply the developing lungs. Blood that passes through the developing pulmonary circulation returns to the left atrium, where it is joined by blood shunting from the right atrium through the foramen ovale. The blood then flows in a normal pattern to the left ventricle, where

TABLE 71–1. Breed Predispositions for Congenital Heart Defects in the Dog

Defect	Breed Predisposition	Defect	Breed Predisposition
Aortic stenosis	Boxer German shepherd German shorthair Pointer Golden retriever Newfoundland	Pulmonic stenosis	Beagle Chihuahua English bulldog German shepherd Giant schnauzer Keeshond Miniature schnauzer Samoyed Terriers
Atrial septal defect	Boxer Old English sheepdog		
Patent ductus arteriosus	Brittany spaniel Cocker spaniel Collie German shepherd Keeshond Pomeranian Miniature poodle Shetland sheepdog	Tetralogy of Fallot	Keeshond Miniature poodle Miniature schnauzer Terriers Wirehaired fox terrier
		Ventricular septal defect	Beagle German shepherd Keeshond Mastiff Miniature poodle Siberian husky
Persistent right aortic arch	Doberman German shepherd Great Dane Irish setter Weimaraner		

it is joined by blood shunting through the ventricular foramen, and is pumped to the aorta. Here the circulation is completed by the additional blood shunted through the ductus (Fig. 71–1). In the late stages of development, or shortly after birth, the shunts (atrial, ventricular, and ductal) close. With inflation of the lungs and reduced resistance to pulmonary blood flow, the right side of the heart becomes the low-pressure circulation and the left side or systemic circulation becomes the high-pressure

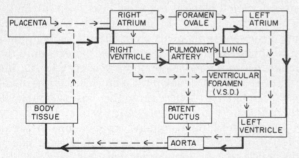

Figure 71–1. The fetal and adult circulation. Partially oxygenated blood from the placenta passes to the right atrium and then through the right ventricle, pulmonary artery, lungs, and left atrium or through the foramen ovale to the left atrium. Blood reaching the right ventricle continues in the normal pattern or passes through the ventricular foramen to the left ventricle. Blood in the pulmonary artery continues to the lung or passes through the ductus arteriosus to the aorta. Because in the fetus the pressures are elevated in the right side of the heart, these three shunts—atrial, ventricular, and ductus—allow blood to bypass the lungs and flow from right to left. In the left side of the heart, blood flows in the normal manner from the left atrium to the left ventricle and aorta, is distributed to the body, and flows back to the placenta for partial oxygenation (broken lines). After birth, with inflation of the lungs, reduced pressure in the right side of the circulation and closure of the shunts, the circulation proceeds in the normal adult manner from the right atrium to the right ventricle, pulmonary artery, lungs, left atrium, left ventricle, aorta, and the body, and back to the right atrium (solid lines).

circuit. The ventricular foramen is filled in and closed. A flap of tissue in the atrium closes over the foramen ovale and is maintained in that position by the high pressure in the left side. Owing to a combination of chemical and physical changes, the ductus closes.[52] The adult cardiovascular system is thus established (Fig. 71–1).

If any of the fetal openings persist, the high pressure in the left side directs the shunt from left to right (Fig. 71–2). (See Table 70–2 for the pressures and oxygen saturations of various heart chambers.)

Malpositioning

Congenital lesions affecting the whole heart are related to specific abnormalities in development. Ectopic cordis, a relatively uncommon anomaly is a malpositioning of the heart, usually in the neck. Occasionally reported in calves, this anomaly is due to the failure of the heart to move into the thorax as the embryo develops.[60] Affected animals are occasionally noted because of the heart can be directly palpated in the neck. There has been no attempt to correct these conditions.

Dextrocardia, or positioning of the heart apex to the right of the thorax rather than the left, is an occasional radiographic finding. Dextrocardia need not be associated with disease, and it is important only as it presents a problem in radiographic diagnosis (Fig. 71–3). The condition is occasionally seen with heart disease but must be differentiated from right-sided heart enlargement. Identification of the pericardial diaphragmatic ligament is helpful in these animals.

The concept of situs with the cardiovascular system relates the heart to body organ positioning. Situs

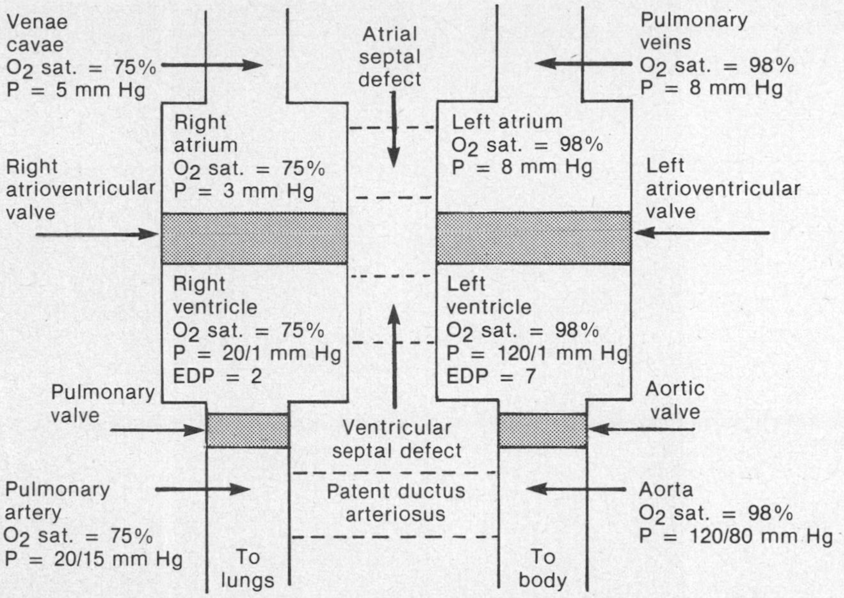

Figure 71–2. The cardiac circulation, showing percent oxygen saturation, pressures, and potential shunts. The blood enters the right side through the vena cava at a pressure (P) 3 to 5 mm Hg and an oxygen saturation (O_2 sat.) of 75%. Right atrial pressures are similar to those of the veins, and the right ventricle systolic pressure is elevated to 20 mm Hg with an end-diastolic pressure (EDP) of 2 to 3 mm Hg. The pulmonary artery pressure is maintained at a mean of 18 mm Hg. Throughout the right side of the heart, saturations are normally 75%. Blood enters the corresponding left side through the pulmonary veins and continues to the aorta with a saturation of approximately 98%. Left atrial pressures are slightly elevated over right atrial pressures, with a mean of 5 to 10 mm Hg. The high (120 mm Hg) systolic pressure in the left ventricle drops to a diastolic pressure of 0 with an end-diastolic pressure of approximately 7 mm Hg. In the aorta, normal blood pressure (120/80 mm Hg) is maintained. Since pressures on the left are normally higher than the corresponding pressures on the right, and the oxygen saturations are higher on the left, shunts at various levels produce flow from the high-pressure left side to the low-pressure right side, with mixing and increasing of the oxygen saturation in the right side.

Venae cavae O_2 sat. = 75% P = 5 mm Hg

Atrial septal defect

Pulmonary veins O_2 sat. = 98% P = 8 mm Hg

Right atrioventricular valve

Right atrium O_2 sat. = 75% P = 3 mm Hg

Left atrium O_2 sat. = 98% P = 8 mm Hg

Left atrioventricular valve

Right ventricle O_2 sat. = 75% P = 20/1 mm Hg EDP = 2

Left ventricle O_2 sat. = 98% P = 120/1 mm Hg EDP = 7

Pulmonary valve

Ventricular septal defect

Aortic valve

Pulmonary artery O_2 sat. = 75% P = 20/15 mm Hg

Patent ductus arteriosus

Aorta O_2 sat. = 98% P = 120/80 mm Hg

To lungs

To body

solitus is the normal relationship, with the heart apex angled toward the left in the thorax; the aorta and arterial tree located on the left side of the body; the venous system to the right side of the body; stomach, spleen, and descending colon predominantly to the left; and liver to the right. Situs inversus is a congenital anomaly, rarely reported in animals but probably much more common than is recognized, in which the body organs are positioned in mirror image. In this condition the heart is tilted to the right, as in dextrocardia; but the arterial tree is to the right; the venous circulation is located to the left; and the stomach, spleen, and descending colon are to the right. Situs inversus is seen in approximately one per 10,000 humans but has only recently been reported in animals (Fig. 71–4).[1,16,43] Frequently associated with situs inversus are other malformations. Branching of the bronchi is altered, and the patient has signs of obstructive pulmonary disease. However, without additional defects most animals with situs inversus have no clinical symptoms.

Venous Anomalies

Major systemic venous anomalies are described in Chapter 79.

The remaining significant venous anomaly associated with cardiovascular disease is persistence of the left anterior cardinal vein or left anterior vena cava. This anomaly causes no physiological problems, but it does produce diagnostic difficulty and is a surgical nuisance. When the developing left anterior vena cava fails to regress and join the right, the vessel continues into the thorax on the left side of the heart and joins the heart at the coronary sinus. Consequently, the left anterior blood reaches the right atrium at the caudal right atrium. This arrangement makes cardiac catheterization from the left jugular vein virtually impossible and venous angiography from the left side confusing. At surgery, the left anterior vena cava may be diminutive or may be a large vessel carrying half the upper body return. Its course is near the vagus nerve across the base of the heart, posterior to the heart and around to the right (Fig. 71–5). When present, therefore, the left anterior vena cava lies lateral to the ductus arteriosus and is frequently associated with the defect. When it is

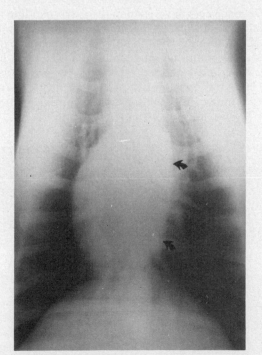

Figure 71–3. Dorsoventral thoracic radiograph of a dog with dextrocardia. Note that the apex is to the right and the aorta (*arrows*) is in its normal position.

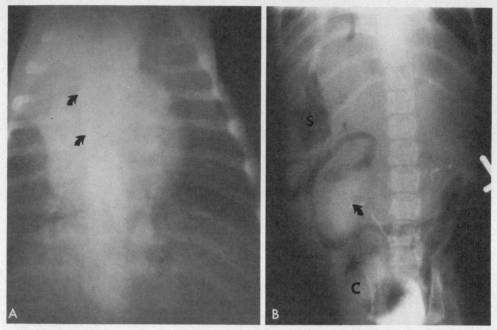

Figure 71–4. A dog with situs inversus. *A*, Dorsoventral thoracic radiograph. Note the abnormal positioning of the aorta (arrows) and reversal of the cardiac silhouette. *B*, Ventrodorsal abdominal radiograph, and intravenous pyelogram. Note the right position of the stomach *(S)*, the abnormal posterior position of the right kidney pelvis *(arrow)*, as well as the right positioning of the colon *(C)*.

present, dissection around and exposure of the ductus is difficult.

Physiology of Left-to-Right Shunts

The most common disease in the area of the right atrium is atrial septal defect (Fig. 71–6). The incidence of atrial septal defect in the dog is considerably less than the literature might lead one to believe.

However, this defect and combination defects involving the atrial septum are more common in the cat. The only dogs showing a predominance are the boxer and Old English sheepdog. Isolated atrial septal defects seldom have signs. Atrial septal defect is a left-to-right shunting disease.

Other left-to-right shunts are ventricular septal defect and patent ductus arteriosus. The pathophysiology of all left-to-right shunts is related to the pressure or flow developed in the corresponding right chambers and lungs. The fetal connections (foramen ovale, interventricular foramen, and ductus arteriosus) allow shunting of blood from the fetal high-pressure right side of the heart to the low-pressure left side and therefore bypassing of the developing lungs. Immediately or shortly after birth, inflation of

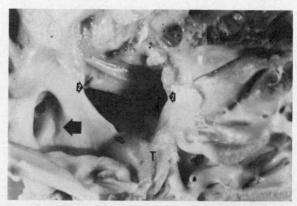

Figure 71–5. Persistent left atrial vena cava *(arrow)* passing from anterior left lateral to the heart across the pulmonary artery *(P)* to enter the right atrium via the coronary sinus at the posterior of the heart (not visible).

Figure 71–6. Atrial septal defect as seen from the right atrium. The tricuspid valve *(T)* is ventral, the coronary sinus *(arrow)* is posterior. The opening of the atrial septal defect is outlined by the small arrows *(2)*.

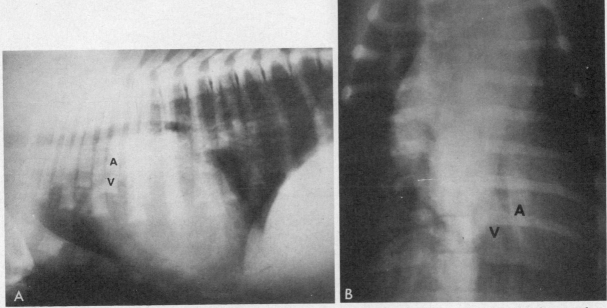

Figure 71–7. A dog with overcirculated lungs due to patent ductus arteriosus. *A,* Lateral thoracic radiograph. The pulmonary densities are caused by increased vascular markings and interstitial edema. The right cranial lobar artery *(A)* and vein *(V)* are enlarged to a greater diameter than the width of the neck of the third rib. There is generalized cardiomegaly. *B,* Dorsoventral thoracic radiograph. The heart is enlarged. The pulmonary densities are due to the increased vasculature and the interstitial edema. The left pulmonary artery *(A)* and vein *(V)* are enlarged.

the lungs reduces pulmonary resistance and decreases the pressure in the pulmonary circulation. As this occurs, the right chambers become lower-pressure chambers than the corresponding left chambers. If persistence of the opening between the two parallel circuits continues, the flow or shunt is from the postnatal high-pressure left side to the low-pressure right, a left-to-right shunt (Fig. 71–2). Because of shunting from the left side to the right, the volume of blood in all chambers of the shunt circuit is increased. This shunt includes the pulmonary arteries, pulmonary capillaries, and pulmonary veins and may be diagnosed by the characteristic radiographic appearance of overcirculated lung (Fig. 71–7). In certain defects, if the left-to-right shunt is great, pressures elevate in the shunt. As a result of pressure elevation in the pulmonary circulation, pulmonary edema may occur, producing the pulmonary signs seen in association with left-to-right shunts.

Atrial Septal Defects

The physical findings with atrial septal defect are related to the shunt from left atrium to right atrium, to right ventricle, to pulmonary vasculature, and the associated pulmonary findings are due to pulmonary overcirculation or pulmonary hypertension. Occasionally, arrhythmias may be associated with atrial septal defect, and syncope or signs of low cardiac output due to arrhythmia may be found.[4,31,75] The development of pulmonary hypertension, a situation probably related to long-standing pulmonary overcirculation, is rare in relatively short-lived animals such as dogs and cats.

Clinical findings in atrial septal defect include a flow murmur associated with the increased blood flow across the pulmonary valve. Because the pressure on the right side is lower than that on the left side, the shunt flow from the left atrium is added to the normal flow through the right side of the heart. This increased volume flow through the normal pulmonary valve produces turbulence. Murmurs are seldom recognized until blood flow through the lungs is more than twice the blood flow through the systemic system. The resultant murmur is similar to the murmur of pulmonary stenosis (discussed later). The second heart sound is frequently split owing to the

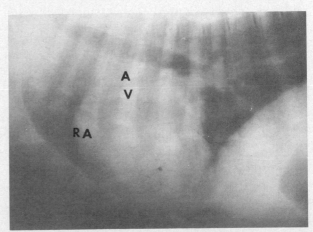

Figure 71–8. Lateral thoracic radiograph of a dog with severe atrial septal defect. The right side of the heart, particularly the right atrium *(RA),* is enlarged. The lungs show an interstitial and vascular density. The right anterior lobar artery *(A)* and vein *(V)* are greatly enlarged.

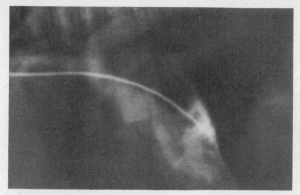

Figure 71–9. Left ventricular angiogram of a dog with atrial septal defect. The catheter has been introduced into the venous circulation and passed into the right atrium across the atrial defect into the left atrium, and the tip has been positioned in the left ventricle. The injection fills the left ventricle and aorta. The catheter is shown in the left ventricle without being present in the left ventricular outflow tract or aorta.

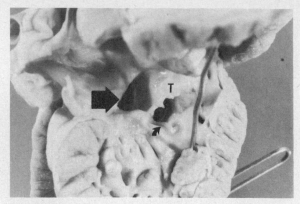

Figure 71–10. Endocardial cushion defect in a cat, from the right side. The dorsal atrium with the atrial defect *(large arrow)* is seen above the tricupid valve *(T)*, which is dorsal to the ventricular defect *(small arrow)*.

delay in closure of the pulmonary valve that results from the increased volume. Electrocardiographic findings with atrial septal defect reflect the amount of additional workload on the right side of the heart. Consequently, as the disease becomes more severe, more right atrial and right ventricular enlargement is recognized on the electrocardiograph. Conduction defects associated with the disease have been reported in the dog.[31,75] Radiographic findings include right heart enlargement and increased vascularity of the lung field (Fig. 71–8).

The diagnosis of atrial septal defect is established by radiographic methods and cardiac catheterization. Radiopaque dye injected into the pulmonary artery outlines the left atrium, left ventricle, right atrium, and right ventricle. The catheter can be positioned across the defect to demonstrate the lesion (Fig. 71–9). Oxygen saturation measurements taken from the anterior vena cava and right atrium demonstrate an oxygen increase from the veins to the atrium (Table 71–2) due to the shunt to the atrium.

Surgical correction of atrial septal defect has been reported once.[31] The patient was symptomatic with syncope, and closure using open heart surgery was successful. Other treatment in animals with clinical signs is medical management of the right-sided heart failure and pulmonary edema, if present.

The prognosis in animals with isolated atrial septal defect is good. In a series at our institution, only 10 per cent of animals with diagnosed atrial septal defect had severe symptoms and only 30 per cent had even minor signs. Careful management of salt level and reduction of activity are adequate for maintenance. However, when atrial septal defect is associated with other lesions that increase right side pressure, right-to-left shunting can be produced at the atrial defect. In these cases severe complications, cyanosis and death are usual. Management of right-to-left shunting disease is extremely difficult, but as yet surgical correction has not been reported.

Endocardial Cushion Defect

In cats, endocardial cushion defect, or atrioventricular canal defect, is the second most common congenital lesion.[54,74] The embryonic endocardial cushions form the ventral portion of the atrial septum, the dorsal portion of the ventricular septum, and portions of the mitral and tricuspid valves. Total endocardial cushion defects, therefore, can produce a butterfly-shaped lesion at the center of the heart, including a low atrial defect, a high ventricular defect, and openings in the atrioventricular valves (Fig. 71–10). Endocardial cushion defects are associated in humans with chromosome abnormalities, but such an association has not yet been demonstrated in animals.

TABLE 71–2. Catheterization Data in Atrial Septal Defect*

Chamber	Pressure (mm Hg)		O_2 Saturation (%)
Vena cava	10/5	Mean 8	75
Right atrium	10/5	Mean 8	85
Right ventricle	25/2	End-diastolic 5	85
Pulmonary artery	22/15	Mean 18	85
Pulmonary artery wedge	10/5	Mean 8	98
Left atrium	10/5	Mean 8	98
Left ventricle	120/0	End-diastolic 6	98
Aorta	120/80	Mean 100	98

*Compare with normal values shown in Table 70–2 (page 1064).

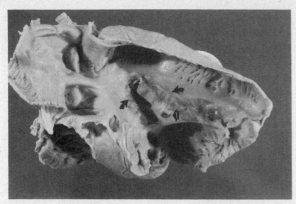

Figure 71–11. Ebstein's anomaly of the tricuspid valve, from the right atrium. The tricuspid valve is abnormal *(curved arrows)*, extending into the ventricle and with abnormal connections to the ventricular wall. There is a cleft in the valve (arrow #1).

The signs of endocardial cushion defect are associated with mitral valve regurgitation and the large left-to-right shunt at the atrial and/or ventricular level, producing extreme pulmonary flows, pulmonary edema, and usually death due to respiratory failure. To date, there has been no report of successful treatment of the lesion in the cat, but pulmonary artery banding (see later) might be effective in reducing the increased pulmonary blood flow.

Tricuspid Valve Disorders

Diseases of the tricuspid valve, once considered a rare entity, are being reported with increasing frequency.[34,55,79] Tricuspid atresia, or absence of the tricuspid valve, is a severe anomaly occasionally seen in animals. Tricuspid dysplasia and Ebstein's anomaly are more commonly seen. In tricuspid dysplasia, the tricuspid valve is abnormally formed, being both stenotic and regurgitant, producing signs of right heart failure. In Ebstein's anomaly, the valve is malpositioned into the ventricle but produces a similar clinical picture (Fig. 71–11).

Animals with tricuspid dysplasia and Ebstein's anomaly have similar signs. Syncopal episodes associated with dysrhythmia may occur. Ascites may be present, and the animal usually has exercise intolerance. A systolic murmur on the right side may also have a diastolic component. On electrocardiograms, a very large P wave suggestive of enlarged right atrium and often evidence of right axis deviation are found. On radiographic examination a gigantic right atrium is seen (Fig. 71–12).

The diagnosis of Ebstein's anomaly or tricuspid dysplasia is established by cardiac catheterization. The catheter is placed in the right atrium, and increased pressure is present. When the catheter is passed into the right ventricle and radiopaque dye is injected, the dye fills the ventricle as well as the right atrium and the posterior vena cava, confirming tricuspid regurgitation.

Surgical treatment for both tricuspid dysplasia and Ebstein's anomaly has been attempted, but results are poor. Medical management of the symptoms appears superior. The prognosis for tricuspid valve lesions is poor. Tricuspid atresia is fatal. Tricuspid dysplasia and Ebstein's anomaly do not respond well to surgery, and animals with these diseases have significantly shortened lives.

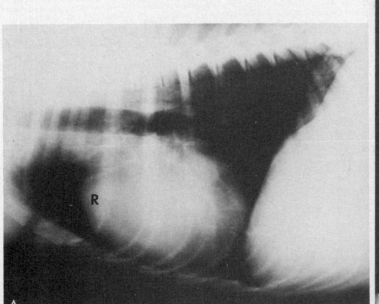
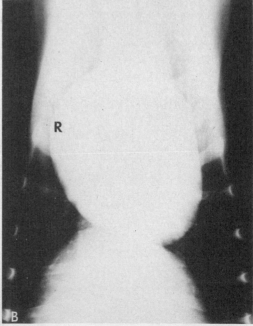

Figure 71–12. Tricuspid dysplasia in a dog. A, Lateral thoracic radiograph. Note the filling of the ventral anterior waist, which represents enlargement of the right atrial appendage (R). B, Dorsoventral radiograph. Note the tremendous enlargement of the cardiac silhouette at the nine to eleven o'clock position, representing enlargement of the right atrium (R).

Ventricular Septal Defect

One of the more common congenital cardiac disorders is ventricular septal defect. The lesion occurs in approximately one per 2,000 live births in dogs.[65] It may be more common in cats, being considered the most common congenital heart defect in cats.[74]

Ventricular septal defects can occasionally be found in the ventricular muscle toward the apex (Fig. 71–13), but much more commonly they are located high in the ventricular septum. When viewed from the right ventricle, the defect is located anterior and just beneath the septal leaflet of the tricuspid valve; when viewed from the left side, it is just beneath the aortic annulus (Fig. 71–14).

Animals with ventricular septal defect exhibit signs associated with pulmonary edema due to increased pulmonary pressure and flow as a result of the shunt from the left to the right ventricle (see Fig. 71–2). Blood flow from the high-pressure left ventricle to the low-pressure right causes increased volume in the right ventricle and the pulmonary circulation. As a result, pulmonary vascular disease and pulmonary hypertension can occur, with signs of cough, shortness of breath, and exercise intolerance. In one short series, 50 per cent of dogs with ventricular septal defect had been treated and referred for chronic mild respiratory and upper respiratory infections.[32]

The pulmonary system is capable of large increases in volume and can be considered a left heart reservoir. Therefore, as in atrial septal defect, signs rarely occur unless pulmonary volume is more than two or three times normal. Thus, a pulmonary-to-systemic flow ratio in excess of 2.5:1 is necessary to produce symptoms and therefore require treatment. With increased pulmonary volume and pulmonary arterial pressure, some right ventricular enlargement may occur. Owing to the increased volume pumped by the left ventricle, left ventricular hypertrophy and dilation may also occur.

The animal with ventricular septal defect has a

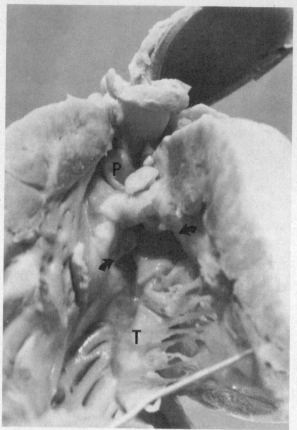

Figure 71–14. Ventricular septal defect *(arrows)* seen from the right ventricle. The tricuspid valve *(T)* is just posterior to the defect. The pulmonary valve *(P)* is anterior and dorsal to the ventricular defect.

murmur associated with the turbulence created at the defect. The sound produced by this turbulence radiates to the right chest wall, as with a lesion of the tricuspid valve. The murmur is pansystolic and

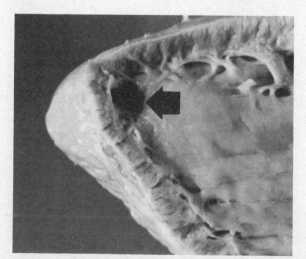

Figure 71–13. Muscular ventricular septal defect, seen from the left ventricle, near the apex *(arrow).*

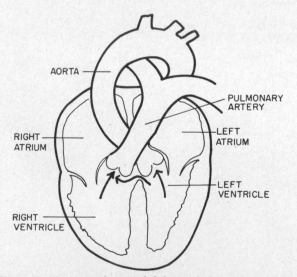

Figure 71–15. Ventricular septal defect with flows depicted. The high-pressure left ventricle ejects blood into both the aorta and the right ventricle via the ventricular septal defect. The jet flow from the ventricle through the defect and its proximity to the tricuspid valve produce turbulence near the tricuspid valve that mimics the murmur of tricuspid regurgitation.

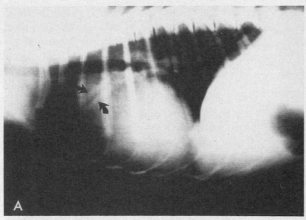
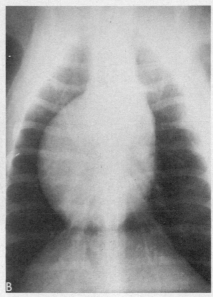

Figure 71–16. A dog with ventricular septal defect. *A,* Lateral thoracic radiograph. The heart is enlarged. Note the enlarged right apical lobar vessels *(arrows)* resulting from overcirculation. *B,* Dorsoventral radiograph. Both ventricles are enlarged. There is evidence of increased vascularity in the lung.

has a slight crescendo-decrescendo quality. Probably because of the approximation of the defect to the aorta, the murmur frequently radiates to the thoracic inlet via the aortic arch and brachiocephalic vessels (Fig. 71–15). If the ventricular defect is severe enough to produce extreme flows to the right side, a crescendo-decrescendo murmur may be heard at the pulmonary valve, as a result of increased flow across the normal pulmonary valve, like the murmur associated with atrial septal defect. The presence of a second murmur in the pulmonary area usually indicates flow severe enough to warrant treatment. The electrocardiographic findings associated with ventricular septal defect include mild left ventricular enlargement and perhaps right ventricular enlargement. Right axis deviation and right ventricular hypertrophy indicate developing pulmonary hypertension and more severe disease. Radiographically, the heart is enlarged on both sides. The pulmonary vasculature is increased (Fig. 71–16). Right and left side enlargement without aortic enlargement and without right atrial enlargement is strong evidence

of ventricular septal defect if there is associated evidence of increased vascularity of the lungs.

The diagnosis of ventricular septal defect is established through the physical findings, the electrocardiographic and radiographic findings plus venous angiogram, with the radiograph taken in the levo phase, which demonstrates the opening between the left and right ventricles (Fig. 71–17). This radiograph must be taken after dye has cleared the right side, and therefore it is imperative that a relatively small injection be made. The dye must be injected over a short period so that the bolus completely clears the right side before dye reaches the left. Cardiac catheterization shows increased oxygen or "step-up" between the right chambers (Table 71–3). Increased oxygen saturation can be used to calculate the left-to-right shunt, as follows:

$$\text{Pulmonary-to-systemic flow ratio} = \frac{\text{Ao} - \text{AVC}}{\text{Ao} - \text{PA}}$$

where Ao is aortic saturation, AVC is anterior vena cava saturation, and PA is pulmonary artery satura-

TABLE 71–3. Catheterization Data in Ventricular Septal Defect*

Chamber	Pressure (mm Hg)		O₂ Saturation (%)
Vena cava	8/1	Mean 4	75
Right atrium	8/1	Mean 4	75
Right ventricle	30/0	End-diastolic 7	85
Pulmonary artery	28/15	Mean 20	85
Pulmonary artery wedge	12/6	Mean 8	98
Left atrium	15/5	Mean 8	98
Left ventricle	120/0	End-diastolic 8	98
Aorta	120/80	Mean 100	98

*Compare with normal values in Table 70–2 (page 1064).

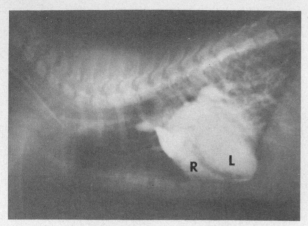

Figure 71–17. Venous angiogram in the levo phase, in a dog with ventricular septal defect. Note the filling of the left ventricle (L) and the presence of dye in the right ventricular outflow tract (R). The recirculated dye indicates the left-to-right shunt.

tion. For example, if Ao is 100 per cent, PA is 90 per cent, and AVC is 70 per cent, the flow ratio is calculated as follows:

$$\text{Pulmonary-to-systemic flow ratio} = \frac{100 - 70}{100 - 90}$$

$$= \frac{30}{10}$$

$$= 3, \text{ or } 3:1.$$

Cardiac catheterization can also be used to demonstrate the severity of the pressure changes (see Table 71–3). The right ventricular and pulmonary artery pressures are increased, depending on the amount of pulmonary vascular change. Most helpful in the diagnosis is a selective left ventricular angiogram, which will demonstrate more clearly than the venous angiogram the left-to-right shunt at the ventricular level (Fig. 71–18). The left ventricular angiogram can be performed regardless of the size of the animal. Cardiac catheterization with selective angiog-

raphy of the left ventricle is much more difficult and time-consuming than venous angiography.

Indications for surgical or medical treatment of ventricular septal defect are (1) an auscultable flow murmur in the pulmonary area, (2) enlargement of the pulmonary artery on dorsoventral radiograph, and (3) a diagnostic venous angiogram. The presence of the greatly enlarged main pulmonary artery and the flow murmur of pulmonary stenosis are strongly associated with large-volume flow and disease severe enough to require therapy.

Surgical Correction of Ventricular Septal Defect. Currently there are several surgical techniques for repair of ventricular septal defect. Open heart surgical repair has been reported.[6] It carries a moderate mortality, repair is total, and the animal can be expected to live a normal life. Hypothermia with inflow occlusion has been reported to have good success but is time-consuming and generally limited to small breeds.[7,80] The palliative procedure, pulmonary artery banding, is effective and safe in both the dog and cat.[32,59] With pulmonary artery banding, right ventricular pressure is increased by the production of a supravalvular pulmonic stenosis (see later). As a result of the increased pressure in the right ventricle, the flow from the left ventricle to the right is decreased and the lungs are protected from increased flow.

The prognosis in ventricular septal defect is good. A small percentage of defects close spontaneously.[8] Approximately 75 per cent of dogs and probably a similar percentage of cats with the defect do not have pulmonary-to-systemic flow ratios greater than 2.5:1 and consequently do not need treatment. In those with large flow ratios results of pulmonary artery banding are good and morbidity is low. The other techniques require extensive time or equipment and although correction is total the mortality associated with these techniques is moderately high.

Pulmonic Stenosis

One of the most common congenital cardiac disorders in all species is pulmonic stenosis.[65] It is seen in approximately one per 1,000 live births in dogs, less frequently in cats[42] and large animals, but it is a common finding with multiple defects such as tetralogy of Fallot.[64] Pulmonic stenosis includes lesions that affect the outflow from the right ventricle to the lungs. The lesion can be supravalvular (in the pulmonary artery), valvular (affecting the valve, usually by fusion of the valve cusps), subvalvular (a very common fibrous lesion just beneath the valve in the right ventricle), or muscular infundibular (frequently a sequel to any of the preceding obstructions in which the physiological response of concentric hypertrophy partially occludes the right ventricular infundibulum) (Fig. 71–19). A term that has become popular in human medicine and well describes the most common complex in the dog is *pulmonary valve*

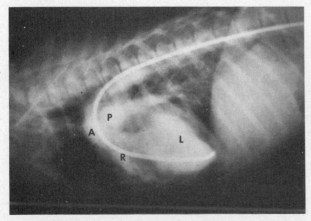

Figure 71–18. Selective left ventricular angiogram of a dog with ventricular septal defect. The left ventricle (L) is filled with dye. Also visualized are the right ventricular outflow tract (R), the pulmonary arteries (P), and the aorta (A).

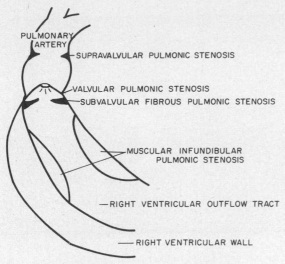

Figure 71-19. Types of pulmonic stenosis.

dysplasia. In this disorder, the obstruction includes the valve and the immediately subvalvular tissue, a combination of valvular and subvalvular pulmonic stenosis.

Supravalvular pulmonic stenosis is extremely rare. Valvular pulmonic stenosis, subvalvular pulmonic stenosis, and combined valve dysplasia are the most common. Pulmonary atresia is rarely diagnosed, as animals with the disease seldom live more than a few weeks. With pulmonary atresia, blood flow to the lungs is maintained by the bronchial arteries and the patent ductus; with closure of the ductus, death quickly ensues. Muscular infundibular pulmonary stenosis is the normal response to obstruction but can occur independently. With pulmonary stenosis, the obstruction to flow to the pulmonary artery is overcome by right ventricular hypertrophy.

If the pulmonary obstruction is not severe, the only finding is the murmur associated with the disease. Signs and physical findings in pulmonary stenosis include a crescendo-decrescendo systolic murmur, heard best at the base of the heart on the left side, which is quite characteristic and tends not to radiate; and findings associated with right-sided heart failure, such as engorged veins, distended liver, and ascites or arrhythmia due to the hypertrophy.

The laboratory findings of pulmonic stenosis include right ventricular hypertrophy and right axis deviation on electrocardiogram and the right-sided cardiac enlargement seen in all views by radiograph. There is usually a post-stenotic dilation of the main pulmonary artery (Fig. 71-20), but the distal pulmonary vessels are normal to reduced in size as in tetralogy of Fallot (see later).

The venous angiogram differentiates pulmonic stenosis from the two lesions that appear similar (Fig. 71-21). Atrial septal defect with the large right ventricle and murmur can be mistaken for pulmonic stenosis, but in the former increased vasculature of the lungs is documented on angiogram. Tetralogy of Fallot may have right-to-left shunting at the ventricular level, and the absence of dye on the left side of the heart three seconds after the injection eliminates the possibility of right-to-left shunt, confirming the diagnosis of pulmonic stenosis. In addition, on the angiogram the approximate location of the obstruction and the severity of the right ventricular hypertrophy can be seen. Electrocardiography can also be used to indicate severity. Right axis deviation generally correlates well with the severity of right ventricular hypertrophy. Right axis shifts to 180 degrees have

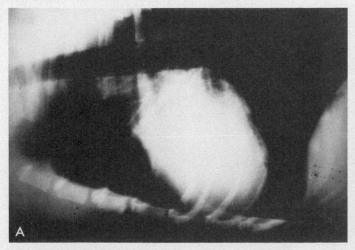

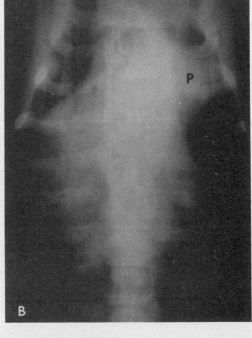

Figure 71-20. A dog with pulmonic stenosis. *A,* Lateral thoracic radiograph. The right side of the heart is enlarged. The pulmonary vessels are small. *B,* Dorsoventral radiograph of a dog with pulmonic stenosis. The right side of the heart is enlarged. The post-stenotic dilation is seen as an enlargement of the main pulmonary artery *(P)* at the one o'clock position.

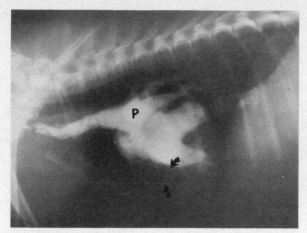

Figure 71–21. Venous angiogram of a dog with pulmonic stenosis, taken at the end of the injection and revealing the thickened right ventrodorsal wall (between *arrows*) and post-stenotic dilation of the pulmonary artery (*P*) indicative of pulmonic stenosis.

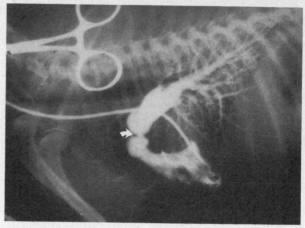

Figure 71–23. Right ventricular angiogram of a dog with supravalvular pulmonic stenosis (*arrow*).

been found consistently in animals that prove by catheterization to be surgical candidates. An animal with demonstrated pulmonic stenosis and right axis deviation greater than 180 degrees or wall thickness more than three times normal is invariably a surgical candidate; however, the surgical severity should be confirmed on cardiac catheterization. The most valuable catheterization information is obtained by right ventricular pressure tracing. The catheter is passed into the right ventricle, and pressures are recorded. If possible, the catheter is passed into the pulmonary artery and withdrawn, demonstrating the point of change of pressure (Fig. 71–22). A selective angiogram confirms the area of obstruction (Figs. 71–23 to 71–27).

The surgical treatment for pulmonic stenosis depends on the specific type. Supravalvular pulmonic stenosis is most easily repaired by a conduit circumventing the obstruction. Valvular or discrete subvalvular pulmonic stenosis or valve dysplasia can be treated in several ways. The preferred method for mature animals at our institution is a modification of the inflow occlusion–pulmonary arteriotomy proce-

dure popularized by Swan.[73] This technique allows direct observation of the pulmonary valve and repair or removal of the valve tissue. It is most effective in mature or nearly mature animals. Immature animals needing surgical repair for pulmonic stenosis at the valve level are most successfully treated with the patch graft technique,[9] in which a redundant patch is fashioned to allow the animal to grow to the size of the patch. The simplest surgical techniques are the bistoury or modified Brock procedures for incising or removing the obstruction,[19,41] but these techniques have the major disadvantage of no direct observation of the valve. Muscular pulmonic stenosis is perhaps the most difficult to manage surgically. Open heart surgical repair has been successful for the muscular type, other techniques having limited success.

Surgery for pulmonic stenosis is recommended if evidence of severe hypertrophy, failure, syncope, or increasing wall thickness is found. An objective criterion for surgery can be obtained by catheterization. In adults, systemic pressure in the right ventricle or

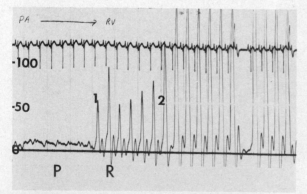

Figure 71–22. Catheter withdrawal from the pulmonary artery (*P*) to the right ventricle (*R*) in pulmonic stenosis. Note the two-step gradient at the valve (*1*) and deeper in the right ventricle, where the ventricular pressure increases (*2*). Scale to the left is in mm Hg.

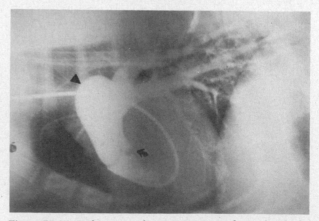

Figure 71–24. Right ventricular angiogram in a dog with valvular pulmonary stenosis. The catheter has been placed in the right ventricle and an injection made. The thickened pulmonic valve (*arrow*) is outlined. The right ventricular wall is thickened. The post-stenotic dilation (*triangle*) in the pulmonary artery distal to the pulmonary valve is seen.

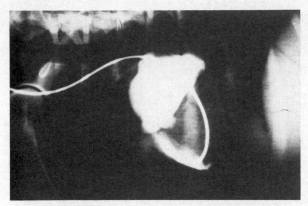

Figure 71–25. Right ventricular angiogram in a dog with discrete subvalvular pulmonic stenosis. Note the area under the normal-appearing valves where there is no dye (the obstructed area).

a gradient of 100 mm Hg across the valve indicates a need for surgical repair. In immature animals, right ventricular pressure greater than 70 mm Hg indicates the need for surgery. Conversely, right ventricular pressure less than 70 mm Hg or a pulmonary artery–to–right ventricle gradient less than 50 mm Hg does not need correction.

Severely affected animals with pulmonic stenosis may live to adulthood but usually die of right-sided heart failure or arrhythmia by one to two years of age. Mildly affected animals with right ventricular pressures less than 70 mm Hg can be expected to live normally. Dogs undergoing surgery have a good prognosis if the lesion is supravalvular, valvular, or immediately subvalvular; fortunately, these represent the majority of cases of pulmonic stenosis. The surgical success rate is higher in dogs reaching adult size before symptoms or pressure changes dictate the need for surgery than in immature animals. Dogs with severe muscular pulmonic stenosis, either primary or secondary to other pulmonic stenosis, have a grave prognosis. Consequently, animals with diagnosed pulmonic stenosis should be monitored frequently, perhaps monthly, until two years of age to ascertain that the hypertrophy is not increasing.

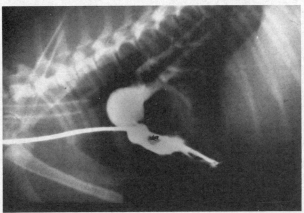

Figure 71–26. Right ventricular angiogram in a dog with secondary muscular pulmonic stenosis. The distal lesions has caused hypertrophy in the outflow tract that is constricting the flow at the portion identified by the *arrow*.

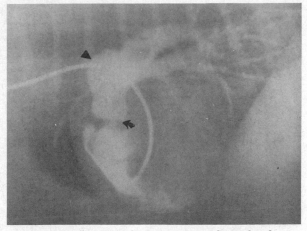

Figure 71–27. Right ventricular angiogram in a dog with pulmonary valve dysplasia. The catheter is introduced into the right ventricle and the injection made. The area of the valve and the immediate subvalvular area *(arrow)* is not filled by contrast media. The post-stenotic dilation *(triangle)* is seen distal to the valve. The right ventricular wall is thickened.

Evidence of increasing hypertrophy is a strong indication for surgical correction. Chapter 73 contains a complete discussion of the surgical procedures and rationale.

Tetralogy of Fallot

The most common cyanotic congenital cardiac disorder seen in the dog and cat is tetralogy of Fallot (tetralogy).[5,18,66] The disorder includes (1) ventricular septal defect; (2) muscular pulmonic stenosis, although any type of pulmonic stenosis is usually included in the group, (3) overriding or rightward positioning of the aorta, although it may not be present in all cases; and (4) right ventricular hypertrophy secondary to the pulmonic stenosis (Fig. 71–28). In humans, 25 per cent of patients with tetralogy have right aortic arches. Cyanosis results from the

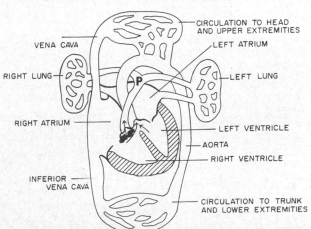

Figure 71–28. Tetralogy of Fallot. The obstruction at the entrance to the pulmonary artery *(P)* causes elevation of the pressure in the right ventricle. Secondarily, the right ventricular muscle thickens. The ventricular septal defect allows an exit from the high-pressure right ventricle, and the overridden aorta allows diversion of blood to the systemic circulation.

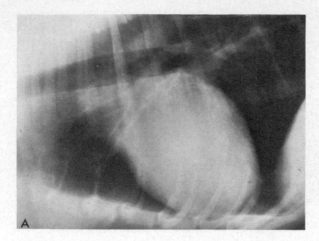

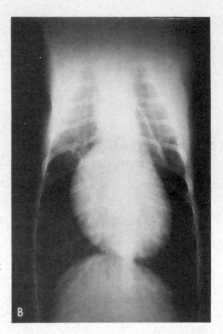

Figure 71–29. Lateral (A) and dorsoventral (B) radiographs of a dog with tetralogy of Fallot. The right side of the heart is considerably enlarged. The lungs are hypovascular.

obstruction of pulmonic stenosis, which produces increased right ventricular pressure and causes venous blood to flow through the ventricular defect and mix with oxygenated blood in the aorta. Tetralogy of Fallot is seen in most breeds of dogs but more frequently in the poodle, Schnauzer, Keeshond, and terriers, particularly the wirehaired fox terrier, and has been reproduced experimentally in beagles.

Animals with tetralogy of Fallot show weakness, failure to thrive and grow, exercise intolerance, and generalized cyanosis. Physical findings include cyanosis and usually a systolic murmur heard at the base of the heart. The murmur may not always be present if the abnormal flow is not turbulent. The presence of severe polycythemia suggests a right-to-

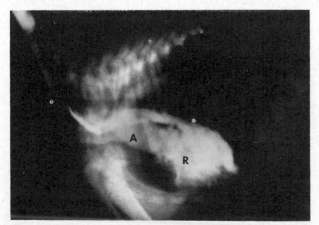

Figure 71–30. Venous angiogram of a dog with tetralogy of Fallot. The dye enters the circulation from the jugular vein and passes through the right side of the heart to the ventricle (R). The dye leaves the heart through the ascending aorta (A) and, to a lesser extent, the pulmonary artery (not shown).

left central shunt. The diagnosis is suggested by the finding of severe right ventricular hypertrophy on electrocardiogram and radiograph. In addition, radiographs show the lungs to be underperfused and clear (Fig. 71–29). Confirmation of the diagnosis is made by a venous angiogram with film taken one to two seconds after injection (Fig. 71–30). Dye in the right atrium, right ventricle, pulmonary artery, ascending aorta, and descending aorta confirms tetralogy of Fallot. Cardiac catheterization helps confirm the systemic to supersystemic pressures in the right ventricle but is not necessary for the diagnosis or selection of therapy.

Treatment for tetralogy is either palliative or curative. Palliative procedures can be medical or surgical. The medical palliation currently used with success in dogs, cats, and humans depends on reduction of the muscular obstruction associated with the pulmonic stenosis.[30] One of the beta-adrenergic blockers, usually propranolol, is used orally two to three times daily to reduce muscle contractility and muscular obstruction, allowing more blood to flow into the pulmonary artery. This therapy is effective in approximately 50 per cent of dogs and cats with tetralogy. Many surgical techniques are used for tetralogy of Fallot, the most commonly used in animals being the Blalock and Potts anastomoses. The Blalock anastomosis allows for return of partially oxygenated arterial blood to the lungs by an end-to-side anastomosis of the left subclavian artery to the pulmonary artery. The Potts anastomosis is a side-to-side anastomosis of the aorta to the pulmonary artery. Total corrective procedures require open heart surgery and resection of the muscular obstruction with closure of the ventricular defect.

Results of treatment with tetralogy are only fair. Medical treatment is effective in about half the patients. The animals are salvaged but usually have limited activity and perform normally as house pets. Either of the surgical anastomoses has good results when performed in dogs greater than 10 kg whose disorder has not responded to medical treatment. In small dogs and cats, the smallness of the subclavian vessel used for the Blalock shunt may cause occlusion or clot. Open heart repair results have been poor at best, with a mortality rate greater than 75 per cent. Because untreated animals with tetralogy of Fallot frequently die at a young age, the diagnosis of the disease mandates medical or surgical management. Without treatment few animals survive to one year of age.

Eisenmenger's Complex

A condition similar to tetralogy of Fallot but much less common is Eisenmenger's complex which consists of ventricular septal defect and severe pulmonary hypertension producing right to left ventricular shunt. Signs are identical to those of tetralogy of Fallot. In Eisenmenger's disease, permanent damage to the pulmonary vasculature causes pulmonary hypertension and right ventricular hypertension, rather than the right ventricular hypertension caused by pulmonic stenosis in tetralogy of Fallot. Classically, Eisenmenger's complex starts as simple ventricular septal defect, but owing to increased pressure and flow and consequent alteration of the pulmonary vasculature, permanent muscular thickening of the pulmonary arterial walls develops and a "malignant pulmonary hypertension" predisposes to the right-to-left shunt. Eisenmenger's complex may be differentiated from tetralogy of Fallot by the presence of systemic or supersystemic pressure in the pulmonary artery, and cardiac catheterization must be done to confirm this pressure (Table 71–4). However, Eisenmenger's complex should be suspected if the main pulmonary arteries are enlarged on radiography.

As a result of permanent pulmonary vascular damage, no treatment is available for animals with Eisenmenger's complex. Recent heart-lung transplants have been attempted in humans with this disease.

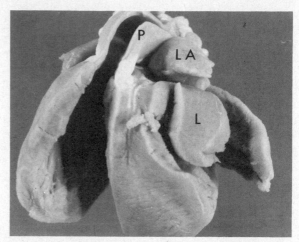

Figure 71–31. Hypoplastic left heart from a cat. The right ventricle is open to the pulmonary artery (*P*). The left ventricle (*L*) is a diminutive chamber attached to the large right heart. The enlarged left atrial appendage (*LA*) is dorsal to the tiny left ventricle.

Animals with Eisenmenger's complex usually die at a young age, although recent evidence suggests the possibility of delaying death with vasodilator therapy.[68]

Anomalous Pulmonary Venous Return

Anomalies of pulmonary venous return are rare in animals. Anomalous pulmonary venous return can be partial, in which only some veins return, usually by a circuitous route, to the right atrium, or total, in which all veins return by an abnormal pathway.

Mitral Valve Abnormalities

Congenital disorders of the mitral valve have occasionally been reported in the dog.[20,28,35,40] In retrospect, many of these cases may have been secondary to congestive cardiomyopathy. Regardless, congenital abnormalities of the mitral valve have signs referable to heart failure with mitral regurgitation, as seen with cardiomyopathy. These conditions are discussed later.

Mitral atresia, associated with poor development of the left ventricle and aortic valve, is a component

TABLE 71–4. Catheterization Data in Tetralogy of Fallot and Eisenmenger's Complex*

| Chamber | Tetralogy of Fallot | | | Eisenmenger's Complex | | |
	Pressure (mm Hg)		O_2 Saturation (%)	Pressure (mm Hg)		O_2 Saturation (%)
Right atrium	10/2	Mean 8	60	10/2	Mean 8	60
Right ventricle	120/0	End-diastolic 10	60	120/0	End-diastolic 10	60
Pulmonary artery	18/5	Mean 8	60	120/80	Mean 10	60
Left atrium	12/4	Mean 5	98	12/4	Mean 5	98
Left ventricle	120/0	End-diastolic 10	92	120/0	End-diastolic 10	88
Aorta	120/80	Mean 100	75	120/80	Mean 100	75

*Compare with normal values in Table 70–2 (page 1064).

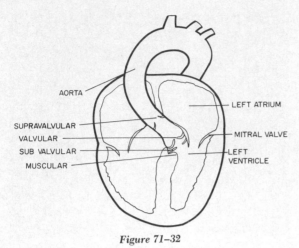

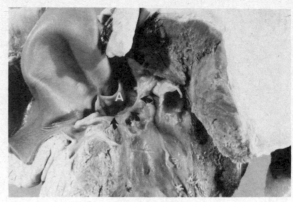

Figure 71–32

Figure 71–33

Figure 71–32. Types of aortic stenosis. Supravalvular and valvular stenoses are quite rare. Subvalvular fibrosis is most commonly seen, but muscular obstructions are reported.

Figure 71–33. The typical fibrous ring *(arrows)* of subvalvular aortic stenosis seen in the dog. The aortic valve *(A)* is slightly thickened just distal to the subvalvular obstruction.

of the hypoplastic left heart syndrome, a rare condition in cats but one not infrequently seen in humans (Fig. 71–31). In mitral atresia–hypoplastic left heart syndrome, the left ventricle develops poorly, the inflow tract to the left ventricle and the outflow tract from the left ventricle are atretic or diminutive, and death occurs within the first few days after birth. At autopsy, which is performed only for concerned breeders, severe pulmonary congestion and a poorly developed left heart are found. There is no treatment for hypoplastic left heart syndrome.

Aortic Stenosis

Left ventricular outflow tract lesions, aortic stenosis, and similar aortic disorders are extremely common in the dog but rarely seen in the cat. Aortic stenosis is hereditary in the dog and affects approximately one per 1,000 live births.[65] Valvular aortic stenosis is rare, but subvalvular fibrous aortic stenosis is hereditary (probably autosomal dominant) and affects the Newfoundland, German shepherd, boxer, golden retriever, and German shorthair pointer (Figs.

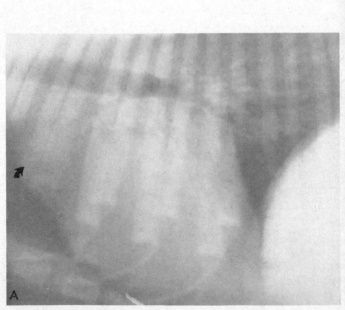

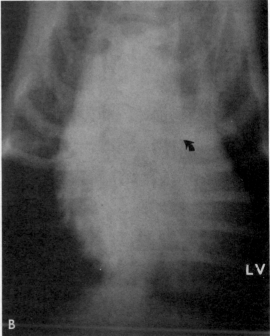

Figure 71–34. A dog with aortic stenosis. *A,* Lateral thoracic radiograph. The heart is greatly enlarged. The anterior waist is filled by the post-stenotic dilation of the ascending aorta *(arrow). B,* Dorsoventral thoracic radiograph of a dog with aortic stenosis. The left ventricle *(LV)* is greatly enlarged, extending nearly to the chest wall. Note that the descending aorta *(arrow)* is not enlarged.

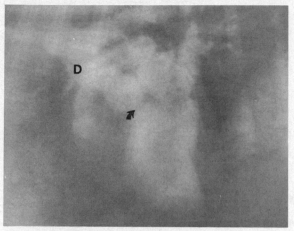

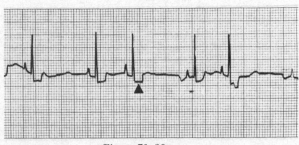

Figure 71–35   *Figure 71–36*

Figure 71–35. Levo phase venous angiogram of a dog with aortic stenosis. The left atrium and left ventricle are filled. The left ventricular wall is slightly thickened. The area of obstruction *(arrow)* represents a narrowing in the outflow from the left ventricle just beneath the aortic valve. The post-stenotic dilation *(D)* is distal to the valve and aortic sinus of Valsalva in the ascending aortic arch.

Figure 71–36. Electrocardiogram demonstrating ST segment depression. The ST segment (above the *triangle*) is depressed from the normal baseline.

71–32 and 71–33). Supravalvular aortic stenosis has been produced in some domestic animals by over-supplementation of vitamins to the pregnant female.[38]

Animals affected with subvalvular aortic stenosis have a history of syncope or a family history of sudden death. On examination, affected dogs have a crescendo-decrescendo systolic murmur, which is heard best at the base of the heart on the left side or in the right anterior thorax near the sternum and radiates into the thoracic inlet and up the neck. If the murmur is extremely intense, it can be heard on the head or down the left dorsal thorax and into the abdomen as far as the femoral arteries. Arterial pulses are weakened. Electrocardiographic findings include left ventricular hypertrophy in approximately half the cases, left axis deviation, and occasional dysrhythmias or ST segment alteration. Radiographic findings include left ventricular enlargement and filling of the anterior waist on the lateral radiograph (Fig. 71–34). The diagnosis of aortic stenosis is simply established by a venous angiogram with the radiograph taken in the levo phase approximately six to eight seconds after

the injection. Post-stenotic dilation of the ascending aorta associated with the obstruction is seen (Fig. 71–35).

If aortic stenosis is mild, animals live normally. (Humans with the disease may have chest pain, which almost certainly also occurs in the dog and is suggested by the ST segment change—Fig. 71–36.) No other signs are seen. If the disease is severe, syncopal episodes, probably related to severe ventricular dysrhythmia, or sudden death occurs. The indications for therapy are syncope, ST segment change on electrocardiograph, and catheterization findings a left ventricular outflow tract gradient of greater than 70 mm Hg (Fig. 71–37). Animals with left ventricular pressures greater than 220 mm Hg (left ventricular–aortic gradients of 100 mm Hg or more) are usually symptomatic and die at an early age. Animals with left ventricular pressures less than 170 mm Hg (left ventricular–aortic gradients of 50 mm Hg or less) are usually asymptomatic.

Several medical treatments suggested for aortic stenosis use beta-adrenergic blockers to lessen the

Figure 71–37. Catheter withdrawal from the left ventricle to the aorta. The left ventricular pressure below the obstruction *(LV1)* exceeds 200 mm Hg. On lead II electrocardiogram at the top are multiple premature ventricular contractions *(top arrow)* and a corresponding low pressure *(bottom arrow)* as the catheter is withdrawn from the ventricle. Just before it passes through the aortic valve, the pressure drops to near normal *(LV2)*. Finally, the catheter is withdrawn across the aortic valve into the aorta *(A)*, with normal arterial pressure.

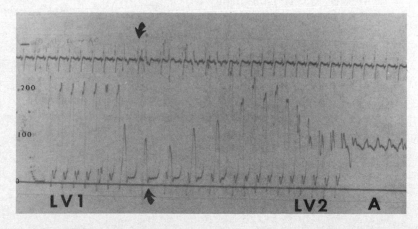

obstruction. This treatment is effective in humans with muscular aortic stenosis but is probably ineffective in dogs with discrete fibrous subvalvular membranous disease. Resection of the obstruction is successful but requires open heart techniques.[24] The procedure is expensive and carries a 25 per cent mortality. Most recently, left ventricular–aortic conduits have been used to bypass the obstruction[10] but also have a high mortality; although these techniques do not require open heart surgery, the valved conduits are expensive. We have attempted a bistoury cut technique to relieve the obstruction in some dogs; the technique carries a high mortality, but it is simple and may be effective.

Aortic Regurgitation

Congenital aortic regurgitation in the dog and cat is rare.[26] It may be associated with aortic stenosis and is then usually trivial. Aortic regurgitation may be a sequel to ventricular septal defect. The proximity of the ventricular defect to the right aortic valve cusp makes support of the root of the aorta depend on some ventricular tissue. Occasionally, animals with ventricular septal defect may develop a prolapse of the right aortic cusp and aortic regurgitation as a result of the Venturi effect of flow through the defect. Animals with this complication reach one to two years of age with a ventricular defect and then develop acute left-sided heart failure and frequently die. The ventricular septal defect murmur continues, but the additional diastolic decrescendo murmur of aortic regurgitation is heard over the left ventricle. The diagnosis of aortic regurgitation is established via a supravalvular aortic dye injection that demonstrates simultaneous filling of the aorta and the left ventricle. There are no reports of repair of this lesion in animals, but surgery would consist of valve replacement and ventricular septal defect closure. There is little likelihood of successful treatment of aortic regurgitation in the dog in the near future.

Transposition of the Great Arteries

An unusual cardiac abnormality that is rarely seen in animals is the transposition complex. Classically, transposition of the great arteries includes switching of the aorta and pulmonary artery to isolate the two vascular circulations (Fig. 71–38). For example, blood returning to the heart through the veins passes through the right atrium into the right ventricle and out via the transposed aorta to the body and back to the heart through the veins. At the same time, blood reaching the left atrium through the pulmonary circulation flows to the left ventricle and out via the transposed pulmonary artery to the pulmonary circulation. Because these two independent circulations are incompatible with life, additional cardiac defects (atrial septal defect, ventricular septal defect, or patent ductus arteriosus) are needed. The transposi-

Transposition

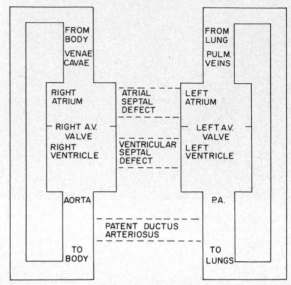

Figure 71–38. Transposition of the great vessels. The blood enters the right atrium from the body via veins and leaves the right side of the heart to the aorta to be returned to the body. Simultaneously, blood enters the left atrium by the pulmonary veins from the lungs and passes to the lungs through the pulmonary artery. This parallel circuit is incompatible with life without mixing by one of the cardiac shunts (atrial septal defect, ventricular septal defect, or patent ductus arteriosus).

tion complex has many variations, associated with variations *in situ* or in the portions of the cardiovascular system involved. This condition is relatively common in human infants but is rarely seen in animals.

One variation of the transposition group that is occasionally seen in dogs is the double-outlet right ventricle (Fig. 71–39).[76] In this disorder, perhaps in association with the transposition complex, both the aorta and pulmonary artery arise from the right ventricle. A ventricular septal defect is present, and affected animals are usually cyanotic, although cyanosis is not a consistent finding. At our institution,

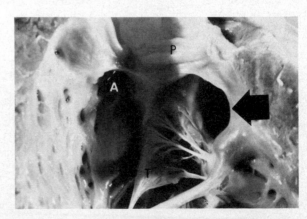

Figure 71–39. Double-outlet right ventricle of the Taussig-Bing variety, seen from the right ventricular outflow tract. The aortic opening (*A*) is transposed above the tricuspid valve (*T*). The ventricular septal defect (*arrow*) is subpulmonic (*P* indicates pulmonic valve).

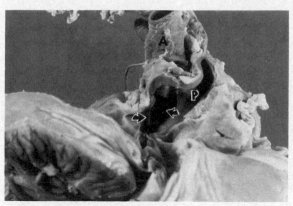

Figure 71–40 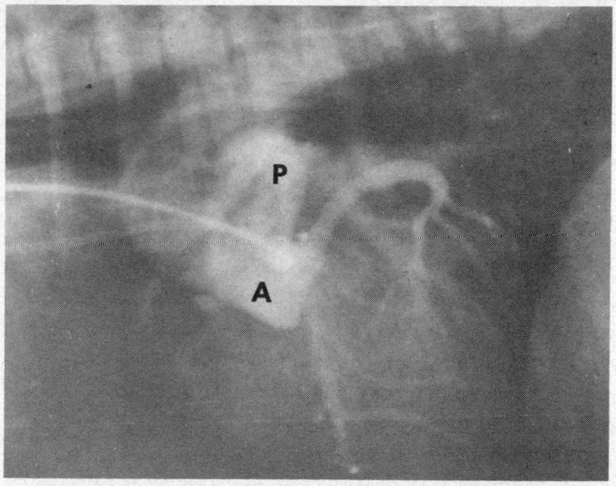   Figure 71–41

Figure 71–40. Aortic pulmonary window. The aorta (A) is at the top of the photograph. The pulmonary artery (P) is open, and the opening between the aorta and pulmonary artery (*arrows*) is identified.

Figure 71–41. Aortic angiogram of a dog with aortic pulmonary window. The catheter is positioned in the aortic arch, and an injection is made, revealing the aorta (A) and pulmonary artery (P). There is no evidence of a patent ductus arteriosus, thus confirming aortic pulmonary window.

two dogs with double-outlet right ventricle have been recognized, both of which died at the hospital under stress or anesthesia induction. The transposition complex in animals is of academic interest only.

Aortic-Pulmonary Window

Several anomalies of the aortic trunk and aortic arch have been reported in animals. Aortic pulmonary window is occasionally reported.[23] The defect is an opening between the aorta and the pulmonary artery at the ascending portion of the aorta (Fig. 71–40). It is like a severe patent ductus arteriosus in a proximal position. Consequently, clinical signs of aortic-pulmonary window are identical to those of severe patent ductus arteriosus (described later). Treatment for aortic-pulmonary window is surgical but has not yet been successful. The severity of the lesion, the proximity to the base of the heart, and the lack of an identifiable vascular connection make repair a difficult surgical exercise. Because of the similarity in appearance and physical findings to

patent ductus arteriosus, the major importance of aortic-pulmonary window is a differential diagnostic consideration in animals suspected of having patent ductus arteriosus (Table 71–5; Fig. 71–41).

Persistent Truncus Arteriosus

Persistent truncus arteriosus is a failure of embryological separation of the aorta and pulmonary artery. Truncus arteriosus may be regarded as a severe form of aortic-pulmonary window. Four major types of truncus have been identified, but the consistent finding in all is a common vascular trunk supporting a portion of both the aorta and the pulmonary artery. Consequently, the pulmonary vascular circulation is subjected to systemic arterial pressures and pulmonary hypertension, pulmonary edema, and resultant abnormal pulmonary function. Truncus arteriosus has been identified in all the major animal species, usually at autopsy.[17,72]

Animals affected with truncus arteriosus usually are cyanotic and unthrifty and seldom live more than

TABLE 71–5. Catheterization Data for Patent Ductus Arteriosus and Aortic-Pulmonary Window*

Chamber	Patent Ductus Arteriosus			Aortic-Pulmonary Window		
	Pressure (mm Hg)		O_2 Saturation (%)	Pressure (mm Hg)		O_2 Saturation (%)
Right atrium	8/1	Mean 5	75	8/1	Mean 5	75
Right ventricle	40/0	End-diastolic 5	75	70/1	End-diastolic 6	75
Pulmonary artery	40/20	Mean 30	85	70/40	Mean 60	90
Left atrium	16/6	Mean 10	98	20/10	Mean 15	98
Left ventricle	120/0	End-diastolic 8	98	120/0	End-diastolic 10	98
Aorta	120/80	Mean 100	98	120/80	Mean 100	98

*Compare with normal values in Table 70–2 (page 1064).

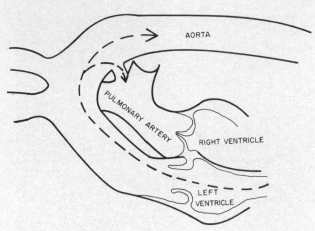

Figure 71–42. The flow in typical left-to-right shunting patent ductus arteriosus. Left ventricular ejection is into the aorta and to the body. A portion of the aortic flow is diverted to the pulmonary artery and lungs via the ductus arteriosus.

several months. Treatment for this disease is surgical but is not performed currently.

Patent Ductus Arteriosus

The most common congenital cardiac disorder is patent ductus arteriosus, which results from failure of closure of the ductus arteriosus, the normal fetal connection between the aorta and pulmonary artery. In dogs and cats, the patent ductus is short, usually 1 cm in width and less than 1 cm in length (Figs. 71–42 and 71–43). The persistence of this embryological connection, which diverted blood from the pulmonary artery around undeveloped lungs to the aorta in the fetus, allows shunting of blood from the high-pressure aorta to the pulmonary artery. As a result, pulmonary hypertension and pulmonary edema may develop. Patent ductus arteriosus is found in approximately one per 750 live births in dogs but is much less common in the cat. In the dog, this disorder is hereditary, is assumed to be polygenic, and affects particularly poodles, German shepherds,

Shetland sheepdogs, collies, Pomeranians, and spaniels as well as other breeds. There is approximately a 4:1 female-to-male distribution.[27]

The diagnosis of patent ductus arteriosus in dogs or cats is usually made via auscultation of the characteristic continuous or so-called machinery murmur in asymptomatic animals presented for vaccination. The murmur is generated by turbulence created as a result of the continuous (systolic and diastolic) gradient and flow between the aorta and the pulmonary artery. If the disease is untreated, signs of pulmonary edema and left-sided heart failure ensue. The signs seem to develop at a younger age in small breeds. The left ventricle, as a result of the large volume it must pump, dilates and hypertrophies, producing dilation of the mitral annulus and mitral regurgitation in approximately half the animals. If mitral regurgitation occurs, development of pulmonary edema is increased, and signs of unthriftiness, exercise intolerance, occasionally cough, and poor growth are exacerbated.

The diagnosis of patent ductus arteriosus can be established by the finding of the continuous murmur. In addition, electrocardiographic evidence of left ventricular hypertrophy and, rarely, late right ventricular hypertrophy can be found. The nearly pathognomonic murmur, in addition to radiographic findings of pulmonary overcirculation, dilation of the descending aorta due to the ductus diverticulum, and left ventricular enlargement (Figs. 71–7 and 71–44), confirms the diagnosis.

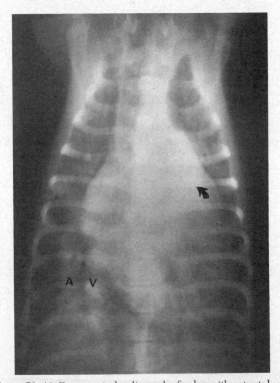

Figure 71–44. Dorsoventral radiograph of a dog with patent ductus arteriosus. Note the increased density throughout the lung field as well as the enlargement of the right pulmonary artery (A) and vein (V). The ductus diverticulum or distension of the descending aorta can be seen (arrow).

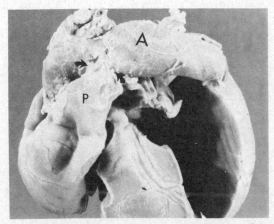

Figure 71–43. The ductus arteriosus (arrows) between the aorta (A) and the pulmonary artery (P). Note the relatively short, thick ductus in the dog.

Patent ductus arteriosus is treated surgically.[27,49] Animals allowed to continue with the disease risk development of mitral regurgitation, left ventricular hypertrophy, permanent pulmonary vascular damage, atrial fibrillation, and death. Large breeds tend to develop atrial fibrillation as a result of left atrial dilation before death. Small breeds seldom live beyond one year, but large breeds may live to five years before severe cardiovascular signs or death ensues.[27]

A small number (1 to 2 per cent) of animals with patent ductus develop a right-to-left shunt.[53] In this group, blood flow is similar to that in the fetus (from the pulmonary artery to the aorta). In some, right-to-left shunts similar to those in Eisenmenger's disease develop as the result of pulmonary hypertension due to increased volume and pressure to the lungs. Some probably never have a left-to-right shunt but continue to have fetal vasculature and circulation after birth. Regardless of the cause of patent ductus arteriosus with right-to-left shunt, the animals have differential cyanosis and weakness in the rear legs. Blood supply and oxygenation to the upper extremities are normal, but blood supplied to the abdomen and lower extremities is incompletely oxygenated (due to the right-to-left mixing posterior to the upper body arteries), thus producing weakness and collapse in the rear legs (Fig. 71–45). Owing to the severely desaturated arterial blood supply to the kidney, erythropoietin is released, and severe polycythemia is found. At our institution packed cell volumes between 70 and 80 per cent in animals with this disease are not uncommon. There is no effective treatment for patent ductus arteriosus with right-to-left shunt. Alteration of the pulmonary vasculature leads to permanent damage to the lungs.

Prognosis in patent ductus arteriosus, if treated early, is excellent. The surgical procedure is simple, requires minimal equipment, and is curative. Animals allowed to proceed into heart failure run a

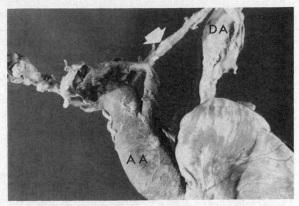

Figure 71–46. Aortic interruption in the dog. The ascending aorta *(AA)* exits from the heart with blood flow anteriorly. The descending aorta *(DA)* supplies the blood to the posterior half of the body via a branch *(arrow)* that was located in the vertebral canal.

slightly higher risk than those operated on earlier, and animals with atrial fibrillation have a 50 per cent mortality.[27] The occasional development of right-to-left shunt may be associated with delay of surgery. Approximately 1.5 per cent of dogs with ligation of the ductus develop rechannelization of the ductus, and a second operation with division of the ductus is needed.[25]

Coarctation of the Aorta

Obstructions of the aortic arch are rare. Aortic interruption with complete absence of a segment of the aortic arch has been reported in the dog and horse (Fig. 71–46).[62,69] In one case, prosthetic surgical reconstruction of an aortic arch in the dog was accomplished.[62] Coarctation of the aorta has been occasionally reported in the dog.[29,63] It is usually a narrow vascular obstruction in the aorta near the left subclavian artery or the ligamentum arteriosum that produces hypertension in the upper extremities and hypotension in the lower extremities (Fig. 71–47). Dogs with the disease develop left ventricular failure, and to date there are no reports of successful treatment. If found early this disease is surgically correctable by resection of the coarctation or plastic repair of the aorta.

Persistent Right Aortic Arch

Vascular anomalies of the aortic arch are common in the dog and occasionally seen in the cat. Included in this group of diseases are anomalous subclavian arteries, double aortic arch, and, most commonly, persistence of the right aortic arch.[2,78] Persistent right aortic arch occurs as the result of failure of the left embryological arch to develop as the dominant and therefore persistent aortic arch. The right arch becomes the permanent aortic arch, but blood flow is physiologically normal. No cardiovascular problems develop. However, the esophagus and trachea are

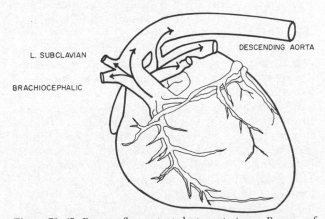

L. SUBCLAVIAN

DESCENDING AORTA

BRACHIOCEPHALIC

Figure 71–45. Reverse-flow patent ductus arteriosus. Because of the high pulmonary artery pressure, blood is diverted from the pulmonary artery to the aorta via the ductus. Since the ductus arteriosus is caudal to the aortic arch vessels supplying the anterior body (brachiocephalic and left subclavian arteries)—most mixing occurs in the descending aorta, and thus the desaturated blood is presented to the caudal half of the body.

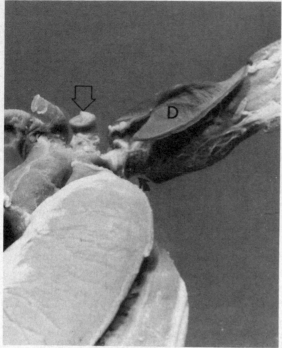

Figure 71–47. Coarctation of the aorta. The coarctation *(arrow)* is located in the aorta just posterior to the left subclavian artery *(open arrow)*. There is a post-stenotic dilation of the aorta distal to the coarctation *(D)*.

trapped in a vascular ring (Fig. 71–48). Persistent right aortic arch is almost certainly hereditary as there is a breed predisposition for the Doberman, Great Dane, Irish setter, and Weimaraner.[2,70]

Animals with persistent right aortic arch have characteristic clinical signs. The animals regurgitate after eating, usually starting at the time of weaning. When the animal begins to eat semi-solid or solid food, the obstruction to the esophagus is manifested by regurgitation. Dogs with this disease may be malnourished and are thin with ravenous appetites. If aspiration pneumonia has occurred, evidence of respiratory difficulty and pneumonia may be present.

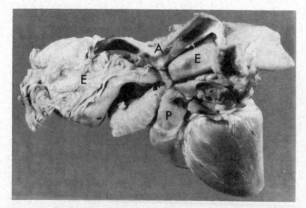

Figure 71–48. Gross specimen of persistent right aortic arch from the dog. The esophagus *(E)* is trapped between and encircled by the vascular ring made up of the aorta *(A)*, the pulmonary artery *(P)*, the base of the heart (not seen) and the ligamentum arteriosum *(arrow)*. The esophagus is dilated anteriorly to the obstruction.

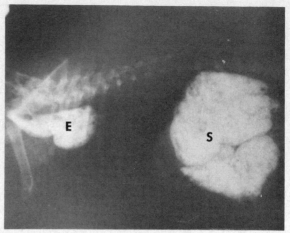

Figure 71–49. Lateral thoracic radiograph of a dog with persistent right aortic arch after barium swallow. The stomach *(S)* is filled with barium. The esophagus *(E)* is filled cranial to the heart. The esophagus is distended cranial to the heart and the barium has stopped just cranial to the heart.

The diagnosis of persistent right aortic arch or other vascular ring anomaly is made via barium swallow study (Fig. 71–49). It is critical that the difference between vascular ring anomalies and megaesophagus be identified early, before permanent damage to the esophagus occurs. The radiographic appearance of vascular ring anomalies on barium swallow radiographs is a bulging of the esophagus anterior to the base of the heart. Posterior to the heart, the esophagus, if filled with radiopaque material, is normal. In megaesophagus the esophagus is dilated throughout its length.

Treatment for vascular ring anomalies and persistent right aortic arch is surgical. Treatment must be instituted before distension of the esophagus becomes so severe as to produce permanent loss of esophageal muscle tone and perhaps destruction of esophageal nerve supply. If surgery is performed shortly after finding of the signs, normal esophageal tone and function can be expected. The longer the delay before surgical relief of the obstruction to the esophagus, the less favorable the results.[70]

Preoperative management of animals with suspected persistent right aortic arch includes liquid diet, feeding on an incline to aid flow of liquid food into the stomach, and frequent small feedings. The surgical treatment is simply division of the ligamentum arteriosum. Postoperative management is identical to preoperative care and should be continued for one to four weeks, depending on the amount of distension of the esophagus at the time of surgery. The patient is slowly returned to a normal diet, frequency of feeding, and consistency and height of food. If regurgitation recurs, a barium swallow radiograph is obtained to ascertain that the esophagus is widely patent, but normal dietary management should be delayed. If the esophagus is not widely patent, exploratory surgery may be necessary. Occasionally, adhesions in the area of the esophageal surgery occur and must be relieved.

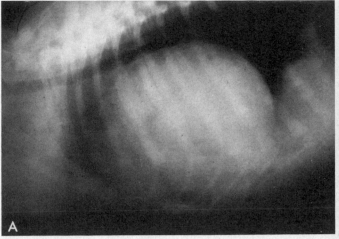

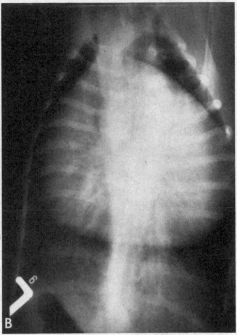

Figure 71–50. A dog with pericardial diaphragmatic hernia. *A,* Lateral thoracic radiograph. The cardiac silhouette is gigantic. The diaphragmatic line is indistinct. *B,* Dorsoventral thoracic radiograph. Note that the diaphragm on the dorsoventral view may appear intact.

Vascular ring anomalies other than persistent right aortic arch are managed on the basis of most favorable anticipated outcome. For example, if an anomalous left subclavian artery is obstructing the esophagus, the left subclavian artery must be divided. If a double aortic arch has trapped the digestive and respiratory tracts, one of the aortic arches is sacrificed, through clamp division and oversewing of the ends. The experience of the surgeon and appropriate exposure determine which structure is to be sacrificed.

Pericardial Diaphragmatic Hernia

One last noncardiovascular disorder manifesting itself as a congenital cardiac defect occasionally found in small animals is congenital pericardial diaphragmatic hernia (see also Chapter 59). With this anomaly, abdominal contents are reflected into the pericardial sac. The developmental defect results from the failure of the transverse septum from the body wall to form the ventral diaphgram. No physiological abnormalities in the heart are necessarily associated, although cardiac defects have been reported.[33]

Signs associated with pericardial diaphragmatic hernia are related to the abdominal contents in the thorax, which may become partially obstructed, respiratory distress associated with the enlarged cardiac silhouette and restriction of respiratory function, and possible alteration of cardiac function. Patients with sternal or umbilical defects often have this disease. The diagnosis of pericardial diaphragmatic hernia is established by radiograph (Fig. 71–50). The radiographic appearance of a *gigantic* cardiac silhouette in a young animal suggests this diagnosis. Other diagnoses include patent ductus arteriosus, which would

cause a murmur, and puppy cardiomyopathy, which would cause heart failure. Celiogram shows dye or air in the pericardial sac. Venous angiograms outline the chambers of the heart, which are smaller than the radiographic size of the pericardial silhouette (Fig. 71–51). Diagnosis is confirmed at surgical repair. The treatment for congenital pericardial diaphragmatic hernia is surgical replacement of the abdominal contents and plastic reconstruction of the pericardium and diaphragm. These techniques are similar to those for repair of other diaphragmatic hernias; however, we believe that median sternotomy is superior for surgical exposure and manipulation. It is important that the re-formed pericardium be separated from the diaphragm, to avoid adhesions to the diaphragm and sternum that may otherwise develop. Surgical results are excellent and complications are few.

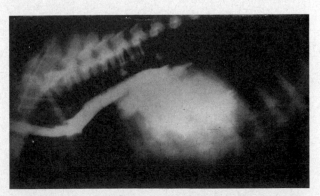

Figure 71–51. Venous angiogram of a dog with pericardial diaphragmatic hernia. The heart is outlined by dye. The additional portion of the cardiac silhouette is due to the abdominal contents in the pericardium.

ACQUIRED CARDIAC DISORDERS

Mitral Regurgitation

Acquired cardiac disorders are fewer in variety but far more common than congenital problems. The vast majority of acquired disorders are associated with mitral valve regurgitation, which affects approximately one out of 12 dogs over five years of age, with a slight preference for males.[21] It affects all breeds but is more commonly found in the small breeds, perhaps owing to the longer lives of smaller dogs. The condition is associated with degenerative changes of the mitral valve leaflets, poor coaptation and eventual dilation of the mitral annulus. Mitral regurgitation develops slowly and often produces no clinical signs for up to five years after the first development of the disease.

The pathophysiology of left heart failure and mitral valve disease described in Chapter 68 should be reviewed. As a result of regurgitation from the left ventricle through the abnormal mitral valve into the left atrium, left atrial pressure is increased. If left atrial pressure and subsequent pulmonary venous pressure exceed about 20 mm Hg, extravasation of fluid from the vascular compartment into the interstitium occurs. The interstitium in this case is the lung, and pulmonary edema results. Pulmonary lymphatics pick up the fluid, and unless the increase is overwhelming, alveolar flooding does not occur. As a result of the increased pressure, the left atrium increases in size and acts as an expansion chamber protecting the lungs from the development of pulmonary edema. As a result of enlargement, the left atrium can produce pressure on the bronchial tree and even cause obstruction of the left main bronchus. Recent experiments in dogs have demonstrated the importance of left atrial and pulmonary vascular pressure elevation before symptoms associated with pulmonary dysfunction can occur.[61] It is doubtful that these pressures are reached in the majority of dogs with spontaneous mitral regurgitation. As a consequence, signs of this disease are related to the left atrial enlargement and subsequent airway obstruction. Recent measurements in spontaneous mitral regurgitation in dogs have demonstrated that a regurgitant fraction (the portion of left ventricular blood ejected to the left atrium) of approximately 60 to 70 per cent is necessary before pulmonary signs and failure develop.[50] Only in severe mitral regurgitation are these volumes attained. Furthermore, there is good evidence to show that the majority of dogs with mitral regurgitation have no abnormalities in ventricular performance, suggesting that there is no need for positive inotrophic support of the heart.[51]

The signs associated with mitral regurgitation in the clinical patient are generally attributed to problems with the lung; the usual presenting complaint is a dry, hacking cough. The animal is elderly, there may or may not be abnormal respiratory sounds, and a pansystolic plateau murmur is present, heard best on the left thorax at about the fourth or fifth rib space. The murmur radiates dorsally. There may be atrial arrhythmias and left ventricular hypertrophy on electrocardiography. The most effective laboratory test for mitral regurgitation is radiography, findings of which are nearly pathognomonic. On the lateral thoracic radiograph there is loss of posterior waist and elevation of the trachea. On the dorsoventral radiograph, similar pulmonary findings are seen, and enlargement of the left atrial appendage is necessary for the diagnosis. Evidence of pulmonary venous engorgement must be present before congestive failure can be diagnosed. Pulmonary venous patterns,

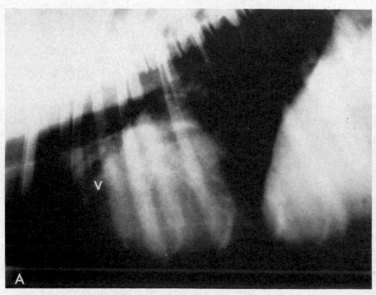
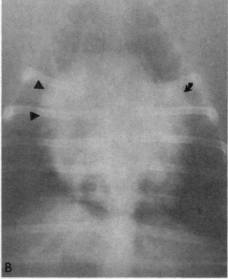

Figure 71–52. A dog with mitral and tricuspid regurgitation. *A,* Lateral thoracic radiograph. The posterior waist is filled. The heart and the pulmonary veins *(V)* are enlarged. *B,* Dorsoventral thoracic radiograph. The enlarged left atrial appendage *(arrow)* is seen at the two to three o'clock position. Distension of the right atrial border *(triangles)* suggests tricuspid regurgitation.

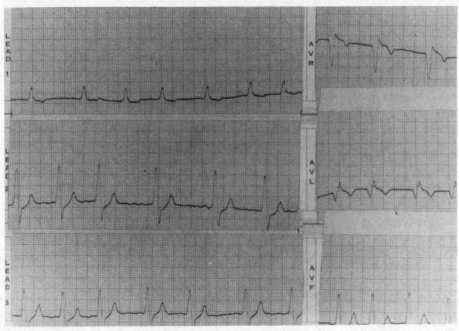

Figure 71–53. Electrocardiogram from a dog with atrial fibrillation. No P-waves are apparent on the electrocardiogram. The rate is irregular.

interstitial patterns, and, in very severe cases, alveolar patterns may be present in the lung (Fig. 71–52). Blood and serum parameters are seldom significantly altered in dogs.

The diagnosis of mitral regurgitation is perhaps the most easily established of all cardiac disturbances. The history of an elderly animal with a loud pansystolic murmur on the left side with radiographic evidence of left atrial enlargement is sufficient for confirmation.

In animals, surgical treatment of significant mitral regurgitation has been successful on few occasions. The mitral valve has been successfully replaced in the dog,[28] and recently, new valved conduits have been successfully used to replace the mitral valve.[11] Mitral valve replacement requires difficult open heart surgery, whereas valved conduit replacement requires expensive prosthetic material. These techniques, although applicable and available, are cost-prohibitive except in the most valuable animals.

The animal with mitral regurgitation seldom has significant problems for several years after the onset of the disease. The delay of onset is due to the fact that degenerative change, dilation of the mitral annulus, enlargement and pressure buffering of the left atrium, and increase in the regurgitant fraction all occur slowly. As a result, animals with the disease show signs only after a long period of the disease or after acute rupture of the chordae tendineae. Medical treatment with diuretics and perhaps vasodilators is used. Since contractility of the ventricle is not affected, digitalization is probably not indicated.

Atrial fibrillation may be a sequel to mitral regurgitation as a result of the enlargement of the left atrium in large breeds. This severe consequence can be fatal and should be aggressively treated. With atrial fibrillation, signs of heart failure are extreme, and the heart rate is fast and irregular. The diagnosis of atrial fibrillation is confirmed by electrocardiography (Fig. 71–53).[3]

Occasionally, as a result of the continuing degeneration of the mitral valve tissues, the chordae tendineae supporting the mitral valve tear (Fig. 71–54). At this time acute increase in left atrial pressure occurs, and subsequent dilation of the left atrium is not sufficient to buffer the pressure, causing acute pulmonary signs. Rupture of the chordae tendineae may be fatal, if large chordae or large numbers of

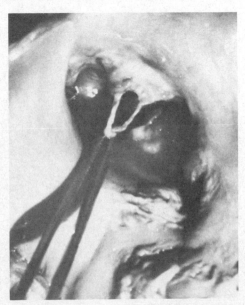

Figure 71–54. Rupture of the chorda tendineae in the dog. Note the torn chorda (in forceps).

chordae rupture, or may resolve with medical therapy, if only small pressure changes occur and the left atrium can dilate, easing the pressure load on the pulmonary vascular system.

The regurgitant stream, as a result of mitral regurgitation, may produce scarring (jet lesions) on the left atrial wall opposite the valve. In rare occasions, tears in these areas can occur, producing pericardial tamponade and death.

Tricuspid Regurgitation

A valvular lesion at the right that is analogous to mitral regurgitation is tricuspid regurgitation. Signs associated with this lesion arise from the systemic veins, particularly the veins of the liver. Tricuspid regurgitation is less common than mitral regurgitation but affects the same groups of animals at an older age. It is invariably present with mitral regurgitation but develops at a slower rate and usually has a later onset; therefore, very old animals with murmurs frequently have both diseases.

The murmur of tricuspid regurgitation is pansystolic, is heard best on the right side at about the fourth intercostal space, and tends not to radiate. Signs of the disease are ascites and previous mitral valve disease. The diagnosis is established by the presence of right atrial enlargement, seen on a lateral radiograph as a filling low in the anterior waist and on the dorsoventral radiograph as an enlargement at approximately the 8 to 11 o'clock position (Fig. 71–52). There are tall P waves on the electrocardiogram.

Treatment for tricuspid regurgitation is similar to that for mitral regurgitation. Diuretics are important in therapy. To date, no surgical intervention has been proposed. Animals with tricuspid and mitral regurgitation usually have signs and symptoms associated primarily with the mitral valve problem. The tricuspid valve disease is less significant.

Dirofilariasis

In some areas, one of the most commonly acquired diseases affecting dogs is dirofilariasis, which is caused by the parasite *Dirofilaria immitis* in the host dog. It affects dogs of all breeds and ages with no sex predilection. Animals at greater risk tend to be shorthaired, spend the majority of their time out of doors, and live in endemic mosquito areas.

The life cycle of the parasite starts with the infection of the host by a mosquito's depositing an infective larva on the skin at the time of a blood meal. After developmental moults, the immature heartworm migrates to the right ventricle and pulmonary artery and matures into an adult. The prepatent period is about six months. Adults then produce microfilaria, which are discharged into the blood and picked up by a mosquito in a blood meal. Microfilaria (not infective to the dog) must undergo developmental moults in the mosquito to become infective larva. The period of development from microfilaria to infective larva in the mosquito is temperature-dependent and can be as little as two weeks. Consequently, the life cycle of *Dirofilaria immitis* is six to nine months.

Dogs have varying responses to the presence of heartworm, from virtually no apparent affect to se-

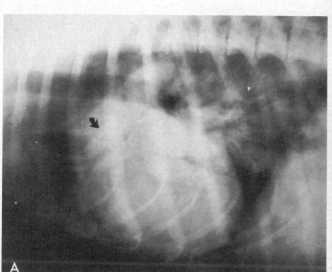
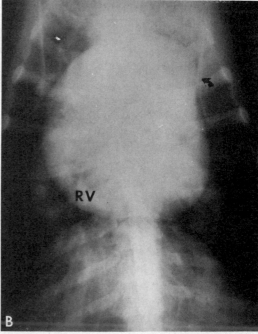

Figure 71–55. A dog with dirofilariasis. *A,* Lateral thoracic radiograph. The lungs are severely congested. The heart is enlarged, primarily on the right side. The increased size of the right anterior lobar artery *(arrow)* is seen when compared to the bronchus and vein. *B,* Dorsoventral thoracic radiograph. The main pulmonary artery is enlarged *(arrow).* The right ventricle (RV) is distended so it is closer to the right chest wall than the left ventricle is to the left chest wall.

vere pulmonary hypertension and right-sided heart failure. The response is not necessarily correlated with the number of heartworms present. The signs are usually associated with respiratory problems. Pulmonary hypertension, embolization of heartworm debris into the lungs, or lung infarction produces irritation and the cough associated with the disease. Pulmonary function may be altered and exercise intolerance may be appreciated. In some cases, owing to either pulmonary hypertension or right ventricular failure, ascites and edema are present.

Diagnosis of dirofilariasis is easily established. The presence on physical examination of a split second heart sound (due to right ventricular emptying delay) and harsh respiratory sounds along with laboratory findings of leukocytosis (particularly eosinophilia) and the presence of microfilaria in the blood (detected by one of the many microfilaria detection laboratory tests) establish the diagnosis. Electrocardiographically, right ventricular hypertrophy is seen in severely reacting patients. Perhaps the best diagnostic and prognostic tool is the thoracic radiograph (Fig. 71–55). Right-sided enlargement, pulmonary artery enlargement, and mild to severe pulmonary change are diagnostic of the disease.[67] The severity of pulmonary hypertension is correlated with the amount of pulmonary artery enlargement.

Dirofilariasis is prevented with diethylcarbamazinc. The methods have been well described elsewhere.[44,45,47] Once infection occurs, medical treatment in mildly to moderately affected dogs is accomplished with arsenicals. In severely affected dogs or dogs with renal or hepatic impairment, surgery may be indicated. At our institution the procedure of preference is inflow occlusion and pulmonary arteriotomy, as for pulmonic stenosis.

The prognosis for recovery from dirofilariasis is good. Mildly affected animals have minimal complications after treatment with arsenical compounds. Severely affected dogs have excellent recovery after heartworms have been removed. Animals with severe right-sided heart failure are at significant risk, but careful technique and monitoring reduces the mortality in these critically ill patients.

An unfortunate sequel to heartworm heart disease is the so-called postcaval syndrome. Postcaval heartworm disease, by definition, is fatal within 72 hours. For some unknown reason, a large migration of heartworms to the posterior vena cava and the right atrium causes vascular blockage, signs of severe failure, and death. Affected animals may be normal before the onset of the syndrome. Signs of postcaval syndrome are acute onset of weakness, collapse and rapid onset of hemolysis with the resultant anemia and hemoglobinuria. The diagnostic signs of postcaval syndrome are similar to those of dirofilariasis, with additional acute signs.

Treatment for postcaval syndrome is emergency surgical removal of the offending worms. Results are good, with greater than 80 per cent survival and return to normal life.[46] It is critical that the procedure be done soon after the onset of the disease, which is otherwise fatal. The postcaval removal (Jackson) technique is a remarkable emergency life-saving procedure.

Cor Pulmonale

In addition to dirofilariasis, one other cause of pulmonary vascular hypertension and right-sided heart disease should be mentioned. Dogs with chronic obstructive lung disease may on rare occasions have signs of right-sided heart failure as a result of pulmonary dysfunction. Cor pulmonale can be seen with any primary or secondary lung disease. Treatment is usually medical. Results of therapy depend on removal of, or recovery from, the original pulmonary lesion or disease.

Acquired Aortic Regurgitation

Aortic valve regurgitation is rare as an acquired disease in dogs. As described previously, it can occur as a secondary complication of ventricular septal defect. It may also be seen in association with bacterial endocarditis or bacterial valvulitis (described later). Aortic regurgitation is the most common acquired cardiac disease in older horses; the etiology is unknown.[71]

If disease of the aortic valve develops such that most of the ejection from the left ventricle into the aorta regurgitates to the left ventricle, signs of serious heart failure develop. The signs of failure associated with aortic regurgitation depend on the amount of regurgitation and the consequent amount of increase in left ventricular end-diastolic volume and pressure. If ventricular filling is excessive or if left ventricular end-diastolic pressure exceeds 20 mm Hg, pulmonary signs of left-sided heart failure develop.

Treatment for aortic regurgitation depends on removal of the cause. If infection is suspected, aggressive medical management must be instituted. Ideally, replacement of the aortic valve should be accomplished. However, this technique is not currently used in animals.

Endocarditis

Infections of cardiac structures produce serious consequences in dogs. Bacterial infections of the heart tend to embolize to other organ systems, most frequently those tissues with the greatest blood supply. Septic emboli from the heart should be considered a possible cause whenever multiple organ infection is suspected or multiple organ pain is detected.

The most common organisms found are Streptococcus and Staphylococcus spp. All dogs appear to be at risk. The signs of bacterial infection of the heart include any or all findings associated with heart disease. If the valves are affected, murmurs are present. If the conduction system is involved, block may be the outcome. If massive portions of the myocardium are involved, cardiac failure may occur. The diagnosis of endocarditis is frequently difficult to establish. The presence of vague and multiple organ system signs should make one suspect cardiac infection, and evidence of septicemia with extremely high white cell counts indicates bacterial endocarditis. The diagnosis is supported if not established by positive blood culture results. Blood culture is negative in a large percentage of the diagnosed cases, especially in animals previously treated with antibiotics.

Treatment for bacterial endocarditis is aggressive antibiotic therapy, preferably with the appropriate antibiotic as established by culture and sensitivity testing. The antibiotic should be bactericidal and administered over a long period. The prognosis depends on the severity of the damage to the myocardium, whether valvular disease is present, and the extent of involvement of other organ systems. Recovery and return to normal activity of animals affected with bacterial endocarditis also depends on the amount of damage to other organ systems.

Complete Heart Block

The major cardiac arrhythmia of surgical significance in dogs is complete heart block. The condition develops as a result of damage to the atrioventricular node or bundle of His such that the conduction from the atrium is completely interrupted. A ventricular rhythm is established, with a heart rate of approximately 40 beats/min. This rate is unacceptable for performance and is a threat to life, and the dog affected with complete heart block is incapable of increasing its ventricular rate. There appears to be little specificity throughout the breeds for complete heart block, but it is seen in older animals.[57]

Signs of complete heart block are sudden onset of exercise intolerance and syncope. Animals with the disease are generally incapable of performing more than minimal activity. The physical findings are heart rate of approximately 40 beats/min and perhaps evidence of right- or left-sided heart failure. The diagnosis is established by electrocardiogram (Fig. 71–56).

The treatment for complete heart block is medical support until surgical implantation of a pacemaker. Medical support includes atropine (usually ineffective) or isoproterenol, which may break the abnormal

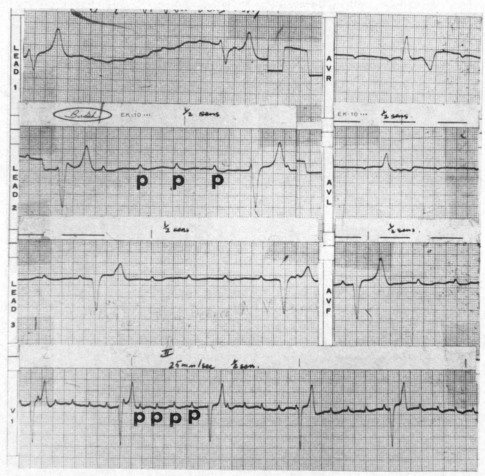

Figure 71–56. Electrocardiogram of complete heart block. The multiple P waves (p) are not associated with QRS complexes.

rhythm or produce a ventricular rhythm at a faster rate. Surgical implantation of a pacemaker should be preceded by placement of a temporary transvenous pacemaker.

The prognosis for therapy with complete heart block is grave unless a pacemaker is inserted. An animal surviving to surgery becomes a major anesthesia risk unless a temporary pacemaker can be used to control the heart rate. With temporary pacing, surgical risk is reduced. Surgical results are good, and generally the animals live more than one year.[57,82] At first impression, this appears to be a poor long-term surgical result, but with the older age of onset of this condition, one year can be considered very good.

Cardiomyopathy

Feline Cardiomyopathy

Recently there has been an increase in the diagnosis of cardiomyopathy in animals. One of the first specific cardiomyopathies recognized was feline cardiomyopathy syndrome.[58] Feline cardiomyopathy has been recognized over the last two decades as a major disease and as the major cause of heart disease in cats. It was first recognized in the northeastern United States and has slowly spread throughout the country. The etiology is unknown, but current speculation is that the disease is a result of a previous viral infection. All cats can be affected, and there is little or no sex predilection.

The feline cardiomyopathy syndrome may encompass as many as four identifiable entities but manifests clinically as one of two basic disease processes: (1) a disease of systolic malfunction, congestive cardiomyopathy, or (2) a disease of diastolic malfunction,

hypertrophic cardiomyopathy. Cats with both types have similar signs: mild to severe respiratory dysfunction, open-mouth breathing, and weakness, along with an occasional cough or sneeze. On physical examination, cats have abnormal respiratory sounds and may have heart murmurs or a diastolic gallop rhythm. The disease is diagnosed on the basis of history, physical findings, abnormal electrocardiographic findings of left ventricular hypertrophy, arrhythmias and incomplete left bundle branch block. The radiographic appearance—pulmonary edema, pleural effusion, and enlargement of the right and left atria, which produces a valentine-shaped heart on dorsoventral radiograph—is nearly pathognomonic (Fig. 71–57).

Differentiation of hypertrophic and congestive cardiomyopathy is difficult without echocardiography. The presence of left ventricular hypertrophy or incomplete left bundle branch block on electrocardiogram strongly indicates hypertrophic cardiomyopathy; a large, globular heart on radiograph with dilation of both right and left ventricles indicates congestive cardiomyopathy. There is, unfortunately, overlap between the two manifestations of cardiomyopathy, and treatment is distinctly different for the two types of disease. In the absence of echocardiographic confirmation, type of cardiomyopathy is most easily determined by venous angiogram. A film taken six to ten seconds after injection demonstrates the wall thickness of the left ventricle and chamber size (Figs. 71–58 and 71–59).

Treatment for feline cardiomyopathy is medical. The hypertrophic condition seems to respond to beta-adrenergic blockade, whereas the congestive form of the disease is helped with digitalization. In either case, diuretics and low-salt diet are recommended.

Prognosis for cats with feline cardiomyopathy syn-

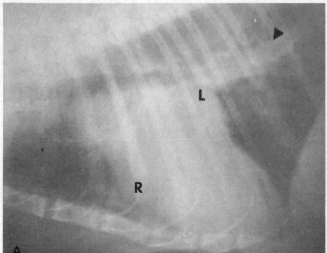

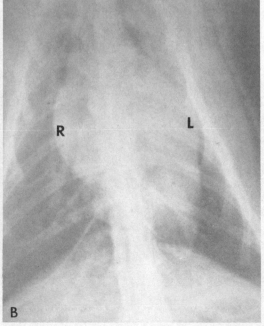

Figure 71–57. A cat with congestive cardiomyopathy. *A,* Lateral thoracic radiograph. The heart is greatly enlarged, particularly the right and left atria (*R* and *L*). The lungs are congested, and increased density represents interstitial and vascular markings *(triangle). B,* Dorsoventral thoracic radiograph of a cat with cardiomyopathy. The "valentine" appearance of the heart is produced by the enlargement of the right and left atria (*R* and *L*).

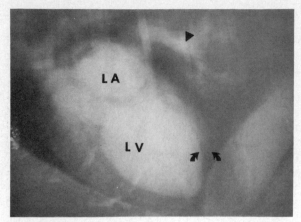

Figure 71–58. Venous angiogram in the levo phase from a cat with congestive cardiomyopathy. The angiogram is taken approximately 8 seconds after the venous injection. The pulmonary veins *(triangle)* are enlarged and tortuous. The large left atrium *(LA)* is outlined. The dilated left ventricle *(LV)* is seen as a rounded chamber. The thin-walled left ventricle (between the *arrows*), along with the large dilated left ventricle, suggests congestive cardiomyopathy.

drome is poor, with the average life expectancy (after signs appear), regardless of therapy, of approximately one year. Animals can be supported with medical treatment and can be made more comfortable. When pulmonary edema and pleural effusion are present, diuretics are important in prolonging the animal's life.

A sequel in one-third of cats with feline cardiomyopathy is embolization. The most common location is at the bifurcation of the aorta, which produces the "saddle thrombus" (Fig. 71–60). Cats with aortic thrombus have signs of acute posterior paralysis and excruciating pain. The rear legs become cold and cyanotic. The toenails do not bleed when cut. The presence of vasoactive substances from the clot blocks development of collateral circulation.[13] Approximately one-third of cats with aortic thrombus die in the acute stages of heart failure or shock, one-third recover, and one-third survive with major deficits of rear leg structure or function. Animals should be

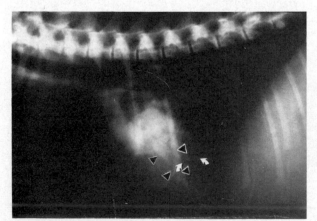

Figure 71–59. Venous angiogram in the levo phase from a cat with hypertrophic cardiomyopathy. The left ventricular cavity is small and funnel-shaped (between *triangles*). The left ventricular wall is thickened (between *arrows*).

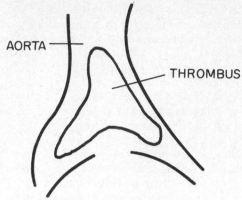

Figure 71–60. "Saddle thrombus" in the descending aorta of the cat with cardiomyopathy.

treated for shock and should be given other symptomatic supportive therapy. Cats surviving aortic embolus average one recurrence within six months.

In cats with an acute onset of aortic thrombus surgical removal of the thrombus should be successful if accomplished within four to six hours (see Chapters 73 and 78).[12] It has been suggested that amputation of the left atrial appendage may eliminate the nidus for clot formation. Mild anticoagulation with aspirin may reduce platelet aggregation and thus decrease the likelihood of future clot formation.[36]

Canine Cardiomyopathy

Congestive Cardiomyopathy. Canine cardiomyopathy can be either hypertrophic or congestive. Congestive canine cardiomyopathy has been recognized only during the last 15 years. The disease affects large and giant breeds, in particular the Doberman.[14] It may be caused by a virus.[15,77] The condition is seen four times more frequently in males and usually occurs in middle age. Dogs with congestive cardiomyopathy have severe heart failure with ascites, pleural effusion, pulmonary edema, reduced exercise tolerance, pale mucous membranes, diastolic sounds, fast heart rates, and arrhythmias. Murmurs may be present. The diagnosis of congestive cardiomyopathy in the dog is established by the following criteria: (1) a large-breed male with a history consistent with heart failure; (2) physical findings of tachycardia, respiratory distress, abnormal lung sounds, and ascites or edema; (3) electrocardiographic evidence of atrial or ventricular arrhythmias; and (4) most importantly, the radiographic appearance of tremendous enlargement of the heart, particularly the atria (Fig. 71–61).[3] If available, echocardiographic findings of poor ventricular wall motion, thin ventricular wall, and poor contractility confirm the diagnosis.[81]

Dogs with congestive cardiomyopathy usually have mitral regurgitation as a result of dilation of the left ventricle and mitral annulus. A mitral regurgitation murmur is frequently heard. The presence of mitral regurgitation accentuates the pulmonary failure. In the past, a large number of animals with congestive

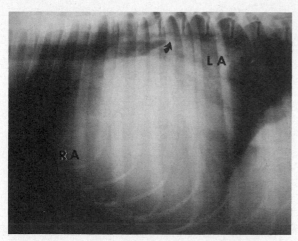

Figure 71–61. Lateral thoracic radiograph of a dog with congestive cardiomyopathy. The cardiac silhouette is grossly enlarged, particularly the right atrial appendage *(RA)* and left atrium *(LA)*. The tremendous enlargement of the left heart, particularly the left atrium, has caused constriction of the left main bronchus *(arrow)*, which could produce signs of cough.

cardiomyopathy were misdiagnosed as having mitral regurgitation, even congenital mitral regurgitation.

The treatment for congestive cardiomyopathy in the dog is medical. At our institution, prior to the understanding of the significance of the myocardial failure, ten animals were operated on for valve replacement, only one of which survived.

The prognosis for dogs with congestive cardiomyopathy is poor. Without therapy, animals live an average of six weeks from the onset of the severe atrial or ventricular arrhythmia.[22] Therapy is effective if the dog's tachycardias are controlled. At our institution, 50 per cent of dogs with congestive cardiomyopathy survived one year and then had a normal life expectancy. Fifty per cent died within the first year, half of these within the first six weeks, regardless of therapy. Recent reports of congestive cardiomyopathy in humans show similar mortality and morbidity rates.[39]

Hypertrophic Cardiomyopathy. Recently, a condition in the dog that is manifested by sudden death and a hypertrophied left ventricle has been described.[56] Hypertrophic cardiomyopathy in the dog is more common than previously anticipated and should be considered in any case of sudden death of an otherwise healthy dog. The boxer is particularly susceptible, and the disease may be inherited as an autosomal dominant trait. Dogs with hypertrophic cardiomyopathy have signs similar to those of aortic stenosis (syncope and sudden death). On physical examination, murmurs may or may not be present, and the dogs appear normal.

Electrocardiographic findings may include left ventricular hypertrophy, conduction disturbances, and ST segment alterations. The thoracic radiograph is not a reliable indicator of disease, but an echocardiogram can be diagnostic. Echocardiographic evidence of abnormal thickening of the septum and free wall or asymmetrical septal hypertrophy with a septum–

free wall ratio greater than 1.3:1 is strong evidence of the disease. A left ventricular angiogram (venous angiogram in small dogs) indicating thickening of the left ventricular free wall can be helpful in making the diagnosis.

Treatment for hypertrophic cardiomyopathy in the dog has not been established. In humans, beta-adrenergic blockade is effective in reducing the frequency of arrhythmia and consequently sudden death.[37] Although this treatment is being used in animals, long-term objective evaluation is not available.

Pericardial Disorders

Disorders of the pericardium in animals are rare. Traumatic pericardial diaphragmatic hernia appears similar to congenital pericardial diaphragmatic hernia, except for the usual history of trauma and absence of sternal abnormalities and history of umbilical hernia. Treatment is similar to that for the congenital lesion.

Pericarditis

Pericarditis, or reactive pericardial disease, is occasionally reported. Animals with pericarditis usually have signs associated with pericardial tamponade. These signs include ascites, pleural effusions, and occasional breathing difficulty. On physical examination, animals with pericardial tamponade may have pericardial friction sounds, but usually the heart sounds are muffled. The diagnosis is established by low-amplitude recording on all leads of the electrocardiogram, echocardiographic signs of effusion, and the radiographic appearance of a circular heart on all views (Fig. 71–62).

The treatment for pericarditis and pericardial disease is pericardiocentesis (see Chapter 74). The tap is both diagnostic and therapeutic. In virtually all cases, the pericardial fluid does not contain pathogenic organisms, but culture should nevertheless be performed. The animal should be followed radiographically to be sure that effusion does not recur. Multiple taps may be necessary to control the continued development of fluid. It is our judgment that if drainage on three separate occasions is not sufficient to halt the development of the disease and control pericardial effusion, pericardectomy should be performed. Pericardectomy is a simple procedure but can be exceedingly difficult if the pericardium is severely thickened and infiltrated with fibrous or granulomatous reactive tissue.

The results of pericardiocentesis for benign pericardial effusions and pericarditis are only fair. Approximately 50 per cent of the animals recover without surgical intervention. In animals requiring pericardectomy, the results are poor. If the lesion is severe, some recurrence of the granulomatous reaction can be expected. If the pericardium is not thickened, results are usually good.

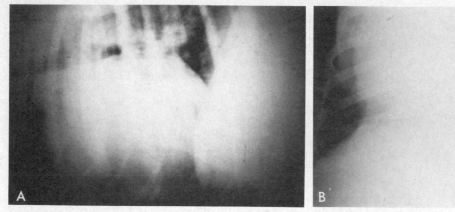

Figure 71–62. Lateral (A) and dorsoventral (B) thoracic radiographs of a dog with pericardial tamponade. The cardiac silhouette is circular in all views. The abdomen is distended by ascites due to heart failure.

TUMORS OF THE HEART

Tumors of the cardiovascular system are extremely uncommon. The two major neoplasms that affect the heart with any frequency, heart base tumor and hemangiosarcoma, are discussed here. Other cardiac tumors are extremely rare, generally metastatic, and disseminated from primary lesions; included in this group is the lymphoma-lymphosarcoma complex. The major discussion of tumors of the cardiovascular system can be found in Chapter 177.

Heart Base Tumor

The so-called heart base tumor is found at the arch of the aorta near the pulmonary artery at the base of the heart (Fig. 71–63). The tumor has been considered to be of thyroid or neural crest origin, but an established cell type has not been consistently found. It is slow-growing and invasive, producing hemorrhage. Animals affected with heart base tumor are almost exclusively brachycephalic, the Boston terrier and boxer making up approximately 90 per cent of

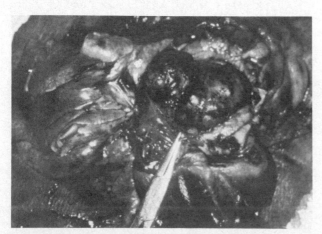

Figure 71–63. Heart base tumor in a Boston terrier. The forceps point to the growth seen dorsal to the heart and beneath the aorta (A).

reported cases.[48] Signs are associated with the hemorrhage into the pericardial sac and pericardial tamponade.

There is no treatment for heart base tumor. Pericardiocentesis can be accomplished to relieve the tamponade, but long-term survival has not been reported.

Hemangiosarcoma

Hemangiosarcoma of the heart, particularly of the right atrium, is either primary or secondary to another hemangiosarcoma, usually of the spleen. The disease is common in animals prone to hemangiosarcoma, particularly the German shepherd. The tumor causes signs similar to those of heart base tumor, because hemorrhage into the pericardial sac produces pericardial tamponade. Although the tumor location is such that resection could be effective, to date no successful surgical removal has been reported.

1. August, J. R., Teer, P. A., and Bartels, J. E.: Kartagener's syndrome in a dog. J. Am. Anim. Hosp. Assoc. *18*:822, 1982.
2. Aultman, S. H., Chambers, J. N., and Vestre, W. A.: Double aortic arch and persistent right aortic arch in two littermates: surgical treatment. J. Am. Anim. Hosp. Assoc. *16*:533, 1980.
3. Bohn, F. K., Patterson, D. F., and Pyles, R. L.: Atrial fibrillation in dogs. Br. Vet. *127*:485, 1971.
4. Boineau, J. P., Moore, E. N., and Patterson, D. F.: Relationship between the ECG, ventricular activation and the ventricular conduction system in ostium primum ASD. Circulation *48*:556, 1973.
5. Bolton, G. R., Ettinger, S. J., and Liu, S. K.: Tetralogy of Fallot in three cats. J. Am. Vet. Med. Assoc. *160*:1622, 1972.
6. Braden, T. D., Appleford, M. D., and Hartsfield, S. M.: Correction of a ventricular septal defect in a dog. J. Am. Vet. Med. Assoc. *161*:507, 1972.
7. Breznock, E. M., Hilwig, R. W., Vasko, J. S., and Hamlin, R. L.: Surgical correction of an interventricular septal defect in the dog. J. Am. Vet. Med. Assoc. *157*:1343, 1970.
8. Breznock, E. M.: Spontaneous closure of ventricular septal defects in the dog. J. Am. Vet. Med. Assoc. *162*:399, 1973.
9. Breznock, E. M., and Wood, G. L.: A patch-graft technique

for correction of pulmonic stenosis in dogs. J. Am. Vet. Med. Assoc. *169*:1090, 1976.

10. Breznock, E. M., Whiting, P., Pendrays, D., et al.: Valved apico-aortic conduit for relief of left ventricular hypertension caused by discrete subaortic stenosis in dogs. J. Am. Vet. Med. Assoc. *182*:51, 1983.

11. Breznock. E. M., Bauer, T., Strack, D., et al.: Prosthetic mitral and tricuspid valve implantation in dogs using deep surface hypothermia (15°C). Abstracts Am. Coll. Vet. Surg., 1983.

12. Buchanan, J. W., Baker, G. J., and Hill, J. D.: Aortic embolism in cats: prevalance, surgical treatment and electrocardiography. Vet. Rec. 79:496, 1966.

13. Butler, H. C.: An investigation into the relationship of an aortic embolus to posterior paralysis in the cat. J. Small Anim. Pract. *12*:141, 1972.

14. Calvert, C. A., Chapman, W. L., and Toal, R. L.: Congestive cardiomyopathy in Doberman pinscher dogs. J. Am. Vet. Med. Assoc. *181*:598, 1982.

15. Carpenter, J. L., Roberts, R. M., Harpster, N. K., and King, N. W.: Intestinal and cardiopulmonary forms of parvovirus infection in a litter of pups. J. Am. Vet. Med. Assoc. *176*:1269, 1980.

16. Carrig, C. B., Suter, P. F., Ewing, G. O., and Dungworth, D. L.: Primary dextrocardia with situs inversus, associated with sinusitis and bronchitis in a dog. J. Am. Vet. Med. Assoc. *164*:1127, 1974.

17. Chen, H. C., Bussian, P., and Whitehead, J. E.: Persistent truncus arteriosus in a dog. Vet. Path. 9:379, 1972.

18. Clark, D. R., Ross, J. N., Hamlin, R. L., and Smith, C. R.: Tetralogy of Fallot in the dog. J. Am. Vet. Med. Assoc. *152*:462, 1968.

19. Custer, M. A., Kantor, A. F., Gilman, R. A., and DeRiemer, R. H.: Correction of pulmonic stenosis. J. Am. Vet. Med. Assoc. *139*:565, 1961.

20. Dear, M. G.: Mitral incompetence in dogs of 0–5 years of age. J. Small Anim. Pract. *12*:1, 1971.

21. Detweiler, D. K., Hubben, K., and Patterson, D. F.: Survey of cardiovascular disease in dogs—preliminary report on the first 1000 dogs screened. Am. J. Vet. Res. *21*:329, 1960.

22. Ettinger, S.: Conversion of spontaneous atrial fibrillation in dogs, using direct current synchronized shock. J. Am. Vet. Med. Assoc. *152*:41, 1968.

23. Eyster, G. E., Daley, J. B., Chaffee, A., et al.: Aorticopulmonary septal defect in a dog. J. Am. Vet. Med. Assoc. *167*:1094, 1975.

24. Eyster, G. E., Hough, J. D., Evans, A. T., et al.: Surgical repair of patent ductus arteriosus, aortic stenosis, and aortic regurgitation in a dog. J. Am. Vet. Med. Assoc. *167*:942, 1975.

25. Eyster, G. E., Whipple, R. D., Evans, A. T., et al.: Rechannelized patent ductus arteriosus in the dog. J. Small Anim. Pract. *16*:743, 1975.

26. Eyster, G. E., Anderson, L. K., and Cords, G.: Aortic regurgitation in the dog. J. Am. Vet. Med. Assoc. *168*:138–141, 1976.

27. Eyster, G. E., Eyster, J. T., Cords, G. B., and Johnston, J.: Patent ductus arteriosus in the dog: characteristics of occurrence and results of surgery in one hundred consecutive cases. J. Am. Vet. Med. Assoc. *168*:435, 1976.

28. Eyster, G. E., Weber, W., Chi, S., et al.: Mitral valve prosthesis for correction of mitral regurgitation in a dog. J. Am. Vet. Med. Assoc. *168*:1115, 1976.

29. Eyster, G. E., Carrig, C. B., Baker, B., et al.: Coarctation of the aorta in a dog. J. Am. Vet. Med. Assoc. *169*:426, 1976.

30. Eyster, G. E., Anderson, L. K., Sawyer, D. C., et al.: Beta adrenergic blockade for management of tetralogy of Fallot in a dog. J. Am. Vet. Med. Assoc. *169*:637, 1976.

31. Eyster, G. E., Anderson, L. K., Krehbiel, J. D., et al.: Surgical repair of atrial septal defect in a dog. J. Am. Vet. Med. Assoc. *169*:1081, 1976.

32. Eyster, G. E., Whipple, R. D., Anderson, L. J., et al.: Pulmonary artery banding for ventricular septal defect in dogs and cats. J. Am. Vet. Med. Assoc. *170*:434, 1977.

33. Eyster, G. E., Evans, A. T., Blanchard, G. L., et al.: Congenital pericardial diaphragmatic hernia and multiple cardiac defects in a litter of collies. J. Am. Vet. Med. Assoc. *170*:516, 1977.

34. Eyster, G. E., Anderson, L., Evans, A. T., et al.: Ebstein's anomaly: a report of 3 cases in the dog. J. Am. Vet. Med. Assoc. *170*:709, 1977.

35. Ford, P. F., Wood, A., Liu, S. K., and Tilley, L. P.: Left ventricular angiocardiography in congenital mitral valve insufficiency of the dog. J. Am. Vet. Med. Assoc. *166*:1069, 1975.

36. Fox, P. R.: Feline myocardial disease. *In*. Kirk, R. W. (ed.); *Current Veterinary Therapy VIII: Small Animal Practice*. W. B. Saunders, Philadelphia, 1983.

37. Frank, M. J., Abdulla, A. M., Canedo, M. I., and Saylors, R. E.: Long-term medical management of hypertrophic obstructive cardiomyopathy. Am. J. Cardiol. *42*:993, 1978.

38. Friedman, W. F., and Roberts, W. C.: Vitamin D and the supravalvular aortic stenosis syndrome. Circulation *34*:77, 1966.

39. Fuster, V., Guiliani, E. R., Gersh, B., et al.: Factors affecting long-term prognosis (5–19 years) of idiopathic dilated cardiomyopathy. Circulation Abstr. *59 & 60* (Suppl. 2):2, 1979.

40. Hamlin, R. L., and Harris, S. G.: Mitral incompetence in Great Dane pups. J. Am. Vet. Med. Assoc. *154*:790, 1969.

41. Hanlon, C. R., Kiaser, G. C., Mudd, J. F. G., and Willman, V. L.: Closed pulmonary valvulotomy. J. Cardiovasc. Surg. 9:496, 1968.

42. Hawe, R. S.: Pulmonic stenosis in a cat. J. Am. Anim. Hosp. Assoc. *17*:777, 1981.

43. Hough, J. D., Carlson, B., Weitkamp, R. A., and McLean, R. T.: Situs inversus and intussusception in a dog. J. Am. Anim. Hosp. Assoc. *15*:335, 1979.

44. Jackson, R. F.: Treatment of heartworm-infected dogs with chemical agents. J. Am. Vet. Med. Assoc. *154*:390, 1969.

45. Jackson, R. F.: Thiacetarsamide for preventive treatment of *Dirofilaria immitis*. J. Am. Vet. Med. Assoc. *154*:395, 1969.

46. Jackson, R. F., Seymour, W. G., Growney, P. G., and Otto, G. F.: Surgical treatment of the caval syndrome of canine heartworm disease. J. Am. Vet. Med. Assoc. *171*:1065, 1977.

47. Jackson, W. F.: Preventative therapy with diethylcarbamazine. J. Am. Vet. Med. Assoc. *154*:396, 1969.

48. Johnson, K. H.: Aortic body tumors in the dog. J. Am. Vet. Med. Assoc. *152*:154, 1968.

49. Jones, C. L., and Buchanan, J. W.: Patent ductus arteriosus: anatomy and surgery in a cat. J. Am. Vet. Med. Assoc. *179*:364, 1981.

50. Kittleson, M. D., Eyster, G. E., Knowlen, G. G., et al.: Myocardial function in small dogs with chronic mitral regurgitation and severe heart failure. J. Am. Vet. Med. Assoc. *184*:455, 1984.

51. Kittleson, M. D., Eyster, G. E., Olivier, N. B., and Anderson, L. K.: Oral hydralazine therapy for chronic mitral regurgitation in the dog. J. Am. Vet. Med. Assoc. *182*:1205, 1983.

52. Knight, D. H., Patterson, D. F., and Milbin, J.: Constriction of the fetal ductus arteriosus induced by oxygen, acetylcholine, and norepinephrine in normal dogs and those genetically predisposed to persistent patency. Circulation *47*:127, 1973.

53. Legendre, A. M., Appleford, M. D., Eyster, G. E., and Dade, A. W.: Secondary polycythemia and seizures due to right to left shunting patent ductus arteriosus in a dog. J. Am. Vet. Med. Assoc. *164*:1198, 1974.

54. Liu, S. K., and Ettinger, S.: Persistent common atrioventricular canal in two cats. J. Am. Vet. Med. Assoc. *153*:556, 1968.

55. Liu, S. K., and Tilley, L. P.: Dysplasia of the tricuspid valve in the dog and cat. J. Am. Vet. Med. Assoc. *169*:623, 1976.

56. Liu, S. K., Maron, B. J., and Tilley, L. P.: Canine hypertrophic cardiomyopathy. J. Am. Vet. Med. Assoc. *174*:708, 1980.

57. Lombard, C. W., Tilley, L. P., and Yoshioka, M.: Pacemaker implantation in the dog: survey and literature review. J. Am. Anim. Hosp. Assoc. *17*:751, 1981.

58. Lord, P. F., Wood, A., Tilley, L. P., and Liu, S. K.:

Radiographic and hemodynamic evaluation of cardiomyopathy and thromboembolism in the cat. J. Am. Vet. Med. Assoc. *164*:154, 1974.

59. Mann, P. G. H., Stock, J. E., and Sheridan, J. P.: Pulmonary artery banding in the cat: a case report. J. Small Anim. Pract. *12*:45, 1971.

60. Milledge, R. D., Eastin, C. E., and Reeves, J. T.: Physiologic and radiographic studies of cervical ectopia cordis in a calf. J. Am. Vet. Med. Assoc. *152*:161, 1968.

61. Miller, J. E., Eyster, G., Robinson, N. E., et al.: Pulmonary function in dogs with mitral regurgitation. Abstracts Am. Coll. Vet. Surg., 1983.

62. Nichols, J. B., Eyster, G. E., Dulisch, M. L., et al.: Aortic interruption in a dog. J. Am. Vet. Med. Assoc. *174*:1091, 1979.

63. Parker, G. W., Jackson, W. F., and Patterson, D. F.: Coarctation of the aorta in a canine. J. Am. Anim. Hosp. Assoc. *7*:353, 1971.

64. Patterson, D. F., Pyle, R. L., Ven Mierop, L., et al.: Hereditary defects of the conotruncal septum in Keeshond dogs: pathologic and genetic studies. Am. J. Cardiol. *34*:187, 1974.

65. Patterson, D. F.: Canine congenital heart disease: epidemiology and etiological hypotheses. J. Small Anim. Pract. *12*:263, 1971.

66. Prickett, M. E., Reeves, J. T., and Zent, W. W.: Tetralogy of Fallot in a thoroughbred foal. J. Am. Vet. Med. Assoc. *162*:552, 1973.

67. Rawlings, C. A., Losonsky, J. M., Lewis, R. E., and McCall, J. W.: Development and resolution of radiographic lesions in canine heartworm disease. J. Am. Vet. Med. Assoc. *178*:1172, 1981.

68. Rich, S., Martinez, J., Lam, W., et al.: Reassessment of the effects of vasodilator drugs in pulmonary hypertension: guidelines for determining a pulmonary vasodilator response. Am. Heart J. *105*:119, 1983.

69. Scott, E. A., Chaffee, A., Eyster, G. E., and Kneller, S. K.: Interruption of aortic arch in two foals. J. Am. Vet. Med. Assoc. *172*:347, 1978.

70. Shires, P. K., and Liu, W.: Persistent right aortic arch in dogs: a long-term follow-up after surgical correction. J. Am. Anim. Hosp. Assoc. *17*:773, 1981.

71. Smetzer, D. L., Bishop, S., and Smith, C. R.: Diastolic murmur of equine aortic insufficiency. Am. Heart J. *72*:489, 1966.

72. Suter, P. F., and Kay, W. J.: Persistent truncus arteriosus in a cat. J. Am. Vet. Med. Assoc. *153*:548, 1968.

73. Swan, H., Zeavin, J., Blount, S. G., Jr., and Virtue, R. W.: Surgery by direct vision in the open heart during hypothermia. J.A.M.A. *153*:1081, 1953.

74. Tashjian, R. J., Das, K. M., Palich, W. E., et al.: Studies on cardiovascular disease in the cat. Ann. N. Y. Acad. Sci. *127*:581, 1965.

75. Troy, G. C., and Turnwald, G. H.: Atrial fibrillation and abnormal ventricular conduction presented as right bundle branch block in a dog with an atrial septum primum defect. J. Am. Anim. Hosp. Assoc. *15*:417, 1979.

76. Turk, J. R., Miller, L., and Hegreberg, G. A.: Double outlet right ventricle in a dog. J. Am. Anim. Hosp. Assoc. *17*:789, 1981.

77. van den Ingh, T. S. G. A. M., van den Linde-Sipman, J. S., and Wester, P. W.: Parvo-virus–like particles in myocarditis in pups. J. Small Anim. Pract. *21*:81, 1980.

78. van den Ingh, T. S. G. A. M., and van der Linde-Sipman, J. S.: Vascular rings in dogs. J. Am. Vet. Med. Assoc. *164*:939, 1974.

79. Weirich, W. E., Blevins, W. E., Conrad, C. R., et al.: Congenital tricuspid insufficiency in a dog. J. Am. Vet. Med. Assoc. *164*:1025, 1974.

80. Weirich, W. E., and Blevins, W. E.: Ventricular septal defect repair. Vet. Surg. *7*:2, 1978.

81. Wood, G. L.: Canine myocardial disease. *In* Kirk, R. W. (ed.): *Current Veterinary Therapy VIII: Small Animal Practice.* W. B. Saunders, Philadelphia, 1983.

82. Yoshioka, M. M., Tilley, L. P., Harvey, H. J., et al.: Permanent pacemaker implantation in the dog. J. Am. Anim. Hosp. Assoc. *17*:746, 1981.

Chapter **72** Principles of Vascular Surgery

Philip Litwak

Vascular surgery deals with blood vessels. These vessels can vary in diameter from 20 mm, e.g., the aorta in a Great Dane, to 1 mm, e.g., the tibial artery of a cat. Vein size can also vary. However, certain surgical principles, instruments, drugs, and prostheses are applicable to all blood vessels. Microvascular surgery and the use of operating microscopes, although a subspecialty of vascular surgery, is not discussed in this chapter.

INSTRUMENTS

Specialized instruments for vascular surgery are not required for many procedures, but their use can lessen the difficulty and improve the results. In some situations they are required. The instruments themselves can be divided into four groups: (1) cutting instruments, (2) grasping instruments, (3) clamps, and (4) needle holders.

Vascular cutting instruments must be sharp and free from imperfections. Rough edges on vessel walls invite deposition of proteins and cells, which can lead to thrombosis. Except for very small incisions for which a No. 11 blade is used, a new No. 15 blade should be used for arteriotomies and venotomies.

There are many configurations of scissors, each especially designed for a particular surgeon or use. The majority of vascular incisions in dogs and cats can be performed using Potts-type scissors with 60- to 90-degree angled points (Fig. 72–1).

Forceps are available in many sizes and shapes.

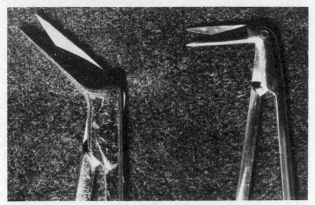

Figure 72–1. Two types of Potts scissors used to extend vascular incisions.

Only atraumatic instruments should be used to grasp vascular tissues. DeBakey vascular forceps have proven the most applicable to a wide range of procedures. Tip widths of 1.5 to 2.0 mm are preferred for all but very large and very small vessels. Extremely fine tips are required for vessels less than 3.0 or 4.0 mm in diameter.

The variety of vascular clamping instruments is tremendous. However, for veterinary vascular surgery, only a few are needed, and in emergencies perhaps only two need be available. In general, clamps either are used to completely block flow or are applied tangentially to partially occlude flow. Except in major vessels such as the aorta and its primary branches and the vena cavae, flow can be totally occluded for 30 to 45 minutes with no apparent effect. Therefore, clamps such as DeBakey ring-handle bulldog clamps are especially useful. They are available in various jaw configurations, but the curved or angled design is most useful. Bulldog clamps can also be used to cross-clamp vessels, but are less

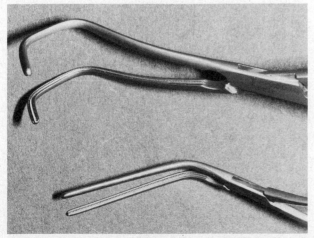

Figure 72–2. Vascular occluding clamps. The instrument at the top is applied tangentially to partially occlude flow, and the instrument at the bottom is applied transversely to totally occlude flow.

versatile for larger arteries. Full-size vascular clamps may be required to reach deep vessels (Fig. 72–2).

Tangential clamps are used to partially occlude a vessel so that a graft or another vessel can be anastomosed to the occluded section. Major vessels whose flow cannot be totally stopped without serious effects require these instruments. Clamps with long distal sections are preferred to get a secure grip on the vessel and still leave enough lumen for blood flow. A clamp with a jaw width of 4 to 5 cm and a depth of 2 to 3 cm is adequate for most uses.

A fine pair of Olsen-Hegar or Mayo-Hegar needle holders suffices for most vascular procedures. However, in procedures involving use of 5-0 or 6-0 suture, a Castroviejo needle holder is helpful; the locking mechanism eliminates the ratchet catch and resulting gross movements necessary with more conventional needle holders.

All of these instruments are available in pediatric sizes and weights. However, these are generally not necessary, since vessels as small as 3 mm can be successfully sutured with the instruments described.

SUTURES

Sutures suitable for vascular procedures are available in a wide range of materials and sizes. Monofilament polypropylene, braided polyester, and silk are most commonly used. Only sutures with swaged-on needles are used to anastomose blood vessels. Diameter of suture used for particular applications depends on the surgeon's preference and the material. Generally, 5-0, 6-0 and 7-0 are sufficiently strong for most peripheral arteries and all feline vascular anastomoses. Aortic grafts in large dogs may require 4-0 sutures.

Monofilament polypropylene is probably the most commonly used vascular suture. It is extremely smooth, strong, and inert. It loses little strength with time when implanted. Its blue color gives high visibility even with 6-0 and 7-0 sizes. Square knots with flat throws should be used and at least five throws should be placed.

Braided polyester suture used for vascular procedures is usually coated with an inert lubricant. This material is strong, inert, and easy to tie. It remains strong for long periods of implantation. Four throws of flat, square knots are required with this suture.

Silk suture continues to be used in vascular surgery. Coating of the braided material results in a suture that passes easily through vessels and grafts, is relatively easy to tie, and is initially strong. Silk loses some tensile strength with duration of implantation, but this loss is not sufficient to preclude its use.

Polyglycolic acid sutures have also been used for vascular anastomoses of autogenous veins to arteries.[12] Where healing occurs between the prosthesis and host vessel, polyglycolic acid sutures retained their strength long enough for healing to occur. There was no higher incidence of aneurysms, dilations, or infection in polyglycolic acid–sutured anastomoses than in polypropylene-sutured anastomoses.

Suture material is a factor in the occurrence of anastomotic false aneurysms and in vascular infection. Failure of monofilament polyethylene and silk sutures was implicated as the cause of more than 60 per cent of the false aneurysms in a large study of peripheral vascular procedures.[16] False aneurysms that occurred when braided Dacron was used were associated not with suture failure but with such factors as arterial wall failure and chronic hypertension.

In an experimental study in rabbits, the effect of suture material in the development of vascular infection was studied.[5] Aortotomy incisions were sutured with a variety of commonly used materials and infected with *Staphylococcus aureus*. Monofilament suture materials had lower suture line bacterial counts than the multifilament materials. Silk had the highest counts, and monofilament nylon and monofilament polypropylene had the lowest.

Many types of needles are swaged to cardiovascular sutures. For most applications in small animal practice, a 3/8-circle or 1/2-circle taper point needle is appropriate. These fine needles must be used with care, as they bend easily unless passed through the tissues with a rotational motion. Care must also be taken not to pull on the needle to draw the suture through the wound, because sutures can be dislodged from the swaged-on needle.

VASCULAR PROSTHESES

Vascular prostheses can be placed in two groups: synthetic, either textile or non-textile; and biological, either fresh or preserved. All grafts currently available function adequately when placed in a high-flow, low-resistance vessel such as the aorta. Graft use in small diameter vessels requires careful selection of type and size. Many prostheses are not suitable for arteries less than 4 mm in diameter, or for most venous applications. However, each type of graft has certain advantages and disadvantages for particular applications.

Synthetic Grafts

All synthetic grafts are fabricated from polymers. Depending on the particular polymer and method of fabrication, a graft can be called a textile or a nonwoven graft. Dacron grafts are examples of the former, and polytetrafluoroethylene (PTFE) and polyurethane grafts are examples of the latter.

Dacron prostheses use knitted, woven, or velour construction. Woven grafts currently have a tight weave and low porosity and are relatively stiff. Preclotting is not required. Owing to low porosity, bleeding is prevented even in heparinized patients,

although woven Dacron does not provide a suitable surface for tissue ingrowth or firm pseudointimal attachment.

Knitted Dacron grafts have a high porosity. They must be preclotted before use.* The high porosity allows ingrowth of fibrous tissue and firm attachment of a pseudointima. Standard and ultra-thin wall thicknesses are available. Ultra-thin grafts are applicable to all vessels in canine and feline practice.

Velour Dacron prostheses are fabricated to allow loops of yarn to extend into the lumen. These loops provide an excellent anchoring substrate for a pseudointima. This graft is porous and must be preclotted prior to use. In general, all types of Dacron prostheses are handled in a similar manner, except that woven grafts do not require preclotting. Textile grafts are easily trimmed, do not fray or tear, and can be autoclaved or ethylene oxide–sterilized. They can be cross-clamped and are kink-resistant.[14]

In humans, Dacron prostheses are the grafts of choice for aortic and aortoiliac replacement. They are not recommended for use below the knee or distal to the axillary artery. Patency rates of virtually 100 per cent are reported for non-aortic replacements with Dacron grafts.[9]

Teflon and polyurethane are the two polymers most commonly used in nonwoven synthetic grafts. Expanded polytetrafluroethylene (PTFE) grafts are fabricated by extrusion and subsequent stretching to produce a microporous tube composed of PTFE nodules connected by PTFE fibrils; thus, these grafts have a microporous structure onto which a pseudointima can form and attach. PTFE's properties—chemical inertness, hydrophobicity and electrical negativity—are thought to be responsible for its lack of thrombogenicity. Despite its porous nature, preclotting is not necessary. An outside additional wrap must be included in the suturing of PTFE grafts to prevent aneurysmal dilation and to provide adequate suture pullout strength. PTFE grafts must be trimmed to the exact length required, as they are virtually noncompliant and nonstretchable. Reported patency rates of PTFE grafts have been variable. As expected, short grafts in high-flow vessels have higher patency rates than longer grafts in low-flow situations. The patency rate of PTFE grafts less than 4 or 5 mm in diameter drops dramatically from that of the larger sizes.

Polyurethane grafts are a recent development.[7] In these devices a liquid polymer solution is deposited on a mandril. A mesh is added externally for additional strength. Apparently these grafts preferentially absorb albumin, an activity that is thought to render

---

*Preclotting is done by filling the grafts with the patient's nonanticoagulated whole blood at least 10 minutes prior to use. The blood is allowed to saturate the graft walls for approximately one or two minutes and is then discarded. Additional blood can be applied to the outside surface to saturate its pores as well. Visible clots are removed with a gauze sponge. After five to eight minutes of drying, the graft should be used without further rinsing.

them nonthrombogenic.[8] Despite their porosity they do not require preclotting. These are the most compliant grafts available and have better patency rates.

Biological Grafts

Biological grafts include both preserved and fresh conduits. The most commonly available prosthesis is glutaraldehyde-tanned human umbilical vein. This prosthesis is externally reinforced with a polyester mesh that should be incorporated into the sutures. These grafts must be thoroughly rinsed with heparinized lactated Ringer's solution (100 mg heparin per liter) prior to use.[3] Following this rinsing, several milliliters of concentrated heparin (100 mg/ml) are instilled directly into the graft, allowed to sit for several minutes, and flushed out just before use. Thromboresistance is apparently enhanced by the heparin bonding to the graft surface.[6] These grafts require special handling owing to the fragile nature of their intimal layers. Metallic vascular clamps are not recommended. Trimming to proper length is necessary, because this prosthesis cannot be stretched. Tanned umbilical veins are only available in diameters between 4 and 7 millimeters. They have been used most extensively in lower limb salvage procedures in humans, in which one-year patency rates exceeding 75 percent have been reported.[4]

A second type of preserved biological vascular graft is the dialdehyde starch–tanned bovine heterograft. After processing of bovine carotid arteries, a tube of essentially nonantigenic collagen is produced. Available sizes are limited to 8 to 11 mm in diameter. Seven-year implants of this graft in dogs have functioned well without dilation or aneurysm formation.[11] Adequate runoff is apparently the key factor required for long-term patency. In humans, the primary use of this graft is to create an arteriovenous interpositional shunt for hemodialysis access.

The most widely used and most successful vascular prosthesis is fresh autogenous vein. The human saphenous vein provides a graft that has sufficient length and diameter for most peripheral uses. Cephalic veins have also been used as prosthetic conduits. Despite their widespread acceptance, autogenous veins undergo morphological histological changes when used as arterial substitutes. Many changes have been related to loss of endothelial viability during harvest and implantation. Heparinized, cold (4°C), whole blood is the preferred storage medium.[1] Preservation in balanced salt solution causes endothelial sloughing, disruption of subendothelial structures, and loss of adventitia.[15] Mechanical hyperdistension of venous grafts causes degenerative changes throughout the wall with increased early thrombosis. A distension pressure of less than 200 mm Hg is recommended to prevent endothelial disruption.[2]

Fresh veins elongate when pressurized in the arterial system. This property must be taken into account when the graft is trimmed. When other veins are considered for use as vascular grafts, it must be remembered that more centrally located vessels are frequently thin and prone to aneurysm formation. Venous branches are ligated rather than cauterized.

ANTICOAGULANT DRUGS

Most vascular procedures involve the use of agents to prevent blood clotting. These drugs may be used before, during, or after operation. They may also be used in combination and can cause serious complications if misused.[13, 17]

Heparin is the most widely used anticoagulant. It can be given subcutaneously but usually is administered intravenously. The anticoagulant actions of heparin are its antithrombin effect, its antithromboplastic effect, and its antiplatelet effect. Large doses of heparin can completely inhibit coagulation, and systemic hemorrhage can occur.

Heparin is sold in various concentrations. One mg of heparin is equal to 100 units. Intravenously, the dose of heparin is 1 to 2 mg/kg of body weight. Subcutaneously, 25 to 50 mg are administered to an average-sized human. This dosage and route, most often used to treat thrombophlebitis and other clotting disorders, are not appropriate for operative use. Heparin activity is usually monitored by measuring the activated clotting time (ACT). Specific instruments are available for this measurement, which is simple to perform. In most animals, 2 mg/kg produces ACT of more than 600 seconds (normal is 80 to 100 seconds), which is considered total anticoagulation. The plasma half-life of heparin is approximately 90 minutes, and the drug is inactivated in the liver.

Heparin can be neutralized with protamine sulfate. The dose of protamine is related to the amount of heparin and the time since heparin was administered. For each mg of heparin, approximately 1 to 1.5 mg protamine is given. If the heparin has been circulating for 30 minutes, only 0.5 mg protamine may be required per mg of heparin.

Dicumarol and warfarin act as anticoagulants by competitive antagonism with vitamin K. Warfarin is more widely used because it is 75,000 times more soluble than dicumarol. Principally, warfarin prevents the synthesis of the vitamin K–dependent clotting factors, especially prothrombin. It does not act on circulating prothrombin.

Warfarin is administered orally. It requires two to five days to achieve its anticoagulant action, and it remains active for up to 14 days after cessation of therapy. For most applications, the dose of warfarin is 1 to 2 mg/kg, usually divided into two doses daily. Because of wide individual variation in the response to warfarin, it must be carefully monitored.

Prothrombin time is the best test to monitor warfarin therapy. If the prothrombin time is kept between 1.5 and 2 times normal, spontaneous hemorrhage is usually prevented. Prothrombin times longer than 3 times normal require the administration of vitamin K. Drugs that affect intestinal production of vitamin K must be carefully monitored during warfarin therapy. These can cause a synergistic potentiation of the warfarin with disastrous effects. Should vitamin K be required, 1 to 10 mg should be given intravenously and the prothrombin time measured in 24 hours. If liver failure is not present and the overdose of warfarin not too great, the prothrombin time should return to normal. Warfarin therapy can then be reinstituted at lower dosages. Whole blood transfusions combined with vitamin K can be used if hemorrhage is severe or prothrombin time is greatly prolonged.

Aspirin acts as an anticoagulant by inhibiting the release of prostaglandins (PGE_2 and PGF_2) from platelets, thus inhibiting platelet aggregation. Bleeding time is prolonged following administration of even single doses of aspirin.

In the cat, aspirin has a long half-life. To produce therapeutic serum levels, it must be administered orally at 25 mg/kg/day. This dose does not produce clinical evidence of toxicosis. In the dog, aspirin given at therapeutic dosages does not cause toxicosis, but it can cause vomiting. Therefore, to maintain adequate blood levels, aspirin must be given every 8 hours at 25 mg/kg.

Dipyridamole prevents platelet aggregation, and adherence and release of platelet factors. When used in combination with aspirin, dipyridamole markedly enhances the patency rates of grafts in canine femoral arteries.[10] In dogs, the dosage is approximately 2 mg/kg twice daily. Generally, dipyridamole therapy is begun three or four days prior to surgery. At this dosage there is little clinical evidence of impaired hemostasis.

1. Abbott, W., Mundth, E., and Austen, W. G.: Autogenous vein grafts: Effects of simple storage on structural properties. Surg. Forum 24:260, 1973.
2. Abbott, W., Weiland, S., and Austen, W. G.: Structural changes during preparation of autogenous venous grafts. Surgery 76:1031, 1974.
3. Dardik, H., Ibraham, I. M., and Sussman, B.: Technical factors in the use of glutaraldehyde-tanned umbilical vein prosthesis for vascular reconstruction in the lower extremity. Vasc. Surg. 15:51, 1981.
4. Dardik, H., Ibraham, I. M., and Dardik, I. I.: Glutaraldehyde-tanned umbilical cord vein: clinical assessment for arterial reconstruction in the lower extremities. In Sawyer, P. N., and Kaplitt, M. J. (eds.): Vascular Grafts. Appleton-Century-Crofts, New York, 1978.
5. Dineen, P.: The effect of suture material in the development of vascular infection. Vasc. Surg. 11:29, 1977.
6. Hufnagel, C.: Heparin bonding in grafts. In Dardik, H. (ed.): Graft Materials in Vascular Surgery. Symposia Specialists, Miami, 1979.
7. Lyman, D. J., Albo, D., and Jackson, R.: Development of small diameter vascular prosthesis. Trans. Am. Soc. Artif. Intern. Organs 23:253, 1977.
8. Lyman, D. J., Metcalf, C., and Albo, D.: The effect of chemical structure and surface properties of synthetic polymers on the coagulation of blood. In vivo absorption of proteins on polymer surfaces. Trans. Am. Soc. Artif. Intern. Organs 22:474, 1974.
9. Noon, G. P., and DeBakey, M. E.: DeBakey Dacron prosthesis and filamentous velour graft. In Sawyer, P. N., and Kaplitt, M. J. (eds.): Appleton-Century-Crofts, New York, 1978.
10. Oblath, R. W., Buckley, F. O., Green, R. M., et al.: Prevention of platelet aggregation and adherence to prosthetic vascular grafts by aspirin and dipyridamole. Surgery 84:37, 1978.
11. Rosenberg, N., Lord, G. H., Henderson, J., et al.: Collagen arterial graft of bovine origin: seven year observations in the dog. Surgery 67:951, 1970.
12. Ross, G., Paulides, C., Long, F., et al.: Absorbable suture materials for vascular anastomoses. Am. Surg. 47:541, 1981.
13. Silver, D.: Blood transfusions and disorders of surgical bleeding. In Sabiston, D. C. (ed.): Textbook of Surgery. W. B. Saunders Co., Philadelphia, 1972.
14. Snyder, R. W., and Botzko, K. M.: Woven, knitted and externally supported Dacron vascular prosthesis. In Sawyer, P. N., and Kaplitt, M. J. (eds.): Vascular Grafts. Appleton-Century-Crofts, New York, 1978.
15. Sottiurai, V. S., and Baston, R. C.: Autogenous vein grafts: experimental studies. In Stanley, J. C., Burkel, W. E., Lindenauer, S. M., et al. (eds.): Biologic and Synthetic Vascular Prosthesis. Grune & Stratton, New York, 1982.
16. Starr, D. S., Weatherford, S. C., Lawrie, G. M., and Morris, G. C.: Suture material as a factor in the occurrence of anastomotic false aneurysms. Arch. Surg. 114:412, 1979.
17. Sxabzniewicz, M., and McCrady, J. D.: Hemostasis, hemostatic, anticoagulant and fibrinolytic agents. In Jones, L. M., Booth, N. H., and McDonald, L. E. (eds.): Veterinary Pharmacology and Therapeutics. Iowa State University Press, Ames, 1977.

Chapter 73

Basic Cardiac Procedures

George E. Eyster and Maralyn Probst

The ability to perform successful cardiovascular surgery depends on excellent anesthesia, understanding of the anatomy of the thorax and cardiovascular structures, surgical skill, understanding of the cardiovascular surgical techniques and procedures, and, most important from the surgical point of view, understanding of the pathophysiology of various cardiac disorders.

Anesthesia for cardiac surgery is described elsewhere (see Chapter 190). Excellent anesthesia is perhaps the single most important factor in successful completion of the cardiac surgical procedure. The surgeon must be in communication with the anesthesiologist before and during the procedure. Fortunately, the surgeon has the ability to monitor two major cardiovascular and anesthesia variables during most procedures, depth of anesthesia (by blood pressure determination) and ventilation (by observation of the left atrium). The majority of cardiac procedures performed in animals are by a left thoracotomy in the fourth intercostal space. From this approach the aorta can be palpated and an approximation of aortic pressure can be made. In general, if the aorta is soft and indents easily, systolic blood pressure is less than 80 mm Hg and the patient is too deeply anesthetized. If the aorta is firm and pushes away when palpated

but still indents, the systolic blood pressure is between 80 and 120 mm Hg and the animal is in a plane of adequate anesthesia. If the aorta pushes away and does not indent, the systolic pressure is greater than 120 mm Hg. The left atrial appendage is pink if the patient is being adequately oxygenated. If the color of the blood transmitted through the thin-walled left atrium or left atrial appendage is darkened, hypoxemia is present, and ventilation should be improved. Two rules are useful for summarizing anesthetic requirements for cardiac procedures. First, the animal should be maintained in as light a plane of anesthesia as possible. Drug administration or other nonphysiologic manipulations should be limited before, during, and after the surgery to the least amount possible.

The anatomy of the heart and cardiovascular system is discussed in Chapter 67. In this chapter, anatomical variations only as related to various disorders are described.

The left lateral thoracotomy in the fourth intercostal space is the technique that can be used for nearly all of the common clinical cardiac surgical procedures (see Chapter 41).

After thoracotomy, the left anterior lung lobe is rotated at its base and is packed posteriorly (Fig.

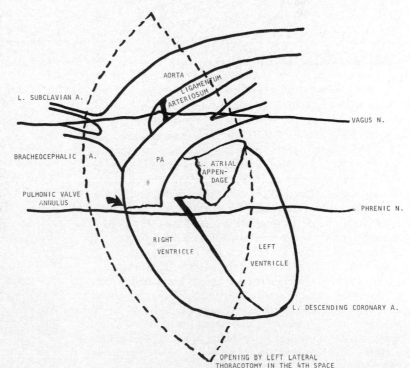

Figure 73–1. Structures seen through a left lateral thoracotomy (lung reflected) in the fourth intercostal space. *Dotted lines,* the edge of the thoracotomy opening; *PA,* pulmonary artery; *arrow,* pulmonic valve annulus.

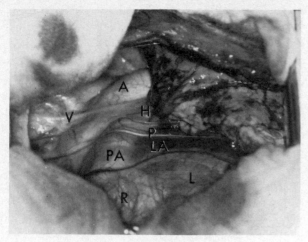

Figure 73–2. After sponges were placed on the wound edge, a Haight rib retractor has been placed and the lung has been rotated caudally to reveal the structures seen through the left lateral thoracotomy in the fourth intercostal space. *A,* aorta; *PA,* pulmonary artery; *V,* vagus nerve; *P,* phrenic nerve; *R,* right ventricle; *L,* left ventricle; *LA,* left atrial appendage; *H,* lung hylus.

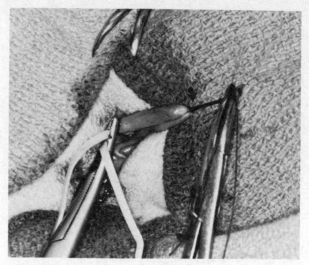

Figure 73–3. An artery is prepared for catheterization. The distal ligation *(arrow)* has been secured with tension on the vessel to stabilize the vessel for manipulation. The proximal ligation, a sterile rubber band, is tightened with a hemostat in preparation for opening the vessel.

73–1). This approach in the left fourth intercostal space reveals the structures of the heart for most of the surgical procedures described in the chapter (Fig. 73–2).

PERICARDIOCENTESIS

Pericardiocentesis, the simplest of the cardiovascular surgical procedures routinely performed in veterinary medicine (see Chapter 74), is a diagnostic and therapeutic (sometimes life-saving) technique. It is easily learned and should be practiced in anticipation of the emergency need.

CARDIAC CATHETERIZATION

The purposes of cardiac catheterization are to measure intracardiac pressures and oxygen saturations and to position the catheter for selective angiograms (see Chapter 70). This procedure requires an invasive maneuver to position the catheter in the appropriate chamber. Cardiac catheterization can be accomplished without the use of fluoroscopy, but fluoroscopy with image intensification should be used. Although fluoroscopic examination is necessary for most catheter manipulation techniques, the image intensifier permits reduced radiation with increased resolution.

Vessels frequently used for intracardiac catheterization in domestic animals are the femoral artery and vein or the carotid artery and external jugular vein. The femoral vessels are easily approached and identified. Femoral artery catheterization allows easier retrograde entry into the left ventricle and left atrium. The femoral vein can be used for entry to the right atrium and ventricle, but catheter manipulation into the pulmonary artery is difficult in small

animals. The neck vessels, carotid and jugular, should always be approached from the right side. Right carotid entry into the left ventricle is less difficult than by left carotid entry. The occasional finding of persistent left anterior vena cava associated with other cardiac defects mandates that the right jugular vein be used for catheterization of the right side of the heart from the anterior.

Percutaneous catheterization can be performed if percutaneous needles and end-hole catheters with wire guides are used. This technique is effective if the vessels are large or if the femoral vessels are used. Because end-hole catheters have distinct disadvantages for pressure injection, percutaneous catheterization is used only in selected patients.

Instead of percutaneous catheterization, direct in-

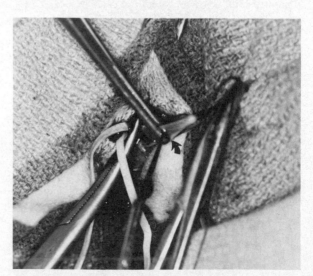

Figure 73–4. Opening of the artery. The occluded vessel is constricted by a forceps. A No. 11 scalpel blade is inserted into the vessel with the cutting edge pointed out *(arrow).* The incision is directed away from the center of the vessel.

troduction of catheters into the vessels is accomplished by an incision over the vessels. The vessels are occluded distally with silk suture (if they are to be sacrificed) or with umbilical tape. Rommel tourniquets or sterile rubber bands are used if preservation of the vessels is to be attempted. The distal stay suture is anchored to the drape with tension. A proximal ligature, preferably a sterile rubber band, is placed around the vessel and the vessel is opened (Fig. 73–3). We prefer not to heparinize (to prevent clots in the occluded vessels) because we routinely sacrifice the arteries and veins. This practice is acceptable in animals because the carotid, jugular, and femoral vessels can be sacrificed without interfering with normal function in dogs.[30] We open the vessels perpendicular to the plane of the vessel, cutting from the midpoint out with a No. 11 blade (Fig. 73–4). The catheters are introduced into the vessel, past the tightened rubber band, and into the heart. The catheter is guided by visualization with fluoroscopy and is positioned in the various chambers. Approach to the left heart from the femoral artery is simple. The catheter is introduced into the femoral vessel and passed anteriorly to the aortic arch. The tip is reflected ventrally, and the catheter is pushed forward. The curve of the aortic arch guides the catheter to and through the aortic valve into the left ventricle. Continued pushing frequently passes the catheter into the left atrium, especially if a large ventricular chamber or mitral regurgitation is present. The femoral vein is entered in a similar manner, and a catheter is passed into the right atrium. The catheter tip is reflected ventrally into the right ventricle, but manipulation into the pulmonary artery is difficult unless the animal is large.

The jugular vein allows easy access into the pulmonary artery. The catheter is passed into the right atrium and turned ventrally into the right ventricle,

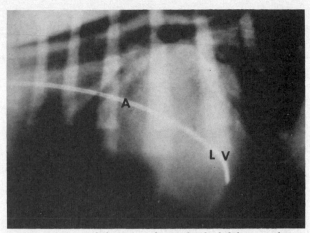

Figure 73–6. Lateral thoracic radiograph of a left heart catheterization. The catheter has been passed down the carotid artery to the ascending aorta (*A*) and across the aortic valve, so that the tip is in the left ventricle (*LV*).

and the curve is continued around and into the pulmonary artery (Fig. 73–5). The carotid artery approach to the left ventricle is slightly more difficult. The catheter must be turned ventrally from the brachiocephalic artery into the ascending aorta. Manipulation across the aortic valve requires patience and gentle probing (Fig. 73–6).

After the studies, catheters are withdrawn, rubber-band ligation is removed, and the vessels are occluded permanently with silk. If the vessels are to be preserved, tourniquets are released, allowing blood to flow and clots to be removed from the vessels. Tourniquets are reapplied, and a continuous suture closure is made in the vessel. If preservation of the vessel is to be accomplished, the opening made in the vessel should be small. Small catheters should be used and the opening should be closed by a purse-string suture. If larger catheters are to be introduced, the vessels are opened parallel to the plane of the vessel and closed in a transverse manner, allowing for slight enlargement of the vessel at the surgical site. In extremely large vessels, the closure can be in the same plane as the incision.

COMMON CARDIAC SURGICAL CONDITIONS

Specific surgical procedures for cardiovascular disorders are divided into two groups: those common conditions that are readily amenable to surgery that can be accomplished without additional major equipment and those fortunately less common complicated surgical procedures that in general require extensive support facilities.

Patent Ductus Arteriosus

The most common cardiovascular surgical procedure is ligation of the patent ductus arteriosus (PDA) (see Chapter 71).[14, 25] Patent ductus is readily corrected by surgical means. Animals with the disease

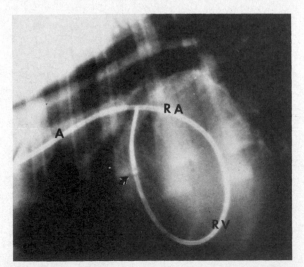

Figure 73–5. Lateral thoracic radiograph of a right heart catheterization. The catheter has been passed down the anterior vena cava (*A*) through the right atrium (*RA*), bent down through the tricuspid valve, rotated through the right ventricle (*RV*), and passed through the pulmonary valve (*arrow*) until the tip of the catheter has reached the pulmonary artery.

die unless it is corrected. The results reported in a large group suggest that the younger the animal, the better the overall success rate.[14] Regardless of size and virtually regardless of age, correction should be performed as soon as the disease is recognized. Although difficult, the procedure can be done in animals weighing as little as 0.5 kg.

Patent ductus arteriosus is approached through a left lateral thoracotomy in the fourth intercostal space. After the lungs have been reflected, the ductus may be seen between the aorta and pulmonary artery. The ductus is ventral to the aorta, dorsal to the pulmonary artery at the point where the vagus nerve crosses between the two vessels, and beneath or medial to the vagus nerve (Fig. 73–7). In obese animals not in cardiac failure, the ductus may not be visible until this dissection has been done to free the mediastinum and pericardium from the ductus. The thrill produced by the continuous turbulence at the ductus can be palpated ventral and anterior to the ductus, at the point where the blood flow from the shunt is reflected off the pulmonary artery near the pulmonary valve. This point corresponds with the position where the murmur is best heard during physical examination, which in large dogs may be 5 cm from the ductus itself. Palpation posterior and dorsal to the heart may reveal a second thrill as a result of mitral regurgitation if left ventricular dilation has occurred. Because of the proximity to and manipulation of the vagus nerve during surgery, animals should be atropinized to protect against vagal slowing of the heart during the dissection around the PDA.

Dissection of the ductus is commenced by opening the pericardium parallel and dorsal to the phrenic nerve. The aorta and pulmonary artery are separated at a natural cleavage point cranial to the ductus. This dissection is carried across the mediastinum (Fig. 73–8). The ductus is approached by looping the vagus nerve in an umbilical tape and reflecting it ventrally. The left recurrent laryngeal nerve passes from the vagus posterior to the PDA. The mediastinum is

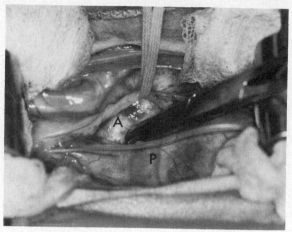

Figure 73–8. Right-angle Lahey bile duct forceps are passed anterior to the ductus across the mediastinum in a natural cleavage plane posterior and ventral to the aorta *(A)* and anterior to the pulmonary artery *(P)*. Extensive dissection on or around the ductus is avoided. The vagus nerve has been elevated with moist umbilical tape.

opened ventral to the aorta, and the pleura and pericardium on the ductus are dissected and lifted away from the ductus with the vagus nerve. Dissection on the right or distal side of the ductus is done with right-angle forceps, preferably a bile duct type with the serrations parallel to the instrument. Owing to the friability of the ductus, the dissection is first done posterior to the ductus near the strong aorta and then continued ventrally along the right wall of the aorta (Fig. 73–9). The tip of the forceps is advanced to the previously opened point anterior to the ductus, and two 2-0 silk sutures are carried behind the ductus to the left lateral side (Fig. 73–10). The suture on the aortic side is tied first. The arterial blood pressure increases dramatically, and usually, as a result of the Branham reflex, the heart rate slows. The pulmonary artery decreases in size, and after a minute or two the suture on the pulmonary

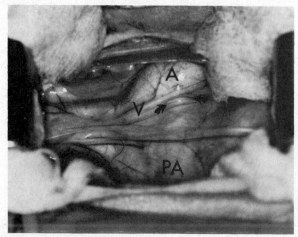

Figure 73–7. Exposure of patent ductus arteriosus. The aorta is dorsal *(A)*, the pulmonary artery is ventral *(PA)*, and the vagus nerve *(V)* courses over the ductus. The ductus is barely visible (between the *arrows*).

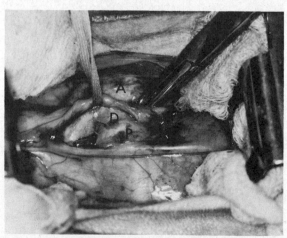

Figure 73–9. The ductus is isolated by passing the right-angle forceps from posterior to anterior beneath the aorta *(A)* and swinging down to the previously opened mediastinum anterior to the ductus. Dissection at the posterior wall of the ductus is reduced to a minimum. The vagus nerve has been elevated with moist umbilical tape. The ductus *(D)* is located coursing between the aorta *(A)* and pulmonary artery *(P)* above the right-angle forceps.

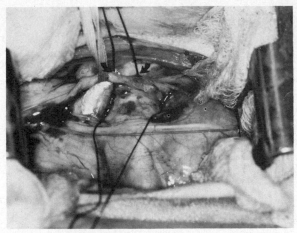

Figure 73–10. Sutures have been carried around the ductus using the right-angle forceps. The suture at the top *(arrows)* is placed dorsal to the vagus nerve on the aortic side, and the ventral suture is placed ventral to the vagus nerve on the pulmonary artery side.

artery side can be tied. Attempts should be made to separate the sutures and allow ductal tissue between them. In small animals this may be difficult.

In animals heavier than 7 kg, safety stay sutures may be placed that would allow occlusion of blood flow to the area if a tear occurred during dissection of the ductus. An umbilical tape is passed around the aorta distal to the ductus in the Blalock manner. This double loop allows one to occlude the aorta by pulling on the free ends. Single umbilical tape loops are passed around the left subclavian and brachiocephalic arteries cranial to the ductus. The pericardium is opened at the transverse pericardial sinus so that a single vascular clamp can be placed to occlude both the aorta and pulmonary artery proximal to the ductus (Fig. 73–11). If during the dissection a tear in the ductus occurs, clamping of the aorta and pulmonary artery and occlusion of the left subclavian and bra-

chiocephalic arteries and distal aorta isolate the ductus from systemic and proximal pulmonary artery blood flow. Occlusion of these vessels should allow two to four minutes to repair the ductus or to clamp it before reestablishment of the circulation must occur. Although blood loss may be severe, animals greater than 7 kg will not exsanguinate in the time it takes to occlude these vessels. However, animals less than 5 kg will exsanguinate in the 10 to 20 seconds needed to occlude the vessels, and therefore in these small animals the safety procedures are not recommended.

Recently, Jackson and Henderson[24] have published a technique for passing the sutures around the ductus in a manner that completely eliminates dissection on the distal right ductal wall. This technique requires passing two sutures around the aorta from dorsal to ventral beneath the aorta and anterior and posterior to the ductus, so that when the sutures are pulled and tied, the loop has included the ductus (Fig. 73–12). The technique is effective and may be safer than the previously described technique. A major disadvantage is that the sutures might not be separated but instead might be aligned in the same groove on the right side of the ductus.

Closure in patent ductus surgery is routine. The suture tag ends are cut, and any safety ligatures are removed. One or two sutures are placed in the pericardium to appose the edges of the pericardium in order to prevent herniation of the left atrial appendage. A chest drain tube is positioned several rib spaces posterior to the opening. Rib sutures are placed, the ribs are drawn together, and the sutures are tied. A three-layer continuous closure including

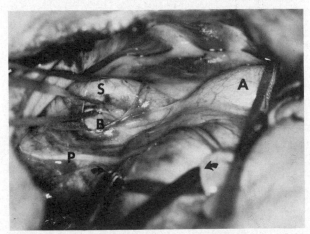

Figure 73–11. Moist umbilical tape is placed around the left subclavian artery *(S)*. Similarly, a tape is placed around the brachiocephalic artery *(B)*. With a Blalock ligation, a moist umbilical tape has been placed around the aorta *(A)* distal to the ductus. The pericardium is open ventral to the phrenic nerve *(P)*, and the clamp is positioned over the pulmonary artery, also including the aorta in the transverse sinus of the pericardium *(arrows)*. Occlusion of these tapes and clamp effectively isolates the ductus, if bleeding should occur.

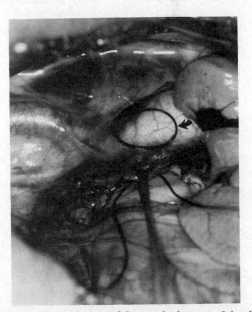

Figure 73–12. The Jackson modification for ligation of the ductus. A loop of suture *(arrow)* has been passed under the aorta from dorsal to ventral with one end anterior and one end posterior to the ductus (not visible beneath the vagus nerve, which has been elevated by the umbilical tape). When traction is applied to both ends of the suture, the loop lies beneath the ductus. A second suture is placed similarly, and the ductus is then double-ligated.

each layer of muscle and the skin is performed. If mild negative pressure is placed on the chest drain throughout the closure, the lungs are usually inflated by the time the skin sutures are complete. The chest is evacuated of air, and the chest drain tube is removed immediately. Sutures are removed in five to seven days, and the animal is denied heavy exercise for 21 days.

Results of PDA correction are excellent. The only precaution is that the animal be neutered, since the disease is hereditary.

Several complications may occur with PDA surgery. The first is the anatomical variation associated with persistent left anterior vena cava (see Chapter 71), which passes across the heart at the ductus, close to the vagus nerve. Consequently, the structure must be moved for adequate exposure and dissection of the ductus. It can be moved with an umbilical tape. The vein is freed from the pericardium on either side of the ductus to allow good exposure and manipulation. Mild retraction on the umbilical tape is used to reflect the vein away from the surgical site. The tape can be the same tape used to reflect the vagus nerve.

Approximately 1.5 per cent of animals with patent ductus ligation have rechannelization of the ductus.[13] With rechannelization, the murmur returns, usually within two months of operation. A rechannelized patent ductus should be divided and sutured. This procedure requires reoperation in the same surgical space and often, owing to adhesions, the left anterior lung lobe must be removed for adequate exposure of the ductus area. If the left anterior lung lobe is not removed, pneumothorax and bleeding from the lung dictates that the chest drain tube be maintained for 12 to 24 hours. The technique for division and suture of rechannelized patent ductus requires additional patent ductus clamps. The surgical approach is identical to that for the ligation technique, but the ductus must be more thoroughly dissected. The clamps are then placed on the ductus at both ends, and the ductus is cut between them. Nonabsorbable 6-0

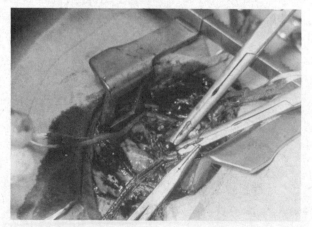

Figure 73–13. The patent ductus arteriosus has been clamped with patent ductus clamps and divided, and the cut ends are being closed with 6-0 vascular suture. Because of the shortness of the ductus, little room is available for placement of the clamps and suture.

vascular suture is placed in a continuous pattern over the ends of the ductus (Fig. 73–13). The clamp on the pulmonary artery side is removed first, and then the clamp on the aortic side is carefully removed. Care should be used in handling the tissues. If bleeding occurs, replacement of the clamps and reinforcement of the suture line may be necessary. Division and suturing of the patent ductus is difficult. The structure is very short, and placement of two clamps with division between them allows little tissue for the suture line. This technique should be performed only by individuals with previous experience in vascular surgery.

Aortic Arch Anomalies

Anomalies of the aortic arch, persistent right aortic arch, double aortic arch, and anomalous arch arteries obstruct the respiratory and gastrointestinal tracts. These diseases constitute the vascular ring anomalies, in which the esophagus is constricted as a result of the anomalous vessel (see Chapter 71).[35]

Persistent Right Aortic Arch

The most common of the aortic arch anomalies is persistent right aortic arch (PRAA), a surgical disease the correction of which at the onset of symptoms gives good results. If the condition persists until esophageal muscle nerve supply has been damaged, results are poor.[32] The pathological anatomy of PRAA is simply the malposition of the aorta to the right of the esophagus and trachea rather than in its usual leftward location. As a result, the trachea and esophagus are encircled by the base of the heart ventrally, the right aortic arch to the right, the dorsal aorta dorsally, and the ligamentum arteriosum and pulmonary artery to the left (Figs. 73–14 and 73–15). Blood flow is normal but tight constriction on the esophagus produces obstruction when solid or large food is eaten.

The surgical correction for persistent right aortic arch is palliative, because the ligamentum is cut, freeing obstruction to the esophagus, but the aortic arch remains to the right of the esophagus. The surgical approach is a left lateral thoracotomy in the fourth intercostal space. The lungs are packed posteriorly, and the dilated esophagus is exposed. If the esophagus has dilated to more than twice its normal diameter, results of surgery are not ideal. An esophageal stethoscope or similar lubricated tube is placed in the esophagus. It will be mobilized through the esophagus once the obstruction has been relieved. Immediately posterior to the distension of the esophagus, the ligamentum arteriosum can be found. It is fibrous in appearance but may be patent. The ligamentum is dissected free from the esophagus throughout its length, double-ligated, and cut (Figs. 73–16 and 73–17). The mediastinal tissue in and around the ligamentum is dissected to free the esophagus and allow it to bulge to the left. The tube

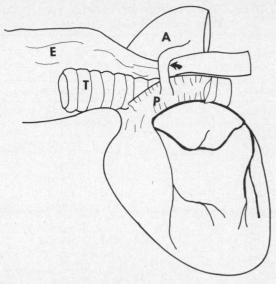

Figure 73–14

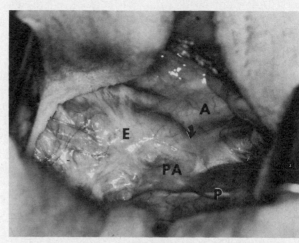

Figure 73–15

Figure 73–14. Persistent right aortic arch. The dilated esophagus (E) is seen anterior to the heart. The ligamentum arteriosum (*arrow*) constricts the esophagus and can be found at the posterior portion of the esophageal dilation. The esophagus and trachea (T) are encircled by the right aorta (A), the ligamentum, the pulmonary artery (P), and the base of the heart.

Figure 73–15. Persistent right aortic arch. Normal structures in the anterior mediastinum are difficult to identify owing to fibrosis and enlargement of the esophagus (E). The phrenic nerve (P) crosses over the heart. A small segment of the aorta (A) is dorsal and to the right of the esophagus. The esophageal constriction (*arrow*) is due to the ligamentum arteriosum. A small portion of the pulmonary artery (PA) can be seen just ventral to the constriction on the esophagus.

previously placed in the esophagus is passed distal to the heart into the stomach. The esophagus is freed of surrounding tissue until the tube can easily pass the obstructed area.

Postoperative management is similar to preoperative management (see Chapter 71). The animal is fed small amounts of liquid diet, placed above the animal to aid movement of food down the esophagus into the stomach, frequently for several weeks. If disten-

sion of the esophagus is minimal, the period of postoperative care can be reduced. If distension is severe, postoperative management should continue for up to two months, the animal slowly returning to normal diet and feeding habits. If regurgitation recurs, radiographs are used to determine whether obstruction is present. Rarely, adhesions around the esophagus may cause slight obstruction, and they may be removed by a second procedure.

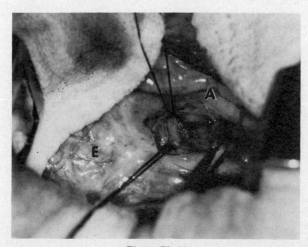

Figure 73–16

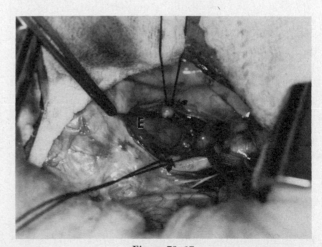

Figure 73–17

Figure 73–16. The ligamentum arteriosum (*arrow*) has been dissected free from the esophagus (E) between the aorta (A) and the pulmonary artery. Two 2-0 silk sutures have been placed around the ligamentum and its fibrous connective tissue sheath in preparation for division of the ligamentum.

Figure 73–17. The ligamentum arteriosum has been divided. The two ends (*arrows*) are seen at the double ligations. The esophagus (E) is freed because the obstruction has been removed.

Double Aortic Arch

Double aortic arch is a rare condition similar to persistent right aortic arch. Both the left and right aortic fetal arches are retained, and they produce a vascular ring around the esophagus. Blood flow is from the heart, to the ascending aortae (both right and left), to the descending aorta. One of the aortic arches must be removed. The approach for surgical resection of double aortic arch is similar to that for persistent right aortic arch. The left aortic arch is exposed, clamped and cut and the ends are sutured. If by radiograph or angiogram the right aortic arch is less developed, a right lateral thoracotomy can be used and the right arch divided. Results of surgical repair of double aortic arch are poor, usually owing to complications.[2] Postoperative management is similar to that for persistent right aortic arch.

Anomalies of Other Vessels

Anomalies of the left subclavian artery or other arch vessels are occasionally reported. Signs are similar to those of persistent right aortic arch. Surgical correction is done by a left lateral thoracotomy in the fourth intercostal space. The offending vessel is recognized just posterior to the bulge in the esophagus, and the vessel is divided. Fortunately, in young animals, loss of the left or right subclavian artery is not associated with vascular insufficiency of the corresponding upper limb, because blood supply through collaterals in the vertebral system is adequate for limb preservation. The surgical site is closed routinely, and postoperative management is similar to that for persistent right aortic arch.

Pulmonic Stenosis

One of the most common cardiac diseases amenable to surgery is pulmonic stenosis. There are several types (see Chapter 71), and each has a preferred surgical correction. Diagnosis and differentiation of the types is important for choice of the most appropriate correction. The diagnosis and, in some cases, determination of types can be established by a venous angiogram. The best method to differentiate types of pulmonic stenosis is direct cardiac catheterization with pulmonary artery–to–right ventricular catheter pullout and selective angiogram, by which the specific lesion can be identified, and the severity of the lesion can be determined.

Diagnosis

Diagnosis of correctable pulmonic stenosis is based on clinical signs, increasing right ventricular hypertrophy, or elevated right ventricular pressure. The symptoms associated with pulmonic stenosis are those of syncope or right-sided heart failure. Evidence of increasing right ventricular hypertrophy can usually be confirmed by electrocardiogram. Right ventricular

TABLE 73–1. Pressure Criteria for Surgery in Dogs with Pulmonic Stenosis

Right Ventricular Pressure (mm Hg)	Right Ventricular to Pulmonary Artery Gradient (mm Hg)	Recommendations
> 120	> 100	Critical pulmonic stenosis; surgery needed immediately
90–120	70–100	If immature, surgery needed immediately If mature, may need surgery
70–90	50–70	If immature, will need surgery; delay if hypertrophy is not severe If mature—no surgery needed unless symptomatic
50–70	< 50	If immature, reevaluate at 9 months of age; surgery if symptomatic If mature, no surgery needed
< 50	< 30	No treatment necessary

pressure greater than 120 mm Hg (systemic pressure) is surgical (Table 73–1). Right ventricular pressure greater than 70 mm Hg in the young animal is an indication for surgery, because growth of the animal with the continued restriction of the pulmonic stenosis gradually increases the pressure. If possible, surgery should be delayed until the animal is mature, but if the criteria listed are met, surgery should be performed. Delay of operation in animals with increasing pulmonic stenosis results in severe right ventricular hypertrophy and hypertrophic cardiomyopathy. With severe right ventricular hypertrophy, results of surgery are poor.

Modified Brock Technique

Several well established techniques can be used to repair or relieve the obstruction in pulmonic stenosis. The Brock or modified Brock procedure is effective in muscular and some subvalvular stenoses.[9] The technique consists of excising fibromuscular obstruction in the right ventricle with a rongeur. It is performed via a left lateral thoracotomy in the fourth intercostal space. The pericardium is opened parallel and ventral to the phrenic nerve. Pericardial basket sutures are placed, and the heart is elevated. A relatively avascular area on the right ventricle is identified, and a deep purse-string suture is placed in the ventricular tissue. A Rommel tourniquet is placed on the purse-string. The epicardium is cut with a sharp blade. The opening is extended to the heart lumen with a blunt instrument, usually a hemostat. Hemorrhage is controlled by tension on the Rommel tourniquet. The infundibular rongeur is introduced into the right ventricle, and muscle is grasped, cut, and removed (Figs. 73–18 and 73–19).

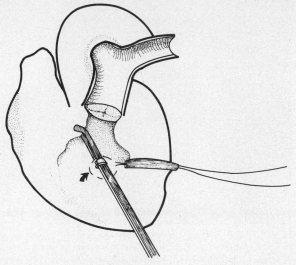

Figure 73–18

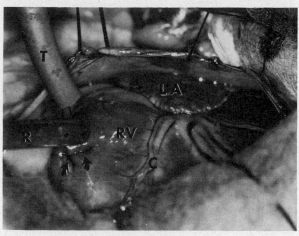

Figure 73–19

Figure 73–18. Brock rongeur removal of right ventricular obstruction. A purse-string suture *(arrow)* has been placed in an avascular portion of the right ventricle. The Rommel tourniquet is placed over the purse-string suture, and the rongeur has been introduced into the right ventricle.

Figure 73–19. The infundibular rongeur *(R)* has been introduced into the right ventricle through a purse-string suture *(arrows)* and a Rommel tourniquet *(T)*. An avascular area of the right ventricular wall is used. The left descending coronary artery *(C)* is just posterior, and the left atrial appendage *(LA)* is posterior and dorsal to the ventriculotomy.

The technique is performed without direct exposure. When the appropriate amount of muscle and fibromuscular tissue has been removed, the purse-string suture is tightened and tied.

The advantage of the Brock procedure is its simplicity. It requires a few additional instruments and is safe. The major disadvantage is the inability to directly observe the tissue being excised. Preoperative and postoperative right ventricular direct pressure measurements can be helpful in determining the amount of reduction of right ventricular pressure.

Bistoury Technique

In veterinary surgery, procedures similar to the Brock technique have remained popular for many years.[10, 26] The bistoury technique for incision of valvular or fibrous subvalvular pulmonic stenosis is safe, simple, and effective. It is performed just like the Brock procedure. Instead of an infundibular rongeur, a teat bistoury is inserted through the purse-string suture into the right ventricle and passed through the obstruction. Cuts are then made in the valvular or fibrous subvalvular ring (Fig. 73–20). Digital manipulation over the obstruction is used to judge the depth of the cut. The instrument is removed, and the closure is similar to that for the Brock procedure. Direct right ventricular pressure measurements before and after incision in the obstructing ring can be used to monitor effectiveness of the surgery. The advantages of the bistoury technique include: extreme simplicity and ease of surgery, minimal cardiac damage, limited need for equipment, and a procedure ideally suited to valvular pulmonic

stenosis. The disadvantage, as in the Brock procedure, is lack of direct observation of the surgical site.

Valve Dilator Technique

If available, valve dilators can be introduced as in the Brock or bistoury technique. Valve dilators designed for use in humans are expensive but are able to spread the tissue as well as make simultaneous multiple cuts (Fig. 73–21).[22] The disadvantages are

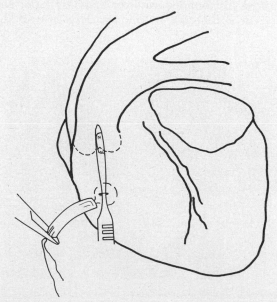

Figure 73–20. Bistoury placement into the right ventricular outflow tract, similar to the Brock procedure. Cuts are made in the stenotic valve.

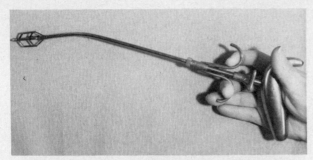

Figure 73–21. The valve dilator with blades extended.

similar to those of the Brock and bistoury techniques, in that the operation is done blind through a stab incision and the intruments are expensive. Valve dilators are used only for fibrous valvular or subvalvular pulmonic stenosis.

Pulmonary Arteriotomy

We prefer a modification of the inflow occlusion pulmonary arteriotomy technique popularized by Swan[33] for valvular, immediate fibrous subvalvular, or dysplastic pulmonic valve stenosis. The Swan procedure requires stopping of blood flow to the heart so that the pulmonary artery can be opened, allowing direct observation. Little additional surgical equipment is needed, but as a result of the inflow occlusion, the surgical risk is higher. Originally, the procedure was done using hypothermia, but we believe that, even though hypothermia allows additional time for observation of the lesion, the time needed for this operation is so short that it can be safely accomplished without hypothermia.

Pulmonary arteriotomy inflow occlusion is performed through a left lateral thoracotomy in the fourth intercostal space. The anterior vena cava is identified, surrounded with an umbilical tape, and placed in a Rommel tourniquet. Exposure of the

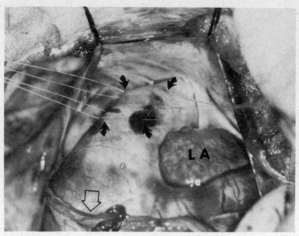

Figure 73–23. A double row of 4-0 sutures are placed in the pulmonary artery *(arrows)*. The incision is made between the rows of sutures. The pulmonary valve is indicated by the *open arrow*. The left atrial appendage *(LA)* is exposed just posterior to the pulmonary artery.

anterior vena cava is difficult, particularly in wide-chested or obese animals. Dissection across the anterior mediastinum to the right anterior vena cava may be tedious. The posterior vena cava is similarly surrounded with tape. The posterior vena cava is identified through the fifth or sixth intercostal space. It is relatively free of excessive connective tissue, but the heart must be rotated anteriorly to see the vena cava from the fourth intercostal space. The mediastinum posterior to the heart is broken by digital manipulation. The heart is rotated anteriorly and to the right, and the vena cava can be exposed and looped in a tourniquet (Fig. 73–22). The pericardium is opened with an incision parallel to and near the phrenic nerve. The dorsal portion of the pericardium is looped in pericardial basket sutures and elevated dorsally. The pulmonary artery, bulging as a result of poststenotic dilation, is easily seen. A double row of 4-0 stay sutures is placed in the pulmonary artery (Fig. 73–23). These sutures are used to manipulate the pulmonary artery during the resection or repair of the pulmonary valve and also to reappose the pulmonary vessel edges for clamping at the end of the repair. The patient is ventilated maximally at this time. At normal temperatures, inflow can be occluded safely for up to four minutes. However, the

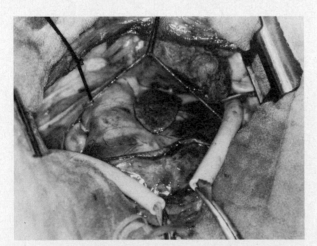

Figure 73–22. Umbilical tape ligations in Rommel tourniquets are placed around the anterior vena cava and posterior vena cava. The tourniquet can be tightened effectively, producing inflow occlusion to the heart.

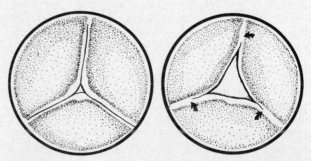

Figure 73–24. Left, a normal semilunar valve. *Right,* a valve with fused cusps *(arrows).* Cuts are made at the fused points to reform the tricuspid valve.

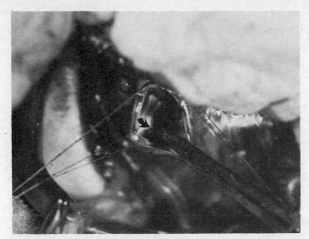

Figure 73–25. The pulmonary artery is opened, and the valve (*arrow*) is grasped prior to repair.

time should be kept to less than three, preferably two, minutes. The tourniquets are tightened, stopping all inflow to the heart except for the azygous and coronary veins. Ventilation is stopped. The heart is allowed to empty (approximately 15 seconds) and a stab incision is made with a No. 11 blade in the pulmonary artery between the stay sutures. The incision may be extended with scissors. Suction is needed to evacuate blood from the pulmonary artery and allow observation of the pulmonic stenosis (Fig. 73–24). With a No. 11 blade or scissors, the pulmonary valve is repaired or excised (Fig. 73–25). Subvalvular obstructive tissue can be cut and removed. The procedure should be performed within three minutes. The stay sutures are used to stabilize and open the pulmonary artery throughout this portion of the procedure. The sutures are then pulled together, bringing the cut edges of the pulmonary artery together, and a Satinsky vascular clamp is placed on the pulmonary artery beneath the stay

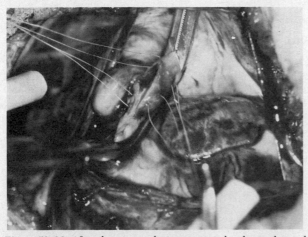

Figure 73–26. After the open pulmonary artery has been elevated with the stay sutures, a Satinsky clamp has been placed over the pulmonary artery opening, effectively closing the pulmonary arteriotomy while still allowing flow to occur through the pulmonary artery beneath the clamp. The tourniquets have been loosened to allow blood to return to the heart.

sutures, effectively closing the arteriotomy (Fig. 73–26). The Rommel tourniquets are released, and circulation and ventilation are reestablished. A double row of continuous 4-0 nonabsorbable sutures is placed in the pulmonary artery to close the arteriotomy; the Satinsky clamp can be removed. The major advantage of this procedure is the ability to directly observe the valvular or subvalvular lesion. If the pulmonic stenosis is valvular alone, the valve frequently can be reformed. In subvalvular stenosis or pulmonary valve dysplasia, the offending tissue is simply removed. Removal or congenital absence of a pulmonary valve is well tolerated by most animals. Pulmonary arteriotomy inflow occlusion is more difficult than the Brock and bistoury techniques, and the results are poorer in young animals. As a result of scarring, the pulmonary valve annulus diameter is fixed at the completion of the pulmonary arteriotomy and does not grow. In very young animals this remaining diameter, though normal at the time, becomes stenotic as the animal grows. Consequently we dilate the annulus with a large Satinsky clamp just before closure of the pulmonary arteriotomy.

Patch Grafting

Recently, a modified patch graft technique for pulmonary outflow tract disease has been recommended by Breznock and Wood[6] for use in veterinary surgery. The patch graft can be large, extending from the pulmonary artery to well down onto the right ventricle. As a result, it can be effective in valvular pulmonic stenosis, pulmonary valve dysplasia, subvalvular pulmonic stenosis, and in some cases of muscular pulmonic stenosis. The technique is the most effective and the preferred technique for young animals that are expected to grow to more than double their size at the time of operation. The patch can be placed so that there is redundant tissue at the time of surgery and the growing animal will not have stenosis when it matures.

The patch graft technique is performed through a left lateral thoracotomy in the fourth intercostal space. The pericardium is incised parallel and ventral to the phrenic nerve with an additional ventral extension of the cut perpendicular to the first incision. Pericardial basket sutures are placed and the heart is elevated.

A patch graft of either pericardium or, preferably, woven Dacron is prepared to act as a substitute right ventricular outflow tract. If Dacron is used, preclotting with the patient's own blood is advised. The graft is cut as a double ellipse to fit from the pulmonary artery across the obstructive lesion to the right ventricle. Pericardium need not be so carefully shaped, because redundant tissue can be sutured in place. A cutting suture or wire is inserted through the right ventricular wall into the right ventricle, up the pulmonary outflow tract to the pulmonary artery, and out of the pulmonary artery (Fig. 73–27). Small 4-0 to 6-0 purse-string sutures are placed around the

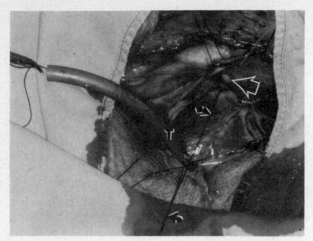

Figure 73–27. A cutting suture *(arrows)* has been passed through the right ventricular wall, into and out of the right ventricle, to the pulmonary artery *(open arrow)*. This cutting suture is used to open the right ventricle, the pulmonary valve, and the pulmonary artery after placement of the patch. Because of the tendency for bleeding at the exit points of the cutting suture, a purse-string suture with a tourniquet *(T)* is placed around the exit point from the ventricle, and a 6-0 vascular suture controls bleeding at the pulmonary artery exit point.

wire entrance and exit holes to control hemorrhage. In patients with moderate to severe right ventricular wall thickening, passing the wire through a large-bore intravenous catheter aids in identifying the lumen of the right ventricle and the outflow tract. If hypertrophy is minimal, a large needle can be used to carry the wire or cutting suture through the right ventricle to the pulmonary artery. The wire or cutting suture is positioned over the right ventricle, and the patch is sutured from the pulmonary artery to the right ventricle over the outside portion of the cutting suture. The patch is placed so that the redundant patch material acts as a portion of the right ventricular wall when the cutting suture is pulled out (Fig. 73–28). The last two sutures at the ventral border of the patch are not completed. The cutting suture is pulled from the pulmonary artery, down through the pulmonary valve area to the right ventricle, and out.

Digital control of bleeding at the ventral border of the patch is used as the last two patch sutures are placed.

The effect of patch graft surgery is to widen the outflow tract by partially diverting blood into the patch. A chest drain tube is maintained in the animal for 12 to 24 hours or until pleural effusion due to presence of foreign material ceases. The advantage of the patch graft technique, and the reason for its preferment, is that a right ventricular outflow tract of any size desired can be produced, allowing for growth in the young animal. The technique is effective in valvular, subvalvular, and muscular stenosis and valve dysplasia. The disadvantages of the technique include: (1) the presence of foreign material on the heart; (2) identification of the lumen in severely hypertrophied ventricles; and (3) placement of the cutting wire without direct observation. Unfortunately, malposition of the wire through the hypertrophied right ventricular wall can occur, so that the wire never reaches the ventricular lumen.

Conduits

Conduit repair of various types of pulmonic stenosis has been reported.[21, 37] Vascular conduit repair may at first seem complicated and expensive, but in fact many of these techniques are relatively simple and inexpensive and may be very effective.

The pulmonary artery–to–pulmonary artery conduit is the most effective method of repair of supravalvular pulmonic stenosis. The technique is performed through a left lateral thoracotomy in the fourth intercostal space, and the pericardium is opened, usually dorsal to the phrenic nerve. The pericardial basket sutures are placed and the heart is elevated. The obstructed area of the pulmonary artery is easily exposed and an appropriate Dacron conduit is chosen and preclotted with the animal's own blood. A partially occluding vascular clamp is

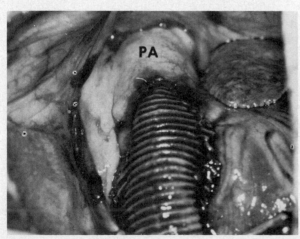

Figure 73–28. Patch graft in place between the pulmonary artery *(PA)* and the right ventricle. The distended patch has become a portion of the right ventricular outflow tract.

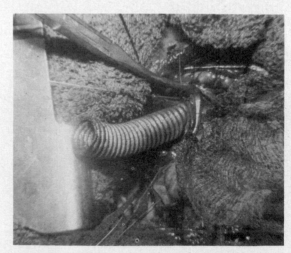

Figure 73–29. The distal end-to-side conduit to pulmonary artery anastomosis is complete. The partially occluding Satinsky clamp is used to isolate a portion of the pulmonary artery, and the anastomosis is made on the isolated, partially occluded segment.

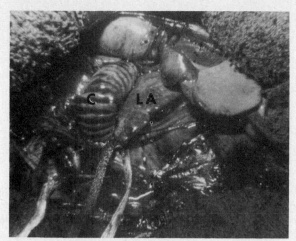

Figure 73–30. Completed pulmonary artery to distal pulmonary artery conduit. The conduit *(C)* is used to bridge the pulmonary artery stenosis. The left atrial appendage *(LA)* is just posterior to the conduit. The vagus nerve is retracted with moist umbilical tape.

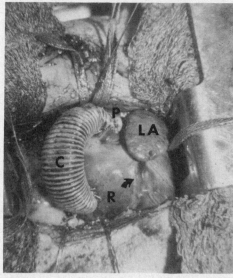

Figure 73–31. Conduit from right ventricle to pulmonary artery. The conduit *(C)* is anastomosed to the right ventricular wall *(R)* and the pulmonary artery *(P)* distal to the obstruction. The left atrial appendage *(LA)* is seen near the distal anastomosis. The left descending coronary artery *(arrow)* identifies the division between the right and left ventricles.

placed on the pulmonary artery distal to the obstruction. The conduit is anastomosed end-to-side to the pulmonary artery with continuous 4-0 to 6-0 sutures. (Fig. 73–29). The conduit is clamped close to the anastomotic site, and the partially occluding clamp is removed from the pulmonary artery distal to the obstruction and replaced on the pulmonary artery proximal to the obstruction. The proximal end of the conduit is anastomosed end-to-side to the proximal pulmonary artery. Air is removed from the conduit by syringe as the clamp on the conduit is removed, allowing the conduit to fill with blood. The partially occluding clamp is removed from the proximal pulmonary artery (Fig. 73–30). The circulation is reestablished around the obstruction, and the pulmonary valve is retained to function normally. Results of pulmonary artery–to–pulmonary artery vascular conduit placement suggest that there are no complicating factors.

Recently, valved or unvalved conduits have been successfully implanted between the right ventricle and the pulmonary artery.[37] Valved conduits are expensive, and the placement of the proximal (right ventricular) anastomosis is difficult and may require an intracardiac cage to prevent obstruction during ventricular contraction. The conduits are placed with the distal end-to-side anastomosis, as in the previous technique. The proximal end of the anastomosis is made by coring a hole in the ventricle. The caged proximal end of the conduit tube is inserted into the hole and then sutured to the ventricular wall (Fig. 73–31). Although still experimental, this technique may prove to be an effective method of repair for all types of pulmonary stenosis.

We have had poor results with placement of conduits from the right atrium to the pulmonary artery (the Fontan procedure). This technique is used for animals with severe obstructive right ventricular disease due to severe muscular hypertrophy or with major obstruction at the tricuspid valve in addition

to abnormalities of the right ventricle. Because the conduit need not be valved, the cost of the material is low. The distal anastomosis is similar to that described for pulmonary artery–to–pulmonary artery conduits, and the proximal anastomosis is end-to-side onto the right atrium, frequently at the right atrial appendage (Fig. 73–32). The Fontan technique as used in humans has many surgical and postoperative problems, and postoperative care is long and difficult. The few attempts in animals have had similar post-

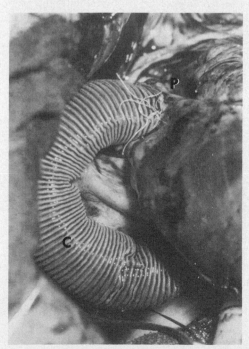

Figure 73–32. A Fontan conduit *(C)* between the right atrium (not visible) and the pulmonary artery *(P)*. The conduit bypasses the right ventricle.

operative complications, including right-sided heart failure and arrhythmia. Success of the technique depends on previous high right atrial pressure, because the right atrium becomes the major pumping chamber for the right side of the heart. Results have been poor, and other surgical intervention should be considered before attempting the Fontan anastomosis.

Open Heart Techniques

Open heart surgical techniques have been used in animals to repair pulmonic stenosis. The techniques of cardiopulmonary bypass are described in Chapter 76. The procedures are time-consuming and expensive and require cardiopulmonary bypass equipment and a team trained in the technique. As a consequence, these procedures are used only at major veterinary institutions or in human hospitals. The open heart techniques are effective in treatment of pulmonic stenosis of any type and have the advantage of direct exposure of the cardiac defect usually with total repair. These techniques, however, are impractical for general use.

Ventricular Septal Defect

Repair or palliation of ventricular septal defect (VSD) has been described for over a decade.[4, 5, 18, 28, 36] The procedures for this disorder are open heart surgery, repair by the use of profound hypothermia, and palliation with pulmonary artery banding.

Open heart surgery for ventricular septal defect gives good results. The problem with the technique, as with its use for pulmonic stenosis, is unavailability of cardiopulmonary bypass machinery and a surgical team. As a result, these techniques are used exclusively at major institutions and have little value to the practitioner. The open heart technique carries with it a 25 per cent mortality, but both anatomic and physiological repairs are possible.

The techniques of deep hypothermia and circulatory arrest for ventricular septal defect are described in Chapter 75. These techniques are effective, enable total anatomic and physiological correction, require minimal additional equipment, but are time consuming. Surgeons should become familiar with the techniques before attempting them on clinical patients.

The currently recommended surgical treatment for ventricular septal defect in the dog and cat is the palliative procedure of pulmonary artery banding.[18, 28] Banding the pulmonary artery creates a supravalvular pulmonary stenosis to increase the right ventricular pressure. In large ventricular defects, the left-to-right shunt flow depends on the pressure gradient between the left and right ventricles. For a given defect, the higher the gradient, the more blood is shunted from the left to the right ventricle and consequently to the lungs, producing pulmonary disease. Surgery for VSD is not necessary unless these

pulmonary symptoms develop (see Chapter 71); they occur when pulmonary-to-systemic flow ratio is greater than 2.5:1. With pressure elevation in the right ventricle, the gradient between the left and right ventricles is decreased, and consequently the left-to-right ventricular shunt is decreased. If pulmonary artery banding is used, the right ventricular pressure elevation must be sufficient to reduce the left-to-right shunt, but not so much as to produce right ventricular failure or, even more seriously, right-to-left shunt.

Pulmonary artery banding is performed through a left lateral thoracotomy in the fourth intercostal space. The lungs are reflected, and the pericardium is incised parallel and dorsal to the phrenic nerve. Pericardial basket sutures are placed and the heart is elevated slightly. The pulmonary artery, enlarged because of increased blood flow, is easily exposed. *Careful* dissection around the main pulmonary artery is made. The dissection is performed close to the pulmonary valve, and extreme care must be taken not to penetrate the right pulmonary artery. Right-angle forceps are passed around the pulmonary artery near the pulmonary valve. An umbilical tape is carried around the pulmonary artery (Fig. 73–33). The tape is brought together and tightened so that the pulmonary artery diameter is reduced to one-third normal (one-third the diameter of the pulmonary artery at its origin, the pulmonary valve annulus). With an instrument holding the tape so it produces a pulmonary artery diameter of one-third, sutures are placed and tied in the tape to maintain the tape diameter (Fig. 73–34), and the tape is tied. Banding the pulmonary artery approximately doubles the pressure in the right ventricle, so the gradient from the left ventricle to the right ventricle is reduced, thus reducing the left-to-right flow. Closure is routine.

Animals with pulmonary artery banding are observed postoperatively for several days. An additional murmur, the pulmonic stenosis, can usually be heard.

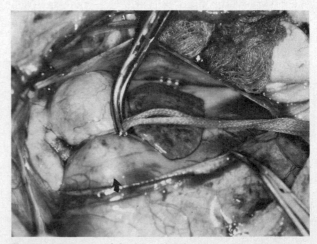

Figure 73–33. An umbilical tape has been positioned around the pulmonary artery close to the pulmonary valve *(arrow)*. The tape has been tightened using right-angle forceps to constrict the pulmonary artery to one-third its normal diameter.

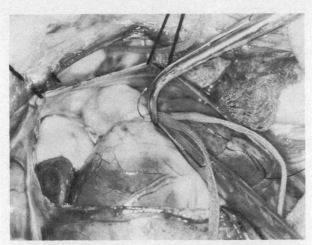

Figure 73–34. A 4-0 nonabsorbable suture ties the umbilical tape edges together with the correct tension. This eliminates the difficulty of having to judge the tension on the knot in the umbilical tape. After the suture is tied, the umbilical tape is secured with a square knot.

The pulmonary signs should decrease. The animal is monitored by observation of the mucous membranes to be certain that cyanosis does not occur. Rare complications occur usually within the first 72 hours. The major complications of pulmonary artery banding are right ventricular failure due to increased pressure load and right-to-left shunt, either of which may result if the band is placed too tightly. If these complications occur, the band must be removed or loosened. Animals with pulmonary artery banding have been followed for up to 10 years. Long-term results are good, and symptoms of pulmonary disease are relieved.

Tetralogy of Fallot

Currently, medical therapy is the most efficacious treatment for tetralogy in the dog (see Chapter 71).[16] In at least 25 per cent of cases the disease does not respond to beta-adrenergic blockage, and surgery should be considered. A wide variety of surgical techniques have been used in animals, including total correction with open heart repair and palliative procedures.

Open heart direct repair using cardiopulmonary bypass has been successfully performed, but the results are extremely poor. Mortality of approximately 75 per cent can be expected. The combination of ventricular septal defect and pulmonary stenosis carries a much more grave prognosis than either of those two diseases alone. The high mortality plus the previously described difficulties of availability in open heart surgery preclude it as a major consideration for clinical practice.

The palliative procedures, Blalock and Potts anastomoses, have been successfully used and should be considered for tetralogy not responsive to medical management.[20] The Blalock anastomosis returns partially oxygenated arterial blood to the lungs to be fully oxygenated, through an end-to-side left subclavian–to–pulmonary artery anastomosis. A similar result is accomplished by the Potts anastomosis, but the pulmonary artery is directly anastomosed side-to-side to the aorta. These two techniques produce increases in pulmonary blood flow and in oxygen content of the blood returning to the left side of the heart and systemic circulation. The increased systemic oxygenation can alleviate signs of the disease. Animals undergoing these palliative procedures still have tetralogy, but the clinical response to hypoxemia and the cyanosis is frequently relieved.

Blalock Anastomosis

The Blalock anastomosis is performed through a left lateral thoracotomy in the fourth intercostal space. The lungs are reflected, and the left subclavian artery is identified. The artery is freed from mediastinal tissue, and the pericardium is opened parallel to and dorsal to the phrenic nerve. The subclavian artery is ligated just proximal to its division. A bulldog or similar small vascular clamp is positioned at the origin of the left subclavian artery, which then is divided proximal to the ligation and reflected posteriorly and ventrally toward the pulmonary artery (Fig. 73–35). A partially occluding vascular clamp is placed on the pulmonary artery so that an end-to-side subclavian artery–to–pulmonary artery anastomosis can be made. The pulmonary artery is opened parallel to the end of the subclavian artery. A double-armed 4-0 to 6-0 vascular suture is placed at each end of the anastomosis through the left subclavian and pulmo-

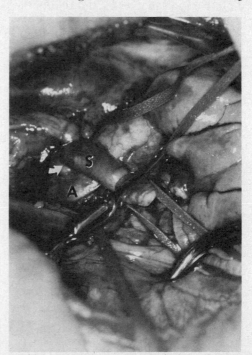

Figure 73–35. The left subclavian artery *(S)* is clamped with a bulldog clamp and divided at its termination. The artery has been reflected posteriorly and ventrally toward the pulmonary artery. Note the kink *(arrow)* in the left subclavian at its reflection from the aorta *(A).*

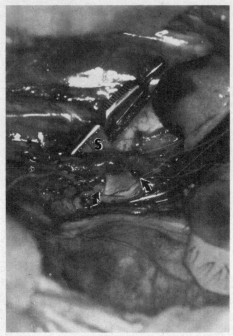

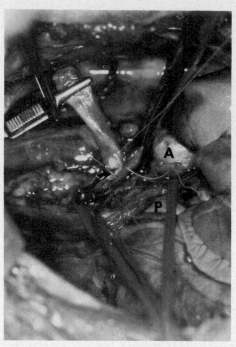

Figure 73–36. The left subclavian artery (S) has been reflected toward the pulmonary artery grasped in the Satinsky clamp. Two 5-0 sutures (arrows) have connected the open end of the left subclavian artery to the incision in the pulmonary artery.

Figure 73–38. Modification of the Blalock method to reduce the kink at the origin of the subclavian artery. A large segment of the aorta (A) has been grasped in the Satinsky clamp. A diamond-shaped segment of arterial tissue, including portions of the aorta and subclavian artery (arrow), was removed at the origin of the subclavian artery to eliminate the redundant arterial tissue as the subclavian artery is positioned toward the pulmonary artery (P). Sutures are placed to approximate the cut edges of the subclavian artery to the aorta.

nary arteries and tied, securing the two vessels to each other (Fig. 73–36). The back of the anastomosis is completed first by passing the suture into the lumen of the vessels and carrying the simple continuous pattern to the opposite end. The suture is then carried out through the vessel and tied to the suture

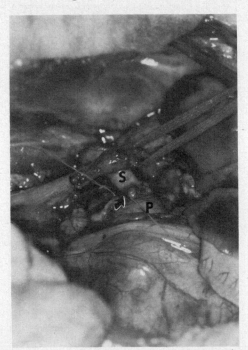

Figure 73–37. The left subclavian artery–to–pulmonary artery anastomosis. Left subclavian artery (S) has been anastomosed with a continuous suture pattern (arrow) to the pulmonary artery (P). The anastomosis is just beneath the vagus nerve which is elevated by umbilical tape.

previously placed at the opposite end of the suture line. The front of the anastomosis is closed in a simple continuous pattern, and the suture is tied to the remaining tag end of the suture at the starting point. The clamp is removed from the pulmonary artery, air is removed from the vessel with a small-bore needle, and the bulldog clamp is removed from the left subclavian artery (Fig. 73–37).

A continuous shunt thrill should be palpated in the left subclavian and pulmonary arteries as a result of flow from the aorta through the left subclavian to the pulmonary artery. Results of Blalock anastomosis in the dog have been poor in animals less than 7 kg and good in animals more than 10 kg. The varying results depend on the size of the vessels at the time of the anastomosis. As in human infants, occlusion and clotting of the vessels occur in the young patient. The usual site of occlusion is at the origin of the left subclavian artery, owing to the 170-degree bend in the vessel. Consequently, a recent modification of the Blalock anastomosis has been used in animals, with some success.[11, 31] With this modification the aorta is partially occluded at the origin of the left subclavian artery, and a diamond-shaped segment of aorta and left subclavian artery is removed at the origin of the subclavian artery (Fig. 73–38). The subclavian artery is then reflected toward the pulmonary artery and anastomosed. The left subclavian–to–aorta anastomosis produces a wider opening and eliminates the kink at the origin of the left

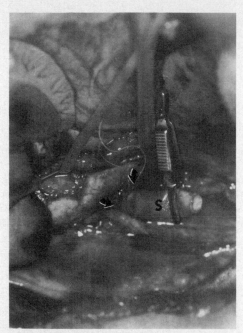

Figure 73–39. The left subclavian artery *(S)* reconstruction at the origin from the aorta (between the *arrows*) has been completed. The left subclavian artery has thus been rotated 90 degrees to better approximate the position in relation to the pulmonary artery.

subclavian artery (Fig. 73–39). The distal Blalock anastomosis is completed in the usual manner. This technique appears to be effective in smaller animals and over a long period may be successful in maintaining the Blalock shunt without occlusion.

Potts Anastomosis

The Potts anastomosis is performed through a left lateral thoracotomy in the fourth intercostal space. The lungs are reflected, and both the aorta and main pulmonary artery are freed from surrounding mediastinal tissue. A partially occluding Potts clamp is placed over the aorta, and a partially occluding vascular clamp is placed on the pulmonary artery (Fig. 73–40). The two vessels are positioned side-to-side and an 8- to 13-mm incision, depending on the dog's size, is made in each vessel. The two vessels are connected at either end of their incision lines by 4-0 to 6-0 double-armed cardiovascular sutures, and the medial side of the anastomosis between the two vessels is performed as in the Blalock technique. The lateral side of the anastomosis is completed, and the pulmonary artery clamp is removed, allowing blood to fill the needle holes. The aortic clamp is slowly released (Fig. 73–41). A profound thrill should be palpated on the pulmonary artery. The Potts anastomosis is a nonregulated anastomosis, because the direct side-to-side shunt produces major flow. The length of the anastomosis is critical to the success of the surgery. An anastomosis site that is greater than 13 mm, even in large dogs, produces pulmonary edema and congestive heart failure as a result of left-to-right shunt, similar to severe patent ductus arteriosis. The Potts anastomosis is effective in dogs in which the Blalock shunt may have a high risk of occlusion. The disadvantages of the Potts anastomosis are surgical difficulty and the cost of the Potts clamps.

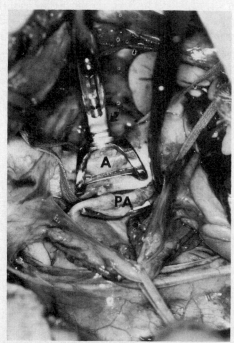

Figure 73–40. The preparation of the aorta *(A)* and the pulmonary artery *(PA)* for the Potts anastomosis. The Potts clamp *(upper arrow)* is placed around the aorta. The Satinsky clamp *(lower arrow)* partially occludes the pulmonary artery.

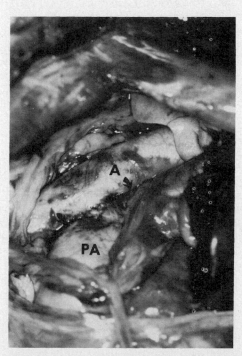

Figure 73–41. The Potts anastomosis is completed. The aorta *(A)* is anastomosed side-to-side to the pulmonary artery *(PA)* (between the *arrows*), thus creating an aorta–pulmonary artery fistula.

Postoperative Management

Postoperative management of animals with either palliative procedure for tetralogy of Fallot is the same. The animal may be given mild anticoagulation (aspirin) for several weeks, but this is usually not necessary. The patient is monitored for continuous shunt murmur and reduction in packed cell volume as the hypoxemia is reduced. Animals surviving for longer than one month may be expected to have good long-term results. The owner of a dog with palliative shunts for this disease should be cautioned that even though the animal is much improved clinically, the underlying disease has not been altered and the dog should not be encouraged to perform heavy activity. At least twice yearly, monitoring of packed cell volume and assessment for evidence of right ventricular hypertrophy or arrhythmia by electrocardiogram is needed. Possible future medical management of arrhythmia may be necessary.

Heartworm Removal

Recently, acquired cardiac conditions have been treated with more aggressive surgical management. Occasionally, surgical removal is the preferred therapy for severe dirofilariasis.[1, 23] The procedures for heartworm removal are varied, depending on the position of the majority of the worms and the physical condition of the animal. Heartworm surgery should be considered if the animal is (1) showing evidence of postcaval syndrome (see Chapter 71), (2) in failure such that the hepatic or renal function is compromised and the routine medical arsenical therapy would be life-threatening, or (3) is not so severely affected but is intended for future major athletic use (for example a hard-working field trial dog). The surgery can be used in any case of heartworms. However, the expense and difficulty, along with a slightly higher mortality than in medical management, makes surgery a second choice.

Pulmonary Arteriotomy

The techniques for surgical removal of the heartworms from the right ventricle or pulmonary artery are performed through a left lateral thoracotomy in the fourth intercostal space. The choice preferred at our institution is a modification of the Swan inflow occlusion pulmonary arteriotomy, as described earlier for pulmonic stenosis. The only difference between the two is that when the pulmonary artery is opened, worms are removed primarily from the pulmonary artery and the right ventricle using bayonet forceps, suction, or long-handled forceps. More blood is lost than in pulmonic stenosis surgery, because the lungs and pulmonary arteries are engorged with blood. The advantages of pulmonary arteriotomy are the direct exposure of the areas most likely to be affected and

the speed of the removal. At least 90 per cent of adult heartworms in the heart and pulmonary arteries can be removed by this technique.

Right Ventricular Removal

A second surgical approach for heartworm removal is through a purse-string–sutured incision in the right ventricle, similar to that used in Brock technique for pulmonary stenosis, described earlier. In this procedure, alligator forceps are inserted into the right ventricle and worms are grasped and removed. The technique is slow and tedious, as only one to two worms can be removed with each pass. Because there is no direct exposure, grasping the worms is difficult. The advantages are limited blood loss and simplicity; but the disadvantage, lack of ability to observe and therefore remove worms in the area, makes this technique a poor choice.

Inflow Occlusion and Right Ventriculotomy

An alternative approach for heartworm removal is by inflow occlusion and opening of the right ventricle via median sternotomy. The vena cavae are more easily located than by left lateral thoracotomy, and tourniquets are placed. The azygous vein can also be temporarily ligated to reduce additional blood loss. Sutures are preplaced in the right ventricle rather than the pulmonary artery, and a portion of the right ventricular outflow tract is opened (Fig. 73–42). The heartworms are directly removed. The preplaced sutures are pulled together, supported if necessary with a partially occluding clamp as in pulmonary arteriotomy, and additional sutures are placed over the preplaced support sutures. The advantage of this technique is direct observation of the right ventricle. However, the disadvantages are related to tearing of the stay sutures in the right ventricle and possible major blood loss before a reinforcement suture line can be completed.

Jugular Venotomy

The other major surgical treatment for dirofilariasis is removal via the jugular vein in the vena cava syndrome (see Chapter 71).[23] The vena cava syndrome is fatal within 72 hours unless heartworms are removed. The animals are critically ill, and removal is performed without general anesthesia. The dog is positioned in left lateral recumbency and a local anesthetic is infiltrated over the right jugular vein. The skin is incised and the right jugular vein is exposed and ligated distally. A tourniquet of umbilical tape is placed proximally. The vein is opened, and long alligator forceps are introduced into the vein and passed into the right atrium (Fig. 73–43). Worms are removed using alligator forceps as described for removal from the right ventricle. The presence of

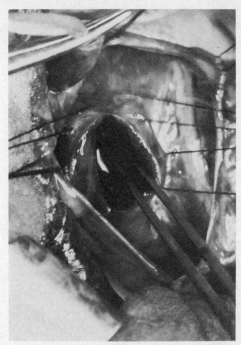

Figure 73–42. The right ventricle is opened and forceps are introduced to remove heartworms.

the worms in the vena cava and right atrium makes them readily accessible. When worms are no longer able to be grasped and removed, the vena cava is ligated and the skin is closed. Results of surgery with vena cava syndrome are good. The disease is fatal without surgery, but long-term survival after surgery is approximately 85 per cent.[23] This dramatic, life-saving technique is the only effective therapy for postcaval dirofilariasis.

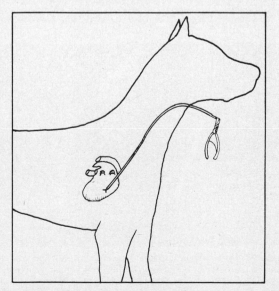

Figure 73–43. Alligator forceps are introduced into the jugular vein and heart for heartworm removal.

Surgical Disorders of the Pericardium

Pericardial Effusion

Surgical diseases of the pericardium include pericarditis and the effusion and granulomatous response to pericarditis (see Chapter 71). The majority of cases of surgical pericarditis can be treated by pericardiocentesis. When this fails, the pericardium can be removed. At our institution, pericardial effusion associated with pericarditis must have been treated unsuccessfully by pericardiocentesis at least twice and usually three times before we resort to pericardectomy.

Pericardectomy can be performed through a lateral thoracotomy in the left or right fifth intercostal space or by a median sternotomy. A disadvantage of lateral thoracotomy is the difficulty in removing the pericardium from the opposite side of the heart. Median sternotomy offers good exposure on both sides up to the heart base. The phrenic nerves, unless incorporated in the granulomatous reaction on the pericardium, can be dissected free of the pericardium, and the pericardium can be removed to the base of the heart. The phrenic nerves are exposed by median sternotomy, and if they are extensively involved in the granulomatous reaction, the pericardectomy can include tissue only from the apex to the phrenic nerves. A disadvantage of median sternotomy is slow healing caused by draining of pleural-pericardial effusion through the ventral midline sternal incision.

In pericardectomy it is important to remove as much pericardium as possible. Removal of a small portion of the pericardium (pericardial window) is usually not satisfactory in canine pericarditis; it alleviates symptoms for a short time, but adhesions to the heart usually form and pericardial effusion returns.

Pericardectomy is frequently extremely hemorrhagic, but electrocautery is helpful in controlling bleeding. Normally small pericardial vessels become major sources of hemorrhage in a thickened, reactive pericardium. When the pericardium has been removed, a chest drain should be placed and left in the thorax until all effusion has ceased, up to five to seven days. Radiographs are taken every other day to confirm removal of pleural fluid and to identify recurrence of pericardial effusion.

The prognosis after treatment for pericardial effusion and pericardial tamponade due to pericarditis is fair. Approximately 50 per cent of animals treated conservatively with pericardiocentesis have a successful long-term result. In the remaining 50 per cent, who undergo pericardectomy, half have a good long-term result; the rest (25 per cent overall) have recurring granulomatous pericarditis at the base of the heart in an area that cannot be resected. Pleural effusion, obstruction to venous return to the heart, and continuing respiratory symptoms usually precede death or request for euthanasia.

Pericardial Diaphragmatic Hernia

Pericardial diaphragmatic hernia, a relatively uncommon condition that may be either congenital or hereditary, can be easily treated surgically.[19] The condition is frequently associated with defects of the sternum or umbilical hernias if congenital and is almost always associated with trauma if acquired. The surgical approach is transabdominal median sternotomy, from mid-sternum to umbilicus. The sternum is divided by heavy scissors or saw, and the pericardial sac–abdomen connection is exposed. The abdominal contents in the pericardial sac are gently returned to the abdomen as the borders of the diaphragm are grasped with Allis tissue forceps and retracted to prevent abdominal contents from entering the thorax. Adhesions are rare but if present must be broken down. The pericardium is incised so that a pericardial sac can be re-formed around the heart. It is separated from the diaphragm and usually can be closed with a single purse-string suture. The heart is allowed to fall freely into the thorax. The remaining portion of the pericardium-diaphragm is closed to form the new diaphragm. The heart and pericardium must be separated from the diaphragm so that adhesions, which may erode through the diaphragm or sternum, do not develop. After closure of the diaphragm, the sternum and abdomen are closed. Chest drains can be removed immediately after operation, and postoperative hospitalization can be limited to 24 hours. The skin sutures are left in place for seven to ten days.

Results of pericardial diaphragmatic hernia repair are excellent. If the repaired pericardium is separated from the diaphragm, adhesions do not occur. However, if sutures are placed so that the pericardium is continuous with the diaphragm, adhesions of the diaphragm and the sternum with the pericardium can occur, and in one instance we have seen resultant erosion of the heart on the sternum.

Feline Aortic Embolism

The major arterial disease in small animals is embolization seen with feline cardiomyopathy (see Chapter 78). Aortic embolectomy is performed to remove the embolus from the distal division of the aorta.[29] Surgery should be performed soon after embolization. If surgery is delayed for six to eight hours, there is little advantage over medical management of the disease. Most recently, clots have been successfully removed with a Fogarty catheter via the femoral arteries.[34]

Complete Heart Block

In the last decade, complete heart block has been effectively treated surgically.[3, 27, 38] Consistently suc-

cessful pacemaker implantation has been accomplished only recently, primarily because of the increased availability of pacemakers.* With low-cost battery-powered, fixed-rate, or demand-rate pacemakers, the procedure has become standard in institutions and is currently being performed in many private practices. Complete heart block is easily diagnosed with an electrocardiogram. Animals with this disease are critical, and surgical therapy is an emergency. Because most animals that develop complete heart block are old, a thorough evaluation of metabolic status should be performed before the heart block surgery is performed. In spite of the relatively low cost of pacemakers, the expense of the procedure is considerable, and animals with end-stage renal disease or diabetes, for example, may be excluded as poor surgical candidates.

In a dog with otherwise good health, the pacemaker is implanted after a transvenous temporary pacemaker is inserted into the right ventricle. The transvenous pacemaker is usually placed percutaneously through the jugular vein in the conscious animal. It is helpful to be able to observe the placement by fluoroscopy, but many pacemaker wires can be inserted without fluoroscopy if they have an inflatable balloon on the tip (Fig. 73–44). The pacemaker wire is placed in the right ventricle and turned on, and the heart is paced at an appropriate rate. (Techniques for introduction of a catheter in the right ventricle are described earlier in this chapter.) After a normal heart rate has been established by temporary pacemaker, the animal can be anesthetized in the usual manner. If temporary pacing is not done before general anesthesia, the animal is atropinized and an intravenous drip is prepared with 0.2 mg isoproterenol per 500 ml of fluid, in order to increase nodal heart rate or to produce ventricular foci if the ventricle is further depressed by anesthesia. Anes-

---

*Medtronics, 1500 N. Dale Blvd. Coon Rapids, MN 55433

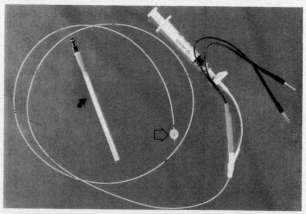

Figure 73–44. A balloon temporary pacing wire set. The stylet and catheter *(arrow)* can be introduced into the jugular vein and the pacing wire passed through the catheter percutaneously. The balloon *(open arrow)* is inflated, and the balloon and electrodes are carried by the blood flow into the right ventricle. The distal end of the catheter arrangement is attached to the pacemaker.

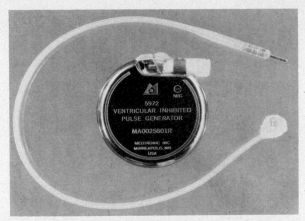

Figure 73–45. A typical unipolar pacemaker and connector wires.

thesia of animals in complete heart block is a high-risk procedure.

The technique for implantation of the pacemaker depends on its type. The unipolar fixed-rate or demand-rate type is most frequently used (Fig. 73–45). The pacemaker battery is usually placed in the flank or in the abdomen. Consequently, two incisions are made, one over the flank area and one for a left lateral thoracotomy in the fifth or, if severe cardiomegaly is present, sixth intercostal space. A pocket for the pacemaker battery pack is made beneath the external abdominal oblique muscles.

The thoracotomy is completed, and the pericardium is opened at the apex. The pacemaker can be attached at the apex of the left ventricle. The newer, easily attached, screw-type wires require no sutures, but some pacemakers may require a suture to attach them to the heart. The wire is carried out through the small opening in the pericardium, the pericardium is loosely closed, and the wire is coiled in the thorax. With the blunt probe usually provided with the pacemaker, a tunnel is made through the dia-

phragm, and the pacemaker wires are carried to the flank. The wire is then connected to the pacemaker, which is inserted into the flank. The temporary pacemaker is turned off or removed. With a satisfactory rhythm established, the permanent battery is secured to the muscles of the flank. The animal is kept in the hospital for at least 48 hours (Fig. 73–46).

The postoperative complications associated with pacemakers include infections associated with foreign bodies, serum pockets near the battery pack, poor pacemaker control of the heart, pleural effusions, and battery failure. Infections associated with foreign material are no greater than in other procedures, but we believe that broad-spectrum antibiotics should be administered preoperatively and one week postoperatively. The serum pocket that may develop around the battery pack can be prevented by making the battery site no longer than the battery pack and suturing the battery pack tightly in place to reduce motion. In some cases, a pressure bandage over the battery pack may also be helpful. The new pacemaker wires at the heart connection have reduced the occasional lack of pacemaker control; however, in some animals this complication may still occur. If so, steroids can be helpful in reducing the inflammation around the pacemaker attachment to the heart, and recontrol can usually be attained. If after 48 hours there is postoperative radiographic evidence of pleural effusion, the fluid should be drained. Battery packs have a life expectancy of five years. If after approximately five years signs of heart block return, the battery must be replaced. Placing the battery in the flank allows replacement under local anesthesia.[3]

The results of pacemaker implantation are fair to good.[27] In the absence of other underlying or additional major metabolic diseases, complete heart block in the dog can be successfully treated with excellent long-term results. Aged animals with multiple organ dysfunction and multiple organ disease have a poorer

Figure 73–46. Lateral thoracic radiograph of a dog with a pacemaker in place. The electrode is attached to the apex of the left ventricle, and the battery pack is positioned in the abdomen.

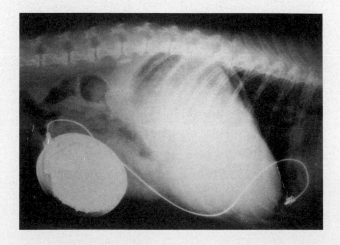

prognosis. The pacemaker battery can usually be expected to outlive these older patients. Results of pacemaker implantation for "sick sinus syndrome" or sinoatrial arrest have not been as good as for complete heart block.[27] Animals with sick sinus syndrome should be carefully evaluated before pacemaker implantation is considered, and medical treatment should be used in preference to pacemaker implantation until it is no longer effective.

COMPLICATED CARDIAC SURGICAL CONDITIONS

Aortic stenosis, atrial septal defect, and mitral and tricuspid valve regurgitation have been corrected in animals but the procedures require major equipment and are time-consuming. These conditions are generally referred to larger veterinary institutions.

Subvalvular Aortic Stenosis

Subvalvular aortic stenosis, a hereditary lesion in the dog, can be corrected by open heart surgical resection, left ventricular–to–aortic conduit, or a closed technique using a valve dilator. Aortic stenosis should be corrected only if the gradient from left ventricle to aorta is severe. Gradients less than 50 mm Hg are minor, and it is unlikely that the animal will ever develop signs associated with the disease. Gradients greater than 100 mm Hg in the dog usually cause death, probably due to arrhythmia, by two years of age. Gradients between 70 and 100 mm Hg have variable results, but we believe that because of the mortality associated with any aortic valve surgery, these animals should not be treated surgically (Table 73–2). Surgical correction of aortic stenosis after six months of age is not effective. Apparently, the myocardial hypertrophy and damage that occur as a result of the obstruction do not regress after surgery, so that animals in which correction was successful develop signs similar to those in animals without sur-

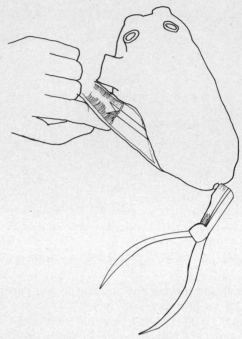

Figure 73–47. The valve dilator is introduced into the left ventricle at the apex and directed to the aorta. The dilator is identified in the aorta by digital palpation before the stenoic subvalvular tissue is incised.

gery. Syncope and sudden death occur. The criteria for surgery for aortic stenosis are (1) the animal must be less than six months of age, (2) the left ventricular–to–aortic gradient must be 100 or greater, and (3) the animal must be large enough that the surgical technique chosen can be effectively accomplished. For open heart surgery, the animal must weigh more than 20 kg. If valve dilation is to be used, the animal must weigh more than 10 kg.

Left ventriculotomy with valvulotomy is similar to the procedure using the valve dilator that was described for pulmonic stenosis. The left ventricle is approached through a left lateral thoracotomy in the fifth or sixth intercostal space. The pericardium is opened, and a pericardial basket is made to elevate the heart. At the left ventricular apex, a purse-string suture is placed deep into the left ventricle. A stab incision is made into the left ventricle, and the valve dilator is inserted into it and advanced until the tip is in the aorta. The dilator is opened and cuts are made in the subvalvular, fibrous, stenotic subaortic ring (Fig. 73–47). The technique is difficult to perform. In tight aortic stenosis, the valve dilator is diverted into the myocardium, and myocardial damage can occur. Occasionally the dilator passes into the aorta around the obstructive ring, producing a second tract and a postoperative aortic insufficiency. Once the first pass has opened the stenosis, multiple passes from the left ventricle to the aorta are easily made, and the opening can be enlarged.

This technique has been used on canine patients less than six months of age, two of which died within the first 24 hours owing to heart failure or arrhythmia. Two animals have survived for longer than one year

TABLE 73–2. Pressure Criteria for Surgery in Immature Dogs with Aortic Stenosis

Left Ventricular Pressure (mm Hg)	Left Ventricular to Aorta Gradient (mm Hg)	Recommendations
> 220	> 100	Critical aortic stenosis; surgery needed immediately
180–220	60–100	Surgery if symptomatic; reevaluate at 6 months of age
140–180	20–60	Reevaluate at 6 months of age
< 140	< 20	No treatment needed

and are normal. A fifth animal was operated on at one year of age, was normal for one year and died suddenly during heavy exercise. Additional work is needed to perfect the technique. The procedure is comparatively simple, and if the operative mortality can be controlled, a simple repair for subvalvular fibrous aortic stenosis in the dog may be available.

Open heart surgical repair has been successful in canine subvalvular aortic stenosis.[12] The animal is connected to cardiopulmonary bypass (see Chapter 76). The aorta is cross-clamped, and a cardioplegic solution is introduced into the heart. When the heart has stopped, the ascending aorta is opened. The subvalvular aortic ring is excised by approaching from the ascending aorta through the aortic valve. Air is evacuated from the left ventricle and ascending aorta. The cross-clamp is removed, the heart is restarted, and cardiopulmonary bypass is ended. The technique carries a mortality of 25 per cent, associated with the cardiopulmonary bypass and its immediate postoperative complications. Animals with repair of this type have done well for up to five years. The advantages of open heart surgical repair are the anatomic removal of the subvalvular fibrous aortic ring and exposure of the stenotic area. The disadvantages are its mortality and the high cost of cardiopulmonary bypass.

Recently, a third method for palliation of subvalvular aortic stenosis has been described.[7] Left ventricular–to–aortic valve conduit is a successful method of decompressing the left ventricle. The offending stenotic fibrous ring is not treated, but the bypass around the obstruction allows ejection of blood into the systemic circulation. The valved conduit is sutured to the descending aorta, the left ventricle apex plug is removed via a method similar to that for pulmonic stenosis, and the conduit is inserted into the apex of the left ventricle. Air is removed from the conduit, and the clamps on the conduit are removed (Fig. 73–48). The procedure is done without cardiopulmonary bypass. Surgical survival is approximately 50 per cent. The advantage of this technique is successful decompression of the left ventricle with-

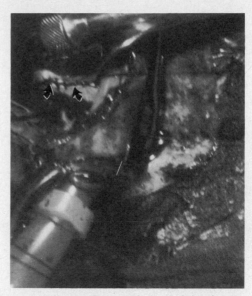

Figure 73–49. Closure of an atrial septal defect by open heart surgery, viewed from the right atrium. The continuous suture line *(arrows)* is nearly complete.

out cardiopulmonary bypass, but the disadvantages are the high mortality and expense of the valved conduits.

Atrial Septal Defect

Atrial septal defect is uncommon in the dog (see Chapter 71), but occasionally animals with the disease are so severely affected that repair is necessary. The only successful operation for atrial septal defect reported in the dog is cardiopulmonary bypass.[17] This condition has a very high success rate in humans, and the one report of its use in an animal also had a successful outcome. The procedure for bypass is described in Chapter 76. The right atrium is opened, and the atrial defect is closed with a continuous or interrupted suture pattern (Fig. 73–49) or with a patch. The bypass time, a major problem in the dog, is short. This technique may be considered in any symptomatic animal with atrial septal defect.

Tricuspid and Mitral Valve Replacement

Tricuspid and mitral valves have been successfully replaced in dogs (Fig. 73–50). Mitral valve disease is the most common acquired canine cardiac disease. Because the myocardium is unaffected, the appropriate treatment is valve replacement. However, this procedure is not routinely done because of extensive surgical problems, cost of prosthetic valves, and the difficulty of cardiopulmonary bypass in the dog. Successful valve replacement is occasionally reported.[8, 15] The mitral valve may be replaced by open heart surgical repair using cardioplegia and insertion of the valve through the left atrium or through the right atrium and across the atrial septum (Fig. 73–51). The

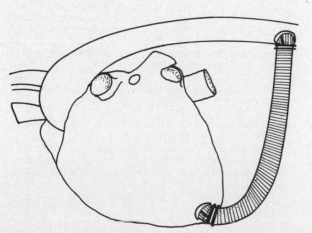

Figure 73–48. Valved conduit from the left ventricle to the aorta.

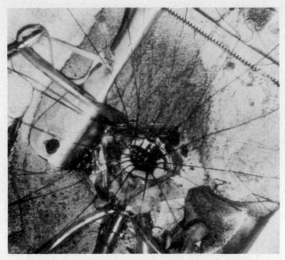

Figure 73–50. Placement of a prosthetic valve in the tricuspid position in a dog. The multiple interrupted sutures are placed and tied.

technique carries a 75 per cent mortality and is generally not recommended. Successful implantation of a prosthetic mitral valve using deep hypothermic-circulatory arrest through the right atrium and atrial septum has been reported.[8] This technique is successful (50 per cent) and may be an effective treatment in the future.

Acquired tricuspid valve disease is usually a secondary condition in animals that have mitral valve disease, and double-valve operations are not successful in animals. The occasional animal with congenital tricuspid valve dysplasia (see Chapter 71) may be helped with the implantation of a prosthetic tricuspid valve. Long-term success is poor. The valved conduit from the right atrium to the pulmonary artery (Fontan procedure) has been performed in animals, but the results are also poor.

Valve replacement by cardiopulmonary bypass,

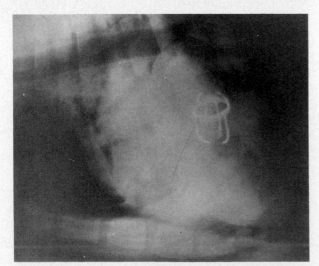

Figure 73–51. Lateral thoracic radiograph of a dog with mitral valve replacement. A ball and cage valve is in the mitral position.

deep hypothermic circulatory arrest, or extracardiac conduits without cardiopulmonary bypass is experimental in dogs. In the future these procedures may be successful enough to merit selected use. The cost of the valves and the procedures, which carry a high mortality, precludes recommendation of these techniques in dogs.

1. Abadie, S. H., Black, E., Dupuy, H. J., and Gonzales, R.: A procedure for the surgical removal of *Dirofilaria immitis*. J. Am. Vet. Med. Assoc. *156*:884, 1970.
2. Aultman, S. H., Chambers, J. N., and Vestre, W. A.: Double aortic arch and persistent right aortic arch in two littermates: surgical treatment. J. Am. Anim. Hosp. Assoc. *16*:533, 1980.
3. Bonagura, D., Helphrey, M. L., and Muir, W.: Complications associated with permanent pacemaker implantation in the dog. J. Am. Vet. Med. Assoc. *182*:149, 1983.
4. Braden, T. D., Appleford, M. D., and Hartsfield, S. M.: Correction of a ventricular septal defect in a dog. J. Am. Vet. Med. Assoc. *161*:507, 1972.
5. Breznock, E. M., Hilwig, R. W., Vasko, J. S., and Hamlin, R. L.: Surgical correction of an interventricular septal defect in the dog. J. Am. Vet. Med. Assoc. *157*:1343, 1970.
6. Breznock, E. M., and Wood, G. L.: A patch-graft technique for correction of pulmonic stenosis in dogs. J. Am. Vet. Med. Assoc. *169*:1090, 1976.
7. Breznock, E. M., Whiting, P., Pendrays, D., et al.: Valved apico-aortic conduit for relief of left ventricular hypertension caused by discrete subaortic stenosis in dogs. J. Am. Vet. Med. Assoc. *182*:51, 1983.
8. Breznock, E. M., Bauer, T., Strack, D., et al.: Prosthetic mitral and tricuspid valve implantation in dogs using deep surface hypothermia (15°C). Abstr. Am. Coll. Vet. Surgeons, 1983.
9. Brock, R. C.: Pulmonary valvotomy for the relief of congenital pulmonary stenosis. Br. Med. J. *1*:1121, 1948.
10. Custer, M. A., Kantor, A. F., Gilman, R. A., and DeRiemer, R. H.: Correction of pulmonic stenosis. J. Am. Vet. Med. Assoc. *139*:565, 1961.
11. de Leval, M. R., McKay, R., Jones, M., et al.: Modified Blalock-Taussig shunt. J. Thorac. Cardiovasc. Surg. *81*:112, 1981.
12. Eyster, G. E., Hough, J. D., Evans, A. T., et al.: Surgical repair of patent ductus arteriosus, aortic stenosis, and aortic regurgitation in a dog. J. Am. Vet. Med. Assoc. *167*:942, 1975.
13. Eyster, G. E., Whipple, R. D., Evans, A. T., et al.: Recanalized patent ductus arteriosus in the dog. J. Small Anim. Pract. *16*:743, 1975.
14. Eyster, G. E., Eyster, J. T., Cords, G. B., and Johnston, J.: Patent ductus arteriosus in the dog: characteristics of occurrence and results of surgery in one hundred consecutive cases. J. Am. Vet. Med. Assoc. *168*:435, 1976.
15. Eyster, G. E., Weber, W., Chi, S., et al.: Mitral valve prosthesis for correction of mitral regurgitation in a dog. J. Am. Vet. Med. Assoc. *168*:1115, 1976.
16. Eyster, G. E., Anderson, L. K., Sawyer, D. C., et al.: Beta adrenergic blockade for management of tetralogy of Fallot in a dog. J. Am. Vet. Med. Assoc. *169*:637, 1976.
17. Eyster, G. E., Anderson, L. K., Krehbiel, J. D., et al.: Surgical repair of atrial septal defect in a dog. J. Am. Vet. Med. Assoc. *169*:1081, 1976.
18. Eyster, G. E., Whipple, R. D., Anderson, L. J., et al.: Pulmonary artery banding for ventricular septal defect in dogs and cats. J. Am. Vet. Med. Assoc. *170*:434, 1977.
19. Eyster, G. E., Evans, A. T., Blanchard, G. L., et al.: Congenital pericardial diaphragmatic hernia and multiple cardiac defects in a litter of collies. J. Am. Vet. Med. Assoc. *170*:516, 1977.
20. Eyster, G. E., Braden, T. D., Appleford, M., et al.: Surgical

management of tetralogy of Fallot. J. Small Anim. Pract. *18*:387, 1977.

21. Ford, R. B., Spaulding, G. L., and Eyster, G. E.: Use of an extracardiac conduit in the repair of supravalvular pulmonic stenosis in a dog. J. Am. Vet. Med. Assoc. *172*:922, 1978.

22. Hanlon, C. R., Kiaser, G. C., Mudd, J. F. G., and Willman, V. L.: Closed pulmonary valvulotomy. J. Cardiovasc. Surg. *9*:496, 1968.

23. Jackson, R. F., Seymour, W. G., Growney, P. G., and Otto, G. F.: Surgical treatment of the caval syndrome of canine heartworm disease. J. Am. Vet. Med. Assoc. *171*:1065, 1977.

24. Jackson, W. F., and Henderson, R. A.: Ligature placement in closure of patent ductus arteriosus. J. Am. Anim. Hosp. Assoc. *15*:55, 1979.

25. Jones, C. L., and Buchanan, J. W.: Patent ductus arteriosus: anatomy and surgery in a cat. J. Am. Vet. Med. Assoc. *179*:364, 1981.

26. Knauer, K. W., Hobson, H. P., and Clark, D. R.: Congenital valvular pulmonic stenosis in the dog: diagnosis and surgical correction. South West. Vet. *Winter*:93, 1970.

27. Lombard, C. W., Tilley, L. P., and Yoshioka, M.: Pacemaker implantation in the dog: survey and literature review. J. Am. Anim. Hosp. Assoc. *17*:751, 1981.

28. Mann, P. G. H., Stock, J. E., and Sheridan, J. P.: Pulmonary artery banding in the cat: a case report. J. Small Anim. Pract. *12*:45, 1971.

29. McCurnin, D. M., and Arp, L. H.: Surgical treatment of aortic embolism in a cat. Vet. Med. Small Anim. Clin. *67*:387, 1972.

30. Perkins, R. L., and Edmark, K. W.: Ligation of femoral vessels and azygous vein in the dog. J. Am. Vet. Med. Assoc. *159*:993, 1971.

31. Rawlings, C. A.: Personal communication, 1983.

32. Shires, P. K., and Liu, W.: Persistent right aortic arch in dogs: a long-term follow-up after surgical correction. J. Am. Anim. Hosp. Assoc. *17*:773, 1981.

33. Swan, H., Zeavin, J., Blount, S. G., Jr., and Virtue, R. W.: Surgery by direct vision in the open heart during hypothermia. JAMA *153*:1081, 1953.

34. Sweetman, J. H., Perry, S. R., and Burke, G.: Personal communication, 1983.

35. van den Ingh, T. S. G. A. M., and van der Linde-Sipman, J. S.: Vascular rings in dogs. J. Am. Vet. Med. Assoc. *164*:939, 1974.

36. Weirich, W. E., and Blevins, W. E.: Ventricular septal defect repair. Vet. Surg. 7:2, 1978.

37. Whiting, P. G., Breznock, E. M., Pendroy, D., and Struck, D.: Double outlet right ventricle for release of pulmonic stenosis in the dog: an experimental study. Abstr. Am. Coll. Vet. Sci., 1982.

38. Yoshioka, M. M., Tilley, L. P., Harvey, H. J., et al.: Permanent pacemaker implantation in the dog. J. Am. Anim. Hosp. Assoc. *17*:746, 1981.

Chapter **74**

Cardiovascular Biopsy Techniques

George E. Eyster

The cardiovascular system is rarely biopsied. Cardiac disorders are usually identified by other diagnostic techniques, and cardiac tumors are rare. Biopsy techniques are primarily used to evaluate the results of research involving myocardial muscle or an assessment of cardiac tissue with the diagnosis of cardiomyopathy.[2] Using biopsy, the clinician should be able to determine the amount and severity of fibrosis in cardiomyopathy or infiltrates from research procedures or a pathogenic process.

The one cardiac biopsy technique that is routinely used clinically is pericardiocentesis for the assessment of pericardial fluid. This procedure is simple and straightforward and a valuable tool for diagnostic as well as therapeutic purposes.

Pericardiocentesis is accomplished at the "cardiac notch," which is found on the right side below the level of the costochondral junction and at the fourth, fifth, or sixth intercostal space (Fig. 74–1). The cardiac notch is the area on the right side where lung does not cover the heart. This relatively unprotected area of the heart has major safety advantages for pericardiocentesis and thoracentesis (the techniques are similar). The cardiac notch area is safe for pericardiocentesis because, first, no coronary arteries

(high-pressure vessels) are located on the heart in that area, and, second, the heart chamber located below the costochondral junction is the moderately thick-walled, relatively low-pressure right ventricle and puncture of the heart at that point will not produce major bleeding. Third, the aforementioned lack of lung in the area obviates the chance of rupturing pulmonary alveoli or major pulmonary vessels.

Pericardiocentesis is performed using a large syringe with a three-way stopcock and a large-bore needle. Low-pressure vacuum tubes can also be used instead of the syringe. The skin in the area of the cardiac notch is clipped and scrubbed. The procedure is performed with the animal standing. Local anesthetic is not necessary. The needle is inserted through the skin at the appropriate point and advanced in the posterior third of the rib space to avoid the intercostal artery, vein, and nerve as they pass just caudal to the ribs. As soon as the pleural space is entered, slight negative pressure is applied to the syringe. The thoracentesis procedure is complete at this point. For pericardiocentesis, the needle is advanced until the heart is felt at the end of the needle or until the pericardium has been entered and peri-

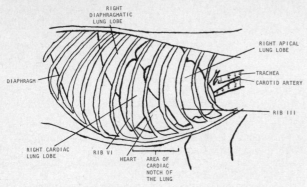

Figure 74–1. Diagram of the "cardiac notch" in the dog from the right. The lungs do not extend ventrally to cover the heart. Thoracentesis, pericardiocentesis, or cardiac tap can be safely performed ventral to the costochondral junction, dorsal to the sternum, in the posterior third of intercostal space 4, 5, or 6.

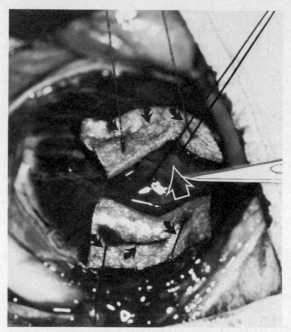

Figure 74–2. Removal of a myocardial biospy. Mattress sutures have been placed outside the biopsy site (*arrows*). A suture has been placed in the proposed biopsy to aid retrieval of tissue (*open arrow*). A No. 11 scalpel has been positioned to cut out the tissue. Support pledgets are shown preplaced to support the mattress sutures.

cardial fluid is removed. In most pathological cases the pericardial fluid is dark red to brown and may appear to be blood. The packed cell volume of the pericardial fluid is usually less than that of blood, and the fluid will not clot. If the needle is advanced, the heart is touched and can be felt moving at the end of the needle. The needle is withdrawn slightly and pericardiocentesis completed. An electrocardiogram may be used to monitor the animal throughout the procedure, but premature beats can be expected when the needle touches the heart.

Pericardiocentesis should remove all fluid from the pericardium. The purpose of pericardiocentesis is to identify the fluid and also relieve the obstruction associated with the fluid of pericardial tamponade. It is helpful to calculate the anticipated fluid volume by estimating the size of the heart as a sphere and the size of the pericardium by radiography. The formula for volume of a sphere is

$$\text{volume} = \frac{4\,(\text{radius})^3}{3}$$

The estimate of the pericardial volume is taken from the spherical appearance on the radiograph. The measurement of the heart volume is taken as an approximation of a sphere similar to the normal heart. The difference between the two volumes equals the amount of pericardial fluid and can be used as a guide for the amount of fluid to remove.

Direct biopsy of the myocardium is done via a routine lateral thoracotomy in the fifth intercostal space. The pericardium is opened and the area for biopsy is prepared. If a large biopsy is needed, a cardiac plug must be taken. Unless specific tissues are needed, the biopsy should be in an avascular area. Deep sutures of a 00 nonabsorbable type are placed into the myocardium using Teflon pledgets. At least two mattress sutures should be placed. The biopsy site is situated between the two sutures so that a deep wedge can be removed. If possible, a suture can be placed in the plug for easy mobilization (Fig. 74–2). Using a #11 blade, deep stab incisions

are made around the plug. The plug is removed and the stay sutures are pulled tight. Digital pressure over the wound controls hemorrhage and the sutures are tied. Additional sutures with pledgets may be necessary to control bleeding from the high-pressure left ventricle. Continuous 4/0 nonabsorbable sutures can be placed in the epicardium. When the bleeding is controlled, the pericardium is loosely closed and the thoracotomy is closed in a routine manner. Postoperative electrocardiographic monitoring for the presence of arrhythmias is instituted using an oscilloscope. If arrhythmias become frequent, lidocaine in an intravenous drip should be used to control the arrhythmias.

If a small biopsy is acceptable, a Tru-cut biopsy needle can be used to obtain the tissue. The approach is similar to plug removal, but only a single purse-string suture 3 to 4 mm in diameter is needed. The needle is introduced inside the purse-string and the sample taken. Digital pressure controls the bleeding, but ligation of the purse-string assures that bleeding does not recur. Postoperative management is similar to that used with the plug technique.

A final cardiac biopsy technique that should be mentioned is the use of a biopsy catheter. Cardiac biopsy catheters have been developed to postoperatively monitor human heart transplant patients for rejection and have recently been advocated for use in the dog.[1] The catheter is introduced into a vein or an artery and passed into the right ventricle or retrograde into the left ventricle. While the catheter is directed under fluoroscopy, a small bite of ventricular wall is taken. The technique in man has proved safe and effective if endocardial change is anticipated.[2] The techniques of cardiac catheterization are described in Chapter 73.

Major vessels can be biopsied by removal of a portion of the vessel. Most of the major vessels in the dog and cat can be safely ligated and small sections of the vessel removed, but it is preferable to save the vessel. A small segment of a major vessel can be excised and the vessel preserved by one of the anastomotic techniques described in Chapter 77.

1. Burk, R. L., Tilley, L. P., Henderson, M. B., and Jones, V. C.: Endomyocardial biopsy in the dog. Am. J. Vet. Res. *41*:2106, 1980.
2. Fenoglio, J. J., Ursell, P. C., Kellogg, C. F., Drusin, R. E., and Weiss, M. B.: Diagnosis and classification of myocarditis by endomyocardial biopsy. N. Engl. J. Med. *308*:12, 1983.

Chapter **75**

Hypothermia

Walter E. Weirich

Reduced body temperature has been used therapeutically for centuries. Folk medicine has included the use of shifts in body temperature for perceived medicinal benefits. The American Indians and the Scandinavians have used heat in a sauna or similar devices in which rocks were heated and placed within a small enclosure. Dry heat caused the patient to sweat. When the sweating was profuse, the patient was plunged into cold water.[10] These treatments may not have been necessary, but some patients must have responded favorably or the practice would not have persisted.

The first documented use of whole-body hypothermia was in 1877, when Dr. James Carrie treated Richard Sutton for acute alcoholism. Cold was used to treat shock and to provide sedation to reduce pain from battle wounds during the American Civil War. At about the same time, several forms of cancer and various dermatologic disorders were also treated with cold.[11] It was not until the mid-1940s that studies were carried out to use cold to reduce the metabolic rate sufficiently that cardiac arrest surgery could be performed. By 1950, enough information had been generated to warrant a conference on hypothermia held in Toronto, Canada.[2] Changes that take place during cooling and rewarming were documented and presented. The first reports of successful use of hypothermia in human heart surgery were published in 1953.[12] At that time, a series of atrial septal defects were repaired using multiple inflow occlusions for up to six minutes.

In the mid-1950s, cardiopulmonary bypass developed as a viable technique for human clinical heart surgery, and hypothermia was temporarily set aside. By the mid-1960s, however, it had been shown that cardiopulmonary bypass was not safe in small infants, whose blood vessels were not large enough to allow adequate flow. Significant damage occurred to formed elements in the blood when normothermic flow requirements were approximated.[8]

It has since been discovered that body surface cooling of infants to between 25 and 30°C followed by thoracotomy for cardiopulmonary bypass allows safe cardiac arrest in the tiny patient. Cardiopulmonary bypass, when used at these lower temperatures, could achieve adequate blood flow for tissue perfusion. The pump was then used to cool the baby to about 20°C and to remove as much blood as possible to allow for a clear dry surgical field. The pump heat exchanger was used to warm the baby to a point at which the heart could be started and could take over and maintain adequate blood flow to vital structures.

The dog presents a significant added problem in cardiopulmonary bypass, in that the canine clotting mechanism is much more active than in humans. The canine red cell is easily damaged by pumping, and subsequent hemolysis leads to accumulation of cellular debris in the filters of the pump as well as in small vessels in the body. The dog, therefore, is not a particularly good subject for the study of cardiopulmonary bypass.[4, ,5]

When a method is sought to provide safe cardiac arrest for the dog, two facts immediately become apparent; first, most cardiac patients requiring cardiac surgery are young animals and therefore small; second, adequate blood flow for tissue perfusion results in damage to red blood cells and in coagulation if cardiopulmonary bypass pumping is attempted. Experience has shown that larger individuals do fairly well with bypass pumping. Dogs less than 15 kg have a significantly increased risk if subjected to cardiopulmonary bypass pumping, because of the technique itself.

Hypothermia for cardiac arrest surgery in the dog was first used clinically by Breznock and colleagues,[3] who successfully closed a ventricular septal defect in a three-month-old beagle puppy in 1971. Others have used the technique with varying degrees of success.

Hypothermia for cardiac arrest surgery can be carried out with a minimum of expense to an institution or private practice. Three elements are required to be successful: personnel, equipment, and training and experience.

Any undertaking of this magnitude requires a team

approach for success. The team should be made up of at least three veterinarians and two technicians. The surgeon and assistant surgeon must be able to concentrate on the surgical manipulations while cardiac arrest is under way. A veterinarian familiar with anesthesia and the use of cardiac drugs is needed to monitor the patient through this procedure, which considerably alters normal homeostatic mechanisms. Blood gas analysis and rapid response to blood gas changes are necessary. The technicians are needed to administer anesthetics and other drugs and to act as operating room nurse.

The equipment needed for hypothermia surgery is minimal, but some basic requirements must be met. First, a good physiologic monitor is needed for ECG, with at least one blood pressure and temperature. Blood gas analysis capability must be rapidly available, so quick reporting of the data can be achieved. No unusual cardiac surgical instruments are needed. If only an occasional hypothermia procedure is to be done, ice can be purchased. A positive-pressure mechanical ventilator is helpful to control the ventilation in patients weighing more than 6 kg. Mechanical ventilators do an outstanding job of providing for uniform ventilation. Patients weighing less than 6 kg should be hand-ventilated, because pediatric ventilators are not usually cost-effective in veterinary practice.

The training and experience of the pesonnel is the most important element in the success or failure of the team's efforts. Veterinarians need to have advanced training, either formal or informal, with a qualified veterinary cardiologist or cardiovascular surgeon. A specific protocol should be established and modified to fit the experience of the team. Table 75–1 is a protocol for hypothermia in the dog with tasks divided according to team member. This protocol represents the tasks that must be done to be consistently successful. Before considering a clinical case, the team should do at least ten successful practice dogs.

Careful diagnosis is required before any cardiac procedure can be considered. The patient should be admitted to the hospital at least 48 hours prior to operation. Nonabsorbable oral antibiotics are given to suppress bowel bacteria. During the period of cardiac arrest no blood will be flowing, possibly leading to vascular changes similar to those in shock. Bacteria and bacterial toxins play an important role when shock becomes irreversible. Therefore, systemic antibiotics are also given to suppress bacterial populations where they might occur within the body and thus perhaps to prevent toxins from being produced when the animal is compromised. The surgical site should be clipped and if the animal has a dense undercoat, consideration should be given to clipping the entire animal. To aid rewarming, the animal should be encouraged to eat to build up glycogen stores in the liver and skeletal muscle. The dog should be given at least 250 mg of vitamin C twice

each day with the oral antibiotics.[7] Vitamin C provides resistance to cold in humans.

On the day of surgery, the dog is premedicated with morphine sulfate and atropine sulfate subcutaneously. When these drugs have taken their full effect, catheters are placed in the jugular and cephalic veins. Phenytoin is given intramuscularly prior to cooling to aid in the prevention of "shock lung" in the postoperative period. Because induced cardiac arrest has similarities to circulatory shock, in which corticosteroids are beneficial,[1] pretreatment with dexamethasone or prednisolone sodium succinate appears to be helpful. Anesthesia is induced with sodium pentothal intravenously. The animal is intubated, and additional pentothal is given until the dog is in the ice bath. The temperature probe is passed deep into the descending colon. The ECG leads are attached to the distal parts of the limbs so that a good upright QRS complex can be seen. The animal is now ready to be placed in the ice bath. If the animal starts to move or shiver, it is immediately paralyzed with succinylcholine to preserve glycogen in the skeletal muscle. The animal breathes a gas mixture of 95 per cent O_2 and 5 per cent CO_2, which causes a dilation of the cerebral vessels, aiding in rapid and complete cooling of the brain.[13] Positive-pressure ventilation will be needed when paralysis is induced or when the animal's rectal temperature reaches 33°C. The water in the ice bath should be deep enough to cover the body of the dog. The water must be constantly stirred to provide maximum cooling rates until the animal is cooled to 27°C. During cooling the blood viscosity increases and the red cells and platelets have an increased tendency to aggregate.[4] To minimize this tendency and maintain optimal blood flow in small vessels, low-molecular-weight dextrans are given during cooling.[8] Dextrans should be delivered by drip and ended when the cooling is complete. When the animal reaches a temperature of 30°C the tendency for the ventricular myocardium to develop arrhythmias is increased.[2] Therefore, lidocaine hydrochloride is administered intravenously. Lidocaine is continued until cardiac arrest is induced. When the animal's rectal temperature drops to 27°C, the animal is removed from the ice bath. The gas is changed to 100 per cent O_2, and the animal is placed on the operating table and prepared for surgery. An after-fall of the temperature occurs, resulting in a temperature of about 23°C when the core equilibrates with the exterior of the body. An arterial catheter should be established in the femoral artery, by cutdown if necessary, for monitoring blood pressure and collecting blood gas samples during rewarming.

Several important physiological changes occur during cooling. The viscosity of the blood increases, as does the tendency for blood cells to aggregate. Blood vessels in the lung and throughout the body become stiff and more like rigid tubes; pulses may be more difficult to palpate. When cooling commences, an intense vasoconstriction occurs. As the animal ap-

TABLE 75–1. Protocol for Hypothermia in Veterinary Cardiac Surgery

Responsible Team Member	Preparation 48 Hours Prior to Cooling	Pre-Cooling on Day of Surgery	Cooling	Arrest	Resuscitation	Warming
Surgeon and assistant surgeon		Catheters in cephalic vein and jugular vein Place temperature probe		Give cold cardioplegic solution (prepare by adding 26 mEq KCl to 1 liter of Ringer's solution) Ringer's slush on heart Surgery	Massage ventricles: abdominal counterpressure Defibrillate 1 watt-sec/kg internal	Flush chest with warm fluids
Anesthesia/medicine DVM		1-hr Preanesthesia Morphine or Atropine (1/4 gr) (.04 mg/kg) Anesthesia: Sodium pentothal IV Pass endotracheal tube Breathing gas (95% O$_2$, 5% CO$_2$)	Monitor ECG	Femoral artery catheter for blood pressure and blood gas Change breathing gas to 100% O$_2$	Monitor ECG and blood pressure Treat arrhythmias and hypotension as needed Blood gas analysis Treat as needed	Monitor ECG and blood pressure Treat as needed Rewarm to 33°C
Anesthesia technician	Clip surgical site Bathe dog Draw blood for crossmatch & transfusion	Attach ECG leads Succinylcholine chloride 20 mg in 60 ml D5W, given to effect	Lidocaine, IV 1 mg/min when temperature below 30°C	Stop lidocaine	Start whole blood Give lidocaine if needed Watch ventilation Keep records	
Medicine technician	Oral antibiotics: Neomycin, 50 mg/kg b.i.d. Erythromycin, 50 mg/kg b.i.d. Systemic antibiotics: Procaine penicillin, 44,000 U/kg s.i.d. Vitamin C, 250 mg b.i.d.	Dilantin, 5 mg/kg IM Dexamethasone, 5 mg/kg IV	Positive-pressure ventilation when temperature below 33°C Keep records LMW 10% Dextran, 10 mg/kg IV Stir water	Keep records	Give epinephrine, 2–5 ml of 1:20,000 IV; calcium Cl 10%, 2 ml/10 kg IV, sodium bicarbonate 2 mEq/kg Keep records	Give drugs as directed Have several gallons of warm fluids ready

proaches 32°C, vasodilation occurs. This is also the point below which the animal cannot rewarm itself by physiologic means. The ECG changes as cooling progresses, and intervals and durations are prolonged. The rate is slow so that at a temperature of 25°C, the heart rate may be less than 40 beats/minute. Because of increased irritability below a temperature of 30°C, ventricular arrhythmias are more likely. Myocardial hypoxia contributes to arrhythmias and can be avoided if ventilation is maintained with a mechanical ventilator. A blood pH less than 7.20 also contributes to ventricular arrhythmias. Serum Ca^{++} tends to increase, and if the pH is allowed to fall (usually owing to poor ventilation), serum K^+ will increase. Levels of both electrolytes return to normal when the animal is rewarmed. Catecholamines are at low levels during cooling but will be at higher than normal levels during rewarming. This is an advantage, as the high levels aid resuscitation.

At 23 to 25°C, a safe cardiac arrest of up to 45 minutes can be commenced. However, the cardiac arrest should be concluded in as short a time as possible. The total time from the beginning of cooling to when the heart is resuscitated should be less than 90 minutes

The azygous vein is ligated and ⅛-inch umbilical tapes are placed on the pre and post cavae to occlude venous inflow. When the heart is stopped, tapes on the vena cavae are drawn tight to prevent blood from entering the heart. The aorta is cross clamped and a near-0°C cardioplegic solution (see Table 72–1) is injected into the ascending aorta.[6] A slush of Ringer's solution is placed around the heart in the pericardial sling, to help preserve the myocardium during the period of cardiac arrest. The ventilator may be turned off while the heart is stopped. When the surgery is complete and all air has been removed from the heart and great vessels, the venous inflow occluders can be released. Epinephrine, calcium, and sodium bicarbonate are given to restart the heart as quickly as possible. Massage, using abdominal counterpressure, is instituted at once. Venous return should be adequate within a few seconds to a minute or more. The abdominal counterpressure (pushing the abdominal contents against the spine as the ventricles are filling) causes a two-fold increase in venous return compared with just ventricular massage.[9] This aids coronary perfusion and allows for rapid and effective defibrillation of the ventricles. As soon as the ventricles are fibrillating briskly, a defibrillation shock of 1 watt-sec/kg is given with internal paddles of adequate size. Once the heart is beating adequately, the process of rewarming can be pursued with vigor. It may be necessary to rewarm with massage before the ventricles can be defibrillated. Rewarming is usually very slow if the heart is not beating spontaneously.

A heating pad (water circulating type is preferred),

which was placed on the table under the dog prior to surgery, is turned on. The chest is warmed by repeated changes of saline or Ringer's solution heated to 43°C. Blood gases should be checked every five minutes during the first 30 minutes after cardiac arrest. After that time, they can be checked at hourly intervals if the cardiac function has been good and the trends in the blood gas values have been in a normal direction. When the deep rectal temperature reaches 33°C, flushing of the chest with warm fluids may be stopped and the incision may be closed. The animal should continue to be warmed by external means until the normal body temperature has been reached. The ECG should be monitored continuously for the first 24 hours. The blood pressure catheter can be removed in the operating room if the pressure has been stable during closure of the chest.

Postoperatively, these animals are usually quite depressed for the first 24 hours because of mild cerebral edema. The CO_2 used in the breathing gas during cooling causes cerebral vascular dilation, and some edema undoubtedly results. Fortunately, after 36 hours the biochemical changes caused by hypothermia and cardiac arrest return to normal, and only the cardiac surgical postoperative problems, if any, should be evident.

1. Adams, H. R., and Parker, J. L.: Pharmacologic management of circulatory shock: cardiovascular drugs and corticosteroids. J. Am. Vet. Med. Assoc. *175*:86, 1979.
2. Bigelow, W. G., Lindsay, W. K., and Greenwood, W. F.: Hypothermia. Its possible role in cardiac surgery: an investigation of factors governing survival in dogs at low body temperature. Ann. Surg. *132*:849, 1950.
3. Breznock, E. M., Vasko, J. S., Hilwig, R. W., et al.: Surgical correction using hypothermia of an interventricular septal defect in the dog. J. Am. Vet. Med. Assoc. *158*:1391, 1971.
4. Ellis, P. R., Kleinsasser, L. J., and Speer, R. J.: Changes in coagulation occurring in dogs during hypothermia and cardiac surgery. Surgery *41*:198, 1957.
5. Gentry, P. A., and Downie, H. G.: Blood coagulation. *In* Swenson, M. J. (ed.): *Dukes Physiology of Domestic Animals.* 9th ed. Cornell University Press, Ithaca, 1977.
6. Jellinek, M., Standven, J. W., Menz, L. J., et al.: Cold blood potassium cardioplegia: effects of increasing concentration of potassium. J. Thorac. Cardiovasc. Surg. *82*:26, 1981.
7. LaBlanc, J.: *Man in the Cold.* Charles C Thomas, Springfield, 1975.
8. Mohri, H., Dillard, D. H., Crawford, E. W., et al.: Method of surface-induced deep hypothermia for open heart surgery in infants. J. Thorac. Cardiovasc. Surg. *58*:262, 1969.
9. Ralston, S. H., Babbs, C. F., and Niebauer, M. J.: Cardiopulmonary resuscitation with interposed abdominal compression in dogs. Anesth. Analg. *61*:645, 1982.
10. Roe, C. F.: Temperature regulation and energy metabolism in surgical patients. Prog. Surg. *12*:96, 1973.
11. Swan, H.: Hypothermia. *In* Gibbon, J. H. (ed.): *Surgery of the Chest.* W. B. Saunders, Philadelphia, 1962.
12. Swan, H., Zeavin, I., Blount, S. G., Jr., and Virtue, R. W.: Surgery of direct vision in the open heart during hypothermia. J. Am. Vet. Med. Assoc. *153*:1081, 1953.
13. Zarins, C. K., and Skinner, D. B.: Circulation in profound hypothermia. J. Surg. Res. *14*:97, 1973.

Chapter 76

Extracorporeal Circulatory Support

David L. Homberg

The use of extracorporeal circulatory support in the correction of cardiac defects in veterinary clinical cases is currently done in few centers. However, cardiac bypass units are available in numerous research institutions and human hospitals. Increasing awareness of the pet-owning public about the availability of such techniques as open-heart surgery should make the use of bypass units more common. The aim of this discussion is to summarize what can be expected from a heart-lung unit, what types of units are available, and what determines their physiological limits.

REQUIREMENTS OF THE EXTRACORPOREAL CIRCULATORY SUPPORT UNIT

The purpose of the extracorporeal unit is to take over the function of the patient's heart and lungs so that these organs may be bypassed while surgical correction of a defect is being performed. To do this, the extracorporeal circulatory support unit (ECSU) must accept the patient's venous blood, modify the soluble gas concentration, and deliver the blood back to the patient in a quantity and physiological form adequate to support life.

Normal oxygen needs of the body are expressed as blood flow in milliliters per square meter body surface area per minute or milliliters per kilogram of body weight per minute[7]: basal flow for a 5-kg animal equals 200 ml/kg/min; basal flow for a 10-kg animal equals 170 ml/kg/min; basal flow for a 20-kg animal equals 135 ml/kg/min. During short-term extracorporeal circulatory support, a low blood flow is acceptable; however, the longer the support, the closer to normal the flow should be. This necessity for normal volumes of blood flow can be modified by the use of hypothermia (see Chapter 75).

The volume that can be delivered by any given oxygenator is usually considered its "rated flow" and is expressed in liters per minute. This is the flow at which normal venous blood can enter the unit and leave with a 95 per cent oxygen saturation.[4] Because oxygen binding to hemoglobin occurs rapidly, the limiting factor to oxygenation is the speed of oxygen diffusion through the plasma. Carbon dioxide removal is almost always more rapid than oxygenation, and therefore it is usually sufficient to consider oxygen efficiency when discussing the oxygenator unit.[4]

The type of blood flow delivered by the ECSU is highly significant. If a constant flow is being delivered to the patient, red blood cells stagnate.[11] In comparisons between continuous and pulsatile flow, urine output is depressed during continuous flow even though the mean arterial pressure is the same as that of the pulsatile flow. Such a depression may be a result of renin release, which is stimulated by a decrease in the peak systolic pressure rather than the mean arterial pressure.[11] Lymph flow also relies on pulsatile arterial pressure even if the peak systolic pressure never exceeds the nonpulsatile flow pressure. The normal pulse massages tissues and helps remove extracellular fluid through the lymphatics.[11] With non-pulsatile flow, fluid accumulates, resulting in a slow reduction in blood volume that necessitates transfusions.[4] The increase in the extracellular fluid space may be as great as 20 per cent.[4]

COMPONENTS OF THE EXTRACORPOREAL CIRCULATORY SUPPORT UNIT

The Prime

Common to all ECSUs is the need to have a minimum volume of fluid within the unit prior to the onset of circulatory support (Fig. 76–1). The makeup and volume of this prime is often a factor limiting the use of cardiac bypass in veterinary medicine. Although whole blood may be the best prime because of its oxygen-carrying ability, its use increases the blood viscosity and the amount of hemolysis occurring with bypass.[4] Conversely, the use of a nonhemic prime (Table 76–1) leads to hemodilution but does have the advantages of reducing blood donor usage, decreasing blood viscosity, and increasing the perfusion of the microcirculation.[7] Decreased damage to blood elements and increased urine output in spite of a decreased glomerular filtration rate occurs with hemodilution.[7] Generally, the volume of nonhemic prime should not exceed 40 ml/kg body weight.[7] The patient's serum total protein should be monitored and should not be allowed to decrease below 4.0 gm/100 ml, because a lower level can result in the development of pulmonary edema. The addition of commercially available albumin* helps minimize fluid loss into the extravascular space.

---

*Canine Albumin, Sigma Chemical Comp., St. Louis, MO.

TABLE 76–1. Components of an Acceptable Nonhemic Priming Solution

Component	Amount
Ringer's solution	500 ml
5% dextrose solution	500 ml
Albumin (globulin-free)	6 gm
Potassium chloride	20 mEq
Sodium bicarbonate	50 mEq

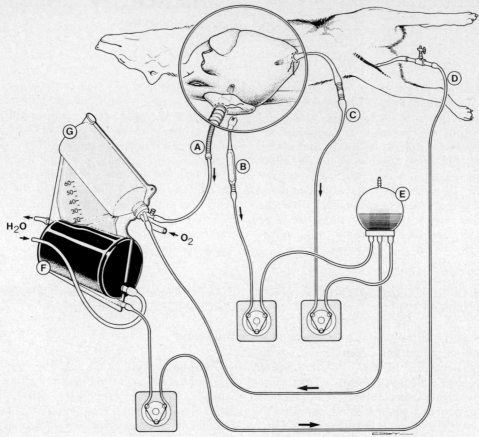

Figure 76–1. Components of the extracorporeal circulatory support unit: *A*, venous cannula inserted into right atrium; *B*, scavenger suction to salvage heparinized blood lost into the operative field; *C*, left ventricular vent; *D*, arterial cannula inserted into femoral artery (stopcock is useful for removing air bubbles and attaching pressure transducers); *E*, reservoir for suction and vent; *F*, heat exchanger; *G*, oxygenator and reservoir.

Gas Exchange Devices or Oxygenators

There are a large number of commercial oxygenators, all of which achieve a large contact area between blood and gas. Two basic types of oxygenators are available on the market: the nonmembrane (bubble) type, in which there is a direct gas-blood interface, and the membrane type, which has an artificial barrier between the gas and blood.

The bubble oxygenator is probably the more common type available to veterinary surgery. It is, unfortunately, the most dangerous type because of foaming and the possibility of air emboli. Also, the gas-blood interface is damaging to the patient's blood and may result in significant physiological changes. The Bentley-Temptrol* disposable oxygenator system is an example of a commercially available bubble oxygenator (Fig. 76–2). It has the advantages of a built-in heat exchanger, low prime volume, and various-sized units for the different flow rates required. The venous blood from the patient enters the unit, and oxygen is bubbled through the blood. (One to five per cent carbon dioxide can also be used to prevent hypocarbia.) Anesthetic agents are added to the gas mixture as needed. The oxygenated blood is

then passed through a defoaming mesh and back to the patient.

The membranous oxygenator has a thin barrier between the patient's blood and the gas mixture. The advantages are less trauma to the formed blood elements, decreased protein denaturation, and lower risk of air emboli. Further, the membrane lung acts as a filter to help remove embolic debris prior to the blood's entry into the patient's arterial system. The success of the membrane lung is demonstrated by its ability to support some human patients on a partial bypass for more than two weeks.[4]

Reservoir

The need to handle prime and to regulate blood flow during the bypass procedure requires the existence of a reservoir in the ECSU. This reservoir is usually located after the oxygenator and is a convenient site for the addition of drugs and banked blood. The volume contained in the reservoir varies with the procedure; in deep hypothermic arrest, the volume equals that of the patient's total blood volume, whereas in short procedures a minimal reserve is kept.[7]

*Bentley Laboratories, Santa Ana, CA.

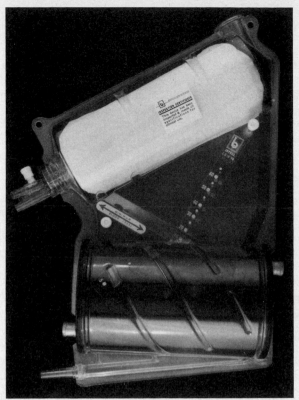

Figure 76–2. Bentley-Temptrol Oxygenator (infant size) showing oxygenator, reservoir, and heat exchanger.

Pumps or Sending Units

The "heart" of the bypass unit is the pump. Its function is to deliver an adequate volume of blood in a form physiologically acceptable to the patient's arterial system. A variable-speed roller pump is usually used to develop the pulsatile flow needed for normal physiological status. Nonocclusive rollers are used because they are less traumatic to red cells than occlusive types. The point of greatest resistance to blood flow is the arterial cannula.[7]

PHYSIOLOGICAL CHANGES IN ORGANS SECONDARY TO CARDIAC BYPASS

Blood

One of the most significant problems in cardiac bypass is damage to the formed elements of the blood. Sheer forces and surface tension encountered by the blood as it passes through the oxygenator, cannulae, and pumping unit either cause hemolysis of red cells or prematurely age cells so that they are removed by the body's reticuloendothelial system. The most traumatic portion of the ECSU is the sending unit. The "trauma index" is the amount of hemoglobin released into the plasma by a pump during a fixed number of strokes.[7] Bubble oxygenators cause the greatest amount of red cell damage

because of the gas-blood interface. White blood cells are also damaged by adhesions with abnormal surfaces. Neutrophils have a decreased killing ability after being passed through a bypass unit.[9]

Platelet function decreases after cardiac bypass.[3] This effect may be due to a decreased packed cell volume and hypoxia and will abate during the postoperative period.[3] Trauma also results in platelet aggregations that can cause ischemia in the microvasculature of the animal. The aggregates are usually temporary and reversible.

Denaturation of plasma proteins and alteration of blood lipids have also occurred secondary to sheer forces and may lead to coating of red blood cells and agglutination.[5, 7] Fats that are normally attached to proteins may be torn free, forming aggregates that produce microemboli.[2]

Alterations in serum electrolyte contents are common during cardiac bypass. Interstitial water content may increase by approximately 12 per cent.[6] The serum sodium level can increase by approximately 10 per cent and the serum potassium level can decrease by a similar amount.[4, 6] Caution must be used with animals that are being maintained on digitalis because spontaneous toxicity may develop secondary to the hypokalemia.

During cardiac bypass, epinephrine is released in increased amounts from the adrenal medulla.[4] Likewise, sympathetic nerve endings release higher amounts of norepinephrine. The combined effect is the shunting of blood away from the skeletal musculature and toward the heart and brain by variations in arteriolar vasoconstriction.[4] This shunting causes muscle hypoxia and a metabolic acidosis.

Heart

Blood, gas, or particulate matter may form microemboli in the arterial supply from the ECSU and cause infarction of the myocardium. Ischemic damage also occurs with cross-clamping of the aorta and with perfusion of an inadequate cardioplegic/hypothermic solution so that the myocardium is anoxic for an excessive period of time. Overfilling of the left ventricle is possible owing to parenchymal or bronchiolar venous drainage from the lungs. Normally prevented by "venting" of the left ventricle, overfilling results postoperatively in excessive stretching of the myocardium and decreased cardiac function.[7] The lactic acidosis that normally occurs with cardiac bypass, when coupled with the sodium and water retention previously discussed, can place an excessive postoperative workload on the heart and result in acute congestive heart failure.

Ventricular fibrillation during cardiac bypass may be either induced or spontaneous and usually is of no significance. Fibrillation makes procedures easier by permitting surgery on a nonmoving organ. It should be pointed out, however, that although ventricular fibrillation does not place significant demands on the cardiac musculature, it has no specific protective effect. Requirements for cardiac defibrillation are coarse fibrillation, good myocardial oxygenation, no pre-existing ventricular dilation or overfilling, normal blood pH, a body temperature above 25° C, and normal electrolyte levels.[7]

Lung

Pulmonary damage is one of the major causes of postoperative death in bypass patients. Pulmonary edema can occur from increased intraventricular pressure due to inadequate left ventricular venting.[7] Right-to-left vascular shunts occur from atelectasis and result in poor postoperative oxygenation of the patient's blood. Emboli released from the ECSU may cause infarction, and the release of vasoactive amines and lysosomal enzymes further damages the pulmonary tissue.[4] "Perfusion lung" is a syndrome characterized by atelectasis, pulmonary edema, and perivascular and alveolar hemorrhage.[10] The occurrence of this condition is extremely serious and usually fatal. Prevention by the use of positive end-expiratory pressure during the bypass procedure and adequate premedication of the patient is the best management.[4, 10]

Liver

Damage to the liver is more common when the bypass is being performed for repair of acquired, rather than congenital heart disease.[8] Damage due to low perfusion rates while the patient is connected to the bypass unit can combine with damage from preoperative or postoperative low cardiac output. The combined effect may result in massive central lobular necrosis.[4] At best, the reticuloendothelial system of the liver has a transient decrease in the activity of the Kupffer cells.[4] The etiology of this decreased activity is unknown.

Brain

The most severe problem with the brain and central nervous system is an embolic crisis.[7] Gas admitted into the left ventricle or particulate matter within the arterial line may be perfused into the nervous tissue, resulting in an infarction or "stroke." The percentage of animals affected by central nervous system dysfunction increases proportionally with the duration of the cardiac bypass.[4] Such dysfunctions may range from severely debilitating or fatal to a mild transitory delirium or disorientation.

Kidney

Although the kidneys can be affected by an embolic infarction, the most common problem is operative or postoperative anuria. Renal blood flow decreases on cardiac bypass, and as the systolic pressure fails, so does urine formation.[7] A mean systolic pressure below 60 mm Hg usually results in no urine formation. The use of mannitol as a premedication or as part of the ECSU prime helps maintain renal blood flow and promote diuresis.[4] Caution should be used, however, because mannitol can produce an operative or postoperative bleeding diathesis that is often uncontrollable.

Gastrointestinal Tract

The major finding in the gastrointestinal tract is a microembolic shower and ischemia to the mucosal lining.[7] The ischema can result in bacterial migration and a gram-negative bacteremia following bypass.

PHARMACOLOGY OF EXTRACORPOREAL CIRCULATORY SUPPORT

Because canine blood clots approximately twice as quickly as human blood when exposed to synthetic polymers, anticoagulant treatment is necessary when considering cardiac bypass in the dog.[7] Heparin, usually given at 200 to 400 units per kilogram of body weight (2 to 4 mg/kg) is given as an initial loading dose. One hundred to 150 units per kilogram per hour are given as maintenance during the bypass procedure. After operation, the heparin is usually neutralized by intravenous administration of an equal amount of protamine sulfate.[1, 4] Clots in the surgical field are evidence of adequate heparin reversal. Prothrombin time and other clotting tests may also be used to determine the completeness of heparin neutralization. Caution should be used when giving protamine sulfate because its vasodilator activity could cause hypotension.[4] Heparin is metabolized rapidly in the dog, and most patients return to normal within four hours. It therefore may be prudent not to use excessive amounts of reversal agents but to let the dog metabolize the heparin.

Drugs that should be considered for the premedication of the cardiac bypass patient are as follows.[4] Alpha-blockers such as acepromazine improve the blood flow to peripheral tissues and decrease the effects of the patient's own catecholamines. Broadspectrum antibiotics used prophylactically minimize the effects of bacteria released from the microscopic gastrointestinal infarcts and clostridial organism proliferation due to poor perfusion of the canine liver parenchyma. Corticosteroids should be used to help stabilize capillary membranes and reduce lysosomal disruption. Valium may be beneficial as a premedication in the prevention of shock or perfusion lung. Diuretics must be used with caution as they may potentiate the hypokalemia normally seen with cardiac bypass. Osmotic diuretics such as mannitol potentiate bleeding owing to increased intravascular pressure.

1. Adkins, J. R., and Hardy, J. D.: Sodium heparin neutralization and the anticoagulant effects of protamine sulfate. Arch. Surg. 94:175, 1967.
2. Allardyce, D. B., Yoshida, S. H., and Ashmore, P. G.: The importance of microembolism in the pathogenesis of organ dysfunction caused by prolonged use of the pump oxygenator. J. Thorac. Cardiovasc. Surg. 52:706, 1966.
3. Ekert, H., and Sheers, M.: Preoperative and postoperative platelet function in cyanotic congenital heart disease. J. Thorac. Cardiovasc. Surg. 67:184, 1974.
4. Ionescu, M. I., and Wooler, G. H.: Current Techniques in Extracorporeal Circulation. Butterworth, Boston, 1967.
5. Lee, W. H., Jr., Krumhaar, O., Fonkalsruo, E. W., et al.: Denaturation of plasma proteins as a cause of morbidity and death after intracardiac operations. Surgery 50:29, 1961.
6. Pacifico, A. D., Digerness, S., and Kirklin, J. W.: Acute alterations of body composition after open intracardiac operations. Circulation 41:331, 1970.
7. Peirce, E. C.: Extracorporeal Circulation for Open-heart Surgery. Charles C Thomas, Springfield, 1969.
8. Sanderson, R. G., Ellison, J. H., and Benson, J. A., Jr.: Jaundice following open-heart surgery. Ann. Surg. 165:217, 1967.
9. Silva, J., Jr., Hoeksema, H., and Fekety, F. R., Jr.: Transient defects in phagocytic functions during cardiopulmonary bypass. J. Thorac. Cardiovasc. Surg. 67:175, 1974.
10. Weedn, R. J., Coalson, J. J., and Greenfield, L. J.: Effects of oxygen and ventilation on pulmonary mechanics and ultrastructure during cardiopulmonary bypass. Am. J. Surg. 120:584, 1970.
11. Wilkens, H., Regelson, W., and Hoffmeister, F. S.: The physiologic importance of pulsatile blood flow. N. Engl. J. Med. 267:443, 1962.

Cardiopulmonary Bypass for Implantation of an Artificial Heart and for Cardiac Transplantation*

Don B. Olsen

Cardiopulmonary bypass (CPB) has been an effective tool for a number of years. The dog has long been used as an experimental model and for teaching CPB techniques in the laboratory. The application of CPB equipment and technology to calves and sheep was made in an effort to use these animals for specific purposes, including the test and evaluation of adult, human-sized devices such as prosthetic heart valves (mechanical and biological) and right or left ventricular assist, biventricular assist, and total cardiac replacement devices. This discussion briefly describes the procedures and special equipment required to put a calf on CPB, to implant a pneumatic total artificial heart and later, to remove it and to transplant a viable natural heart from the calf's twin. Special techniques for operative and postoperative management of the recipients are also presented.

CARDIOPULMONARY BYPASS

Dizygotic chimeric twin calves, three months old, are screened for general health and blood samples are obtained for base-line values.[1, 5, 10] After being housed for a minimum of three to five days in the laboratory, the larger of the two animals is held off feed for 18 hours and off water for 12 hours before induction of anesthesia. Fermentation gases within the rumen are controlled by administering two grams of neomycin sulfate orally four to six hours before anesthesia. An indwelling intravenous cannula is placed in the left jugular vein, and 4 mg of atropine and approximately 750 mg of pentothal are administered. The calf is placed in left lateral recumbency, intubated with a cuffed tracheal tube and protected with a biting block, and its mouth is taped shut. The tracheal tube is connected to a Bird Mark 14, pressure-regulated respirator at 80 per cent to 20 per cent air–oxygen mix, and fluothane is administered at between 0 and 0.75 per cent. The previously placed intravenous cannula is fixed with a silk dermal suture, and lactated Ringer's solution is administered as an intravenous drip.

The right rear leg is tied in a spread fashion, exposing the saphenous artery and vein in the medial aspect of the thigh of the left leg. The animal is clipped, with the hair removed from the area of the saphenous artery and vein, the right jugular furrow, and extensively over the right thorax. This area is prepared with soap and water followed by liberal amounts of iodoform solution. The excess solution used in the surgical preparation of the skin is carefully removed from the surgery table to avoid subsequent chemical burns. A large pad approximately 10 to 12 centimeters thick is placed between the calf and the table at the sixth rib, to flex the spine and facilitate exposure through the right chest wall. The animal is draped with sterile linen drapes, with a Steridrape

*Editor's Note: Dr. Olsen's historic efforts were instrumental in the development of the first artificial heart implanted in a human. He contributed this part of Chapter 76 by special request. The material is included here as an example of the application of surgical science, in the hope that the philosophy and some of the findings may be useful in clinical practice and research.

This work was supported in part by grants from the National Institutes of Health via the National Heart, Lung, and Blood Institute's grant No. HL 24419.

placed over the chest incision site. Epidermal cannulae are placed in the saphenous artery and vein, and the venous catheter is advanced into the abdomen at approximately the level of the renal veins. Venous blood pressure measurements obtained here are referred to as central venous pressure. These catheters are fixed and a suture is placed around the vessel (allowing the catheters to be withdrawn on day one or two postoperatively), and tied percutaneously, obliterating the vessel to avoid any hemorrhage.

A midcervical incision is made over the right jugular furrow, exposing the carotid artery and jugular vein. Umbilical tape tourniquets are placed proximally and distally on the exposed vessels in preparation for cannulation for cardiopulmonary bypass. The skin is incised over the rib, extending from approximately 12 cm from the dorsal midline to slightly below the costochondral junction. The skin incision is made with a sharp blade, and the subsequent incision is made with electrocautery for optimum hemostasis. After the skin and cutaneous trunci muscle are incised, the incision is manipulated cranially and continued through the musculature onto the rib. Subcuticular and subcutaneous trunci tunnels are made, extending from the seventh intercostal space at the costochondral junction dorsally to almost ten to 12 centimeters from the dorsal midline for the left pneumatic drive line. A similar tunnel is made from the sixth intercostal space, extending to approximately five to seven centimeters cranially from the exit of the left drive line. This tunnelling and perforation of the skin are done prior to the administration of anticoagulants. Umbilical tapes are threaded through these tunnels to lead the respective drive lines. The periosteum over the fifth rib is incised and scraped free of the rib, which is cut at the dorsal aspect of the incision and snapped free at the costochondral junction at the distal end of the incision. The incision is continued through the periosteal bed and the adhered pleura into the thorax. The incision is extended ventrally in the fourth interspace, approximately two to three centimeters, the internal thoracic artery and vein being avoided.

The phrenic nerve is lifted from the right lateral aspect of the cranial vena cava, and an umbilical tape tourniquet is passed around the cranial vena cava to avoid encompassing the phrenic nerve. The tourniquet around the cranial vena cava is placed caudal to the azygous vein. If this is not possible, an additional tourniquet is placed around the azygous vein. A similar tourniquet is placed beneath the phrenic nerve on the caudal vena cava. The entire right lateral wall of the pericardium is removed, with the dorsal incision just inferior to the phrenic nerve. Care is taken to avoid entry into the left pleural space. The calf has an intact mediastinum, which prevents cross-contamination of any blood or air into the left hemithorax. An incision is made through the right lateral aspect of the pleural pouch surrounding the intermediate lobe of the right lung that communicates with the right chest between the aorta and the caudal vena cava. A rayon umbilical tape is placed around the aorta by dissecting the pulmonary artery free from the cranioventral aspect of the aorta and blindly placing a Favaloro clamp around the aorta through the cardiac sinus. The calf has a very short ascending aorta; therefore, care should be taken in placing this tourniquet so that the brachiocephalic trunk is not the only vessel within the tourniquet. Careful inspection is made throughout all incisions, and stringent hemostasis is established for administration of heparin (3 mg/kg).

The components of the cardiopulmonary priming solution are listed in Table 76–2. A multiple-head cardiopulmonary bypass unit is used and facilities for hypothermia are available. Bubble oxygenators have been effective in the calf; however, membrane oxygenators are superior and are absolutely essential for cardiopulmonary bypass in the sheep. The cardiopulmonary bypass circuit is established as follows:

The arterial return cannula is placed retrograde in the right carotid artery, to which a tourniquet has been applied previously. Preparation is made for reanastomosis of the incision into the carotid artery, and the cannula is fixed. Care is taken to assure this cannula fixation in order to avoid a blowout under the high pressures of the flow, 6 liters/min., used in the calf. It is also advisable to use the largest-bore catheter for the carotid artery. The carotid cannula remains cross-clamped until the initiation of partial bypass. A large-bore 30F venous cannula is passed via the jugular vein into the cranial vena cava. The catheter tip is positioned two to four centimeters cranially from the previously placed cranial vena cava tourniquet. This cannula remains cross-clamped until initiation of partial bypass. The venous blood from the caudal vena cava is collected by a 30F catheter introduced through an atriotomy of the right auricular appendage and passed into the caudal vena cava. With great consistency, this cannula enters the coronary venous sinus, but with transmural digital manipulation, the tip of the catheter can be directed into the posterior vena cava. The tip of the catheter is positioned right at the vena cava hiatus of the diaphragm. All of the cardiopulmonary bypass lines and placed cannula must be primed. Small amounts of air in the venous cannula are not serious; however, large amounts of air cause an airlock in the venous return. Air must be avoided in the arterial line.

The arterial return cannula cross-clamp is removed, as are both cross-clamps on the cranial and

TABLE 76–2. Priming Solution for Cardiopulmonary Bypass in the Calf

Component	Amount
Lactated Ringer's solution	2.5 liters
Dextran 40	500 ml
Sodium bicarbonate	50 mEq
Cephalosporin	2 gm
Beef lung heparin	10,000 units

caudal vena caval lines. Partial bypass is maintained for approximately three to four minutes to permit dilution of the priming solutions with the circulatory blood volume of the calf. Because 100 per cent of the cardiopulmonary bypass return goes directly to the brain of the calf, it is not desirable to have a rapid influx of priming solutions. It is not uncommon to find hypotension at this time. Hypotension can be eliminated by alerting the pump technician to avoid removing too much blood from the calf to the venous reservoirs of the circuit. It is advisable not to use vasoconstrictive agents, but rather to manage the hypotension with volumes and flows.

During this interim of partial bypass, two things are accomplished:

1. Any source of hemorrhage subsequent to total anticoagulation of the calf is located and corrected.

2. The apex of the heart is tipped out of the pericardial sac and a 2-0 braided-silk suture is passed twice around the hemiazygous vein as it traverses the left lateral aspect of the left atrial wall, slightly posterior to the left atrium.

Total cardiopulmonary bypass is established by tightening the caudal and the cranial vena caval tourniquets. Careful monitoring of the central venous pressure is important to establish the efficacy of the venous return from the caudal part of the animal to the circuit. The femoral artery pressure, monitored via the saphenous arterial catheter, is also important in assuring adequate pressure through the arterial system. Induction of hypothermia is started through the heat exchanger in the membrane oxygenator to approximately 30°C. Care is taken to avoid temperature differential greater than 10°C in the heat exchange system.

IMPLANTATION OF THE PNEUMATIC TOTAL ARTIFICIAL HEART

Residual left ventricular blood is manually expressed from the ventricle while the aortic tourniquet is tightened. When the aortic tourniquet is closed, the right ventricular wall and septum are quickly opened to accommodate blood returning to the left ventricle via the bronchial arteries. The volume of left-to-left shunt through the bronchial veins has never been quantitated in the calf, but our estimates indicate that it is approximately six per cent of the cardiac ouput. Early venting of the closed left ventricular cavity avoids pulmonary edema associated with high left atrial pressures from blood entering from an arterial source. The ventricular myocardium is transected from the atria at the atrial-ventricular groove, leaving the leaflets of the tricuspid and mitral valves with the atria. These leaflets are trimmed, leaving the valvular annular ring to which the atrial cuff anastomoses may be sutured. The coronary venous sinus is occluded by placing a suture circumscribing the orifice as it enters the right atrium.

The pulmonary artery with its intact pulmonary valve is freed from the cranial margin of the right atrium and the aorta. The previous incision separating the pulmonary artery from the aorta for the tourniquet is continued toward the pulmonary valve, and the pulmonary artery is separated from the cranial margin of the right atrium by an incision through the supraventricular crest in the right ventricular outflow tract. The right coronary artery, remaining on the aorta that was separated from the pulmonary artery, is used as a landmark. Approximately three to four millimeters of right ventricular outflow tract remain subvalvular.

The aorta stays attached to the cranial left atrium. The right coronary artery is ligated, and any small auxiliary branches forming the right coronary artery system are oversewn with fine sutures. The left main coronary artery is ligated. When needed, the left coronary artery is an ideal port of entry for the placement of a chronically indwelling, open-port, pressure-monitoring and sampling catheter. For this and subsequent manipulations of the aorta, the tourniquet is replaced by a Satinski clamp.

Suturing of the atrial cuffs and the aortic vascular graft has been described previously in detail.[7] In summary: The aorta is sutured to the vascular graft with a continuous mattress suture, and the left atrial cuff and aorta are sewn, encompassing the anterior leaflet of the mitral valve by a continuous suture using 3-0 prolene. The atrial septum is included in a mattress suture joining the right and left atria. The remaining parts of the atrial cuffs are sutured in a simple continuous suture pattern. The pulmonary artery vascular graft is secured with a continuous mattress suture, and all anastomoses are tested and evaluated for leaks. Any hemorrhage under pressure is corrected with carefully placed interrupted sutures, some of which may be pledgeted.

The left ventricle is brought to the thoracic incision, and the drive line is passed into the chest through the incision and then through the thoracic wall at the costochondral junction of the seventh interspace. This drive line is passed along the subcutaneous tunnel and leaves the previously perforated skin in the right lateral thoracic wall via the stress-relief, percutaneous skin button (a device at the skin–drive line interface).

The left pneumatic drive line is passed off the table to the heart driver. The aortic quick connector is snapped onto the valveless outflow tract of the artificial ventricle and the left atrial quick connector to the inlet port of the left ventricle. The ventricle is primed, all air being removed. Air removal is facilitated by starting the respirator, and removing the Satinski clamp from the aorta, and distorting the aortic valve annulus to permit retrograde flow of arterial blood into the left ventricle, giving assurance that all air has been removed from the aorta. The left ventricle is pumped at 40 beats/min., with sufficient driving pressure to overcome the aortic pressure as demonstrated by a synchronous pulse wave in the femoral artery pressure monitor.

The aortic and left atrial anastomoses suture lines are inspected for leaks. The respirator is turned on, and the previously collapsed lungs are gently and rhythmically reinflated. The left ventricle is positioned in the most ventral caudal space of the pericardial sac—resulting in optimum alignment of the aortic outflow tract without reducing the left atrial space—and the excessive line is pulled from the thorax and exteriorized. The severed edges of the remaining pericardium are carefully inspected for hemorrhage, and hemostasis is established using electrocautery. A thorough inspection of the chest is made for any hemorrhage, and the accessible suture lines are again inspected for leaks. The right ventricle is brought into the field; the drive line is passed off to the heart driver. The pulmonary artery is brought into apposition with the right ventricular outflow port of the artificial ventricle, care being taken that no torsion exists in the pulmonary artery vascular graft, a common source of increased pulmonary vascular resistance due to constriction of the outflow tract. The connection is made, and the right atrium is connected to the tricuspid inflow valve of the right ventricle. The tourniquet around the caudal vena cava is released, permitting venous blood to fill the right atrium and the right ventricle during the primary procedure. After assurance that all air has been removed from the right side, the pumping of the right heart is initiated.

At this point, both ventricles are pulsing at 40 beats. Approximately 35 per cent of the duty cycle is systole. The air driving pressures of the right and left side are tuned for full ejection. The cardiopulmonary bypass machine supplies approximately 75 per cent of the total body perfusion. The respirator is adjusted for approximately 18 to 22 breaths/min., with peak inflation pressure of 22 to 24 cm H_2O using 100 per cent oxygen. Any potential bleeding sites are carefully evaluated, and necessary corrections are made. The tourniquet around the cranial vena cava line is loosened, and the tourniquets of the cranial and caudal vena cavae are removed. The caudal return cannula is clamped, the cannula is removed, a Satinski clamp is applied across the right auricular appendage, and a ligature is placed to secure this aperture. The heart rate is gradually increased weaning the calf from the cardiopulmonary bypass machine. At this juncture, the artificial ventricles could quickly take over the total circulatory support for the animal. However, in most cases, additional oxygenation of the blood is required, and bypass is maintained at approximately two to 2.5 liters/min. over the next ten to 15 minutes. Ventilation-perfusion shunts are common in the laterally recumbent calf, after flow returns through the previously apneic lungs. Pulmonary shunting persists in some cases until the calf is placed in sternal recumbency. Pulmonary function improves dramatically in all calves when sternal recumbency is attained.

Two chest drains are placed, one cranial and one caudal to the artificial ventricle, perforating the skin on the right lateral thorax. The rib spreader is removed, and the periosteal bed of the excised fifth rib is approximated with chromic gut. Care is taken to achieve good apposition with the use of the periosteal bed as a good suture medium for the first layer of closure. In the young calf, there is a remarkable regeneration of the fifth rib in the periosteal bed, with near-total replacement by three months. The muscle layers are closed separately using hemostatic techniques during closure. The skin over the thorax is closed, and the jugular CPB line is removed. Most of the priming blood from the bypass unit is returned via the carotid artery, depending on individual needs. The carotid arteriotomy and jugular venotomy are closed with 6-0 prolene, and the neck incision is closed.

Protamine sulfate, 3 mg/kg, is administered to neutralize the heparin. The calf is placed in the recovery cart. Primary treatment consists of maintaining normothermia by a warm-water blanket and normovolemia by monitoring the chest drainage volume. This volume is replaced with blood transfusions obtained from slaughterhouse donors to maintain normal hematocrit. During the first 8 hours after cardiopulmonary bypass, 90 mEq of potassium chloride is administered routinely. Frequently, the serum potassium levels do not indicate the need for additional potassium; however, when potassium is not given, the calf develops hypokalemia in the early part of the second day after cardiopulmonary bypass.

The saphenous artery catheter is used to measure arterial pressure and obtain samples for arterial blood gases. The saphenous vein catheter is used to monitor central venous pressure and mixed venous blood gases. The respirator is adjusted accordingly, with a gradual weaning from 100 per cent O_2 toward 40 per cent O_2, and early extubation is accomplished.[2, 8]

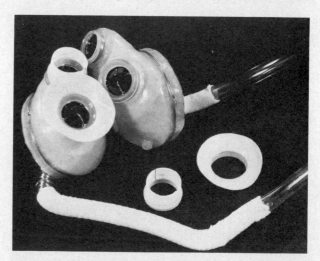

Figure 76–3. A pneumatic total artificial heart. The right ventricle is shown with the atrial cuff and pulmonary artery vascular grafts' quick connectors removed. The pneumatic drive lines are covered with velour on those portions remaining intrathoracically and through the thoracic wall. The stroke volume of this heart is 165 ml.

THE ARTIFICIAL HEART

The Jarvik-5 pneumatically powered total artificial heart is fabricated from a segmented, polyether-polyurethane (Biomer). The ventricles consist of a rigid base fastened into a semi-rigid housing with an inflow and outflow port. Each ventricle has an atrial quick connector that is sutured to the remnant atria of the recipient. The atrial cuff snaps onto a rigid valve-holding ring mounted in the ventricle (Fig. 76–3). Low-profile, 29-mm tilting-disc, mechanical valves are used. There are four thin, flexible polyurethane diaphragms, with graphite lubrication between them, separating the blood chamber from the air chamber.[9] The air chamber is connected to a two-meter plastic drive line. These drive lines have a velour covering on their intrathoracic and transthoracic segments, and then a specially designed percutaneous device referred to as a skin button. The skin button is movable along the drive line to facilitate surgical implantation. The outflow port of the ventricle has a rigid quick connector that fastens to a Dacron vascular graft, which is anastomosed end-to-end to either the aorta or the pulmonary artery. The outflow valve-holding ring can be fitted with 27-mm tilting-disc, mechanical valves, or the natural aortic and pulmonary artery valves can be retained *in situ*.[7]

The pneumatic drive lines are connected to an artificial heart driver which delivers pulsatile air into the ventricles. The Utah heart driver is operated at fixed rate with manually-selected left and right driving pressures and heart rate. The cardiac cycle is adjusted according to the percentage of the cycle in systole, which is approximately 35 to 40 per cent. The cardiac performance is monitored by using a specially designed and built cardiac output monitor and diagnostic unit (COMDU).[6] This device quantitates the amount of blood entering each ventricle by extracorporeally measuring the amount of air exhausted from the pneumatic driver. The COMDU also simultaneously displays the rate of fill of the right and left ventricles. The display is a valuable monitor of stroke volume, filling rate, and cardiac output. Changes in any of these parameters aid in diagnosis.

POSTOPERATIVE MANAGEMENT

Each calf is housed in an individual cart,[10] which is designed to permit the calf to stand up, lie down, and take one or two steps forward or backward. The front panel swings away and permits the calf to be led forward onto a treadmill, and then back off into its cart. The heart driver is placed on a platform suspended on the top of the wheeled calf cart (Fig. 76–4).

No anticoagulants have been given in this series of experiments. Most commonly, the animals receive only the five days of postoperative antibiotics. The calves are offered *ad libitum* water and alfalfa hay

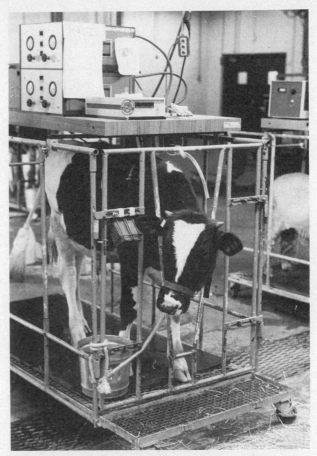

Figure 76–4. A total artificial heart recipient calf. The calf is housed in a cage on wheels with a platform on top of the cage. The platform holds two pneumatic heart drivers and a time-lapse clock. The central air supply, power, and monitoring lines are overhead to keep the floor uncluttered.

and a high-protein supplement. Usually by the second postoperative day they have healthy appetites.

The recovered calves are walked on the treadmill three times per week for up to one hour per exercise period and are kept in a good state of health, growing at a rate quite comparable to that of calves with natural hearts. All blood chemistry and hematological valves return to normal within seven to ten days postoperatively; these values are monitored frequently in the early postoperative course and then weekly thereafter.

CARDIAC TRANSPLANTATION

The calves are maintained on the total artificial heart for 40 to 70 days, and then undergo reoperation. Cardiopulmonary bypass and explantation procedures were previously developed on calves with total artificial hearts used for ventricular replacement or excision of pannus in the inflow tracts.[3]

The techniques successfully developed by the Stanford group are used for the preparation and removal of the donor heart with the appropriate cardioplegia and hypothermia.[4] The transplant recipient is prepared by exposure of the right artificial ventricle through a right lateral thoracotomy. Strong adhesions between the previous suture line and the lung are more easily managed by entering the thorax in the fourth periosteal bed. The lung is reflected dorsally with exposure of the right atrium and pulmonary artery. Heparin is given because the calf has not been given anticoagulants. Cardiopulmonary bypass is established with the same configuration as for implantation of the artificial heart: arterial return retrograde into the right carotid artery, with one venous uptake in the cranial vena cava through the right jugular vein and the other in the caudal vena cava via the caudal roof of the right atrium. A fine purse-string suture is placed in the main right pulmonary vein for a left ventricular vent cannula. Cardiopulmonary bypass is started, the anterior and posterior vena cava tourniquets are occluded, the right ventricle is turned off and the atrial and pulmonary artery quick connectors are released. The air drive line between the chest wall and subcutaneous tissues is transected, and the right ventricle is removed. The left ventricle is pulsed at 40 beats/min., while the pseudopericardium, pulmonary artery, and aorta are debrided. The left ventricle is turned off, the atrial and aortic connectors are released, the drive line is transected, and the ventricle is removed. The intact natural aortic valve does not leak, and with the ventricle removed, the aorta is more easily cross-clamped with a Satinski clamp.

The atrial quick connectors are excised with the appropriate amount of atrial wall. The aortic and pulmonary artery connectors and their valves are excised for a cardiac recipient, as described for clinical cardiac transplantation.[4] The suturing order of the transplant is modified from the human (transsternal approach) to the calf (right lateral thoracotomy).

The donor heart, in which cardioplegia has been induced with crystalloid via the coronary artery, is kept cool with multiple changes of iced saline. The left ventricle is vented via the purse-string–sutured pulmonary vein, and the aortic cross-clamp is removed after the left-side anastomosis is completed. The first coronary venous blood is discarded, to eliminate the residual cardioplegic (hyperkalemic) solution. Care is taken to eliminate all air from the chambers. Spontaneous sinus rhythm occurs in some cases, but 100 to 200 watt-sec. (joules) of counter shock are used when needed. Left ventricular decompression is maintained via the vent for 20 to 30 minutes before the left myocardium is permitted to work. The left ventricular vent is occluded, and the caval tourniquets are released to increase the ventricular myocardial workload gradually. Isoproterenol is given in increments for optimal heart rate, and the calf is weaned from cardiopulmonary bypass. Hemostasis is attained by neutralizing the heparin with protamine, and the chest is closed in the manner described for the implantation of the total artificial heart.

After the thoracotomy closure is completed, the percutaneous drive line leads are removed by making an elliptical incision around the cutaneous interface and manual retraction. The calf is removed from the table, and the previously placed saphenous arterial and venous catheters (for measuring arterial and central venous pressures) and the electrocardiogram are monitored. Antibiotics and isoproterenol are the only drugs administered.

RESULTS

The first two attempted cardiac transplantations in twin calves were unsuccessful. The problem was in obtaining adequate cardiac output from the transplanted hearts. When the bypass unit was removed, the ventricles dilated and repeatedly fibrillated. It was concluded that inadequate cardioplegia and hypothermic cardiac preservation were attained. Furthermore, the blood entering the left atrium distended the left heart and had to be expelled into the aorta by manual massage. This process bruised the myocardium and caused extravasation of the anticoagulated blood.

In subsequent cases, more topical cooling was used, with frequent changes of iced saline over the donor heart. More importantly, a left ventricular vent was placed via a pulmonary vein. This eliminated the need to periodically empty the accumulated blood manually. These techniques were perfected successfully in a pair of twin calves in which the recipient had not received a total artificial heart.

The results of blood typing tests on all twins clearly identified them as chimeric, dizygotic twins. The females all had hermaphroditic (freemartin) genital tract development. Post-transplantation hemorrhage was the cause of death in one case, and a small cerebral thromboembolus caused death in another.

Cardiac transplantation was successfully done in one calf after 44 days on the total artificial heart. This calf (Fernando) lived for 12 months on the heart transplanted from its brother. It died from pulmonary thromboemboli as a result of repeated cardiac catheterization and thermodilution cardiac output determinations. There was no cardiac rejection.

The final experiment in the series was a pair of twin calves (Charley and Diane) of which the male was kept on a total artificial heart for 74 days and then successfully given its sister's heart. This animal had five days of antibiotic therapy and no immunosuppressives. At the time of writing, Charley had lived 27 months after transplantation and was the herd sire for 125 dairy cattle, with the first calves expected in 30 days.

Cardiac transplantation had never previously been achieved in calves; however, their immunotolerance has long been known.[1, 5, 7, 10] Figure 76–5 shows the cardiac output for several calves as they grew and gained in weight. Measurements were made on calves with a natural heart, a total artificial heart, and

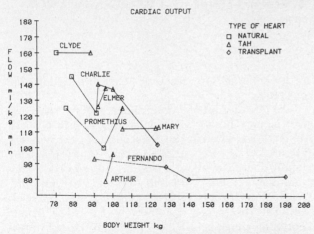

Figure 76–5. The cardiac output (ml/kg-min) plotted against the body weight in kilograms. The decline of cardiac output is not related to the type of the heart implanted but rather is a function of body size. *TAH*, total artificial heart.

a transplanted heart. The blood chemistry and coagulation profiles remained within the normal values for calves of similar age and weight.

DISCUSSION AND CONCLUSIONS

The calf, currently the most commonly used animal for artificial heart research, presents some unique features for tissue or organ transplantation. Anatomically, the side-to-side compressed chest creates slightly different heart and great vessel placement within the chest. These alterations are much more easily handled with a trans-sternal surgical approach. However, the thickness of the sternum and the attending stress associated with the early postoperative ambulation essential to the calf's well being negates the sternal approach.[8]

The most extensive work on transplantation in calves was reported in 1965 by Stone and colleagues.[11] They reported that skin grafts were completely rejected by cattle twins in from 122 to 468 days, with a mean rejection time of 229 days. This chronic rejection was not affected by irradiation. The conclusions drawn from these studies would suggest that the immunological tolerance of the dizygotic twins was not permanent.[11] The results of cardiac transplantation suggest that the rejection of transplanted skin is not a true rejection but more probably an expulsion or crowding out of the transplanted germinal layers by the recipient during the normal growth and cellular dynamics of stratified squamous epithelium.

Explantation of the total artificial heart was also best accomplished via right lateral thoracotomy.[3] The cardiac transplantation techniques developed in humans were modified slightly for the calf. Removal of the prosthesis was simplified by the use of the previously developed quick connector system. Very little encapsulation of the ventricles was encountered,

but the adhesions of the lung to the chest wall and pulmonary artery outflow tract were severe. Venting the left ventricle to avoid dilation and the associated cardiac massage was necessary for success. It was important to permit the ventricles to beat without a workload (no blood) for ten to 25 minutes, to avoid fibrillation and allow reconstitution of the high-energy phosphate bonds (ATP). All monozygotic twins are tissue-compatible in all species of animals. Dizygotic twins in cattle exhibit a high percentage (more than 93 per cent) of free martinism. However, it was found through blood typing in my laboratory that chimerism occurred in 100 per cent of the twins. It occurs from the intraplacental anastomosis of the fetal vascular systems. Each fetus was therefore inoculated with the circulating stem cells of the opposite twin to preclude the necessity for immunosuppression. Stone and colleagues[11] demonstrated that this tissue compatibility was not permanent, and twins eventually rejected skin grafts over six to 18 months. The cardiac-transplanted calves, however, have not shown rejection after nine, ten, 12, and 25 months.

The calves with total artificial hearts and with transplanted hearts continued to grow at a rate comparable to that of normal calves. Of greater importance, the transplanted bovine hearts with severed nerves continued to grow in all proportions to an adult size.

1. Billingham, R. E., and Lampkin, G. H.: Further studies in tissue homotransplantation in cattle. J. Embryol. Exp. Morphol. 5:351, 1957.
2. Fukumasu, H., Iwaya, F., Olsen, D. B., et al.: Surgical implantation of the Jarvik-5 total artificial heart in a calf. Trans. Am. Soc. Artif. Intern. Organs 25:232, 1979.
3. Fukumasu, H., Olsen, D. B., Lawson, J., et al.: Reoperative surgery in calves with a total artificial heart. J. Artif. Organs 3:24, 1980.
4. Griepp, R. B., Stinson, E. B., Bieber, C. P., et al.: Human heart transplantation: current status. Ann. Thorac. Surg. 22:171, 1976.
5. Lillie, F. R.: The theory of the freemartin. Science 53:611, 1916.
6. Nielsen, S. D., Willshaw, P., Nanas, J., and Olsen, D. B.: Non-invasive cardiac monitoring and diagnostics for pneumatic pumping ventricles. Trans. Am. Soc. Artif. Intern. Organs 29:(in press), 1983.
7. Olsen, D. B., Kilff, J., Lawson, J., et al.: Saving the aortic and pulmonary artery valves with total artificial heart replacement. Trans. Am. Soc. Artif. Intern. Organs 22:468, 1976.
8. Olsen, D. B., Fukumasu, H., Kolff, J., et al.: Implantation of the total artificial heart by lateral thoracotomy. J. Artif. Organs 1:92, 1977.
9. Olsen, D. B., Kessler, T. R., Pons, A. B., et al.: Fabrication, implantation and pathophysiology of the total artificial heart in calves for six months. *In* Pierce, W. S. (ed.): *USA-USSR Joint Symposium on Circulatory Assistance and the Artificial Heart, Tbilisi, USSR.* (N.I.H. No. 80-2032.), National Institutes of Health, Washington, D. C., 1981.
10. Owen, R. D.: Immunogenetic consequences of vascular anastomoses between bovine twins. Science 102:400, 1947.
11. Stone, W. H., Cragle, R. G., Swanson, E. W., and Brown, D. G.: Skin grafts: delayed rejection between pairs of cattle twins showing erythrocyte chimerism. Science 148:1335, 1965.

Chapter 77

Basic Peripheral Vascular Procedures

Philip Litwak

ARTERIOTOMY

Arteriotomy is the act of incising an artery. It is the basic procedure in vascular surgery. The care with which the arteriotomy is made can influence the ultimate outcome of the procedure.

If the vessel is to be totally occluded for an arteriotomy, the patient should be heparinized. If partial occlusion is to be used, heparinization may be required. Either appropriate clamps or umbilical tape and traction can be used to occlude the vessel (Fig. 77–1). Arteriotomy incisions are generally made parallel to the long axis of the vessel (Fig. 77–2). Transverse arteriotomies are used when catheters are being introduced, because there is less diminution of diameter when a transverse incision is closed (Fig. 77–3). A scalpel is used initially to incise the artery, and the incision is lengthened with sharp scissors. The incision should be made perpendicular to the vessel wall to prevent necrotic edges that can result from a bevelled incision. Loosely adherent adventitia should be removed so as not to be dragged into the vessel lumen with the suture material. During handling of the vessel edges, care should be exercised not to pinch them in the forceps' jaws, as pinching can damage endothelium and precipitate thrombosis. Arteriotomies are closed with either a simple continuous suture or simple interrupted sutures. The needle penetrates the vessel wall perpendicular to the surface, and the holes are directly across the incision from each other. This practice results in the strongest bite of vessel wall with the least amount of suture material within the lumen. A slight outward rolling of the cut edges is desirable to ensure endothelial apposition.

Size of the artery determines suture size and placement. The aorta of a large dog is sutured with 4-0 material, whereas the distal aorta of a cat requires 6-0 or 7-0 suture. An aortotomy in a large dog requires sutures about every 2 mm placed 2 mm from the cut edge. At the opposite extreme, the distal feline aorta is sutured at about 1-mm intervals with sutures placed 1 mm from the edge. Knots should be snug against the vessel wall but not drawn down tightly, so as to avoid necrosis and subsequent aneurysm or hemorrhage. The proximal occluding clamp or suture is released before the final suture is tied, to allow air and thrombi to be flushed out of the vessel. After distal occlusion is released, pressure over the incision controls bleeding. The temptation to stop leakage with additional sutures should be avoided, unless the leak is severe. Extra sutures can lead to further leakage and weakening of the vessel. Even spurting wounds can usually be stopped with five minutes of direct pressure.

VENOTOMY

Venotomy is rarely indicated in veterinary surgery. When required, it is done like an arteriotomy. However, for suturing of a vein, it is unusual to use larger than 5-0 or 6-0 material. The suture pullout strength of veins is almost twice that of comparably sized arteries, unless excess adventitia has been removed from the vein.

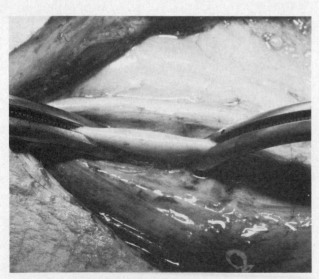

Figure 77–1. Application of DeBakey vascular clamps to the carotid artery. Closure is just tight enough to occlude flow. Slippage of complete occlusion clamps is usually not a problem.

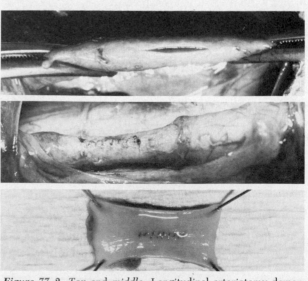

Figure 77–2. *Top* and *middle*, Longitudinal arteriotomy demonstrating typical diminution of diameter that occurs with this procedure. *Bottom*, The luminal side of the suture line.

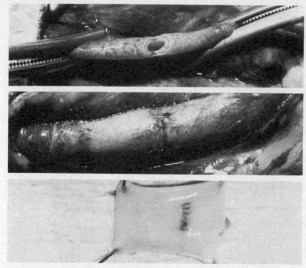

Figure 77–3. *Top* and *middle,* Transverse arteriotomy demonstrating the preservation of vessel diameter using this technique. *Bottom,* The luminal side of the suture line.

ANASTOMOTIC TECHNIQUES

The most common anastomotic techniques are end-to-end and end-to-side, with specific indications for each. Most prosthetic grafts are sewn end-to-side.

End-to-end direct reconnection of vessels is the procedure of choice only when they can be approximated without tension. There are many variations of the basic technique, depending on the location, size, and condition of the vessel.

With the patient heparinized and the two ends occluded, a test fit should be made to ensure the lack of tension. The exposed ends must be cleanly cut, with no adventitia covering them. Excess adventitia can be stretched over and cut flush with the end (Fig. 77–4). When released it usually retracts several millimeters from the end.

Using a suture with needles on each end, the surgeon passes one needle through each of the vessel ends from inside to outside, to keep knots outside

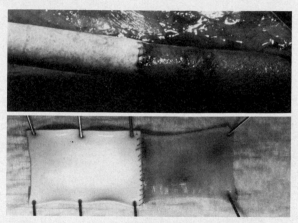

Figure 77–5. *Top,* Completed end-to-end anastomosis illustrating proper graft-to-vessel size matching and equidistant suture placement, which prevents gaps in the suture line. *Bottom,* The same anastomosis from the luminal side.

the vessel lumen. A second suture is similarly placed 180 degrees from the first. These two corner sutures are tied. It may be necessary for an assistant to hold the vessel ends together by the occluding clamps, thus removing all stress from these two sutures. The anterior wall is sutured in a simple continuous pattern, with all bites equidistant and the vessel edges everted. Extreme care must be taken to ensure equal-sized bites of vessel, because severe leakage can result from the mismatched ends. Each suture is tied as the anastomosis proceeds. There should be no obvious crimping of the vessel walls by sutures that are pulled too tight. The first suture end is tied to one end of the other suture when the anterior wall is completed. The back wall is exposed by passing one of the remaining sutures under the vessel to turn it over. The posterior wall is sutured as the anterior wall was. Tension on the unused suture end keeps the vessel turned to provide adequate visibility. The last loop of suture is left loose, and the proximal clamp is released. When all apparent air and thrombi have been flushed out, the last suture is tied. Direct pressure may be required if there is leakage (Fig. 77–5).

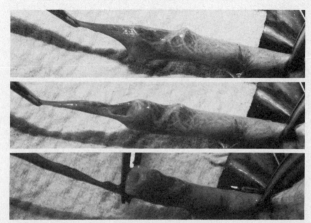

Figure 77–4. Removal of excess adventitia from the end of a severed vessel. Care must be taken not to cut the vascular wall when cutting the stretched adventitia.

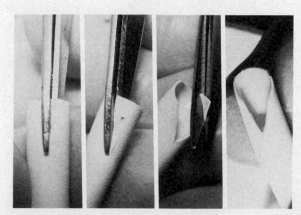

Figure 77–6. Traditional steps in trimming the end of a prosthetic graft in preparation for a "cobra-head" end-to-side anastomosis. Sharp scissors are used to prevent frayed edges.

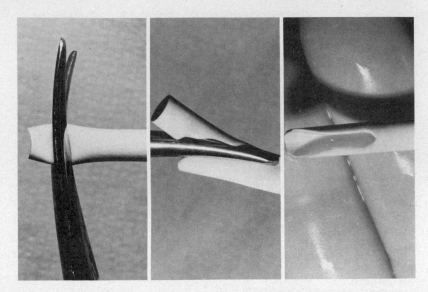

Figure 77–7. Modified steps in trimming the end of a prosthetic graft in preparation for a "cobra-head" end-to-side anastomosis. One motion is employed for the entire cut to prevent an irregular edge.

Variations of the procedure are required if a vessel such as the aorta cannot be rotated. In this case anastomosis begins with a single suture in the middle of the posterior wall. Each end is used to suture halfway around the circumference and tied together on the anterior wall (Fig. 77–5).

Simple interrupted sutures can be used to reconnect a severed vessel. This technique offers the advantage of allowing the suture line to expand and contract, rather than being constrained by the continuous suture. In practice, other than in very small arteries (less than 3–4 mm), continuous suturing is usually the method of choice. If a graft is to be anastomosed interpositionally end-to-end, the occluding clamps should not be released until both anastomoses are completed. The proximal clamp is removed first to let the pressure force out any residual air.

End-to-side suture is most often used to anastomose grafts to vessels. It offers the advantages of not necessarily total flow occlusion, a longer anastomosis

(lessening the possibility of thrombosis), and an enlarged lumen at the anastomotic site. To minimize turbulence, the graft is attached at an angle of about 30 degrees to the vessel. The length of the anastomosis should be at least twice the diameter of the involved vessel.

The end of the graft is trimmed in such a way that the lumen is enlarged over the anastomosis. This is frequently called a "cobra-head" anastomosis (Fig. 77–6). A longitudinal cut whose length is about twice the graft diameter is made in one end. Narrow triangular pieces of graft are removed by additional angled longitudinal cuts on either side of the first. The edge of the graft is further trimmed to fit by removal of small triangular pieces from the corners. A second method can be used to produce the same effect but with smooth rounded edges. With the walls of the graft pinched together, and using straight sharp scissors, one begins by cutting the prosthesis transversely for about half its circumference. With one smooth motion, one rotates the angle of the cut 90 degrees so that it is now parallel to the longitudinal plane. The cut in the longitudinal plane should remove a narrow sliver of graft wall. One should continue in this direction for about twice the diameter and again rotate the scissors 90 degrees to release the piece of graft wall to be removed. Figure 77–7 illustrates the steps in this process.

Once the graft has been prepared, the artery can be isolated and the patient given anticoagulant. A longitudinal arteriotomy is made with a scalpel to cut through the wall, layer by layer. Potts scissors are usually required to finish the arteriotomy (Fig. 77–8). Its length should closely match that of the prepared end of the graft. Two double-armed sutures, one at each end of the cut edge, are passed from outside to inside through the graft and then from inside to outside through the vessel wall. Both are tied to secure the graft to the vessel. Suturing can begin from either end on either side at the surgeon's discretion. However, the acute corner angles are the

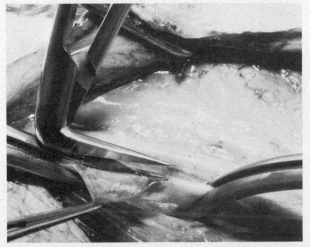

Figure 77–8. Use of Potts scissors to complete a longitudinal arteriotomy. Note that the vessel is held by its adventitia, never by grasping the cut edge of the wall.

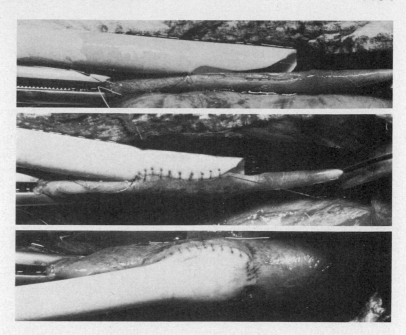

Figure 77–9. Steps in accomplishing a "cobra-head" end-to-side anastomosis. The suture is first tied in the acute angle and then run along both sides. The flared anastomosis can be seen in the lower view.

most difficult areas to suture properly and can be most accurately approximated when sewn first. Many surgeons suture the entire length of one side and then tie that end to one of the unused ends. A preferred technique is to suture halfway along one side with one suture end and then begin at the other end with another suture end. The two sutures meet along the side of the anastomosis and are tied to each other. This method offers three advantages: maximum exposure of the corners, placement of knots where they can be observed for proper tension and flatness of throws, and equal use of all needles, which prevents excessive roughening of two needles and non-use of the other two needles.

A second, equally acceptable method of end-to-side anastomosis requires only one double-armed suture. The graft and artery are prepared as previously described. One end of the suture is passed from inside to outside at the acute angle end of the prosthesis. The other end of the suture is also passed

from inside to outside in the corresponding end of the arteriotomy. These ends are knotted to appose the graft and vessel. One side of the anastomosis is sewn for about two-thirds of its length. The other side of the anastomosis is sewn with the second suture end. This second suture line is carried around the obtusely angled end to the anastomosis and tied to the first suture end. Maximum exposure of the acute angle, where most leaks occur, is the primary advantage of this method. However, care must be taken to ensure even bites of artery and graft, or there will be a mismatch near the end of the second suture line (Fig. 77–9).

The graft is cross-clamped close to the anastomosis before blood is allowed to flow, in order to prevent blood from sitting in the graft while the second end is anastomosed. Upon completion of the second anastomosis, the cross-clamp is released to drive air and thrombi out of the graft. Only then are the vascular occluding clamps removed.

Chapter **78** # Peripheral Vascular Disorders

Philip Litwak

There are very few primary disorders of the peripheral vasculature in dogs and cats. Most clinical cases are presented as secondary manifestations. Although the primary condition may be obvious, the vascular damage may not be so evident. Therefore, the veterinary surgeon must frequently be prepared

to repair blood vessels without the extensive workup usually available for human clinical cases.

All injuries involve some vascular trauma, which may be signified by hemorrhage or hematoma. However, in some cases, major vessels such as the jugular vein can be severed with little bleeding. This occurrence is usually attributable to retraction and vasospasm. Indirect damage to blood vessels can cause obstruction of flow. Contusion over an artery and compression by fractured or displaced bones are examples of indirect vascular trauma. Foreign objects such as bullets and pellets can lodge in blood vessels and cause thrombosis. Arteriovenous fistulas can result from untreated vascular injuries.

Even the most severe hemorrhage from peripheral vessels can often be temporarily stopped with direct pressure. Exploration of these wounds is required to ascertain the location and extent of damage. Inflatable pressure cuffs proximal to the lesion may prove helpful because they can be temporarily released during surgery to find the bleeding. Most vascular injuries can be repaired by either direct suturing, end-to-end anastomosis, or implantation of a prosthetic conduit.

End-to-end direct reanastomosis of severed vessels is often very difficult. It must be done with complete lack of tension on the suture line. Severed vessels frequently retract, and suturing should be attempted only in healthy vascular tissue, conditions that make reapproximation difficult. If there is any doubt about the amount of tension required to hold the ends together, a prosthesis should be considered. The saphenous vein is usually of adequate size to be used for most peripheral arteries.

When major vessels are traumatized, repair should be considered. Arteries such as the femoral, axillary, and carotid can be cross-clamped during anastomosis. Serious complications can result from total occlusion of the larger arteries and veins such as the aorta and vena cava; tangential occlusion should be used on these vessels. Temporary intraluminal shunts have also been used to prevent flow disruption during repair.[10]

Repair of major vessels usually involves a prosthetic conduit. Peripheral veins are not large enough to bridge disruptions of large arteries unless the damage occurs near the distal end. Both end-to-end and end-to-side anastomotic techniques are satisfactory.

Arteriovenous (AV) fistula (see Chapter 69) is an abnormal communication between an artery and vein that does not involve a capillary bed. It can be congenital or traumatic. Extravascular injection of irritant drugs such as pentobarbital and thiobarbiturates has been reported to produce AV fistula. Untreated arterial injuries, bite wounds, and onychectomy have also been implicated as causes.

All types of AV fistulas are uncommon in dogs and rare in cats. The vast majority involve the extremities. Fistulas have been reported to involve the flank,[4] and the liver,[5,11,15] and an aortocaval fistula was reported in a three-month-old kitten.[1] Hepatic fistulas usually form between the hepatic artery and portal vein and may cause reversed flow in the portal vein. Ascites and presinusoidal portal hypertension may also occur.

Even moderate-sized fistulas can cause a serious overloading of the heart, with only slight diminution of flow to the distal limb, in response to the greatly lowered total peripheral resistance due to the low shunt resistance and normal arteriolar peripheral resistance. Total arterial flow above the shunt and venous return from the shunt can increase dramatically.[3] The decrease in total peripheral resistance increases cardiac output as reflexes attempt to maintain arterial pressure.

In addition, there can be serious effects on the venous system distal to a fistula. Increased venous pressure can result in dilation and incompetence of venous valves. As a consequence, blood flow may be reversed in peripheral veins.

Blood flow distal to a fistula can vary from slightly less to much less than normal. These variations can result in a limb that is warm or cold with or without ulcerations and ischemia. Most often in small to moderate-sized fistulas, there are only slight distal physical changes.

Diagnosis of AV fistula in the extremities is usually not difficult. The affected limb may be slightly swollen. A continuous murmur, similar to that of patent ductus arteriosus, can be heard at the fistula site. A thrill may be present. Pulsation of veins in the area is an inconsistent finding. Very large fistulas cause more severe symptoms. Sudden digital occlusion of a large fistula causes a drop in heart rate, increased diastolic pressure, and disappearance of the murmur and thrill. This phenomenon is known as Branham's sign. Depending on location, additional signs may imply local change in blood supply. Neurological deficit, exophthalmos, and ascites have been reported.[16]

Plain radiographs of the affected area may be unrevealing. Periosteal proliferation has been seen in animals with large fistulas. Cardiomegaly, left atrial enlargement, and increased vascularity of lung may also be seen with large fistulas (Fig. 78–1). Intra-arterial contrast radiographs are helpful for definitive diagnosis and determination of extent prior to surgery. Contrast medium should be injected proximal

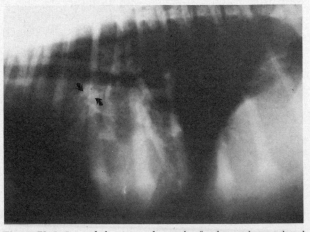

Figure 78–1. Lateral thoracic radiograph of a dog with peripheral arteriovenous fistula. There is cardiomegaly. Note the overcirculated lungs, indicated by the enlarged right anterior lung lobe vessels (*arrows*).

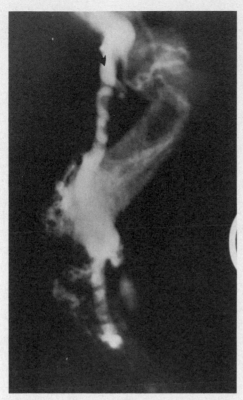

Figure 78–2. Angiogram from the leg of a dog with multiple peripheral arteriovenous fistulas. Note the mass of vessels and the large vein draining from the fistulas (*arrow*).

to the suspected fistula. The increased flow rate necessitates multiple exposures during or shortly after injection (Fig. 78–2). Radiographic appearance of fistula is variable. Usually, a mass of tortuous vessels is apparent, but in small fistulas of short duration, only a few vessels may be seen. Rapid filling of the veins and decreased contrast medium in the distal artery are good indications of a fistula. Often the exact site of communication cannot be identified.

Treatment of AV fistulas is surgical separation of the arterial and venous systems and interruption of the arterial supply. The separation must be complete or the fistula will gradually re-establish itself. If the exact site of the fistula cannot be located, the arterial supply and venous drainage must be ligated and divided both above and below the area. Incomplete closure or partial interruption of the arterial supply can result in a condition worse than the original.

Closure of large fistulas in main arteries may require prosthetic conduits to bypass the affected area and supply blood to the distal tissues. All branches that could somehow communicate with the fistula must be ligated and divided. This communication may involve circuitous routes.

Ideally, if the connection can be identified, the artery and vein are separated and repaired individually. This is difficult to do even in fistulas involving a large artery such as the femoral or carotid. Often the vein can be sacrificed to save the artery by leaving a patch of vein attached to the artery and ligating the remaining vein above and below. The venous patch can then be oversewn to create a "patch angioplasty" of the arterial wall. The carotid artery or the femoral artery distal to the deep femoral artery can be safely ligated without endangering structures distal to the ligation. Sudden closure of large AV fistulas can cause hypertension and bradycardia.

Small fistulas and fistulas located distally on a limb are best treated by either ligation of the arterial supply or arterial embolization. The latter technique involves the use of tissues such as muscle and fat or nonabsorbable materials such as polyvinyl alcohol foam (Ivalon), Dacron felt, and silicone microspheres to cause thrombosis of the supply artery. The tissues or materials are usually placed via an arterial catheter in fistulas that are difficult to approach surgically.

Concomitant with the increased use of prosthetic grafts is an increased incidence of complications. These can be disastrous, especially when infection is involved. In the human incidences of infection have been reported to be between 0.25 and 6 per cent.[9,17] Vein grafts have also become infected, suggesting that more than a foreign body response may be involved.

Direct contamination from the skin overlying a graft is a common cause of infection. Poor surgical technique resulting in devitalized tissue, hematoma, scroma, or lymphocele predisposes to wound infection. Local lymph node infection has also been implicated.

As is the case with most disastrous situations, prevention is the best course. In veterinary medicine, vascular procedures are generally performed on an emergency basis, precluding postponement of operation in febrile or malnourished animals, for example. However, these factors should alert the surgeon to potential complications, and other factors that can be controlled, such as surgical technique, must be meticulously attended to.

Prophylactic antibiotics are indicated in all vascular procedures. Both systemic and topical preparation should be considered. Parenteral penicillin, cephalosporin, and gentamicin are the most commonly used drugs. Topical antibiotics have included penicillin, neomycin, polymyxin, and bacitracin. In no case can antibiotics substitute for a carefully executed operation. Good operative technique is the single most important preventive measure.

Despite the most careful precautions, a small proportion (approximately one per cent) of grafts will become infected. Any patient with a vascular graft and signs of sepsis should be considered to have an infected graft unless proven otherwise. In the patient with a graft in the abdomen, gastrointestinal bleeding could be a sign of prosthetic-enteric fistula.

Untreated graft infections have a very high mortality rate, perhaps 100 per cent if the aorta is involved. Amputation is often necessary when grafts in major peripheral arteries become infected. Once a diagnosis of graft infection is made, the patient should be prepared for surgical exploration of the area and probable graft removal.

When an infected graft is excised, the remaining vessels should be closed in two layers and this suture line covered by viable tissue. Complete debridement of the surrounding tissues also accompanies prosthesis removal. When the entire area is clean and well irrigated, revascularization can be considered. The replacement prosthesis is not placed in the same location as the one that was removed. Anastomoses are placed in healthy portions of the vessels even if a long shunt is required. Careful technique combined with intensive antibiotic therapy offers the best chance of salvage in these cases.

The most common vascular disorder requiring surgical intervention is aortic embolism due to feline cardiomyopathy. Feline aortic embolism is secondary to underlying cardiac disease.[7] It is a widespread, though relatively uncommon condition. Cats of all ages and both sexes are affected equally.[6] The condition was described in 1930, but it was not until 1955 that a series of cases were reported.[8] Since that time, less than 50 reports have appeared in the literature.[2,6,12,13]

Clinically, cats with aortic embolism are usually presented with a sudden onset of pain and posterior lameness or paralysis. Upon examination the animal is in obvious distress, frequently in shock, and constantly crying as if in pain. One or both femoral pulses are diminished or absent. The affected hindlimb is cooler than normal and possibly swollen. Cyanosis can be observed in cats with light-colored foot pads. The gastrocnemius muscles may be in spasm, and more general signs of shock (pale mucous membranes, dyspnea, weakness) are usually present. Cardiac auscultation frequently reveals abnormal heart sounds or murmurs.

Laboratory findings are usually not remarkable. Serum potassium and bicarbonate are decreased.[14] Total white blood cell and differential counts are within normal limits. Hematocrit may be slightly increased. Routine radiographs do not aid diagnosis other than to eliminate trauma as a possible cause. Cardiomegaly may be seen if the thoracic cavity is included in the radiographs. Angiography, though not always advised, would demonstrate embolus at the termination of the aorta involving one or both iliac vessels (Fig. 78–3).

Aortic embolism must be differentiated from other acute causes of posterior pain and paresis. Conditions to be eliminated include traumatic injuries, spontaneous fractures, bite wounds, spinal lesions, intervertebral disc prolapse, and urethral calculi. Each of these usually has several symptoms that make a diagnosis of complete aortic occlusion relatively obvious. In less obvious cases, constant crying, relatively cold extremities, and posterior paresis are most useful in diagnosis. Venous angiograms in the levo phase are diagnostic.

Treatment of aortic embolism is surgical removal. This should be done as quickly as possible after the

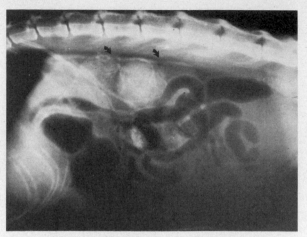

Figure 78–3. Angiogram from a dog with multiple aortic thromboembolism (*arrows*).

animal's overall condition has been stabilized. In animals presented more than six hours after signs appeared, medical therapy alone has been advocated. When surgical treatment is not begun within six hours, there is little chance for improvement, and almost certainly there will be secondary complications. Even when successful treatment is given within several hours of onset, there is only about a 50 per cent chance of long-term (greater than one year) survival owing to the underlying heart disease.

Atropine should be the only preanesthetic drug. Sedatives and tranquilizers are not advised. Anesthesia can be induced intravenously with thiobarbiturates, but because the animal's response may be exaggerated, they must be administered cautiously. Inhalation anesthetics can also be used for induction, although they are best used for maintenance during the surgical procedure. Methoxyflurane and halothane are suitable agents. Fluids are administered intravenously and contain additional sodium bicarbonate (e.g., 1 mEq/10 ml).

The cat is positioned in dorsal recumbency with its back arched by a pack placed beneath the lumbar vertebrae. The termination of the aorta is approached via a ventral midline incision that extends from the brim of the pelvis to the umbilicus. Intestines are packed off with saline-soaked gauze pads. Incision of the parietal peritoneum exposes the aorta and origin of the iliac arteries. Gentle palpation of the aorta aids in estimating the extent of the embolus. Either vascular clamps or loops of umbilical tape can be used to occlude blood flow. Before opening the aorta, the cat is heparinized (2 mg/kg). Heparin reduces the rate at which additional emboli form and lessens the amount of thrombus on the aortotomy suture line. The aorta is opened longitudinally over the embolus, which can usually be removed easily with fine forceps (Fig. 78–4). Theoretically, a horizontal aortotomy incision causes less diminution of lumen diameter when sutured, but it is difficult to remove a long embolus from this incision without damaging endothelium. When all visible embolus has been re-

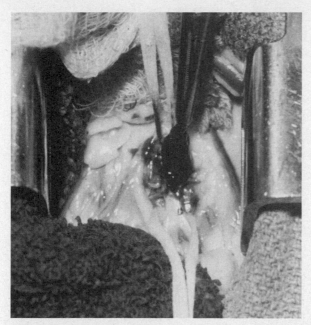

Figure 78–4. Aortic embolism being removed from the aorta of a cat. Note the tapered end suggesting that the whole embolus is being removed.

moved, each occlusion is temporarily released to flush out remaining tiny emboli. The aortotomy is sutured with 6-0 or 7-0 monofilament polypropylene in either a simple continuous or an interrupted suture pattern. Blood flow to the hindlegs is re-established slowly to dilute the amount of acidic hyperkalemic blood suddenly entering the circulation. Mild pressure over the aortic incision stops blood leakage. After palpation to confirm the presence of femoral pulses, the abdomen may be closed routinely.

Immediately postoperatively, diuresis is encouraged by the administration of dextrose in water. Additional heparin is administered subcutaneously (10 to 15 mg every 8 hours) for the first 48 hours. Antibiotics are administered for at least 14 days. Once the animal has recovered from embolectomy, a long-term treatment plan aimed at the underlying cardiac disease must be instituted. In all cases, anticoagulants must be continued for the life of the animal. Despite its potential side effects, aspirin is excellent in preventing platelet aggregation. It is given intermittently and in low doses (75 mg every 72 hours); this dosage is well below the toxic level for cats. Underlying cardiac disease should be investigated and aggressively treated with diuretics, digoxin, or beta-adrenergic blocking agents.

If occlusion of the aorta has been present for an extended time before embolectomy, irreversible necrosis of hindlimb structures may occur despite complete re-establishment of blood flow. This occurrence can be manifested as permanent paresis or paralysis, gangrene of the toes, and localized areas of necrosis and suppuration. Long-term prognosis for cats surviving aortic embolism is poor. Recurrence is high despite treatment, although recent reports are encouraging.

1. Bolton, G. R., Edwards, J. J., and Hoffer, R. E.: Arteriovenous fistula of the aorta and caudal vena cava causing congestive heart failure in a cat. J. Am. Anim. Hosp. Assoc. *12*:463, 1976.
2. Buchanan, J. W., Baker, G. J., and Hill, J. D.: Aortic embolism in cats: prevalence, surgical treatment and electrocardiography. Vet. Rec. 79:496, 1966.
3. Burton, A. C.: *Physiology and Biophysics of the Circulation.* Year Book Medical Publishers, Inc., Chicago, 1972.
4. Butterfield, A. B., Hix, W. R., Pickrel, J. C., and Johnson, K. E.: Acquired peripheral and arteriovenous fistula in a dog. J. Am. Vet. Med. Assoc. *176*:445, 1980.
5. Easley, J. C., and Carpenter, J. L.: Hepatic arteriovenous fistula in two Saint Bernard pups. J. Am. Vet. Med. Assoc. *165*:167, 1975.
6. Evans, M. G.: Aortic thromboembolism in a cat. Vet. Med./ Small Anim. Clin. 75:1150, 1980.
7. Harpster, N. K.: Acquired heart disease in the cat. Proc. Anim. Hosp. Assoc. *40*:118, 1973.
8. Holzworth, J., Simpson, R., and Wind, A.: Aortic thrombosis with posterior paralysis in the cat. Cornell Vet. *45*:468, 1955.
9. Hamieson, G. G., DeWeese, J. A., and Rob, C. G.: Infected arterial grafts. Am. J. Surg. *181*:850, 1975.
10. Kolata, R. J., Cornelius, L. M., Bjorling, D. E., and Mahaffey, M. B.: Correction of an obstructive lesion of the caudal vena cava in a dog using a temporary intraluminal shunt. Vet. Surg. *11*:100, 1982.
11. Landers, E. A., and Mitten, R. W.: Intrahepatic arteriovenous fistula with portosystemic communications: a case report. J. Am. Vet. Radiol. Soc. *19*:70, 1978.
12. Lord, P. F., Wood, A., Tilley, L. P., and Liu, S. K.: Radiographic and hemodynamic evaluation of cardiomyopathy and thromboembolism in the cat. J. Am. Vet. Med. Assoc. *164*:154, 1974.
13. McCurnin, D. M., Sceli, D. E., and Arp, L. H.: Surgical treatment of aortic embolism. Vet. Med./Small Anim. Clin. 67:387, 1972.
14. Robins, G. M., Wilkinson, G. T., Menrath, V. H., et al.: Long-term survival following embolectomy in two cats with aortic embolism. J. Small Anim. Pract. *23*:165, 1982.
15. Rogers, W. A., Suter, P. F., Breznock, E. M., et al.: Intrahepatic arteriovenous fistulae in a dog resulting in portal hypertension, portacaval shunts and reversal of portal blood flow. J. Am. Anim. Hosp. Assoc. *13*:470, 1977.
16. Suter, P. F.: Diseases of the Peripheral Vessels. *In* Ettinger, S. J. (ed.): *Textbook of Veterinary Internal Medicine.* 2nd ed. W. B. Saunders, Philadelphia, 1983.
17. Talkington, C. M., and Thompson, J. E.: Prevention and management of infected prosthesis. Surg. Clin. North Am. *62*:515, 1982.

79 Portacaval Shunts and Anomalies

Eugene M. Breznock and Pamela G. Whiting

NORMAL ANATOMY

The common hepatic artery arises from the celiac artery in the dog and cat. The hepatic artery of the dog divides into one to five branches, which supply the various liver lobes, and into the right gastric and gastroduodenal arteries. The gastroduodenal artery terminates as the right gastroepiploic and cranial pancreaticoduodenal arteries. In the cat, the hepatic artery usually divides into three branches supplying the right, left, and middle hepatic divisions.

In the dog and cat, the portal vein originates from the inferior (caudal) mesenteric vein, the superior (cranial) mesenteric vein, and the splenic vein. In dogs, the right gastroepiploic vein enters the gastroduodenal vein, which then enters the portal vein. The portal vein divides extrahepatically into right and left major divisions prior to the right division bifurcating to the caudal and right lateral liver lobes. The left main portal division divides into five branches: to the papillary process of the caudate lobe and the left lateral, left medial, quadrate, and right medial liver lobes. In the cat, usually three branches of the portal vein divide into the right, central, and left divisions of the liver.

The left hepatic vein is the largest and most consistent in the dog and drains most of the liver; it is the most cranial and ventral. Other inconsistent hepatic veins usually drain from the right and caudate lobes.

In the dog, the left liver lobe (subdivided into the left lateral and left medial lobes) forms one-third to one-half of the total liver mass. The remaining lobes are the quadrate, right medial, right lateral, and caudate.

For most mammalian species, the liver receives 20 per cent of the total cardiac output. In normal dogs and humans, the hepatic artery carries 20 to 25 per cent and the portal vein carries 75 to 80 per cent of the total hepatic blood flow. The blood flow is similar in both species (humans and dogs), with the portal venous blood and hepatic arterial blood mixing in the sinusoids. The hepatic veins in dogs, however, have smooth muscle "sphincters" that are absent in the thin-walled human hepatic veins.[15, 46, 57, 79]

ABNORMAL ANATOMY*

The abnormal hepatic vasculature in dogs, cats, and humans may be divided into recognized macrovascular and presumed microvascular patterns (Table

*Frequency of signs and variations based on 120 cases seen at the University of California.

79–1). Macrovascular patterns are either single (80 per cent) or multiple portacaval shunts (20 per cent). Single intrahepatic or extrahepatic portacaval shunts are presumed to exist as congenital anomalies. Of the portacaval vascular anomalies observed in companion animals, less than 2 per cent were observed in cats.

Intrahepatic single portacaval communications (28 per cent) exist when the fetal ductus venosus remains patent or other portal to hepatic vein or vena caval communications exist. The majority of these communications drain into the left hepatic vein, often with a tortuous sinusoidal dilation as the anomalous vessel leaves the left medial or lateral liver lobes prior to entering the hepatic vein or vena cava. The other prominent location for intrahepatic shunts is as the portal vein enters the right liver lobes. The majority of single intrahepatic shunts are found in large-breed dogs (Doberman, golden retriever, Labrador, Irish setter, Samoyed, Irish wolfhound). In dogs, the ductus venosus usually closes shortly after birth (two to three days).[44] Newborn lambs have been used to investigate intrahepatic shunting, as their ductus venosus remains open for the first few days of life.[56, 84]

Single extrahepatic portacaval anomalies comprised 50 per cent of cases observed and included (1) portal vein to azygos vein (5 per cent), or (2) direct portal vein or other splanchnic veins anastomosing with the vena cava, totally bypassing the portal vein (45 per cent). Most extrahepatic portacaval shunts are observed in small breeds (miniature schnauzer, Yorkshire terrier, poodle, dachshund). Rarely has total

TABLE 79–1. Hepatic Vascular Defects

Recognized Macrovascular
    SINGLE
        Venous-venous
            Ductus venosus, intrahepatic
            Extrahepatic
                Portosystemic (referred to as "portacaval" in text)
                    portacaval
                    porta-azygous
                Splanchnic-systemic
                  splanchnic-caval
                  splanchnic-azygous
        Arteriovenous
    MULTIPLE
        Splanchnic-caval
        Renal-vertebral
        Esophageal-azygous
        Esophageal-caval
        Hemorrhoidal-caval
Microvascular (investigational)

absence of portal vein entry into the liver been observed (1.5 per cent).

Extrahepatic multiple portacaval shunts may be acquired as a result of a generalized increase in hepatic portal venous resistance and subsequent mild transient portal hypertension (12 to 15 mm Hg). Multiple venous communications in the dog are usually splanchnic; human multiple portacaval shunts are frequently esophageal. Multiple extrahepatic portacaval shunts are most commonly observed in the German shepherd (7 of 21) and Doberman pinscher (5 of 21) and are frequently accompanied by ascites. Single intrahepatic and extrahepatic portacaval shunts may be congenital because, unlike the multiple extrahepatic shunts, they usually are diagnosed in young animals (less than one year). A geographic variation in distribution of single portacaval shunts exists, suggesting the shunts may be acquired *in utero* as a result of exposure to some inciting agent.

Portacaval shunts occur rarely in cats. Like the dog, insignificant portosystemic communications exist in the normal cat, and a gradual increase in feline portal venous pressure results in formation of dilated portacaval communications. Single extrahepatic portacaval shunts and multiple extrahepatic portacaval shunts have been observed in cats; multiple shunts are often observed in cats with generalized intrahepatic portal obstruction (hepatic lymphosarcoma).[75]

Arteriovenous communications (1.5 per cent) may be either intrahepatic or extrahepatic. Hepatic arteriovenous fistulae of the liver may be congenital or acquired. They are probably secondary to penetrating or blunt trauma, surgical procedures, or degeneration and rupture of arteries into accompanying veins. The artery may communicate with either the hepatic or portal venous systems. With hepatic artery–portal vein fistulae, large, tortuous vessels extend from the affected liver surfaces. Fremitus can be palpated in these large, tortuous vessels. Auscultation over the area of the fremitus usually reveals a continuous

murmur. Temporary occlusion of the hepatic arteries supplying the tortuous shunt vessels may decrease or eliminate the fremitus. Most cases of hepatic artery to portal vein fistulae cause transient portal hypertension that results in the formation of multiple extrahepatic portacaval shunts and ascites.

Hepatic microvascular shunts have been described in cirrhotic human patients and exist both as portal vein to hepatic vein and hepatic artery to portal vein communications. An increase in the ratio of hepatic arterial perfusion to portal venous perfusion may occur in conditions of hepatic dysfunction.[27]

PATHOPHYSIOLOGY

Most cases (93 per cent) of portacaval vascular anomalies in companion animals are seen with some degree of neurological dysfunction related to hepatic encephalopathy (Table 79–2).

Clinicopathological data contribute to establishing the definitive diagnosis of portacaval shunt. Hematological values often indicate anemia (34 per cent), microcytosis (72 per cent),[25] hypoproteinemia (64 per cent), leukocytosis (30 per cent), and coagulation abnormalities.

Anemia with hepatic disease is frequent in humans but not well documented in dogs. Anemia may result from blood loss secondary to coagulopathies, destruction of erythrocytes, or production abnormalities (decreased erythropoietin described in human cirrhosis; decreased transferrin observed in dogs with portacaval shunts). Hypoproteinemia results from decreased hepatic metabolism and albumin production as well as loss of protein in ascitic fluid owing to altered hepatic vascular and tissue pressures. Microcytosis may result from the effects of toxins, e.g., ammonia altering heme synthesis, or from hepatic metabolic defects. The leukocytosis in portacaval anomalies may be related to intestinal bacteria in the systemic cir-

TABLE 79–2. Clinical Findings Associated with Portasystemic Abnormalities (in Decreasing Order of Frequency)

Neurological (93%)	Gastrointestinal (75%)	Other Abnormalities (80%)
Depression	Vomiting	Weight loss, 53%
Vague CNS signs	Ptyalism	Polydipsia, 35%
Stupor	Diarrhea	Relationship of signs to meals, 23%
Pacing and/or circling	Anorexia	Ascites, 19%
Staggering and/or ataxia	Foreign body	Polyuria, 18%
Amaurotic blindness	ingestion	Abdominal pain, 15%
Collapse and/or weakness	Voracious appetite	Fever, 13%
Personality changes		Poor coat, 13%
Seizures		Epistaxis, bleeding gums, 3%
Head pressing		Pleural effusion, 2%
Long tract deficits		Prolonged anesthetic recovery period
Hyperactivity		noted in 18 (of 120) cases that had
Head held down		undergone anesthetic procedures
Head and/or muscle tremors		prior to referral
Acting deaf		
Coma		

TABLE 79–3. Biochemical Abnormalities Associated with Portacaval Anomalies

Increased Serum Chemistry Values (% of Patients)		Decreased or Subnormal Serum Chemistry Values (% of Patients)	
Serum alkaline phosphatase (65%)		BUN (70%)	
SGOT (55%)		Cholesterol (57%)	
SGPT (48%)		Albumin (41% low, 32% low normal)	
Total bilirubin (16%)		Potassium (44%)	
Fasting ammonia	93%		
Postammonia tolerance	100%	Branched chain aromatic amino acids	
BSP	93%		100%

culation that normally would be filtered by the liver via the portal circulation. Serum biochemical abnormalities are listed in Table 79–3.

Increased SGPT and SGOT levels occur with either liver necrosis or increased hepatocyte membrane permeability. Serum alkaline phosphatase is also elevated in hepatocellular disease. Although less common, bilirubinemia indicates severe hepatocellular disease and biliary stasis. Cholesterol levels are often depressed because the liver is the main source of its production. Due to depressed hepatic function in converting ammonia to urea via the Krebs cycle, a decreased blood urea nitrogen (BUN) level has been a consistent finding. Sulfobromophthalein dye (bromsulphalein, BSP) retention is a sensitive test of liver function or liver blood flow, since it requires uptake and conjugation by the liver for excretion. Since hepatic blood flow and metabolism are affected in patients with portacaval shunts, BSP retention is increased. Ammonia is produced by the bacterial breakdown of intestinal protein, especially in the colon. If blood bypasses the liver or if liver metabolism is depressed, ammonia conversion to urea is impaired and elevated ammonia levels may be observed.* Plasma aminograms also indicate hepatic dysfunction. Hypokalemia has been described as a result of gastrointestinal loss, diuretics, or urinary loss.[25, 28, 60, 65]

Abnormal urological findings of bilirubinuria (64 per cent), urobilinogen (58 per cent), ammonium biurate crystalluria (52 per cent), low specific gravity (44 per cent), and uric acid calculi (cystic 13 per cent, renal 3 per cent) may exist in dogs with portacaval shunts. The incidence of bilirubinuria is slightly higher than that reported in normal dogs. The presence of bilirubin in conjunction with the low urine specific gravity often indicates hepatocellular disease. Urobilinogen is removed from plasma by the liver and little should be excreted in the urine; increased urobilinogen is observed in hepatic disease. The

presence of ammonium biurate crystalluria has been considered pathognomonic for portacaval shunts. The predisposition to uric acid calculi often results from high ammonium, hydrogen ion, and uric acid levels in the urine.

Hepatic arteriovenous fistula (whether hepatic artery to hepatic vein or hepatic artery to portal vein) may result in systemic signs that include tachycardia, decreased diastolic pressure, and wide pulse pressure. Laboratory data usually reveal an increased blood volume and increased cardiac output. Large, chronic fistulae may lead to cardiomegaly and high-output left heart failure (see Chapter 69). These shunts usually cause transient portal hypertension, a concomitant development of multiple extrahepatic portacaval communications.

HEPATIC ENCEPHALOPATHY

Metabolic encephalopathy occurs frequently in patients with severe hepatic dysfunction. Hepatic encephalopathy or hepatic coma is not uncommon in patients with hepatic decompensation resulting from a portacaval shunt. Hepatic encephalopathy is associated with metabolic changes that must be differentiated from or recognized concurrently with other causes of metabolic encephalopathy that may synergistically affect a patient with hepatic disease. Hypoglycemic encephalopathy may occur in chronic liver disease because of decreased liver glycogen and impaired gluconeogenesis, especially when coupled with fasting. Other metabolic causes of encephalopathy (acid-base, osmolar, electrolyte, and renal abnormalities) must be considered in the comatose patient regardless of the functional status of the liver; these abnormalities may occur simultaneously with hepatic encephalopathy.

The clinical appearance of hepatic encephalopathy is similar to that of other metabolic encephalopathies. Generally the patient is depressed, demented, or stuporous. Respiratory changes with hyperventilation and respiratory alkalosis are common in humans. Peripheral oculomotor responses are generally intact.

*Blood ammonia is subject to significant fluctuations if not properly transported. Minor alterations in handling of the sample may invalidate the test.

Although pupils may be small, they are usually responsive to light. Muscle tremors have been reported in dogs with hepatic encephalopathy and hepatic disease. Motor abnormalities of strength, tone, and reflexes may be involved. Focal and generalized seizures have been observed in dogs with portacaval shunts.[50]

The specific metabolic causes of hepatic encephalopathy are equivocal. Several theories account in part for the metabolic abnormalities that accompany hepatic encephalopathy. The predominant hypothesis recognizes toxins with a coma-producing potential that interact with other nonspecific metabolites to exacerbate the effects of the toxins. The synergistic interactions produce neurological signs disproportionate to their individual effects. Ammonia is a primary pathogenic factor in this theory; it is produced in the colon and small intestine and to a lesser extent by the kidney. Urease-producing bacteria in the colon hydrolyze intestinal urea; other bacteria deaminate dietary amino acids to produce ammonia. Normally, the ammonia in the colon is absorbed into the portal circulation, taken to the liver, and converted via the Krebs cycle to urea, which is excreted in the urine. In hepatic encephalopathy, increased ammonia and decreased urea production are usually present. Increased ammonia can be measured in the blood, cerebrospinal fluid, and brain. Feeding large amounts of protein or other ammonia-generating substances can produce hepatic encephalopathy in patients with portacaval shunts. Repeated experimental ammonia intoxication results in Alzheimer type II astrocytes, indistinguishable from those in patients in hepatic coma.[19–21, 60, 83]

The correlation of ammonia and hepatic encephalopathy is not direct. The concentration of blood ammonia does not correlate well with the severity of clinical signs, although blood ammonia is not proportional to brain ammonia. Brain and spinal fluid glutamine concentrations may be more reliable indicators of the severity of hepatic encephalopathy.[19, 83]

Ammonia intoxication produces a hyperkinetic preconvulsive or convulsive state. Hyperammonemia in the comatose hepatic patient is usually a hypokinesive state, due in part to the small amount of ammonia necessary to produce clinical signs in a patient with other metabolic abnormalities.[50, 83]

Other endogenous toxins implicated in hepatic coma are mercaptans and fatty acids. Synergism exists among ammonia, mercaptans, fatty acids, hypoglycemia, and hypoxia, increasing each factor's encephalopathy-producing potential.[83]

Hepatic encephalopathy may involve an imbalance of plasma amino acids. Increases in the aromatic amino acids (tryptophan, phenylalanine, and tyrosine) and decreases in the branched-chain amino acids in both plasma and brain may result in alterations in brain neurotransmitters. Ammonia plays a secondary role in contributing to plasma amino acid imbalance and the increased uptake of aromatic amino acids in the brain. The aromatic amines result in excess serotonin (an inhibitory neurotransmitter), accumulation of false neurotransmitters, and a reduction in the excitatory neurotransmitters dopamine and norepinephrine. Although ratios of branched-chain to aromatic amino acids

$$\left(\frac{\text{valine} + \text{isoleucine} + \text{leucine}}{\text{tyrosine} + \text{phenylalanine}} \right)$$

have been reported to indicate the severity of hepatic disease, these amino acid imbalances by themselves have not been consistent in predicting the production or magnitude of central nervous system dysfunction (normal ratio = 3.5 to 5, significant if <2; dogs with a portacaval shunt often have ratios of <1). Reversal of signs of hepatic coma with L-dopa has been cited as evidence for this theory (since L-dopa alters the amino acid ratio), but L-dopa also results in increased renal excretion of ammonia and urea.[67, 83]

Hepatic encephalopathic patients usually have increased levels of brain gamma-aminobutyric acid (GABA), an inhibitory neurotransmitter bound to increased numbers of GABA receptors. Impaired energy metabolism of the brain resulting from hepatic dysfunction will result in encephalopathy.[12, 14, 18, 19, 50, 60, 67, 83]

The causes of hepatic encephalopathy are numerous, and synergism between causative agents exists. Although the therapeutic approach for dogs with portacaval shunts is surgery, recognition of the causes of encephalopathy is essential in development of therapeutic regimens for hepatic encephalopathy.

PATHOLOGY

Hepatic histopathology in dogs with portacaval shunts is not identical to that of human hepatic cirrhosis with secondary collateral circulation. Histopathological descriptions in dogs are similar regardless of the location of the shunt vessel: diffuse atrophy, lobular collapse, and proliferation of the small vessels or lymphatics. Close proximity of the portal triads, compressed hepatic cords, and inconspicuous portal veins indicate atrophy of hepatic lobules. Occasional cytoplasmic clear vacuoles in hepatocytes are observed. The peripheral lobular sinusoidal and venular dilation and congestion suggest intrahepatic vascular obstruction. The walls of the central veins are often thickened and surrounded by fibrous connective tissue. The sinusoidal and venular dilations may be secondary to the same changes that cause mild portal hypertension or may be related to the fibrosis around the central veins (i.e., postsinusoidal intrahepatic obstruction). However, these same changes may be the result of sluggish hepatic perfusion at another intrahepatic location (sinusoidal or presinusoidal in origin). More than 25 per cent of dogs with naturally occurring multiple portacaval shunts have ascites and mild depression of total protein, suggesting an intrahepatic etiology.

LIVER HEMODYNAMICS

The liver receives one-fourth of the total cardiac output, three-fourths of which is transported in the portal vein and the remainder in the hepatic artery. In most mammals, portal venous and hepatic arterial pressures are 6 to 12 and 80 to 100 mm Hg, respectively. The portal venous blood of dogs has a lower oxygen tension and contains bacteria, whereas in cats and humans it has a high oxygen tension and is sterile. Ligation of the portal vein of the dog and cat causes severe portal hypertension (>40 mm Hg), splanchnic congestion with stagnant hypoxia, and death within a few hours. Death does not occur if complete obstruction of the portal vein is performed slowly over several weeks. Slow intrahepatic or extrahepatic obstruction of the portal venous system (hepatic cirrhosis, tumors, iatrogenic obstruction) results in mild portal hypertension (<20 mm Hg) and the development of multiple collateral portacaval communications. Multiple extrahepatic portacaval communications develop in normal dogs with moderate portal hypertension within three weeks of banding the extrahepatic portal vein.

The many portacaval communications (from portal vein to vena cava or to renal, gonadal, and hemorrhoidal veins) shunt splanchnic blood from the liver into the systemic venous circulation. Usually, these venous collateral pathways are insignificant and nonfunctional but become important in mild portal venous hypertension. Unlike the case in humans, in whom collateral portosystemic pathways originate from gastric and esophageal veins (esophageal varices), most of the collateral pathways in dogs and cats are at or distal to the renal veins. Single or multiple portacaval shunts in dogs and cats reduce portal blood flow and result in hepatic atresia, hypoplasia, or atrophy. Although hepatic arterial flow may compensate for the decreased portal flow, portacaval shunts

probably diminish hepatic regenerative, detoxification, metabolic, and immunological capacities. Nonetheless, hepatic parenchymal function is usually adequate to sustain life, albeit under restricted conditions.[13, 16, 38, 45, 52, 53, 73, 81]

In dogs and cats common hepatic artery ligation ordinarily is not fatal, since efficient collateral flow exists from the gastroduodenal and pancreaticoduodenal arteries. Elevated hepatic arterial oxygen tension probably prevents anaerobic organism overgrowth in the dog; high doses of antibiotics (for hepatic anaerobes) should be administered following ligation of the proper hepatic artery. Since the cat has a higher portal blood oxygen tension than the dog, antibiotics probably do not have to be administered following hepatic ligation.[29, 45]

Since the hepatic portal system consists of a myriad of elastic vessels, laws describing hydrodynamic events in rigid tubes cannot be applied to blood vessels in the splanchnic venous bed. Draining one portal vessel should not necessarily drain others, and functionally separate sectors could exist. The complexity of hepatic circulation can be approximated by the Wheatstone bridge analogue (Fig. 79–1). In this model, the blood supply to the hepatic sinusoids is derived from the hepatic artery and the portal vein, and the volume of flow contributed by each vessel depends on the pressures and resistances in each limb of the system.[6]

Clinical observations and experimental data suggest that the splanchnic circulation in humans and dogs is compartmentalized. Splanchnic compartmentalization has been documented in dogs, and the proximal canine portal circulation has compartments that do not overflow into one another until a pressure of 70 cm H$_2$O occurs. Huge spontaneous collateral veins secondary to portal hypertension are sometimes present between the splanchnic vein and the renal vein in human patients who bleed from splanchnic

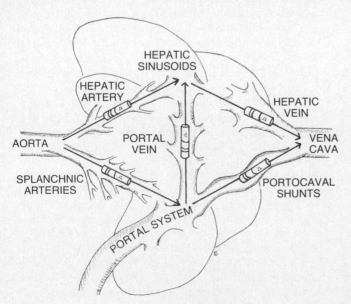

Figure 79–1. Schematic diagram of Wheatstone bridge analogy of hepatic circulation.

varices. Varices can be decompressed with a gastric vein–caval shunt without changing the portal vein pressure. The pattern of splanchnic shunting varies widely among cirrhotic human patients with portal hypertension.

The measurements of portal venous pressure, total hepatic flow, and the direction and magnitude of portal venous flow do not correlate with morbidity or mortality from any shunt. Blood flow in the portal vein is often sluggish and relative flows to different shunts bear no relation to the cross-sectional area of the shunt. Bidirectional blood flow in branches of the portal system has been demonstrated in unanesthetized cirrhotic human patients; however, spontaneous reversal of the portal flow in cirrhosis is probably uncommon. In dogs, reversible portal flow has been demonstrated angiographically.

Animal models with iatrogenic portacaval shunts have demonstrated improved hepatic function, following increased total hepatic blood flow and sinusoidal pressure by channelling new arterial blood into the liver; in human patients with portal hypertension and a palliative iatrogenic portacaval shunt, liver function has not improved. In human patients subjected to hepatic revascularization procedures, the methods used to estimate hepatic blood flow have been equivocal in that statistical analyses were difficult to evaluate, and too much dependence had been placed on mitotic counts of DNA synthesis as an indicator of hepatic growth. Mitotic counts could as well be attempts to repair hepatic cellular damage from unaccustomed perfusion pressures. It is doubtful whether arterialization can restore hepatotrophic factors lost when the splanchnic venous circulation to the liver is interrupted by a portacaval shunt. Dogs with multiple portosystemic shunts subjected to liver revascularization techniques do not improve clinically.[1, 4, 6, 17, 37, 47–49, 76]

Dogs that develop mild portal hypertension (16 to 18 mm Hg) following portacaval shunt attenuation or occlusion usually have normal portal vein pressure within several weeks of surgery. Evidence suggests that a decrease in the intrahepatic portal vascular resistance occurs in initially portal hypertensive dogs because all the dogs (1) clinically improve, (2) have cineangiographic and scintigraphic evidence of improved hepatoportal circulation, with a marked decrease in shunt blood flow, and (3) have a functional shunt ligature.

Third space (ascites) and interstitial (edema) fluid accumulates from attenuation or obstruction of portacaval shunt blood flow; it is probably a primary result of venous hypertension. Edema does not form with relatively small (<10 mm Hg) reductions in plasma osmotic pressure (decreases in plasma protein) or similar small elevations in venous pressure. Protective mechanisms exist that limit the shift of fluids over a range of ± 10 mm Hg around the normal hydrostatic and colloidal osmotic pressure found in capillaries; edema does not occur until venous pressure exceeds 10 to 15 mm Hg. When the venous pressure is increased beyond 20 mm Hg, interstitial volume increases markedly, tissue hydrostatic pressure increases nearly fivefold, and reabsorption is converted to filtration. Similarly, some dogs with moderate portal hypertension (16 to 18 mm Hg) develop ascites after attenuation or occlusion of their single, extra-, or intrahepatic shunts; this ascites disappears in one to three weeks, at the same time that portal vein pressure returns to normal.[38, 73, 80]

Attenuation of the caudal vena cava may result in ascites and rear limb edema. As collateral veins (vertebral, caudal, epigastric, azygos) dilate, hind limb edema usually disappears simultaneously with the ascites (within three weeks).

DIAGNOSIS

Portacaval shunt can be diagnosed tentatively by history, clinical signs, and biochemical abnormalities (Fig. 79–2). Abdominal radiographs may demonstrate a small liver, enlarged kidneys, and cystic or renal calculi. Kidney enlargement may occur as a compensatory response to decreased liver function, since both kidney and liver are involved in excretory functions.

A definitive diagnosis of portacaval shunt may be obtained through cranial mesenteric angiography (cranial mesenteric arterial portography), jejunal venography (intraoperative mesenteric portography), transabdominal splenoportography, or ^{99m}Tc sulfur colloid nuclear hepatic scintigraphy. Nuclear scintigraphy is the least invasive of these procedures and does not require anesthesia. Technetium sulfur colloid (^{99m}Tc) is normally taken up by the reticuloendothelial (mononuclear phagocytic, Kupffer cells) system of the liver of dogs and humans. Extrahepatic uptake of ^{99m}Tc sulfur colloid occurs with liver dysfunction, in the spleen and bone marrow in humans and spleen and lungs in dogs. In humans, lung uptake has been interpreted as a prognostic indicator of severe liver disease. In dogs with portacaval shunts, lung uptake of sulfur colloid is a reversible condition; less lung uptake occurs within a day or two following surgical attenuation or occlusion of the vascular defect. Extrahepatic uptake by the reticuloendothelial system in the canine lung is in part a preferential uptake phenomenon, since lung uptake is noted in the first-pass study prior to the appearance of radioactivity in the liver.

First-pass nuclear scintigraphic studies with ^{99m}Tc sulfur colloid also provide hepatic perfusion information (the arterial-venous ratio). The ratio derived through analysis of time/activity curves is highly reliable for diagnosing portacaval shunt (A-V ratio of a normal dog = 0.9 to 1.7; A-V ratio of a dog with a portacaval shunt = >2). Animals subjected to liver scans must be isolated for approximately 24 hours because of the 6-hour half-life of ^{99m}technetium. The amount of radiation exposure to the patient, however,

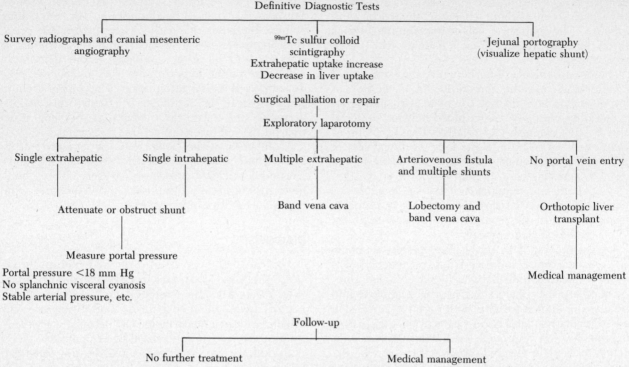

Figure 79–2. Algorithm for management of portacaval shunt. See Table 79–2 for history of abnormal behavior, CNS signs, and gastrointestinal signs. See Table 79–3 for biochemical abnormalities and specific liver function test abnormalities (BSP, NH₃ tolerance, amino acid ratios) compatible with portacaval shunt.

is less than that in a routine radiographic procedure such as cranial mesenteric angiography.[5, 22, 30, 39, 40]

Parenchymal uptake of ^{99m}Tc varies in different species. The liver in dogs and humans is the primary organ for uptake of ^{99m}Tc sulfur colloid. In cats, extrahepatic uptake of ^{99m}Tc sulfur colloid occurs in the lung, overshadowing the information gained from hepatic uptake because of the much poorer images of the liver. Biliary uptake agents may be considered for first-pass hepatic scintigraphic studies in cats.

Conventional radiographic procedures (cranial mesenteric angiography or jejunal venography) require general anesthesia and have been the standard method of diagnosis for portacaval shunt. Injection of intravenous contrast medium into the cranial mesenteric artery outlines the portal system via the venous drainage of the splanchnic viscera. Direct cannulation of a mesenteric vein and injection of contrast medium outlines the portal system without the arterial phase. Transabdominal splenoportography has been used to demonstrate the portal system, but the risks of hemorrhage (especially with hepatic dysfunction) may preclude its routine use.[31, 58, 59, 68, 69]

Other radiographic techniques (dynamic computed tomography, digital subtraction techniques, and videodensitometry) and nuclear scintigraphic techniques (inert gas washout, macroaggregated albumin) aid in understanding the components of hepatic blood flow. Currently these techniques are research tools and are not used clinically. Dynamic computed tomography (dynamic CT scans) involves serial cross-sec-

tional analysis of hepatic perfusion following injection of contrast medium into the portal vein or cranial mesenteric artery. Digital subtraction removes all background structures, resulting in a clarified image of portal blood flow following contrast medium injection. Videodensitometry relies on computerized analysis of the concentration of contrast media detected in the hepatic vasculature.[41]

By direct or indirect techniques, a variety of nuclear scintigraphic agents has been used to distinguish total hepatic flow from nutritional or functional hepatic flow and for evaluation of intrahepatic microvascular shunt blood flow. Inert gases such as ^{81m}krypton and ^{133}xenon have been injected into both portal vein and hepatic parenchyma, and clearance or washout curves have been inscribed to differentiate between total and nutritional hepatic flow. ^{81m}Krypton can be used during surgery to determine whether manipulation alters portal perfusion. Macroaggregated albumin labelled with ^{99m}Tc has been used to demonstrate intrahepatic microvascular shunts. Particles of macroaggregated albumin (20 to 50 μ in diameter) will not pass through the presinusoidal capillaries and hepatic sinusoids. When microvascular shunts bypass the sinusoids, macroaggregated albumin is trapped in the capillaries of the lung instead of the liver. Lung activity compared with liver activity then yields a quantitation of shunt flow. Hepatic arterial injections of ^{131}I macroaggregated albumin have demonstrated hepatic arteriovenous shunts in humans with liver cirrhosis.[26, 34, 55, 71]

MEDICAL MANAGEMENT

Medical management of portacaval anomalies should be instituted prior to surgery. If surgical intervention is unsuccessful, medical management may alleviate clinical signs.[14, 28, 65, 78]

Prevention of signs of hepatic encephalopathy is the major concern of medical management. Low-protein (6 per cent in dogs, 12 per cent in cats) purified diets with reduced aromatic to branched-chain amino acid ratios are recommended. Oral aminoglycoside antibiotics (neomycin sulfate) initially will alter the urealytic and proteolytic bacterial flora in the intestine, but their long-term effectiveness is equivocal. Lactulose also inhibits the metabolism of amino acids by enteric bacteria. The mechanism by which lactulose lowers the blood ammonia levels is not entirely understood; an intracolonic ammonia-trapping mechanism has been proposed in addition to its known cathartic action.[78]

When severe signs of portacaval shunt encephalopathy exist, cleaning enemas reduce potential encephalopathic agents in the colon. Warm water enemas with neomycin, lactulose, or other carbohydrates may reduce morbidity.

Whether sodium benzoate will prove clinically useful in lowering blood ammonia levels in animals with a portacaval shunt is unknown. Early clinical trials with sodium benzoate have not consistently decreased blood ammonia. Sodium benzoate has been used to lower blood ammonia levels in children with hepatic urea cycle enzymopathies.[2, 3, 36]

The administration of 3,4-dihydroxyphenylalanine (L-dopa) and bromocriptine has decreased blood ammonia in patients with chronic hepatic encephalopathy. L-dopa, a neurotransmitter precursor, and bromocriptine, a dopamine receptor agonist, may act either by direct neurotransmitter mechanisms or by other pathways such as augmented renal excretion of ammonia.[83]

Supportive care of the encephalopathic patient necessitates monitoring and adjustments of blood gases, electrolytes, glucose, and osmolality. Intravenous fluids should be maintained until the patient is capable of oral maintenance. Antibiotics should be administered if septicemia exists or if active liver enzyme elevations indicate hepatic necrosis. Penicillins are the antibiotics of choice for hepatic anaerobes (Clostridia). Intestinal bacterial septicemias do occur with an anomalous portacaval shunt. Blood cultures and sensitivity studies should be made if septicemia is suspected.

ANESTHESIA AND DRUG RESPONSE IN LIVER DISEASE

By hepatic conjugation, drugs are changed from lipid-soluble to water-soluble compounds for biliary and urinary excretion. Drug effects may be categorized as those that produce liver damage and those for which the responses are altered in liver disease. Drug damage to the normal liver may occur with many substances. Predictable drug injury is often a dose-related phenomenon. Nonpredictable drug injury to the liver probably affects only a small percentage of patients. With impaired liver function, drug injury becomes a critical issue.

Changes in drug response in liver disease may result from a number of different causes. The bioavailability of the drug may be altered by portacaval shunting. The first-pass effect responsible for extraction and biotransformation is altered if drugs bypass the liver because of abnormal portal circulation (portacaval shunt).

The volume of distribution of the drug to the liver and other organs is influenced by perfusion of these organs. Drugs heavily bound to plasma proteins are affected by low albumin concentrations in liver disease. Therefore, therapeutic and pharmacological effects of the free (unbound) drug may be enhanced as distribution is enhanced. Absorption, metabolism, and clearance of drugs also may be reduced, thereby increasing the half-life of those drugs in the circulation.

The effects of many tranquilizers and analgesics are prolonged with impaired liver function; diazepam and barbiturates especially are affected by low albumin concentrations. Certain neuromuscular blocking agents have a prolonged duration of action in the presence of hepatic disease. Halothane has been reported to induce hepatotoxicosis. Dogs with portacaval shunts frequently are anesthetized with balanced anesthesia (narcotic with muscle relaxant) combined with a low concentration of halothane or methoxyflurane. The doses of anesthetic agents should be carefully titrated to the cardiovascular response of the patient; systemic arterial pressure should be monitored throughout the surgical procedure.

Penicillin or its analogues are frequently utilized antibiotics for liver disease. Despite their metabolism by the liver, most are rapidly excreted by the kidneys and therefore normal doses of penicillins can be used. Chloramphenicol, clindamycin, lincomycin, and erythromycin may reach toxic levels with impaired liver metabolism. All drugs employed with hepatic disease should be evaluated for their potential toxicity as well as therapeutic concentration.[23, 51, 82]

SURGERY OF EXTRAHEPATIC AND INTRAHEPATIC SINGLE PORTACAVAL SHUNTS

Whether single extrahepatic or intrahepatic shunts are congenital or acquired is equivocal. Medical and dietary management of the renal, gastrointestinal, and central nervous system dysfunction (hepatic encephalopathy) caused by portacaval shunts is invaluable but is presently palliative rather than curative. All forms of macrovascular portacaval shunting may be approached surgically. The surgical procedure varies, depending on the location and type of the shunt.

Single portacaval shunts should be surgically attenuated or obstructed. In many cases, a single portacaval shunt can only be attenuated; complete obstruction of such a shunt will result in fatal acute portal hypertension. Portal vein pressure should be measured during shunt manipulation; an increase of portal vein pressure above 20 to 23 cm H_2O (18 mm Hg)* when the portacaval shunt is completely occluded indicates that the anomalous vessel can only be attenuated. Partial occlusion of single intrahepatic portacaval shunts may predispose to portal vein thrombosis and death.

As a rule, small dogs have entrahepatic shunts and large dogs have single intrahepatic portacaval shunts. Although bizarre single extrahepatic shunts occur (portal-azygos, portal-internal thoracic vein), most single extrahepatic portacaval shunts originate from the gastrosplenic or splenic vein prior to the splanchnic vein entering the portal vein. The anomalous shunting vessel usually terminates in the caudal vena cava between the left phrenicoabdominal and renal veins.

Although never observed by us, when present, small venous tributaries from a single extrahepatic portacaval shunt should be ligated. Prior to attenuation or ligation of the single portacaval shunt, the portal vein or splenic vein is catheterized to measure portal venous pressure (Fig. 79–3). A purse-string suture (5–0, 6–0 silk) can be placed in the portal vein and a needle incision made within the purse-string suture. Catheterization is made through the needle venotomy incision. A segment of mesenteric vein

*All pressure measurements are made with an arterial transducer or water manometer standardized at the level of the femoral triangle; i.e., the transducer rests in the inguinal area during measurements.

may be sacrificed and the catheter placed through a venotomy incision into this portal vein tributary. With the portal vein catheterized, the anomalous shunt is identified and isolated as close to the vena cava as possible. A silk ligature is passed around the anomalous shunt and the ligature gradually tightened, attenuating shunt blood flow.

Normal portal venous pressure is equal to approximately 8 to 12 mm Hg; attenuation or obstruction of the anomalous vessel should not increase portal venous pressure above 18 mm Hg. Portal venous pressure above 20 mm Hg may reduce splanchnic perfusion and result in severe portal hypertension and death. Dogs and cats cannot survive complete, acute obstruction of the portal vein, and some dogs cannot survive even acute, moderate portal hypertension (25 mm Hg) following attenuation or obstruction of the anomalous shunt; several patients have died with a measured portal venous pressure of only 20 mm Hg. With the anomalous portocaval shunt attenuated or obstructed, the portal vein catheter can be removed and the purse-string suture tied. If the catheter has been placed in a mesenteric vein, the surgeon can completely obstruct the mesenteric vein (or shunt vessel) below the venotomy incision.

In addition to measured portal venous pressure, other important parameters to be monitored are heart rate, central venous pressure, systemic arterial pressure, and color of the splanchnic viscera (especially pancreas). However, observing the splanchnic viscera for signs of stagnant hypoxia (cyanosis) as the only measure in deciding whether to completely obstruct or attenuate the anomalous shunt probably should not be done. Canine patients have died 12 to 24 hours following surgery from severe splanchnic congestion even though the splanchnic viscera had an apparently normal circulation as judged by the color of the serosal surface of the abdominal viscera.[7, 8, 24, 66]

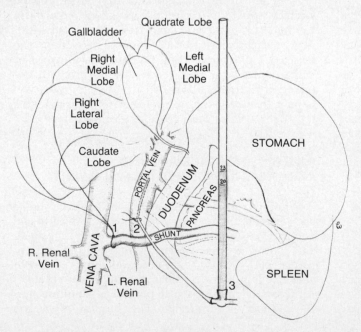

Figure 79–3. Single extrahepatic portacaval shunt. The anomalous vein is usually as large as the renal vein. The shunt usually originates from a splenic or mesenteric vein and usually enters the vena cava between the phrenicoabdominal and renal veins. A ligature is placed around the shunt (*1*), near the vena cava. A purse-string suture is placed in the portal vein with a catheter for portal pressure (*2*). Pressure is measured with a water manometer (*3*) (maximum pressure not to exceed 20 to 23 cm H_2O) or with a pressure transducer (maximum pressure not to exceed 18 mm Hg).

Surgical manipulation of intrahepatic single portacaval shunts (including patent ductus venosus) is technically more difficult than that of the extrahepatic single shunt. The intrahepatic shunt in the dog may be completely (360°), nearly completely (270°), or partially (180°) surrounded by hepatic parenchymal tissues. When completely surrounded by parenchymal tissue, the intrahepatic shunt may be located in the right or left liver lobes. Shunts incompletely surrounded by hepatic parenchyma are usually closely associated with the left lateral liver lobe. Shunts incompletely surrounded by the hepatic parenchyma usually originate from extrahepatic portal veins (most commonly from the area of the gastroduodenal vein), and the shunt usually traverses the abdominal cavity as a free vessel before becoming partially enveloped by hepatic parenchymal tissue. The free vessel portion of the shunt is probably the fetal vestige of the left umbilical vein.

Three surgical techniques are employed to attenuate or obstruct blood flow through intrahepatic portacaval shunts in dogs. Two are extravascular techniques: one involves identification and isolation of the branch of the portal vein supplying the liver lobe containing the shunt (Fig. 79–4), and the other isolation of the shunt where it communicates with the hepatic vein prior to the hepatic vein communicating with the prehepatic caudal vena cava (Fig. 79–5). A third approach involves an intravascular (within the prehepatic vena cava) technique (see Fig. 79–6); this method does not compromise portal blood flow to the liver.

The first procedure involves isolating the extrahepatic portal vein prior to the portal vein tributary entering specific liver lobes (see Fig. 79–4). The small livers of these patients make identification of the portal branches possible. The ductus venosus or intrahepatic shunt may arise from the left (most common) or right main branch of the portal vein and

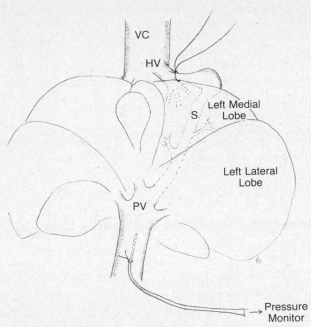

Figure 79–5. Intrahepatic portacaval shunt: extrahepatic hepatic vein approach. A ligature is placed around the shunt (S) vessel as it enters the hepatic vein (HV) prior to entering the vena cava (VC). Note the aneurysmal dilatation of the shunt as it exits the liver. A catheter is placed in the portal vein (PV) to measure portal venous pressure.

may communicate with a hepatic vein draining the left, central, and right hepatic divisions. Because of its variable location, the intrahepatic shunt may be difficult to locate. Segmental isolation and obstruction of portal vein branches while monitoring portal pressure usually indicate the area of the shunt. Hepatic portal resistance is negligible in large intrahepatic shunts, and portal venous pressure is near or equal to central venous pressure (3 to 5 cm H_2O). Obstructions of a portal vein branch not intimately connected with the shunt result in no change in portal pressure. When the portal vein intimately connected with the shunt is obstructed, portal vein pressure increases to normal (8 to 15 cm H_2O) or above normal. Additionally, the appearance of a large prehepatic bulbous aneurysm near the hepatic vein or the presence of a palpable hepatic parenchymal "soft spot" indicates the location of the intrahepatic portacaval shunt.

Blind probing with a portal vein catheter (a side-hole catheter or infant feeding tube) into the intrahepatic portal circulation frequently results in the catheter being slipped through the shunt defect and into the prehepatic caudal vena cava. Palpation of this catheter as it passes between liver lobes and through the shunt identifies the path through the intrahepatic portacaval shunt.

Once the shunt is located, the portal vein supplying this area is isolated. Every attempt should be made to isolate only that portion of the portal vein that supplies the portacaval shunt, taking care to avoid portal vein branches not associated with the shunt and hepatic arteries and biliary ducts of all liver lobes.

The second site of intrahepatic portacaval shunt

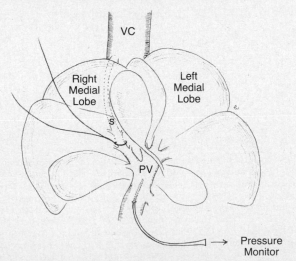

Figure 79–4. Intrahepatic portacaval shunt: extrahepatic portal vein approach. A ligature is placed around the shunt (S) vessel before its entry into the liver. The shunt empties into the vena cava (VC). A catheter for measuring portal venous pressure is placed into the portal vein (PV).

manipulation is performed extravascularly and cranial to the liver where the shunt joins the hepatic venous system (see Fig. 79–5). This location is usually chosen only when the hepatic parenchymal tissue does not completely encircle the shunt. In our experience, this site involves only the left medial or lateral liver

lobe. Incision of the left triangular ligaments frees the left lateral liver lobe; retraction of this lobe to a right, cephalic position improves the exposure of the junction between the anomalous shunt and the left hepatic vein. Following careful sharp and blunt dissection, a ligature can be passed around the anoma-

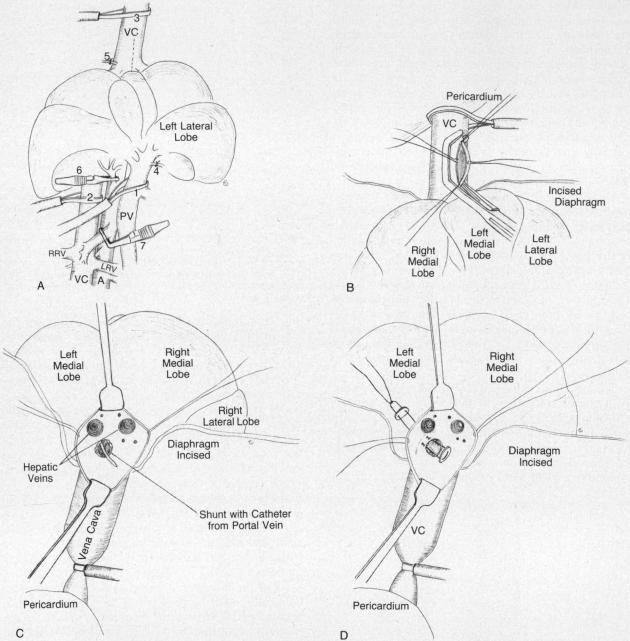

Figure 79–6. Intrahepatic portacaval shunt: intravascular repair. *A*, Vascular occlusion. Temporary venous occlusion is accomplished by placing moistened umbilical tape ligatures around the: (*1*) portal vein (*PV*), (*2*) caudal vena cava (*VC*) caudal to liver, and (*3*) caudal vena cava, cranial to the liver, leaving adequate space for the partial occlusion clamp and venotomy incision (dotted line). The umbilical tape ligatures are passed through rubber tubing for temporary occlusion. The phrenicoabdominal veins are ligated if their flow contributes to hepatic flow during occlusion; variable entry of the phrenicoabdominal veins into the portal vein (*4*) or vena cava cranial to the liver (*5*) is noted in the illustration. (If the phrenicoabdominal vein enters the vena cava near the real veins [*RRV* or *LRV*], ligation is not necessary.) Temporary arterial occlusion is accomplished with bulldog clamps placed on the celiac artery (*6*) and the cranial mesenteric artery (*7*). If isolation of these arteries is not possible, an arterial clamp may be temporarily placed across the aorta (*A*). *B*, A partial tangential occlusion clamp is applied and an incision into the vena cava (*VC*) is made. Retraction sutures are placed to aid intravascular exposure. *C*, Diaphragmatic view. Retraction sutures and Cushing vein retractors allow exposure of the intrahepatic defect. The normal hepatic veins have a tunnelled appearance with smooth margins. In contrast, the anomalous shunt vessel has irregular margins. The shunt may enter either a hepatic vein or the vena cava. *D*, Suture pattern. The attenuating suture is placed through a felt pledget outside the vena cava (*VC*), through the vena cava, across the shunt opening, and into an intraluminal felt pledget.

Illustration continued on opposite page

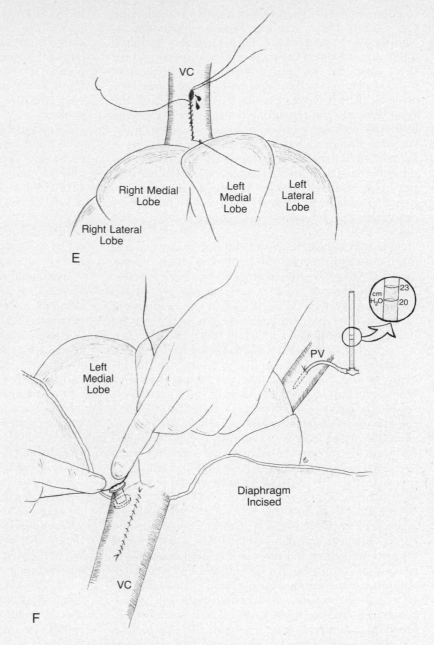

Figure 79–6 Continued. E, Closure of the vena cava. A continuous suture pattern closes the venotomy incision. Trapped air and blood are allowed to escape from the venotomy prior to final suture placement. The temporary occlusion tape on the vena cava cranial to the liver is removed last. *F*, The shunt is attenuated with the preplaced suture while the portal venous pressure is monitored. The pressure should not exceed 20 to 23 cm H_2O or 18 mm Hg.

lous vessel at its junction with the hepatic vein. A single silk ligature is used to attenuate or obstruct the anomalous vessel.

The third method for closure of the intrahepatic portacaval shunt is an intravascular technique that does not compromise portal blood flow to the liver lobes. A medial epigastric incision is performed that extends into a medial sternotomy with the incision of three to four sternebrae. The diaphragm is incised down to the vena cava hiatus; this incision is continued partially around the vena cava. Umbilical tapes are passed around the thoracic caudal vena cava near the border of the pericardial sac, the posthepatic caudal cava proximal to the renal veins, and the portal vein just proximal to the first hepatic branch. The umbilical tapes are passed through rubber tubing for obstruction of vessel flow when needed.

The phrenicoabdominal veins are identified, isolated, and ligated. The celiac and cranial mesenteric arteries are isolated and prepared for obstruction by vascular occlusive instruments (bulldog clamps) (Fig. 79–6A). Regional hypothermia of the splanchnic viscera with an ice slush of lactated Ringer's solution or saline may protect abdominal organs during venous occlusion. Moderate hypothermia should be included in the anesthetic regimen at this stage of the surgical procedure; i.e., heating blankets turned off, intravenous fluids cooled.

Traction sutures (3-0 silk) are placed in the prehepatic caudal vena cava at the left hepatic vein. With slight elevation of the traction sutures, the vena cava wall is elevated and a partial occluding vascular clamp placed as close to the liver as possible (Fig. 79–6B). Between the partial occluding clamp and traction sutures, a longitudinal incision is made with scalpel and Potts' scissors. Hepatic blood flow is completely obstructed by tightening the umbilical tapes around the prehepatic and posthepatic caudal vena cava and the portal vein and placement of bulldog clamps on the celiac and cranial mesenteric arteries. The vascular clamp is removed from the vena cava and the remaining hepatic blood aspirated from the venotomy incision. Exposure of the intravascular defect, which is variable in location, is evident by its sharp, irregular border; hepatic veins typically have a "tunnelled" appearance. If a catheter has been threaded through the defect into the prehepatic caudal vena cava, the defect is readily apparent where the venous catheter emerges through the defect (Fig. 79–6C).

Although partial suture of the defect with simple interrupted or cruciate stitches is commonly recommended, we presently recommend one large mattress suture buttressed with a Dacron pledget passed through opposite walls of the defect and brought out through the vena cava wall near the border of the hepatic parenchymal vein wall (Fig. 79–6D). This suture is not tied until normal hepatic blood flow and pressure occur. Slight traction is placed on the sutures in the vena cava, and the partial occluding vascular clamp is placed to confine the limits of the venotomy incision. The clamp is placed loosely over the caudal cava to allow escape of air from the vascular channels of the liver and vena cava when the portal vein and the abdominal caudal vena cava tapes and the celiac and cranial mesenteric bulldog clamps are released (Fig. 79–6E). The thoracic caudal vena cava tape is released last.

Hepatic blood flow can be interrupted safely for periods of up to 20 minutes. During shunt manipulation, however, splanchnic blood flow is interrupted for no longer than ten minutes. If additional time is needed to complete the technique, the partial occluding clamp may be replaced and the caudal vena cava and the vascular obstructing tapes and instruments released for a 10- to 15-minute period. Once blood pressure and flow are stable, the splanchnic circulation can again be obstructed and intracaval manipulation of the shunt performed a second time. During obstruction of the splanchnic circulation, systemic arterial and abdominal caudal vena caval pressure decrease and increase to a mean of 30 and 25 mm Hg, respectively. Autoregulatory vasodilation of hypoxic splanchnic and distal peripheral circulations may require the administration of a large volume of fluid or an alpha-stimulating drug (phenylephrine, 200 to 400 µg) to increase systemic arterial pressure following the removal of the obstructing tapes and instruments.

With the vascular occluding clamps in place and vascular pressures at levels equal to those that existed prior to the obstruction of hepatic blood flow, the preplaced, buttressed mattress suture across the defect is tied slowly while portal venous pressure is monitored (Fig. 79–6F). Portal pressure should not exceed 18 mm Hg. Following attenuation or obstruction of the defect, the caudal vena caval incision is closed with a simple continuous suture pattern using one of the preplaced traction sutures. The diaphragm, median sternotomy, and median epigastric abdominal incisions are repaired in a routine manner. The portal vein pressure catheter is treated as previously described.

Intravascular obstruction of portacaval shunts by total interruption of the liver circulation is a difficult technique, and the small patient size (<10 kg) probably precludes adequate venotomy length and exposure of the defect within the liver. Which technique to use for surgical manipulation of the single intrahepatic portosystemic shunt depends on the location of the shunt, the accessibility of the extrahepatic portal venous system, the size of the liver and patient, and the accessibility of the hepatic venous system.

Intrahepatic portacaval shunts are most easily attenuated or occluded cranial to the liver where the shunt joins the hepatic venous system; this technique is usually best suited for those shunts only partially encircled by hepatic parenchymal tissue. Although most of the shunts that are only partially encircled by hepatic parenchymal tissue exist as free vessels and could be more easily attenuated or occluded at this extrahepatic site, it is impossible to determine whether a second or third small intrahepatic shunt communicates from the normal intrahepatic portal system and the large anomalous shunt just before the larger shunt drains into the hepatic vein. Preoperative angiography does not often identify a complete intrahepatic portal system in dogs with large single portacaval shunts. If the surgeon elects to attenuate or occlude a shunt that is partially or completely surrounded by hepatic parenchymal tissue at a location free of hepatic tissue, portal angiography should be performed during surgery and following shunt attenuation.

Another theoretical technique for correction of the intrahepatic portosystemic shunt is placement of a special "umbrella" vascular catheter to partially or completely obstruct the shunt window. This occlusive catheter may be placed by fluoroscopy or during surgery. The umbrella web, opened within the ductus venosus, slowly closes over several weeks to completely or nearly completely obstruct shunt blood flow. If the liver is unable to handle the increased portal blood flow, mild portal hypertension and multiple portosystemic shunts may develop. However, if the umbrella web thromboses acutely and the liver is unable to accept the increased portal blood flow, the patient may die from severe splanchnic congestion.

Theoretically, direct portal vein catheterization with the presently available intravenous catheter tip filters and occluders makes it possible to decrease shunt flow during the catheterization procedure, thus eliminating the need for major surgery for attenuation or occlusion of intrahepatic portosystemic shunts. Because potentially fatal portal hypertension usually develops when the intrahepatic portacaval shunt is completely occluded, intravascular catheter tip attenuation of the intrahepatic shunt would probably require determining portal pressure at the time of attenuation and partially obstructing blood flow that would preclude acute thrombosis. The large diameter of most single extrahepatic or intrahepatic shunts accounts for portal hypotension prior to surgery; transient portal hypertension (16 to 18 mm Hg) is the usual sequela to surgical attenuation or obstruction of the shunt.[8, 9]

SURGERY OF MULTIPLE EXTRAHEPATIC PORTOSYSTEMIC SHUNTS

In the past, dogs with extrahepatic multiple portacaval shunts have been subjected to surgical techniques that attempted to increase hepatic blood flow and included (1) peritonealization of a raw liver surface with a segmental intestinal neurovascular pedicle, (2) an end-to-end splenic artery, portal-vein arteriovenous anastomosis, (3) multiple obstruction of a large number of the portacaval shunts, and (4) a combination of these treatments. No alterations in clinicopathological data nor improvement in patient symptoms has been observed following previous surgical manipulations. Clinical improvement has been observed in more than 60 per cent of the dogs with multiple extrahepatic shunts following suture atten-

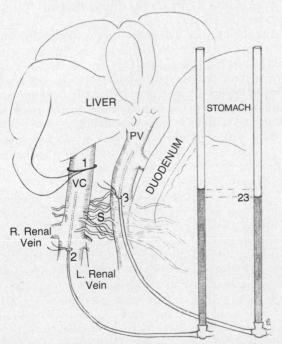

Figure 79–7. Multiple extrahepatic portacaval shunts. When multiple shunts (*S*) are identified, a ligature (*1*) is placed around the vena cava (*VC*) between the shunts and the liver. Catheters are placed in the vena cava (*2*) and portal vein (*3*) to measure venous pressure. The ligature around the vena cava is tightened until the vena caval pressure exceeds the portal venous pressure by 1 to 2 mm Hg and the maximum portal venous pressure does not exceed 20 to 23 cm H_2O or 18 mm Hg.

uation of the caudal vena cava just behind the hepatic hiatus (Fig. 79–7). Incomplete ligation of the vena cava is performed with a silk suture until a gradient of 1 or 2 mm Hg pressure is established from the posthepatic caudal vena cava to the portal vein. Posthepatic vena caval attenuation results in a minimal elevation in portal vein pressure (from 10 to 12 to 14 to 17 mm Hg) and a marked elevation in posthepatic vena caval pressure (from 0 to 4 to 16 to 18 mm Hg). Central venous pressure and systemic arterial pressure usually remain unchanged. During posthepatic vena caval occlusion, intravenous glucagon (which reduces hepatic vascular resistance) does not alter portal, posthepatic vena caval, right atrial, or systemic arterial pressures.

ARTERIOVENOUS FISTULA

Both hepatic artery to portal vein and hepatic artery to hepatic vein communications may exist. Resection of the liver lobe is performed if the arteriovenous shunt involves a single liver lobe. Because of the extensive arterial supply to the affected lobes, lobectomy is best performed by vascular occlusion (see Fig. 79–6A) as for intravascular intrahepatic shunt repair. Although current texts often describe finger fractionation techniques for lobectomy, in the A-V fistula patient this technique increases the possibility of fatal hemorrhage. Prior to vascular occlusion, all easily isolated vessels and biliary ducts of the involved lobe are ligated. To minimize blood loss that would ensue from blunt finger dissection techniques, the occlusion tapes are applied and the lobes excised with rapid sharp dissection. Vascular defects are oversewn with 4-0 or 5-0 vascular suture prior to release of the venous and arterial occluders.

If hepatic lobe resection cannot be performed, selective dearterialization of the affected lobe should be performed. Dearterialization involves identification, isolation, and ligation of the hepatic arterial supply to the specific lobe containing the A-V fistula. Although suture material can be used for the arterial ligatures, arterial vascular hemoclips are easier to use. If dearterialization rather than hepatic lobectomy is performed, systemic arterial collateral vessels may persist, resulting in recurrence of the disease. Selected dearterialization for embolization through an angiocatheter may be effective for hepatic A-V fistula. Acrylic, gel, foam, muscle, polyurethane foam, or similar substances may be injected through an angiocatheter to effectively obliterate the A-V shunt.

The multiple portosystemic shunts that usually accompany the hepatic artery–portal venous fistula require banding of the vena cava (see surgery for multiple extrahepatic portacaval shunts). During manipulation of these shunts, portal venous pressures are monitored and should not exceed 18 mm Hg. If portal hypertension persists following partial hepatectomy of the involved liver lobes, manipulation of the multiple shunts at the time of surgery is not advised. This portal hypertension may regress over the first two to three weeks postoperatively, at which time the caudal caval banding procedure for multiple shunts may be considered.

OTHER SURGICAL CONSIDERATIONS

Cases with cystic or renal calculi are managed according to the severity of the urinary tract involvement and the length of time involved for the primary liver procedure. If the surgical time has been brief and the patient is stable, urinary calculi are removed from the bladder or one kidney at the time of the shunt surgery. However, if the surgery has been lengthy, the urinary calculi may be left for a second operation several weeks later. If the urinary calculi are jeopardizing the recovery of the patient because of recurring urinary obstruction, treatment is mandatory. Biurate crystals do not resorb; if they exist in the kidney or bladder they should be removed at the initial or a second operation.

Following all extensive hepatic manipulations, the abdomen is lavaged with several liters of warm saline. A liver biopsy specimen is taken prior to abdominal closure. Should a second operation be necessary for urinary calculi, a second liver biopsy study provides an indication of progression of the disease process.

In the rare cases in which the portal vein empties directly into the vena cava, completely bypassing the liver, orthotopic liver transplantation may be an alternative. Immunosuppressive agents are necessary to avoid rejection of canine liver allografts.[64]

RESULTS AND COMPLICATIONS

Prior to 1976, medical palliation was the only treatment for portacaval shunts.[14, 18, 63, 74] Presently, single shunts are surgically identified, isolated, and attenuated or obstructed depending on portal pressure. For single extrahepatic shunts, surgical treatment has resulted in minimal mortality and excellent prognosis. Clinical improvement is generally noted within the first postoperative day. Signs of hepatic encephalopathy generally disappear. Immediate postoperative biochemical evaluation of the liver and pancreas (serum enzymes, BSP clearance, ammonia tolerance) is like that of dogs undergoing other types of major abdominal surgery. Most of these animals do very well in terms of weight gain, reversal of central nervous system and gastrointestinal signs, decrease in susceptibility to disease, and increase in life expectancy. Nuclear scans with ^{99m}Tc sulfur colloid taken one to two days postoperatively reveal improved liver uptake and reduced extrahepatic uptake of the colloid. Time/activity curves show hepatic arterial and portal venous uptake slopes similar to those in normal dogs.[40]

Single intrahepatic portacaval shunts present a technically more difficult problem. Identification and isolation of the anomalous communication are more difficult, and surgical risks are increased. Hemorrhage is of critical concern in patients with low hematocrits, hypoproteinemia, and coagulation defects. Transfusions of whole blood or plasma may be necessary. When hepatic blood flow is interrupted by the surgical technique, the duration of splanchnic occlusion is critical to the survival of the patient. Complete hepatic circulatory stasis should not last longer than 10 to 12 minutes at any one time. Previous mortality studies in dogs subjected to hepatic circulatory occlusion of less than 20 minutes duration indicated 100 per cent survival. Splanchnic visceral ischemia can result in release of potent vasoactive vasodilator substances. Patients subjected to temporary splanchnic circulatory arrest may develop mild arterial hypotension or peripheral and splanchnic venous hypertension. Alpha-adrenergic drugs may be administered intravenously to reverse the systemic arterial hypotension that may occur following splanchnic circulatory arrest.

Postoperative fatal portal vein thrombosis has been observed in one dog with a partially attenuated intrahepatic shunt (within two hours). If manipulation of the liver and shunt have been extensive, a single anticoagulant dose of heparin may be advisable at the time of shunt ligation. Should hemorrhage become an overriding concern, protamine sulfate may be administered. Although the majority of patients with intrahepatic shunts do well following surgery, the incidence of complications, including postoperative hepatic failure, is higher than for animals with single extrahepatic shunts.

Although the overall prognosis for single intra- and extrahepatic shunts is excellent, the prognosis for multiple extrahepatic shunts is not as favorable. At present, no criteria are available to predict which cases of hepatic dysfunction with multiple shunts will benefit from surgical intervention. In the past, we attempted a number of salvage surgical procedures in dogs with multiple extrahepatic portacaval shunts that could not be controlled by dietary palliation. Although the salvage procedures did not result in mortality, patients were not improved.

Currently, the surgical method of choice for multiple extrahepatic shunts is partial attenuation of the caudal vena cava posterior to the liver but anterior to the splanchnic varices. The ligature is tightened until a caval-to-portal gradient of 1 to 2 mm Hg exists (pressure not to exceed 20 mm Hg). Ascites and pelvic limb edema are not uncommon sequelae in these dogs with partially attenuated posterior vena cava and mild portal hypertension. Ascites generally disappears within two to three weeks of surgery, suggesting a decrease in portal pressure and splanchnic resistance. Occasionally ascites occurs with single shunt ligation with mild portal hypertension as well. However, no dogs with single shunts and transient ascites developed multiple extrahepatic shunts postoperatively.

Clinical improvement is generally noted within the

first two days postoperatively. Nuclear scintigrams two days postoperatively are similar to postoperative scans of single shunts; increased liver uptake and decreased extrahepatic uptake are noted. Subtle balances may exist among portal hypertension, functional or nutritional hepatic flow, microvascular intrahepatic shunting, and extrahepatic uptake. Approximately 60 per cent of dogs with multiple shunts and an attenuated caudal vena cava have improved clinically. Long-term follow-up reports are not yet available.

All animals with portosystemic shunts should be considered surgical candidates. Clinical, biochemical, and nuclear scintigraphic improvement indicate reversibility of poor liver function in most cases. When biopsy samples from single portacaval shunts have been obtained several months postoperatively, the histopathological description resembles that of normal liver. When surgery has not been curative, medical management is indicated.

RESEARCH IMPLICATIONS

Although pathological changes in the livers of dogs with portosystemic shunts vary from those in humans, a number of clinical as well as pathophysiological changes are similar.

Medical management and dietary alterations in the percentage of protein and the composition of amino acids are being investigated in both species. Compared with humans, the branched-chain to aromatic amino acid ratio in plasma decreases in animals with hepatic dysfunction and is extremely low in portosystemic shunts. This same altered aminogram is seen in human cerebrospinal fluid and has been implicated in pathogenesis of portosystemic encephalopathy. The metabolism of the increased numbers of aromatic amino acids to potentially toxic intermediates and its relationship to decreased synthesis of central neurotransmitters are active areas of current research. Initial results of studies using essential amino acid diets in both humans and dogs have been equivocal in reversing amino acid ratios. Clinical improvement on these low-protein purified diets is observed in both species.

Alternate pathways of ammonia excretion are also being investigated in humans and dogs. Infants with urea cycle enzymopathies and hyperammonemia have shown clinical improvement and reduced ammonia levels following administration of sodium benzoate. Sodium benzoate should promote the excretion of nitrogen as hippurate rather than as urea. Hippurate nitrogen is derived from glycine or ammonium ion. Whether sodium benzoate, which relies on a liver pathway, would be useful in reducing ammonia levels in hepatic encephalopathy is unknown. Whether a reduction in ammonia would result in reversibility of encephalopathic signs is also unknown.

Nuclear scintigraphic methods for investigations of extrahepatic uptake with ^{99m}Tc sulfur colloid, macroaggregated albumin, and inert gas washout studies have all suggested a difference between total blood flow and total nutritional or functional blood flow. Improvement of hepatic function by altering pressure gradients and decreasing shunt percentages is currently under investigation. Determinations of microvascular shunt fraction to total nutritional blood flow may yield information regarding the severity of hepatic disease and may be a prognostic indicator for particular surgical treatment or medical intervention.[10-12, 32, 33, 35, 42, 43, 54, 61, 62, 70, 72, 77]

1. Adamsons, R. J., Arif, S., Babich, A., Butt, K., Lam, A., and Minkowitz, S.: Arterialization of the liver in combination with a porta-caval shunt in the dog. Surg. Gynecol. Obstet. *140*:594, 1975.
2. Batshaw, M. L., and Brusilow, S. W.: Treatment of hyperammonemic coma caused by inborn errors of urea synthesis. J. Pediatr. 97:893, 1980.
3. Batshaw, M. L., Painter, M. J., Sproul, G. T., Schafer, I. A., Thomas, G. H., and Brusilow, S.: Therapy of urea cycle enzymopathies: Three case studies. Genetics Clinics of the Johns Hopkins Hospital. Johns Hopkins Med. J. *148*:34, 1981.
4. Bennett, T. D., and Rothe, C. F.: Hepatic capacitance responses to changes in flow and hepatic venous pressure in dogs. Am. J. Physiol. *240*:H18, 1981.
5. Biersack, H. J., Torres, J., Thelen, M., Monzon, O., and Winkler, C.: Determination of liver and spleen perfusion by quantitative sequential scintigraphy: Results in normal subjects and in patients with portal hypertension. Clin. Nucl. Med. *16*:218, 1981.
6. Bradley, S. E.: Methods of evaluation of the splanchnic circulation. *In* McMichael, J. (ed.): Circulation. Proceedings of the Tercentenary Congress. Blackwell, Oxford, 1958, p. 255.
7. Breznock, E. M.: Surgical manipulation of portosystemic shunts in dogs. J. Am. Vet. Med. Assoc., *174*:819, 1979.
8. Breznock, E. M.: Surgery of the liver. *In* Bojrab, M. J. (ed.): *Current Techniques in Small Animal Surgery*, 2nd ed. J. B. Lippincott, Philadelphia, 1981.
9. Breznock, E. M., Berger, B., Pendray, D., Wagner, S., Manley, P., Whiting, P., Hornof, W., and West, D.: Surgical manipulation of intrahepatic portacaval shunts in dogs. J. Am. Vet. Med. Assoc. *182*:798, 1983.
10. Burchell, A. R.: Hemodynamic evaluation of shunting techniques. *In* Orloff, M. J., Stipa, S., and Ziparo, V. (eds.): *Medical and Surgical Problems of Portal Hypertension*. Academic Press, London, 1982.
11. Burchell, A. R., Moreno, A. H., Panke, W. F., and Nealon, T. F.: Hepatic artery flow improvement after portacaval shunt: A single hemodynamic clinical correlate. Ann. Surg. *184*:289, 1976.
12. Charters, A. C., Brown, B. N., Sviolka, S. C., Knox, D. G., and Orloff, M. J.: The influence of portal perfusion on the response to portavacal shunt. Am. J. Surg. *310*:226, 1975.
13. Christie, J. H., and Chaudburi, T. K.: Measurement of hepatic blood flow. Semin. Nucl. Med. *2*:97, 1972.
14. Cornelius, L. M., Thrall, D. E., Halliwell, W. H., Grank, G. M., Kern, A. J., and Woods, C. B.: Anomalous portosystemic anastomoses associated with chronic hepatic insufficiency in six young dogs. J. Am. Vet. Med. Assoc. *167*:220, 1975.
15. Crouch, J. E.: *Atlas of Cat Anatomy*. Lea & Febiger, Philadelphia, 1969.
16. Delin, N. A., Ekestrom, S., Lindahl, J., Nylander, G., and Sundblad, R.: Immediate changes in blood flow and oxygen metabolism of the cirrhotic liver following portacaval shunt operations. Surg. Gynecol. Obstet. *144*:499, 1977.
17. Elias, E. G., and Evans, J. T.: Segmental revascularization of the liver. J. Surg. Res. *12*:346, 1972.

18. Ewing, G. O., Suter, P. F., and Bailey, C. S.: Hepatic insufficiency associated with congenital anomalies of the portal vein in dogs. J. Am. Anim. Hosp. Assoc. 10:463, 1974.

19. Fischer, J. E.: Portosystemic encephalopathy. In Wright, R., Alberti, K. G. M. M., Karran, S., and Millward-Sadler, G. H. (eds.): Liver and Biliary Disease. W. B. Saunders, Philadelphia, 1979, pp. 973–1001.

20. Fischer, J. E., Funovics, J. M., Aguirre, A., James, J. H., Keane, J. M., Wesdorp. R. I. C., Yoshimura, N., and Westmau, T.: The role of plasma amino acids in hepatic encephalopathy. Surgery 78:276, 1975.

21. Fischer, J. E., Rosen, H. M., Ebeid, A. M., James, J. H., Keane, J. M., and Soeters, P. B.: The effect of normalization of plasma amino acid on hepatic encephalopathy in man. Surgery 80:77, 1976.

22. Fleming, J. S., Humphries, N. L. M., Karran, S. J., Goddard, B. A., and Ackery, D. M.: In vivo assessment of hepatic-arterial and portal-venous components of liver perfusion: Concise communications. J. Nucl. Med. 22:18, 1981.

23. George, C. F., and Watt, P. J.: The liver and response to drugs. In Wright, R., Alberti, K. G. M. M., Karran, S., and Millward-Sadler, G. H. (eds.): Liver and Biliary Disease. W. B. Saunders, Philadelphia, 1979, pp. 344–377.

24. Gofton, N.: Surgical ligation of congenital portosystemic venous shunts in the dog: A report of three cases. J. Am. Anim. Hosp. Assoc. 14:728, 1978.

25. Griffiths, G. L., Lumsden, J. H., and Valli, V. E. O.: Hematologic and biochemical changes in dogs with porto-systemic shunts. J. Am. Anim. Hosp. Assoc. 17:205, 1981.

26. Gross, G., Goldberg, H. I., and Shames, D. M.: A new approach to evaluating hepatic blood flow in the presence of intrahepatic portal systemic shunting. Invest. Radiol. 11:146, 1976.

27. Groszmann, R. J., Kravetz, D., and Parysow, O.: Intrahepatic arteriovenous shunting in cirrhosis of the liver. Gastroenterology 73:201, 1977.

28. Hardy, R. M.: Diseases of the liver. In Ettinger, S. J. (ed.): Textbook of Veterinary Internal Medicine: Diseases of the Dog and Cat. W. B. Saunders, Philadelphia, 1975, 1219–1246.

29. Hockerstedt, K., Nieminen, J., and Scheinin, T. M.: Liver blood flow after liver hilus dearterialization. Ann. Chir. Gynaecol. Fenn. 67:224, 1978.

30. Hornof, W. J., Koblick, P. D., and Breznock, E. M.: Radio-colloid scintigraphy as an aid to the diagnosis of congenital portacaval anomalies in the dog. J. Am. Vet. Med. Assoc. 182:44, 1983.

31. Hornof, W. J., and Suter, P. F.: The use of prostaglandin E₁ and Tolazoline to improve cranial mesenteric arterial portography in the dog. J. Am. Vet. Radiol. Soc. 20:15, 1979.

32. Huet, P. M., Chartrand, R., and Marleau, D.: Extrahepatic uptake of ^{99m}Tc-phytate: Its mechanism and significance in chronic liver disease. Gastroenterology 78:76, 1980.

33. Huet, P. M., Lavoie, P., Legare, A., and Viallet, A.: Combined hepatic vein, umbilicoportal vein, and superior mesenteric artery catheterization in portal hypertension: Estimation of the portal fraction of total hepatic blood flow in cirrhotic patients. Yale J. Biol. Med. 48:55, 1975.

34. Huet, P. M., Marleau, D., Lavoie, P., and Viallet, A.: Extraction of 1251-Albumin microaggregates from portal blood. An index of functional portal blood supply in cirrhotics. Gastroenterology 70:74, 1976.

35. Huet, P. M., Villeneuve, J. P., Marleau, D., and Viallet, A.: Hepatic circulation: Applicable human methodology. In Lautt, W. W. (ed.): Hepatic Circulation in Health and Disease. Raven Press, New York, 1981, pp. 57–86.

36. Humphreys, D. J.: Benzoic acid poisoning in the cat. Vet. Rec. 98:219, 1976.

37. Inokucki, K., Kobayashi, M., Ogawa, Y., Saku, M., Nagasue, N., and Iwaki, A.: Results of left gastric vena-caval shunt for esophageal varices: Analysis of one hundred clinical cases. Surgery 78:628, 1975.

38. Kershner, D., Hooton, T. C., and Shearer, E. M.: Production of experimental portal hypertension in the dog. Arch. Surg. 53:425, 1946.

39. Koblick, P. D., Hornof, W. J., and Breznock, E. M.: Quantitative hepatic scintigraphy in the dog. Vet. Radiol., 24:226, 1983.

40. Koblick, P. D., Hornof, W. J., and Breznock, E. M.: Use of quantitative hepatic scintigraphy to evaluate spontaneous portosystemic shunts in 12 dogs. Vet. Radiol., 24:232, 1983.

41. Lantz, B. M. T., Link, D. P., Holcroft, J. W., and Foerster, J. M.: Video dilution technique: Angiographic determination of splanchnic blood flow. In Granger, D. N., and Buckley, G. B. (eds.): Measurement of Blood Flow: Applications to the Splanchnic Circulation. Williams & Wilkins, Baltimore, 1981, 425–438.

42. Leiberman, D. P., Mathie, R. T., Harper, A. M., and Blumbart, L. H.: An isotope clearance method for measurement of liver blood flow during portosystemic shunt in man. Br. J. Surg. 65:578, 1978.

43. Lindberg, B. O., and Clowes, G. H.: An experimental method for study of liver blood flow and metabolism in intact animals. J. Surg. Res. 31:156, 1981.

44. Lohse, C. L., and Suter, P. F.: Functional closure of the ductus venosus during early postnatal life in the dog. Am. J. Vet. Res. 38:839, 1977.

45. Markowitz, J., Archibald, J., and Downie, H. G.: Surgery of the liver. In Markowitz, J., et al.: Experimental Surgery, 5th ed. Williams & Wilkins, Baltimore, 1964, pp. 507–562.

46. Miller, M. E., Christensen, G. C., and Evans, H. E.: Anatomy of the Dog. W. B. Saunders, Philadelphia, 1964.

47. Moreno, A. H., Burchell, A. R., Reddy, R. V., Stean, J. A., Panke, W. F., and Nealon, T. F.: Spontaneous reversal of portal blood flow: The case for and against its occurrence in patients with cirrhosis of the liver. Ann. Surg. 181:346, 1975.

48. Moreno, A. H., Burchell, A. R., Rousselot, L. M., Panke, W. F., Slafsky, F., and Burke, J. H.: Portal blood flow in cirrhosis of the liver. J. Clin. Invest. 46:436, 1967.

49. Nabseth, D. C., Widrich, W. C., O'Hara, E. T., and Johnson, W. C.: Flow and pressure characteristics of the portal system before and after splenorenal shunts. Surgery 78:739, 1975.

50. Plum, F., and Posner, J. B.: The Diagnosis of Stupor and Coma. F. A. Davis, Philadelphia, 1972.

51. Read, A. E.: The liver and drugs. In Wright, R., Alberti, K. G. M. M., Karran, S., and Millward-Sadler, G. H. (eds.): Liver and Biliary Disease. W. B. Saunders, Philadelphia, 1979, pp. 822–847.

52. Richardson, P. D. I., and Withrington, P. G.: Liver blood flow: I. Intrinsic and nervous control of liver blood flow. Gastroenterology 81:159, 1981.

53. Richardson, P. D. I., and Withrington, P. G.: Liver blood flow: II. Effects of drugs and hormones on liver blood flow. Gastroenterology 81:356, 1981.

54. Rigotti, P., Zanchin, G., Vassanelli, P., Bettineschi, F., Dussini, N., and Battistin, L.: Cerebral amino acid levels and transport after portacaval shunt in the rat: Effects of liver arterialization. J. Surg. Res. 33:415, 1982.

55. Rikkers, L. F.: Radiocolloid technique for quantitation of portosystemic shunting of intestinal blood flow. In Granger, D. N., and Bukley, G. B. (eds.): Measurements of Blood Flow, Applications to the Splanchnic Circulation. Williams & Wilkins, Baltimore, 1981.

56. Rothuizen, J., Van Den Ingh, T. S.: Voorhout, G., Van der Luer, R. J. T., and Wouda, W.: Congenital porto-systemic shunts in sixteen dogs and three cats. J. Small Anim. Pract. 23:67, 1982.

57. Schmidt, S., Lohse, C. L., and Suter, P. F.: Branching patterns of the hepatic artery in the dog: Arteriographic and anatomic study. Am. J. Vet. Res. 41:1090, 1980.

58. Schmidt, S., and Suter, P. F.: Angiography of the hepatic and portal venous system in the dog and cat: An investigative method. Vet. Radiol. 21:57, 1980.

59. Schmidt, S., and Suter, P. F.: Indirect and direct determination of the portal vein pressure in normal and abnormal dogs and normal cats. Vet. Radiol. *21*:246, 1980.

60. Sherding, R. G.: Hepatic encephalopathy in the dog. Comp. Cont. Ed. *1*:55, 1979.

61. Sherriff, S. B., Smart, R. C., and Taylor, I.: Clinical study of liver blood flow in man measured by ^{133}Xe clearance after portal vein injection. Gut *18*:1027, 1977.

62. Simert, G., Persson, T., and Vang, J.: Factors predicting survival after portacaval shunt: A multiple linear regression analysis. Ann. Surg. *187*:174, 1978.

63. Simpson, S. T., and Hribernick, T. N.: Portosystemic shunt in the dog: Two case reports. J. Small Anim. Pract. *17*:163, 1976.

64. Starzl, T. E., Marchioro, T. L., Porter, K. A., Tayler, P. D., Faris, T. D., Hermann, T. J., Hlad, C. J., and Waddell, W. R.: Factors determining short- and long-term survival of orthotopic liver homotransplantation in the dog. Surgery *58*:131, 1965.

65. Strombeck, D. R.: *Small Animal Gastroenterology.* Stonegate Publishing, Davis, CA, 1979.

66. Strombeck, D. R., Breznock, E. M., and McNeal, S.: Surgical treatment for portosystemic shunts in two dogs. J. Am. Vet. Med. Assoc. *170*:1317, 1977.

67. Strombeck, D. R., and Rogers, Q.: Plasma amino acid concentrations in dogs with hepatic disease. J. Am. Vet. Med. Assoc. 173:93, 1978.

68. Suter, P. F.: Portal vein anomalies in the dog: Their angiographic diagnosis. J. Am. Vet. Radiol. Soc. *16*:84, 1975.

69. Suter, P. F.: Radiographic diagnosis of liver disease in dogs and cats. Vet. Clin. North Am. *12*:153, 1982.

70. Thiel, H.: Liver hemodynamics and portacaval shunt. Surg. Gynecol. Obstet. *150*:587, 1980.

71. Thorne, J., Bennett, R., Shields, R., Johnson, J., and Taylor, F.: A comparison of Xe-133 clearance with electromagnetic flowmeters and an indicator dilution method for measurement of liver blood flow. Br. J. Surg. *66*:385, 1979.

72. Ueda, H.: Blood flow shunt and dual blood supply of liver studied with scintillation camera coupled with computer and digital color analyzer. *In* Leevy, C. M. (ed.): *Diseases of the Liver and Biliary Tract.* S. Karger, Basel, 1976, pp. 8–9.

73. Volwiler, W., Grindlay, J., and Bollman, J. L.: The relation of portal vein pressure to the formation of ascites—an experimental study. Gastroenterology *14*:40, 1950.

74. Vulgamott, J. C.: Hepatic encephalopathy associated with acquired portacaval shunt in a dog. J. Am. Vet. Med. Assoc. *175*:724, 1979.

75. Vulgamott, J. C., Turnwald, G. H., King, G. K., Herring, D. S., Hansen, J. F., and Boothe, H. W.: Congenital portacaval anomalies in the cat: Two case reports. J. Am. Anim. Hosp. Assoc. *16*:915, 1980.

76. Waddell, W. G., Bouchard, A. G., Wellington, J. L., and Ewing, J. B.: Functional relations of the proximal components of the portal system: A preliminary report. J. Surg. Res. *12*:281, 1972.

77. Warren, W. D., Millikan, W. J., Henderson, J. M., Wright, L., Kutner, M., Smith, R. B., Fulenwider, J. T., and Salam, A. A.: Ten years' portal hypertensive surgery at Emory: Results and new perspectives. Ann. Surg. *195*:530, 1982.

78. Weber, F. L.: Therapy of portal systemic encephalopathy: The practical and the promising. Gastroenterology *81*:174, 1981.

79. Wheaton, L. G., Sarr, M. G., Schlossberg, L., and Bulkley, G. B.: Gross anatomy of the splanchnic vasculature. *In* Granger, D. N., and Bukley, G. B. (eds.): *Measurements of Blood Flow: Applications to the Splanchnic Circulation.* Williams & Wilkins, Baltimore, 1981, pp. 9–46.

80. Wiederheilm, C. A.: Dynamics of transcapillary fluid exchange. J. Gen. Physiol. *52*:29, 1968.

81. Wiles, C. E., Schenk, W. G., and Lindenberg, J.: The experimental production of portal hypertension. Ann. Surg. *136*:811, 1952.

82. Wright, R., Strunin, L., Davies, G. E., Sipes, I. G., Hempel, V., Davis, M., Neuberger, J. M., et al.: Part IV. Halothane-associated hepatitis. *In* Davis, M., Tredger, J. M., and Williams, R. (eds.): *Drug Reactions and the Liver.* Pitman Medical, Ltd., London, 1981, pp. 205–256.

83. Zieve, L.: The mechanism of hepatic coma. Hepatology *1*:360, 1981.

84. Zink, J.: The fetal and neonatal hepatic circulation. *In* Lautt, W. W. (ed.): *Hepatic Circulation in Health and Disease.* Raven Press, New York, 1981, pp. 227–248.

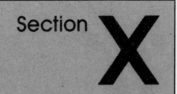

Section **X**

Hemolymphatic System

Anthony Schwartz
Section Editor

Chapter 80

Physiology and Pathophysiology of the Hematopoietic System

Susan M. Cotter and Julia Blue

HEMATOPOIESIS

Hematopoiesis is the process of formation and maturation of the various types of blood cells. The site of hematopoiesis in the embryo is the yolk sac. Stem cells migrate from the yolk sac to the liver near the end of the first third of gestation,[27] and the liver becomes the major site of hematopoiesis in mid-fetal life. The spleen and bone marrow begin to produce hematopoietic cells at about the same time. By the end of gestation the marrow of all bones is hematopoietically active and replaces the liver as the primary organ of blood cell production. The organization of the bone marrow for this purpose is discussed in Chapter 83. The liver and spleen gradually cease to produce hematopoietic cells after birth but retain the capacity to revert to active production throughout adult life.

The red pulp of the spleen is a major site of hematopoiesis during early fetal development, but after the appropriate microenvironment is established in the marrow, hematopoiesis shifts to that tissue. In some species, e.g., the mouse, splenic hematopoiesis may persist throughout life, but hematopoietic activity of the spleen is greatly diminished in postnatal dogs and cats. Megakaryocytes and a few foci of erythropoiesis usually are present in the spleen of normal dogs and cats.

As an animal reaches maturity and its blood volume ceases to expand, active marrow diminishes in the long bones and is replaced by inactive, fatty marrow.[3] If, later in life, there is a strong stimulus to increase blood cell production, as in severe hemolytic anemia, active marrow may expand again into areas that are fatty in normal animals. In patients with congenital hemolytic anemia, the active marrow in the long bones does not involute. In human patients with some types of congenital hemolytic anemia, hematopoietic tissue may expand even beyond the normal limits of the medullary cavity by eroding cortical bone or escaping to the outside of the bones.[11] The rate of erythropoiesis in such patients can be ten times normal or even greater, so the erythrocyte life span sometimes must decrease to one-tenth of normal before anemia becomes evident.

The only sign of shortened erythrocyte survival time in such patients may be reticulocytosis. In Basenji dogs with hereditary pyruvate kinase deficiency, the long bones are filled with hematopoietic marrow into adulthood.[37] However, in many affected dogs, the hematopoietic marrow is replaced progressively by collagen and thickened bone trabeculae (myelofibrosis and osteosclerosis), resulting in hematopoietic failure and death.[2,31] In dogs and cats (especially the latter) with chronic anemia, extramedullary hematopoiesis may develop in organs such as the spleen, liver, or lymph nodes. This response may not be exclusively of benefit to the host. For example, in some feline myeloproliferative disorders, such as erythroleukemia, extramedullary hematopoiesis may be so extensive as to replace the normal architecture of the liver and spleen, yet anemia persists. Thus, ineffective erythropoiesis may accompany damage to the liver and spleen.

Observations of the physical associations between stromal cells and hematopoietic cells and the results of various experimental studies have demonstrated that nonhematopoietic cells of the marrow, including reticular cells, macrophages, endothelial cells, and lymphocytes, provide a special environment necessary for appropriate function of the hematopoietic cells.[12, 44, 46, 47] This hematopoietic microenvironment most likely is the result of complex cell to cell interactions and the local production of regulatory substances. The hematopoietic microenvironment seems to support and regulate the proliferative responses of stem cells, committed precursor cells, and differentiating cells but probably does not determine the cell line to which a stem cell becomes committed. Anemia induced in mice by lethal irradiation can be treated by engraftment of syngeneic marrow stromal elements[32] (see Chapter 15, Transplantation Immunology). Hereditary anemia caused by defective marrow stroma in mice can also be treated by engraftment of normal syngeneic stroma.[32]

The marrow contains pluripotent stem cells that give rise to all red and white cells and platelets[32] (Fig. 80–1). The stem cell, which resembles a small lymphocyte, divides to produce one stem cell and one cell that becomes committed to differentiate along a specific line, depending on the stimulus it receives. Thus, the number of stem cells remains constant unless some are destroyed by a disease or toxin. There is independent control of circulating numbers of each cell lineage. However, when there is active production of red cells, e.g., stimulated as a result of acute blood loss or hemolysis, leukocytosis or thrombocytosis also may occur from concomitant general bone marrow stimulation. In normal individuals the number of circulating cells remains remark-

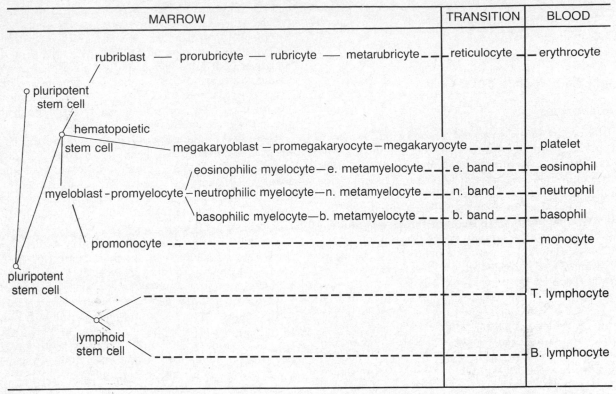

Figure 80–1. A model of hematopoiesis. The stem cell compartment replenishes itself and serves as a source of cells that differentiate as shown. The early stages of differentiation and maturation occur in the marrow. Some immature cells appear in the blood when the system is driven to the left by depletion of mature cells or other stimuli to increase production of given cell types and, in cases of malignancy, of cells of a given lineage.

ably constant owing to homeostatic control mechanisms.

Production of Red Blood Cells

The stem cell pool in the marrow produces rubriblasts, which undergo four additional divisions to become reticulocytes in about three to four days.[13] The nucleus is lost and the cell matures through the reticulocyte stage to become a mature red cell. Thus, one rubriblast gives rise to 16 red cells, if all survive. Apparently, there is some loss of maturing red cells in the marrow. This normal attrition of red cell precursors may provide a reserve capacity should an increased need arise.[35] During maturation the erythrocyte cytoplasm changes from deep blue to red on Wright-Giemsa stain as the hemoglobin content increases. The nucleus becomes smaller and the chromatin more condensed and pyknotic until, finally, the nucleus is extruded. The reticulocyte has no nucleus but does contain many polyribosomes that can be stained with new methylene blue, allowing their enumeration. When stained with Wright-Giemsa stain, the reticulocyte appears slightly larger and more basophilic than the mature red cell. Maturation of canine and human reticulocytes takes one to two days. There has been dispute as to the maturation time and significance in cats, of punctate

reticulocytes, the presence of which may reflect a prolonged reticulocyte maturation time.[9] In normal dogs about 1 per cent of circulating red cells are reticulocytes. In cats, up to 10 per cent of red cells contain some RNA, but only about 1 per cent are young reticulocytes containing aggregates of stainable polyribosomes. The rest of the reticulocytes contain only punctate stained material.

Most maturing erythrocytes enter the blood as reticulocytes. In cats and dogs, even following moderate blood loss or hemolysis, nucleated red cells do not enter the circulating blood. In situations of severe erythrocyte loss, however, increased immature reticulocytes and some circulating nucleated red cells may appear in the blood. The presence of circulating nucleated red cells, *without* the concomitant appearance of reticulocytes, does not indicate a regenerative marrow. Rather, the existence of disorders such as lead poisoning, hemangioendothelioma, and myeloproliferative diseases should be considered.

The rate of erythropoiesis is governed by the rate of oxygen transport to the tissues, which, in turn, depends on both oxyhemoglobin concentration and cardiac output. Hypoxia causes erythropoietin to be produced by the kidney, which causes more erythroid precursors to differentiate. The rate of maturation of erythroid precursors is independent of the degree of anemia. The life span of the red cell varies from 80 to 90 days in the cat and from 110 to 120 days in the dog.[33] For this reason, when bone marrow failure occurs, anemia develops more quickly in cats than in dogs.

Production of White Blood Cells

Granulocytes

In contrast to erythrocytes, granulocytes are present in the blood only while in transit from the marrow to the tissues, where they function primarily in areas of inflammation or bacterial infection. Once neutrophils enter the tissues they do not return to the blood. The stimulus for granulocyte production is less well-defined than that for erythroid cell production. A granulocyte colony–stimulating factor apparently is produced by endothelial cells, fibroblasts, and monocytes.[32] Eosinophils and basophils proliferate in response to parasitic or allergic stimuli, and their life span in the circulation appears to be several days. The half-life of segmented neutrophils in the circulating blood is about six to seven hours, and the entire circulating granulocyte pool is replaced at least twice daily.[3] In man, approximately 1×10^{11} neutrophils, with a packed volume of 66 ml, are produced per day.[3] The time it takes for a progenitor cell committed to differentiate along the myeloid line to become a mature segmented neutrophil is approximately two weeks.[45] Two cell divisions are needed for maturation from myeloblast to promyelocyte to myelocyte. A pool of myelocytes remains in the marrow to produce more myelocytes, i.e., not every one is committed to differentiate.[10] The myelocyte is the most mature cell still capable of cell division. At the myelocyte stage of maturation specific granules of neutrophils, eosinophils, and basophils first become evident. In times of stress or infection, increased numbers of myelocytes begin to divide at the same time that segmented and band neutrophils leave the marrow for the inflammation site. Maturation from myelocyte to neutrophil takes 8 to 14 days. Myelocytes continue to proliferate and provide a reserve supply of granulocytes as the need continues.[45] Granulocyte cell division and maturation times are fixed, regardless of the need. An increase in the number of cells stimulated to replicate allows for rapid and sustained leukocytosis.

Reserves of granulocytes are present in the marrow and on the inner endothelial surfaces of blood vessels. The latter reserve of cells is called the *marginal pool*. The rapid release of the marrow granulocyte pool and utilization of the circulating marginal pool are the first responses to chemotactic stimuli. Epinephrine mobilizes the marginal pool, explaining the leukocytosis that may occur when blood is drawn from a frightened but otherwise normal animal.[33] In dogs, a sterile inflammatory stimulus can deplete marrow stores of granulocytes and cause rapid peripheral granulocytosis within 16 hours.[10] Granulo-

cytosis follows a one- to two-hour period of neutropenia, which occurs as circulating neutrophils leave the blood to approach the inflammatory site. Within 24 hours the myeloid:erythroid (M:E) ratio of the marrow quadruples, associated with a rapid increase in myelocytic replication and DNA synthesis. Thus, it appears that granulopoiesis results when an intramedullary sensing system somehow responds to depletion of neutrophils from the marrow.

Granulocyte Function. Granulocytes rid the body of particulate material, such as bacteria, through phagocytosis (cellular engulfment of an organism). Effective phagocytosis involves chemotaxis, opsonization, ingestion, degranulation, and killing by mechanisms including H_2O_2 and superoxide production and release of lysosomal enzymes.[36] The body has many ways of signalling for help from neutrophils. Such signals, referred to as chemotactic factors, include complement-related factors such as C_3 and C_5 fragments; endogenous enzymes, such as plasminogen activator; fibrin degradation products; bacterial factors such as N-formyl methionine peptides; cellular products, such as lymphokines and products of neutrophil granules; denatured proteins; and foreign proteins.[36] Chemotaxis is defined as migration of a cell against an increasing concentration gradient of such factors. Neutrophils are capable of ameboid motility, which allows them to reach the source of chemotactic stimuli.

Both adherence of complement and specific binding of antibody of the IgG class to an organism can facilitate its phagocytosis by the arriving neutrophils. This process is called *opsonization*. As a neutrophil phagocytizes an organism, the outer layer of the neutrophil cell membrane becomes the inner layer of the resultant phagocytic vacuole (phagosome).[30] Within 30 minutes of phagocytosis, the products of the neutrophil's lysosomal granules are released into the phagosome, which then becomes a *phagolysosome*. At the time of "degranulation," the neutrophil becomes stimulated to undergo a respiratory burst.[1] In the resting neutrophil the major source of energy is anaerobic glycolysis. After stimulation, increased oxygen consumption occurs with production of oxygen radicals, such as superoxide, hydroxyl radicals, hydrogen peroxide, and hypochlorite.[1] These radicals are important for the killing of microorganisms but they can also be toxic to host tissues when released from dying neutrophils. Several mechanisms in the tissues protect against tissue damage by oxygen radicals, including superoxide dismutase, catalase, glutathione, ascorbic acid, and vitamin E.

Defects in chemotaxis, phagocytosis, and degranulation are harmful to the host. Such defects can be iatrogenic. For example, corticosteroids may increase the release of granulocytes from the marrow, but they also decrease chemotaxis and inhibit the exit of neutrophils from the blood into a tissue site of inflammation. Thus, corticosteroids given in the presence of an infection may give the clinician a false sense of security because the white cell count becomes elevated (implying a response to the infection). However, because these circulating cells are not functioning normally, the infection may be under poorer control than if steroids had not been used.

Because of the short life span of circulating granulocytes, they cannot be supplied in a clinically useful way, even by fresh, whole blood transfusion. In man, white blood cell transfusions are used in some specialized centers as part of the short-term therapy of septic neutropenic patients. However, it has been shown that it would require the buffy coat derived from 40 units of whole blood to raise the granulocyte count in human peripheral blood by 1000/μl.[26] More recently, leukapheresis has been utilized in man to obtain white cells for transfusion, but this technique is not yet practical in animals.

Monocytes

These cells arise from myeloblasts, so stimuli for granulocyte production may also result in increased monocyte production (see Fig. 80–1).[21] Mature monocytes may be produced in as short a time as nine to ten hours and are released quickly from the marrow.[41] Their circulatory half-life is 22 hours in the mouse. Monocytes respond more slowly than neutrophils to chemotactic stimuli. They are able to ingest larger particles than granulocytes and persist for months in the tissues as macrophages. Cells of monocyte lineage also "process" antigens for presentation to lymphocytes (see Chapter 15).

Megakaryocytes

Bone marrow megakaryocytes are large cells with multilobed nuclei containing up to 64 times the diploid number of chromosomes. Stimulation for differentiation of stem cells toward megakaryocytes probably is via a humoral factor, thrombopoietin.[32] Platelets form by fragmentation of megakaryocytes (see hereafter). They enter the circulation, where they remain for eight to nine days under ordinary circumstances.[33] Platelets are active in the first stage of coagulation. They aggregate in response to endothelial damage and release factors that activate the clotting mechanism (see Chapter 81).

Lymphocytes

Lymphocyte precursors originally are formed in the marrow but are processed differently to mature into one of several types. They survive, depending on the type, from a few days to years. Some (T cells) are processed in the thymus and are responsible for cell-mediated responses and for helping or suppressing the humoral immune response. Some (B cells) are processed in the bursa of Fabricius in birds or its equivalent in mammals. B cells produce humoral antibodies. Other lymphoid cells (null cells) apparently are processed by neither the bursal equivalent

nor the thymus. Lymphocyte differentiation is covered in more depth in Chapter 15.

Release of Blood Cells From the Marrow

The interplay of several factors leads to release of the various blood cells into the circulation at an appropriate stage of maturity. Megakaryocytes extend strips of cytoplasm, called protoplatelets, through endothelial cells into the sinus lumen, where the strips break free. Subsequently, perhaps in the lungs, the protoplatelets mature further and fragment into as many as 1,200 platelets.[39] Release of reticulocytes and granulocytes from the hematopoietic cords seems to be determined chiefly by the maturity of the cell and the integrity of the sinus wall. These cells must migrate to the outer surface of the sinus, penetrate the cytoplasm of the endothelial cell, and squeeze through the newly formed aperture to gain entry to the sinus lumen.[43] During normal transendothelial passage, the cells are remarkably deformed. Therefore, motility and deformability are prerequisites for passage through an intact sinus wall. Maturation in the granulocyte series is accompanied by increases in both motility and deformability.[22] The reticulocyte, after extrusion of its nucleus, can propel itself the short distance to the sinus wall.[4] Although less deformable than mature red cells, reticulocytes manage to squeeze through the endothelium with little difficulty.[20] Depending on the rate of blood flow through a particular sinus, cells in the lumen may remain there for a variable period of time or be carried away rapidly, into the peripheral blood.

As a cell crosses a sinus wall by pushing through the cytoplasm of the endothelial cell, a temporary aperture is created that closes following its passage.[43] Cell passage takes place only at areas of the sinus wall that are not covered by reticular cell cytoplasm (see Chapter 83). In circumstances of increased cell traffic, less of the endothelium is covered.[6,38] Some evidence suggests that reticular cells may retract their cytoplasm, thereby exposing more of the endothelium. Both endotoxin and erythropoietin can decrease the adventitial cover of the sinus and increase the number of reticulocytes and granulocytes released.[6,19,43] This effect is early and direct and is independent of any stimulatory effect on hematopoiesis.[6] The marked increase in circulating segmented and band neutrophils, often associated with the early stages of acute, severe anemia may well be due to the ability of erythropoietin to enhance the release of not only marrow reticulocytes but granulocytes as well. Leukocytosis is often more severe in acute hemolytic anemia than in acute blood loss. This may be due to stimulation of granulocyte production by breakdown products of damaged red cells. The endothelium itself can be profoundly altered in hyperplastic marrow.[44] In addition, large gaps can develop in the lining of the sinuses, perhaps created by the passage of so many cells that the endothelium is unable to repair itself. Such a change would permit the nonselective release of immature cells of both series.

SURGICAL CONSIDERATIONS IN THE ANEMIC PATIENT

Some anemic patients require surgery for diagnosis or treatment. These patients are discussed relative to the classification of the anemia.

Regenerative Anemia

Included in the category of regenerative anemia are "blood loss" and "hemolytic" anemias. The cause of most blood loss anemia is obvious, although slow or intermittent gastrointestinal blood loss may be hard to diagnose. In the initial stages of acute blood loss, monitoring the packed cell volume (PCV) is not helpful in determining the degree of anemia, because loss of plasma occurs as well and the PCV remains constant. An animal might bleed to death and yet have a normal PCV, because the extravascular to intravascular fluid shift that occurs to maintain circulating blood volume requires several hours before a decrease in the PCV is detectable.[18] There is a delay of about four days after hemorrhage before reticulocytosis occurs. Therefore, the anemia resulting from acute hemorrhage initially is normochromic and normocytic. Signs of shock from decreased circulatory volume include tachycardia, hypotension, pale mucous membranes out of proportion with the drop in PCV, and slow capillary refill time. A refill time of longer than 2 seconds is prolonged and indicates poor peripheral perfusion.[18] The extremities may be cold, and respiration may be rapid and shallow. Monitoring arterial blood pressure by direct or indirect means and central venous pressure may provide useful measurements of the response to fluid or blood therapy.

Acute massive internal or external hemorrhage often requires emergency surgical intervention, whereas less severe traumatic internal hemorrhage due to blunt trauma to the chest or abdomen may cease spontaneously. However, in the case of a penetrating wound to the thorax or abdomen, exploratory surgery usually is necessary, partially for control of hemorrhage and partially for examination for other injuries. Except for acute loss of more than one-third of the circulating blood volume, a blood transfusion normally is not needed.[18] Rather, blood volume may and should be replaced rapidly with IV crystalloid fluids such as lactated Ringer's solution. If surgery is necessary to stop bleeding, oxygen should be administered to the patient to maximize oxygen delivery to tissues. Optimal oxygen transport occurs at a PCV of 35 to 45 per cent.[14] However, because blood viscosity is lower after hemorrhage and volume replacement with IV fluids, the oxygen-carrying ca-

pacity of the blood may remain adequate as long as the PCV remains approximately 25 per cent or more.

If *bleeding persists or occurs from multiple sites*, the existence of a coagulopathy should be considered (see Chapter 81). Persistent blood loss is associated, initially, with macrocytosis, polychromasia, and reticulocytosis. Later, as iron stores are depleted, reticulocyte numbers decline and the red cells become microcytic and hypochromic.[3] Animals with chronic blood loss should be given supplemental iron while the underlying problem is being treated.

If *gastrointestinal blood loss* occurs, one must first rule out medically treatable causes of bleeding, such as parasites, or chronic inflammatory diseases, such as eosinophilic gastroenteritis. A positive stool guaiac test indicates the presence of blood. If a weak positive test is obtained, meat should be eliminated from the diet for about three days and a stool sample retested to avoid false positive results from meat pigments. A radiographic barium contrast study of the upper or lower gastrointestinal tract or endoscopy for examination and biopsy may supplement the medical work-up. If medical causes are eliminated, surgery might be indicated for diagnosis or therapy. In older dogs, intestinal tumors, such as leiomyomas, may ulcerate and cause significant blood loss. Other gastrointestinal tumors include adenocarcinomas, lymphomas, leiomyosarcomas, and mast cell tumors. Ulceration from foreign bodies, infections, or other inflammatory disorders also are causes of gastrointestinal bleeding.

Urinary tract hemorrhage can result from tumors of the bladder or kidney or from calculi, polyps, cystitis, or trauma. Welsh Corgis with familial hamartomas of the kidney, often with significant chronic blood loss, have been presented at the Angell Memorial Animal Hospital. The latter lesions are not likely to be surgically resectable, as they are frequently multiple. Renal tumors, such as renal cell carcinomas or nephroblastomas (Wilm's tumor), also may be associated with hematuria. However, because renal lymphomas are associated with interstitial infiltrates, they are not likely to cause hematuria.

Epistaxis is a frequent manifestation of a coagulopathy because the fragile nasal mucous membranes are vulnerable to bleeding. This is especially likely if platelets are decreased, as in immune-mediated thrombocytopenia, or dysfunctional, as in myeloma. Epistaxis, with or without a purulent discharge, also may occur owing to nasal tumors or, less frequently, fungal infections such as aspergillosis, in which the fungus invades blood vessels.

Hemangioendothelioma (hemangiosarcoma) is one of the major causes of sudden or recurring internal hemorrhage in older dogs, especially German shepherds.[17] The two most common sites for such tumors are the spleen and the right auricular appendage. Splenic tumors have abnormal vascular spaces that may rupture and that cannot contract as do normal vessels, so bleeding may be severe. A splenic mass associated with intra-abdominal hemorrhage is an indication for exploratory laparotomy as soon as the animal's clinical condition is stabilized. Unfortunately, rupture often results in seeding of the abdomen with tumor cells. Splenectomy is indicated in the absence of gross metastases because the mass may be benign and surgery is of at least palliative benefit in the case of malignancy. Although less common than in dogs, splenic hemangioendotheliomas with rupture have also been diagnosed in cats.

Hemangioendotheliomas of the right auricular appendage in dogs grow without clinical signs until rupture causes bleeding into the pericardium and cardiac tamponade.[17] This can result in sudden death, or, if the hemorrhage is slow, the pericardial sac may fill and cause increased vena caval pressure and ascites. In the acute form, the typical findings of a large, round cardiac shadow, visible on chest radiographs, and a decreased amplitude of the QRS complex on an electrocardiogram may *not* be present. However, the central venous pressure usually is quite elevated in such cases. Pericardiocentesis is indicated for diagnostic purposes and to provide temporary therapeutic benefit. This should be followed by thoracotomy, since evaluation of the pericardial fluid usually does not distinguish between inflammatory and neoplastic causes.[17] An hemangioendothelioma located in the subcutaneous tissue may be confused with a bruise or hematoma. Hemangioendotheliomas also may be associated with disseminated intravascular coagulation, because activation of the clotting cascade may occur at the walls of abnormal vessels of the tumor. Microangiopathic hemolysis (direct trauma to red cells in abnormal vessels) may also occur. In this condition, fragmented red cells (schistocytes) may be evident on a blood smear (see Chapter 84). Nucleated red cells may appear in the circulation out of proportion to the degree of anemia[23] because the spleen is not functioning properly to remove the nuclei or because of increased release of these cells from the marrow due to increased hematopoiesis in response to a hemolytic process.

Congenital porphyria has been reported as a red cell defect in cats, sometimes associated with mild hemolysis. In this disorder animals have brown pigmented teeth that fluoresce bright pink when exposed to ultraviolet light. The urine contains uroporphyrins that may also flouresce. Humans with porphyria often have an exacerbation of clinical signs after exposure to barbiturates and thus are poor surgical risks.[42] It is not known if this sensitivity also occurs in feline porphyria, although at least one such cat has been anesthetized with thiamylal sodium and maintained on halothane for an ovariohysterectomy without complications (S. Cotter, unpublished observation).

Splenectomy as a Treatment for Hemolytic Anemia

The spleen is the major organ involved in removal of senescent red cells and is responsible for anemia associated with extravascular hemolysis (removal of antibody-coated erythrocytes by fixed macrophages) as seen in IgG-mediated immune hemolytic anemia (see Chapter 84).[40] When this type of anemia is recurrent or unresponsive to immunosuppressive drugs, splenectomy may be of benefit, especially if splenomegaly is present.[40] In myeloproliferative disorders associated with splenomegaly, the spleen may become "overactive" (hypersplenism) and may remove excessive numbers of normal red cells, resulting in anemia. This condition also might benefit from splenectomy if the underlying cause of splenomegaly is otherwise controllable. Myeloproliferative diseases of cats are difficult to manage because they are resistant to current chemotherapeutic protocols. Therefore, it is doubtful that splenectomy would be of enough benefit in such conditions to justify the additional morbidity associated with surgery (see Chapter 84 for an in-depth discussion of the involvement of the spleen in anemia).

Nonregenerative Anemia

Anemia associated with bone marrow failure usually is not amenable to surgical treatment. Examination of a sample of bone marrow is required to determine the cause and prognosis (see Chapter 83). Unexplained nonregenerative anemia may accompany chronic illness of many causes. In such situations the anemia usually is not severe.

One specific cause of aplastic anemia (decrease in myeloid, erythroid, and platelet precursors) that may be surgically correctable is hyperestrogenism associated with a *Sertoli cell tumor* in the dog.[34] Therefore, a search for a testicular tumor should be made when aplastic anemia occurs in a male dog. Conversely, if a dog is presented with a testicular tumor, especially if other clinical signs of hyperestrogenism exist, a complete blood count and a platelet count should be done preoperatively to avoid the unexpected complications of bleeding due to thrombocytopenia or infection due to granulocytopenia. Bone marrow suppression secondary to hyperestrogenism may reverse only weeks to months following removal of the tumor. During the period of marrow recovery, anemia is not a major problem, since red cell transfusions are easy to provide. However, white cell and platelet recoveries are critically important to avoid bleeding or infection, since their replacement is difficult and expensive. If marrow suppression or feminization recur after castration, metastasis of the Sertoli cell tumor should be suspected. An elevated serum estradiol level may be detectable as well.

Preparation of Anemic Patients for Surgery

A presurgical blood transfusion is indicated to increase the oxygen-carrying capacity of the blood in severely anemic patients. The PCV does not have to be raised to normal but probably should be brought to at least 25 per cent. In anemic patients a degree of hemodilution will decrease peripheral resistance and aid cardiac output. Oxygen therapy preoperatively and administration of a 30 per cent or more oxygen-containing gas mixture during inhalation anesthesia allow for maximal oxygenation of the blood. In patients with chronic anemia, oxygenation of the tissues is already increased because of compensatory mechanisms, including increased cardiac output and a shift of the oxyhemoglobin dissociation curve to the right (decreasing the affinity of hemoglobin for oxygen).[2] Factors causing this shift to the right include (1) increased levels of 2,3-diphosphoglycerate (2,3 DPG), (2) increased body temperature, and (3) decreased pH of the blood. The oxyhemoglobin dissociation curve of canine or human red cells is more sensitive than that of the cat to changes in 2,3-DPG levels.[24] Levels of 2,3-DPG tend to rise more in anemic cats than in other species, possibly compensating for this lower sensitivity.

One must avoid overhydration during treatment of chronically anemic patients, because cardiac enlargement, especially left ventricular hypertrophy, may occur as a component of the compensatory response. Therefore, high output cardiac failure may ensue if large volumes of intravenous fluids or whole blood are given during surgery. Cats are especially prone to developing acute pulmonary edema under such circumstances.[7] This dangerous problem can be prevented by carefully controlling the volume and rate of administration of fluids and monitoring the central venous and/or arterial blood pressures (see Chapter 9).

SURGICAL CONSIDERATIONS IN LEUKOPENIC OR IMMUNOSUPPRESSED PATIENTS

Infections and poor wound healing may be encountered in immunosuppressed patients or those with granulocytopenia.[16] Some dogs with granulocytopenia due to an acute parvovirus infection have clinical signs resembling those of intestinal obstruction. In addition, upper gastrointestinal contrast study findings, such as a prolonged gastric emptying time, and dilated loops of small intestine may be detected on radiographic studies. In such cases, exploratory surgery of the abdomen, especially if accompanied by enterotomy, may be associated with a high rate of post-operative complications.

Immunosuppressive Drugs

Animals receiving immunosuppressive drugs, particularly corticosteroids, are at risk for post-operative complications, including an increased risk of infection and poor wound healing. However, surgical procedures sometimes must be performed on animals receiving corticosteroids, e.g., splenectomy for treatment of immune-mediated hemolytic anemia or thrombocytopenia. By poorly understood mechanisms, corticosteroids inhibit fibrin deposition and capillary and fibroblast proliferation in a wound and also interfere with collagen deposition, so the tensile strength of connective tissue is decreased.[16] Therefore, nonabsorbable sutures should be used throughout such procedures, and skin sutures should be left in place for three to four weeks, even if healing appears to be complete prior to that time.

When corticosteroids are administered, intestinal surgery is associated with an increased risk of dehiscence or infection. Sometimes, surgery is required anyway, e.g., in cases of feline eosinophilic enteritis unresponsive to corticosteroids, in which case a biopsy or excision of the affected areas of intestine is performed. Because the chance of complications is high, when faced with a surgical patient receiving corticosteroids, the surgeon must weigh the risks and benefits of immediate surgery versus stopping corticosteroid therapy and postponing surgery for one to two weeks.

Hematopoietic Neoplasia

Hematopoietic neoplasia, especially of the bone marrow, renders patients more prone to complications following surgery.[16] Surgery may be necessary to diagnose the malignancy or correct an associated problem. Animals with leukemia, lymphoma, and myeloma are often immunologically abnormal as well as granulocytopenic or thrombocytopenic. Animals with myeloma may have a bleeding tendency because platelets may become coated with abnormal immunoglobulins and may fail to aggregate normally. An additional concern in dogs with lymphoma is hypercalcemia (pseudohyperparathyroidism). Hypercalcemia is present at the time of diagnosis in approximately 25 per cent of such dogs.[28] Clinical signs may be noted but are not always evident. Hypercalcemia may result in renal tubular damage and failure. Ventricular arrhythmias also may be present and can be exacerbated by anesthesia. For these reasons, in addition to a complete blood count, serum calcium and BUN or creatinine concentrations should be determined prior to surgery. In dogs suspected of having lymphoma, the serum calcium level can sometimes be corrected by saline diuresis prior to surgery. Corticosteroids also will decrease calcium levels but should be avoided prior to histological confirmation of the diagnosis, because necrosis of the tumor may occur, rendering the biopsy material nondiagnostic.

Surgery in Cats Infected with Feline Leukemia Virus

Approximately 1 to 2 per cent of apparently healthy cats are infected with feline leukemia virus (FeLV).[8] The presence of the virus can be detected in blood smears by immunofluorescence or in plasma or serum by the ELISA technique. Viremic cats are prone to the development of leukemia or lymphoma, bone marrow suppression, immune deficiency, and other disorders such as glomerulonephritis or reproductive disorders.[8] Approximately one-half of healthy FeLV-positive cats develop some fatal disease within two years, and most of these cats die from nonmalignant disorders.[25] The virus exerts most of its immunosuppressive effects on T lymphocytes, but this immunosuppression may coexist with neutropenia, making these cats susceptible to a broad range of infections (see Chapter 15).[29]

Indications for surgery of FeLV-positive cats include diagnostic procedures, such as the biopsy of suspected tumors; therapeutic procedures, such as excision of tumors, debridement or drainage of infections, or treatment of oral or dental disease; and elective procedures, such as neutering. A complete blood count should be done before surgery, with special attention paid to the PCV and granulocyte and platelet numbers. This is especially important in cats with severe stomatitis or dental disease. These conditions may be a result of pre-existing marrow suppression or may be a presenting problem of cats with leukemic infiltration of the marrow. Because of viral immunosuppression, any infection must be treated aggressively. If surgery is necessary, the risks should be considered, but necessary procedures should be performed. For example, routine surgery, such as castration or ovariohysterectomy, can be performed on FeLV-positive cats as long as the owner is informed of the decreased chance of a normal life span. Hospitalization should be for as short a period of time as possible to minimize the risk of exposing the FeLV-positive cat to cats that may be carrying other communicable diseases. The risk of transmission of FeLV from positive cats to healthy cats in the hospital is small, since FeLV is not likely to be an airborne infection and the virus is easily killed by drying, soaps, or disinfectants.[15] Obviously, however, endotracheal tubes used for FeLV-positive cats should be discarded or thoroughly disinfected before use on another cat.

1. Babior, B. M.: Oxygen-dependent microbial killing by phagocytes. N. Engl. J. Med. 298:659, 1978.
2. Bannerman, R. M., Edwards, J. A., and Pinkerton, P. H.: Hereditary disorders of the red cell in animals. In Brown, E. B. (ed.): Progress in Hematology, Vol. 8. Grune and Stratton, New York, 1973, pp. 131–179.
3. Beck, W. S.: Hematology, Harvard Pathophysiology Series. MIT Press, Cambridge, 1973.
4. Bessis, M.: Blood smears reinterpreted. Springer-International, Berlin, 1977.
5. Bishop, C. R., Athens, J. W., Boggs, D. R., Warner, H. R., Cartwright, G. E., and Wintrobe, M. M.: Leukokinetic studies XIII. J. Clin. Invest. 47:249, 1968.
6. Chamberlain, J. K., Leblond, P. F., and Weed, R. I.: Reduction of adventitial cell cover: an early direct effect of erythropoietin on bone marrow ultrastructure. Blood Cells 1:655, 1975.
7. Cotter, S. M.: Anemia associated with feline leukemia virus infection. J. Am. Vet. Med. Assoc. 175:1191, 1979.
8. Cotter, S. M., Hardy, W. D., and Essex, M.: Association of feline leukemia virus with leukemia and other diseases in the cat. J. Am. Vet. Med. Assoc. 166:449, 1975.
9. Cramer, D. V., and Lewis, R. M.: Reticulocyte response in the cat. J. Am. Vet. Med. Assoc. 160:61, 1972.
10. Cronkite, E. P.: Kinetics of granulocytopoiesis. Clin. Hematol. 8:351, 1979.
11. Crosby, W. H.: The limits of erythropoiesis: How much can the marrow produce with total recruitment? Blood Cells 1:497, 1975.
12. Dexter, T. M.: Stromal cell associated haemopoiesis. J. Cell Physiol. (Suppl. 1):87, 1982.
13. Erslev, A. J.: Production of erythrocytes. In Williams, W., et al. (eds.): Hematology. McGraw Hill, New York, 1972, pp. 162–177.
14. Erslev, A. J.: General effects of polycythemia. In Williams, W., et al. (eds.): Hematology. McGraw Hill, New York, 1972, pp. 204–206.
15. Francis, D. P., Essex, M., and Gayzagian, D.: Feline leukemia virus: Survival under home and laboratory conditions. J. Clin. Microbiol. 9:154, 1979.
16. Harvey, H. J.: Principles of cancer surgery. In Ettinger, S. (ed.): Textbook of Veterinary Internal Medicine. W. B. Saunders, Philadelphia, 1983, pp. 405–416.
17. Kleine, L. J., Zook, B. C., and Munson, T. O.: Primary cardiac hemangiosarcomas in dogs. J. Am. Vet. Med. Assoc. 157:326, 1970.
18. Kolata, R. J., Burrows, C. F., and Soma, L. R.: Shock: pathophysiology and management. In Kirk, R. (ed.): Current Veterinary Therapy VII. W. B. Saunders, Philadelphia, 1980, pp. 32–48.
19. Leblond, P. F., Chamberlain, J. K., and Weed, R. I.: Scanning electron microscopy of erythropoietin-stimulated bone marrow. Blood Cells 1:639, 1975.
20. Leblond, P. F., LaCelle, P. L., and Wees, R. I.: Cellular deformability: A possible determinant of the normal release of maturing erythrocytes from the bone marrow. Blood 37:40, 1971.
21. Leder, L. D.: The origin of blood monocytes and macrophages: A review. Blut 16:86, 1967.
22. Lichtman, M. A.: Cellular deformability during maturation of the myeloblast. Possible role in marrow egress. N. Engl. J. Med. 283:943, 1970.
23. Madewell, B. R., and Feldman, B. F.: Characterization of anemias associated with neoplasia in small animals. J. Am. Vet. Med. Assoc. 176:419, 1980.
24. Mauk, A. G., Whelen, H. T., Putz, G. R., and Taketa, F.: Anemia in domestic cats—effect on hemoglobin components and whole blood oxygenation. Science 185:442, 1974.
25. McClelland, A. J., Hardy, W. D., Jr., and Zuckerman, E. E.: Prognosis of healthy feline leukemia virus infected cats. In Hardy, W. D., Jr., Essex, M., and McClelland, A. J. (eds.): Feline Leukemia Virus. Elsevier North Holland Inc., New York, 1980, pp. 121–131.
26. McCredie, K. B., and Freireich, E. J.: Blood component therapy. In Holland, J., and Frei, E. (eds.): Cancer Medicine. Lea & Febiger, Philadelphia, 1974, pp. 1115–1129.
27. Moore, M. A. S., and Metcalf, D.: Ontogeny of the hematopoietic system: yolk sac origin of in vivo and in vitro colony forming cells in the developing mouse embryo. Br. J. Haematol. 18:279, 1970.
28. Osborne, C. A., and Stevens, J. B.: Pseudohyperparathyroidism in the dog. J. Am. Vet. Med. Assoc. 162:125, 1973.
29. Perryman, L. E., Hooever, E. A., and Yohn, D. S.: Immunosuppression in experimental feline leukemia. J. Natl. Cancer Inst. 49:1357, 1972.
30. Prasse, K. W.: White blood cell disorders. In Ettinger, S. (ed.): Textbook of Veterinary Internal Medicine. W. B. Saunders, Philadelphia, 1983, pp. 2001–2045.
31. Prasse, K. W., Crouser, D., Beutler, E., Walker, M., and Schall, W. D.: Pyruvate kinase deficiency anemia with terminal myelofibrosis and osteosclerosis in a Beagle. J. Am. Vet. Med. Assoc. 166:1170, 1975.
32. Quesenberry, P., and Levitt, L.: Hematopoietic stem cells. N. Engl. J. Med. 301:755, 819, 868, 1979.

33. Schalm, O. W., Jain, N. C., and Carroll, E. J.: *Veterinary Hematology*, 3rd ed., Lea & Febiger, Philadelphia, 1975.
34. Sherding, R. G., Wilson, G. P., and Kociba, G. J.: Bone marrow hypoplasia in eight dogs with sertoli cell tumors. J. Am. Vet. Med. Assoc. *178*:497, 1981.
35. Stohlman, F. Jr., Howard, D., and Beland, A.: Hormonal regulation of erythropoiesis, kinetics of red cell production. Ann. N.Y. Acad. Sci. *149*:156, 1968.
36. Stossel, T. P.: Phagocytosis. N. Engl. J. Med. *290*:717, 1974.
37. Tasker, J. B., Severin, G. A., Young, S., and Gillette, E. L.: Familial Anemia in the Basenji Dog. J. Am. Vet. Med. Assoc. *154*:158, 1969.
38. Tavassoli, M.: Adaptation of marrow sinus wall to fluctuations in the rate of cell delivery: studies in rabbits after bloodletting. Br. J. Haematol. *35*:25, 1977.
39. Tavassoli, M.: Megakaryocyte-platelet axis and the process of platelet formation and release. Blood *55*:537, 1980.
40. Tizard, I.: *An Introduction to Veterinary Immunology*. 2nd ed. W. B. Saunders, Philadelphia, 1982.
41. Van Furth, R., and Cohn, Z. A.: The origin and kinetics of mononuclear phagocytes. J. Exp. Med. *128*:415, 1968.
42. Waldenstrom, J. G.: Neurological symptoms caused by so-called acute porphyria. Acta Psychiat. Neurol. *14*:375, 1939.
43. Weiss, L.: Transmural cellular passage in vascular sinuses of rat bone marrow. Blood *36*:189, 1970.
44. Weiss, L.: The haemopoietic microenvironment of bone marrow: an ultrastructural study of the interactions of blood cells, stroma, and blood vessels. *In: Blood Cells and Vessel Walls: Functional Interactions* (Ciba Foundation Symposium 71). Excerpta Medica, Amsterdam, 1979, pp. 3–19.
45. Wintrobe, M. M., Lee, R. G., et al.: *Clinical Hematology*. Lea & Febiger, Philadelphia, 1975, pp. 244–262.
46. Wolf, N. S.: The haemopoietic microenvironment. Clin. Haematol. 8:469, 1979.
47. Wolf, N. S., and Trenton, J. J.: Hematopoietic colony studies. V. Effect of hemopoietic organ stroma on differentiation of pleuripotent stem cells. J. Exp. Med. *127*:205, 1968.

Chapter **81**

Blood Dyscrasias Affecting the Surgical Patient—Hemostatic and Thrombotic Disorders

W. Jean Dodds

INTRODUCTION

The fundamentals of hemostasis (discussed in Chapter 6) are important to veterinary surgeons, as are the more common hereditary and acquired causes of bleeding. The surgeon must develop a practical approach to the diagnosis, management, and treatment of animals with hemostatic defects.[7, 10] The following information is intended as a summary of this continually advancing field. Most of the diseases listed and their causes and mechanisms have been reported in man and in several animal species.

The fundamentals of preventing or minimizing hemorrhagic complications during or after surgery can be divided into three categories. The first is *clinical evaluation* of the patient, which includes a complete medical and family history and a thorough physical examination. This assessment should determine whether the patient has a pre-existing bleeding tendency or is at risk for operative or postoperative hemorrhage. Elective procedures should be avoided or discouraged in animals with a previous or current history of bleeding.

The second consideration is *laboratory evaluation* by appropriate preoperative hemostatic tests. Depending on the age and medical history of the patient, these tests should include measurement of the bleeding time (e.g., cuticle bleeding time[15]), a platelet count, and screening tests of coagulation and fibrinolysis. Elective and major surgical procedures should be avoided, if possible, in animals with a known history of bleeding or markedly abnormal bleeding time and laboratory test results. If a diagnostic or therapeutic surgical procedure is unavoidable, it should be undertaken with caution in animals in these categories. Large surface swellings should not be incised until careful assessment has differentiated between a hematoma and other causes of swellings, such as a seroma, cyst, tumor, or abscess.

The final basic principle for prevention of excessive surgical bleeding in animals with hemorrhagic tendencies involves the use of *blood or blood component replacement* prior to surgery. The form of treatment used depends on the cause of bleeding. Such therapy may have to be continued during and after the operation.

Supported in part by research grants HL09902 and HL07173, awarded by the National Heart, Lung, and Blood Institute, PHS/DHHS, and by grants from the Geraldine R. Dodge Foundation and the American Kennel Club.

HEMOSTATIC DISORDERS

The bleeding disorders of animals are classified as inherited and acquired. Acquired problems are more common, although the inherited diseases are seen more often than is generally realized because of the selected inbreeding practiced within certain animal populations, e.g., in purebred dogs.[10–12, 18] Hereditary bleeding diseases are encountered most often as a consequence of inbreeding, especially in rare breeds of dogs, which, by necessity, are inbred, and in breeds in which particular dog show winners are used extensively for breeding. Both transmission and recognition of genetic defects are facilitated by inbreeding. An effective mechanism to discover and eventually control the frequency of such genetic defects is the development of large-scale screening programs for the identification of affected or carrier animals (by "gene-dosage" effects in heterozygotes) within the population. Screening programs of this type have been used successfully in humans for many years (e.g., for Tay-Sachs disease and phenylketonuria) and have recently been applied to animals (e.g., for mannosidosis in cattle, hip dysplasia, and eye and blood diseases in dogs).[10–12, 18] The following discussion provides a brief review of the hereditary and acquired bleeding disorders of animals.

Hereditary Defects[8, 9, 16, 24]

Clotting Factor Deficiencies

Factor VII Deficiency. This trait is autosomal and incompletely dominant. It has been reported in beagles in North America, Scandinavia, and Europe[24] and has also been studied in a family of Alaskan malamutes[9] and in a group of colony-bred mongrels.[19]

Factor VII deficiency results in a mild disease characterized by easy bruising and an apparent predisposition to demodicosis. The condition is often discovered fortuitously during routine coagulation screening of beagles in commercial breeding stock before their use in research studies. Homozygotes have less than 3 per cent of the normal level of factor VII activity and a prolonged prothrombin time (PT) but normal Stypven time. Heterozygotes have about 50 per cent factor VII activity but are asymptomatic and usually have a normal PT.

Hemophilia A (Factor VIII: Coagulant Deficiency; Classical Hemophilia). This is an X chromosome–linked recessive disease that is carried by females and manifested in males. Female hemophiliacs (homozygotes) can be produced, however, by the mating of hemophilic males (hemizygotes) to carrier females (heterozygotes). This is the most commonly reported severe inherited coagulation defect of animals. It has been recognized in most breeds of dogs as well as in mongrels, in standardbred and thoroughbred horses, and is quite often seen in cats (five cases were referred to our laboratory in 1982).[8]

The degree of clinical disease may be severe, moderate, or mild. Mild cases frequently are undetected until after the animal reaches young adulthood and is old enough to reproduce. Therefore, in inbred dog families with a mild form of hemophilia, affected females can be produced. Laboratory diagnosis is based on the same methods as those used to detect hemophilia in man. Findings include a prolonged whole blood clotting time and activated partial thromboplastin time (APTT), but the PT, thrombin clotting time (TCT), and platelet count are normal. The APTT clotting defect *is not* corrected by the addition of normal serum. Affected animals have very low factor VIII coagulant activity (FVIII:C) but normal or elevated levels of factor VIII-related antigen (FVIIIR:Ag) (a measurement of the von Willebrand's factor [VWF] protein). Heterozygous, carrier females have FVIII:C levels about 40 to 60 per cent of normal and normal or elevated FVIIIR:Ag levels. Thus, the ratio of FVIII:C to FVIIIR:Ag in hemophilic carriers is about 1:2, a finding that has been used successfully in human and animal families in the identification of potential carriers. Genetic counselling for animal breeders based on these carrier detection tests is an important responsibility of veterinary clinicians.[11, 18]

Hemophilia B (Factor IX Deficiency; Christmas Disease). This disorder is inherited as an X chromosome–linked recessive trait, as is hemophilia A. It has been reported in only 11 breeds of dogs—Cairn terriers, black and tan coonhounds, St. Bernards, American cocker spaniels, French bulldogs, Shetland sheepdogs, Alaskan malamutes, Scottish terriers, old English sheepdogs, Labrador retrievers, and bichons frise—and in short-haired cats in Britain. All affected families have moderate to severe disease. Results of diagnostic screening tests are the same as those described for hemophilia A, except that the APTT defect *is* corrected by addition of normal serum (because serum contains factor IX activity [FIX] but not FVIII:C, and the plasma defect is in FIX and not FVIII:C). Affected dogs have FIX levels less than 10 per cent and usually less than 1 per cent, and carrier females have about 40 to 60 per cent of the normal level.

von Willebrand's Disease (VWD). VWD is the most common, mild inherited bleeding disorder of man and animals. It is an autosomal trait with two forms of clinical and genetic expression:[11] (1) a disease with autosomal recessive expression in which clinically affected individuals are homozygous for the VWD gene and have two asymptomatic, heterozygous (carrier) parents; and (2) a disease with an autosomal, incompletely dominant expression (variable penetrance), in which both homozygotes and heterozygotes have a bleeding tendency. Homozygosity is often lethal in the latter form of VWD. The recessive form of disease has been recognized in Poland-China swine, Scottish terriers, and Chesapeake Bay retrievers. The incompletely dominant form of the disease is much more common and has been recognized in 29 breeds of dogs to date. These include German shepherd dogs, golden retrievers, miniature schnauzers, Doberman pinschers, Pembroke Welsh corgis, and standard Manchester terriers, which, along with Scottish terriers, have a high prevalence of the disease (15 to 60 per cent gene frequency), as well as English springer spaniels, Cairn terriers, Lakeland terriers, rottweilers, Labrador retrievers, great Danes, boxers, basset hounds, Afghan hounds, Irish setters, standard and miniature poodles, standard and miniature dachshunds, Lhasa apsos, Vizslas, Shetland sheepdogs, Airedale terriers, and toy Manchester terriers.

High morbidity and low mortality are associated with VWD. Generally, there is a mild to severe bleeding diathesis that unusually involves mucosal surfaces. Bleeding is exacerbated by physical, emotional, and physiological stresses as well as by other concomitant diseases. Typical clinical signs include recurrent gastrointestinal hemorrhage with or without diarrhea; recurrent hematuria; epistaxis; gingival, vaginal, and penile bleeding; lameness that mimics eosinophilic panosteitis; stillbirths or neonatal deaths ("fading pups") with evidence of bleeding at necropsy; prolonged estrual or postpartum bleeding; hematoma formation on the surface of the body, limbs, or head; excessive umbilical cord bleeding at birth; and excessive bleeding from toenails cut too short or after tail docking, ear cropping, and dewclaw removal. Affected dogs may bleed to death from surgical procedures.

Diagnostic tests for canine VWD are similar to those used for human VWD. Specialized VWF assays are required. Screening coagulation tests (APTT, PT, and TCT) are not diagnostic. Affected individuals have prolonged bleeding times, abnormal platelet retention *in vitro*, and variable FVIII:C levels (normal to moderately reduced). Definitive diagnosis is made by finding reduced or undetectable levels of FVIIIR:Ag or the platelet-related assays for VWF. Animals affected with the genetically recessive form of the disease are homozygotes and have no FVIIIR:Ag/VWF, whereas their heterozygous parents have reduced levels (15 to 60 per cent of normal). Animals with the incompletely dominant form of the disease have reduced but measurable FVIIIR:Ag/VWF (less than 7 to 59 per cent of normal).

Factor X Deficiency. This is an autosomally inherited disease that has been recognized only in American cocker spaniels and a crossbred Labrador-shepherd–type dog. It produces a severe bleeding diathesis in neonatal and young dogs but only a mild condition in mature adult dogs, unless they are subjected to surgery. The condition is lethal in the homozygous state. Surviving affected heterozygotes have a prolonged APTT, PT, and Stypven time but a normal TCT. Factor X levels are reduced to 18 to 70 per cent of normal. In fatal cases (in which the dogs are presumed to be homozygous for the gene), FX levels are less than 15 per cent of normal.

Factor XI (PTA) Deficiency. PTA deficiency is an autosomally inherited disease reported in Holstein cattle, English springer spaniels, great Pyrenees,

Kerry blue terriers, bulldogs, and Weimaraners. This is a mild, spontaneous bleeding disorder (i.e., characterized by hematuria, gingival bleeding, or epistaxis), but severe, protracted bleeding usually occurs 12 to 24 hours after even minor surgical procedures. Homozygotes have a prolonged APTT, normal PT and TCT, and very low factor XI activity (less than 20 per cent); heterozygotes have 40 to 60 per cent FXI.

Factor XII Deficiency (Hageman Trait). Factor XII deficiency is inherited as an autosomal trait. It occurs quite frequently in cats (six cases were recognized by our laboratory in 1982), and one case has been recognized in a standard poodle. This condition is *not* associated with a bleeding diathesis. A similar deficiency is a normal clinicopathological characteristic of marine mammals, reptiles, and birds (domestic fowl and wild birds). The defect is recognized in homozygotes by finding a markedly prolonged APTT, a normal PT and TCT, and very low levels (usually less than 5 per cent) of factor XII. Heterozygotes have about half the normal level of FXII activity.

Dysfibrinogenemia. This disease is inherited as an autosomal trait. It was discovered recently in a family of inbred borzois (Russian wolfhounds). Affected dogs showed a mild bleeding disorder characterized by body surface hematomas, lameness, epistaxis, and excessive bleeding following trauma or surgery. Diagnostic tests reveal a markedly to slightly prolonged APTT, PT, and TCT but normal amounts of fibrinogen measured by physical or immunological methods. This represents the first finding of an inherited functional fibrinogen defect in animals other than man.[9]

Other Defects. Two dog families (boxer and otterhound) have been discovered with defects in the vitamin K–dependent synthesis or regulation of prothrombin-complex clotting factors.[9] One case of prothrombin (factor II) deficiency has been described in an English cocker spaniel.[17] A family of Saanen dairy goats with afibrinogenemia and a St. Bernard family with hypofibrinogenemia also have been reported,[8] but these have not been maintained for research purposes. Other breeds recognized to have hypofibrinogenemia are the collie and Viszla. To date, there have been no animals recognized with either factor V or factor XIII deficiencies.

Platelet Function Defects

Thrombasthenia (Glanzmann's Disease). This is an autosomal disorder recognized in otterhounds. The specific platelet defect is a mixed thrombasthenic-thrombopathia with functional and biochemical characteristics of human Glanzmann's disease but some morphological features similar to those of Bernard-Soulier syndrome of man. Homozygotes express a mild to moderate bleeding diathesis with symptoms like those seen in VWD. Heterozygotes are asymptomatic but have a partial reduction in platelet function. The platelet defect is characterized by long bleeding times, abnormal clot retraction and platelet retention, markedly reduced platelet aggregation induced by ADP and other agonists, and abnormal platelet membrane glycoproteins IIb and IIIa.[9]

Thrombopathia ("Storage Pool Disease"). The inherited thrombopathias include a variety of platelet function defects, other than thrombasthenia, that have been recognized in American foxhounds and basset hounds, several cats, and in fawn-hooded (FH) rats. Frequently, these defects are caused by a deficiency in the constituents of platelet storage granules (i.e., nucleotides and serotonin), hence the term "storage pool disease." These are autosomal traits. Affected animals have a mild to moderate bleeding diathesis with signs similar to those associated with VWD. Abnormalities in platelet function depend on the specific type of thrombopathia and vary from mild to severe. These disorders are characterized by long bleeding times, abnormal platelet retention on glass bead columns, platelet aggregation, and platelet release of secretable constituents with a variety of inducers. Usually clot retraction is normal. The disease in basset hounds appears to be widespread among North American breeding stock.[9]

Acquired Diseases[4-9, 16]

Platelet Function Defects

Quantitative Abnormalities
Thrombocytopenia

Increased Platelet Destruction, Utilization, or Sequestration. This type of thrombocytopenia results from immunological and nonimmunological causes. *Immunological causes* include (1) primary idiopathic thrombocytopenic purpura (ITP) and (2) secondary disease from such conditions as incompatible blood transfusions, autoimmune diseases, allergies, drugs, toxic agents, live virus vaccines, and hemolytic disease of the newborn. *Nonimmunological causes* include severe infections, malignancy, drugs (e.g., heparin), disseminated intravascular coagulation, hemolytic-uremic syndrome, splenomegaly, and hypothermia.

Most cases of chronic recurrent thrombocytopenia in dogs are immune-mediated.[8, 9] Similar disorders also have been recognized in horses and cats. Antiplatelet activity can be demonstrated by specialized assays such as the platelet factor 3 (PF3) release test. Because antiplatelet antibodies disappear rapidly (within 24 to 48 hours) from the circulation after steroid therapy, it is important to collect a small (1 to 2 ml) pretreatment sample for the PF3 test.

Decreased Platelet Production. Causes of this condition in man and animals include marrow depression (drugs, anemias); marrow infiltration; infections, especially with viruses; drugs (diuretics, estrogens); cyclic thrombocytopenia; and paroxysmal nocturnal hemoglobinuria.

Thrombocytosis

Increased Platelet Production. Causes of increased platelet production in man and animals include mye-

loproliferative disorders such as polycythemia vera, chronic leukemia, and thrombocythemia; chronic inflammatory disorders such as autoimmune diseases, cirrhosis, granulomatosis, tuberculosis, sarcoidosis, chronic pneumonitis, and osteomyelitis; malignancy (lymphomas, carcinomas); and miscellaneous causes such as acute infection, acute hemorrhage, iron deficiency, postoperative rebound, and osteoporosis.

Release from Tissue Stores (spleen, lung). This can be a response to exercise or can be caused by drugs such as adrenalin and vincristine.

Qualitative Abnormalities

Qualitative abnormalities of platelet function are important but commonly overlooked causes of a bleeding tendency. Causes include uremia, in which the accumulation of nitrogenous wastes inhibits platelet function; myeloproliferative disorders; macroglobulinemia; liver disease, which inhibits platelet function by some unknown mechanism; fibrinolysis; thrombocytopenia; systemic lupus erythematosus; congenital heart disease; anemias; and leukemias. A wide variety of drugs also produces platelet dysfunction by several different mechanisms.[6] The drugs most commonly associated with platelet dysfunction are aspirin (a long-lasting effect), phenylbutazone, promazine-derivative tranquilizers, estrogens, plasma expanders (dextran, hydroxyethyl starch), nitrofurans, sulfonamides, anti-inflammatory drugs, penicillin compounds, local anesthetics, phenothiazines, and live virus vaccines (during the period of viremia, three to ten days postvaccination).

Bleeding associated with either quantitative or qualitative platelet dysfunctions mimics that seen in VWD and is commonly expressed as petechiae and/or ecchymoses of the skin and mucous membranes. In thrombocytopenia, platelet counts are usually below 100,000/mm^3 but may be less than 10,000/mm^3. Clinical signs include fever, pallor, depression, lethargy, and evidence of regenerative erythropoiesis and nonspecific neutrophilia.

Vitamin K Deficiency[6, 21]

Vitamin K is required for hepatic synthesis of the prothrombin-complex clotting factors (factors II, VII, IX, and X). Deficiencies occur as a result of poisoning with warfarin (D-Con), diphacinone (Diphacin), brodifacoum (Talon), and chlorophacinone (Rozol) rodenticides. Other causes include physiological hypoprothrombinemia of the newborn due to hepatic immaturity, gastrointestinal conditions associated with impaired absorption, antibiotic sterilization of the bowel, and hepatic insufficiency. In vitamin K–deficient states, the liver synthesizes biologically inactive precursors of the prothrombin-complex clotting factors. The rapidity of their appearance and the decrease in their respective biological activities are directly proportional to the half-lives of the clotting factors involved, i.e., factor VII first, followed by factors IX, X, and II.

The most common causes of vitamin K deficiency in animals are rodenticidal poisonings.[21] Prolonged use of antibiotics that may cause sterilization of the bowel also may cause similar results. The so-called first generation rodenticides (warfarin and the indandiones diphacinone and pindone) were developed over 30 years ago and are still used today. More recently, second generation rodenticides (brodifacoum) have been produced that have increased potency and faster action than their earlier counterparts. The various types of rodenticides require different treatment regimens to control toxicity.[21] The routine treatment for warfarin (D-Con) poisoning, which consists of vitamin K_1 (0.25 to 2.5 mg/kg body weight for four to six days) and blood or plasma transfusions as needed (6 to 10 ml/kg body weight), is insufficient for the more potent or long-lasting rodenticides. For indandione poisoning, the inhibition of vitamin K–dependent pathways can last three to four weeks because these compounds are very slowly metabolized by the liver. To treat the latter toxicity, it has been recommended that oral vitamin K_1 be used for three weeks at 5 mg/kg.[21] Much higher doses have also been given, but prolonged use of high doses can induce Heinz-body hemolytic anemia in human beings and dogs.[6]

The latest and most potent (10 to 15 times more active) rodenticide in use is brodifacoum (Talon). This product has been associated with intractable, fatal bleeding. In successfully treated cases, serial blood transfusions and the usage of vitamin K_1 for up to six weeks have been necessary to reverse the inhibitory effects on hepatic vitamin K–dependent protein synthesis.

Liver Disease[2, 3, 6, 13]

Because the liver is the primary site of synthesis of blood coagulation factors, acute or chronic generalized liver disease often produces a bleeding tendency. Although spontaneous bleeding is rarely encountered,[2] surgical patients may bleed excessively. The primary detectable clotting defect is a prolonged PT, but other tests (fibrinogen, APTT, platelet count and function) also may be abnormal. Hepatic disease also can produce disseminated intravascular coagulation (e.g., in infectious canine hepatitis virus infection). In some patients with liver disease the thrombin clotting time is prolonged out of proportion to both the level of fibrinogen-fibrin degradation products and the decrease of plasma fibrinogen, thus suggesting the presence of an abnormal fibrinogen.[6] The coagulation defects in liver disease are so complicated that it may not be possible to state unequivocally why a particular clotting factor is decreased. The decrease could be due to lack of synthesis, increased destruction from intravascular coagulation, or fibrinolysis. Furthermore, the assays may be inaccurate because of the presence of inhibitors. Indeed, it may be impossible either to identify the factors responsible for bleeding or to predict which patients with liver disease will have a bleeding disorder.[6] Coagulation studies can give some prognostic indication,[2, 3, 14] however, and have been used as an index of the diseased liver's synthetic capacity. As factor VII has the shortest half-life of all clotting factors (about four hours), patients with acute hepatic failure and very low levels of factor VII have a poor prognosis, whereas those capable of maintaining factor VII levels above 8 per cent of normal usually survive.[14]

In a study of 32 dogs with four types of naturally occurring hepatic diseases (degeneration, inflammation, cirrhosis, and neoplasia), two-thirds of the animals had abnormal APTT and PT coagulation screening tests.[2] A more recent follow-up study[3] of another 28 dogs with the same types of hepatic diseases showed that all affected dogs had at least one abnormal specific coagulation factor and fibrinolytic test and that most had several abnormalities. Some assays, such as FVIIIR:Ag, were consistently elevated in patients with cirrhosis or neoplasia.[3]

Other Diseases

Dysproteinemias. A nonspecific bleeding diathesis occurs in association with monoclonal gammopathies (myeloma, macroglobulinemia). The abnormal protein appears to coat platelets and clotting factors, thus impairing their functions. Epistaxis is a common sign of these diseases.[6, 8]

A bleeding tendency associated with amyloidosis in man and animals most often causes factor X deficiency, although factor IX deficiency and thrombocytopenia can also occur.[8]

Impaired Vascular Integrity. Collagen diseases such as Ehlers-Danlos syndrome, scurvy (vitamin C deficiency), diabetes mellitus, and hyperadrenocorticism cause a bleeding tendency by impairment of vascular integrity.[6]

THROMBOTIC DISORDERS[4-6]

Intravascular Coagulation with Fibrinolysis[4-6, 20, 22, 23, 25]

Intravascular coagulation, or thrombosis, can occur as an acute or chronic, localized or disseminated condition. The etiology and pathophysiological changes involved and the methods of treatment vary depending on the severity of the problem and the type and severity of the underlying precipitating cause.

Localized Thrombosis

Tissue inflammation and necrosis, vascular stasis, and ischemia all induce localized thrombosis as part of the normal pathophysiological process of repair. The concomitant red blood cell, platelet, endotoxin, or antigen/antibody–mediated endothelial damage initiates hemostasis. Thrombin, thus formed, accelerates fibrin formation and cellular damage at the microvascular level. This self-perpetuating process stimulates fibrinolysis and activates the complement cascade. Kinins are also generated, which cause increased vascular permeability, pain, and vasodilation, which further promote coagulation, vascular stasis, and tissue ischemia. When this process remains restricted to a tissue, organ, or part such as a limb, the patient often can handle the stress with appropriate local corrective measures. If the problem becomes generalized, a more serious situation develops.

Disseminated Intravascular Coagulation (DIC)

Other common names for this serious syndrome are consumption coagulopathy and defibrination syndrome. DIC is not a primary disease entity but is secondary to some underlying cause. The more common causes of DIC include the following:

Obstetrical Complications. Eclampsia, dystocia, amniotic fluid embolism, cesarean section, and retained fetus or placenta.

Malignancy. Mammary, ovarian, testicular, pulmonary, pancreatic, gastric, gallbladder, colonic and prostatic carcinomas; malignant melanoma; and the leukemia-lymphoma complex.

Infections. In man and animals, gram-negative sepsis; systemic rickettsial or bacterial diseases; and viral diseases such as fowl plague, hog cholera and related diseases, African swine fever, epizootic hemorrhagic disease of deer, Rocky Mountain spotted fever, infectious canine hepatitis, and feline infectious peritonitis; as well as several systemic parasitic diseases (trypanisomiasis, piroplasmosis, canine heartworm disease) also can cause DIC.

Miscellaneous Causes. Shock; severe stress; surgery; liver disease, especially hepatic necrosis and cirrhosis; heat stroke; incompatible blood transfusions; amyloidosis; snake bites; cardiomyopathy with iliac saddle embolism in cats; and parasitic mesenteric artery embolism in horses.

Fulminating cases of DIC usually are fatal, whereas moderate or low-grade chronic DIC may be a continuing entity in older animals with chronic malignancy or infection. Diagnosis of DIC may be difficult, depending on which stage of the process is present at the time. In the later or consumption coagulopathy stage, there is usually thrombocytopenia; a prolonged APTT, TCT, and perhaps PT; reduced factors V and VIII activities; enhanced fibrinolysis; and the presence of circulating fibrinogen-fibrin degradation products (FDP). Significant levels of FDP are considered diagnostic of DIC.

Acute DIC.[20] The acute form of DIC was first identified in association with obstetrical emergencies in women but has since been recognized in animals. Acute DIC also is seen as a complication of massive infections, shock, severe trauma, major and lengthy operations, generalized hepatic disease, and malignancy. Other causes were listed previously. Most patients with acute DIC are critically ill and die of either acute renal or respiratory failure.[20, 23] About one-third of patients experience significant bleeding, primarily from wounds, the gastrointestinal tract, and lungs. Clinically significant acute DIC thus has a dismal prognosis.

Chronic DIC.[4–7] The chronic syndrome is much more common than the acute form of DIC, although it is not recognized as readily because the alarming bleeding or striking changes in coagulation tests associated with the acute form do not occur. In many cases the patient is not suspected of having the condition, as there may be no unusual bleeding or thrombosis. Such patients are at risk should they require major surgery. Therefore, it is important to perform presurgical coagulation tests on animals with diseases that predispose to thrombosis, the most common of which is malignancy.[25]

DIAGNOSIS, MANAGEMENT, AND TREATMENT OF THE BLEEDING SURGICAL PATIENT

Diagnosis[2–5, 7, 8, 13, 14, 23, 25, 26]

General Principles

Diagnostic blood tests not only can identify the specific disease affecting an animal but, in the case of inherited disorders, can provide useful information about the genetic status of their apparently healthy relatives. Thus, diagnostic screening of relatives for the carrier or asymptomatic heterozygous state of such disorders is a practical and feasible goal.[11, 12, 18] Carriers should be bred only if they are critical to a particular breeding program or to a study of the genetic defect involved, e.g., its clinical signs, inheritance pattern, and the most effective treatment methods. Offspring of such planned matings can be blood tested and/or test mated for the defect in question. Normal puppies from these matings can be kept for breeding to maintain the genetic line. Because of these laboratory tests, the occurrence of serious genetic defects, like hemophilia, within an otherwise desirable bloodline need not destroy that line.

Routine screening tests of clotting activity, such as the APTT, PT, and TCT, usually do not detect individuals that carry or are mildly or even moderately affected with these genetic diseases.[11, 18] The diagnostic tests required are quantitative assays for specific clotting factors, and the results are meaningful only if the tests are performed by specialized coagulation laboratories experienced with coagulation assays of animal plasma. There are defined species differences in coagulation activities; thus, homologous, species-specific assays must be used. Most human coagulation laboratories do not have the experience of the homozygous standards for assays of dog or cat samples. Fortunately, plasma samples can be processed locally and, following special instructions, shipped frozen in dry ice to specialized laboratories for the required tests.

For most platelet function disorders, the tests cannot be performed on shipped specimens.[8] The blood must be tested immediately after collection, as platelets are labile and cannot be preserved for this purpose. Therefore, the animals must be shipped or brought to the closest testing laboratory. This is a serious disadvantage because there are only a few places that measure platelet function in animal blood. An up-to-date list of these can be obtained from the author. A practical field test for basset hound thrombopathia is under final evaluation in the author's laboratory.

Presurgical Work-up

Medical History.[7, 10] A complete medical history should include information about the current bleeding problem, previous bleeding problems, family history, environmental influences; and when and whether any drugs had been administered to the animal. Any previous illness should be re-evaluated to identify a possible association with the current clinical signs. Bleeding problems, especially internal ones, can mimic a variety of other disease states.

The information to obtain about the current bleeding episode should include: (1) the location of the hemorrhage (internal and/or external); (2) whether bleeding was spontaneous or induced by trauma or surgery (the most common causes of excessive surgical bleeding are listed in Table 81–1); (3) whether the hemorrhage is characterized as profuse bleeding or oozing and seeping; (4) the duration of bleeding; and (5) how it was controlled.

If previous bleeding episodes are known to have occurred, additional information should include: the type and site of bleeding; the patient's age at the time of the first bleed (hereditary defects usually occur in early life, whereas acquired problems are likely to affect adults); the frequency of episodes; the presence of underlying disease that could compromise hemostasis (liver disease, uremia, autoimmune disease, malignancy, systemic infections); and whether the patient has had previous surgery *without* bleeding complications (this would suggest that the current problem is recently acquired and not hereditary).

A thorough family history should be obtained whenever possible. For example, has there been a bleeding tendency in any immediate relatives, and, if so, was the problem spontaneous or secondary to trauma or surgery? Have both sexes been affected or have only males been involved? Have elective procedures such as ovariohysterectomy been performed without problems?

Environmental factors and drugs could be contributing factors. Pertinent information includes exercise habits (whether the patient roams freely or is restricted to a yard, leash, or house), any rodenticides available or used in or near the home, and any drugs recently administered that are known to interfere with hemostasis or platelet production.

Physical Examination.[7, 10] A thorough physical examination is essential to determine the location, severity, and nature of the bleeding and to identify the underlying disease that may be present. The type and site of bleeding should be considered carefully. Is the hemorrhage superficial or deep? Is there epistaxis, hematuria, melena, petechiation, or ecchymosis on mucosal surfaces or hematoma formation in soft tissues or body cavities? Certain findings may point to a specific diagnosis. For example, chronic mucosal surface bleeding suggests a platelet disorder or VWD, whereas large hematomas are more commonly caused by clotting factor disorders. Other findings, which suggest acquired rather than inherited causes, are splenomegaly, hepatomegaly, and lymphadenopathy.

Laboratory Evaluation.[8] Proper collection and preparation of blood samples for laboratory diagnosis is crucial if meaningful results are to be obtained. Blood should contact only clean, smooth surfaces to prevent activation of factor XII and platelets. Therefore, plastic or siliconized glassware, syringes, and test tubes should be used in all sample preparation. Blood must be drawn by careful venipuncture to minimize contamination with tissue juices, which can activate coagulation within 10 seconds. Even a small clot in a specimen activates and consumes enough clotting activity to invalidate the interpretation of results. Because the blood from most animals coagulates more rapidly than human blood, it is advisable to add the anticoagulant to the syringe beforehand or to use an anticoagulant-filled vacuum collection tube (Vacutainer) for obtaining samples. Trisodium-citrate (one part of 3.8% citrate to nine parts of blood) is the anticoagulant of choice for coagulation and platelet function studies. Sodium oxalate can be used but only if the control or normal specimens are also collected in this anticoagulant. Heparin and EDTA should not be used for hemostatic studies, as the former inhibits thrombin and factor IX activation and the latter prevents platelet reactivity.

Reference and control reagents needed for hemostatic tests include fresh-frozen, pooled citrated plasmas deficient in specific clotting factor activities to be used as substrates in specific coagulation assays and a fresh-frozen, pooled plasma from healthy animals of the species being studied. The deficient substrate plasma need not be obtained from the same

TABLE 81–1. The Most Common Causes of Excessive Surgical Bleeding

Surgical accident
Thrombocytopenia
Von Willebrand's disease
Thrombopathia—renal disease, drugs (see text)
Liver disease
Chronic intravascular coagulation

species as the reference standard and test samples. For practical reasons, general screening and specific assays usually are performed on fresh-frozen patient and reference plasmas. Results obtained with fresh plasma differ from those obtained with frozen samples, and so comparison of fresh patient plasma with a frozen reference plasma is misleading. There is a relatively wide normal range for most coagulation assays, which varies not only with the individual plasmas studied but also with the specific method, reagents, and laboratory involved. Results, therefore, cannot be compared directly between laboratories. For each laboratory, a range of normal values needs to be established by testing at least 20 healthy individuals of the species. Without this information, the comparison of results from a fresh patient sample with that of an individual, fresh control plasma is unadvisable, as mildly or moderately abnormal results easily can be masked if the control specimen reads close to the upper or lower limits of the normal range.

Table 81–2 summarizes the practical screening tests commonly used for diagnosis of bleeding diseases. An additional important *in vivo* presurgical screening test is the *cuticle bleeding time*.[15] While the animal is under anesthesia and is being prepared for surgery, one or more toenails are cut short enough to cause bleeding. If hemostasis is normal, the bleeding should stop within five to six minutes in most dogs, provided that the foot is left undisturbed. Although a normal cuticle bleeding time does not preclude the existence of a mild underlying hemostatic or thrombotic defect, it does indicate that the surgeon should be able to operate without encountering significant bleeding. Recent experience has shown this technique to be valuable in determining those patients at risk during elective surgery (e.g., Doberman pinschers with VWD).

In a recent review of 346 human patients with

DIC,[23] the most valuable diagnostic tests were concluded to be those for FDP, fibrin monomer (ethanol or protamine sulfate gelation tests), and antithrombin III. The most frequently decreased clotting factors were II, V, VII, and X. In contrast to the prevailing dogma, the factor VIII:C level was decreased in only 9 per cent of these patients, and, in fact, it was elevated in most patients, as was factor VIIIR:Ag.

Postsurgical Follow-up for Problem Cases

The surgeon needs to be familiar with the recognized effects of surgical operations on tests used to diagnose bleeding tendencies and DIC. Elective, uncomplicated surgical procedures have been associated with changes in platelet count (both increases and decreases). In addition, an increase in plasma fibrinogen level and a significant increase in FDP have been associated with surgical procedures. Both of the latter changes peak on the third and fourth postoperative days.[14] Fibrin monomer levels also increase postoperatively.

Animals with either postsurgical hemorrhage or thrombosis need to be monitored serially by hemostatic tests. Supportive therapeutic measures should be given to control bleeding as indicated. It is important for the surgeon to be aware of the expected changes in laboratory parameters induced by surgery alone so that the status of the patient may be assessed accurately.

Management and Treatment[1, 4, 10, 20–22]

General Considerations

Proper management and treatment of patients with bleeding disorders cannot be achieved without an appropriate physiological and physical environment for hemostasis, tissue repair, and prevention of recurrence. An extremely important aspect of medical management is to avoid the use of the drugs, listed previously, that are known to interfere with hemostasis. These are contraindicated for patients with moderate or severe hemostatic defects, since they impair platelet function and further compromise the stability of the hemostatic plug.

Any live-virus vaccine or viral infection can impair platelet or endothelial synthesis and cell turnover. The effect occurs during the viremic phase after vaccination or exposure (usually at five to ten days) and results in a relative thrombocytopenia or endothelial injury, which may prolong the bleeding time and predispose the animal to hemorrhage. Platelet reductions of $100,000/mm^3$ can occur. During this period animals with hemostatic defects are at risk and should be evaluated carefully for signs of bleeding. Elective surgical procedures such as ear cropping, ovariohysterectomy, castration, and dental surgery either should be performed within 48 hours after vaccination or should be postponed for 10 to 14 days. In most cases, animals admitted for elective

TABLE 81–2.   Summary of Practical Screening Tests for Diagnosis of Bleeding Disease

Test	Function Measured
Platelet count	Platelet contribution to hemostasis
Dilute whole blood clot retraction and lysis test	Platelet function and fibrinolysis
Prothrombin time (PT)	Extrinsic coagulation
Activated partial thromboplastin time (APTT) or activated clotting time (ACT)	Intrinsic coagulation
Thrombin clotting time (TCT)	Fibrinogen
Fibrinogen-fibrin degradation products (FDP), e.g., ThromboWellco test (Wellcome Reagents, Greenville, NC)	Intravascular coagulation

surgery are vaccinated immediately or within 24 hours of surgery, which may account for the relatively few vaccine-related bleeding problems.

Once bleeding has been controlled by appropriate systemic therapy (see hereafter), one may be tempted to drain large external hematomas. However, this should be avoided because rebleeding and infection can occur. Healing and resorption of large hematomas may take several weeks. Hemoglobinuria, from renal clearance of blood pigments from the resorbing lesion, is often observed during the first week. If the skin overlying the hematoma becomes necrotic and drainage occurs, it should be treated topically and allowed to heal as an open wound. If the wound becomes infected, topical antibiotics should be used. If profuse hemorrhage occurs, the lesion should be packed with topical hemostatic agents, such as topical thrombin,* absorbable microfibrillar collagen (Avitene†), or absorbable gelatin sponge (Gelfoam‡), and antibiotic ointment or cream and bandaged tightly. High oral doses of broad spectrum, systemic antibiotics should be given for seven to ten days. Antibiotics known to impair platelet function (sulfonamides, nitrofurans, and some penicillin compounds) are not recommended.

Hemophiliacs or other severe bleeders should be given medications by the oral, intravenous, or subcutaneous route but never by intramuscular injection. Large hematomas frequently occur at the site of intramuscular injections. Affected animals are best housed individually in pens or cages with smooth, vertical bars to minimize trauma. Chain link fencing is not recommended for enclosures. If the patient is a house pet, it should not be left unattended with another animal. Elimination of external and internal parasites is another important adjunct to good management.

Oral iron and vitamin supplements should be given during and after bleeding episodes. High-quality, softened diets are recommended to avoid injury to the gingiva or gastrointestinal tract; excessive development of tartar has not been a problem in these animals. Bones, biscuits, and hard toys should not be offered.

Specific Therapy

Topical Therapy. Microfibrillar collagen (Avitene†) has recently been developed as a topical hemostat.[1] This material has been shown to be useful during cardiovascular surgery and has been found to be superior, hemostatically, to pressure alone or absorbable gelatin sponge (Gelfoam‡) or topical thrombin.*

Blood or Blood Component Replacement. This subject is covered in detail in Chapter 7. The type and volume of blood or blood products recommended to treat moderate or severe bleeding disorders is outlined in Table 81–3. The preferred anticoagulants for collection of whole blood for transfusion are acid-citrate-dextrose (ACD) or citrate-phosphate-dextrose. Heparin is not recommended because it activates platelets, causing them to clump. Blood products used to control and treat bleeding should be as fresh as possible or fresh-frozen, because coagulation factors and platelets are labile. As mentioned previously, animals with bleeding disorders are likely to require repeated transfusions during their lifetime and thus are at risk for transfusion incompatibilities. The use of unmatched whole blood, therefore, is contraindicated except in life-threatening emergencies. The appropriate therapy involves fresh, typed universal donor blood or crossmatching (see Chapter 7). It is wise to determine the blood type of patients that need recurrent transfusions to know whether they can safely receive random, unmatched blood.

Because platelets and coagulation factors have relatively short in vivo half-lives (e.g., 4 hours for factor VII; 8 to 12 hours for factor VIII:C; 2 to 3 days for fibrinogen, prothrombin, and platelets),[8] the control of bleeding episodes requires that the daily amount be divided and given at regularly spaced intervals (see Table 81–3). This regimen also reduces the risk of circulatory overload.

Thrombocytopenia. The treatment of choice for thrombocytopenia, whatever the cause, is adrenal corticosteroids. Standard dosage regimens start with prednisone at 2 to 4 mg/kg body weight or an equivalent dose of dexamethasone (approximately eight times more potent), given for five to seven days or until the platelet count rises to at least 100,000/mm³. In our experience severe cases respond better to initial therapy with dexamethasone, followed by dexamethasone or prednisone after the first week. The dosage of steroids is then gradually reduced by giving 50 per cent of the initial dose for three to five days, then reducing that amount by 50 per cent for another three to five days, and so on. It is not necessary to normalize the platelet count. The aim is to maintain the platelet count at or above 80,000/mm³ until the patient goes into remission. In nonresponsive animals, high doses of steroids should not be given for more than 10 to 14 days because of the risk of side effects. Refractory cases may have to be treated with more drastic measures, as indicated, such as splenectomy or immunosuppressive drugs. However, the conservative regimen previously outlined is usually successful.

Once in remission, the patient should be monitored by a platelet count every two to three months to detect recurrent episodes before there is a relapse with clinical signs. This is especially important because, in unmonitored cases, spontaneous central nervous system hemorrhage can be a fatal complication of chronic ITP.

Vitamin K Deficiency. Therapy with vitamin K only is beneficial in cases in which a bleeding disorder is attributable specifically to its deficiency; it will not control other types of bleeding problems.

---

*Parke-Davis, Detroit MI.
†Avicon, Fort Worth, TX.
‡The Upjohn Co., Kalamazoo, MI.

TABLE 81–3.   Transfusion Therapy of Bleeding Disorders

All Types*	Inherited Disorders†	
PCV less than 20% and platelet defects Fresh, preferably typed and/or crossmatched homologous whole blood—12 to 20 ml/kg body weight repeated as necessary once or twice during first 24 hr	Factor VII deficiency	Mild condition; treatment not required
	Factor VIII deficiency (Hemophilia A) Von Willebrand's disease	Fresh or fresh-frozen plasma, plasma cryoprecipitates,‡ or special FVIII concentrates
Plasma defects with PCV at or above 20% Fresh or fresh-frozen homologous plasma—6 to 10 ml/kg body weight every 6 to 8 hr until bleeding stops; 6 to 10 ml/kg body weight once or twice daily for next 3 to 5 days if required	Factor IX deficiency (Hemophilia B; Christmas disease)	Fresh or fresh-frozen plasma supernatant from plasma cryoprecipitates‡ or special FIX concentrates
	Factor X deficiency Factor XI deficiency	Fresh or fresh-frozen plasma
Platelet defects with PCV at or above 20% Fresh, homologous, platelet-rich plasma—6 to 10 ml/kg body weight 1 to 3 times daily until bleeding stops	Fibrinogen deficiencies	Fresh or fresh-frozen plasma, plasma cryoprecipitates, or fibrinogen concentrates
	Prothrombin deficiencies	Fresh or fresh-frozen plasma or prothrombin concentrates
	Platelet function defects	Fresh platelet-rich plasma

*Transfusion not to exceed 4 to 6 ml/min.

†If PCV is less than 20%, treat with fresh, matched whole blood as listed above *or* with packed red blood cells and plasma and/or platelet components. If PCV is at or above 20%, treat with plasma and/or platelet components as listed above.

‡The treatment of choice for severe hemostatic defects is concentrate therapy. Method for preparation of plasma cryoprecipitates is found in References.

Note: Drugs that impair hemostasis are contraindicated for management and treatment of inherited bleeding disorders (see text).

The natural form of this vitamin (K_1) (e.g., Aqua-Mephyton*) is the most active therapeutically; other forms of vitamin K are either not as effective or completely ineffective. The standard dose of vitamin K_1 for treating a deficiency is 0.25 to 0.5 mg/kg body weight given for four to six days. Anaphylaxis may be a side effect of intravenous administration of vitamin K_1, so this route is not recommended. In severe cases of rodenticidal poisoning it is usually advisable to give the patient one or two transfusions of fresh, compatible whole blood or plasma 10 to 12 hours apart. As mentioned earlier, poisoning with the diphacinone or brodifacoum rodenticides usually requires three to five weeks of aggressive therapy. Once the toxicant has been metabolized by the liver, the bleeding tendency and clotting test defects may still persist for a few days or longer, since it takes time for the liver to replace the depleted clotting factors. Therefore, it is recommended that the patient remain in the hospital or be kept as quiet as possible at home to avoid further bleeding complications during the immediate posttreatment period.

Disseminated Intravascular Coagulation. Recommendations for the management and treatment of DIC are as numerous and controversial as are the causes of this syndrome.[4, 20, 22] The most important point is that early diagnosis and appropriate treatment may prevent a fatal outcome.

An extremely important adjunct to treatment of DIC is continuous fluid replacement, which helps to maintain tissue perfusion, keeps the vasculature patent, and avoids stasis or sludging. This minimizes the chances for further release of thromboplastic materials from injured or ischemic tissues and, by maintaining blood flow, helps to dilute the effects of locally accumulated thromboplastins. Fluids used for volume replacement include routine intravenous fluids such as saline-dextrose, albumin in saline-dextrose, and plasma expanders such as dextran. Secondary complications of DIC such as polycythemia, hemoconcentration, metabolic acidosis, hypoxia, dehydration, and hemolytic anemia should be corrected or reversed as soon as possible.

Other replacement fluids that may be needed in the early stages of DIC or when the fibrinogen level is very low include fresh, compatible whole blood (only if red cells are essential), fresh or fresh-frozen plasma, and fibrinogen concentrates. These transfusions should be given once or twice, 12 hours apart, very slowly, and at the low dosage rate of 6 to 10 ml/kg body weight. Since there is considerable risk of promoting further thrombosis by giving the patient

---

*Merck Sharp & Dohme, West Point, PA.

additional platelets or clotting factors, blood or plasma replacement must be used with caution, preferably in conjunction with anticoagulant and/or antiplatelet therapy.

One of the best platelet function inhibitors is aspirin (150 to 300 mg daily or every second day for up to ten days), which blocks platelet prostaglandin metabolism via the cyclooxygenase pathway. When used in conjunction with anticoagulants, there is a synergistic antihemostatic effect, so the dosage of anticoagulant must be reduced accordingly.

The anticoagulant of choice for treatment of DIC is heparin, a potent thrombin inhibitor.[4, 20, 22] The dosage is variable, but, ideally, the patient's APTT or whole blood clotting time should be maintained between 1.5 and 2 times the normal for the species. Dicumarol has not been shown to be particularly effective for treating DIC and, therefore, is not recommended.[4, 20] If it is chosen, it is desirable to achieve 1.5 to 3 times prolongation of the PT.

Anticoagulation is much more effective if a constant, rather than a fluctuating, level of anticoagulant activity can be maintained throughout the day. This is especially important because of the rebound phenomenon that occurs when anticoagulation is waning. During this period, coagulation tends to increase, and platelet adhesiveness and clotting tests may become accelerated. The best way to achieve a constant level of anticoagulation is to administer repeated small doses, subcutaneously, every four to six hours.

Fibrinolytic drugs, such as streptokinase and urokinase, are not recommended for routine use in animals with DIC because of species-specific differences in their effects as compared with those in man. Inhibitors of fibrinolysis are contraindicated for treatment of DIC because they accelerate thrombosis by preventing dissolution of pre-existing clots.

Most animals with DIC are presented to the veterinarian in the later stages, when bleeding due to consumption coagulopathy is the main complaint. Therefore, it is very difficult for the clinician to assess the exact status of the patient and initiate appropriate therapy. Furthermore, because cases of DIC are seen infrequently, most veterinarians are not experienced in the management or treatment of the disease. They also lack access to the wide variety of specialized laboratory tests required for accurate diagnosis. Because of this, the most appropriate way for them to manage and treat DIC is via a conservative approach, i.e., by combined fluid replacement and platelet function inhibitors such as aspirin. Only those clinicians experienced with heparin should attempt to treat DIC with this drug because of the risk of complications from its usage (excessive bleeding[20] or heparin rebound with acceleration of thrombosis[4]).

1. Abbott, W. M., and Austen, W. G.: The effectiveness and mechanism of collagen-induced topical hemostasis. Surgery 78:723, 1975.
2. Badylak, S. F., and Van Vleet, J. F.: Alterations of prothrombin time and activated partial thromboplastin time in dogs with hepatic disease. Am. J. Vet. Res. 42:2053, 1981.
3. Badylak, S. F., Dodds, W. J., and Van Vleet, J. F.: Plasma coagulation factor abnormalities in dogs with naturally-occurring hepatic disease, in press.
4. Bick, R. L.: Disseminated intravascular coagulation and related syndromes: etiology, pathophysiology, diagnosis, and management. Am. J. Hematol. 5:265, 1978.
5. Bick, R. L.: The clinical significance of fibrinogen degradation products. Sem. Thromb. Hemost. 8:302, 1982.
6. Bowie, E. J. W., and Owen, C. A., Jr.: Hemostatic failure in clinical medicine. Sem. Hematol. 14:341, 1977.
7. Bowie, E. J. W., and Owen, C. A., Jr.: The significance of abnormal preoperative hemostatic tests. In Spaet, T. H. (ed.): Progress in Hemostasis and Thrombosis, Vol. 5. Grune and Stratton, New York, 1980, pp. 179–209.
8. Dodds, W. J.: Hemostasis and coagulation. In Kaneko, J. J. (ed.): Clinical Biochemistry of Domestic Animals, 3rd ed. Academic Press, New York, 1980, pp. 671–718.
9. Dodds, W. J.: Second international registry of animal models of thrombosis and hemorrhagic diseases. ILAR News 24:R3, 1981.
10. Dodds, W. J.: Management and treatment of hemostatic defects. In Bojrab, M. J. (ed.): Pathophysiology in Small Animal Surgery. Lea and Febiger, Philadelphia, 1981, pp. 475–477.
11. Dodds, W. J.: Detection of genetic defects by screening programs. Am. Kennel Gazette 99:56, 1982.
12. Dodds, W. J., Moynihan, A. C., Fisher, T. M., and Trauner, D. B.: The frequencies of inherited blood and eye diseases as determined by genetic screening programs. J. Am. Anim. Assoc. 17:697, 1981.
13. Dymock, I. W., Tucker, J. S., Woolf, I. L., Paller, L., and Thomson, J. M.: Coagulation studies as a prognostic index in acute liver failure. Br. J. Haematol. 29:385, 1975.
14. Egan, E. L., Bowie, E. J. W., Kazmier, F. J., Gilchrist, G. S., Woods, J. W., and Owen, C. A., Jr.: Effect of surgical operation on certain tests used to diagnose intravascular coagulation and fibrinolysis. Mayo Clin. Proc. 49:658, 1974.
15. Giles, A. R., Tinlin, S., and Greenwood, R.: A canine model of hemophilic (factor VIII:C deficiency) bleeding. Blood 60:727, 1982.
16. Greene, C.: Hemorrhagic disorders. In Bojrab, M. J. (ed.): Pathophysiology in Small Animal Surgery. Lea and Febiger, Philadelphia, 1981, pp. 463–474.
17. Hill, B. L., Zenoble, R. D., and Dodds, W. J.: Prothrombin deficiency in a cocker spaniel. J. Am. Vet. Med. Assoc. 181:262, 1982.
18. Jolly, R. D., Dodds, W. J., Ruth, G. R., and Trauner, D. B.: Screening for genetic diseases: principles and practice. Adv. Vet. Sci. Comp. Med. 25:245, 1981.
19. Landi, M. S., and Higson, J. E.: Factor VII deficiency in colony bred mongrels. Lab. Anim. Sci. 32:429, 1982.
20. Mant, M. J., and King, E. G.: Severe, acute disseminated intravascular coagulation: a reappraisal of its pathophysiology, clinical significance and therapy based on 47 patients. Am. J. Med. 67:557, 1979.
21. Mount, M. E., and Feldman, B. F.: Vitamin K and its therapeutic importance. J. Am. Vet. Med. Assoc. 180:1354, 1982.
22. Ruehl, W., Mills, C., and Feldman, B. F.: Rational therapy in disseminated intravascular coagulation. J. Am. Vet. Med. Assoc. 181:76, 1982.
23. Spero, J. A., Lewis, J. H., and Hasiba, U.: Disseminated intravascular coagulation: findings in 346 patients. Thromb. Haemost. 43:28, 1980.
24. Spurling, N. W.: Hereditary disorders of haemostasis in dogs: a critical review of the literature. Vet. Bull. 50:151, 1980.
25. Sun, N. C. J., McAfee, M., Hum, G. J., and Weiner, J. M.: Hemostatic abnormalities in malignancy: a prospective study of 108 patients. Part I. Coagulation studies. Am. J. Clin. Pathol. 71:10, 1979.

Chapter 82

Canine and Feline Blood Groups

W. Jean Dodds

Like man, all domestic animal species have a blood group system identified by specific antigens on the surface of their red blood cells.[1-4, 7-11] However, important differences exist between the blood group antigens of animals and man that affect the clinical relevance of antigen/antibody reactivities observed *in vitro*.[7] First, although many red cell antigens of animals have been given the same letter designations as the human ABO system, these were used for convenience and do not signify related blood group specificities.[4, 8-11] Second, unlike the ABO system of man, animals with erythrocytes bearing one alloantigen of an allelic blood group system usually do not have naturally occurring isoantibodies of significant titer directed against the other, absent antigens of the system. Thus, in contrast to man, animals, with the possible exception of cats (see hereafter),[2] rarely exhibit acute transfusion reactions when first given incompatible blood.[7, 11] However, because sensitization of the recipient to future incompatible transfusions can occur in such instances, the use of typed and crossmatched compatible blood is always preferable. Crossmatched compatible blood not only avoids sensitization but allows for maximum survival time of the transfused cells in an already compromised host. An additional discussion of the biological consequences of incompatibility is found in Chapter 7.

CANINE RED BLOOD CELL GROUPS

The blood group system of dogs has been one of the most thoroughly characterized in animals.[3, 4, 7-11] As early as 1936, Wright[12] observed serological incompatibilities during plasmapheresis experiments in dogs that were associated with transfusion reactions *in vivo* and hemagglutination of the red cells of one animal by the serum of the other. This was followed by the systematic studies of Young and colleagues[11, 13] that identified eight alloantigenic determinants in canine blood and provided the foundation for current knowledge about canine blood groups.

Nomenclature

The nomenclature of the canine blood group system has undergone two changes and one proposed change since the original designations were introduced by Young and colleagues.[11, 13] Originally, the

blood groups were designated by the letters A through G in the order of their discovery. Two types of A-positive red cells were recognized; a strongly reacting subtype A_1 and a more weakly reacting subtype A_2.[11] Antibodies to group E and G specificities are no longer available (the immunized dogs have died), and the newer factors Tr and He have been added to the list. Thus, the original letter nomenclature for the dog blood groups has largely persisted and is in common usage today.

In 1973, a new nomenclature was adopted at the First International Workshop on Canine Immunogenetics.[9] Each factor was labelled by the acronym CEA for canine erythrocyte antigen and a number from 1 to 8. In 1976 the term CEA was replaced by DEA for dog erythrocyte antigen to avoid confusion with carcinoembryonic antigen, which shared the original acronym. Since then yet another nomenclature was proposed[9] to account for the failure of the CEA and DEA designations to distinguish between genetically independent blood group systems. This system has not been officially adopted and is confusing to some readers because it uses a capital letter for each genetic system and a lower case letter for each factor within that system (e.g., DEA 1 and DEA 2, subtypes of the same system, become Aa and Aa_1).

An alternative and simpler system has been used by Bull and associates and myself[4] since 1978. The 1976 designation is used with a slight modification to indicate the subtype relationship between the DEA 1 (A_1) and DEA 2 (A_2) loci. These are renamed as DEA 1·1 and DEA 1·2 for A_1 and A_2, respectively (Table 82–1).

TABLE 82–1. Canine Blood Groups*

New Nomenclature†	Common Name	Incidence (%)‡
DEA 1·1	A_1 ⎫	40–45
DEA 1·2	A_2 ⎭	20
DEA 3	B	5
DEA 4	C	98
DEA 5	D	20–25
DEA 6	F	98
DEA 7	Tr	45–50
DEA 8	He	40

*Data from Stormont, C., and Suzuki, C. Y.: Canine blood groups. *In* Shifrine, M., and Wilson, F. D. (eds.): *The Canine as a Biomedical Research Model: Immunological, Hematological, and Oncological Aspects.* Natl. Tech. Inform. Svc., DOE/TIC-10191, US Dept. Com., Springfield, VA, 1980.

†Dog erythrocyte antigen system as designated in 1976 and modified by Bull and associates[4] (see text).

‡In random populations.

Supported, in part, by research grants HL09902 and HL07173, awarded by the National Heart, Lung, and Blood Institute, PIIS/DIIIIS.

Serology and Genetics of Canine Blood Groups

Whereas the blood groups A through G originally described had no relationship to the human ABO system, the more recently discovered canine Tr antigen is serologically related to the human A blood group.[10] Canine Tr is also similar to the A-like specificities of other species (e.g., J of cattle, R of sheep, and A of pigs) because it is a soluble tissue substance adsorbed onto red cells from plasma and not an intrinsic component of the red cell.[9] Tr is closely associated with canine secretory antigen (CSA-A), which is also serologically related to human A. A new antibody called anti-O has been discovered in the Tr system that permits identification of three phenotypes: Tr, O, and absence of both Tr and O.[9]

The canine He blood group factor is found in saliva but not on red cells.[8, 10] Additional information about this and other canine erythrocyte antigens such as E and G; the 4, 5, 6, and 7 factors of Suzuki and associates (6 and 7 are related to the human MN and cattle FV types); and the five other nonallelic factors of Colling and Saison is not available.[9]

The incidence of the eight named blood factors is listed in Table 82–1. These figures were obtained from and were similar to those of random dog populations in several countries.[4, 8] About 60 per cent of random animals are positive at the A antigen (DEA 1) locus, 40 per cent are positive for the A_1 allele, and 20 per cent are positive for the A_2 allele. Thus, the remainder of the population (about 40 per cent) is negative at the DEA 1 locus, and, for practical purposes, these animals are "universal" donors (see Chapter 7 for clinical relevance and transfusion recommendations). Surveys of over 100 randomly selected animals from the United States, Australia, and France have produced similar findings.[8]

Specific family data concerning the inheritance of the canine blood factors are limited.[9] From the studies available, it appears that each blood factor is inherited as a simple autosomal dominant with the DEA 1·1 and 1·2 factors (A_1 and A_2) presumably being controlled by allelic genes. Segregation data have shown the A system to be independent of B and C and B to be independent of D. The other less well-defined factors may be either codominant autosomal alleles (6 and 7 of Suzuki and coworkers) or nonallelic (Colling and Saison),[9] whereas the remaining factors have been assigned to separate genetic systems largely on the basis of population incidence data.

Blood Typing and Crossmatching

Blood Typing

Alloantibodies raised in dogs against erythrocytes bearing recognized canine blood groups are used as blood-typing reagents.[4, 7, 9–11] Fresh autogenous serum is added to the anti-DEA 1 (A) reagent because it enhances the agglutination and thereby the recognition of A-positive red cells. The other typing sera are used as in-saline agglutinins, as the presence of serum has no effect on the reactivity to these specificities. The DEA 1·1 (A_1) and 1·2 (A_2) alleles are distinguished by rapid hemagglutination and hemolysis of A_1 cells in the presence of anti-A and complement from fresh autologous serum. By contrast, A_2 cells are weakly reactive and are not hemolyzed by anti-A and complement. Some A_2 subtypes are difficult to detect in a standard saline agglutination test and require the addition of canine Coombs' reagent (rabbit anti-dog globulin) to enhance the reaction.

Another situation that can present problems for typing dog alloantigens is the spontaneous, progressive hemolysis exhibited by dog red cells in the presence of autologous or any other normal dog serum.[9] This phenomenon is poorly understood and is neither complement-mediated nor abolished by heating the serum to 56°C. Thus, to be significant, hemolytic activity demonstrated by canine red cells in the presence of complement should appear within 15 to 20 minutes after addition of the reagents.

Interpretation of hemolytic reactions obtained with typing antisera of low titer or weak avidity may be difficult. A way to solve the problem of spontaneous hemolysis is to absorb the typing serum with red cells, specifically those derived from the dog that produced the serum to avoid removal of the desired alloantibodies.[9] Two serial 20-minute absorptions are used with the undiluted, heated (30 minutes at 56°C) antiserum and a 1:2 ratio of thrice-washed red cells to serum for each absorption. The typing reactions with the absorbed reagent can be allowed to develop for several hours before reading, permitting evaluation of weakly reacting specificities. In some cases, the sensitivity of agglutination reactions can be improved by addition of dextran and bovine serum albumin.[9]

Crossmatching

Table 82–2 outlines the technique for crossmatching blood from any species. The importance of crossmatching canine donor and recipient bloods has been emphasized by several authors.[3, 4, 7, 14] This is especially true when the facilities or reagents for blood typing are unavailable.

When a recipient has been transfused with incompatible blood, isoantibodies develop within seven to ten days.[3] These isoantibodies can decrease the survival of subsequently transfused red blood cells and can result in a severe transfusion reaction if the incompatibility involves the DEA 1 locus, specifically its DEA 1·1 (A_1) allele. By choosing donors and recipients at random, the incidence of isosensitization at the DEA 1 locus is about 25 per cent.[14] The chance of a transfusion reaction on a repeat transfusion for random donors and recipients is about 15 per cent.[14] Thus, if typed, compatible donors are unavailable, a crossmatch must be done to identify a suitable donor before the recipient receives a second transfusion.

Crossmatching should be performed on fresh blood, since many blood group antibodies (e.g., anti-DEA 1) are complement-fixing. The donor's red cells must be compatible in the major crossmatch (donor's cells in recipient's serum) at all three temperatures and should be compatible in the minor crossmatch (recipient's cells in donor's serum) at least at 37°C.[4] It is important to perform these tests at all three temperatures because isoantibodies can be reactive over a wide temperature range.[3, 4, 7] Despite this generally accepted principle, the clinically significant isoantibodies of man and animals nearly always react at 37°C, with just a few being cold reactive (4°C).[6] Furthermore, very few room temperature–reacting antibodies present a clinical problem.[6]

Once the appropriate mixtures of donor and recipient specimens and their respective controls are incubated for 15 minutes at each temperature (see Table 82–2), the tubes are centrifuged and the supernatants examined for hemolysis. The tubes are gently tapped against the hand or finger to check for agglutination as the red cell button leaves the bottom of the tube. Compatible crossmatches show neither agglutination nor hemolysis. If no agglutination is noted grossly, a small amount of the suspension is transferred to a microscope slide and examined at low power for agglutination. Compatibility must be present in the major crossmatch, but slight hemolysis or agglutination in the minor crossmatch usually means that the donor's blood can be used on an emergency basis with appropriate precautions. The latter situation applies because the weakly reacting antibodies present in the donor's plasma are rapidly diluted by the recipient's plasma volume.

If the crossmatch produces a questionable reaction, a nonagglutinating amount of antibody might have become bound to the test cells. Trace canine DEA 1 incompatibility reactions can be enhanced by performing an indirect Coombs' test on the crossmatch mixtures.[3, 7] The tubes should be recentrifuged and the red cells washed three times in saline. Two drops are placed in an empty test tube. Two drops of canine Coombs' (antiglobulin) serum are added and mixed, and the mixture is centrifuged and examined for agglutination or hemolysis. If this mixture is nonreactive it can be remixed, incubated at room temperature for 15 minutes, recentrifuged, and examined again.

Safety and Efficacy of Compatibility Tests

A recent review by Masouredis[6] discussed safety and efficacy for pretransfusion compatibility testing in man. Many of the same principles apply to animals, although the veterinarian is severely hampered in carrying out the recommended procedures because of the poor availability of blood reagents and testing laboratories. Pretransfusion tests are intended to guarantee the normal survival of transfused red cells at minimum cost. The long-standing debate about what constitutes safe and cost-effective compatibility testing while providing blood in a timely manner would be obviated if there were more reliable and effective in vitro methods for predicting in vivo red cell survival.[6] In the late 1960s human blood banking technology expanded to the point where methods were developed to detect all antibodies present in both donor and recipient bloods. Consequently, overzealous testing revealed reactivities with little clinical relevance and complicated the interpretation and significance of compatibility testing results. Thus, prudent testing designed to be predictive of potential clinical problems is essential.

Incompatibilities revealed by crossmatching indicate prior sensitization of the recipient. However, the use of crossmatched, compatible blood does not preclude sensitization of the recipient for future transfusions if the donor cells contain alloantigens not present on recipient red cells. Thus, animals in need of repeated transfusions, such as those with autoimmune hemolytic disease, should be given blood from donors with which they are blood type and crossmatch compatible.[4]

FELINE RED BLOOD CELL GROUPS

Relatively little is known about the blood groups of cats. Several blood group systems have been described,[1–3, 5] but transfusion reactions rarely occur, and crossmatching, while advocated by one group,[2] is not routinely used and may be of limited value.[3] One possible explanation for the failure of clinicians in North America to observe transfusion reactions in cats, despite the predictions of the Australian group,[1, 2] may be that those cats requiring transfusions for treatment of feline leukemia virus–induced anemia are immunosuppressed and thus fail to respond to the red cell alloantigens.

TABLE 82–2. Blood Crossmatching*

	Donor (vol ml)		Recipient (vol ml)	
	Red cells	*Serum*	*Red cells*	*Serum*
Major crossmatch	0.1	—	—	0.1
Minor crossmatch	—	0.1	0.1	—
Donor control	0.1	0.1	—	—
Recipient control	—	—	0.1	0.1

*Performed after incubation for 15 minutes at 37°C, room temperature, and 4°C (see text).

The original reports of feline blood groups[5] described several specificities; three were named O, F, and EF by Holmes, and four were designated as A through D by Euquem and Podliachouk. Groups E and F were described as isoantigens associated with red cells, and the counterpart isoagglutinins were present in serum. The incidence of these alloantigens was listed as 3.8 per cent for type O, 0.97 per cent for F, and 95.2 per cent for EF.[5] Agglutination with the isoantibodies was most active at room temperature, inactive at 56°C, and weakly reactive with some cold sera.

The question remains whether the specificities described by Euquem and Podliachouk were the same as or distinct from those of Holmes.[5] The weak agglutinin found in the serum of EF cats by Holmes was called anti-B by the other investigators, and they also observed an anti-A agglutinin that contained both the anti-E and anti-F of Holmes. Euquem and Podliachouk described A and B antigens present in 85 and 15 per cent of random cats, respectively, and designated antigens C and D that were frequently associated with B.

More recently, Auer and coworkers[1, 2] have defined the AB blood group system of cats. The incidence of these antigens in nearly 2000 cats from Brisbane, Australia, was 73.3 per cent for group A, 26.3 per cent for B, and 0.4 per cent for AB. Group B cats had high titers of anti-A in their sera, whereas anti-B was infrequently present and of very low titer in sera from those of group A. The anti-A reactivity was a strong agglutinin and hemolysin and the anti-B was a weak agglutinin but strong hemolysin. These investigators pointed out the potential clinical importance of the widespread distribution of naturally occurring isoantibodies (3 in 16), especially in group B cats.[2]

Although severe reactions could be induced experimentally by a single incompatible transfusion,[2] the probability of encountering transfusion reactions in clinical situations in cats remains to be determined. In addition to the clinical case suggestive of but unproved to be caused by transfusion incompatibility (the recipient was not typed),[2] two other authors have described transfusion reactions in cats.[2, 5] According to Ditchfield, red blood cell and tissue contaminants in homologous tissue panleukopenia vaccines produced isoimmunization of queens and contributed to red cell destruction and the fading kitten syndrome in their offspring.[5] As cited by Auer and colleagues,[2] Thornton has reported complications after single and multiple transfusions in cats, although these were not documented.

Should crossmatching be advisable or required for cats, as has been proposed by Auer and colleagues,[2] the same technique as that previously described for dogs can be used. In any event, it would be wise to pay closer attention to the question of blood compatibility for transfusion replacement in all species. Certainly, transfusion reactions, although minor in most cases, present an additional physiological stress to the debilitated patient.

1. Auer, L., and Bell, K.: The AB blood group system of cats. Anim. Blood Groups: Biochem. Genet. 12:287, 1981.
2. Auer, L., Bell, K., and Coates, S.: Blood transfusion reactions in the cat. J. Am. Vet. Med. Assoc. 180:729, 1982.
3. Buening, G. M.: Transfusions. In Bojrab, M. I. (ed.): Pathophysiology in Small Animal Surgery. Lea & Febiger, Philadelphia, 1981, pp. 478–482.
4. Dodds, W. J., and Bull, R. W.: Canine blood groups and blood banking. Pure Bred Dogs-Am. Kennel Gaz. 96:68, 1979.
5. Gorham, J. R., Henson, J. B., and Dodgen, C. T.: Basic principles of immunity in cats. J. Am. Vet. Med. Assoc. 158:846, 1971.
6. Masouredis, S. P.: Pretransfusion tests and compatibility: questions of safety and efficacy. Blood 59:873, 1982.
7. Michel, R. L.: Blood groups, typing and cross-matching of animal blood. Bull. Am. Soc. Vet. Clin. Pathol. 4:3, 1975.
8. Spurling, N. W.: Haematology of the dog. In Archer, R. K., and Jeffcott, L. B. (eds.): Comparative Clinical Haematology. Blackwell Scientific Publications, London, 1977, pp. 414–417.
9. Stormont, C., and Suzuki, C. Y.: Canine blood groups. In Shifrine, M., and Wilson, F. D. (eds.): The Canine as a Biomedical Research Model: Immunological, Hematological, and Oncological Aspects. Natl. Tech. Inform. Svc., DOE/TIC-10191, US Dept. Com., Springfield, VA, 1980, pp. 127–133.
10. Swisher, S. N., Bull, R., and Bowdler, J.: Canine erythrocyte antigens. Tissue Antigens 3:164, 1973.
11. Swisher, S. N., and Young, L. E.: The blood group system of dogs. Physiol. Rev. 41:495, 1961.
12. Wright, A.: Isohemolysins and isoagglutinins occurring in dogs. Proc. Soc. Exp. Biol. Med. 34:440, 1936.
13. Young, L. E., Ervin, D. M., and Yuile, C. L.: Hemolytic reactions produced in dogs by transfusion of incompatible dog blood and plasma. 1. Serologic and hematologic aspects. Blood 4:1218, 1949.
14. Young, L. E., O'Brien, W. A., Swisher, S. N., Miller, G., and Yuile, C. L.: Blood groups in dogs: their significance to the veterinarian. Am. J. Vet. Res. 13:207, 1952.

Chapter 83

The Bone Marrow

Susan M. Cotter and Julia Blue

ORGANIZATION OF THE BONE MARROW

The principal hematopoietic tissue in postnatal dogs and cats is sheltered within the medullary cavities of various bones. This tissue, the bone marrow, produces nearly all the red cells, granulocytes, monocytes, and platelets that circulate in the peripheral blood. It is the bone marrow, with its special arrangement of stromal cells and vessels, that most effectively supports the proliferation and differentiation of hematopoietic stem cells and their progeny and delivers the end products of hematopoiesis into the blood (see Chapter 80). The marrow is rich in macrophages and filters blood.

In normal adult animals, hematopoietic marrow persists in the bones of the axial skeleton and in the ends of some long bones.[3] The ilium and the proximal ends of the femur and the humerus are accessible sites in dogs and cats of any age for sampling bone marrow by aspiration or core biopsy techniques (see hereafter). The slight differences in cellularity among these sites are not great enough to be diagnostically significant.[3,8] Unless the marrow is markedly fibrotic, a sample containing flecks of hematopoietic tissue can nearly always be aspirated from one of these sites.

Gross Characteristics of Marrow

Normal marrow is soft and semisolid and tends to spread when removed from bone and placed on a smooth surface. In general, red marrow is hematopoietically active owing to its content of hemoglobin-containing red cell precursors. Inactive, fatty marrow is usually yellow. Paradoxically, in diseases such as feline panleukopenia, the marrow sample is red, although depleted of hematopoietic cells. This is because, following rapid depopulation of differentiating hematopoietic cells, whether due to viruses, radiation, or cytotoxic drugs, the small vessels in marrow expand with blood and some tear. Congestion and hemorrhage produce the red color. In contrast, in hypoplastic or aplastic anemia in which hematopoietic cell numbers are reduced gradually, lipid-filled stromal cells increase in volume and marrow architecture is preserved. Areas normally filled with red marrow thus contain yellow marrow in patients with hypoproliferative anemia. Marrow that is markedly infiltrated with nonerythroid neoplastic cells is often gray. Marrow that contains an excessive amount of extracellular material, whether collagen or reticulin, is firm and rubbery, although it may still be red.

Microscopic Organization of Marrow

Hematopoietically active marrow is composed of irregular cords of hematopoietic tissue separated by thin-walled venous vessels called *sinuses*.[15] The blood supply to the marrow is derived from branches of the nutrient arteries to the bone. Arterioles from cortical bone enter the marrow and link with venous sinuses. Sinuses subsequently drain into larger veins, which conduct blood away from the marrow. Because of these vascular arrangements, blood flowing through the marrow is retained within vessels and does not percolate through the hematopoietic cords. Nevertheless, blood flowing through the marrow is partly cleared of particles and effete cells by macrophages lying within the lumena of sinuses and by pseudopodia extended into the lumen by perisinusal macrophages.

The hematopoietic cords consist of a framework of branched connective tissue cells, called *reticular cells*, which are similar to those of the spleen. The scaffolding formed by reticular cells supports the hematopoietic cells, macrophages, plasma cells, and lymphocytes of active marrow. Extracellular fibers are few, but a delicate network of extracellular material, called *reticulin,* can be demonstrated in sections of normal marrow by staining with silver nitrate. The reticular cells extend sheetlike cytoplasmic processes that not only form a supporting framework for cells but also extend around sinuses to partly cover the outer surface of the endothelium. Reticular cells can accumulate lipid to become the fat cells of active marrow.[14] Fat cells occupy approximately 50 per cent of the volume of normal hematopoietic marrow. The lipid in these cells contains a higher proportion of unsaturated fatty acids than does the lipid in extramedullary body fat.[14] This lipid is rapidly mobilized when hematopoiesis is accelerated, and the reticular cells assume a flatter configuration. The decrease in reticular cell volume allows for an increase in volume of hematopoietic cells within the confines of the medullary cavity.

Differentiating hematopoietic cells are not distributed randomly through the cords but preferentially occupy certain locations.[13] Megakaryocytes lie against the outer surface of the sinuses. Erythroblasts are concentrated around the sinuses. Granulocytes mature in areas distant from the sinuses. Maturing erythroblasts and granulocytes are found in physical association with different stromal cells of marrow. Erythroblasts differentiate to the point of nuclear extrusion within units called *erythroblastic islets*,[2] which consist of a central macrophage surrounded by concentric tiers of erythroblasts embedded in the velamentous cytoplasmic extensions of the macrophage. The macrophage phagocytizes defective erythroblasts and extruded nuclei and may transfer iron in the form of ferritin granules to the erythroblasts. Developing granulocytes typically cluster around reticular cells rather than macrophages.[16]

EXAMINATION OF THE BONE MARROW

Indications for Examination and Interpretation of Marrow Samples

Anemia

Examination of the bone marrow provides important information to supplement the hemogram when evaluating hematopoietic problems. The marrow may give a preview of coming events. For example, in aplastic anemia, a better prognosis can be given if increased marrow cellularity is present, whereas a relatively nonreactive and acellular marrow indicates that no significant response can be expected in the blood within the next five to six days. When anemia is caused by blood loss or hemolysis, the hemogram usually shows signs of bone marrow regeneration after the first few days, including reticulocytosis, polychromasia, macrocytosis, anisocytosis, and, sometimes, the presence of spherocytes, nucleated red cells, or leukocytosis. If the hemogram does show such changes, evaluation of the marrow is not likely to give enough additional information to warrant performing the procedure. However, if, from the results of a hemogram, the anemia is classified as nonregenerative, examination of the marrow is indicated, because primary marrow failure may exist (see Chapter 80). This condition is called *red cell aplasia* if only erythroid precursors are decreased and *aplastic anemia* if there is pancytopenia. Normal or increased numbers of erythroid precursors in the bone marrow of an animal with a hemogram giving the appearance of nonregenerative anemia indicate either that improvement is impending or that destruction or a maturation arrest is occurring earlier than the reticulocyte stage. A decrease in erythroid precursors is the most common bone marrow finding in nonregenerative anemia. Occasionally, infiltration of the marrow with leukemic cells may cause nonregenerative anemia in the absence of circulating leukemic cells.

Abnormal White Cells in the Peripheral Blood

The presence of atypical lymphocytes in the peripheral blood implies either the existence of an active immune response or leukemia. If any abnormal lymphocytes are present in the blood of a patient with lymphadenopathy, a marrow aspirate may circumvent the need for a lymph node biopsy.

Generally, immature granulocytes circulate in the peripheral blood (i.e., a "left shift") in response to certain acute bacterial infections, especially those with "pyogenic" organisms. In the latter case, normally mature granulocytes still predominate over immature forms. If the left shift is severe, myelocytes may appear in the circulation. This has been called a *leukemoid response* because of the similarity of the hemogram to that found in granulocytic leukemia. With acute granulocytic or monocytic leukemia, a majority of the circulating white cells are immature and sometimes include blast forms. Examination of the marrow may help differentiate a leukemoid reaction from leukemia.[1] In granulocytic leukemia, the marrow is replaced with myeloblasts or promyelocytes, whereas in a leukemoid reaction increased granulocytic precursors are present while other cells are normal.

Unexplained Leukopenia

Increased numbers of normal myeloid precursors in the bone marrow of an animal with peripheral leukopenia are indicative of either impending improvement or excessive consumption of granulocytes by severe infection. A decreased number of myeloid precursors in the bone marrow is an adverse prognostic sign associated with aplastic anemia of various causes. In small animals the most common cause of peripheral blood leukopenia concomitant with decreased marrow myeloid elements is infection of cats with feline leukemia virus (FeLV).[5] Suppression of granulocytes, lymphocytes, platelets, or red cell precursors singly or in various combinations may occur as a direct effect of FeLV infection.

Thrombocytopenia

Examination of a marrow aspirate may allow the prediction of whether thrombocytopenia is reversible. Evidence of reversibility, as demonstrated by increased numbers of megakaryocytes in the bone marrow, would be observed, for example, in immune-mediated thrombocytopenia. On the other hand, decreased megakaryocytes are seen on bone marrow preparations in conditions such as aplastic anemia, FeLV infection, erlichiosis, endogenous or exogenous estrogen toxicity, leukemia, or the effects of toxic chemicals, such as benzene, cytotoxic chemotherapeutic agents, or drugs such as phenylbutazone.

Posterior Paresis in Cats

Occasionally, domestic cats develop lymphoma in the lumbar extradural space. Approximately 50 per cent of such cats also develop leukemic infiltrates in the marrow even without circulating abnormal cells.[4] Therefore, examination of a bone marrow aspirate is indicated in cats with posterior paresis if other causes, such as trauma or aortic embolism, have been ruled out.

Unexplained Hypercalcemia or Monoclonal Gammopathy

Hypercalcemia in dogs, in most cases, is associated with lymphoma or another malignancy. If a tumor cannot be found elsewhere, the marrow should be examined for evidence of leukemia. In dogs or cats with monoclonal gammopathy, myeloma should be considered. Even in the absence of radiographic evidence of bone lesions, myeloma sometimes may be diagnosed by examination of the marrow.

Mast Cell Neoplasia

Systemic mastocytosis is more common in cats than in dogs, although it can occur in members of either species. In cats, a common manifestation is massive splenomegaly (see Chapter 84), sometimes in the absence of other signs.[5] Occasionally circulating mast cells are present in the circulating blood and are best detected by examination of the buffy coat. Although some of these malignant mast cells originate in the spleen, the marrow may be involved as well. Examination of the bone marrow allows the clinician to "stage" the disease and decide on a prognosis by determining the extent of the disease.

Techniques of Examination of the Bone Marrow

Bone Marrow Aspirate Versus Biopsy

A *bone marrow aspirate* is a sample obtained by inserting a needle into the marrow and applying negative pressure via a syringe, resulting in aspiration of a cell suspension. This suspension is examined as a smear or squash preparation or may be allowed to clot and is then fixed in formalin, sectioned, and examined histologically. Aspirates can allow the clinical pathologist to estimate the number of cells per unit volume of marrow (i.e., the cellularity). The finding of low bone marrow cellularity may be an artifact if the sample is contaminated with blood, which may occur if excessive negative pressure is applied during aspiration. An aspirate is the sample of choice for evaluation of cell type and morphology. Because most disease processes detectable by study of canine and feline bone marrow are diffuse, an aspirate usually gives a representative picture of the entire marrow.

A *bone marrow biopsy* is a core sample, taken with architecture intact and fixed in formalin. Such samples provide more information than do formalin-fixed clots taken with an aspiration needle. The bone marrow architecture is disrupted in the latter but not in the former method. For the diagnosis of patchy lesions, marrow biopsies give a better indication of cellularity and are more useful than aspirates. Also, they provide additional information when few or no cells are present in an aspirate. Aplastic anemia and myelofibrosis are associated with hypocellular aspirates. Patchy lesions appear to be much less common

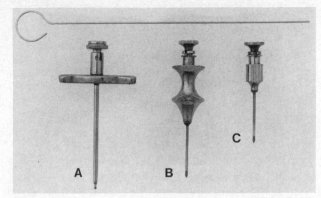

Figure 83–1. Three types of needles used for biopsy and aspiration of bone marrow from dogs and cats. All needles have stylets in place. *A*, Jamshidi infant marrow biopsy needle (13 gauge, 2 inch). The probe above the needle is inserted retrograde into the pointed tip of the needle to push the specimen out of the needle and into formalin. *B*, Rosenthal bone marrow aspirate needle (18 gauge, 1 inch). *C*, Osgood bone marrow aspirate needle (18 gauge, 1 inch).

in dogs and cats than in human beings, in whom metastatic neoplasms or granulomatous infections such as tuberculosis are more likely to invade the marrow.

Needles

All needles for aspiration of bone marrow have stylets that are held in place during insertion into the bone. An 18-gauge, 1-inch needle may be used for cats or small dogs (Fig. 83–1). Osgood needles are adequate for cats and are less expensive than the more sturdy Rosenthal needles. Osgood needles should be discarded after a few uses because they are difficult to sharpen. These needles are less suitable for use in dogs owing to the potential for breakage at the hub when the needles are embedded deeply in the pelvis. Therefore, for the iliac crest an 18-gauge, 1-inch Rosenthal needle is best for most medium-sized dogs. A one and one-half–inch needle is also available for large or obese dogs. To obtain a femoral marrow sample from large or obese dogs, a three- or four-inch needle may be more useful when aspirating marrow via the greater trochanter.

Selection of Sites

The sites from which bone marrow samples are most commonly obtained in dogs and cats are the anterior iliac crest and the proximal femur. The iliac crest is more superficial and therefore more accessible than the proximal femur. Difficulty is sometimes encountered in obtaining an adequate sample from this site in cats because of the small size of the marrow space; the femur should be used in this species, especially if more than a few drops of marrow are needed. The rib may be used in large, obese dogs when difficulty is encountered finding landmarks.

The Iliac Crest. If the iliac crest is selected as the bone marrow aspiration site, patients are positioned in sternal recumbency. Sedation usually is not re-

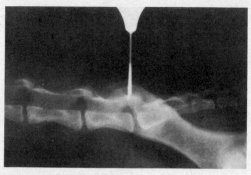

Figure 83–2. Lateral radiograph of the posterior lumbosacral spine and pelvis of a cat. An 18-gauge, 1-inch needle is in the proper location in the anterior iliac crest for aspiration of marrow. (Reprinted with permission from Cotter, S. H.: Feline leukemia virus induced disorders in the cat. Vet. Clin. North Am. 6:367, 1976.)

quired for dogs, but cats often are given an agent such as ketamine (40 to 50 mg IM). Hair is removed, and the area is prepared for aseptic surgery. In both dogs and cats, 2 per cent xylocaine is infiltrated intradermally and down to the periosteum of the iliac crest. With a #12 scalpel blade, a small skin incision no larger than the diameter of the needle to be used is made. The needle is held firmly and, with the stylet in place, is driven through the soft tissue into the bone. Care should be taken to assure that the stylet is not dislodged during this procedure to prevent bending the tip of the needle or plugging the needle with bone. The ilium is entered perpendicular to the center of the dorsal aspect of the iliac crest (Fig. 83–2). The needle is rotated clockwise and then counterclockwise repeatedly as it is advanced. In dogs, but not in cats, a decrease in resistance may be felt as the needle enters the marrow cavity. In cats, the needle is assumed to be in the cavity when it is firmly embedded in the bone for a distance of about 1.0 to 1.5 cm.[4] At this point the stylet is removed, and a 12-cc syringe without anticoagulant is tightly attached. Approximately 5 to 8 cc of negative pressure is applied, and the neck of the syringe is watched. The negative pressure is stopped and the needle is removed as soon as any marrow is observed at the hub of the needle. If no marrow is seen, the needle is slowly withdrawn while the vacuum is maintained, and any contents of the needle are expressed onto a slide. Sufficient marrow is usually in the needle to make adequate smears. If marrow is easily obtained, the smears should be made with the first few drops to avoid contamination with blood. Marrow cells and, especially, neoplastic cells are easily traumatized by excessive pressure or agitation, resulting in enough cell damage (e.g., smudge cells) to obscure the diagnosis. Excessive negative pressure may also rupture venous sinuses, causing the marrow to be contaminated with blood, complicating interpretation. It is noteworthy that a pain reaction often occurs when negative pressure is applied to the marrow because local anesthesia extends no deeper than the level of the periosteum.

If additional marrow is needed for other procedures, a second syringe, rinsed with heparin, can be attached to the needle. Up to several ml of marrow can usually be obtained from the iliac crest of the dog but not the cat. Heparin may interfere with cellular detail and should be avoided if the sample is to be examined cytologically. Failure to obtain marrow from the iliac crest may be caused by myelofibrosis, aplastic anemia, severe packing of the marrow with malignant cells, and, occasionally in cats, lack of a marrow cavity.

The Femur. The proximal end of this bone is preferred by some clinicians as an aspiration site for bone marrow samples from both cats and dogs. The animal is placed in lateral recumbency, and the area of the greater trochanter is prepared for aseptic surgery. Care should be taken to stay sufficiently lateral to avoid the sciatic nerve, although this nerve is not likely to be close enough to the site of the needle entry to be damaged. However, temporary sciatic paralysis has occurred following infiltration of the area with a local anesthetic. The marrow cavity is entered just medial to the greater trochanter, with the needle directed toward the center of the long axis of the shaft of the femur. Larger volumes of marrow can be obtained from the femur than from the iliac crest of cats and small dogs. Marrow is most plentiful near the metaphysis. The distal long bones of adult animals normally contain little marrow.

Bone Marrow Biopsy Technique

Both aspirates and biopsies may be obtained during the same procedure by using a 13-gauge, 2-inch infant Jamshidi needle[6] (see Fig. 83–1). The interior diameter of the cutting portion of the needle is tapered toward the tip to prevent occlusion of the needle with the bone plug. The hub of the stylet interlocks with the hub of the needle to prevent it from becoming dislodged, and it projects beyond the cutting end to protect the needle tip.

To perform a biopsy, the patient and the surgical site are prepared as for an aspirate. The needle, with stylet in place, is advanced into the marrow cavity via a small skin incision. The stylet is then removed and an aspirate taken. With the stylet removed, the needle is advanced deeper into the bone marrow, using a clockwise motion. After the needle is advanced about 1 cm, it is rotated in a counterclockwise and then clockwise direction and withdrawn. The core is removed by inserting a probe retrograde into the tip of the needle. Bone marrow biopsy specimens generally are fixed in 10 per cent buffered formalin, sectioned, stained with hematoxylin and eosin, and examined microscopically. After marrow is obtained no suture should be necessary. If severe thrombocytopenia exists, local pressure should be applied for one to two minutes, although bleeding is rarely encountered. Post biopsy complications are extremely rare.

Preparation of Bone Marrow Samples

The marrow aspirate may be prepared for examination in several ways, depending on personal preference. (1) Slide preparations may be made and stained in a manner similar to blood smears. Such slides should be made quickly to prevent clotting of the specimen. (2) Coverslip preparations sometimes are preferred. In this case, a drop of marrow is placed on one coverslip. A second coverslip is placed on top of the first and is rotated 45°. The two coverslips are pulled apart, so that two slides are obtained from one drop. If the sample appears dilute, several drops may be placed at the top end of a slanted slide. The red cells and plasma run down the slide, leaving marrow spicules at the top. A second slide or coverslip may then be pulled across this area as described previously. One slide can be stained with a quick stain such as new methylene blue and examined immediately to be sure the sample has adequate cellularity and detail for examination. In most cases the marrow should be examined by a hematologist or someone with experience in marrow examination. Additional information on techniques and equipment may be found elsewhere.[10–12]

Evaluation of Results

Stained marrow samples are examined first for cellularity, cellular detail, and staining quality. If the sample is hypocellular, a core biopsy or several aspirates from different sites should be submitted. The next step is to determine if erythroid, myeloid, and megakaryocytic elements are represented in expected proportions and if maturation is normal in all cell lines. Lymphocytes should be mature and should make up less than 15 per cent of the cells in normal marrow.[12] A relative lymphocytosis may exist in some hypocellular samples, and a transient increase of lymphocytes may occur in some cats carrying FeLV. In leukemia or myeloproliferative diseases the marrow is composed predominantly of one abnormal cell type (greater than 50 per cent) with a depletion of other cell types.

The sample is also examined for asynchronous maturation of the nucleus and cytoplasm. This is most often associated with hematopoietic malignancies. In man, this may also be seen in cases of folate or vitamin B_{12} deficiency or in Pelger-Huët anomaly, conditions that have not been documented in dogs or cats.

The myeloid:erythroid (M:E) ratio in the marrow is also important. In hemolytic or blood loss anemia the M:E ratio may be greatly reduced. Conversely, it may be increased in nonregenerative anemia or acute bacterial infections with increased granulocyte production. Thus, the M:E ratio must be interpreted in light of the knowledge of whether the change represents an increase of one cell type, a decrease in another, or both. This can be ascertained by estimating the overall cellularity of the sample. Megakaryocytes are usually distributed mainly along the edges of the slide, so they should be examined under low power magnification (100×). Determination of increased or decreased numbers of megakaryocytes requires experience because they normally comprise less than 1 per cent of the nucleated cells. Megakaryocytes are increased in conditions of increased platelet utilization or destruction, such as immune-mediated trombocytopenia, and are often decreased in disorders such as aplastic anemia and leukemia.

In some situations, several examinations of the marrow may be required over a period of time to arrive at a diagnosis. For example, an anemic animal may have a low peripheral blood reticulocyte count in the presence of massive numbers of early erythroid precursors in the marrow. This could represent an impending physiological response to anemia or an early erythroleukemia. If peripheral blood reticulocytosis and a rising hematocrit do not occur within a two-week period, a second marrow aspirate should be obtained for study. Early malignant infiltration may be confirmed or ruled out. The marrow also may be used to monitor the efficacy of chemotherapy in neoplastic disorders, because clearing of neoplastic cells from the marrow is necessary before repopulation with normal cells can occur. An aplastic blood picture may occur two weeks after myelosuppressive chemotherapeutic drugs are given as initial therapy for leukemia. Remission is predicted if the marrow, at that time, shows the return of normal elements. The prognosis is poor if the marrow still remains filled with blast forms. Additional information on normal values and interpretation of bone marrow samples are available elsewhere.[7,9,12]

1. Bernard, J., and Tanyer, J.: Chronic myelocytic leukemia. *In* Holland, J., and Frei, E. (ed.): *Cancer Medicine.* Lea & Febiger, Philadelphia, 1974.
2. Bessis, M.: *Blood Smears Reinterpreted.* Springer-International, Berlin, 1977.
3. Calvo, W., Fliedner, T. M., Herbst, E. W., and Fache, I.: Regeneration of blood-forming organs after autologous leukocyte transfusion in lethally irradiated dogs. I. Distribution and cellularity of the bone marrow in normal dogs. Blood *46*:453, 1975.
4. Cotter, S. M.: Feline leukemia virus induced disorders in the cat. Vet. Clin. North Am. 6:367, 1976.
5. Cotter, S. M.: Disorders of the hematopoietic system. *In* Holzworth, J. (ed.): *Feline Medicine and Surgery.* W. B. Saunders, Philadelphia (in preparation).
6. Jamshidi, K., and Swaim, W. R.: Bone marrow biopsy with unaltered architecture: A new biopsy device. J. Lab. Clin. Med. 77:334, 1971.
7. Lewis, H. B., and Rebar, A. H.: *Bone Marrow Evaluation in Veterinary Practice.* Ralston Purina Co., St. Louis, 1979.
8. Penny, R. H. C., and Carlisle, C. H.: The bone marrow of the dog: a comparative study of biopsy material obtained from the iliac crest, rib and sternum. J. Small Anim. Pract. *11*:727, 1970.
9. Penny, R. H. C., Carlisle, C. H., and Davidson, H. A.: The blood and bone marrow of the cat. Br. Vet. J. *126*:459, 1970.

10. Perman, V., Osborne, C. A., and Stevens, J. B.: Bone marrow
    biopsy. Vet. Clin. North Am. *4*:293, 1974.
11. Schalm, O. W.: Bone marrow cytology as an aid to diagnosis.
    Vet. Clin. North Am. *11*:383, 1981.
12. Schalm, O. W., Jain, N. C., and Carroll, E. J.: *Veterinary
    Hematology,* 3rd ed. Lea & Febiger, Philadelphia, 1975.
13. Weiss, L.: Bone marrow. *In* Weiss, L., and Greep, R. (eds.):
    Histology, 4th ed. McGraw-Hill Book Co., New York, 1977,
    pp. 487–502.
14. Weiss, L., and Brookoff, D.: Anatomy of the marrow. *In*

Lichtman, M. A. (ed.): *The Science and Practice of Clinical
    Medicine,* Vol. 6 (Hematology and Oncology). Grune and
    Stratton, New York, pp. 1–6, 1980.
15. Weiss, L., and Chen, L.: The organization of hematopoietic
    cords and vascular sinuses in bone marrow. Blood Cells
    1:617, 1975.
16. Westen, H., and Bainton, D. F.: Association of alkaline-
    phosphatase-positive reticulum cells in bone marrow with
    granulocytic precursors. J. Exp. Med. *150*:919, 1979.

84 The Spleen

Chapter

Alan J. Lipowitz, Julia Blue, and Victor Perman

The spleen has multiple and diverse functions, many of which can be assumed by other organs in its absence. Although not essential to life or health, the spleen is a highly structured organ that is well designed to perform its important functions. The splenic parenchyma, or pulp, is comprised of two tissue components with separate functions. The white pulp, which is a lymphatic tissue, is a major site of trapping and immunological recognition of blood-borne antigens and subsequent antibody production (see Chapter 15). The red pulp is a vast, highly efficient filter that clears the circulating blood of particulate material such as bacteria and aged or damaged blood cells. In domestic animals the red pulp also serves as a reservoir of red cells and platelets. Unique vascular and stromal arrangements provide the basis for splenic function.

GROSS ANATOMY

The spleen lies in the left anterior quadrant of the abdomen, typically in a dorsoventral orientation. The dorsal tip is relatively fixed near the midline beneath the last rib. The rest of the spleen is freely moveable and may vary in location, so that at times it lies nearly longitudinally along the dorsal left flank.[87] Often, its contour conforms to the greater curvature of the stomach. The spleen is attached to the greater omentum along a ridge, called the *hilus*, that runs the length of its visceral surface. The parietal surface is convex.

Arterial vessels and sympathetic nerves enter the spleen and venous vessels and lymphatics leave the spleen through the hilus (Fig. 84–1). The splenic artery arises from a branch of the celiac artery, which, before reaching the spleen, gives off branches that are the main arterial supply to the left part of the pancreas.[40,87] Similarly, the venous drainage from the left hemipancreas is through vessels that join the splenic vein. Just prior to reaching the spleen, the splenic artery divides into many branches that pen-

etrate the capsule along the hilus. Multiple short venous branches leave the spleen through the hilus and join to form the splenic vein. Venous blood from the spleen empties into the portal vein and subsequently flows through the liver. The spleen has efferent but no afferent lymphatic vessels.[36] Therefore, all extracellular fluid, soluble antigens, cells, and other particles that reach the spleen are conveyed there by blood vessels. Efferent lymphatics, which

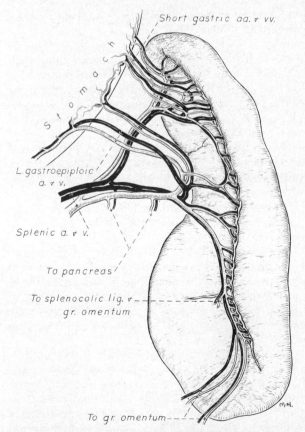

Figure 84–1. Blood supply of the spleen. (The cranial border is reflected laterally.) (Reprinted with permission from Evans, H. E., and Christensen, G. C.: *Miller's Anatomy of the Dog,* 2nd ed. W. B. Saunders, Philadelphia, 1979.)

follow large arteries, carry away a portion of the plasma and lymphocytes brought to the spleen by the blood. Smooth muscle cells in the blood vessels, capsules, and trabeculae are innervated by sympathetic fibers from the celiac ganglion. The spleen has no parasympathetic nerve supply.

The splenic pulp in dogs and cats is enclosed in a capsule of smooth muscle cells and connective tissue. Branches from the inner surface of the capsule form a rich network of muscular trabeculae that carry vessels and nerves throughout the spleen. The abundance of smooth muscle cells in the spleen of dogs and cats enables it to contract, a property not shared by the human spleen. The spleen in a resting dog or cat contracts and relaxes rhythmically.[2] Relaxation of smooth muscle is induced by anesthetics such as barbiturates or tranquilizers such as acetylpromazine. This allows congestion of the red pulp with blood and results in marked splenic enlargement. A congested spleen is dark red and has a smooth capsule and rounded edges. Stimulation of contraction by mental or physical stress or injection of catecholamines shrinks the spleen, expelling free blood cells and plasma from the red pulp. The contracted spleen is flattened, bluish purple, and has a wrinkled capsule.

The cut surface of the spleen appears as dark red tissue interrupted by scattered gray foci and irregular gray streaks. The red tissue is red pulp, the gray foci are part of the white pulp, and the gray streaks are branches of the trabecular system.

MICROSCOPIC ANATOMY

White Pulp

The lymphatic tissue of the spleen consists primarily of lymphocytes and macrophages supported by a scaffolding of branched connective tissue cells called *reticular cells*. The meshwork of supporting cells and extracellular fibers produced by them is called the *reticulum*. The white pulp is distributed along the course of arterial vessels. Within the white pulp are zones rich in T lymphocytes and zones of B lymphocyte predominance.[95] The former are designated *periarterial lymphatic sheaths* (PALS) and the latter *nodules* (follicles). A PALS is a cylinder of lymphatic tissue that surrounds an artery after it leaves a trabecula.[99] Nodules are spherical collections of B lymphocytes distributed along the length of a PALS. Some nodules contain germinal centers, which are areas of B lymphocyte proliferation and differentiation and high-level antibody production. Germinal centers develop in the nodules in response to antigenic stimulation (see Chapter 15).[14] Capillary branches from the central artery of the PALS supply the white pulp with nutrients. Plasma and soluble antigen tend to be skimmed off into the white pulp capillaries, whereas cells remain within the artery until it terminates in the red pulp.

The white pulp is separated from the surrounding red pulp by a region called the *marginal zone*. In rodents and rabbits, the marginal zone is densely populated with macrophages and receives blood from many arterial endings. It is, therefore, a major site of blood filtration in these species. The marginal zone is less highly developed in dog and cat spleen, and its role in filtration is minor compared with that of the red pulp.[7,9]

Red Pulp

The red pulp consists mainly of arterial capillaries, small venous vessels, and a reticulum filled with macrophages and blood.[7,10] Blood is delivered into the red pulp reticulum from the terminal segments of arterial capillaries, which are continuations of the central arteries of the white pulp. After a PALS tapers out, its artery enters red pulp as a penicillar artery, which then branches, loses its muscle coat, and forms arterial capillaries. The arterial capillaries are surrounded by a sheath composed of reticular cells and highly intertwined macrophages. This structure is the *periarterial macrophage sheath* (PAMS), or ellipsoid.[8] The endothelium of the arterial capillary within the sheath is porous. Plasma, particles, and some cells are squeezed out of the lumen into the PAMS through interendothelial slits. Particles such as bacteria are caught in the sheath and are phagocytized by the PAMS macrophages. Judging from studies using intravenous injections of inert particles such as carbon or thorium dioxide, the PAMS is the primary particle filter in the spleen of dogs and cats.[7,10]

In dogs and cats, the terminal portion of each arterial capillary leaves its PAMS and opens into the red pulp reticulum.[7,8,10,90] Blood cells and plasma discharged from arterial terminations flow through the reticulum to reach and enter venous vessels. The spaces in the red pulp reticulum constitute vascular pathways of an intermediate circulation interposed between arterial and venous vessels; these nonendothelial lined channels of blood flow are unique to the spleen. Much of the blood flowing through the red pulp is in fast-moving streams, but a portion of the blood moves slowly, allowing prolonged contact of cells and particles with the many macrophages that are spread out on the reticular cell framework. This arrangement provides ample opportunity for recognition and phagocytosis.

The major anatomical difference, and therefore the basis for the major functional difference, between the spleen of dogs and cats is the structure of the venous vessels in the red pulp.[7,10] The venous vasculature in the dog's red pulp, as in the human spleen, consists of an anastomosing system of venous sinuses. Sinuses are composed of long, sturdy, rod-shaped endothelial cells that lie parallel to one another and to the longitudinal axis of the vessel. Rings of basement membrane and reticular cell branches incompletely cover the outer surface of the endothelium, an arrangement that can be likened to staves of a barrel encircled by hoops. Sinuses are closed and blunt at their origins. They terminate by converging to form larger veins that drain into veins within the trabeculae. To leave the spleen, blood cells must squeeze between adjacent endothelial cells and enter the sinus lumen. Normal red cells accomplish this feat easily by deforming and narrowing to a remarkable degree, but abnormally rigid red cells pass through interendothelial slits with difficulty, if at all. Many fragment as they do.

In contrast, venous vessels in the cat's red pulp, called *pulp venules*, are thin-walled and lined by flat, squamous-shaped endothelial cells. At many points contiguous endothelial cells are pulled apart to form large apertures through which blood cells may enter the lumen without changing shape.[10] Furthermore, pulp venules are open-ended at their origins. Pulp venules, like sinuses, drain into trabecular veins.

SPLENIC FUNCTIONS

The Reservoir Function

Ninety per cent of the red cells entering the spleen of a resting dog or cat pass through it as quickly as do red cells flowing through a conventional capillary bed.[88,89] The transit time for these red cells is about 30 seconds.[88,89] Red cells in the remaining 10 per cent of total spleen blood flow move more slowly and traverse the spleen in seven or eight minutes.[88,89] Due to the longer transit time, the red cells in the slowly moving component of spleen flow accumulate and constitute a pool of red cells in the red pulp. At any time, the spleen contains a volume of red cells amounting to 10 per cent or more of the total red cell mass of a resting dog or cat.[78,88,89] Contraction of the spleen ejects this reservoir of red cells from the spleen and raises the packed cell volume (PCV) of blood in the rest of the circulation.[35] Thereafter, as long as the spleen remains contracted, 98 per cent of spleen blood flow is in rapid transit and the reservoir pool is eliminated until the spleen again relaxes.[42]

The presence of a readily available splenic reservoir of red cells has physiological importance. In response to strenuous exercise, contraction of the spleen adds sufficient volume of red cells to prevent a reduction in blood flow to the kidney and other visceral organs.[94] The reservoir also protects against the effects of acute blood loss. A decrease in PCV after acute hemorrhage may not be evident for several hours owing largely to the infusion of the splenic pool of red cells, which subsequently is diluted by movement of tissue fluid into the vasculature as a compensatory measure to restore blood volume. Furthermore, exercise or mental stimulation, even pleasurable, can raise the PCV, whereas sedation or anesthesia lowers the PCV by promoting excessive pooling in the red

pulp.[3,44,79] Therefore, the effect of splenic contraction should be considered when interpreting the PCV of peripheral blood.

A pool of slowly moving platelets is also maintained in the red pulp.[1,45] Approximately one-third of the total platelet mass is in the spleen at any time. The platelet pool, like the red cell pool, turns over slowly and is in equilibrium with other circulating platelets. Platelet transit time through the spleen is about eight minutes.[1] The platelet pool likewise can be expelled by splenic contraction, raising the platelet count in a blood sample.[1]

Reticulocyte Sequestration and Surface Remodeling

Reticulocytes released from the marrow are transiently sequestered in the red pulp.[88,89] While there, they lose some of their surface membrane to acquire the shape and size of mature red cells. The loss of ribosomes (the "reticulum" demonstrated by new methylene blue staining) is independent of the spleen, but surface remodeling seems to occur only in the spleen.[18,24,48] The loss of membrane may be the result of attachment of reticulocytes to splenic macrophages.[10] Despite a report that epinephrine injection raises the reticulocyte count of peripheral blood in the cat, other studies have indicated that reticulocytes in the spleen are not dislodged by contraction induced by adrenergic stimulation.[5,37,42]

Red Cell Testing, Culling, and Pitting

Among the most important functions of the red pulp are the recognition and removal or modification of aged or damaged red cells.[98] The complete removal of a red cell from the circulation is called *culling;* *pitting* is the selective removal of intraerythrocytic inclusions.[23] In pitting, rigid intracellular inclusions such as nuclei, Howell-Jolly bodies (nuclear remnants), Heinz bodies (precipitated hemoglobin), and intracellular parasites are pinched from a red cell as it squeezes between endothelial cells of the sinus wall.[57,101] The red cell, freed of its inclusion, may continue to circulate unless it is severely damaged during pitting. Pitting is a function of sinusal spleens only.

Red cells in the red pulp, especially those exposed for prolonged periods to the red pulp milieu, are beset by conditions that test their viability and deformability. The rhythmic contractions of the spleen alternately pack an area of the reticulum with red cells, and send a wave of plasma to dislodge them and carry them on toward venous vessels.[10] These packed red cells are temporarily subjected to low pH and low glucose and cholesterol concentrations, conditions that tend to reduce membrane pliancy.[97,101] Although temporary exposure to this environment probably does no irreversible harm to normal red cells, aged red cells or those with existing defects in membranes or glycolytic enzymes are vulnerable to the biochemical hazards of stasis. Obstruction of blood flow, due either to intra- or extrasplenic abnormalities, can result in increased red cell pooling, prolonged exposure to red pulp conditions and, consequently, shortened red cell life. Red cells with reduced pliancy may be trapped in the red pulp until phagocytized or may fragment into smaller pieces that re-enter the circulation.[100]

The reticulum of the red pulp is crowded with macrophages that have receptors for the Fc portion of IgG and for complement (C3b). Red cells passing by macrophages are subjected to close scrutiny, and those bearing even small amounts of IgG or complement are likely to become bound to macrophages. Partial or complete phagocytosis often follows recognition. Partial phagocytosis removes some membrane, and the freed red cell is then a spherocyte.[63,83] The spleen, then, is the site of removal of minimally damaged or coated red cells.[20,22] The liver, although it receives a greater blood flow, does not provide the same degree of contact between red cells and macrophages or the same conditions of stasis and hemoconcentration. In the presence of the spleen, the liver is a less sensitive filter; in the absence of the spleen, the phagocytic capacity of Kupffer cells increases and the liver becomes a more efficient site of blood clearance.[50,52]

Normal red cells at the end of their life span are culled from the circulation by macrophages in the spleen, liver, and bone marrow.[17] Recognition apparently is mediated by immunoglobulins. As red cells age in the circulation, they acquire small amounts of IgG on their surface.[41,53] This antibody, when eluted, can re-attach to young red cells that have been treated with neuraminidase. It is postulated that this IgG is a "physiological autoantibody" that binds to determinants on the red cell that are exposed during normal aging.[53]

The only known difference in function between dog and cat spleens is the inability of the cat spleen to pit intracellular bodies from the red cell. The wall of the pulp venule in cat spleen, with its larger apertures, poses no barrier to the exit of inclusion-bearing red cells from the spleen.[10] In the dog spleen, the sinus wall is the final and most demanding test of red cell deformability.[7] The lack of pitting ability accounts in part for the frequent finding of Heinz bodies in red cells of nonanemic cats. Heinz bodies are aggregates of oxidatively denatured hemoglobin. In other species, Heinz body formation usually is the result of exposure to oxidant drugs. Cat hemoglobin, however, is particularly susceptible to oxidative denaturation, and Heinz bodies may form even in the absence of exogenous agents.[6,47,84] Red cells containing small, seemingly nonpathological Heinz bodies can circulate freely through the cat spleen without being subjected to culling or pitting.[51,84] In any species, Heinz bodies large enough to severely reduce

red cell pliancy are trapped and destroyed within the red pulp, resulting in hemolytic anemia.[15,80]

Although the cat spleen inefficiently removes intraerythrocytic inclusions, it nevertheless can free red cells of the epicellular parasite *Hemobartonella felis*. During the clinical phase of hemobartonellosis, the parasitemia and PCV fluctuate, although not always together. A decrease in the number of parasitized cells can be followed by a sharp rise in PCV.[46] This increase in parasite-free red cells indicates that organisms were selectively removed and that the red cells were released to circulate again. Macrophages in the spleen seem able to pluck organisms from the red cell surface.[64] Later, in the carrier phase, parasitemia usually is kept to such a low level as to be undetectable as long as the cat has a fully functional spleen. Removal of the spleen or concurrent diseases that suppress macrophage function permit the *Hemobartonella* to rise to detectable levels and reveal the latent infection. Although *Hemobartonella canis* usually does not produce clinically apparent hemolytic anemia, splenectomy of infected dogs likewise promotes detectable parasitemia.[84] Blood donors should be splenectomized and checked for parasitemia to avoid transmission of *Hemobartonella* to already diseased patients. Splenectomy of dogs infected with *Babesia canis* may also permit recrudescence of clinical anemia.[84] The spleen confers no protection against *Ehrlichia canis*, so splenectomy does not change the course or manifestations of the disease.[81]

Immune Responses and Protection in Septicemia (see also Chapter 15)

The red pulp, marginal zone, and white pulp act in concert in defense against blood-borne bacteria and in response to blood-borne antigens.[25] Bacteria and particulate antigens that are deposited at arterial terminations in the red pulp and marginal zone are phagocytized by macrophages. In dogs and cats, as in other species with well-developed PAMS, much of the particle load is filtered and phagocytized in these structures and thereby removed from circulation. Even bacteria not coated with specific antibody are efficiently removed in the spleen, whereas well-opsonized bacteria are readily phagocytized by macrophages throughout the vascular system. Thus, the spleen is a front line of defense against blood-borne bacteria during the first exposure of the animal to the organism. The spleen is both the main site of clearance of blood-borne bacteria at the first exposure and the first site of production of specific IgM antibody in such infections.[34] In human patients, one of the most serious complications of splenectomy is overwhelming septicemia involving one of the many strains of *Streptococcus pneumoniae* (pneumococci). These bacteria are encapsulated and are resistant to phagocytosis unless type-specific antibody is present as a result of either vaccination or prior exposure. Fortunately, postsplenectomy sepsis is not common in dogs and cats.

Some of the blood-borne particulate antigens deposited in the marginal zone appear to be transported into lymphatic nodules, resulting in stimulation of B lymphocyte proliferation, formation of germinal centers, and antibody production.[68,93] In the event of prior exposure to the antigen, an accelerated germinal center response occurs.[68] Stromal dendritic cells in the nodules retain antigen on their surface, making it available for continued stimulation of the immune response.[20]

In the absence of exposure to an appropriate antigen in the spleen, members of the recirculating lymphocyte pool pass through the spleen and reenter blood or lymph. Lymphocytes deposited at arterial terminations either cross red pulp with other blood cells and regain the circulation via venous vessels or migrate through marginal zone and white pulp to leave via lymphatic vessels.[100] During their travels through the white pulp, lymphocytes are sorted into B and T lymphocyte zones. In the rat, passage through white pulp takes about four hours for T lymphocytes and six to eight hours for B lymphocytes.[100]

Hematopoiesis

The splenic red pulp is a site of blood cell production during fetal development and to a limited extent postnatally. Splenic hematopoiesis in dogs and cats becomes more prominent in certain diseases (see also Chapter 80).

Mechanisms of Splenomegaly

Splenomegaly can be symmetrical or asymmetrical.[13] Symmetrical enlargement is generally due to congestion or infiltration of the spleen. Asymmetrical enlargement is most frequently caused by nonhemic neoplasia or trauma.

Symmetrical Splenomegaly

Purely congestive splenomegaly, the result of vascular disorders, is rarely encountered in small animals. In people, hepatic cirrhosis associated with portal hypertension frequently results in blood pooling in the red pulp and massive splenomegaly. This finding is less consistent in dogs with hepatic cirrhosis.[33] Liver cirrhosis with portal vein obstruction (Banti's syndrome) has been reported in a dog.[65]

Congestive splenomegaly due to splenic torsion often accompanies gastric dilation-volvulus, although it may occur in the absence of gastric involvement.[60,66,71] Splenic pedicle torsion obstructs venous outflow more completely than arterial inflow, since arterial walls are muscular and less easily com-

pressed. Consequently, blood accumulates in the red pulp.

Symmetrical splenomegaly with increased sequestration and destruction of blood cells may be secondary to macrophage recruitment and proliferation in infectious diseases, especially those caused by organisms that infect macrophages and stimulate mononuclear phagocytes. Histoplasmosis, cryptococcosis, leishmaniasis, trypanosomiasis (Chaga's disease), and tuberculosis are diseases of man and animals in which splenomegaly and shortened red cell life span may result from obstruction of vascular pathways and enhanced phagocytic capacity of activated macrophages.[46,70] Lymphoid hyperplasia in patients with bacterial or viral diseases may be of sufficient magnitude to cause splenic enlargement, but this does not result in hemolysis or congestion.

Splenomegaly may be associated with hemolytic anemia in patients in whom the spleen is a major site of red cell destruction. In some types of autoimmune hemolytic anemia, the arrival of antibody-coated red cells in the red pulp induces the local recruitment of blood monocytes that subsequently become macrophages. The spleen enlarges as macrophages accumulate (work hypertrophy), and flow through red pulp is impeded. In anemias in which decreased red cell pliancy is the initial insult, e.g., Heinz body hemolytic anemia, congestive splenomegaly due to blockage of intrasplenic vascular channels by rigid red cells is complicated by splenic expansion due to recruitment of macrophages.[15,16] In contrast, splenomegaly usually is not prominent in patients with immune-mediated thrombocytopenia, even though the spleen may be the main site of platelet destruction.

Neoplasia of hemic tissue may occur in a myeloid form affecting bone marrow or in a lymphoid form affecting lymphoid tissues.[43] In myeloid neoplasia the splenic red pulp is infiltrated with neoplastic cells, the degree of symmetrical splenomegaly depending on the extent and course of the disease. Neoplasia of lymphoid tissue affects the spleen in varied ways; splenic white pulp involvement may lead to symmetrical or asymmetrical splenic enlargement.

Mast cell sarcoma of the dog may produce symmetrical or asymmetrical splenomegaly. In the cat, mast cell neoplasia involving the spleen is symmetrical and the enlargement is massive.[62]

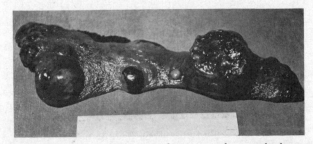

Figure 84–2. Hemangiosarcoma of a canine spleen; multiple neoplastic nodules creating asymmetrical splenomegaly. The largest nodule has ruptured, causing hemoperitoneum.

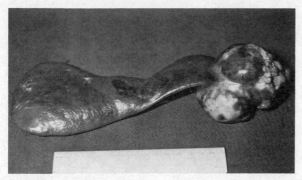

Figure 84–3. Asymmetrical splenomegaly in a dog caused by a fibrosarcoma.

In the past, the term *hypersplenism* was used to designate a syndrome including splenomegaly, peripheral cytopenia, cellular bone marrow, and correction of the cytopenia after splenectomy.[41] Due to a better understanding of the disease processes mentioned in the preceding paragraphs, it has become evident that hypersplenism is not a state of unprovoked splenic hyperfunction. Instead, splenomegaly and sequestration or destruction of blood cells are secondary to conditions that induce changes in the blood cells or the phagocytic cells or in the circumstances in which they are brought together. That is, hypersplenism, like anemia, is a sign of disease rather than a diagnosis.

Asymmetrical Splenomegaly

Primary tumors of vascular cells, connective tissue, or smooth muscle tend to produce single or multiple nodular growths on the spleen. Subcapsular splenic hematoma due to trauma usually produces a single focal enlargement, whereas nodular hyperplasia frequently occurs as multiple nodules of varied size.

Hemangiosarcoma is the most common primary tumor of the spleen.[13] This neoplasm is composed of a poorly developed vascular stroma that leads to hematoma formation. The associated hematoma may be very large and is prone to rupture (Fig. 84–2). Metastasis occurs by seeding of the peritoneum and autotransfusion of the resultant peritoneal effusion.

Fibrosarcomas and leimyosarcomas are solid splenic tumors that occur less frequently than hemangiosarcomas (Fig. 84–3). Fibrosarcomas are prone to metastasis.[13]

REGENERATION OF THE SPLEEN

The spleen has a remarkable capacity to regenerate from fragments of splenic tissue. After traumatic rupture of the spleen, multiple splenules may be found throughout the abdomen, a condition called *splenosis*.[76] Spleen regrowth rarely occurs after surgical removal of an intact spleen. In studies of splenic autotransplantation, it has been found that slices of the original spleen, when laid on omentum or peritoneum, first degenerate and then regrow the stromal meshwork and blood vessels.[92] Later, the newly formed reticulum is populated with lymphocytes and macrophages and filled with circulating blood. The form and function of the regenerated tissue are equivalent to those of the original organ, but the total filtration capacity is dependent on the volume of regenerated tissue and the volume of blood flow through the splenules.[55]

HEMATOLOGICAL CHANGES AFTER SPLENECTOMY

Postsplenectomy hematological changes may differ from one species to another. In humans, changes indicative of an absent or hypofunctional spleen include persistent increases in neutrophil, lymphocyte, and monocyte counts; transient thrombocytosis; and increased numbers of Howell-Jolly bodies, target cells, and red cells with pocked surfaces.[24,76] The effect of splenectomy on peripheral blood findings has not been studied as extensively in dogs and cats as it has in humans. In dogs, the number of Howell-Jolly bodies and nucleated red cells tends to be higher after splenectomy, reflecting the loss of pitting.[84] There may be increased numbers of target cells in blood smears from splenectomized dogs. These red cells have a target appearance because they contain slightly more surface membrane than red cells that have undergone normal surface remodeling in the spleen. Platelet counts in dogs may rise and remain elevated for prolonged periods after splenectomy.[84] Neither anemia nor erythrocytosis should follow removal of the spleen if bone marrow erythropoiesis is normal. No change has been detected in red cell life span after splenectomy of normal animals.

Clinical Evaluation of Splenomegaly

Splenomegaly may frequently be detected by abdominal palpation. However, in some cases of localized rather than diffuse enlargement the abnormal size or shape of the spleen may not be palpable. Radiographs of the abdomen may be necessary to confirm the presence of splenic enlargement; interpretation is based on the size, shape, location and density of the spleen as well as the position of adjacent viscera.[69] Special radiographic procedures such as pneumoperitoneum, splenic arteriography, and splenoportography may also be used.[69] Radioisotopic scans, tomography, and ultrasonography are used to evaluate the spleen in humans.[54] Ultrasonography is now being used to evaluate splenic enlargement in dogs and cats.[38]

The cause of splenic enlargement may be reflected in the results of other diagnostic evaluations. For example, alterations of packed cell volume; hemoglobin concentration; erythrocyte, leukocyte and platelet counts and the changes in the morphology of these cells frequently accompany diseases that involve the spleen and may aid in diagnosis.[4,77]

Splenic Biopsy

Histological evaluation of splenic tissue is necessary to definitively establish a diagnosis in cases of splenomegaly. Malignant lymphoma, myelogenous leukemia, and nonvascular tumors such as fibrosarcoma and leiomyosarcoma may be diagnosed by percutaneous splenic biopsy.[72] This procedure should not be performed if vascular tumors of the spleen, such as hemangiosarcoma, are suspected because of the possibility of life-threatening hemorrhage or peritoneal metastasis.[72] Similarly, patients with blood clotting disorders should not be subjected to percutaneous biopsy regardless of the cause of the splenomegaly.

Percutaneous Biopsy

Common techniques for performing percutaneous splenic biopsy include punch biopsy, needle aspiration, and fine needle aspiration. The last-named technique, using a 25-gauge tuberculin needle or the longer Franzeen needle, is preferred.[73] If unsuccessful, punch biopsy may be considered using a modified Franklin-Silverman needle, a Vim Tru-cut punch needle, or a Jamschidi soft tissue needle. Fine needle aspiration is recommended because of its simplicity and because the cytological preparations of spleen made with this technique are as good as those made from samples obtained by punch biopsy.

Fine needle aspiration biopsy of the spleen is usually done without anesthesia. For punch biopsy, either local or general anesthesia is used. Local anesthesia combined with tranquilization produces sufficient restraint and analgesia in most situations. A line block of the lateral abdominal wall, as described for emergency lateral gastrostomy, may also be used.[74,96]

The patient is placed in right lateral recumbency, and the spleen is located by palpation. Normally it lies in the cranial left quadrant of the abdomen. An area of skin overlying the spleen is surgically prepared. A biopsy needle attached to a syringe is gently passed into the spleen through the overlying skin and abdominal musculature. The spleen is held in position by palpation as the needle penetrates its parenchyma. As the needle penetrates the spleen, negative pressure is created and maintained in the syringe by gentle, steady withdrawal of the syringe plunger. When the needle has penetrated the spleen to a sufficient depth, the negative pressure within the syringe is terminated by slowly returning the plunger to its original resting position. The needle and attached syringe are then withdrawn from the patient. Biopsy sample contamination by peripheral elements is avoided if the negative pressure in the syringe is released before the needle leaves the spleen. Processing of the biopsy material should be immediate. If the sample clots, processing and interpretation may be difficult.

Complications have not been observed following percutaneous fine needle aspiration of the spleen. Potential complications include persistent hemorrhage, damage to other abdominal viscera, and peritonitis.[73]

Splenic Biopsy at Celiotomy

The spleen may be biopsied easily during celiotomy. Needle or punch biopsy is indicated when gross examination suggests splenic metastasis from a neoplasm such as an hepatic or pancreatic carcinoma. Incisional splenic biopsy is indicated when diffuse splenomegaly is present. Primary splenic neoplasms should be removed by total splenectomy; incisional biopsy is not recommended in such cases, particularly for tumors of vascular origin. Hemorrhage from the biopsy site may be difficult to control, or it may occur after the abdomen has been closed. An incisional biopsy is the surgical removal of a portion of a lesion or tissue.[72] Depending on the location, incisional splenic biopsy may be performed in one of two ways.

If a sample from the margin of the spleen is desired, the section to be removed may be delineated by mattress sutures placed through the parietal and visceral surfaces. The splenic parenchyma is sharply transected between the mattress sutures and the edge of the spleen. This leaves the mattress sutures in place to control hemorrhage.

A more centrally located region may be biopsied as follows. Two parallel incisions of sufficient length and depth to remove a representative sample are made (one on each side of the lesion). Two additional, shorter incisions are then made at 90° to the first pair of incisions. Then, the resulting rectangular piece of spleen is removed. Hemorrhage from the parenchymal defect is controlled with absorbable sutures placed in a cruciate or vertical mattress pattern across the biopsy site. Any subsequent seepage of blood from the biopsy site is controlled by digital pressure.

The most obvious and severe complication of incisional biopsy is persistent hemorrhage. This may be controlled by more sutures, digital pressure, or a combination of both. The abdomen should not be closed until hemorrhage has ceased. Patients with blood clotting disorders are not good candidates for splenic biopsy.

Surgical Disease of the Spleen Amendable to Splenectomy

Primary splenic neoplasia is the most common indication for total splenectomy.[13] Splenic torsion also frequently requires total removal of the spleen; however, attempts to salvage the spleen by rotation of the twisted vascular pedicle should first be attempted

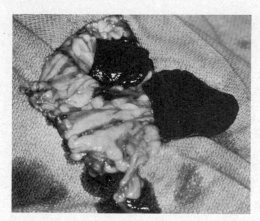

Figure 84–4. Two separate portions of a canine spleen found at celiotomy. The spleen was probably damaged by previous trauma.

(see hereafter). Similarly, severe splenic trauma frequently leads to total splenectomy. Trauma to the spleen does not necessarily justify total splenectomy; e.g., lacerations may be sutured, or a partial splenectomy may be done to remove the severely damaged portion. In addition, it is likely that even severe trauma to the spleen often heals spontaneously (Fig. 84–4).

Therapeutic removal of a spleen enlarged because of myeloproliferative or lymphoproliferative neoplasia has little justification in dogs or cats, except perhaps in cases of disseminated mastocytoma in cats. In such cases, if the spleen is the major site of involvement, splenectomy may prolong life for several years.[62]

Life-threatening destruction of peripheral blood cells by the spleen may be an indication for total splenectomy. In addition, immune-mediated hemolytic anemia or thrombocytopenia not controlled by long-term corticosteroid or immunosuppressant therapy may benefit from splenic removal.

Torsion of the Spleen

Splenic torsion occurs when there is twisting or rotation of the spleen on its vascular pedicle. This results in occlusion of the vessels leading to the splenic hilus. The condition frequently accompanies gastric dilation-volvulus (see Chapter 49),[103] but it may occur alone. Only the latter, isolated occurrence of splenic torsion is discussed here. Splenic torsion typically occurs in large or giant breed dogs. Males and females are equally affected. The age of affected animals varies, although it has not been reported in the very young. Although the etiology is unknown, it has been suggested that splenic displacement and then torsion are preceded by gastric dilation. The gastric distension then subsides, leaving the spleen in its abnormal state.[66] Congestive splenomegaly follows due to complete occlusion of the thin-walled splenic vein and partial occlusion of the thicker-walled splenic artery. Thus, blood inflow is maintained, outflow is inhibited, and the spleen enlarges to accommodate its increase in blood volume.[60] Splenic vein thrombosis may occur if the torsion persists, and areas of splenic infarction may develop if the arterial supply also becomes occluded.

Clinically, splenic torsion may present in two

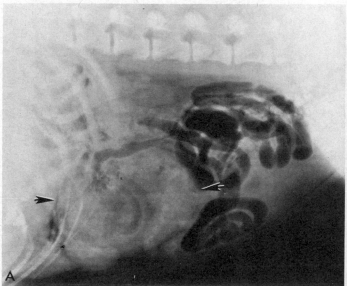
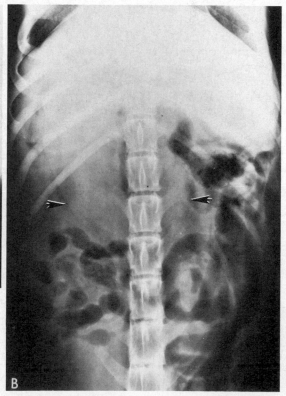

Figure 84–5. Lateral (A) and ventrodorsal (B) radiographic views of the abdomen of a dog with splenic torsion. The enlarged spleen is characterized by a cranioventral, centrally located soft tissue density (arrows). Displacement of viscera, particularly gas-filled intestines, is present.

forms. The less severe form may mimic a mild gastrointestinal disturbance, whereas cardiovascular collapse and shock are the hallmarks of the acute form.

Acute Isolated Splenic Torsion

Signs of acute splenic torsion are similar to those of acute gastric dilation-volvulus, except that the abdomen is not greatly distended. Patient discomfort is manifested by pacing and frequent changes in body position while sitting or lying down. Excessive salivation, drooling, gagging, or retching may occur. Physical weakness rapidly becomes obvious, and mental alertness decreases. Within several hours signs of cardiovascular collapse and shock develop. Rapid pulse rate, pale to congested oral mucous membranes, and an increased capillary refill time are frequent physical findings. Respiratory rate is usually increased. Delineation of abdominal viscera by palpation may be difficult owing to abdominal wall tenseness. In some cases the enlarged spleen may be palpable. Laboratory findings usually do not contribute to a diagnosis. Hemoglobin and packed cell volume values may be low but still within normal limits; mild leukocytosis with neutrophilia may be present. Splenic enlargement and visceral displacement may be present on plain radiographs of the abdomen (Fig. 84–5).

The differential diagnosis should include conditions that cause acute abdominal discomfort such as gastric dilation-volvulus, rupture and hemorrhage from a splenic or other neoplasm, intestinal volvulus, acute gastrointestinal obstruction, peritonitis, pancreatitis, torsion of the uterus, torsion of an intra-abdominal testicular tumor, and poisoning.

Treatment involves cardiovascular resuscitation and exploratory celiotomy. Intravenous fluids, shock doses of glucocorticoids, and perhaps whole blood should be administered. If possible, the patient should be stabilized physiologically prior to anesthesia and exploratory surgery.

A ventral midline abdominal approach is used with the incision long enough to allow easy manipulation of the grossly enlarged spleen. Caution is required when entering the abdomen to avoid laceration of the enlarged and frequently displaced spleen. In many cases the splenic pedicle, including the gastrosplenic ligament, greater omentum, and accompanying vessels, are caught in a confusing labyrinth of twisted tissues (Fig. 84–6). Occasionally, in this condition, the spleen tears through the greater omentum, adding further confusion to the anatomical arrangement of the displaced structures.

Torsions of greater than 360° may occur. It is frequently difficult to determine the direction required to untwist the splenic pedicle. However, if the pedicle can be untwisted, the splenic artery and vein and their branches should be examined for thrombosis. If thrombosis is present, total splenectomy is necessary. In the absence of thrombosis,

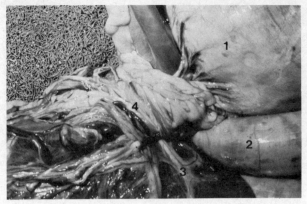

Figure 84–6. Twisted vascular pedicle and mesenteric attachments of the spleen of a dog with splenic torsion. Necropsy specimen: stomach (1), intestine (2), spleen (3), twisted pedicle (4).

several minutes are allowed to determine if restoration of splenic blood flow will relieve the organ of its entrapped blood. Gentle, firm digital pressure may aid in the emptying process. Intrasplenic injection of epinephrine has been suggested to hasten splenic emptying.[13] However, because cardiac dysrhythmia may result, careful patient monitoring is necessary if epinephrine is used.

Subacute-Chronic Isolated Splenic Torsion

Anatomical derangements and surgical management of the less acute clinical form of splenic torsion are similar to those described for the acute form, although the less acute type frequently occurs with clinical signs and a history of vague abdominal discomfort, usually of several days duration. Lethargy, anorexia, occasional vomiting or retching, and salivation are common.[60,66] In some cases historical information, such as a recent whelping or the administration of anthelmintics, may cloud the clinical picture.

Physical findings include an increased heart rate and slightly increased respiratory rate. Body temperature is usually elevated. The abdomen may be distended, and a large intra-abdominal mass may be palpated. Some patients may resist palpation, and without tranquilization or anesthesia, palpation of abdominal viscera is difficult. During the examination, the patient should be placed in right and left lateral recumbency as well as in a standing position with the forequarters elevated for thorough abdominal palpation. A large homogeneous soft tissue density in the midventral area of the abdomen is a frequent radiographic finding.[60,69,71,82] The mass may cause displacement of the stomach, duodenum, and other viscera.

Anemia and dehydration often develop after several days of splenic pedicle obstruction.[66] The packed cell volume may reach 20 per cent with a commensurate drop in hemoglobin and erythrocyte count. White blood cell counts may range between 15,000 and 50,000 cells/μL, manifested primarily as a neutrophilia. Proteinuria, hemoglobinuria, and bilirubinuria are frequently detected in more chronic cases of splenic torsion. Urine may be dark amber to reddish brown.[66] These findings, in conjunction with anemia, indicate extensive red cell destruction within the spleen. Blood urea nitrogen and serum creatinine levels are usually within normal limits. The slight increases that may occur, barring pre-existing renal disease, are prerenal in origin, most likely due to patient dehydration. The serum alkaline phosphatase level may be elevated, but this is not a consistent finding.[13,60,66] Experimental splenic artery ligation in dogs produces splenic infarcts and, in some cases, an increase in serum alkaline phosphatase.[49] All dogs studied developed splenic infarcts, but not all dogs with infarcts had increased levels of serum alkaline phosphatase. Only alkaline phosphatase of osseous origin is found in the serum of normal dogs.[21] The most common cause of clinical increases of serum alkaline phosphatase levels is cholestasis, in which the enzyme arises from the hepatic tissue. The origin of the elevated level of serum alkaline phosphatase in cases of splenic torsion is not known.

Pancreatitis is a potential complication of splenic torsion. Blood supply to the left limb of the pancreas is from branches of the splenic artery in the greater omentum. Pancreatic ischemia and pancreatitis may occur because of splenic artery occlusion and twisting of its pancreatic branches, as the greater omentum becomes involved in the twisted splenic pedicle.

Response to treatment is usually rapid in both forms of clinical presentation once the spleen has been removed or the splenic vessels are untwisted. Administration of antibiotics before or after surgery is a matter of personal preference; their use is recommended because of the potential alteration of the patient's defense mechanisms. Postoperative care may include whole blood administration if anemia is severe. Patients with cardiovascular collapse require intensive monitoring. Cardiomyopathy, frequently seen in large and giant breed dogs, may be exacerbated by the stress of splenic torsion. If cardiac dysrhythmias occur, their vigorous control is essential.

Splenic Trauma

Splenic trauma is unusual in the dog. For example, in one study of 600 dogs hit by cars, only 3 had splenic injuries.[56] However, in a series of patients selected because of suspected abdominal organ injury, 3 of 20 had splenic rupture.[26]

Splenic injuries may be classified as mild, moderate, or severe. Intra-abdominal hemorrhage is the major clinical problem associated with severe splenic injury. Large deep parenchymal lacerations and extensive crush injuries without tearing of hilar vessels may produce life-threatening hemorrhage. Another source of severe splenic hemorrhage is the spontaneous rupture of a large subcapsular hematoma. Although rare in small animals, this is a frequent occurrence in humans who have sustained abdominal trauma.[19]

Severe splenic trauma is most often associated with motor vehicle accidents or falls from heights. The presenting signs and laboratory and radiographic findings depend on the rate and amount of blood loss prior to presentation as well as the presence of concomitant injuries. Rapid exsanguination rarely occurs from a traumatized spleen. Splenic hemorrhage is usually characterized by a steady loss of blood, producing signs of hypovolemia within several hours of injury.

Abdominal pain or discomfort may be produced by palpation. Depending on the amount of blood loss and the type of splenic injury, palpation of a soft enlargement may indicate a large clot or hematoma, and free fluid may be detected by ballottement.[28] Tachycardia, increased capillary refill time, distended abdomen and increased respiratory rate and effort are frequent accompanying signs. Hypovolemia and shock occur in association with continued hemorrhage. Although not pathognomonic for severe splenic trauma, these signs and findings are indicative of intra-abdominal hemorrhage, for which splenic hemorrhage is the most likely cause.

Radiographic findings vary with the type and extent of splenic injury and the amount of blood and free fluid within the abdomen.[69,82] Excessive intra-abdominal blood or fluid obliterates much of the normal radiographic appearance of the viscera. Larger hematomas may appear as a well-marginated localized splenic enlargement; pre-existing asymmetrical splenic enlargement, such as in benign hyperplasia, neoplasia, or abscesses, may have a similar radiographic appearance.

Intra-abdominal hemorrhage may be confirmed by abdominal paracentesis. The use of a multiperforated semiflexible catheter, inserted through the abdominal wall on the ventral midline midway between the xyphoid cartilage and pubis, is the preferred technique.[26,55] Results are far superior to those obtained by paracentesis performed with a needle and syringe inserted in the upper and lower abdominal quadrants.

Clinical laboratory findings may or may not contribute to a diagnosis of severe splenic injury; they must be interpreted in conjunction with other findings and historical information. A normal packed cell volume may indicate either a mild injury or one of greater severity that had occurred a short time before the sample was obtained.[19]

During the initial assessment of a traumatized patient, splenic injury and intra-abdominal hemorrhage may be overlooked. It should be suspected in patients without significant external hemorrhage that do not respond well to initial shock therapy and in those that do respond initially but have a relapse within a very short period of time. Persistent hemorrhage requires surgical intervention. Selective ligation and partial splenectomy are preferred, with the goals of stopping the hemorrhage while preserving splenic function.

Splenic capping is another surgical procedure designed to treat severe splenic lacerations.[29] A woven polyglycolic acid mesh is stretched snugly over the injured bleeding spleen and sutured in place. The secure fit of the mesh aids in hemostasis by tamponade; the mesh also provides a network of material to support sutures, which may also be needed for hemostasis, as well as a surface for the development of a pseudocapsule. To date, the capping procedure has only been used experimentally in dogs, but it appears to have potential as a method of treating splenic trauma and preserving splenic function.

Mild splenic injuries are rarely diagnosed by signs, radiographic evidence, or abdominal paracentesis. Usually, small subcapsular hematomas exist that may be accompanied by a few torn hilar vessels. Clinically significant signs rarely occur, and unless celiotomy is performed these injuries usually remain undetected.

Moderate splenic injuries may include tearing of some hilar vessels and small parenchymal lacerations. Hemoperitoneum frequently occurs, but the hemorrhage ceases spontaneously and surgical intervention is rarely necessary. Injuries of this type should be suspected in a traumatized patient with hemoperitoneum that responds to therapy and in which the hemoperitoneum rapidly subsides as determined by repeated abdominal paracentesis.

Total Splenectomy

The spleen is exposed via a midline abdominal incision, and laparotomy sponges moistened with warm saline are placed over the abdominal viscera. A self-retaining abdominal wall retractor may aid in exposure. Beginning at the free or distal end of the spleen and ending at its head or proximal end, the splenic hilar vessels are all doubly ligated and transected.[40] Folds of the thin gastrosplenic ligament must also be severed. Absorbable sutures may be used for vessel ligation; monofilament nonabsorbable sutures may be preferred in cases complicated by peritonitis. Metallic vascular clips may also be used.

Although not particularly difficult, total splenectomy may be tedious because of the many ligations required. Difficulty may occur if the spleen is grossly enlarged and the abdominal incision is not long enough to expose the spleen. The spleen should not be forced or squeezed through an insufficient opening; the incision should be lengthened. This is particularly important when performing splenectomy for splenic hemangiosarcoma or hematoma.

Intrasplenic injection of epinephrine has been suggested to reduce the size of an enlarged spleen and facilitate its removal.[13] Others disagree.[40] In cats, splenic contraction occurs within two minutes after intravenous injection of epinephrine.[11,12] However, splenic relaxation and resequestration of red blood cells begin 1 minute later, and nearly 20 per cent of the maximum circulating packed cell volume created by the splenic contraction has returned to the spleen within 20 minutes of injection. Thus, it appears that the effect of epinephrine on splenic contraction, at least in cats, is transitory. In addition to the transitory splenic emptying, intravenous epinephrine in the face of certain inhalation anesthetics (e.g., halothane) may predispose the patient to cardiac dysrhythmias. For these reasons intravenous epinephrine to induce splenic contraction prior to splenectomy is not recommended.

Partial Splenectomy

Partial splenectomy is recommended whenever possible[31,39,94] and especially in cases of splenic trauma in which only one portion of the spleen is in-

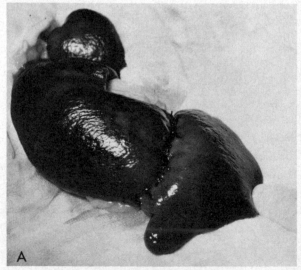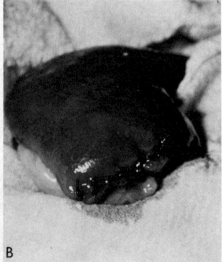

Figure 84–7. Partial splenectomy in a dog. *A,* Mattress sutures placed through the parietal and visceral surfaces. *B,* Spleen following removal of portion distal to sutures.

volved.[32,40] It is not recommended for splenic neoplasia even though the obvious tumor mass may grossly involve only one portion of the spleen.

The obvious advantage of partial splenectomy is the retention of some splenic function, which, as indicated previously, is important in dogs and cats that are latent carriers of *Hemobartonella* and *Babesia* organisms.[13,46,64,77] In addition, negative effects on hematological values are less extreme in dogs that undergo partial splenectomy versus those that undergo complete splenectomy.[27,58,61]

Several partial splenectomy techniques have been described; they differ primarily in the method by which the splenic parenchyma is transected and

handled to prevent hemorrhage. Regardless of the method used, hilar vessels that supply the portion of spleen to be removed are doubly ligated and transected. This results in an obvious color difference between ischemic and perfused splenic tissue. This line of demarcation is used as the guideline for splenic transection. In one method of partial splenectomy, the spleen is squeezed between thumb and forefinger and splenic pulp is "milked" toward the ischemic side along the line of color demarcation.[27,32] Forceps are placed across the flattened portion, and the spleen is divided between forceps. The cut surface of the spleen adjacent to the remaining forceps is closed with absorbable suture material in a continuous pat-

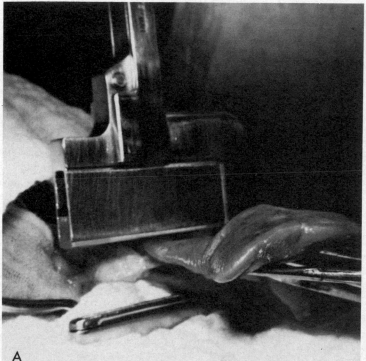

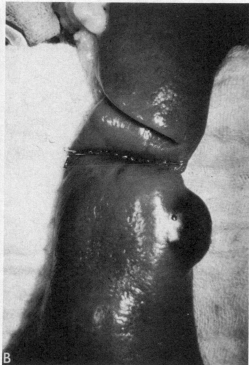

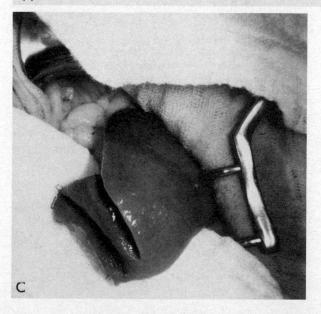

Figure 84–8. Partial splenectomy in a dog. *A,* Stapling machine positioned across the spleen. *B,* Double row of staples placed through parenchyma. *C,* Spleen following removal of portion distal to staples.

tern. Digital pressure is used to control any hemorrhage following forceps removal.

In another technique, mattress sutures of absorbable suture material are placed through the parietal and visceral surfaces of the spleen along the line of color demarcation.[40] The spleen is then transected distal to the sutures (Fig. 84–7). Hemorrhage is controlled by further suture placement or digital pressure.

Automatic stapling devices may be used for partial splenectomy. The stapling machine is placed across the spleen near the line of color demarcation. It is important to place the double row of staples in the perfused nonischemic portion of the spleen. The spleen is transected distal to the row of staples; hemorrhage, if it occurs, may be controlled by digital pressure (Fig. 84–8).

Finally, a partial splenectomy technique has been described in the dog that employs an ultrasonic cutting device.[30] Following hilar vessel ligation, the instrument is used to transect the spleen along the line of color demarcation. Parenchyma and smaller vessels are easily cut, and hemorrhage is controlled by cauterization. Vessels larger than 2 mm are not easily cut; they are identified, occluded with metal clips, and transected. (This instrument has also been used for partial hepatic lobectomy and partial pneumonectomy.)

Splenic Re-implantation

In spite of efforts to preserve the spleen, there are circumstances, such as severe trauma or splenic torsion with vessel thrombosis, when only total splenectomy is sufficient. Splenic function can be maintained in these situations by autotransplantation of splenic tissue.[59,67,75,85,86,92,102]

Following removal of the entire spleen, the area is prepared for re-implantation. Two to five cross sections of tissue are harvested, preferably from the mid portion of the spleen. Each section should be approximately 3 mm thick. The greater omentum is spread out and its distal margin folded back and sutured, forming a pocket large enough to receive the pieces of spleen. The harvested slices are placed side by side in the pocket, which is closed with additional sutures. The omentum, with the implanted tissue, is then returned to its usual anatomical location.

Autotransplantation of the spleen to the omentum has been clinically effective in maintaining normal splenic function in humans. However, all other splenic tissue must be removed and only the slices of splenic tissue returned to the patient. The implanted pieces fail to regain function if other splenic tissue remains; re-implantation is not effective in conjunction with partial splenectomy. Re-implantation of the spleen has not been reported in dogs or cats, except experimentally. It appears to have many advantages and should be attempted under the appropriate circumstances.

Complications of Splenectomy

Hemorrhage, although rarely life-threatening, is the major complication of partial and total splenectomy. All vessels occluded with ligatures or hemostatic clips must be examined for hemorrhage before the abdomen is closed. Following partial splenectomy, the splenic remnant must also be examined. Additional ligatures are placed as needed. Persistent hemorrhage following total or partial splenectomy is unusual. If it occurs, clinical signs are similar to those of severe splenic trauma. Fresh whole blood transfusions and re-operation may be indicated. Splenic torsion following partial splenectomy has not been described.

Ischemic pancreatitis is a potential complication of partial or total splenectomy. Vascular supply to the left limb of the pancreas arising from branches of the splenic artery may be accidentally transected, resulting in disruption of pancreatic blood flow. Performing all ligations at the splenic hilus prevents this problem.

As noted previously, sepsis following splenectomy is not a problem in small animals as it is in humans. However, subclinical hemobartenellosis or babesiosis may be exacerbated in dogs and cats that have undergone splenectomy, although this rarely occurs.

1. Aster, R. H.: Pooling of platelets in the spleen: role in the pathogenesis of hypersplenic thrombocytopenia. J. Clin. Invest. 45:645, 1966.
2. Barcroft, J., and Nisimaru, Y.: Cause of rhythmical contraction of the spleen. J. Physiol. 74:229, 1932.
3. Barcroft, J., and Stephens, J. G.: Observations on the size of the spleen. J. Physiol. 64:1, 1927.
4. Barton, C. L.: The spleen: Pathophysiology of disease. In Bojrab, M. J.: Pathophysiology in Small Animal Surgery. Lea & Febiger, Philadelphia, 1981.
5. Berendes, M.: The proportion of reticulocytes in the erythrocytes of the spleen as compared with those of circulating blood, with special reference to hemolytic states. Blood 14:558, 1959.
6. Beretic, T.: Studies on Schmauch bodies. I. The incidence in normal cats (Felis domestica) and the morphologic relationships to Heinz bodies. Blood 25:999, 1965.
7. Blue, J., and Weiss, L.: Electron microscopy of the red pulp of the dog spleen including vascular arrangements, periarterial macrophage sheaths (ellipsoids) and the contractile, innervated reticular meshwork. Am. J. Anat. 161:189, 1981.
8. Blue, J., and Weiss, L.: Periarterial macrophage sheaths (ellipsoids) in cat spleen—an electron microscope study. Am. J. Anat. 161:115, 1981.
9. Blue, J., and Weiss, L.: Species variation of the structure and function of the marginal zone—an electron microscope study of cat spleen. Am. J. Anat. 161:169, 1981.
10. Blue, J., and Weiss, L.: Vascular pathways in nonsinusal red pulp—an electron microscope study of the cat spleen. Am. J. Anat. 161:135, 1981.
11. Breznock, E. M., and Strack, D.: Blood volume of nonsplenectomized and splenectomized cats before and after acute hemorrhage. Am. J. Vet. Res. 43:1811, 1982.
12. Breznock, E. M., and Strack, D.: Effects of the spleen,

epinephrine, and splenectomy on determination of blood volume in cats. Am. J. Vet. Res. 43:2062, 1982.

13. Brodey, R. S.: The spleen. In Archibald, J. (ed.): Canine Surgery, 2nd ed. American Veterinary Publications, Inc., Santa Barbara, CA, 1974.

14. Chen, L. L., Adams, J. C., and Steinman, R. M.: Anatomy of germinal centers in mouse spleen, with special reference to "follicular dendritic cells." J. Cell Biol. 77:148, 1978.

15. Chen, L. T., and Scheffel, U.: Blood flow and phagocytic activity of the spleen of the rat with hemolytic anemia. J. Reticuloendothel. Soc. 22:507, 1977.

16. Chen, L. T., and Weiss, L.: The role of the sinus wall in the passage of erythrocytes through the spleen. Blood 41:529, 1973.

17. Clark, C. H., and Woodley, C. H.: The absorption of red blood cells after parenteral injection at various sites. Am. J. Vet. Res. 20:1002, 1959.

18. Come, S. E., Shohet, S. B., and Robinson, S. H.: Surface remodeling vs. whole-cell hemolysis of reticulocytes produced with erythroid stimulation or iron deficiency anemia. Blood 44:817, 1974.

19. Cooney, D. R.: Splenic and hepatic trauma in children. Surg. Clin. North Am. 61:1165, 1981.

20. Cooper, R. A., and Shattil, S. J.: Mechanisms of hemolysis—the minimal red-cell defect. N. Engl. J. Med. 285:1514, 1971.

21. Cornelius, C. E.: Liver function. In Kaneko, J. J. (ed.): Clinical Biochemistry of Domestic Animals, 3rd ed. Academic Press, New York, 1980.

22. Crome, P., and Mollison, P. L.: Splenic destruction of Rh-sensitized and of heated red cells. Br. J. Haematol. 10:137, 1964.

23. Crosby, W. H.: Normal functions of the spleen relative to blood cells: a review. Blood 14:399, 1959.

24. Crosby, W. H.: Splenic remodeling of red cell surfaces. Blood 50:643, 1977.

25. Crosby, W. H.: Structure and functions of the spleen. In Williams, J. J., Beutler, E., Erslev, A. J., and Rundles, R. W. (eds.): Hematology, 2nd ed. McGraw-Hill, New York, 1977.

26. Crowe, D. T., Jr., and Crane, S. W.: Diagnostic abdominal paracentesis and lavage in the evaluation of abdominal injuries in dogs and cats: Clinical and experimental investigations. J. Am. Vet. Med. Assoc. 168:700, 1976.

27. deBoer, J., Sumner-Smith, G., and Dounie, H. G.: Partial splenectomy: technique and some hematological consequences in the dog. J. Ped. Surg. 7:378, 1972.

28. DeHoff, W. D., Green, R. W., and Greiner, T. P.: Surgical management of abdominal emergencies. Vet. Clin. North Am. 2:301, 1971.

29. Delany, H. M., Porreca, F., Mitsuda, S., Solanki, B., and Rudersly, A.: Splenic capping: An experimental study of a new technique for splenorrhaphy using woven polyglycolic acid mesh. Ann. Surg. 196:187, 1982.

30. Derderian, G. P., Walshaw, R., and McGehee, J.: Ultrasonic surgical dissection in the dog spleen. Am. J. Surg. 143:269, 1982.

31. Dillon, A. R., Hanken, G. H., Nachreiner, R. F., and Redding, R. W.: Experimental hemorrhage in splenectomized and nonsplenectomized dogs. Am. J. Vet. Res. 41:707, 1980.

32. Dingwall, J. S.: Surgical management of abdominal trauma. J. Am. Vet. Med. Assoc. 159:1406, 1971.

33. Doige, C. E., and Furneaux, R. W.: Liver disease and intrahepatic portal hypertension in the dog. Can. Vet. J. 16:209, 1975.

34. Eichner, R. R.: Splenic function: Normal, too much and too little. Am. J. Med. 66:311, 1979.

35. Eisenberg, S., Klein, G. F., and Wolf, P. S.: Dynamics of the splenic erythrocyte reservoir in the dog. J. Surg. Res. 9:595, 1969.

36. Evans, H. E., and Christensen, G. C.: The lymphatic system. In Miller's Anatomy of the Dog, 2nd ed. W. B. Saunders, Philadelphia, 1979.

37. Fan, L. C., Dorner, J. L., and Hoffman, W. E.: Reticulocyte

response and maturation in experimental acute blood loss anemia in the cat. J. Am. Anim. Hosp. Assoc. 14:219, 1978.

38. Feeney, D. A., Johnston, G. R., and Hardy, R. M.: The role of two-dimensional gray scale ultrasound in the assessment of liver and splenic neoplasia in the dog and cat. J. Am. Vet. Med. Assoc., submitted for publication.

39. Ffoulken-Crabbe, D. J. O., Creighton, R. E., Volgyesi, G. A., Steward, D. J., and Nisbet, H. I. A.: The effect of splenectomy on circulatory adjustments to hypoxemia in the anesthetized dog. Br. J. Anaesth. 48:639, 1976.

40. Furneaux, R. W.: Surgical techniques for the spleen and liver. Vet. Clin. North Am. 5:363, 1975.

41. Gill, F. M.: Hematologic indications for splenectomy in pediatrics. Am. J. Pediatr. Hematol. Oncol. 2:41, 1980.

42. Groom, A. C., and Song, S. H.: Effects of norepinephrine on washout of red cells from the spleen. Am. J. Physiol. 221:255, 1971.

43. Groopman, J. E., and Golde, E. W.: The histiocytic disorders: A pathophysiologic analysis. Ann. Intern. Med. 94:95, 1981.

44. Hahn, P. F., Bale, W. F., and Bonner, J. F.: Removal of red cells from active circulation by sodium pentobarbital. Am. J. Physiol. 138:415, 1943.

45. Harker, L. A.: The role of the spleen in thrombokinetics. J. Lab. Clin. Med. 77:247, 1971.

46. Harvey, J. W., and Gaskin, J. M.: Experimental feline haemobartonellosis. J. Am. Anim. Hosp. Assoc. 13:28, 1977.

47. Harvey, J. W., and Kaneko, J. J.: Oxidation of human and animal haemoglobins with ascorbate, acetylphenylhydrazine, nitrite, and hydrogen peroxide. Br. J. Haematol. 32:193, 1976.

48. Heath, C. W., and Daland, G. A.: The life of reticulocytes—experiments on their maturation. Arch. Intern. Med. 46:533, 1930.

49. Highman, B., Thompson, E. C., Boshe, J., and Altand, P. D.: Serum alkaline phosphatase in dogs with experimental splenic and renal infarction and with endocarditis. Proc. Soc. Exp. Biol. Med. 95:109, 1957.

50. Jacob, H. S., MacDonald, R. A., and Jandl, J. H.: Regulation of spleen growth and sequestering function. J. Clin. Invest. 42:1475, 1963.

51. Jain, N. C.: Studies on the occurrence and persistence of Heinz bodies in erythrocytes of the cat. Folia Haematol. (Leipzig) 99:28, 1973.

52. Jandl, J. H., Files, N. M., Barnett, S. B., and MacDonald, R. A.: Proliferative response of the spleen and liver to hemolysis. J. Exp. Med. 122:299, 1965.

53. Kay, M. M. B.: Role of physiologic autoantibody in the removal of senescent human red cells. J. Supramol. Struct. 9:555, 1978.

54. King, D. R., Lobe, T. E., Haase, G. M., and Bolen, E. T., Jr.: Selective management of injured spleen. Surgery 90:677, 1981.

55. Kolata, R. J.: Diagnostic abdominal paracentesis and lavage: experimental and clinical evaluation in the dog. J. Am. Vet. Med. Assoc. 168:697, 1976.

56. Kolata, R. J., and Johnston, D. E.: Motor vehicle accidents in urban dogs: A study of 600 cases. J. Am. Vet. Med. Assoc. 167:938, 1975.

57. Koyama, S., Aoki, S., and Deguchi, K.: Electron microscopic observations of the splenic red pulp with special reference to the pitting function. Mie Med. J. 14:143, 1964.

58. Krumbhaar, E. B.: The changes produced in the blood picture by removal of the normal mammalian spleen. Am. J. Med. Sci. 184:215, 1932.

59. Kusminsky, R. E., Chang, H., Hossino, H., Zehan, S. M., and Boland, J. P.: An omental implantation technique for lavage of the spleen. Surg. Gynecol. Obstet. 155:407, 1982.

60. Lipowitz, A. J., Todoroff, R. F., and Mero, K. N.: Clinicopathologic conference: Splenic torsion. J. Am. Vet. Med. Assoc. 170:65, 1977.

61. Lipson, R. L., Bayrd, E. D., and Watkins, C. H.: The

postsplenectomy blood picture. Am. J. Clin. Pathol. 32:536, 1959.

62. Liska, W. B., MacEwen, E. G., Zoki, F. A., and Garvey, M.: Feline systemic mastocytosis: A review and results of splenectomy in seven cases. J. Am. Anim. Hosp. Assoc. 15:589, 1979.

63. LoBuglio, A. F., Cotran, R. S., and Jandl, J.: Red cells coated with immunoglobulin G: binding and sphering by mononuclear cells in man. Science 158:1582, 1967.

64. Maede, Y.: Sequestration and phagocytosis of *Haemobartonella felis* in the spleen. Am. J. Vet. Res. 40:691, 1979.

65. Marshake, R. M.: A probable case of Banti's syndrome in a dog. J. Am. Vet. Med. Assoc. 123:125, 1953.

66. Maxie, M. G., Reed, J. H., Pennock, P. W., and Hoff, B.: Splenic torsion in three great danes. Can. Vet. J. 11:249, 1970.

67. Millikan, J. S., Moore, E. E., Moore, G. E., and Stevens, R. E.: Alternatives to splenectomy in adults after trauma: Repair, partial resection, and reimplantation of splenic tissue. Am. J. Surg. 144:711, 1982.

68. Nossal, G. J. V., Austin, C. M., Rye, J., and Mitchell, J.: Antigens in immunity. XII. Antigen trapping in the spleen. Int. Arch. Allergy 29:368, 1966.

69. O'Brien, T. R.: *Radiographic Diagnosis of Abdominal Disorders in the Dog and Cat.* W. B. Saunders, Philadelphia, 1978, pp. 450–458.

70. Odom, L. F., and Tubergen, D. G.: Splenomegaly in children. Identifying the cause. Postgrad. Med. 65:191, 1979.

71. Orman, M. E., and Lorenz, M. D.: Torsion of the splenic pedicle in a dog. J. Am. Vet. Med. Assoc. 160:1099, 1972.

72. Osborne, C. A.: General principles of biopsy. Vet. Clin. North Am. 4:213, 1974.

73. Osborne, C. A., Perman, V., and Stevens, J. B.: Needle biopsy of the spleen. Vet. Clin. North Am. 4:311, 1974.

74. Pass, M. A., and Johnston, D. E.: Treatment of gastric dilation and torsion in the dog. Gastric decompression by gastrostomy under local analgesia. J. Small Anim. Pract. 14:131, 1973.

75. Patel, J., Williams, J. S., Shmigel, B., and Hinshaw, J. R.: Preservation of splenic function by autotransplantation of traumatized spleen in man. Surgery 90:683, 1981.

76. Pearson, H. A., Johnston, D., Smith, K. A., and Touloukian, R. J.: The born-again spleen. Return of splenic function after splenectomy for trauma. N. Engl. J. Med. 298:1389, 1978.

77. Perman, V., and Schall, W. D.: Diseases of red blood cells. In Ettinger, S. J. (ed.): *Textbook of Veterinary Internal Medicine,* 2nd ed. W. B. Saunders, Philadelphia, 1982.

78. Prankerd, T. A. J.: The spleen and anemia. Br. J. Med. 2:517, 1963.

79. Reeve, E. B., Gregersen, M. U., Allen, T. H., and Sear, II.: Distribution of cells and plasma in normal and splenectomized dog and its influence on blood volume estimates with p²² and T-1824. Am. J. Physiol. 175:195, 1953.

80. Rifkind, R. A.: Heinz body anemia: An ultrastructural study. II. Red cell sequestration and destruction. Blood 26:433, 1965.

81. Ristic, P., and Small, E.: Canine ehrlichiosis: The role of the spleen in protection against the disease. Vet. Med. Sm. Anim. Clin. 74:1469, 1979.

82. Root, C. R.: Interpretation of abdominal survey radiographs. Vet. Clin. North Am. 4:763, 1974.

83. Rosse, W. F., and de Boisfleury, A.: The interaction of phagocytic cells and red cells modified by immune reactions. Blood Cells 1:345, 1975.

84. Schalm, O. W., Jain, N. C., and Carroll, E. J.: *Veterinary Hematology,* Lea & Febiger, Philadelphia, 1975.

85. Schwartz, A. D., and Goldthorn, J. F.: "Born-again spleens" and resistance to infection. N. Engl. J. Med. 299:832, 1978.

86. Sherman, R.: Rationale for and methods of splenic preservation following trauma. Surg. Clin. North Am. 61:127, 1981.

87. Sisson, S.: Spleen. In Getty, R. (ed.): *Sisson and Grossman The Anatomy of the Domestic Animals,* Vol. 2, 5th ed. W. B. Saunders, Philadelphia, 1975.

88. Song, S. H., and Groom, A. C.: Storage of blood cells in spleen of the cat. Am. J. Physiol. 220:779, 1971.

89. Song, S. H., and Groom, A. C.: The distribution of blood cells in the spleen. Can. J. Physiol. Pharmacol. 49:734, 1971.

90. Suzuki, T., Furusata, M., Takasaki, S., Shimizu, S., and Hataba, Y.: Stereoscopic scanning electron microscopy of the red pulp of dog spleen with special reference to the terminal structure of cordal capillaries. Cell Tiss. Res. 182:441, 1977.

91. Szymanski, I. O., Odgren, P. R., Fortier, N. L., and Snyder, L. M.: Red blood cell associated IgG in normal and pathologic states. Blood 55:48, 1980.

92. Tavassoli, M., Ratzan, R. J., and Crosby, W. H.: Studies on regeneration of heterotopic splenic autotransplants. Blood 41:701, 1973.

93. Van Rooijen, N.: Immune complexes in the spleen: Three concentric follicular areas of immune complex trapping, their interrelationships and possible function. J. Reticuloendothel. Soc. 21:143, 1977.

94. Vatner, S. F., Higgins, C. B., Millard, R. W., and Franklin, D: Role of the spleen in the peripheral vascular response to severe exercise in untethered dogs. Cardiovasc. Res. 8:276, 1974.

95. Veerman, A. J. P., and van Ewijk, W.: White pulp compartments in the spleen of rats and mice. A light and electron microscope study of lymphoid and non-lymphoid cell types in T- and B- area. Cell Tiss. Res. 156:417, 1975.

96. Walshaw, R., and Johnston, D. E.: Treatment of gastric dilatation—volvulus by gastric decompression and patient stabilization before major surgery. J. Am. Anim. Hosp. Assoc. 12:162, 1976.

97. Weed, R. I.: The importance of erythrocyte deformability. Am. J. Med. 49:124, 1970.

98. Weed, R. I., and Weiss, L.: The relationship of red cell fragmentation occurring within the spleen to cell destruction. Trans. Assoc. Am. Physic. 79:426, 1966.

99. Weiss, L.: The white pulp of the spleen. The relationships of arterial vessels, reticulum, and free cells in the periarterial lymphatic sheath. Bull. Johns Hopkins Hosp. 115:99, 1964.

100. Weiss, L.: The spleen. In Weiss, L. and Greep, R. (eds.): *Histology,* 4th ed. McGraw-Hill, New York, 1977.

101. Weiss, L., and Tavassoli, M.: Anatomical hazards to the passage of erythrocytes through the spleen. Sem. Hematol. 7:372, 1970.

102. Williams, J. S., Patel, J. M., and Hinshaw, J. R.: Omental pouch technique for reimplantation of the spleen. Surg. Gynecol. Obstet. 155:730, 1982.

103. Wingfield, W. E., and Hoffer, R. E.: Gastric dilation-torsion complex in the dog. In Bojrab, M. J., (ed.): *Current Techniques in Small Animal Surgery.* Lea & Febiger, Philadelphia, 1975.

The Tonsils

Chapter **85**

Mary L. Dulisch

ANATOMY

The paired palatine tonsils are masses of lymphoid tissue in the lateral walls of the oropharynx caudal to the palatoglossal arch and ventral to the soft palate. The tonsil is divided into two parts: a large portion that variably protrudes into the pharynx and a smaller part that lies under mucosa, which forms the anterior part of the lateral wall of the tonsillar sinus (crypt). The smaller portion is exposed when the main portion is retracted from the crypt. The base of the tonsil is in the dorsolateral aspect of the tonsillar crypt (Fig. 85–1). In young dogs, much of the tonsil may protrude from the tonsillar crypt and be exposed to the pharynx. This is rare in cats.

The blood supply to the tonsil is from the tonsillar artery, derived from the lingual artery. Sensory innervation to the tonsil is via a branch of the glossopharyngeal nerve. There are no afferent lymphatics to the tonsil. The efferent lymph vessels drain to the medial retropharyngeal and submandibular lymph nodes.[7,8]

PHYSIOLOGY AND PATHOPHYSIOLOGY

The tonsillar crypts of normal dogs and cats contain a diverse bacterial flora, including potential pathogens such as *Erysipelothrix insidiosa*, hemolytic *Streptococcus*, *Pasteurella* spp., and *Corynebacterium pyogenes*.[10] The normal host immune mechanisms can effectively deal with a small number of these pathogens, but larger numbers may lead to

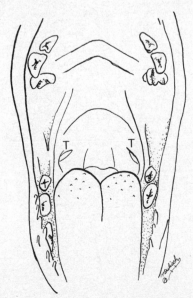

Figure 85–1. The tonsils (*T*) are located in the lateral walls of the oropharynx.

clinical infection. Therefore, the tonsil may serve as a portal of entry for these or other bacterial or viral pathogens. For example, the tonsil is probably the most common natural entry site of enteric viruses, such as infectious canine hepatitis, canine distemper, and feline panleukopenia.[1] From this site of initial multiplication, hematogenous or lymphatic spread may occur.[10] The tonsil can also act as a reservoir for pathogens during an inapparent infection or convalescence or when the host is an asymptomatic carrier of infection. Viruses can multiply in the epithelial cells and macrophages of the lymphoid tissue prior to viremia and systemic infection. Viruses may also predispose the host to bacterial invasion by damaging the local phagocytic and humoral defense mechanism.[10] The most common bacteria to infect the tonsils of the dog are the hemolytic streptococci and coliforms. Leptospirae may also enter through this portal. Abscesses of the tonsil seldom occur.

DISEASES

Figure 85–2 presents an algorithm useful for approaching the differential diagnosis of the more common tonsillar lesions.

Tonsillitis

Primary tonsillitis is usually a bilateral inflammation of the tonsillar tissue that can be either acute or chronic in nature. This condition appears to be more frequent in dogs than in cats, is often seen in small breeds of dogs, and is uncommon in dogs over one year of age.[4]

In acute bacterial tonsillitis, the tonsils are erythematous, endematous, and enlarged, so they often protrude further from their crypts into the pharynx. The clinical history frequently includes dysphagia, coughing, pawing at the base of the ears, hypersalivation, anorexia, and listlessness. On physical examination, the body temperature may be elevated and the mandibular lymph nodes may be enlarged and painful. The surface of the tonsils may have areas of punctate hemorrhages, necrosis, or white plaques of inflammatory exudate. The tissue is friable and bleeds easily on manipulation. Treatment in these cases often consists of penicillin or broad spectrum antibiotics but should depend on the results of bacterial culture and sensitivity testing. Supportive care includes fluid replacement therapy and mild analgesics as indicated. Tonsillectomy is not suggested for treatment during an episode of acute tonsillitis, because this may result in further spread of the infection to adjacent or distant tissues.[5]

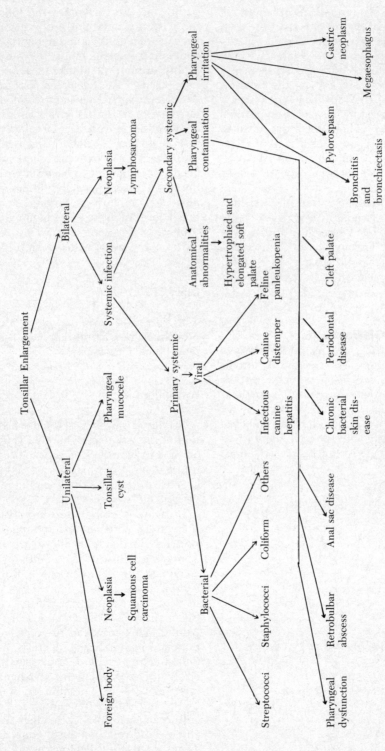

Figure 85–2. Differential diagnoses for common tonsillar lesions.

Chronic Tonsillitis

Chronic bacterial tonsillitis is usually observed in young dogs as an intermittent disease that recurs at intervals of weeks or months and lasts several days at each episode.

ETIOLOGY OF TONSILLITIS

Primary causes of tonsillitis include bacteria, viruses, and foreign bodies. As mentioned previously, a variety of potential bacterial pathogens partially comprise the normal flora of the tonsillar crypt. The most common pathogenic bacteria isolated from cases of tonsillitis, however, are α and β hemolytic streptococci, staphylococci, and coliforms in both the dog and cat.[4]

Secondary tonsillitis can occur as a result of other disease processes. One category of such diseases includes the causes of pharyngeal irritation, such as recurring vomition or regurgitation due to disorders such as megaesophagus, pylorospasm, or gastric neoplasia. Other chronic bacterial diseases also can lead to tonsillitis; for example, periodontal disease and distant infections, such as bacterial skin diseases and chronic anal sacculitis, which lead to chronic contamination of the mouth with pathogens owing to licking. Similarly, a chronic productive cough, resulting from bronchitis or bronchiectasis, cleft palate (by chronic exposure of the nasopharynx to contamination), or pharyngeal dysfunction (as in cricopharyngeal achalasia or from a retropharyngeal abscess) can also cause secondary tonsillitis.[4] In addition, anatomical abnormalities, including elongated soft palate and hypertrophied soft palate, observed in brachycephalic breeds (boxers, Boston terriers, and English bulldogs), can result in chronic pharyngitis and tonsillitis.

Tumors of the tonsil, such as squamous cell carcinoma or tonsillar lymphosarcoma should always be part of a differential diagnosis when enlarged or otherwise abnormal tonsils are found (see Fig. 85–2). Although squamous cell carcinoma is usually unilateral, lymphosarcoma frequently is bilateral, leading to potential confusion of the latter tumor with infectious tonsillitis.[3] Although pharyngeal mucoceles do not directly affect the tonsils, this entity should be ruled out if dysphagia is a primary presenting complaint. A foreign body, such as a grass awn or a piece of wood, lodged in a tonsil or crypt may cause inflammation and swelling. Tonsillar cysts should also be considered when enlargement of the organ is observed.

DIAGNOSIS AND CASE SELECTION

When an animal is presented with tonsillar enlargement, a complete physical examination and a complete blood count and serum chemistry profile should be evaluated to determine if there is an underlying systemic disease and if the animal is a good surgical risk. The three main indications for tonsillectomy are (1) chronic recurrent tonsillitis that is unresponsive to antibiotics, (2) acute tonsillar enlargement causing mechanical interference with swallowing or air flow, and (3) neoplasia.[8] Acute tonsillitis is usually not an indication for surgery, because surgical intervention may lead to spread of the infection.

ANESTHETIC TECHNIQUE

The choice of anesthetic is dependent on the health of the animal and the anesthetist's preference; there is no specific regimen. However, regardless of the technique, endotracheal intubation is essential if the swallowing reflex is to be eliminated. To further prevent aspiration of blood or discharges, the pharynx should be packed with gauze.[9]

TONSILLECTOMY

Several techniques are used to perform a tonsillectomy. The objectives with each are complete removal

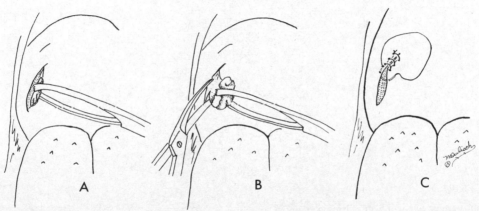

Figure 85–3. Tonsillectomy technique 1. *A*, An Allis tissue forceps is used to grasp the tonsil and evert it from the crypt. *B*, The tonsil is excised using scissors. *C*, After removal of the tonsil, the tonsillar fold can be sutured over the tonsillar crypt.

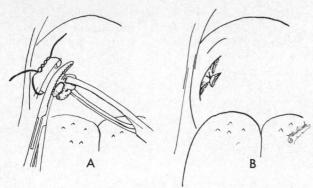

Figure 85–4. Tonsillectomy technique 2. *A*, After clamping the tonsillar base, en mass ligation of the base is performed. *B*, The tonsil is excised.

of the tonsillar tissue, minimal tissue trauma, and maximal hemostasis.

Techniques

1. The tonsil is grasped with an Allis tissue forcep, a tonsillar forcep, or a vulsellum forcep and is gently retracted from the tonsillar crypt. All deeper tonsillar tissues are exposed. These tissues and the tonsil may then be excised with Metzenbaum scissors, beginning rostrally and cutting caudally (Fig. 85–3). Bleeding is controlled by individual ligation of blood vessels, digital pressure, or electrocoagulation. Another technique is to inject a small amount of epinephrine, diluted 1:10,000 or 1:100,000, deep to the tonsil. However, because some inhalation anesthetics, such as halothane, can sensitize the myocardium to epinephrine-induced arrhythmias, it might be best to avoid this combination completely; at the least, extreme care should be taken when using this technique; i.e., the heart should be monitored closely.[6] The tonsillar fold may also be sutured over the crypt using a simple continuous pattern of a fine absorbable suture material, such as 4-0 chromic gut.

2. Another technique involves clamping the tonsillar base with a curved Kelly hemostat prior to excision. Clamping facilitates control of hemorrhage. The base is ligated en mass or transfixed using 2-0 or 3-0 chromic gut, or the tonsillar fold can be sutured closed (Fig. 85–4). Some surgeons employ a Parker-Kerr (Cushing pattern) or a simple continuous oversew of the hemostat for hemostasis and crypt closure.

3. A tonsil snare, with or without diathermy, can also be used. The snare is placed around the base of the tonsil and closed. The crushing action contributes to hemostasis. The diathermy snare works in a similar manner but has the advantage of electrocoagulation to prevent hemorrhage (Fig. 85–5).

4. Another technique involves the use of a raspatory to scrape the tonsillar lymphoid tissue from supporting structures until it is only partially attached to the mucous membranes. These last attachments are then severed with scissors, sometimes preceded by vascular ligation as necessary (Fig. 85–6).

5. Finally, another instrument that has been used in veterinary medicine is a tonsillotome, which cuts and crushes the base of the tonsil while simultaneously excising tissue beyond the crushed area. Care must be taken to ensure complete removal of the lymphoid tissue. The instrument should be left on for about five minutes to obtain maximum hemostasis (Fig. 85–7).

Once removed, the tonsil should be divided and submitted for bacterial culture and antibiotic sensitivity testing, impression smears, or scrapings, and histopathological examination. If a tumorous tonsil extends into the pharyngeal wall, so that excision is not possible, three different biopsy techniques may be utilized for diagnostic purposes: (1) needle aspiration of involved tissue or (2) guillotine biopsy can be performed as described in Chapter 86 (p. 1224) for use with lymph nodes. For the guillotine biopsy, 2-0 chromic catgut is looped over a segment of the tonsil and tied. The tissue distal to the ligature then can be excised and divided for the different diagnostic procedures (Fig. 85–8). (3) Finally, partial excision of tonsillar tissue can be accomplished by the use of electrosurgery, which also provides hemostasis. A large enough piece should be removed so that some tissue that is not coagulated, and thereby rendered useless, is available for histological evaluation.

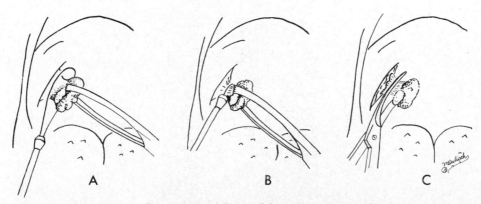

Figure 85–5. Tonsillectomy technique 3. *A*, After eversion of the tonsil from its crypt, a tonsil snare is applied. *B*, The tonsil snare is closed to crush the base of the tonsil. *C*, Remaining tissue strands must be cut with scissors.

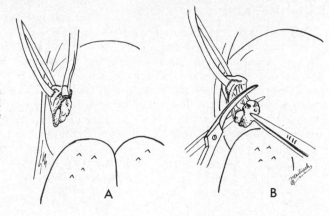

Figure 85–6. Tonsillectomy technique 4. *A,* The tonsillar base is exposed and a raspatory is used to scrape the tonsillar lymphoid tissue from supporting elements. *B,* The last attachments at the base are severed with scissors.

HISTOPATHOLOGY

In bacterial tonsillitis, the tonsillar crypts become filled with debris, white blood cells (especially neutrophils in pyogenic infections), bacteria, and desquamated epithelium. There may be edema and follicular hyperplasia or ulceration of the epithelial lining of the crypts.

PROGNOSIS

For cases of mechanical pharyngeal obstruction due to tonsillar enlargement and chronic tonsillitis, the prognosis for complete recovery after resection is excellent. The prognosis after resection of tumors varies with the neoplasm in question (see Chapter 178).

AFTERCARE

Hemorrhage or hypersalivation after tonsillectomy may lead to aspiration of fluids and resultant pneumonia or hypoxia. To help prevent these complications, the endotracheal tube should be left in place until the animal is making voluntary attempts at swallowing. The systemic antibiotic of choice should be administered for five to seven days. Animals should not be fed for 24 hours after surgery, so intravenous fluids are given as required. Corticosteroids may be required to reduce severe pharyngeal edema and inflammation, which occur postoperatively in some patients. After 24 hours, soft food and liquids may be offered, and the animal's normal diet can be started on the fourth or fifth postoperative day. Complete healing of the area should occur by ten days to two weeks after surgery.

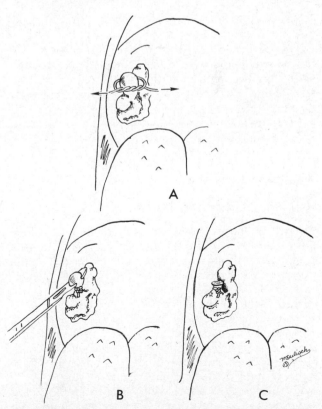

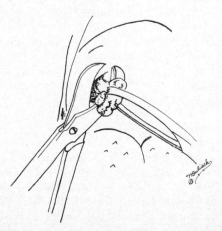

Figure 85–7. Tonsillectomy technique 5. A tonsillotome is used to cut and crush the base of the tonsil. The instrument should be left on for about five minutes to obtain maximal hemostasis.

Figure 85–8. A tonsillar biopsy using the "guillotine" technique. *A,* The ligature should compress but not cut completely through the tissue. *B,* The ligature is tied. *C,* Tissue distal to the ligature is severed.

COMPLICATIONS

Hemorrhage may occur during the first 24 hours after surgery. A blood transfusion or anesthesia to obtain hemostasis is rarely necessary. Aspiration pneumonia also is a rare occurrence. Localized pharyngitis present prior to surgery may persist. This usually can be controlled by administration of antibiotics. Regrowth of incompletely removed tonsillar tissue is possible, requiring subsequent removal if clinical signs persist.

1. Anderson, N. V.: Disorders of the small intestine, *In* Ettinger, S. J. (ed.): *Textbook of Veterinary Internal Medicine*, 2nd ed., W. B. Saunders, Philadelphia, 1983, Chap. 42.
2. Baker, G. J.; Surgery of the pharynx and larynx, J. Small Anim. Pract, 13:505, 1972.
3. Brodey, R. S.; Differentiating tonsillar lesions in the dog, Mod. Vet. Pract, 47:58, 1966.
4. Harvey, C. and O'Brien, J: Disorders of the oropharynx and salivary glands, *In* Ettinger, S. J. (ed.): *Textbook of Veterinary Internal Medicine*, 2nd ed. W. B. Saunders, Philadelphia, 1983, Chap. 39.
5. Johnson, J. H., Hull, B. L., and Dorn, A. S.: The mouth, *In* Anderson, N. V.: *Veterinary Gastroenterology*, Lea & Febiger, Philadelphia, 1980, Chap. 20.
6. Kaplan, B.; A technic for tonsillectomy in the dog, Vet. Med. Small Anim. Clin, 64:805, 1969.
7. Leighton, R. L.; *In* Archibald, J.: *Canine Surgery*, 2nd ed. American Veterinary Publications, Inc., Santa Barbara, CA, 1974, Chap. 8.
8. Miller, M. E., Christensen, G. C., and Evans, H. E.: *In Miller's Anatomy of the Dog*, 2nd ed. W. B. Saunders, Philadelphia, 1979, pp. 453–454.
9. Peiffer, R. L.: The lymph nodes and vessels, *In* Bojrab, M. J.: *Current Techniques in Small Animal Surgery I*, Lea & Febiger, Philadelphia, 1975, Chap. 35.
10. The tonsils in the pathogenesis of disease, Vet. Rec. 95:234, 1974.

Chapter **86**

Lymph Nodes and Lymphatics

K. Ann Jeglum and Mary Dulisch

EMBRYOLOGY

The formation of the lymphatic system begins in the six-week embryo. Paired jugular sacs enlarge and, together with endothelial pockets, form the lymphatics. By nine weeks, the lymphatic channels develop. Protrusions from the lymphatics coalesce with connective tissue to form lymph nodes with afferent and efferent lymph vessels.

ANATOMY

Peripheral Lymphatic System

True lymphatic vessels, bearing one-way valves, exist only in vertebrate animals.[16] Each lymphatic drains via as many as eight to ten regional lymph nodes to major channels that empty into the thoracic duct and, ultimately, into the major veins, which return blood to the heart. The terminology applied to the lymphatic system is similar to that applied to the blood vascular system. There are three major components of the lymphatic system: capillaries, collecting vessels, and lymph nodes. A capillary network collects fluid (lymph) from interstitial spaces of the body and empties it into collecting vessels that act as conduits to the lymph nodes (a filtering system) and, thence, to the venous system. The thoracic duct, originating as a cranial continuation of the cisterna chyli between the crura of the diaphragm in the sublumbar region, is the chief vessel returning lymph from the body. As the thoracic duct passes along the lumbar vertebrae and aorta, its major drainage into the venous system is into the jugular vein and cranial vena cava. Large lymphatic vessels are enveloped in smooth muscle and adventitia. They may also contain neural elements. A major force for the flow of lymph is supplied by adjacent muscular contraction. The lymphatic vessels generally are satellites of the venous system except within the central nervous system, splenic pulp, bone marrow, skeletal muscle, eye, and inner ear cartilage, where lymphatics do not exist. Lymphatic vessels have a marvelous ability to regenerate. The tissues most richly supplied with lymphatics are the dermis and the mucous membranes of the digestive and respiratory systems. A free flap between the tissue space and the interior of the terminal lymphatic vessel allows drainage of the tissue spaces.

Lymph Nodes

Lymph nodes are variable in size and are dispersed throughout the lymphatic system. They are bean-shaped and encapsulated in connective tissue.[16] Afferent lymph vessels draining from the periphery enter the convex surface of the lymph node. Lymph flows through the capsule into the cortex and medullary sinuses and leaves at the hilus, via one or several efferent vessels. Trabeculae extending from the capsule create cavities lined by reticular tissue.

Histologically, the lymph node is poorly divided into a cortex with lymph nodules or cortical follicles and a medulla of cords of tissue and sinuses (see Chapter 15). The major cell of the lymph node is the lymphocyte. Lymph nodes are sites of lymphocyte generation, B lymphocytes and T lymphocytes being produced in different parts of each node. Lymphocyte proliferation as well as "trapping" of lymphocytes during recirculation can result in increased cellularity and size of nodes following antigenic stimulation (see Chapter 15). The medullary cords contain small lymphocytes, plasma cells, and macrophages. Many factors, including age, diet, and hormones, influence the cellularity of lymph nodes. The regional anatomy of the lymphatic vessels and lymph nodes is discussed elsewhere under specific organs and systems.[24, 30]

PHYSIOLOGY

One of the major functions of the lymphatics is to carry proteinaceous fluid and large particulate matter away from interstitial tissue spaces into the blood.[16] Interstitial fluid that becomes lymph constitutes one-tenth of the volume of the arterial capillary filtrate. Owing to its high protein content, lymph cannot be absorbed readily by the blood.

The content of the lymphatic fluid is approximately the same as that of the tissue fluid of the area it is draining. For example, the protein content of interstitial space lymph is approximately 1.8 gm/dl, whereas that of liver lymph is about 6 gm/dl, and that of intestinal lymph is 3 to 4 gm/dl protein. Intestinal lymph also contains a high percentage of fat as chylomicrons. Lymph draining from infected tissues may carry bacteria to the regional lymph node, where they are removed from the circulation. Lymph return to the blood stream is important in maintaining the circulating blood volume. If there is an obstruction of the peripheral lymphatics, paralymphatic channels can transport the fluid. Fluids that accumulate in tissue spaces are reabsorbed via pathways that are not lined by endothelium. These include interstitial, submucosal, subendothelial, perivascular, and perineural fluid spaces as well as spaces within the peritoneal and pleural body cavities.

Another important function of the lymphatic system, especially the lymph nodes, is defensive. Lymph nodes act as filtration barriers to foreign material and particulate agents such as bacteria, which are phagocytized by macrophages within the nodes. The lymph nodes also participate in humoral and cell-mediated immune responses to foreign antigens (see Chapter 15) and in extramedullary cytopoiesis.

The regional lymph nodes that drain tumor sites may serve important functions in the outcome of neoplasia,[6, 11-15] by acting as primary barriers to further metastasis, and by initiating systemic immunity to solid tumors. Once a lymph node is overwhelmed by a tumor infiltrate, however, its function as a barrier ceases. It may then serve as a source of tumor cells for distant metastases.

DISORDERS OF THE PERIPHERAL LYMPHATIC VESSELS

Lymphangitis

Lymphangitis is inflammation of a lymphatic vessel. It is most often caused by a bacterial or fungal infection. Streptococci and staphylococci are the most commonly involved bacteria. The causative agent may be introduced via the skin or mucous membranes into subcutaneous or submucosal tissues by bite wounds, foreign bodies, lacerations, abrasions, and so on. Extension to lymphatic vessels occurs because of their intimate association with the skin and mucous membranes. Generally, superficial rather than deep lymphatics are involved in lymphangitis. The tissues surrounding affected lymphatic vessels become hyperemic and infiltrated with inflammatory cells such as neutrophils. The vessels eventually may become plugged with inflammatory cells, desquamated endothelial cells, and coagulated lymph. If the draining lymph nodes cannot contain the infection, there may be systemic spread, i.e., bacteremia or septicemia. Draining lymph nodes may enlarge and become painful. This secondary inflammatory response is termed lymphadenitis. Secondary lymphatic obstruction and subsequent edema may result from inflamed lymphatics and activated lymph nodes. The involved area, such as a limb, may swell, become hot and painful, and lose function.

In humans, an erythematous tract may be seen, running from the site of infection to the draining lymph node (e.g., in cat scratch fever). The erythema in animals may not be visible owing to overlying hair. In severe cases, ulceration and drainage of pus occurs along the course of the lymphatic, and the draining lymph node may become abscessed. If a limb is involved, lameness may result. The patient also may become ill, demonstrating clinical signs including fever, anorexia, and lethargy. In acute cases, neutrophilic leukocytosis may occur. In some instances, the entire process may be subclinical, with the regional node containing the infection.

Treatment

The treatment of acute lymphangitis includes immobilization, antibiotics, and "hot packing" of the involved areas. Hot packing helps improve drainage and reduce swelling. Systemic broad-spectrum antibiotics are initiated and changed according to the results of bacterial culture and antibiotic sensitivity testing. Surgical intervention is rarely necessary but may be required if abscess formation occurs, fistulous tracts develop, or foreign bodies are involved. An incision may aggravate the inflammatory process. The main purposes of surgery include drainage to improve removal of the organism and removal of a foreign body. Complete recovery, with eventual restoration of lymphatic drainage, usually results.

Chronic lymphangitis may result in permanent damage to the lymphatic system and lymphedema. The skin and subcutaneous tissues may be indurated and thickened, from treatment failure or inadequate treatment of acute lymphangitis, foreign bodies, reactive hyperplasia, or granulomatous disease. Treatment of chronic forms of lymphangitis often involves surgical exploration.

Primary Lymphedema

Lymphedema is associated with congenital absence or acquired destruction of lymphatic vessels resulting in an abnormal interstitial accumulation of lymph. The edema occurs primarily in the distal extremities, although it may move proximally, occasionally becoming generalized. The two major classifications of lymphedema are primary and secondary.

Primary or idiopathic lymphedema occurs when no other underlying disease is present to cause the obstruction of lymphatic vessels. There are several subclassifications of primary lymphedema. It may be hereditary or nonhereditary, and congenital or developing later in life. There are different forms of primary lymphedema based on morphological abnormalities found on lymphangiography.

The clinical signs of all forms of primary lymphedema are similar. In the congenital form, owners often notice swelling in the extremities shortly after birth. Pitting edema is often confined to the hind legs, especially the distal aspects. The limbs may be painless, and lameness is uncommon. In humans, lymphedema is associated with a dull, mild pain. There may be transient edema or progressive obstruction leading to generalized edema of head, body, and all limbs. The severity of the edema may fluctuate, and premature death may result. In severe cases, irreversible damage to skin and subcutaneous tissue occurs. Secondary fibrosis may impair drainage, resulting in permanent edema. Differential diagnoses for primary lymphedema include thrombophlebitis, trauma, hypoproteinemia, venous or lymphatic inflammation, neoplasia, arteriovenous fistula, swelling from a clotting abnormality, and, rarely, congestive heart failure. The results of a complete blood count, plasma protein measurements, and serum electrophoresis are generally within normal ranges. Survey radiographs show no bony changes.

In congenital and early forms of primary lymphedema, most likely both quantity and quality of healthy lymphatic vessels are deficient. If the deficiency is marginal, repeated trauma with age may cause the lymphedema later in life. In humans, primary lymphedema is divided into subgroups on the basis of age of occurrence. The congenital form, *lymphedema congenita*, is present at birth or shortly thereafter (less than 10 per cent of primary lymphedema pa-

tients). The largest proportion of patients develop lymphedema between early childhood and 30 years of age, and the disorder is termed *lymphedema praecox*. Women are affected three times as often as men. Patients who develop lymphedema after 30 years of age have *lymphedema tarda*. The three age groups probably represent an artificial separation of similar pathophysiologic events.

The congenital, hereditary type of primary lymphedema (lymphedema congenita) in man is called Melroy's disease. It is extremely rare in both humans and animals, and has not been reported in cats. Patterson and colleagues[27] reported congenital hereditary lymphedema in dogs in 1967. One affected dog and her descendants were studied. Genetic studies indicated that the developmental abnormality of the peripheral lymphatic system was inherited as an autosomal dominant characteristic. Extreme variability in the severity of lymphedema was noted among the genetic carriers. Three types of edema were seen in 24 affected offspring: edema of rear limbs only, edema of rear and forelimbs, and edema of all four limbs, trunk, and tail. Lymphangiography was used to examine the morphological disorders. The four types of lymphatic abnormalities seen were: aplasia, hypoplasia, hyperplasia, and lymphangiectasia.

In hereditary lymphedema in dogs, lymphatic obstruction occurs in the hind limbs at the level of the popliteal lymph nodes.[22] In one report, the popliteal lymph nodes were not detectable by lymphangiography or at necropsy, i.e., they were aplastic. When forelimb edema was present, axillary lymph nodes were absent, but the central body lymph nodes were present. The most distal lymphatics were dilated and increased in number, size, and tortuosity. These changes were compatible with lymphangiectasia. (Some forms of lymphangiectasia in other diseases are due to an absence of valves within the lymphatic.) The major distal lymphatics of the hind limbs terminated in the popliteal fossa with no major lymphatics evident above the femorotibial joint. There was also an extensive plexus of fine lymphatic vessels in the metatarsal and digital regions.[22] Pups that had edema of trunk and limbs died. In those that survived the neonatal period, the edema decreased with time, perhaps via continued morphogenesis after birth, so that abnormal lymphatics became adequately functional to allow drainage of the limb. Regional lymph nodes were not present, even though edema subsided. Necropsy studies demonstrated an unexplained skeletal and cardiac myopathy. Aplasia or hypoplasia of lymph nodes in the affected limbs was thought to be a component of the developmental abnormality of the peripheral lymphatic system rather than a cause of the lymphedema.[22]

Secondary Lymphedema

Secondary lymphedema is obstruction of normal lymphatic vessels. The causes of obstruction include trauma, pressure bandages, inflammatory lesions, and neoplasms. The obstruction causes an increased accumulation of fluid in the interstitial spaces drained by the lymphatics. A considerable number of lymphatic vessels or several sequential lymph nodes must be blocked to cause edema. Both afferent and efferent lymph vessels in the lymph nodes must be blocked. Otherwise, collateral lymphatics and veins compensate for the obstruction. In small animals, secondary lymphedema is more common than primary lymphedema.

Experimental models of chronic, secondary lymphostasis have been studied to determine the pathophysiology of lymphatic obstruction and lymphedema.[1] During the latent phase of lymphedema, the collecting terminal lymphatics develop intracellular edema and become massively dilated; endothelial junctions of the collecting lymphatics open; endothelial and smooth muscle cells in the walls of the lymphatics become edematous; smooth muscle cells in the lymph collectors produce collagen and are transformed into fibroblast-like cells; thrombi of fibrinoid material form within the lymph capillaries; and inflammatory cells migrate into the area of thrombi and the walls of the lymphatics. Because the vessels are extremely dilated, the valves within the lymphatics do not function normally. The sinuses of the lymph nodes dilate, medullary tissue is reduced, and germinal follicles are absent. The surrounding blood vessels in the area also undergo changes, e.g., their smooth muscle may transform into fibroblast-like cells and thrombi may form within the blood vessels.

During chronic lymphedema, the lymphatic capillaries remain extremely dilated. The basement membrane of these vessels becomes continuous, so that larger molecular substances cannot cross. The endothelial anchoring filaments increase, lymphatic collectors become lymphangioma-like, and vessels lose their elasticity. The lymphatic vessels, small and large, become fibrotic. Thrombi within vessels become organized, and the medullary sinuses of lymph nodes are less dilated because of sclerosis of trabeculae. Venous obstruction also worsens, so that tissue fluid resorption does not occur. The arteries and veins undergo different degrees of sclerosis. Atypical proliferative tissue accumulates in subcutaneous tissue. Chronic inflammatory cells may be found. The overlying epidermis becomes thinned. Subepidermal cysts containing erythrocytes, granulation tissue, and cell debris may form and ulcerate through the epidermis.

The clinical signs of secondary lymphedema vary from intermittent swelling of a limb to severe systemic illness. Signs may include lethargy, fever, anorexia, and weight loss. Owners may relate the edema to trauma or a surgical procedure. If only one limb is edematous, the obstruction is usually in the proximal limb. The etiology and location of the obstruction determine the severity of the lymphedema; e.g., bilateral hindlimb edema usually signifies an obstruction in the pelvis or in the sublumbar or retroperitoneal regions. Forelimb, neck, and thoracic edema may be due to obstruction in the prescapular and axillary region or mediastinum. Palpation of enlarged regional lymph nodes shows an absence of pain. Differential diagnoses for secondary lymphedema are similar to those for primary lymphedema. Regional obstruction should be investigated and ruled out.

The clinicopathological findings vary according to the cause. If the etiology is infection or if secondary inflammation is present, the white blood cell count may show neutrophili, leukocytosis, and a left shift. Debilitation of the animal can be associated with anemia. Hypoproteinemia may be present to complicate the severity of edema.

Survey radiographs of the affected areas show evidence of aggressive bone lesions, suggesting inflammatory or infectious processes. Soft tissue masses causing the obstruction may be seen. Regional contrast studies of the involved areas, such as angiography and an esophogram, may help define the obstruction. Lymphangiography is the primary diagnostic tool for locating and determining the extent of the causative lesion. The technique of lymphangiography is discussed later in this chapter. Water-soluble dyes are recommended in lymphedema that may have an inflammatory component, because oily media further aggravate the condition, and because the oil may embolize to the peripheral pulmonary arteries.

Lymphangiography demonstrates changes that are, in many cases, similar to those discussed under "Primary Edema"; e.g., in both forms of lymphedema, there are dilated, tortuous lymphatics. An obstructive mass may be visible that was not seen on survey radiographs. There may be bidirectional lymph flow due to obstruction of lymphatic valves. Collateral lymph channels circumvent obstructed areas. Partial filling or absence of filling of lymph nodes may be seen. Such filing defects may outline a tumor or the site of inflammation. Dermal backflow or the peripheral flow of dye outlining dermal lymphatic capillaries occurs in both primary and secondary lymphedema. If rupture of lymphatics and perivascular channels occurs, the tissue spaces may become filled with dye.

The causes of secondary lymphedema are varied. The most common cause in humans is acute filariasis due to a mosquito-borne nematode, *Wuchereria bancrofti*. The most common causes in small animals are related to surgery, trauma, and neoplasia. Any surgical procedure or trauma that interrupts or removes a large area of lymphatic tissue may initiate lymphedema, with concomitant compromise of venous return. Radical lymph node dissections due to malignant disease are a common cause of lymphedema. The presence of a primary or metastatic tumor within a lymph node may cause swelling. Lymphedema associated with neoplasia, without discrete lymph node involvement, may signify disseminated neoplastic involvement with lymphatic and vascular plugging. The most common tumors in dogs and cats causing edema include mammary adenocarcinoma and lymphoma. The inflammatory type of mammary adenocarcinoma commonly causes edema of the extremities. Lymphedema may also develop with an infectious disease that involves the lymphatics, lymph nodes, or veins, especially when recurrent and severe lymphangitis and lymphadenitis result in fibrosis or sclerosis. Wound healing may be interrupted by lymphedema. Radiation therapy of animals may rarely injure lymphatic endothelium and result in secondary lymphedema.

Treatment

The treatment of secondary lymphedema involves removing the cause, although under many circumstances, this may be impossible. Symptomatic treatment including antibiotics, anti-inflammatory drugs, diuretics, bandaging, massage, and mild exercise may be beneficial in traumatic or postsurgical edema. In infectious processes causing lymphedema, long-term broad-spectrum antibiotics may be needed. Neoplastic disease requires aggressive treatment, usually involving anticancer drugs.

In humans, the surgical forms of treatment for secondary lymphedema are required for only a small number of patients.[34] The indications for surgery in humans are: (1) increasing size of limb despite aggressive medical treatment; (2) functional impairment; (3) serious skin changes; (4) recurrent infection resistant to antibiotics; and (5) emotional disturbance.

Three surgical procedures have been used to correct lymphedema.[5] First, subcutaneous threads or tubes of foreign material have been implanted to stimulate new lymphatic growth; this procedure has not been effective and is no longer used. In the second procedure, large amounts of the diseased tissue are resected to improve physical appearance of the patient and to attempt anastomosis of remaining superficial lymphatics and deeper vessels below the excision site. Neither of these procedures has shown consistent success. The final method involves attempted transposition of healthy lymphatic tissue to the diseased area. Dermal flaps have been implanted into subcutaneous tissue with hopes of their acting as a conduit for lymphatic drainage. Another procedure involves implanting a piece of intact omentum into the edematous tissue. The omentum has a rich, centripetal lymphatic flow and blood supply. Connections between omental lymphatics and deeper lymphatics in patients treated this way have been visible on lymphangiography, and one-third to one-half of the patients treated have developed successful drainage. None of these procedures has been reported in dogs or cats other than experimentally.

Intestinal Lymphangiectasia

Intestinal lymphangiectasia is characterized by increased enteric protein loss, hypoproteinemia, edema, lymphocytopenia, malabsorption, and abnormally dilated lymphatics in the small intestine.[33] In humans, intestinal lymphangiectasia can be part of a generalized congenital disorder of the lymphatic system.[35] In these patients, there is a high incidence of chylous effusions as well as structurally abnormal peripheral, retroperitoneal, and thoracic lymphatics. A suggested mechanism for the occurrence of intestinal lymphangiectasia is that hypoplastic visceral lymphatics obstruct lymph flow.[25] An increase in intestinal lymphatic pressure leads to dilation of lymphatic vessels throughout the small intestine and mesentery. The enteric protein loss, resulting in hypoproteinemia and steatorrhea, is due to the rupture of lymphatics and leakage of chyle into the intestinal lumen and serous cavities. The size of the lymphatic vessels does not correlate with the degree of protein loss. In some cases of intestinal lymphangiectasia, the protein may diffuse from the intestinal capillaries and enter the lumen through an intact epithelium. The absorption of long-chain triglycerides stimulates the flow of lymph and increases protein leakage. Because long-chain triglycerides are transported by the lymphatics, steatorrhea occurs.

Intestinal lymphangiectasia in the dog may be congenital or acquired.[7, 26] In the congenital form, there is malformation or hypoplasia of the lymphatic vessels. In the acquired type, there is obstruction of intestinal lymphatics by inflammation, including granulomatous disease, or by neoplasia. The obstruction is usually a central block of the lacteal at the level of the regional lymph nodes. Lymphangiectasia is one of the most common causes of protein-losing enteropathy in the dog. Other diseases in the dog associated with protein-losing enteropathy include congestive heart failure, neoplasia, immunodeficiency, and parasites.

The clinical signs of intestinal lymphangiectasia include varying degrees of diarrhea, edema, ascites, and weight loss.[2, 4, 8, 10, 23, 26] The primary laboratory finding is hypoproteinemia, especially hypoalbuminemia and low levels of the immunoglobulins IgG, IgA, and IgM. Other significant laboratory tests include hypocholesterolemia, lymphopenia, hypocalcemia, and one or more abnormal intestinal absorption tests. Lymphopenia may be due to the loss of T lymphocytes into the intestinal lumen. This phenomenon could lead to deficient cellular immune responses. The presence or absence of lymphopenia may be helpful in differentiating lymphangiectasia from other causes of protein-losing enteropathies. In humans and dogs, increased protein loss into the intestinal tract has been demonstrated by measuring fecal excretion of ^{51}Cr- and ^{125}I-labelled canine or human albumin.[2]

Radiographs of the small bowel may show mucosal edema and a malabsorption pattern. Lymphangiography may demonstrate dilation of mucosal and submucosal lymphatics in the small intestine. Hypoplastic peripheral and visceral lymphatics, with absence of retroperitoneal lymph nodes, may indicate a more generalized disorder. On exploratory laparotomy, grossly dilated mesenteric lymphatics may be evident. The definitive diagnosis of intestinal lymphangiectasia is based on: histopathology of the involved bowel and demonstration of increased enteric protein loss. Biopsy reveals dilated and telangiectatic lymphatic vessels in the lamina propria and submucosa. The villi may be club-shaped owing to the grossly dilated lymphatics. These histological findings are reversible with successful treatment.

The primary goal in treating intestinal lymphangiectasia is to decrease the amount of protein loss via the gastrointestinal tract. In a majority of cases, dietary management is required. Antibiotics, corticosteroids, and other, nonspecific pharmacological treatments are unsuccessful. In the rare case of a localized lesion causing the lymphangiectasia, surgical excision may be indicated. However, most cases cannot be approached surgically, except via biopsy, because of the diffuse nature of intestinal disease.

Dietary treatment involves lowering fat intake and minimizing long-chain triglycerides because they increase lymph flow and promote steatorrhea.[19] The diet consists of high levels of carbohydrates and medium-chain triglycerides and provides adequate protein intake. Medium-chain triglycerides are absorbed by the portal circulation rather than by the lacteals. Suggested foods include macaroni, rice, bread, spaghetti, and low-fat canned dog foods.

The prognosis in canine intestinal lymphangiectasia is guarded to unfavorable. There are mixed reports in the veterinary literature of success and failure of dietary management.

Other Disorders of the Peripheral Lymphatic Vessels

Neoplasia

Lymphangioma and lymphangiosarcoma, primary tumors arising from the lymphatic vessels, are rare in domestic animals, having no known rate of incidence. An unusual late complication in women who have undergone radical mastectomy is the development of a lymphangiosarcoma of the ipsilateral arm.[17, 36] This is a secondary tumor that develops in association with limb edema between five and 25 years after mastectomy. This infrequent complication has not been reported in dogs and cats subjected to radical mastectomy. Lymphangiomas are also rare tumors of the small intestine in humans. Surgical excision of a lymphangioma or a lymphangiosarcoma is usually unsuccessful owing to the invasiveness of the lesion. If such a tumor is present in a limb, the treatment of choice is amputation.

The most common metastatic tumors involving the lymphatic system are carcinomas. Inflammatory mammary carcinomas result from diffuse infiltration of the draining lymphatics and have an extremely poor prognosis. Carcinomas may also metastasize to the lymphatics in the lungs, causing a peribronchial infiltrate on thoracic radiographs. Tumors that metastasize to or involve lymphatic vessels are associated with a high potential for systemic involvement.

Chylous Effusions

Chylous effusions may represent a segment of a generalized lymphatic vessel disorder or may be due to rupture of the thoracic duct (see Chapter 42).

DISORDERS OF LYMPH NODES

Lymph nodes respond dynamically to pathophysiological changes. Biopsy followed by histological examination is required to obtain a definitive diagnosis of lymph node abnormalities. Immunosuppression due to chronic disease, drugs, congenital immune deficiency disease, malnutrition, age, and stress may cause lymph node hypoplasia. This is a histological diagnosis that is not usually detected clinically. Atrophy of the lymphoid nodule may occur after stress.

The most common change in the lymph node is enlargement (lymphadenopathy). The diagnosis, etiology, and classification of lymph node enlargement depends on the type of cellular infiltrate discovered by histopathological examination (Table 86–1). Because of the complexity of lymph node morphology, it is important to submit the entire lymph node for histopathological examination whenever possible. There are two basic mechanisms of lymphadenopa-

TABLE 86–1. Classification of Lymph Node Enlargement

Lymphadenitis	Reactive lymphoid hyperplasia
	Bacterial lymphadenitis
	Viral lymphadenitis
	Parasitic lymphadenitis
	Toxoplasma-induced lymphadenitis
	Filarial lymphadenitis
	Fungal lymphadenitis
	Coccidioidal lymphadenitis
	Histoplasma-induced lymphadenitis
	Traumatic lymphadenitis
Lymphadenopathies	Autoimmune lymphadenopathies
	"Collagen-vascular" diseases
	Systemic lupus erythematosus–associated lymphadenopathy
	Rheumatoid lymphadenopathy
	Hydantoin lymphadenopathy
	Tumor-reactive lymphadenopathy
Tumor	Primary
	Lymphomas
	Secondary
	Leukemias
	Metastatic (especially carcinomas)

thy: an increase in the number and size of lymphoid follicles with proliferation of lymphocytes and reticuloendothelial cells (immune stimulation) and infiltration with cells (tumor) not normally found in lymph nodes.

In immune stimulation, there is a wide spectrum of changes in lymph node morphology, based on the amount and nature of antigenic stimuli. The result is a proliferation of reticuloendothelial cells resulting in increased phagocytic activity. The increased population of cells include T and B lymphocytes, macrophages, and plasma cells. This histological response within a lymph node is called *reactive hyperplasia*.

Lymphadenopathy may result from an infiltration with tumor cells. As yet unknown stimuli cause malignant transformation in primary neoplasia of the lymph node, termed lymphoma. Nonlymphoid tumors may metastasize to regional and distant lymph nodes, causing loss of normal architecture and cellularity. Recent evidence suggests that the regional lymph node in tumor-bearing animals and humans may act as the initiator of systemic immunity.[9] Carcinomas are the most common solid tumors to metastasize to draining lymph nodes. In the dog and cat, the most common tumor to spread via lymphatics is mammary adenocarcinoma. However, most tumors do not metastasize exclusively via lymphatics or blood vessels. Approximately 15 per cent of dogs with osteosarcoma have a metastasis to the regional lymph node in addition to hematogenous spread to the lungs.[29]

Although the definitive diagnosis of lymph node disease is based on histological findings, there are some clinical changes characteristic of specific types of lymphadenopathy. Many of the superficial lymph nodes of adult animals are not palpable unless they are diseased. Lymphadenopathy is more common in animals less than one year of age than in older animals, because the lymph nodes of young animals respond with greater intensity to antigenic stimuli. Biopsy is often unnecessary in a young animal with lymphadenopathy unless signs of disease exist. Histological examination of these lymph nodes usually shows reactive lymphoid hyperplasia. Acute inflammation within lymph nodes, known as lymphadenitis, causes asymmetrically enlarged and painful nodes. The skin overlying superficial lymph nodes may become erythematous. Lymph nodes infiltrated with a metastatic tumor are painless, firm, usually asymmetrical, and immovable. Lymphoma or lymphosarcoma causes generalized lymphadenopathy consisting of painless, firm, symmetrical, and movable nodes.

APPROACH TO LYMPHADENOPATHY

A thorough history and physical examination are the first steps in diagnosing lymphadenopathy. The external lymph nodes are palpated to determine whether the lymphadenopathy is generalized or regional. Generalized lymphadenopathy represents systemic disease. In regional lymphadenopathy, the area drained by those lymph nodes should be examined carefully for primary disease. The most readily palpable external lymph nodes are submandibular, retropharyngeal, prescapular, axillary, inguinal, and popliteal. Some lymph nodes (e.g., popliteal) are often enclosed in fatty deposits that may be difficult to distinguish from an enlarged node. Lymph nodes occur in clusters, and several nodes may be palpable in each anatomic site. The consistency of the enlarged nodes is an important aid to diagnosis. A lymph node infiltrated with tumor cells is firm, but an enlarged, reactive lymph node is usually soft. One should note erythema, skin swelling, and whether a draining tract exists over the lymph node (which would suggest lymphadenitis).

There are sites where enlarged lymph nodes cannot be palpated, e.g., mediastinal, hilar, sternal, and hepatic, and, usually, mesenteric, para-aortic, and external iliac. In cats, intra-abdominal lymph nodes may be palpable. Massive mediastinal lymphadenopathy may decrease the compressibility of the cranial chest wall in cats, and other clinical signs (e.g., dyspnea) may suggest internal lymphadenopathy. Hepatosplenomegaly may also suggest lymphoma.

The age and sex of an animal should be considered in diagnosing lymphadenopathy. For example, neoplasia is less likely in young animals than in middle-aged to old animals. Some sex-associated tumors (mammary, prostatic, testicular, or ovarian) may cause secondary regional lymphadenopathy. Knowledge of any recent exposure to trauma or infectious agents is important. Clinical signs, including fever, malaise, and weight loss, may accompany lymphoreticular or hematological malignancies and systemic infections. The duration of lymphadenopathy may be significant. Neoplastic lymph nodes are detectable longer than enlarged lymph nodes secondary to infection or inflammation.

Radiographic and hematological studies are important to diagnosis. Chest radiographs may provide evidence of metastatic tumors or intrathoracic lymphadenopathy associated with infection. Intra-abdominal lymph nodes in the dog can often be evaluated by radiography only, unless they are massively enlarged and palpable. Hematology may reveal leukemia with abnormal circulating blood cells. Leukocytosis with neutrophilia corroborates other findings suggesting infection.

Cytological examination of needle aspirates of enlarged lymph nodes may provide a definitive diagnosis. Certain malignancies such as mast cell tumors are easily diagnosed cytologically, but lymphoma is difficult to diagnose by cytological methods alone. In infectious, bacterial, or fungal lymphadenitis, the procedure may reveal neutrophils, reactive lymphocytes, macrophages, plasma cells, fungi, or bacteria.

Culture of involved lymph nodes may be indicated to identify specific organisms, and blood cultures, in systemic infections associated with fever and leuko-cytosis. Serological tests for specific infectious agents also may be helpful. Appropriate skin tests for such disorders as histoplasmosis and coccidioidomycosis may confirm a tentative diagnosis.

Biopsy of an enlarged lymph node is often required for definitive diagnosis of primary lymph node tumors (lymphoma) or metastatic tumors such as carcinomas.[18] It is best to sample the most easily accessible abnormal lymph node. Lymphadenitis, regardless of etiologic organism, is characterized by a leukocytic infiltrate primarily of mature and band forms of neutrophils as well as with macrophages and plasma cells. Lymphoblasts may be found in such nodes.

Histological differentiation between tumor and lymphoid/reactive hyperplasia may be difficult. For example, a lymph node undergoing malignant transformation with lymphoma may be interpreted as reactive in the prodromal stages. In addition, early tumor metastasis may induce activation of the lymph node prior to detectable tumor cell infiltration and loss of architecture.

Lymphangiography

Kinmouth first used an intralymphatic injection of contrast material in the distal limbs of dogs to visualize lymphatic vessels and lymph nodes.[21] Previous attempts at injecting dye into the lymph nodes had been unsuccessful. Although developed in dogs, lymphangiography is now used more in humans than in domestic animals.

Technique

Lymphangiography must be performed with the patient under anesthesia. Evans blue dye is injected intradermally in the web between the toes in the front or hind feet. The total dose (0.5 ml in cats and up to 1 ml in dogs) is divided between two or three injections. Immediately, the dye is taken up selectively by the lymphatics. This take-up is usually not visible through the skin. A small "cutdown" is done on the dorsum of the paw along the bifurcation of the cephalic veins. A 30-gauge lymphangiography needle with an attached polyethylene catheter is placed in the lymphatic vessel and secured with a loop of 4-0 silk. The contrast material used for radiographic visualization is Ethiodol, an iodine compound dissolved in an ester of poppy seed oil. Serial radiographs are taken to visualize the lymphatic vessels, the flow of lymph, and the lymph nodes.

Application

The major application of lymphangiography in the dog has been to study lymphedema. In humans, the technique is used for the diagnosis and staging of lymphomas, and intra-abdominal, pelvic, and thoracic masses. Other lymphatic disorders, including infectious and granulomatous diseases, also have been evaluated.[31]

The intralymphatic route of administration also has been used: to deliver isotopes to selectively identify microscopic foci of tumor cells; to inject immune adjuvants, such as Bacillus Calmette-Guerin (BCG) or *Corynebacterium parvum* directly into the reticuloendothelial system; and to inject autochthonous tumor cell vaccines to treat canine lymphoma and feline mammary adenocarcinoma.[20] Further applications of this route of administration are currently being explored.

Diagnostic Evaluation of Lymph Nodes

The main indications for evaluating a lymph node histologically are: to determine the cause of localized or generalized lymphadenopathy; to help stage a neoplastic disease, i.e., to determine whether a tumor has metastasized to a regional lymph node; and to evaluate an immune-mediated disease. The lymph nodes most frequently sampled via biopsy (in decreasing order) are the popliteal, inguinal, and prescapular (MLD), because of their ready accessibility.

The three principal methods of obtaining tissue are fine-needle aspiration, incisional biopsy, and excisional biopsy. Fine-needle aspiration causes the least morbidity and is rapid and easily performed, often without anesthesia. Because incisional and excisional biopsies allow evaluation of nodal architecture, they are more reliable.

Fine-Needle Aspiration

Fine-needle aspiration is used most often for subcutaneous lymph node biopsy. Occasionally, enlarged deeper lymph nodes, e.g., sublumbar, may be aspirated to provide definitive diagnosis of metastatic tumors such as a circumanal gland adenocarcinoma. The surgical site is clipped and prepared in a routine manner. A subcutaneous node is stabilized between the thumb and index finger of one hand. A 22- to 25-gauge needle attached to a 5 ml syringe is directed into the node and at least three aspirations are made at 90 degrees to one another. The center of the node is avoided because it may be necrotic. As the needle is partially removed and redirected from one area of the lymph node to another, negative pressure is maintained. However, prior to withdrawal of the needle from the lymph node, negative pressure is released. After three positionings, the needle is withdrawn. Air is slowly drawn into the syringe, and the aspirated tissue is expelled from the needle onto glass slides. A thin smear of the sample is then made. After air drying, the sample is stained with new methylene blue or Wright's stain. Depending on the disease state, other aspirates may be obtained for bacterial culture and sensitivity testing. This technique is particularly useful in suspected lymphosarcoma.

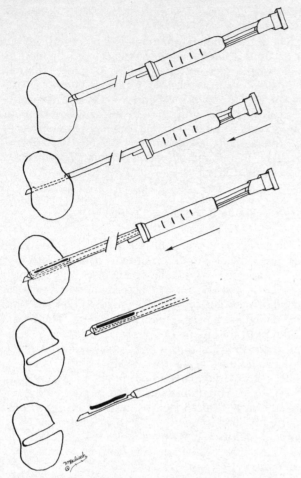

Figure 86–1. Lymph node biopsy using a Tru-cut needle.

Incisional Biopsy

Incisional biopsy is indicated if the node cannot be totally removed with ease, because of either size or location (e.g., in the sublumbar region). Some common techniques include needle biopsy (using a Franklin-modified Vim Silverman or a Tru-cut* needle), ligation and proximal resection (guillotine technique), and a wedge biopsy. Franklin-modified Vim Silverman and Tru-cut needles provide samples that are usually 1 to 2 mm wide and 5 to 10 mm long (Fig. 86–1). The Tru-cut instrument is a single unit and may be easier to manipulate than the multiple-component Vim Silverman needle.

The guillotine method consists of placing a loop of suture material, such as 2-0 chromic gut, over a portion of the lymph node and slowly compressing the node with the loop. The suture is tied, and the tissue distal to the ligature is excised with a scalpel blade (Fig. 86–2).

A scalpel blade is used for wedge biopsy. The cut edges of the lymph node are apposed with horizontal mattress sutures of 2-0 or 3-0 chromic gut (Fig. 86–3).

*Tru-cut, Travenol Laboratories, Inc., Deerfield, Ill.

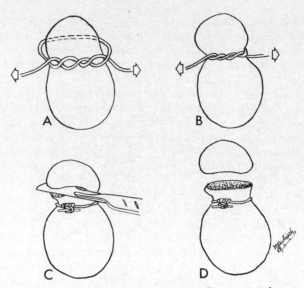

Figure 86–2. Guillotine biopsy of a lymph node using 2-0 chromic gut.

Excisional Biopsy

An excisional biopsy provides the largest amount of tissue. The entire node can be evaluated histologically. The lymph node should be manipulated and freed from its loose attachments to the surrounding tissue, using blunt dissection with a hemostat or scissors. Afferent and efferent lymphatics are usually friable and do not require ligation. Blood vessels supplying the lymph node, however, should be ligated or electrocoagulated.[28]

Comparison of Impression Smears and Scrapings

Slides prepared from biopsies allow cytological in addition to histological examination. With impression

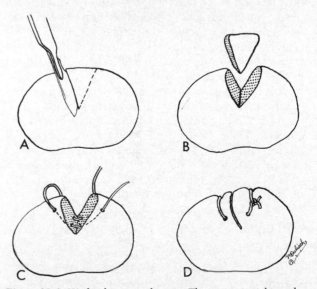

Figure 86–3. Wedge biopsy technique. The suture is tightened so that the lymph node edges are apposed but the suture does not cut into the node.

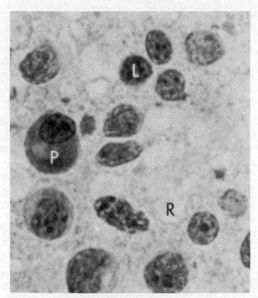

Figure 86–4. Tissue from a dog lymph node obtained by aspiration biopsy. The distribution of plasma cells (P) and small lymphocytes (L) is indicative of benign lymphoid hyperplasia. R = red blood cell. (New methylene blue stain; × 1000.) (Reprinted with permission from Perman, V., Stevens, J., Alsaker, R., and Osborne, C.: Lymph node biopsy. Vet. Clin. North Am. *4*:281, 1974.)

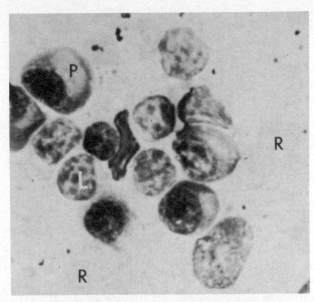

Figure 86–6. Aspiration biopsy smear from an enlarged lymph node of a dog wih benign lymphoid hyperplasia. P = plasma cells; L = small lymphocytes; R = red blood cells. (Wright's stain; × 1000.) (Reprinted with permission from Perman, V., Stevens, J., Alsaker, R., and Osborne, C.: Lymph node biopsy. Vet. Clin. North Am. *4*:281, 1974.)

smears, an inadequate number of cells may adhere to the slide. To avoid this possibility, a scalpel blade can be scraped over the cut surface of a node and the cells may be smeared onto the slide.

Cytological Examination

The primary cell type in normal and hyperplastic lymph nodes is the small lymphocyte (Figs. 86–4 and

86–5). Less than five per cent of the cell population are large lymphoblasts. In addition, hyperplastic lymph nodes contain plasma cells and their precursors (Fig. 86–6). Stromal cells are found infrequently.

Although neoplastic lymphoid cells from different species or different individuals within the same species vary morphologically, from small to large, neoplastic cells obtained from an individual may be similar in appearance (all small, all large, or all blastic)

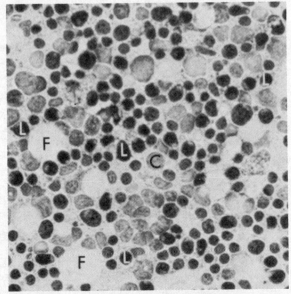

Figure 86–5. Aspiration biopsy smear from an enlarged lymph node of a dog with benign lymphoid hyperplasia. L = small lymphocytes; C = pale-staining cells, which are damaged lymphocytes; F = fat droplets. (New methylene blue stain; × 400.) (Reprinted with permission from Perman, V., Stevens, J., Alsaker, R., and Osborne, C.: Lymph node biopsy. Vet. Clin. North Am. *4*:281, 1974.)

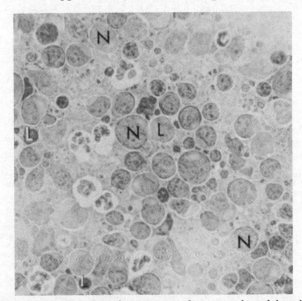

Figure 86–7. Aspiration biopsy smear from an enlarged lymph node of a dog with malignant lymphoma. Neoplastic lymphocytes (N) are as large or larger (12 to 18 microns) than polymorphonuclear leukocytes. The neoplastic lymphocytes have large nuclei and prominent nucleoli. L = small lymphocytes. (New methylene blue stain; × 400.) (Reprinted with permission from Perman, V., Stevens, J., Alsaker, R., and Osborne, C.: Lymph node biopsy. Vet. Clin. North Am. *4*:281, 1974.)

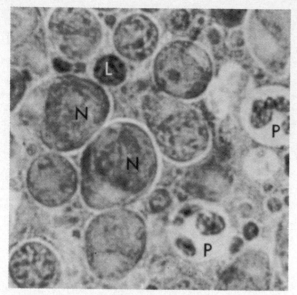

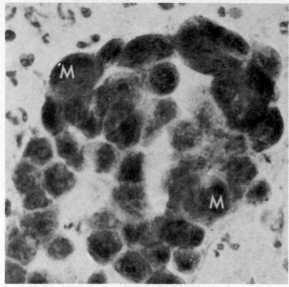

Figure 86–8

Figure 86–9

Figure 86–8. Aspiration biopsy smear from an enlarged lymph node of a dog with malignant lymphoma. N = neoplastic lymphocytes; L = small lymphocytes; P = polymorphonuclear leukocytes. (New methylene blue stain; × 1000.) (Reprinted with permission from Perman, V., Stevens, J., Alsaker, R., and Osborne, C.: Lymph node biopsy. Vet. Clin. North Am. 4:281, 1974.)

Figure 86–9. Aspiration biopsy from an enlarged lymph node of a cat. The lymph node contains clusters of metastatic carcinoma cells (M). Compare the size of these epithelial-like cells to the polymorphonuclear leukocytes. (New methylene blue stain; × 400.) (Reprinted with permission from Perman, V., Stevens, J., Alsaker, R., and Osborne, C.: Lymph node biopsy. Vet. Clin. North Am. 4:281, 1974.)

(Figs. 86–7 and 86–8). When neoplastic cells are present in low numbers, differentiation from non-neoplastic cell types may be impossible either cytologically or histologically. Metastatic neoplastic cells usually can be identified easily in a biopsy specimen (Fig. 86–9).[28]

Aftercare

There should be little postoperative care, other than skin suture removal ten to 14 days following an incisional or excisional biopsy. There is no specific postoperative care after needle aspiration.

Complications and Contraindications to Biopsy

The type of complication varies with the area from which the node is taken and the method of sampling. The major complication of fine-needle aspiration of a subcutaneous lymph node is hemorrhage or bruising. If there is a possibility or suspicion of a bleeding disorder, it should be evaluated prior to any surgical procedure. Hemorrhage also is a possible complication following excisional or incisional biopsy. If lymphadenitis is present, extension of infection to surrounding tissue may occur following an incisional biopsy or if the node is traumatized during excision. Because of this problem, aspiration biopsy might be preferred in the presence of infection.[32] Local spread of malignant cells or distant metastasis after needle aspiration may occur, but is unsubstantiated.[3]

1. Altorfer, J., Hedinger, C., and Clodius, L.: Light and electron microscopic investigation of extremities of dogs with experimental chronic lymphostasis. Folia Angiol. 25:141, 1977.
2. Barton, C. L., Smith, C., Troy, G., et al.: The diagnosis and clinicopathological features of canine protein-losing enteropathy. J. Am. Anim. Hosp. Assoc. 14:85, 1978.
3. Brodey, R. S.: Surgery. In Theilen, G. H., and Madewell, B. R. (eds.): Veterinary Cancer Medicine. Lea & Febiger, Philadelphia, 1979.
4. Campbell, R. S. F., Brobst, D., and Bisgard, G.: Intestinal lymphangiectasia in a dog. J. Am. Vet. Med. Assoc. 153:1050, 1968.
5. Clodius, L.: The experimental basis for the surgical treatment of lymphedema. In Clodius, L. (ed.): Lymphedema. Georg Thieme, Stuttgart, 1977.
6. Ellis, R. J., Wernick, G., Zabriskie, J. B., and Goldman, L. I.: Immunologic competence of regional lymph nodes in patients with breast cancer. Cancer 35:655, 1975.
7. Fadell, E. J., Dame, R. W., and Wolford, J.: Chronic hypoalbuminemia and edema associated with intestinal lymphangiectasia. J. Am. Vet. Med. Assoc. 194:917, 1965.
8. Farrow, B. R. H., and Penny, R.: Protein-losing enteropathy in a dog. J. Small Anim. Pract. 10:513, 1969.
9. Fidler, J., Gersten, M., and Hart, I. R.: The biology of cancer and metastasis. Adv. Cancer Res. 28:150, 1978.
10. Finco, D. R., Duncan, J. R., Schall, W. D., et al.: Chronic enteric disease and hypoproteinemia in 9 dogs. J. Am. Vet. Med. Assoc. 163:262, 1973.
11. Fisher, B., and Fisher, E. R.: Studies concerning the regional lymph node in cancer. I: Initiation of immunity. Cancer 27:1001, 1971.
12. Fisher, B., and Fisher, E. R.: Studies concerning the regional lymph node in cancer. II: Maintenance of immunity. Cancer 29:1496, 1972.
13. Fisher, B., Saffler, E., and Fisher, E. R.: Studies concerning the regional lymph node in cancer. IV: Tumor inhibition by regional lymph node cells. Cancer 33:631, 1974.
14. Fisher, B., Wolmark, N., Coyle, J., et al.: Studies concerning the regional lymph node in cancer. VIII: Effects of two

asynchronous tumor foci on lymph node cell cytotoxicity. Cancer 36:521, 1975.

15. Goldfarb, P. M., and Hardy, M. A.: The immunologic responsiveness of regional lymphocytes in experimental cancer. Cancer 35:778, 1975.

16. Guyton, A. C.: The lymphatic system, interstitial fluid dynamics and edema. *In: Textbook of Medical Physiology.* 4th ed. W. B. Saunders Co., Philadelphia, 1971.

17. Harris, J. R., and Hellman, S.: Local and regional management of carcinoma of the breast. *In* Carter, S. K., Glatstein, E., and Livingston, R. B. (eds.): *Principles of Cancer Treatment*, New York, McGraw-Hill, 1982.

18. Ioachim, H. L.: Lymph Node Biopsy. J. B. Lippincott Co., Philadelphia, 1982.

19. Jeffries, G. H., Chapman, A., and Sleisenger, M. H.: Low-fat diet in intestinal lymphangiectasia. N. Engl. J. Med. 270:761, 1964.

20. Jeglum, K. A.: Unpublished results.

21. Kinmouth, J. B., Taylor, G. W., and Harper, R. M. E.: Lymphangiography: technique for its clinical use in lower limbs. Br. Med. J. 1:940, 1952.

22. Luginbuhl, H., Chacko, S. K., Patterson, D. F., et al.: Congenital herditary lymphoedema in the dog. Part II: Pathological studies. J. Med. Genet. 4:153, 1967.

23. Matthews, D., DeRick, A., Thoonan, W., and Van der Stock, J.: Intestinal lymphangiectasia in a dog. J. Small Anim. Pract. 15:757, 1974.

24. Miller, M. E.: The lymphatic system. *In Anatomy of the Dog.* W. B. Saunders Co., Philadelphia, 1964.

25. Munro, D. R.: Route of protein loss during a model protein-losing gastropathy in a dog. Gastroenterology 66:960, 1974.

26. Olson, N. C., and Zimmer, J. F.: Protein-losing enteropathy secondary to intestinal lymphangiectasia in a dog. J. Am. Vet. Med. Assoc. 173:271, 1978.

27. Patterson, D. F., Medway, W., Luginbuhl, H., et al.: Congenital hereditary lymphoedema in the dog. Part I. Clinical and genetic studies. J. Med. Genet. 4:145, 1967.

28. Perman, V., Stevens, J., Alsaker, R., and Osborne, C.: Lymph node biopsy. Vet. Clin. North Am. 4:281, 1974.

29. Pool, R. R.: Tumors of bone and cartilage. *In* Moulton, J. E. (ed.): *Tumors in Domestic Animals.* 2nd ed. University of California Press, Berkeley, 1978.

30. Ratzloff, M. H.: The superficial lymphatic system of the cat. Lymphology 3:151, 1970.

31. Schaffer, B., Koehler, P. R., Daniel, C. R., et al.: A critical evaluation of lymphangiography. Radiology 80:917, 1963.

32. Stoll, S. G.: Lymph node biopsy. *In* Bojrab, M. J. (ed.): *Current Techniques in Small Animal Surgery I.* Lea & Febiger, Philadelphia, 1975.

33. Strombeck, D. R.: Protein-losing enteropathy. *In Small Animal Gastroenterology.* Stonegate Publishing, Davis, Ca., 1979.

34. Thompson, N.: The surgical treatment of chronic lymphedema of the extremities. Surg. Clin. North Am. 47:445, 1967.

35. Waldman, T. A.: Protein-losing gastroenteropathies. *In* Bockus, H. L. (ed.): *Gastroenterology.* 3rd ed. W. B. Saunders, Philadelphia, 1976.

36. Woodward, A. H., Ivins, J. C., and Soule, E. H.: Lymphangiosarcoma arising in chronic lymphedematous extremities. Cancer 30:562, 1972.

Chapter 87

The Thymus

Sharon Stevenson

INTRODUCTION

Surgery of the thymus of dogs and cats has been performed primarily as an immunological research method; however, the clinical significance of the thymus and its diseases in small domestic animals is rapidly becoming apparent. Since 1970 at least 50 canine and feline thymomas have been reported in the veterinary literature. In addition, these thymomas have been associated with other diseases (e.g., myasthenia gravis, autoimmune disorders, and neoplasia), as in human beings. This chapter summarizes the current knowledge of thymic anatomy and physiology and discusses the pathophysiology of various diseases in relation to clinical syndromes, surgical indications, and techniques.

ANATOMY[12, 19, 45]

The thymus is relatively large at birth and continues to grow rapidly thereafter, reaching its maximum size before sexual maturity, or between the fourth and fifth postnatal months. It then begins to involute, probably under the influence of adrenal corticoste-roids. Initially, the process of involution is rapid and the gland is replaced by fat as it decreases in size and loses its lymphoid structure. It does not, however, disappear completely, as remnants are visible histologically, even in old age.

The canine and feline thymus share many gross and microscopic features. The thymus lies cranioventrally in the thoracic cavity, enclosed in the precardial mediastinal septum. It extends from the thoracic inlet in the dog and from 1 cm cranial to the first rib in the cat to approximately the fifth rib in both species. It is divided into left and right lobes, the left of which is slightly larger. The lobes are separated by connective tissue, although they appear to be fused cranially on gross examination. Slightly cranial to the anterior border of the heart the lobes divide, the left lobe extending further caudally than the right lobe and lying between the thoracic wall and the left ventricle (Fig. 87–1). The thymus is contiguous with the phrenic nerve, the cranial vena cava, and the trachea. In addition, when the thymus reaches its maximum size, lateral impressions on the gland are caused by the cranial lung lobes. The major blood supply to each lobe is from the ipsilateral internal thoracic artery via one or two thymic

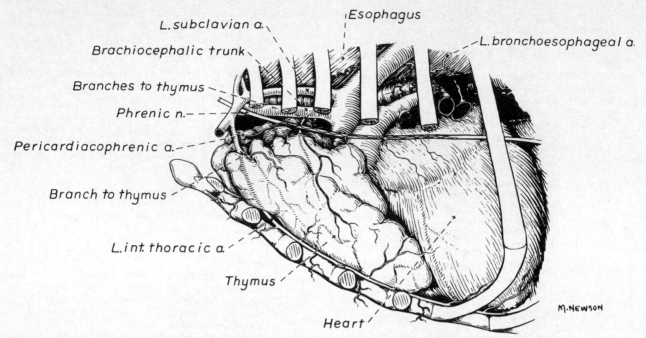

Figure 87–1. Anatomy of the thymus gland in a young dog, showing its blood supply. (Reprinted with permission from Evans, H. G., and Christensen, G. C.: *Miller's Anatomy of the Dog.* 2nd ed. W. B. Saunders, Philadelphia, 1979.)

branches. From a surgical standpoint, the internal thoracic arteries are closely associated with the cranioventral portion of the thymus and are often embedded in the glandular parenchyma. Occasionally, an additional thymic branch leaves the brachiocephalic artery on the right side and/or the subclavian artery on the left side. Thymic veins parallel the arteries. Lymph drains via four to six vessels that empty into the cranial mediastinal and sternal lymph nodes. The thymus has both sympathetic and parasympathetic (vagal) innervation.

HISTOLOGY[26, 41]

The thymus consists of an epithelial network derived from the endoderm of the third and fourth pharyngeal pouches intermeshed with lymphoid cells of bone marrow origin. Anatomically, the thymus is divided into an outer cortex, an inner cortex, and a medulla, all of which are contained within a thymic capsule consisting of one to two layers of fibroblasts. Delicate fibrous septae extend from the capsule into the parenchyma, often accompanied by small arteries, arterioles, capillaries, and veins. The supporting matrix of the thymus is formed by anastomosing cords of epithelial cells and their basement membranes. The outer cortex consists of a high proportion of large lymphocytes and epithelial-reticular cells, whereas the inner cortex consists of medium and small lymphocytes. The medulla consists of epithelial cells and fewer lymphocytes than the cortex. The medulla also contains Hassall's corpuscles—concentrically arranged degenerating, keratinized epithelial cells. Eosinophils, mast cells, neutrophils, and macrophages

may be found throughout the thymus, most commonly in perivascular locations.

Lymphocytes move gradually from the cortex to the medulla and on to the blood stream and peripheral lymph nodes ("peripheralization" in the fetus). This movement is associated with maturation and takes place under the influence of humoral factors produced by thymic epithelial cells (see Chapter 15).

PHYSIOLOGY

The major contribution of the thymus to the animal is its influence on the maturation of undifferentiated lymphocytes of bone marrow origin into mature, functioning "thymus-derived lymphocytes" (T cells). A normal, functioning thymus gland is necessary for the development and regulation of cell-mediated immunity. The development and maturation of B lymphocytes (bursa-dependent, responsible for humoral immunity) are relatively independent of the thymus, but their activity is regulated by subpopulations of T cells (helper or suppressor cells) (see Chapter 15).

The exact cellular or molecular mechanism by which the thymus influences the maturation of T cells is not known. It has been shown that precursor cells acquire specific, defined antigens and functions during their differentiation in the thymus.[6] This maturation is probably due to interaction with a polypeptide(s) produced by thymic epithelial cells. In addition, thymic hormones may modify T cell function in sites far removed from the thymus. Thymosin is a major thymic hormone that enhances the response of mouse thymocytes and lymph node cells to T cell mitogens and allogeneic spleen cells *in vitro* and *in vivo*.[23] Thymosin administration has also increased both the percentage and absolute number of E-rosette–forming cells (T cells that bind to certain erythrocytes) in the peripheral blood of human patients with immunodeficiency and autoimmune diseases (e.g., thymic hypoplasia and systemic lupus erythematosus) but not of those from normal individuals.[23] In addition, thymosin has augmented cell-mediated immunity in human beings with thymic hypoplasia, combined immunodeficiency disease, and terminal neoplasia.[24] Other thymic factors include thymin I and II[25]; thymic humoral factor and circulating thymic factor, which act similarly to thymosin[5]; lymphocyte-stimulating hormone[34]; and homeostatic thymus hormone, a glycopeptide that acts antagonistically toward ACTH, TSH, thyroxine, and gonadotropins but synergistically with growth hormone.[10] It is not clear whether these factors are really different hormones or various molecular forms of the same hormone with different effects.

The effect of thymectomy on the host seems to depend on the state of immunological development at the time of thymectomy.[15] For example, in rodents, in which thymic and lymphoid development is incomplete at birth, neonatal thymectomy leads to impairment of T cell functions associated with a wasting disease syndrome. In contrast, in several species in which thymic and lymphoid development is advanced before birth (e.g., the ox, dog, cat, sheep and pig), adverse effects have not been associated with early postnatal thymectomy.[15, 28]

Peripheralization of thymus-derived lymphocytes occurs by about the fortieth day of gestation in the cat[1] and by the forty-eighth day in the dog.[31] In contrast to the minimal effect of thymectomy on the neonatal dog, thymectomy of a 48-day-old canine fetus produces defective cell-mediated immunity when measured at birth and at 75 days post partum.[15] Adult thymectomy in all species does not affect the immune system severely, but there is evidence in mice indicating a decrease in most T cell functions measured from one month to one year after adult thymectomy.[5]

The thymus is also intimately involved in a network of immune-neuroendocrine interactions.[7, 44] These interactions are bidirectional and affect the development of both systems.

PATHOPHYSIOLOGY

Aplasia or *hypoplasia* of the human thymus generally occurs as part of a general embryopathy of the third and fourth pharyngeal pouches.[8] There is a decrease in the number of T cells, and both humoral and, particularly, cellular immunity are impaired. Associated problems include hypoparathyroidism, abnormal facies, and cardiovascular abnormalities. Hypoplasia of the human thymus is termed DiGeorge

syndrome; a corresponding condition has not been reported in the dog or cat.

Thymic atrophy of unknown etiology has been reported in seven of eight members of a litter of Weimaraner pups.[48] Each affected pup had a small thymus with a marked absence of thymic cortex, normal humoral immunity, normal white blood cell count, histologically normal peripheral lymphoid tissue, and decreased thymus-dependent cell-mediated immunity. Two of eight pups developed a wasting syndrome, which responded to thymosin treatment, and all had a decreased growth hormone response to clonidine HCl stimulation. Thymic atrophy may occur in dogs as a consequence of infection with canine distemper virus or parvovirus.[22, 47] Multiple, small cysts lined with ciliated columnar epithelium, probably remnants of the branchial pouch, have also been described in dogs.[29]

Atrophy of the thymus and depletion of other lymphoid tissues have been described in cats infected with feline leukemia virus post partum.[2] Most affected kittens were runts, and several had concurrent infections. Also of interest was an increased susceptibility to alimentary lymphosarcoma and lymphoblastic leukemia. Thymic atrophy has also been reported in association with feline panleukopenia virus infection.[2]

Myasthenia Gravis and the Thymus

Acquired myasthenia gravis is a neuromuscular disorder manifested by weakness of voluntary (skeletal) muscles.[17] Myasthenia gravis is associated with an antibody-mediated autoimmune response to the acetylcholine receptor that results in a decreased sensitivity of the postsynaptic membrane to the neurotransmitter acetylcholine.[55] Congenital myasthenia gravis is not discussed here, since it is not associated with thymic disorders or autoantibody. Congenital myasthenia gravis is due to a primary lack of acetylcholine receptors in the dog.[32] Approximately 75 per cent of humans with acquired myasthenia gravis have thymic abnormalities. Of these, 85 per cent show hyperplasia and 15 per cent show gross or microscopic thymomas.[17] Human thymic lymphocytes[21] and thymic myoid cells of many species display cell-surface markers that may crossreact with antigenic determinants on the acetylcholine receptor.[53] In addition, there is evidence that thymus from humans with myasthenia may contain thymocyte-bound, acetylcholine receptor–like material and/or receptor-specific helper T cells that can augment receptor-specific antibody production by peripheral lymphocytes.[39] These findings suggest that a dysfunction of immunoregulation exists in myasthenia gravis. One hypothesis is that there is a deficiency of suppressor T cells specific for acetylcholine receptors, which would normally suppress the autoimmune response. Another possibility, perhaps related to the first, is an increased production of helper T cells that promote the synthesis of antibodies to acetylcholine receptors. Irrespective of the precise mechanism, about 50 per cent of human myasthenics are aided by thymectomy.[3] Anticholinesterases, glucocorticosteroids, immunosuppressive therapy, and plasmapheresis (presumably by removal of autoantibody) also are clinically beneficial.[3, 14] Although 4 of 31 dogs with acquired myasthenia gravis also had a thymoma,[20, 30, 42] the nature and degree of the association of thymic abnormalities with myasthenia gravis in the

dog and cat are not well defined. Likewise, there are insufficient data to determine the efficacy of thymectomy in the treatment of myasthenia gravis in the dog and cat.

Thymomas occur with or without an associated paraneoplastic syndrome, which in human beings may include myasthenia gravis, polymyositis, hypogammaglobulinemia, eosinopenia, anemia, disorders of cell-mediated immunity, and an increased frequency of other tumors.[8, 49] The prevalence of associated paraneoplastic syndromes in human thymoma

TABLE 87–1. Thymomas in Dogs

Case No.	Reference No.	Breed	Age (yrs)	Clinical Findings	Other Findings
1	13	Labrador retriever	5	Salivation, weight loss	Megaesophagus, myasthenia gravis
2	13	Mixed	12	N/A*	Megaesophagus
3	20	German shepherd	6	Weakness, dyspnea	Myasthenia gravis
4	27	Labrador cross	6	Weakness, dyspnea	Megaesophagus, myasthenia gravis
5	36	Dachshund	13	Dyspnea	
6		Niederlaufhund	15	Dyspnea, coughing	
7	38	Old English sheepdog	8	Depression, dysphagia	Thymoma in esophagus
8	46	Wire-haired terrier	8	Dyspnea, coughing	
9	50	Mixed	8	Dyspnea	
10	51	German shepherd cross	10	Dyspnea, weight loss	
11	54	Boxer	6	Dyspnea, weight loss	
12	4	Labrador retriever	3	Lethargy, dysphagia	
13	4	Collie	12	Forelimb edema	Mammary adenocarcinoma
14	4	Doberman Pinscher	6	Dyspnea, weight loss	Myasthenia gravis, megaesophagus, lymphoma
15	4	Beagle cross	7	Lethargy, weight loss	
16	4	Great Dane	5	Weakness, myositis	Megaesophagus, myasthenia gravis
17	4	Labrador retriever	11	Vomiting	Adenocarcinoma
18	4	Poodle cross	11	Weakness	Megaesophagus, myasthenia gravis
19	4	Golden retriever	10	Aspiration pneumonia, dyspnea, weight loss	Megaesophagus, myasthenia gravis, myositis
20	4	German shepherd	9	Forelimb edema, dyspnea, pleural effusion	
21	4	Basset hound	10	Pleural effusion, dyspnea, coughing	Pheochromocytoma
22	4	Golden retriever	9	Pneumonia, weakness, coughing	Myasthenia gravis
23	4	Collie cross	13		Myasthenia gravis
24	4	Labrador retriever	9	Weight loss	
25	4	Border collie	7		
26	43	German shepherd	10	N/A	
27	43	German shepherd	8	N/A	
28	43	German shepherd	8	N/A	
29	43	German shepherd	10	N/A	
30	43	German shepherd	8	N/A	
31	43	German shepherd	14	N/A	
32	32	German shepherd	7	N/A	Megaesophagus, myasthenia gravis

*Not available.

TABLE 87–2. Thymomas in Cats

Case No.	Reference No.	Breed	Age (yrs)	Clinical Findings	Other Findings
1	9	Siamese	18	Coughing, pleural effusion	
2	9	DSH*	N/A†	Lethargy, weakness	Myositis, myocarditis
3	9	DSH	N/A	Lethargy, weakness	Myositis, myocarditis
4	9	DSH	8		Dermatitis
5	9	DSH	N/A	Lethargy, weakness	Myositis
6	9	DSH	N/A	Dyspnea, pleural effusion	
7	9	DSH	N/A	Dyspnea, pleural effusion	
8	9	DSH	N/A	Dyspnea, pleural effusion	
9	9	DHS	N/A	Dyspnea	Diabetes mellitus
10	9	DSH	N/A	Dyspnea	
11	9	DSH	N/A		
12	18	DSH	11	Dyspnea	
13	13	DSH	11	Dyspnea	
14	33	Siamese	6	Anorexia, dermatitis	
15	56	Siamese	10	Dyspnea, pleural effusion	
16	56	DSH	N/A	Cough, pleural effusion	
17	11	N/A	N/A		
18	36	DSH	9	Dyspnea, pleural effusion	
19	36	DSH	8	Dyspnea, cough	

*Domestic short-haired cat.
†Not available.

patients is 71 per cent with myasthenia gravis occurring in 44 per cent.[49] Some of the previously mentioned paraneoplastic disorders have been described in case reports of dogs and cats with thymomas. A summary of 32 dogs with thymoma (Table 87–1) indicates that 31 per cent had myasthenia gravis, 10 per cent had myositis, and 13 per cent had other tumors. Of 19 cats with thymoma (Table 87–2), one had reduced esophageal motility, three had myositis, and one had hypogammaglobulinemia.[9] Megaesophagus was present in eight dogs and one cat with thymomas and was almost always accompanied by signs of myasthenia gravis. In another study, 11 of 14 dogs with acquired myasthenia gravis had documented megaesophagus.[32] The most logical explanation for this finding is that the canine esophagus contains striated muscle throughout its length,[19] which is affected by myasthenia. Megaesophagus may be present and may cause clinical signs before generalized muscular weakness is noted.

SURGICAL DISORDERS

In general, the only surgical disorder of the canine or feline thymus is the thymoma.* Although thymectomy is employed routinely to treat human myasthenia gravis at certain medical centers,[40] it is not often performed in animals for that purpose. Neonatal or intrauterine thymectomy of dogs and cats has been employed in immunological research.[15, 16, 52]

Thymoma

Thymomas are tumors composed of both thymic epithelial cells and lymphocytes in varying proportions. Although both cell types are present, epithelial cells are the essential neoplastic component.[37]

The prevalence of thymoma in the dog and cat is low. To the best of our knowledge, only 32 dogs and 19 cats with thymomas have been reported. The dogs were all members of medium to large breeds (see Table 87–1) and ranged in age from 3 to 15 years (average 8.9 years). The male:female ratio was 1:1. Cats ranged in age from 6 to 18 years (average 10 years) with a male:female ratio of 11:1 (see Table 87–2).

Clinical Signs. Dogs and cats with thymomas demonstrate a wide variety of clinical signs. Thymomas may be clinically silent and found only incidentally at necropsy or after routine chest radiography. When clinical signs are present they may be due to the space-occupying nature of the mass (dyspnea, coughing, muffled heart sounds, forelimb edema, and pleural effusion in the cat) or an associated paraneoplastic syndrome (e.g., muscle weakness and megaesophagus). Nonspecific signs include depression, lethargy, weight loss, and vomiting. In a recent series of 14 canine thymomas, 6 dogs had neurological signs (skeletal weakness, megaesophagus, and a decremen-

---

*The occurrence of branchial cysts of the thymus recently has been reported in 15 dogs and two cats.[57] These cysts arise from vestiges of fetal structures, most likely the branchial duct II, pharyngobranchial duct II, and cervical vesicle. The main clinical sign was dyspnea, and radiographic signs included pleural effusion and a cranial mediastinal mass. The most consistent histopathological finding was multiple cysts embedded in a stroma of fibrous connective tissue, adipose tissue, and vessels. Thoracotomy and resection were performed on seven dogs; three survived at least 18 months.

tal electromyographic response) compatible with myasthenia gravis.[4] In four of these six dogs, the diagnosis of myasthenia was confirmed by administration of an anticholinesterase (edrophonium chloride), which ameliorated the signs. It should be noted that megaesophagus, dysphagia, and increased salivation may occur without generalized skeletal muscle weakness. Three of 11 cats[9] had myositis and/or megaesophagus, but the diagnosis of myasthenia was not confirmed with cholinesterase inhibitors. Muscular weakness and, particularly, megaesophagus predispose to vomiting or regurgitation and subsequent aspiration pneumonia, which can complicate both the diagnosis and treatment.

Laboratory Findings. The laboratory findings in animals with thymoma have been either unremarkable or due to secondary problems such as aspiration pneumonia. Radiographically, an anterior mediastinal mass of varying size is present. A definitive diagnosis is made by aspiration or incisional or excisional biopsy. A careful evaluation of the biopsy material must be made because the admixture of epithelial cells and lymphocytes varies considerably from one area to another and a mistaken diagnosis of thymic lymphosarcoma is possible (particularly in the cat). The absence of lymphoid neoplasia in adjacent lymph nodes or elsewhere is an important differentiating factor, as is the mature appearance of the lymphocytes in thymoma compared with that of thymic lymphosarcoma. The histological appearance of the tumor is of little help in determining malignancy; cells are usually slightly anaplastic and mitotic figures are uncommon.[37] The histological appearance of thymomas that recur or metastasize does not differ significantly from that of benign thymomas, with rare exceptions.[4, 43]

Diagnosis. A presumptive diagnosis of thymoma is indicated by the presence of myasthenic signs and/or megaesophagus and an anterior mediastinal mass. Thymic lymphosarcoma, tumors of the aortic body or ectopic thyroid tissue, and cranial mediastinal metastases from carcinomas[37] must be ruled out. Of the 32 known reported canine thymomas, one metastasized to multiple distant sites[43] (lungs, spleen, liver, diaphragm, bronchial and mediastinal lymph nodes, and pericardium) and two invaded adjacent structures (anterior vena cava, pleura).[4, 27]

Therapy. Because of the small number of thymomas reported, it is difficult to recommend a course of therapy. In two dogs, thymomas were diagnosed by biopsy during exploratory thoracotomy; the mass was not resected and chemotherapy (vincristine, cytoxan, adriamycin) was administered for two to three months.[4] Unfortunately, both dogs were lost to follow-up. Thymectomies were attempted in three dogs; one died intraoperatively, one died after surgical correction of gastric dilatation/volvulus that occurred two days after the thoracotomy, and one survived the surgery only to have the tumor recur after four months. A thymectomy was performed on one cat after diagnosis of a thymoma by aspiration biopsy.

The tumor recurred two months postoperatively and was treated with cytosine arabinoside, cyclophosphamide, vincristine and prednisone. Chemotherapy eliminated the clinical signs, and the cat was reported to be improved one year later.[56] Thymectomy with follow-up chemotherapy is the most rational approach. The prognosis in cases of thymoma is guarded to poor. Since anticholinesterases, glucocorticosteroids, immunosuppressive therapy, and plasmapheresis are beneficial in humans with thymoma and myasthenia, they may be considered in dogs and cats with myasthenia gravis and thymoma.

Thymectomy—Thymoma

Preoperative evaluation includes a complete blood count, routine blood chemistry, and thoracic radiographs. Most affected animals are middle-aged to old individuals and thus are prone to multisystemic problems. The animal should be examined thoroughly for concurrent tumors that may affect treatment and prognosis. Megaesophagus, if present, predisposes to aspiration pneumonia, especially during and after surgery.

A thymoma is best approached through a left or right third intercostal space thoracotomy, depending on the location of the thymoma. A sternal splitting approach also may be used if the tumor is extensive.

Thymomas are quite friable and vascular. Often, they surround the cranial vena cava, from which they must be dissected with great care. Extensive hemorrhage may occur, so crossmatched blood should be available for immediate transfusion. Hemorrhage results from tearing of the tumor and its blood supply and from adherent pleural surfaces. Hemostatic clips have been used to facilitate hemostasis. Because of the friable nature of the tumor, it is extremely difficult to remove without seeding the thoracic cavity with tumor cells. This seeding probably accounts for many of the recurrences noted clinically and is an indication for postoperative chemotherapy. Pre- and postoperative antibiotics are given at the discretion of the surgeon. Aftercare and complications are those of any thoracic surgical procedure. If present, signs of myasthenia gravis should gradually recede after thymectomy, sometimes requiring several months to regress completely.

1. Ackerman, G. A.: Developmental relationship between the appearance of lymphocytes and lymphopoietic activity in the thymus and lymph nodes in the fetal cat. Anat. Rec. *158*:387, 1967.
2. Anderson, L. J., Jarrett, W. F. H., Jarrett, O., and Laird, H. M.: Feline leukemiavirus infection of kittens: Mortality associated with atrophy of the thymus and lymphoid depletion. J. Nat. Canc. Inst. *47*:807, 1971.
3. Arnason, B. G.: Myasthenia gravis. *In* Parker, C. W. (ed.): *Clinical Immunology.* W. B. Saunders, Philadelphia, 1980, pp. 1088–1105.
4. Aronsohn, M., Stevenson, S., Schunk, K., and Carpenter, J.: Thymoma in the dog. Submitted to the J. Am. Vet. Med. Assoc., 1984.

5. Bach, J. F.: The mode of action of thymic hormones and its relevance to T-cell differentiation. Trans. Proc. 8:243, 1976.

6. Bach, J. F.: Thymic hormones: Biochemistry, biological, and clinical activities. Ann. Rev. Toxicol. 17:281, 1977.

7. Besedovsky, H., and Sorkin, E.: Network of immune-neuroendocrine interactions. Clin. Exp. Immunol. 27:1, 1977.

8. Blaese, R. M.: T and B cell immuno-deficiency diseases. *In* Parker, C. W. (ed.): *Clinical Immunology*. W. B. Saunders, Philadelphia, 1980, pp. 334–336.

9. Carpenter, J. L., and Holzworth, J.: Thymoma in eleven cats. J. Am. Vet. Med. Assoc. 180:248, 1982.

10. Comsa, J.: Homeostatic thymic hormone. *In* Luckey, T. D. (ed.): *Thymic Hormones*. University Park Press, Baltimore, 1973.

11. Cotchin, E.: Neoplasms in cats. Proc. Roy. Soc. Med. 45:671, 1952.

12. Crouch, J. E.: *Text-Atlas of Cat Anatomy*. Lea and Febiger, Philadelphia, 1969, pp. 260–262.

13. Darke, P. G. G., McCullagh, K. G., and Geldart, P. H.: Myasthenia gravis, thymoma and myositis in a dog. Vet. Rec. 97:392, 1975.

14. Dau, P. C., Lindstrom, J. H., Cassel, C. K., Denys, E. H., Shen, E. E., and Spitler, L. E.: Plasmapheresis and immuno-suppressive drug therapy in myasthenia gravis. N. Engl. J. Med. 297:1134, 1977.

15. Dennis, R. A., Jacoby, R. O., and Griesemer, R. A.: Intra-uterine techniques for studying development of the immune response of the fetal dog. Lab. Anim. Care 18:561, 1968.

16. Dixit, S. P., and Coppola, E. D.: Intrauterine thymectomy in the canine fetus. Can. J. Surg. 13:170, 1970.

17. Drachman, D. B.: Myasthenia gravis. N. Engl. J. Med. 298:136, 186, 1978.

18. Dubielzig, R. R., and DeLaney, R. G.: A thymoma in a cat. Vet. Med./Sm. Anim. Clin. 75:1270, 1980.

19. Evans, H. F., and Christensen, G. C.: *Miller's Anatomy of the Dog*, 2nd ed. W. B. Saunders, Philadelphia, 1979, pp. 838–40.

20. Fraser, D. C., Palmer, A. C., Senior, J. E. B., Parkes, J. D., et al.: Myasthenia gravis in the dog. J. Neurol. Neurosurg. Psychiat. 33:431, 1970.

21. Fuchs, S., Schmidt-Hopfeld, I., Tridente, G., and Tarral-Haydai, R.: Thymic lymphocytes bear a surface antigen which cross-reacts with acetylcholine receptor. Nature 287:162, 1980.

22. Gibson, J. P., Griesemer, R. A., and Koestner, A.: Experimental distemper in the gnotobiotic dog. Pathol. Vet. 2:1, 1965.

23. Goldstein, A. L., Cohen, G. H., Rossio, J. L., Thurman, G. B., et al.: Use of thymosin in treatment of primary immunodeficiency diseases and cancer. Med. Clin. North Am. 60:591, 1976.

24. Goldstein, A. L., Thurman, G. B., Cohen, G. H., and Rossio, J. L.: The endocrine thymus: Potential role for thymosin in the treatment of autoimmune disease. Ann. N.Y. Acad. Sci. 244:390, 1976.

25. Goldstein, G.: Isolation of bovine thymin: A polypeptide hormone of the thymus. Nature 247:11, 1974.

26. Gorgollon, P., and Ottone-Anaya, M.: Fine structure of canine thymus. Acta Anat. 100:136, 1978.

27. Hall, G. A., Howell, J. McC., and Lewis, D. G.: Thymoma with myasthenia gravis in a dog. J. Pathol. 108:177, 1972.

28. Hoover, E. A., Krakowka, S., Cockerell, G. L., and Olsen, R. G.: Thymectomy in preweanling kittens: Technique and immunologic consequences. Am. J. Vet. Res. 39:99, 1978.

29. Jubb, K. V. F., and Kennedy, P. C.: *Pathology of Domestic Animals*, 2nd ed. Academic Press, New York, 1970, pp. 366–367.

30. Kelly, M.: Myasthenia gravis—a receptor disease. Comp. Cont. Ed. Pract. Vet. 3:544, 1981.

31. Kelly, W. D.: The thymus and lymphoid morphogenesis in the dog. Fed. Proc. 22:600, 1963.

32. Lennon, V. A., Lambert, E. H., Palmer, A. C., et al.: Acquired and congenital myasthenia gravis in dogs—A study of 20 cases. *In* Japan Medical Research Foundation (ed.): *Myasthenia Gravis. Pathogenesis and Treatment*. University of Tokyo Press, Tokyo, 1981.

33. Loveday, R. K.: Thymoma in a Siamese cat. J. S. Afr. Vet. Med. Assoc. 30:33, 1959.

34. Luckey, T. D.: Lymphocyte-stimulating hormone. *In* Luckey, T. D. (ed.): *Thymic Hormones*. University Park Press, Baltimore, 1973.

35. Mackey, L.: Clear-cell thymoma and thymic hyperplasia in a cat. J. Comp. Pathol. 85:367, 1975.

36. Mettler, F.: Thymome bei Hund und Katze. Schweiz. Arch. Tierheilk. 117:577, 1975.

37. Moulton, J. E., and Dungworth, D. L.: Tumors of the lymphoid and hemopoietic tissues. *In* Moulton, J. E. (ed.): *Tumors in Domestic Animals*. University of California Press, Berkeley, 1978, pp. 177–178.

38. McNeil, P. H.: A thymoma as a cause of oesophageal obstruction in a dog. N.Z. Vet. J. 28:143, 1980.

39. Newsom-Davis, J., Willcox, N., and Calder, L.: Thymus cells in myasthenia gravis selectively enhance production of anti-acetylcholine-receptor antibody by autologous blood lymphocytes. N. Engl. J. Med. 305:1313, 1981.

40. Olanow, C. W., Wechsler, A. S., and Roses, A. D.: A prospective study of thymectomy and serum acetylcholine receptor antibodies in myasthenia gravis. Ann. Surg. 196:113, 1982.

41. Pack, F. D., and Chapman, W. L.: Light and electron microscopic evaluations of thymuses from feline leukemia virus-infected kittens. Exp. Pathol. 18:96, 1980.

42. Palmer, A. C., and Barker, J.: Myasthenia in the dog. Vet. Rec. 95:452, 1974.

43. Parker, G. A., and Casey, H. W.: Thymomas in domestic animals. Vet. Pathol. 13:353, 1976.

44. Pierpaoli, W., Kopp, H. G., Mueller, J., and Keller, M.: Interdependence between neuroendocrine programming and the generation of immune recognition in ontogeny. Cell. Immunol. 29:16, 1977.

45. Reichard, J., and Jennings, H. S.: *Anatomy of the Cat*. Henry Holt and Co., New York, 1935, p. 254.

46. Robinson, M.: Malignant thymoma with metastases in a dog. Vet. Pathol. 11:172, 1974.

47. Robinson, W. F., Wilcox, G. E., and Flower, R. L. P.: Canine parvoviral disease: Experimental reproduction of the enteric form with a parvovirus isolated from a case of myocarditis. Vet. Pathol. 17:589, 1980.

48. Roth, J. A., Lomax, L. G., Hampshire, J., Kaeberle, M. L., et al.: Thymic abnormalities and growth hormone deficiency in dogs. Am. J. Vet. Res. 41:1256, 1980.

49. Souadjian, J. V., Enriquez, P., Silverstein, M. N., and Pepin, J.: The spectrum of disease associated with thymoma. Arch. Intern. Med. 134:374, 1974.

50. Swalley, J.: Thymoma and food-bolus choke in a dog. Vet. Med./Sm. Anim. Clin. 76:347, 1981.

51. Talerman, A., and Gwynn, R.: Epithelial thymoma in a dog. J. Pathol. 101:62, 1970.

52. Tilney, N. L., and Economou, S. G.: The technique of transternal thymectomy in the puppy. Transplantation 8:79, 1969.

53. Van de Velde, R. L., and Friedman, N. B.: Thymic myoid cells and myasthenia gravis. Am. J. Pathol., 59:347, 1970.

54. Watson, A. D., and Farrow, B. R. H.: True thymoma in a dog: A case report. Vet. Rec. 89:460, 1971.

55. Weiner, H. L., and Hauser, S. L.: Neuroimmunology I: Immunoregulation in neurological disease. Ann. Neurol. 11:437, 1982.

56. Willard, M. D., Tvedten, H., Walshaw, R., and Aronson, E.: Thymoma in a cat. J. Am. Vet. Med. Assoc. 176:451, 1980.

57. Liv, S. K., Patnaik, A. K., and Burk, R. L.: Thymic branchial cysts in the dog and cat. J. Am. Vet. Med. Assoc. 182:1095, 1983.

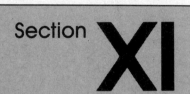

Section **XI**

Nervous System

Stephen T. Simpson
Section Editor

Chapter 88

Anatomy and Physiology

Stephen T. Simpson

The nervous system enables an organism to perceive its internal and external environment, analyze all sensory information, and, through other functional organs, perform necessary adjustments to maintain homeostasis. The various sensory systems are constantly sampling the internal and external environment and sending that information centripetally to different levels of the central nervous system (CNS). At each level, there is a degree of assimilation and processing of the accumulated information. When processing is completed, an appropriate response is initiated. The response occurs within the CNS, and its effects are observed through skeletal muscle, smooth muscle, cardiac muscle, or glands. The responses that occur may be initiated at spinal cord levels, as in spinal reflexes; at brain stem levels, as in respiratory regulation; or at cerebral levels, as in an animal's response to environmental changes.

GENERAL STRUCTURE AND FUNCTION

The neuron is the functional and structural unit of the nervous system. Its principal function is to conduct nerve impulses from one site to another and affect another neuron, muscle, or gland. Neurons are usually classified in one of the following categories: (1) afferent (sensory) neuron, (2) interneuron, and (3) efferent (motor) neuron (Fig. 88–1).

Axons are neuronal cell processes that conduct an impulse to another site. They are covered with support cells that produce a lipid insulation called myelin. These support cells are Schwann cells in the peripheral nervous system and oligodendroglia in the central nervous system. The myelin insulates nerve fibers and enhances nerve conduction velocities.

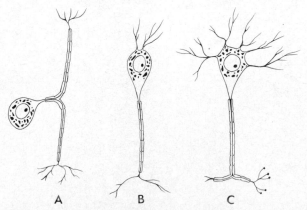

Figure 88–1. Schematic drawing of vertebrate neurons. *A,* Sensory neuron. *B,* Interneuron. *C,* Motor neuron. (Reproduced with permission from Redding, R. W.: Neurological examination. *In:* Hoerlein, B. F. (ed.): *Canine Neurology: Diagnosis and Treatment.* 3rd ed. W. B. Saunders, Philadelphia, 1978.)

Some thinly myelinated or unmyelinated nerve fibers do exist. The myelin sheath allows the axon to conserve energy and facilitates the action potential propagation. Nerve conduction velocity is directly proportional to the amount of myelin around an axon.

Afferent neurons conduct sensory information to the central nervous system. Heavily myelinated sensory fibers conduct such modalities as position sense (proprioception) and light touch. Less myelinated fibers conduct temperature and some pain (nociceptive) information. Other pain responses are conducted by unmyelinated, slow conducting fibers.[12]

Efferent neurons conduct different neural impulses to skeletal muscle, smooth muscle, or glands. Nerves to skeletal muscle are well myelinated, whereas nerves to smooth muscle and glands are unmyelinated nerves.[12]

The motor system consists of two major components, the upper motor neuron (UMN) and the lower motor neuron (LMN). The UMN is a collective set of neurons located in several levels of the brain. The neurons influence one another, and some descend the nervous system to directly or indirectly influence neurons in the spinal cord, cerebellum, or brain stem. The descending neuronal systems are generally considered to constitute the UMN system.

The LMN is a neuronal pool that resides in gray matter nuclei of the brain stem or gray matter cell columns of the spinal cord. The LMN affects an end organ that is skeletal muscle, cardiac or smooth muscle, or a gland. This effect is accomplished by a neurotransmitter at the synapse with the end organ (Fig. 88–2). The chemical transmitter is released by the nerve ending. The transmitter causes an electrical depolarization of the muscle membrane before being destroyed.

The LMN receives afferent information from UMN systems and from the sensory nerves that are continuously sampling sensory information. The LMN and its muscle are known as the motor unit. The motor unit is the motor output mechanism for the entire nervous system. Because of this relationship, the LMN may be considered the final common pathway[18] of the entire nervous system.

SPINAL CORD

A butterfly-shaped column of neurons occupies the central portion of the spinal cord. This column of cells is the gray matter of the spinal cord and is divided into three cell columns: (1) dorsal cell column, (2) ventral cell column, and (3) intermediate

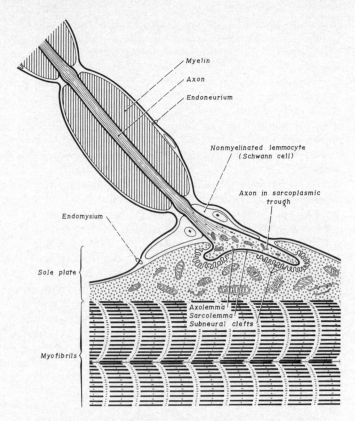

Figure 88–2. Neuromuscular junction of a motor end-plate. (Reprinted with permission from de Lahunta, A.: *Veterinary Neuroanatomy and Clinical Neurology.* W. B. Saunders, Philadelphia, 1977.)

cell column (Fig. 88–3). The dorsal cell column receives dorsal root afferents and is concerned with sensory reception. The ventral cell column contains the LMN for skeletal muscle and is concerned with muscle tone and motor function. The intermediate cell column contains the preganglionic autonomic nerve cells. The thoracolumbar spinal cord segments provide sympathetic innervation, and the sacral spinal cord segments provide parasympathetic innervation. The remaining parasympathetic innervation originates in the brain stem.

The gray matter of the spinal cord is surrounded by the white matter containing the cell processes of both ascending and descending neurons. The white matter is divided into four funiculi (see Fig. 88–3). The ventral half of the white matter contains most of the descending (motor) tracts of the UMN system. Ascending (sensory) tracts largely reside in the dorsal half of the white matter.[4]

Meninges

The spinal cord is ensheathed within three meningeal layers. The outermost and strongest layer is the dura mater. The middle layer is the arachnoid, and the innermost membrane is the pia mater. A potential space exists between the dura mater and the arachnoid. The subarachnoid space contains the cerebrospinal fluid. The pia mater is the most delicate of the three membranes and is tightly adherent to the central nervous system parenchyma. The men-

ingeal coverings provide a protective cushion and part of the blood-brain barrier.

Spinal Cord: Functional Anatomy

The spinal cord has four distinct longitudinal segments: (1) cervical spinal cord (C_1 to C_5), (2) brachial intumescence, or cervicothoracic (C_6 to T_1), (3) thoracolumbar (T_2 to L_3), and (4) lumbosacral intumescence (L_4 to S_3).

The cervical spinal segment gray matter contains the LMN cell bodies to abaxial muscles of the neck, and the white matter contains ascending and descending fiber tracts to all limbs. Contained within the ventral gray column of the brachial intumescence are the LMN cell bodies to the pectoral limb. The cervicothoracic spinal cord also contains the ascend-

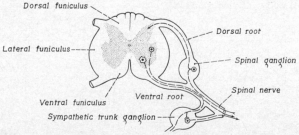

Figure 88–3. Schematic of cross section of the canine spinal cord. (Reprinted with permission from de Lahunta, A.: *Veterinary Neuroanatomy and Clinical Neurology.* W. B. Saunders, Philadelphia, 1977.)

ing and descending fiber tracts to the trunk and pelvic limbs. The thoracolumbar spinal cord contains primarily ascending and descending fiber tracts to the pelvic limbs and the LMN cell bodies to thoracic and lumbar abaxial musculature. The lumbosacral spinal cord provides the neuronal cell bodies for nerves to the pelvic limbs and perineal region. Neurons for bladder and sphincter control are contained here also.

Functionally, the cervical spinal cord can be considered to relay neuronal information rostrally and caudally to affect function in all four limbs. The brachial intumescence provides LMN function to the pectoral limb and relays UMN function to the pelvic limbs. The thoracolumbar spinal cord has little effect on the pectoral limbs and relays the UMN function to the pelvic limbs. It also gives rise to the preganglionic sympathetic neurons to the entire body. The lumbosacral spinal cord provides somatic LMN function to the pelvic limbs and the urethral and anal sphincters and provides parasympathetic neurons to the pelvic viscera.

PERIPHERAL NERVOUS SYSTEM: STRUCTURE

The peripheral nervous system consists of all neurons and cell processes that exist outside the brain or spinal cord. Major components are autonomic ganglia, dorsal root ganglia, all spinal nerves including named appendicular nerves, peripheral cranial nerves, and all dorsal (sensory) and ventral (motor) nerve roots.

BRACHIAL PLEXUS

The nerve supply to the pectoral limb arises from spinal cord segments C_6 through T_2. The brachial plexus is derived from a network formed by the ventral branches of the sixth, seventh, and eighth cervical nerves and the first two thoracic nerves.[1, 7] The nerve root origin and major motor function of each of the major pectoral limb nerves are given in Table 88–1. The rostral portions of the brachial plexus form the nerves for the shoulder muscles and the

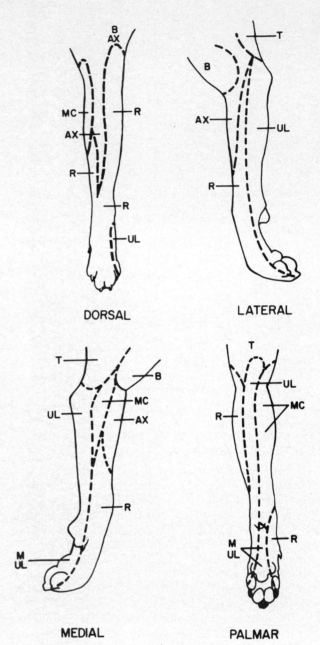

DORSAL   **LATERAL**

MEDIAL   **PALMAR**

Figure 88–4. Peripheral nerve innervation of the skin of the left thoracic limb of the dog. *B,* brachiocephalic; *AX,* axillary; *MC,* musculocutaneous; *R,* radial; *UL,* ulnar; *T,* thoracic roots.

TABLE 88–1. Nerves of the Brachial Plexus, Roots of Origin, and Function of Muscles Innervated

Nerve	Roots of Origin*	Function of Muscles
Suprascapular	C_6, (C_7)	Shoulder extension (supraspinatus)
		Shoulder flexion or extension (infraspinatus)
Subscapular	C_6, (C_7)	Shoulder extension
Axillary	(C_6), C_7, C_8	Shoulder flexion and abduction
Musculocutaneous	(C_6), C_7, C_8	Elbow flexion (biceps brachii and brachialis)
		Shoulder extension and adduction (coracobrachialis)
Radial	C_7, C_8, T_1, T_2	Elbow, carpal, and digital extension
Median	C_8, T_1, (T_2)	Carpal and digital flexion
Ulnar	C_8, T_1, (T_2)	Carpal and digital flexion

*( ) = variable occurrence.

elbow flexors. The caudal brachial plexus innervates the elbow extensor muscles and the carpal flexors and extensors.

The cutaneous sensory distribution of the pectoral limb is different from the motor distribution of this limb. The sensory distribution is illustrated in Figure 88–4. The rostral brachial plexus and other cervical nerves provide sensory function for the craniolateral portion of the brachium and a thin cutaneous strip on the medial surface of the antebrachium to the carpus via the musculocutaneous nerve. The lateral surface of the brachium is innervated by the mid region of the brachial intumescence via the axillary nerve. The caudal portion of the brachium is innervated by the intercostal nerves. The brachial plexus provides sensory innervation to the remainder of the antebrachium but not to the brachium (see Fig. 88–4).

LUMBOSACRAL PLEXUS

Like the brachial plexus, the lumbosacral plexus is the network of nerves from the ventral branches of the last five lumbar nerves and all three sacral nerves. The rostral portion of the lumbosacral plexus provides the innervation for hip flexion, stifle extension, and hip adduction. The caudal lumbosacral plexus provides hip abduction and extension, stifle flexion, and both extension and flexion of the tarsus and digits (Table 88–2).

The cutaneous sensory distribution of the lumbosacral plexus is different from the motor distribution of this plexus. The lateral cutaneous femoral nerve branches from the ventral branch of L_4 where the femoral nerve arises and provides cutaneous sensation to the cranial and lateral aspects of the proximal rear limb. The caudal cutaneous sensation of the proximal pelvic limb is provided by the caudal cutaneous femoral nerve, a branch of the first two sacral spinal nerves.[7] The sensory modalities of the crus are supplied by the peroneal nerve (cranially and crani-

olaterally), the tibial nerve (caudally and caudolaterally), and the saphenous nerve (medially, craniomedially, and caudomedially) (Fig. 88–5). The saphenous nerve is a branch of the femoral nerve (L_4, L_5).[7] Considerable overlap in cutaneous innervation has been demonstrated in the pectoral and pelvic limbs.[1, 15]

Spinal nerves other than those involved in a plexus provide motor function to abaxial musculature and sensory function to the truncal skin in a dermatomic distribution (Fig. 88–6). The thoracic motor neurons provide LMN function to the intercostal nerves, thereby providing much of the LMN function to the respiratory musculature. The phrenic nerve innervates the diaphragm, providing the remainder of LMN respiratory function.

The autonomic nervous system comprises the sympathetic system of the thoracic, and part of the lumbar, spinal cord and the parasympathetic nervous system of the sacral spinal cord and the cranial nerves. The first three thoracic cord segments provide the sympathetic supply to the head, neck, and eyes. Sympathetic innervation to the eye causes mydriasis, protrusion of the globe to a proper point, and retraction of the lids and the third eyelid.[3] The remaining sympathetic nervous system provides sympathetic function to the viscera, cardiovascular system, and the skin.

The parasympathetic nervous system is represented in the intermediate cell column of the sacral spinal cord. The sacral spinal cord provides parasympathetic autonomic function to the pelvic viscera (bladder and colon) through the pelvic nerves and plexus.

CRANIAL ANATOMY

The brain develops from the rostral end of the neural tube. First, three vesicles are formed that later develop into a five-vesicle brain. The vesicular lumens develop into the ventricular system of the

TABLE 88–2. Nerves of the Lumbosacral Plexus, Roots of Origin, and Function of Muscles Innervated

Nerve	Roots of Origin*	Function of Muscles
Femoral	(L_3), L_4, L_5	Stifle extension Coxofemoral flexion
Obturator	(L_4), L_5, L_6	Coxofemoral adduction
Cranial gluteal	L_6, L_7, S_1	Coxofemoral abduction
Caudal gluteal	L_7, (S_1, S_2)	Coxofemoral extension
Sciatic	L_6, L_7, S_1	Stifle flexion Coxofemoral extension
Peroneal	L_6, L_7, S_1	Hock flexion Digital extension
Tibial	L_6, L_7, S_1	Hock extension Digital flexion
Pudendal	S_1, S_2, (S_3)	Anal and external urethral sphincters

*( ) = variable occurrence.

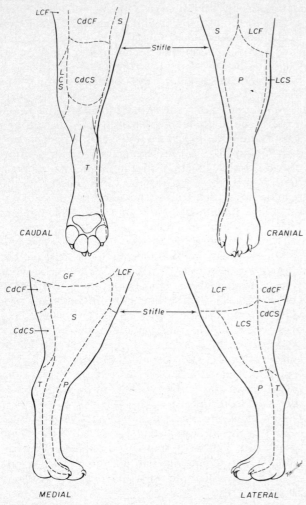

Figure 88–5. Peripheral nerve innervation of the skin of the left pelvic limb of the dog. *CdCF*, Caudal cutaneous femoral; *CdCS*, caudal cutaneous sural; *GF*, genitofemoral; *LCF*, lateral cutaneous femoral; *LCS*, lateral cutaneous sural; *P*, peroneal; *S*, saphenous; *T*, tibial. (Reprinted with permission from Evans, H. D., and de Lahunta, A.: *Miller's Guide to the Dissection of the Dog.* 2nd ed. W. B. Saunders, Philadelphia, 1980.)

brain. Table 88–3 outlines vesicle and ventricular development.

The rhombencephalon develops closest to the spinal cord. It is also called the hindbrain, and its final structures occupy the floor of the caudal fossa of the skull. The medulla develops most caudally and the pons more rostrally. The cerebellum develops later in gestation from cells that originate in the pons. The fourth ventricle develops from the lumen of the rhombencephalon. Cranial nerves 5 through 12 are associated with the rhombencephalon.

The rhombencephalic structures supply motor function and coordination. Several nuclei of the extrapyramidal UMN system reside in this area. Generally, motor function of tracts originating in the medulla or pons affect ipsilateral motor activity.[2, 4] In addition, vestibular function is centered in the pons and medulla, and damage to the caudal brain stem usually causes some vestibular signs. Cardiovascular and respiratory regulatory centers as well as other visceral reflex centers are located in the reticular substance of the medulla and pons.

The cerebellum develops from a dorsal outcropping in the pons.[5] By receiving motor signals from UMN structures and current afferent input from proprioceptive and vestibular systems, the cerebellum coordinates the ultimate motor output of the brain. The cerebellum generally functions to inhibit most motor activity. By this modulating, the movements become smooth and fluid and more functional. Damage or disease to the cerebellum usually produces exaggerated motor movements, excessive muscle tone, and a characteristic tremor (see Chapter 89).

The mesencephalon, or midbrain, develops into a cylindrical shape. The mesencephalic aqueduct connects the third ventricle with the fourth ventricle. The midbrain has three layers: (1) the tectum (roof), (2) tegmentum (body), and (3) basis (floor). The tectum of the midbrain serves as an auditory and visual reflex center. The tegmentum contains the nerve cell bodies of the third and fourth cranial nerves. The reticular formation of the midbrain is responsible for maintaining consciousness and attention via the reticular activating system.[13] Significant lesions within the reticular formation of the midbrain cause loss of consciousness (coma). The primary motor function at this level is represented largely by the red nucleus. The rubrospinal tract originates in the midbrain, decussates immediately, and descends as an extensor inhibitor. Bilateral motor disturbances in the midbrain cause a postural attitude known as decerebrate rigidity. The limbs are maintained in extreme extensor rigidity due to the removal of most extensor inhibition and the continued extensor facilitation from lower brain stem motor nuclei.[14] This is a release phenomenon.

The diencephalon develops from the prosencephalon. It becomes the major relay center for most sensory information. The afferent information, in-

TABLE 88–3. Ventricular Development of the Brain

Three-Vesicle Brain	Five-Vesicle Brain	Related Ventricle
Rhombencephalon	Myelencephalon	Fourth ventricle
	Metencephalon	Fourth ventricle
Mesencephalon	Mesencephalon	Mesencephalic aqueduct
Prosencephalon	Diencephalon	Third ventricle
	Telencephalon	Lateral ventricles

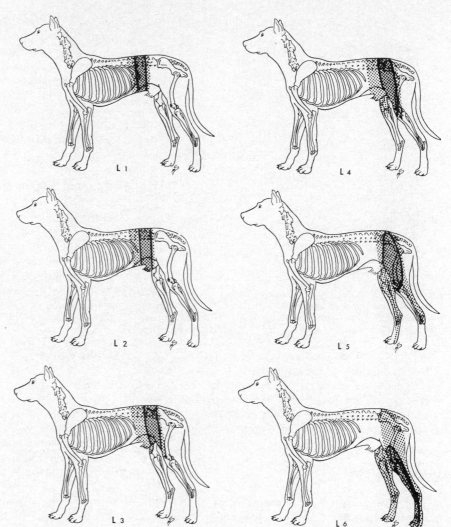

Figure 88–6. Tactile dermatomes relative to skeletal landmarks in the dog. Darker areas represent maximal innervation for the dermatome. (Reprinted with permission from Fletcher, T. F., and Kitchell, R.: The lumbar, sacral, and coccygeal dermatomes of the dog. J. Comp. Neurol. *128*:171, 1966.)

cluding conscious proprioception, enters both specific and nonspecific thalamic nuclei. Some degree of integration occurs at the thalamic level, and the information is relayed to the cerebral cortex. Specific nuclei transfer sensory information to areas of cerebral cortex designated for sensory recognition. Nonspecific nuclei including the reticular activating system project sensory information to several areas of the cerebral cortex.

The hypothalamus is the ventral portion of the diencephalon. The hypothalamus functions to control many visceral and autonomic functions. Among these functions are many neuroendocrine relationships including growth, thyroid, adrenal, reproductive, and other hormones and enkephalins. Body temperature regulation, glucose metabolism, and visceral function, including cardiovascular, respiratory, and gastrointestinal function, are regulated at the hypothalamic level. The rostral portion of the hypothalamus is involved with sympathetic autonomic regulation and the caudal hypothalamus with parasympathetic autonomic regulation.

The diencephalon is connected to the hemispheres of the telencephalon by white matter stria known as the internal capsule. Almost all sensory information is relayed from the thalamus to the cerebrum through the internal capsule. Also, all cerebral output impulses descend to thalamic or lower levels through the internal capsule.

The cerebral cortex is the final development of the telencephalon. The surface of the cerebral cortex of domestic animals is marked by convolutions that allow for a large increase in surface area. The cerebral cortex is regionalized by function (Fig. 88–7). The visual areas are in the caudal and central occipital regions. The temporal regions are primarily involved with audition. Removal of the auditory cortex does not render a dog deaf but may raise the auditory threshold and alter responses to previous auditory conditioning. The motor cortex lies in the frontal area immediately caudal to the cruciate sulcus. The somatosensory cortex lies immediately caudal to the motor cortex. The prefrontal cortex is the rostral pole of the cerebral cortex. Little is known of its major function, but it is involved with memory and social, psychic, and emotional responses. There is a functional connection between olfaction and the prefrontal area via the limbic system.

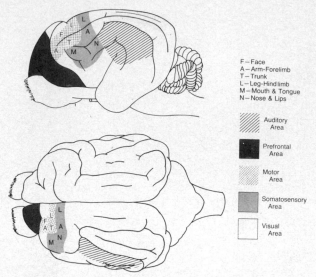

F—Face
A—Arm-Forelimb
T—Trunk
L—Leg-Hindlimb
M—Mouth & Tongue
N—Nose & Lips

Auditory
Area

Prefrontal
Area

Motor
Area

Somatosensory
Area

Visual
Area

Figure 88–7. Motor and sensory areas of the cerebral cortex of the dog. (Reprinted with permission from Redding, R. W.: Neurological examination. *In:* Hoerlein, B. F. (ed.): *Canine Neurology Diagnosis and Treatment.* 3rd ed. W. B. Saunders, Philadelphia, 1978.)

Located deep in the subcortex, the basal nuclei are aggregates of neurons involved in fine motor movement. They are part of the extrapyramidal system. Lesions within the basal nuclei produce paresis, circling movements, and other motor disabilities.

LIMBIC SYSTEM[11, 19]

The limbic system is a neuronal network represented in the cerebral cortex, subcortical structures, and the hypothalamus. Connections with the midbrain are also present. The limbic system, through its connections, provides an animal's basic emotional responses to stimuli. Disease within the limbic system is usually observed by changes in a patient's behavior and seizures. Depending on the portion of limbic system affected, clinical signs may include changes in temperament, eating, drinking, sleeping, or activity level and purposeless movements.

CRANIAL NERVE ANATOMY AND FUNCTION

Olfactory Nerve

The olfactory nerves are exclusively sensory for smell. Chemoreceptors within the olfactory mucosa produce impulses that are transmitted to the olfactory bulbs over numerous bundles of nerves through the cribriform plate.[16]

Optic Nerve

The second cranial nerve, the optic nerve, supplies nerve impulses generated by light. The retina perceives light and transmits the nerve impulses over the optic nerve. The nerve cell body for the optic nerve is in the ganglion cell layer of the retina. The optic nerve forms at the caudal pole of the globe and proceeds through the retrobulbar tissue through the optic foramen (Fig. 88–8) to the optic chiasm. The optic nerve is surrounded by meninges and contains cerebrospinal fluid. At the chiasm most fibers decus-

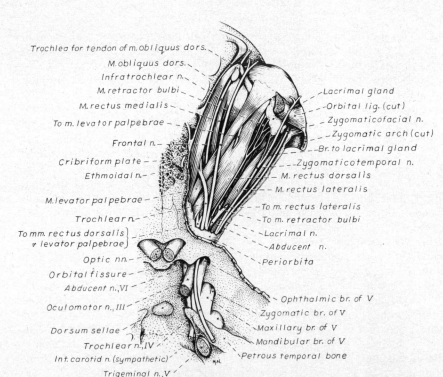

Trochlea for tendon of m. obliquus dors.
M. obliquus dors.
Infratrochlear n.
M. retractor bulbi
M. rectus medialis
To m. levator palpebrae
Frontal n.
Cribriform plate
Ethmoidal n.
M. levator palpebrae
Trochlear n.
To mm. rectus dorsalis
v levator palpebrae
Optic nn.
Orbital fissure
Abducent n., VI
Oculomotor n., III
Dorsum sellae
Trochlear n., IV
Int. carotid n. (sympathetic)
Trigeminal n., V

Lacrimal gland
Orbital lig. (cut)
Zygomaticofacial n.
Zygomatic arch (cut)
Br. to lacrimal gland
Zygomaticotemporal n.
M. rectus dorsalis
M. rectus lateralis
To m. rectus lateralis
To m. retractor bulbi
Lacrimal n.
Abducent n.
Periorbita
Ophthalmic br. of V
Zygomatic br. of V
Maxillary br. of V
Mandibular br. of V
Petrous temporal bone

Figure 88–8. Distribution of the nerves of the eye. Dorsal aspect. (Reprinted with permission from McClure, R. C.: The cranial nerves. *In:* Evans, H. E., and Christensen, G. C. (eds.): *Miller's Anatomy of the Dog.* 2nd ed. W. B. Saunders, Philadelphia, 1979.)

sate and continue to the lateral geniculate as the contralateral optic tract. Some fibers remain ipsilateral.

Oculomotor Nerve

The oculomotor, or third cranial, nerve is the primary motor nerve to the eye. The fibers originate in the midbrain, exit the ventral surface of the midbrain, and course intracranially in a rostral direction within the cavernous sinus. Each nerve exits the cranial cavity through the orbital fissure (see Fig. 88–8) to enter the retrobulbar area within the periorbital fascia. Two types of fibers are contained in the oculomotor nerve. The parasympathetic fibers arise from the parasympathetic nucleus in the midbrain and pass with the oculomotor nerve to the ciliary ganglion immediately behind the caudal pole of the globe. This portion of the nerve supplies the parasympathetic function of pupillary constriction. The somatic nerve fibers arise from a somatic nucleus in the midbrain, pass with the oculomotor nerve, and supply innervation to the dorsal, ventral, and medial rectus muscles and the ventral oblique muscle of the eye.

Trochlear Nerve

The fourth cranial nerve is the trochlear nerve. It is a pure motor nerve and the smallest of all cranial nerves. It originates in the gray matter of the midbrain ventral to the mesencephalic aqueduct. Fibers course in a dorsal direction within the midbrain to leave the midbrain on the dorsal surface, where they decussate in the rostral medullary velum. The trochlear nerve follows the dural reflections and emerges from the cranium through the orbital fissure (see Fig. 88–8) within the periorbital fascia. It functions to rotate the eye on its longitudinal axis so that the dorsum of the eye moves medially.

Trigeminal Nerve

The trigeminal, or fifth cranial, nerve is the thickest of all cranial nerves. It supplies motor function to the muscles of mastication and tactile sensory function for the head from the external auditory canal rostrally. The trigeminal nerve has three major branches: the ophthalmic branch, the maxillary branch, and the mandibular branch.

The ophthalmic branch, the smallest of the three, arises from the trigeminal ganglion and emerges from the cranium through the orbital fissure (see Fig. 88–8) in close association with the oculomotor and trochlear nerves. It is the principle sensory nerve for the orbit, dorsum of the nose, and portions of the nasal and sinus mucosa.[16]

The maxillary branch arises from the trigeminal ganglion and travels in the dura mater to leave the skull through the round foramen and rostral alar canal (see Fig. 88–8). It supplies tactile sensation for the skin of the muzzle, nasal mucosa, maxillary sinuses, mucous membrane of the nasopharynx, soft and hard palates, and the teeth and gingiva of the maxilla.[16]

The mandibular branch follows a similar course except that it passes from the skull through the oval foramen (see Fig. 88–8). It is a mixed nerve containing efferent fibers to the muscles of mastication. Its tactile sensory distribution extends from the rostral side of the ear ventrally to include the mandible, mandibular teeth and gingiva, and tongue.[16] It also supplies parasympathetic nerves to the sublingual and parotid salivary glands. The cutaneous areas of each branch of the trigeminal nerve overlap considerably.[20]

Abducens Nerve

The abducens (sixth cranial nerve) is a motor nerve to the retractor bulbi and the lateral rectus muscles. It leaves the brain stem ventrally immediately caudal to the pons, and passes rostrally to enter the cavernous sinus and continue rostrally. It leaves the cranial vault through the orbital fissure (see Fig. 88–8) to enter the orbital fascia. The abducens nerve moves each eye laterally around its polar axis and retracts the globe into the orbit.

Facial Nerve

The seventh cranial nerve is the facial nerve (Fig. 88–9). It is a mixed nerve that contains both autonomic efferent and afferent fibers, special afferent fibers, and efferent fibers to the muscles of facial expression. The parasympathetic fibers arise from the salivatory nucleus in the medulla and are distributed through petrosal nerves and the chorda tympani nerves. The taste function of the seventh nerve is similarly distributed to the cranial third of the tongue.[16]

The muscle (efferent) fibers of the facial nerve arise from the motor nucleus of the facial nerve in the rostroventral medulla, pass dorsorostrad around the abducens nucleus, and leave the lateral side of the medulla.[17] There they become associated with the vestibulocochlear nerve and accompany it into the internal acoustic meatus.[16] The facial nerve has three terminal branches: auriculopalpebral branch, ventral buccal nerve, and dorsal buccal nerve (see Fig. 88–9).[16]

The auriculopalpebral branch supplies motor function to the orbicularis oculi to close the eyelids. It continues to supply muscles of facial expression to the proximal and dorsal muzzle.

The ventral buccal branch supplies muscular branches to the muscles of the ear that depress the

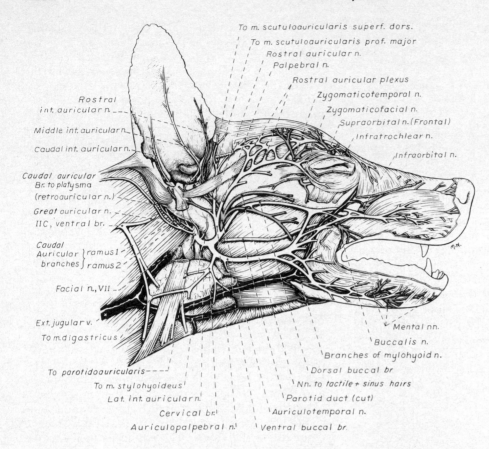

To m. scutuloauricularis superf. dors.
To m. scutuloauricularis prof. major
Rostral auricular n.
Palpebral n.
Rostral auricular plexus
Zygomaticotemporal n.
Zygomaticofacial n.
Supraorbital n.(Frontal)
Infratrochlear n.
Infraorbital n.

Rostral int. auricular n.
Middle int. auricular n.
Caudal int. auricular n.
Caudal auricular Br. to platysma (retroauricular n.)
Great auricular n.
IIC, ventral br.
Caudal Auricular branches {ramus 1, ramus 2}
Facial n., VII
Ext. jugular v.
To m. digastricus
To parotidoauricularis
To m. stylohyoideus
Lat. int. auricular n.
Cervical br.
Auriculopalpebral n.

Mental nn.
Buccalis n.
Branches of mylohyoid n.
Dorsal buccal br.
Nn. to tactile + sinus hairs
Parotid duct (cut)
Auriculotemporal n.
Ventral buccal br.

Figure 88–9. Superficial branches of the facial nerve. Lateral aspect. (Reprinted with permission from McClure, R. C.: The cranial nerves. *In*: Evans, H. E., and Christensen, G. C. (eds.): *Miller's Anatomy of the Dog.* 2nd ed. W. B. Saunders, Philadelphia, 1979.)

ear. By anastomosis with the dorsal buccal nerve, it supplies some of the orbicularis oris muscle.

The dorsal buccal nerve supplies the remainder of the orbicularis oris muscle as well as the muscles around the end of the muzzle.

Vestibulocochlear Nerve

The vestibulocochlear nerve is the eighth cranial nerve. It serves to provide the senses of balance and hearing. Two nerve bundles comprise this nerve: the vestibular nerve and the cochlear (auditory) nerve.

The cochlear portion is stimulated by the hair cells of the spiral organ of the inner ear. The vestibular portion is stimulated by hair cells associated with the maculae, saccules, and semicircular canals. The nerve passes through the internal acoustic meatus to enter the brain stem caudal to the pons on the lateral side.

Glossopharyngeal Nerve

The glossopharyngeal nerve (ninth cranial nerve) is a mixed nerve providing motor function to glands and muscle and sensation to the pharynx, a portion of the tongue, and the carotid sinus. It contains preganglionic fibers from the salivatory nuclei in the medulla and provides innervation to the parotid and

zygomatic salivary glands. Motor function is provided to pharyngeal and laryngeal muscles. Taste sensation and tactile sensation are accomplished in the caudal third of the tongue and pharyngeal region by the glossopharyngeal nerve.

Vagus Nerve

The vagus nerve provides the major visceral parasympathetic efferent function. The vagus nerve supplies parasympathetic function to the heart, smooth muscles, and glands of the thoracic and abdominal viscera. In addition, motor innervation to esophageal and laryngeal musculature is provided by the vagus nerve. These muscles are derived from the last three branchial arches of the embryo.

Visceral afferent information from tongue, esophagus, larynx, pulmonary parenchyma, heart, and other viscera is transmitted centrally by the vagus nerve. The vagus supplies some taste function in the pharyngeal area and provides some tactile sensation to the external ear canal.

The vagus forms from a series of fine rootlets and passes into the jugular foramen. As it passes through the jugular foramen it enters the petro-occipital fissure and accompanies the spinal accessory nerve to exit the skull. Multiple branching occurs to form nerves to the vagosympathetic trunk, the recurrent laryngeal nerves, and nerves to a pharyngeal plexus.[17]

Spinal Accessory Nerve

The eleventh cranial nerve, the spinal accessory, is formed from rootlets that emerge from the lateral side of the cervical spinal cord (C_1 through C_7) and converge rostrally, entering the cranium through the foramen magnum. There they are joined by rootlets from the nucleus ambiguus in the medulla. The spinal accessory nerve exits the skull with the vagus nerve to provide motor innervation to the cleidomastoideus, sternomastoideus, omotransversarius, and trapezius muscles.

Hypoglossal Nerve

The hypoglossal nerve provides motor innervation to the tongue on each side. It supplies all the extrinsic muscles of the tongue as well as the intrinsic tongue muscles.

It arises from rootlets from the ventrolateral surface of the medulla oblongata and leaves the cranium through the hypoglossal foramen. From its exit caudal to the osseous bulla, it passes rostromedially in close association with the lingual artery and lateral to the hyoid apparatus. It is vulnerable to injury from

external trauma or surgery near the osseous bulla or hyoid apparatus.

PARACRANIAL ANATOMY

Arterial Blood Supply

The major arterial supply to the brain is provided by the internal carotid and vertebral arteries. The vertebral arteries anastomose at the foramen magnum to form the basilar artery. The basilar artery is slightly tortuous along the ventral surface of the brain stem. Along its course it gives rise to several superficial arteries that supply the ventral and lateral surfaces of the brain stem. In addition, deep arteries penetrate to the core of the brain stem. At the level of the caudal midbrain, the basilar artery bifurcates into a pair of caudal cerebral arteries (Fig. 88–10).

The internal carotid artery branches off the common carotid artery and enters the skull through the jugular foramen and the carotid canal, emerging in the cranium in the caudal portion of the cavernous sinus. It courses rostrally within the cavernous sinus to the level of the optic chiasm. An anastomotic branch to the external ethmoidal artery is given off

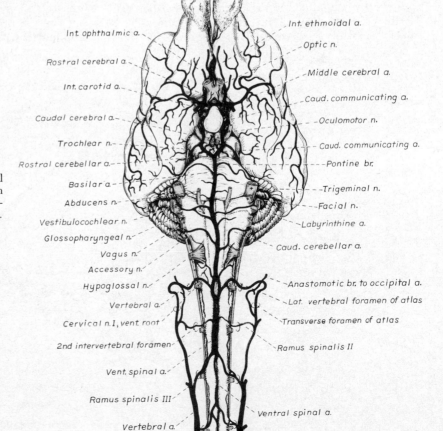

Figure 88–10. Arteries of the brain and cervical spinal cord. Ventral aspect. (Reprinted with permission from Evans, H. E., and Christensen, G. C. (eds.): *Miller's Anatomy of the Dog.* 2nd ed. W. B. Saunders, Philadelphia, 1979.)

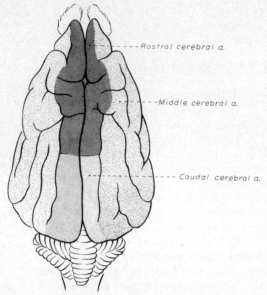

Rostral cerebral a.

Middle cerebral a.

Caudal cerebral a.

Figure 88–11. Areas of the brain supplied by the cerebral arteries. Dorsal aspect. (Reprinted with permission from Evans, H. E., and Christensen, G. C. (eds.): *Miller's Anatomy of the Dog,* 2nd ed. W. B. Saunders, Philadelphia, 1979.)

while within the cavernous sinus. The internal carotid artery turns dorsally and penetrates the dura mater and provides anastomosis to the arterial circle of the brain. Caudal communicating arteries anastomose with the previously described caudal cerebral artery to form the caudal half of the circle (see Fig. 88–10).

The middle cerebral artery branches from the lateral side of the circle. The cerebrum is thus supplied by the rostral cerebral, the caudal cerebral, and the middle cerebral arteries (Fig. 88–11).[8] The cerebellum is supplied by paired caudal cerebellar arteries, branches of the basilar artery, and the rostral cerebellar arteries.

Venous Drainage of the Brain

The venous return from the brain is provided by large vascular conduits that are thin-walled and encased in the dura mater and/or bone. The drainage routes are called venous sinuses and occur in a dorsal and ventral set (Fig. 88–12).

The dorsal set drains to the single sagittal sinus that lies on the dorsal midline where the falx cerebri attaches. The sagittal sinus collects the dorsal cerebral and diploic venous drainage and joins the straight sinus caudally. The straight sinus is shorter and deeper and drains blood from the corpus callosum and the great cerebral vein. It enters the sagittal sinus near its termination. The transverse sinuses are a pair of sinuses that begin within the dorsal portion of the occipital bone by receiving the sagittal sinus and any aberrant sinus drainage not received by the sagittal sinus.

The ventral set of sinuses are formed by more but smaller sinuses. The sigmoid sinus is a slightly bent caudoventral continuation of the transverse sinuses. The dorsal petrosal sinus drains a large portion of the brain stem and ventral cerebrum. The cavernous sinus is the most significant of the ventral set. It is an important route of drainage for the ventral part of

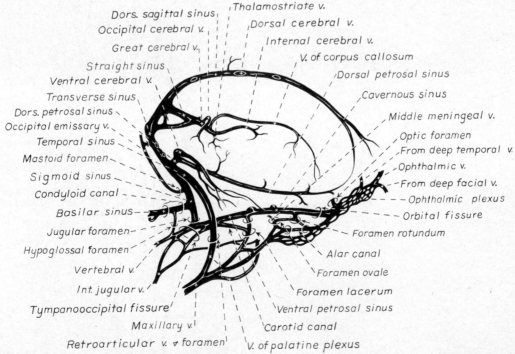

Dors. sagittal sinus
Occipital cerebral v.
Great cerebral v.
Straight sinus
Ventral cerebral v.
Transverse sinus
Dors. petrosal sinus
Occipital emissary v.
Temporal sinus
Mastoid foramen
Sigmoid sinus
Condyloid canal
Basilar sinus
Jugular foramen
Hypoglossal foramen
Vertebral v.
Int. jugular v.
Tympanooccipital fissure
Maxillary v.
Retroarticular v. & foramen

Thalamostriate v.
Dorsal cerebral v.
Internal cerebral v.
V. of corpus callosum
Dorsal petrosal sinus
Cavernous sinus
Middle meningeal v.
Optic foramen
From deep temporal v.
Ophthalmic v.
From deep facial v.
Ophthalmic plexus
Orbital fissure
Foramen rotundum
Alar canal
Foramen ovale
Foramen lacerum
Ventral petrosal sinus
Carotid canal
V. of palatine plexus

Figure 88–12. Diagram of the cranial venous sinuses. Lateral aspect. (Reprinted with permission from Reinhard, K. R., Miller, M. E., and Evans, H. E.: The craniovertebral veins and sinuses of the dog. Am. J. Anat. *111*:67, 1962.)

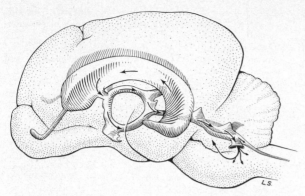

Figure 88–13. The canine ventricular system. (Reprinted with permission from de Lahunta, A.: *Veterinary Neuroanatomy and Clinical Neurology.* W. B. Saunders, Philadelphia, 1977.)

the brain.[9] It begins by receiving the orbital plexus. It then receives the middle meningeal vein and numerous smaller ventral veins. The internal carotid artery travels through much of the cavernous sinus. The pair of sinuses surround the pituitary stalk and the dorsum sellae.

Cerebrospinal Fluid

The production of cerebrospinal fluid (CSF) occurs at many sites. The choroid plexuses of all four ventricles are prominent sites of production. Other sites include the ependymal lining of the ventricular surfaces, the pia-glia membrane on the surfaces of the CNS, and the blood vessels of the pia-arachnoid. Approximately 40 per cent of CSF is produced outside the ventricular system.[6]

Cerebrospinal fluid circulates from sites of production to sites of absorption. From the ventricular system CSF must pass to the lateral apertures of the fourth ventricle to reach the subarachnoid space.

Within the ventricular system CSF flows from the site of production caudally to the lateral apertures. In a cranial to caudal direction CSF follows this sequence: lateral ventricle through the interventricular foramen to the third ventricle through the mesencephalic duct to the fourth ventricle through the lateral apertures (Fig. 88–13). Most of the CSF passes dorsally and rostrally to the major sites of absorption. In the spinal cord CSF flow is bidirectional.[6]

Flow is accomplished by blood pulsation causing minute yet acute changes in CSF pressure, surging CSF to the lateral apertures. Ependymal cilia may also play a role.

Absorption of CSF occurs mainly at the arachnoid villi located in venous sinuses or major cerebral veins. Arachnoid villi act as one-way valves, allowing fluid flow in one direction. When CSF pressure is greater than venous pressure, the arachnoid villi remain open and functional. When venous pressure exceeds CSF pressure, the arachnoid villi collapse (Fig. 88–14).

1. Bailey, C. S., Kitchell, R. L., and Johnson, R. D.: Spinal nerve root origins of the cutaneous nerves arising from the canine brachial plexus. Am. J. Vet. Res., *43*:820, 1982.
2. Chrisman, C. L.: Head tilt, circling, nystagmus and other vestibular deficits. *In: Problems in Small Animal Neurology.* Lea and Febiger, Philadelphia, 1982.
3. de Lahunta, A. (ed.): Spinal cord disease. *In Veterinary Neuroanatomy and Clinical Neurology.* W. B. Saunders, Philadelphia, 1977.
4. de Lahunta, A. (ed.): Upper motor neuron system. *In: Veterinary Neuroanatomy and Clinical Neurology.* W. B. Saunders, Philadelphia, 1977.
5. de Lahunta, A. (ed.): Cerebellum. *In Veterinary Neuroanatomy and Clinical Neurology.* W. B. Saunders, Philadelphia, 1977.

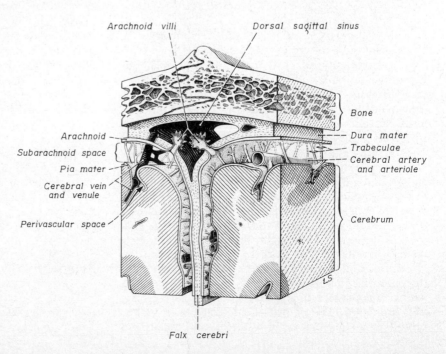

Figure 88–14. Cerebral meninges and arachnoid villi. (Reprinted with permission from de Lahunta, A.: *Veterinary Neuroanatomy and Clinical Neurology.* W. B. Saunders, Philadelphia, 1977.)

6. de Lahunta, A. (ed.): Cerebrospinal fluid and hydrocephalus. *In Veterinary Neuroanatomy and Clinical Neurology.* W. B. Saunders, Philadelphia, 1977.

7. Evans, H. E., and Christensen, G. C. (eds.): The spinal nerves. *In Miller's Anatomy of the Dog,* 2nd ed. W. B. Saunders, Philadelphia, 1977.

8. Evans, H. E., and Christensen, G. C. (eds.): The heart and arteries. *In Miller's Anatomy of the Dog,* 2nd ed. W. B. Saunders, Philadelphia, 1977.

9. Evans, H. E., and Christensen, G. C. (eds.): Veins of the central nervous system. *In Miller's Anatomy of the Dog,* 2nd ed. W. B. Saunders, Philadelphia, 1977.

10. Fletcher, T. F.: Spinal cord and meninges. *In* Evans, H. E., and Christensen, G. C. (eds.): *Miller's Anatomy of the Dog,* 2nd ed. W. B. Saunders, Philadelphia, 1977.

11. Guyton, A. C. (ed.): Behavior functions of the brain: The limbic system, role of the hypothalamus, and control of vegetative functions of the body. *In Textbook of Medical Physiology,* 6th ed. W. B. Saunders, Philadelphia, 1981.

12. Guyton, A. C. (ed.): Sensory receptors and their basic mechanism of action. *In Textbook of Medical Physiology,* 6th ed. W. B. Saunders, Philadelphia, 1981.

13. Guyton, A. C. (ed.): Activation on the brain—the reticular activating system; the generalized thalamocortical system; brain waves; epilepsy; wakefulness and sleep. *In Textbook of Medical Physiology,* 6th ed. W. B. Saunders, Philadelphia, 1981.

14. Guyton, A. C. (ed.): Motor functions of the spinal cord and the cord reflexes. *In Textbook of Medical Physiology,* 6th ed. W. B. Saunders, Philadelphia, 1981.

15. Haghighi, S. T., Spurgeon, T. L., and Kitchell, R. L.: Electrophysiological studies of the cutaneous innervation of the pelvic limb of the male dog. Anat. Histol. Embryol. 9:93, 1980.

16. McClure, R. C.: The cranial nerves. *In* Evans, H. E., and Christensen, G. C. (eds.): *Miller's Anatomy of the Dog,* 2nd ed. W. B. Saunders, Philadelphia, 1977.

17. Meyer, H.: The brain. *In* Evans, H. E., and Christensen, G. C. (eds.): *Miller's Anatomy of the Dog,* 2nd ed. W. B. Saunders, Philadelphia, 1977.

18. Palmer, A. C.: *Introduction to Animal Neurology.* F. A. Davis, Philadelphia, 1965.

19. Redding, R. W.: Anatomy and physiology. *In* Hoerlein, B. F. (ed.): *Canine Neurology Diagnosis and Treatment,* 3rd ed. W. B. Saunders, Philadelphia, 1978, pp. 47–51.

20. Whalen, L. R., and Kitchell, R. L.: Electrophysiological studies of the cutaneous nerves of the head of the dog. Anat. Histol. Embryol. 9:96, 1980.

Chapter **89**

Localization in Clinical Neurology

Kyle G. Braund and
Stephen T. Simpson

Localization of a central nervous system (CNS) or peripheral nervous system (PNS) lesion is usually determined by an objective, *constant* combination of signs that are obtained from historical information and neurological examination and which are accepted as localizing syndromes in neurological pathology.[4, 9, 15] Lesions in any structure of the nervous system will result in a predictable combination of clinical signs (structure versus function).

In general, neurological signs result from an organic lesion or physiological dysfunction in the CNS or PNS that produces stable or progressive deficits. However, several symptomatic disorders of the nervous system are causally related to diseases not primarily neurological, such as hypoglycemia, hepatic encephalopathy, paraneoplasia, and hyperviscosity states. These disorders are often episodic or paroxysmal, and animals are usually neurologically normal between attacks. A detailed physical examination helps to rule out disorders of other body systems, such as cardiopulmonary and skeletal systems, that may produce signs similar to those of a neurological dysfunction in CNS or PNS.

Lesions of the nervous system may be classified as degenerative, anomalous, autoimmune, allergic, metabolic, neoplastic, nutritional, inflammatory, toxic, and traumatic. The nature of a lesion can be determined by a combination of historical and signalment data and objective neurological findings. The actual cause of a problem is confirmed by ancillary data from laboratory tests and pathologic examinations. The majority of neurological problems in clinical practice can be diagnosed and managed without detailed knowledge of neuroanatomy and neurophysiology. The aim of this chapter is to aid localization based on recognition of clinical syndromes. For the purpose of this discussion, syndromes have been tabulated for 12 different areas of the CNS and PNS.

NEUROMUSCULAR SYNDROMES

Diseases of the neuromuscular system include disease processes of peripheral nerves, neuromuscular junctions, and muscles. These diseases can be present in a regional or restricted distribution or they can be diffuse and generalized. The disease progression can vary from an explosive onset and rapid progression to an insidious onset with very slow to no progression.

Neuropathic Syndrome

The most dramatic clinical findings in neuropathies relate to dysfunction of the structures innervated by motor nerves. Motor nerves represent the lower motor neuron, because they are the final common pathway between the CNS and their target organs. In the voluntary (somatic) nervous system, these organs are skeletal muscles. The target organs of the autonomic nervous system are the smooth muscles associated with blood vessels and visceral structures, glands, and cardiac muscle.

Peripheral neuropathies result in lower motor neuron signs, including flaccid muscle weakness or paralysis, significant muscular atrophy, and reduction or absence of muscle tone (hypotonia, atonia) and reflexes (hyporeflexia, areflexia).[1, 3, 11, 13, 14] Because most spinal nerves contain motor and sensory components, a variable degree of sensory loss is detected in cutaneous (dermatomal) testing.[11] Peripheral neuropathies may involve a single or a few nerves (regional neuropathy) or a large number of nerves (polyneuropathy). Regional neuropathies are most likely to be asymmetrical and to involve only one limb or one or two cranial nerves. Their clinical signs are more likely to have both motor and sensory components, but there may be only motor deficits. Common causes of regional neuropathy are trauma, such as brachial plexus avulsion, and iatrogenic intraneural injection.

In generalized neuropathies the pattern of distribution is more diffuse, involving multiple segments if not the entire peripheral nervous system. These disorders are usually symmetrical and may be proximal (e.g., hereditary spinal muscular atrophy in Brit-

TABLE 89–1. Spinal Nerve Lesions and their Associated Deficits

Nerve	Muscles	Clinical Signs of Dysfunction
Suprascapular (C6–C7)	Supraspinatus Infraspinatus	Loss of shoulder extension (muscle atrophy with prominent spine of scapula).
Musculocutaneous (C6–C8)	Biceps brachii Brachialis Coracobrachialis	Reduced elbow flexion; loss of biceps reflex; reduced sensation over medial surface of forearm.
Axillary (C7–C8)	Deltoideus Teres major Teres minor	Reduced shoulder flexion; deltoid atrophy.
Radial (C7–T1)	Triceps brachii Extensor carpi radialis Ulnaris lateralis Lateral digital extensor Common digital extensor	Reduced extension of elbow, carpus, and digits; loss of extensor postural thrust and limb support (with high radial damage; i.e., above elbow); loss of triceps reflex; reduced sensation over dorsal surface of forearm.
Median (C8–T1)	Flexor carpi radialis Superficial digital flexor	Reduced flexion of carpus and digits.
Ulnar (C8–T1)	Flexor carpi ulnaris Deep digital flexor	Reduced flexion of carpus and digits; reduced sensation over caudal surface of forearm.
Femoral (L4–L5)	Iliopsoas Quadriceps Sartorius	Inability to extend stifle and inability to bear weight; loss of patellar reflex; reduced sensation over medial surface of paw, hock, stifle, and thigh (saphenous nerve).
Obturator (L5–L6)	External obturator Pectineus Gracilis	Inability to adduct hip and thigh (animal "does the splits" on smooth surface).
Sciatic (L6–L7–S1)	Biceps femoris Semimembranosus Semitendinosus	Inability to flex stifle and other functions along its branches (tibial and common peroneal nerve); loss of flexor reflex.
Tibial	Gastrocnemius Popliteus Deep digital flexor	Inability to extend hock and flex digits; reduced sensation over plantar surface of paw.
Common peroneal	Peroneus longus Lateral digital extensor Long digital extensor Cranial tibial	Inability to flex hock and extend digits; knuckling of dorsal paw; reduced sensation over dorsocranial surface of the paw, hock, and stifle.
Pudendal (S1–S2–S3)	External anal sphincter Striated urethral	Loss of perineal reflex; loss of bulbocavernosus reflex.
Pelvic (S2–S3)	Smooth muscle of bladder, rectum	Detrusor muscle paralysis.

TABLE 89–2. Cranial Nerve Lesions and their Associated Deficits

Nerve	Clinical Signs of Dysfunction	Clinical Tests	Normal Response	Abnormal Response
I. Olfactory	Hyposmia or anosmia	Smell of food or nonirritating volatile substance	Food: interest or attempt to eat Volatile substance: sniffing, recoil, and nose lick	No reaction
II. Optic*	Visual impairment, hesitancy in walking	Obstacle test Visual placing test Menace reaction Following movement (Ophthalmoscopic examination)	Avoidance of obstacle Visual placing of limbs Eye blink Follows motion of objects	Bumping objects No reaction No reaction No reaction
	Anisocoria, mydriasis	Point source of light in each eye	Direct and consensual pupillary reflexes	On affected side, direct and consensual pupillary reflexes absent; on unaffected side, direct and consensual pupillary reflexes present
III. Oculomotor	Anisocoria, mydriasis, ptosis, esotropia and exotropia (ventrolateral)	Point source of light in each eye	Direct and consensual pupillary reflexes	On affected side, direct pupillary reflex absent, consensual reflex present; on unaffected side, direct pupillary reflex present, consensual reflex absent
		Observation of eye movements when following a moving object in horizontal/vertical planes	Normal medial, dorsoventral ocular movement	Impaired ocular movement in vertical plane and impaired ocular adduction in horizontal plane (unable to follow upward, downward, or medially)
IV. Trochlear	Esotropia and exotropia (dorsomedial)	None	None	None
V. Trigeminal (motor) (sensory)	Masseteric and temporalis muscle atrophy; inability to open and close jaws	Jaw tonus	Resistance to opening jaws	Lack of resistance or supranormal resistance
		Palpation of masseter and temporalis muscle	Normal contour/muscle resilience	Hypotonia, atrophy
		Palpebral reflex Corneal reflex	Eye blink Globe retraction	No reaction; intense discomfort recoil, vocalization
VI. Abducens	Esotropia and exotropia (medial)	Observation of eye when following moving object in horizontal plane	Normal lateral ocular movement	Impaired ocular abduction (unable to follow laterally)
VII. Facial	Asymmetry of facial expression, inability to close eyelids, lip commissure paralysis, auricular paralysis	Palpebral reflex Menace reflex Handclap	Eye blink	No reaction
		Tickle ear	Auricular contraction	No reaction
VIII. Vestibulocochlear (cochlear)	Deafness	Handclap	Startle reaction, blink, auricular contraction	No reaction
		EEG alerting	EEG alert recordings	No reaction

Table continued on opposite page

TABLE 89–2. Cranial Nerve Lesions and their Associated Deficits *Continued*

Nerve	Clinical Signs of Dysfunction	Clinical Tests	Normal Response	Abnormal Response
(Vestibular)	Circling, head tilt, nystagmus, loss of balance	Rapid head movement in horizontal/vertical planes	Physiologically induced nystagmus	No reaction; spontaneous/ positional nystagmus; esotropia and exotropia (ventrolateral upon dorsal head extension)
		Caloric test		
		Rotatory test	Postrotatory nystagmus	
		Righting reactions	Normal righting	
IX. Glosso- pharyngeal	Dysphagia	Gag reflex	Swallow	No reaction
X. Vagus	Dysphagia	Gag reflex	Swallow	No reaction
		Laryngeal reflex	Cough	No reaction
		Oculocardiac reflex	Bradycardia	No reaction
XI. Spinal accessory	Dorsolateral neck muscle atrophy; torticollis	Palpation of cervical musculature	Normal contour/muscle resilience	Hypotonia, muscle atrophy
XII. Hypoglossal	Deviation of tongue (animal licks only affected side)	Tongue stretch	Retraction	No retraction

*The optic nerve is not a true nerve developmentally, structurally, or in its pathology. It is a tract of the central nervous system. It is surrounded by meninges, including a subarachnoid space.

tany spaniels), or distal (e.g., giant axonal neuropathy in German shepherds). Pelvic limbs are usually first affected in generalized polyneuropathies. Whereas some neuropathies may be acute (e.g., traumatic, ischemic) or subacute (e.g., coonhound paralysis) in onset, the majority are insidious and have a chronic course. Signs of autonomic nerve dysfunction are rarely observed in animals with diffuse polyneuropathies. Similarly, cranial nerve dysfunction is uncommon, with the exception of the facial nerve (VII) in coonhound paralysis and occasionally in hypothyroid neuropathy, and the vagus (X) (dysphagia, megaesophagus) in giant axonal neuropathy.

In contrast to generalized or diffuse muscle atrophy that occurs secondary to chronic spinal cord disease or systemic diseases that produce cachexia (and may take several months to develop), neurogenic atrophy occurs only in those muscles innervated by the injured nerve (segmental atrophy), and it becomes clinically apparent after one to two weeks.[1, 3, 11, 13] Chronic neurogenic atrophy may result in fibrosis and limited joint movement from contractures.

Certain disorders of the neuromuscular junction (junctionopathies), namely botulism and tick paralysis, produce signs that mimic those of diffuse peripheral neuropathy. Electrodiagnostic testing helps to differentiate a junctionopathy from a polyneuropathy.

The veterinary surgeon is most often challenged by the regional neuropathies, since some of them require surgical intervention. The generalized neuropathies are not diseases of concern to surgeons other than from a differential diagnostic viewpoint. Likewise, most diseases of the neuromuscular junction are of only diagnostic significance to the surgeon and have no surgical indications. The singular excep-

tion is acquired myasthenia gravis and its association with thymoma (see Chapter 87).

Specific clinical deficits in spinal and cranial nerves are listed in Tables 89–1 and 89–2. Signs associated with the neuromuscular syndrome are outlined in Table 89–3.

Myopathic Syndrome

Generalized muscle disease is characterized by muscle weakness and fatigue with reduced exercise tolerance. Muscle strength may return with rest. The

TABLE 89–3. Signs of the Neuromuscular Syndromes*

Signs	Neuropathic	Myopathic
Flaccid paresis to paralysis	+	+
Exercise intolerance	+	+ +
Stiff/stilted gait	+	+ +
Muscle atrophy	+ + +	+
Muscle hypertrophy	−	+
Hyporeflexia/hypotonia	+ +	+/−
Dimple contracture	−	+/−
Hypalgesia	+/−	−
Hyperesthesia	+/−	+/−
Limited range of motion	+ (late)	+/−

*+ = positive finding (graded). − = negative finding. +/− = variable finding.

gait is often stiff and stilted, possibly because many muscle diseases cause muscles to be slow to relax (myotonia). As a result of the muscle weakness, animals learn to support themselves and walk reluctantly by locking joints into extension. Clinical signs are often episodic.

Selected muscles may be increased in size because of inflammation, hypertrophy, or spasm. More frequently, muscle mass is reduced as a result of nerve damage (neurogenic atrophy) or because of fiber degeneration and necrosis. A dimple contracture in a muscle (e.g. limb or tongue) may be elicited in myotonic myopathies following a sudden tap with a percussion hammer.[7] Muscle pain, induced by palpation, is often recorded in animals with polymyositis. In general, primary myopathies are uncommon. Tendon reflexes are usually preserved but may be reduced or absent, and sensory perception of pain is not impaired.

A junctionopathy that produces signs very similar to those of the myopathic syndrome is myasthenia gravis. Clinical signs of the myopathic syndrome are incorporated in Table 89–3.

SPINAL CORD SYNDROMES

As discussed in Chapter 88, the spinal cord is functionally divided into four segments: the lumbosacral, thoracolumbar, cervicothoracic, and cervical, each of which produces a distinctive syndrome in diseased states. Some clinical signs are common to all segments of spinal cord disease and are used to determine presence of spinal cord disease, e.g., presence of bilateral, and often symmetrical, clinical signs, whereas other clinical signs are useful to specify the spinal cord segment involved.

Upper motor neuron (UMN) is a collective term given to motor systems in the brain that control lower motor neurons. The UMN system is responsible for maintaining body tone and posture and for initiating and coordinating voluntary movement. Lesions of the UMN system produce a characteristic set of clinical signs caudal to the lesion, including increased extensor tone and exaggerated reflexes. In spinal cord disease, lower motor neuron signs mask UMN signs if the lesion is at the level of cervical or lumbar intumescences.

Signs of the various spinal cord syndromes are summarized in Table 89–4.

Lumbosacral Syndrome (L4–S3)

Signs of lumbosacral disease are associated with lesions involving the lumbosacral (LS) intumescence or the lumbosacral nerve roots. The spinal cord components of this segment are in an anatomical relationship with the L4, L5, and L6 vertebrae.[5] The nerve roots traverse the spinal canal from the cord segment of origin caudally to the intervertebral foramen, which they exit. Therefore, the sacral nerve roots arise within the vertebral canal at about L6 and proceed to the S1, S2, or S3 foramen.[1, 3] Disease involving the cord segments of origin appears the same as a lesion involving the nerve roots. A lesion in the lumbosacral intumescence involves the nerves originating from L4–S3 cord segments, namely the femoral, obturator, sciatic, pudendal, and pelvic nerves, and reflects various degrees of lower motor neuron involvement of the pelvic limbs or bladder, anal and urethral sphincters, and tail. Accordingly, depending on the level and extent of the lesion, clinical signs may range from flaccid paraparesis and ataxia of pelvic limbs and tail to paraplegia with normal thoracic limb function. Occasionally, lesions of the rostral lumbosacral intumescence produce a posture characterized by flaccid paraplegia with hypertonic extensor function in the thoracic limbs (Schiff-Sherrington posture).

Pelvic limb postural reactions are depressed or absent. Flexor, patellar, and perineal reflexes (and

TABLE 89–4. Signs of Spinal Cord Syndromes

Syndrome	Paresis/ Paralysis	Lower Motor Neuron Signs	Upper Motor Neuron Signs	Sensory Loss	Postural Reactions	Other Signs
Lumbosacral (L4–S3)	Flaccid paresis to paralysis of pelvic limbs	Pelvic limbs, anal sphincter, tail, bladder, and urethral sphincter	—	In pelvic limbs, anal sphincter, tail, bladder, and urethral sphincter	Depressed or absent in pelvic limbs, normal in thoracic limbs	Passive urinary incontinence
Thoracolumbar (T3–L3)	Spastic paresis to paralysis in pelvic limbs	—	In pelvic limbs (hyperreflexia, hypertonia, no significant muscle atrophy)	Hypalgesia to analgesia caudal to lesion site; hyperalgesia at or immediately above lesion site	Depressed or absent in pelvic limbs, normal in thoracic limbs	+/– Schiff-Sherrington posture
Cervicothoracic (C6–T2)	Hemiparesis to tetraplegia	In thoracic limbs	In pelvic limbs	Same as thoracolumbar	Depressed in all limbs, esp. thoracic	+/– Horner's syndrome (T1–T2) Unilateral or bilateral absence of panniculus reflex (C8–T1)
Cervical (C1–C5)	Hemiparesis to tetraplegia	Same as thoracolumbar	In thoracic and pelvic limbs	Same as thoracolumbar	Depressed in thoracic and pelvic limbs	Cervical pain and rigidity

bulbocavernosus reflex in males) are depressed or absent. Tone in pelvic limb muscles is reduced (hypotonia) or absent (atonia), with weak or no resistance to pelvic limb manipulation. Clinical neurological deficits in pelvic limbs may be symmetrical or asymmetrical. Muscle atrophy due to denervation is observed in chronic disorders.[1, 3, 11, 13] Pain perception in pelvic limbs, tail, and perineum may be reduced (hypalgesia) or absent (analgesia).

Other clinical signs of a lesion in the sacral segments or in lumbosacral roots within the cauda equina result in a denervated bladder with urine retention and passive incontinence. (Refer to discussion of thoracolumbar syndrome for comparison with upper motor neuron or automatic spinal cord bladder.) Anal sphincter paralysis results in fecal incontinence.[1, 3, 12, 13]

Thoracolumbar Syndrome

A spinal cord lesion between cervical and lumbar enlargements (intumescences), i.e., between T3 and L3, produces clinical signs of the thoracolumbar syndrome, which is the most commonly encountered spinal cord syndrome in the dog and cat.

When upper motor neurons are damaged by disease processes, the overall effect is release of lower motor neurons from upper motor inhibitory influences,[3] which results in exaggerated myotatic (tendon) reflex responses (hyperreflexia) and, sometimes, clonus (spasms in which contraction and relaxation alternate in rapid succession).[11] Flexor reflexes may show a prolonged after-discharge, which is observed as repetitive flexion of the limb in absence of repeated stimuli. Another example of release of lower motor neurons is the crossed extensor reflex,[1, 3, 11] which may be elicited in the laterally recumbent animal when the flexor reflex is stimulated. A crossed extensor reflex is present when pinching a toe produces a rapid and complete extension of the opposite limb. The leg that extends is released from the upper motor neuron inhibition. Muscle tone usually is heightened, with increased resistance to passive manipulation of the limbs. This release is known as spasticity. Pelvic limb weakness (paraparesis) or paralysis, is usually spastic. Pain perception is often depressed (hypalgesia) or absent (analgesia) in areas caudal to the lesion site. In contrast, pain response may be increased (hyperalgesia) at or immediately above the level of the lesion.

Urinary incontinence is a typical complication of the thoracolumbar syndrome. However, in contrast to lower motor neuron incontinence (see "Lumbosacral Syndrome"), the incontinence of thoracolumbar syndrome is associated with a "spastic bladder" or "spinal bladder." Immediately following spinal cord trauma the bladder is atonic and overfills. With time, the bladder regains tone and has a reduced filling volume, and a reflex bladder contraction occurs. The external urinary sphincter may also become spastic, characterized by hyperreflexia and increased tone. The clinician may find it difficult if not impossible (and dangerous) to express the bladder manually. This sphincter spasticity is particularly evident in male patients.[1, 12]

Acute, compressive lesions of the thoracolumbar spinal cord may be accompanied by the Schiff-Sherrington posture, which is observed as rigid extension of the thoracic limbs and pelvic limb hypotonia (pelvic limb reflexes are normal or exaggerated). Voluntary movement and postural reaction testing, however, are normal in the thoracic limbs.

Cervicothoracic Syndrome (C6–T2)

The cervicothoracic cord segments that extend from C6 through T2 form the cervical intumescence. A lesion in this location produces signs of cervicothoracic syndrome.

Clinical signs may range from weakness in all four limbs (tetraparesis) to paralysis of all limbs (tetraplegia). Thoracic and pelvic limbs on the same side of the body may be involved (hemiparesis, hemiplegia).

Because nerves from the cervical intumescence innervate thoracic limb muscles, a lesion in the cervicothoracic region of the spinal cord usually results in lower motor neuron signs in the thoracic limb(s) and upper motor neuron signs in the pelvic limb(s).[3, 11] Accordingly, paresis or paralysis in thoracic limbs is flaccid, whereas in the pelvic limbs it is spastic. Postural reactions may be depressed in all limbs, especially thoracic limbs. Reflexes and muscle tone are depressed in thoracic limbs (reflecting the lower motor neuron signs) and exaggerated in pelvic limbs (reflecting the upper motor neuron signs). Neurogenic muscle atrophy is restricted to the thoracic limb(s). Occasionally, in early stages of chronic, slow-onset diseases such as cervical malformation-malarticulation in Great Danes and Doberman pinschers, the white matter is affected more selectively, causing limited thoracic limb signs and marked pelvic limb signs.[1] There may be a unilateral or bilateral absence of the panniculus reflex, since the efferent limb of the reflex is mediated via the lateral thoracic nerve, which originates in cord segments C8–T1.

Horner's syndrome may occur with lesions of cord segments T1–T3. This syndrome is characterized by miosis, ptosis, and enophthalmos, with passive prolapse of the third eyelid. In some instances of traumatic avulsion of the brachial plexus, a partial Horner's syndrome may result, with only miosis observed (see Chapter 95).

Cervical Syndrome (C1–C5)

The cervical syndrome is observed when a spinal cord lesion occurs between the first and fifth cervical cord segments. Clinical signs range from weakness in all four limbs (tetraparesis) to weakness in thoracic and pelvic limbs on the same side as the lesion (hemiparesis) to complete paralysis (hemiplegia or tetraplegia). A lesion in this region of the spinal cord results in upper motor neuron signs in thoracic and pelvic limbs such as hyperreflexia, hypertonia, and spastic paresis or paralysis. Postural reactions are depressed to absent in all four limbs.[1, 3, 11] Pain perception is normal or depressed caudal to the site of the lesion. At the level of or immediately above the lesion, palpation or cervical manipulation may induce pain. The animal may manifest cervical rigidity.

Horner's syndrome, characterized by miosis, ptosis, enophthalmos, and passive prolapse of the third eyelid, is observed infrequently, and then only with severe destructive lesions of the cervical spinal cord.

BRAIN STEM SYNDROMES

Because the brain stem serves many functions, brain stem disease may result in several syndromes of clinical findings: pontomedullary, vestibular, cerebellar, and midbrain syndromes.

Pontomedullary Syndrome

Diseases involving the pons and medulla oblongata are represented in this syndrome. Clinical signs of disease in this segment of the nervous system include motor deficits similar to those of the cervical syndrome with the addition of signs of involvement of the cranial nerves (trigeminal, abducens, facial, glossopharyngeal, vagus, spinal accessory and hypoglossal) (see Table 89–1) and possible disturbance of consciousness and autonomic function.[1, 11]

Upper motor neuron signs associated with lesions of the caudal brain stem resemble cervical cord disease. Gait, posture, and postural reactions are noticeably altered (tetraparesis, hemiparesis, tetraplegia, etc.). Spasticity is usually present, resulting in extensor hypertonus and exaggerated myotatic reflexes.

Trigeminal nerve (V) deficits are detected by reduced sensation to the face (facial hypesthesia) or atrophy or flaccid paralysis of the muscles of mastication (Fig. 89–1).[11]

A lesion involving the abducens nucleus or nerve (VI) results in estropia and impaired ability to abduct the eye (ipsilateral).

Facial nerve (VII) deficits include paresis or paralysis to the lips, eyes, and ears and are more clearly observed when only one side of the face is affected, producing marked asymmetry. Figure 89–2 shows both chronic and acute facial nerve paralysis. Signs of dysphagia may be detected by history or neurological examination and suggest dysfunction of cranial nerves IX and X (glossopharyngeal and vagus, respectively). The spinal accessory nerve (XI) is rarely affected, but when it is, the presenting appearance

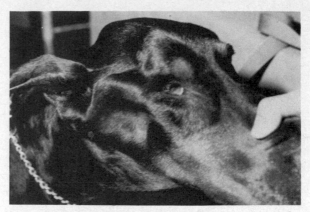

Figure 89–1. Atrophy of the muscles of mastication in a mature Doberman pinscher. The eye is severely sunken owing to atrophy of the pterygoid muscle, which forms the major support for the floor of the orbit. The trigeminal nerve was destroyed by pressure necrosis from a slowly growing meningioma in the right caudal fossa.

may be a scoliosis or torticollis of a nonorthopedic cause. The hypoglossal nerve (XII) innervates the extrinsic and intrinsic muscles of the tongue. As a result of paralysis of this nerve, the animal is unable to protrude the tongue properly and can lick only the affected side.[1] Atrophy of the tongue muscles occurs in chronic cases.

Disturbances of consciousness (depression) can occur with lesions of the pontine area because of dysfunction in the reticular activating system. Lesions of the more caudal reticular formation produce signs of autonomic (urinary incontinence) and respiratory (irregular respiration) dysfunction more than signs of conscious disturbances.[1, 3, 11] Signs of the pontomedullary syndrome are summarized in Table 89–5.

Vestibular Syndrome

Vestibular signs may be present with either pontine or medullary lesions[8] or with lesions of the eighth cranial nerve or its end organ, the membranous labyrinth. Signs of vestibular disease may be so dominant that signs of upper motor neuron disease may be obscured.

The vestibular system is responsible for maintaining and integrating posture of head, eyes, and body. Vestibular disorders result in a loss of equilibrium, leading to imbalance and ataxia. Clinical signs such as head tilt, broad-based stance, deviation of the trunk, falling, rolling, and walking in tight circles reflect postural imbalance that occurs with vestibular system dysfunction.

Abnormal ocular posture is manifested as *vestibular exotropia*, which may be elicited by elevating the head (Fig. 89–3), and is characterized by a ventrolateral deviation of the ipsilateral eye, and as *nystagmus*, an involuntary rapid movement of the eyes. Spontaneous nystagmus, present in the acute stages of most vestibular disease, is usually jerking or rotational with fast and slow components. The fast phase of horizontal or rotational nystagmus is in a direction

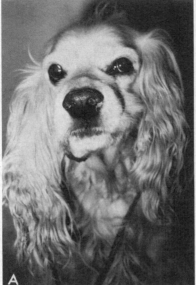

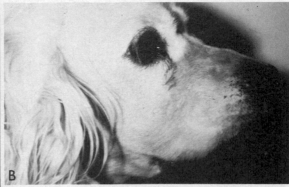

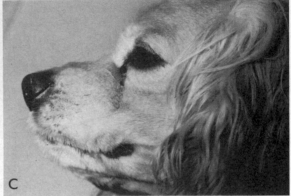

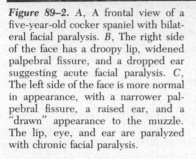

Figure 89–2. A, A frontal view of a five-year-old cocker spaniel with bilateral facial paralysis. *B,* The right side of the face has a droopy lip, widened palpebral fissure, and a dropped ear suggesting acute facial paralysis. *C,* The left side of the face is more normal in appearance, with a narrower palpebral fissure, a raised ear, and a "drawn" appearance to the muzzle. The lip, eye, and ear are paralyzed with chronic facial paralysis.

away from the side of the lesion. Sometimes, abnormal nystagmus can be initiated by moving and holding the head in a different position (*positional nystagmus*). Normal physiological nystagmus can be induced by rapid head movements in vertical or horizontal planes. The fast phase of the nystagmus is in the direction of the head movement. This response is depressed in an animal with vestibular disease when the head is moved toward the side of the lesion. Other procedures that have been used to induce nystagmus include the post-rotary test and the caloric test. Both procedures are cumbersome and may produce equivocal results.

The vestibular syndrome may occur with central

TABLE 89–5. Signs of the Pontomedullary Syndrome

Spastic hemiparesis to tetraplegia
Upper motor neuron signs in thoracic and pelvic limbs
Postural reactions depressed in thoracic and pelvic limbs
   (ipsilateral)
+/– Mental depression
+/– Irregular respiration
+/– Hypalgesia of trunk and limbs
+/– Facial hypalgesia, masticatory muscle paralysis
   (cranial nerve V)
+/– Esotropia (VI)
+/– Facial paresis/paralysis (VII)
+/– Pharyngeal paresis (IX, X)
+/– Torticollis (XI)
+/– Tongue paresis (XII)

or peripheral vestibular disease. Signs of central vestibular disease include vertical nystagmus and nystagmus that changes with different positions of the head, change in mental status, paresis, and

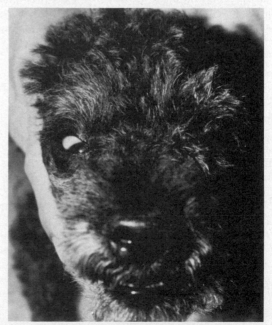

Figure 89–3. A ventromedial positional extropia in a dog with acute right vestibular syndrome due to head trauma. A fracture line was demonstrated in the right temporal bone in the area of the inner ear.

TABLE 89–6. Signs of Peripheral or Central Vestibular Syndrome

Sign	Central Disease	Peripheral Disease
Head tilt	Present	Present
Falling, rolling	Present	Present
Nystagmus		
Horizontal	Present	Present
Rotary	Present	Present
Vertical	Present	Absent
With change in position	Yes	No
Esotropia and exotropia	Yes	Yes
Cranial nerve lesions	V, VI, VII	VII
Horner's syndrome	No	Yes
Gait dysfunction	Severe ataxia, ipsilateral hemiparesis	Mild ataxia
Cerebellar signs	Possible	Not possible

evidence of other cranial nerve (e.g. trigeminal) dysfunction (Table 89–6). A pontine lesion may involve vestibular nuclei and fibers of the facial nerve, producing vestibular signs in combination with facial paralysis.

Horner's syndrome and facial nerve paralysis may occur with peripheral vestibular disease associated with otitis media or externa, since both nerves pass through the middle ear.

A paradoxical vestibular syndrome occurs with a lesion in the confluence of the cerebellar peduncles. It causes ipsilateral UMN paresis and contralateral head tilt. The direction of the head tilt is opposite to the side of the lesion, hence the term paradoxical.[3, 13]

Cerebellar Syndrome

The cerebellum is a reinforcing and coordinating organ that plays an important role in harmonizing muscular contraction, both voluntary movement and maintenance of posture. Cerebellar disease results in an inadequate response and, thus, an inability to regulate the rate, range, and force of a movement. Clinical signs include exaggerated limb response (hypermetria) when a movement is initiated, such as "goose-stepping" when walking or during postural reaction testing, and overshooting a food bowl when attempting to eat. All motor responses are clumsy, faltering, and jerky. Animals have no loss of voluntary strength. The animal assumes a broad-based stance at rest, and swaying of the trunk (truncal ataxia) may be observed when the animal is walking. Initiation of movements is delayed and often accompanied by tremors (intention tremors). This is especially noticeable in the head. Intention tremors disappear at rest.

TABLE 89–7. Signs of the Cerebellar Syndrome

Dysmetria (usually hypermetria)

Intention tremor (head)

Wide-based stance

Truncal ataxia

+/− deficit in menace response

+/− eye tremors

Fine pendular or oscillatory ocular movements may also be seen.

Menace response may be absent in animals with cerebellar disease. If the lesion involves only one side of the cerebellum, the menace deficit is ipsilateral. Vision is unaffected.

Infrequently observed signs with dysfunction of specific areas of the cerebellum include opisthotonus and extensor rigidity (with a lesion involving the rostral lobe), and vestibular signs (with involvement of the flocculonodular lobe). Signs of the cerebellar syndrome are listed in Table 89–7.

Midbrain Syndrome

Lesions involving midbrain structures produce a syndrome characterized by opisthotonus with rigid extension of all limbs (decerebration), spastic hemiparesis (contralateral) or tetraparesis, and mentation change (depression, stupor, or coma). Hypalgesia of the head, trunk, and limbs may be detected. Signs of cranial nerve III deficits are ventrolateral exotropia, mydriasis, and nonreactive pupil (ipsilateral).

Lesions at the level of and caudal to the midbrain result in noticeable gait disturbances (compare with the cerebral/diencephalic syndrome). Signs of the midbrain syndrome are listed in Table 89–8.

Cerebral/Diencephalic Syndrome

Lesions that affect the cerebral cortex and diencephalon (thalamus/hypothalamus) produce a readily

TABLE 89–8. Signs of the Midbrain Syndrome

Opisthotonus

Spastic hemiparesis (contralateral) or tetraplegia

Postural reactions depressed in thoracic and pelvic limbs (contralateral)

Mental status change:
  Depression
  Stupor
  Coma

Ventrolateral exotropia

Mydriasis

+/− Hypalgesia of head, trunk, and limbs

identifiable syndrome. Alterations in mental status or behavior are usual. Wakefulness and full consciousness are maintained by activity of a network of neurons throughout the brain stem. These neurons form the *ascending reticular activating system.* They receive information from all conscious projections and relay it to the cerebral cortex via the thalamus. Dysfunction of this system results in disturbances of consciousness ranging from hyperexcitability, depression, and stupor (semicoma) to coma.

Emotion and behavior are controlled primarily by the limbic system. Aggression and psychomotor epilepsy are hallmarks of limbic dysfunction.

In addition to altered mental status or behavior, animals with the cerebral/diencephalic syndrome commonly manifest seizures that may be partial, with localizing signs such as head turning or spasms in one limb without loss of consciousness, or generalized, with loss of consciousness and uncontrolled visceral (salivation, urination, defecation, pupillary dilation, and chewing movements) and somatic activity (muscular rigidity followed by running and paddling movements of the limbs).

Animals usually have contralateral deficits in postural reaction testing without severe gait abnormality. Affected animals may stand with head and trunk twisted (pleurothotonus) toward the side of the lesion. Pacing and head pressing may be seen, and circling may occur, with head and eyes directed toward the side of the lesion. Wide circling toward the lesion may be seen.

Contralateral visual deficits with normal pupillary function, are common. The particular vulnerability of the central visual pathways stems from their long course from thalamus to visual cortex. Papilledema may be observed as a result of elevated intracranial, and hence cerebrospinal fluid, pressure. Motor, sensory, and visual deficits are contralateral to the lesion.

Rarely, a *hypothalamohypophyseal* syndrome is

TABLE 89–9. Signs of the Cerebral Diencephalic Syndrome

Behavioral/mental status change:
   Apathy
   Disorientation
   Hyperexcitability
   Aggression

Abnormal posture/movement
   Circling (ipsilateral)
   Pacing
   Head pressing
   Pleurothotonus

Postural reactions depressed (contralateral)

+/− Visual impairment (contralateral)

+/− Seizures

+/− Papilledema

+/− Hypothalamohypophyseal signs

seen. This syndrome, which can occur with pituitary neoplasia compressing or infiltrating the overlying hypothalamus, is characterized by disorders of body temperature, glucose metabolism, appetite control, autonomic nervous system, water balance, and gonadal/thyroidal/adrenal function. If the tumor extends rostrally to involve the optic chiasma, visual deficits with pupillary abnormalities may ensue. Signs of, and common diseases associated with, the cerebral diencephalic syndrome are listed in Table 89–9.

PAROXYSMAL SYNDROMES

The term paroxysmal syndromes refers to a group of disorders that occur sporadically. Each syndrome has distinctive clinical signs, and the animal is usually normal (i.e., without neurological deficits) between episodes.

Seizures were mentioned briefly in the discussion of cerebral/diencephalic syndrome. This group of disorders is most commonly associated with seizures. The terms seizure, convulsion, epilepsy, and fit are synonyms for brain dysfunction expressed as a paroxysmal cerebral dysrhythmia that has a sudden onset, ceases spontaneously, and has a tendency to recur. The actual attack is called the ictus. Sometimes, a pre-ictal aura may occur seconds to minutes before the seizure, during which time the animal may appear apprehensive and restless and may seek out the owner or hide and act fearful. The post-ictal period is the interval during which recovery occurs.[13] It is often manifested as depression, visual impairment, protracted sleep, or other disturbances of behavior and may last from an hour to a day or more. With the exception of post-traumatic brain scarring, the many causes of seizures in animals that are neurologically normal beween attacks are extracranial.

Episodic weakness consists of paroxysmal attacks of muscular weakness and fatigue usually precipitated by exercise. The animal, at rest, is neurologically normal. Episodic weakness often signals neurological, neuromuscular, metabolic, or cardiopulmonary disease.[3]

Episodic sleep, or narcolepsy, is characterized by excessive sleepiness in people. In dogs, however, the only clinical sign is cataplexy, which is characterized by sudden, paroxysmal attacks of flaccid paralysis that may last from a few seconds to several minutes. The attacks may be induced by excitement. The frequency of attacks may vary from one every other day to several hundred per day. The most common electrophysiologic finding associated with narcolepsy/cataplexy in dogs is the REM (rapid eye movement) onset sleep with a shortened sleep cycle.[10]

Syncope (fainting) is a sudden loss of consciousness resulting from paroxysmal episodes of cerebral deprivation of oxygen or glucose. Syncope most commonly occurs secondary to decreased cerebral perfusion (cardiopulmonary disease).

Episodic cramping may occur in greyhounds in

association with lack of physical fitness, excessive excitement, or hot, humid climate.[6] The most characteristic is pelvic limb rigidity of sudden onset. Cramping may also occur in Scottish and Cairn terriers ("Scotty cramp").[2] Scotty cramp is due to a genetically determined deficiency of serotonin. Attacks are precipitated by excitement and exercise. Affected animals may develop a slight abduction in the thoracic limbs, arching of the lumbar spine, and hyperflexion of the pelvic limbs. The head may be drawn between the front legs as a result of spasm of the ventral cervical musculature, and the dog may somersault forward and lie motionless. Recovery usually occurs within 15 to 20 seconds.

1. Chrisman, C. L.: *Problems in Small Animal Neurology.* Lea & Febiger, Philadelphia, 1982.
2. Clemmons, R. M., Peters, R. I., and Meyers, K. M.: Scotty cramp: a review of cause, characteristics, diagnosis and treatment. Comp. Contin. Ed. 2:385, 1980.
3. de Lahunta, A.: *Veterinary Neuroanatomy and Clinical Neurology.* 2nd ed. W. B. Saunders, Philadelphia, 1983.
4. de Recondo, J.: *Principaux Syndromes Neurologiques.* Roussel Laboratories, Paris, 1976.
5. Fletcher, T. L., and Kitchell, R. L.: Anatomical studies on the spinal cord segments of the dog. Am. J. Vet. Res. 27:1759, 1966.
6. Gannon, J. R.: Exertional rhabdomyolysis (myoglobinurea) in the racing greyhound. *In* Kirk, R. W. (ed.): *Current Veterinary Therapy VII: Small Animal Practice.* W. B. Saunders, Philadelphia, 1980.
7. Griffiths, I. R., and Duncan, I. D.: Myotonia in the dog: a report of four cases. Vet. Rec. 93:184, 1973.
8. Hoerlein, B. F.: The brain and related disorders. *In* Hoerlein, B. F. (ed.): *Canine Neurology—Diagnosis and Treatment.* 3rd ed. W. B. Saunders, Philadelphia, 1978.
9. McGrath, J. T.: *Neurologic Examination of the Dog.* 2nd ed. Lea & Febiger, Philadelphia, 1960.
10. Mitler, M. M., Soave, O., and Dement, W. C.: Narcolepsy in seven dogs. J. Am. Vet. Med. Assoc. 168:1036, 1976.
11. Oliver, J. E., Jr.: Localization of lesions in the nervous system. *In* Hoerlein, B. F. (ed.): *Canine Neurology—Diagnosis and Treatment.* 3rd ed. W. B. Saunders, Philadelphia, 1978.
12. Oliver, J. E., Jr., and Selcer, R. R.: Neurogenic causes of abnormal micturition in the dog and cat. Vet. Clin. North Am. 4:517, 1974.
13. Palmer, A. C.: *Introduction to Animal Neurology.* 2nd ed. Blackwell Scientific Publications, Oxford, 1976.
14. Redding, R. W., and Braund, K. G.: Neurological examination. *In* Hoerlein, B. F. (ed.): *Canine Neurology—Diagnosis and Treatment.* 3rd ed. W. B. Saunders, Philadelphia, 1978.
15. Vinken, P. J., and Bruyn, G. W.: *Handbook of Clinical Neurology: Localization in Clinical Neurology.* Vol. 2. North-Holland Publishing Co., Amsterdam, 1969.

Chapter **90**

Pathogenesis of Diseases of the Central Nervous System

Joe N. Kornegay

THE BRAIN

Anatomy

The skull and dural septae protect the brain but limit its ability to adjust to increases in intracranial volume. These constraints are expressed by the Monro-Kellie doctrine: the brain, cerebrospinal fluid (CSF), and cerebral blood volume are virtually incompressible, and their total volume remains relatively constant.[77] An increase in volume of any one of these three compartments is accompanied by a reciprocal decrease in another, or intracranial pressure increases. In this regard, the cranial vault demonstrates low compliance (volume added per change in pressure).

Intracranial space-occupying lesions initially may be accommodated through transfer of CSF to the spinal subarachnoid space or reduction in cerebral blood volume. These compensatory mechanisms are eventually overcome if the lesion becomes too large or interferes with either CSF or venous outflow. Resultant increased intracranial pressure (>200 mm H_2O or 15 mm Hg) may impede cerebral blood flow (see "Cushing Response") or lead to displacement (herniation) of portions of the brain through foramina or ventral to dural septae.[77, 102]

Four forms of brain herniation have been identified in animals: (1) cingulate gyrus herniation ventral to the falx cerebri (subfalcial herniation) (Fig. 90–1A), (2) herniation of portions of the temporal cortex ventral to the tentorium cerebelli (caudal transtentorial herniation) (Fig. 90–1B), (3) caudal cerebellar vermis herniation through the foramen magnum (foramen magnum herniation) (Fig. 90–1C), and (4) herniation of the rostral cerebellar vermis ventral to the tentorium cerebelli (rostral transtentorial herniation) (Fig. 90–1D).[72] Caudal transtentorial and fora-

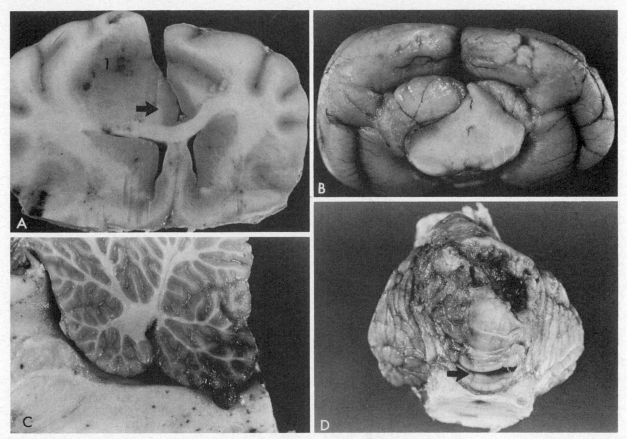

Figure 90–1. Forms of brain herniation in animals. *A*, Coronal section at the basal nuclei from a ten-year-old female English setter with chronic, progressive neurological dysfunction referable to the left forebrain. A mass in the left frontal cortex (1) compresses adjacent tissue, resulting in displacement of the left cingulate gyrus medially *(arrow)*. A diagnosis of left subfalcial brain herniation secondary to a metastatic sarcoma was made. *B*, Caudal view from a three-year-old male domestic cat with acute, progressive neurological dysfunction. The brain has been transected between the midbrain and pons. There is caudal displacement of the parahippocampal gyri with compression of the midbrain and collapse of the mesencephalic aqueduct. A diagnosis of caudal transtentorial brain herniation secondary to cerebral phaeohyphomycosis was made. See Figures 90–2 and 90–14. *C*, Sagittal section from a two-year-old male German shepherd with acute, progressive neurological dysfunction. The caudoventral cerebellar vermis (uvula and nodulus lobules) is discolored and malacic. There are petechiae in the underlying medulla oblongata. A diagnosis of foramen magnum brain herniation secondary to a pituitary carcinoma was made. *D*, Rostral view from a nine-year-old female Vizsla with acute, progressive neurological dysfunction. The dorsal cerebellar vermis is discolored and malacic. Folia of the rostral cerebellar vermis are flattened and grooved ventrally *(arrow)*. A diagnosis of rostral transtentorial brain herniation secondary to a cerebellar abscess was made. (*A* and *D* reprinted with permission from Kornegay, J. N., et al.: Clinicopathologic features of brain herniation in animals. J. Am. Vet. Med. Assoc. *182*:1111, 1983.)

men magnum herniation are the most detrimental forms. Both often cause tetraplegia and coma because of involvement of motor pathways and the reticular activating system, respectively. Animals with caudal transtentorial herniation also may have pupillary dilation owing to oculomotor nerve compression (Fig. 90–2); those with foramen magnum herniation usually are apneic because of involvement of medullary respiratory centers or pathways. Either form may be associated with additional cranial nerve deficits if herniation continues.

The speed of onset of the inciting lesion is an important determinant of both the likelihood of brain herniation and the severity of resultant neurological dysfunction. Slowly expanding lesions allow time for spacial accommodation and physiological regulation (see later). These protective mechanisms are circumvented by acute lesions and, therefore, both the risk of brain herniation and the severity of its consequences are increased.[72] Factors that may precipitate

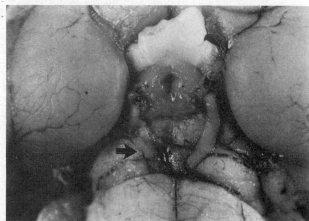

Figure 90–2. Ventral view of the cat in Figure 90–1*B*. The right oculomotor nerve (arrow) is grooved and distorted. A diagnosis of oculomotor nerve compression secondary to caudal transtentorial brain herniation was made. (Reprinted with permission from Kornegay, J. N., Oliver, J. E., and Gorgacz, E. J.: Clinicopathologic features of brain herniation in animals. J. Am. Vet. Med. Assoc. *182*:1111, 1983.)

herniation in animals with brain disease include the administration of volatile anesthetic agents and aspiration of CSF. Most volatile anesthetics cause cerebral vasodilation, which increases the cerebral blood volume and intracranial pressure.[36] Removal of CSF increases the pre-existing pressure gradient between the cranial and spinal compartments.[31]

The protective effects of the skull and dural septae are obvious. However, unique microscopic vascular features are equally important in protecting the brain from injury. One such feature is the continuity of the cerebral capillary endothelium; fenestrations found in the capillaries of certain other organs are not present in the brain.[64] The most important factor, however, is the blood-brain barrier, which is formed collectively by the endothelial cells and basement membranes of the cerebral capillaries and astrocytic processes (end-feet) that invest the vessel wall. The blood-brain barrier is readily penetrated by only water, oxygen, and carbon dioxide. Other substances such as glucose also penetrate the barrier, but at a much slower rate than elsewhere in the body. Thus, the brain is physically insulated from blood-borne injurious agents such as microorganisms and certain chemicals. Although the blood-brain barrier protects the healthy brain, it also impedes delivery of therapeutic agents. In treating brain disease, therefore, the degree of penetration of any drug becomes an additional factor that must be considered together with its efficacy and side effects.[71] The problem of penetration is partially countered by the fact that the blood-brain barrier is disrupted by infection and tumor involvement. As such, certain drugs that might otherwise be impeded may gain entrance in therapeutic concentrations.[51] Other drugs are excluded from the brain even when it is inflamed.[41]

Physiology

The brain largely depends upon oxidative metabolism of glucose for its unusually high energy requirements. To ensure uninterrupted supply of oxygen and glucose, cerebral blood flow must be maintained at a relatively constant rate. The level of cerebral blood flow is determined by cerebral perfusion pressure (mean arterial pressure minus intracranial pressure). Factors causing either a reduction in mean arterial pressure or an increase in intracranial pressure may impede the brain's blood supply. Fortunately, intrinsic safeguards insulate cerebral blood flow from routine fluctuations in both mean arterial pressure and intracranial pressure. Blood supply to the brain is also adjusted to meet changes in cerebral metabolic requirements and to avoid the injurious effects of both systemic hypoxia and hypercapnia. Mechanisms responsible for these essential safeguards and their limitations are discussed in the following sections.

Pressure Autoregulation

Coupling of cerebral blood flow and mean arterial pressure is termed pressure autoregulation (Fig. 90–3). This process maintains the brain's blood supply at a constant rate despite fluctuations in mean arterial pressure between 50 and 160 mm Hg.[77] Several mechanisms have been proposed to explain this phenomenon. The myogenic theory attributes pressure autoregulation to pressure-sensitive smooth muscle in cerebral vessel walls.[7] Studies supporting this theory indicate that the tone of this muscle varies directly with the intraluminal pressure.[38] Increased mean arterial pressure causes vasoconstriction, resulting in diminution of cerebral blood flow. A decrease in intraluminal pressure has the opposite effect. Other theories attribute pressure autoregulation to changes in local tissue pressure[132] and sympathetic innervation of cerebral blood vessels.[8]

Pressure autoregulation is impaired by brain disease.[77, 102] Hypoxia, trauma, cerebral infarction, vasospasm, and seizures are among the disorders that may have such an effect. With loss of pressure autoregulation, cerebral blood flow becomes passively dependent on mean arterial pressure. Widespread vasodilation and associated congestion and edema almost invariably occur,[102] causing a further increase in intracranial pressure, and thus potentiating the risk of brain herniation, which in turn intensifies the degree of ischemia. The process becomes self-perpetuating, and rapid neurologic deterioration (decompensation) ensues.

Cushing Response

Increased intracranial pressure evokes a corresponding increase in systemic arterial pressure (Cushing response) that maintains cerebral blood flow.[87] Although mechanisms responsible for this phenomenon are unclear, experiments suggest a role for intracranial receptors sensitive to differences in pressure between the intravascular space and the cerebrospinal fluid.[107] Evidently, increased intracranial pressure is perceived by these receptors as a decrease in intravascular pressure, thus eliciting sympatheti-

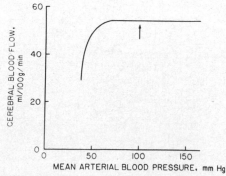

Figure 90–3. Effect of mean arterial blood pressure (*arrow* denotes normal value) on cerebral blood flow. Cerebral blood flow is relatively constant despite moderate hypotension and severe hypertension. (Reprinted with permission from Jensen, D. J.: *Principles of Physiology.* Appleton-Century-Crofts, New York, 1980.)

cally mediated peripheral venous constriction. Impairment of this response during brain disease exposes the brain to the deleterious effects of increased intracranial pressure (brain ischemia and herniation). The Cushing response is more resilient than pressure autoregulation, at least with regard to hypoxia.[87]

Metabolic Autoregulation

Cerebral blood flow also varies according to the metabolic needs of brain tissue. Increased neural activity such as occurs subsequent to seizures increases cerebral blood flow,[116] and decreased activity causes diminution.[85] Coupling of cerebral metabolism and blood flow is termed metabolic autoregulation. Although its physiological basis is unproven, accumulation of metabolic by-products, including hydrogen, potassium and adenosine, is thought to contribute.[77] Metabolic autoregulation is impaired by head injury.[15]

Chemical Regulation

Cerebral vessels are also sensitive to the arterial partial pressures of oxygen (Pa_{O_2}) and carbon dioxide (Pa_{CO_2}).[75] Systemic hypoxia induces cerebral vessel dilation, leading to increased cerebral blood flow. Brain tissue oxygenation is maintained until Pa_{O_2} falls to 20 mm Hg.[77] Further reduction in oxygen tension necessitates anaerobic glycolysis, and energy requirements are no longer met. The effect of Pa_{O_2} on cerebral vessels is not well defined but appears to be mediated, at least in part, through the action of tissue pH on vascular smooth muscle.[77] Fluctuations in Pa_{CO_2} have an even more potent effect on cerebral vessel tone. Systemic hypercapnia causes cerebral vessel dilation. Resultant enhancement of blood flow prevents cerebral acidosis. Reduction of Pa_{CO_2} through hyperventilation has an opposite effect and is useful in controlling hemorrhage during brain surgery. The effect of Pa_{CO_2} either is due to a direct effect on vascular smooth muscle[114] or occurs through a reflex mediated by chemoreceptors in the aortic and carotid areas.[63] Chemical regulation is also disrupted by intracranial disease. However, it appears to be more resistant to impairment than pressure autoregulation.[102]

Response to Disease

Neural tissue reactions are limited. Most brain diseases cause glial proliferation, proliferation and congestion of vessels, and at least some edema. In addition, many result in necrosis (malacia), hemorrhage, and infiltration of inflammatory cells. The distribution and progression of these lesions vary with the disease (Table 90–1). However, regardless of their type, cause, and location, many of these changes eventually interfere with physiological regulation, resulting in brain herniation and a final common clinical course. Frequently encountered

TABLE 90–1. Major Categories of Brain Disease in Dogs and Cats*

Etiology	Lesion Distribution	Onset	Progression
Inflammatory	Diffuse	Insidious	Gradual
Degenerative	Diffuse	Insidious	Gradual
Metabolic	Diffuse	Insidious	Gradual
Vascular	Focal	Acute	None
Neoplastic	Focal	Insidious	Gradual
Toxic	Diffuse	Acute or insidious	None or gradual
Traumatic	Focal or diffuse	Acute	None or gradual

*The table describes the typical course of each category.

brain lesions and their potential causes are discussed in the following sections.

Malacia

Brain necrosis (encephalomalacia) is liquefactive and can be focal or diffuse. Diffuse lesions preferentially may involve either gray matter (polioencephalomalacia) or white matter (leukoencephalomalacia). Principal causes of encephalomalacia in dogs and cats are depletion of brain oxygen or glucose, trauma, and inflammation.

Ischemia, Hypoxia, and Hypoglycemia. Reduction of either brain oxygen or glucose causes malacia. Causes of cerebral hypoxia include diminution of Pa_{O_2} (hypoxic hypoxia), depletion of blood hemoglobin (anemic hypoxia), impaired tissue utilization of oxygen (histotoxic hypoxia), and reduction of the brain's blood supply (cerebral ischemia) due to either selective impairment of cerebral blood flow (oligemic hypoxia) or reduced cardiac output (stagnant hypoxia).[12] Reduction of brain glucose may occur because of either cerebral ischemia or systemic hypoglycemia.

The malacic effects of cerebral ischemia are well documented.[14] Mechanisms involved, however, remain poorly defined. Classic studies provide indisputable evidence of irreversible neuronal injury following four to six minutes of cerebral ischemia.[43] Some brain function may return after periods of complete ischemia lasting as long as 60 minutes.[61] This finding suggests that variables other than the duration of ischemia contribute to the severity of injury. One such variable is the quality of cerebral blood flow after the initial ischemic insult. There is general agreement that brain blood supply remains impaired for a variable period after removal of the offending lesion. Known as the "no-reflow phenomenon," this process of postischemic hypotension was originally believed to occur because of ischemia-induced endothelial cell swelling and associated narrowing of the vascular lumen. Although a recent

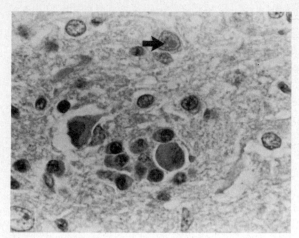

Figure 90–4. Thalamus from a one-year-old male Pekingese with cervical hyperesthesia and stupor of three days duration. The two neurons at the center of the picture are ischemic. Their cell bodies are shrunken and surrounded by inflammatory cells. The nucleus of the neuron to the top of the picture *(arrow)* contains an inclusion body. A diagnosis of polioencephalomalacia secondary to canine distemper virus infection was made. H & E ×252.

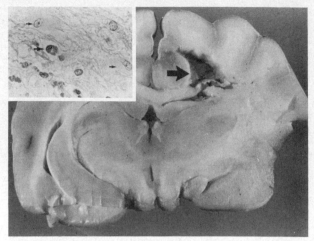

Figure 90–5. Transverse section of brain at the thalamus from a ten-year-old female domestic cat with seizures of recent onset. Note the cavity in the right parietal cortex dorsal to the corpus callosum *(arrow)*. Focal ischemic encephalopathy was suspected and confirmed by microscopic examination. *Inset,* Photomicrograph from the edge of the infarct. Note the extravasated erythrocytes at the lower left and the hemosiderin-laden macrophage *(large arrow)* flanked by two gemistocytic astrocytes *(small arrows)* toward the center of the picture. H & E ×252.

study questions this explanation of its origin,[34] the detrimental effects of postischemic hypotension on brain function have been substantiated by others.[60] Accordingly, measures taken to improve the quality of postischemic perfusion facilitate return of function.[110] An additional factor contributing to the severity of ischemic injury is the completeness of the insult. Surprisingly, experimental data suggest that complete cessation of cerebral blood supply may be less injurious than incomplete ischemia.[60] Simple failure of cellular metabolism owing to hypoxia and hypoglycemia is no longer an adequate explanation for cell injury. Pathological processes that require glucose (lactic acidosis) or oxygen (lipid peroxidation) have been proposed.[24, 86] Regardless of the exact pathogenesis, the metabolic effects of ischemia are manifested morphologically within 12 hours by neuronal shrinkage and eosinophilia (ischemic cell change)[12] (Fig. 90–4). Neurons in cerebrocortical layers having higher metabolic demands are involved initially, often resulting in a characteristic laminar (single layer) or pseudolaminar (multiple layers) pattern of cerebrocortical neuronal necrosis. When there is diffuse cerebral ischemia, the patient may die prior to the development of other lesions. Such is often the case in animals dying following cardiac arrest.[99] A similar pattern of cerebrocortical necrosis has also been seen in dogs with canine distemper, presumably because of ischemia subsequent to vascular changes induced by the virus.[79] In cases of focal cerebral ischemia, there usually is long-term patient survival, and these neuronal changes are followed by fragmentation of axons and myelin, proliferation of macrophages, gliosis, and eventual cavitation (Fig. 90–5). Such lesions of focal cerebral infarction are common in humans because of their high incidence of cerebral atherosclerosis but occur infrequently in dogs (Fig. 90–6) and cats (see Fig. 90–5). An ischemic encephalopathy syndrome has been identified in cats.[21]

Although the cause and pathogenesis of this syndrome are not clear, some cats have had unexplained middle cerebral artery thrombosis, and one had concomitant lesions compatible with feline infectious peritonitis.[134]

The occurrence of ischemic cell change in association with nonischemic forms of cerebral hypoxia and systemic hypoglycemia suggests that these conditions have pathogenetic mechanisms similar to those of ischemia.[13] There usually is selective neuronal involvement with limited white matter degeneration, resulting in laminar or pseudolaminar cerebrocortical necrosis similar to that seen after cardiac arrest.[11] Documented causes of nonischemic cerebral hypoxia

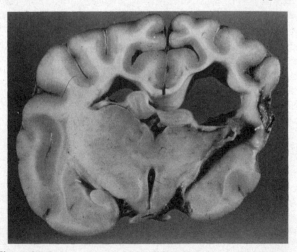

Figure 90–6. Transverse section of brain at the thalamus from a three-year-old female Yorkshire terrier with neurological dysfunction referable to the right forebrain. Note the atrophy of the right thalamus and temporal cortex and the consequent enlargement of the right ventricle (hydrocephalus *ex vacuo*). On the basis of these features and histological evidence of cholesterol clefts and previous hemorrhage, a diagnosis of cerebral atrophy subsequent to infarction was made.

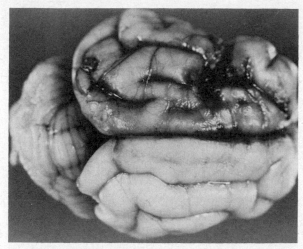

Figure 90–7. Brain from a one-year-old female domestic cat with acute, progressive deterioration of neurological function after cranial trauma. The left frontal cortex is lacerated, and there is associated hemorrhage and malacia. There was concomitant caudal transtentorial and foramen magnum brain herniation.

in dogs include cyanide poisoning (histotoxic hypoxia)[52] and lead poisoning (undefined mechanism).[138] Systemic hypoglycemia has been reported subsequent to hyperinsulinism.[73]

Trauma. Traumatic brain injury is common in cats but relatively infrequent in dogs because of the protective effects of their heavy temporal musculature and thick calvarium.[68, 93] Many animals with traumatic neurological dysfunction have no demonstrable brain lesion (concussion) or only focal subpial hemorrhage with minimal malacia (contusion). Others, however, have extensive malacia (Fig. 90–7), intracranial hemorrhage (see under "Hemorrhage") or both subsequent to the combined effects of brain laceration and vascular tears. Neurological dysfunction resulting from focal traumatic encephalomalacia may be due largely to concomitant edema and hemorrhage and may gradually resolve, particularly if the

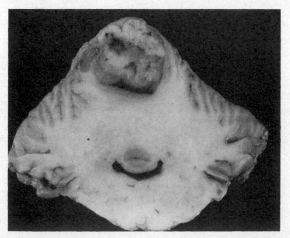

Figure 90–8. Transverse section of brain at the medulla oblongata from the dog in Figure 90–1D. The dorsal cerebellar vermis contains a roughly circular area of caseous necrosis. On microscopic examination, there was a marked infiltrate of neutrophils. *Enterobacter* sp. was cultured from the lesion. A diagnosis of focal cerebellar abscess was made.

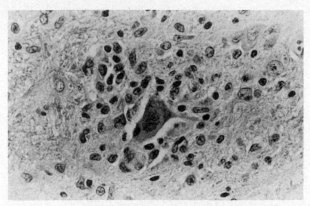

Figure 90–9. Spinal cord from a four-year-old male domestic cat with ascending lower motor neuron paralysis. Clinical signs occurred after inoculation with an approved rabies vaccine. The neuron at the center of the picture is degenerating and is surrounded by numerous microglial cells (neuronophagia). Fluorescent antibody testing of brain tissue from the cat was positive for rabies. A diagnosis of vaccine-induced rabies was made.

lesion is rostral to the midbrain. These primary effects of trauma often cause physiological deregulation leading to brain herniation within 12 hours.[72] Animals that recover after cranial trauma may have residual seizure foci.

Inflammation. Release of lysosomal enzymes by degenerating neutrophils and macrophages results in malacia. Lesions may occur focally as with bacterial abscess formation (Fig. 90–8) or diffusely owing to disseminated encephalitis. Diffuse inflammatory processes often have a perivascular distribution, especially if there is concomitant vasculitis. There may be selective involvement of either gray matter (polioencephalitis) or white matter (leukoencephalitis). Examples of polioencephalitis include a poorly defined condition of apparent viral origin in cats,[120] a syndrome associated with canine distemper virus infection[79] and rabies.[33] The classic lesion of polioencephalitis is neuronal degeneration and subsequent phagocytosis (neuronophagia) (Fig. 90–9). Leukoencephalitis and attendant lymphocyte-mediated demyelination are the hallmarks of canine distemper virus infection.[122, 127] An apparent variant of this disease occasionally produces cerebrocortical leukoencephalomalacia (Fig. 90–10). Animals with inflammatory brain disease are especially prone to brain herniation, probably because of the tendency for extensive concomitant edema,[72] and particularly if there is vascular involvement.

Hemorrhage

Intracranial hemorrhage may be extradural, subdural, subarachnoid, or intracerebral. Subarachnoid hemorrhage and associated cardiac arrhythmias account for four to five per cent of all natural sudden deaths in humans.[101] Dysfunction of both the parasympathetic and sympathetic nervous systems have been implicated. Experimental data indicate that subarachnoid hemorrhage may induce cardiac arrhythmias in animals as well.[92] The other forms of intracranial hemorrhage also may induce myocardial

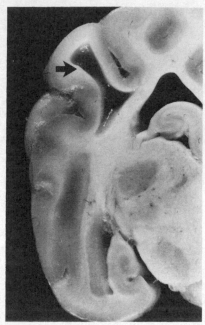

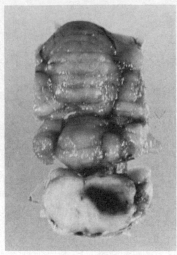

Figure 90–12. Transverse section of brain at the caudal medulla oblongata from a six-year-old male Maltese terrier with acute neurological dysfunction after cranial trauma. The right medulla oblongata contains a focal area of hemorrhage.

Figure 90–10. Transverse hemisection of brain at the thalamus from an adult female Chihuahua with seizures. The white matter of a gyrus of the parietal cortex at the top of the picture is malacic *(arrow).* White matter elsewhere in the corona radiata was similarly affected. On microscopic examination, there was an associated mononuclear inflammatory cell infiltrate. Virus-induced leukoencephalomalacia was suspected.

changes.[62] A greater potential danger, however, is the risk of increased intracranial pressure and consequent diminution of cerebral blood flow and brain herniation. The principal causes of intracranial hemorrhage in dogs and cats are trauma and vascular disease.

Trauma. All cranial trauma probably causes at least minimal subclinical intracranial hemorrhage. The incidence of hematoma formation in dogs and cats, however, is low. Epidural and subdural hematomas usually occur when the injury induces either rapid acceleration or rapid deceleration of the entire head.[86]

Both types of hematoma usually are formed shortly after trauma but may not be manifested clinically until hours or days later, when brain edema further increases intracranial pressure, resulting in herniation. Most epidural hematomas are associated with linear skull fractures that tear meningeal vessels, particularly the middle meningeal artery. Subdural hematomas usually form either subsequent to tearing of a surface vein or because of exteriorization of intracerebral hemorrhage (Fig. 90–11). The cause and clinical manifestations of intracerebral hematomas (Fig. 90–12) are different.[87] Most are associated with focal application of force as occurs with missile injuries and depressed skull fractures. Neurological dysfunction is related to the area of involvement, occurs acutely, and may be static or may even improve unless the hematoma enlarges or herniation occurs.

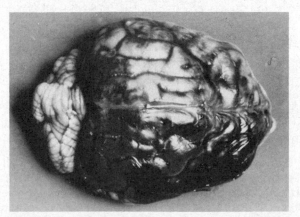

Figure 90–11. Dorsal view of brain from a one-year-old female Australian shepherd with acute, progressive deterioration of neurological function after cranial trauma. The dura covering the cerebellum was removed but is intact over the cerebral hemispheres. There is diffuse subarachnoid hemorrhage, and a focal area of subdural hemorrhage overlies the right frontal and parietal cortices. Evidence of caudal transtentorial brain herniation was also found.

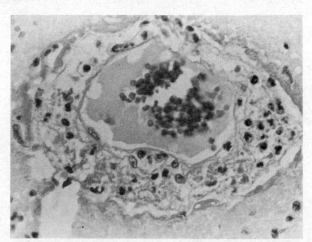

Figure 90–13. Cerebral brain from a one-year-old female domestic cat with acute, progressive neurological dysfunction and gross evidence of caudal transtentorial and foramen magnum brain herniation. The vessel wall contains neutrophils and is undergoing fibrinoid necrosis. Extravascular vacuoles are compatible with vasogenic edema. A diagnosis of cerebral vasculitis and edema was made. Feline infectious peritonitis virus infection was suspected. H & E ×160.

Vascular Disease. Cerebrovascular disease is uncommon in dogs and cats. Feline infectious peritonitis causes vasculitis (Fig. 90–13) and associated petechial or ecchymotic cerebral hemorrhage.[115] Vasculitis involving the central nervous system also has been described in dogs.[59] Degenerative vascular diseases such as atherosclerosis are rare in both species.

Edema

Brain edema occurs subsequent to most cerebral diseases. Its gross morphological features include flattening of cerebrocortical gyri and loss of distinction between gray and white matter (Fig. 90–14). Diffuse involvement increases intracranial pressure, resulting in brain ischemia and herniation. Forms of edema that have been identified are vasogenic, cytotoxic, and interstitial.[35, 65] They often occur concomitantly.

Cytotoxic Edema. The principal cause of cytotoxic edema is hypoxia-induced failure of the cellular sodium pump.[35] Sodium accumulates intracellularly, necessitating imbibition of water to maintain osmotic equilibrium. Neurons, glia, and endothelial cells are all affected. Causes of cerebral hypoxia were discussed previously.

Vasogenic Edema. Vasogenic brain edema occurs when any factor increases cerebrovascular permeability, allowing escape of fluid into the extracellular space. Fluid accumulates chiefly within white matter, through which it is transported to other areas of the brain by bulk transport.[106] Mechanisms responsible for fluid exudation include enhanced pinocytosis,[126] penetration of endothelial cell tight junctions,[6] and transmembranal flooding.[6] Principal causes of vasogenic brain edema in dogs and cats include encephalitis, head injury, and brain tumors. Brain herniation is most likely to occur subsequent to this form of edema.

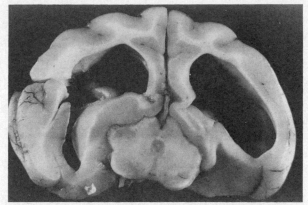

Figure 90–15. Transverse section of brain at the midbrain from an eight-month-old male Siamese cat with chronic neurological dysfunction referable to diffuse brain involvement. The lateral ventricles are dilated bilaterally. The surrounding cerebrocortical tissue is atrophic. The midbrain is compressed bilaterally because of concomitant caudal transtentorial brain herniation. On microscopic examination, there was evidence of chronic meningoencephalitis, ventriculitis, and choroiditis. A diagnosis of hydrocephalus subsequent to decreased cerebrospinal fluid absorption was made. Feline infectious peritonitis virus infection was suspected.

Interstitial Edema. Hydrocephalus is the lone cause of interstitial brain edema. Increased intraventricular hydrostatic pressure results in transependymal movement of CSF into the extracellular space of the periventricular white matter. Despite expansion of the extracellular space, however, rapid dissolution of myelin lipids actually decreases the volume of periventricular white matter (Fig. 90–15). Obstruction to CSF outflow and defective absorption of CSF at the arachnoid villi are the principal causes of hydrocephalus. Outflow obstruction may occur at either the lateral apertures (Fig. 90–16) or the mesencephalic aqueduct (Fig. 90–17), owing to anomalous development, neoplasia, or inflammation.[58] Potential causes of defective absorption of CSF at the arachnoid villi include malformation[58] and arachnoiditis.[74]

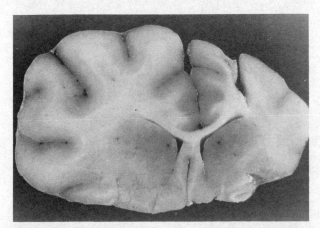

Figure 90–14. Transverse section of brain from the cat in Figures 90–1B and 90–2. The cerebrocortical gyri are flattened and there is expansion of the white matter of the corona radiata on the left side. The left cingulate gyrus and thalamus are displaced medially. There also was evidence of caudal transtentorial and foramen magnum herniation. On microscopic examination of adjacent sections, there was evidence of a fungal encephalitis. A diagnosis of cerebral phaeohyphomycosis and associated edema was made.

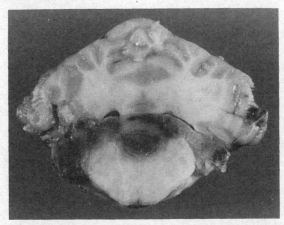

Figure 90–16. Transverse section of brain at the medulla oblongata from a three-year-old male domestic cat with chronic wasting and vague neurological dysfunction. The fourth ventricle and lateral apertures contain fibrinopurulent material and associated hemorrhage. On microscopic evaluation, there was evidence of an acute necrotizing ventriculitis and choroiditis. Feline infectious peritonitis virus infection was suspected.

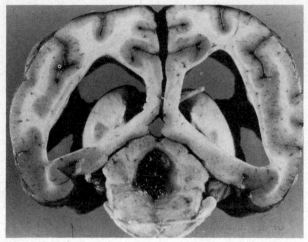

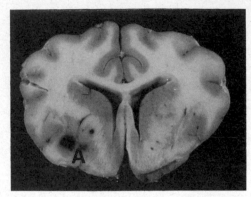

Figure 90–17   *Figure 90–18*

Figure 90–17. Transverse section of brain at the midbrain from a six-year-old male Boston terrier with cervical hyperesthesia and vague neurological dysfunction referable to the brain stem. Brain stem involvement occurred acutely within 12 hours of death. The mesencephalic aqueduct is poorly defined and the periaqueductal tissue is discolored. Both lateral ventricles are dilated and the surrounding cerebrocortical tissue is atrophic. Microscopic features of the periaqueductal lesion were compatible with an oligodendroglioma. Similar tissue extended into the fourth ventricle. Ventricular enlargement was presumed owing to obstructive hydrocephalus. There was concomitant foramen magnum brain herniation.

Figure 90–18. Transverse section of brain at the thalamus from a 12-year-old male Boston terrier with neurological dysfunction referable to the left forebrain of four weeks duration. A poorly defined astrocytoma *(A)* and associated hemorrhage are evident in the left temporal cortex lateral to the internal capsule.

Neoplasia

Recent reviews have established the incidence, morphology and topography of primary intracranial neoplasms of dogs and cats (Table 90–2) (Figs. 90–17 to 90–20).[32, 55, 81, 133] Most of these tumors develop as solitary masses that grow primarily by expansion and seldom metastasize to points either within or outside the central nervous system. That these are biological features of a benign neoplasm is ironic, in that brain tumors are among the most catastrophic of all illnesses. Nevertheless, this course of growth does account for the typically insidious onset and progression of clinical signs of most intracranial neoplasms. Occasional variation from this clinical pattern also may be explained by the tumor's biological behavior. Dedifferentiation (anaplasia) of cells composing the tumor generally is associated with rapid growth, local invasiveness, and an increased likelihood of metastasis. Tumors fulfilling these criteria are malignant and cause neurological dysfunction that is both acute in onset and rapidly progressive.

Most types of extracranial neoplasms occasionally metastasize to the brain (Fig. 90–21). These secon-

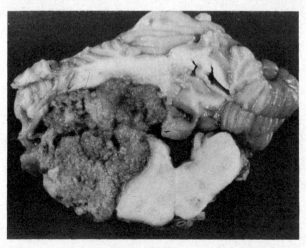

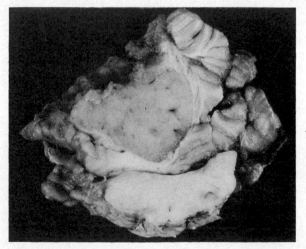

Figure 90–19   *Figure 90–20*

Figure 90–19. Transverse section of brain at the medulla oblongata from an eight-year-old male Irish setter with progressive neurological dysfunction referable to a left central vestibular lesion of eight weeks duration. A large, pedunculated, well-demarcated choroid plexus papilloma compresses the left medulla oblongata and cerebellum.

Figure 90–20. Transverse section of brain at the medulla oblongata from a four-year-old Old English sheepdog with neurological dysfunction of six months duration referable to the cerebellum. A large, well-demarcated meningioma compresses the cerebellum and medulla oblongata.

TABLE 90–2. Neoplasms of the Central Nervous System of Dogs and Cats

Tumor Type	Incidence (Dogs)	Breed Predilection (Dogs)	Age Predilection	Gross Morphological Features	Histological Features	Location	Biological Behavior
Astrocytoma (Fig. 90–18)	Common	Brachycephalic	Old	Solid, gray-white, poorly demarcated	Variable depending on cell origin: protoplasmic, fibrillary, gemistocytic, pilocytic	Cerebrum, thalamus	Benign
Oligodendroglioma (Fig. 90–17)	Common	Brachycephalic	Old	Friable, red, poorly demarcated; hemorrhage	Small hyperchromatic nuclei; perinuclear halos	Cerebrum	Ventricular invasion
Choroid plexus papilloma (Fig. 90–19)	Common	None	Middle-aged to old	Papillary, gray-white to red, well-demarcated	Papilliform; resembles choroid plexus	Cerebellopontine angle, third and fourth ventricles	Benign
Meningioma (Figs. 90–10, 90–22)	Common	Dolicho-cephalic	Old	Solid, gray-white, multilobulated, well-demarcated	Variable: endotheliomatus, fibromatous	Cerebrum (dogs and cats), cerebellum and spinal cord (dogs)	Benign
Reticulosis	Common	None	Middle-aged to old	Poorly demarcated	Variable: granulomatous, neoplastic, microgliomatous	Cerebrum, brain stem	Locally invasive
Pituitary adenoma	Common	Brachycephalic	Old	Gray-white to red, well-demarcated; hemorrhage, necrosis	Adenomatous	Pituitary, third ventricle, thalamus	Locally invasive
Glioblastoma	Infrequent	Brachycephalic	Old	Solid, gray-white to red, poorly demarcated; hemorrhage, necrosis	Cellular pleomorphism, hemorrhage, necrosis	Cerebrum, thalamus	Locally invasive
Ependymoma (Fig. 90–27)	Infrequent	None	Middle-aged to old	Soft, bulging, gray-white, poorly demarcated; hemorrhage, necrosis	Small hyperchromatic nuclei, rosettes and pseudorosettes	Lateral ventricle, spinal cord	Locally invasive; ventricular invasion
Medulloblastoma	Infrequent	None	Young to middle-aged	Soft, bulging, gray-red, well-demarcated	Small hyperchromatic nuclei, pseudorosettes	Cerebellum	Ventricular invasion; CSF metastasis
Epidermoid or dermoid cyst	Infrequent	None	Young	Soft, caseous, gray-white, well-demarcated	Cyst, squamous epithelium, keratin	Cerebellopontine angle, fourth ventricle	Benign
Metastatic (Figs. 90–21, 90–28)	Common	None	Middle-aged to old	Variable depending on primary; usually solid, well-demarcated	Variable: sarcoma, carcinoma, melanoma	Cerebrum	Variable

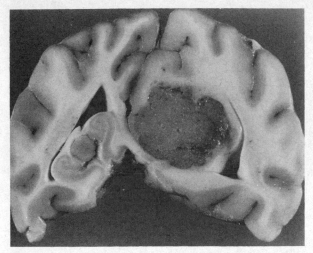

Figure 90–21. Transverse section of brain at the occipital cortex from a 11-year-old male Shih Tzu with seizures of recent onset. The right occipital cortex contains a large, well-demarcated metastatic pheochromocytoma that compresses adjacent tissue and the lateral ventricle.

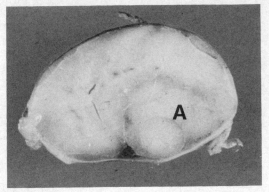

Figure 90–22. Transverse section of spinal cord at the seventh cervical spinal cord segment from an 11-year-old male German shepherd with progressive right-sided hemiparesis. A lobulated, well-demarcated subdural meningioma (A) compresses the spinal cord.

dary brain tumors usually are associated with acute, progressive neurologic dysfunction referable to the site of metastasis. Because the primary tumor often is subclinical, neurological dysfunction may be the initial clinical sign. Aspiration or biopsy of unexplained dermal or abdominal masses can assist in diagnosis.

The clinical effects of intracranial neoplasms are due primarily to compression of adjacent tissue. However, secondary effects may be equally detrimental. Brain tumors tend to disrupt the blood-brain barrier, resulting in vasogenic edema, may cause vessel wall necrosis and associated hemorrhage, and can obstruct CSF outflow. Increases in intracranial pressure produced by any or all of these factors may lead to brain herniation.[72]

THE SPINAL CORD

Anatomy

Acute and chronic diseases of the spinal cord are distinct clinicopathological syndromes. Anatomic restrictions placed on the spinal cord are particularly important in the pathogenesis of chronic compression, in contrast to acute injury, which is largely a physiological phenomenon (see "Physiology").

Movement of the spinal cord in response to compressive extramedullary lesions is restricted not only by the surrounding vertebrae and meninges but also by the nerve roots as they leave the spine. The spinal cord often becomes trapped between one of these structures and the offending lesion (Fig. 90–22). Less frequently, extradural masses encircle the spinal cord, because their growth follows the route of least resistance (Fig. 90–23). The gradual onset of many of these lesions allows time for spinal cord accommodation, so there may be minimal initial neurological

dysfunction. With continued compression, however, neural function is lost in a predictable sequence. Conscious proprioception is lost first, followed by voluntary motor activity, superficial (primary) pain sensation, and deep (secondary) pain sensation.[117]

Mechanisms responsible for the effects of chronic spinal cord compression are not clear. The sequence of neurological deterioration appears to reflect greater sensitivity to pressure of large, heavily myelinated fibers that convey position sense and motor function, compared with the lightly or nonmyelinated polysynaptic pathways responsible for pain sensation.[117] A similar effect of pressure has been demonstrated in peripheral nerves, in which larger A fibers are more pressure-sensitive than C fibers.[104] Anatomic changes accounting for this apparent mechanical effect of pressure have been identified in affected nerves.[91] Analogous lesions, however, have not been clearly documented after experimental chronic spinal cord compression. One study showed that histological

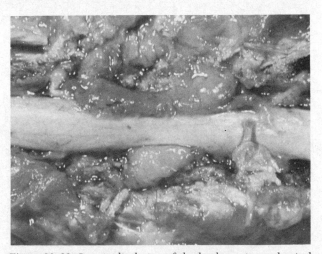

Figure 90–23. Longitudinal view of the lumbar spine and spinal cord. At the center of the picture, the spinal cord is compressed bilaterally by an extradural mass. Similar neoplastic tissue was present ventral to the spinal cord and in the underlying vertebral body. The tumor was a bile duct carcinoma with vertebral body metastasis.

changes occurring after seven hours of slow, graded compression were consistent with those of ischemia[113] (see "Malacia"). Other studies, though, indicate that mechanical factors are more important than ischemia.[50, 117] Spinal cord lesions following weeks of compression due to spontaneous disease also seem more compatible with mechanical injury. These changes usually are consistent with wallerian degeneration with minimal gray matter involvement (see "Demyelination"). Discrepancies between clinical and experimental findings probably reflect the mode and duration of compression. Lesions induced by only hours of experimental compression do not necessarily equate with those incurred after weeks of gradual compression due to spontaneous disease.

Physiology

An appreciation of the intricacies of spinal reflexes and autoregulation of spinal cord blood flow is necessary to fully understand the syndrome of acute spinal cord injury.

Spinal Reflexes

Spinal reflex activity is mediated locally and occurs independent of thought. Nevertheless, spinal reflexes are influenced considerably by both descending and ascending pathways. These interactions are responsible for spinal shock, hyperreflexia, mass reflex, the crossed extensor reflex, and the Schiff-Sherrington phenomenon.

Spinal Shock. Areflexia caudal to a lesion following acute functional spinal cord transection is termed spinal shock.[57, 109] It occurs because of sudden interruption of facilitory brain stem and forebrain input to spinal neurons. This supraspinal facilitory input alone is not adequate to initiate a reflex but adds considerably to the excitability of the neuron. When the facilitation is removed, the stimulus provided through the afferent arc of the reflex may be inadequate for neuronal depolarization.

Spinal shock is a transient condition that varies in depth and duration with the degree of cerebral dominance over the brain stem (encephalization).[57, 109] It may extend for months in humans and anthropoid apes but lasts only hours in carnivores. Responsible spinal pathways also vary with the degree of encephalization. The reticulospinal and vestibulospinal tracts in cats[39] and the corticospinal tracts in monkeys[57] have been incriminated.

Mechanisms responsible for recovery from spinal shock are not clear. Dorsal root axon sprouting could replenish the lost facilitory synaptic contacts.[109] This process, however, would require days and would not account for the rapidly reversible nature of spinal shock in carnivores. An alternate theory suggests that functional changes are induced in spinal neurons by supraspinal denervation.[109] These changes may contribute to the occurrence of spinal shock and may be reversible, thus accounting for recovery.

Hyperreflexia. Most dogs and cats with acute spinal cord injury have recovered from spinal shock when first examined and exhibit either normoreflexia or hyperreflexia. Extensor reflexes are especially prone to hyperactivity. Several factors may contribute to extensor hyperreflexia.[109] The most plausible explanation is that there is loss of supraspinal inhibition to extensor spinal neurons concomitant with the loss of facilitation responsible for spinal shock. With recovery from spinal shock, loss of inhibition would supervene, resulting in hyperreflexia and increased extensor muscle tone. These inhibitory spinal pathways are in the ventral funiculi in cats.[78] Another mechanism that may contribute to hyperreflexia is denervation hypersensitivity. Motor neurons partially denervated by spinal transection are overly sensitive to acetylcholine[16] and, therefore, may overreact to routine afferent stimulation. Dorsal root axonal sprouting initiated to replenish lost supraspinal input may produce an excess of synaptic contacts.[80] This excess would increase the magnitude of a reflex elicited by peripheral stimulation.

Mass Reflex. Spinal reflex activity in dogs and cats may become markedly exaggerated several months after functional spinal transection. In affected animals, peripheral stimulation induces bilateral, rapid limb flexion and tail twitching. Bowel and bladder evacuation also may occur. Advanced effects of those mechanisms causing hyperreflexia are responsible.

Crossed Extensor Reflex. Movements in all four limbs are normally coordinated through ascending and descending spinal tracts and neurons of the propriospinal system.[57] Noxious stimuli, applied peripherally, induce reflex responses in all four limbs (Fig. 90–24). These so-called long spinal reflexes are normally suppressed by descending supraspinal input. With experimental spinal transection, this inhibitory influence is removed, and hindlimb flexion is

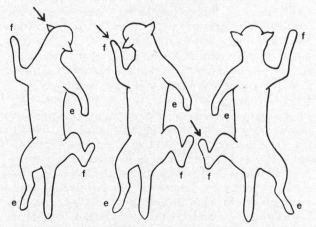

Figure 90–24. Reflex activity initiated in a cat with cranial cervical spinal cord transection when a noxious stimulus is applied at the point indicated by the arrow. *e*, Leg extended in response; *f*, leg flexed in response. (Reprinted with permission from Henneman, E.: Neural control of the spinal cord and its reflexes. *In* Mountcastle, V. B. (ed.): *Medical Physiology*, 14th ed. C. V. Mosby, St. Louis, 1980; after Sherrington, C. S.: Decerebrate rigidity and reflex coordination of movements. J. Physiol. 22:319, 1897–1898.)

accompanied by extension of the opposite hindlimb (crossed extensor reflex). The pattern is reversed in the contralateral limbs. The crossed extensor reflex is also seen clinically in animals with either complete functional spinal cord transection or chronic, incomplete lesions.

Schiff-Sherrington Phenomenon. Ascending spinal tracts in the ventral funiculi exert an inhibitory influence on the extensor muscles of the forelimbs.[26] Functional transection of these pathways causes forelimb extension, resulting in a characteristic posture. This process is termed the Schiff-Sherrington phenomenon.[108]

Spinal Cord Blood Flow

Normal spinal cord blood flow to gray matter (50 to 60 ml/100 gm/min) is approximately five times that of white matter (10 to 15 ml/100 gm/min.) in dogs and cats.[30, 45, 76] This level of spinal cord blood flow is maintained despite fluctuations in mean arterial pressure in a way analogous to cerebral blood flow pressure autoregulation.[28, 97] One study found that hypovolemic hypotension affects spinal cord blood flow more adversely than cerebral blood flow, suggesting that cerebral pressure autoregulation is more efficient.[66] Spinal cord blood flow was reduced by approximately 50 per cent when mean arterial pressure fell to 50 mm Hg and completely stopped at 30 mm Hg. Another study found that spinal cord blood flow was unchanged at mean arterial pressures of 70 to 80 mm Hg.[50] Spinal cord blood flow also varies directly with the Pa_{CO_2}.[30] Both chemical regulation and pressure autoregulation are impaired by spinal cord trauma.[50, 97]

Histopathological effects of spinal cord ischemia[19] are similar to those induced by acute impact injury.[30] Both are characterized by central hemorrhagic necrosis, suggesting that ischemia may contribute to the pathogenesis of acute spinal trauma. This supposition has been verified by studies showing that spinal cord blood flow is reduced for up to 24 hours after acute spinal cord injury.[25, 67, 112] That the reduction of blood flow is more pronounced and more prolonged centrally correlates with the sequence of histopathological changes seen after experimental ischemia and impact injury. Initial lesions of both are restricted to the gray matter; white matter is markedly involved only after either prolonged ischemia or extreme impact. Reasons for preferential gray matter involvement are not clear. However, the relative compactness of white matter and gray matter probably contributes. In contrast to the tightly packed fibers of white matter, neurons and their processes are loosely arranged and, therefore, are more easily separated by hemorrhage and edema.[30] Increases in post-traumatic spinal intramedullary pressure also are more concentrated centrally, thus predisposing this area to greater injury.[83] The increased metabolic demand of gray matter in comparison with white matter is an additional factor, particularly during periods of ischemia.

Two principal mechanisms have been proposed to explain the reduction of spinal cord blood flow after acute injury: vascular and neurovascular. The vascular theory attributes ischemia to direct effects of trauma on vessel walls, resulting in vasospasm,[2] vascular tears,[25] endothelial cell swelling,[25] and thrombi.[42] Most investigators agree that these effects of trauma contribute to spinal cord ischemia. However, some believe that the most important factor is vasospasm induced by vasoactive agents such as norepinephrine[95] and its precursor, dopamine.[89] Potential sources of these neurotransmitters include local hemorrhage[123] and severed spinal sympathetic nerve endings.[119] Although some studies have shown increased spinal cord tissue concentrations of either dopamine or norepinephrine after spinal trauma,[89, 95, 123] another study failed to demonstrate increased levels of either neurotransmitter.[105] Beneficial effects of alpha methyl tyrosine, an agent that blocks norepinephrine synthesis, are also controversial.[56, 96]

Response to Disease

Responses to spinal cord and brain disease are similar. This discussion is confined mainly to lesions that are more commonly associated with spinal disorders.

Malacia

Acute spinal cord injury often results in central hemorrhagic necrosis in dogs and cats. The most common cause is acute intervertebral disc herniation (Fig. 90–25).[44, 94] Factors contributing to the evolution of this lesion include ischemia (see previous discussion), mechanical distortion,[118] vascular damage,[90] and release of lysosomal enzymes.[131] The severity of histological changes varies directly with the force of impact.[30] With moderate impact, microvascular tears and associated hemorrhage and edema occur in the

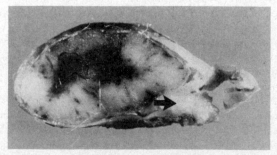

Figure 90–25. Transverse section of spinal cord at the sixth cervical segment from a five-year-old female Doberman pinscher with acute tetraplegia. The gray matter is malacic and hemorrhagic. A small amount of intervertebral disc material is seen ventrolaterally on the right side (arrow). A diagnosis of central hemorrhagic necrosis subsequent to acute intervertebral disc herniation was made.

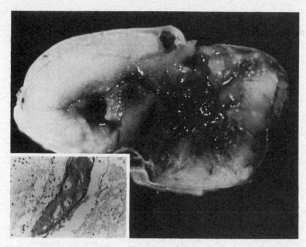

Figure 90–26. Transverse section of spinal cord at the lumbar intumescence from an adult Great Dane with acute paraplegia. All funiculi on the right side of the spinal cord are malacic and contain blood. Ischemic myelopathy subsequent to fibrocartilaginous embolism was suspected and confirmed by microscopic examination. *Inset*, A large fibrocartilaginous embolus occludes the vessel at the center. PAS-hematoxylin ×160.

gray matter within 15 minutes, neuronal degeneration is seen at one to four hours, and edema and focal axonal swelling occur in the white matter between four and six hours.[30, 124] Lesions resulting from intense impact are more severe and more widely distributed, often resulting in central cavitation with sparing of only a peripheral rim of white matter five to six days after injury.[30] Measures directed at reversing this process may be beneficial in treating acute spinal cord injury in dogs and cats.[84]

Myelomalacia also occurs subsequent to ischemia induced by vascular occlusion due to fibrocartilaginous emboli originating from the intervertebral disc.[20] This syndrome typically involves large dogs,[123] but smaller dogs[70] and cats[137] also may be affected. These emboli may originate from the nucleus pulposus and then gain access to the spinal cord microvasculature by penetrating either the vertebral venous sinuses[135] or arteries of the annulus fibrosus.[54]

Resulting myelomalacia often is lateral and usually involves both gray and white matter (Fig. 90–26). Emboli can be demonstrated histologically in most affected animals (Fig. 90–26, *inset*).

Demyelination

Loss of myelin without preceding axonal injury is termed primary demyelination. The most common cause of primary demyelination in small animals is canine distemper virus infection. In this disease, myelin is stripped from axons by invading lymphocytes as a result of a poorly defined immune-mediated process.[122, 127] Lesions usually involve the brain but may selectively affect the spinal cord, resulting in neurological signs indistinguishable from those caused by compressive spinal cord disease.

Loss of myelin secondary to axonal injury is termed secondary demyelination. The process of concomitant degeneration of the axon and its myelin sheath distal to the point of separation from the neuronal cell body, called wallerian degeneration, is the most common form of demyelination in dogs and cats. It is particularly marked after chronic spinal cord compression (see "Anatomy"). Histological lesions of wallerian degeneration begin within 30 hours after axonal severence and gradually progress over a period of six months.[10] Axons and their myelin sheaths are fragmented into a series of ovoid segments referred to as ellipsoids. The axonal fragments and myelin debris gradually are removed by macrophages, leaving residual vacuoles throughout the white matter. The anatomical distribution of these lesions in the spinal cord reflects the organization of afferent (sensory; cell bodies caudal to lesion) and efferent (motor; cell bodies cranial to lesion) pathways of the spinal cord. Vacuoles and degenerating axons are more prominent in the dorsolateral columns (primarily afferent) cranial to the lesion and in the ventrolateral columns (primarily efferent) caudal to the lesion. Near the site of injury, axonal endings that are still attached to the cell body become distended with axoplasm, forming bulbous axonal spheroids.

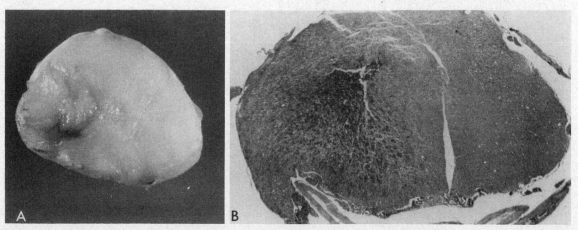

Figure 90–27. Transverse gross (A) and microscopic (B) sections of spinal cord at the thirteenth thoracic segment from an 11-year-old female bichon frise with progressive paraparesis of two months duration. The left ventral and lateral funiculi are largely replaced by a densely cellular ependymoma.

TABLE 90–3. Degenerative and Demyelinating Central Nervous System Diseases of Dogs and Cats

Disease	Breed Predilection	Age of Onset	Neurological Sign(s)*	Lesion(s)	Anatomical Distribution	Pathogenesis
Chronic degenerative radiculomyelopathy[3, 47, 125]	German Shepherd	5 to 10 yrs	Paraparesis	Demyelination, axonal degeneration	Midthoracic spinal cord (all funiculi) and nerve roots	Immunological
Hereditary myelopathy[4, 18]	Afghan	3 to 8 mo	Paraparesis progressing to tetraparesis	Demyelination, cavitation	Spinal cord; cervical (dorsal funiculi), thoracic (all funiculi), lumbar (ventral funiculi)	Hereditary (autosomal recessive), unknown defect
Progressive axonopathy[49]	Boxer	3 to 6 mos	Paraparesis progressing to tetraparesis, hyporeflexia	Axonal swelling and degeneration	Spinal cord (lateral and ventral funiculi), brain stem, peripheral nerves	Hereditary, unknown defect
Demyelinating myelopathy[27]	Miniature poodle	2 to 4 mos	Paraparesis progressing to tetraparesis	Demyelination	Spinal cord (all funiculi), brain stem	Hereditary, unknown defect
Hereditary ataxia[9, 53]	Smooth-haired fox terrier, Jack Russell terrier	2 to 6 mos	Posterior ataxia, forelimb hypermetria	Wallerian degeneration	Spinal cord (dorsolateral and ventromedial)	Hereditary, unknown defect
Feline hereditary neuroaxonal dystrophy[125]	Domestic cats	5 wks	Ataxia	Axonal swelling, neuron loss, cerebellar vermis atrophy	Brain stem, cerebellum	Hereditary (autosomal recessive), unknown defect
Leukoencephalomyelopathy[40]	Rottweiler	2 to 3 yrs	Tetraparesis, hypermetria	Demyelination, axonal degeneration	Spinal cord (most pronounced in cervical area)	Unknown defect
Globoid cell leukodystrophy[37]†	Cairn and West Highland White terriers, domestic and Siamese cats	3 to 6 mos	Paraparesis progressing to tetraparesis, blindness, tremor	Demyelination, globoid cells	Spinal cord (all funiculi), cerebral cortex	Hereditary (autosomal recessive), β-galacto-cerebrosidase deficiency

Disease	Breed/Species	Age	Clinical Signs	Pathology	Location	Etiology
Gangliosidoses[5]† (GM$_1$ and GM$_2$)	German short-haired pointer (GM$_2$), beagle (GM$_1$), domestic (GM$_1$, GM$_2$) and Siamese (GM$_1$) cats	2 to 3 mos	Ataxia, hypermetria, tetraparesis, tremor	Neuronal distension with ganglioside	Diffuse CNS	Hereditary (autosomal recessive), β-galactosidase (GM$_1$), hexosaminidase (GM$_2$) deficiency
Neuronal ceroid-lipofuscinosis[69, 121]	English setter, dachshund, chihuahua	12 to 15 mos (English setter, chihuahua), adulthood (dachshund)	Dullness, seizures, ataxia	Neuronal distension with ceroid-lipofuscin	Diffuse CNS	Hereditary (autosomal recessive), unknown enzymatic defect (English setter); unknown defect (dachshund, chihuahua)
Hereditary canine spinal muscular atrophy[17]	Brittany spaniel	4 to 6 mos	Crouching atactic gait, proximal limb muscle atrophy, hyporeflexia	Neuron loss, neurogenic muscle atrophy	Spinal cord (most pronounced in lumbar area), brain stem	Hereditary (autosomal recessive), unknown defect
Hereditary quadriplegia and amblyopia[10]	Irish setter	Birth to 5 wks	Tetraplegia, tremors, nystagmus, seizures	Purkinje cell loss, wallerian degeneration	Diffuse CNS	Hereditary (autosomal recessive), unknown defect
Hereditary neuronal abiotrophy[111]	Swedish Lapland	5 to 7 wks	Ataxia progressing to tetraplegia, distal limb muscle atrophy, hyporeflexia	Neuronal loss	Diffuse CNS	Hereditary (autosomal recessive), unknown defect
Hereditary cerebellar cortical and extrapyramidal nuclear abiotrophy[22]	Kerry Blue terrier	9 to 16 wks	Ataxia, hypermetria, tremor, hypertonus	Neuronal loss	Cerebellum, brain stem	Hereditary (autosomal recessive), unknown defect
Hereditary cerebellar cortical abiotrophy[23]	Gordon setter	6 to 24 mos	Ataxia, dysmetria	Neuronal loss	Cerebellar cortex	Hereditary (autosomal recessive), unknown defect

*Neurological signs of all of these diseases progress over a period of months, usually causing incapacitation or necessitating euthanasia.
†Globoid cell leukodystrophy and the gangliosidoses are two of the many lysosomal storage diseases described in dogs and cats.

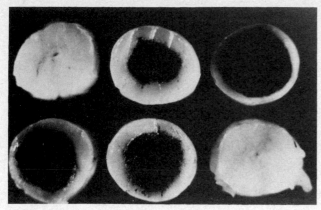

Figure 90–28. Transverse sections of spinal cord at the tenth thoracic segment from a ten-year-old male mixed breed dog with chronic, progressive paraparesis. The segment at the upper left is most cranial and that to the lower right is most caudal. A malignant melanoma replaces most of the spinal cord parenchyma in the central sections. The primary tumor was in the skin.

Dogs and cats have numerous diseases in which myelination is either delayed or faulty or in which myelin, axons, or both degenerate late in life (Table 90–3). Many of these conditions selectively involve the spinal cord, resulting in neurological signs indistinguishable from those caused by spinal cord compression. The veterinary surgeon, therefore, is obligated to be familiar with these diseases. Unnecessary diagnostic procedures or surgery might otherwise be performed.

Edema

Vasogenic edema is an integral component of the process of central hemorrhagic necrosis.[48, 129] Fluid exudation occurs initially through vascular tears induced by trauma[25] and later because of loss of vascular continuity subsequent to the necrotizing effects of ischemia.[30] This fluid is concentrated in the central gray matter at first but gradually spreads peripherally to involve the white matter. Although one study indicated that extravasation of proteinaceous fluid had largely stopped by six hours after injury,[48] another showed increased spinal cord water content for up to 20 days after trauma.[130] Edema increases intraluminal spinal cord pressure, causing further compression of its vascular and neural structures. Therapeutic measures directed at the removal of edema are important in the resolution of spinal injury.

Neoplasia

In dogs and cats, approximately 50 per cent of spinal tumors are extradural (see Fig. 90–23), 30 per cent are intradural-extramedullary (see Fig. 90–22), and 20 per cent are intradural-intramedullary[52, 103, 129] (Figs. 90–27 and 90–28). Most extradural tumors are primary vertebral tumors, including osteosarcoma, fibrosarcoma, and chondrosarcoma. These tumors usually grow rapidly, resulting in acute, progressive

paresis. Meningioma (see Fig. 90–22) and neurofibroma, the most common intradural-extramedullary tumors, often initially involve or compress a single nerve root with associated monoparesis but usually ultimately compress the spinal cord, causing either paraparesis or tetraparesis. Intradural-intramedullary tumors may be either primary neural (see Fig. 90–27) or metastatic (see Fig. 90–28) tumors. Their clinical course varies from acute to insidious.

1. Ames, A., Wright, R. L., Kowada, M., et al.: Cerebral ischemia. II. The no-reflow phenomenon. Am. J. Pathol. 52:437, 1968.
2. Assenmacher, D. R., and Ducker, T. B.: Experimental traumatic paraplegia. The vascular and pathological changes seen in reversible spinal cord lesions. J. Bone Joint Surg. 53A:671, 1971.
3. Averill, D. R.: Degenerative myelopathy in the aging German Shepherd Dog: clinical and pathologic findings. J. Am. Vet. Med. Assoc. 162:1045, 1973.
4. Averill, D. R., and Bronson, R. T.: Inherited necrotizing myelopathy of Afghan Hounds. J. Neuropathol. Exp. Neurol. 36:734, 1977.
5. Baker, H. J., Reynolds, G. D., Walkley, S. U., et al.: The gangliosidoses: comparative features and research applications. Vet. Pathol. 16:635, 1979.
6. Baker, R. N., Cancilla, P. A., Pollock, P. S., and Frommes, S. P.: The movement of exogenous protein in experimental cerebral edema. An electron microscopic study after freeze-injury. J. Neuropathol. Exp. Neurol. 30:668, 1971.
7. Bayliss, W. M.: On the local reactions of the arterial wall to changes of internal pressure. J. Physiol. (London), 28:220, 1902.
8. Bill, A., and Linder, J.: Sympathetic control of cerebral blood flow in acute arterial hypertension. Acta Physiol. Scand. 96:114, 1976.
9. Bjorck, G., Mair, W., Olsson, S. E., and Sourander, P.: Hereditary ataxia in Fox Terriers. Acta Neuropathol. Suppl. I:45–48, 1962.
10. Blackwood, W.: Normal structure and general pathology of the nerve cell and neuroglia. In Blackwood, W., and Corsellis, J. A. N. (eds.): Greenfield's Neuropathology. Year Book Medical Publishers, Chicago, 1976.
11. Braund, K. G., and Vandevelde, M.: Polioencephalomalacia in the dog. Vet. Pathol. 16:661, 1979.
12. Brierley, J. B.: Cerebral hypoxia. In Blackwood, W., and Corsellis, J. A. N. (eds.): Greenfield's Neuropathology. Year Book Medical Publishers, Inc., Chicago, 1976, pp. 43–85.
13. Brierley, J. B., Brown, A. W., and Meldrum, B. S.: The nature and time course of the neuronal alterations resulting from oligaemia and hypoglycaemia in the brain of Macaca mulatta. Brain Research, 25:483–499, 1971.
14. Brierley, J. B., Meldrum, B. S., and Brown, A. W.: The threshold and neuropathology of cerebral "anoxic-ischemic" cell change. Arch. Neurol., 29:367–374, 1973.
15. Bruce, D. A., Langfitt, T. W., Miller, J. D., et al.: Regional cerebral blood flow, intracranial pressure and brain metabolism in comatose patients. J. Neurosurg. 38:131, 1973.
16. Cannon, W. B., and Haimovici, H.: The sensitization of motoneurones by partial "denervation." Am. J. Physiol. 126:731, 1939.
17. Cork, L. C., Griffin, J. W., Munnell, J. F., et al.: Hereditary canine spinal muscular atrophy. J. Neuropathol. Exp. Neurol. 38:209, 1979.
18. Cummings, J. F., and de Lahunta, A.: Hereditary myelopathy of Afghan Hounds, a myelinolytic disease. Acta Neuropathol. (Berl.) 42:173, 1978.
19. DeGirolami, U., and Zivin, J. A.: Neuropathology of experimental spinal cord ischemia in the rabbit. J. Neuropathol. Exp. Neurol. 41:129, 1982.
20. de Lahunta, A.: Feline ischemic encephalopathy—a cerebral

infarction syndrome. *In* Kirk, R. W. (ed.): *Current Veterinary Therapy VI*. W. B. Saunders Co., Philadelphia, 1977.

21. de Lahunta, A., and Alexander, J. W.: Ischemic myelopathy secondary to presumed fibrocartilaginous embolism in nine dogs. J. Am. Anim. Hosp. Assoc. *12*:37, 1976.

22. de Lahunta, A., and Averill, D. R.: Hereditary cerebellar cortical and extrapyramidal nuclear abiotrophy in Kerry Blue Terriers. J. Am. Vet. Med. Assoc. *168*:1119, 1976.

23. de Lahunta, A., Fenner, W. R., Indrieri, R. J., et al.: Hereditary cerebellar cortical abiotrophy in the Gordon Setter. J. Am. Vet. Med. Assoc. *177*:538, 1980.

24. Demopoulos, H. B., Flamm, E., and Ransohoff, J.: Molecular pathology and CNS membranes. *In* Jobsis, F. F. (ed.): *Oxygen and Physiological Function. 60th FASEB Annual Meeting*. Dallas, Professional Information Library, 1977.

25. Dohrmann, G. J., Wagner, F. C., and Bucy, P. C.: The microvasculature in transitory traumatic paraplegia. An electron microscopic study in the monkey. J. Neurosurg. *35*:263, 1971.

26. Dougherty, M., Shea, S., Liu, C. N., and Chambers, W. W.: Effects of spinal cord lesions on cutaneously elicited reflexes in the decerebrate cat. Tonic bulbospinal and spinobulbar inhibitory systems. Exp. Neurol. *26*:551, 1970.

27. Douglas, S. W., and Palmar, A. C.: Idiopathic demyelination of brain-stem and cord in a Miniature Poodle puppy. J. Pathol. Bacteriol. *82*:67, 1961.

28. Ducker, T. B., and Kindt, G. W.: The vasomotor control of the spinal cord circulation. *In*: Proceedings of the 17th Spinal Cord Injury Conference, 1969.

29. Ducker, T. B., and Perot, A. L.: Spinal cord blood flow compartments. Trans. Am. Neurol. Assoc. *96*:229, 1971.

30. Ducker, T. B., Kindt, G. W., and Kempe, L. G.: Pathological findings in acute experimental spinal cord trauma. J. Neurosurg. *35*:700, 1971.

31. Duffy, G. P.: Lumbar puncture in the presence of raised intracranial pressure. Br. Med. J. *1*:407, 1969.

32. Fankhauser, R., Luginbuhl, H., and McGrath, J. T.: Tumours of the nervous system. Bull. W.H.O. *50*:53, 1974.

33. Farrow, B. R. H., and Love, D. N.: Infectious diseases. *In* Ettinger, S. J. (ed.): *Textbook of Veterinary Internal Medicine*. W. B. Saunders Co., Philadelphia, 1975.

34. Fischer, E. G., and Ames, A.: Studies on mechanisms of impairment of cerebral circulation following ischemia: effect of hemodilution and perfusion pressure. Stroke *3*:538, 1972.

35. Fishman, R. A.: Brain edema. N. Engl. J. Med. *293*:706, 1975.

36. Fitch, W., and McDowall, D. G.: Effect of halothane on intracranial pressure gradients in the presence of intracranial space-occupying lesions. Brit. J. anaesthesiol. *43*:904, 1971.

37. Fletcher, T. F., Zee, D. G., and Hammer, R. F.: Ultrastructural features of globoid-cell leukodystrophy in the dog. Am. J. Vet. Res. *32*:177, 1971.

38. Folkow, B.: Intravascular pressure as a factor regulating the tone of small vessels. Acta. Physiol. Scand. *17*:289, 1948.

39. Fulton, J. F., Liddell, E. G. T., and Rioch, D. M.: The influence of experimental lesions of the spinal cord upon the knee jerk. I. Acute lesions. Brain *53*:311, 1930.

40. Gamble, D. A., and Chrisman, C. L.: Leukoencephalomyelopathy in two Rottweiler dogs. *In: Proceedings of the 33rd Annual Meeting of the American College of Veterinary Pathologists*, 1982.

41. Goitein, K., Michel, J., and Sacks, T.: Penetration of parenterally administered gentamicin into the cerebrospinal fluid in experimental meningitis. Chemotherapy *21*:181, 1975.

42. Goodman, J. H., Bingham, W. G., and Hunt, W. E.: Platelet aggregation in experimental spinal cord injury. Ultrastructural observations. Arch. Neurol. *36*:197, 1979.

43. Grenell, R. G.: Central nervous system resistance. I. The effects of temporary arrest of cerebral circulation for periods of two to ten minutes. J. Neuropathol. Exp. Neurol. *5*:131, 1946.

44. Griffeths, I. R.: A syndrome produced by dorsoventral "explosions" of the cervical intervertebral discs. Vet. Rec. *87*:737, 1970.

45. Griffeths, I. R.: Spinal cord blood flow in dogs. I. The "normal" flow. J. Neurol. Neurosurg. Psychiatry *36*:34, 1973.

46. Griffeths, I. R.: Vasogenic edema following acute and chronic spinal cord compression in the dog. J. Neurosurg., *42*:155, 1975.

47. Griffeths, I. R., and Duncan, I. D.: Chronic degenerative radiculomyelopathy in the dog. J. Small Anim. Pract. *16*:461, 1975.

48. Griffeths, I. R., and Miller, R.: Vascular permeability to protein and vasogenic oedema in experimental concussive injuries to the canine spinal cord. J. Neurol. Sci. *22*:291, 1974.

49. Griffeths, I. R., Duncan, I. D., and Barker, J.: A progressive axonopathy of Boxer dogs affecting the central and peripheral nervous systems. J. Small Anim. Pract. *21*:29, 1980.

50. Griffeths, I. R., Trench, J. F., and Crawford, R. A.: Spinal cord blood flow and conduction during experimental cord compression in normotensive and hypotensive dogs. J. Neurosurg. *50*:353, 1979.

51. Harter, D. H., and Petersdort, R. F.: A consideration of the pathogenesis of bacterial meningitis: review of experimental and clinical studies. Yale J. Biol. Med. *32*:280, 1960.

52. Hartley, W. J.: Polioencephalomalacia in dogs. Acta Neuropathol. (Berl.) *2*:271, 1963.

53. Hartley, W. J., and Palmer, A. C.: Ataxia in Jack Russell Terriers. Acta Neuropathol. *26*:71, 1973.

54. Hayes, M. A., Creighton, S. R., Boysen, B. G., and Nolfeld, N.: Acute necrotizing myelopathy from nucleus pulposus embolism in dogs with intervertebral disk degeneration. J. Am. Vet. Med. Assoc. *173*:289, 1978.

55. Hayes, H. H., Priester, W. A., and Pendergrass, T. W.: Occurrence of nervous-tissue tumors in cattle, horses, cats, and dogs. Int. J. Cancer *15*:39, 1975.

56. Hedeman, L. S., Shellenberger, M. K., and Gordon, J. H.: Studies in experimental spinal cord trauma. Part 1: Alterations in catecholamine levels. J. Neurosurg. *40*:37, 1974.

57. Henneman, E.: Organization of the spinal cord and its reflexes. In Mountcastle, V. B. (ed.): *Medical Physiology*. Vol. 1. C. V. Mosby Co., St. Louis, 1980.

58. Hoerlein, B. F., and Gage, E. D.: Hydrocephalus. *In* Hoerlein, B. F. (ed.): *Canine Neurology*. W. B. Saunders Co., Philadelphia, 1978.

59. Hoff, E. J., and Vandevelde, M.: Case report: necrotizing vasculitis in the central nervous systems of two dogs. Vet. Pathol. *18*:219, 1981.

60. Hossmann, K.-A., and Kleihues, P.: Reversibility of ischemic brain damage. Arch. Neurol. (Chicago), *29*:375, 1973.

61. Hossmann, K.-A., and Zimmerman, V.: Resuscitation of the monkey brain after one hour's ischemia. I. Physiological and morphological observations. Brain Res. *81*:59, 1974.

62. Hunt, D., and Gore, L.: Myocardial lesions following experimental intracranial hemorrhage: prevention with propranolol. Am. Heart J. *83*:232, 1972.

63. James, I. M., and MacDonnell, L. A.: The role of baroreceptors and chemoreceptors in the regulation of the cerebral circulation. Clin. Sci. Mol. Med. *49*:465, 1975.

64. Jensen, D. J.: *Principles of Physiology*. Appleton-Century-Crofts, New York, 1980.

65. Klatzo, I.: Neuropathological aspects of brain edema. J. Neuropathol. Exp. Neurol. *26*:1, 1967.

66. Kobrine, A. I., Doyle, T. F., and Martins, A. N.: Local spinal cord blood flow in experimental traumatic myelopathy. J. Neurosurg. *42*:144, 1975.

67. Kobrine, A. I., Evans, D. E., and Rizzoli, H. V.: Relative vulnerability of the brain and spinal cord to ischemia. J. Neurol. Sci. *45*:65, 1980.

68. Kolata, R. J., Kraut, N. H., and Johnston, D. E.: Patterns of trauma in urban dogs and cats: a study of 1,000 cases. J. Am. Vet. Med. Assoc. *164*:499, 1974.

69. Koppang, N.: Neuronal ceroid-lipofuscinosis in English Setters. Juvenile amaurotic familial idiocy (AFI) in English Setters. J. Small Anim. Pract. *10*:639, 1970.

70. Kornegay, J. N.: Ischemic myelopathy due to fibrocartilaginous embolism. Comp. Contin. Educ. Small Anim. Pract. 2:402, 1980.

71. Kornegay, J. N., Lorenz, M. D., and Zenoble, R. D.: Bacterial meningoencephalitis in two dogs. J. Am. Vet. Med. Assoc. 173:1334, 1978.

72. Kornegay, J. N., Oliver, J. E., and Gorgacz, E. J.: Clinicopathologic features of brain herniation in animals. J. Am. Vet. Med. Assoc. 182:1111, 1983.

73. Krook, L., and Kenney, R. M.: Central nervous system lesions in dogs with metastasizing islet cell carcinoma. Cornell Vet. 52:385, 1962.

74. Krum, S., Johnson, K., and Wilson, J.: Hydrocephalus associated with the noneffusive form of feline infectious peritonitis. J. Am. Vet. Med. Assoc. 167:746, 1975.

75. Lambertsen, C. J.: Chemical control of respiration at rest. In Mountcastle, V. B. (ed.): Medical Physiology. Vol. I. C. V. Mosby Co., St. Louis, 1980.

76. Landau, W. M., Freygang, W. H., Roland, L. P., et al.: The local circulation of the living brain; values in the unanesthetized and anesthetized cat. Trans. Am. Neurol. Assoc. 80:125, 1955.

77. Langfitt, T. W.: Increased intracranial pressure and the cerebral circulation. In Youmans, J. R. (ed.): Neurological Surgery. Vol. 2. W. B. Saunders Co., Philadelphia, 1982.

78. Liddell, E. G. T., Matthes, K., Oldberg, E., and Ruch, T. C.: Reflex release of flexor muscles by spinal section. Brain 55:239, 1932.

79. Lisiak, J. A., and Vandevelde, M.: Polioencephalomalacia associated with canine distemper virus infection. Vet. Pathol. 16:650, 1979.

80. Liu, C.-N., and Chambers, W. W.: Intraspinal sprouting of dorsal root axons. Arch. Neurol. Psychiatry (Chicago) 79:46, 1958.

81. Luginbuhl, H., Fankhauser, R., and McGraft, J. T.: Spontaneous neoplasms of the nervous system in animals. Prog. Neurol. Surg. 2:85, 1968.

82. Luttgen, P. J., Braund, K. G., Brawner, W. R., and Vandevelde, M.: A retrospective study of twenty-nine spinal tumours in the dog and cat. J. Small Anim. Pract. 21:213, 1980.

83. McVeigh, J. F.: Experimental cord crushes with especial reference to the mechanical factors involved and subsequent changes in the areas of the cord affected. Arch. Surg. 7:573, 1923.

84. Mendenhall, H. V., Litwak, P., Yturraspe, D. J., et al.: Aggressive pharmacologic and surgical treatment of spinal cord injuries in dogs and cats. J. Am. Vet. Med. Assoc. 168:1026, 1976.

85. Meyer, J. S., and Hunter, J.: Effects of hypothermia on local blood flow and metabolism during cerebral ischemia and hypoxia. J. Neurosurg. 14:210, 1957.

86. Miller, J. D., and Becker, D. P.: General principles and pathophysiology of head injury. In Youmans, J. R. (ed.): Neurological Surgery. Vol. 4. W. B. Saunders Co., Philadelphia, 1982.

87. Miller, J. D., Stanek, A., and Langfitt, T. W.: Concepts of cerebral perfusion pressure and vascular compression during intracranial hypertension. Progr. Brain Res. 35:411, 1971.

88. Myers, R. E., and Yamaguchi, M.: Effects of serum glucose concentration on brain response to circulatory arrest. J. Neuropathol. Exp. Neurol. 35:301, 1976.

89. Naftchi, N. E., Demeny, M., DeCrescito, V., et al.: Biogenic amine concentrations in traumatized spinal cords of cats. Effect of drug therapy. J. Neurosurg. 40:52, 1974.

90. Nelson, E., Gertz, D., Rennels, M., et al.: Spinal cord injury. The role of vascular damage in the pathogenesis of central hemorrhagic necrosis. Arch. Neurol. 34:332, 1977.

91. Ochoa, J., Fowler, T. J., and Gilliatt, R. W.: Anatomical changes in peripheral nerves compressed by a pneumatic tourniquet. J. Anat. 113:433, 1972.

92. Offerhaus, I., and Van Gool, J.: Electrocardiographic changes and tissue catecholamines in experimental subarachnoid hemorrhage. Cardiovasc. Res., 3:433, 1969.

93. Oliver, J. E.: Intracranial injury. In Kirk, R. W. (ed.): Current Veterinary Therapy VI. W. B. Saunders Co., Philadelphia, 1977.

94. Olsson, S.-E.: The dynamic factor in spinal cord compression. A study on dogs with special reference to cervical disc protrusions. J. Neurosurg. 15:308, 1958.

95. Osterholm, J. L., and Mathews, G. J.: Altered norepinephrine metabolism following experimental spinal cord injury. Part 1: Relationship to hemorrhagic necrosis and postwounding neurological deficits. J. Neurosurg. 36:386, 1972.

96. Osterholm, J. L., and Mathews, G. J.: Altered norepinephrine metabolism following experimental spinal cord injury. 2. Protection against traumatic spinal cord hemorrhagic necrosis by norepinephrine synthesis blockade with alpha methyl tyrosine. J. Neurosurg. 36:395, 1972.

97. Palleske, H.: Experimental investigations on the regulation of the spinal cord circulation. III. The regulation of the blood flow in the spinal cord altered by edema. Acta Neurochir. 21:319, 1969.

98. Palleske, H., and Herrmann, H.-D.: Experimental investigations on the regulation of the blood flow of the spinal cord. I. Comparative study of the cerebral and spinal cord blood flow with heat clearance probes in pigs. Acta Neurochir. 19:73, 1968.

99. Palmer, A. C., and Walker, R. G.: The neuropathological effects of cardiac arrest in animals: a study of five cases. J. Small Anim. Pract. 11:779, 1970.

100. Palmer, A. C., Payne, J. E., and Wallace, M. E.: Hereditary quadriplegia and amblyopia in the Irish Setter. J. Small Anim. Pract. 14:343, 1973.

101. Parizel, G.: On the mechanism of sudden death with subarachnoid hemorrhage. J. Neurol. 220:71, 1979.

102. Plum, F., and Posner, J. B.: The Diagnosis of Stupor and Coma. F. A. Davis Co., Philadelphia, 1982.

103. Prata, R. G.: Diagnosis of spinal cord tumors in the dog. Vet. Clin. North Am. 7:165, 1977.

104. Price, D. D.: Characteristics of second pain and flexion reflexes indicative of prolonged central stimulation. Exp. Neurol. 37:371, 1972.

105. Rawe, S. E., Roth, R. H., Boadle-Biber, M., and Collins, W. F.: Norepinephine levels in experimental spinal cord trauma. Part 1: Biochemical study of hemorrhagic necrosis. J. Neurosurg. 46:342, 1977.

106. Reulen, H. J.: Vasogenic brain edema. New aspects in its formation, resolution and therapy. Br. J. Anaesthesiol. 48:741, 1976.

107. Rodbard, S., and Stone, W.: Pressor mechanisms induced by intracranial compression. Circulation 12:883, 1955.

108. Ruch, T. C.: Transection of the spinal cord. In Ruch, T. C., and Patton, H. D. (eds.): Physiology and Biophysics. I. The Brain and Neural Function. W. B. Saunders Co., Philadelphia, 1979.

109. Ruch, T. C., and Watts, J. W.: Reciprocal changes in reflex activity of the forelimbs induced by post-brachial "cold-block" of the spinal cord. Amer. J. Physiol. 110:362, 1934.

110. Safer, P., Stezoski, W., and Nemoto, E. M.: Amelioration of brain damage after 12 minutes' cardiac arrest in dogs. Arch. Neurol. (Chicago) 33:91, 1976.

111. Sandefeldt, E., Cummings, J. F., de Lahunta, A., et al.: Hereditary neuronal abiotrophy in the Swedish Lapland dog. Cornell Vet. 63:Suppl. 3, 1973.

112. Sandler, A. N., and Tator, C. H.: Effect of acute spinal cord compression injury on regional spinal cord blood flow in primates. J. Neurosurg. 45:660, 1976.

113. Schramm, J., Hashizume, K., Fukushima, T., and Takahashi, H.: Experimental spinal cord injury produced by slow, graded compression. J. Neurosurg. 50:48, 1979.

114. Shalit, M. N., Shimojyo, S., and Reinmuth, O.: Carbon dioxide and cerebral circulatory control. I. The extravascular effect. Arch. Neurol. (Chicago) 17:290, 1967.

115. Slauson, D. O., and Finn, J. P.: Meningoencephalitis and panophthalmitis in feline infectious peritonitis. J. Am. Vet. Med. Assoc. 160:729, 1972.

116. Sokoloff, L.: Circulation and energy metabolism of the brain.

In Albers, R. W., Siegel, G. J., Katzman, R., and Agranoff, B. W. (eds.): *Basic Neurochemistry.* Little, Brown and Co., Boston, 1972.

117. Tarlov, I. M.: Spinal cord compression studies. III. Time limits for recovery after gradual compression in dogs. Arch. Neurol. Psychiatry 70:813, 1953.

118. Tarlov, I. M.: Acute spinal cord compression paralysis. J. Neurosurg. 36:10, 1972.

119. Tibbs, P. A., Young, B., Ziegler, M. G., and McAllister, R. G.: Studies of experimental cervical spinal cord transection. Part II: Plasma norepinephrine levels after acute cervical spinal cord transection. J. Neurosurg. 50:629, 1979.

120. Vandevelde, M., and Braund, K. G.: Polioencephalomeylitis in cats. Vet. Pathol. 16:420, 1979.

121. Vandevelde, M., and Fatzer, R.: Neuronal ceroid-lipofuscinosis in older Dachshunds. Vet. Pathol. 17:686, 1980.

122. Vandevelde, M., Kristensen, F., Kristensen, B., et al.: Immunological and pathological findings in demyelinating encephalitis associated with canine distemper virus infection. Acta Neuropathol. (Berlin) 56:1, 1982.

123. Vise, W. M., Yashon, D., and Hunt, W. E.: Mechanisms of norepinephrine accumulation within sites of spinal cord injury. J. Neurosurg. 40:76, 1974.

124. Wagner, F. C., Dohrmann, G. J., and Bucy, P. C.: Histopathology of transitory traumatic paralegia in the monkey. J. Neurosurg. 35:272, 1971.

125. Waxman, F. J., Clemmons, R. M., Johnson, G., et al.: Progressive myelopathy in older German Shepherd dogs. I. Depressed response to thymus-dependent mitogens. J. Immunol. 124:1209, 1980.

126. Westergaard, E.: Ultrastructural permeability properties of cerebral microvasculature under normal and experimental conditions after application of tracers. *In* Cervos-Navarro, J., and Ferszt, R. (ed.): *Advances in Neurology.* Vol. 28 (Brain Edema). Raven Press, New York, 1980.

127. Wisniewski, H., Raine, C. S., and Kay, W. J.: Observations on viral demyelinating encephalomyelitis. Canine distemper. Lab. Invest. 26:589, 1972.

128. Woodard, J. C., Collins, G. H., and Hessler, J. R.: Feline hereditary neuroaxonal dystrophy. Am. J. Pathol. 74:551, 1974.

129. Wright, J. A., Bell, D. A., and Clayton-Jones, D. G.: The clinical and radiological features associated with spinal tumours in thirty dogs. J. Small Anim. Pract. 20:461, 1979.

130. Yashon, D., Bingham, W. G., Faddoul, E. M., and Hunt, W. E.: Edema of the spinal cord following experimental impact trauma. J. Neurosurg. 38:693, 1973.

131. Yashon, D., Bingham, W. C., Freedman, S. S., and Faddoul, E. M.: Intracellular enzyme liberation in primate spinal cord injury. Surg. Neurol. 4:43, 1975.

132. Youmans, J. R.: Cerebral blood flow in clinical problems. *In* Youmans, J. R. (ed.): *Neurological Surgery.* Vol. 2. W. B. Saunders Co., Philadelphia, 1982.

133. Zaki, F. A.: Spontaneous central nervous system tumors in the dog. Vet. Clin. North Am., 7:153, 1977.

134. Zaki, F. A., and Nafe, L. A.: Ischaemic encephalopathy and focal granulomatous meningoencephalitis in the cat. J. Small Anim. Pract. 21:429, 1980.

135. Zaki, F. A., and Prata, R. G.: Necrotizing myelopathy secondary to embolization of herniated intervertebral disk material in the dog. J. Am. Vet. Med. Assoc. 169:222, 1976.

136. Zaki, F. A., Prata, R. G., and Kay, W. J.: Necrotizing myelopathy in five Great Danes. J. Am. Vet. Med. Assoc. 165:1080, 1974.

137. Zaki, F. A., Prata, R. G., and Werner, L. L.: Necrotizing myelopathy in the cat. J. Am. Vet. Med. Assoc. 169:228, 1976.

138. Zook, B. C.: The pathologic anatomy of lead poisoning in dogs. Vet. Pathol. 9:310, 1972.

Chapter **91**

Diagnostic Methods

Andy Shores, Kyle G. Braund, Steven L. Stockham, and Stephen T. Simpson

HISTORY, PHYSICAL, AND NEUROLOGICAL EXAMINATIONS

The objectives in the diagnosis of neurological disorders are (1) localization of the lesion, (2) determination of the extent (severity) of the lesion, and (3) determination of the cause of the lesion. The approach to the management of patients with neurological disorders is outlined in Table 91–1. The problem-oriented medical record system is useful in attaining these objectives. Disorders of the nervous system require a detailed examination; however, by approaching the neurological patient in a logical, organized fashion, an accurate list of differential diagnoses can be prepared in the examination room. The use of a neurological examination form (Fig. 91–1) is an important part of the procedure, since its use precludes the omission of important testing procedures.

The form can be designed to meet the individual clinician's needs.

Minimum Data Base

Signalment and History

The signalment consists of the animal's breed, age, sex, and use. Certain neurological and physical disorders occur with increasing frequency in each of these categories. Clinical disorders do not always fall into their proper category. Table 91–2 lists several items that should be included in the history.

Three types of neurological cases are most often seen: seizure disorders, cranial or spinal cord trauma, and spinal cord compression (cervical or thoracolumbar) without a history of trauma. Additional historical facts and detailed descriptions of the onset and previous episodes of similar problems are helpful.

The course of the disease process is determined by the history, and its patterns (acute, chronic, progressive, paroxysmal) are often charted on a sign-time graph (Fig. 91–2). The severity of the signs (rapidity of onset, frequency of occurrence, and progression) are plotted as a function of time.[33]

Physical Examination

A good physical examination is essential in every case. The examination should be thorough and conducted in a logical, organized manner. The vital signs (heart rate, respiratory rate, temperature, mucous membrane color) and all organ systems should be evaluated. In trauma cases in which a spinal fracture or luxation is possible, manipulation of the patient is minimal.

It is not within the scope of this chapter to discuss the entire physical examination; however, certain aspects of the neurological examination may be accomplished during the routine physical examination.

The techniques employed in a physical examination include observation, palpation, percussion, and auscultation. Observation is the oldest diagnostic tool and, consciously or subconsciously, the most utilized diagnostic method. The patient is observed as it enters the examination room; attitude, facial expression, breathing patterns, posture, gait, incoordina-

---

A. MENTAL STATUS
B. GAIT & POSTURE
C. CRANIAL NERVES
  1. Olfaction
  2. Optic   OD   OS
    a. Menace
    b. Following
    c. Obstacle Course
  3. Oculomotor
    a. Intraocular   OD   OS
      Pupillary
        direct
        consensual
    b. Extraocular   OD   OS
      Strabismus
    c. Sympathetic   OD   OS
      Horner's Syn.
  4. Trochlear   OD   OS
  5. Trigeminal
    a. Motor   R   L
    b. Sensory
      Ophthalmic
        corneal reflex   OD   OS
        direct
        consensual
        palpebral   OD   OS
        direct
        consensual
      Maxillary   R   L
      Mandibular   R   L
  6. Abducens   R   L
    Corneal reflex
  7. Facial   R   L
  8. Vestibulocochlear
    a. Cochlear   R   L
    b. Vestibular   R   L
      Head tilt
      Nystagmus   OD   OS
        physiological
        spontaneous
        positional

  9. Glossopharyngeal   R   L
  10. Vagus   R   L
  11. Spinal Accessory   R   L
  12. Hypoglossal   R   L
D. POSTURAL REACTIONS
  1. a. Wheelbarrowing   RF   LF
    b. Wheelbarrowing with extended
      neck   RF   LF
  2. Hemistanding/Hemiwalking R   L
  3. Hopping   RF LF RH LH
  4. Conscious Proprioception
               RF LF RH LH
  5. Extensor Postural Thrust   RH LH
  6. Righting Response   R   L
  7. Tonic Neck/Eye
E. MUSCLE TONE   LF RF LH RH
F. SEGMENTAL REFLEXES
  1. Myotatic
    a. Biceps   R   L
    b. Triceps   R   L
    c. Patellar   R   L
    d. Cranial tibial   R   L
    e. Gastrocnemius   R   L
  2. Flexor
    a. Thoracic limb   R   L
    b. Pelvic limb   R   L
  3. Crossed Extensor RF LF RH LH
  4. Panniculus
  5. Hyperpathic Response
  6. Anal Sphincter
G. SENSATION
  1. Thoracic Limbs
  2. Pelvic Limbs
  3. Perineum
  4. Tail
  5. Head
H. COMMENTS

GRADING SCALE:
  0 = absent
  1 = decreased
  2 = normal
  3 = exaggerated
  4 = very exaggerated

SYNDROME:

LOCALIZATION:

ADDITIONAL TESTS:

CLINICIAN _____

Figure 91–1. Neurological examination form.

TABLE 91–1. Diagnosis of Neurological Disorders

1. Minimum Data Base
   a. Signalment and History
   b. Physical Examination
2. Neurological Examination
   a. Mental Status
   b. Locomotion
   c. Cranial Nerves
   d. Postural Reactions
   e. Spinal Reflexes
   f. Sensory Perception
   g. Localization of the Lesion
3. Differential Diagnosis List and Client Education
4. Ancillary Tests
   a. Clinical Pathology (hematology, serum chemistries, urinalysis, CSF analysis)
   b. Radiology
   c. Electrodiagnostics
   d. Other Diagnostics (e.g., biopsy)
5. Diagnosis, Prognosis, and Client Education
6. Therapy

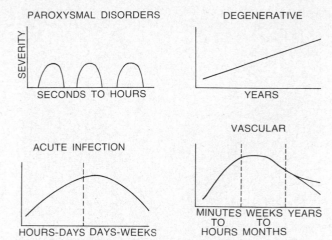

Figure 91–2. Patterns of disease progression as demonstrated with a sign-time graph. (Reprinted with permission from Oliver, J.E., Jr., and Hoerlein, B. F.: Localization of lesions in the nervous system. *In* Hoerlein, B. F. (ed.): *Canine Neurology: Diagnosis and Treatment*, 3rd ed. W.B. Saunders, Philadelphia, 1978.)

tion, obvious fractures, and so on should all be noted.[30] After observing the patient, the clinician proceeds with evaluation of the face and head. A cursory cranial nerve examination is performed at this time; a more detailed evaluation is made during the neurological examination.

Certain orthopedic problems must be considered among the differential diagnoses of spinal problems. All bony structures and joints should be palpated and the range of motion for each joint evaluated and compared with the contralateral side.

The order of the physical examination is not as

TABLE 91–2. Anamnesis

Each history should include all of the following:
1. Reason for presentation (chief complaint)
2. Onset of the problem (description, acute vs. chronic)
3. Duration of the problem and subsequent signs
4. Status of the problem (static, progressive, improved)
5. Previous therapy and response
6. Past episodes of this problem
7. Any history of trauma
8. Previous anesthesia, surgery, or medical problems
9. Description of the animal's environment
10. Diet
11. Complete vaccination history
12. Reproductive status

Additional historical facts necessary with certain neurological disorders:
1. Seizure Disorders
   a. Description of the seizure (prodromal, ictal, and postictal phases)
   b. Age when first seizure occurred
   c. Frequency and total number of seizures
   d. Any alterations in personality
   e. Associated occurrences (environmental and physiological)

2. Cranial or Spinal Cord Trauma
   a. Time since trauma occurred
   b. Type and description of trauma
   c. Status immediately post trauma (conscious? ambulatory?) and subsequent signs
   d. Method and manner of transport to the clinic

3. Spinal Cord Compression Without History of Trauma
   a. Previous episodes of pain, paresis, or paralysis
   b. Activity at onset of problem (climbing stairs, jumping off furniture, etc.)
   c. Evidence of urinary or fecal incontinence

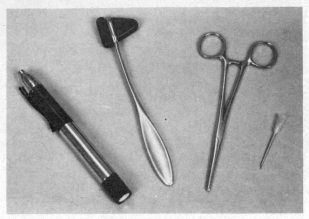

Figure 91–3. Equipment required for a complete neurological examination. *Left to right,* Bright penlight, reflex hammer (pleximeter), large hemostatic forceps, blunted 18-gauge needle.

TABLE 91–3. Disorders That Alter Gait and Posture

1. Motor
   Dysmetria, hypotonia, paresis: cerebrum and brainstem (upper motor neuron)
   Paresis, paralysis: brainstem, spinal cord, or peripheral nerves
2. Visual
   Hesitancy to move, collision with objects: retinal and optic pathways, cerebrum
3. Vestibular and Cerebellar
   Hypermetria, hypometria, incoordination: cerebellum
   Circling, loss of balance: vestibular system
4. Proprioceptive/Motor
   Dysmetria, ataxia, paresis, or paralysis, dragging or knuckling of toes

important as the consistency in which the order is followed, which facilitates the recognition of abnormalities and precludes the deletion of any portion of the examination. The recording of the examination results (normal/abnormal and a description of the abnormal) is essential.

Neurological Examination

Special equipment needed for neurological examinations is shown in Figure 91–3. The neurological examination should be conducted with an open mind; all results are first recorded and then a determination of the severity of the lesion and its location is made by reviewing the results. When assessing the results, an attempt is made to explain all clinical signs by the presence of one lesion; when all such possibilities are exhausted, multifocal or diffuse causes of disease are considered. If the results are questioned by the examiner, repeat examinations are performed.

Mental Status

The mental status and level of consciousness are the first evaluations in the examination. They are influenced by the functional integration of higher cortical centers and the reticular activating system of the brainstem. The normal animal is bright, alert, and responsive to its environment and all external stimuli. Animals with an altered mental status may be depressed, stuporous, disoriented, delirious, comatose, hysterical, or irritable.[36] Sedatives or tranquilizers alter the mental status, and their possible influence should be noted on the record.

Gait and Posture

Normal gait and posture require integration of activity from the motor cortex, vestibular system, cerebellum, brainstem, spinal cord, peripheral nerves, and proprioceptors in the joints, muscles, and tendons. In addition, the visual system assists ambulation in unfamiliar surroundings.[36] Disorders that alter gait and posture affect the motor, visual, vestibular, cerebellar, or proprioceptive system[36] (Table 91–3).

Cranial Nerve Examination

The cranial nerve examination evaluates specific areas of the brainstem and the peripheral nerve component of each cranial nerve (CN). Cranial nerve function is first evaluated during the physical examination by a general observation of the position of the head, facial expression, eye and ear movement, and pupillary size and symmetry. Any abnormalities are recorded and evaluated in detail during the neurological examination.

The *olfactory nerve (CN I)* is evaluated by observing the patient entering the room (smelling objects in the room) or by blindfolding the animal and placing food or a nonirritating, volatile substance such as cloves under the nose. Hyposomia or anosomia is an abnormal finding but may be difficult to evaluate[14, 36] and may represent cerebrocortical disease as well as CN I dysfunction.

Evaluation of the *optic nerve (CN II)* and associated pathways includes the pupillary light reflex (CN II and III), the menace response test (CN II and VII), an obstacle test, visual following, visual placing reactions, and an ophthalmoscopic examination.

The pupillary light reflex is assessed by shining a penlight directly into the eye (Fig. 91–4). The normal reflex (constriction of both pupils) requires a functional retina, optic nerve, optic tract, pretectal area, parasympathetic nucleus of the oculomotor nerve (Edinger-Westphal nucleus), and oculomotor nerve.[36] The opposite pupil (consensual reflex) also constricts since 65 to 75 per cent of the optic nerve fibers decussate at the optic chiasm and in the pretectal area in the cat and dog. A dilated, unresponsive pupil is abnormal. A dilated pupil with an absent direct pupillary light reflex and a normal consensual reflex indicates a lesion in the visual pathway of that eye.[13] Absence of a consensual reflex indicates a lesion in

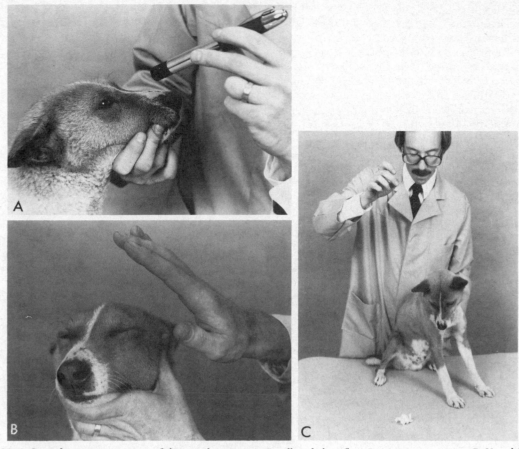

Figure 91–4. Cranial nerve examination of the visual system. *A*, Pupillary light reflex. *B*, Menace response. *C*, Visual following.

the oculomotor nerve. Lens opacities and iris disease may also alter the pupillary light reflex.

The menace response is evaluated by covering one eye and vigorously petting the animal over the other eye with a cupped hand and then withdrawing the hand and returning it to a position close to the eye and within the visual field (see Fig. 91–4). The animal should blink and move its head away from the hand. The absence of a blink response is abnormal and indicates vusual deficits or facial nerve (CN VII) dysfunction. When performing this test, it is important that excessive air currents are not created when returning the hand to a position close to the eye. The air currents stimulate the surface of the cornea (CN V, sensory) and may initiate a blink response.[36]

The obstacle test is performed by placing objects in the pathway of the patient and observing its ability to avoid them. This test should be performed in both brightly and dimly lit areas. A blind animal is reluctant to move and cannot avoid the objects in its path.

Visual following is evaluated by dropping a cotton ball from behind the animal so that it passes through the visual field of one eye. The normal response is for the animal to see and look toward the object as it falls to the floor (See Fig. 91–4).[36]

Visual placing tests the animal's ability to perceive the edge of a table and place its front feet on the table as the examiner moves the animal toward the table. This test is discussed later with the postural reactions.

An ophthalmoscopic examination is an important part of any evaluation of the visual system; however, it is usually performed following the neurological examination, since the pupils should be properly dilated for examination.

Ventrolateral strabismus and ptosis of the eyelid result from damage to the somatic portion of the *oculomotor nerve (CN III)*. The parasympathetic portion is evaluated by the pupillary light reflex previously discussed.

Bilaterally dilated, unresponsive pupils result from damage to the midbrain, specifically to the oculomotor parasympathetic (Edinger-Westphal) nucleus. This sign is indicative of a grave prognosis in patients with a decreased level of consciousness following cranial trauma. Retinal disease or a lesion involving the optic chiasm must be differentiated when these signs are seen.

Unilateral miosis results from a decrease in sympathetic tone as seen with Horner's syndrome. Its clinical signs include miotic pupil, ptosis of the eyelid, enophthalmos and protrusion of the third eyelid.

Bilateral miotic pupils can result from a lack of sympathetic stimulation, as seen with bilateral Horner's syndrome, or from exposure to parasympathomimetic agents (e.g., organophosphate toxicity).[13, 36]

Clinical signs associated with dysfunction of the *trochlear nerve (CN IV)* are rare; however, a slight dorsolateral rotational strabismus may be seen with acute trochlear paralysis or a dorsomedial rotational strabismus may be seen with chronic disease and resultant muscle contracture.[36]

Sensory tests for the *trigeminal nerve (CN V)* are (1) the corneal reflex (retraction of the globe after the cornea is lightly touched), (2) the palpebral reflex (Fig. 91–5), (3) the maxillary/ophthalmic reflex (a blink response following stimulation of the maxillary and periorbital areas with a blunted 18- to 20-gauge needle), (4) mandibular cutaneous sensory response (evaluation of sensation to the mandibular area with a blunted 18- to 20-gauge needle), and (5) sensory testing of the nasal mucosa with a blunt instrument such as a small hemostat (see Fig. 91–5). Trigeminal motor function is determined by evaluating jaw tonus and palpating the masseter and temporalis muscles for atrophy.[36]

Medial strabismus and a failure to retract the globe in response to stimulation of the cornea with a moistened cotton ball (sensory CN V) are associated with dysfunction of the *abducens nerve (CN VI)*.

Function tests for the *facial nerve (CN VII)* (see

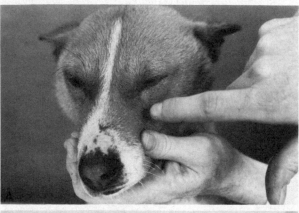

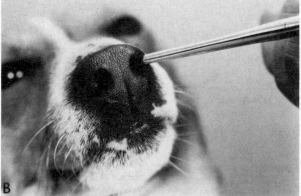

Figure 91–5. Cranial nerve examination for tactile sensation. *A*, Palpebral reflex. *B*, Sensory examination of the nasal mucosa.

Figs. 91–4 and 91–5) are the menace response (visual CN II, blink response CN VII), the trigeminal sensory reflexes (sensory CN V, blink response CN VII), and movement of the ear in response to light stimulation ("tickling") of the inside of the ear. If the facial nerve is damaged, there will be no blink response and there may be drooping of the face or ear on the affected side.[36]

The vestibular portion of the *vestibulocochlear nerve (CN VIII)* is special-proprioceptive[14] for equilibrium and posture. The cochlear portion is sensory for hearing. Vestibular lesions may be central (involving the vestibular nuclei) or peripheral.

A head tilt toward the side of the lesion is the most common sign associated with vestibular dysfunction and is caused by a deficiency in antigravity tone of the ipsilateral side via the descending medial longitudinal fasciculus and vestibulospinal tracts. The animal often falls and has a curvature of the trunk toward the affected side.[39]

Nystagmus, a rhythmic oscillation of the eyes, is often seen with vestibular disease. Spontaneous nystagmus may be observed as a resting nystagmus (occurring while the animal is at rest) or positional nystagmus (occurring when the animal's head is placed in an unusual position, e.g., upside down or extended). Any signs of spontaneous nystagmus are abnormal. Spontaneous nystagmus is also characterized by the direction of its fast phase, which is away from the affected side.[39]

Induced nystagmus includes vestibular nystagmus (tonic eye or oculocephalic reflex) and postrotatory nystagmus. Vestibular (physiological) nystagmus occurs when the animal's head is moved from side to side or up and down. This form of nystagmus is normal and should be in the direction of the head movement.[36, 39] Postrotatory nystagmus is evaluated by rotating the patient rapidly and observing the speed, character, and direction of the induced eye movements immediately after rotation is abruptly stopped. During rotation, the nystagmus should initially occur in the direction of the rotation and in the opposite direction for a brief period when the rotation is stopped.[39] Both directions are tested, and the response should be symmetrical.

Any form of induced nystagmus is normal. The absence of induced nystagmus suggests a central vestibular lesion or involvement of the ascending medial longitudinal fasciculus. Asymmetry of the induced nystagmus suggests a central vestibular lesion and a normal medial longitudinal fasciculus.[39]

In peripheral vestibular disease, the nystagmus is horizontal or rotatory but never vertical. Nystagmus due to central vestibular disease may be horizontal, vertical, or rotatory. Central vestibular disease may also accompany ipsilateral deficits with CN V, VI, and VII. Table 91–4 is a summary of central vestibular and peripheral vestibular signs.[39]

Bilateral vestibular disease results in ventral flexion of the head and neck and possibly nystagmus in the acute phase. In the chronic state, ataxia and wide

TABLE 91–4. Neurological Signs Associated With Central and Peripheral Vestibular Dysfunction

Central	Possible Signs	Peripheral
+	Head tilt	+
+ +	Circling	+
+ +	Falling, rolling	+
	Spontaneous nystagmus	
	Resting or positional nystagmus	
+	Horizontal	+
+	Rotary	+
+	Vertical	−
	Positional	
+	change of direction	−
	Induced nystagmus	
+	Failure to induce	−
+	Induced abnormally	+

TABLE 91–5. Cranial Nerve Function Testing

1. Olfaction: CN I
2. Eyes:
   a. Pupillary light reflex, pupil size and symmetry: CN II, III, sympathetic nerve supply
   b. Menace response: CN II, VII, cerebral, cerebellar
   c. Position (strabismus): CN III, IV, VI, VIII
   d. Corneal reflex (retraction of the globe) and palpebral reflex: CN V, VI, VII
   e. Nystagmus: CNS VIII, vestibular system
3. Facial symmetry, sensation: CN V, VII
4. Head position, startle reflex: CN VIII, XI
5. Tongue, swallowing: CN IX, X, XII
6. Neck muscles: CN XI

excursions of the head from side to side occur and nystagmus may be difficult to induce.[13, 39]

Cochlear nerve function is tested by the auditory startle and the electroencephalographic auditory evoked response tests. Historical evidence of hearing loss and the patient's response to auditory stimuli and its environment during the initial examination period are usually sufficient to determine hearing function. Partial dysfunctions are difficult to evaluate; however, frequency ranges can be evaluated with the aid of an electroencephalogram.[36]

The gag reflex is used to test the *glossopharyngeal nerve (CN IX)* and the *vagus nerve (CN X)*, both of which are sensory and motor for swallowing. External pressure on the caudal pharyngeal area or direct digital stimulation of the pharynx should cause the animal to swallow (Fig. 91–6).[13, 36] Any change in laryngeal tone as determined by palpation indicates CN IX dysfunction. Changes in vocalization may also be associated with CN X dysfunction. Cardiovascular and gastrointestinal signs are not prominent unless bilateral vagus nerve involvement is present,[36] and the oculocardiac reflex is not practical unless electrocardiographic monitoring is performed simultaneously.

The *spinal accessory nerve (CN XI)* is tested by evaluating muscle tone of the trapezius, sternomastoid, cleidomastoid, omotransversarius, and cleidocervicalis muscles. Severe cervical scoliosis can occur with unilateral CN XI dysfunction; however, dysfunction of this nerve is not common.[36]

Motor innervation to the tongue is supplied by the *hypoglossal nerve (CN XII)*. It can be evaluated by manual stretching of the tongue, palpation of the tongue, and observation of the tongue for evidence of atrophy or deviation to one side. Acute CN XII damage results in deviation of the tongue to the side opposite the lesion. Eventually, atrophy of the tongue muscles occurs on one side and the tongue deviates toward the affected and atrophied side.[36] In either case, the patient can lick only the maxillary region of the affected side.

To the novice examiner, a cranial nerve examination may seem difficult to perform and very time-consuming; however, with experience, abnormalities are quickly recognized. Table 91–5 is a simplified summary of cranial nerve function testing.

Postural Reactions

When performing this part of the neurological examination, it is helpful to evaluate the animal on a surface that offers adequate traction (e.g., carpeting, grass). The important postural reactions to evaluate are discussed here.

Wheelbarrow. The pelvic limbs are picked up and the animal is moved forward on the pectoral limbs (Fig. 91–7). Any difficulty in performing this exercise is abnormal and may include failure to hold the head up, weakness of one or both limbs, and conscious proprioceptive deficits. The animal is also tested in the same manner with the neck extended (see Fig. 91–7). Excessive difficulty in performing this exercise suggests a subtle lesion. The wheelbarrow test is useful in paraparetic patients to differentiate diseases

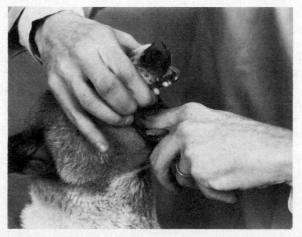

Figure 91–6. The gag reflex demonstrates the normal function of cranial nerves IX and X.

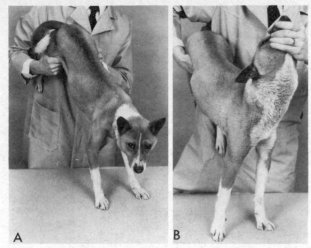

Figure 91–7. Wheelbarrow postural reactions. *A,* Normal posture. *B,* With extended neck.

of the cervical spinal cord or brachial plexus from diseases of the thoracolumbar spinal cord.

Hemistanding and Hemiwalking. The pectoral and pelvic limbs of one side are held off the floor to evaluate the animal's ability to stand and move laterally and forward on the contralateral pectoral and pelvic limbs. The test is then repeated on the opposite side (Fig. 91–8). Abnormalities include incoordination, weakness (paresis), or an inability to support weight on the affected limb. This test evaluates the symmetry of the neurological deficit and determines the functional integrity of the motor system.

Hopping Response. This test evaluates the neurological function of each limb individually. One pectoral limb is tested first by holding up the contralateral pectoral limb and both pelvic limbs and then hopping the animal on the one forelimb in forward, lateral, and craniomedial directions (see Fig. 91–8). The evaluation proceeds to the opposite pectoral limb and then to each pelvic limb. Any abnormalities in the motor control of the limbs are noted. Abnormal findings include collapse of the patient, a delayed response, and overshooting. The hopping response is very complex, involving the function of the cerebrum, cerebellum, brainstem, spinal cord, and touch-pressure/pressure-stretch receptors in the joints, muscles, and tendons.[36]

Extensor Postural Thrust. This response is tested by holding the animal in an upright position with the hind limbs off the floor and slowly lowering the animal until the rear feet touch the floor (see Fig. 91–8). The normal response is an orderly backward stepping of the pelvic limbs. This reflex is mediated by the cervical spinal cord and the cerebellum/ vestibular system.[24]

Placing Reaction. This test further evaluates the proprioceptive and motor abilities of each limb and the visual system. The test is conducted in two parts: tactile placing (animal is blindfolded) and visual placing. Each limb is evaluated separately by holding the

animal and moving it toward the edge of a table or counter (see Fig. 91–8). In the tactile placing test, the dorsal surface of the paw is touched to the surface edge, stimulating tactile receptors. The normal response is for the animal to pick the limb up and place the foot on the surface. With visual placing, the animal should observe and recognize the edge of the table and initiate an appropriate response. Abnormal responses may indicate deficits in sensation, motor ability, or the visual system.[36]

Conscious Proprioception. This test is performed on each limb and consists of placing the dorsum of the paw in contact with the floor (Fig. 91–9). The normal response is a quick return of the foot to its normal position. Stoic animals may not return the paw to a normal position for several seconds and may be difficult to evaluate. Proprioception is also evaluated when the animal walks, by inspecting the dorsal surface of the nails for excessive wear, and during several of the other postural reactions.

Another test of conscious proprioception often useful in cats is performed by placing a sheet of paper or towelling under the foot and slowly pulling the paper or towelling laterally, thereby displacing the foot laterally (see Fig. 91–9). The normal response is a quick return of the foot to a normal position.

With either method, a delayed or absent response is abnormal and may involve the afferent system (loss of position sense) or the efferent system (decreased motor control or paresis) or both.

Righting Response. This tests the animal's ability to right itself to sternal recumbency from lateral recumbency. The limbs on the recumbent side should flex; the opposite limbs should extend. A normal response requires a functional vestibular system, visual pathway, and proprioceptive abilities.[24, 36]

Spinal (Segmental) Reflexes

Myotatic and flexor reflexes are the two types of spinal reflexes commonly examined. Spinal reflexes are elicited through a reflex arc that includes the receptor, afferent peripheral nerve pathway, the spinal cord synapses, efferent peripheral nerve pathway, and effector muscles. Spinal reflexes are evaluated in the pectoral and pelvic limbs and aid in localization of spinal cord disease. Reflex responses are normal, hyperreflexic, hyporeflexic, or areflexic.

Before conducting reflex evaluations, muscle tone in each limb is recorded. Muscle tone may be absent (atonia), decreased (hypotonia), normal, or exaggerated (hypertonia).[36]

Myotatic Reflexes. When conducting myotatic reflex evaluations, the tendons and muscles involved must be stretched (loaded) to produce the proper response. For example, when testing the biceps reflex, the pectoral limb should be pulled caudally, stretching the biceps muscle and tendon. In addition, the pleximeter should be held to allow it to swing like a pendulum as it strikes the tendon. The plex-

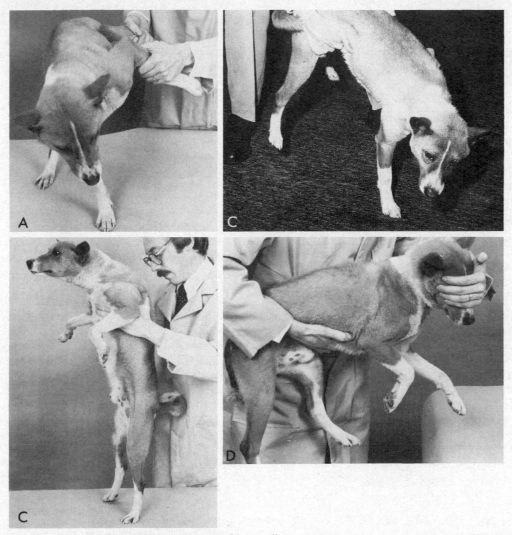

Figure 91–8. Postural reaction testing in the dog. *A,* Hemistand/hemiwalk. *B,* Hopping response. *C,* Extensor postural thrust. *D,* Placing reaction.

imeter should not be held and swung in the same manner as that used with a hammer to drive nails.

In the forelimbs, the biceps and triceps muscle reflexes are evaluated. At times, it may be difficult to evaluate pectoral limb reflexes (e.g., in long-haired or obese dogs); however, if the muscles are palpated during the evaluation, the contractions can be felt.

The biceps reflex test is performed by placing the

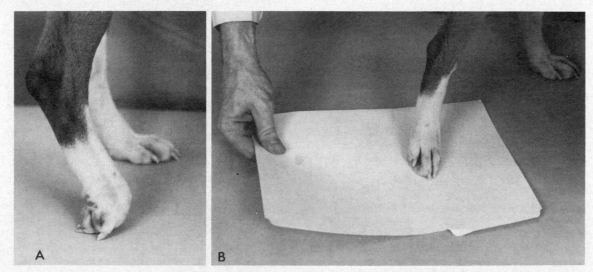

Figure 91–9. Methods of examining for conscious proprioceptive function. *A,* Dorsal knuckling. *B,* Stepping response.

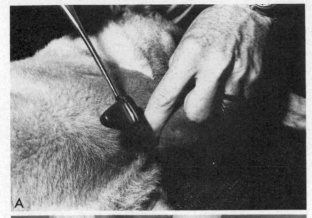

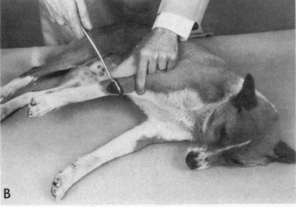

Figure 91–10. Myotatic reflexes of the pectoral limb. *A,* Triceps reflex. *B,* Biceps reflex.

index finger over the distal end of the biceps and brachialis tendons at the level of the elbow and tapping the finger with the pleximeter. The normal response is slight flexion of the elbow and contraction of the biceps muscle proximal to the examiner's finger (Fig. 91–10). Increased or decreased reflexes (hyper- or hyporeflexia) are abnormal. This test evaluates the musculocutaneous nerve and the C_{7-8} spinal cord segment.[36]

The triceps reflex is evaluated by placing the index finger over the tendon of insertion of the triceps muscle just proximal to the olecranon while holding the elbow in flexion and the shoulder in extension. Again, the finger is tapped with the pleximeter (see Fig. 91–10). A slight extension of the elbow and contraction of the triceps muscle should be seen. Increased or decreased reflexes are abnormal. This reflex evaluates the radial nerve and the C_{7-8}, T_{1-2} spinal cord segments.[14, 36]

The pelvic limb reflexes include the patellar reflex and the sciatic nerve reflexes. The patellar reflex is used to evaluate the femoral nerve (spinal cord segments L_{4-6})[36] and is the most reliable pelvic limb reflex. The test is performed by placing the limb in a slightly flexed position and lightly tapping the straight patellar ligament with the pleximeter (Fig. 91–11). The normal response is an extension of the stifle that is "just brisk."

The sciatic nerve and its branches can be evaluated

at three different levels. One test is to tap between the greater trochanter and the ischiatic tuberosity with the pleximeter. The expected response is flexion of the limb.

The cranial tibialis reflex is tested by tapping the limb directly below the lateral tibial condyle while extending the stifle and extending the tibiotarsal joint (see Fig. 91–11). The normal response is slight flexion of the tibiotarsal joint.[13]

The gastrocnemius reflex is performed by placing the index finger over the gastrocnemius tendon directly above the hock while holding the hock flexed and sharply tapping the finger with the pleximeter (see Fig. 91–11). The normal response is a quick extension of the hock, followed by flexion of the hock.[36]

The three sciatic reflex tests evaluate the sciatic nerve and spinal cord segments L_{5-7} and S_1. Abnormalities are the same as those listed for other myotatic reflexes.

Flexor Reflexes. The flexor reflexes are used to evaluate the animal's ability to withdraw the limb in response to a stimulus. A test of this reflex evaluates cervical or lumbar intumescent function and should be performed in each limb. The digits of the limb to be tested are first pinched with the fingers; a hemostat may be used if additional stimulus is needed to produce a reflex (see Fig. 91–11). Complete physiological or physical transection of the spinal cord above the level of this reflex may result in upper motor neuron signs and a rapid or repetitive withdrawal of the limb in response to stimuli. This should never be confused with the ability to perceive pain.

Other Spinal Reflexes. The crossed extensor reflex is tested at the same time the flexor reflexes are evaluated. The "toe pinch" is applied and the contralateral limb is observed. The reflex is present if the contralateral limb extends in response to flexion (withdrawal) of the ipsilateral limb. This test must be performed with the patient in lateral recumbency, and gross attempts by the patient to right itself invalidate the results. The presence of this reflex demonstrates a lack of contralateral inhibition (release phenomenon) in the spinal cord and is an upper motor neuron sign.[36] It is frequently seen in severe spinal cord damage; however, its presence does not constitute irreparable damage to the spinal cord.

The anal sphincter (perineal) reflex evaluates the pudendal nerve and spinal cord segments S_{1-3}. Stimulation of the perineal area should result in contraction of the external anal sphincter (Fig. 91–12). A decrease in anal tone is abnormal.

A test of the panniculus reflex and the hyperpathia test are used to localize spinal cord lesions. The panniculus reflex test is performed by lightly stimulating the skin on each side of the dorsal midline with a blunted 18- to 20-gauge hypodermic needle (Fig. 91–13). The reflex evaluation is begun in the lumbosacral area and proceeds cranially. A normal response is contraction or "rippling" of the subcutaneous muscle at the point of stimulation and forward

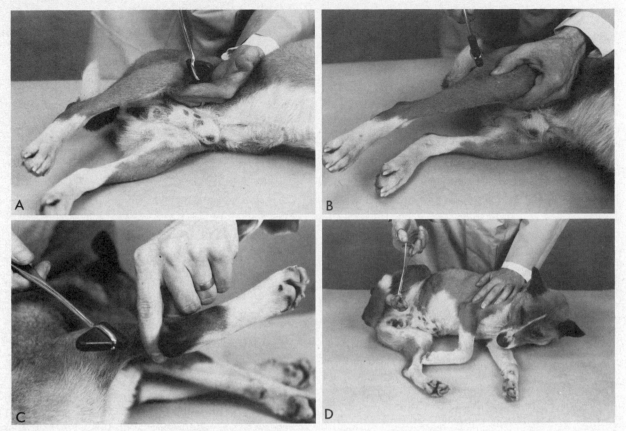

Figure 91–11. Segmental reflexes of the pelvic limb. *A*, Patellar reflex. *B*, Cranial tibial reflex. *C*, Gastrocnemius reflex. *D*, Flexor reflex.

to the cervicothoracic region. An abnormal response is the absence of this reflex. Because of the dermatomic distribution of the spinal nerves. the reflex often begins one or two spinal segments caudal to a spinal cord lesion. A painful or exaggerated response may be present over the lesion. The panniculus reflex arc involves an afferent pathway consisting of the cutaneous thoracolumbar innervation and an efferent

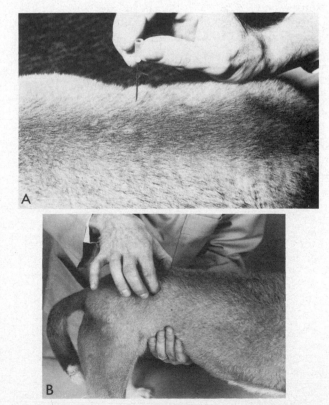

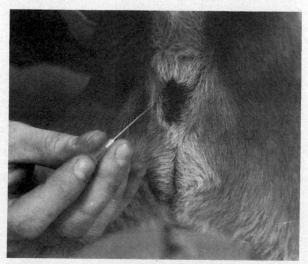

Figure 91–12. Perineal reflex.

Figure 91–13. *A*, Panniculus reflex. *B*, Testing for hyperpathia.

pathway mediated by the C8 spinal cord segment and motor nerve. This reflex may be helpful in localizing the level of a spinal cord lesion; however, it is not always a reliable reflex.

Hyperpathia is the response of the animal to pressure on the transverse processes or the dorsal spinous processes of the lumbar and thoracic vertebrae. Abdominal muscle tone is palpated while the pressure is applied. A reflex tightening of the abdominal muscles is expected when pressure is exerted over the vertebrae at the level of spinal cord involvement (see Fig. 91–13).[52] This test may be valuable in localizing a spinal lesion; however, it should be used with caution if a spinal fracture or luxation is suspected.

Sensory Perception

This is often the most important test prognostically and is a good indicator of the functional integrity of the spinal cord. The test is performed on each limb and the tail by applying painful stimuli to the digits or the distal end of the tail. The initial test should be performed with the flexor reflexes with a toe pinch stimulus. With sensory impairment, the use of Carmalt forceps may be necessary to produce a pain response. The normal response is withdrawal of the limb and crying, turning the head toward the painful stimulus, or vigorous attempts to pull away or bite the examiner. The results of this test must be evaluated carefully, since they often determine the prognosis in spinal cord compression cases.

Additional sensory testing can include cutaneous sensory evaluation of the head and face (cranial nerves) and peripheral nerve function in the pectoral or pelvic limbs by needle pricks and observation of the conscious responses.

TABLE 91–6. Localization of Neurological Lesions

1. Cerebrum, brainstem: cranial nerve abnormalities
2. Cerebellum: coordination, hypermetria, central vestibular signs
3. Upper cervical (vertebrae C1–C5):
   a. Hyperreflexic pectoral limbs
   b. Hyperreflexic pelvic limbs
4. Lower cervical (vertebrae C6–T1):
   a. Hyporeflexic pectoral limbs
   b. Hyperreflexic pelvic limbs
5. Thoracic and upper lumbar (vertebrae T2–L3):
   a. Normal forelimbs
   b. Hyperreflexic pelvic limbs
6. Lower lumbar (vertebrae L4–L7):
   a. Normal pectoral limbs
   b. Hyporeflexic pelvic limbs*
7. Lumbosacral (vertebrae L7–S3):
   a. Normal pectoral limbs and patellar reflexes
   b. Hyporeflexic sciatic nerve reflexes with a L7–S1 lesion
   c. Normal pelvic limbs with a lesion at S1–S3
   d. Anal sphincter dysfunction

*Lesions caudal to L4–L5 vertebrae may result in normal patellar reflexes and hyporeflexic sciatic nerve reflexes.

Interpretation/Localization

Localization of the lesion is the primary goal of the neurological examination. Localization is discussed in detail in Chapter 89; however, an outline is provided in Table 91–6.

By conducting a complete, organized examination of the patient with neurological disease, diagnostic efforts are rewarding. Making the diagnosis helps to provide the more detailed information needed in discussing the prognosis and therapeutic measures available with the client and initiating the appropriate therapy.

CEREBROSPINAL FLUID

Collection

Cerebrospinal fluid (CSF) is best evaluated when collection techniques are standardized. Anesthetic agents, positioning, and methods of withdrawal can affect total CSF evaluation.

A 1 1/2-inch, 22-gauge spinal needle is used on most dogs and cats. Large breed dogs may require a 2 1/2-inch needle. Sterile gloves should be worn if the collector palpates the site of the skin prick. If the tap can be made without such palpation and the needle is handled only by the hub, gloving is not necessary. A manometer and three-way valve are used for measuring CSF pressure.

The anesthetic agent of choice is a short-acting thiobarbiturate, although other neuroanaleptic agents can be used. A knowledge of the effects of anesthetic agents on CSF pressure is necessary to interpret CSF pressure recordings. If longer anesthesia is needed for other diagnostic or surgical procedures, gas anesthesia should be administered after the CSF pressure has been recorded.

CSF can be collected with the patient in sternal or lateral recumbency. Pressure recordings can be made with the animal in a lateral position only. With the patient in lateral recumbency, the head is flexed

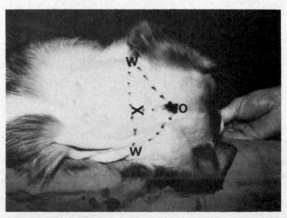

Figure 91–14. Landmarks and location for a cisterna magnum spinal tap. *W*, Wings of atlas; *O*, occipital protuberance; *X*, site for needle insertion.

gently toward the sternum to achieve an approximate 90° angle with the spine. The nose is held with its long axis parallel to the surface of the table. The head is held firmly so that the animal does not move or slide on the table.

Palpable landmarks are the occipital protuberance and the most prominent position of the wings of the atlas. Imaginary lines are drawn from the occipital protuberance down the midline and across the midline connecting the two wings of the atlas. The point of intersection is the site of entry of the spinal needle (Fig. 91–14). If bone is encountered, the needle is withdrawn about half the distance and the tip redirected more caudally. When the dura mater is penetrated the needle often snaps through, which can be felt by the collector. The stylet is withdrawn and the hub of the needle observed for fluid.

Pressure Recording

A previously assembled manometer and three-way valve are inserted into the hub of the spinal needle. Care must be taken not to move the needle. Fluid rises into the manometer for several seconds. When the fluid level becomes stable, the elevation of the fluid is read as the opening pressure and is recorded in millimeters of CSF (Fig. 91–15). A syringe is then attached to the three-way valve and 1 to 2 ml of CSF slowly withdrawn. An optional and possibly safer method is to allow CSF to drip from the three-way valve into a collection tube until a sufficient quantity is obtained. After CSF is collected the three-way valve is again directed to the manometer and the CSF falls to a new level (closing pressure).

Opening CSF pressures[14, 29, 31, 34, 41, 46] are normal up to 170 mm in the dog. Closing pressures are more

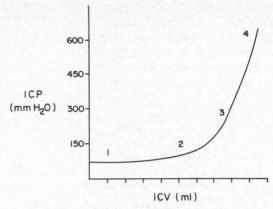

Figure 91–16. Idealized CSF pressure–volume relationship. 1 to 2 = Normal pressure, good compliance; 2 to 3 = normal pressure, poor compliance; 3 to 4 = elevated pressure, poor compliance. ICP, Intracranial pressure; ICV, volume of intracranial contents.

variable and depend on opening pressures. Closing pressures should not fall by more than 25 to 30 per cent of the opening pressure. Elevated opening pressures or a precipitous drop in closing pressures indicates increased intracranial pressure or a decrease in CSF compliance (Fig. 91–16).

Evaluation

CSF is frequently difficult to analyze in veterinary medicine because of three major potential problems: (1) collection of CSF free of blood; (2) collection of a sufficient volume for routine or special analytical techniques; and (3) access to a laboratory with appropriate instrumentation, skilled personnel, and analytical techniques needed for accurate CSF analysis. If quality collection, handling, and analysis are accomplished, results can help detect, confirm, or better define neurological disorders. Reference or standardized methods have not been established for CSF analysis; thus, results from different laboratories vary. Specific methods used and their indications and limitations can be found elsewhere.[2–4, 22, 25, 27, 32, 37]

Subjective assessment of CSF color and turbidity is especially important for observing differences between traumatic (collection) and pathological hemorrhage (Table 91–7). Objective assessment of xanthochromia may have better analytical sensitivity and specificity and thus be of more diagnostic value.[23, 28, 45] A recognition of the fragility of cells in CSF and optimal sample handling are required for proper interpretation of xanthochromia.

All procedures for determining cell numbers and preparing slides for cytology must be accomplished within one hour after collection, as cells rapidly deteriorate in the low protein and lipoprotein environment. Manual cell-counting procedures (nucleated cells and erythrocytes) are prone to relatively poor accuracy and poor reproducibility because of the low numbers usually present. All cell counts should be confirmed by finding similar cell ratios on concentrated CSF preparations. Traumatic hemor-

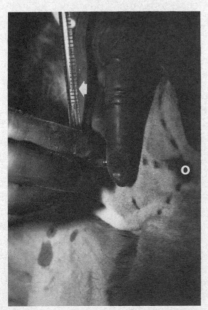

Figure 91–15. Technique for measuring CSF pressure using a column manometer. *O,* Occipital protuberance. CSF meniscus level is indicated by *arrow.*

TABLE 91–7. Abnormal CSF Findings

1. Turbidity
   a. > 200 nucleated cells/mm³ (2.0 × 10⁸/L)
   b. > 400 erythrocytes/mm³ (4.0 × 10⁸/L)
   c. Other: microorganisms, contrast media, other foreign material
2. Xanthochromia (pink to orange to yellow)
   a. Bilirachia (yellow)
      1. Degradation of hemoglobin within CSF one to two days after *in vivo* hemolysis
      2. Bilirubinemia (systemic jaundice) (conjugated or unconjugated)
   b. Free oxyhemoglobin (pale orange to pale pink)
      1. *In vivo* hemolysis two to four hours after hematorrhachis
      2. *In vitro* hemolysis one to four hours after traumatic tap
   c. > 150 mg/dl (1.5 gm/L) protein
   d. Melanin: consider metastatic melanoma
3. Red to pink CSF
   a. Traumatic or technique hemorrhage
      1. CSF is initially red but clears with continued aspiration
      2. Supernatant crystal clear in centrifuged CSF (must be centrifuged within one hour of collection)
   b. Hematorrhachis
      1. CSF is red throughout collection
      2. Xanthochromic supernatant (pale orange to yellow) if erythrocytes were present in CSF for at least two to four hours
4. Pleocytosis (elevated total nucleated cell count)
   a. Infectious: bacterial, fungal, viral, parasitic, protozoal
   b. Inflammatory (noninfectious): tissue necrosis (traumatic, metabolic, degenerative, toxic, neoplasia, foreign body, vascular abnormality)
   c. Neoplasia: lymphoid neoplasia, primary or metastatic neoplasia
5. Elevated protein concentration
   a. Increased blood–CSF barrier permeability (primarily inflammation; also endocrine, metabolic, and toxic disorders)
   b. Froin's syndrome (lumbar collection) obstruction in CSF flow in vertebral canal
   c. Increased production of proteins (immunoglobulins) by B-lymphocytes and/or plasma cells
   d. Tissue degeneration
   e. Traumatic tap (CSF contamination with plasma)

TABLE 91–8. "Correction" of CSF Leukocyte Count and Protein Concentration for Leukocytes or Protein Added to CSF as a Result of Traumatic Tap (Technique Hemorrhage)

$$\text{Corrected WBC} = \text{WBC}_{csf} - \text{WBC added}$$

$$\text{Corrected TP} = \text{TP}_{csf} - \text{TP added}$$

$$\text{WBC added} = \frac{\text{WBC}_b \times \text{RBC}_{csf}}{\text{RBC}_b}$$

$$\text{TP added} = \frac{\text{TP}_b \times \text{RBC}_{csf}}{\text{RBC}_b}$$

Notes: WBC_{csf} (usually stated as number of nucleated cells/mm³ [or L] [as determined by hemocytometer] in the CSF)

= leukocytes/mm³ (or L) determined by subtracting macrophages, pia-arachnoid cells, plasma cells, and other non blood cells from total nucleated cell count quantitated in CSF

WBC_b = leukocytes/mm³ (or L) in blood
RBC_{csf} = erythrocytes/mm³ (or L) in CSF
RBC_b = erythrocytes/mm³ (or L) in blood
TP_{csf} = total protein (mg/dl or gm/L) measured in CSF

TP_b (usually stated as protein concentration quantitated in plasma or serum [incorrect])

= total protein concentration in blood (mg/dl or gm/L), which equals $(\text{TP}_{serum} + \text{fibrinogen}_{plasma}) \times \frac{(1 - \text{PCV})}{100}$ or

$$\text{TP}_{plasma} \times \frac{(1 - \text{PCV})}{100}$$

Measured factors could be in error by 10 per cent (method dependent). PCV (packed cell volume) expressed as volume per cent.

rhage contaminates collected CSF and alters cellular and chemical concentrations.

Correction formulas or factors have been proposed to establish "true" CSF leukocyte counts (WBC) and total protein concentrations (TP) (Table 91–8). The correction formulas are based on several assumptions, including (1) erythrocyte counts (RBC) are accurate; (2) pathological hematorrhachis was not present; and (3) the cell and protein concentrations in peripheral venous blood are identical to those of the blood contaminating the CSF. The proportional ratios that are most frequently stated do not include other correction factors, such as (1) subtraction of "resident" nucleated cells (macrophages, pia-arachnoid meso-

thelial cells, ependymal cells, plasma cells, and so on) from the total nucleated cell count (TNCC) to obtain the leukocyte number in the CSF; (2) conversion of serum or plasma total protein (TP) concentration to whole blood TP concentration based on packed cell volume; and (3) recognition of the variable precision in measurements. As a result, a common correction formula is considered unreliable in clinical CSF samples.[57] It should be noted that reported methods do not include cytological confirmation of erythrocyte/nucleated cell ratios, correction of WBC counts for "resident" nucleated cells, and clarification of blood total protein concentration versus plasma total protein concentration. Based on the number of assumptions and necessary correction factors, it is difficult to substantiate that any correction factor (based on erythrocytes present) yields consistently valid conclusions. Finding crenated erythrocytes in the counting chamber or on cytological preparations is not a reliable indicator of hematorrhachis.

Nucleated cell differentiation and morphological evaluation are necessary for routine CSF analysis, but satisfactory results can be obtained only from special techniques that concentrate cells without causing cell lysis or distortion. Hemocytometer chamber differentials are not recommended. Blood film techniques (e.g., push slide) using unconcentrated CSF frequently result in either no cells found or cell lysis. Routine centrifugation in clinical centrifigues and smears made from resuspended sediment frequently yield low cell numbers and poor morphology. Several cytological preparatory techniques have been developed for CSF, and each has its advantages and limitations.[2, 22, 25, 32] In our experience, the cytocentrifuge* preparations have yielded satisfactory results for most CSF.

Varied cell numbers and cell types have been reported for normal dog and cat CSF[48, 50, 53] owing to varied techniques and lack of standardized cell terminology. Small lymphocytes and monocytes (synonyms: reticulomonocytes, meningeal histiocytoid cells, pia-arachnoid [PAM] cells) are frequently observed in cytocentrifuge preparations of normal CSF.

Neutrophils (occasionally with cytoplasmic vacuolation), reactive lymphoid cells (plasmacytoid lymphocytes, immunocytes), plasma cells, macrophages, and eosinophils are seen in a variety of pathological processes (see Table 91–8). Erythrophages (macrophages with phagocytized erythrocytes) indicate that erythrocytes have been present in the CSF for a few hours (in vivo or in vitro). Siderophages (macrophages with iron pigment, hemosiderin, or hematoidin crystals) indicate hematorrhachis several days to weeks before sampling. Lipophages (macrophages with lipid droplets) are seen with neural tissue necrosis. Neoplastic cells are not commonly observed. Neoplastic lymphoid cells (or other hematopoietic cells in cats) are seen. Sarcomatous or carcinomatous cells may be suspected on routine preparations but may require special techniques or other diagnostic procedures to confirm their presence.[37]

Microorganisms (bacteria, fungi, protozoa) may be seen, but their absence on morphological studies should not rule out infectious processes when suspected. Microbiological cultures are more likely to detect low numbers of organisms.

Elevated total protein concentrations indicate a disease process affecting central nervous tissue or meninges. As there is no single method for total protein quantitation, one must expect results to vary among laboratories if different methods and different protein standard solutions are utilized. The method used should be minimally affected by albumin/globulin ratios[18, 38] and require minimal sample volume. Several procedures are clinically useful.[3, 22, 27] The Pandy test is frequently mentioned as a useful qualitative procedure for detecting globulins; however, the turbidity seen with the addition of phenol to CSF can occur with globulins and albumin,[4, 35] and the test is not recommended as a substitute for quantitative procedures.[26, 40]

An assessment of creatine kinase (CK) (creatine phosphokinase/CPK) activity in CSF has been proposed for routine CSF analysis.[20] Increased total CK activity appears to have good diagnostic sensitivity for neurological disease, but increased activity has been found in a variety of disorders.[21, 49] One must expect different CSF CK activity measurements if different assay methods or reaction temperatures are used. It may be necessary to modify the procedure used for serum CK activity quantitation, as the CSF CK activity may be below the assay's analytical sensitivity or near the bottom of the assay's linear range. Both analytical properties may lead to poor analytical precision and low reproducibility. Erythrocytes or hemolysis may lead to false CK activity measurements because erythrocyte adenylate kinase, glucose-6-phosphate, or ATP may interfere by participating in coupled or side reactions. Creatine kinase activity is less stable in CSF than in serum, and analysis should be done as soon as possible.[42]

BIOPSY TECHNIQUES

The application of new methods of processing, staining, and microscopically examining tissue samples has contributed enormously to our understanding of disease processes. Furthermore, histochemistry and electron microscopy have aided the recognition of a number of new diseases. Biopsy techniques as applied to skeletal muscle, peripheral nerve, and brain are described.

Skeletal Muscle Biopsy

Muscle biopsies are important in confirming clinical and electrophysiological evidence of neuromuscular disease, and may also provide an etiological diagnosis.

The following criteria are suggested when choosing a muscle for biopsy:

1. The muscle is affected by the myopathy. In acute disease, a more severely involved muscle should be chosen. However, in a chronic disease process, a muscle that is only moderately affected may afford better recognition of the disease process than one in which the disease process is well advanced.

2. The muscle is readily accessible and easily identified.

3. The muscle sampling site is in an area where biopsy will not jeopardize peripheral nerves, blood vessels, tendons, or joints.

4. The sampling is limited to selected proximal and distal muscles in thoracic and pelvic limbs. Biopsies are taken from muscles for which normal, statistically evaluated distribution of fiber types and fiber sizes is available. The sampling site in any muscle should also be standardized, since distribution of fiber types may vary within a muscle.

5. The sampling site permits combined muscle and nerve biopsy.

6. Postoperative discomfort is minimal.

*Cytospin, Shandon Southern Products Ltd., Cheshire, England.

Biopsy Technique[6, 15]

Skeletal muscles that are routinely biopsied include the following:

From the pelvic limb:
  Biceps femoris (distal third)
  Vastus lateralis (distal third)
  Lateral head of gastrocnemius (proximal third)
  Cranial tibial (proximal third)

From the thoracic limb:
  Long head of triceps brachii (distal third)
  Medial head of triceps brachii (distal third)
  Superficial digital flexor (proximal third)

The site for biopsy of the common peroneal and ulnar nerves (see Nerve Biopsy) permits sampling of the biceps femoris and gastrocnemius muscles in the pelvic limb and of the medial head of the triceps brachii and superficial digital flexor muscles in the thoracic limb.

In most instances, muscle biopsies are performed immediately after electrodiagnostic procedures (electromyography, nerve conduction velocity determinations, and so on), during which time the animal is under general anesthesia. In older or high risk animals, oxymorphone hydrochloride and acepromazine are used for sedation, followed by local infiltration of the skin at the biopsy site with 2% lidocaine. The biopsy site is surgically prepared and an incision (approximately 5 cm in length) is made through the skin and fascia to expose the muscle. A segment of muscle is grasped with toothed forceps and a sample removed by cutting a cylinder with a pair of sharp scissors. Multiple samples may be taken from the same area (to reduce the chances of missing a focal pathological change). After the biopsy, the fascia and subcutaneous tissues are sutured with absorbable material and the skin is closed.

No attempt is made to maintain the muscle under stretch for routine histology and histochemistry. However, maintaining the muscle in a slightly stretched length is very important for electron microscopy. For this purpose, special biopsy clamps are used.

In contrast to percutaneous needle biopsy, this muscle procedure permits adequate tissue sampling and facilitates orientation for freezing and sectioning.

Processing[6, 15]

Muscle samples removed at biopsy are placed on and covered with a slightly moistened gauze sponge. Portions of muscle that were grasped by forceps are removed with a sharp blade, and the sample is divided and oriented for cutting in transverse and longitudinal planes.

Histological and histochemical studies are performed on frozen sections. Limited information is derived from samples fixed in formalin solution. The specimens are frozen within one hour of biopsy to avoid loss of soluble enzymes; in emergencies, interpretable muscle histochemistry is obtained in samples refrigerated (4°C) overnight.

We use the gum tragacanth/isopentane/liquid nitrogen method of freezing. It is a reliable method and results in the production of the fewest artifacts. The trimmed muscle cube (approximately 1 cm square) is embedded in the tragacanth, mounted on thin slices of cork, and oriented for cutting in a transverse or longitudinal plane.

The muscle sample mounted on the cork is immersed (using long forceps) in the isopentane and precooled to $-160°C$ for approximately ten seconds. Too short a period of freezing creates artifacts in the muscle, and too long a period may produce fissures in the sample. Long-term storage is at $-70°C$.

When sections are required, the muscle sample is transferred from the deep freeze to the interior of a cryostat maintained at -20 to $-25°C$. The cork is mounted onto a standard chuck in the cryostat chamber by freezing with a drop of water. Sections are cut at 8 μm and mounted directly onto glass slides. Unstained sections may be mailed to a laboratory with facilities for histochemistry. If the sections are stained within four days, interpretation of the histochemistry can be made.

Histochemistry

Enzyme histochemical techniques applied to skeletal muscle have resulted in the recognition of fiber types, have demonstrated abnormalities in fibers that appear to be normal by routine staining procedures, and have made possible the diagnosis of specific enzyme deficiencies.

In the past, the classification of fiber types in skeletal muscle has been complicated by the use of various enzymatic techniques and physiological-histochemical correlations. In an attempt to satisfy the suggested guidelines of Dubowitz and Brooke relating to a more simplified system of classification, the fiber types in canine skeletal muscle have been classified according to the human nomenclature.[6] This is based on adenosine triphosphatase (ATPase) reactivity with ATPase substrate under acidic and alkaline preincubation conditions to inactivate different ATPase systems.

Three fiber types are found in mature canine muscle based on ATPase staining: types I, IIA, and IIC (Table 91–9, Figs. 91–17 and 91–18). ATPase is more stable than other metabolic enzymes for the differentiation of fiber types in muscles affected by diverse pathological or physiological states. There is a clear differentiation of fiber types using alkaline (routine) ATPase. The type I fibers are more lightly stained and the type II fibers (both type A and type C) are more heavily stained. The pattern of the ATPase reaction is markedly altered by incubating sections at pH 4.3 (see Table 91–9; Figs. 91–17 and 91–18). Under these conditions, the type IIA fibers

TABLE 91–9. Histochemical Profile of Fiber Types in Canine Appendicular Skeletal Muscle

Histochemical Procedure	Staining Intensity According to Fiber Type		
	Type I	Type IIA	Type IIC
ATPase, preincubation pH 9.4	Low to moderate	High	High
ATPase, preincubation pH 4.5	High	Low to negative	Moderate
ATPase, preincubation pH 4.3	High	Low to negative	Moderate
NADH-TR	High	Moderate	Moderate
PAS	Low	High	High
Glycine-formaldehyde*	Low to negative	Moderate	Moderate

*Glycine-formaldehyde, preincubation pH 7.25, followed by standard ATPase incubation.

no longer stain, whereas the type I fibers stain darkly. Type IIC fibers stain with a moderate intensity.

Additional histochemical stains routinely employed include the following.

Reduced Nicotinamide Adeninedinucleotide Tetrazolium Reductase (NADH-TR). This is an oxidative enzyme with a reciprocal relationship to alkaline ATPase activity. Accordingly, type I fibers stain darkly and type II fibers lightly (see Table 91–9). The NADH-TR staining intensity is used as an index of mitochondrial presence and, hence, aerobic metabolism.

Periodic Acid Schiff (PAS). This stain is frequently used to demonstrate glycogen in muscle. The PAS reaction stains type II fibers more strongly than type I fibers (see Table 91–9).

Other histological stains that are used routinely include hematoxylin and eosin and the modified Gomori's trichrome. These stains demonstrate muscle fibers, nerves, blood vessels, connective tissue, adipose tissue, and nuclei.

Morphometry

Quantitative morphological procedures on skeletal muscle include fiber type percentages and fiber diameter determinations. Both factors vary between, and sometimes within, individual muscles of the same animal. A range of normal morphometric values has been established in various muscles of the dog, against which changes occurring as a result of disease may be judged.[7, 10]

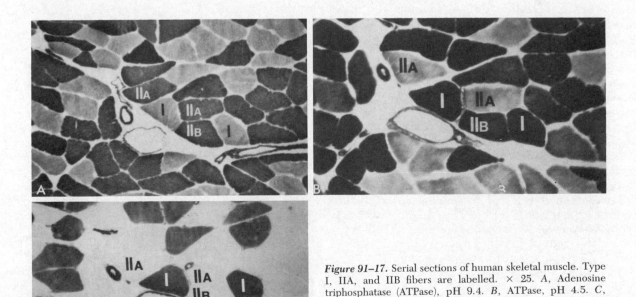

Figure 91–17. Serial sections of human skeletal muscle. Type I, IIA, and IIB fibers are labelled. × 25. *A,* Adenosine triphosphatase (ATPase), pH 9.4. *B,* ATPase, pH 4.5. *C,* ATPase, pH 4.3.

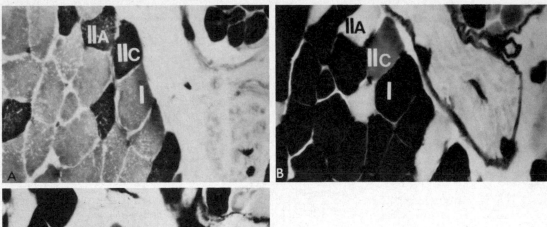

Figure 91–18. Serial sections of canine skeletal muscle. Type I, IIA, and IIC fibers are labelled. ×40. *A*, ATPase, pH 9.4. *B*, ATPase, pH 4.5. *C*, ATPase, pH 4.3.

For each muscle biopsy, the following morphometric parameters may be evaluated:

Mean Lesser Fiber Diameter. This is defined as the maximum diameter across the lesser aspect of the muscle fiber and is designed to overcome the distortion that occurs when a muscle fiber is cut obliquely. In any muscle section, 200 fibers of each type are measured (type IIC fibers usually are not included, since they represent less than 2 per cent of the fibers in mature canine muscle). The mean diameter range in dogs weighing more than 15 kg is 40 to 50 μm, and in dogs weighing less than 15 kg the range is 30 to 40 μm (Table 91–10).

Percentage of Fiber Types. Type I fibers predominate in the medial head of triceps brachii and superficial digital flexor muscles, whereas type IIA fibers are more numerous in biceps femoris, the long head of the triceps brachii, and cranial tibial muscles. An approximately equal ratio is present in the gastrocnemius muscle. Percentages of fiber types are determined from a random count of approximately 1000 fibers in transverse sections.

Percentage of Internal Nuclei. In normal mature canine appendicular muscle, the number of fibers with internal nuclei usually does not exceed 1 per cent. The number is determined from a random count of 1000 fibers in transverse sections.

Variability Coefficient. This factor is calculated as follows:

$$\frac{\text{Standard deviation} \times 1000}{\text{Mean fiber diameter}}$$

Any fiber type with a variability coefficient of greater than 250 is considered to demonstrate abnormal variability in fiber size.

Atrophy and hypertrophy factors. These factors are derived from histograms and are an expression of the number of abnormally small or large fibers in the biopsy. These factors may be useful in detecting the presence of atrophy or hypertrophy that is not readily apparent microscopically.

All of these statistical parameters may be programmed for rapid results using a video display image-analysis system interfaced with a computer.*

Nerve Biopsy

In conjunction with clinical and electrophysiological evaluation, nerve biopsies are being increasingly used for the investigation of neuromuscular disorders. The complete examination of a nerve biopsy specimen is a complex and time-consuming procedure that is best performed at centers where there is an interest in peripheral nerve disorders.

Fascicular nerve biopsies are used whenever possible, leaving the majority of the nerve trunk intact.[12] This technique preserves the neurological and electrophysiological integrity of the parent nerve and permits data to be compiled on histological, ultrastructural, biochemical, and teased-fiber studies. The following criteria are suggested in choosing a nerve for biopsy:[17]

1. The nerve is affected by the neuropathy. The clinical signs of peripheral neuropathies are listed in Chapter 89.

2. The nerve is constant in its location and readily

---

*Optomax Semi-Automatic Image Analysis System, Optomax Inc., Hollis, NH.

TABLE 91–10. Total Group Means for Fiber Diameter, Variability Coefficient, and Fiber Percentage of Types I, IIA, and IIC Fibers in Various Canine Skeletal Muscles

Muscle	Fiber Type	Group A*				Fiber Type	Group B†				Significance‡
		Mean Fiber Diameter ± S.D.	Variability Coefficient	Fiber Percentage	Number of Muscles in Which a Given Fiber Type Was Present		Mean Fiber Diameter ± S.D.	Variability Coefficient	Fiber Percentage	Number of Muscles in Which a Given Fiber Type Was Present	
Biceps femoris	I	40.64±8.92	220	41.0	19	I	33.75±9.06	260	33.0	9	$p < 0.005$
	IIA	42.99±8.93	206	58.0	19	IIA	31.34±7.64	240	66.1	9	$p < 0.0003$
	IIC	35.36±6.35	180	1.0	17	IIC	25.57±5.34	204	0.9	7	$p < 0.002$
Gastrocnemius	I	47.48±9.02	186	49.0	19	I	37.32±6.69	170	50.0	9	$p < 0.005$
	IIA	44.49±8.89§	196	49.4	19	IIA	33.08±6.74	200	48.6	9	$p < 0.0001$
	IIC	41.81±8.45	200	1.6	15	IIC	32.70±7.12	210	1.4	6	$p < 0.001$
Medial head of the triceps brachii	I	50.60±9.64	184	88.0	18	I	36.47±7.43	200	77.0	6	$p < 0.003$
	IIA	42.07±8.50	192	11.1	14	IIA	30.76±6.32	200	21.6	6	$p < 0.004$
	IIC	37.24±7.46	200	0.9	10	IIC	28.04±5.37	190	1.4	4	$p < 0.05$
Long head of the triceps brachii	I	40.89±9.00	220	31.0	19	I	32.22±8.24	250	28.0	7	$p < 0.007$
	IIA	42.06±8.84	210	67.9	19	IIA	31.05±7.49	240	70.8	7	$p < 0.0002$
	IIC	34.29±6.96	200	1.1	13	IIC	29.83±5.50	170	1.2	6	$p < 0.01$
Superficial digital flexor	I	46.65±9.58	210	73.0	19	I	31.68±7.47	230	72.0	8	$p < 0.0001$
	IIA	43.65±8.78	200	25.5	18	IIA	29.35±7.03	230	26.9	8	$p < 0.0001$
	IIC	39.24±7.14	180	1.5	12	IIC	26.81±5.71	210	1.1	6	$p < 0.005$

*Dogs > 15 kg (n = 19).

†Dogs < 15 kg (n = 9).

‡Significance level comparing mean fiber diameters of fiber types from group A and group B.

§Mean fiber diameter in 15 dogs less than 7 years of age = 47.32±9.09; mean fiber diameter in four dogs 7 to 15 years of age = 36.03±9.12.

accessible to identification and nerve conduction velocity determinations.

3. The nerve is located in an area where biopsy will not jeopardize blood vessels, tendons, or joints.

4. The nerve is protected from areas of entrapment and not exposed to recurrent trauma.

5. Postoperative discomfort and neurological deficits are minimal.

6. Normal statistically evaluated morphometric data (histological and teased-fiber measurements) are available for the nerve in question.

7. The nerve is either pure motor or pure sensory. In this laboratory, mixed nerves are routinely sampled because electrophysiological data are available for these nerves in the dog and cat. Control studies indicate that fascicular biopsy of common peroneal and ulnar nerves does not produce clinical sensory or motor deficits.[12]

Common Peroneal Nerve

This is a mixed nerve with motor fibers innervating muscles that flex the hock and extend the digits. It is sensory to the skin of the dorsocranial surface of the paw, hock, and stifle. When combined nerve and muscle biopsy is desired, biopsy of the nerve at the stifle provides exposure for biopsy of the underlying gastrocnemius muscle (lateral head) and distal biceps femoris muscle.

The common peroneal nerve is the nerve favored for biopsy. It is a flat nerve in which individual fascicles are easily identified. Its long subcutaneous course over the stifle, without branching, allows removal of ample lengths (2 to 5 cm), if needed. In addition, well-established, normal electrophysiological,[5, 12, 44, 47] and normal age-related, statistically evaluated morphometric data[8, 9] are available. However, the superficial location of the nerve as it crosses the lateral aspect of the stifle joint renders it vulnerable to trauma.

Biopsy Technique

Following general anesthesia, the animal is positioned in lateral recumbency, and the stifle area is surgically prepared. A 10-cm oblique skin incision is made over the lateral femoral condyle (Fig. 91–19). The nerve is located as it crosses the lateral head of the gastrocnemius muscle and is carefully isolated from surrounding areolar tissue. A 5–0 silk suture with a swaged-on noncutting needle is placed in the nerve at its caudal border to include approximately one-third of its width. A 1-gm weight (we use a 42-gauge stainless steel orthopedic screw that is wrapped with 3–0 stainless steel suture with needle) is hooked into the caudal border of the nerve approximately 3 to 5 cm distal to the previously placed suture. After gentle retraction of the suture, a pair of fine, sharp scissors is used to longitudinally divide 30 per cent of the nerve fascicles from the parent trunk to a point immediately distal to the weight. The nerve fascicles

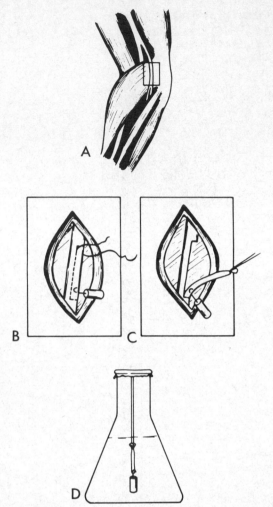

Figure 91–19. Fascicular nerve biopsy technique of the peroneal nerve. *A*, The nerve is isolated as it crosses the lateral head of the gastrocnemius muscle (inset). *B*, A suture is placed in the proximal portion of the nerve to be excised, and a weight is secured 3 to 5 cm distally. *C*, The suture is tied and the nerve is divided to a point distal to the weight. *D*, The nerve biopsy sample is suspended in fixative solution.

are removed from the parent trunk by a transverse incision and are suspended immediately in fixative (see Fig. 91–19). The fascial and subcutaneous tissues are closed with absorbable suture and skin closure is completed. A dry dressing is applied and held in place with a 10-cm elastic bandage. Activity of the animal is limited during the immediate postoperative period.

Ulnar Nerve

This is a mixed nerve with motor branches to the flexors of the carpus and digits. Sensory branches supply the caudal surface of the antebrachium. When combined nerve and muscle biopsy is desired, a combination biopsy of ulnar nerve at the elbow with biopsy of the medial head of the triceps brachii and superficial digital flexor muscles has proven satisfactory. There are no muscular branches that leave the ulnar nerve as it traverses the brachium. This nerve has been used for quantitative electrophysiological[5, 12, 44, 47] and morphometric[8, 9] studies.

There are a few disadvantages to the use of the ulnar nerve for biopsy: (1) it is closely associated with the collateral ulnar vessels; (2) individual fascicles cannot be identified; and (3) fascicles are difficult to separate in this cylindrical nerve.

Biopsy Technique

Following general anesthesia and positioning, the medial surface of the thoracic limb is surgically prepared, extending from the axilla to the metacarpal region. A 10-cm long skin incision centered midway between the point of the olecranon and the medial condyle of the humerus is made in a slightly oblique fashion. The incision is continued by blunt dissection to expose the ulnar nerve as it crosses parallel to the medial head of the triceps brachii muscle. The nerve is isolated from adipose tissue, fascia, and accompanying collateral ulnar artery and vein. A fascicular biopsy may be obtained by using the technique described for the common peroneal nerve. The wound is closed with close attention to hemostasis and accurate approximation of the fascia, subcutaneous tissue, and skin.

Tibial Nerve and Plantar Branches

In some instances, sampling of more distal nerves may be indicated (e.g., distal axonopathies). In this situation, biopsy of the distal tibial nerve and its branches (medial and lateral plantar nerves) enables comparison of distal and proximal changes. All three nerves may be sampled from a single incision.

The mixed tibial nerve supplies motor branches to muscles that extend the hock and flex the digits. It is sensory to the skin and footpads of the plantar surface of the paw and metatarsus. At about the middle of the crus near the medial surface, the tibial nerve lies near the plantar branch of the saphenous artery and vein. Approximately 1 cm proximal to the tibiotarsal joint, the tibial nerve bifurcates into medial and lateral plantar nerves. The medial plantar nerve is smaller and more medial and superficial than the lateral plantar nerve.

There are several disadvantages to the use of these nerves for biopsy: (1) potential bleeding from the branches of the saphenous vessels; (2) insufficient morphometric (histological and teased-fiber measurements) data[11] and no electrophysiological data available for the plantar nerves; (3) plantar nerves are not readily accessible to conduction velocity determinations; (4) fascicles of tibial nerve are difficult to separate; and (5) the lateral plantar nerve is deeper than a cutaneous nerve and it is difficult to obtain adequate lengths of nerve for special study.

Biopsy Technique

The caudomedial surface of the pelvic limb is surgically prepared from the stifle to the digits. A 10-cm long skin incision centered midway between the tuber calcanei and the medial malleolus of the tibia is made. The incision is continued by blunt dissection to expose the distal tibial nerve and its bifurcation into medial and lateral plantar nerves. The tibial nerve is isolated from dense fascia and closely associated plantar branches of the saphenous artery and vein. A fascicular biopsy is performed as for the common peroneal nerve. The plantar branches are isolated from their respective plantar vessels and, at a level approximately 2 to 3 cm distal to the bifurcation of the tibial nerve, whole nerve biopsies of each nerve are performed. This procedure does not result in clinical sensory or motor deficits. The entire nerve is removed as described for the fascicular biopsy.

Processing[1, 8, 9, 16]

Fresh nerve samples may be frozen in liquid nitrogen and stored for biochemical studies. For routine light microscopy, nerve samples may be fixed in buffered 10% formalin for three days and divided into three 1-cm segments. One segment is processed for paraffin embedding and routine histological staining. A second segment is washed overnight in Millonig's phosphate buffer (pH 7.3) at 4°C. This sample is postfixed in 1% osmium tetroxide for one hour, washed in phosphate buffer, transferred through graded ethanol solutions, and processed for embedding in epon. Semithin sections (1 to 2 μm) are cut transversely and stained with paraphenylenediamine or toluidine blue. For electron microscopy, silver to gray ultrathin sections are cut and stained with uranyl acetate and lead citrate (fixation of nerve samples in 2.5% glutaraldehyde solution produces better sections for electron microscopy). The third sample of nerve is postfixed in 1% osmium tetroxide for three to four hours. The nerve is placed in 66% glycerin for 48 hours and in 100% glycerin for 24 hours for teased-fiber preparations. With this procedure, the nature of myelin and axon changes along the course of the nerve can be studied.

The nerve sample, along with several drops of glycerin, is placed on a glass slide. Fascicles are pulled apart using curved, pointed forceps and epineurium/perineurium stripped off under a dissecting microscope. Small strands of nerve fibers are pulled apart, and, from each strand, single fibers are stripped off and slid onto a clean slide adjacent to the slide on which the teasing is done. The friction of the fiber on the glass straightens the fiber and causes it to pull loose from the tips of the forceps. Up to ten teased fibers are placed in the center of each glass slide. Coverslips are applied using standard mounting medium.

In our laboratory, technicians can prepare 200 to 300 teased fibers per day. For any given nerve biopsy, 100 fibers per nerve sample are teased randomly from all fascicles, without preselection for size or abnormality, with each fiber containing at least four to six internodes.

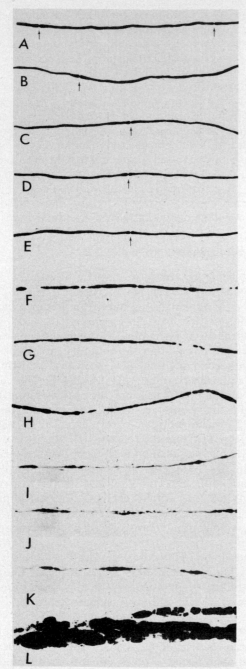

Figure 91–20. Single teased fibers of plantar nerves from a dog with diabetes mellitus. *A–E,* Single continuous teased fiber with normal internodal length and myelin thickness. Nodes of Ranvier (arrows). *F–H,* Single continuous teased fiber with myelin irregularity and multiple regions of nodal lengthening and internodal myelin absence. *I–K,* Single continuous teased fiber with linear rows of myelin balls. *L,* Teased fibers showing segmentation into myelin ovoids. Osmium tetroxide × 40 *(A–K);* ×160 *(L).*

Teased-fiber preparations identify demyelination and fiber degeneration (Fig. 91–20). Normal teased fibers show little variation in diameter and internodal length. Fibers with segmental demyelination are characterized by regions of nodal lengthening or internodal myelin absence. The hallmark of axonal degeneration is long linear rows of myelin ovoids or balls. Short intercalated internodes with inappro-priately thin myelin sheaths suggest fiber remyeli-nation.

Morphometry

Quantitative morphological procedures are neces-sary to identify subtle changes and to characterize patterns of nerve fiber loss seen in some neuropa-thies. Myelinated fiber diameters, areas, and densi-ties are determined from semithin preparations of cross-sectioned nerve. Alterations in nerves resulting from incomplete regeneration and repair are best recognized by quantitative studies on teased fibers. Following axonal degeneration and successful regen-eration, internodal lengths are uniformly short. In contrast, fibers with segmental demyelination fol-lowed by remyelination are characterized by inter-nodes of variable lengths. In this laboratory, mor-phometry is accomplished using a video display, semiautomatic, image-analysis system interfaced with a preprogrammed computer.*

The results of quantitative studies depend on sev-eral variables, including type and duration of fixation used, particular nerve selected, sampling site on the nerve, and species and age of animal.

Brain Biopsy

Evaluation of brain function in veterinary medicine continues to rely on clinical and electrophysiological studies. Although techniques for brain surgery have been decribed for approximately 20 years, its practi-cal application in clinical neurology has been limited to decompression following head injury. With the possible exception of experimental research in infec-tious, toxic, and metabolic diseases, brain biopsy procedures in dogs and cats probably will not become a routine adjunct to other diagnostic aids. The reasons for this stem not only from financial and emotional considerations but also from inadequate training in surgical competency and almost complete uncertainty about sequelae of brain biopsy in relation to site of sampling. Furthermore, clinical encephalopathies of infectious (e.g., canine distemper virus encephalitis), toxic (e.g., lead poisoning), and metabolic (e.g., he-patic encephalopathy) origin can usually be diagnosed by alternative ancillary techniques, and brain biopsy for suspected focal lesions (e.g., infarcts, tumors) usually is not indicated. Brain biopsy may have potential value in experimental studies necessitating sequential tissue sampling.

Biopsy Technique

The following procedures are derived mainly from a recent report[43] in which brain biopsy techniques were evaluated. Cerebral biopsies were performed on 12 dogs, and cerebellar biopsies were done on a

---

*Optomax Inc.

second group of 12 dogs. No clinical neurological deficits occurred (during a two-month postsurgery observation period) in the cerebral group; however, in the cerebellar group, two dogs exhibited temporary vestibular and cerebellar clinical signs.

Cerebral Biopsy

The dorsal and lateral areas of the head are prepared for surgery. With the animal in lateral recumbency, a vertical skin incision is made midway between the lateral canthus of the eye and the rostral border of the base of the ear extending from the dorsal midline of the skull to the zygomatic arch. The palpebral nerve, which lies superficially and perpendicular to the incision line, is avoided. With blunt dissection, the bone is exposed and a 12- to 16-mm diameter craniotomy defect is made using either a pneumatic craniotome* or a manual skull trefine.† The dura is incised with a No.11 scalpel blade about halfway around the circumference of the defect in an area free of meningeal vessels. The dura is reflected and, with a No.11 blade, a pyramidal wedge of cerebrocortical tissue (approximately $3\times3\times4$ mm) is removed using a sterile applicator stick. Hemorrhage is controlled using gelatin foam. When the bleeding has ceased, the foam is removed and the dural flap replaced but not sutured. The fascia of the temporal muscle and subcutaneous tissues are closed with absorbable material. The skin is sutured with 5–0 stainless steel.

Cerebellar Biopsy

The dorsal areas of the skull and cervical spine are surgically prepared. The animal is placed in sternal recumbency with the head flexed and the nose perpendicular to the table. The area is draped and a midline incision made from just cranial to the occipital protuberance to the level of the atlas. Superficial fascia and dorsal cervical musculature are incised on the midline. With blunt dissection using a surgical sponge, the occipital bone is exposed. A 12- to 16-mm defect is made in the occipital bone with either the pneumatic drill or the manual trefine. The dura mater is incised, the caudal portion of the vermis of the cerebellum is biopsied, and the wound is closed in the same fashion as for the cerebrum.

1. Asbury, A. K., and Johnson, P. C.: *Pathology of Peripheral Nerve.* W. B. Saunders, Philadelphia, 1978.
2. Barrett, D. L., King, E. B., and Hasson, P. L.: Collection and cytopreparatory techniques for serous effusions and cerebrospinal fluids. Part 1. Lab. Med. 9:9, 1978.
3. Barsanti, J. A., and Duncan, J. R.: Determination of the concentration of protein in cerebrospinal fluid with a dye-binding method. Vet. Clin. Pathol. 7:6, 1978.
4. Bauer, J. D., Ackerman, P. G., and Toro, G.: Examination of biologic fluids (serous fluids, cerebrospinal fluid, synovial fluid, amniotic fluid, sputum, pus). *In* Bauer, J. D., et al. (eds.): *Clinical Laboratory Methods,* 8th ed. C. V. Mosby, St. Louis, 1974, pp. 602–611.
5. Bowen, J. M.: Peripheral nerve electrodiagnostics, electromyography, and nerve conduction velocity. *In* Hoerlein, B. F. (ed.): *Canine Neurology — Diagnosis and Treatment,* 3rd ed. W. B. Saunders, Philadelphia, 1978, p. 254.
6. Braund, K. G., Hoff, E. J., and Richardson, K. E. Y.: Histochemical identification of fiber types in canine skeletal muscle. Am. J. Vet. Res. 39:561, 1978.
7. Braund, K. G., and Lincoln, C. E.: Histochemical differentiation of fiber types in neonatal canine skeletal muscle. Am. J. Vet. Res. 42:407, 1981.
8. Braund, K. G., McGuire, J. A., and Lincoln, C. E.: Age-related changes in peripheral nerves of the dog. I. A morphologic and morphometric study of single-teased fibers. Vet. Pathol. 19:365, 1982.
9. Braund, K. G., McGuire, J. A., and Lincoln, C. E.: Age-related changes in peripheral nerves of the dog. II. A morphologic and morphometric study of cross-sectional nerve. Vet. Pathol. 19:379, 1982.
10. Braund, K. G., McGuire, J. A., and Lincoln, C. E.: Observations on normal skeletal muscle of mature dogs : A cytochemical, histochemical, and morphometric study. Vet. Pathol. 19:577, 1982.
11. Braund, K. G., and Steiss, J. E.: Distal neuropathy in spontaneous diabetes mellitus in the dog. Acta Neuropathol. 57:263, 1982.
12. Braund, K. G., Walker, T. L., and Vandevelde, M.: Fascicular nerve biopsy in the dog. Am. J. Vet. Res. 40:1025, 1979.
13. Chrisman, C. L.: *Problems in Small Animal Neurology.* Lea & Febiger, Philadelphia, 1982, pp. 39–58.
14. de Lahunta, A.: *Veterinary Neuroanatomy and Clinical Neurology.* W. B. Saunders, Philadelphia, 1977, pp. 48, 344–354.
15. Dubowitz, V., and Brooke, M. H.: *Muscle Biopsy : A Modern Approach.* W. B. Saunders, Philadelphia, 1973.
16. Dyck, P. J.: Pathologic alterations of the peripheral nervous system of man. *In* Dyck, P. J., Thomas, P. K., and Lambert, E. H. (eds.): *Peripheral Neuropathy.* W. B. Saunders, Philadelphia, 1975, p. 296.
17. Dyck, P. J., and Lofgren, E. P.: Method of fascicular biopsy of human peripheral nerve for electrophysiologic and histologic study. Mayo Clin. Proc. 41:778, 1966.
18. Henry, R. J., Sobel, C., and Segalove, M.: Turbidimetric determination of proteins with sulfosalicylic and trichloracetic acids. Proc. Soc. Exp. Biol. Med. 92:748, 1956.
19. Hoerlein, B. F., and Oliver, J. E.: Brain surgery. *In* Hoerlein, B. F. (ed.) : *Canine Neurology — Diagnosis and Treatment,* 3rd ed. W. B. Saunders, Philadelphia, 1978, p. 697.
20. Hoffman, W. E., and Dorner, J. L.: Creatine phosphokinase: Current concepts and speculation regarding its use in veterinary medicine. J. Am. Anim. Hosp. Assoc. 11:451, 1975.
21. Indrieri, R. J., Holliday, T. A., and Keen C. L.: Critical evaluation of creatine phosphokinase in cerebrospinal fluid of dogs with neurologic disease. Am. J. Vet. Res. 41:1299, 1980.
22. Kjeldsberg, C. R., and Knight, J. A.: *Body Fluids, Laboratory Examination of Cerebrospinal, Synovial, and Serous Fluids: A Textbook Atlas.* American Society of Clinical Pathologists, Chicago, 1982.
23. Kjellin, K. G., and Soderstrom, C. E.: Diagnostic significance of CSF spectrophotometry in cerebrovascular diseases. J. Neurol. Sci. 23:359, 1974.
24. Knecht, C. D.: Clinical neurologic examination of the dog: The spinal cord. Norden News *Winter*:18, 1969.
25. Kölmel, H. W.: *Atlas of Cerebrospinal Fluid Cells.* Springer-Verlag, New York, 1976.
26. Krawowka, S., Fenner, W., and Miele, J. A.: Quantitative determination of serum origin cerebrospinal fluid proteins in the dog. Am. J. Vet. Res. 42:1975, 1981.
27. Krieg, A. F.: Cerebrospinal fluid and other body fluids. *In* Henry, J. B. (ed.): *Clinical Diagnosis and Management by Laboratory Methods,* 16th ed. W. B. Saunders, Philadelphia, 1979, pp. 635–656.

---

*Craniotome 30, Model C-100, 3M Company, Santa Barbara, CA.
†Galt Trefine, J. Sklar Mfg. Co., Long Island, NY.

28. Kronholm, V., and Lintrup, J.: Spectrophotometric investigations of the cerebrospinal fluid in the near-ultraviolet region. Acta Psychiatr. Neur. Scand. *35*:314, 1960.

29. Leonard, J. L. and Redding, R. W.: Effects of hypertonic solutions on cerebrospinal fluid pressure in the lateral ventricle of the dog. Am. J. Vet. Res. *34*:213, 1973.

30. Low, D. G., Osborne, C. A., and Finco, D. R.: The pillars of diagnosis: History and physical examination. *In* Ettinger, S. J. (ed.): *Textbook of Veterinary Internal Medicine*. W. B. Saunders, Philadelphia, 1975, pp. 36–40.

31. Lund, L. O., Beckwitt, H. J., Grover, R. F., and Virtue, R. N.: Effect of urea on circulation and cerebrospinal fluid pressure in the dog. Anesthesiology *26*:45, 1965.

32. Oehmichen, M.: *Cerebrospinal Fluid Cytology, An Introduction and Atlas*. W. B. Saunders, Philadelphia, 1976.

33. Oliver, J. E., Jr.: Localization of lesions in the nervous system. *In* Hoerlein, B. F. (ed.): *Canine Neurology—Diagnosis and Treatment*, 3rd ed. W. B. Saunders, Philadelphia, 1978, pp. 98–100.

34. Parker, A. J.: The diagnostic uses of cerebrospinal fluid. J. Small Anim. Pract. *13*:607, 1972.

35. Ravel, R.: Cerebrospinal fluid examination. *In* Ravel, R. (ed.): *Clinical Laboratory Medicine, Application of Laboratory Data*, 2nd ed. Year Book Medical Publishers, Chicago, 1973, pp. 203–211.

36. Redding, R. W., and Braund, K. G.: Neurological examination. *In* Hoerlein, B. F. (ed.): *Canine Neurology Diagnosis and Treatment*, 3rd ed. W. B. Saunders, Philadelphia, 1978, pp. 53–70.

37. Roszel, J. F.: Membrane filtration of canine and feline cerebrospinal fluid for cytologic evaluation. J. Am. Vet. Med. Assoc. *160*:720, 1972.

38. Schriever, H., and Gambino, S. R.: Protein turbidity produced by trichloroacetic acid and sulfosalicylic acid at varying temperatures and varying ratios of albumin and globulin. Am. J. Clin. Pathol. *44*:667, 1965.

39. Simpson, S. T.: Diseases of the vestibular system. *In* Kirk, R. W. (ed.): *Current Veterinary Therapy VIII*. W. B. Saunders, Philadelphia, 1983, pp. 54–59.

40. Sorjonen, D. C., Warren, J. N., and Schultz, R. D.: Qualitative and quantitative determination of albumin, IgG, IgM and IgA in normal cerebrospinal fluid of dogs. J. Am. Anim. Hosp. Assoc. *17*:833, 1981.

41. Spano, J. S., and Hoerlein, B. F.: Laboratory examinations. *In* Hoerlein, B. F. (ed.): *Canine Neurology—Diagnosis and Treatment*, 3rd ed. W. B. Saunders, Philadelphia, 1978, pp. 138–140.

42. Stockham, S. L., and Franklin, R. T.: Unpublished data, 1983.

43. Swaim, S. F., Vandevelde, M., and Faircloth, J. C.: Evaluation of brain biopsy techniques in the dog. J. Am. Anim. Hosp. Assoc. *15*:627, 1979.

44. Swallow, J. S., and Griffiths, I. R.: Age-related changes in the motor nerve conduction velocity in dogs. Res. Vet. Sci. *23*:29, 1977.

45. Van Der Muelen, J. P.: Cerebrospinal fluid xanthochromia: an objective index. Neurology *16*:170, 1966.

46. Verdura, J., White, R. J., and Albin, M.: Chronic measurements of cerebrospinal fluid pressure in the dog. J. Neurosurg. *21*:1047, 1964.

47. Walker, T. L., Redding, R. W., and Braund, K. G.: Motor nerve conduction velocity and latency in the dog. Am. J. Vet. Res. *40*:1433, 1979.

48. Wilson, J. W.: Canine cerebrospinal fluid: Normal composition. Minn. Vet. *16*:25, 1976.

49. Wilson, J. W.: Clinical application of cerebrospinal fluid creatine phosphokinase determination. J. Am. Vet. Med. Assoc. *171*:200, 1977.

50. Wilson, J. W.: Cerebrospinal fluid analysis. *In* Kirk, R. W. (ed.): *Current Veterinary Therapy VII*. W. B. Saunders, Philadelphia, 1980, pp. 769–773.

51. Wilson, J. W., and Stevens, J. B.: Effects of blood contamination on cerebrospinal fluid analysis. J. Am. Vet. Med. Assoc. *171*:256, 1977.

52. Withrow, S. J.: Localization and diagnosis of spinal cord lesions in small animals (part I). Comp. Cont. Ed. *2*:473, 1980.

53. Wright, J. A.: Evaluation of cerebrospinal fluid in the dog. Vet. Rec. *103*:48, 1978.

Chapter **92**

Electrodiagnostic Methods

R. W. Redding and S. T. Simpson

Since orthopedic and soft tissue trauma is associated with some concomitant injury or compression of nervous tissue structures, evaluation of the functional status of nerve tissue aids in the diagnosis and prognosis of the condition.

Electromyography, electroencephalography, cystometrography, and evaluation of motor and sensory nerve conduction, H and F wave reflexes, spinal and brain stem–evoked responses, and somatosensory responses may be used to assess neurological damage. The following discussion of these techniques is limited to those most applicable to the field of surgery. Metabolic, toxicological, and infectious diseases have been omitted or limited for differential diagnostic purposes. The reader is referred to other textbooks on the specific subjects for further details.

ELECTROMYOGRAPHY[4, 7, 34]

Electromyography (EMG) is the recording and interpretation of characteristic patterns of electrical activity of striated muscle. Pathological processes that may be detected using electromyography include (1) peripheral nerve injury, (2) ventral nerve root injury, (3) plexus injury, (4) myoneural junction disease, (5) muscle fiber disease, and (6) ventral horn cell disease.

Electromyograms record motor unit and individual skeletal muscle fiber activity by means of an electrode inserted into the muscle to be evaluated. The electrical activity is characterized by the presence or absence of wave forms at rest and during voluntary effort. The wave forms are evaluated for configuration and intensity. The electromyograph consists of an

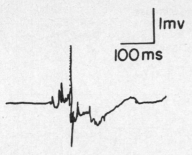

Figure 92–1. Normal insertion potentials. Note the cessation of electrical activity when the needle is not moved.

electrode system, amplifier with filters, cathode ray oscilloscope, and audio system for listening to the sounds produced by the muscle.

Normal EMG

Electromyographic activity consists of insertion potentials, rare spontaneous waves, and motor unit potentials. Insertional activity is brief bursts of electrical activity that do not continue for more than a fraction of a second after cessation of the needle movement (Fig. 92–1). The electrical potentials seen and heard on the EMG are induced by mechanical stimulation, injury to muscle fibers, and activation of intrafascicular nerve branches by the needle electrode. Movement of the electrode induces another burst of activity of short duration. The potentials associated with needle insertion have amplitudes of from 50 to 10,000 microvolts (μV) and durations between 1 and 20 milliseconds (msec). Large positive waves may be seen.

Spontaneous activity, with the exception of end-plate noise, should not be seen in normal skeletal muscle. Occasionally the electromyogram of normal muscle reveals a low-amplitude (10 to 50 μV), 0.5- to 2.0-msec activity when the electrode is very near an end-plate region. The auditory component is a soft rushing noise. It is important not to confuse this end-plate noise with fibrillation potentials, which are abnormal.

Motor unit potentials are seen in voluntary muscle contraction and when a motor nerve is stimulated (evoked potentials) and are called "M" responses or potentials; a normal muscle at rest is electrically silent. The M response is the summation of individual muscle fiber activity belonging to a motor unit within the recording range of the electrode. Motor units are characterized by voltages of from 200 μV to 1.5 mVolts and a duration of 2.0 to 10.0 msec with two to three phases.

Abnormal Electromyographic Activity

Insertional Activity

When a needle electrode is inserted into a muscle and prolonged discharges are seen and heard, hyper-

excitability of the muscle fibers is present and is considered abnormal. This response is most prominent 6 to 10 days following severe peripheral nerve injury. After this time it decreases, and after 20 days it can no longer be recorded.[2]

Fibrillation Potentials

Fibrillation potentials are spontaneous, repetitive action potentials of a single or a few muscle fibers not elicited by nerve impulses. These abnormal potentials are a result of instability of the muscle cell membrane potential in the end-plate region following denervation (Fig. 92–2). The time of appearance of fibrillation potentials after denervation depends on the species and size of the animal. Small rodents show fibrillation potentials as early as two to three days post denervation, whereas dogs and cats have an onset of five to seven days post denervation.[10] After onset, fibrillation increases for several weeks and then decreases until the muscle fibers have undergone atrophy. If re-innervation of the muscle occurs, the fibrillation potentials decrease in number about two weeks before motor unit potentials can be recorded.[2] Fibrillation potentials are characterized by monophasic or biphasic wave forms that have a duration of 0.5 to 5.0 msec (average 1 to 2 msec) with an amplitude of 50 to 300 μV. The sound associated

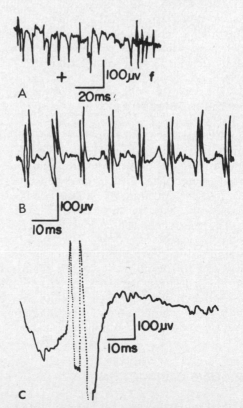

Figure 92–2. *A*, Fibrillation potentials (*f*) and positive sharp waves (+) suggest recent denervation. *B*, Myopathic potentials consisting of two-tone musical tone of continuous nature. *C*, Giant, polyphasic motor unit potential suggests re-innervation.

with fibrillation potentials has been described as similar to that made by crackling cellophane, frying eggs, or rain on a tin roof.

Positive Sharp Waves (Positive Potentials)

Positive sharp waves are frequently associated with denervation and occasionally with myopathic diseases. These are slower waves than fibrillation potentials. They show an initial potential change in the positive direction followed by a slower negative component (see Fig. 92–2).[6] The duration of a wave may be 10 msec or longer, with a variable amplitude of from 100 μV to 4 mV. The frequency of discharge is usually consistent in an area of muscle, usually 5 to 20 Hertz (Hz). The sound varies depending on the frequency. Sounds similar to musical tones, an idling motor boat, and a continuous dive bomber roar may be heard.

Myopathic Potentials

Myopathic potentials are less consistent than the waves usually observed with denervation. In general, myopathic wave forms consist of continuous tones that may vary in pitch (dive bomber sound). There may be more than one sound (see Fig. 92–2). With inflammatory muscle disease there may be nerve involvement, which would give rise to fibrillation potentials and positive sharp waves. There are many other myopathic potentials related to nonsurgical muscle disease. The reader is referred to an electromyography text for further information.[12]

Re-innervation Potentials

Re-innervation of a denervated muscle produces motor unit potentials that tend to be polyphasic (i.e., five or more phases) and of low amplitude initially, then later greater than normal (giant potentials) (see Fig. 92–2). The appearance of these potentials is a good prognostic sign in the recovery from nerve trauma. The shorter the time period following injury, the better the prognosis.

The surgeon will find electromyography an aid in diagnosis and prognosis in suspected traumatic peripheral nerve lesions, herniated intervertebral disc disease, and avulsion of nerve root lesions. EMG combined with motor and sensory determinations and H and F reflexes is also helpful.

MOTOR NERVE CONDUCTION[1, 20, 34]

Peripheral motor nerves conduct impulses to skeletal muscle. This important function may be reduced or abolished by disease. Therefore, a working knowledge of nerve conduction is important in diagnosis

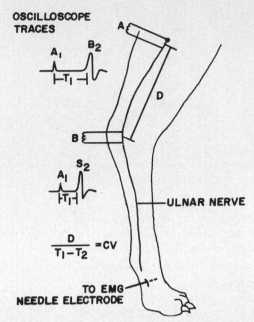

Figure 92–3. Technique and waveforms for recording motor nerve conduction velocity. (Reprinted with permission from Steinberg, H. S.: A review of electromyographic and motor nerve conduction velocity techniques. J. Am. Anim. Hosp. *15*:613, 1979.)

and prognosis. The surgeon is frequently confronted with a traumatic disorder in which peripheral motor nerves may be damaged. Calculation of the conduction velocity and comparison with normal data indicate the functional status of the nerves evaluated. Motor nerve conduction studies aid the surgeon in his surgical procedure, advice to the client, and prognosis.

Motor nerve conduction studies can be undertaken using a standard electromyograph with a nerve stimulator connected to the recorder. Most commonly a recording needle is inserted into the muscle being examined. The motor nerve of the muscle is stimulated with a supramaximal stimulus at two points along its course. Measurements are taken of the time (latency) between stimulus onset and the evoked skeletal muscle potential (M response). The two latencies are used to calculate the time between the two stimulating points. This is divided into the distance the nerve impulses travelled, resulting in a conduction velocity in meters per second (Fig. 92–3).

Evaluation of the wave form, amplitude, and duration of the M response gives information relative to the status of the muscle itself and the function of the motor nerve. Normal data for each nerve and muscle of the dog are available for comparison.[1, 3, 20] Motor nerve conduction velocities are altered by a combination of nonpathogenic metabolism, age, and temperature variations.[32, 35] In patients in which a nerve has been severed or severely traumatized, an M response cannot be elicited when the stimulus is applied above the injury site.

Reduced conduction velocity or reduced amplitude of the M response indicates peripheral nerve damage or a pathological process characterized by segmental

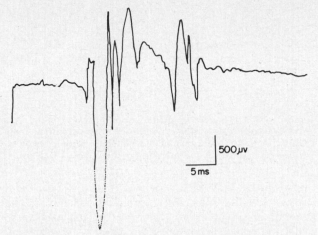

Figure 92–4. Polyphasic evoked motor unit potential from a dog with segmental demyelination.

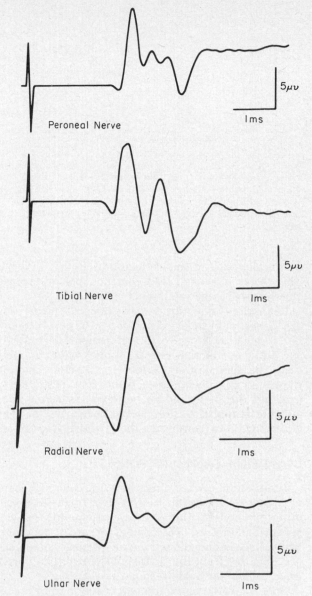

Figure 92–5. Sensory nerve conduction potentials from various nerves of the dog.

demyelination. Figure 92–4 demonstrates a polyphasic evoked motor unit potential from a dog with generalized peripheral demyelination.

Re-innervation following nerve repair can be evaluated by electromyography, evoked M response, and nerve conduction velocity determination.

SENSORY NERVE CONDUCTION

Sensory nerve conduction studies consist of stimulating a cutaneous nerve field and recording the afferent impulses as they pass a recording site along the course of the nerve. Sensory nerve conduction studies probably have less value than motor nerve studies for orthopedic surgeons; however, such studies may be indicated in special cases.

The amplitude of the evoked sensory nerve impulse is very small, and special averaging equipment is required to accurately measure the nerve impulse to calculate the conduction velocity. Some electromyographs have an averaging computer connected to the recording system to evaluate sensory nerves.

Reference values for sensory nerve conduction velocities of the dog and cat have been published[14, 29] (Fig. 92–5).

H WAVE REFLEX

The H wave is a compound muscle action potential that results from activation of a monosynaptic reflex. The reflex results from orthodromic conduction of afferent sensory impulses from the site of nerve stimulation to the spinal cord, where alpha motor neurons are activated.

Since H wave reflex determination involves afferent, central connections and efferent pathways, it is of value in determining the functional status of the spinal cord segment as well as the dorsal and ventral roots and mixed peripheral nerve. The surgeon may

be interested in spinal cord radicular and peripheral nerve function in certain cases.

H waves can be recorded using standard electromyographic equipment. Special techniques and skill are required to record this wave form. Reference values for H wave reflexes have been published for the dog[17, 33] (Fig. 92–6).

F WAVE REFLEX

The F wave is a compound muscle action potential that has a longer latency than the M wave and a slightly shorter latency than the H wave. It is considered to be due to antidromically conducted motor nerve action potentials, which are initiated peripherally at the stimulus electrode. The impulse proceeds up the motor neuron and then passes ortho-

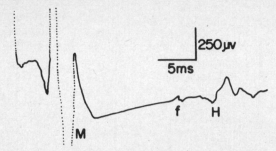

Figure 92–6. Evoked potentials from the dog demonstrating the motor unit potential (M), H wave reflex (H), and the F wave (f). (Reprinted with permission from Knecht, C. D., and Redding, R. W.: Stimulating techniques and response characteristics of the M and F waves and H reflex in dogs. Vet. Res. Commun. 6:123, 1983.)

dromically back to the skeletal muscle.[11, 36, 38] The F wave can be evoked and recorded using standard electromyographic equipment (see Fig. 92–6).

Reference values for F wave latencies of the dog have been published.[18] The surgeon probably would not request an F wave determination, since EMG and nerve conduction velocity studies would, in most cases, be sufficient. F wave determinations may be requested in special cases when it is desirable to evaluate the motor nerve between the spinal cord and the stimulation site. Nerve root avulsions may be evaluated by combining the H and F wave tests.

BRAIN STEM–EVOKED RESPONSES

Brain stem–evoked responses are computer-averaged signals recorded from various brain stem synaptic junctions in the auditory, visual, and somatosensory pathways. The potentials are exceedingly small, in the nanovolt and microvolt range; since they are recorded from the surface of the scalp, they have been called "far field" responses.[5, 9, 21]

Special averaging equipment is required to record these small potentials. Some electromyographic equipment can be combined with an averaging system to record such data.

There are occasions when a surgeon may be interested in the functional status of the brain stem, and such tests would prove valuable for diagnostic and prognostic purposes. Atlantoaxial luxations and cervical and head trauma cases may benefit from such tests.

AUDITORY EVOKED RESPONSES[5, 37]

Auditory evoked responses are the most complex of the brain stem responses and probably the most useful in the location of brain stem lesions, since more synaptic junctions and anatomical areas are involved.

To average auditory evoked potentials with a computer, an auditory stimulus consisting of a click sound lasting 1 or 2 msec with an amplitude of 65 to 75 decibels is delivered to each ear of the patient at the

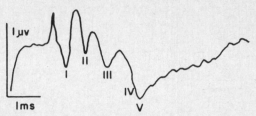

Figure 92–7. The brain stem auditory evoked response in the dog. Negative polarity is upward. (Reprinted with permission from Whidden, S. J.: Evaluation of the far field averaged auditory evoked responses in the canine. Dissertation, Auburn University, 1979.)

onset of each averaging period. In auditory evoked responses the averaging period is 10 msec. The stimuli are given every 100 msec, or 10 clicks/sec, so that the responses do not interact with one other.

The recordings are made by placing one electrode over the auditory cortex and the other over the vertex of the skull. The electrodes are connected to the input of the amplifier with a high gain, and the output of the amplifier is connected to the input of the computer and usually to a monitoring oscilloscope as well. To record an averaged response to be stored in the memory of the computer, 256 to 512 stimuli are sufficient. The memory is then displayed on the oscilloscope, and a permanent record is made for analysis.

A sequence of five to six component waves can be recorded in the dog, cat, and horse (humans usually have seven waves), all of which occur in 10 msec. The waves are believed to be generated by: I, cochlea and acoustic nerve; II, cochlear nuclei; III, dorsal nucleus of the trapezoid body; IV and V, caudal colliculus area; VI, medial geniculate and auditory radiation; and VII, seen in man in the auditory cortex. See Figure 92–7 for canine responses.[37]

A lesion in one of these structures produces an abnormality of the response starting at the component, which represents excitation of that structure. The latency and amplitude of the component waves are increased and reduced, respectively.

The location of a suspected lesion in the brain stem may be determined using auditory evoked recordings. In addition, evoked potentials are used to evaluate hearing in animals (electrical response audiometry)

VISUAL EVOKED RESPONSES

Visual stimulation excites retinal pathways and initiates impulses that are conducted through the brain stem to the primary visual cortex. Through these pathways, a visual stimulus to the eyes can be recorded over the occipital regions. Four or five wave forms can be recorded from the dog and cat over a time period of 300 msec. The first wave is a volume-conducted electroretinogram (ERG) and optic nerve potentials. The remaining three or four waves are visual pathways: optic tract, lateral geniculate, and optic radiation, or visual cortex.[27]

A flash response is elicited by delivering a bright

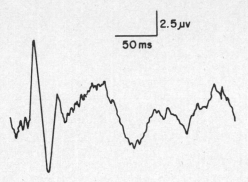

Figure 92–8. Visual cortical evoked response in the dog.

flash of diffused light (one to three cycles per second [cps]) at a distance of 40 to 60 cm from the patient's eyes. This produces a series of potential changes as described previously. As in auditory evoked responses, it is necessary to use an averaging computer system to delineate the wave forms.

A visual evoked response (Fig. 92–8) is more difficult to record in the dog and cat than auditory evoked responses. Because of the anatomy of the cortical visual system, two types of abnormalities may be distinguished: (1) prechiasmal defects and (2) postchiasmal defects.[27] Very little work has been reported on visual evoked responses in animals. Future investigation may develop reference data, which will be useful in the diagnosis of brain stem lesions.

SOMATOSENSORY EVOKED RESPONSES

Somatosensory evoked responses are measurements of the conduction of impulses through the somatosensory system. Electrical stimuli are applied to the radial or ulnar nerve at rates of up to 10 Hz. Recordings are made over the cervical vertebrae (very difficult), cysterna magna, and sensory cortex.

Many hundreds to thousands of stimuli must be computer averaged to record potentials. There is little agreement as to the latency, shape, and origin of the individual components recorded.[19, 23, 24] Additional investigations are necessary regarding recording techniques, methods of restraint, and interpretation before somatosensory evoked responses are useful in veterinary medicine. Conceivably this technique would be of value to the surgeon diagnosing cervical cord disease.

SPINAL EVOKED POTENTIALS[15]

These potentials can be recorded with computer-averaging systems by inserting one needle electrode against a vertebral body or interarcuate space and a reference electrode over the vertebra. Stimulation of the tibial nerve in the hind limb or the ulnar nerve of the forelimb allows recording of potentials at various spinal cord levels. The potentials are compound action potentials of all sensory afferents ascending in the spinal pathways. When the potentials are recorded near the stimulus sites the compound action potential is diphasic or triphasic. As it is recorded more cephalad, individual components with different conduction velocities can be distinguished by their different latencies, producing compound action potentials that become polyphasic and of longer duration. To record spinal evoked potentials in the dog and cat, 128 to 512 stimuli are sufficient.

This technique holds promise for the surgeon, because it can evaluate any area of the spinal sensory pathways. The blockage of impulses beyond a certain vertebra can locate a lesion definitively. The conduction velocity of the pathways can be calculated by dividing the distance between the recording points by the difference in onset or peak recorded at specific points. The spinal evoked potential may be of use in spinal trauma patients or surgery patients to establish a more accurate prognosis. The normal conduction

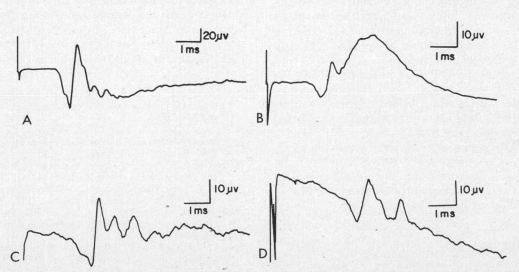

Figure 92–9. Spinal evoked potentials in the cat. The stimulus is applied to the tibial nerve. Recordings are made from A, L7; B, L5; C, L2; and D, T13.

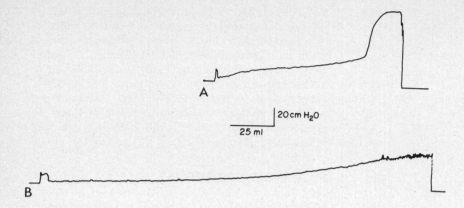

Figure 92–10. Canine cystometrograms. *A,* From a normal dog. *B,* From a dog with a lumbosacral cord disease. (Courtesy of Dr. John E. Oliver, Jr.)

velocity for cats and dogs is 55 to 100 m/sec (Fig. 92–9).[15, 28, 31]

ELECTROENCEPHALOGRAPHY[13, 16, 25, 26, 30]

The electroencephalogram (EEG) is a graphic recording of the electrical activity of the cerebral cortex obtained by means of electrodes attached to the scalp of an animal. This electrical activity varies depending on the age of the animal, the state of awareness from very alert to deep sleep, the presence or absence of external stimuli, and the influence of drugs on the nervous system.

The electrical potentials recorded are highly complex when compared with all other potentials discussed in this chapter. The frequency varies from 1 to 50 Hz, with amplitudes of 5 to 200 μV. These frequencies and amplitudes may be superimposed on each other or may occur in paroxysms. Certain states of awareness may be characterized by dominant activity and amplitudes. Likewise, the age of the animal has a marked effect on frequency and amplitude characteristics.

The EEG is recorded using an electroencephalograph containing eight or more channels, each composed of amplifiers, filters, and direct writing units. It is necessary to simultaneously record different areas of the cerebral cortex to localize abnormal activity in a particular cortical area.

The electroencephalogram is primarily used in the diagnosis of cerebral diseases such as hydrocephalus, epilepsy, the various encephalidites, toxicosis, posttraumatic cases, focal mass lesions, brain edema, and metabolic encephalopathies.

Although the neurologist frequently uses the EEG, a surgeon occasionally uses it to evaluate the brain following skull fractures and during postoperative recovery. The EEG frequently indicates the rate of recovery following brain trauma.[8]

CYSTOMETROGRAPHY[22]

Although the cystometrogram is not a direct recording of the electrical activity of the reflex involved in bladder contraction, it is a direct recording of bladder function and is included in this chapter for reference purposes. The cystometrogram is useful in detecting the location of a neurological deficit in a patient with urinary disabilities.

It is a recording of the pressure changes in the urinary bladder and the reflex response (micturation reflex) that occurs when a certain intraluminal volume and pressure are attained. Since the reflex centers are in the lumbosacral segments of the spinal cord, surgeons may be interested in the evaluation of this region following trauma to the pelvic area. If these reflex centers are severely damaged, the prognosis is poor. Even though the body structure may be successfully repaired, the patient may not be a desirable household pet because of urinary or fecal incontinence.

The cystometrograph uses a pressure transducer attached to a urinary catheter inserted into the bladder. The pressure and flow rate of gas or fluid into the bladder are regulated so that a reflex response occurs in a normal manner. If the animal responds normally it is assumed that the reflex center and the spinal afferent and efferent pathways are intact. No response seen at threshold volume indicates a malfunction of the reflex center in the lumbosacral spinal segments. An unsustained reflex suggests a disturbance within spinal afferent or efferent systems that are involved with the micturition response. Figure 92–10 illustrates normal and abnormal responses.

1. Bowen, J. M.: Electromyographic analysis of evoked potentials of canine muscle motor points. J. Am. Vet. Med. Assoc. *164:*509, 1974.
2. Bowen, J. M.: Quantitative EMG analysis of the time course of denervation in the canine pectineus muscle. Arch. Phys. Med. Rehabil. 58:339, 1977.
3. Bowen, J. M.: Peripheral nerve electrodiagnostics, electromyography, and nerve conduction velocity. *In:* Hoerlein, B. F. (ed.): *Canine Neurology: Diagnosis and Treatment,* 3rd ed. W. B. Saunders, Philadelphia, 1978.
4. Brown, N. O., and Zaki, F. A.: Electrodiagnostic testing for evaluation of neuromuscular disorders in dogs and cats. J. Am. Vet. Med. Assoc. *174:*86, 1979.
5. Buchwald, J. S., and Huang, C.: Far field acoustic response: Origins in the cat. Science *189:*382, 1975.
6. Chrisman, C. L.: Special ancillary investigations. *In: Problems in Small Animal Neurology.* Lea and Febiger, Philadelphia, 1982.

7. Chrisman, C. L., Burt, J. K., Wood, E. T., and Johnson, E. W.: Electromyography in small animal clinical neurology. J. Am. Vet. Med. Assoc. 160:311, 1972.
8. Croft, P. G.: Electroencephalography in canine head injury. J. Small Anim. Prac. 11:473, 1970.
9. Davis, H.: Principles of electric response audiometry. Ann. Otol. Rhinol. Laryngol. 85(Suppl.):3, 1976.
10. Feinstein, B., Pattle, R. E., and Weddell, G.: Metabolic factors affecting fibrillation in denervated muscle. J. Neurol. Neurosurg. Psychiatry 8:1, 1945.
11. Gassel, M. M., and Wiesendanger, M.: Recurrent and reflex discharges in plantar muscles of the cat. Acta Physiol. Scand. 65:138, 1965.
12. Goodgold, J., and Eberstein, A.: *Electrodiagnosis of Neuromuscular Diseases*. Williams and Wilkins, Baltimore, 1972.
13. Herin, R. A., Puriton, P. T., and Fletcher, T. F.: Electroencephalography in the unanesthetized dog. Am. J. Vet. Res. 29:329, 1968.
14. Holliday, T. A., Ealand, B. G., and Weldon, N. E.: Sensory nerve conduction velocity. Technical requirements and normal values for branches of the radial and ulnar nerves of the dog. Am. J. Vet. Res. 42:975, 1981.
15. Holliday, T. A., Weldon, N. E., and Ealand, B. G.: Percutaneous recording of evoked spinal cord potentials of dogs. Am. J. Vet. Res. 40:326, 1979.
16. Klemm, W. R.: Subjective and quantitative analysis of the electroencephalogram of anesthetized normal dogs: Control data for clinical diagnosis. Am. J. Vet. Res. 29:1267, 1968.
17. Knecht, C. D., and Redding, R. W.: Monosynaptic reflex (H wave) in clinically normal and abnormal dogs. Am. J. Vet. Res. 42:1586, 1981.
18. Knecht, C. D., and Redding, R. W.: Stimulating techniques and response characteristics of the M and F waves and H reflex in dogs. Vet. Res. Commun. 6:123, 1983.
19. Kornegay, J. N., Marshall, A. E., Purinton, P. T., and Oliver, J. E.: Somatosensory evoked potential in clinically normal dogs. Am. J. Vet. Res. 42:70, 1981.
20. Lee, A. F., and Bowen, J. M.: Evaluation of motor nerve conduction velocity in the dog. Am. J. Vet Res. 31:1361, 1970.
21. Marshall, A. E., Byars, T. D., Whitlock, R. H., and George, L. W.: Brainstem auditory evoked response in the diagnosis of inner ear injury in the horse. J. Am. Vet. Med. Assoc. 178:282, 1981.
22. Oliver, J. E., Jr., and Young, W. O.: Air cystometry in dogs under xylazine-induced restraint. Am. J. Vet. Res. 34:1433, 1973.
23. Parker, A. J.: Comparison of the averaged evoked cisterna cerebellomedullaris potential, cortical potential, and neurologic examination in the diagnosis of spinal cord injury of the dog. Am. J. Vet. Res. 39:1816, 1978.
24. Parker, A. J., Marshall, A. E., and Sharp, J. G.: Study of the use of evoked cortical activity for clinical evaluation of spinal cord sensory transmission. Am. J. Vet. Res. 35:673, 1974.
25. Prynn, R. B., and Redding, R. W.: Electroencephalographic continuum in dogs anesthetized with methoxyflurane and halothane. Am. J. Vet. Res. 29:1913, 1968.
26. Redding, R. W.: Canine electroencephalography. *In* Hoerlein, B. F. (ed.): *Canine Neurology: Diagnosis and Treatment*, 3rd ed. W. B. Saunders, Philadelphia, 1978.
27. Redding, R. W.: Visual evoked responses in the canine. Unpublished data.
28. Redding, R. W.: Spinal evoked responses in the cat. Unpublished data.
29. Redding, R. W., Ingram, J. T., and Colter, S. B.: Sensory nerve conduction velocity of cutaneous afferents of the radial ulner, peroneal, and tibial nerves of the dog: Reference values. Am. J. Vet. Res. 43:517, 1982.
30. Redding, R. W., and Knecht, C. D.: *An EEG Atlas of the Dog and Cat*. Praeger Scientific, Philadelphia, in press.
31. Sarnowski, R. J., Cracco, R. Q., Vogel, H. B., and Mount, F.: Spinal evoked response in the cat. J. Neurosurg. 43:329, 1975.
32. Sims, M. H., and Redding, R. W.: Maturation of nerve conduction velocity and the evoked muscle potential in the dog. Am. J. Vet. Res. 41:1247, 1980.
33. Sims, M. H., and Selcer, R. R.: Occurrence and evaluation of a reflex-evoked muscle potential (H reflex) in the normal dog. Am. J. Vet. Res. 42:975, 1981.
34. Steinberg, H. S.: A review of electromyographic and motor nerve conduction velocity techniques. J. Am. Anim. Hosp. 15:613, 1979.
35. Swallow, J. S., and Griffith, I. R.: Age related change in the motor nerve conduction velocity in dogs. Res. Vet. Sci. 23:29, 1977.
36. Thorne, J.: Central responses to electrical activation of the peripheral nerves supplying the intrinsic hand muscles. J. Neurol. Neurosurg. Psychiatry 28:482, 1965.
37. Whidden, S. J.: Evaluation of far field averaged auditory evoked responses in the canine. Dissertation, Auburn University, 1979.
38. Yates, S. K.: Characteristics of the F response: A single motor unit study. J. Neurol. Neurosurg. Psychiatry 42:161, 1979.

Chapter **93** # Neuroradiology

William R. Brawner, Robert D. Pechman, and Jan E. Bartels

SKULL AND BRAIN

Radiographic Technique and Patient Positioning

Diagnostic radiographs of the skull require precise patient positioning and excellent radiographic technique. High-contrast radiographs, made with high-mAs and low-kVp techniques, aid in detecting osseous abnormalities. Low-mAs techniques may be occasionally helpful for soft tissues surrounding the skull. Radiographic detail is enhanced by using non-screen x-ray film or x-ray cassettes with slow-intensifying screens. A grid is used to reduce the image-degrading scatter radiation reaching the x-ray film.

Radiographs of the skull are made with the patient heavily sedated or under general anesthesia. Patient positioning is facilitated by sedation or general anesthesia, so the long exposure times necessary for high MAS techniques can be achieved without patient movement. Chemical restraint may be contraindicated in some patients that require skull radiographs,

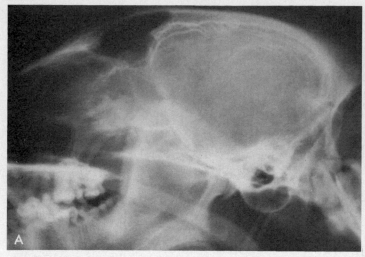

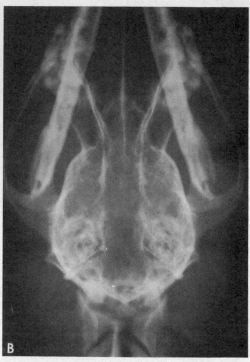

Figure 93–1. Lateral (A) and ventrodorsal (B) radiographs of the dog skull. The bilateral symmetry to the calvarium is clearly demonstrated on the ventrodorsal view. Structures on one side of the skull can be compared with those on the other side to evaluate abnormalities. Positioning is ideal on the lateral view, with superimposition of the two sides of the calvarium.

most notably after trauma. The safety of the patient should not be compromised to obtain skull radiographs. A number of references describe positioning for skull radiography.[26,29,35]

Radiographic examination of the skull includes at least a lateral view and a ventrodorsal or dorsoventral view (Fig. 93–1). The ventrodorsal projection is more difficult to position than the dorsoventral projection but is preferred because there is less distortion of the cranial vault.[2] The dorsoventral projection is easier to position, because the mandibular shafts can be used as supports on which the skull can rest for symmetrical positioning. In either projection, precise positioning achieves the bilateral symmetry that aids interpretation of skull radiographs.

Exact positioning of the skull for the lateral view is just as important as for the ventrodorsal or dorsoventral projection and is more difficult. The necessary time and care must be taken to achieve a precise lateral view with superimposition of the opposing sides of the skull. Oblique lateral views make interpretation considerably more difficult and predispose to errors in interpretation.

Additional radiographic views can be made to evaluate specific regions of the skull. Oblique projections may be helpful to outline clinically apparent masses and to assess the extent of bony involvement beneath the mass. The skull is positioned with the area of interest tangential to the x-ray beam and the exposure is made. Oblique views must be properly identified to avoid confusion in interpretation. Frontal views of the skull are helpful in assessing the foramen magnum and the dorsal and lateral walls of the cranial vault. Frontal views are especially helpful in patients with suspected cranial fractures.

Radiographic Anatomy of the Skull

The skull is bilaterally symmetrical, greatly aiding interpretation of skull radiographs. Structures on one side of the skull may be compared with their counterparts on the other side. However, comparative evaluation is not adequate for accurate interpretation of skull radiographs. A thorough knowledge of the radiographic anatomy of the skull is required.[33]

The brain is surrounded by the bones of the cranium and is normally invisible on skull radiographs. The convoluted surface of the brain is reflected by bony ridges on the inner surface of the cranial vault. These ridges are variable among breeds of dogs, but departure from the expected normal may indicate intracranial disease.

Indications for Skull Radiographs

The most common indications for skull radiographs are trauma and seizure disorders. Radiographs of the skull are also indicated in patients with clinical signs of middle or inner ear disease or with palpable masses associated with the calvarium. Sudden changes in temperament or neurologic signs suggesting a central neurologic lesion may also indicate a need for skull radiographs.

Radiographs are always indicated in patients with trauma to the skull. Fractures of the skull are not uncommon and must be searched for carefully. The majority of skull fractures appear as thin, radiolucent lines disrupting the normally continuous surface of the calvarium (Fig. 93–2). Displacement of the fracture segments is usually minimal, although in some

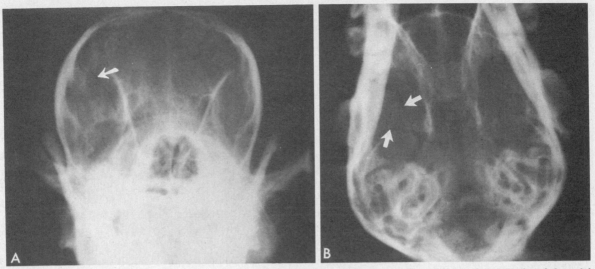

Figure 93–2. Frontal view (A) and ventrodorsal view (B) of the skull of a dog with fractures of the right parietal and frontal bones (*arrows*). Note the minimal displacement of the fractures. These fractures should not be misinterpreted as cranial suture lines.

cases there is great displacement and the fractures are obvious (Fig. 93–3). Skull fractures are seen best when the x-ray beam is perpendicular to the fracture line; multiple views of the skull may be required to detect fractures of the calvarium. Frontal projections are especially helpful in detecting fractures involving the frontal or occipital bones and in determining whether fractures of the temporal or parietal bones are depressed into the cranial vault.

Differentiation of skull fractures from normal cranial sutures is vital in young patients with cranial trauma. Thorough knowledge of the location and appearance of normal cranial sutures is important in making this decision. Fortunately, most skull fractures do not follow the course of the suture lines, but care must be exercised to avoid misinterpretation.

Traumatic injury of the brain cannot be detected on routine radiographs. Intracranial hemorrhage, subdural hematoma, or contusion of the brain may occur following skull trauma. Profound neurological disease in the absence of skull fractures may suggest such injuries, but diagnosis must be made by techniques other than radiography.

Patients with seizure disorders rarely have abnormal skull radiographs. Radiographs are indicated, however, because occasionally an abnormality is found that suggests a cause of the seizures. Neoplastic or inflammatory disease of structures surrounding the brain, such as neoplasia or infection of the nasal passages or frontal sinuses or osseous neoplasia of the calvarium, may cause seizures in some patients (Fig. 93–4). Occipital dysplasia and open fontanelles have been detected in patients with seizures due to hydrocephalus.[30] Occipital dysplasia, however, is also seen in clinically normal toy dogs and may be normal.

Disorders of the brain parenchyma responsible for seizures are not usually detected on routine radiographs of the skull. Idiopathic epilepsy, encephalitis, metastatic tumors, and hereditary or congenital

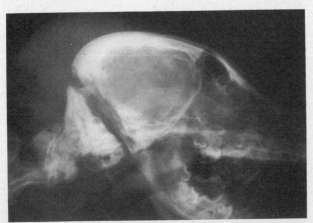

Figure 93–3. A lateral radiograph of the skull of a dog with fractures of the occipital and temporal bones. Fracture displacement is great, and diagnosis is straightforward.

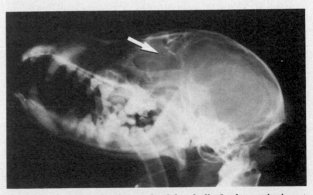

Figure 93–4. A lateral radiograph of the skull of a dog with chronic nasal discharge and convulsions. The dorsal portion of the ethmoid bone is not visible (*arrow*). (Compare with Figure 93–1A.) Nasal adenocarcinoma had eroded through the ethmoid bone, invaded the cerebral tissue, and caused the convulsions.

anomalies of the brain, which may cause seizures, do not cause abnormalities on survey radiographs. Brain neoplasia is usually not seen on routine radiographs. Hydrocephalus affects the cerebral ventricular and aqueduct system and may cause seizures. Because the cerebrospinal fluid in the enlarged ventricles and the brain parenchyma are equal in radiographic density, the enlarged ventricles are not visible radiographically. In some severe cases of hydrocephalus, there may be thinning of the bones of the calvarium or effacement of the normal gyral ridges on the inner surface of the cranial vault. These radiographic changes strongly suggest hydrocephalus but are not diagnostic for the disease.

Skull radiographs of patients with inner or middle ear disease may indicate the extent of involvement of the osseous bullae and petrous temporal bones in the disease process. Changes in density or margination of the petrous temporal bone can be detected in some chronic infections. Thickening of the osseous bulla is common in chronic otitis media. Occasionally, fluid may be detected within the osseous bulla, requiring surgical intervention.[8] Soft tissue or osseous neoplasia may cause erosion of the petrous temporal bone or bony proliferation along the margins of the bone.[32]

Neoplastic, degenerative, metabolic, or inflammatory diseases of the brain may produce changes in temperament or other clinical signs indicating a central neurological lesion. In rare cases the diseased areas of the brain may become mineralized and therefore visible radiographically.[17] Skull radiographs are indicated in patients with central neurological lesions, but only rarely is an abnormality related to the underlying disease found.

Special Radiographic Techniques

Since most brain diseases responsible for clinical signs cannot be detected on survey radiographs, other radiographic procedures may be required. A number of radiographic contrast studies can be performed to delineate diseased areas of the brain. The most common contrast procedures are cerebral arteriography, cavernous sinus venography, and ventriculography. Cerebral scintigraphy and computed axial tomography may also be helpful. Radiographic contrast studies are discussed briefly in this section; alternative imaging methods are described later in the chapter.

Cerebral Arteriography

Cerebral arteriography requires injection of radiopaque contrast material into an artery supplying blood to the brain. The arterial blood supply is opacified and can be examined for displacement or other abnormalities. Changes in the pattern of arterial supply to the brain may indicate masses within the brain or abnormal arteriovenous communications.

The venous drainage from the brain can be assessed on radiographs made late in the study.

Arterial catheters may be inserted into the internal carotid artery through a surgical approach to the common carotid artery. An alternative method is the transfemoral approach to the internal carotid or vertebral arteries, by which the arterial catheter is inserted into the femoral artery and advanced up the aorta and into the desired artery supplying the brain. This latter technique is preferred by some because of the available access to both vertebral and both internal carotid arteries with a single arterial puncture. Expensive and sophisticated radiographic equipment is required for cerebral arteriography, restricting its use to large teaching institutions.[2,9]

Interpretation of cerebral arteriograms is difficult and frequently frustrating (Fig. 93–5). Tremendous breed variation in the size and shape of the calvarium makes precise determination of normal arterial position difficult. Subtraction techniques can help in visualizing the cerebral vasculature, but small changes in arterial position, indicating displacement by a mass, are easily missed. Large parenchymal masses and highly vascular masses can usually be detected. Masses that are smaller or have poor blood supply are usually not detectable.

Cavernous Sinus Venography

This contrast procedure requires injection of radiopaque contrast medium into a vein that drains into the cavernous sinus. The angularis occuli veins are easily accessible and may be used. These are superficial veins located rostral to the orbit. Cannulation of the veins bilaterally and simultaneous injection of contrast medium into both veins provides good opacification of the entire cavernous sinus.

Cavernous sinus venography may be helpful in detecting masses involving the optic chiasm, pituitary gland, and brain stem. A firm command of the complex anatomy of the cavernous sinus is necessary for accurate interpretation (Fig. 93–6). Special equipment is usually not required. A complete description of the technique, anatomy, indications, and interpretation is available.[28]

Ventriculography

Ventriculography may be performed with either positive or negative contrast medium. The procedure is most useful for confirming a diagnosis of hydrocephalus and determining the extent of ventricular enlargement (Fig. 93–7).[2,27]

With the patient under general anesthesia, a small hole is made in the dorsal calvarium. In some patients with open fontanelles, the already existing opening may be used. A spinal needle is passed into the brain 1 cm lateral to the midline midway between the orbit and occipital crest. The needle is advanced until the

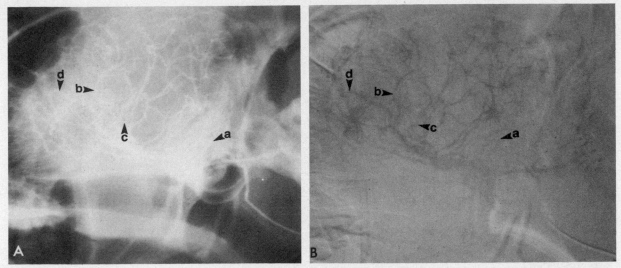

Figure 93–5. *A,* A lateral radiograph of a cerebral arteriogram. *B,* A subtraction radiograph of the same contrast examination. Many of the vessels are more clearly seen on the subtraction radiograph, because the image of the overlying calvarium has been photographically removed. *a,* internal carotid artery; *b,* rostral cerebral artery; *c,* middle cerebral artery; *d,* ethmoid artery.

lateral ventricle is penetrated. Cerebrospinal fluid is removed and is replaced with an equal volume of air or positive contrast material. Vertical and horizontal beam radiographs are made with the patient's head in a variety of positions to determine the severity of ventricular enlargement. In most cases the entire extent of the lateral ventricles can be determined. In many cases the third ventricle can be filled and the cerebral aqueducts identified. Masses within the lateral ventricles may also be identified.

THE SPINE

Spinal anatomy and radiography of companion animals are complex. The vertebral segments and radiographic anatomy are identified similarly in both dogs and cats. The anatomical nomenclature of the vertebral column conforms to *Nomina Anatomica Veterinaria*[11,33] and is the same for both species. The morphology of individual vertebrae differs markedly

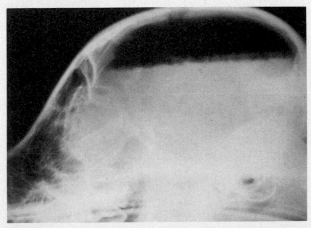

Figure 93–6. A normal cavernous sinus venogram. The venous structures are opacified with contrast medium. Note that the larger arteries on the floor of the calvarium appear as linear, lucent, filling defects in the cavernous sinus. *a,* internal carotid artery; *b,* orbital plexus; *c,* cavernous sinus; *d,* ventral petrosal sinus; *e,* external maxillary vein; *f,* anastomosis of ophthalmic veins.

Figure 93–7. A horizontal beam lateral radiograph of a pneumoventriculogram in a dog with severe hydrocephalus. An air-fluid interface is evident where the injected air has risen above the remaining cerebrospinal fluid in the lateral ventricles. Only a thin shell of cerebral tissue surrounds the greatly dilated lateral ventricles.

TABLE 93–1. Normal Sagittal and Frontal Diameters (mm) of the Canine Vertebral Canal in Selected Breeds

Breeds*	No. Dogs	Cervical Spinal Canal					Thoracic Spinal Canal			Lumbar Spinal Canal				
		Sagittal Diameter			Ventrodorsal Diameter		Sagittal Diameter		Ventrodorsal Diameter	Sagittal Diameter		Ventrodorsal Diameter		
		C2	C3	C5-C6	C2	C5-C6	T2	T11-T13	T11-T13	L1-L2	L4	L1-L2	L4	L6
Small Breeds														
Pekingese	9													
Mean		9.78	7.25	7.5	8.29	7.5	7.0	6.13	7.29	6.12	6.67	7.25	7.78	8.5
SD		.67	.89	1.07	.95	.58	.63	.99	.76	.83	.87	.71	.97	1.05
Cocker spaniel	7													
Mean		11.5	8.57	9.71	10.4	9.75	8.0	7.14	8.17	7.5	8.14	8.33	9.67	10.
SD		1.22	.53	.76	1.14	.95	0	.38	.41	.84	.69	.52	.52	.77
Dachsund	23													
Mean		10.0	7.83	8.09	9.89	9.0	6.9	5.91	7.68	6.05	6.64	7.7	8.57	9.74
SD		1.02	1.65	1.08	1.32	1.57	.94	.75	.99	.79	.66	.86	1.03	.99
Miniature Dachsund	8													
Mean		9.85	7.86	8.18	9.86	8.83	6.33	5.86	7.75	6.0	6.67	7.88	8.63	9.5
SD		.69	1.07	.75	.69	1.17	.52	.90	.46	.58	.52	.35	.52	.53
Chihuahua	7													
Mean		8.57	6.83	7.33	7.67	7.0	6.5	4.86	5.86	5.29	5.57	6.14	6.86	7.17
SD		.98	.75	1.03	1.15	.82	.55	.69	.69	.76	.53	.37	.90	1.17
Poodle	7													
Mean		10.0	7.71	8.57	9.33	9.2	7.0	6.0	6.57	6.14	7.0	6.8	8.17	8.6
SD		1.15	.49	1.13	.82	.45	1.15	.89	.79	1.07	.63	.84	.75	.55
Large Breeds														
German shepherd	20													
Mean		16.3	11.38	12.38	15.78	14.77	11.67	11.22	12.24	10.45	11.11	12.6	14.19	15.87
SD		1.53	.89	1.09	1.72	1.42	1.75	1.35	1.03	1.28	.99	1.24	1.47	1.48
Pointer	9													
Mean		14.67	11.6	11.8	14.4	13.5	10.83	11.0	11.67	10.13	10.57	11.57	13.33	14.17
SD		1.21	1.14	1.10	.55	2.09	.75	2.09	1.51	1.25	.53	.79	1.37	1.17
Great Dane	13													
Mean		18.23	16.67	13.69	19.17	16.17	13.75	12.89	14.6	13.27	13.36	14.67	16.55	18.0
SD		2.24	1.44	1.75	2.58	2.29	1.16	1.76	1.17	2.32	1.96	.71	2.11	1.49
Doberman	21													
Mean		15.33	11.62	11.29	15.44	13.9	16.32	11.56	12.94	11.21	11.58	12.67	14.76	15.68
SD		1.71	1.28	1.52	1.34	1.52	1.29	1.42	1.11	1.03	1.26	1.08	1.25	1.2

*SD = standard deviation.

from other bones in the skeleton. The spine consists of approximately 50 irregularly shaped vertebrae: seven cervical (C), 13 thoracic (T), seven lumbar (L), three sacral (S), and a variable number of caudal (Cd) vertebrae.

Normal Spine

The normal development and ossification centers of the vertebrae provide an important base for neurological diagnosis. Multiple osseous defects may occur during development. A knowledge of normal anatomy and the variations of the respective vertebral bodies and their appearance is necessary for radio-

graphic interpretation of abnormalities.[33,38] Individual segments throughout the vertebral column differ in shape, and both diarthrodial and amphiarthrodial joints are present.[11,33]

Each spinal segment has unique anatomical features. There are approximately 30 vertebral bodies (not including caudal vertebrae) and 26 intervertebral discs. The C1-C2 articulation is a diarthrodial joint and contains no intervertebral disc. The sixth cervical vertebra is unique in appearance because of the large ventral projection of its transverse processes. In the thoracic region, a normal complement of 13 paired ribs is often varied by agenesis or supernumerary ribs. The discs from T1 to T11 rarely herniate because ligaments connect paired rib heads (the intercapital

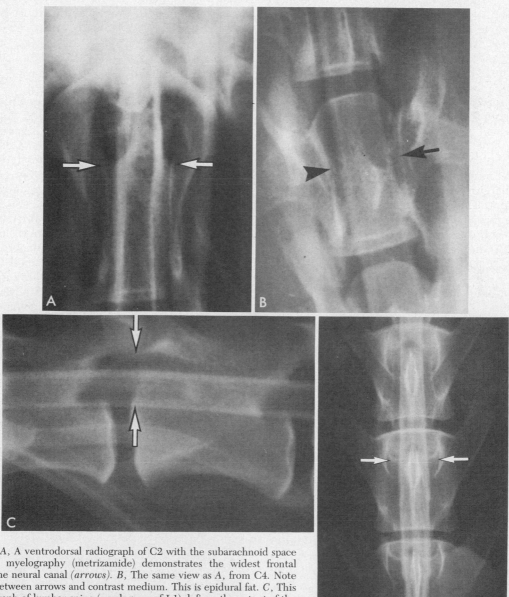

Figure 93–8. *A,* A ventrodorsal radiograph of C2 with the subarachnoid space enhanced by myelography (metrizamide) demonstrates the widest frontal diameter of the neural canal *(arrows). B,* The same view as *A,* from C4. Note the lucency between arrows and contrast medium. This is epidural fat. *C,* This lateral radiograph of lumbar spine (myelogram of L1) defines the extent of the subarachnoid space *(upper arrow)* compared with the neural canal containing epidural fat dorsally *(lower arrow). D,* This ventrodorsal radiograph of lumbar spine (L4), with subarachnoid space enhanced by myelography, defines the neural canal in a frontal plane. *Arrows* indicate intersection of lamina. Note the normal widened segment of cord corresponding to the lumbar enlargement (intumescentia lumbalis of L4-S2) and respective nerve roots.

ligaments).[11] The T10-T11 intervertebral space shows a transition in spinous process direction and provides a good landmark. In dogs, the ratio of lumbar spinous process height to vertical diameter of the neural canal is approximately 2:1; in cats, this ratio is 1:1. In the dog, the lumbar transverse processes are directed cranially and present a rounded or club-shaped cranial peripheral border. The spinal cord diameter and its relationship to the vertebral canal diameter vary throughout the spinal canal (Table 93–1).

The articular processes, neural arch, dorsal and ventral borders to the neural canal, cranial and caudal vertebral end-plates, spinous process, transverse processes, and vertebral body have a distinctive radiographic appearance (Fig. 93–8). Canine vertebral bodies are nearly square. In the ventrodorsal projection, the spinous processes are rounded. The lumbar vertebrae are generally longer than the thoracic vertebrae. Although longer and more massive, the pedicles and laminae of the lumbar vertebrae resemble those of the thoracic and cervical vertebrae.

The radiographic appearance of the feline spine differs from that of the canine spine. The vertebral bodies are generally more elongated and rectangular. The laminae and pedicles of the articular facets are less distinct. The lumbar spinous processes are approximately the same height as the spinal canal. The intervertebral foraminae are difficult to assess along the dorsal margin. The transverse processes sweep in a cranioventral direction and have a pointed peripheral margin. The vertebral bodies of T12, T13, and L1 consistently have angular cranial endplates. Caudal to L1, the vertebral end-plates are aligned more perpendicularly. The neural arch is consistently indistinct.

Indications for Diagnostic Spinal Radiography

Diagnosis of spinal disease requires staged clinical investigation. Neurological examination, including electrodiagnostic evaluation, clinical assessment, and other ancillary tests should be completed prior to radiographic examination, except in acute trauma cases. Radiography is not an appropriate method to "search" for a lesion. It is utilized to confirm a presumptive clinical diagnosis. The involved anatomic segment can usually be determined when radiographic examination is indicated by neurological findings.

Complete clinical evaluation of the patient is mandatory. In approximately 40 per cent of spinal radiographic examinations, no lesions can be seen.[3] Differential diagnoses must be formulated, considering all clinical parameters and using radiology as a diagnostic aid. Definitive diagnosis of spinal lesions can be made on radiography alone only 55 per cent of the time, even when contrast procedures are employed.[3]

In many instances, acute spinal trauma is mimicked by chronic underlying spinal disease. If survey radiographs of a patient with suspected acute spinal cord trauma are normal, other neurological diseases should be considered. Those that may cause acute signs include: fibrocartilaginous embolization or infarction; acute intervertebral disc herniation; neoplastic processes of the cord, nerve roots, or vertebrae; transverse myelopathies; and cord concussion. In such cases, a careful neurological examination is usually more useful than radiography. Survey radiographs are usually normal, suggesting that further diagnostic techniques be employed.

The incidence of disease is related to the population surveyed or radiographed, e.g., the incidence of congenital inflammatory, neoplastic, and traumatic disease of the spine in the cat is lower than in the dog.[18,25] Spinal radiography and contrast procedures are not indicated as frequently in the cat.

Spinal Radiography

The necessity for optimum film quality in spinal radiography cannot be overemphasized. Lesions may be obscure and are often masked by other structures. Survey radiography of the spine allows detection of lesions where there is lysis, proliferation, or displacement of osseous structures. Significant osseous disease may occur before it is visible radiographically; loss of 30 per cent of bone mineral must occur before lysis can be seen on radiographs. Minor, seemingly insignificant lesions may cause profound clinical signs because of the rigid nature of the spinal canal.

Optimum film quality can be attained only when the patient is anesthetized so that there is complete relaxation of the axial musculature. The spine should be radiographed in multiple short segments, because distortion of anatomic relationships increases with distance from the central beam. Radiographs of the entire spine on a single exposure are not acceptable for evaluation of intervertebral disc spaces and other

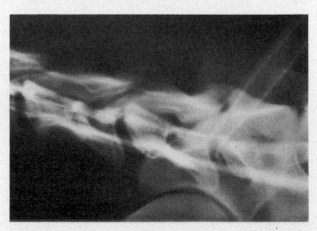

Figure 93–9. A lateral radiograph of the cervical spine. The ventral venous sinus is demonstrated by injection of contrast medium via cervical vertebral body (venogram). Notice the location and extent of the venous sinus relative to neural canal size.

critical assessments. Narrow collimation is essential to prevent scatter radiation from obscuring fine detail. Precise patient positioning is absolutely necessary for accurate radiographic diagnosis. Radiolucent positioning pads are used to prevent sagging or rotation of the spine and subsequent positional artifacts. Optimum radiographic detail of spinal structures is attained with high mAs and low kVp to increase radiographic contrast.

Many screen-film combinations have been used for

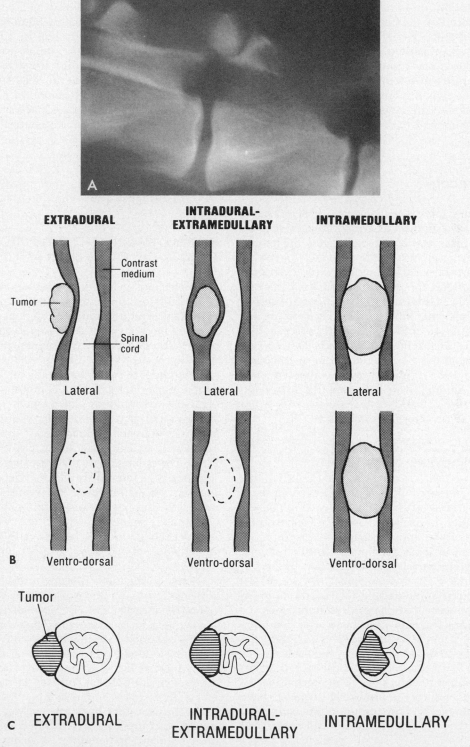

Figure 93–10. *A,* A lateral radiograph myelogram of L3–L4, demonstrating the characteristic obstruction to contrast flow due to an intramedullary mass. *B* and *C,* Diagrammatic portrayals of the locations and compressive features (projections) of mass lesions as defined on subarachnoid myelography. (Reprinted with permission from Suter, P. F., et al.: Myelography in the dog. J. Am. Vet. Radiol. Soc. *12:*40, 1971.)

spinal radiography. The imaging system must provide adequate detail at an acceptable radiation dose and exposure time. Developments in rare earth phosphors have received much attention.[21] Rare earth technology has allowed the production of faster intensifying screens that also maintain good detail. These faster imaging systems combined with higher-output radiography units allow shortened exposure times and reduced motion artifact. Rare earth screens may be of particular benefit in large dogs. High-quality spinal examinations can also be made with conventional (calcium tungstate) imaging systems. The cost of rare earth screens is nearly twice that of conventional screens. It is prudent when considering the purchase of intensifying screens to test them with the x-ray machine and darkroom for which they are being bought.

Linear Tomography

Linear tomography is valuable in spinal radiography. It provides a method whereby the body may be radiographed in a series of selected planes. Structures out of the plane of interest are blurred owing to motion of the tube head during the x-ray exposure. Tomography allows the portrayal of certain lesions with elimination of superimposed structures such as rib heads and articular processes, resulting in precise imaging at the depth of the pathological process. The procedure requires general anesthesia and special diagnostic radiographic equipment. Linear tomography should not be confused with computed axial tomography. Although the latter may be extremely valuable in neurological diagnosis, the system is too expensive for most veterinary practices.

Contrast Radiography of the Spine

Contrast radiographic procedures, including myelography, epidurography, venography (Fig. 93–9), and discography have been used to demonstrate abnormalities of the spinal canal.[18] Myelography is the most useful of these techniques in small animal neurology. Compressive spinal lesions may be located and characterized by myelography. Figure 93–10 shows the myelographic patterns of extradural, intramedullary, and extramedullary-intradural lesions.

Several contrast agents have been used for myelography. Metrizamide (Amipaque)* is currently the contrast agent of choice in veterinary medicine. Available since 1975, it is the most practical contrast agent for myelographic techniques. The technique of administration and the neurological sequelae have been documented.[1,3,18] Some neurologists, surgeons, and radiologists recommend injection of contrast at the cisterna magna, whereas others prefer lumbar administration.

Neurological reactions to intrathecal injection of metrizamide may occur but usually are not severe. Less than 15 per cent of animals exhibit significant neurological sequelae.[1,3] Adverse sequelae include fasciculations and motor activity, which may culminate in partial or generalized motor seizures. These reactions occur approximately 90 minutes after myelography and can be controlled by administration of diazepam (Valium).* If the animal remains anesthetized for a surgical procedure immediately after myelography, prolonged general anesthesia may mask adverse sequelae of metrizamide.

Because metrizamide does possess a potential for neurological sequelae, pharmaceutical manufacturers are continuing their efforts to produce an inert contrast agent to be utilized in the subarachnoid space. Currently, agents such as iogulaide, a nonionic intrathecal agent, iohexol, and iopamidol are being investigated for possible clinical application.[6]

NUCLEAR IMAGING AND COMPUTED TOMOGRAPHY OF THE BRAIN AND SPINE

The technology of diagnostic imaging has advanced remarkably in the last decade.[19] Improvement in existing procedures and development of entirely new imaging methods offer increased diagnostic accuracy with reduced patient risk. Radionuclide brain imaging was perfected in the mid-1970s but has since largely been replaced in human medicine by computed tomography.[37] The computed image reconstruction techniques developed for computed tomography[14] have been refined further for use in positron emission tomography,[19] nuclear magnetic resonance (NMR) imaging,[31] and digital radiography.[24] Ultrasonographic diagnosis has developed rapidly but is of limited use in disorders of the central nervous system, because the brain and spinal cord are encased in bone, which alters sound transmission and inhibits sonographic imaging.[19] Very small ultrasound probes are now being made that may allow examination of the brain through burr holes in the skull.

Many of the new imaging procedures are noninvasive; i.e., they require no catheterization or operative intervention. Because they are safer than angiography or myelography, diagnostic information can be obtained with lower morbidity and mortality. Patient discomfort is minimal, usually limited to venipuncture for administration of radiopharmaceuticals or organic iodine contrast agents.

The high cost of buying and maintaining the equipment necessary for the new imaging procedures has limited the application of this technology in animals. Conventional radiography remains the primary

---

*Amipaque, Winthrop Laboratories, 90 Park Avenue, New York, NY.

*Valium, Hoffman–LaRoche, Inc., Nutley, NJ.

method of diagnostic imaging in veterinary neurology. Survey radiographs, however, yield limited information in neurological cases without osseous involvement. Contrast procedures improve diagnostic accuracy but may be technically difficult or dangerous, especially when evaluating brain disease. Newer imaging methods should be considered when there is clinical evidence of a focal brain lesion or spinal lesion that cannot be seen on conventional radiographs. Facilities for radionuclide scans are available at many veterinary colleges. Some of these colleges also have access to computed tomography equipment at nearby medical centers. Positron emission tomography, nuclear magnetic resonance imaging, and digital radiography show great promise for neurological diagnosis but currently are less accessible for animal patients.

Radionuclide Imaging

Nuclear medicine may be defined broadly as any use of radioactive materials in diagnosis and treatment of disease. Radionuclide imaging (scintigraphy) is the application of gamma-emitting radiotracer techniques to organ or organ system visualization in living organisms.[15] Radionuclide images are obtained by administering a tracer dose of a radiolabelled compound (radiopharmaceutical), which is selectively accumulated in or excluded from certain organs or tissues. A gamma camera or rectilinear scanner is used to obtain a visual image of the pattern of radionuclide accumulation in the patient. The gamma camera detector is a collimated scintillation crystal that allows precise determination of the number and location of gamma emissions. Each detected gamma ray is displayed as a dot on a cathode ray tube from which an image can be recorded on film.

Radionuclide imaging complements the information obtained by conventional radiography. Anatomical detail is far superior on radiographs, but the radionuclide images offer physiological or functional information because the pattern of radioactivity in the patient's body depends on physiological distribution of the radiopharmaceutical.

Technetium-99m has become the radionuclide of choice for clinical nuclear imaging because of its short half-life (6.0 hr), monoenergetic gamma emission (140 keV), absence of beta emission, and ready availability from commercially produced generators. Radiopharmaceutical kits allow easy preparation of technetium-99m-labelled compounds. A variety of these kits are available so that imaging agents can be conveniently prepared for most organ systems.

Animals that have been given technetium-99m radiopharmaceuticals emit measurable radioactivity for 36 to 72 hours and, by federal regulation, must be confined during that time. Technetium-99m is eliminated in the urine and feces, which must be collected and held for radioactive decay. Because of the agent's short half-life, the radioactivity decays to negligible levels in 72 hours or less.

Nuclear imaging is often useful in neurological diagnosis even though no radiopharmaceuticals are specifically accumulated by nerve cells. Radionuclide brain imaging and bone imaging of the spine are the techniques most often employed in veterinary neurology. Radionulcide cisternography is used to evaluate CSF dynamics in humans[15] but has not been reported in veterinary practice.

Radionuclide Brain Imaging

Radionuclide brain imaging for clinical diagnosis in animals was first reported in 1970.[36] Subsequent reports have described the technique and have shown its efficacy in demonstrating focal brain lesions in dogs and cats.[10,20]

Brain tumors and abcesses are rarely seen on skull radiographs because the lesions are the same radiographic density as the surrounding normal brain parenchyma. Some brain lesions may be located by cerebral angiography, but the procedure is technically difficult and often unrewarding in dogs and cats. Radionuclide brain imaging is a safe, noninvasive technique that is sensitive in detecting lesions larger than 1 cm in diameter.[20] The technique does not allow differentiation of the nature of the lesion, however, because radionuclide accumulation is not specific for tumors or inflammatory lesions. Abnormalities are detected as a result of deficits in normal physiological function rather than unique metabolic properties of the lesion. The rationale for radionuclide brain imaging is based on the function of the blood-brain barrier. The barrier excludes the radiopharmaceutical from the brain parenchyma, causing the brain to be represented in images as an area of low activity. Tumors and other lesions cause "breakdown" of the blood-brain barrier with deposition of radiopharmaceutical in the lesion and surrounding tissue. The lesions appear as areas of increased activity ("hot spots") on images made with the gamma camera (Fig. 93–11).

Brain imaging may be performed using technetium-99m pertechnetate, or technetium-99m–labelled glucoheptonate (^{99m}TcGH) or diethylene-triamine-penta-acetic acid (^{99m}TcDTPA). Animal patients are sedated or anesthetized so that they can be accurately positioned and do not move during the imaging procedure. Approximately 10 millicuries (mCi) of radiopharmaceutical are injected intravenously. Rapid sequential images may be made immediately after injection to demonstrate the distribution of blood flow to the brain (radionuclide angiography). Radionuclide angiography is particularly useful in the diagnosis of vascular abnormalities and highly vascular tumors.

Acquisition of final images is delayed until one to three hours after radiopharmaceutical administration. The delay allows time for distribution of the tracer

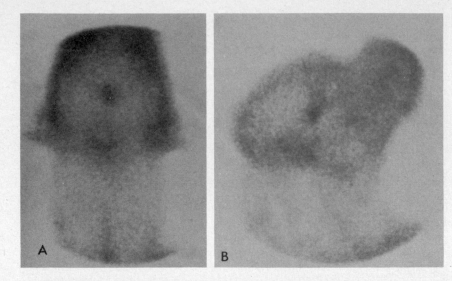

Figure 93–11. Dorsal (A) and right lateral (B) radionuclide brain images of a boxer dog with a pituitary tumor causing blindness. The brain is seen as an area of decreased activity because radionuclide is excluded from brain parenchyma by the blood-brain barrier. Accumulation of radionuclide in the tumor results in the "hot spot" seen at the base of the brain.

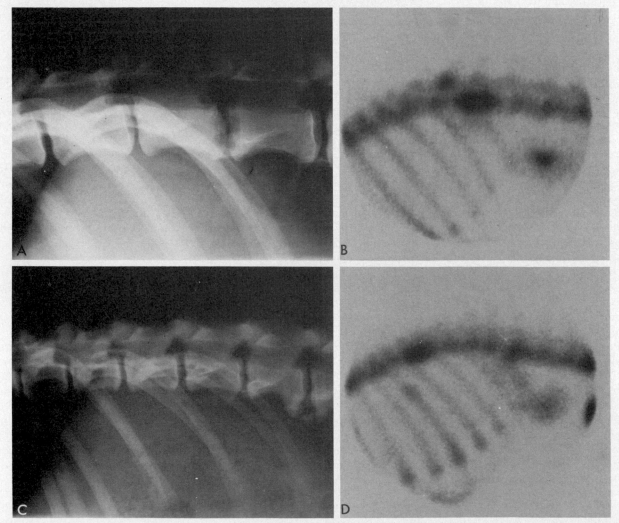

Figure 93–12. Lateral radiograph (A) and lateral radionuclide bone image (B) of the thoracolumbar region of a dog with discospondylitis. Lysis of vertebral end-plates at L1-L2 and fracture at the base of the caudal articular process of T13 seen on the radiograph correlate well with sites of increased radionuclide accumulation on the bone scan. Radionuclide in the pelvis of the right kidney can be seen ventral to the lumbar spine. Lateral radiograph (C) and lateral radionuclide bone image (D) of another dog with discospondylitis. In this case there was intense radionuclide activity at T11-T12 on the bone scan with no corresponding radiographic lesion. Because of the bone scan abnormality, T11-T12 was explored surgically and the diagnosis of discospondylitis was made. There was also increased radionuclide activity associated with the spondylitic lesion at L2-L3 and a small fracture callus on the tenth rib.

into the interstitial fluid space and for clearing of radioactivity from the vascular pool by renal excretion. Some lesions that cannot be seen on images made at one hour may be detected at two to three hours after radiopharmaceutical injection. The delay is especially important in dogs and cats because of the need to allow clearing of radioactivity from the thick masseter and temporal muscles overlying the calvarium. [99m]TcGH and [99m]TcDTPA are superior to pertechnetate for brain imaging in dogs because they are more rapidly excreted into the urine.[5]

For accurate anatomical localization of brain lesions, images must be made in more than one plane. A thorough scintigraphic examination of the brain should include dorsal, left lateral, right lateral, and caudal (occipital) images.[5]

Radionuclide Bone Imaging

No nuclear imaging technique enables visualization of the spinal cord itself, but indirect information can be obtained from bone imaging of the osseous spinal column. Radionuclide bone imaging is a sensitive but nonspecific technique.[4] Technetium-99m-labeled phosphate compounds are administered intravenously and accumulate in bone. All bone shows some accumulation of the tracer, but higher accumulation occurs at sites of increased bone turnover. Radiographic evidence of bone lysis or sclerosis cannot be seen until there is a change of 30 per cent or more in the mineral content of a focal area of bone, but radionuclide bone images show bone lesions much earlier in the course of disease. The scans usually

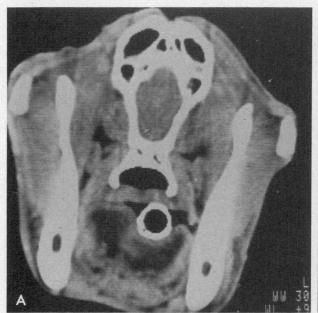

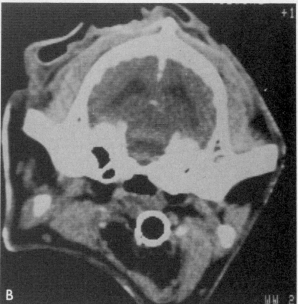

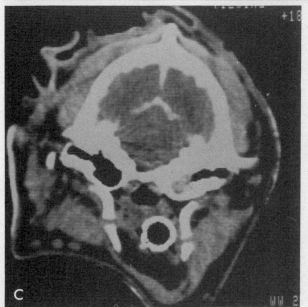

Figure 93–13. Computed tomographic images of the skull of a dog show cross-sectional anatomy in the transverse plane. *A,* Rostral. The frontal sinuses and rostral extent of the brain can be identified below the dorsal midline. Cross-sections of the mandibular rami and zygomatic arches can also be seen. *B,* Central. A transverse section through the central portion of the calvarium shows the brain parenchyma as a homogenous density. The lateral ventricles can be identified as chevron-shaped areas of lesser density. *C,* Caudal. This image of the cerebellum shows a cross-section of the osseous tentorium. An air-filled auditory bulla is seen at the base of the calvarium, and hyoid bones extend ventrally. The dense circular structure seen ventrally in all three images is the endotracheal tube.

show "hot spots" or increased tracer accumulation at sites of disease but may also show "cold spots" (photon-deficient lesions), where there is bone destruction without repair.[7] The scans do not allow differentiation of traumatic, inflammatory, and neoplastic lesions without additional clinical or laboratory information. In humans bone scans are frequently used to detect early evidence of bone metastasis in malignant neoplasia. Metastatic sites may be detected several months earlier on radionuclide scintigraphy than on radiography.[4]

Radionuclide bone imaging is a safe, noninvasive procedure. Technetium-99m methylene diphosphonate (^{99m}TcMDP) is administered intravenously. The radiopharmaceutical is initially distributed in the blood pool. Gamma camera images made just after injection may show areas of increased vascularity in soft tissue as well as bone. Static images of the areas of interest are made three hours after injection. The delay allows time for localization of radiotracer in bone and urinary elimination of background activity.

Because of the rapid urinary excretion of methylene diphosphonate, there is considerable radioactivity in the urinary bladder at the time of imaging, causing a large "hot spot" that may obscure the spine. For critical evaluation of the lumbar and sacral spine, it is often necessary to catheterize the patient and remove the radioactive urine; proper safety precautions are imperative in this procedure.

Bone scintigraphy may be used to locate vertebral lesions not seen on conventional radiography (Fig. 93–12). Radionuclide bone imaging may be particularly useful in locating vertebral neoplasia, spinal osteomyelitis or discospondylitis, and nondisplaced fractures. If a single site of inflammatory or neoplastic disease is seen on survey radiography, scintigraphy may be used to find additional lesions. Radionuclide bone imaging also may aid in distinguishing chronic, resolved lesions from active, progressive ones.

Computed Tomography

Computed tomography generates cross-sectional head or body images with excellent anatomic detail. A narrow x-ray beam is passed through the patient, and a radiation detection device on the far side of the patient measures attenuation of the beam. The x-ray tube and detector are rotated around the patient as thousands of measurements from different directions are obtained. It is this rotation of the x-ray beam around the axis of the patient that gave the procedure its original name, *computerized axial tomography*. The attenuation measurements are recorded as digital information by a computer. The computer is then used to reconstruct gray-scale image projections in which 0.5- to 1.0-mm^2 video picture elements (pixels) are assigned levels of gray relative to the x-ray attenuation (density) of the tissue examined.[14,19] Computed tomography can resolve structures as small as 1 mm and can distinguish density differences of 0.3 to 0.5 per cent.

A number of cross-sectional images or "slices" are made at intervals of 0.3 to 1.0 mm to examine a given area of the body. The resultant series of images provides the antemortem equivalent of a serial-section anatomy specimen. The cross-sectional nature of the images allows anatomical structures to be seen without the superimposition that occurs on conventional radiographs.

Animal patients must be heavily sedated or anesthetized for computed tomography. Modern CT units require 2 to 10 seconds to accumulate the information for each image and the patient must remain motionless during that time. A complete examination of the brain of a dog may require an hour or longer. Images of the canine brain are usually made in the transverse plane, but those in sagittal and frontal planes may also be obtained by repositioning the dog or by computed reconstruction of the image.

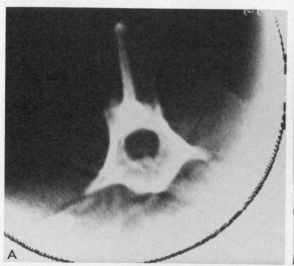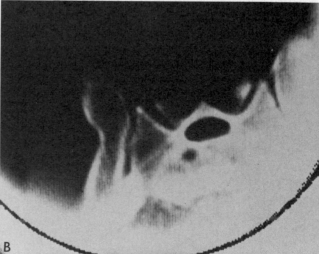

Figure 93–14. Computed tomographic images of the spine show transverse sections of the fourth lumbar vertebra (A) and the sacrum (B) in a normal dog. The spinal canal is clearly seen in both images. The sacroiliac joints can be seen in B.

Computed tomography allows excellent visualization of anatomical structures of the skull and brain (Fig. 93–13) and may also be used to obtain cross-sectional images of the spine (Fig. 93–14). It is an excellent method to diagnose brain tumors in dogs and cats[12,13,22,23] but has not been employed frequently in diagnosis of spinal disorders.

Mass lesions of the brain can be detected on computed tomographic images by changes in density and by displacement or distortion of other intracranial structures, especially the ventricles. Most brain tumors are best seen with contrast enhancement, a technique in which images are made after intravenous administration of organic iodine contrast medium. The contrast medium accumulates in the tumor (because of increased vascularity and/or breakdown of the blood-brain barrier) and markedly increases the density of the lesion. The degree of contrast enhancement may be characteristic for certain tumor types and grades, allowing more specific diagnosis.[13]

Computed tomography is currently the most accurate method for locating mass lesions of the brain in dogs and cats. It is useful in planning surgery or radiotherapy for definitive treatment of brain tumors. Expense and limited availability in veterinary institutions are the primary impediments to routine clinical application of computed tomography in veterinary neurology. At present, radionuclide brain imaging may be employed as a screening procedure for mass lesions of the brain, because gamma cameras are available at many veterinary colleges and the cost of this procedure is usually much less than that of computed tomography. Computed tomography should be considered for more definitive localization of lesions found on radionuclide imaging when surgery or other definitive treatment is contemplated. If readily available and economically feasible, computed tomography should be the primary imaging procedure for suspected brain lesions.

1. Bartels, J. E., Braund, K. G., and Redding, R. W.: An experimental evaluation of a non-ionic agent—Amipaque (metrizamide) as a neurologic medium in the dog. J. Am. Vet. Rad. Soc. 28:117, 1977.
2. Bartels, J. E., Hoerlein, B. F., and Boring, J. G.: Neuroradiology. In Hoerlein, B. F.: Canine Neurology: Diagnosis and Treatment. 3rd ed. W. B. Saunders, Philadelphia, 1978.
3. Bartels, J. E.: Unpublished data. Presented at 6th International Congress on Veterinary Radiology, University of California, Davis, California, August, 1983.
4. Bassett, L. W., Bold, R. H., and Webber, M. M.: Radionuclide bone imaging. Radiol. Clin. North Am. 19:675, 1981.
5. Brawner, W. R., Jr.: Static and dynamic radionuclide brain imaging in the normal canine: technique and appearance. Dissertation, Auburn University, Auburn, Alabama, 1981.
6. Bryan, R. N., Centero, R. S., Hershkowitz, N., et al.: Neurotoxicity of iohexol: a new non-ionic contrast medium. Radiology 145:379, 1982.
7. Charkes, N. D.: Mechanisms of skeletal tracer uptake. J. Nuclear Med. 20:794, 1979.
8. Chrisman, C. L.: Disease of peripheral nerves and muscles. In Ettinger, S. J. (Ed.): Textbook of Veterinary Internal Medicine. W. B. Saunders, Philadelphia, 1975.
9. Conrad, C. R., and Oliver, J. E., Jr.: Cerebral arteriography. In Ticer, J. W.: Radiographic Technique in Small Animal Practice. W. B. Saunders, Philadelphia, 1975.
10. Dijokshoorn, J. A., and Rijnberk, A.: Detection of brain tumors in dogs by scintigraphy. J. Am. Vet. Rad. Soc. 18:147, 1977.
11. Evans, H. E., and Christensen, J. C. (eds.): Miller's Anatomy of the Dog. 2nd ed. W. B. Saunders, Philadelphia, 1979.
12. Fike, J. R., LeCouteur, A. A., and Cann, C. E.: Anatomy of the canine brain using high resolution computed tomography. Vet. Radiol. 22:236, 1981.
13. Fike, J. R., LeCouteur, R. A., Cann, C. E., et al.: Computerized tomography of brain tumors of the rostral and middle fossas in the dog. Am. J. Vet. Res. 42:275, 1981.
14. Gordon, R., Gabor, T. H., and Steven, J. J.: Image reconstruction from projections. Sci. Am. 233:56, 1975.
15. Gottschalk, A., and Potchen, E. J. (eds.): Diagnostic Nuclear Medicine. Williams & Wilkins, Baltimore, 1976.
16. Hare, W. C. D.: The age at which epiphyseal union takes place in the limb bone of a dog. Wien. Tierarztl., Mchr., Festschrift, Schreiber, 1960.
17. Hause, W. R., Helphrey, M. L., Green, R. W., and Stromberg, P. C.: Cerebral arteriovenous malformation in a dog. J. Am. Anim. Hosp. Assoc. 18:601, 1982.
18. Hoerlein, B. F.: Canine Neurology: Diagnosis and Treatment. 3rd ed. W. B. Saunders, Philadelphia, 1978.
19. Jaffe, C.: Medical imaging. Am. Sci. 70:576, 1982.
20. Kallfelz, F. A., deLahunta, A., and Allhands, R. V.: Scintigraphic diagnosis of brain lesions in the dog and cat. J. Am. Vet. Med. Assoc. 172:589, 1978.
21. Koblik, P. D., Hornof, W. J., and O'Brien, R. R.: Rare earth intensifying screens for veterinary radiography: an evaluation of two systems. Vet. Radiol. 21:224, 1980.
22. LeCouteur, R. A., Fike, J. R., Cann, C. E., et al.: X-ray computed tomography of brain tumors in cats. J. Am. Vet. Med. Assoc. 183:301, 1983.
23. LeCouteur, R. A., Fike, J. R., Cann, C. E. Pedroia, V. G.: Computed tomography of brain tumors in the caudal fossa of the dog. Vet. Radiol. 22:244, 1981.
24. Mistretta, C. A., Crummy, A. B., and Strother, C. D.: Digital angiography: a perspective. Radiology 139:273, 1981.
25. Morgan, J. P.: Radiology and Veterinary Orthopedics. Lea & Febiger, Philadelphia, 1979.
26. Morgan, J. P., and Silverman, S.: Techniques of Veterinary Radiography. 3rd ed. Veterinary Radiology Associates, Davis, 1982.
27. Oliver, J. E., Jr., and Conrad, C. R.: Cerebral ventriculography. In Ticer, J. W.: Radiographic Technique in Small Animal Practice. W. B. Saunders, Philadelphia, 1975.
28. Oliver, J. E., Jr.: Cranial sinus venography in the dog. J. Am. Vet. Rad. Soc. 10:66, 1969.
29. Owens, J. M.: Radiographic Interpretation for the Small Animal Clinician. Ralston Purina, St. Louis, 1982.
30. Parker, A. J., and Park, R. D.: Occipital dysplasia in the dog. J. Am. Anim. Hosp. Assoc. 10:520, 1974.
31. Pykett, I. L., Newhouse, J. H. Buonanno, F. S., et al.: Principles of nuclear magnetic resonance imaging. Radiology 143:157, 1982.
32. Rendano, V. T., deLahunta, A., and King, J. M.: Extracranial neoplasia with facial nerve paralysis in two cats. J. Am. Anim. Hosp. Assoc. 16:921, 1980.
33. Schebitz, H., and Wilkins, H.: Atlas of Radiographic Anatomy of the Dog and Cat. 3rd ed. Verlag Paul Parey/W. B. Saunders, Philadelphia, 1980.
34. Sumner-Smith, G.: Observation of epiphyseal fusion of the canine appendicular skeleton. J. Small Anim. Pract. 7:303, 1966.
35. Ticer, J. W.: Radiographic Technique in Small Animal Practice. W. B. Saunders, Philadelphia, 1975.
36. Ullrich, K., Klemm, J., and Berg, G.: Hirnszintigraphie beim hund, eine neue methode in der diagnostik von intracerebralen krankheitsprozessen. Kleintier-Prax. 15:235, 1970.
37. Weiss, L., Gilbert, H. A., and Posner, J. B. (eds.): Brain Metastasis. G. K. Hall, Boston, 1978.
38. Wright, J. A.: A study of radiographic anatomy in the cervical spine of the dog. J. Small Anim. Pract. 18:341, 1970.

94 Instruments and General Principles

Charles D. Knecht

INTRODUCTION

The opportunity to heal by surgical intervention is one of the joys of veterinary practice. The likelihood of full recovery, the decreased time from treatment to recovery, and even the challenge of increased risk under the surgeon's control are common to most nonelective surgical procedures but are rarely more essential than to the decision for surgical rather than medical treatment of neurological diseases.[10, 11, 13] Even a cursory review of the veterinary literature reveals that diseases of the nervous system suffer from categorization into three disciplinary types: (1) those in which the diagnosis is paramount because no treatment exists (pathology), (2) those in which medical therapy is used to delay progression, lessen clinical signs, and possibly effect a cure (medicine), and (3) those that may respond rapidly to repair, decompression, or stabilization (surgery).

It is no wonder that the early veterinary clinical neurologists were neuropathologists or neurophysiologists. Nor should it surprise us that the second generation was composed nearly entirely of surgeons. The improved percentage and rate of recovery after surgery for intervertebral disc disease reported by Hoerlein,[7] Redding,[17] Fundquist,[4] and others encouraged each of us to learn to diagnose and treat, not just confirm, the disease entity. For nearly 20 years the emphasis in veterinary neurology remained neurosurgical and the literature abounded with old, new, and modified surgical techniques reported by veterinary surgeons.[5, 18, 20, 23] Each of us defended our techniques with a series of anecdotal reports or clinical retrospective studies.[1, 11, 13, 16] In the exchange of personal views and provincialism, a serious reader of the recent veterinary literature might miss the original truths that early decompression increases the recovery in compressive and traumatic diseases of the spinal cord and brain, that stabilization of fractured spinal vertebrae prevents further disruption of the spinal cord, and that peripheral nerves will heal if properly aligned and fixed.

Were it not for a phenomenon of organized veterinary medicine, the origination of the neurology subspecialty under the umbrella of internal medicine, the students of the history of veterinary medicine might wonder that so many could stray from the surgical track to study anew the diagnosis and treatment of known neurological diseases and define the existence and characteristics of "new" diseases.

The new neurology is propounded by persons interested in internal medicine, anatomy, physiology, pathology, therapeutics, and immunology and by those veterinary neurosurgeons who know, by experience, that most of neurosurgery is medicine. It is these persons who are represented by the authors in these chapters on neurosurgery. It is these persons who meld a knowledge of structure and function with the goals, methods, and prognostic probabilities of medical and surgical treatment. They come at an appropriate time to remind us what we know but do not always recall, that the risks of therapy should not exceed those of the disease.

The indications and surgical therapy for specific diseases of the nervous system are defined. The few pages that follow will, it is hoped, provide an overview of the general principles of neurosurgery including those factors that might reduce the risk.

PREOPERATIVE CONSIDERATIONS

The surgical treatment of many nervous system disorders is within the province of the practicing veterinarian who is willing to determine the anatomical and functional peculiarities of the nervous system, develop thorough techniques in neurological and neuroradiographical examination, maintain strict asepsis, and practice the surgical approaches. Some diseases require neurophysiological testing (electroencephalograms, electromyograms, sensory or motor nerve conduction velocities, and so on) or cerebrospinal fluid analysis for diagnosis or require surgery so rarely done in practice as to prohibit competency (such as craniotomy). The appropriate referral center should be consulted in such cases.

The brain and spinal cord are soft, friable tissues supported by relatively weak connective tissue but surrounded by meninges and the rigid osseous cranium and vertebrae, respectively. The central nervous system (CNS) is vascular but very sensitive to blood or oxygen deficiency and equally subject to congestion and degenerative changes from these deficiencies. The central nervous system is also subject to physiological failure in response to minimal trauma and to irreversible damage if severely traumatized. Although peripheral nerves can regenerate, regeneration of the central nervous system has not been confirmed.

Although the central nervous system has a vascular supply, most neural tissue is protected from rapid alterations in environment by the blood brain barrier. The barrier is not only protective but prevents many chemotherapeutic agents from reaching neural tissues in effective levels. Aseptic techniques are therefore essential in neurosurgery. If antibiotics are needed, those that penetrate the blood brain barriers should be used.

The clinical signs and progression of neurological diseases are varied and complicate the preoperative assessment. The manner in which specific signs affect the prognosis and treatment of specific diseases is discussed elsewhere (see Chapters 95 to 99). Certain features of neurological disease imply important anesthetic considerations (see Chapter 191).

Preoperative Evaluation and Anesthesia

The considerations for anesthesia in diseases of the nervous system differ little from those of soft tissue or orthopedic surgery. Salient requirements are total immobilization of the axial and appendicular muscles but not the muscles of respiration, profound analgesia, and adequate oxygenation.

The use of specific anesthetic agents varies with the patient, procedure, effects of the anesthetic, and the surgeon's experience. Short procedures, such as cerebrospinal fluid collection, are usually performed using short-acting barbiturate anesthetics. More complex procedures may require inhalation anesthetics or combined anesthesia/analgesia. A detailed discussion of anesthetic for neurosurgery is found in Chapter 191.

Animals presented to referral centers for spinal surgery have frequently been treated with adrenocorticosteroids. The effects of such therapy on the liver and on hematology are well known.[2] Serum alanine amino transferase (ALT or SGPT) levels may be markedly elevated. When elevated ALT levels are accompanied by neutrophilia, lymphopenia, and eosinopenia, response to adrenocorticosteroid therapy may reasonably be suspected. The elevation of ALT levels is a response to liver cell damage and is not an artifact of the drug itself. For this reason, liver function tests such as BSP retention and ammonia tolerance may be indicated if surgery can be delayed. In acute onset paralysis, delay in surgery may be unwarranted. These patients should not be anesthetized with barbiturates. Induction of inhalation anesthesia by mask or, in toy animals and cats, an induction chamber is a safe alternative. Elevation of the serum pancreatic lipase level is also common after adrenocorticosteroid therapy. Recent studies indicate that an elevation of this serum enzyme level after corticosteroids is not necessarily an indication of pancreatitis.[15]

Animals with disease of the central nervous system should be carefully monitored during anesthesia. To avoid repeated anesthesia and to effect early decompression, a single anesthetic episode is usually used for radiography, myelography, and surgery. The duration of anesthesia is long in such circumstances and may result in acidosis if the patient is not carefully monitored and ventilated.

Respiratory assistance is important in paraplegic animals because the abdominal musculature may be flaccid. Assisted respiration is essential in quadraplegic patients whose thoracic musculature is affected. If the tests are available, blood gases should be sampled at least every 30 minutes and adjusted by respiratory assistance and intravenous sodium bicarbonate as required.

Respiratory assistance is no less important in cranial injury and surgery. Depressed function of the central nervous system frequently leads to reduced respiratory rate, volume, and character, and respiratory acidosis is common. However, presumptive use of sodium bicarbonate is not warranted. The cerebral vasculature is responsive to carbon dioxide rather than oxygen deficiency. An excess of sodium bicarbonate may reduce CO_2 and the apparent need to maintain vascular dilation and may result in a secondary hypoxia. Hypoxia increases cerebral edema; hyperoxygenation by hyperventilation is used to reduce cerebral edema and remove carbon dioxide.

The patient with cerebral disease is a poor candidate for routine monitoring. Pupillary and corneal response, eye position, jaw tone, and swallowing may be reduced or absent. Auditory, electrocardiographical and, if available, electroencephalographical monitoring of the animal's condition is essential.

Similar monitoring of auditory and electrophysiological parameters is indicated in head or cervical surgery because the anesthetist cannot observe the reaction of the eye and head. In any patient, frames may be used to reduce the tendency of the surgeon to place pressure on the thorax and to permit better observation of the patient by the person monitoring anesthesia.

The tendency to cause shock is not unique to surgery of the central nervous system. Nevertheless, extensive manipulation of muscles and pressure on the abdomen and thorax are common. Capillary refill time and pulse rate and character are valuable indicators of the development of shock. Monitors of arterial and central venous pressures are better. Every animal undergoing major surgery should have balanced electrolytes administered through an indwelling catheter, but overhydration should be avoided.

POSITIONING

The patient should be placed in a position that makes the surgical site easily approachable and is comfortble for the surgeon and safe for the patient. Specific positions are described with individual surgical procedures; a few general comments are appropriate here. The central nervous system is not easily approached surgically. Exploration of the cranium requires trephination or construction of a bone flap in the skull. Both require rigid immobilization whether performed by hand or with power equipment. Although the lower jaw and neck may be taped to a sandbag and the sandbag to the table, a head-holding device is more convenient and safer (Chapter 99). Properly positioned, the device elevates the head to facilitate removal of venous blood and edema from the brain, permits endotracheal intubation without compression by incisors or sandbags, permits the anesthetist to examine the mucous membranes and evaluate jaw tone, and provides a comfortable and rigid working area for the surgeon.

For spinal surgery, the animal's torso should not be stretched or distorted unnecessarily. If the forelimbs are stretched forward and outward, thoracic movements are reduced. Minimal distraction or caudal displacement of the limbs is preferable. Similarly, the limbs should not be abducted laterally to prevent rolling in ventral or dorsal recumbency. This position fatigues the muscles and is less effective than sandbags or styrofoam vacuum bags placed adjacent to the thorax and abdomen.

The animal is placed on towels or similar clean padding to prevent pressure on bony prominences. A water bath heating pad* is used to prevent hypothermia in small dogs and cats. Sandbags or rolled towels are commonly placed under the neck with the animal in dorsal recumbency to increase the width of the disc space. The nose may be fixed close to the table with the lower jaw free. This position appears to cause minimal stress. The endotracheal tube is frequently retracted cranially in this position, leaving a portion of trachea, without endotracheal tube enclosed, in the caudal surgical site. Careless manual or self-retaining retraction may partially occlude the tracheal lumen. The end of the endotracheal tube should be palpated. Retractors should not be placed on the trachea without adequate internal support.

In the past, surgeons placed towels or sandbags under the abdomen to facilitate the approach for hemilaminectomy or laminectomy. This technique may cause sufficient abdominal pressure during surgery to (1) reduce the motion of the diaphragm and abdomen essential for respiration, (2) encourage esophageal reflux of stomach contents, (3) occlude venous return via the postcava and compromise circulating volume, (4) increase venous return via the vertebral sinuses and therefore encourage hemorrhage at the operative site, and (5) reduce urinary output via occlusion of the ureters. A sandbag under the abdomen does not aid the surgeon without undue hazard to the patient.

In recent years, trephination has been replaced by dissection at the articular facet in hemilaminectomy. The laminae are closely apposed at this point. Elevation of the caudal spinous process with towel clamps or forceps opens the articulation slightly and facilitates hemilaminectomy. This maneuver also narrows the intervertebral disc space, creates the most pressure ventrally, and encourages extrusion of the remaining nucleus. The surgeon may elevate the spinous process minimally, using moderate tension and smooth motions. The procedure should never be used to approach a possible fracture or fracture luxation unless the cord and surrounding bone can be adequately observed to prevent additional damage.

INSTRUMENTS

An experienced neurosurgeon can perform most thoracolumbar decompressive procedures using a standard soft tissue surgery pack, adequate drapes for towelling-in, several specialized rongeurs, a large-bore metal hypodermic needle or claw scraper, a Gelpi retractor, adequate lavage and suction, and an optional trephine. The pack is relatively inexpensive but provides minimal exposure and no latitude should complications arise.

The typical neurosurgery pack of the academic surgeon (Table 94–1) may be faulted for redundancy and cost and is inadequate for laminectomies, hemilaminectomies in large dogs, and ventral cervical decompressions without the addition of power equipment and a controllable electrosurgery unit. It is inadequate for peripheral nerve surgery and craniotomies.

The typical pack consists of a soft tissue surgery pack plus instruments for neurosurgery. The instruments are readily available from surgical supply houses and are depicted in several available texts.[8, 12] Several comments about the choice of instruments are needed.

The large number of towel clamps is beneficial for four-corner draping, towelling-in after skin incision, and attachment of suction tubing and electrosurgical

---

*Gorman-Rupp Industries Division, Bellville, OH.

TABLE 94–1. Neurosurgery Pack

1 Michele trephine	Assorted skin sutures
1 Stille-Ruskin double-action rongeur	1 Senn hand retractor
1 Lempert double-action rongeur (very small)	2 Gelpi retractors
1 Adson tissue forceps	1 periosteal elevator (thin)
12 Backhaus towel clamps, 3¼ in.	Frazier suction tips (#80 Fr., #10 Fr.)
8 Halsted mosquito forceps	1 needle holder
2 Allis tissue forceps	2 #3 Bard-Parker scalpel handles
1 Metzenbaum scissors	2 claw tartar scrapers
1 Mayo scissors	1 14-gauge needle (straight with stylette)
1 suture scissors	1 14-gauge needle (curved with stylette)
1 saline bowl	1 22-gauge spinal needle with stylette
4 disposable drapes	Curette, size 3-0
4 cloth towels	

wires to the drapes. A thin periosteal elevator is very helpful in approaching the vertebrae for decompression and as an aid in retraction during disc fenestration. The Michele trephine is a straight-walled trephine useful for penetrating the vertebral pedicles at the articular facets. Approach without trephination or power equipment has been described.[21] Either technique can be excessively traumatic to the spinal cord in the hands of an inexperienced surgeon. Practice is important.

Gelpi retractors are effective in most neurosurgical procedures, but the sharp points dictate care in application. A ball stop on each tine is partially effective in the tissues around the vertebral column. Inclusion of a thick and thin dental claw* is helpful for fenestration and for removal of disc material from beneath the spinal cord. A small curette is alternatively used for the latter purpose. I prefer large-gauge needles for lateral fenestration after hemilaminectomy because they penetrate the annulus, are replaced frequently, and thus remain sharp, and are less likely to force nucleus dorsally through a weakened annulus.

The shape and type of rongeurs depend on the

preference of the surgeon (Fig. 94–1). Friedman, Reiner, or other rongeurs may be substituted for Stille-Ruskin rongeurs. Small, double-action Lempert rongeurs are recommended for laminectomy and hemilaminectomy in toy animals but are not strong enough for use in large dachshunds. Frazier suction tips may be attached to suction tubing or replaced by other suction apparatus with variable and controllable vacuum.

Several other instruments are beneficial in specific patients and may be packed separately. A bulb syringe is useful for maintaining lavage of the surgical site without damaging neural tissue with the moistened sponge.[22] In larger breeds and in ventral decompression, Love-Kerrison bone-cutting forceps are helpful. The instrument may be 6 to 8 mm for large dogs but small (2 to 3 mm) and with a very thin foot plate for small animals.

Several companies manufacture power drills.* The equipment for neurosurgery should be air- or nitrogen-driven and of high speed. Power packs that convert for use as high-speed drills and that have reduction gears for orthopedic drill bits and screw-

---

*Swaim Fenestration Instrument, Richards Instruments Co.

*Stryker, Zimmer Manufacturing Co., Warsaw, IN; 3M Company, Santa Barbara, CA.

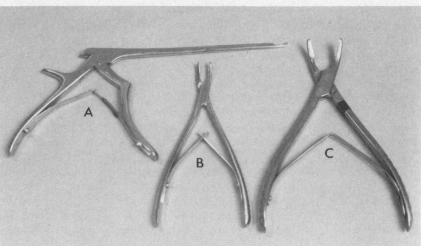

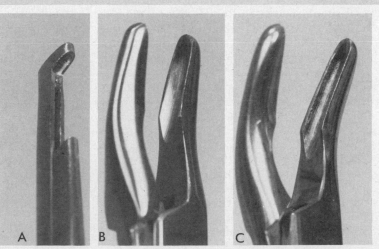

Figure 94–1. Representative rongeurs used in neurosurgery. *A,* Kerrison. *B,* Lempert. *C,* Ruskin.

drivers are available and provide a dual purpose at minimal added cost.[8] Conversions are similarly available for craniotomy instruments. At least two sizes of burrs are needed if power equipment is used for laminectomy: a pineapple-shaped 3- to 4-mm burr and a 1.5- to 2-mm round burr. Burrs should not be reused because of the potential of added heat and trauma to the spinal cord.

Specific fixation devices needed for repair of fractures and dislocations are described in Chapter 97.

Craniotomies are rarely performed on the dog and cat (see Chapter 99). The additional instruments needed for craniotomy *per se* are used for retraction of the brain and meninges. Craniotomy may be performed with a cranial drill (Stille or comparable) to preplace four holes; the flap is made with a Gigli wire saw and handles. A grooved director is essential to pass the Gigli wire from one drill hole to the next. The animal's head must be firmly fixed in a head holder. When power equipment is available, a craniotome or craniotomy adapter may be used through a craniotomy burr hole to form the bone flap. The power equipment is also used to drill wire holes at the sides of the flap and craniotomy incisions so that the flap may be repositioned during closure.

Other items needed in addition to the standard neurosurgery pack are a dura hook, 4-0 or 5-0 sutures, a smooth blade retractor, and cotton flannel for hemostasis. Some surgeons prefer to use silver microvascular clips for ligation of meningeal and cortical vessels. An electroscalpel with output intensity controls and a needle blade are nearly essential for incision of the brain parenchyma.

The surgical instruments necessary for peripheral nerve repair are described in Chapter 95. They are small and lack teeth in the tines to reduce trauma. Microvascular instruments are excellent if available.

POSTOPERATIVE CARE

Vertebral and cranial immobilization is rarely needed after fenestration or decompression. A firm bandage providing moderate support is indicated for two to three days. The bandage should not be too tight and should not extend under the mandible so as to cause dyspnea. Such immobilization is necessary for 7 to 14 days after repair of fracture-dislocation of the vertebral column and may occasionally be the only immobilization needed.

The main postoperative concerns other than immobilization are physical therapy and care of urinary function. The latter is the most important. Urinary retention and secondary cystitis are common in paralyzed animals. The bladder must be palpated and, if necessary, expressed or catheterized at least three times daily. Many paralyzed animals develop a bladder that evacuates automatically five to seven days after the onset of paralysis. This reflex phenomenon results in apparent urination when sufficient urine expands the bladder wall or when abdominal pressure is applied. The volume expelled may suggest voluntary emptying; incomplete emptying and retention of more than 15 to 20 cc of urine indicate that the urination is reflexive and not voluntary.[14]

Partial reflex urination also occurs as a delayed phenomenon in lesions of the sacrum or pelvic plexus. The animal may have overflow incontinence or may urinate in "spurts," particularly in response to manual pressure on the bladder. The volume excreted, however, is always small, with a large volume retained.

Frequent and thorough emptying of the bladder is accompanied by frequent bathing to prevent urine scalds and administration of systemic antibiotics to prevent or treat urinary tract infection. In some paraplegic animals, urinary retention may be accompanied by difficulty in expressing the bladder. This form of dyssynergia results from centrally or peripherally mediated parasympathetic deficiency and abnormal urethral tone. Recent evidence suggests that the latter results from alpha-adrenergic stimulation of the urethral continence zone and skeletal muscle and not from excessive pudendal nerve stimulation.[3, 9] The unique innervation of skeletal muscle by autonomic sympathetic fibers is supported by clinical and experimental reduction in urethral tone with alpha-adrenergic blocking agents (phenoxybenzamine).[3, 9, 14] Fecal retention should be treated by enema.

Physical therapy consists of repeated passive manipulation of the paretic limbs and encouragement of voluntary activity. The former should be performed for five to ten minutes three times daily and should include the full range of joint motions. Active and passive motion are encouraged by a water bath, whirlpool, or sling support until the animal stands and takes a few steps. The warm-water whirlpool or bath is beneficial because it facilitates passive movement, encourages active movement by reducing the weight born by paretic limbs, cleanses the skin, and reduces scalding and the tendency to form pressure sores. Whirlpool therapy can begin two to three days after surgery if the incision is covered with collodion. An effective and safe germicide, such as povidone iodine, is used routinely in the whirlpool.

Sling supports and walking with the rear limbs and trunk supported by a towel are also useful in maintaining muscle mass and joint mobility and encouraging walking. Some clinicians encourage the use of a paraplegic cart* during recovery[19]; the mobility achieved without exercise of the affected limbs appears to contradict this recommendation.

Other forms of physical therapy include diathermy, heating pads or warm towels, and ultrasound. None is curative, but the proper use of each may add to the physical comfort of the patient.

Lastly, the patient should be observed for signs of gastrointestinal distress. Spinal trauma in the form of fracture or disc herniation, decompressive laminectomy, or hemilaminectomy and adrenocorticoste-

---

*K-9 Cart Company, Berwyn, PA.

roids, particularly in high and prolonged doses, may produce gastric irritation and ulceration. Treatment for this complication should be instituted as soon as diarrhea or vomiting occurs and should be vigorously pursued. Treatment for shock may be necessary in severely affected patients. Because this complication is more likely with high and repeated doses of corticosteroids, I prefer a single injection of dexamethasone (0.5 to 1.0 mg/kg body weight) once at the time of surgery only, unless serious complications occur.

1. Brown, N. O., Helphrey, M. L., and Prata, R. G.: Thoracolumbar disc disease in the dog: A retrospective analysis of 187 cases. J. Am. Anim. Hosp. Assoc. 13:665, 1977.
2. Dillon, A. R., Sorjonen, D. C., Power, R. D., and Spano, J. S.: Effect of dexamethasone and surgical hypotension on hepatic enzyme and morphology of dogs. Am. J. Vet. Res. in press.
3. Elbadawi, A., and Schenk, E.: New theory of innervation of bladder musculature. IV. Innervation of vesicourethral junction and external urethral sphincter. J. Urol. 111:613, 1974.
4. Fundquist, B.: Decompressive laminectomy in thoraco-lumbar disc protrusion with paraplegia in the dog. J. Small Anim. Pract. 11:445, 1970.
5. Gage, E. D.: Modifications in dorsolateral hemilaminectomy and disc fenestration in the dog. J. Am. Anim. Hosp. Assoc. 11:407, 1975.
6. Hoerlein, B. F.: The treatment of intervertebral disc protrusions in the dog. Proc. Am. Vet. Med. Assoc., 1952, p. 206.
7. Hoerlein, B. F.: Canine Neurology, 3rd ed. W. B. Saunders, Philadelphia, 1978, p. 209.
8. Hurov, L.: Handbook of Veterinary Surgical Instruments and Glossary of Surgical Terms. W. B. Saunders, Philadelphia, 1978.
9. Khanna, O. P., Heber, D., and Gonick, P.: Cholinergic and
10. Knecht, C. D.: Results of delayed hemilaminectomy in intervertebral disc protrusion. J. Am. Anim. Hosp. Assoc. 7:346, 1971.
11. Knecht, C. D.: Results of surgical treatment for thoracolumbar disc protrusion. J. Small Anim. Pract. 13:449, 1972.
12. Knecht, C. D., Allen, A. R., Williams, D. J., and Johnson, J. H.: Fundamental Techniques in Veterinary Surgery, 2nd ed. W. B. Saunders, Philadelphia, 1981.
13. Martin, J. G.: The feasibility of delayed surgery in intervertebral disc protrusion causing paraplegia and paresis. Proc. 36th Ann. Mtg. Am. Anim. Hosp. Assoc., 1969, p. 423.
14. Moreau, P. M.: Neurogenic disorders of micturition in the dog and cat. Comp. Cont. Ed. 4:12, 1982.
15. Parent, J.: Effects of dexamethasone on pancreatic tissue and on serum amylase and lipase activities in dogs. J. Am. Vet. Med. 108:743, 1982.
16. Prata, R. G.: Neurosurgical treatment of thorocolumbar disks: The rationale and value of laminectomy with concomitant disk removal. J. Am. Anim. Hosp. Assoc. 17:17, 1981.
17. Redding, R. W.: Laminectomy in the dog. Am. J. Vet. Res. 12:123, 1951.
18. Shores, A.: Intervertebral disc syndrome in the dog. Part III. Thoracolumbar surgery. Comp. Cont. Ed. 4:1, 1982.
19. Short, T. R.: Experiences with a mobile support for paraplagic dogs. J. Am. Vet. Med. Assoc. 152:973, 1968.
20. Swaim, S. F.: Ventral decompression of the cervical spinal cord in the dog. J. Am. Vet. Med. Assoc. 162:276, 1973.
21. Swaim, S. F.: A rongeuring technique for performing thoracolumbar hemilaminectomy. Vet. Med. Small Anim. Clin. 71:172, 1976.
22. Tator, C. H., and Deeke, L.: Value of normothermic perfusion, hypothermic perfusion and durotomy in the treatment of experimental acute spinal cord trauma. J. Neurosurg. 19:52, 1973.
23. Trotter, E. J., Brasmer, T. H., and de Lahunta, A.: Modified deep dorsal laminectomy in the dog. Cornell Vet. 65:402, 1975.

adrenergic neuroreceptors in urinary tract of female dogs. J. Urol. 5:616, 1975.

Chapter **95** # Surgical Diseases of Peripheral Nerves

Stephen T. Simpson, Joe N. Kornegay, and Marc R. Raffe

AVULSION AND TRAUMATIC LESIONS OF PERIPHERAL NERVES

Brachial Avulsion

Brachial plexus lesions resulting from trauma are relatively common complex neuropathies in the dog and less common in the cat.[20] Traumatic radial nerve paralysis is the most common diagnosis made. Radiographs of the affected limb often reveal no abnormalities.

The traumatic injury is usually abduction. A caudoventral displacement of the dorsal border of the scapula results in severe abduction of the brachial plexus.[63] In humans, a severe anterior and inferior displacement of the scapulohumeral joint results in

brachial root avulsion by stretching of the brachial plexus across the humeral head.[146] In dogs, this same directional displacement (caudoventral) of the shoulder joint usually results in avulsion of the caudal brachial plexus roots.

Penetrating injuries of the brachial plexus are rare but when present may have less severe neurological findings. Major blood vessels in the axilla are often concurrently affected, resulting in extensive hemorrhage that may be of more immediate concern than the neuropathy.

Trauma to the shoulder may result in severe traction of the brachial plexus. The traction causes axonal fragmentation within an intact perineural sheath or tearing of the perineural sheath. The tension on the brachial plexus is directed through the intervertebral

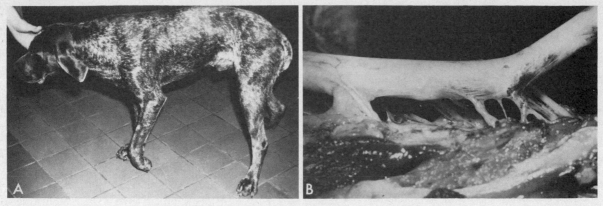

Figure 95–1. *A*, A mature German short-haired pointer after receiving a severe abducting traction injury to the left forelimb exhibiting the typical stance of a complete brachial avulsion. *B*, Dissected spinal cord of same dog demonstrating the absence of nerve roots of the left brachial plexus.

foramen, resulting in nerve root avulsion. Nerve root avulsion may cause transient spinal cord damage, which is reflected in the other limbs. The spinal cord signs usually resolve within one to three days.

Brachial plexus damage may manifest as partial or complete functional loss of one limb. The most common presentation is a complete plexus lesion. If any portion of the plexus remains intact, the rostral portion is more often spared, leaving a functional suprascapular or musculocutaneous nerve.[142] Occasionally the rostral end of the plexus is more severely affected, leaving a partially functional caudal brachial plexus.

Brachial avulsion patients are presented with or without a history of trauma. Physical findings supportive of an automobile accident include grease, scrapes, or road burns, and abraided toe nails. More complex injuries such as open wounds, internal injuries, and fractures provide the diagnosis of trauma.

In evaluation of a patient with a traumatic brachial plexus lesion, many physical examination techniques must be used. Careful palpation of the axillary region

of the affected limb ensures that no primary orthopedic disease is present. A neurological examination will reveal distinct findings indicative of brachial avulsion. The most obvious neurological defect is the profound loss of motor function of the limb. Typically, there is no ability to extend the carpus and digits and the elbow is "dropped" below its usual level. If the rostral portion of the brachial plexus is relatively spared, the elbow may be sufficiently flexed to hold the paw above the ground. If the brachial plexus lesion is more severe, the dorsum of the paw touches the ground and the paw is dragged (Fig. 95–1). Some forward movement of the shoulder joint may be evident when the patient uses the brachiocephalic muscle.

The sensory deficits are less obvious. The extent of the sensory deficits depends on the extent of the root lesions. Most cases of brachial avulsion produce anesthesia in the antebrachium below the elbow (Fig. 95–2A). If the musculocutaneous nerve roots are spared, a thin strip of innervated skin may be detected on the medial surface of the antebrachium

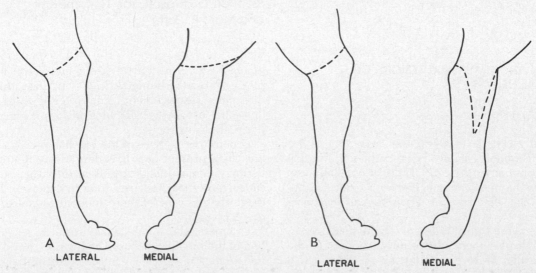

LATERAL   MEDIAL   LATERAL   MEDIAL

Figure 95–2. Areas of densensitized skin (hatched). *A*, complete brachial avulsion. *B*, Partial brachial avulsion (sparing of the musculocutaneous nerve).

distally to a level just above the carpus (Fig. 95–2). This area of skin is usually hypesthetic or anesthetic, depending on the degree of brachial root avulsion. The caudolateral aspect of the brachium is not desensitized in brachial avulsions.[57] This portion of skin is innervated by thoracic nerve roots not involved with avulsion lesions. The lateral aspect of the brachium may exhibit hypesthesia or anesthesia when the axillary nerve is affected.

Additional neurological signs include defects in nerves that supply the motor limb of the panniculus reflex and the sympathetic nerves to the face and eyes. The lateral thoracic nerve innervates the cutaneous trunci muscle. If the C8 and T1 nerve roots are avulsed, the lateral thoracic nerve is involved, and the panniculus reflex is absent on the affected side. A contralateral reflex may be observed when the affected side is stimulated. The first and second thoracic nerve roots also supply a large portion of sympathetic preganglionic fibers to the eye. An avulsion involving these nerve roots causes a partial sympathetic paralysis to the ipsilateral eye known as a partial Horner's syndrome. Miosis (constriction) of the ipsilateral pupil occurs. Enophthalmus and narrowed orbital fissure are other signs of sympathetic paralysis, but they are not always observed with brachial avulsions.

Penetrating injuries to the brachial plexus are usually not as severe or complete as avulsion injuries, because only a few nerves may be affected. The lateral thoracic and sympathetic nerves are not as likely to be affected, so the panniculus reflex and sympathetic function usually remain intact.

Electrodiagnostic testing is often useful in determining the extent of a brachial avulsion. A high index of suspicion is present when clinical signs of distal limb anesthesia, ipsilateral sympathetic paralysis to the eye, and an ipsilateral panniculus deficit concurrent with typical motor signs are found. Nearly all animals with brachial avulsion have nonfunctional radial, median, and ulnar nerves.[142] Axillary and musculocutaneous nerves are frequently, but not always, involved. In those patients with musculocutaneous sparing, an electromyogram (EMG) can determine satisfactory function within the biceps brachii and brachialis muscles, even though triceps muscles and carpal extensors and flexors are not functional.

Nerve conduction studies are not as valuable in brachial avulsions, but they can help to determine whether any integrity remains in median or ulnar nerves or the sensory radial nerves.[57] Inexcitable radial nerves indicate a poor prognosis for spontaneous return of neurologic function.[5] H wave reflex evaluation may be helpful in some cases. Spinal-evoked potentials can be employed to determine return of sensory function. These determinations may be of value, particularly in stoic patients or in ones that are long standing and when it is necessary to know the full extent of the lesion to decide on surgical techniques.

Salvage Procedures for Brachial Avulsion

Attempts to salvage the limb can be made in patients with incomplete brachial avulsions. In most avulsion patients, the elbow and carpal extension function is totally lost, but if elbow flexion is adequate the patient may be a candidate for surgery.

It is necessary to fix the carpus in a walking position. Carpal anthrodesis[72] is described in Chapter 160.

To reestablish some function to the elbow it is necessary to provide extension or supporting ability with the musculature that remains functional. Brachial avulsions that spare musculocutaneous function may be salvagable with surgery. The musculocutaneous nerve innervates the flexors of the elbow, the biceps brachii, and the brachialis muscles. Treatment involves tendon transposition of one of the muscle insertions to provide some extension stability to the elbow.

Brachialis tendon transposition has been described.[84] From a lateral approach, the tendon of insertion of the brachialis muscle is located and severed deep to the region of the extensor carpi radialis. The tendon and muscle are partially elevated from the spiral groove and redirected beneath the lateral head of the triceps (Fig. 95–3). The tendon is attached to the olecranon through a preplaced hole by stainless steel wires.

Partial extensor function may be regained by transposition of the biceps brachii tendon[10, 73, 84] through a medial approach parallel to the humerus to expose the biceps brachii. The tendon of insertion is located deeply between the extensor carpi radialis and pronator teres muscles. Care must be exercised to avoid the brachial artery, median veins, and several collateral branches of each. Part of the tendon of insertion of the biceps brachii is in common with the brachialis tendon, which is left intact. After the tendons of attachment are severed, the muscle is carefully freed

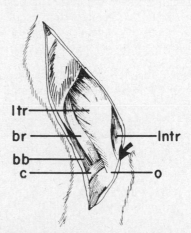

Figure 95–3. Transplantation of the brachialis tendon to the olecranon. Lateral approach. *br,* Brachialis muscle; *bb,* biceps brachii muscle; *o,* olecranon; *lntr,* long head, triceps muscle; *ltr,* lateral head, triceps muscle; *c,* extensor carpi radialis muscle. Site of attachment (*arrow*).

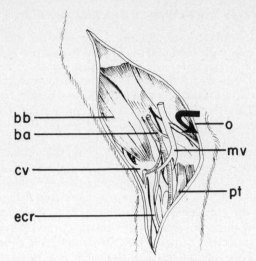

Figure 95–4. Transplantation of the biceps brachii tendon of insertion. Medial approach. *bb*, Biceps brachii; *ba*, brachial artery; *cv*, cephalic vein; *ecr*, extensor carpi radialis; *pt*, pronator teres; *mv*, median vein; *o*, olecranon. Site of attachment (*arrow*).

and redirected more caudally, to overlie the brachial artery and median vein (Fig. 95–4), and is attached to the olecranon by stainless steel wire. Both methods of tendon transposition require external support for two weeks and then light range-of-motion exercises and gradual increases in limb use over the following two weeks.

Postoperative care includes preservation of muscle and skin that has been denervated. Denervated skin loses tensile strength and ability to respond to abrasions. Massage of muscle and skin and prompt attention to minor skin lesions is important in the postoperative care of any denervated skin.

Complications resulting from the avulsion or surgery are considerable and probably are responsible for the high failure rate. Patient selection is of paramount importance. Operations performed on avulsions that involve the entire plexus including the musculocutaneous nerve will fail. The best patient is one with a partial avulsion with musculocutaneous innervation. If sensory function distal to the elbow is spared, surgical intervention may afford better success.

Apart from routine complications associated with tendon surgery, such as dehiscence and infection, the avulsion causes sensory dennervation in the distal limb. Same patients can successfully reinnervate the distal limb and develop adequate sensory perception in the limb. Many patients fail to reinnervate and never develop sensory perception. Failure to innervate produces a limb that is susceptible to severe laceration with hemorrhage, fracture, or crushing without the animal's knowledge.

Self-mutilation is another complication related to denervation. It frequently begins one to three weeks following injury. Occasionally, it may begin after a longer delay. Early self-mutilation probably represents early neuroma formation and aberrant sensation or reinnervation of sensory nerves. Later self-mutilation probably occurs because of the so-called phan-

tom limb syndrome or the perception of abnormal referred sensation, which is probably due to neuroma formation or delayed aberrant reinnervation.

Distal Radial Nerve Paralysis

The distal radial nerve is commonly injured when the humerus is fractured. Because of the fracture and resultant paralysis of carpal extension this injury appears quite similar to and may occur simultaneously with a brachial avulsion. Specific differences from avulsions of the brachial plexus include the lack of Horner's syndrome and the presence of a panniculus reflex. Sensory deficits are not as severe. Median and ulnar nerve function is retained, allowing for reflex and conscious sensory preception from the palmar and lateral portions of the antebrachium and paw.

If these clinical signs remain, radial nerve damage should be suspected. Primary repair of the severed nerve is the optimal surgical treatment. Peripheral nerve anastomosis is discussed later in this chapter.

If the injury is too severe for anastomosis or if anastomosis fails, salvage techniques to supply carpal extension have been described, including (1) anastomosis of the functional flexor carpi radialis tendon with the nonfunctional common digital extensor, (2) transposition of the flexor carpi radialis with a side-to-side anastomosis to the common digital extensor[10] and (3) transposition of both tendons with end-to-end anastomosis.[143]

Fibular Nerve Paralysis

The fibular (peroneal) nerve is a distal branch of the ischiatic nerve. It is susceptible to injury either as a fascicle of the ischiatic nerve or as the fibular nerve more distally. Common causes of fibular nerve injury include trauma associated with fractured pelvis, dislocated coxofemoral joint, and fractured femur, and iatrogenic injury due to intramuscular injections. Entrapment of the ischiatic or fibular nerve as a result of injury may also occur. Signs of entrapment usually are more progressive and chronic and have a delayed onset.

Signs of fibular paralysis include gait abnormalities such as dorsal knuckling of the affected limb, and dragging and abrading the foot, often without knowledge of any wound. Sensory deficiencies can usually be detected over the dorsum of the metatarsal and phalangeal area, and decreased sensation may be evident over the dorsolateral aspect below the stifle joint.

As with radial nerve paralysis, surgical intervention is directed to the location of the nerve injury or entrapment. If anastomotic techniques fail, tendon transposition may salvage the limb. Techniques for tendon transposition for fibular and ischiatic nerve damage have been described.[10, 91, 163] When fibular nerve damage exists alone, the long digital flexor tendon can be transferred to extend its force to the long digital extensor tendon by a side-to-side anastomosis.[10] If both fibular nerve and tibial nerve are injured in an ischiatic nerve palsy, the long digital flexor muscle is no longer innervated, and its transposition provides no useful function. A technique of tranposing the origin of the long digital extensor muscle to the vastus lateralis tendon of insertion has been described.[91] This procedure allows transfer of the vastus lateralis force to the long digital extensor and causes extension of the digits and partial flexion of the hock. Because extension of the digits is the primary result intended, talocrural immobilization or anthrodesis of the hock is recommended.[163]

LESIONS OF THE LUMBOSACRAL INTUMESCENCE AND CAUDA EQUINA

Lesions of the lumbosacral intumescence or cauda equina cause a characteristic clinical syndrome.[117, 156] Affected animals usually have paraspinal hyperesthesia, paraparesis, pelvic limb and perineal hyporeflexia, and urinary and fecal incontinence. Recognition of these clinical signs provides insight regarding their underlying etiology, as several diseases selectively involve the lumbosacral area.[117, 156, 158, 169] Because these diseases have a common neuroanatomic basis and share many diagnostic features,[46] they are discussed collectively. The pathogenesis, treatment, and distinguishing clinical and radiographic features of each disease are discussed separately.

Anatomy

Embryological development of the vertebral column and spinal cord are closely linked in all species.[68] However, the vertebral column grows at a slightly greater rate than the spinal cord. As a result, the spinal cord ends at the level of the vertebral body of L6 in dogs[75] and at L7 in cats.[104] Its terminal tip, the conus medullaris, is connected to the dural sac by a thread-like band, the filum terminale.

Because of the difference in their growth rates, a distinction is made between vertebral and cord segment numbers. Spinal cord segments generally are slightly cranial to the corresponding vertebrae.[46, 75, 104] This tendency is particularly pronounced in the lumbosacral area, where caudal lumbar, sacral, and coccygeal segments are closely clustered. In dogs, the last three lumbar segments are at the level of the body of L4; the sacral segments overlie the body of L5; and the coccygeal segments are at the level of the body of L6 (Fig. 95–5).[34, 46] Spinal cord segments are located slightly more caudally in cats.[104]

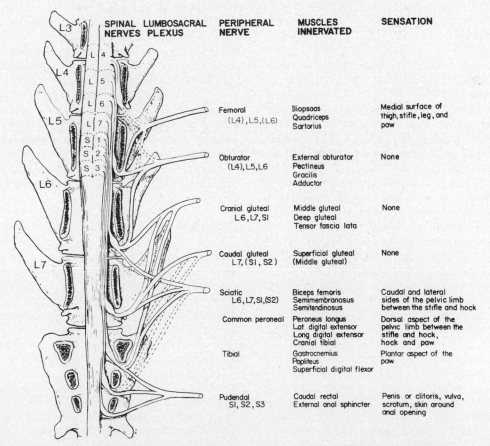

Figure 95–5. Muscles innervated by nerves of the dog's lumbosacral plexus and the sensory distribution of these nerves. (Modified from de Lahunta, A.: *Veterinary Neuroanatomy and Clinical Neurology*, 2nd ed. W. B. Saunders, Philadelphia, 1977.)

Spinal cord nerve roots are formed by axons that originate from spinal motor neurons (ventral roots) or peripheral sensory neurons (dorsal roots). A pair of roots demarcates each spinal cord segment. Roots from the lumbar, sacral, and coccygeal segments leave the spinal canal at the intervertebral foramina caudal to the vertebrae of the same number.[34, 46, 75, 104] Therefore, nerve roots that originate from cord segments positioned considerably cranial to the corresponding vertebrae must pass a considerable distance before exiting. The collection of spinal roots that occupy the vertebral canal caudal to the point of termination of the spinal cord is termed the cauda equina.

The swollen area of spinal cord from which the nerve roots of the lumbosacral plexus originate is referred to as the lumbosacral intumescence. Nerves of the lumbosacral plexus are responsible for innervation of the somatic musculature of the pelvic limb, urethra, and perineum (see Fig. 95–5).[34, 64] Deficits referable to the femoral, sciatic, and pudendal nerves or the spinal cord segments and nerve roots from which they originate are commonly encountered.[64] The femoral nerve is formed primarily by the fourth and fifth lumbar roots, the sciatic from the sixth and seventh lumbar and first sacral roots, and the pudendal from the sacral roots.[34] Muscles innervated by these nerves and their sensory distribution are shown in Figure 95–5.

Clinical Syndrome

Clinical signs of lesions of the lumbosacral intumescence or cauda equina vary according to the severity of the lesion.[117, 156, 158, 170] Mild compression or meningitis usually causes only paraspinal hyperesthesia. With further compression or extension of the inflammatory process to neural tissue, paraparesis, hyporeflexia and urinary-fecal incontinence occur. The nature of these additional deficits varies with the site of the lesion and whether or not the spinal cord, nerve roots, or both are affected. There often is concomitant lower and upper motor neuron paresis, i.e., the same lesion might cause lower motor neuron dysfunction referable to the origins of the femoral nerve and upper motor neuron dysfunction referable to the origins of the sciatic nerve.

Functional obliteration of the fourth and fifth lumbar spinal cord segments causes paraplegia, quadriceps femoris areflexia, complete anesthesia of the pelvic limbs, and loss of the micturition reflex. An identical lesion at the level of the seventh lumbar and first sacral segments spares the origins of the femoral nerve, so affected animals still have voluntary and reflex quadriceps femoris motor function and medial pelvic limb pain sensation. Nevertheless, this lesion is incapacitating because of loss of both voluntary and reflex biceps femoris motor function, lateral pelvic limb anesthesia, and loss of the micturition reflex. Functional obliteration of the second

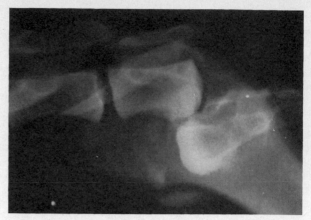

Figure 95–6. Lateral radiograph of the caudal vertebral column of a five-year-old male golden retriever with paraparesis and urinary incontinence that occurred after being hit by a car. There is dorsocaudal displacement of the L7 vertebra with respect to the sacrum. On neurological examination, the flexion reflex was absent bilaterally in the hind limbs and the patellar reflex was absent in the right leg. Involvement of the patellar reflex was attributed to the combined effects of hemorrhage and edema within spinal cord segments cranial to the vertebral luxation.

and third sacral spinal cord segments spares the origins of both the femoral and sciatic nerves, but loss of urinary and fecal continence due to urethral and anal sphincter denervation debilitates the animal.

Spinal nerve roots are often also affected by lesions of the lumbosacral spine. In fact, a spinal nerve root may be selectively compressed, resulting in radicular hyperesthesia and monoparesis. Therefore, in assessing the potential consequences of a vertebral lesion, consideration must be given to both the overlying spinal cord segments and the nerve roots. An additional factor that must be weighed is the potential concussive effects of the inciting injury. Traction placed on the spinal cord or nerve roots by sudden trauma may cause hemorrhage within segments cranial to the injury. As such, fractures of the sacrum or coccygeal vertebrae may be associated with deficits referable to lumbar spinal cord segments (Fig. 95–6).

Diagnosis

Radiography is the most important diagnostic tool for identifying lesions of the lumbosacral intumescence or cauda equina. However, care must be taken when interpreting survey radiographs of this area, as subclinical anomalies and developmental lesions of the lumbosacral spine are common.[115, 173] When results of radiography and neurological examination are incompatible, the radiographic lesion is of questionable significance, and positive contrast studies should be done. Contrast material may be injected into either the subarachnoid space (myelography),[174] epidural space (epidurography),[45] or intraosseous vertebral venous sinuses (vertebral venography.)[106] Myelography is restricted primarily to lesions at or cranial to the spinal cord termination.[174] Lesions overlying

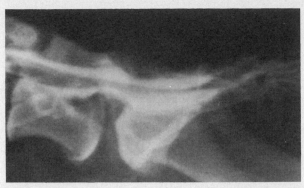

Figure 95–7. Epidurogram of the lumbosacral spine of a 12-year-old male dachshund with a two-month history of tail biting. The ventral dye column overlying the L7–S1 disc space is displaced dorsally. Herniated intervertebral disc material was recovered from this site at surgery.

the sacrum or coccygeal vertebrae may be delineated by epidurography[45] (Fig. 95–7) or venography.[106] However, results of both of these procedures may be falsely positive and therefore must be interpreted cautiously.[45, 106]

Electromyography is not essential but is an extremely helpful procedure for identification of lesions of the lumbosacral intumescence or cauda equina.[29, 58] When interpreted with clinical findings, the electromyographic pattern of denervation usually predicts the site of involvement correctly. This information is invaluable when there are no radiographic abnormalities or the clinical and radiographic findings are in conflict.

Diseases

Intervertebral disc herniation, vertebral neoplasia, and discospondylitis may involve the lumbosacral intumescence or nerve roots. Principles of diagnosis and treatment of these conditions are covered in their respective sections. This section deals only with those diseases that are unique to the lumbosacral area.

Syndromes referred to as lumbosacral malarticulation-malformation and lumbosacral stenosis are discussed separately even though they may represent the same entity. This is justified because they differ with regard to clinical signs and radiographic features, suggesting that they may differ in pathogenesis. Whereas lesions of lumbosacral malarticulation-malformation are acquired, the syndrome of lumbosacral stenosis may be developmental.

Lumbosacral Malarticulation-Malformation

Etiology and Pathogenesis. Neurological deficits due to lumbosacral malarticulation-malformation result from compression of nerve roots at the lumbosacral junction due to ventral displacement of the dorsal lamina of S1, proliferation of surrounding ligamentous tissue, or spondylosis at the L7-S1 intervertebral foramina.[117] Some dogs have concomitant

dorsal protrusion of the L7-S1 intervertebral disc. These changes presumably occur secondary to instability of the lumbosacral articulation. Although mechanisms responsible for this instability are not clear, the prevalence of lumbosacral malarticulation-malformation in large dogs suggests that stresses placed on the spine by increased size may play a role. This idea probably accounts for disproportionate involvement of German shepherds. However, a genetic basis for their predilection to this disease cannot be excluded.

Clinical Features. Lumbosacral malarticulation-malformation occurs in large dogs, particularly German shepherds. Thirteen of the 20 affected dogs in the only published series of cases were males.[117] Neurological deficits, which are related primarily to nerve roots contributing to the sciatic and pudendal nerves, include paraspinal hyperesthesia, paresis, flexor and perineal hyporeflexia, and urinary-fecal incontinence. The hindlimbs may be affected equally or asymmetrically. These signs usually are insidious in onset and progression.

Radiography. Affected dogs have variable changes at the lumbosacral junction (Fig. 95–8).[117] Most have evidence of spondylosis ventral or lateral to the vertebral bodies, some have ventral displacement of the body of S1 relative to L7, and some have dorsoventral narrowing of the sacral spinal canal. However, neurological deficits cannot automatically be attributed to these changes, because all are recognized in clinically normal dogs.[115, 173] Emphasis has been placed on the potential diagnostic value of calculating the *sacrovertebral* angle, formed at the point of

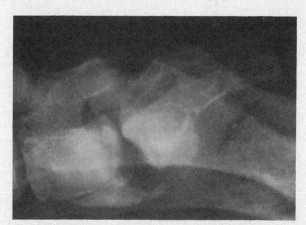

Figure 95–8. Lateral radiograph of the lumbosacral spine of a one-year-old male German shepherd with lumbosacral hyperesthesia and paraparesis. There is a new bone proliferation ventral to the L7 and sacral vertebral bodies. Evidence of sclerosis adjacent to the disc space suggests there may be new bone proliferation laterally as well. Narrowing and wedging of the L7–S1 disc space indicates disc protrusion. The ventral portion of the caudal end plate of L7 is misshapen, indicating maldevelopment or degenerative bone disease. Slight irregularity of the cortical surfaces of the L7 and S1 vertebral end plates is compatible with early discospondylitis. At necropsy, the right L7 spinal nerve root was trapped at the L7–S1 intervertebral foramina and there was no evidence of bone infection. When interpreted jointly, radiographic and pathological findings were consistent with lumbosacral malarticulation and malformation.

intersection of lines drawn parallel to the *dorsal* aspects of L7 and sacral vertebral bodies.[45, 117] In normal dogs of variable age and weight, the mean sacrovertebral angle was 160 degrees when the hindlimbs were positioned perpendicular to the spine and 154 degrees when they were extended caudally.[45] This angle reportedly approaches 180 degrees in dogs with neurological deficits referable to lumbosacral malarticulation-malformation.[117] However, this supposition was not verified by results of another study in which the *lumbosacral* angle formed at the point of intersection of lines drawn parallel to *ventral* aspects of the vertebral bodies of L7 and the sacrum was calculated.[173] The investigators of the latter study found no significant difference between the mean values for dogs with and without deficits referable to the cauda equina. All changes on survey radiographs, therefore, must be interpreted cautiously. Cauda equina compression must be verified by either exploratory surgery or contrast radiography.

Electromyography. Fibrillation potentials or other evidence of denervation may be identified in muscles innervated by nerves arising from the L7, sacral, and coccygeal roots.[117]

Treatment. Restriction of exercise and occasional administration of analgesics may result in temporary remission of clinical signs. However, most affected dogs have progressive cauda equina compression, so do not have lasting improvement subsequent to medical management. These dogs are treated most effectively with lumbosacral dorsal laminectomy in combination with foramenotomy at L7–S1, if an L7 root is trapped.[117] The approach to a lumbosacral dorsal laminectomy is described in Chapter 96. The dorsal laminae are removed with an air drill and bone rongeurs, with the vertebral pedicles and facets left intact if possible. After the cauda equina is exposed, the roots are gently dissected with a nerve root retractor, and fibrous adhesions should be removed. The L7 roots are followed to the L7–S1 foramina. If either nerve is trapped by bone or fibrous connective tissue, foramenotomy is needed. Foramenotomy at L7–S1 is done by removing the caudal articular facet and part of the pedicle of L7 so that the root is completely exposed as it leaves the spinal canal.[117] Removal of bone ventral to the foramen is restricted by the wing of the ilium.

Dogs with concomitant intervertebral disc herniation at L7–S1 may benefit from dorsal laminectomy alone.[117] To ensure recovery, however, the protruded disc should be removed. The cauda equina is retracted laterally with umbilical tape, and the dorsal longitudinal ligament and annulus fibrosus overlying the space are excised. Protruding nucleus pulposus is removed using a dental tartar scraper together with sharp excision. The laminectomy defect should be covered with an autologous fat graft to reduce the likelihood of cicatrix formation.[76] Stabilization is not required.

Postoperative Care. Antibiotics may be needed if there is bacterial cystitis. They should be selected according to bacterial sensitivity and continued for at least two weeks or longer if infection persists. The bladder is emptied at least three times daily if micturition is absent. Bladder emptying is usually accomplished manually, because urethral sphincter tone is decreased. The animal usually regains motor and urinary control at approximately the same time. The period that elapses before return of these functions varies directly with the duration of clinical involvement. Some return of function should occur within two to four weeks.

Lumbosacral Stenosis

Etiology and Pathogenesis. Although mechanisms responsible for lumbosacral stenosis are not clear, congenital vertebral lesions that restrict the diameter of the spinal canal at L6–L7, L7–S1, or both may contribute.[156] Vertebral changes that are presumably present at birth in affected dogs include shortening of the pedicles and thickening of the laminae and articular facets (Fig. 95–9). Although these changes initially may be subclinical, resultant attentuation of the spinal canal predisposes the cauda equina to compression by otherwise clinically insignificant proliferation of bone or fibrous tissue.

Similar developmental stenotic lesions occur at L4–L5 and L5–S1 in man.[16, 53, 59, 169] Selective involvement of these articulations in affected human patients has been attributed to stresses placed on the caudal lumbar spine because of lordosis. These stresses may cause enlargement and subluxation of the articular processes and ligamentum flavum hypertrophy. That affected dogs have similar proliferative lesions suggests that a similar pathogenetic mechanism may be responsible for their disproportionate lumbosacral involvement.[156]

Factors that may exacerbate clinical signs of lumbosacral stenosis in both affected dogs and man are extension of the lumbar spine[59, 156] and exercise.[156, 170] Extension of the lumbar spine displaces redundant

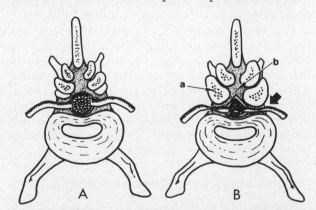

Figure 95–9. Transverse sections of normal (*A*) and stenotic (*B*) vertebrae. The spinal canal in *B* is narrowed because of thickening of the articular facets (*a*) and dorsal lamina (*b*). This has caused compression of both the spinal cord and an exiting spinal nerve root (arrow). (Reprinted with permission from Tarvin, G., and Prata, R. G.: Lumbosacral stenosis in dogs. J. Am. Vet. Med. Assoc. 177:154, 1980)

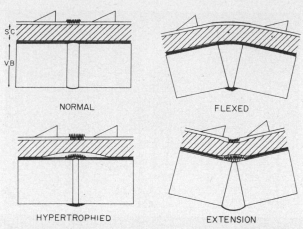

Figure 95–10. Effects of flexion and extension of the vertebral column when the spinal cord is compressed by hypertrophied ligamentous structures. Flexion stretches these structures, thus relieving the compression. The compressive effect of this redundant tissue is augmented by extension. The relative widths of the spinal canal (SC) and vertebral body (VB) may be used to assess the degree of stenosis. (Reprinted with permission from Tarvin, G., and Prata, R. G.: Lumbosacral stenosis in dogs. J. Am. Vet. Med. Assoc. *177*:154, 1980.)

ligamentous tissue into the spinal canal, causing further spinal cord or cauda equina compression (Fig. 95–10). The effect of exercise is attributed to a vascular phenomenon referred to as neurogenic intermittent claudication.[169] Exercise increases spinal cord blood flow, necessitating dilation of vessels that pass through the intervertebral foramina. Because the foramina already are narrowed, the dilation evidently causes further compression of the nerve roots and exacerbation of clinical signs.

Clinical Features. Unlike lumbosacral malarticulation-malformation, lumbosacral stenosis often affects small dogs. Of the 15 dogs included in the only published series of cases, four were toy or miniature poodles and two were beagles.[156] The nine males and six females were between three and eight years old. Clinical signs were similar to those of lumbosacral malarticulation-malformation with two exceptions: Lameness in dogs with lumbosacral stenosis worsened with exercise, and eight of these dogs had paresthesia as evidenced by self-mutilation of the tail or pelvic limbs.

Radiography. Findings on radiography usually were inconclusive.[156] Dorsoventral stenosis of the spinal canal at L6–L7 or L7–S1 or both often was apparent. Measurements of the ratio of spinal canal to vertebral body were not significantly different from those of a matched group of normal dogs. Results of myelography and intraosseous venography from one dog were reported. Myelography was inconclusive; compression at L7–S1 was demonstrated by venography.

Treatment. The preferred treatment is dorsal laminectomy and foramenotomy as for lumbosacral malarticulation-malformation.[156] Decompression may be necessary at both L6–L7 and L7–S1.

Anomalies

Animals are affected by numerous spinal anomalies. Those occurring from faulty closure of the neural tube are referred to collectively as spinal dysraphism.[50, 52, 89] Dysraphic lesions most commonly affect the caudal vertebral column and spinal cord,[51, 74, 88, 100, 120, 135, 170] so are discussed here. These lesions often cause severe incapacitation, necessitating euthanasia of the affected puppy or kitten. Others are subclinical, strictly cosmetic, or associated with only mild neurologic dysfunction. Neurological deficits caused by spinal dysraphism are not amenable to surgery. However, the veterinary surgeon may be asked to correct cosmetic defects or to close open lesions that predispose the affected animal to infection.

Embryology. The central nervous system develops from specialized ectoderm (neuroectoderm) that lies dorsal to the notochord throughout the axis of the embryo.[3] This neuroectoderm differentiates to form the neural tube, from which the ventricular system and central canal of the spinal cord develop. Neural tube development requires three phases: neurulation, caudal canalization, and regression.[89] *Neurulation* entails formation and subsequent fusion of the neural folds to form the neural tube cranial to the cranial lumbar area. The neural tube caudal to this point is formed through *canalization* of a mass of undifferentiated neuroectoderm called the tail bud. This process is less precise than neurulation, accounting for the preponderance of spinal anomalies involving the caudal lumbar, sacral, and coccygeal spine. The final phase, *regression,* occurs because of the combined effects of dedifferentiation of some cells of the caudal neural tube and the disproportionate growth rates of the vertebral column and the neural tube. As a result, the caudal neural tube migrates cranially to assume its permanent position within the spinal canal.

The vertebrae and epaxial musculature develop from mesoderm surrounding the notochord.[4] This mesoderm is condensed to form paired segments termed somites. The dorsomedial portion of each somite (myotome) forms the paravertebral skeletal muscles. Vertebrae are formed from the ventromedial portion of the somite (sclerotome). Normal differentiation of these mesodermal tissues and the overlying skin depends on proper development of the neural tube.[68] Therefore, defective neural tube formation is often associated with dermal clefts and vertebral anomalies.

Pathogenesis. Theories of abnormal embryogenesis proposed to explain dysraphic lesions involve two mechanisms: (1) overgrowth of neural tube cells, resulting in eversion of the neural folds and failure of neural tube closure, and (2) reopening of the formed neural tube due to either increased intraluminal pressure (hydrodynamic theory)[52] or development of a cleft on the dorsal midline of the neural tube for unexplained reasons (neuroschisis theory).[119]

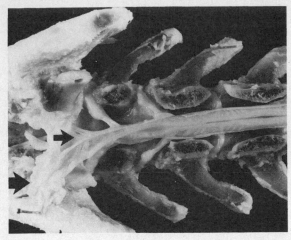

Figure 95–11. Caudal vertebral column, spinal cord, and cauda equina from a two-month-old English bulldog with urinary-fecal incontinence since birth. Portions of the cauda equina extend dorsally into a meningeal sac (large arrow); sacral roots on the left side are hypoplastic (small arrow); and a dorsal longitudinal spinal cord cleft is present. A diagnosis of meningomyelocele with associated myeloschisis was made.

Both mechanisms probably contribute to spinal dysraphism.

Clinicopathological Features. The most common expression of spinal dysraphism in animals is protrusion of meninges alone (meningocele) or together with spinal cord (meningomyelocele) through a defect in the overlying vertebral arches (Fig. 95–11).[74, 120, 170] Defective closure of the vertebral arches with meningeal or spinal herniation is called spina bifida aperta (cystica, manifesta).[170] The herniated tissue may be covered by skin or exposed to the environment. Communication between the cyst and subarachnoid space usually can be demonstrated radiographically (Fig. 95–12). When the vertebral defect occurs alone, the lesion is termed spina bifida occulta.[100] Sacrococcygeal vertebral agenesis is often identified with spina bifida, particularly in the Manx cat.[74, 88, 135]

Additional dysplastic spinal lesions often occur with

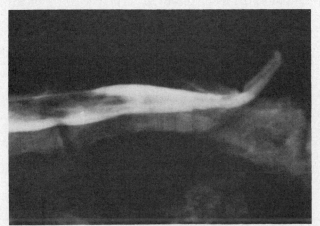

Figure 95–12. Lateral myelogram of the caudal vertebral column of a kitten with urinary-fecal incontinence since birth. Contrast material extends dorsally into the subcutis because of communication between the subarachnoid space and a meningomyelocele. The L7 and sacral vertebral bodies are fused.

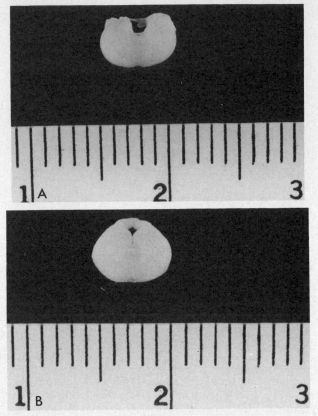

Figure 95–13. Transverse section of spinal cord from the dog in Figure 95–11. *A,* Area of myeloschisis. The dorsal cleft extends to the level of the central canal (centimeter scale). *B,* Cranial to area of myeloschisis. There is a syrinx within the dorsal funiculi (centimeter scale).

spina bifida in animals. Spinal clefts resulting from faulty neural tube closure (myeloschisis) extend cranially for a considerable distance (Figs. 95–11 and 95–13), and may communicate with a dilated central canal (hydromyelia)[88, 170] or cystic spaces within the spinal parenchyma (syringomyelia) (see Fig. 95–13).[88, 100, 170] Caudal lumbar, sacral, and coccygeal spinal cord segments and nerve roots are often malformed or misdirected.[88, 135] The spinal cord may also extend further caudally in the spinal canal because of faulty regression. Division of the spinal cord into halves by a bony spicule or fibrous band (diastematomyelia) commonly occurs in humans with spina bifida[50] and was reported in one Manx cat.[74] Some affected animals have had hydrocephalus in addition to their spinal lesions. However, cerebral features of the Arnold-Chiari syndrome[50] that often accompany spina bifida aperta in humans have not been identified in animals.

Spina bifida occulta/aperta and associated dysplastic spinal cord lesions occur most commonly in English bulldogs[120, 170] and Manx cats.[74, 88, 100] Affected animals often are paraparetic and have urinary or fecal incontinence. Further examination usually reveals evidence of hyporeflexia and loss of sensation over the dermal distribution of the affected spinal cord segments or nerve roots. There may be a cleft in the overlying skin,[51] or the hair at this site may be whorled.[170] The musculature adjacent to the caudal spine and that of the pelvic limbs usually is atrophic.[51, 170]

An additional syndrome attributed to spinal dysraphism occurs in Weimaraners.[105] Affected puppies usually are atactic by four to six weeks of age. The ataxia is usually manifested by symmetrical advancement of the hindlimbs at gait referred to as "bunny-hopping." These signs usually are static and not debilitating. At necropsy, the neural tube is closed but there often is evidence of hydrosyringomyelia.

Treatment. Neurological deficits due to spinal dysraphism do not respond to treatment. When given this information, most owners request euthanasia of severely affected animals. To do otherwise is impractical, because long-term management of these animals is extremely difficult. Hence, surgical management of animals with spina bifida aperta has not been reported. Operative procedures used in the treatment of affected human infants involve return of the herniated neural tissue to the spinal canal, reconstruction of the dural sac, and closure of the overlying dermal cleft.[50]

Animals with subclinical or nondebilitating dysraphic lesions usually do not need therapy. However, spinal meningocele may require removal if the dural sac is exposed or is objectionable to the owner. Techniques for management of meningoceles of human infants are applicable.[50] The meningocele sac should be opened to expose the interior of the spinal canal and to allow careful dissection of adherent neural tissue. Redundant dura is removed, and the dural edges are closed with 5–0 nylon suture using a continuous pattern. The apposed dura is covered with a layer of paraspinous fascia to insure a tight junction. Skin closure is routine.

Sacrococcygeal Fractures and Luxations

Etiology and Pathogenesis. Vertebral fractures usually occur adjacent to points of rigid spinal stability such as the sacroiliac articulation. Lumbosacral and sacrococcygeal luxations and fractures of the sacrum and first three coccygeal vertebrae collectively accounted for 27.3 per cent of traumatic vertebral lesions of dogs and cats in one study.[44] Several factors contribute to neurological deficits subsequent to these lesions. Vertebral displacement may sever or compress the terminal spinal cord or nerve roots. Vessels are torn, and extradural hemorrhage and further compression occur. Traction on the spinal cord as a result of sudden nerve root avulsion may also cause parenchymal hemorrhage and edema both at and distal to the injury. Therefore, animals with vertebral fractures occasionally have neurological deficits that cannot be explained by injury of either overlying spinal cord segments or nerve roots (Figs. 95–6 and 95–14).

Clinical Features. Neurological deficits resulting from fractures in this area are acute and usually static, unless further displacement occurs.[158] Verte-

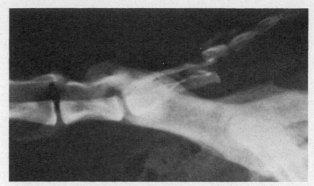

Figure 95–14. Lateral radiograph of the caudal vertebral column of a two-year-old female domestic cat. The cat had been hit by a car and had paraplegia and hind limb and perineal areflexia. There is sacrococcygeal luxation. Involvement of the hind limbs was attributed to the combined effects of hemorrhage and edema within spinal cord segments cranial to the site of vertebral luxation.

bral malalignment is usually apparent on radiographic evaluation (see Fig. 95–14). The distribution of lower motor neuron and sensory deficits usually reflects the radiographic level of injury. However, parenchymal hemorrhage and edema distant to the vertebral lesion may cause additional deficits. Caudal lumbar fractures and lumbosacral subluxations usually cause pelvic limb motor deficits and urinary incontinence, because of either interference with the micturition reflex or urethral sphincter denervation or both. Fractures of the sacrum produce urinary incontinence and may also cause pelvic limb paresis, if the S1 nerve root is involved or there is parenchymal hemorrhage. Coccygeal fractures often cause only paralysis of the tail; however, urinary incontinence and pelvic limb deficits may occur if severe traction has been placed on the terminal spinal cord, causing avulsion of sacral nerve roots.

Treatment. Management of caudal lumbar fractures, lumbosacral luxations, and sacroiliac separations is discussed in Chapter 97. Animals with sacrococcygeal fractures may be candidates for surgery.[158] Neurological deficits resulting from these lesions are often irreversible regardless of therapy. However, dorsal laminectomy allows observation of the extent of injury and removal of extradural hemorrhage and bone fragments. The approach to the sacral spinal column is similar to the lumbosacral approach described in Chapter 96. Extra precautions must be taken to avoid damage of nerve roots due to displacement of unstable bone fragments. The dorsal laminae of affected vertebrae are removed using either bone rongeurs or an air drill. Nerve roots are observed, and compressive bone fragments and hemorrhage are removed. If the nerve roots are intact, fractures may be stabilized (see Chapter 97). When the coccygeal roots are severed, the involved vertebra(e) still may be stabilized and the tail preserved. However, proximal denervation impedes retraction of the tail during defecation, and there is soiling of the tail and perineum. Paresthesia also may develop distal to the point of injury, resulting in self-mutilation. For these reasons, the denervated tail should be amputated at the time of initial surgery (see Section 18).

Postoperative Care. When the tail is amputated distally, the stump should be bandaged for several days. If the micturition reflex is absent, the bladder is emptied manually at least three times daily, because urethral sphincter tone is decreased. The owner should be cautioned about potential irreversibility of neurological deficits, especially if lumbar and sacral nerve root severance has been documented at surgery.

SURGICAL REPAIR OF PERIPHERAL NERVES

General Principles

Successful results in peripheral nerve surgery come from familiarity with technical surgical concepts, an understanding of tissue biology, appropriate surgical instruments, practice, and patience. Attention to detail and the desire to spend a few extra moments to obtain technical perfection are rewarded by a higher rate of success and less time lost in repeat exploratory procedures.

The decisions most important to the surgeon and the patient are whether or not surgery should be performed and when surgery should be done. Exploratory surgery is justified in five instances: (1) to establish an accurate diagnosis in cases when ancillary clinical diagnostic methods have been inconclusive or contradictory, and to observe the extent and severity of the lesion; (2) when incomplete loss of function has occurred, but no clinical improvement is evident; (3) when injury has occurred more than three weeks prior to surgery and no function has returned; (4) to improve function of the nerve by surgical means, and (5) to establish a prognosis.[131, 145, 151]

Judgment as to probable etiology of the lesion aids in deciding whether surgery is justified. Penetrating external wounds that transect nerve trunks in a focal area and fractures that lacerate nerve tissue are examples of injuries amenable to surgical intervention. Surgical exploration may not be appropriate for injuries to extensive areas of nerve by traction to a nerve trunk or blunt injury to a large zone of soft tissue.[151]

Classification of the injury may include clinical assessment of the extent of anatomical disruption. The extent of injury may be deduced from history, physical examination, and ancillary diagnostic techniques, and the information may be used to judge whether the injury is amenable to surgical exploration. Mild functional injury from blunt trauma is usually classified as neuropraxia. No physical disturbance of neural subunits can be noted, and functional recovery occurs in seven to 21 days. If physical disruption of a variable number of axons without stromal disturbance is noted, the lesion is classified as axonotmesis. The axoplasm and cell membrane are

disrupted, but the Schwann cell and connective tissue elements remain intact. Examination shows incomplete neurological deficits distal to the injured nerve tissue. Disparity in functional loss between motor and sensory elements may be noted. Complete severance of neural and connective tissue elements is classified an neurotmesis. Total functional loss to regions distal to the injury site is clinically apparent.

The timing of surgical repair after injury depends on the type of injury and the facilities available at initial presentation. Two time schemes for surgical repair have been advocated in the literature—immediate (primary) repair, in which definitive surgery is performed eight to 12 hours after injury, and early delayed (secondary) repair, which is performed two to six weeks after initial injury. Immediate repair is indicated in cases of transection of a nerve trunk related to a clean sharp wound such as a glass cut. If partial transection of a nerve trunk has occurred, immediate repair of the injured tissue is also indicated.[134, 150, 151] Advantages of immediate suture repair include earlier return to function, better funicular observation for more accurate realignment of tissue, and decreased tension upon the suture line due to stump contraction. Disadvantages to primary repair include specific types of injury, some of which are not amenable to immediate surgical correction; no advantage in ultimate functional recovery over early secondary repair; potential for suture line dehiscence due to delayed necrosis; and increased epineural friability. If primary repair is not performed but nerves are observed at initial surgery, placement of fine (6-0) metallic sutures in the epineurium and attachment to surrounding tissue allows radiographic evaluation and minimizes stump retraction until definitive repair is performed.[81, 123, 140, 151, 161]

Delayed (secondary) repair is preferred when major trauma and contamination are associated with nerve damage. Abolition of wound contamination and inflammatory response results in a better environment for nerve regeneration. The delay is also biologically compatible with changes in peripheral nerve metabolism and nerve cell body changes. Phagocytosis of neurotubular debris and hypertrophy of connective tissue elements allow immediate peripheral regrowth of the proximal stump. Advantages of delayed definitive repair for two to six weeks after injury include hypertrophy of epineurium for easier suturing and greater tensile strength, demarcation of injured nerve elements at the site of injury for easier resection of neuroma, and changes in cell physiology related to regrowth. Disadvantages of secondary repair are stump retraction and neuroma debridement, both of which contribute to increased tension at the site of the suture line, increased tissue fibrosis and hemorrhage in the surgical field, and later return of function. Delaying definitive repair beyond six to eight weeks can result in poor clinical results. Progressive stromal fibrosis and narrowing of Schwann cells in the distal stump decrease successful axoplasmic recannulation. Atrophy and fibrosis of denervated skeletal muscle impair clinical recovery. Surgical identification of anatomical structures is impeded. Finally, stump retraction and healing may produce large nerve gaps.[54, 87, 107, 134, 140, 151, 154]

Instruments for peripheral nerve surgery can be procured from several manufacturers of ophthalmic and microsurgical instruments. Generally, ophthalmic instruments are adequate for all but sophisticated repair procedures and are generally less expensive. General surgical instruments are appropriate for the initial surgical approach. Suggested instrumentation for peripheral nerve surgery can include a small ophthalmic needle holder, two pairs of jeweler's forceps, 4-inch strabismus scissors, 4-inch iris scissors, mouse-tooth Adson forceps, and a razor blade holder. Disposable supplies include lint-free sponges such as Gelfoam* or Weck-Cel,† wooden tongue depressors, double-edge razor blades or scalpel blade, silicone nerve cuffs, and suture material. Suture material should preferably be monofilament with low tissue reaction. Polypropylene or nylon (5-0 to 7-0) with a swaged, taper-point needle is adequate for most surgical techniques. Funicular repair may dictate 8-0 to 10-0 suture.

Preparation of surgical instruments is critical to ensure success. Cleaning in a detergent-free soap solution is recommended. Ultrasonic bathing may be used as a final cleaning process. Good instrument cleaning is essential to remove tissue debris, blood, dust, lint, and cutaneous secretions, any or all of which could contribute to excessive fibroplasia at the suture line with blockage of axonal migration. Instruments should be placed on a tray lined with a lint-free towel material. Disposable dental napkins may be used for this purpose. Sterilization should be by dry heat or ethylene oxide. Repeated use of moist heat may cause corrosion and dull the working edges of delicate instruments. Sharp edges of razor or scalpel blades may also be dulled after moist heat application.[151]

Preparation of the patient for surgery is important for successful results. Standard clipping and preparation for aseptic surgery must be rigidly followed, and the use of skin drapes such as incorporating the limb in a stockinette is helpful. The stockinette may be fixed to the subcutis with suture material or wound clips to aid exclusion of surface debris and tissue fragments.[125, 128]

Tissue dissection should be along anatomical lines of separation. If exposure requires separation of muscle tissue, the muscle is split in the direction of its fibers. If this is not possible, transection of a muscle at its ligamentous attachment is recommended; reattachment is made at the conclusion of the surgical procedure. Surgical goals are hemostasis and minimal tissue damage, because bleeding and tissue debris promote excessive scarring, which attenuates the results of the surgical procedure. Lavage of the surgical site to remove tissue debris is helpful if not excessively done. Hemostasis can be expedited by the usage of low-voltage electrocoagulation on transected vascular beds.[150, 151]

After exposure, the nerve is mobilized from surrounding tissues. Each nerve is surrounded by an adventitial tissue (mesoneurium) that contains collateral vessels. Some of this tissue must be incised and stripped from the nerve trunk. Although the amount of tissue that can be safely removed is controversial, it appears that six to eight centimeters can be stripped without adverse effects. This amount is usually sufficient to give adequate mobilization of the nerve trunk.[116, 138]

Manipulation of the nerve trunk should be done with great care. Nerve tissue can be safely handled by one of three methods. Gentle handling of the epineurium with jeweler's forceps may be used, but care must be exercised to avoid incorporating funiculi with the forceps and creating additional tissue injury. Manipulation using the incised mesoneurium may also be done. More commonly, placement of traction sutures through the epineurium with manipulation of the sutures is performed. These sutures, in addition to traction, provide landmarks for alignment if resection and anastomosis of the nerve trunk are required.[116, 124, 151]

At this point, examination of the nerve and assessment of damage are important to planning for corrective techniques. If anatomical continuity of the nerve trunk is present, electrical stimulation with microelectrodes and observation of response may provide information about the level of the lesion. One may also note the presence of a swollen, indurated area within the substance of nerve trunk. This area is classified as a neuroma and requires surgical judgment as to disposition prior to surgical repair (Fig. 95–15).[58, 69, 70, 80, 83, 151]

Neuroma formation indicates axonotmesis or neurotmesis. The shape and location of the neuroma may give an estimation of the prognosis. A fusiform neuroma (Fig. 95–15A) indicates integrity of some fascicles in the area of injury. If the neuroma is firm, fibrosis has occurred at the point of injury. Spontaneous recannulation of neurotubules by regenerating axoplasm is unlikely. If consistency is softer, a spontaneous healing is more likely.[127, 134, 151]

Location of the neuroma within the nerve trunk may also aid in judging lesion severity. Lateral neuromas (Fig. 95–15C) indicate partial neurotmesis with functional tissue remaining. If the injury does not exceed 50 per cent of the width of the nerve trunk, spontaneous recovery may occur without surgical intervention. However, if more than 50 per cent is involved, resection and neurorrhaphy are indicated. Bulbous and dumbbell-shaped neuromas (Fig. 95–15B and D) suggest widespread neurotmesis with poor prognosis for spontaneous recovery. Excision of the neuroma and neurorrhaphy are indicated.[30, 80, 83, 134, 150]

If a neuroma is encountered at exploration, it

---

*Gelfoam, Upjohn Co., Kalamazoo, MI.
†Weck-Cel, Edward Weck Co., New York, NY.

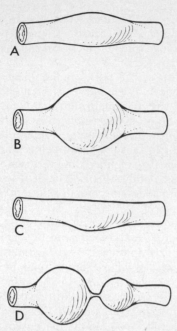

Figure 95–15. Neuromas that may be noted during exploration. *A,* Fusiform. *B,* Bulbous. *C,* Lateral. *D,* Dumbbell. (Reprinted with permission from Raffe, M. R.: Peripheral nerve injuries, Parts I and II. Comp. Cont. Ed. *1*:207, 269. 1979.)

should be classified as described, and a decision should be made for or against surgical resection. If uncertainty exists, electrical stimulation and recording of the evoked response may be beneficial. Fine platinum electrodes are directly applied to the nerve above and below the lesion. An electrical stimulus is produced and the response (nerve action potential) is recorded on an oscilloscope. This examination allows estimation of electrical transmission through the lesion and may aid in differentiating axonotmesis from neurotomesis. Alternatively, trial section of the neuroma may be performed by one of three common methods. Internal neurolysis may be performed by longitudinal incision through the epineurium only. Careful dissection and separation of individual nerve fascicles with removal of excess fibrous tissue can be performed. If more than one-half to three-quarters of the nerve is disrupted, resection and anastomosis are performed. Alternately, trial section of a neuroma by either of two transverse methods may be used. In one procedure, the neuroma is supported by a wooden tongue depressor acting as an anvil. A transverse incision is made at the point of greatest induration and is deepened 0.5 millimeters at a time until normal nerve tissue is seen. If more than one-half to three-quarters of the diameter of the nerve trunk is involved, resection of the neuroma and anastomosis of the nerve are indicated. In an alternate method, a collar of polyethylene surgical drape is placed around the nerve trunk and fixed with right-angle forceps. Trial incision is performed with use of a razor edge in a fashion similar to that previously described.[21, 30, 80, 83, 129, 150]

The neuroma is transected back to normal tissue.

Serial transverse sections of one millimeter are removed from the incised edge of the neuroma until tissue is seen. This procedure is done on both the proximal and distal stumps. Constant inspection of the excised tissue and maintenance of adequate length without undue tension are necessary. Wide and extensive tissue excision must be avoided so that anastomosis is without undue tension.[30, 136, 150]

Inadequate hemostasis following resection causes excessive fibrosis and distortion of nerve architecture. Only lint-free ophthalmic sponges or absorbable gelatin sponges should be used. The degree of intraneural vasculature is surprising, and if excessive hemorrhage is encountered, the sponges may be dipped in a 1:100,000 epinephrine solution, or bipolar electrocoagulation may be used.[125]

Suture placement is critical. Suture material is passed through the epineurium only. Incorporation of neural elements by suture material results in scar tissue formation proportional to the amount of fibrous invasion from the suture. All sutures should be tied with equal tension. The tension applied should be just enough for alignment and contact of the neural bundles. Excessive tension may result in crushing and misalignment of the nerve bundles, predisposing to poor recannulation of distal nerve tubules and neuroma formation at the surgical site.[11, 116]

Optical magnification and supplemental lighting are beneficial to achieve optimum results. A binocular magnifying loupe similar to one used in ophthalmic surgery is helpful. Interchangeable eye pieces allow 2.5- to 5.0-power magnification. Supplemental lighting may be provided from spot-type surgical lamps, fiberoptic headlamps, or flexible neck lights. As techniques of surgical repair and tissue transplantation have improved, use of operating microscopes has increased. The operating microscope should have a magnification range 10 to 25, and usually has an auxiliary light source built into it. Such an instrument is helpful in identification and dissection of nerve elements from a neuroma and in discrimination of normal from distorted nerve architecture. It is also useful in repair techniques involving suture of subunits of the nerve trunk and can increase accuracy in suture placement and rotational alignment of the nerve stumps. Equal applications of tension at the suture line can also be observed.[1, 77, 150, 151]

Surgical Techniques

The simplest surgical repair is an end-to-end anastomosis. In this procedure, the entire nerve trunk is sutured as a unit by sutures placed in the epineurium or by placement of a single suture through the axial center of the injured nerve trunk.[150, 151]

The most common technique of nerve repair (neurorrhaphy) involves placement of a series of simple interrupted sutures through the epineurium (Fig. 95–16). Low-power magnification from a five-power binocular loupe, as described, may help in distin-

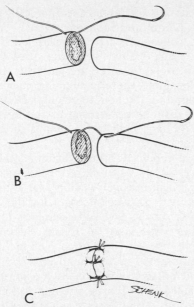

Figure 95–16. Placement of epineural sutures for neurorrhaphy. *A* and *B*, Care must be exercised to incorporate only epineurium in suture placement. *C*, All sutures are preplaced prior to tying to ensure even suture line tension. (Reprinted with permission from Raffe, M. R.: Peripheral nerve injuries, Parts I and II. Comp. Cont. Ed. *1*:207, 269, 1979.)

guishing structures and ensuring suture passage through the epineurium only. The epineurium is grasped and tensed with jeweler's forceps. Because the tissue has elastic fibers, the epineurium may be slightly stretched to facilitate suture placement. Prior to suture placement, peripheral nerve stumps should be realigned correctly.[123–125, 150, 151]

Sutures should be approximately 0.5 to 1.0 mm from the incised edge. The suture material is placed from the surface of the nerve and emerges just beneath the epineurium. It is brought out to the free edge and the process is repeated in the opposing nerve stump. The number of sutures required for adequate alignment of stumps varies, depending on the diameter of the nerve. The smallest number of sutures possible is desirable so that inflammatory reaction to the suture material is minimized. However, adequate alignment is paramount for the success of the surgical procedure. Swaim states that four equidistant sutures generally provide sufficient alignment for healing. Depending upon the size of the nerve, more may be required for adequate alignment.[25, 28, 123, 124, 150, 151]

It is advisable to preplace all sutures and then to tie them all to minimize excess traction and prevent the suture from tearing through tissue. To begin, two sutures are placed in the nerve trunk 180 degrees apart. These sutures maintain alignment of the nerve stumps. Additional suture or sutures are placed in the upper portion of the nerve. Several or all of these sutures may be tied to obtain adequate alignment. The suture ends may be carefully grasped and the nerve trunk rotated to expose the underside of the nerve. An additional suture or sutures are then placed

and tied to complete apposition of the nerve trunk. All knots are inspected to ensure that equal tension is present. The goal of epineural suturing is to provide funicular alignment for rapid growth into the distal segment. The epineural placement of sutures does not invade neural elements but, in a sense, provides a coaptation "splint" of the connective tissue elements, enabling realignment and stabilization. Excessive suture tension induces malalignment and compression of neurotubular elements, with unfavorable results.[19, 25, 28, 123, 124, 150, 151]

An alternate suture technique for end-to-end anastomosis involves placing a single suture aligned with the longitudinal axis of the nerve trunk and securing the two ends of the suture by means of small buttons on the outside of the nerve trunk (Fig. 95–17). This may be performed in one of two ways. In the first method, the suture is begun seven to eight millimeters from the transection site and is directed perpendicularly to the longitudinal axis into the center of the nerve trunk. The suture is then redirected to follow the central axis of the nerve trunk and to emerge at the center of the transection site. It is then carried to the opposing stump and is inserted in the central axis. It is advanced for seven to eight millimeters and then redirected to emerge 180 degrees opposite the initial suture placement. The end result has the appearance of the letter Z.[54, 139, 150, 151]

In the second method, a double-armed suture is used. Each needle is inserted centrally into one of the two nerve stumps. They are each directed down the longitudinal axis and redirected so that each emerges 180 degrees from its counterpart. This mod-

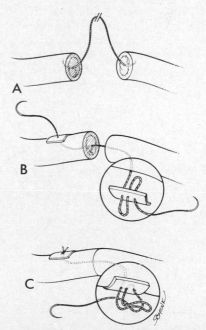

Figure 95–17. Intraneural neurorrhaphy. *A*, Central placement of intraneural suture is critical to prevent rotational misalignment. *B*, Attachment of suture of fascial buttons. *C*, Triple suture passage technique for tying suture. (Reprinted with permission from Raffe, M. R.: Peripheral nerve injuries, Parts I and II. Comp. Cont. Ed. *1*:207, 269, 1979.)

ification increases the likelihood of central suture placement, which is critical for proper alignment.[124, 125]

Fascial or silicone buttons approximately three millimeters square are prepared. Each end of the suture is attached to a button, which acts as an anchor. One end is secured by placement of a square knot on top of the button. The other button is affixed by use of a slip knot, which applies tension for alignment and apposition of the nerve trunks. The slip knot involves a triple suture passage and use of a loop and suture strand to tie a square knot. This method provides good alignment and knot security.[54, 124, 125]

The main advantage of this suture technique for anastomosis is that less postsurgical neuroma formation and ingrowth of scar tissue occur. However, it is technically more difficult, and there is the potential for severe complications. The most common complication is stump rotation and instability unless the suture is carefully centered in the nerve trunk.[54, 124, 125]

As microsurgery has progressed, suture repair of peripheral nerve subunits (Fig. 95–18) has increased. Placement of one or two sutures of 10-0 suture material in the perineurium to anastomose individual funiculi has found favor in the past 10 years. With this type of surgical repair, definitive anastomosis of funiculi occurs without the potential for aberrant centrifugal regrowth that is possible with epineural sutures. An additional refinement of this technique used electrical stimulation of individual funiculi in acute injury to match both stumps of a transected funiculus by positive identification. Clinical results showed no superiority with the use of electrical stimulation over anatomic repair of nerve stumps. Funicular repair may be combined with epineural suture to aid in strength of the suture line at the site of repair. Controversy still remains as to which method gives better clinical function.

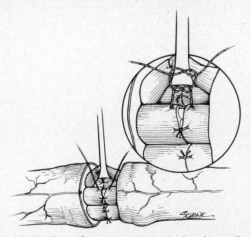

Figure 95–18. Funicular nerve repair. Each subunit (funiculus, fascicle) is sutured within the nerve trunk. Epineural sutures may be added. (Reprinted with permission from Raffe, M. R.: Principles of peripheral nerve repair and regeneration. *In* Newton, C. D., and Nunamaker, D. M. (Eds.): *Textbook of Small Animal Orthopedics,* J. B. Lippincott, Philadelphia, in press.)

An interesting technique incorporating principles of both epineural and funicular repair, reported by Tsuge and colleagues,[160] has been called the anchor funicular suture. This technique uses horizontal mattress sutures to incorporate both the epineurium and perineurium, thereby aligning major funiculi and incorporating the holding strength of the epineurium. The major disadvantage of this technique is the lack of approximation gained in all funiculi.[1, 14, 17, 37, 56, 71, 82, 118, 149, 159, 160, 172]

Ideally, a repair technique using methods other than sutures would be preferred. All suture material evokes an inflammatory reaction that can result in excess granulation tissue. Recognizing the advantage of sutureless repair, several researchers have evaluated various techniques of repair. Several groups reported on the use of plasma clot techniques in repair of transected nerve stumps.[18, 101, 153, 154, 175] The major disadvantages of this technique were technical difficulty and lack of tensile strength in a position of traction to the nerve. Later groups investigated the use of hydrocarbon-chain cyanacrylate cements for tissue repair and found excessive tissue reaction and actual neural damage, which precluded clinical use.[47–49, 78, 86] The most promising implanted synthetic material was a micropore adhesive tape composed of rayon fabric with a polymer adhesive, which was used as a coaptation splint at the site of surgical repair. Favorable healing with minimal tissue reaction has been reported with this technique. The material is nearly reabsorbed with little tissue response 28 days after implantation. The major drawback, like that of plasma clot techniques, is tissue dehiscence under low tension, which has prevented widespread clinical use of this repair technique.[78, 86]

Nerve Cuffs

Two of the major difficulties in achieving optimum surgical results are ingrowth of connective tissue from neighboring regions and prevention of misguided axon migration. Many biological and synthetic materials have been employed as ensheathing cuffs to shield the surgical site. Tantalum, plasma clots, gold, autografted and homografted blood vessels, muscle, Surgicel, surgical tape, liquid plasticiers, collagen, sheets and tubes of Millipore and Silastic, and copolymeric polylactic and polyglycolic acid have been used. The most acceptable have been plasma clot, Millipore, Silastic and copolymeric acid sheaths.[78, 126, 134, 151]

Millipore showed promise as a sheath material. With a pore size of 0.45 microns, normal flow of extracellular tissue fluid without tissue migration could be obtained. This aided in meeting nutritional requirements for regenerating epineural tissue. The prevention of early ingrowth of connective tissue allowed early epineural continuity to be reformed, and subsequent linear regeneration via the "contact guidance" phenomenon. The disadvantage of Millipore is subsequent dystrophic calcification and fragmentation about eight weeks after implantation. Micropore tape, similar to that used for sutureless repair, was also evaluated as a nerve cuff material. Disruption of the adhesive surfaces led to impaired healing and neuroma formation.[27, 47–49, 107, 150]

Currently, silicone rubber compounds (Silastic) are used clinically as shielding implants. Silicone rubber is relatively inert, flexible, thin-walled, and uniform in diameter. Assorted diameters and lengths are commercially available.[41, 109, 110]

Experiments in dogs suggest favorable results using co-polymeric polyglycolic acid sheaths. Histological evaluation of experimentally induced transection and repair of peroneal and ulnar nerves ensheathed with this material showed biological degradation of the cuffs by the eighth postoperative week. Increased epineural fibrosis was noted during evaluation, but, protection of intraneural elements and preservation of neural element alignment was demonstrated. In eight of 18 samples, less epineural fibrosis was noted on the cuff repair than with standard techniques.[126]

Certain guidelines must be followed if a nerve cuff is to be used. The cross-sectional area of the cuff should be two to three times that of the nerve trunk. A cuff smaller than this may create constriction at the anastomotic site as nerve swelling occurs and predisposes to neuroma formation. A larger cuff may invaginate and constrict the nerve trunk. Also, ingrowth of connective tissue may predispose to neuroma formation. The length of the cuff should not exceed eight to ten millimeters. Greater length may inhibit collateral circulation to the nerve trunk. Adequate length should be used, however, because a short cuff may not provide sufficient shielding at the surgical site. A neuroma may be formed at the edge of the cuff, but the surgical site should remain protected.[39–43, 166]

Placement of the cuff onto a nerve stump prior to anastomosis is required. The cuff is placed onto a jeweler's forceps or small hemostat. The epineurium is gently grasped and the cuff is slipped onto the nerve stump. After the end-to-end anastomosis, the cuff is centered over the anastomotic site and fixed in position into the epineurium with sutures. One suture at each end of the cuff provides sufficient anchorage and prevents cuff distortion.[110, 150, 151]

Complications result from improper cuff size. A recent report of this procedure in humans suggests that reevaluation of the guidelines for cuff sizing may be required.[23]

Nerve Grafts

In extensive injuries, loss of tissue may result in a nerve gap. This gap may be surgically irreducible, and alternative management techniques are required to aid return of function. Numerous techniques have been used to obtain reapposition of severed nerve ends. These include stretching of the nerve stumps by mobilizing the mesoneurium and surrounding tissues, joint flexion to shorten nerve course, transposition of nerve route, osseous resection and limb shortening, nerve pedicle flaps, gap tubulation with a variety of materials, direct neurotization of muscle, and nerve grafting. All of these methods have been applied clinically, with reported success rates depending on the species operated on and the expertise of the reporting authors.

Nerve stumps my be stretched to a limited extent to attain apposition, with surgical factors being course of the nerve, vascular supply, and species involved. Any degree of stretching may decrease healing of the nerve. Generally, enough length is present to overcome a gap of two to three centimeters. Stretching or mobilization in excess of this length endangers the extrinsic vascular supply to the nerve as well as predisposes to failure of the repair through increased suture line tension. In experimental studies, regeneration rate through a suture line under tension was no slower than that in a properly utilized nerve graft.[12, 28, 35, 60, 61, 65, 79, 111, 113, 114, 168]

Tubulation of nerve gaps to promote healing has been proposed by several authors. Use of various biological and synthetic materials has been reported, and the success rates varied with author and species. Successful clinical use of this technique for nerve gaps in primates has been reported. Other alternate procedures to obtain apposition of nerve ends without grafting have met with variable success.[8, 13, 102, 150, 164, 165]

Much research effort has been expended to develop techniques for suppression of the immune reaction in grafted tissue. Currently, freezing, irradiation, and immunosuppressive drugs appear to overcome detrimental effects of homograft and heterograft procedures.[9, 93–99, 137, 167]

The autograft is most easily available for grafting in clinical veterinary medicine. The question of fresh grafts *versus* preserved grafts *versus* predegenerated grafts remains unsolved. From a practical viewpoint, fresh grafts are probably most frequently used in veterinary medicine. Free graft donor sites in the dog are the lateral cutaneous nerve of the thigh and the median nerve of the forearm. In addition, nerve transposition to restore function by anastomosis of a viable proximal stump to the distal stump of another nerve has been documented. The decision to use a nerve graft is based on the diagnosis of irreducible nerve gap at surgery. Anatomical mapping experiments have shown that funiculi are not distinct subunits but undergo continuous division and integration with neighboring fascicles. The pattern of funiculi changes every 0.5 cm along the course of a peripheral nerve; therefore, unless individual funiculi are united by microsurgical techniques (cable grafting), interposition of a nerve graft segment does not guarantee perfect axonal migration and cannulation of the distal stump.[11, 112, 130, 147, 148, 162, 175]

The diameter of the graft closely approximates that of the nerve trunk to be grafted. Inadequate graft diameter may predispose to incomplete axonal regrowth because an insufficient number of Schwann tubes is provided by the graft. The graft length should be 15 to 25 per cent longer than the gap to be spanned, in order to allow for graft shrinkage and to release tension on suture lines at anastomotic sites.[11, 65, 133, 150]

There are several causes of failure in autograft procedures, including inadequate training and instrumentation, failure of matching graft diameter and length to the injured nerve, and improper matching of donor and host funiculi. Nerve grafts are similar to other devascularized tissue implants. Regeneration of blood supply must be provided by surrounding tissues to provide nutrition for neurilemma. Revascularization proceeds axially from the surgical site of the graft and abaxially from the epineurial surface in a centripetal direction. The danger of ischemic necrosis of the central graft core is increased, particularly in a poorly vascularized tissue bed. Necrosis could result in destruction of Schwann tubules and failure of axonal regeneration through the graft. This danger is compounded in allografts and heterografts, in that patency of Schwann tubes is threatened not only because of the vascular supply but also by the tissue-mediated immune response. There is always a race between regeneration of axons across a free graft and destruction of patent Schwann tubes.[7, 31, 32, 96, 101, 128, 141, 148, 155]

Recent advances hold promise in nerve grafting. Microsurgical techniques have been used for reconstruction of microvasculature with a free nerve graft, which allows live graft tissue and prevents degeneration of the graft due to lack of vascularity.[157] Further work in microsurgery has demonstrated that reversing the polarity of free graft has no effect.[71, 144] Cable grafting of funiculi may give faster return of function when pre-degenerated funicular grafts are used. Tissue typing of grafts may improve survival rate in the recipient.[62, 137] The use of nerve cuffs at anastomotic sites of nerve grafts continues to remain controversial. Proponents recognize decreased tissue reaction at surgical sites in the early postoperative period. Opponents point to the dangers of shielding vascular ingrowth with degeneration of the graft. Cuffs eight to nine millimeters in length at the anastomotic sites may be used with good results.[27, 41, 108, 110]

Nerve Gaps

On occasion, a short irreducible gap may be encountered without immediate provision for graft repair as described. In these cases, an alternate approach may be to bring the nerve stumps as close as possible in a dry tissue bed and tack the cut ends to the tissue bed with two epineural sutures in each stump, creating a nerve gap without continuity. This technique may be used for defects not exceeding one to two centimeters. Successful regeneration across nerve gaps has been reported in the dog and in children. However, factors discussed previously must be overcome to obtain success. In addition, increased regeneration time should be expected.[90]

Factors Influencing Success of Surgical Repair

Application of surgical techniques for repair of peripheral nerve injuries only mechanically sets the stage for orderly progression of healing. Unfortunately, complications often arise and failure often occurs in operative repair. Most failures can be attributed to technical errors or postoperative management.

The type of nerve involved can determine the course of healing. Pure motor or sensory nerve usually has a more uncomplicated recovery. Mixed nerves have the potential for transposition of axons during regeneration and therefore the potential for improper end organ reinnervation, which can result in patient disorientation and a lower level of ultimate functional recovery. This complication can be minimized by careful matching, and in some cases suturing, of funicular bundles.[22, 70, 85]

The age of the patient may determine return of function. Younger patients recover more completely, and in a shorter time. This difference can be attributed to several factors. The length covered in the course of regeneration is shorter owing to shorter limb length. There appears to be a faster degeneration in distal nerve stumps, which can contribute to a quicker and more satisfactory regrowth of axons. Biosynthetic processes are already present, thereby decreasing the lag phase for prebiosynthesis. Finally, adaptability and compensatory sensory and motor reeducation are greater in young patients.[22, 70, 85, 90]

As previously discussed, the degree of injury is an important consideration in functional return. Proximal injuries require greater metabolic biosynthesis for functional recovery. The requirement may exceed the capabilities of the nerve cell body and result in cell death. If this occurs on a widespread basis in the nerve, regeneration will fail.[22, 39, 70]

The extent of the injury is also important. Lesions in continuity or those with focal neuroma formation or small gaps respond better than injuries with irreducible gaps or long defects. The difference is related to segmental vascular supply, suture line tension, and biological considerations of nerve grafting. In addition, large defects interrupt funicular architecture and increase the potential for functional cross-innervation in mixed nerves. Appearance of surrounding soft tissue is also important. Clean vascular beds for regeneration decrease neuroma formation and suture line failure related to motion of tendons, joints, and regional bones. Rerouting of the nerve may be required to achieve the best site for regeneration. Tension at the suture site to gain length in the trunk may result in failure of regeneration. Minimum tension increases the potential for nerve healing.[12, 22, 122, 150]

Associated injury may superimpose additional burdens on nerve regeneration. Polysystemic trauma or massive deep wounds may damage the vascular supply to superficial and deep soft tissues. Orthopedic disease may superimpose management complications. Sepsis, scar formation, and wound contraction as well as all the previously listed factors interfere with physical, medical, and surgical management of the patient. Recognition of the wound biology of individual tissue types also aids in formulation of a management plan.[22, 55, 141]

Timing of surgical intervention is important in successful management. Previous discussion on the merits and indications for immediate *versus* early secondary repair are familiar to the reader. However, as time increases from injury to surgical intervention, irreversible changes occur in the distal segment of the nerve trunk. In addition, neurogenic atrophy and fibrosis of denervated muscle segments complicates functional recovery. Therefore, early repair of nerve injury is advocated, with the time of repair depending on other surgical factors.[22, 67, 70, 134, 140, 172]

Postoperative Care

Routine closure is performed after nerve repair. If tension at the suture line is evident at surgery, the limb should be splinted or cast in a relaxed position for no less than two weeks. After this time, passive motion of the limb may be slowly begun, and the goal is to obtain full range of motion by the sixth postoperative week.[6, 124, 150, 151]

The denervated limb must be protected from mutilation, until evidence of reinnervation is apparent, by padded bandages, splints, or moldable cast material. In some cases, self-mutilation of the denervated portion may be attempted and may be correlated with early stages of axon growth and reinnervation of sensory-deprived areas. Conservative management is usually sufficient to prevent further damage, using a protective bandage, side brace, bucket collar, or muzzling.

Serial clinical examination and electrodiagnostic evaluation provides evidence of the degree of progress. Although 100 per cent function will not be regained, the goal is for restoration of enough function to allow for adequate daily locomotion and activity.

Assessment of Nerve Repair

Postoperatively, healing ideally proceeds at a rate of one to three millimeters per day. Given the initial tissue reaction to the surgical procedure, the inflammatory reaction and tissue resorption of the initial

injury, and the biochemical changes in the ventral cell body, a delay of several weeks may occur until axoplasmic migration invades the distal stump and maximum rate of regrowth occurs. The level of injury also determines ultimate time of recovery, as well as other factors previously described.[39, 70]

In humans, accurate records of regional reinnervation may be elicited from patient observations and physical examination. Migration down the affected nerve trunk of an uncomfortable "pins and needles" sensation (referred to as a Tinel's sign) is used to measure postoperative progress. Alternate methods must be used in veterinary medicine. Qualitative return of sensory function has been measured by dermatone examination and recorded for assessment of functional recovery. Recently, evoked nerve potentials (motor nerve conduction velocity) has been used as an early indicator of functional recovery (see Chapter 92).[2, 5, 96]

When peripheral nerve lesions and surgical repair are assessed by electrophysiological methods, several points should be remembered. Prognosis of functional recovery in the postsurgical patient may be aided by the use of evoked potentials. Compound motor nerve action potentials may precede return of clinical function and can be used as an index of reinnervation. Additionally, evoked potentials may aid in determination of medical or surgical therapy in questionable cases. Compressive lesions in continuity show functional recovery by 12 to 16 weeks after injury. If electrophysiological evaluation reveals no progress by this time, surgical exploration is indicated. In similar fashion, partial transection of a nerve trunk may reveal the presence of evoked potentials with diminished amplitude. Comparison of the amplitude immediately after and again ten days after injury allows an estimate of the percentage of surviving motor fibers.[15, 24, 26, 33, 39, 66, 122]

1. Alivisi, C., Ambrosetto, P., and Leghissa, S.: Microsurgical repair of small nerves. J. Neurosurg. Sci. *18*:181, 1974.
2. Almquist, E., and Eeg-Olofsson, O.: Sensory nerve conduction velocity and two-point discrimination in sutured nerves. J. Bone Joint Surg. *52A*:791, 1970.
3. Arey, L. B.: The histogenesis of nervous tissues. In: *Developmental Anatomy*. 7th ed., revised. W. B. Saunders Co., Philadelphia, 1974.
4. Arey, L. B.: Morphogenesis of the skeleton. In: *Developmental Anatomy*. 7th ed., revised. W. B. Saunders Co., Philadelphia, 1974.
5. Assmus, H.: Somatosensory evoked cortical potentials (SSEP) in regenerating nerves following suture. Z. EEG, EMG *9*:167, 1978.
6. Babcock, W. W.: A standard technique for operations on peripheral nerves. Surg. Gynecol. Obstet. *45*:364, 1927.
7. Barnes, R., Bacsich, P., Wyburn, G. M., and Kerr, A. S.: A study of the late nerve homografts in man. Br. J. Surg. *34*:34, 1947.
8. Bassett, C. A., Campbell, J. B., and Husby, J.: Peripheral nerve and spinal cord regeneration: factors leading to success of a tubulation technique employing millipore. Exp. Neurol. *1*:386, 1959.
9. Bellanti, J. A.: *Immunology*. W. B. Saunders Co., Philadelphia, 1971.

10. Bennett, D., and Vaughan, L. C.: The use of muscle relocation techniques in the treatment of peripheral nerve injuries in dogs and cats. J. Sm. Anim. Pract. 17:99, 1976.

11. Bentley, F. H., and Hill, M.: Nerve grafting. Br. J. Surg. 24:368, 1936.

12. Berger, A., and Millesi, H.: Nerve grafting. Clin. Orthop. and Related Res. 133:49, 1978.

13. Binns, J. H., Johnston, G. A., and Zamick, P.: Lypholised corium grafts in peripheral nerve repair. Br. J. Plast. Surg. 29:251, 1976.

14. Bora, F. W.: A comparison of epineural perineural and epiperineural methods of nerve suture. Clin. Orthop. 133:91, 1978.

15. Bowen, J. M.: Peripheral nerve electrodiagnostics, electromyography and nerve conduction velocity. In Hoerlein, B. F. (ed.): Canine Neurology. 3rd ed. W. B. Saunders Co., Philadelphia, 1978.

16. Bowen, V., Shannon, R., and Kirkaldy-Willis, W. H.: Lumbar spinal stenosis. Child's Brain 45:257, 1978.

17. Bratton, B. R., Kline, D. G., Coleman, W., and Hudson, A. R.: Experimental interfascicular nerve grafting. J. Neurosurg. 51:323, 1979.

18. Braun, R. M.: Comparative studies of neurorrhaphy and sutureless peripheral nerve repair. Surg. Gynecol. Obstet. 122:15, 1966.

19. Braun, R. M.: Epineural nerve suture. Clin. Orthop. Related Res. 163:50, 1982.

20. Bright, R. M., Crabtree, B. J., and Knecht, C. D.: Brachial plexus neuropathy in the cat: a case report. J. Am. Anim. Hosp. Assoc. 14:612, 1979.

21. Brown, B. A.: Internal neurolysis in traumatic peripheral nerve lesions in continuity. Surg. Clin. North Am. 52:1167, 1972.

22. Brown, P. W.: Factors influencing the success of the surgical repair of peripheral nerves. Surg. Clin. North Am. 52:1137, 1972.

23. Buch, R.: Silicone rubber cuffs—a cause for nerve compression. Hand 2:211, 1979.

24. Buchthal, F., and Kuhl, V.: Nerve conduction, tactile sensibility, and the electromyogram after suture or compression of peripheral nerve: a longitudinal study in man. J. Neurol. Neurosurg. Psychiatry 42:436, 1978.

25. Buncke, H. J., Jr.: Digital nerve repairs. Surg. Clin. North Am. 52:1267, 1972.

26. Burke, P. F., and O'Brien, B. McC.: A comparison of three techniques of micro nerve repairs in dogs. Hand 10:135, 1978.

27. Campbell, J. B., Bassett, C. A., and Bohler, J.: Frozen-irradiated homografts shielded with microfilter sheaths in peripheral nerve surgery. J. Trauma 3:303, 1963.

28. Campbell, J. B.: Peripheral nerve repair. Clin. Neurosurg. 17:77, 1968.

29. Chrisman, C. L., Burt, J. K., Wood, P. K., and Johnson, E. W.: Electromyography in small animal clinical neurology. J. Am. Vet. Med. Assoc. 160:311, 1972.

30. Clark, W. K.: Surgery for injection injuries of peripheral nerves. Surg. Clin. North Am. 52:1325, 1972.

31. Comtet, J. J., and Revillard, J. P.: Peripheral nerve allografts. Transplantation 28:103, 1978.

32. Davis, L., and Ruge, D.: Functional recovery following the use of homogenous nerve grafts. Surgery 27:102, 1950.

33. Davis, L. A., Gordon, T., Hoffer, J. A., et al.: Compound action potentials recorded from mammalian peripheral nerves following ligation or resuturing. J. Physiol. 285:543, 1978.

34. de Lahunta, A.: Veterinary Neuro-anatomy and Clinical Neurology. W. B. Saunders Co., Philadelphia, 1977.

35. Denny-Brown, D., and Doherty, M. M.: Effects of transient stretching of peripheral nerve. Arch. Neurol. Psych. 54:116, 1945.

36. Dickson, R. A., Dinley, J., Rushworth, G., and Colwin, A.: Delayed (degenerate) interfascicular nerve grafting: a new conception in peripheral nerve repair. Br. J. Surg. 64:698, 1977.

37. Dolenc, V., Trontelj, J. V., and Janko, M.: Neurophysiological evaluation of microsurgically implanted grafts bridging peripheral nerve defects. Acta Neurochirurg. Suppl. 28:608, 1979.

38. Donoso, R. S., Ballantyne, J. P., and Hansen, S.: Regeneration of sutured human peripheral nerves: an electrophysiological study. J. Neurol. Neurosurg. Psychiatry 42:97, 1979.

39. Ducker, T. B., Kempe, L. G., and Haytes, G. J.: The metabolic background for peripheral nerve surgery. J. Neurosurg. 30:270, 1966.

40. Ducker, T. B., and Hayes, G. J.: A comparative study of the technique of nerve repair. Surg. Forum 28:443, 1967.

41. Ducker, T. B., and Hayes, G. J.: Experimental improvements in the use of Silastic cuff for peripheral nerve repair. J. Neurosurg. 28:582, 1968.

42. Ducker, T. B., and Hayes, G. J.: Peripheral nerve injuries: a comparative study of the anatomical and funetional results following primary repair in chimpanzees. Military Med. 133:298, 1968.

43. Ducker, T. B.: Metabolic factors in surgery of peripheral nerves. Surg. Clin. North Am. 52:1109, 1972.

44. Feeney, D. A., and Oliver, J. E.: Blunt spinal trauma in the dog and cat: Neurologic, radiologic and therapeutic correlations. J. Am. Anim. Hosp. Assoc. 16:664, 1980.

45. Feeney, D. A., and Wise, M.: Epidurography in the normal dog: technic and radiographic findings. Vet. Radiol. 22:35, 1981.

46. Fletcher, T. F.: Dissertation, University of Minnesota, 1964.

47. Freeman, B. S.: Adhesive anastomosis techniques for fine nerves: experimental and clinical techniques. Am. J. Surg. 108:529, 1964.

48. Freeman, B. S.: Adhesive neural anastomosis. Plast. Reconstr. Surg. 35:167, 1965.

49. Freeman, B. S., Perry, J., and Brown, D.: Experimental study of adhesive surgical tape for nerve anastomosis. Plast. Reconstr. Surg. 43:174, 1969.

50. French, B. N.: Midline fusion defects and defects of formation. In Youmans, J. R. (ed.): Neurological Surgery. 2nd ed. W. B. Saunders Co., Philadelphia, 1982.

51. Frye, F. L., and McFarland, L. Z.: Spina bifida with rachischisis in a kitten. J. Am. Vet. Med. Assoc. 146:481, 1965.

52. Gardner, W. J.: The Dysraphic States from Syringomyelia to Anencephaly. Excerpta Medica, Amsterdam, 1973.

53. Getty, C. J. M.: Lumbar spinal stenosis. The clinical spectrum and the results of operation. J. Bone Joint Surg. 62B:481, 1980.

54. Gourley, I. M., and Snyder, C. C.: Peripheral nerve repair. J. Am. Anim. Hosp. Assoc. 12:613, 1976.

55. Grabb, W. C.: Management of nerve injuries in the forearm and hand. Orthop. Clin. North Am. 1:419, 1979.

56. Grabb, W. C., Bement, S. L., Koepke, G. H., and Green, R. A.: Comparison of methods of peripheral nerve suturing in monkeys. Plast. Reconstr. Surg. 46:31, 1970.

57. Griffiths, I. R., Duncan, I. D., and Lawson, D. D.: Avulsion of the brachial plexus—two clinical aspects. J. Small Anim. Pract. 15:177, 1974.

58. Griffiths, I. R., and Duncan, I. D.: The use of electromyography and nerve conduction studies in the evaluation of lower motor neurone disease or injury. J. Small Anim. Pract. 19:329, 1978.

59. Hancock, D. O.: Congenital narrowing of the spinal canal. Paraplegia 5:89, 1967.

60. Hassler, O.: Vascular reactions after epineural nerve section, suture, and transplantation. Acta Neurol. Scand. 45:335, 1968.

61. Highet, W. B., and Saunders, F. K.: The effects of stretching nerves after suture. Br. J. Surg. 30:355, 1943.

62. Hirasawa, Y., and Marmor, L.: The protective effect of

irradiation combined with ensheathing methods on experimental nerve heterografts: Silastic, autogenous veins and heterogenous arteries. J. Neurosurg. 27:401, 1967.

63. Hoerlein, B. F., and Bowen, J. M.: Clinical Disorders of Nerve and Muscles. *In* Hoerlein, B. F. (ed.): *Canine Neurology—Diagnosis and Treatment.* 3rd ed. W. B. Saunders Company, Philadelphia, 1978.

64. Hoerlein, B. F.: Peripheral nerve distribution and function. *In: Canine Neurology—Diagnosis and Treatment.* W. B. Saunders Co., Philadelphia, 1978.

65. Hoen, T. I., and Brackett, C. E.: Peripheral nerve lengthening. J. Neurosurg. 13:43, 1956.

66. Holliday, T. A., Ealand, B. G., and Weldon, N. E.: Sensory nerve conduction velocity: technical requirements and normal values for branches of the radial and ulnar nerves of the dog. Am. J. Vet. Res. 38:1543, 1977.

67. Holmes, W., and Young, J. Z.: Nerve regeneration after immediate and delayed suture. J. Anat. 77:63, 1942.

68. Holtzer, H., and Detwiler, S. R.: An experimental analysis of the development of the spinal column. III. Induction of skeletogenous cells. J. Exp. Zool. 123:335, 1953.

69. Howard, F. M.: The electromyography and conduction studies in peripheral nerve injuries. Surg. Clin. North Am. 52:1343, 1972.

70. Hubbard, J. H.: The quality of nerve regeneration. Factors independent of the most skillful repair. Surg. Clin. North Am. 52:1099, 1972.

71. Hudson, A. R., Hunter, D., Kline, D. G., and Bratton, B. R.: Histological interfascicular graft repairs. J. Neurosurg. 51:333, 1979.

72. Hurov, L. I., Lumb, W. V., Hankes, G. H., and Smith, K. W.: Wedge grafting of the canine carpus. J. Am. Vet. Med. Assoc. 148:260, 1966.

73. Hussain, S., and Pettit, G. D.: Tendon transplantation to compensate for radial nerve paralysis in the dog. Am. J. Vet. Res. 28:335, 1967.

74. James, C. C. M., Lassman, L. P., and Tomlinson, B. E.: Congenital anomalies of the lower spine and spinal cord in Manx cats. J. Pathol. 97:269, 1969.

75. Jenkins, T. W.: *Functional Mammalian Neuroanatomy.* Lea & Febiger, Philadelphia, 1972.

76. Keller, J. T., Dunsker, S. B., McWhorter, J. M., et al.: The fate of autogenous grafts to the spinal dura. An experimental study. J. Neurosurg. 49:412, 1978.

77. Khodadad, G.: Microsurgical techniques in repair of peripheral nerves. Surg. Clin. North Am. 52:1157, 1972.

78. Kline, D. G., and Hayes, G. J.: An experimental evaluation of the effect of a plastic adhesive methyl 2-cyanocrylate on neural tissue. J. Neurosurg. 20:647, 1963.

79. Kline, D. G., Hackett, E. R., Davis, G. D., and Myers, B.: Effect of mobilization on the blood supply and regeneration of injured nerves. J. Surg. Res. 12:254, 1972.

80. Kline, D. G., and Hulsen, F. E.: The neuroma in continuity: its preoperative and operative management. Surg. Clin. North Am. 52:1189, 1972.

81. Kline, D. G., Hackett, E. R., and LeBlanc, H. J.: The value of primary repair for bluntly transected nerve injuries: physiological documentation. Surg. Forum 25:436, 1974.

82. Kline, D. G., Hudson, A. R., and Bratton, B. R.: Experimental study of fascicular nerve repair with and without epineural closure. J. Neurosurg. 54:513, 1981.

83. Kline, D. G.: Timing for exploration of nerve lesions and evaluation of the neuroma-in-continuity. Clin. Orthop. Related Res. 163:142, 1982.

84. Knecht, C. D.: Radial-brachial paralysis. *In* Kirk, R. W. (ed.): *Current Veterinary Therapy V.* W. B. Saunders Co., Philadelphia, 1974.

85. LaBelle, J. J., and Allen, D. E.: The peripheral nerve repair: a review. J. Maine Med. Assoc. 63:164, 1972.

86. Lehman, R. A. W., Hayes, G. J., and Leonard, F.: Toxicity of alkyl-2-cyanoacrylates. I. Peripheral nerve. Arch. Surg. 93:441, 1966.

87. Lehman, R. A. W., and Hayes, G. J.: Degeneration and regeneration in peripheral nerve. Brain 90:285, 1967.

88. Leipold, H. W., Huston, K., Blauch, B., and Guffy, M. M.: Congenital defects of the caudal vertebral column and spinal cord in Manx cats. J. Am. Vet. Med. Assoc. 164:520, 1974.

89. Lemire, R. J.: Variations in development of the caudal neural tube in human embryos (horizons XIV–XXI). Teratology 2:361, 1969.

90. Leonard, M. H.: Return of skin sensation in children without repair of nerves. Clin. Orthop. 95:273, 1973.

91. Lesser, A. S.: The use of a tendon transfer for the treatment of a traumatic sciatic nerve paralysis in the dog. J. Vet. Surg. 7:85, 1978.

92. Lesser, A. S., and Soliman, S. S.: Experimental evaluation of tendon transfer for the treatment of sciatic nerve paralysis in the dog. Vet. Surg. 9:72, 1980.

93. Levinthal, R., Brown, W. J., and Rand, R. W.: Preliminary observation on the immunology of nerve allograft rejection. Surg. Gynecol. Obstet. 146:57, 1978.

94. Marmor, L.: The repair of peripheral nerves by irradiated homografts. Clin. Orthop. 34:161, 1964.

95. Marmor, L.: Regeneration of peripheral nerves by irradiated homografts. J. Bone Joint Surg. 46A:383, 1964.

96. Marmor, L.: *Peripheral Nerve Regeneration Using Nerve Grafts.* Charles C Thomas, Springfield, 1967.

97. Marmor, L., and Hirasawa, Y.: Further studies of irradiated nerve heterografts in animals with Imuran immunosuppression. J. Trauma 8:32, 1968.

98. Marmor, L.: Peripheral nerve grafts. Clin. Neurosurg. 17:126, 1969.

99. Marmor, L.: Nerve grafting in peripheral nerve repair. Surg. Clin. North Am. 52:1177, 1972.

100. Martin, A. H.: A congenital defect in the spinal cord of the Manx cat. Vet. Pathol. 8:232, 1971.

101. Matras, H., Dinges, H. P., Mamoli, B., and Lassman, H.: Non-sutured nerve transplantation. J. Maxillofacial Surg. 1:37, 1973.

102. Matson, D. D., Alexander, E., and Weiss, P.: Experiments on the bridging of gaps in severed peripheral nerves of monkeys. J. Neurosurg. 5:230, 1948.

103. McClure, R. C.: The spinal cord and meninges. *In* Miller, M. E., Christensen, G. C., and Evans, H. E. (eds.): *Anatomy of the Dog.* W. B. Saunders Co., Philadelphia, 1969.

104. McClure, R. C., Dallman, M. J., and Garrett, P. G.: *Cat Anatomy.* Lea & Febiger, Philadelphia, 1973.

105. McGrath, J. T.: Spinal dysraphism in the dog. With comments on syringomyelia. Pathol. Vet. *Suppl.* 2, 1965.

106. McNeel, S. V., and Morgan, J. P.: Intraosseous vertebral venography: a technic for examination of the canine lumbosacral junction. J. Am. Vet. Radiol. Soc. 19:168, 1978.

107. McQuillan, W.: Nerve repair—the use of nerve isolation. Hand. 2:19, 1970.

108. Meta, R., and Seeger, W.: Collagen wrapping of nerve homotransplants in dogs; a preliminary report. Europ. Surg. Res. 1:157, 1969.

109. Midgeley, R. D., and Woolhouse, F. M.: Silastic sheathing technique for the anastomosis of nerves and tendons: a preliminary report. Can. Med. Assoc. J. 98:550, 1968.

110. Midgeley, R. D., and Woolhouse, F. M.: Silicone rubber sheathing as an adjunct to neural anastamosis. Surg. Clin. North Am. 48:1149, 1968.

111. Millesi, H.: Reconstruction of transected peripheral nerves and nerve transplantation. Munch. Med. Wochen. 111:2669, 1968.

112. Millesi, H., Meissl, G., and Berger, A.: The interfascicular nerve-grafting of the median and ulnar nerves. J. Bone Joint Surg. 54A:727, 1972.

113. Miyamoto, Y.: Experimental studies on repair for peripheral nerves. Hiroshima J. Med. Sci. 28:87, 1979.

114. Miyamoto, Y., Watari, S., and Tsuge, K.: Experimental

studies on the effects of tension on intraneural microcirculation in sutured peripheral nerves. Plast. Reconstr. Surg. 63:398, 1979.

115. Morgan, J. P., Ljunggren, G., and Read, R.: Spondylosis deformans (vertebral osteophytosis) in the dog. A radiographic study from England, Sweden and U.S.A. J. Small Anim. Pract. 8:57, 1967.

116. Naffziger, H. C.: Methods to secure end-to-end suture of peripheral nerves. Surg. Gynecol. Obstet. 32:193, 1921.

117. Oliver, J. E., Selcer, R. R., and Simpson, S.: Cauda equina compression from lumbosacral malarticulation and malformation in the dog. J. Am. Vet. Med. Assoc. 173:207, 1978.

118. Orgel, M. C., and Terzis, J. K.: Epineural vs. perineural repair. An ultrastructural and electrophysiological study of nerve regeneration. Plast. Reconstruct. Surg. 60:80, 1977.

119. Padget, D. H.: Neuroschisis and human embryonic maldevelopment: new evidence on anencephaly, spina bifida and diverse mammalian defects. J. Neuropathol. Exp. Neurol. 29:192, 1970.

120. Parker, A. J., Park, R. D., Byerly, C. S., and Stowater, J. L.: Spina bifida with protrusion of spinal cord tissue in a dog. J. Am. Vet. Med. Assoc. 163:158, 1973.

121. Patten, B. M.: Embryological stages in the establishing of myeloschisis with spina bifida. Am. J. Anat. 93:365, 1953.

122. Payan, J.: Anterior transposition of the ulnar nerve: an electrophysiological study. J. Neurol. Neurosurg. Psychiatry 33:157, 1970.

123. Peacock, E. E., and Van Winkle, W.: *Wound Repair.* W. B. Saunders Co., Philadelphia, 1972.

124. Raffe, M. R.: Electrodiagnostic assessment of peripheral nerve surgery. Thesis, Purdue University, 1978.

125. Raffe, M. R.: Peripheral Nerve Injuries, Parts I and II. Comp. Cont. Ed. Sm. Anim. Pract. 1:207, and 269, 1979.

126. Reid, R. L., Cutright, D. E., and Garrison, J. S.: Biodegradable cuff as an adjunct to peripheral nerve repair: a study in dogs. Hand 10:259, 1978.

127. Rizzoli, H. V.: Treatment of peripheral nerve injuries *In: Neurosurgical Surgery of Trauma.* U.S. Govt. Printing Off., Washington, D.C., 1965.

128. Roberts, R. S.: Fate of frozen irradiated allogenic nerve graft. Surg. Form 18:445, 1967.

129. Rydevik, B., Lundborg, G., and Nordberg, C.: Intraneural tissue reactions induced by internal neurolysis. Scand. J. Plast. Reconstr. Surg. 10:3, 1976.

130. Sanders, F. K., and Young, J. Z.: The degeneration and reinnervation of grafted nerves. Anatomy 76:143, 1942.

131. Seddon, H. J.: Three types of nerve injury. Brain 66:238, 1943.

132. Seddon, H. J., and Holmes, W.: The late condition of nerve homografts in man. Surg. Gynecol. Obstet. 79:342, 1943.

133. Seddon, H. J.: Nerve grafting. J. Bone Joint Surg. 45B:447, 1963.

134. Seddon, H. J.: Nerve injuries. J. Univ. Mich. Med. Center 31:4, 1965.

135. Segedy, A. K., Yano, B. and Jeraj, K.: Sacral spinal cord agenesis in a kitten. J. Am. Vet. Med. Assoc. 174:510, 1979.

136. Sims, M. H., and Redding, R. W.: Failure of neuromuscular transmission after complete nerve section in the dog. Am. J. Vet. Res. 40:931, 1979.

137. Singh, R., Vriesendorp, H. M., Mechelse, K., et al.: Nerve allografts and histocompatibility in dogs. J. Neurosurg. 47:737, 1977.

138. Smith, J. W.: Factors influencing nerve repair. I: Blood supply of peripheral nerves. Arch. Surg. 93:335, 1966.

139. Snyder, C. C., Webster, H., Pickens, J. E., et al.: Intraneural neurrorhaphy: a preliminary clinical and histological evaluation. Ann. Surg. 167:691, 1968.

140. Spurling, R. C., and Woodhall, B.: Experiences with early nerve surgery in peripheral nerve injuries. Ann. Surg. 123:731, 1946.

141. Starkweather, R. J., Neviaser, R. J., Adams, J. P., and Parsons, D. B.: The effect of devascularization on the regeneration of lacerated peripheral nerves: an experimental study. J. Hand Surg. 3:163, 1978.

142. Steinburg, H. S.: The use of electrodiagnostic techniques in evaluating traumatic brachial-plexus root injuries. J. Am. Anim. Hosp. Assoc. 15:621, 1979.

143. Sterner, W., and Moller, A. W.: Tendon transplantation–a surgical approach to radial paralysis in the dog. J. Am. Vet. Med. Assoc. 137:71, 1960.

144. Stromberg, B. V., Vlastou, D., and Earle, A. S.: Effect of nerve graft polarity on nerve regeneration and function. J. Hand Surg. 4:444, 1979.

145. Sunderland, S.: A classification of peripheral nerve injuries producing loss of function. Brain 74:491, 1951.

146. Sunderland, S.: Brachial plexus lesions due to compression, stretch and penetrating injuries. *In: Nerve and Nerve Injuries.* E. and S. Livingstone, Edinburgh, 1968.

147. Sunderland, S.: Anatomical features of nerve trunks in relation to nerve injury and repair. Clin. Neurosurg. 17:38, 1969.

148. Sunderland, S.: The restoration of median nerve function after destructive lesions which preclude end-to-end repair. Brain 97:1, 1974.

149. Sunderland, S.: The pros and cons of funicular nerve repair. J. Hand Surg. 4:201, 1979.

150. Swaim, S. F.: Peripheral nerve surgery in the dog. J. Am. Vet. Med. Assoc. 161:905, 1972.

151. Swaim, S. F.: Peripheral nerve surgery. In Hoerlein, B. F. (ed.): *Canine Neurology.* 3rd ed. W. B. Saunders Co., Philadelphia, 1978.

152. Tallis, R., Stamforth, P., and Fisher, R.: Neurophysiological studies of autogenous sural nerve grafts. J. Neurol. Neurosurg. Psychiatry 41:677, 1978.

153. Tarlov, I. M., Denslow, C., Swarz, S., and Pineles, D.: Plasma clot suture of nerves. Arch. Surg. 47:44, 1943.

154. Tarlov, I. M., and Benjamin, B.: Plasma clot and silk suture of nerves. Surg. Gynecol. Obstet. 76:366, 1943.

155. Tarlov, I. M., and Epstein, J. A.: Nerve grafts: The importance of an adequate blood supply. J. Neurosurg. 2:49, 1945.

156. Tarvin, G., and Prata, R. G.: Lumbosacral stenosis in dogs. J. Am. Vet. Med. Assoc. 177:154, 1980.

157. Taylor, G. I.: Nerve grafting with simultaneous microvascular reconstruction. Clin. Orthop. 133:56, 1978.

158. Taylor, R. A.: Treatment of fractures of the sacrum and sacrococcygeal region. Vet. Surg. 10:119, 1981.

159. Terzis, K. J., and Strauch, B.: Microsurgery of the peripheral nerve: a physiological approach. Clin. Orthop. 133:39, 1978.

160. Tsuge, K., Ikuta, Y., and Sakane, M.: A new technique for nerve suture: the anchoring funicular suture. Plast. Reconstr. Surg. 56:496, 1975.

161. Van Beek, A., and Glover, J. L.: Primary versus delayed primary neurrorhaphy in rat sciatic nerve. J. Surg. Res. 18:335, 1975.

162. Vasconez, L. O., Mathes, S. J., and Grau, G.: Direct fascicular repair and interfasicular nerve grafting of median and ulnar nerves in the rhesus monkey. Plast. Reconstr. Surg. 58:482, 1976.

163. Walker, T. L.: Ischiadic nerve entrapment. J. Am. Vet. Med. Assoc. 178:1284, 1981.

164. Weiss, P.: Nerve reunion with sleeves of frozen-dried artery in rabbits, cats, and monkeys. Proc. Soc. Exp. Biol. Med. 54:274, 1943.

165. Weiss, P.: Functional nerve regeneration through frozen-dried nerve grafts in cats and monkeys. Proc. Soc. Exp. Biol. Med. 54:277, 1943.

166. Weiss, P.: The technology of nerve regeneration: a review. Sutureless tubulation and related methods of nerve repair. J. Neurosurg. 1:400, 1944.

167. Weiss, P., and Taylor, A. C.: Repair of peripheral nerves by grafts of frozen-dried nerve. Proc. Soc. Exp. Biol. Med. 52:326, 1943.

168. Whitcomb, B. B.: Separation at the suture site as a cause of

failure in regeneration of peripheral nerves. J. Neurosurg. 3:399, 1046.

169. Wilson, C. B., Ehni, G., and Grollmus, J.: Neurogenic intermittent claudication. Clin. Neurosurg. 18:62, 1971.

170. Wilson, J. W., Kurtz, H. J., Leipold, H. W., and Lees, G. E.: Spina bifida in the dog. Vet. Pathol. 16:165, 1979.

171. Wise, A. J., Topuzlu, C., Davis, P., and Kaye, I. S.: A comparative analysis of macro- and microsurgical neurrorhaphy techniques. Am. J. Surg. 117:566, 1968.

172. Woodhall, B., and Lyons, W. R.: Peripheral nerve injuries. I: The results of early nerve sutures. Surgery 19:757, 1946.

173. Wright, J. A.: Spondylosis deformans of the lumbo-sacral joint in dogs. J. Small Anim. Pract. 21:45, 1980.

174. Wright, J. A., and Jones, D. G. C.: Metrizamide myelography in sixty-eight dogs. J. Small Anim. Pract. 22:415, 1981.

175. Young, J. Z., and Medawar, P. B.: Fibrin suture of peripheral nerves. Lancet 2:126, 1940.

176. Zachary, R. B., and Holmes, W.: Primary sutures of nerves. Surg. Gynecol. Obstet. 82:632, 1946.

Chapter **96** # Surgical Approaches to the Spine

James Tomlinson and Kay L. Schwink

The surgical approaches to the spinal column discussed in this chapter cover the cervical, thoracolumbar, and sacral regions. The anatomical exposure of the vertebrae is described so that appropriate surgical procedures can be performed. The surgical procedure for correction of a specific neurological disease is described in the appropriate chapter within the neurosurgery section.

A successful approach to the spine or any bone depends on a thorough knowledge of the anatomy of the area, gentle tissue handling, and aseptic technique. A thorough knowledge of the regional anatomy is necessary so that the approach can be made quickly and efficiently without damage to surrounding muscle, blood vessels, or other soft tissue. Gentle soft tissue handling is of paramount importance for rapid tissue healing without excessive fibrous tissue, decreased chance of sepsis, and decreased pain and discomfort for the patient. A thorough knowledge and practiced use of the principles of aseptic surgery are mandatory. Infection, though unwanted in any surgery, is a disaster when associated with the spinal cord and vertebrae.

The surgical approaches start with the cervical spine and proceed in a cranial to caudal direction to end at the sacrum. Most of the figures depict the removal of the muscle from only one side of the spine, as performed in hemilaminectomy or disc fenestration. Laminectomy and other procedures require exposure of both sides of the spine at the surgeon's discretion.

VENTRAL APPROACH TO THE CERVICAL VERTEBRAE[2]

This approach is indicated for ventral slot decompression and disc fenestration. The dog is placed in dorsal recumbency with the legs tied back along the body (Fig. 96–1). A sandbag is placed under the neck to extend the neck. Care must be taken to place the dog vertically.

A ventral midline incision is made from the larynx to the sternum. The incision is deepened to expose the paired sternomastoideus and sternohyoideus muscles (Fig. 96–2). Midline separation of these muscles exposes the trachea (Fig. 96–3). Dissection is continued along the right side of the trachea, exposing the carotid sheath (Fig. 96–4). Care must be used to avoid damage to the recurrent laryngeal nerve and carotid sheath. Reflection of the trachea to the left side protects the esophagus and exposes the longus colli muscle (Fig. 96–5). The disc spaces

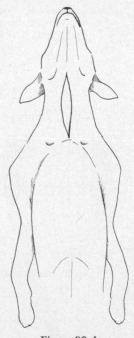

Figure 96–1.

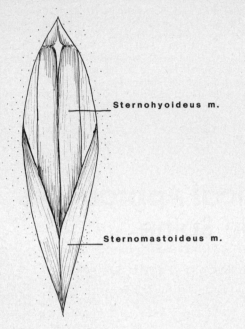

Sternohyoideus m.

Sternomastoideus m.

Figure 96–2.

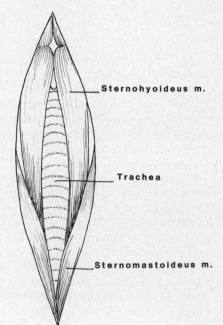

Sternohyoideus m.

Trachea

Sternomastoideus m.

Figure 96–3.

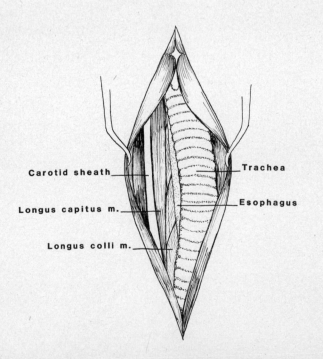

Carotid sheath

Trachea

Longus capitus m.

Esophagus

Longus colli m.

Figure 96–4.

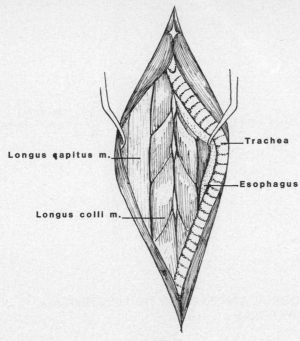

Longus capitus m.

Trachea

Esophagus

Longus colli m.

Figure 96–5.

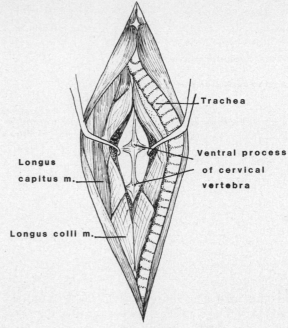

Trachea

Longus capitus m.

Ventral process of cervical vertebra

Longus colli m.

Figure 96–7.

are located just caudal to the midline ventral processes of the vertebrae. Longitudinal separation and blunt dissection of the longus colli muscle expose the disc space for fenestration (Fig. 96–6). Further blunt dissection of the longus colli muscle provides the exposure necessary for a ventral slot decompression (Fig. 96–7).

In closing, the longus colli muscle is sutured if it has been extensively elevated from the vertebrae. The sternohyoideus and sternomastoideus are su-

tured along the midline with a simple continuous suture pattern. The subcutaneous tissue and skin are closed in a routine fashion.

DORSAL APPROACH TO THE FIRST AND SECOND CERVICAL VERTEBRAE[1]

This approach is indicated for repair of atlantoaxial luxations and fractures of the first and second cervical vertebrae and for hemilaminectomy for tumors associated with spinal cord segments C_1 and C_2.

A dorsal midline incision is made from the external occipital protuberance to the dorsal process of the fourth cervical vertebra (Fig. 96–8). The incision is deepened through the subcutaneous tissue to the level of the underlying muscle fascia. The incision is continued on the midline between the paired bellies of the cervicoscutularis, cervicoauricularis superfici-

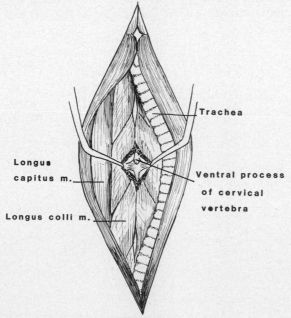

Trachea

Longus capitus m.

Ventral process of cervical vertebra

Longus colli m.

Figure 96–6.

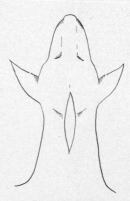

Figure 96–8.

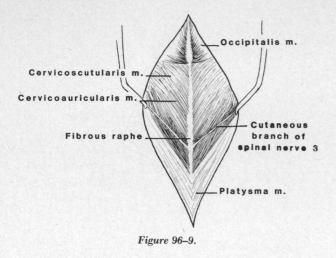

Occipitalis m.

Cervicoscutularis m.

Cervicoauricularis m.

Fibrous raphe

Cutaneous branch of spinal nerve 3

Platysma m.

Figure 96–9.

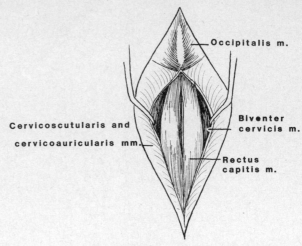

Occipitalis m.

Cervicoscutularis and cervicoauricularis mm.

Biventer cervicis m.

Rectus capitis m.

Figure 96–10.

alis, and platysma muscles (Fig. 96–9). Lateral retraction of these muscles exposes the biventor cervicis and rectus capitis dorsalis major muscles (Fig. 96–10). At this point, the dissection can be continued on one or both sides of the vertebrae, depending on the exposure needed. Separation of the paired bellies of the biventor cervicis and rectus capitis dorsalis major exposes the dorsum of C_1 and the dorsal process of C_2. The rectus capitis dorsalis major is sharply elevated from the dorsal spinous process of C_2 to provide further exposure of C_1 and C_2 (Fig. 96–11). The vertebral artery lies in the muscle ventrolateral to the articular process of C_1 to C_2 and must be avoided as the dissection is continued laterally. The interarcuate ligament between C_1 and C_2 is carefully excised to expose the spinal cord.

Closure is accomplished by suturing the respective muscles together at the midline with simple interrupted sutures. Subcutaneous tissue and skin are closed in a routine manner.

DORSAL APPROACH TO THE MIDCERVICAL VERTEBRAE[1]

This approach is indicated for repair of fractures and luxations of vertebrae C_2 through C_5 and for dorsal laminectomy or hemilaminectomy of vertebrae C_2 through C_5. The animal is placed in sternal recumbency with padding placed under the neck to flex and elevate the neck.

A dorsal midline incision is made from the base of the skull to the first thoracic vertebra (Fig. 96–12). The incision is continued on the dorsal midline through the subcutaneous tissue and fibrous median raphe derived from the aponeurosis of the platysma, cleidocervicalis, and trapezius muscles until the nuchal ligament is exposed (Fig. 96–13). The platysma, cleidocervicalis, and trapezius are retracted laterally. An incision is made along one side of the nuchal ligament and between the paired bellies of the rectus capitis dorsalis major (cranially) and the spinalis et

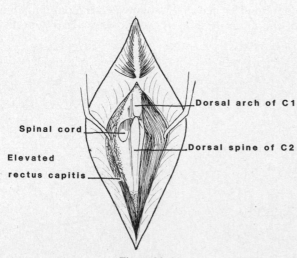

Spinal cord

Elevated rectus capitis

Dorsal arch of C1

Dorsal spine of C2

Figure 96–11.

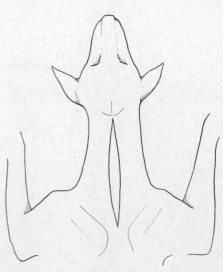

Figure 96–12.

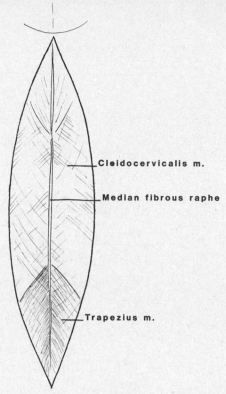

Figure 96–13.

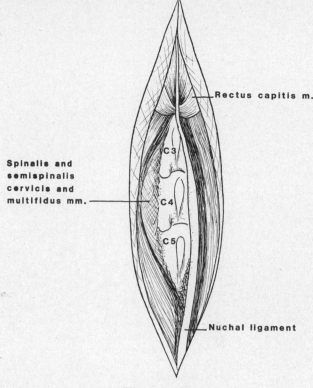

Figure 96–15.

semispinalis cervicis and multifidus cervicis (caudally) (Fig. 96–14). A periosteal elevator is used to remove these muscles from the dorsal lamina of the vertebrae (Fig. 96–15). Branches of the vertebral artery are located in the muscle near each articular process and bleed profusely if the dissection is carried past the articular processes. The insertion of the nuchal ligament may be elevated from the spinous process of the axis if needed.

Closure is started by suturing the fascia of the deep muscles (rectus capitus dorsalis major, spinalis et semispinalis cervicis, and multifidus cervicis) to the nuchal ligament. The fibrous median raphe is sutured next, followed by the subcutaneous tissue. The skin is closed routinely.

DORSAL APPROACH TO THE CAUDAL CERVICAL VERTEBRAE[3]

This approach is indicated for dorsal laminectomy or hemilaminectomy of C_5 through T_3 and open reduction of fractures or luxations of C_5 through T_3. The animal is placed in sternal recumbency with the front legs pulled in close to the body or the front legs crossed to abduct the scapulas. Sandbags are used to maintain the animal in this position.

A dorsal midline skin incision is made from the midcervical area to the dorsal spines of T_4 (Fig. 96–16). An incision through the subcutaneous tissue will reveal the midline tendinous raphe of the aponeurosis of the trapezius muscle cranially and the rhomboideus muscle caudally (Fig. 96–17). An incision is made through tendinous raphe slightly to one side of the midline. The subscapularis, splenius, and serratus

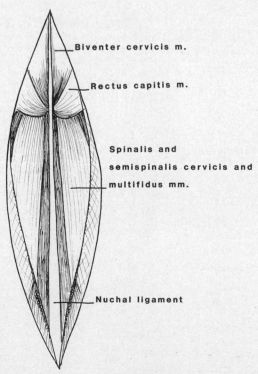

Figure 96–14.

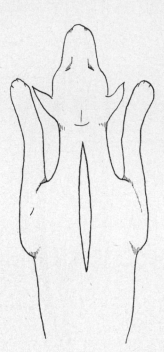

Figure 96–16.

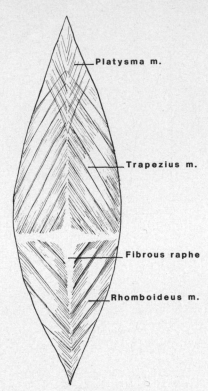

- Platysma m.
- Trapezius m.
- Fibrous raphe
- Rhomboideus m.

Figure 96–17.

dorsalis muscles are exposed by lateral retraction of the trapezius and rhomboideus muscles and scapula (Fig. 96–18). The incision is continued through the attachment of the splenius and serratus dorsalis mus-

cles on the tendinous raphe. Lateral retraction of the splenius and serratus dorsalis muscles exposes the semispinalis capitus and longissimus cervicis muscles, the nuchal ligament, and dorsal spines of the verte-

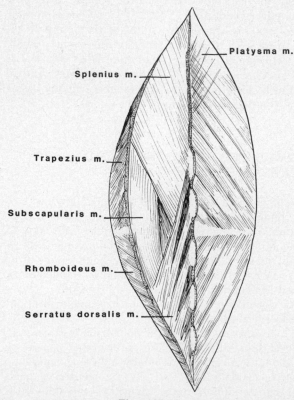

- Platysma m.
- Splenius m.
- Trapezius m.
- Subscapularis m.
- Rhomboideus m.
- Serratus dorsalis m.

Figure 96–18.

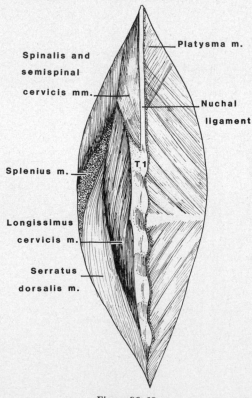

- Spinalis and semispinal cervicis mm.
- Platysma m.
- Nuchal ligament
- Splenius m.
- T 1
- Longissimus cervicis m.
- Serratus dorsalis m.

Figure 96–19.

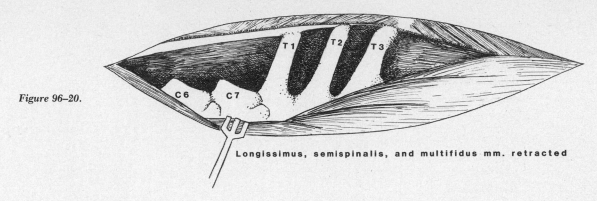

Figure 96–20.

Longissimus, semispinalis, and multifidus mm. retracted

brae (Fig. 96–19). Sharp and blunt dissection is used to elevate the semispinalis capitus, longissimus cervicis, and multifidus cervicis from the dorsal spine and lamina of the vertebrae (Fig. 96–20). The deep cervical artery runs through the semispinalis capitus muscle and bleeds profusely if severed. The dorsal spines of T_1 through T_3 can be removed for dorsal laminectomy because the nuchal ligament is continuous with the supraspinous ligament. The interarcuate ligament between C_6 through C_7 and C_7 through T_1 can be excised with a #11 scalpel blade to expose the spinal cord.

The muscles are sutured to the tendinous raphe or nuchal ligament in their respective layers. The sub-

cutaneous tissue and skin are closed in a routine fashion.

DORSAL APPROACH TO THE THORACOLUMBAR VERTEBRAE[5]

This approach is indicated for dorsal laminectomy and hemilaminectomy, fenestration of the thoracolumbar discs, and reduction of thoracolumbar fractures and luxations.

The skin incision is made slightly off the dorsal midline and extends three vertebrae cranial and caudal to the vertebrae to be exposed (Fig. 96–21).

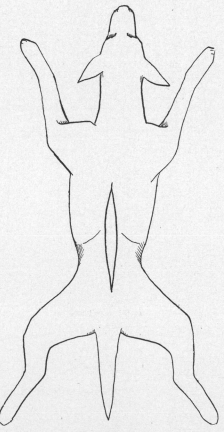

Figure 96–21.

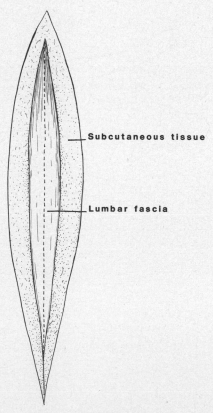

— Subcutaneous tissue

— Lumbar fascia

Figure 96–22.

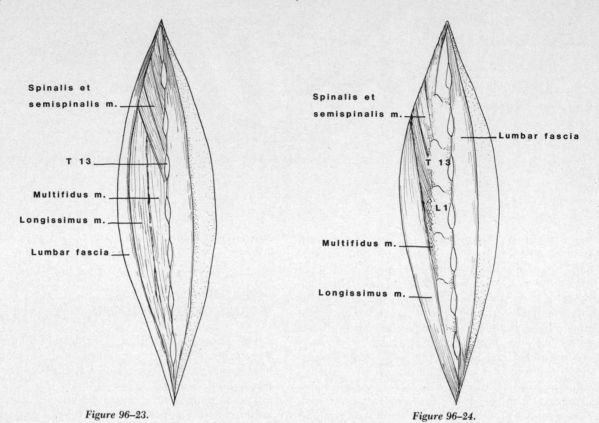

Figure 96–23.

Figure 96–24.

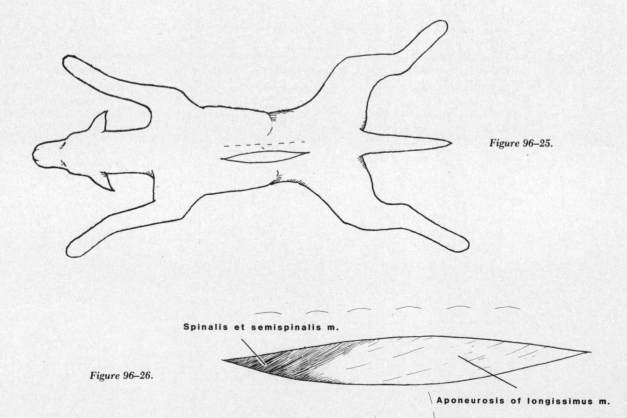

Figure 96–25.

Figure 96–26.

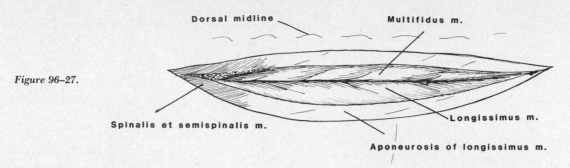

Figure 96–27.

The subcutaneous tissue is incised to the muscle fascia, undermined from the tough muscle fascia, and retracted laterally with the skin. the supraspinous ligament is incised along the top and between the dorsal spinous processes (Fig. 96–22). Lateral retraction of the lumbar fascia exposes the longissimus lumborum and multifidus caudally and the spinalis et semispinalis muscle cranially (Fig. 96–23). The multifidus, interspinalis, and rotatores longi muscles are elevated from the spinous processes and vertebral arches one vertebrae cranial and caudal to the affected vertebrae with a periosteal elevator. The muscle elevation is continued to the lateral aspect of and slightly ventral to the articular processes (Fig. 96–24). This allows sufficient exposure for dorsal laminectomy. Exposure for fenestration and hemilaminectomy requires further ventral elevation of the muscles. Care must be taken to protect the dorsal branch of the spinal nerve, which exits from the intervertebral foramina just cranial and ventral to the insertion of the longissimus thoracis et lumborum muscle on the accessory process of the vertebrae. A small blood vessel is severed at each articular process. This dissection is performed unilaterally for fenestration and hemilaminectomy and bilaterally for dorsal laminectomy.

Closure is started by suturing the dorsal fascia of the thoracolumbar musculature. The subcutaneous tissue and skin are closed in separate layers.

DORSOLATERAL APPROACH TO THE THORACOLUMBAR DISKS[6]

This approach is indicated for fenestration of intervertebral discs from T_9 through L_7. The animal is positioned in sternal recumbency with a sandbag placed under the abdomen to maintain the normal curvature of the thoracolumbar spine.

A dorsal incision is made 1 cm off the midline extending two vertebrae cranial and caudal to the segment of the spine to be fenestrated (Fig. 96–25). The subcutaneous tissue is incised and reflected from the deep external fascia of the trunk for 1 cm to either side of the incision (Fig. 96–26). The incision is continued through the deep external fascia of the lumbar trunk 5 to 10 mm lateral and parallel to the dorsal midline of the spine. As the fascial incision is extended cranially to the spinalis et semispinalis muscle, the incision is directed medially so that the spinalis et semispinalis muscle is incised 1 to 2 mm from the spinous processes (Fig. 96–27). The multifidus and longissimus muscles are separated by blunt dissection from caudal to cranial. The first distinct muscle division lateral to the dorsal spinous process in the lumbar region is the division between the multifidus lumborum and longissimus lumborum. As the muscles are separated, small tendons cross the surgical field in a rostromedial direction toward the spine. These are fascicles of the longissimus thoracis et lumborum muscle that attach to the accessory process of the vertebrae (Fig. 96–28). In the thoracic region, these fascicles divide and also attach to the ribs. The dorsal branches of the spinal nerves are located just ventral to these tendinous insertions. The intervertebral disc space is located caudoventral to these muscle insertions. A small blunt periosteal elevator is used to expose the disc space. A nerve root retractor is used to retract the nerve cranially during the fenestration.

The surgical incision is closed in three layers. The deep external fascia of the trunk is closed with a row

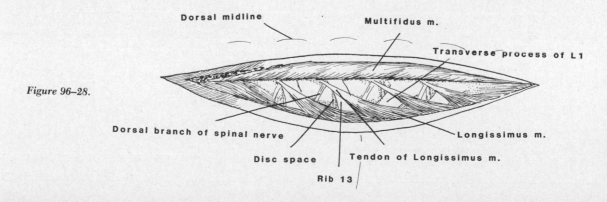

Figure 96–28.

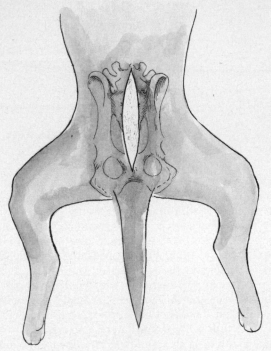

Figure 96–29.

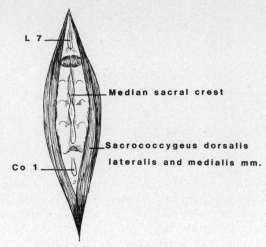

Figure 96–31.

of simple interrupted sutures of absorbable material. Subcutaneous tissues and skin are closed separately.

DORSAL APPROACH TO THE SACRUM[4]

This approach is indicated for dorsal laminectomy for cauda equina syndrome, disc ruptures, and spinal

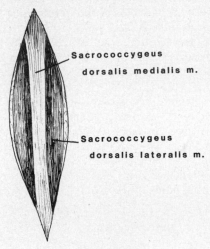

Sacrococcygeus
dorsalis medialis m.

Sacrococcygeus
dorsalis lateralis m.

Figure 96–30.

cord tumors and repair of fractures and luxations of the sacrum and seventh lumbar vertebra. The animal is placed in sternal recumbency, with care taken to ensure that the animal is placed vertically.

A skin incision is made on the dorsal midline from the dorsal process of the seventh lumbar vertebra to the first coccygeal vertebra (Fig. 96–29). The subcutaneous tissue is incised to the muscle fascia, undermined, and retracted with the skin. An incision is made through the deep fascia on the midline between the sacrococcygeus dorsalis medialis (Fig. 96–30) and is continued to the spinous processes of the sacrum. A sharp periosteal elevator is used to reflect the muscle from the dorsum of the vertebrae, and the muscle is retracted laterally (Fig. 96–31).

Closure is accomplished by suturing the fascia of the sacrococcygeus dorsalis medialis with a simple interrupted suture pattern. The subcutaneous tissue and skin are closed in a routine fashion.

1. Funkquist, B.: Decompression laminectomy for cervical disk protrusion in the dog. Acta Vet. Scand. 3:88, 1962.
2. Olsson, S. E.: On disk protrusion in the dog. Acta Orthop. Scand. Suppl. VIII, 1951.
3. Parker, A.: Surgical approach to the cervicothoracic junction. J. Am. Anim. Hosp. 9:374, 1973.
4. Piermattei, D. L., and Greeley, R. G.: *An Atlas of Surgical Approaches to the Bones of the Dog and Cat.* W. B. Saunders, Philadelphia, 1974, p. 54.
5. Redding, R. W.: Laminectomy in the dog. Am. J. Vet. Res. 12:123, 1951.
6. Yturraspe, D. J., and Lumb, W. V.: Dorsolateral muscle separating approach for thoraco-lumbar intervertebral disk fenestration in the dog. J. Am. Vet. Med. Assoc. 162:1037, 1973.

Chapter 97

Diseases of the Spinal Column

Tom L. Walker, James Tomlinson, Jr.,
Donald C. Sorjonen, and Joe N. Kornegay

FRACTURES AND LUXATIONS OF THE SPINAL COLUMN

The assessment of traumatic spinal injuries requires a rational, multidisciplinary approach based on sound neurological localization and an appreciation of spinal orthopedics. A proportion of traumatic injuries produce permanent or fatal neurological consequences, whereas others of similar origin allow remarkable ambulatory function and rapid recovery. It is those cases between the extremes that must be diagnosed, assessed for their potential for recovery, and treated accordingly. This diagnostic and therapeutic dilemma is most rationally handled when one has a working knowledge of the pathophysiology of spinal injury and the current concepts of surgical treatment.

Biomechanics of Spinal Fractures and Luxations

Spinal fractures and luxations occur most commonly at the junction of a mobile and an immobile portion of the spine.[35,73] The majority of traumatic injuries are localized to the body of the axis in the cervical area, the lower thoracic spine in the thoracolumbar region, and the lumbosacral junction in the lumbar segment.[35,68,73] Each region is predisposed to specific types of fractures in response to the forces of hyperflexion, hyperextension, compression (axial loading), and rotation. Five areas of the affected vertebrae may be involved: the body, the pedicles, the laminae, the spinous, articular, and transverse processes, and the intervertebral space.[73]

A stable spinal fracture or luxation is one in which the fragments are not likely to move and thereby cause damage during healing. When instability and neural damage are likely, the spinal segment is unstable, whether the displacement occurred immediately or occurred progressively during an extended healing process. The stability of a spinal fracture or luxation is governed in part by the mechanism involved in the vertebral injury. The infrequent hyperextension injury is usually stable, but flexion injuries (e.g., a blow to the head or pelvis with the spine arched dorsally) may be quite unstable and may require internal fixation. Therefore, consideration must be given to these mechanisms when spinal injuries are grouped for classification and treatment.

Extension Injuries

Hyperextension injury to the spine of a small animal most frequently results from a blow to the dorsum of the spine. Rather than the vertebral body fracturing, the dorsal articular facets are collapsed together, and the ventral portion of the annulus fibrosus tears. The nucleus pulposus is harmlessly extruded ventrally, while the residual stability provided by the interspinous and supraspinous ligaments, the ligamentum flavum, and the joint capsule of the articular facets maintains stability.

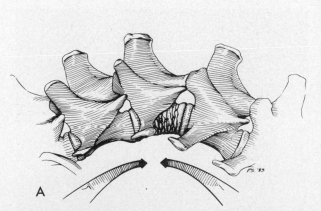

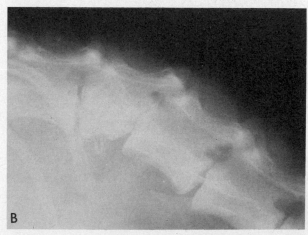

Figure 97–1. A, Wedge compression fractures result when compressive forces load the vertebral column while the spine is in flexion (*arrows*). B, A wedge compression fracture of L2 vertebra.

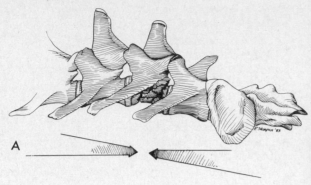

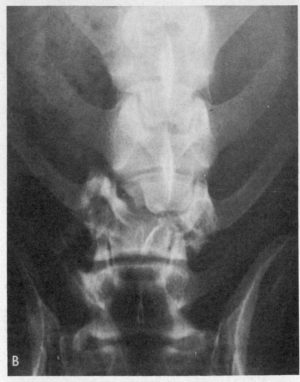

Figure 97–2. *A,* Bursting compression fractures result when compressive forces load the vertebral column while the spine is straight *(arrows)*. *B,* A "burst" fracture of L6 vertebra.

Flexion Injuries

Compression Fractures

In general, most vertebral injuries involve flexion with compression and longitudinal shortening of the vertebral body or interspace.[79] When a significant flexion load is applied, the excessive compression is absorbed by the vertebral body. The distribution of shearing forces fractures the vertebrae ventrally but usually allows the dorsal supporting complex to remain intact. When pure hyperflexion injuries result in mildly displaced vertebral body fractures, the residual stability provided by the dorsal interspinous ligaments and the joint capsule of the articular facets

frequently allows conservative management.[38,63] When hyperflexion is more severe or is combined with rotation, the resulting instability may require internal stabilization.

A wedge compression fracture occurs when cancellous and cortical bone along the ventral aspect of the vertebral body is crushed by a more severe flexion force applied to the head or pelvic area (Fig. 97–1). The narrow part of the wedge is located ventrally, with the intact dorsal ligamentous support acting as a fulcrum.[14,73] These fractures most commonly occur in the lower cervical, thoracolumbar, and lumbar spinal regions.

The bursting compression fracture occurs when compressive forces act along a straightened segment

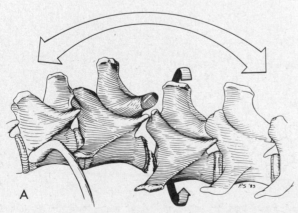

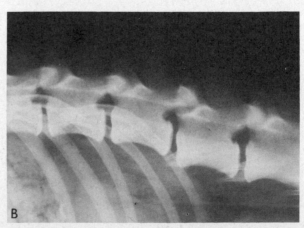

Figure 97–3. *A,* An intervertebral subluxation results when a predominant flexion force is accompanied by simultaneous rotation of the vertebra *(arrows)*. *B,* A subluxation at L1-L2 vertebrae.

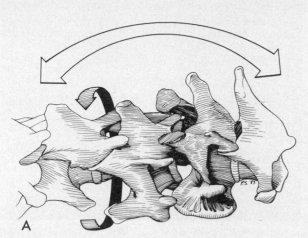

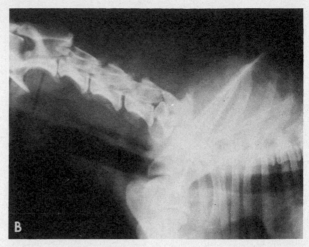

Figure 97–4. A, Cervical vertebral subluxations result from flexion and rotary forces that cause unilateral or bilateral facet dislocation and interlocking *(arrows)*. B, A C5-C6 spinal subluxation with both facets dislocated and interlocked. Bilateral facet dislocation is usually accompanied by serious spinal cord compression or transection.

of vertebral bodies (Fig. 97–2). As the vertebrae collide, a comminuted fracture develops. The intervertebral disc may be extruded or simultaneously forced into the adjacent vertebral body. Bone fragments may be driven outward from the fracture and may cause direct cord trauma or compression.[14,73] In these cases, the stability provided by spinous processes and ligaments, which varies, determines the need for internal fixation.[79]

An uncommon atlas fracture resulting from axial compression of the atlas against the occipital condyles has been described in the dog. This fracture resembles the Jefferson fracture described in humans, which is caused by a forward displacement of the

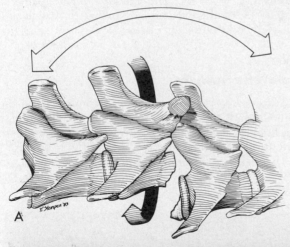

Figure 97–5. A, Vertebral fracture dislocations result when a predominantly rotary force is applied with flexion to crush one vertebral body against the one cranial or caudal to it *(arrows)*. B, A fracture dislocation at L6-L7 vertebrae. Note the "teardrop" portion that has been fractured from the L6 vertebral body. C, A "teardrop" type fracture dislocation at L3-L4 vertebrae illustrates more severe flexion than shown in B.

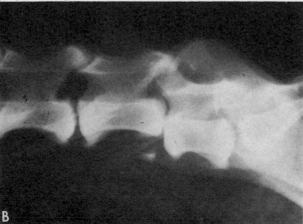

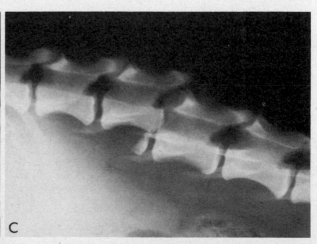

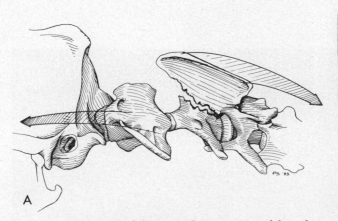

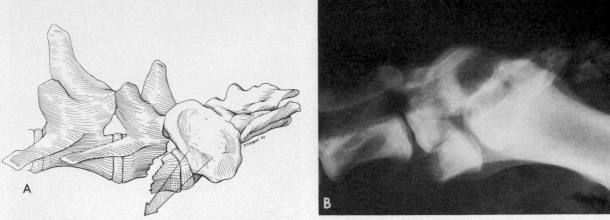

Figure 97–6. A, Fracture-dislocation at L4-L5, demonstrating the cranioventral displacement of the caudal vertebral segments *(arrows)*. *B*, Vertebral fracture dislocation at L7.

dens and widening of the arches of the atlas at the fracture lines.[79] It represents a particular type of bursting fracture.[68]

Luxation and Fracture Luxation

Spinal displacement (luxation) at the intervertebral space results when flexion occurs as the primary traumatic force is applied with simultaneous rotation to the vertebral segment. A minor displacement is termed subluxation (Fig. 97–3). In the cervical area, flexion and rotary forces result in subluxation with unilateral or bilateral articular facet dislocation. The facets interlock and prevent normal alignment of the articular processes (Figure 97–4).[73]

When a predominantly rotary force is applied with flexion in other areas of the spine, a "teardrop" type fracture-dislocation results (Fig. 97–5). A "teardrop" fracture dislocation occurs from the crushing of one vertebral body by the vertebral body cranial or caudal to it. A portion of the involved vertebra not only is compressed but is frequently broken away from the major portion. The fragment resembles a drop of water dripping from the vertebral body. The importance of the injury is the displacement of the margin of the fractured vertebral body into the spinal canal and the resulting instability.[34,79]

Luxations and fracture-dislocation of the lumbosacral area are usually the result of trauma to the pelvic area. The spinal deformity results from either an oblique fracture of the seventh lumbar vertebra or a subluxation of L7-S1. The caudal spinal segment is luxated ventrally and cranially owing to weight and muscle action of the sacral and pelvic unit (Fig. 97–6).[16]

Transverse Fractures

Transverse fractures occur most commonly on the spinous and transverse processes as a result of a direct blow, flexion, or hyperextension injury to these structures or of muscular avulsion of the process.[14]

The axis is a common site for a transverse or oblique type fracture. The anatomy of the cervical

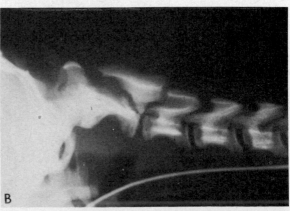

Figure 97–7. A, Flexion and distraction forces transmitted from the cervicocranium (skull, dens, and body of the axis) and remainder of the cervical spine culminate at the axis and lead to fracture *(arrows)*. *B*, A "distraction" fracture of the axis.

area accounts for the disproportionate involvement of the axis in trauma. The skull, atlas, and body of the axis form a relatively stable unit called the cervicocranium.[68] The dorsal spinous process of the axis and the remainder of the lower cervical spine are secured by attachments of the nuchal ligament, the spinalis and semispinalis muscles, and their articular facets. Flexion and distraction forces transmitted through the axis act at the transition point to create a transverse fracture (Fig. 97–7).[68] These fractures may be comminuted and may involve either the pedicles or the vertebral body. The degree of comminution and the obliquity of the fracture are determined by the dynamic forces of distraction, flexion, and possible rotation at the time of the injury.

Pathophysiology of Spinal Cord Trauma

The role of the spinal cord vasculature and the dramatic reduction in spinal cord blood flow after injury are important in the pathophysiology of acute spinal cord trauma.[7] Under normal conditions, spinal cord blood flow is primarily responsive to P_{CO_2} and the cord vasculature's autoregulation mechanism. The normal response to hypercapnia and hypoxia is lost in the traumatized vessels of an injured spinal cord. The retarded blood flow exacerbates the hypoxia and leads to the characteristic histopathological effects of spinal cord ischemia.[65]

In general, after the spinal cord is severely injured and a fall in blood flow begins, the spinal cord gray matter becomes severely affected within one to two hours. At this point, central gray matter necrosis with edema and petechial hemorrhages of the white matter is present. Within hours, the petechiae enlarge and polymorphonuclear and microglial reactions are evident. Coagulation necrosis involving up to 40 per cent of the central gray matter and adjacent white matter may be evident by four hours, with complete necrosis plus cavitation of the involved cord segment within 24 hours.[65,68] These irreversible pathological sequelae, in general, are directly related to the severity of impact injury and therefore do not always go to completion.

When an injury producing transient paralysis is sustained, white matter blood flow returns to normal or an elevated level even though gray matter blood flow may remain depressed. This recovery in white matter blood flow may be the initial factor in determining clinical recovery of cord function.[7] Therefore, if the mechanisms by which these pathological changes occur can be checked early in their development, adequate cord function may be preserved by ensuring the integrity of the all important ascending and descending fiber tracts that traverse the injury. The mechanism of traumatic microcirculatory failure as well as a detailed description of its histological effects is discussed further in Chapter 90.

Initial Examination and Management of Spinal Injuries

The routine emergency management of trauma patients must be supplemented with special considerations when spinal trauma is suspected. The animal should be placed on a makeshift stretcher and secured in place with tape or a blanket in all cases of suspected spinal instability.[69] Whenever clinical signs of cranial trauma are apparent, associated cervical or thoracolumbar trauma may be present. Excessive manipulation of the neck to maintain a patent airway or for intubation could aggravate a cervical fracture.[5,65]

Shock and other life-threatening disorders must be corrected and stabilized. If sedation is necessary for the control of pain or prevention of further injury, a limited neurological examination should be performed first. Serial changes in neurological status are important for an accurate prognosis and for delineation of appropriate therapy. The most important of these tests is to determine the ability of the animal to perceive deep pain by applying a stimulus to the digits or tail. This perception may be exhibited by dilation of the pupils, barking, or attempts to bite the examiner. All limbs should be compared for differences in response. When the perception of pain is absent, the prognosis is guarded.[65]

Spinal shock has been described as a transient syndrome demonstrating stages of (1) immediate and complete flaccid paralysis with suppression of reflex activity caudal to the lesion and (2) loss of sensibility. Although the occurrence in humans and anthropoid apes is common, when it occurs in dogs or cats it is transient and has subsided by the time the animal is examined or has recovered from the cardiovascular shock associated with the trauma. Therefore, its clinical importance in the dog and cat is questionable.[2,5,35]

The localization of a spinal cord lesion by neurological examination and the physiology involved with its interpretation are reviewed in Chapter 89 and elsewhere.[5,12,35] In spinal trauma, the examiner mainly uses spinal reflexes and forgoes most postural and attitudinal reactions until the vertebral column is assessed as stable. One common manifestation of an acute traumatic spinal injury that requires comment is the Schiff-Sherrington phenomenon. The result of an acute, severe traumatic lesion to the ventral funiculi of the thoracolumbar cord, this phenomenon is characterized by pelvic limb musculature atony or flaccidity and pectoral limb extensor rigidity with frequent opisthotonos. The integrity of pelvic limb reflexes depends on the location of the lesion in relation to the lumbosacral plexus. The animal usually demonstrates upper motor neuron signs owing to the preponderance of T13-L1 fractures. Whether or not the lesion is irreversible depends on the severity of the compressive myelopathy and the ability of the animal to perceive pain from the pelvic limbs and tail. Presence of the Schiff-Sherrington phenomenon usually implies a lesion so severe that a cord transection has occurred, but it should not be considered diagnostic of transection or any irreversible lesion.[12,35,65]

Radiography is performed on an emergency basis to specifically localize a lesion, assess the degree of vertebral damage, and aid in the overall prognosis. Whenever possible, general anesthesia should be initially avoided to allow protection of the spine by the animal's normal physiological stabilizing mechanisms. Anesthesia may allow excess movement, especially of cervical fractures, which could exacerbate the original injury. The spine should be kept as stable as possible without flexion or extension until a lateral view is examined. Dorsoventral or ventrodorsal views should be carefully positioned and are always necessary to evaluate the spine.

Radiographic signs should correlate with neurological findings. The radiograph of the vertebrae represents their position at the time of the radiograph only. A spinal subluxation that has been reduced may show subtle clinical signs or may have severed the spinal cord prior to reduction. Multiple fractures of the spine often allow one fracture to mimic or mask signs of a second fracture (Fig. 97–8). When an animal presented with acute paraplegia displays upper motor neuron lesions that localize caudal to T2, evaluation of the *entire* thoracic and lumbar spine to the level of L3, rather than just the thoracolumbar junction, is required. This statement also applies to lower lumbar fractures that cause lower motor neuron signs and mask the upper motor neuron signs of a concurrent fracture between T2 and L3.[5]

The neurological assessment of the animal should be based on the results of the neurological examination, never on the interpretation made from a radiograph. When the neurological and clinical examinations indicate spinal trauma, yet no gross abnormalities can be delineated, myelography may be necessary to confirm a lesion. Spinal cord contusion often occurs without evidence of vertebral damage.

The initial emergency treatment of acute spinal injury has been based on results of experimental trauma models and includes a variety of treatments to overcome some of the recorded biochemical changes in CNS trauma. The use of corticosteroids to stabilize damaged capillary membranes and thus prevent edema has been advocated for years. Doses of 1 to 10 mg/kg body weight repeated at 4- to 6-hour intervals have been reported. This extreme dosage is decreased to a third of the initial amount within three days. Corticosteroid treatment should not be used in a massive dose for more than 72 hours.[35,65] The deleterious effects of gastrointestinal hemorrhages, ACTH suppression, and delayed wound healing have been well documented.[35,75]

Anticatecholamine therapy using alpha-methyltyrosine, reserpine, phenoxybenzamine, and adrenergic receptor agonists significantly alters cord injury in experimental models but has questionable clinical significance.[47,48,51–53,86] DMSO (dimethyl sulfoxide) has

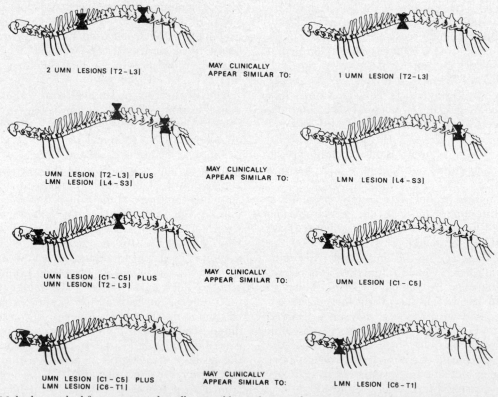

2 UMN LESIONS (T2–L3)   MAY CLINICALLY APPEAR SIMILAR TO: 1 UMN LESION (T2–L3)

UMN LESION (T2–L3) PLUS LMN LESION (L4–S3)   MAY CLINICALLY APPEAR SIMILAR TO: LMN LESION (L4–S3)

UMN LESION (C1–C5) PLUS UMN LESION (T2–L3)   MAY CLINICALLY APPEAR SIMILAR TO: UMN LESION (C1–C5)

UMN LESION (C1–C5) PLUS LMN LESION (C6–T1)   MAY CLINICALLY APPEAR SIMILAR TO: LMN LESION (C6–T1)

Figure 97–8. Multiple vertebral fractures may clinically resemble single sites of compression. (Modified from Bailey, C. S., and Morgan, J. P.: Diseases of the spinal cord. *In* Ettinger, S. J. (ed.): *Textbook of Veterinary Internal Medicine.* 2nd ed. W. B. Saunders Co., Philadelphia, 1983.)

been advocated for its anti-inflammatory, anti-edemic, vasodilatory, and diuretic properties.[62] Hyperosmolar diuretics (urea, mannitol, glycerol, 50 per cent glucose or sucrose) are not particularly useful in cord edema.[7,80] Recently, opiate antagonists have shown promise, but they have not undergone extensive clinical testing.[18]

Cervical Fractures and Luxations

Although a number of cervical spine injuries lead to sudden death secondary to respiratory paralysis, a high proportion have signs of transient neurological deficits with good potential for recovery. The cervical spine maintains a spacious anatomical relationship between the diameter of the cervical cord and the corresponding epidural space even though the cranial cervical segments and brachial intumescence have large cord diameters. This accommodation allows remarkable vertebral displacements without severe cord compression in some cases, but underscores the seriousness of cord damage when clinical neurological deficits and unstable vertebral fractures or luxations are present.

Diagnosis

The most common clinical signs of cervical trauma are neck pain and proprioceptive deficits.[10] The severity of spinal segmental reflex and postural reaction deficits can vary from subtle changes to presenting signs of acute quadriplegia or quadriparesis. Patients with severe head injuries or coma due to trauma are also candidates for cervical evaluation to prevent iatrogenic trauma.

Clinical neurological examination to assess neurological function and delineate painful or swollen areas over fractured vertebrae should be done with caution. Once trauma is suspected, the vertebrae should be maintained in a neutral position to prevent flexion and extension. When intubation and cervical radiography are performed, care must be taken not to stress the fracture site. Bulky support bandages should be considered whenever instability is suspected.

Anesthesia will eventually be required for accurate radiographic evaluation. One must study oblique views carefully to understand the type of injuries present. Because of the potential for disruption of the respiratory centers located in the medullary areas as well as the potential for permanent quadriplegia, positioning for stress views must not aggravate an unstable area. Myelography may be indicated whenever multiple fracture sites are involved or when soft tissue compression is suspected.

Conservative Management

Conservative management of cervical spinal fractures and luxations, in the form of external supports, is relatively ineffective. Logistical difficulties prevent closed reduction using skull and skeletal traction, and because the dog lacks well-developed clavicles, neck braces do not maintain stable reduction once it is achieved.[10]

Supports such as braces, casts, bandages, and splints may be useful in protecting nondisplaced fractures with minimal neurological deficits but also require strict confinement to a small area. The one instance in which closed reduction and casting has been effective is the treatment of atlanto-occipital dislocation. Two reported patients progressed well with this treatment.[29]

Surgical Management

In the traumatized cervical spine, decompression of the spinal cord via some form of laminectomy is indicated only in cases of irreducible displacement, bone or disc fragments in the spinal canal, or exploration of a subarachnoid block identified on myelography.[38] The previous belief that decompression of the cervical spine routinely improved recovery has been disproven by the finding that in some cases the laminectomy increased morbidity and mortality because of additional spinal cord trauma and vertebral instability.[6] Cervical decompression should be accomplished by reduction of the displacement and adequate internal fixation.

Stable internal fixation in this area is hindered by its small spinous processes and by the lateral location of the vertebral artery. Fractures of the atlas, axis, and C3-C7 must be stabilized according to the type of fracture or instability occurring and the availability of bone for fixation.

Atlantoaxial Instability

Anatomy

The atlantoaxial joint is a multifaceted diarthrodial articulation formed by the first two cervical vertebrae.[17,21,27,49,85] The atlas arises from three centers of ossification but the axis (Fig. 97–9) may develop from up to seven centers.[31] A schedule of times for the formation and union of the centers of ossification of the atlas and axis is given (Table 97–1). The accessory center of ossification for the apex of the dens is present in many dogs. Failure of this latter center to unite may account for many atlantoaxial subluxations in small breeds of dogs.[35]

The atlas and axis are joined together by external and internal ligaments. Externally, the dorsal atlantoaxial ligament joins the atlas and axis dorsally and limits ventrodorsal flexion of the atlantoaxial joint.[21,27,49] The dens projects from the rostral aspect of the axis below the spinal cord and lies on the floor of the atlas.[27,49] Internally, the dens is attached to the central arch of the atlas by a transverse ligament, to the occipital bone by the apical ligament, and to the occipital condyles by the alar ligaments (Fig. 97–

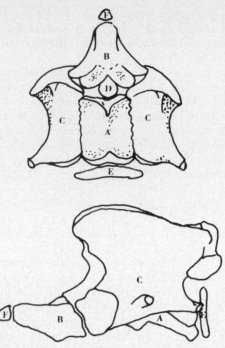

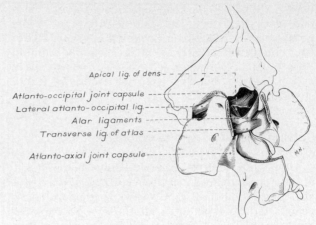

Figure 97–10. The ligaments of the occiput, atlas, and axis. (Reprinted with permission from Evans, H. E., and Christensen, G. E. (eds.): *Miller's Anatomy of the Dog.* 2nd ed. W. B. Saunders, Philadelphia, 1979.)

Figure 97–9. Ventral *(top)* and lateral *(bottom)* views of the axis, illustrating centers of ossification: body *(A)*, dens *(B)*, arch *(C)*, cranial epiphysis *(D)*, caudal epiphysis *(E)*, accessory center for apex of dens *(F)*. (Reprinted with permission from Oliver, J. E., Jr., and Lewis, R. E.: Lesions of the atlas and axis in dogs. J. Am. Anim. Hosp. Assoc. 9:305, 1973.)

10).[17,27,49] The atlantoaxial joint allows rotation and lateral movement of the head.

Pathology

Atlantoaxial instability results from luxation or fracture of the atlantoaxial spine and is characterized by dorsal displacement of the axis into the spinal canal and varying degrees of spinal cord compression.

TABLE 97–1. Schedule of Formation and Union of the Centers of Ossification of the Atlas and Axis

Center	Formation (weeks from birth)	Union (months from birth)
Atlas		
Ventral arch	Birth	4
Lateral mass/dorsal arch	Birth	4
Axis		
Body	Birth	3
Arch	Birth	3
Dens	Birth	7–9
Cranial epiphysis	3	4
Caudal epiphysis	3	7–9
Accessory center for apex of dens	9–12	3

(Adapted from Hare, W. C. D.: Radiographic anatomy of the cervical region of the canine vertebral column. Part II: Developing vertebrae. J. Am. Vet. Med. Assoc. 139:217, 1961.)

Atlantoaxial luxation occurs with intact or congenitally abnormal dens. Luxation with an intact dens results from acute traumatic rupture of the dorsal atlantoaxial, alar, and transverse ligaments (Fig. 97–11). The apical ligaments may remain intact.[49] Affected animals usually have severe spinal cord compression that results in respiratory failure and death. With congenital abnormality, the hypoplastic or agenetic dens produces insufficient internal support between the axis and atlas or occipital bones. Luxation occurs when any force causes sufficient flexion of the atlantoaxial joint to rupture the dorsal atlantoaxial ligament and remaining internal ligaments (Fig. 97–12). Dogs with congenital abnormalities of the dens may remain asymptomatic if the dorsal atlantoaxial ligament and any internal liga-

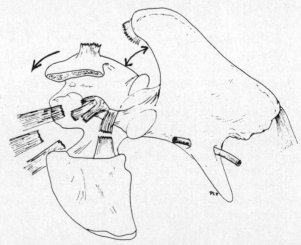

Figure 97–11. Rupture of ligaments of the dens (alar and transverse ligaments) causes stress on the dorsal atlantoaxial ligament resulting in rupture and subluxation. (Reprinted with permission from Gage, E. D.: Atlantoaxial subluxation. *In* Bojrab, M. J. (ed.): *Current Techniques in Small Animal Surgery I.* Lea & Febiger, Philadelphia, 1975.)

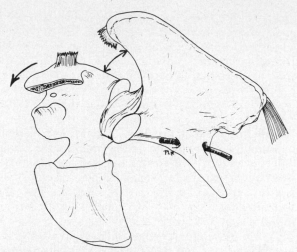

Figure 97–12. A cause of atlantoaxial subluxation is the congenital hypoplasia or agenesis of the dens resulting in insufficient ligamentous support of the dens and leading to subluxation. (Reprinted with permission from Gage, E. D.: Atlantoaxial subluxation. *In* Bojrab, M. J. (ed.): *Current Techniques in Small Animal Surgery I.* Lea & Febiger, Philadelphia, 1975.)

ments present remain intact. Clinical signs become evident as the ligaments stretch. Consequently, congenital abnormalities of the dens may produce a chronic, progressive condition. Clinical signs range from cervical pain to motor dysfunction, including mild ataxia, tetraparesis, and total tetraplegia. In some cases cervical deviation over the atlantoaxial joint may be palpated. Acute trauma may precipitate clinical signs in animals with previously undetected congenital abnormality of the atlantoaxial joint.

Atlantoaxial instability can occur with fracture of the dens, body of the axis, or epiphysis. With fracture of the dens, there is separation of the dens from the body of the axis. The internal ligaments remain intact, but the dorsal atlantoaxial ligament ruptures, resulting in atlantoaxial luxation (Fig. 97–13). In mature animals, atlantoaxial luxation most commonly results

from a fracture of the dens, although it may also be caused by fracture of the body of the axis. In the immature animal, atlantoaxial luxation usually results from epiphyseal separation. With fractures that result in atlantoaxial luxation, severe neurological deficits are usually noted.

Abnormal angulation of the dens is another suspected congenital abnormality of the dens. In reported cases, motor dysfunction noted clinically was the result of spinal cord compression from upward angulation of the dens.[54,72] Evidence of a fracture, nonfusion of the dens, or abnormality of the dens ligaments was not found on necropsy. Evidence from both cases suggests odontoid abnormality but without the usual atlantoaxial luxation.

Diagnosis

The diagnosis of atlantoaxial instability is based on history and physical, neurological, and radiographic examinations. Atlantoaxial luxation occurs most frequently in miniature or toy breeds of dogs between 6 and 18 months of age. The disorder may occur without age or breed predisposition when associated with trauma. In most instances, the onset is sudden. History of trauma is not always present. In congenital atlantoaxial luxation without a history of trauma, the onset may be slowly progressive. The clinical signs are cervical pain and upper motor neuron deficits that range from thoracic or pelvic paresis to total tetraplegia. Dyspnea and respiratory failure may be seen when trauma or acute spinal cord compression is involved. Pain and motor dysfunction can be aggravated by slight flexion of the high cervical region. Excessive manipulation of the cervical spine must be avoided at all times. Palpation over the atlantoaxial area may reveal dorsal displacement of the axis if luxation has occurred, or crepitus and compression of the wings of the atlas if fractures are present.

Definitive diagnosis of atlantoaxial instability is made on radiographic examination. In cooperative patients, preliminary views may be taken without anesthesia. To maximize radiographic detail of the lesion and to minimize the chance for further injury to the spinal cord, general anesthesia should be used.

Atlantoaxial luxation, fractures of the body of the axis, and epiphyseal separation are best diagnosed by a lateral view. Atlantoaxial luxation is characterized by dorsal displacement of the axis and widening of the dorsal atlantoaxial space (Fig. 97–14). If preliminary views are nondiagnostic, slight flexion of the head may allow radiographic demonstration of the luxation. Increased flexion may be required to demonstrate atlantoaxial luxation when the dens has remained intact.[49] Care should be taken not to overflex the anesthetized patient, who can no longer maintain muscle tension. The ventrodorsal view may appear normal in animals with ligamentous rupture only; however, fractures or congenital absence of the dens may be well visualized on this view. An oblique lateral or open-mouth view may demonstrate abnor-

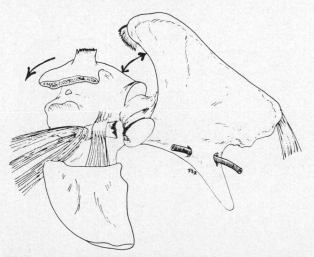

Figure 97–13. If the dens is fractured, the dorsal atlantoaxial ligament may rupture, resulting in subluxation. (Reprinted with permission from Gage, E. D.: Atlantoaxial subluxation. *In* Bojrab, M. J. (ed.): *Current Techniques in Small Animal Surgery I.* Lea & Febiger, Philadelphia, 1975.)

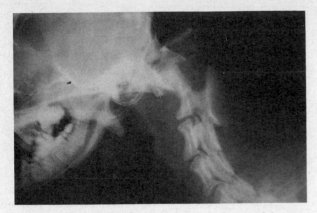

Figure 97–14. Lateral radiograph showing atlantoaxial luxation. Note the dorsal displacement of the axis and the widening of the dorsal atlantoaxial space.

mal development of the dens. However, absence or abnormalities of the dens alone should not be considered sufficient evidence of atlantoaxial luxation.

Because spastic paresis or -plegia observed with atlantoaxial instability may mask the neurological signs of certain spinal cord lesions below the atlantoaxial area, lateral and ventrodorsal views of the entire vertebral column should be made.

Prognosis

The degree and duration of the spinal cord injury determine the prognosis. Absence of cortical recognition of a noxious stimulus applied caudal to the suspected lesion signals a poor prognosis. The prognosis is good to guarded if pain pathways are intact and there is no severe muscular spasticity, contracture, or atrophy.[21,49]

Treatment

Atlantoaxial Luxation. Immobilization of the atlantoaxial joint by external splinting for three to four weeks is a reported treatment.[1, 35, 76] Surgical intervention is generally necessary for permanent correction. Operative techniques include reduction and stabilization of the vertebral fracture or luxation. Spinal cord decompression by hemilaminectomy is performed in case of acute onset. In less severe cases reduction of the displacement provides adequate decompression.[35, 49]

Following anesthetic induction, the patient is carefully intubated and maintained on an inhalent anesthetic. Severe cases of spinal cord compression may benefit from dexamethasone (2.2 mg/kg IV) and mannitol (1 gm/kg IV). Parenteral broad spectrum antibiotics may also be started.

Dorsal Approach. The dorsal approach for atlantoaxial instability is performed with the patient in ventral recumbency and the head supported in a moderately flexed position or in a head stand.[49] During positioning, one must avoid compressing the external jugular veins, since occlusion may cause

exaggerated hemorrhage if the cervical vertebral sinuses are ruptured.[76] The approach to the dorsal atlantoaxial joint has been described in Chapter 96. Dissection of the cranial and caudal margins of the arch of the atlas free of periosteum and adjacent fibrous tissue exposes the spinal cord. Any adhesions of the dura mater to the arch of the atlas are gently removed.

Spinal cord decompression, if performed, is done by carefully removing the lateral lamina of the caudal aspect of atlas and the rostral aspect of the atlas. Care is taken to avoid the vertebral and cerebrospinal arteries, the anastomotic veins, and the first and second cervical nerves. Two small holes are drilled in the rostral half of the axis.

Gently grasping the spine of the axis with a hemostatic forceps and depressing it ventrally reduces the atlantoaxial luxation. Reduction should be maintained throughout the procedure. Vertebral stabilization can be maintained by using a double strand of 20- or 22-gauge orthopedic stainless steel wire. A wire loop is passed rostrally beneath the arch of the atlas (Fig. 97–15A). One strand of the wire should lie on either side of the axis. Wire passage must be performed carefully to avoid trauma to the spinal cord. Flexion of the head and removal of the caudal aspect of the occipital bone or cranial arch of the atlas with rongeurs may facilitate passage of the wire.

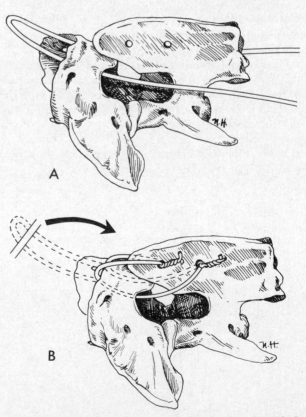

Figure 97–15. A, A loop of wire is passed under the atlas with the caudal strands on opposite sides of the axis. *B,* The cranial and caudal pairs of strands are tied together in their respective predrilled holes. (Reprinted with permission from Swaim, S. F.: Surgical approaches to spinal cord diseases of small animals. Proc. Am. Anim. Hosp. Assoc. *1*:317, 1975.)

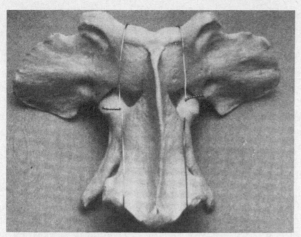

Figure 97–16. Dorsal view of two individual loops of fixation wire on either side of the spine of the axis created by passing the wire loop under the dorsal lamina of the axis and the dorsal arch of the atlas. (Reprinted with permission from Cook, J. R., and Oliver, J. E. Jr.: Atlantoaxial luxation in the dog. Compend. Contin. Educ. Pract. Vet. 3:242, 1981.)

The wire loop is retrieved from the atlantooccipital space, folded back to the axis, and cut in the center. The strands of wire from the atlantoaxial space are tightened through the caudal hole, and the strands of wire from the atlantooccipital space are tightened through the cranial hole (Fig. 97–15*B*). The tissues are approximated in individual layers for closure.

Modifications to the dorsal wiring technique are numerous. Methylmethacrylate bone cement has been used successfully to repair an atlantoaxial luxation after the original dorsal wiring techniques had failed.[60] If the dorsal spine of the axis cannot be used in the fixation, a wire loop can be started at the caudal lamina of the axis and passed cranially under the axis and atlas to be withdrawn from the atlantooccipital space.[11] The loop is cut on either side of the axis, and the cranial and caudal ends of each wire are tightened to form 2 separate loops (Fig. 97–16). To avoid passing the fixation wire under the arch of the atlas, small holes can be drilled on either side of the arch of the atlas.[35] A loop of wire is passed transversely through the drilled holes. The loop is

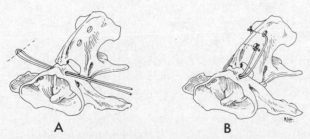

Figure 97–17. Wire is placed transversely through predrilled holes. Trauma to the cord is minimized in this procedure; however, the bony support of the atlas may not be as great as with the longitudinal wire placement. (Reprinted with permission from Hoerlein, B. F. (ed.): *Canine Neurology: Diagnosis and Treatment.* 3rd ed. W. B. Saunders, Philadelphia, 1978.)

cut, and the individual strands that result are tightened through holes drilled in the spine of the axis (Fig. 97–17).

Nonmetallic suture material and the nuchal ligament have been used to stabilize atlantoaxial luxation.[8,45] Nonmetallic suture material is used in dogs with epidural spaces too small to safely manipulate a wire loop. The nonmetallic suture is tied through holes in the spine of the axis or around the dorsal arches of the atlas and axis, as described for the wiring technique. Similarly, after the nuchal ligament is transected from the dorsal spine of the first thoracic vertebra, it can be reflected cranially and split in half lengthwise, and the two halves can be passed under the arch of the atlas. The paired halves are sutured together and secured to a notch in the dorsal spine of the axis.[45]

Ventral Approach. A ventral approach for the repair of atlantoaxial luxation has been described that utilizes decompression by odontoidectomy, fixation with orthopedic pins, and fusion with a medullary bone graft.[67] Atlantoaxial fusion is the treatment of choice for atlantoaxial instability in humans.[30] The ventral approach provides: (1) odontoidectomy in those cases in which the dens is abnormal or has remained intact, (2) good surgical alignment of the atlantoaxial joint, (3) adequate bony mass and mechanical strength to prevent short-term failure of the surgical repair, and (4) joint fusion by medullary bone graft to prevent long-term failure of the surgical repair.

With the patient in dorsal recumbency, a surgical approach to the ventral cervical region is much as described in Chapter 96. Additionally, the right proximal humerus is aseptically prepared for later harvest of a cancellous bone graft. The longus colli muscle is separated and retracted laterally from the underlying bone, from the base of the occipital bone to the third cervical vertebra. Exposure of the luxated vertebra reveals a step deformity of the atlantoaxial interface; the axis is displaced dorsally and slightly cranially. The joint capsule is completely removed to expose the articular surface of the atlantoaxial joint. If a periosteal elevator or similar instrument is placed in the atlantoaxial joint, the luxated vertebrae can be levered into alignment. A slot is created with rongeurs in the caudal half of the ventral arch of the atlas. The dens, if present, is removed with rongeurs or a high-speed drill at its junction with the axis. The dens is reflected rostrally, and any ligamentous structures attached to the apex are incised. This procedure can also be used for odontoidectomy in dogs with abnormal angulation of the dens without atlantoaxial instability.

The atlantoaxial joint is scarified with a No. 15 scalpel blade and dental tarter scraper to remove all articular cartilage. If a bone graft is taken, the right proximal humerus is surgically exposed, and harvested cancellous bone is transferred to the scarified atlantoaxial joint space. The atlas and axis are aligned

VD VIEW OF ATLANTO-AXIAL JOINT

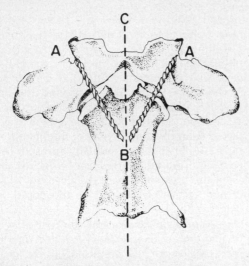

Figure 97–18. Line drawing showing the ideal pin placement. *BC* is a line drawn on the midline. *A* is the medial border of the alar notch of the atlas. (Reprinted with permission from Sorjonen, D. C., and Shires, P. M.: Atlantoaxial instability: a ventral surgical technique for decompression, fixation, and fusion. Vet. Surg. 10:22, 1981.)

and held with small fragment forceps. Nonthreaded Kirschner wires (11.4-mm or 15.9-mm [0.45-inch or 0.625-inch]) are placed bilaterally from the body of the axis, through the atlantoaxial joint, and into the atlas. The best placement is achieved when the pins are started close to the midline on the caudoventral body of the axis. The pins are directed medially toward the alar notch on the cranial edge of the atlas, and they should be advanced as parallel as possible to the ventral surface of the axis (Fig. 97–18). A hand or gas-powered drill can be used for pin placement. The vertebral artery laterally and the spinal cord medially should be avoided during placement of the pins. The tissues are approximated in individual layers for closure.

Atlantoaxial Fracture. Animals with atlantoaxial fractures should be manipulated, radiographed, and anesthetized as are animals with atlantoaxial luxation. Surgical repairs of atlantoaxial fractures are generally performed within 24 to 48 hours of trauma and consist of spinal cord decompression and vertebral stabilization.[19, 20, 49] As with atlantoaxial luxations, the prognosis and preoperative and postoperative medical therapy in atlantoaxial fracture are determined by the severity of the neurological signs.

A fracture of the atlas similar to the Jefferson fracture in humans has been described in the dog. The atlantal arches are split, leaving the vertebra in equilateral halves and requiring wiring of both dorsal and ventral arches for repair.[68] Atlantal wing fractures are treated conservatively.

The junction of the axial body and the cranial articular facets is the area of the cervical spine most commonly fractured.[68] The flexion-distraction forces make reduction difficult from a dorsal approach and prevent dorsal wiring from adequately stabilizing the fracture.[68, 76]

Dorsal Approach. When dorsal structures can be used to support fixation devices, the dorsal approach can be used for repair of fractures of the dens, body of the atlas and axis, or axial endplates. The hemilaminectomy is performed over the area of greatest spinal cord compression. Any bone fragments or blood clots are gently removed. The area is flushed with a suitable isotonic solution. In animals with severe neurological deficits, a durotomy provides meningeal decompression of the spinal cord and an opportunity to evaluate for myelomalacia. Vertebral reduction and stabilization are performed using the techniques described for atlantoaxial luxation repair by the dorsal approach. A fracture of the occiput and dorsal arch of the atlas with atlantoaxial luxation in a dog has been reported; surgical stabilization used a strand of stainless steel wire connecting the external occipital protuberance to the dorsal spine of the axis.[20]

Ventral Approach. The ventral approach is applicable when damaged dorsal structures cannot support fixation devices or when dorsal repair has failed. The approach is identical to that for ventral repair of atlantoaxial luxation. The fracture segments are identified, and the fracture is reduced with a periosteal elevator. Gentle traction on the head aids reduction. One or two finger plates are molded to fit the axis.[28] The single plate is applied on the midline, after the medial ridge is removed flush with the vertebral body, so that two screws can be placed on either side of the fracture line. When two plates are employed, they are applied to each side of the medial ridge of the axis. Fracture stability is improved when two screws per plate are used on either side of the fracture line. Each plate is held in place with a hemostat until it can be secured with screws. Screws should engage inner cortical bone but should not enter the spinal canal. Preoperative radiographs may be used to ensure proper screw depth.

In breeds too small for plates, or when the fracture leaves insufficient bone for proper plate application (e.g., fracture of the dens), odontoidectomy and ventral fixation with pins or screws and bone fusion can be used.

Postoperative Treatment

Postoperative treatment consists of broad-spectrum antibiotics. Patients with severe spinal cord damage may require corticosteroids and hyperosmolar diuretics. A metal splint extending from the dorsal aspect of the skull to the caudal cervical area is generally applied for five to seven days. In nonsurgical corrections, the splint should remain for 14 to 21 days. Isometric exercises or hydrotherapy beginning the third day after surgery should continue until the patient is ambulatory. Recovery generally begins within 10 to 14 days, depending on the interval from onset to surgery and the degree of permanent spinal cord damage.

Complications

Spinal cord injury resulting from passage of fixation materials under the atlas, stabilization failures secondary to insufficient bone support for fixation devices, bone weakening following hemilaminectomy, and breakage of fixation materials are complications reported with the dorsal approach.[8,60]

Complications encountered with the ventral approach include stabilization failures from screw migration when plates are used. If pins are improperly angulated, they enter the neural canal or puncture the vertebral artery, and inadequate bony purchase may cause pin migration and joint instability.[67]

Fractures of C3-C7

Compression fractures with possible subluxation of the vertebral body should be approached ventrally. In these cases, decompression may be difficult but it can be accomplished by a cervical slot procedure. When the decompression produces additional instability in the area, the aim of repair includes reduction of the fracture and stabilization with ventrally attached (metal or plastic) body plates or pins incorporated in methylmethacrylate.[10] When screws are placed through a plate into the vertebral body they should not penetrate two cortices owing to the risk of iatrogenic cord trauma from a screw's penetrating the spinal canal. Acutely lateral angulation of a screw may aid in securing two cortices; however, when this maneuver is not possible, a number of screws will loosen and the fixation could fail before adequate callus formation occurs. Early fusion of the fracture site can be aided by use of autogenous cancellous or corticocancellous bone grafts in all defects, including a decompression slot.[10]

Luxations involving locked, overriding, and fractured articular facets are best approached dorsally. Luxations must be cautiously reduced when facets are "locked," in order to prevent further cord trauma. When facet fractures are not present, routine closure and neck splintage may be all that is required for stabilization. When facet fractures are involved, fusion should be attempted with some form of fixation. In these cases, the loss of stability by the dorsal supporting complex indicates internal fixation. The spinous processes of C3-C7 are not strong or large enough for pin or plate fixation, but small pins can be laid alongside the process and secured with wires to the dorsal spinous processes. Strips of corticocancellous bone have been used in a similar manner in humans to facilitate fusion, in preparation of a "bed" at the base of the spinous and articular processes and attachment of the strips of graft with wires. Care must be exercised, if wire is passed under the dorsal arch, to prevent cord trauma in all cases. When dorsal stabilization is not accomplished, ventral fixation and grafting may be necessary, but its benefit must be weighed against the increased instability of a combined dorsal and ventral approach.[3,10]

Thoracic and Lumbar Fractures and Luxations

The most common site of trauma to the vertebral column of the dog is the thoracolumbar spine. Regardless of the type of fracture or combination of fractures, whether fixation and decompression are necessary is determined by five factors: (1) neurological findings, (2) stability of the fracture and assessment of cord compression, (3) size of the animal, (4) integrity of the vertebral spinous processes and vertebral body, and (5) location of the fracture.

Diagnosis

The diagnosis of trauma begins with the history of any traumatic event leading to increased thoracic or lumbar pain, paraparesis, or paraplegia. The necessity of a neurological examination and the clinical interpretation of segmental reflexes cannot be overemphasized. The principle that in multiple fractures of the thoracic and lumbar area one fracture may mimic or mask signs of the second fracture must be followed in every case. Special care is required to minimize iatrogenic trauma during manipulation of the spine during diagnostic radiography. Anesthesia is mandatory, with stress and ventrodorsal views being used only after stability has been confirmed. Any radiographic or palpable evidence of vertebral movement must be considered a serious instability. The location and biomechanics involved in the specific fracture aid the choice of conservative or surgical treatment.

Conservative Management

A large number of thoracic and lumbar spinal fractures do not require surgery. Stable, mildly displaced fractures or subluxations with minimal neurological deficits are often handled conservatively. In these cases, the fragments are not likely to move or cause neural damage during the healing phase. Strict confinement to a cage for four to 12 weeks and good nursing care will often allow satisfactory recovery. Excessive movement during this early, critical period may cause the healing callus to enlarge and result in secondary cord compression after initial clinical improvement. Splints or casts will not stabilize an unstable spinal segment but will aid in preventing lateral as well as dorsoventral movement, which could aggravate a stable fracture. Although they may well be indicated to prevent worsening an animal's condition while working with the patient early in the recovery stage, heavy, loose casts do little more than add weight and cause discomfort. The unique requirements for body casting or splinting have been outlined and are generally as follows: (1) the cast is applied with the animal under profound sedation or anesthesia; (2) appropriate support material of thin plywood, yucca board, or aluminum splint rod is cut to correct length; (3) the material is heavily padded on each end of support to prevent pressure on the dorsal spines; (4) the entire area to be splinted is wrapped with cast padding and roll gauze; and (5) the entire area is covered with heavy tape or light cast material.[35]

Cast material should fit snugly in the flank area and requires cranial anchoring, to the hair. A wedge or triangle is cut from the cast to free the prepuce when necessary. Many casts are excessively loose soon after application owing to emptying of gas from the stomach or poor coaptation to the caudal abdomen. Heavy taping of the splint material often provides a fixation that is more secure fixation and more amenable to modification as necessary. A body cast or splint applied securely over the thoracic area must not impair respiration; it is modified until the desired effect is attained.[35]

Surgical Management

Not all thoracic or lumbar fractures require decompression via some form of laminectomy. The hemilaminectomy is indicated when it allows for the removal of traumatically extruded disc material or depressed bone fragments, redirection of the spinal cord around an abnormal contour of the vertebral canal, prognostic exploration of a swollen cord, or removal of epidural hemorrhage or other foreign materials. Decompression can also be performed prior to fixation if it will help prevent iatrogenic trauma during manipulation. The dorsal laminectomy has these features but requires removal of the vertebral spinous processes, which may be needed in the fixation and for postoperative protection. When unilateral hemilaminectomies do not provide adequate spinal decompression, bilateral hemilaminectomies may be indicated.

When decompression is used, the spinal cord is inspected. On the basis of the amount of edema present, meningeal decompression may be instituted. A durotomy is used to allow direct visual inspection of the cord substance, to facilitate cord decompression,[56] and to allow midline myelotomies to be performed. A myelotomy is accomplished via a dorsal laminectomy by longitudinal transection of the cord along its midline to at least the level of the central canal. Recent reports have advocated this radical form of treatment in severe cases of spinal cord trauma.[61,62,65,74]

Stabilization of the thoracolumbar spine involves plating or pinning either the vertebral spinous processes or the vertebral bodies. Although good anatomical alignment is optimal, absolute reduction of the fracture may not be necessary or possible in some cases. The exact form of fixation depends upon the size of the dog, the degree of vertebral body comminution, the intregrity of the spinous processes and the location of the vertebra fractured.[35,71]

When the vertebral spinous processes are used for fixation, all the vertebral spinous processes used must be intact. The dorsal approach is modified to reflect muscle from both sides of the vertebral spines after

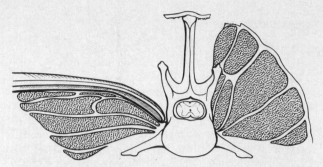

Figure 97–19. A 1- to 2-cm band of lumbodorsal fascia is left attached to the spinous processes to cover the plates after they are applied. (Reprinted with permission from Swaim, S. F.: Thoracolumbar and sacral spine trauma. *In* Bojrab, M. J. (ed.): *Current Techniques in Small Animal Surgery I.* Lea & Febiger, Philadelphia, 1975.)

a broad band of thoracolumbar fascia is retained to cover the plates (Fig. 97–19). When the vertebral body is used for immobilization, the standard dorsolateral approach allows adequate exposure for decompression and implant application.

Spinous Process Stabilization
Metal Plates. Metal plates* are best fitted for transverse and compression vertebral body fractures as well as luxations and subluxations of the lower thoracic and the entire lumbar spine. In dogs weighing more than 10 kg, these vertebrae have spinous processes wide enough to support a bolt† placed through their base. The plates range in length from

---

*Auburn Spinal Plates, Richards Mfg. Co., Memphis, TN.
†Attachment bolts for Auburn Spinal Plates, Richards Mfg. Co., Memphis, TN.

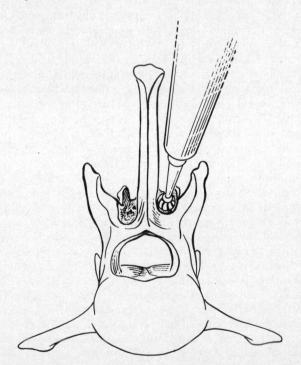

Figure 97–20. Removal of the ridge of laminar bone between the articular and spinous processes with a burr or rongeur allows the plate to fit more ventrally against the spinous process.

3.5 to 12.4 cm (1⅜ to 4⅞ inches) and are selected so that two spinous processes cranial and two caudal to the fracture are included. The plates should be positioned as low on the spinous processes as possible to gain maximum purchase of bone when the holes are drilled. Adjusting the plate along the long axis of the spine will align most holes with the center of the process, and rongeurs can be used to create a groove in the ridge of laminar bone between the articular and spinous processes for more ventral seating (Fig. 97–20).

With one plate held in place, a hole is drilled with a drill bit to allow easy movement of the bolt through the plate and spinous processes. After each hole is drilled, a bolt is placed to engage a plate, the spinous process, and a second plate. When all bolts are in place, they are secured with a washer and nut and firmly tightened without crushing or breaking the spinous process (Fig. 97–21). Excess bolt material is cut off adjacent to the nut.[35,83]

Plastic Plates. The indications and basic approach for the application of plastic plates* to the thoracic and lumbar spinous processes are identical to those described for metal plates. The plates are made of a vinylidine fluoride resin and have one smooth surface and one roughened, friction-grip surface. Four plate sizes, ranging from small to extra large, allow incorporation of two to three spinous processes on each side of the fracture. The plastic can be contoured to some degree with rongeurs, high-speed burrs, or a scalpel to maintain better contact of the plate to the base of the spinous processes. Vitallium nuts and bolts† engage both plates between the spinous processes rather than through them.[87] Stainless steel bolts similar to those described for metal plates can be

---

*Lubra Plates, The Lubra Company, Fort Collins, CO.
†Vitallium, Howmedica, Rutherford, NJ.

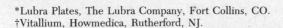

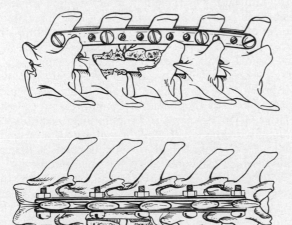

Figure 97–21. Lateral *(top)* and dorsoventral *(bottom)* views of metal spinal plates in place with at least two spinous processes cranial and two caudal to the site of instability. The plates are placed as low as possible on the spinous processes to provide a greater purchase of cortical bone by the bolts.

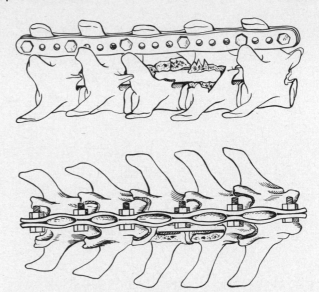

Figure 97–22. Plastic plates "hold" the spinous processes between their surfaces. The bolts and nuts are placed between the spinous processes.

used but may loosen if not applied with a nut and washer on each side of the plate.[35] Tightening the bolts apposes the plates and holds them to the spinous process by friction and compression (Fig. 97–22).

These plates are more useful in the thoracic area than the stainless steel plates, because a hole drilled through the base of the narrow thoracic spinous processes predisposes them to fracture. The plastic plates are available in longer lengths for use in larger breeds and may be more practical than their stainless steel counterparts.

Their disadvantages lie in the means of establishing fixation. The pressure required for the plate to "hold" or "sandwich" the spinous processes can cause some necrosis of bone along the points of plate-bone contact. As the fracture stabilizes and the dog becomes more active, necrosis combined with more active spinal flexion and extension tends to loosen the grip on the cranial and caudal spinous processes. The resultant movement instigates a seromatous response, which often requires plate removal for resolution.[35]

Stainless Steel Pins and Wires. Spinal "staples" are used in cats and in dogs weighing less than 12 kg as an excellent means of fixation in the thoracic, lumbar, and sacral spine. Small holes are drilled at the base of the spinous processes of the fractured vertebra and the two vertebrae on either side of the fracture. The diameter of the end-holes should be the same as that of the pin used for fixation. The fixation pin is selected (.045 to .062 inches [1.1 to 1.5 mm] in diameter) according to the size of the animal. The pin is bent at 90-degree angles with exactly the length between the most cranial and caudal hole. The ends of the pin are left long and inserted through the holes until the pin lies against the base of the spinous processes. The long ends are then bent back toward the fracture and can be cut off 2 to 3 cm from the bend (Fig. 97–

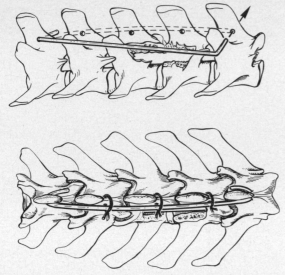

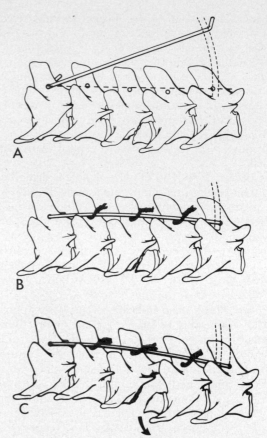

Figure 97–23. Spinal "stapling" method as described by Gage. The 1.6-mm (0.62-in.) stainless steel intramedullary pin is bent at right angles to span the distance between the predrilled cranial and caudal spinous processes. The ends are cut 2 to 3 cm from the bend, inserted into the holes, and crimped as shown.

23) or may be left long to allow double strength (Fig. 97–24).[35] Final crimping is performed to secure both sides of the fixation pin against the most cranial and caudal spinous processes. Orthopedic wire (22 to 24 gauge) is passed through the holes and around the pin to secure the intervening spines. In compression fractures, the pin may be bent at a length one to two millimeters longer than the distance between the cranial and caudal holes to allow for distraction of the fracture. Allowing too much distraction or using a shorter length to compress the fracture can lead to disastrous results by aggravating spinal cord compression or creating instability (Fig. 97–25).[38]

Figure 97–25. A and B, A spinal staple may be bent 1 to 2 mm longer than the distance between the cranial and caudal holes to allow for distraction of a compressed fracture. C, Bending the pin too long so that the segments are over-distracted creates instability or a possible subluxation.

Vertebral Body Stabilization

Vertebral Body Plating. A vertebral fracture in a medium to large dog in which a majority of the vertebral body has remained intact may be repaired by small bone plates* applied to the dorsolateral vertebral body surfaces. Exposure and vertebral size limit the technique to the caudal thoracic area and the cranial lumbar region (T12-L4). The approach is less extensive but otherwise identical to that described for the dorsolateral hemilaminectomy, which may be used as the means of decompression prior to plate fixation. It may also be helpful to position the animal with the left side slightly elevated in order to place the vertebral body at an elevated 30-degree angle, which facilitates screw hole placement.

The plate is positioned so that it rests at the transverse process–vertebral body junction just ventral to the hemilaminectomy defect (Fig. 97–26). The spinal nerve exiting the involved interspace is located and is severed to prevent entrapment by the plate or future osteophytes. Therefore, plates cannot be applied where roots of the lumbosacral plexus are present (L4-L5 through L7-S1). The correct plate

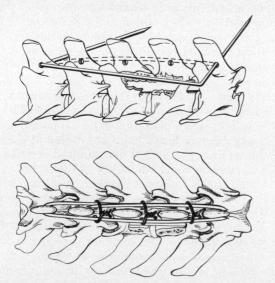

Figure 97–24. Spinal "stapling" modification as described by Hoerlein. Doubling the pin provides additional strength.

*Vertebral Body Plates, Richards Mfg. Co., Memphis, TN.

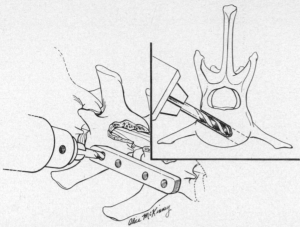

Figure 97–26. The vertebral body plate is placed at the transverse process–vertebral body junction in the lumbar area. The spinal nerves are usually severed at the site of placement, complicating utilization of a plate at the L4–L7 interspace. *Inset,* The proper path of the drill through the vertebral body to supply maximum purchase of cortical bone is demonstrated. (Reprinted with permission from Swaim, S. F.: Thoracolumbar and sacral spine trauma. *In* Bojrab, M. J. (ed.): *Current Techniques in Small Animal Surgery I.* Lea & Febiger, Philadelphia, 1975.)

size (1¼, 1½, or 1¾ inches [32, 38, or 44 mm]) is selected so that two holes are located cranial and two holes caudal to the fracture or subluxation. Comminuted and transverse fractures that do not allow adequate purchase in bone by the screws are not candidates for this type of fixation.

A 2-mm (5/16-inch) drill bit is used to drill through cranial or caudal plate holes in a ventrolateral direction to allow thread engagement in the maximum amount of bone possible. A depth gauge is used to measure the depth of the hole, and the appropriate self-tapping screw* is secured in the hole. The remaining screws are placed. It is important to cover the hemilaminectomy defect with a finger to prevent the screwdriver from slipping off the screw and injuring the cord.

Application of the plates to the caudal thoracic area requires temporary dislocation of the rib heads from their costovertebral articulation. A small K-wire is used to drill a dorsoventral hole in the head of each rib to be separated from its vertebrae. The rib heads are separated with bone cutters and retracted ventrally, allowing plate application as previously described. A pneumothorax is sometimes unavoidable when rib disarticulation is performed and should be considered in the anesthetic management of the case prior to surgery. In a severely traumatized area, tissues must be dissected and handled carefully to facilitate closure of the thoracic wall defect.

When decompression and plating are complete, approximation of the ribs to their original position allows for more cosmetic closure. Stainless steel orthopedic wire passed from the predrilled rib head to the corresponding spinous process is used to elevate the rib. Concurrent stabilization with a spi-

nous process plating technique is often helpful. Closure is as for hemilaminectomy.[70]

Vertebral Body Pinning. This method of fixation is most useful in the repair of subluxations, particularly in the lumbar area. It is frequently employed when other methods have been exhausted owing to fractured spinous processes, vertebrae too small for bone plating, or immature bone too soft for traditional fixation. It is not used in the thoracic area because of limited exposure and rib location.

The standard hemilaminectomy approach and decompression are used. Pins from 1.1 to 1.5 mm (0.045 to 0.062 inch) in diameter are used most frequently, and larger pins have been suggested in larger breeds. In most cases the subluxation is immobilized by cross-pinning of the vertebral bodies involved. One pin is introduced into the vertebral body cranial to the lesion, to a point midway along the vertebral body but just dorsal to the transverse processes in the lumbar area or to the ribs in the caudal thoracic area. The pin is aimed in a caudoventral direction to cross the involved disc space and seat in the next caudal vertebral body. A second pin is introduced into the caudal vertebra and directed to assume a similar diagonal course, resulting in the cross-pinning configuration (Fig. 97–27). It may be necessary to introduce the pin through the paravertebral musculature and direct it into the vertebral body to achieve the proper angle of insertion.

Vertebral body pinning has been described in cases of transverse vertebral fractures. Each pin is anchored in adjacent normal vertebral bodies. This type of fixation is difficult and may require spinous process immobilization.[22]

Postoperative Care. In most cases, external support with splints for seven to 14 days is indicated. An immature or large dog with internal fixation may fracture the spinous processes if the fixation is not supplemented with external support. Body casting or splinting was outlined previously.

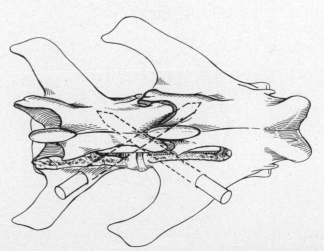

Figure 97–27. A "crossed pin" technique is used to span a single intervertebral space or fracture.

*Richards Bone Screw, Richards Mfg. Co., Memphis, TN.

Lumbosacral Fracture or Luxation

Diagnosis

Luxation of the lumbosacral joint presents a unique problem. The clinical presentation of an animal that has proprioceptive deficits of the rear limbs but potentially severe urinary and fecal incontinence is often puzzling. Because the roots of the femoral nerve (L4-L6) are not involved with the fracture and because approximately 40 to 50 per cent of sciatic nerve roots are unaffected, these patients usually show marked improvement in gait after the initial injury. The major clinical signs in lumbosacral luxation are directly related to the nerve roots passing through the lumbosacral junction. These roots—S1, S2, and S3—are vital not only for conscious urinary and fecal control but also for normal reflex urination and defecation. When the roots are severed, irreversible changes occur that may make fracture or luxation fixation academic. A thorough neurological examination to document remaining sensory or reflex integrity of the S1–S3 nerve roots is mandatory prior to surgery.[66] Any reflex response or conscious pain perception in the anal or tail area is an indication for fracture fixation. When these responses are absent, the operation should be performed on an exploratory basis to confirm irreversible root damage, if possible. Radiography reveals the involvement of L7 and the amount of luxation but does not alter the plan of therapy.

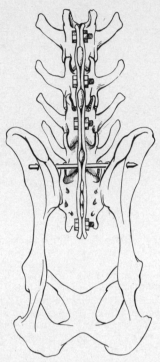

Figure 97–29. Transilial pin used in conjunction with dorsal plates provides additional support for lumbar or lumbosacral fractures.

Conservative Management

The lumbosacral luxation or fracture-luxation is not amenable to closed reduction and external fixation. Although some patients recover without reduction, surgery is the only reliable treatment.[66]

Surgical Management

Exposure of the L7 sacral region is via a dorsal approach (see Chapter 96). Exact reduction of the luxation is accomplished by caudal and dorsal distraction of the pelvic-sacral unit until the articular facets of L7 are properly located on their sacral articulations.[66] At that time, a limited dorsal laminectomy between the L7 and sacral articular facets may be done to examine the cauda equina.[50] If the procedure is being done with poor prognostic criteria, the establishment of root severing will confirm the irreversibility of the lesion and eliminate the need for further stabilization techniques.

Once the luxation is reduced, the use of a transilial pin either by itself (Fig. 97–28) or in conjunction with a plate (Fig. 97–29) provides the extra fixation necessary. The pin contacts the dorsal surface of L7 to prevent the pelvic-sacral unit from luxating ventral to it. The transilial pin can be secured by bending its ends flush with the ilium or by using a threaded pin and nut to secure one end of the pin and making a 90-degree bend at its cut end.[16,66]

Dorsal spinal plates (metal or plastic) have been placed from the lower lumbar spines to the sacral

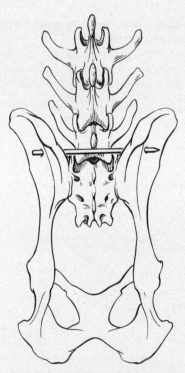

Figure 97–28. Transilial pin used to stabilize a fracture of the body of L7 or a lumbosacral subluxation.

spinous processes for fixation.[71] In small dogs and in cats, the sacral processes are too small to hold a bolt and too small for use of plastic plates. In large dogs, a plate large enough to secure the lumbar spines may be too large for the sacrum. A transilial pin through the plate augments this fixation.

CERVICAL MALFORMATION AND MALARTICULATION

Cervical malformation and malarticulation (CMM) is one of many names used to describe a common disease syndrome in the Great Dane, Doberman pinscher and other large breeds*. Thirteen other breeds with this syndrome are the basset hound, Scottish deerhound, golden retriever, chow chow, bullmastiff, Pyrenian Mountain dog, boxer, Weimaraner, German shepherd, St. Bernard, Irish setter, Siberian husky, and Rhodesian ridgeback.[37,55] The condition is characterized by a slowly progressive ascending tetraparesis and ataxia. Hindlimb ataxia is usually the earliest clinical sign and may be the presenting complaint.

Males generally are reported to be affected with CMM more commonly than females, with cited ratios of 2:1,[64] 3:1,[9] and 4:1.[37,59] However, one report of 57 cases revealed an equal sex distribution.[77] The age range for affected dogs is seven weeks to ten years.[9,37,59,64] Most commonly, CMM is seen in young growing Great Danes and in middle-aged adult Doberman pinschers.

Pathophysiology

The etiology of CMM is unknown. Overnutrition, genetic predisposition, conformation, and degenerative disc disease have all been suggested as causes. CMM has been induced in young Great Danes by feeding a diet high in protein, energy, calcium, and phosphorus. The accelerated growth induced various skeletal abnormalities, including changes in the cervical vertebrae consistent with CMM.[32]

Genetic predisposition to CMM has been suggested as an important factor in the development of the disease.[13,46,58] Littermates were affected in four cases, and in one instance three members of the same litter were affected. A single sire appeared often and in the recent background on both sides of the pedigrees of these dogs.[46]

Conformation of affected breeds may also be significant. These dogs have long slender necks with large heavy heads. The proposed theory is that the neck cannot handle the stresses induced by the head and that consequently the spinal column abnormali-

ties are induced by the increased stress applied to the growing cervical spine.

In the young dog affected with CMM, various pathological changes will be seen in the spinal column. Multiple interspaces may be involved, but the abnormalities are generally limited to one or two disc spaces. Cervical vertebral interspaces 4-5, 5-6, and 6-7 are most commonly involved. Pathological changes seen in the vertebrae include:

1. Bony malformation, which results in a narrow cranial vertebral canal orifice (Fig. 97–30), medial ingrowth of the articular processes, dorsoventral flattening of vertebral canal, and plowshare shape of the vertebral body.[64]

2. Soft tissue changes, including enlargement of the dorsal annulus fibrosa (ventral compression), enlargement of the interarcuate ligament (dorsal compression), and enlargement of the joint capsule (lateral compression).

3. An abnormal relationship of one vertebra to another (vertebral tipping). This abnormal relationship may be stable or unstable. The vertebral tipping may be misleading in that it is not always associated with a spinal cord lesion.[64]

Various combinations of these different lesions may be seen in affected dogs.

In the middle-aged Doberman pinscher, the disease is associated with chronic degenerative disc disease.[61] It is not known whether the disc disease is primary or is caused by the vertebral instability. In these dogs, the dorsal annulus fibrosus compresses the spinal cord from hyperplasia, hypertrophy, or collapse of the disc space with redundancy of the

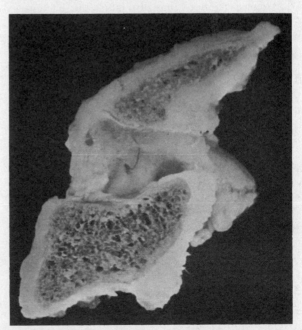

Figure 97–30. Sagittal section of C7 showing severe coning and subsequent narrowing of the spinal canal. (Reprinted with permission of the American Animal Hospital Association from Seim, H. B., and Withrow, S. J.: Pathophysiology and diagnosis of caudal cervical spondylo-myelopathy with emphasis on the Doberman pinscher. Am. Anim. Hosp. Assoc. *18:*248, 1982.)

---

*Other names are: caudal cervical spondylo-myelopathy,[64] cervical vertebral instability,[37] caudal cervical vertebral malformation-malarticulation,[77] cervical vertebral malformation,[59] caudal cervical spondylopathy,[9] caudal cervical subluxation,[24] and spondylolisthesis.[15]

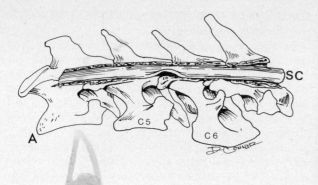

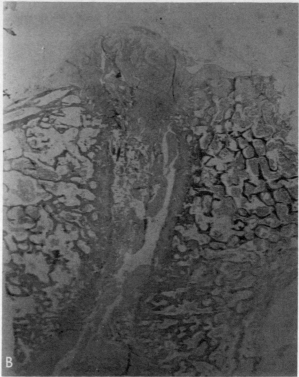

Figure 97–31. *A,* Spinal cord *(SC)* compression caused by enlargement of the dorsal annulus fibrosus between C5 and C6 with the neck in normal extension in dogs with CMM. *B,* Sagittal section taken through C5 and C6 demonstrating the enlarged dorsal annulus fibrosus in a middle-aged Doberman pinscher with CMM.

annulus (Fig. 97–31). When the neck is flexed, the annulus is stretched, relieving the spinal cord compression (Fig. 97–32); this is probably why these dogs prefer to keep their necks flexed. When the neck is hyperextended, the annulus causes increased compression of the spinal cord (Fig. 97–33). The interarcuate ligament may also cause dorsal compression of the spinal cord in this position. With linear traction, spinal compression is relieved by stretching the dorsal annulus flat (Fig. 97–34).

The end result of the bony and soft tissue changes in the vertebrae is spinal cord compression. Spinal cord lesions occur from interference with the blood supply to this region of the spinal cord. Myelin degeneration is the most prominent lesion. At the site of injury to the spinal cord, myelin degeneration is usually seen in all funiculi. Cranial to the lesion, degeneration is limited to the ascending tracts of the dorsal and dorsolateral funiculi. Caudal to the injury,

lesions are confined to the descending tracts of the ventral and deep portions of the lateral funiculi.[77]

History

Often, the predominant presenting complaint of CMM is a slowly progressive incoordination of the hindlimbs. Most patients are presented with a history of insidious onset, and it is difficult for the owners to pinpoint when the problem started. In one report concerning 45 dogs, the average length of time that dogs were symptomatic was 4.5 months, with a range from two days to 24 months; 29 of these dogs had a slowly progressive onset, nine dogs a slowly progressive onset with an acute exacerbation, and seven dogs an acute onset only.[64] The owner may report that the dog has a stiff, stilted gait in the front legs. A number of affected dogs keep their necks flexed. Cervical pain is rarely observed by the owner.

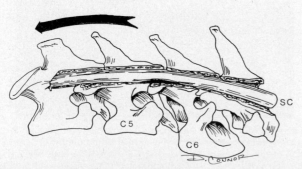

Figure 97–32. Decrease in spinal cord *(SC)* compression at disc space C5-C6 with the neck in flexion in a dog with CMM caused by enlargement of the dorsal annulus fibrosus.

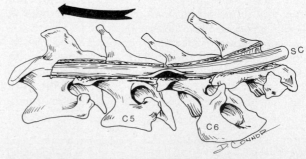

Figure 97–33. Increase in spinal cord *(SC)* compression at C5-C6 with the neck in hyperextension caused by further redundancy of the dorsal annulus fibrosus due to enlargement of the dorsal annulus fibrosus.

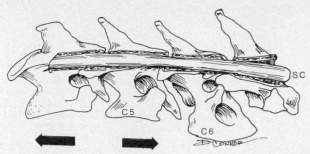

Figure 97–34. Linear traction applied to the neck results in flattening of the enlarged dorsal annulus fibrosus and decompression of the spinal cord *(SC)* at disc space C5-C6.

Clinical Signs

On general physical examination, the principal clinical signs of CMM are bilateral paresis and ataxia of the pelvic limbs and occasionally of the thoracic limbs.[77] A broad-based stance is often noted in the rear legs of affected dogs. These dogs walk with an awkward swaying movement of the hindquarters owing to a pelvic limb stride that is longer than normal and asymmetric. On turning, the pelvic limbs cross or abduct widely. The dogs will sometimes drag their toe nails or step on the dorsal surface of the paw.[77] Palpation often reveals atrophy of the scapular muscles. Cervical pain is rarely elicited by cervical manipulation, although often these dogs prefer to keep their necks flexed and they resist manipulation.

The degree of neurological deficit varies from mild ataxia to tetraparesis. In one study of 45 dogs, 13 were mildly ataxic, 12 were moderately ataxic, nine were severely ataxic, and eight could not walk.[64] Neurological deficits are usually more pronounced in the rear limbs, in which upper motor neuron reflexes are often present. Proprioception (tested by knuckling and hopping postural reactions) is often slow and sometimes absent completely. Neurological signs may be mild or absent in the front limbs. Thoracic limb reflexes are generally normal or only mildly affected. Weight-bearing postural reactions such as "wheelbarrowing" and hopping are often affected. Proprioceptive deficits may be difficult to elicit from the front legs. Mild proprioceptive deficits or paresis may be revealed by extending the dog's neck and "wheelbarrowing" the dog. Care must be exercised in extending the dog's neck because the cervical spinal cord may be acutely injured. Neurological signs are due to cervical spinal cord white matter lesions involving ascending proprioceptive tracts and descending motor tracts.[77]

Diagnosis

A tentative diagnosis of CMM is based on history and physical findings. Clinical signs of CMM are similar to those seen with cervical disc extrusions, vertebral fractures, congenital vertebral malformations (hemivertebrae), ischemic myelopathy, distemper, and spinal cord or column tumors. A definitive diagnosis of CMM requires cervical radiographs with myelography. (Myelography is discussed in more detail in Chapter 93.) The dog must be anesthetized for optimal technique and positioning for cervical radiographs. Plain films should be taken in both ventrodorsal and lateral positions of the entire cervical spine. Flexed and extended positional films may be taken to demonstrate changes in the relative position of the vertebral bodies. Care must be exercised in cervical manipulation because any manipulation, especially hyperextension, may exacerbate neurological deficits. Contrast studies should include ventrodorsal and lateral views and a lateral traction view. The linear lateral traction view is taken while firm, steady linear traction is applied to the cervical spine by grasping the dog by the base of the skull or maxilla and the forelegs and trunk and gently pulling in opposite directions.

The most commonly affected vertebral interspaces are C4-C5, C5-C6, and C6-C7.[37,59,64] The reported incidence of multiple lesions varies. In a study mainly of Doberman pinschers (35 Dobermans of 45 subjects), only seven dogs had myelographic lesions at two interspaces.[64] In two reports of 52 dogs (12 breeds) combined, 39 dogs had multiple lesions; however, no mention was made of myelographic documentation of the lesions.[37,59] The middle-aged Doberman pinscher generally has one lesion, and the immature Great Dane or Doberman tends to have multiple lesions.

The diagnostic radiographic features of this disease are:

1. Abnormal relationships of one vertebrae to an adjacent vertebra. The abnormal relationship may be unstable or stable and is best evaluated on the lateral flexed and normal extended views. Care must be exercised in interpreting vertebral "tipping" as the site of spinal cord injury. In one study, 25 per cent of dogs with tipping on plain films did not have compression at that site on the myelogram.[64]

2. Coning of the vertebral canal with stenosis of the cranial orifice of the vertebral canal. This change is most often seen in the young (less than 2 years) Great Dane and Doberman pinscher.

3. Remodelling of the cranial aspect of the vertebral body. This gives the vertebral body a "plowshare" conformation.

4. Spondylosis of the ventral aspect of the vertebral body with degenerative disc disease. In the middle-aged Doberman pinscher, this finding most accurately reflects the site of the lesion.[64]

5. Periarticular and articular process abnormalities. The periarticular changes are arthritic changes of the articular process probably due to abnormal stress. Asymmetry of the position, size, and shape of the articular process is seen but may be difficult to assess because of the effects of minor positional changes on the appearance of these structures.

Myelography is required for definitive diagnosis of the affected interspace(s). In a study of 45 dogs, the plain film interpretation missed the actual lesion in 14 dogs and missed one of two lesions in four other

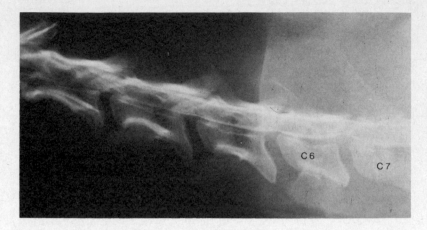

Figure 97–35. Myelogram of the cervical spine showing ventral compression of the spinal cord at C6-C7 (normal extended lateral view). This is the typical myelographic lesion seen in the middle-aged Doberman pinscher with CMM.

dogs.[64] Myelography demonstrates soft tissue compression of the spinal cord due to enlargement of the interarcuate ligament (dorsally), the dorsal annulus fibrosus and dorsal longitudinal ligament (ventrally), and of the joint capsule and facets (laterally). Spinal cord compression from the annulus fibrosus and interarcuate ligament is best seen on the lateral film, and compression from the facets and joint capsule is best seen on the ventrodorsal projection.

In the middle-aged Doberman pinscher, in which spinal cord compression is caused mainly by enlargement of the dorsal annulus fibrosus (Fig. 97–35), a flexion myelogram (lateral view) will eliminate or at least greatly alleviate spinal cord compression (Fig. 97–36). In contrast, the hyperextension myelogram exaggerates the compression ventrally and causes dorsal compression from the interarcuate ligament. Linear traction shows at least partial or complete relief of the spinal cord compression (Fig. 97–37). Spinal cord compression caused by bony lesions or disc extrusion is altered by linear traction.

Treatment

Conservative treatment of dogs with CMM has generally consisted of restriction of activity and corticosteroids. Overall success with conservative treatment has been poor, yielding either temporary or no improvement. The principles of surgical treatment of CMM are decompression of the spinal cord and stabilization of unstable vertebral segments. Patients are divided into two categories: Group I is characterized by the immature or young adult, giant dog such as the Great Dane. These dogs generally have bony malformation as well as soft tissue compression of the spinal cord. Group I has both soft tissue and bony compression of the spinal cord. The group also tends to have involvement of multiple vertebrae. Dorsal laminectomy is the treatment of choice for these dogs, since it is the only procedure that will allow adequate decompression of the spinal cord. Stabilization of the vertebrae can be obtained either by wiring or by screwing the articular processes.

The surgical approach to the affected vertebrae is by the dorsal approach to the caudal cervical vertebrae (see Chapter 96). The dog is premedicated with dexamethasone (2 mg/kg IM), one to two hours prior to surgery. The antibiotic of choice is also administered preoperatively and during the surgery as needed. After exposure of the cervical vertebrae, the dorsal spines of the affected vertebrae are excised with a bone rongeur. The laminectomy defect is

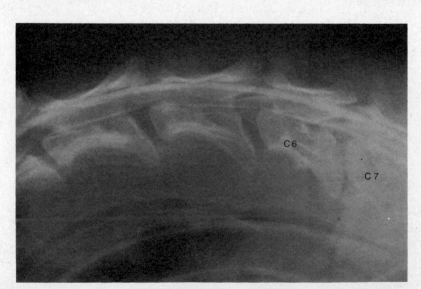

Figure 97–36. Lateral flexion myelogram of the cervical spine demonstrating the relief of compression at C6-C7 caused by flattening of the enlarged dorsal annulus fibrosus in this position.

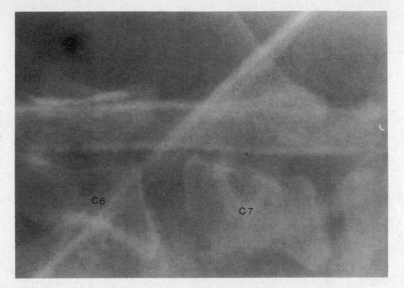

Figure 97–37. Lateral myelographic radiograph of the cervical spine demonstrating the absence of spinal cord compression at C6-C7 after linear traction has been applied to the neck in a middle-aged Doberman pinscher.

outlined with a high-speed air drill. The width of the laminectomy is limited by the medial aspect of the caudal articular processes of the cranial vertebra. The length of the defect is three-quarters the length of each vertebra but can extend the whole length if needed. The lateral groove is deepened through the cortex and cancellous bone ventrally as far as possible before breaking into the spinal canal. The dorsal groove connecting the lateral grooves is drilled through to the spinal canal. Incision of the interarcuate ligament and joint capsule allows *en bloc* resection of the vertebral arch. Further undercutting of the cancellous bone and inner cortical layer of the vertebral pedicles is continued if needed to just above the vertebral sinus (Fig. 97–38). Great care must be exercised during the undercutting. Any hypertrophied joint capsule, interarcuate ligament, or medial ingrowth of the articular processes is removed.[77]

If stabilization is needed, a 1.5-mm (0.625-inch) K wire is used to drill a hole through the articular processes. The articular cartilage is removed from the articular processes with a high-speed drill, and a cancellous bone graft is placed. An 18-gauge orthopedic wire is placed through the hole and tightened (see Fig. 97–38). A lag screw can be used instead of the wire. The laminectomy site is copiously lavaged with saline. The laminectomy defect is filled with a free fat graft, and the incision is closed.

Postoperative care includes administration of dexamethasone in decreasing doses, antibiotics, and good nursing care. A well-padded neck brace or body cast should be worn by the animal for four to six weeks. Such a dog is generally worse neurologically after the surgery and represents a management problem because of its size. It must be kept clean and dry and in a well-padded cage. A walking cart is the best means of rehabilitation if the animal cannot walk. One postoperative complication is breakage of the articular wires with a decline in the neurological status. Replacement of the broken wire is then required. The prognosis for a Group I dog as a functional pet is fair because of the multiple defects, the size of the animal, and the postoperative care and rehabilitation required.

The second group of CMM dogs (Group II) is represented primarily by the middle-aged Doberman pinscher. Group II has compression of the spinal cord caused mainly by enlargement of the dorsal annulus fibrosus. Compression can be relieved by placement of linear traction on the cervical spine, and the surgical procedure for this group is based on this principle. The goal is to arthrodese the vertebrae in linear traction.

As with Group I surgery, dexamethasone (2 mg/kg) is given one to two hours before surgery, and prophylactic antibiotic therapy is also recommended. The animal is placed in dorsal recumbency, and care is taken that the cervical spine is straight and not rotated. The front legs are extended back along the body so that the proximal end of the humerus is readily accessible for cancellous bone collection.

A ventral approach to the vertebral canal is made (see Chapter 96). By means of a high-speed air drill, an ellipse centered over the disc space is drilled (Fig. 97–39A). The elliptical hole is drilled dorsally, 75 per cent of the height of the vertebral body (usually 12–

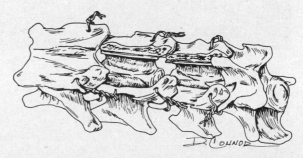

Figure 97–38. A dorsal laminectomy performed over C5-C6 with undercutting of the vertebral arches to decompress the spinal cord. The articular processes have been wired to provide stability between the vertebrae.

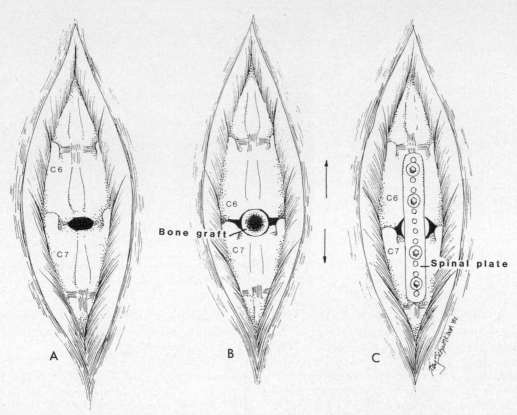

Figure 97–39. *A,* Ventral aspect of cervical vertebrae 6 and 7 with an elliptical hole drilled over the disc space. *B,* A tibial allograft 1 cm in diameter has been placed in the hole after linear traction has been applied to the cervical spine, thus enlarging the elliptical hole into a circle. *C,* A straight plastic spinal plate is attached to the ventral aspect of the vertebrae on either side of the tibial allograft with cortical bone screws. The main function of the spinal plate is to hold the bone graft in place.

16 mm). The width (lateral direction) of the ellipse should be approximately 1 cm.

A previously collected distal tibial allograft (0.8 to 1.0 cm in diameter by 12 to 16 mm long) is placed in the elliptical hole. This graft is collected aseptically from the distal tibia of a 7- to 10-kg dog. The bone is stored in a double-container system (two jars) and frozen until needed. At the time of surgery the graft

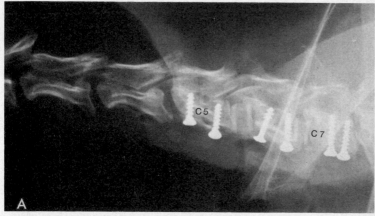

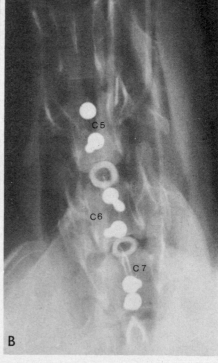

Figure 97–40. Lateral (A) and ventrodorsal (B) radiographs taken postoperatively after tibial allographs were inserted at C5-C6 and C6-C7. The lateral radiograph demonstrates the correct screw lengths and extension of the bone grafts 75 per cent of the height of the vertebral body. The ventrodorsal radiograph demonstrates that the screws have been angled to the left and right to avoid entering the spinal canal.

is warmed in sterile saline, and all periosteum and medullary canal contents are removed.

Linear traction is applied to the dog's neck by two nonsterile assistants. One assistant applies traction on the head, and the second on the forelimbs. The linear traction turns the elliptical hole into a circle, and the tibial allograft is slipped into the hole so that the vertebrae are maintained in linear traction (Fig. 97–39*B*). Cancellous bone is collected from the proximal humerus and packed in and around the allograft. A straight plastic plate* is applied to the ventral aspect of the vertebrae on either side of the affected disc space. Two cortical bone screws (3.5 mm in diameter by 12 to 18 mm long) are used to fix the plate to the vertebral bodies (Fig. 97–39*C*). The screw holes are drilled dorsolaterally in alternating directions to prevent entering the spinal canal. Screw length is estimated from the radiographs (Fig. 97–40). The screws are inserted without tapping the holes. Cancellous bone is placed around the edge of the plate over the disc space. The surgical area is lavaged and closed in a routine manner. The dog's postoperative neurological status should be the same as its preoperative status.

Postoperatively, the dog is placed in a body cast that incorporates the neck and thoracic cavity. Dexamethasone is generally stopped one to two days after surgery, and antibiotics are continued for one week. Good nursing care is required until the dog learns to walk with the cast. For animals that are nonambulatory before surgery, a walking cart is extremely useful for rehabilitation. The dog is radiographed at monthly intervals, and the cast is removed three months after operation. Prognosis is good for Group II dogs treated with this procedure.

DISCOSPONDYLITIS

Discospondylitis is among the most common spinal cord diseases in dogs.

Etiology and Pathogenesis

Staphylococcus aureus is the most common organism isolated from either bone or blood of dogs with discospondylitis.[42,43] *Brucella canis*,[33] *Streptococcus* spp.[36,43] and other bacteria[36] and fungi[36,57,84] are cultured less frequently. These organisms may reach the involved disc or vertebrae after foreign body migration.[4,39,44] However, most infections originate elsewhere in the body and spread hematogenously to the vertebrae.[42] Urinary tract infections,[42] bacterial endocarditis,[36] and orchitis[33,42] have been identified as potential primary sources of infection in affected dogs. Organisms localize in the vertebral body because subchondral vascular loops in the vertebral epiphysis slow circulation, allowing colonization of blood-borne bacteria.[78,82] These bacteria diffuse through the cartilaginous end plate of the vertebral body to reach the disc. Infection is further disseminated to the adjacent vertebra(e) through freely communicating venous sinuses.

Factors that may predispose vertebrae to infection are trauma[25] and disc surgery.[43] Fifty per cent of affected dogs in one series had suffered trauma prior to developing discospondylitis.[25] However, affected dogs evaluated in another study rarely had a history of trauma.[42,43] Nevertheless, the prevalence of discospondylitis in large male dogs indicates that stresses placed on the spine by increased size and activity may be important. Three dogs in one study developed discospondylitis subsequent to disc fenestration.[43] However, the rarity of this disease in dachshunds suggests that neither disc disease nor disc surgery significantly predisposes dogs to its occurrence.

Neurological deficits seen in dogs with discospondylitis occur primarily because of spinal cord compression by new bone and fibrous connective tissue (Figs. 97–41 and 97–42). Less frequently, instability may occur, leading to vertebral subluxation and additional compression (Fig. 97–43). Although extension of infection to the spinal cord and meninges was reported in one study as a common sequel of discospondylitis,[4] affected dogs evaluated in another study did not have evidence of suppurative meningitis on cerebrospinal fluid evaluation.[42] This discrepancy might reflect a difference in pathogenesis of the lesions studied; whereas discospondylitis in dogs in the second study was hematogenous in origin,[42] lesions in dogs of the first study often occurred subsequent to foreign body migration.[4]

Clinical Findings

Discospondylitis usually affects large, middle-aged male dogs.[42,43] German shepherds[42] and Great

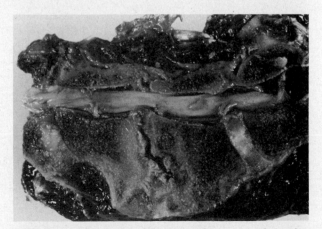

Figure 97–41. Lateral view of the C6-C7 disc space and vertebrae from a six-year-old male Great Dane. Vertebral lysis has caused erosion of portions of the end-plates at C6-C7. Fibrous tissue and new bone dorsal to the disc space compress the spinal cord ventrally. The intervertebral disc at C6-C7 is absent. Considerable new bone is seen ventral to the C6-C7 disc space, and both vertebral bodies are sclerotic adjacent to it. A diagnosis of discospondylitis was made. (Reprinted with permission from Kornegay, J. N.: Canine diskospondylitis. Comp. Cont. E. Pract. Vet. *1*:930, 1979.)

---

*Lubra Company, 1905 Mohawk, Fort Collins, CO.

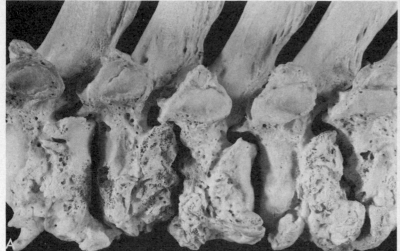

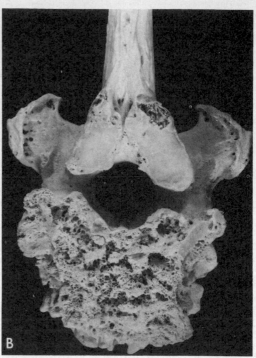

Figure 97–42. Vertebrae from a five-year-old male Great Dane with spinal hyperesthesia and paraparesis of nine days' duration. *A,* Lateral view of the fourth through the eighth thoracic vertebrae. There is subtle lysis of the vertebral end-plates at T4-T5 and more pronounced lysis at T5-T6 and T7-T8. Note the new bone ventral and lateral to the affected disc spaces. *B,* The cranial vertebral end-plate of T6. Note marked erosion of cortical bone that results in a honeycomb pattern. (Reprinted with permission from Kornegay, J. N.: Musculoskeletal infections. *In* Greene, C. E. (ed.): *Clinical Microbiology and Infectious Diseases of the Dog and Cat.* W. B. Saunders Co., Philadelphia, 1984.)

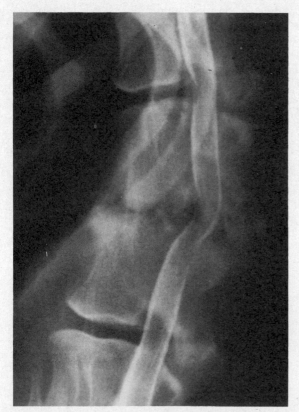

Danes[36] are affected disproportionately. Affected dogs may have clinical evidence of systemic illness, neurological dysfunction, or both.[36,42,43] Clinical signs directly related to the vertebral lesion include spinal hyperesthesia, lameness, stilted gait, and paresis caudal to the affected disc. These deficits are subtle initially and are often overlooked or misinterpreted by the client. The dog's illness may be attributed

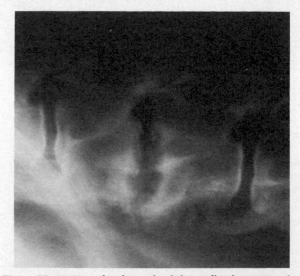

Figure 97–43. Lateral myelogram from a six-year-old male German shepherd with paraplegia and spinal hyperesthesia. Vertebral lysis has caused ersion of portions of the cranial aspect of the vertebral body of L2 and the caudal aspect of the vertebral body of L1. the vertebral body of L1 is displaced dorsally in relation to the vertebral body of L2. The intervertebral disc space and foramen are decreased in size. A diagnosis of vertebral subluxation secondary to discospondylitis was made.

Figure 97–44. Lateral radiograph of the midlumbar spine of an eight-year-old male Labrador retriever with pelvic limb ataxia and spinal hyperesthesia. The L2-L3 disc space is at the center of the picture. There is lysis of the caudal end-plate of L2 and the cranial end-plate of L3. The intervertebral foramen, disc space, and facet space are narrowed at L2-L3. New bone formation is evident ventral to the L2 and L3 vertebral bodies. There is evidence of spondylosis deformans at L1-L2 and L3-L4.

TABLE 97–2. Antibiotic Sensitivity of Bacteria from Blood or Bone of Dogs with Discospondylitis

	Bacterium		
	S. aureus	B. canis	β-Hemolytic streptococcus
No. of isolates	30	5	2
Antibiotic efficacy (%)			
Ampicillin	27	100	100
Cephalothin	97	60	100
Chloramphenicol	83	100	100
Cloxacillin	93	20	100
Erythromycin	77	100	100
Gentamicin	83	100	0
Lincomycin	46	20	100
Penicillin	20	100	100
Streptomycin	60	100	0
Sulfadimethoxine	11	0	0
Tetracycline	57	100	100
Trimethroprim	65	40	100
Triple sulfa	10	0	0

(Adapted from Kornegay, J. N.: Diskospondylitis. *In* Kirk, R. W. (ed.): *Current Veterinary Therapy VIII.* W. B. Saunders, Philadelphia, 1983.)

incorrectly to a visceral lesion because of the presence of abdominal tenseness, anorexia, depression, and pyrexia.

Solitary or multiple lesions may be identified.[36,42,43] Multiple involvement often occurs in adjacent discs, suggesting local extension of the causative organism. Other affected dogs have widely separated lesions, indicating probable multifocal hematogenous dissemination of the pathogen. The midthoracic spine, C6–C7, and L7–S1, are affected most commonly.[43]

Diagnosis

Radiographic changes of vertebral osteomyelitis may not occur until four to six weeks after the onset of infection.[26,40] Animals with discospondylitis initially have radiographic evidence of focal lysis of one or both vertebral end-plates followed by sclerosis, spondylosis, and further lysis (Fig. 97–44).[25,36,42] Both the intervertebral disc space and intervertebral foramen are decreased in size.

Leukocytosis is infrequently present in dogs with discospondylitis.[42] Pyuria (>8 WBC/hpf), bacteriuria, or both occur in about 50 per cent.[42] Results of cerebrospinal fluid evaluation usually are normal except for mild elevation of protein.[42]

Bacterial cultures of bone, blood, or urine often yield the causative organism. *S. aureus* is isolated most commonly; *B. canis* and *Streptococcus* spp. are cultured less frequently.[42] Other bacteria found are contaminants unless cultured directly from bone or multiple blood cultures.

The agglutination test for *B. canis* also should be performed, particularly if bacterial culture results are negative. Titers from 1:250 to 1:500 indicate bacteremia; titers between 1:50 and 1:100 suggest exposure; a titer of 1:25 may occur because of cross-agglutination with another organism.

Treatment

Factors to be considered in choosing a therapeutic regimen include (1) degree of neurological dysfunction, (2) results of *B. canis* titer and blood cultures, (3) multiplicity of lesions, and (4) surgical accessibility of the lesion(s).[42]

Dogs with little or no neurological dysfunction usually respond to an antibiotic selected through results of serology or blood cultures.[42] If such results are negative, the causative organism is assumed to be *S. aureus* and the antibiotic is chosen accordingly (Table 97–2). Antibiotics are administered parenter-

TABLE 97–3. Antibiotics and Dosages for Treatment of Discospondylitis in Dogs

Bacterium	Antibiotic and Dosage
S. aureus*	Cephradine, 20 mg/kg t.i.d. PO for 4–6 weeks† Cloxacillin, 10 mg/kg q.i.d. PO for 4–6 weeks
B. Canis	Tetracycline hydrochloride, 20 mg/kg t.i.d. PO for 3 weeks‡ Streptomycin, 20 mg/kg b.i.d. IM for 5 days at start of tetracycline regimen Skip for 3 weeks and repeat this regimen.
β-Hemolytic streptococcus*	Ampicillin, 20 mg/kg t.i.d. PO for 4–6 weeks Penicillin, 40 mg/kg q.i.d. PO for 4–6 weeks

*Dogs with acutely progressive clinical signs should be treated parenterally for five days and then orally for at least four to six weeks. The antibiotic listed first is preferred.

†A number of cephalosporins are available. Cephradine (Velosef) is used because of its availability and low cost. Cephalexin (Keflex) also has been used.

‡Minocycline hydrochloride also has been used and may be more efficacious. However, it is also more expensive. (Reprinted with permission from Kornegay, J. N.: Diskospondylitis. *In* Kirk, R. W. (ed.): *Current Veterinary Therapy VIII.* W. B. Saunders, Philadelphia, 1983.)

ally for the first five days and continued orally for four to six weeks (Table 97–3). Most dogs treated with an appropriate antibiotic show almost immediate clinical improvement and do not have relapse. Dogs in which signs worsen after antibiotic therapy or that fail to improve within five days are reassessed. Those with a solitary, readily accessible lesion are operated on, at which time the lesion is curetted and sampled for culture. Dogs with multiple, widely spaced lesions or lesions that are not readily accessible are treated with a different antibiotic.

Dogs with pronounced paresis or paralysis have spinal cord compression that is amenable only to surgery.[25,36,41,42] A myelogram may be helpful to determine the extent of the compression prior to surgery. Hemilaminectomy is the preferred approach, because the dorsal spines are preserved for stabilization, if needed. Offending bone and fibrous tissue should be carefully dissected from the spinal canal. The involved disc space and contiguous vertebrae are curetted, and portions of the necrotic bone are submitted for histopathological evaluation and culture. Use of a cancellous bone graft is desirable if curettage produces a large defect.[41] Spinal immobilization may be indicated if there is marked lysis of the vertebral end-plates, particularly if the infection has extended to the articular facets. Dorsal spinal plating, spinal stapling, and vertebral body plating have been used.[25] Antibiotic therapy is instituted parenterally, on the basis of either blood or bone culture results, and is continued orally for four to six weeks after surgery.

Dogs with discospondylitis due to *B. canis* should be treated with a staged regimen using tetracycline and streptomycin (see Table 97–3). Decompressive surgery also is indicated if the dog has pronounced paresis or paralysis. Intact dogs should also be neutered. It is difficult to eliminate *B. canis*, so repeated treatment may be required. Most dogs can be kept relatively free of clinical signs with periodic treatment. Owners should be advised of the potential public health significance of such an infection.

1. Archibald, J., Pennock, P. W., and Cawley, A. J.: Trauma of the vertebral column in dogs. Vet. Med. *54*:518, 1959.
2. Archibald, J., Holt, J. C., and Sokolovsky, V.: *Management of Trauma in Dogs and Cats.* American Veterinary Publications, Santa Barbara, 1981.
3. Babcock, J. L.: Introduction to symposium on cervical spine injuries. Arch. Surg. *3*:637, 1976.
4. Bailey, C. S., and Holliday, T. A.: Diseases of the spinal cord. *In* Ettinger, S. J. (ed.): *Textbook of Veterinary Internal Medicine.* W. B. Saunders Co., Philadelphia, 1975.
5. Bailey, C. S.: Diseases of the spinal cord. *In* Ettinger, S. J. (ed.): *Textbook of Veterinary Internal Medicine.* W. B. Saunders Co., Philadelphia, 1983.
6. Bohlman, H. H.: Acute fractures and dislocations of the cervical spine. J. Bone J. Surg. *61-A*:1119, 1979.
7. Braund, K. G.: Acute spinal cord traumatic compression. *In* Bojrab, M. J. (ed.): *Pathophysiology in Surgery.* Lea & Febiger, Philadelphia, 1981.
8. Chambers, J. N., Betts, C. W., and Oliver, J. E.: The use of nonmetallic suture material for stabilization of atlantoaxial subluxation. J. Am. Anim. Hosp. Assoc. *13*:602, 1977.
9. Chambers, J. N., and Betts, C. W.: Caudal cervical spondy-lopathy in the dog: a review of 20 clinical cases and the literature. J. Am. Anim. Hosp. Assoc. *13*:571, 1977.
10. Chambers, J.: Surgery of the cervical spine. *In* Archibald, J. (ed.): *Canine and Feline Surgery.* American Veterinary Publications, Santa Barbara, in press.
11. Cooke, J. R., Jr., and Oliver, J. E., Jr.: Atlantoaxial luxation in the dog. Compend. Cont. Ed. *3*:242, 1981.
12. de Lahunta, A.: *Veterinary Neuroanatomy and Clinical Neurology.* W. B. Saunders, Philadelphia, 1977.
13. Denny, H. R., Gibbs, C., and Gaskell, C. J.: Cervical spondylopathy in the dog—a review of thirty-five cases. J. Small Anim. Pract. *18*:117, 1977.
14. De Palma, A. F.: *The Management of Fractures and Dislocations, An Atlas.* 2nd ed. W. B. Saunders, Philadelphia, 1970.
15. Dueland, R., Furneaux, R. W., and Kaye, M. M.: Spinal fusion and dorsal laminectomy for midcervical spondylolis-thesis in a dog. J. Am. Vet. Med. Assoc. *162*:366, 1973.
16. Dulisch, M. L., and Nichols, J. B.: A surgical technique for management of lower lumbar fractures: case report. Vet. Surg. *10*:90, 1981.
17. Evans, H. E., and Christensen, G. C. (eds.): *Miller's Anatomy of the Dog.* 2nd ed. W. B. Saunders, Philadelphia, 1979.
18. Faden, A. I., Jacobs, T. P., and Holaday, J. W.: Thyrotropin-releasing hormone improves neurologic recovery after spinal trauma in cats. N. Engl. J. Med. *305*:1063, 1981.
19. Gage, E. D.: Surgical repair of a fractured cervical spine in the dog. J. Am. Vet. Med. Assoc. *153*:1407, 1968.
20. Gage, E. D.: Surgical repair of fractured occiput, atlas, and axis in a dog. J. Am. Vet. Med. Assoc. *158*:1951, 1971.
21. Gage, E. D., and Smallwood, J. E.: Surgical repair of atlantoaxial subluxation in a dog. Vet. Med./Small Anim. Clin. *65*:583, 1970.
22. Gage, E. D.: A new method of spinal fixation in the dog. Vet. Med./Small Anim. Clin. *64*:295, 1969.
23. Gage, E. D.: Surgical repairs of spinal fractures in small breed dogs. Vet. Med./Small Anim. Clin. *66*:1095, 1971.
24. Gage, E. D., and Hall, C. L.: Surgical repair of caudal cervical subluxation in a dog. J. Am. Vet. Med. Assoc. *160*:424, 1972.
25. Gage, E. D.: Treatment of discospondylitis in the dog. J. Am. Vet. Med. Assoc. *166*:1164, 1975.
26. Garcia, A., and Grantham, S. A.: Hematogenous pyogenic vertebral osteomyelitis. J. Bone J. Surg. (Am.) *42*:429, 1960.
27. Geary, J. C., Oliver, J. E., and Hoerlein, B. F.: Atlanto-axial subluxation in the canine. J. Small Anim. Pract. *8*:557, 1967.
28. Gendreau, C. L., and Cawley, A. J.: Repair of fractures of the axis. Can. Vet. J. *10*:297, 1969.
29. Greenwood, K. W., and Oliver, J. E.: Traumatic atlanto-occipital dislocation in two dogs. J. Am. Vet. Med. Assoc. *173*:1324, 1978.
30. Griswold, D. M., Albright, J. A., Schiffman, E., et al.: Atlantoaxial fusion for instability. J. Bone J. Surg. *60-A*:285, 1978.
31. Hare, W. C. D.: Radiographic anatomy of the cervical region of the canine vertebral column. Part II. Developing vertebrae. J. Am. Vet. Med. Assoc. *139*:2117, 1961.
32. Hedhammar, A., Fu-Ming, W., Krook, L., et al.: Overnutrition and skeletal disease. An experimental study in growing Great Dane dogs. Cornell Vet. *64* (Suppl. 5), 1974.
33. Henderson, R. A., Hoerlein, B. F., Kramer, T. T., and Meyer, M. E.: Discospondylitis in three dogs infected with *Brucella canis.* J. Am. Vet. Med. Assoc. *165*:451, 1974.
34. Heppenstall, R. B.: *Fracture Treatment and Healing.* W. B. Saunders Co., Philadelphia, 1980.
35. Hoerlein, B. F. (ed.): *Canine Neurology, Diagnosis and Treatment.* 3rd ed. W. B. Saunders, Philadelphia, 1978.
36. Hurov, L., Troy, G., and Turnwald, G.: Diskospondylitis in the dog: 27 cases. J. Am. Vet. Med. Assoc. *173*:275, 1978.
37. Hurov, L. I.: Treatment of cervical instability in the dog. J. Am. Vet. Med. Assoc. *175*:279, 1979.
38. Jacobs, B.: Cervical fractures and dislocations (C3-7). Clin. Orthoped. Rel. Res. *109*:18, 1975.
39. Johnston, D. E., and Summers, B. A.: Osteomyelitis of the

lumbar vertebrae in dogs caused by grass-seed foreign bodies. Aust. Vet. J. *47*:289, 1971.

40. Kemp, H. B. S., Jackson, J. W., Jeremiah, J. D., and Hall, A. J.: Pyogenic infections occurring primarily in intervertebral discs. J. Bone J. Surg. (Br.) 55:698, 1973.

41. Kornegay, J. N., Barber, D. L., and Earley, T. D.: Cranial thoracic diskospondylitis in two dogs. J. Am. Vet. Med. Assoc. *174*:192, 1979.

42. Kornegay, J. N., and Barber, D. L.: Diskospondylitis in dogs. J. Am. Vet. Med. Assoc. *177*:337, 1980.

43. Kornegay, J. N.: Diskospondylitis. *In* Kirk, R. W. (ed.): *Current Veterinary Therapy VIII*. W. B. Saunders, Philadelphia, 1983.

44. LaCroix, J. A.: Vertebral body osteomyelitis: A case report. J. Am. Vet. Radiol. Soc. *14*:17, 1973.

45. LeCouteur, R. A., McKeown, D., Johnson, J., and Eger, C. E.: Stabilization of atlantoaxial subluxation in the dog using the nuchal ligament. J. Am. Vet. Med. Assoc. *177*:1011, 1980.

46. Mason, T. A.: Cervical vertebral instability (wobbler syndrome) in the Doberman. Aust. Vet. 53:440, 1977.

47. Mendenhall, H. V., Litwak, P., Yturraspe, D. J., et al.: Aggressive pharmacologic and surgical treatment of spinal cord injuries in dogs and cats. J. Am. Vet. Med. Assoc. *168*:1026, 1976.

48. Naftchi, N. E.: Functional restoration of the traumatically injured spinal cord in cats by clonidine. Science *217*:1042, 1982.

49. Oliver, J. E., and Lewis, R. E.: Lesions of the atlas and axis in dogs. J. Am. Anim. Hosp. Assoc. 9:304, 1973.

50. Oliver, J. E., and Selcer, R. R.: Decompression of the lumbosacral spinal cord and nerve roots. *In* Bojrab, J. M. (ed.): *Current Techniques in Small Animal Surgery I*. Lea & Febiger, Philadelphia, 1975.

51. Osterholm, J. L.: The pathophysiological response to spinal cord injury: The current status of related research. J. Neurosurg. *40*:5, 1974.

52. Osterholm, J. L., and Matthews, G. L.: Altered norepinephrine metabolism following experimental spinal cord injury. Part I: relationship to hemorrhagic necrosis and post-wounding neurological deficits. J. Neurosurg. 36:386, 1972.

53. Osterholm, J. L., and Matthews, G. L.: Altered norepinephrine metabolism following experimental spinal cord injury. Part II: protection against traumatic spinal cord hemorrhagic necrosis by norepinephrine synthesis blockade with alpha-methyltyrosine. J. Neurosurg. 36:395, 1972.

54. Parker, A. J., and Cusick, P. K.: Abnormal odontoid process angulation in a dog. Vet. Rec. *93*:559, 1973.

55. Parker, A. J., Park, R. D., and Henry, J. D.: Cervical vertebral instability associated with cervical disc disease in two dogs. J. Am. Vet. Med. Assoc. *162*:1369, 1973.

56. Parker, A. J., and Smith, C. W.: Functional recovery from spinal cord trauma following incision of spinal meninges in dogs. Res. Vet. Sci. *16*:276, 1974.

57. Patnaik, A. K., Liu, S. K., Wilkins, R. J., et al.: Paecilomycosis in a dog. J. Am. Vet. Med. Assoc. *161*:806, 1972.

58. Raffe, M. R., and Knecht, C. D.: Cervical vertebral malformation in bull mastiffs. J. Am. Anim. Hosp. Assoc. *14*:593, 1978.

59. Raffe, M. R., and Knecht, C. D.: Cervical vertebral malformation—a review of 36 cases. J. Am. Anim. Hosp. Assoc. *16*:881, 1980.

60. Renegar, W. R., and Stoll, S. G.: The use of methylmethacrylate bone cement in the repair of atlantoaxial subluxation stabilization failures. Case report and discussion. J. Am. Anim. Hosp. Assoc. *15*:313, 1979.

61. Riulin, A. S., and Tator, C. H.: Effect of vasodilators and myelotomy on recovery after spinal cord injury in rats. J. Neurosurg. *50*:349, 1979.

62. Rucker, N. A., Lumb, W. V., and Scott, R. J.: Combined pharmacologic and surgical treatments for acute spinal cord trauma. Am. J. Vet. Res. *42*:1138, 1981.

63. Ruge, D.: Spinal cord injuries. *In* Ruge, D., and Wiltse, L. (eds.): *Spinal Disorders*. Lea & Febiger, Philadelphia, 1977.

64. Seim, H. B., and Withrow, S. J.: Pathophysiology and diagnosis of caudal cervical spondylo-myelopathy with emphasis on the Doberman pinscher. J. Am. Anim. Hosp. Assoc. *18*:241, 1982.

65. Selcer, R. R.: Trauma to the central nervous system. Vet. Clin. North Am. *10*:619, 1980.

66. Slocum, B., and Rudy, R. L.: Fracture of the seventh lumbar vertebra in the dog. J. Am. Anim. Hosp. Assoc. *11*:167, 1975.

67. Sorjonen, D. C., and Shires, K. P.: Atlantoaxial instability: a ventral surgical technique for decompression, fixation, and fusion. Vet. Surg. *10*:22, 1981.

68. Stone, E. A., Betts, C. W., and Chambers, J. N.: Cervical fractures in the dog: a literature and case review. J. Am. Anim. Hosp. Assoc. *15*:463, 1979.

69. Swaim, S. F.: Spinal cord trauma in the canine: initial management and examinations. Auburn Vet. *27*:36, 1970.

70. Swaim, S. F.: Vertebral body plating for spinal immobilization. J. Am. Vet. Med. Assoc. *158*:1683, 1971.

71. Swaim, S. F.: Thoracolumbar and sacral spine trauma. *In* Bojrab, M. J. (ed.): *Current Techniques in Small Animal Surgery I*. Lea & Febiger, Philadelphia, 1975.

72. Swaim, S. F., and Greene, C. E.: Odontoidectomy in a dog. J. Am. Anim. Hosp. Assoc. 11:663, 1975.

73. Swaim, S. F.: Biomechanics of cranial fractures, spinal fractures, and luxations. *In* Bojrab, M. J. (ed.): *Pathophysiology in Surgery*. Lea & Febiger, Philadelphia, 1981.

74. Teague, H. D., and Brasmer, T. H.: Midline myelotomy of clinically normal canine spinal cord. Am. J. Vet. Res. *39*:1584, 1978.

75. Toombs, J. P., Caywood, D. D., Lipowitz, A. J., et al.: Colonic perforation following neurosurgical procedures and corticosteroid therapy in four dogs. J. Am. Vet. Med. Assoc. *177*:68, 1980.

76. Trotter, E. J.: Surgical repair of fractured axis in a dog. J. Am. Vet. Med. Assoc. *161*:303, 1972.

77. Trotter, E. J., deLahunta, A., Geary, J. C., and Brasmer, T. H.: Caudal cervical vertebral malformation-malarticulation in Great Danes and Doberman pinschers. J. Am. Vet. Med. Assoc. *168*:917, 1976.

78. Trueta, J.: The three types of acute hematogenous osteomyelitis. A clinical and vascular study. J. Bone J. Surg. (Br.) *41*:671, 1959.

79. Urbaniak, J. R.: Fractures of the spine. *In* Sabiston, D. C. (ed.): *Textbook of Surgery*. 12th ed. W. B. Saunders Co., Philadelphia, 1981.

80. Vandervelde, M.: Spinal cord compression. *In* Bojrab, M. J. (ed.): *Pathophysiology in Surgery*. Lea & Febiger, Philadelphia, 1981.

81. Wagner, F. C., Dohrmann, G. I., and Bucy, P. C.: Histopathology of transitory traumatic paraplegia in the monkey. J. Neurosurg. 35:272, 1971.

82. Waldvogel, F. A., Medoff, G., and Swartz, M. N.: Osteomyelitis: a review of clinical features, therapeutic considerations and unusual aspects. Part 1. N. Engl. J. Med. *282*:198, 1970.

83. Walker, T. L.: Surgery of the thoracolumbar spine. *In* Archibald, J. (ed.): *Canine and Feline Surgery*. American Veterinary Publications, Santa Barbara, in press.

84. Wood, G. L., Hirsh, D. C., Selcer, R. R., et al.: Disseminated aspergillosis in a dog. J. Am. Vet. Med. Assoc. *172*:704, 1978.

85. Wortzman, G., and Dewar, F. P.: Rotary fixation of the atlantoaxial joint: rotational atlantoaxial subluxation. Radiology 90:479, 1968.

86. Wurtman, R. J., and Zervas, N. T.: Monoamine neurotransmitters and the pathophysiology of stroke and central nervous system trauma. J. Neurosurg. *40*:34, 1974.

87. Yturraspe, D. J., and Lumb, W. V.: The use of plastic spinal plates for internal fixation of the canine spine. J. Am. Vet. Med. Assoc. *161*:1651, 1972.

98 Intervertebral Disc Disease

Tom L. Walker and C. W. Betts

Intervertebral disc disease results in the most common neurological syndrome in animals. Disc degeneration has been reported in 84 breeds, with particular susceptibility in those labeled "chondrodystrophoid" (e.g., dachshund, Pekingese, and beagle). These breeds have a characteristic skeletal enchondral ossification and a predisposition for degenerative intervertebral disc morphology.[7,41,45,47,71]

ANATOMY

The intervertebral discs in the cervical through lumbar spine of the dog constitute the 26 major amphiarthrodial joints of the vertebral column. Each disc consists of two anatomical regions: the gelatinous nucleus pulposus and the annulus fibrosus, which encircles the central nucleus. The nucleus pulposus originates from embryonic notochord and rests in an eccentric position between vertebral end-plates (Fig. 98–1). It is primarily composed of mesenchymal cells with a gel-like matrix of poorly differentiated collagen fibrils and glycosaminoglycans, which absorb shock.[5,22]

The fibrocartilaginous annulus fibrosus is formed by bands of 25 to 30 concentrically placed fibrous bundles (lamellae) that form a lace-like pattern between adjacent vertebrae.[41] The inner lamellae are attached to the cartilaginous end-plates of the vertebral body, and the outer ones are a continuation of Sharpey's fibers of the vertebral epiphyses. The thickness of the ventral aspect of the annulus, being two to three times that of its dorsal aspect, results in the eccentric position of the nucleus and plays an important part in the pathogenesis of disc extrusion.[45]

The ligamentous structures adjacent to the disc include the dorsal and ventral longitudinal ligaments. The dorsal longitudinal ligament unites the vertebral bodies by strong attachment to the median ridge of bone on the floor of the vertebral canal. It fans out at each disc space to intermingle with the dorsal annulus. The ventral longitudinal ligament spans the ventral surfaces of the vertebrae. A series of intercapital ligaments extend from each rib head, over the dorsal annulus, to the opposite rib head (see Fig. 98–1), blending their fibers with the dorsal longitudinal ligament and annulus fibrosus. Their presence from T1-T2 to T10-T11 is largely responsible for the decreased occurrence of disc rupture in the thoracic area.[22]

The vertebral venous plexuses (sinuses), which lie on the floor of the vertebral canal, are valveless bilateral veins continuous with the dorsal sinuses of the cranium. In the cervical region, the veins are large and lie against the pedicles of the vertebral arches. They take a more medial course in the thoracolumbar area, diverging slightly at each intervertebral disc space. Hemorrhage from these plex-

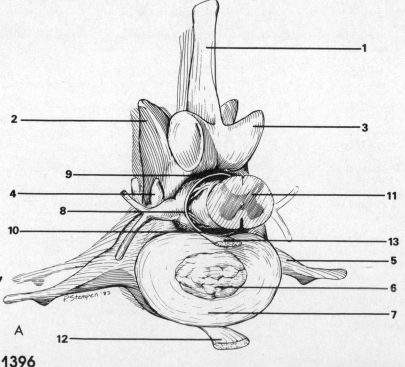

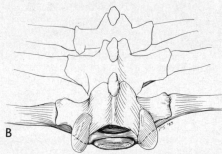

Figure 98–1. A, Thoracolumbar spine in the dog through an intervertebral disc and associated structures. *1,* Spinous process; *2,* cranial articular process; *3,* caudal articular process; *4,* accessory process; *5,* transverse process; *6,* nucleus pulposus; *7,* annulus fibrosus; *8,* dura mater and arachnoid; *9,* epidural space; *10,* subarachnoid space; *11,* spinal cord; *12,* ventral longitudinal ligament; *13,* dorsal longitudinal ligament. *B,* Dorsal aspect of thoracic spinal canal illustrating the intercapital ligament.

uses during surgery is the major technical problem in ventral cervical and dorsolateral thoracolumbar spinal decompression techniques.[28]

The meninges surrounding the spinal cord consist of dura mater, arachnoid, and pia mater. The subarachnoid space, between the pia mater and arachnoid, contains cerebrospinal fluid and an extensive vascular network. These anatomical relationships are an important consideration when durotomy or myelography is performed. The epidural fat surrounding the neural elements within the spinal canal and the spinal fluid of the subarachnoid space cushion the neuraxis and provide room for displacement during physiological motion.[22,28]

PATHOPHYSIOLOGY OF DISC DISEASE

Degeneration

Discs lose their resilient, shock-absorbing qualities by metaplastic degeneration. In the classic work by Hansen,[41] two distinctly different types of metaplastic changes were identified in the pathogenesis of degenerative disc disease. A chondroid metaplasia occurs in chondrodystrophoid dogs between eight months and two years of age, with 75 to 100 per cent of all intervertebral discs having undergone the degenerative change by one year of age. Chondroid degeneration is characterized by an increase in collagen content, a change in the specific glycosaminoglycan concentrations of the nucleus, concurrent degeneration of the annulus, and a decrease in the disc's water content. The disc becomes progressively more cartilaginous, and its nucleus takes on a granular consistency. These alterations impair the hydroelastic properties of the disc, thereby reducing its ability to absorb shock and distribute loading forces. Nuclear nutrition is decreased owing to inefficiency of the pumping mechanism that normally feeds the avascular disc. The degenerate nucleus pulposus becomes progressively mineralized, further aggravating the disc's condition.[6,7,30,31,45] Hansen postulated that degeneration and loss of functional integrity of the disc resulted in increased incidence of intervertebral disc disease in chondrodystrophoid breeds. He termed the process "systemic disc disease" and described the resultant massive mechanical rupture of these discs as Hansen Type I protrusions (Fig. 98–2).[40,41]

The second type of degenerative disc, classified as a Hansen Type II, occurs in nonchondrodystrophoid breeds. It is a partial rupture of the annular bands and a dome-like bulging of the dorsal annulus (see Fig. 98–2). The degeneration is a result of fibrinoid metaplasia—a maturing or geriatric process. The slow, insidious process leaves the disc with a higher glycosaminoglycan level and lower collagen content than the comparable chondrodystrophic disc. These discs maintain a more gel-like consistency because of the higher water content of the nucleus pulposus and rare mineralization. The dogs are usually eight to ten

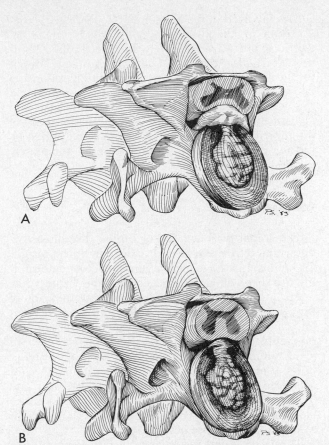

Figure 98–2. Hansen's classification of disc protrusions. *A,* The Type I (chondrodystrophoid) disc is a clinical rupture with massive extrusion of the nucleus compressing the spinal cord. *B,* The Type II disc is a small dome-shaped protrusion seen in older dogs of the nonchondrodystrophoid breeds.

years of age when significant degenerative fibroid changes occur. Massive ejection of the nucleus pulposus is not seen in Type II discs, but rather a fibrous mass slowly encroaches on the neural structures.[40,41,45]

The causes of disc degeneration remain obscure and speculative. Trauma has been considered the important factor in disc herniation. Although the presence of a traumatic incident may be a factor in the precipitation of disc herniation, it is not important in the initiation of disc degeneration. Endocrine abnormalities (e.g., hypothyroidism) are important in disc degeneration, although they are detected infrequently.[36,60] An autoimmune phenomenon has also been suggested as the initiating factor of the degenerative process.[57] This phenomenon may induce a cycle of events whereby released lysosomal enzymes derange the proteoglycan complex of the disc. The isolation of a species-specific antigen and at least two antigenic determinants from canine, bovine, and human discs lends credence to this theory but does not determine whether the autoimmune response initiates the degeneration or results from a post-inflammatory response.[3,61] Also, the initiation of lysosomal activity is not necessarily limited to autoimmunity, because low-grade mechanical insults can elicit lysosomal rupture in the fibrocartilaginous cells.[5] Genetic factors involved in the accelerated degenerative process seen in chondrodystrophoid breeds cannot be ignored, but they remain to be specifically identified.[2,32] The fact that the chondroid change is limited to the spine suggests a complex interrelationship between the pathogenic processes just described and the pathological alterations in the disc's cellular and glycoprotein matrix content. The ultimate control of disc nutrition and lysosomal enzyme activity must be further studied before disc disease is completely understood.

Pathogenesis

The initial pathogenesis of canine disc disease is determined by the type of disc degeneration present. The clinical pathogenesis is due to factors determining the disc's effect on adjacent nervous tissue.

An intervertebral disc herniation is a protrusion of the nucleus pulposus or annulus fibrosus.[20] In general, a disc *protrusion* is one in which the nuclear elements are displaced dorsally or laterally, with some annular lamellae remaining intact. The annular bulging may place pronounced pressure on the cord or nerve roots and may cause significant pain and hyperesthesia. When the annulus ruptures, and nuclear material is forced out, a disc *extrusion* (expulsion) or disc prolapse occurs.

The basic lesion resulting from disc extrusion is a compressive myelopathy (a nonspecific, functional disturbance of the spinal cord) or a compressive radiculopathy (disturbance of nerve roots).[20,45] Because the disc protrusion or extrusion results in focal involvement, the term transverse myelopathy generally applies.

The pain of disc protrusion or extrusion may originate from a number of sources. Direct inflammation or compressive ischemia of a nerve root by protruding or extruded disc material has been termed "radicular pain." The intense cervical muscle spasms that accompany root entrapment are frequently recognized. The meningeal response to compression and inflammation is well-documented as "meningeal pain." A third source thought to exist in the dog involves "discogenic pain" arising from receptors supplying the annulus fibrosus. A so-called sinovertebral nerve is described in humans that carries sensory impulses from the annulus fibrosus to elicit a referred cervical pain complex. Therefore, symptoms of pain from the head, neck, and shoulder area can be seen with degenerative cervical discs that are not producing radicular or meningeal irritation but are in fact early Type I degenerative protrusions.[45]

The location of disc lesions along the spinal canal also influences the pathogenesis of the clinical syndrome. The cervical spine enjoys a spacious spinal canal relative to the diameter of the cervical cord. Therefore, relatively large masses within the canal may not cause significant compression of the cord. A thoracolumbar disc, on the other hand, has little room to extrude until significant filling of the small epidural space has occurred. Although the termination of the cord in the L5 vertebral area allows space for larger amounts of disc material to occupy the spinal canal, extrusions caudal to L5 trap the delicate nerve roots of the lumbosacral plexus. The location as well as severity of the disc lesion determines the integrity of clinical reflexes and postural responses evaluated during the neurological examination. The localization of lesions, based on these responses, is discussed in Chapter 89 and is of primary importance in diagnosing disc disease.

The degree to which Type I discs protrude or extrude, along with the dynamics of disc eruption, has a pronounced effect on the clinical symptoms that follow. Although the volume of mechanical compression a disc places on a neural element is responsible for certain histological changes, it is the dynamic force with which any amount of disc material hits the cord that accounts for the acute and most severe pathological changes.[80] Thus, Type I discs that rupture slowly (over days to weeks) allow adaptation by the displaced nervous system until significant impingment is achieved. Acute, severe extrusions, called "blowouts," result in cord vasculature changes more deleterious and progressive than changes associated with mechanical distortion of the cord. The severity of the changes is in fact proportional to the disc's force of impact. The range of nervous tissue response to dynamic compression includes hematomyelia, malacia, demyelination, and edema.[45] A more detailed description of the pathological alterations is given in Chapter 90.

Degenerative nuclear material itself may initiate much of the extradural inflammatory reaction in disc extrusion.[44,45] When Type I discs begin to extrude mineralized material, a substantial inflammatory reaction ensues that causes a fibrous adhesion between the material and the dura. Simultaneous rupture of the vertebral venous sinuses and even penetration of the dura mater by the exploding nucleus pulposus can occur. Polymorphonuclear leukocytes, red cells, fibroblasts, and large mononuclear and polynuclear giant cells are found throughout the inflammatory debris. Remodeling and attempted absorption of the debris frequently leave a calcified fibrous or cartilaginous mass. When the disc repeatedly extrudes small amounts of material, the consolidated mass may grow quite large or may extend over several vertebral lengths.

Another syndrome associated with intervertebral disc disease results in spinal cord infarction due to emboli originating from a degenerative nucleus pulposus.[16,35,38,42,90,91] The occlusion of arterioles, venules, or both within the spinal cord microvasculature results in an acute, nonprogressive, often lateralized paresis or paralysis. The manner and site of entry of the nucleus pulposus into the vascular system have been postulated by several theories. Venous embolization has been observed when direct herniation of nuclear material into the overlying longitudinal venous sinus is encountered. Embolization at the site of disc extrusion would have to be driven retrograde into meningeal and intramedullary veins during periods of increased intra-abdominal or intrathoracic pressure. There are three proposals for arterial embolization:[4,42,56]

1. A lateral extrusion of degenerative annulus fibrosus with spontaneous tearing of the adjacent radicular artery allows fragments of the nucleus to enter the cord's microvasculature.

2. Persistent embryonal arteries or an anomalous vascular supply travels to or lies within the disc.

3. The annulus fibrosus is generally considered avascular at maturity but can undergo vascularization following senile disc degeneration in humans and nonchondrodystrophoid dogs. After initial fissure development, the splitting annulus is penetrated by blood vessels. An acute increase in disc pressure could allow the dissection and injection of semifluid nuclear material into these small vessels, with retropulsion delivering the material into the radicular artery. Intradisc pressure can reach levels of 1.5 kg/cm², much higher than arterial pressure (0.1 kg/cm²). Such a pressure gradient would allow penetration of arteries and movement of emboli in either direction.[42]

The last explanation is the most likely pathogenesis for arterial embolization by the nucleus pulposus. To date, reported cases have occurred in nonchondrodystrophoid breeds, in which Hansen Type II discs occur. The nucleus remains gel-like in the early stages of degeneration, and displaced nucleus pulposus is generally confined within the annulus fibrosus. Pathological findings include chronic disc protrusion with vascularization of the annulus, concurring with an acute injection of material following a chronic, degenerative course. Trauma and exertion may increase intradisc pressure and may contribute to sudden embolus extrusion into the arterial or venous system.[42]

The most commonly encountered syndrome remains compression of the spinal cord or its roots by displaced nucleus pulposus and/or annulus fibrosus in the chondrodystrophoid dog. The variety and severity of clinical signs that follow intervertebral disc protrusion or extrusion depend on: (1) the type of disc degeneration present (Type I or Type II discs), (2) the location of the lesion, (3) the "dynamic force" with which the degenerative nucleus is driven against the cord, (4) the inflammatory, mechanical, and vascular sequences of cord lesions that follow compression, and (5) the duration of marked cord compression.

CERVICAL DISC DISEASE

Incidence

Cervical lesions account for approximately one-fifth of all intervertebral disc problems. The syndrome is seen primarily in chondrodystrophoid and other small breeds, with the dachshund, beagle, and toy poodle accounting for over 80 per cent of the cases. Incidence in the sexes is approximately equal.[27,34,39,45] Although the median age at presentation is five years, Gage[27] noted a nearly uniform incidence of cervical disc disease from four through eight years. Female dachshunds with cervical disc disease were significantly older than those with thoracolumbar involvement, but no other such relationship between sex and breed was found.[34]

The most common site of disc involvement for all breeds is at the smallest disc, C2-C3, where 50 per cent of cervical herniations are reported. The frequency of involvement decreases from C3-C4 through C7-T1.[17,34,47,66] The Doberman pinscher is the only large nonchondrodystrophoid breed commonly affected with cervical disc disease.[27,39,47] The degenerative process does not become clinically significant until middle age or later. The special relationship between this Type II degenerative disc disease and the cervical vertebral instability of the Doberman's caudal cervical region is described in Chapter 97.

Clinical Signs

Most animals are presented with neck pain as the first and most constant clinical sign.[17,45] The head and neck are held in a "tense" position and the animal shows reluctance to extend or elevate the cervical vertebral segment for negotiating stairs or even lifting its muzzle over a bowl to eat or drink. Hyperpathia is common, with deep palpation causing excruciating pain or extreme cervical muscular tensing. Spontaneous whining with cervical guarding, evidenced by periodic elevation of the ears or spasms of the shoulder and cutaneous cervical musculature, is often seen.

Because cervical discs by nature extrude slowly, the intensity and consistency of pain from the discogenic, radicular, or meningeal sources can be variable. Frequently, an insidious history of recurrent pain is noted. The spacious spinal canal allows a chronic protrusion to deteriorate and extrude large amounts of material into the epidural space before sufficient pressure produces a clinical motor deficit. The disc consolidates to form a dense calcific mass, which mechanically distorts the cord without the acute "blowouts" more commonly seen in the thoracolumbar segment. When a compressive myelopathy does occur, postural reaction and motor deficits vary from paresis to a slow progressive motor paralysis. These signs are often more severe on one side. When the process is allowed to progress, bilateral involvement ultimately becomes evident.

Chronic progression of the syndrome can be accompanied by acute onset of signs. Stoic dogs or dogs kept on analgesics may appear with acute, profound paresis. Segmental reflex responses show upper motor neuron signs due to the location of disc rupture

TABLE 98–1. Differential Diagnosis of Diseases that Mimic the Cervical Intervertebral Disc Syndrome

Classification	Examples
Degenerative	Spinal osteoarthritis
	Ossifying pachymeningitis
	Cervical vertebral instability
Anomalous	Atlantoaxial subluxation
	Hemivertebrae
Immunological	Polyarthritis
	Polymyositis
Nutritional	Hypervitaminosis A
	Nutritional secondary hyperparathyroidism
Neoplastic	Slow compression or acute pathological fracture
Infectious	Meningitis
	Myelitis
	Discospondylitis
Traumatic	Fracture
	Luxation
	Blunt trauma
Vascular	Fibrocartilaginous emboli*

*Disc disease plays an integral part in this more complex differential diagnosis.

(C2-C3 through C4-C5), with an occasional caudal cervical lesion producing characteristic lower motor neuron reflex changes.

Diagnosis

The initial diagnosis of cervical disc disease must be confirmed, the extent of protrusion or extrusion evaluated, and the location specifically identified prior to treatment. The age, breed, history, physical findings, and clinical neurological findings are all primary indicators of the cervical syndrome. The common differential diagnoses must be eliminated in a systematic fashion, through the use of hematologic and blood chemistry evaluation along with a cerebrospinal fluid examination when necessary (Table 98–1). Lateral and ventrodorsal survey radiographs are taken using anesthesia with the neck held in extension. Mineralization of the nucleus indicates dehydration, chondroid degeneration, and calcium deposition. Its presence is merely a sign of a degenerative Type I disc or an occasional chronic Type II degeneration. Annular mineralization indicates progressive disease with a higher susceptibility to expulsion.[45] Discogenic pain may often be the source of hyperpathia when mineralized nuclear material is forced between the fibrous bundles of the annulus. Narrowing, wedging, or collapse of the disc spaces without radiographic evidence of disc material in the canal is significant whenever accompanied by compatible clinical neurological signs. This occult Type I disc extrusion represents once compact and dense nuclear material that is thinned and extruded to the point of radiolucency.[1] Normally, cervical discs consolidate within the epidural space to form a radiopaque mechanical obstruction. The mineralized density is rarely accompanied by traumatic rupture of the venous sinus or an edematous cord response. The typical Type II disc shows no radiographic evidence of a mineralized mass within the spinal canal. In these cases or any occult or equivocal disc extrusion without radiographic (plain film) documentation, a myelogram must be considered to determine the extent, location, and number of discs involved. The

TABLE 98–2. Stages of Cervical Disc Disease

Hansen Type	Stage	Radiographic Signs	Clinical Signs	Treatment
Type I (*chondro-dystrophoid breeds*)	I	Nuclear mineralization	None	None
	II	Nuclear mineralization with/without annular mineralization (protrusion present)	Intermittent hyperesthesia	1. Medical 2. Fenestration
	III	Mineralized mass extruded into canal (myelogram necessary to delineate an occult mass when survey radiographs indicate wedged or narrowed IV space)	Hyperesthesia ± motor deficits	Ventral decompression (slot)
Type II (*nonchondro-dystrophoid breeds*)	I	No disc lesion; possible spondylosis	None	None
	II	Minimal narrowing or wedging of IV space	Intermittent hyperesthesia	1. Medical 2. Fenestration
	III	Collapsed or wedged IV space; significant fibrous mass evident on myelogram	Hyperesthesia ± motor deficits	Ventral decompression (slot)

specific techniques for myelography are described in Chapter 93.

Staging

Degenerative cervical disc disease is not in itself painful. When a disc's pathological state is classified or staged, a rational treatment regimen can be established. Such a general staging system for disc disease is summarized in Table 98–2 for Type I and Type II cervical disc disease.[17,44–46,61,68,76]

On the basis of previous discussion of cervical anatomy and the insidious sequence of compressive events, it is understandable why most cases of cervical disc disease are given a good prognosis. To arrive at that prognosis as effectively as possible, a concerted effort must be made to correlate the current state of disc involvement in each patient with the correct treatment plan.[11,45,46,78]

Treatment

Conservative (Medical) Treatment

The principle of conservative or medical management is strict confinement for seven to 14 days and the cautious use of anti-inflammatory drugs to control pain and hyperesthesia. When discogenic pain accompanies radiographic evidence of Type I or Type II disc protrusion (stage II), conservative therapy can work well as an initial treatment. The disc remains in its original location and returns to a quiescent state if allowed time for healing of annular fissures or mechanical reorganization of nuclear protrusion.[45] Any cervical pain experienced by the dog aids in limiting activity and should be treated only when severe. Absolute confinement is necessary when anti-inflammatory drugs are used if recurrence or intractable clinical signs are to be prevented.[17,45,66] Treatment of stage III cervical disc disease (extrusion) by conservative means may transiently relieve or improve the clinical signs but is not a rational correction. The temporary euphoria of pain relief often leads to a worsening extrusion.

The first anti-inflammatory drugs to consider are the prostaglandin inhibitors (e.g., aspirin, phenylbutazone, flunixin meglumine). However, corticosteroids such as dexamethasone and prednisolone are frequently chosen for therapy. Because treatment of spinal cord trauma or edema is not involved in cervical protrusions, low anti-inflammatory doses of the steroids are recommended in all cases.[45] The drugs are administered for no longer than 72 hours to prevent side effects.[55,82] Muscle relaxants and vitamin E–selenium preparations have been used with mixed results.[45,52] Although any of these drugs can curb hyperesthesia, conservative treatment relies on forced rest and strict confinement to allow "resolution" of inflammation. After the seven to 14 days of confinement, limited physical activity, with the ani-

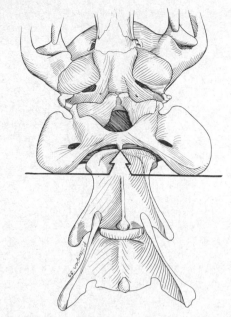

Figure 98–3. The cranial landmark for identifying the intervertebral disc spaces is the ventral prominence of C1, found cranial to a line joining the caudal borders of the wings of the atlas.

mal on a harness or in a small enclosure, may be gradually increased.[45]

Surgery

Surgical correction of cervical disc disease involves removal of the degenerative disc material from its inciting position. An accurate anatomical descent to the paired longus colli muscles, which attach diagonally to the ventral prominence of each vertebra, marks the initial step in either disc fenestration or cord decompression. This ventral approach is described in Chapter 96.

Identification of the exact disc space through the longus colli muscle is by using two landmarks. The cranial reference point is located by palpating the caudal borders of the wing of the atlas. An imaginary line connecting these caudal points passes over the body of the axis (Fig. 98–3). The often sharp ventral prominence palpated cranial to this line as located

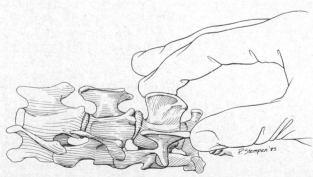

Figure 98–4. The transverse processes of C6 are followed to their vertebral body. C5–C6 and C6–C7 intervertebral spaces are easily identified.

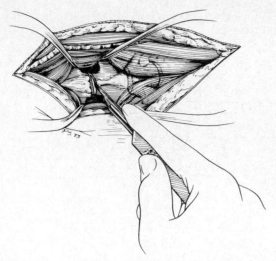

Figure 98–5. An elliptical wedge of ventral annulus is removed with a No. 11 scalpel blade.

on C1 with the C1-C2 synovial joint immediately adjacent to it. The first disc space (C2-C3) is located by moving caudally along the midline to the next ventral prominence, which is located on C2. Each succeeding disc space is located immediately caudal to the ventral prominence. The caudal landmarks are the large, paired transverse processes of C6 (Fig. 98–4). They are readily palpable lateral and ventral to the midline. The ventral prominence of C5 lies centrally between the cranial borders of these transverse processes. Specific intervertebral spaces can be accurately confirmed by counting from both cranial and caudal directions.

Fenestration. The ventral annulus of disc spaces C2-C3 through C6-C7 is exposed by placing closed hemostatic forceps or scissors just caudal to the ventral prominence of the respective vertebral body and spreading the paired tendons of the longus colli muscle. The white fibrous ventral annulus and ventral longitudinal ligament are exposed as the instrument is opened.[12] Exposure can be maintained by careful placement of a small Gelpi retractor into the muscular trough. Incising the tendons of the longus colli mus-

cle at their point of attachment to the ventral prominence increases exposure but often leads to unnecessary hemorrhage. Fenestration is accomplished by creating a slit with a No. 11 Bard-Parker scalpel blade, or a window with a small (2-mm) burr, in the ventral annulus (Fig. 98–5). When a scalpel blade is used, the sharp surface of the blade is directed away from the surgeon, and the tip is inserted into the ventral annulus no more than one-half the estimated depth of the disc. The blade is advanced across the disc to incise the ventral annulus. A small wedge of annulus can be removed for nuclear extraction.[12] The nucleus is withdrawn with a 4-0 bone curette or a thin-blade tartar scraper (Fig. 98–6). Even though degenerative disc material is considered inflammatory, nuclear material that remains after fenestration is not removed by the animal's normal defense mechanisms.[74] Therefore, repeated passes with the curette or tartar scraper are required until all discs from C2-C3 thru C6-C7 (inclusive) are free of nucleus pulposus. When C7-T1 disc degeneration is present, the site is fenestrated.

Ventral Decompression. Identification of the offending disc space is done as described for disc fenestration. Tendons of the longus colli muscle are incised at their periosteal attachments to the ventral prominence. The muscle is then reflected from the vertebral body cranial and caudal to the involved disc space by subperiosteal elevation. Gelpi retractors are placed at the caudal and cranial aspects of the opening to establish exposure and aid hemostasis.

The ventral slot is initiated by removing the ventral prominence cranial to the disc space and a portion of the ventral annulus with a rongeur. Either a pneumatic[76,77] or an electric drill[85,86] and burr may be used to create an opening approximately one-third the length of the vertebral body on each side of the disc space. Slot width is limited to the center one-third to one-half of the vertebral body (Fig. 98–7).[33,77] The slot should be uniformly oval without "funnelling" toward the spinal canal. A sharp round or pineapple-shaped burr is used in a paintbrush fashion to remove a thin layer of bone with each pass of the drill. Saline is intermittently dropped on to the burr

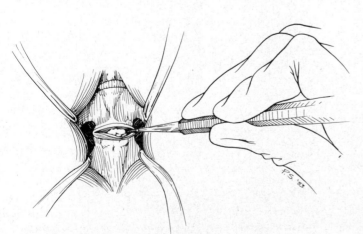

Figure 98–6. Curettage of the nucleus is accomplished with a tartar scraper.

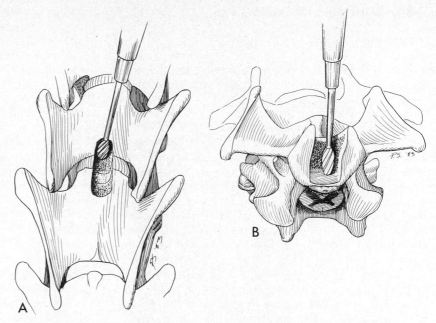

Figure 98–7. *A*, An oblong burr is used to cut a slot into the vertebral bodies adjacent to the extruded disc. *B*, The depth of the slot is monitored until a thin, inner cortical layer remains.

site for cooling and to aid removal of bone dust and small bone chips.[30,75,77]

The landmarks for determining the depth of the slot are critical. The dense outer cortical layer is first encountered, followed by the trabecular cancellous layer, and finally by a thin inner crust of dense, white cortical bone adjacent to the spinal canal. When a vertebral nutrient artery is encountered in the cancellous layer, bone wax may be necessary to control hemorrhage. A 2-mm round burr may be used to thin the final cortical layer with greater accuracy.

Final entry into the spinal canal is initiated using a blunt, thin-blade tartar scraper or small bone curette and continued with fine rongeurs. A burr should never be used to enter the canal, because of the potential for iatrogenic cord damage. Remnants of the dorsal annulus and dorsal longitudinal ligament may be carefully removed with sharp rongeurs or the tartar scraper. Herniated Type I disc material has a cottage cheese–like consistency and is removed in small increments.[77] A Type II disc is more fibrous and tough, requiring delicate rongeuring or fine-thumb forceps and hemostats to grasp the material for excision with a No. 11 scalpel blade.[76]

When the disc extrudes on the midline, the venous sinuses are deviated to a dorsolateral position with the cord elevated. These extrusions can often be removed without lacerating the displaced but fragile venous structures. When the disc surrounds the sinuses, or when the chronic inflammatory response to the extruded material forms adhesions between sinuses and the periosteum, dorsal annulus, or dorsal longitudinal ligament, removal of the extruded material via the slot elicits bleeding. The bleeding is profuse and is most easily controlled by packing the slot with a gelatin sponge for several minutes and

relieving all pressure from the jugular veins. If bleeding persists, suction or localized packing of the slot allows completion of decompression. Overzealous suction can result in hypovolemic shock. Adequate monitoring of cardiovascular status and fluid therapy are therefore of vital importance.[45,77,86]

When dura mater is observed through the site, adequate decompression has been achieved, and the slot is copiously lavaged with saline to remove all bone dust and disc material. A gelatin sponge is packed into the site. Vertebral fusion can be expected without autogenous bone grafting.[33,76,77] The author recommends fenestration of all remaining cervical discs as previously described. It can be accomplished while awaiting hemostasis from a lacerated venous sinus or immediately after successful completion of the decompression.

Aftercare. The vast majority of animals with cervical disc disease can walk immediately after surgery and will require limited activity for adequate healing. Two to three weeks of confinement to a small room or pen with exercise for urination and defecation only is optimal. Excessive exercise results in hyperesthesia, requiring forced cage rest and occasional low-dose anti-inflammatory therapy. Routine postoperative analgesic administration should be discouraged. Owners tend to allow exercise until hyperesthesia occurs rather than restrict exercise and allow a full, uncomplicated recovery. The animal should be fitted with a harness and should discontinue wearing a neck collar of any kind.

When fenestration has been used as the sole treatment, any signs of severe or recurrent hyperesthesia after three weeks should be investigated for an undiagnosed extrusion.[77] The possibility of a concurrent disease process must never be overlooked when neurological recovery does not occur after surgery.

THORACOLUMBAR DISC DISEASE

Incidence

Intervertebral disc disease involving the thoracolumbar spine causes the majority of spinal neurological cases in small animals.[10,18,24,26,45,71] In 654 dogs with thoracolumbar disc disease, 72 per cent were dachshunds,[27] and in a separate study of 8,117 cases, dachshunds accounted for nearly half the cases, with the Pekingese, beagle, Welsh corgi, Lhaso apso, and Shih Tzu also at a significantly increased risk (P < 0.01).[71] Hoerlein's study of 2,395 cases reported a similar breed involvement with 73.1 per cent of the dogs seen for thoracolumbar disc disease being between three and six years of age.[27,45] In nonchondrodystrophoid breeds, the peak age is around six to eight years.[71] The different studies have shown that the incidence of intervertebral disc disease is approximately equal in males and females.[45] A subtle but significant risk factor was found in within-breed weight increases—i.e., risk in males > risk in spayed females > risk in females. This finding may be explained by a weight factor as well as by a protective effect of estrogen against disc degeneration.[71]

The location of intervertebral discs most prone to rupture has been well documented. Over 65 per cent of the lesions are between T11-T12 and L1-L2, with the T12-T13 interspace the most common site of rupture.[10,27,45,59] The spinal cord region involved determines many of the clinical signs and the type of peripheral elicitable reflexes.

Clinical Signs

The neurological signs vary tremendously, depending on the severity of the spinal cord involvement and the acuteness with which it developed. The signs generally are characteristic of lesions in thoracolumbar or lumbosacral spinal segments, but they differ greatly in magnitude from animal to animal. Small lesions or extrusions confined to the lateral aspects of the spinal canal cause a radiculopathy. Because the irritation to the nerve roots and meninges can cause severe pain and hyperesthesia when the vertebral column is manipulated,[59] even ambulatory animals with disc disease should be handled carefully. If the lesion is cranial to spinal cord segment L3-L4, the clinical signs reflect upper motor neuron (UMN) damage.[45] A demarcating painful response to a pinprick, hemostat pinch, or deep palpation and pressure over the transverse processes helps localize the lesion. If the panniculus response is positive and consistent, the lesion is one or two cord segments cranial to the point of response.[59] The panniculus reflex may be vague or inconsistent, and testing of peripheral reflexes should always be done. Normal or hyperreflexic quadriceps reflex, flexor reflex, and perineal reflex are expected. Conscious perception of pain is evaluated with the flexor reflex by using the minimal noxious stimulus possible to obtain an appreciable response. Lesions at or distal to spinal cord segment L3-L4 cause lower motor neuron (LMN) signs. For the nonambulatory dog, the surgeon should always determine the level of sensory perception, whether the lesion is causing UMN or LMN signs, and, most important, whether the dog consciously perceives pain. When other causes of disease have been ruled out, accurate localization of the lesion and knowledge of the animal's sensory status are combined with the results of the general physical examination and history to establish a surgical prognosis and plan.

Diagnosis

A minimum data base for suspected cases of thoracolumbar disc disease includes packed cell volume and BUN measurements and a urinalysis, with additional tests as indicated by the physical findings or a concomitant systemic illness. Changes in the hemogram, blood chemistry, or urinalysis results are often secondary to paresis. Reluctance to eat and drink and inability to posture for defecation and urination may be significant. Animals in pain often pant excessively, causing an increased insensible fluid loss.

A strong index of suspicion must be maintained when a chondrodystrophoid dog in a high-risk age group is presented with signs of thoracolumbar intervertebral disc disease. In nonchondrodystrophic breeds with signs, intervertebral disc disease is still an important differential diagnosis to consider. In both instances, other potential causes of spinal cord compression must be evaluated. An accurate history helps to define or eliminate some of these possible diagnoses, such as fractures and luxations, vertebral instabilities, osteocartilaginous exostoses, extradural and meningeal tumors, and discospondylitis or vertebral body osteomyelitis. The history may suggest some congenital or breed problems, including malformations of the spine or spinal cord seen with spina bifida, dysraphism, syringomyelia, hemivertebra, and block vertebrae. Traumatic cord disorders ranging from contusion and concussion to myelomalacia may simulate disc disease, and vascular disorders such as fibrocartilaginous embolism have been confused with intervertebral disc disease.[35,37,38,42,47,59,69,90,91] The extensive list of possible differential diagnoses emphasizes the importance of a thorough history and a careful complete physical examination.

Radiographic confirmation of the neurological diagnosis is the essential diagnostic aid in confirming thoracolumbar disc disease. Unless the dog is cooperative and not in pain, radiographs of the unanesthetized animal are seldom diagnostic. Radiographic examination is justified for cases treated conservatively, if necessary, to confirm the diagnosis of degenerative disc disease. The radiographic findings must be correlated with the lesion localization as determined on neurological examination. In a series of 187 cases, the radiographic disc lesion was confirmed at surgery in 75.4 per cent of the cases. Clinical neurological localization correlated with the surgical localization in only 40 per cent of the cases, but the correlation increased to 75 per cent if an error of two interspaces was allowed.[10] Radiographic signs of an intervertebral disc rupture are discussed elsewhere.[10, 45] If a well-defined lesion is not evident on the survey films, or if more than one lesion is apparent in the suspect cord region, myelography should be performed.[47] If two lesions are seen within one to two interspaces, it is often easier on the spinal cord and more efficient to explore both areas surgically than to subject the dog to a myelogram. If referral for surgery is contemplated, radiographs taken with the dog sedated or under a short-acting barbiturate are not recommended prior to referral. The radiographs are usually repeated at the referral institution, and the depressant effect of the drug may negatively influence the neurological findings.

In humans, the sensitivity of lumbar myelography in detecting ruptured lumbar discs is about 75 per cent. Approximately 90 per cent of patients free of lumbar disc herniation have a normal myelogram. The indications for myelography in humans are applicable in dogs. Myelograms are done for (1) accurate localization of disc herniation, (2) multiple disc herniations, (3) ruling out of spinal neoplasms, and (4) clarification of a questionable diagnosis of herniated lumbar disc. Some of the complications of myelography include septic meningitis, aseptic meningitis, encystment of dye, avulsion of nerve roots, neurological deficit, headache, extra-arachnoid injection of dye, and intravasation of dye with pulmonary hemorrhage.[13,58,72]

Selective ascending lumbosacral venography in the assessment of lumbar disc herniation was 98 per cent diagnostically accurate, compared with 90 per cent for myelography in a group of 50 patients with no previous disc surgery. Venography was of limited value in patients that had one or more prior disc operations, because it did not distinguish between scarring and recurrent disc hernation.[53] Lumbosacral vertebral sinus venography via transjugular catheterization in the dog, for identification of lesions compressing the caudal lumbar and sacral nerve roots, has been less successful than in humans because of difficulty in consistently locating the canine median sacral vein.[50]

Discography in humans has been a useful adjunct to myelography to help determine the specific disc that has degenerated. This technique requires percutaneous puncture and is best done with the aid of image intensification. With simple degeneration without an annular tear, the nucleus pulposus is no longer regular, and there is a shredding and tearing of the contrast medium.[13] Technical difficulties with performing this procedure in dogs have so far precluded successful use of the technique.[45]

Recently, herniated lumbar discs have been diagnosed with the use of computed tomography. Computed tomography is the procedure of choice for diagnosing lumbar stenosis and facet joint disease.[58] This procedure is available through cooperative efforts with selected medical institutions.

Staging

Staging of thoracolumbar intervertebral disc disease is necessary to establish guidelines for the most beneficial therapy for different groups of problems. A successful method is to divide dogs with intervertebral disc disease into four groups: *Group I* dogs exhibit pain only with their first episode and do not have a neurological deficit. *Group II* dogs exhibit recurrent pain and/or mild to moderate paresis. *Group III* dogs have severe paraparesis. *Group IV* dogs are paraplegic and are divided into subgroups; *Group IVA* dogs are paraplegic but retain deep pain sensation, and group IVB dogs are paraplegic and analgesic.

Dogs in group I are acceptable candidates for medical therapy. A study by Funkquist[26] supports the use of fenestration in these dogs as well, because of a 48 per cent recurrence rate in similar cases treated conservatively.[26] Group II dogs are candidates for fenestration at the majority of institutions. Groups III and IVA should undergo decompression,[10,29,43,49] with or without fenestration.[25,45,59] Group IVB dogs are treated medically if the deep pain response has been absent 48 hours or longer[59] or with decompression if it has been absent less than 36 hours.[29] Dogs with acute paralysis and no deep pain should be operated as soon as possible, preferably within two to four hours (see Table 98–3).[38,45,59]

Historically, the decision whether to treat a given case medically or surgically varies tremendously among individuals, and the type and timing of surgical procedure recommended vary even more among

TABLE 98–3. Guidelines for Therapy of Canine Thoracolumbar Intervertebral Disc Disease in the Dog

Group	Treatment
I	Medical therapy
II	
Multiple episodes of pain	Fenestration
Mild ataxia and paresis	Medical therapy
Paresis and ataxia—second episode	Decompression with fenestration
III	Decompression with fenestration
IV	
A	Decompression with fenestration
B	
Less than 48 hours	Decompression, durotomy, lavage, plus intensive medical therapy
After 48 hours	Medical therapy

clinicians.[10,18,23,24–26,29,43,45,49,59,70,83] The ability of the animal to demonstrate conscious pain perception on the pedal reflex is, however, a point of universal agreement.[45] At Auburn University, surgical intervention is recommended for the following situations: (1) recurrent attacks of neurological dysfunction due to disc protrusion, each attack being more severe than the previous one, (2) pain and paresis that are unresponsive to nonsurgical care, and (3) moderate paresis to profound paralysis with fecal and urinary dysfunction produced by a local compression.

Prognosis

The prognosis for each animal differs depending on its neurological status and the treatment regimen chosen. There is good evidence to support surgical therapy over medical therapy for the majority of cases. Funkquist[26] published a comparative study of conservative treatment versus intervertebral disc fenestration for thoracolumbar disc disease in the dog. Recurrence was 48 per cent in dogs managed conservatively versus 17 per cent in dogs receiving fenestration. She concluded that without surgical prophylaxis, a recurrence could be expected within a three year period in about 50 per cent of the dogs suffering one or more attacks. There was no significant difference in mean recovery time between the two groups, a finding that supports the contention of most surgeons that fenestration should be regarded primarily as a prophylactic technique.[26] Funkquist emphasized that if the discs with radiographic evidence of degeneration are evacuated, there should be a nearly 100 per cent freedom from recurrence for several years. Also, numerous dogs in groups III and IVA respond in three to four days after disc fenestration, occasionally in a dramatic manner. The fact that the offending disc material is still in the spinal canal lends credence to the beliefs of those who support Olson's "dynamic factor" theory.[23] However, total recovery for all categories takes six to 12 weeks,[23] contradicting any major therapeutic effect of fenestration. Dogs that retain deep pain perception have a 50 to 90 per cent chance of recovering with conservative therapy. The greater percentage results from a thorough, well-designed medical and physical therapy program for dogs that have the least severe signs. Clients should be warned that at least three to five per cent of dogs in groups I to III will continue to deteriorate and progress into paraplegia, whereas almost 50 per cent of the ones that recover will suffer a recurrence. The prognosis for recovery after surgical fenestration for all groups collectively has been reported as high as 90 to 95 per cent.[18,23]

Decompressive surgery is usually done for Groups III and IVA. Time is a very important factor in these categories, with success rates of 80 to 96 per cent reported when operation is performed in less than 48 hours. Up to a 50 per cent success rate has been reported for Group IVB dogs operated on within 36 hours of the loss of ability to walk, under standard protocol and by experienced surgeons.[29] After 48 hours, the chance for recovery is probably less than 5 per cent.[59] Hoerlein[45] and Oliver and Lorenz[59] advocate decompression and fenestration as a therapeutic and prophylactic measure for Group III and IVA dogs, whereas Brown and colleagues[10] and Prata[70] advise decompression alone because the incidence of disc extrusion at a second site in their series was only 2.67 per cent (5 of 187). In a series of 99 cases treated by hemilaminectomy, dogs with paresis, pain, or both recovered generally at the same rate whether or not surgery was delayed. Group IVA dogs responded favorably if operated on within four days of onset. However, dogs in Group IVB did not respond.[49]

The overall prognosis for recovery is good as long as the dog retains conscious pain perception. Recovery time and quality are proportional to severity and duration of neurological impairment. If surgery is to be done, the sooner the better, especially for dogs in Group IV. Clients who opt for conservative management should be warned that the dog's neurological status may deteriorate and that there is a high recurrence rate in dogs treated conservatively. Other factors influencing the prognosis include the dog's general health, willingness of the owner to work diligently on rehabilitation of the dog, and whether the dog is overweight. For surgical cases, the skill and experience of the surgeon must be considered in addition to these other factors.[25]

Treatment

Conservative (Medical) Treatment

Nursing Care. As described, medical treatment is reserved for animals that are experiencing an initial episode of pain or mild neurological dysfunction, and those that have had no deep pain response for longer than 48 hours.[59] Medical therapy may be the only recourse available for other categories if a surgical referral is not practical or surgery is economically prohibitive. The key element for a successful outcome is strictly enforced rest. Ambulatory dogs should not be placed in an open baby crib or playpen, as they often attempt to jump out. Close confinement in a small airline crate in a quiet room to minimize disturbances is preferable, with exercise restricted to leash walks away from other animals twice a day.[59] The owner should provide a comfortable area for the dog to lie on, such as blankets over foam rubber pads or sheep wool mats. Nonambulatory dogs must be watched more closely to prevent decubital ulcers, dehydration, and soiling.

Dogs in Groups I and II respond well to confinement and supervised exercise. Those in Groups III and IV require considerably more nursing care and physical therapy. In addition to preventing decubital ulcers, one must minimize urinary tract infections and muscle atrophy.[45,59] Urine retention from UMN or LMN disease causes a stagnation cystitis and may result in overstretching of the detrusor muscle, further impairing urination. Manual expression of the bladder is effective in females, and the client can be instructed to express the dog's bladder at least three times a day. Male bladders are much more difficult to express and often require catheterization. Soft, atraumatic catheters are used to lavage the bladder with sterile warm saline. When cystitis is present, dilute nitrofurazone or neomycin can be instilled into the bladder after the lavage until culture and sensitivity testing establish the correct antibiotic treatment. The majority of clients are capable of properly catheterizing male dogs. Female dogs that need catheterization are best hospitalized and treated by a veterinarian. Retention catheters may be used and the dog may be sent home, but the client must be diligent about keeping the dog's perineum and the catheter as clean as possible; the increased risk of ascending infections associated with retention catheters as well as client dissatisfaction from the urine leakage generally precludes this option. Warm-water enemas, mineral oil in the food, or pediatric glycerin suppositories are recommended when the dog needs assistance with bowel movements.

Water intake is monitored to assure adequate hydration and renal function. Many paraplegics develop a negative nitrogen balance and a secondary anemia. To maintain good nutrition, a well-balanced diet such as P/D,* supplemented with iron and liver, is desirable. All B-complex vitamins should be provided in therapeutic amounts. Injections of vitamin B_{12} and calcium may be beneficial for selected animals. K/D† diet is recommended for dogs with evidence of poor renal function.[45]

Physiotherapy is an integral part of the care and provides mental stimulus as well as aiding neuromuscular function. Warm water baths for dogs with acute pain are beneficial for relaxing muscle spasms. For the paraplegic dog that is not in too much pain to be manipulated, alternate sitting-standing motions can be provided for the dog with walking motions. Muscle massage while bathing the dog or using a whirlpool promotes circulation, and bathing helps prevent urine dermatitis. These treatments should be the responsibility of an employee who is interested, gentle, and reliable. The client is often the best nurse but must be instructed to never leave a paraplegic animal unattended in a tub of water because of the danger of drowning.

Tail-up exercises, belly band support, and exercise carts can all be beneficial. A comfortable sling devised for the dog so that the client can stand erect while exercising the dog encourages therapy. Exercise carts are useful to get the dog up and can be used to provide exercise that needs indirect supervision. However, passive rather than active rear limb exercise and the dog's dependency on the cart can impede a complete recovery.

To summarize, nursing care includes: (1) rest, (2) access to water and food and monitoring of intake, (3) comfortable bedding to help prevent decubital ulcers, (4) supervision, assistance, and monitoring of urination and defecation, and (5) a thorough, consistent physical therapy program. Paraplegic dogs that are clean, exercised correctly, eating and drinking, and taken outside for fresh air and sunshine seem to respond the best.

Drug Therapy. The drugs most commonly used in the medical management of thoracolumbar disc disease are the adrenocorticosteroids and phenylbutazone. Group I and II dogs usually respond well to prednisolone, 0.5 mg/kg every 12 hours for 72 hours and discontinued. It is advisable to keep the dog hospitalized or crated for one week. Three weeks of cage confinement at home is recommended, followed by three more weeks of house confinement and leash exercise. The client should be advised of the 50 per cent chance of recurrence.[59] Dexamethasone can be used at 0.2 mg/kg for an anti-inflammatory effect,[45] with doses of 2 mg/kg intravenously recommended during the early preoperative period for Group III and IV dogs, followed by a dose of 0.1 to 0.2 mg/kg every 12 hours for 48 hours.[45,59] There is considerable disagreement among surgeons about dose levels for dexamethasone. Dosages from as low as 0.06 mg/kg twice a day for two days after disc fenestration,[23] which is below the anti-inflammatory level, to a total of 0.25 to 0.50 mg three times a day, tapering over seven to 10 days, are recommended for treatment of back pain.[70] The latter dose is combined with methocarbamol* at 15 mg/kg body weight divided three times a day for seven to 10 days for relief of muscular spasm. The level of steroid administration is dictated by the severity of the neurological loss, not by whether medical or surgical management will be employed. Gastrointestinal hemorrhage and ulceration and melena are anticipated side effects of high doses or of prolonged use of any dose. Phenylbutazone and indomethacin are used less commonly.[45]

Comments. Emphasis has been placed initially on the general nursing and rehabilitative care of the dog with intervertebral disc disease. A common mistake is to rely primarily on anti-inflammatory products to provide symptomatic relief and not follow through with complete care. A surprising number of referral calls are instigated by overzealous corticosteroid administration and inadequate client education. A typical history is as follows: A group I or II dog has an initial episode one day, for which it receives a steroid injection and is sent home on oral steroids. The next day the dog feels much better, and the day after that the dog's activity level precipitates an acute nuclear expulsion, placing the dog in group III or IV. The client is upset and the prognosis is worse,

---

*P/D Prescription Protein Diet, Hill Dog Food, Topeka, Kansas.
†K/D Prescription Kidney Diet, Hill Dog Food, Topeka, Kansas.

*Robaxin. A. H. Robins Co. Richmond, Va.

often precipitating an emergency referral. Even worse, sometimes the dog is treated medically one more day to see if it improves and then referred the next day. Sometimes this scenario is unavoidable, but judicious use of corticosteroids tempered with exercise restriction or confinement is highly recommended and will prevent many such situations.

Surgery

Fenestration. The value of fenestration done properly is the complete prophylaxis achieved against future herniation or rupture of the operated discs. The ventral abdominal and dorsolateral approaches and the lateral muscle–separating techniques have all been advocated.[18,23,45,89] The dorsolateral approach is covered in Chapter 96. The indications for fenestration include dogs in groups I and II. Dogs that are primarily experiencing back pain, with or without mild paresis, especially of an unrelenting or recurrent nature are satisfactory candidates for fenestration. The goal in this instance is to relieve intradisc pressure and evacuate the remaining nuclear material. This procedure eliminates the danger of an acute extrusion, which might drastically alter the dog's neurological status, and stops the ongoing extrusion of disc contents, thus removing the "dynamic factor." The proponents of fenestration for therapeutic reasons acknowledge that disc material already in the spinal canal is not removed, a situation that is easily documented by taking postoperative radiographs. Therefore, the only value for fenestration in group III and IV dogs is the prevention of ongoing inflammation, i.e., the "dynamic factor," or the beneficial effect of surgically "firing" the area. The latter enhances circulation and promotes arrival of phagocytes and resorption of cellular debris. Some group III dogs inexplicably respond quickly after fenestration, even with very low doses of preoperative and postoperative corticosteroids. However, in the only comparative study,[23] which also included significant numbers in the conservative treatment and fenestration groups, there was no significant difference in the mean recovery times. In a report of 67 cases encompassing all four grades of spinal cord involvement, a 95 per cent success rate was achieved, but the majority of cases took from six to 12 weeks to recover totally.[23] Twenty-seven of 30 dogs in a comparable study achieved complete recovery within an average period of 3½ weeks after surgery.[18] It is difficult to ascribe more than a prophylactic effect to the procedure with these recovery times. Fenestration may be totally unrewarding in dogs experiencing severe radiculopathy. A second operation aimed at mass removal and nerve root decompression has been necessary in some cases.[70] The prophylactic value of fenestrating adjacent, high-risk discs has also been questioned, because the incidence of disc extrusion at a second interspace occurred after definitive laminectomy and disc removal is only 2.67 per cent.[70] Regardless of the surgical approach, once adequate

surgical exposure is achieved, a window or perforation (fenestration) is made in the annulus fibrosus to create a pathway to the nucleus pulposus. If a normal disc is fenestrated, there is sufficient hydrostatic pressure within the nucleus that a spontaneous extrusion of the mucinous nuclear material usually occurs as the annular plug is removed. This does not occur in the dehydrated, degenerated disc undergoing chondroid metaplasia. A generous window should be made with the location of the spinal cord and the vertebral sinuses borne in mind.[23] A sharp clean entry into the disc is made using a No. 11 scalpel blade. Cores of annulus and nucleus may also be taken by fenestrating with a large hypodermic needle. Forcible puncture of the annulus with a tartar scraper is to be discouraged, because the sudden displacement of the mass of the scraper may result in further extrusion of nucleus dorsally into the spinal canal at the offending site. A tartar scraper, hypodermic needle, small bone curette, or pituitary rongeur may be used to remove the nuclear contents. Adequate surgical exposure and hemostasis are requisites for successful surgery. Fenestrating the T11-T12 through L3-L4 discs includes the sites with high risk for rupture and can usually be done with minimal chance of inflicting iatrogenic cord or nerve root trauma. The low incidence of disc rupture caudal to L3-L4 and the consequences of damaging nerve roots that contribute to essential peripheral nerves in this area preclude routine fenestration and warrant careful surgical technique when fenestration is performed.

Muscle Separation Technique. The muscle separation techniques have gained popularity and are now used extensively in preference to other techniques.[18,23,74,89] When fenestration is the only objective of the operation, the muscle separation approach is quick, atraumatic, and effective, and hemorrhage is seldom a problem. The technique is easily combined with decompression, obviating the extensive exposure employed for decompression plus fenestration. The dorsolateral approach is used for the lumbar discs and the lateral approach for the thoracic discs. This combination provides good exposure with minimal dissection, is bloodless, and is easily combined with a dorsal decompression or hemilaminectomy. The incision through the lumbodorsal fascia is made over the mammillary process of the articular facets of the lumbar vertebrae, to ensure a dissection plane between the multifidus complex medially and the longissimus muscle laterally. The last rib is palpated through the incision, and the mammillary process just caudal to the rib is identified; it should be the T13-L1 articular process. Dissection is started at the L2-L3 interspace by pressing the smooth side of a periosteal elevator against the dorsolateral aspect of the articular process. The musculature is elevated subperiosteally in a ventral direction to the accessory process (Fig. 98–8), which stops the progress of the elevator. The elevator is moved laterally two to three millimeters over the accessory process and slightly caudal three to five millimeters, and then is carefully

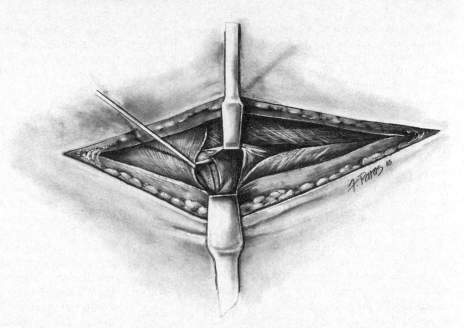

Figure 98–8. Dorsolateral approach for intervertebral disc fenestration exposes an opening to observe the lateral surface of the disc. The multifidus muscle (dorsally) and longissimus muscle (ventrally) are bluntly dissected and retracted. The neurovascular bundle is retracted dorsally (small retractor).

directed ventrally to the transverse process. The lateral step prevents laceration of the vessel associated with the tendon of insertion of the longissimus muscle on the accessory process, and the caudal adjustment prevents passing of the elevator cranial and ventral to the transverse process. The longissimus muscle is elevated laterally following the transverse process and then is retracted with an Army-Navy or small Myerding retractor. The tissue is elevated from the junction of the transverse process with the vertebral body dorsally to the accessory process, and the insertion of the longissimus muscle on the accessory process is retracted with a Senn retractor. The connective tissue is bluntly elevated from the lateral aspect of the intervertebral disc, which is just cranial to the junction of the body of the vertebra and the transverse process. The neurovascular bundle emerges from the intervertebral foramen along the craniodorsal margin of the disc. This tissue can be retracted with the elevator or a nerve root retractor (Fig. 98–9). The disc is then fenestrated.

The lumbar discs are fenestrated, and a new dissection plane is established just ventral to the thoracic part of the longissimus muscle over each rib. The dorsolateral aspect of the rib is exposed to the level of the costotransverse ligament, and dorsal retraction is maintained on the longissimus muscle. The levator costae muscle is separated from the rib. Disc is exposed just cranial to the head and neck of the rib. The surgeon must be familiar with the location, in both the lumbar and thoracic areas, of the intervertebral foramen in respect to other landmarks. Sharp dissection at the level of the costotransverse ligament results in a lacerated venous sinus or spinal cord. To define the ventral limit of the disc, a small periosteal elevator can be eased along the ventrolateral aspect of the disc and carefully placed under the vertebral body. The aorta and the sympathetic chain are just ventral to the vertebral bodies, but not immediately adjacent to the bone. The elevator can be used as a retractor for the intercostal muscles by application of careful downward pressure. The pleural cavity is so close that the excursion of the lungs often may be seen through the pleura. Placing the elevator beneath the disc has provided a measure of security previously lacking before a definite ventral boundary was established.

The dorsolateral approach for hemilaminectomy is often extensive enough that fenestration can be done by minimal additional dissection. The muscle insertions on each adjacent articular process cranial and caudal to the intervertebral disc have to be released to facilitate the necessary ventral exposure and lateral retraction from this approach. The offending disc can easily be fenestrated in this manner after the hemilaminectomy even when the exposure is minimal for the decompression.

Anti-inflammatory Medication. Because of the inherent manipulation of the spinal column during anesthesia, positioning, and surgery, the dog is given an anti-inflammatory injection of dexamethasone (1mg/10kg) preoperatively and postoperatively. If the neurological status has not deteriorated from preoperative levels 24 hours after surgery, the dexameth-

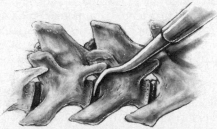

Figure 98–9. After an incision is made in the lateral side of the lumbar disc, a tartar scraper is used to extract as much nucleus pulposus as possible.

asone is discontinued. The dog's neurological condition is rarely worsened by the procedure.

Aftercare. The care of dogs after fenestration is similar to that for dogs with similar signs that are treated medically. The incision should be checked daily for any sign of swelling or discharge and should be kept clean and dry. Protective support bandages are left to the discretion of the surgeon. Dogs are routinely released to the clients the day after surgery. They should be strictly confined and restricted to leash walks for a minimum of three to four weeks. There should be few, if any, complications if the operation was done atraumatically. Seromas form occasionally but are easily managed.

Most dogs progress well without repeated episodes of back pain. However, when entrapment of the affected nerve root by the extruded disc material is not relieved and dogs experience postoperative radicular pain, mass removal and nerve root decompression are indicated.[37]

Decompression. Decompression, whether by hemilaminectomy[9,45,49,59,79] or dorsal laminectomy,[10, 25, 29, 43, 58, 65, 70, 83] is the procedure of choice for dogs in groups III and IV, because pressure on neural tissue or vascular supply to the spinal cord cannot be relieved by fenestration alone.[15,19,21,63,67,70,88] In humans, the available space in the spinal canal is a highly significant factor in the symptomatology of disc lesions and in the response to treatment.[67] The dog has a much smaller spinal canal relative to cord size than the human, with approximately 80 per cent of the thoracolumbar spinal canal occupied by the spinal cord.[47]

Studies on blood supply to the spinal cord and tension on the cord and vasculature associated with cord elevation from mass intrusion emphasize the importance of decompression and mass removal.[15,19,21,63] Simulated acute anterior (ventral) epidural masses were created in monkeys. When posterior (dorsal) decompression restored normal arterial and venous hemodynamics, neurological integrity was maintained even with considerable mechanical cord distortion. When either the anterior (ventral) spinal artery or the posterior (dorsal) spinal vein remained obstructed following laminectomy, the monkeys were paraplegic. The conclusion was that acute ventral epidural masses larger than 4 mm in diameter could not be adequately decompressed with a dorsal approach. Only minor dorsal displacement of the cord is seen following laminectomy in the presence of large ventral masses.[21] Besides its effect on circulation, the anterior mass causes an axial tension in the spinal cord that increases with vertical distance and may reach a critical degree on the posterior (dorsal) surface of the cord; decompressive laminectomy will not relieve this tension.[65]

The role of the dentate ligaments in the pathogenesis of myelopathy secondary to disease conditions that alter the normal biomechanics of the spinal canal was studied in dogs and also in human cadavers. At levels of dorsal elevation usually within the confines of the canine canal, the dentate ligaments were the most significant element increasing tension and somatosensory evoked potential requirements. In the human cadaver studies, a reduction in force of approximately 50 per cent was shown after dentatotomy. Seemingly, after dentate ligament section, the applied tension is distributed over a longer segment of the cord, with a reduction in tension and disruption of axonal conduction where the force was applied.[15] This finding supports decompression for mass removal and relief of nerve root or spinal cord compression.[70] Unfortunately, few cases of thoracolumbar cord compression respond rapidly to decompression, even with mass removal. There are studies comparing medically treated cases with surgically treated cases, but none comparing fenestration with decompression in similarly involved animals. The comparison of hemilaminectomy *versus* dorsal laminectomy for group III and IV animals needs to be done. Are better results obtained when decompression plus mass removal is effected, whether by hemilaminectomy or dorsal laminectomy?

Some surgeons advocate fenestration,[18,23] others decompress with dorsal laminectomy and mass removal but never fenestrate,[10,29,43,70] and yet others decompress with hemilaminectomy[9,45,59] and also fenestrate. There is no support for preferring medical over surgical therapy, although clinical and experimental studies emphasize the need for decompression in group III and IVA cases.[10,19,21,25,26,29,43,45,49,59,70,83] The question that needs to be resolved is whether it is essential or worthwhile to fenestrate adjacent high-risk discs when the problem disc site has been decompressed and mass removal has been accomplished. Is a two to three per cent incidence of disc rupture at a second interspace[10,70] too high, and would routine prophylactic fenestration lower it?

In Hoerlein's series,[45] there is overwhelming support for surgical over nonsurgical therapy, although the surgical group was approximately five times larger. Results in both groups are divided into good, fair, and poor for dogs with paralysis, paresis, and pain, respectively. The surgery consisted of hemilaminectomy and multiple fenestrations done by a number of surgeons. Good results, defined as complete recovery of motor and urinary function, were 87, 90.5, and 82.7 per cent for the paralysis, paresis, and pain groups, respectively. Although a lack of recurrence was noted, the percentage and time of recurrence were not provided.[45] Funkquist[26] maintains that following total "clearing" of the back, a nearly 100 per cent freedom from recurrence could be expected for several years. Because of unforeseen problems during operation and varying ability between surgeons, it is impossible to rely on total clearing or complete fenestration of all adjacent discs at risk. A 17 per cent recurrence rate was seen in the fenestrated series, versus 48 per cent in conservatively treated dogs that were still ambulatory.[26] Would the recurrence rate have been less if decompression and mass removal were done, but no fenestrations?

On the basis of preceding information, decompression is indicated for dogs in groups III and IVA and is recommended to be performed as soon as possible. The operation is seldom of benefit after seven days.[45] An occasional animal, even in group IVB, responds in a significantly short time to decompression, even after having been paraplegic for several weeks prior to surgery. In these cases, the distortion of the neural elements and demyelination from chronic pressure and ischemia are reversible once the mass is removed. There is no benefit to these dogs from a fenestration, especially in chronic cases, because the recovery is due to remyelination, which would not be enhanced by a fenestration. In the group IVB dog that has been paraplegic for several weeks, it is extremely unlikely that the dynamic factor is an important consideration. Dogs that have been unresponsive to medical therapy or fenestration and still suffer back pain are also candidates for a decompressive procedure.

Dorsal laminectomy and hemilaminectomy are the two standard techniques used to decompress the spinal cord. It is apparent from the experimental data and clinical surgical experience of many that a "deroofing" procedure without mass removal is inadequate.[10,21,45,65,69] The dorsal laminectomy procedure is more readily extended to accommodate lesions on either side of the cord than the hemilaminectomy, as the lesions seem to occur on the right and left sides with equal frequency.[70] If a dog has strong historical and neurological evidence of lateralizing disease that is confirmed radiographically, a hemilaminectomy on the affected side is preferred.

Dorsal decompression techniques can be divided into three basic groups: the Funkquist type A, the Funkquist type B, and the modified deep dorsal laminectomy.[83] Slight variations used by different surgeons are usually intermediate between the Funkquist type B and the modified deep dorsal techniques.[29,43,70,79]

Because the Funkquist type B laminectomy does not provide reasonable access to the spinal canal for mass removal, except for dorsolaterally and the more uncommon dorsally located extrusions, it is not recommended for other lesions. Bilateral facetectomy and foramenotomy at the site of disc extrusion, combined with a laminectomy over two vertebral bodies with variable amounts of bilateral pedicle removal, has been recommended.[70] This combination assures adequate visual access to the ventrolateral gutter and eliminates the need to manipulate the cord to remove the extruded disc. A dorsal midline or slightly elliptical off-midline incision, for dogs with prominent dorsal spines, is made and the lumbodorsal fascia is incised adjacent to the dorsal spines. The affected interspace is identified by palpating the last rib and the adjacent dorsal spine and is confirmed as addi-

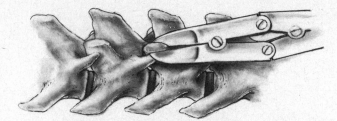

Figure 98–10. The articular facet is removed by using bone-cutting forceps or rongeurs. The decompressive hemilaminectomy is completed by using rongeurs, trephine, or power equipment.

tional dissection is done. Other means of identifying landmarks include premarking a dorsal spine with sterile new methylene blue, and inserting a Kirschner wire in a dorsal spine and identifying the needle and wire location radiographically. A foolproof method is to expose the costotransverse ligament of the 13th rib. The epaxial muscles are elevated subperiosteally from the dorsal spines and articular facets and held with self-retaining retractors. The decompression is done with an air drill and burrs, rongeurs, or both after the dorsal spines have been removed.

The technique for hemilaminectomy is similar, but the dissection is confined to one side, usually the left, for right-handed surgeons. The epaxial muscles are released to the level of the transverse processes and retracted laterally, usually with two Gelpi retractors. Additional exposure can be gained by severing the insertion of the longissimus muscle on the accessory process or by fracturing the accessory process at its base, facilitating retraction. The articular facets are removed with a bone cutter or rongeurs (Fig. 98–10), and the decompression is performed (1) with rongeurs after cranial traction on the cranial dorsal spine to open the articular facet space for entry of the rongeur, (2) with a trephine and rongeurs,[45] or (3) with an air drill with burrs and then rongeurs (Fig. 98–11). When the window is created with an air drill, careful attention must be paid to the color changes as one progresses toward the spinal canal. As the depth of the defect decreases, the outer white cortical bone is brushed away, and the inner red medullary bone appears. The next layer is the inner white cortical bone, followed by the appearance of

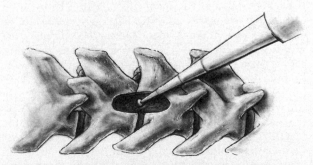

Figure 98–11. The power drill is used to produce a hole in the dorsolateral lamina to allow access to the vertebral canal.

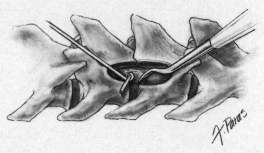

Figure 98–12. Any extruded nuclear material may be removed by using a small tartar scraper and teasing material from beneath the spinal cord. Occasionally, a bilateral hemilaminectomy must be performed.

the translucent inner periosteum. The periosteum may appear black if a sinus clot from the disc rupture is immediately adjacent to it, or the cord and dural vessels may be visible through the periosteum if a contralateral disc is displacing the cord toward the operative defect. Rongeurs can be used at the level of the inner cortical bone or at the periosteal level, depending on the surgeon's skill with the air drill. Every precaution must be made not to touch the spinal cord with the rongeur. The jaw of the rongeur placed toward the spinal cord should not be inserted inside the canal unless there is sufficient room to accommodate it without displacing the spinal cord. These guidelines apply to both the dorsal laminectomy and hemilaminectomy. The defect created usually extends from the cranial and caudal aspects of the articular facets on either side of the involved interspace. The presence of normal epidural fat indicates sufficient decompression.

The extruded nuclear material is carefully removed with a mosquito hemostat, nerve root retractor, tartar scraper, or small bone curette (Fig. 98–12). The canal can be carefully flushed with sterile lactated Ringer's solution or saline to remove small particles. A 3½F Brunswick rubber feeding catheter is easily inserted up or down the canal and occasionally under the spinal cord. A gentle flushing pressure is used to dislodge small particles of disc material and to float debris from the canal. Too much pressure can displace the spinal cord out of the defect. The catheter can be passed under and lifted through disc material entrapped in a sinus clot. Once the clot is fragmented, the flushing action helps dislodge the amorphous mass. Small amounts of disc material adhering to but not penetrating the dura should not be removed forcibly. Hemilaminectomy is effective for removing ipsilateral lesions or decompressing a swollen edematous cord.[45] It can be used in conjunction with fusion and spinal fixation techniques if the disc material is firm and the extrusion is large. Contralateral lesions are difficult to remove without excessive cord manipulation; in this instance, the hemilaminectomy should be converted to a dorsal laminectomy, or a bilateral hemilaminectomy should be done.[79]

A durotomy is not done except as a diagnostic aid in group IVB dogs to determine the integrity of the nervous tissue. It is not indicated for dogs with deep pain sensation. When a durotomy is done, the incision should be extensive enough that a swollen, edematous cord would not protrude through the dural opening, thus focusing pressure at that junction. A durotomy is a relatively innocuous procedure when done on a normal spinal cord and may be beneficial when done immediately after trauma.[62,64] A midline myelotomy can be performed to check for central hemorrhagic necrosis. Myelotomy has been recommended, in conjunction with the use of certain drugs that are effective against vasoactive substances released subsequent to spinal trauma, for the arrest of central hemorrhagic necrosis, but it is not an innocuous procedure. A full-thickness midline myelotomy was found to cause severe necrosis of spinal gray matter.[81]

Prior to closure, a pedicle or free fat graft should be placed over the cortical defect to prevent adhesions.[70] Processed gelatin sheets are clinically acceptable and have been used for years.[45,51] Closure is routine for both procedures, but a thorough closure of the thoracolumbar fascia and subcutaneous dead space is important (see Chapter 96).

Aftercare and Complications. The postoperative care of dogs that have had a decompression is similar to that of dogs treated medically for the same neurological deficit. Physical therapy should be started as soon after surgery as the dog can tolerate it. The incision is protected and evaluated as described for fenestration. The dog is sent home in the client's care as soon as micturition is spontaneous and effective, or earlier if the client can adequately monitor and manage bladder function, perhaps as soon as 48 to 72 hours after surgery. Almost without exception, dogs receive better nursing care and respond more quickly when treated at home.

Serious complications seldom arise but vary from wound infection to decubital ulcers, cystitis, and partial or no neurological recovery. Repeat operations after an unsatisfactory result are unrewarding,[84] and a decision to reoperate should not be made hastily.

Preoperative and postoperative antibiotic therapy directed at suspect bacteria reduces the incidence of wound infections. An extensive study in humans determined that administering specific antistaphylococcal agents for one or two doses immediately preoperatively and intraoperatively was the equivalent of 40 doses of a broad-spectrum antibiotic administered over the first 10 days postoperatively.[48]

An area that is receiving more support and gaining popularity in treatment of intervertebral disc disease in humans is chemonucleolysis.[87] This procedure is the injection of chymopapain into affected discs, where the proteolytic component of papaya latex rapidly dissolves portions of the water-insoluble, noncollagenous components of nucleus pulposus. Earlier investigations in dogs were inconclusive because of technical difficulties and variable results.[45]

1. Bailey, C. S., and Morgan, J. P.: Diseases of the spinal cord. *In* Ettinger, S. J. (ed.): *Textbook of Veterinary Internal Medicine*. W. B. Saunders, Philadelphia, 1983.

2. Ball, M. V., McGuire, J. A., Swaim, S. F., and Hoerlein, B. F.: Patterns of occurrence of disc disease among registered dachshunds. J. Am. Vet. Med. Assoc. *180*:519, 1982.

3. Bisla, R. S., Marchisello, P. J., Lockskin, M. D., et al.: Autoimmunological basis of disc degeneration. Clin. Orthop. Rel. Res. *121*:207, 1976.

4. Bots, A. M., Wattendorf, A. R., Buruma, O. J. S., et al.: Acute myelopathy caused by fibrocartilaginous emboli. Neurology *31*:1250, 1981.

5. Braund, K. G.: Canine intervertebral disc disease. *In* Bojrab, M. J. (ed.): *Pathophysiology in Small Animal Surgery*. Lea & Febiger, Philadelphia, 1981.

6. Braund, K. G., Ghosh, P., Taylor, T. K. F., and Larsen, L. H.: Morphological studies of the canine intervertebral disc. The assignment of the beagle to the achondroplastic classification. Res. Vet. Sci. *19*:167, 1975.

7. Braund, K. G., Ghosh, P., Taylor, T. K. F., and Larsen, L. H.: The qualitative assessment of glycosaminoglycans in the canine intervertebral disc using a critical electrolyte staining technique. Res. Vet. Sci. *21*:314, 1976.

8. Braund, K. G., and Larsen, L. H.: Genetic factors in the maturation of the canine intervertebral disc. Res. Vet. Sci. *19*:304, 1975.

9. Braund, K. G., Taylor, T. K. F., Ghosh, P., and Sherwood, A. A.: Lateral spinal decompression in the dog. J. Small Anim. Pract. *17*:583, 1976.

10. Brown, N. O., Helphrey, M. L., and Prata, R. G.: Thoracolumbar disk disease in the dog: a retrospective analysis of 187 cases. J. Am. Anim. Hosp. Assoc. *13*:665, 1977.

11. Chambers, J. N., Oliver, J. E., Kornegay, J. N., and Malnati, G. A.: Ventral decompression for caudal cervical disk herniation in large and giant breed dogs. J. Am. Vet. Med. Assoc. *180*:410, 1982.

12. Cechner, P. E.: Ventral cervical disk fenestration in the dog: a modified technique. J. Am. Anim. Hosp. Assoc. *16*:167, 1980.

13. Collins, H. R.: An evaluation of cervical and lumbar discography. Clin. Orthop. *107*:133, 1975.

14. Colter, S. B.: Fenestration, decompression, or both? Vet. Clin. North Am. *8*:379, 1978.

15. Cusick, J. F., Ackmann, J. J., and Larson, S. J.: Mechanical and physiological effects of dentotomy. J. Neurosurg. *46*:767, 1977.

16. deLahunta, A., and Alexander, J. W.: Ischemic myelopathy secondary to presumed fibrocartilaginous embolism in nine dogs. J. Am. Anim. Hosp. Assoc. *12*:37, 1976.

17. Denny, H. R.: The surgical treatment of cervical disc protrusions in the dog: a review of 40 cases. J. Small Anim. Pract. *19*:251, 1978.

18. Denny, H. R.: The lateral fenestration of canine thoracolumbar disc protrusions: a review of 30 cases. J. Small Anim. Pract. *19*:259, 1978.

19. Dommisse, G. F. The blood supply of the spinal cord: a critical vascular zone in spinal surgery. J. Bone J. Surg. *56B*:225, 1974.

20. *Dorland's Illustrated Medical Dictionary*, 26th ed., W. B. Saunders, Philadelphia, 1981.

21. Doppman, J. L., and Girton, M.: Angiographic study of the effect of laminectomy in the presence of acute anterior epidural masses. J. Neurosurg. *45*:195, 1976.

22. Evans, H. E., and Christensen, G. C. (eds.): *Miller's Anatomy of the Dog*. 2nd ed. W. B. Saunders, Philadelphia, 1979.

23. Flo, G. L., and Brinker, W. O.: Lateral fenestration of thoracolumbar discs. J. Am. Anim. Hosp. Assoc. *11*:619, 1975.

24. Friedman, S. B., Simon, A. M., and Shaw, B. M.: The surgical approach to canine intervertebral disc disease. J. S. Afr. Vet. *44*:421, 1973.

25. Funkquist, B.: Decompressive laminectomy in thoracolumbar disc protrusion with paraplegia in the dog. J. Small Anim. Pract. *11*:445, 1970.

26. Funkquist, B.: Investigations of the therapeutic and prophylactic effects of disc evacuation in cases of thoraco-lumbar herniated discs in dogs. Acta Vet. Scand. *19*:441, 1978.

27. Gage, E. D.: Incidence of clinical disc disease in the dog. J. Am. Anim. Hosp. Assoc. *11*:135, 1975.

28. Gage, E. D., and Hoerlein, B. F.: The vertebral column. *In* Archibald, J. (ed.): *Canine Surgery*. 2nd ed. American Veterinary Publications, Santa Barbara, 1974.

29. Gambardella, P. C.: Dorsal decompressive laminectomy for treatment of thoracolumbar disc disease in dogs: a retrospective study of 98 cases. Vet. Surg. *9*:24, 1980.

30. Ghosh, P., Taylor, T. K. F., and Braund, K. G.: The variation of the glycosaminoglycans of the canine intervertebral disc with ageing. Gerontology *23*:87, 1977.

31. Ghosh, P., Taylor, T. K. F., Braund, K. G., and Larsen, L. H.: A comparative chemical and histological study of the chondrodystrophoid and non-chondrodystrophoid canine intervertebral disc. Vet. Pathol. *13*:414, 1976.

32. Ghosh, P., Braund, K. G., Taylor, T. K. F., et al.: Genetic factors in the maturation of the canine intervertebral disc. Res. Vet. Sci. *19*:304, 1975.

33. Gilpin, G. N.: Evaluation of three techniques of ventral decompression of the cervical spinal cord in the dog. J. Am. Vet. Med. Assoc. *168*:325, 1976.

34. Goggins, J. E., Li, A. S., and Franti, C. E.: Canine intervertebral disk diseases: characterization by age, sex, breed, and anatomical site of involvement. Am. J. Vet. Res. *9*:1687, 1970.

35. Greene, C., and Higgins, R. J.: Fibrocartilaginous emboli as the cause of ischemic myelopathy in a dog. Cornell Vet. *66*:131, 1976.

36. Greene, J. A., Knecht, C. D., and Roesel, O. F.: Hypothyroidism as a possible cause of canine intervertebral disc disease. J. Am. Anim. Hosp. Assoc. *15*:199, 1979.

37. Griffiths, I. R.: The extensive myelopathy of intervertebral disc protrusions in dogs ("the ascending syndrome"). J. Small Anim. Pract. *13*:425, 1972.

38. Griffiths, I. R.: Spinal cord infarction due to emboli arising from the intervertebral discs in the dog. J. Comp. Pathol. *83*:225, 1973.

39. Griffiths, R. C., and Russell, W. W.: Recurrence of cervical disk syndrome in surgically and conservatively treated dogs. J. Am. Vet. Med. Assoc. *153*:1412, 1968.

40. Hansen, H. J.: A pathologic-anatomical interpretation of disc degeneration in dogs. Acta Orthop. Scand. *20*:280, 1951.

41. Hansen, H. J.: A pathologic-anatomical study on disc degeneration in dogs. Acta Orthop. Scand. Suppl. 11, 1952.

42. Hayes, M. A., Creighton, S. R., Boysen, B. G., and Holfeld, N.: Acute necrotizing myelopathy from nucleus pulposus embolism in dogs with intervertebral disc degeneration. J. Am. Vet. Med. Assoc. *173*:289, 1978.

43. Henry, W. B.: Dorsal decompressive laminectomy in the treatment of thoracolumbar disc disease. J. Am. Anim. Hosp. Assoc. *11*:627, 1975.

44. Hoerlein, B. F.: Intervertebral disc protrusions in the dog. Am. J. Vet. Res. *19*:260, 1953.

45. Hoerlein, B. F.: Intervertebral disks. *In*: *Canine Neurology: Diagnosis and Treatment*. 3rd ed. W. B. Saunders, Philadelphia, 1978.

46. Hoerlein, B. F.: The status of the various intervertebral disc surgeries for the dog in 1978. J. Am. Anim. Hosp. Assoc. *14*:563, 1978.

47. Hoerlein, B. F.: Comparative disk disease: man and dog. J. Am. Anim. Hosp. Assoc. *15*:535, 1979.

48. Horwitz, N. H., and Curtin, J. A.: Prophylactic antibiotics and wound infections following laminectomy for lumbar disc herniation. J. Neurosurg. *43*:727, 1975.

49. Knecht, C. D.: Results of surgical treatment for thoracolumbar disc protrusion. J. Small Anim. Pract. *13*:449, 1972.

50. Koblik, P. D., and Suter, P. F.: Lumbo-sacral vertebral sinus venography via transjugular catheterization in the dog. Vet. Radiol. *22*:69, 1981.

51. La Rocca, H., and McNab, I.: The laminectomy membrane. J. Bone J. Surg. *56B*:545, 1974.

52. Lecht, L., Bostic, J. B., and Stevenson, R.: The use of selenium-tocopherol in treatment of orthopedic cases. Vet. Med./Sm. Anim. Clin. 5:494, 1968.

53. McNab, I., St. Louis, E. L., Grabias, S. L., and Jacob, R.: Selective ascending lumbosacral venography in the assessment of lumbar disc herniation: an anatomical study and clinical experience. J. Bone Jt. Surg. 58A:1093, 1976.

54. Meyer, G. A., Haughton, V. M., and Williams, A. L.: Diagnosis of herniated lumbar disk with computed tomography. N. Engl. J. Med. 301:1166, 1979.

55. Moore, R. W., and Withrow, S. J.: Gastrointestinal hemorrhage and pancreatitis associated with intervertebral disc disease in the dog. J. Am. Vet. Med. Assoc. 180:1442, 1982.

56. Naiman, J. L., Donohue, W. L., and Prichard, J. S.: Fatal nucleus pulposus embolism of spinal cord after trauma. Neurology 11:83, 1961.

57. Naylor, A.: The biophysical and biochemical aspect of intervertebral disc herniation and degeneration. Ann. Roy. Coll. Surg. Engl. 31:91, 1962.

58. Naylor, A.: The late results of laminectomy for lumbar disc prolapse: a review after ten to twenty-five years. J. Bone J. Surg. 56B:17, 1974.

59. Oliver, J. E., and Lorenz, M. D.: *Handbook of Veterinary Neurologic Diagnosis*. W. B. Saunders, Philadelphia, 1983.

60. Paatsama, S., Rissanen, P., and Rokkanen, P.: Effect of estradiol testosterone, cortisone acetate, somatotropin, thyrotropin, and parathyroid hormone on the lumbar intervertebral disc in growing dogs. J. Small Anim. Pract. 10:351, 1969.

61. Pankovitch, A. M., and Korngold, L.: A comparison of the antigenic properties of the nucleus pulposus and cartilage polysaccharide complexes. J. Immunol. 99:431, 1967.

62. Parker, A. J., and Smith, C. W.: Functional recovery following incision of spinal meninges in dogs. Res. Vet. Sci. 13:418, 1972.

63. Parker, A. J.: Distribution of spinal branches of the thoracolumbar segmental arteries in the dog. Am. J. Vet. Res. 34:1351, 1973.

64. Parker, A. J., and Smith, C. W.: Functional recovery from spinal cord trauma following incision of spinal meninges in dogs. Res. Vet. Sci. 16:276, 1974.

65. Patterson, R. H., and Arbit, E.: A surgical approach through the pedicle to protruded thoracic discs. J. Neurosurg. 48:768, 1978.

66. Pettit, C. D.: The surgical treatment of cervical protrusions in the dog. Cornell Vet. 50:259, 1960.

67. Porter, R. W., Hibbert, C. S., and Wicks, M.: The spinal canal in symptomatic lumbar disc lesions. J. Bone Jt. Surg. 60B:485, 1978.

68. Prata, R. G., and Stoll, S. G.: Ventral decompression and fusion for the treatment of cervical disc diseases in the dog. J. Am. Anim. Hosp. Assoc. 9:462, 1972.

69. Prata, R. G., Stoll, S. G., and Zaki, F. A.: Spinal cord compression caused by osteocartilaginous exostoses of the spine in two dogs. J. Vet. Med. Assoc. 166:371, 1975.

70. Prata, R. G.: Neurosurgical treatment of thoracolumbar disks: the rationale and value of laminectomy with concomitant disk removal. J. Am. Anim. Hosp. Assoc. 17:17, 1981.

71. Priester, W. A.: Canine intervertebral disc disease—occurrence by age, breed, and sex among 8,117 cases. Theriogenology 6:293, 1976.

72. Rothman, R. H., Campbell, R. E., and Menkowitz, E.: Myelographic patterns in lumbar disc degeneration. Clin. Orthop. 99:18, 1974.

73. Shores, A.: Intervertebral disc syndrome in the dog. III: Thoracolumbar disk surgery. Comp. Cont. Educ. 4:24, 1982.

74. Shores, J. A.: Structural changes in the intervertebral discs following lateral fenestration: a study of the radiographic, histologic and histochemical changes in the chondrodystrophoid dog. Thesis, Purdue University, 1982.

75. Swaim, S. F.: Ventral decompression of the cervical spinal cord in the dog. J. Am. Vet. Med. Assoc. 162:276, 1973.

76. Swaim, S. F.: Use of pneumatic surgical instruments in neurosurgery. Part I: Spinal surgery. Vet. Med./Small Anim. Clin. 68:1404, 1973.

77. Swaim, S. F.: Ventral decompression of the cervical spinal cord in the dog. J. Am. Vet. Med. Assoc. 164:491, 1974.

78. Swaim, S. F., and Hyams, D.: Clinical observations and client evaluation of ventral decompression for cervical intervertebral disc protrusion. J. Am. Vet. Med. Assoc. 181:259, 1982.

79. Swaim, S. F., and Vandevelde, M. Clinical and histological evaluation of bilateral hemilaminectomy and deep dorsal laminectomy for extensive spinal cord decompression in the dog. J. Am. Vet. Med. Assoc. 170:407, 1977.

80. Tarlov, I. M., Klinger, H., and Vitale, S.: Spinal cord compression studies. I. Experimental techniques to produce acute and gradual compression. Arch. Neurol. Psych. 70:813, 1950.

81. Teague, H. D., and Brasmer, T. H.: Midline myelotomy of the clinically normal canine spinal cord. Am. J. Vet. Res. 39:1584, 1978.

82. Toombs, J. P., Caywood, D. D., Lipowitz, A. J., and Stevens, J. B.: Colonic perforation following neurosurgical procedures and corticosteroid therapy in four dogs. J. Am. Vet. Med. Assoc. 177:68, 1980.

83. Trotter, E. J., Brasmer, T. H., and deLahunta, A.: Modified deep dorsal laminectomy in the dog. Cornell Vet. 65:402, 1975.

84. Waddell, G., Kummell, E. G., Lotto, W. N., et al.: Failed lumbar disc surgery and repeat surgery following industrial injuries. J. Bone Jt. Surg. 61A:201, 1979.

85. Walker, T. L.: Hobby drill techniques. Proceedings, 48th Annual Meeting Am. Anim. Hosp. Assoc., 1981.

86. Walker, T. L., Roberts, R. E., Kincaid, S. A., and Bratton, G. R.: The use of electric drill as an alternative to pneumatic equipment in spinal surgery. J. Am. Anim. Hosp. Assoc. 17:605, 1981.

87. Weir, B. K. A.: Prospective study of 100 lumbosacral discectomies. J. Neurosurg. 50:283, 1979.

88. Worthman, R. P.: The longitudinal vertebral venous sinuses of the dog. Am. J. Vet. Res. 17:341, 1956.

89. Yturraspe, D. J., and Lumb, W. V.: A dorsolateral muscle-separating approach for thoracolumbar disk fenestration in the dog. J. Am. Vet. Med. Assoc. 162:1037, 1973.

90. Zaki, F. A., and Prata, R. G.: Necrotizing myelopathy secondary to embolization of herniated intervertebral disc material in the dog. J. Am. Vet. Med. Assoc. 169:222, 1976.

91. Zaki, F. A., Prata, R. G., and Kay, W. J.: Necrotizing myelopathy in five Great Danes. J. Am. Vet. Med. Assoc. 165:1080, 1974.

Chapter 99

Intracranial Surgery

Richard J. Indrieri and Stephen T. Simpson

Indications for decompressive brain or intracranial surgery are: removal of a rapidly expanding mass lesion such as neoplasm or hemorrhage, decompression of a swollen, edematous brain following trauma, elevation of a depressed skull fracture, and shunting of CSF in hydrocephalus. Additionally, post-traumatic infection (including meningitis, encephalitis, and ventriculitis) is a common sequel to head injury in which the skin and skull have been penetrated. Prompt medical and surgical interventions to protect the brain may be essential to prevent such an infection.

NEOPLASIA

Incidence

The incidence of primary and metastatic intracranial tumors in companion animals, as well as their histologic classification, has been reviewed extensively.[11, 37, 38, 39, 40, 60] The subject is also reviewed in Chapter 179.

Clinical Signs and Course

The biological activity of specific intracranial tumors in companion animals is unknown. Some tumors produce a short terminal illness, others a protracted illness that ends in death after a year or more,[25, 40] whereas extensive neoplasms may be found at autopsy in animals with no history or clinical evidence of neurological disturbance.[39, 40] Generally, the neurological dysfunction and the clinical course associated with intracranial tumors are slowly progressive (Fig. 99–1).

The signs associated with intracranial tumor usually reflect its anatomical location. As time passes, however, tumor growth and necrosis, brain swelling and edema, hemorrhage, ischemia, hydrocephalus, and brain herniation produce more complex signs that make accurate localization more difficult. Although his scheme is quite simplified, McGrath classified intracranial tumors on the basis of clinical syndromes they produce.[40] Thus, a variety of syndromes may be caused by tumors in particular regions of the brain (see Chapter 89 for localization).

Pathophysiology

Pathophysiological mechanisms of intracranial tumors include an increase in intracranial pressure, altered neuronal metabolism and function resulting in abnormal activity (i.e., seizures), loss of neuronal function due to cell death, and abnormal endocrine function.[7] These mechanisms are discussed in more detail in Chapter 90.

LABORATORY FINDINGS

Intracranial tumors are rarely associated with hematologic or serum abnormalities.

Cerebrospinal Fluid

Changes in CSF produced by an intracranial tumor are variable and are influenced by size, location, histological type, and the duration of a tumor. For the most part these changes are nonspecific. Spinal fluid pressure and CSF protein are more frequently abnormal than cytological values.[8, 14, 54] Increases in creatine kinase (CK) and lactic dehydrogenase (LDH) in CSF may occur but usually reflect entry from the serum.[12] In one study, no consistent increase in CK in CSF from animals with intracranial tumors was found.[24] See Chapter 91 for more detailed information about CSF characteristics.

CSF Pressure

The range in CSF pressures reported is variable. Normal pressures published have been between 60 and 170 mm H_2O. In our experience, pressure readings in animals with intracranial tumors have been mostly between 200 and 300 mm H_2O. Less than half of all dogs with intracranial tumors confirmed by surgical exploration or necropsy have had an increase in CSF pressure.

CSF pressure is a reflection of intracranial pressure. Intracranial pressure is determined by volume-pressure relationships, which are defined by the terms *compliance* and *elastance*.[14, 32] Compliance is the amount of "give" in the intracranial compartment.

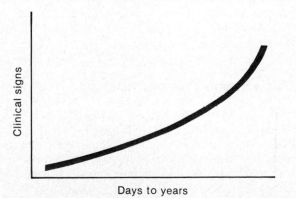

Figure 99–1. Sign-time graph of neoplasia of the brain. Clinical signs may not be apparent until relatively late in the course of the disease.

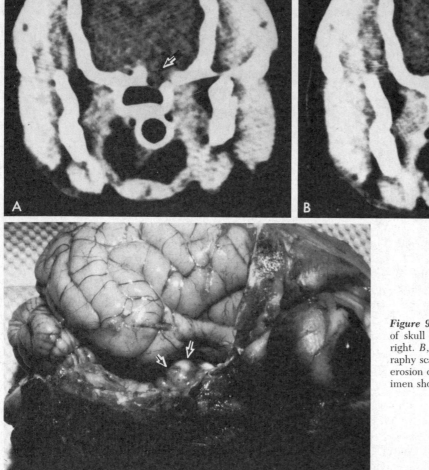

Figure 99–2. *A*, Computerized tomography scan of skull showing defect in bone *(arrow)* on the right. *B*, Contrast-enhanced computerized tomography scan showing tumor *(arrow)* associated with erosion of bone observed in *A*. *C*, Necropsy specimen showing the tumor *(arrows)*.

Compliance is great during early tumor growth, when a large increase in the mass or volume of the tumor produces only a small or no increase in intracranial pressure. Elastance is the "resistance" to expansion of intracranial mass or volume. Elastance is high when a small increase in tumor mass causes a large increase in intracranial pressure. Thus, as an intracranial tumor expands, intracranial compliance decreases, elastance increases, CSF pressure is elevated, and intracranial decompensation occurs. See Chapter 91 for further discussion of CSF pressure.

Radiography

Routine, noncontrast radiographs of the skull rarely help identify a tumor unless it arises from the skull, erodes away part of the skull, or contains significant calcification. Confirmation of an intracranial tumor usually requires special diagnostic procedures, including cerebral angiography,[9, 10, 26] cranial sinus ve-

nography,[4, 44] cerebral ventriculography,[18] brain imaging, radionuclide or isotope scanning or scintigraphy,[29, 47] optic thecography or optic nerve opacification,[34] and computerized tomography[13, 33] (Fig. 99–2). These procedures not only confirm but also localize the tumor. They also help determine whether or not surgical exploration might be of benefit and indicate the best surgical approach.

Electroencephalography (EEG)

The EEG may be helpful in the diagnosis of an intracranial tumor. Changes observed on the EEG depend upon the location of the tumor. Abnormalities described include low-frequency, high-amplitude waves[30, 51] with occasional bursts of high-frequency spike discharges.[51] Although nonspecific in themselves, these EEG changes, along with history, clinical signs, and other diagnostic tests, may confirm the presence of tumor.

Surgical Methods

Approach

The diagnosis of intracranial tumor usually warrants a guarded prognosis. However, surgical intervention may be an alternative to euthanasia or doing nothing at all. Refinement in diagnostic techniques, such as those previously discussed, frequently permits localization of the tumor. If the tumor can be localized, precise surgical exposure is possible and the potential for greater neural damage by the exploration can be eliminated.

The surgical approach employed is dictated by the location and extent of the lesion. From a practical standpoint, a topographical classification of intracranial tumors is helpful in deciding on the approach that will give the greatest exposure and will facilitate tumor removal. The cranial cavity consists of rostral fossa, middle fossa, and caudal fossa. Several surgical approaches to the brain have been described.[19, 20, 41, 43, 45, 57]

Cerebral Lobe and Deep Hemispheric Tumors. Maximum surgical exposure of unilateral hemispheric tumors of the middle and caudal extents of the rostral fossa is achieved by rostrotentorial (lateral) craniotomy. Although Hoerlein and colleagues[19] were concerned about restricted exposure to the caudal poles of the occipital lobes using this approach, Oliver[43] achieved very adequate exposure of this area. He believed that lateral craniotomy was the simplest, safest, and most useful of surgical approaches to the cerebral hemispheres. Most cerebral structures, including the lateral ventricle, caudate nucleus, and hippocampus as well as the pituitary gland and middle cranial fossa, can be exposed through this approach. On the other hand, exposure of the remainder of the rostral fossa is restricted by the frontal sinuses.[43, 45] A transfrontal craniotomy through the sinus is required to examine the rostral fossa.[45] The major drawback of this procedure is the potential for postoperative infection and drainage of CSF into the sinus.

Midline, Hemispheric Tumors. Rostrotentorial, midline hemispheric tumors are difficult to expose. Oliver[43] used a bilateral rostrotentorial craniotomy and carefully preserved the integrity of the sagittal sinus, to gain access to the corpus callosum.[43] The dorsal aspect of the third ventricle lies directly beneath this structure and is exposed by incising it. Transient neurological dysfunction occurs after callosal transection.[35]

Transbuccal,[41] transtemporal,[22] and ventral cervical[57] approaches to the sella turcica and pituitary gland have been described. The ventral approaches are extremely difficult and require considerable surgical precision and judgment. They give limited exposure, and the risk of hemorrhage from the cavernous and intercavernous sinuses is great. Postoperative infection is a potential danger of the transbuccal approach. Oliver[43] exposed the pituitary gland from a lateral craniotomy by extending the craniotomy ventrally to the floor of the middle cranial fossa with rongeurs and by gently retracting the brain. Low lateral craniotomy[43] is preferred to ventral craniectomy to expose the pituitary gland and to facilitate exploration of the cranial floor.[19]

Tumors Straddling the Middle and Caudal Fossae. Tumors of the tentorium or tumors that involve the middle and caudal fossae are extremely difficult to expose and remove. A combination of lateral craniotomy, suboccipital craniectomy, and removal of the tentorium may be necessary to obtain sufficient exposure. The potential danger in this procedure is interruption of any of the venous sinuses (sagittal sinus, the confluens sinuum, transverse sinus, straight sinus, and sigmoid sinus) that are encountered. Hemorrhage from these sinuses is profuse and difficult to control. Ligation or occlusion of flow through the sinuses can result in severe brain swelling[42] or death.[43]

Caudal Fossa Tumors and Tumors Crossing into the Spinal Canal. Suboccipital craniectomy is used to expose the structures of the caudal fossa. Midline cerebellar tumors and caudal medullary tumors can be removed by this approach. The suboccipital approach is also best for tumors straddling the spinal canal and caudal fossa. Exposure of the rostral aspects of the cerebellum, the fourth ventricle, and the medulla, however, is limited by the tentorium cerebelli.

Preoperative Preparation

Preoperative evaluation should include an assessment of hydration and electrolyte balance. If any abnormalities exist, they should be corrected before surgery. Animals are frequently given diuretics, mannitol, or steroids to reduce cerebral edema (to "dehydrate" the brain) or to reduce intracranial pressure. Repeated doses of these agents can cause clinically evident dehydration and significant electrolyte disturbances.[42, 46, 55] Laboratory determination of the hematocrit and serum sodium, potassium and protein levels is helpful in correcting existing imbalances. Overhydration, as well as dehydration, should be avoided, because it potentiates edema and brain swelling.[42] Normal hydration can be maintained by keeping serum osmolality between 275 and 300 mOsm.[55]

Steroids. Steroids are more effective in preventing cerebral edema than in eliminating it.[53] The clinical benefit of steroid administration to humans with intracranial tumors (which is supposedly due to a reduction in edema) is dramatic.[15, 28, 32] We have also observed clinical improvement following steroid use in animals with intracranial tumors. Dexamethasone, the drug most commonly used in human[3] and veterinary medicine,[21] may be given a day or two prior to surgery to reduce edema and brain swelling. The dosage range is wide, between 1 and 10 mg/kg;[21]

however, on the basis of the results reported in one study, a dose of 1.0 to 2.0 mg/kg/day is recommended.[53]

Antibiotics. Prolonged operating time, wound contamination, the presence of devitalized or ischemic tissue, and the use of steroids are factors that may justify the use of antibiotics for antimicrobial prophylaxis. As a rule, the antibiotic used should be available in the tissues from the systemic circulation at the time of surgery, in order to provide maximal suppression of infection by bacteria introduced at that time.[1, 36] Antibiotics are started a day or two before operation, and as long as there has been no contamination or break in asepsis, they are discontinued 72 hours following operation to prevent the development of resistant flora.[1] Antibiotics should not be used indiscriminately, and one should not be lulled into a false sense of security, believing that antibiotics will provide an "umbrella" of protection against infection. The importance of assessing the actual need for antibiotics is emphasized by the results of a study that demonstrated an increased incidence of postoperative infection in a series of human patients who had received antibiotic prophylaxis.[48] It is clear that careful, judicious use of antibiotics is paramount.[56]

Selection of an appropriate antibiotic for use in preoperative prophylaxis depends on the knowledge of which bacteria are most likely to produce infection, to which antibiotics these organisms are most sensitive, and which drugs are most likely to reach effective concentrations in the brain and CSF. The blood-CSF and blood-brain barriers are not the same. In general, antibiotics traverse the blood-CSF barrier more readily than they do the blood-brain barrier.[16]

TABLE 99–1. Relative Diffusion of Antimicrobial Agents From Blood Into Cerebrospinal Fluid

Excellent with or without inflammation	Chloramphenicol
	Sulfonamides
	Trimethoprim/ sulfamethoxazole
Good only with inflammation	Ampicillin
	Penicillin G
	Methicillin
	Carbenicillin
	Cephalothin
	Tetracycline
	Kanamycin
Minimal even with inflammation	Streptomycin
	Gentamicin
	Erythromycin
None even with inflammation	Benzathine–penicillin G
	Lincomycin
	Polymyxin G
	Bacitracin

(Taken from Neurosurgery Conference, University of California Medical School, Davis, California, and Medical Teaching Hospital, Sacramento, California, 1977.)

TABLE 99–2. Blood and Brain Concentrations of Antibiotics, and Blood-Brain Ratio of Antibiotics Up to Four Hours After Administration

Antibiotic	Average Blood Level (μg/ml)	Average Brain Level (μg/ml)	Ratio
Chloramphenicol	4.0	36.0	1:9
Cephalothin	11.7	1.6	7:1
Ampicillin	21.3	0.4	56:1
Penicillin	7.5	0.32	23:1
Cephaloridine	18.04	0.90	20:1

(Reprinted with permission from Kramer, P. W., Griffith, R. S., and Campbell, R. L.: Antibiotic penetration of the brain: a comparative study. J. Neurosurg. 31:295, 1969.)

Chloramphenicol is the only antibiotic that enters the brain[31] and the CSF[59] in significant concentrations. Table 99–1 shows the relative diffusion of various antibiotics from blood into the CSF of humans. Table 99–2 shows human blood and brain concentrations of five antibiotics that reach sufficient levels to inhibit sensitive bacteria within four hours of administration.

Ninety per cent of bacterial cultures from canine hair around the head yield pure growths of *Staphylococcus aureus*.[58] This organism, however, is only an occasional inhabitant of canine skin, which is primarily colonized by micrococci.[23] Cutaneous insult, including surgery, creates a shift in resident populations that permits *S. aureus*, *Pseudomonas*, and *Proteus* to colonize the skin. These are pathogenic bacteria, and *S. aureus* is the major cutaneous pathogen in dogs.[23] *S. aureus*, as well as some other pathogens, is the organism most likely to produce postcraniotomy infection. Many pathogenic staphylococci are resistant to penicillin and ampicillin but are sensitive to chloramphenicol. If antimicrobial prophylaxis is to be employed preoperatively, chloramphenicol is the drug of choice.

Mannitol. Mannitol is the osmotic drug of choice to reduce brain swelling due to edema and to reduce

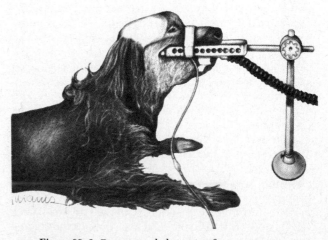

Figure 99–3. Recommended position for craniotomy.

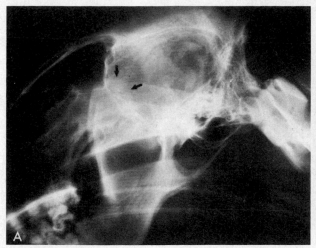
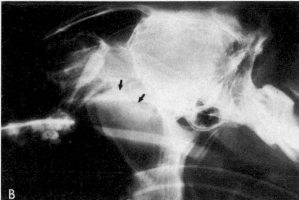

Figure 99-4. Position of the coronoid processes of mandible with mouth closed. *B*, Position of the coronoid processes with the mouth held widely open.

intracranial pressure. It is indicated preoperatively to facilitate operation and prevent cerebral swelling. The optimal dose of mannitol is between 1 and 3 gm/kg of a 20 to 25 per cent solution intravenously.[46] A reduction in intracranial pressure begins within 15 to 20 minutes of its use,[17] and a single dose may reduce CSF pressure by 30 to 60 per cent for two to four hours.[27] The drug is given slowly over 10 to 20 minutes.[27, 46] Mannitol therapy can be repeated two or three times over a 24-hour period postoperatively with benefit. Beyond this, however, its use is of doubtful value, because the brain adapts to plasma hyperosmolality by increasing cellular osmolality. To be effective, plasma osmolality must be raised higher each time mannitol is given, eventually leading to severe systemic acidosis and renal failure.[28] If mannitol is used, an indwelling urinary catheter should be used to monitor fluid loss and to accurately determine fluid replacement.

Anesthesia

The anesthetic agents and techniques to be used need careful consideration to minimize the risk of acute increases in intracranial pressure, and to reduce the potential for swelling of the brain during surgery. (See Chapter 191 for detailed anesthetic considerations.)

Patient Positioning

Poor positioning of the animal for surgery may reduce surgical exposure and hinder the surgeon's progress. It is recommended that a frame be used to support the head (Fig. 99-3).[42, 43] This posture facilitates venous drainage from the head as well as drainage of fluid and blood from the surgery site. It is imperative that the neck not be draped over sandbags or towels, because such a position would occlude the jugular veins, reduce venous drainage of the head, and tend to increase intracranial pressure.

For the same reasons, use of indwelling jugular catheters should be avoided if possible.

With the head placed in the support frame, it may be inclined obliquely to the right or left, depending on which side the craniotomy is to be performed. Maximum exposure to the temporal fossa can be achieved by opening the mouth widely. Lateral retraction of the temporalis muscle is restricted by the coronoid process of the mandible with the mouth closed (Fig. 99-4). Forward and downward flexion of the head (with the nose pointed toward the table) provides maximum exposure of the occipital and suboccipital areas for surgery of the caudal fossa.

Surgical Approach

Lateral Craniotomy. A horseshoe-shaped skin incision is made (Fig. 99-5). Cutaneous hemorrhage is controlled by ligation or electrocautery. The skin is undermined and is reflected laterally by gently rolling it over a skin towel or gauze sponge to prevent interruption of its vascular supply along the base of the pedicle. The superficial preauricular and postauricular muscles are incised to expose the temporalis

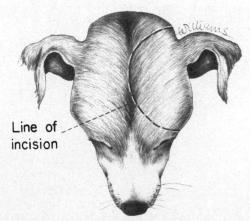

Figure 99-5. Horseshoe-shaped skin incision used for lateral craniotomy.

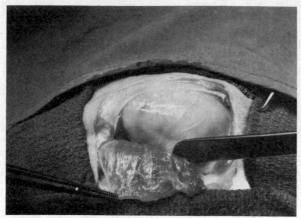

Figure 99–6. Elevation of temporalis muscle away from the lateral aspect of the skull.

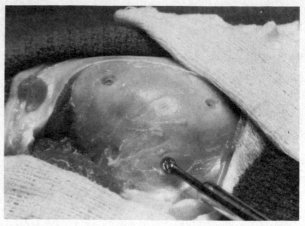

Figure 99–7. Placement of burr holes through the skull to the dura mater.

muscle and fascia. The temporalis fascia and muscle are incised close to their attachments, with sufficient margin left for suturing and reattachment of the muscle fascia.

The temporalis muscle is easily elevated away from the temporal fossa using a scalpel handle, osteotome, or periosteal elevator (Fig. 99–6). Blunt dissection of the muscle is carried as far ventrally as possible. Lateral reflection of the muscle is limited by the zygomatic arch, which can be transected to achieve greater exposure.[43]

The next step is to create the skull or bone flap. There are several ways of proceeding, depending upon the instruments available. A single burr hole is required if a craniotome is used. The hole is made with a power drill and burr (or trephine) and is large enough to accommodate the footplate and dural guard of the craniotome. With the upper surface of the dural guard held firmly against the inner cranial surface the caudal, dorsal and rostral edges of the bone flap are slowly and carefully cut. The ventral edge is left uncut to preclude injury to the middle meningeal artery. A shallow groove cut along the ventral margin of the flap using the power drill and small burr facilitates even breakage of the bone along

the groove when the flap is gently elevated from the skull.

Four holes are drilled if a Gigli saw or power drill is used to cut the flap (Fig. 99–7).

Burr holes penetrate to the inner cranial surface to expose but not lacerate the dura mater. Burr holes also define the width of bone in each quadrant of the skull. Use of the Gigli saw to cut the flap is difficult and usually results in laceration and damage to the dura mater. Separation of the dura mater from the inner cranial surface and passage of the Gigli saw between burr holes are also extremely difficult. For these reasons, when a craniotome is not available, a power drill and burr is preferred.

With the power drill, grooves are placed in the skull, connecting each burr hole and defining the boundaries of the bone flap (Fig. 99–8). The grooves are carefully drilled through the bone along the edges of the flap except ventrally, where the groove is shallow and does not penetrate to the dura mater. Frequent irrigation and use of bone wax to control diploic hemorrhage permit excellent exposure.

The boundaries of the skull flap are limited by important anatomical structures. The rostral border is limited by the frontal sinus, which should be

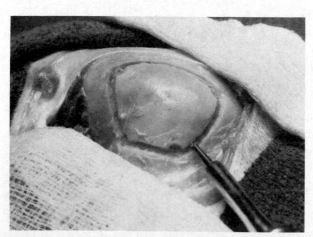

Figure 99–8. Limits of craniotomy flap are defined using air drill and small burr.

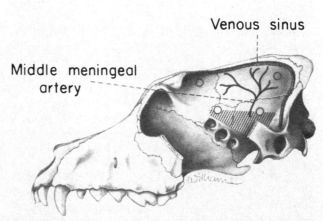

Figure 99–9. Relationship of burr holes to the sagittal sinus, the transverse sinus, and the middle meningeal artery.

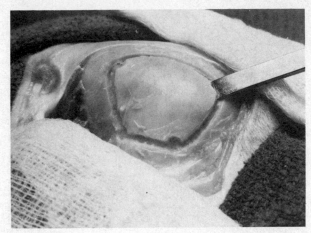

Figure 99–10. The craniotomy flap is gently pried free.

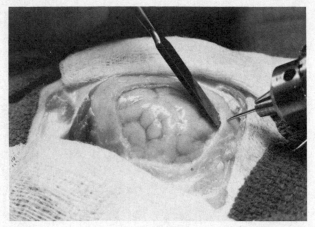

Figure 99–11. Preplacement of holes for repair of craniotomy at the completion of the procedure.

avoided. Postoperative contamination and infection may result if the sinus is entered and the brain and dura mater are exposed to the sinus. The dorsal border is cut about one centimeter from the midline to avoid laceration and severe hemorrhage from the sagittal sinus. The caudal border is cut about 0.5 cm rostral to the nuchal crest, which indicates the location of the tentorium cerebelli and transverse sinus (Fig. 99–9).

The ventral boundary is formed by a line connecting the two ventral burr holes. The reflected temporalis muscle is an obstacle and determines the ventral boundary. Once the craniotomy flap is removed, the craniotomy may be extended ventrally with rongeurs more easily.

When the limits of the craniotomy flap are defined and all drilling is completed, the ventral border of the flap is broken by gently prying it away from the skull (Fig. 99–10). This is usually accomplished easily because the bone is relatively thin. The break occurs along the shallow groove created in the bone. As the craniotomy flap is gently lifted from its position, the underlying dura mater is teased free of any attachments to the inner cranial surface. This step is important to prevent avulsion of the arborizations of the middle meningeal artery, which arise from a point approximately opposite the caudal base of the zygomatic arch. In young dogs, removal of the flap without injury to the dura mater and middle meningeal artery is relatively easy. In mature dogs, the dura mater may be more adherent and in some cases cannot be dissected free. In this case, the surgeon must be prepared to remove the flap and quickly identify, clamp, and ligate or clip the artery as far ventrally as possible.

If the bone flap is to be replaced at the end of the procedure, the skull and bone flap are prepared at this point. Small holes are placed through the skull at the corners of the craniotomy site using a .045-inch stainless steel K-wire and hand chuck. The underlying dura mater and brain are protected during placement of the holes by insertion of the tip of a scalpel handle or osteotome between the dura mater

and inner cranial surface, beneath the point being drilled (Fig. 99–11). Matching holes are carefully placed in the four corners of the bone flap. The holes in the skull are used for preplacement of stainless steel sutures that will be used in closure (Fig. 99–12). Sutures are retracted from the field with hemostats. The bone flap is placed in a saline-moistened sponge or preserved in warm saline until needed again. When the bone flap is removed, during the preparation just described and during the operation it is essential to keep the dura mater moist. Frequent irrigation is absolutely essential for this reason.

Before the dura mater is incised to expose the brain, the middle meningeal artery must be ligated or clipped as far ventrally as possible to prevent significant hemorrhage when its branches are cut by the dura mater incision.

A dural hook is used to nick the dura mater and elevate it away from the brain (Fig. 99–13). A No. 11 scalpel blade is used to incise the dura sufficiently to introduce the tip of the dural scissors. The dural flap is cut relatively close to the borders of the skull rostrally, dorsally, and ventrally. A rim of dura mater

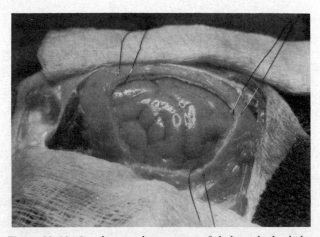

Figure 99–12. Stainless steel sutures are fed through the holes and are retracted from the surgical site with hemostats.

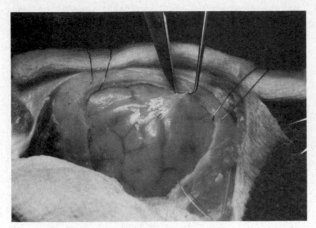

Figure 99–13. A sharp dural hook is passed through the dura mater and is placed under gentle upward tension. A No. 11 scalpel blade is used to incise the dura mater. Once the initial dural incision is made, it can be continued using dural scissors.

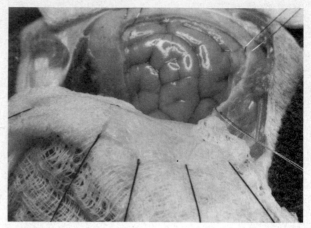

Figure 99–14. The dural flap is placed under tension, retracted over a moist saline sponge, and "sandwiched" between moist 4 × 4 sponges. The cerebral gyri and sulci are prominent and easily identified.

is left beyond the bone edge to facilitate closure at the end of the exploration.

When the dural flap has been cut, stay sutures are placed at the corners or at several more places around the periphery of the flap (Fig. 99-14). Hemostats are used to grasp these sutures. The flap is placed under tension, is retracted over a moist saline sponge, and "sandwiched" between moist 4 × 4 sponges. The need for frequent irrigation cannot be overemphasized.

With the brain surface exposed, sulci and gyri can be easily identified. The brain can be palpated for tumors that lie beneath the surface by light digital palpation. Such areas may be more firm than adjacent normal brain.

The brain can be retracted to examine the cranial and middle fossae more thoroughly. The more the cerebral tissues are handled and manipulated, however, the more swelling occurs.

If a parenchymal tumor is present and the cortex is to be incised, the pia mater and superficial cortex are cauterized first. The cortical incision is made

through the gyrus, the more highly vascular sulci being avoided. The cortex is retracted to exposure the underlying white matter, which is relatively soft and avascular. Tumor tissue can be gently teased or aspirated from the brain. Samples should be submitted for pathological evaluation and tumor identification. Hemostasis is maintained by the use of moist cotton balls or cottonoid to tamponade the vessels. When the tumor is removed and hemorrhage is controlled, the incised cortical edges are freed and allowed to appose.

Whether or not intramedullary exploration and tumor removal are performed, the dura mater must be closed. The use of 5-0 or 6-0 silk with an atraumatic needle is acceptable. A continuous or simple interrupted suture pattern can be used (Fig. 99–15). The most frequently encountered problem is operative swelling that prevents closure of the dura mater. If it happens, a graft of temporalis fascia can be sewn into position. Regardless of which tissue is used (dura mater or temporalis fascia), the closure should be watertight to prevent leakage of CSF. Closure over

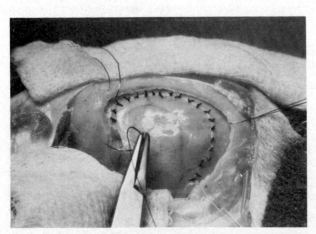

Figure 99–15. An interrupted or continuous suture pattern is used to close the dura mater and make it "watertight."

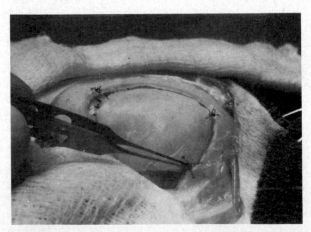

Figure 99–16. The craniotomy flap is wired back into position. The ventral aspect of the craniotomy was extended using rongeurs (*arrows*).

the dura mater minimizes outward cerebral herniation and the formation of a cortical scar.

With the dura mater closed, the bone flap is replaced and wired into position using the preplaced steel sutures (Fig. 99–16). The temporalis muscle and fascia are sutured and the skin is closed in routine fashion.

If a tumor involves the skull, samples are obtained for pathological evaluation, and the remaining tissue is excised and discarded. Extensive areas of the skull can be removed without adverse effect, because the prominent temporalis muscles provide some protection. The potential for injury is greater with a direct blow to the head, however. A synthetic cranial prosthesis* can be formed to cover and protect the brain if wide areas of the skull have been removed. However, the potential for infection is increased when a prosthesis is used.

Suboccipital Craniectomy. Adequate surgical exposure of the occipital and rostral cervical areas is achieved with the animal's head flexed at the atlanto-occipital articulation. A midline incision extends from one to two centimeters rostral to the external occipital protuberance to the caudal aspect of the dorsal spine of the axis. After the skin has been towelled off, the cervical musculature is dissected on the midline down to the occipital bone and dorsal arch of the atlas. An osteotome or scalpel handle is used to elevate the musculature from the bone and reflect it laterally. The cervical muscles are transected perpendicular to their longitudinal attachment along the caudal border of the nuchal crest to gain more exposure. Hemorrhage may be encountered during this procedure if the occipital emissary vein is cut, but hemostasis is

---

*Codman Cranioplastic Kit, Codman & Shurtleff, Inc., Randolph, MA.

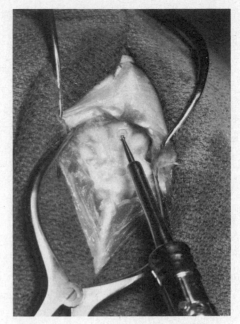

Figure 99–18. Burr hole in occipital bone.

achieved using ligatures or electrocautery. Gelpi or other suitable retractors are used to maintain distraction of the musculature (Fig. 99–17).

A power drill and small burr are used to create a small window in the relatively thin occipital bone (Fig. 99–18). Care is taken not to lacerate the dura mater. A suitable small rongeur is used to remove bone and expose the cerebellum (Fig. 99–19). Frequently, the dura mater is tightly adhered to the occipital bone and is removed along with the bone as the craniectomy site is extended with rongeurs.

To prevent severe hemorrhage and preserve the

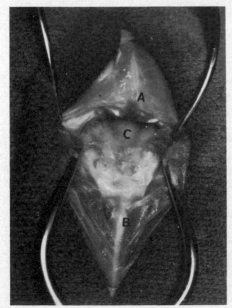

Figure 99–17. Surgical approach to the occipital area. *A*, external occipital protuberance; *B*, dorsal spinous process; *C*, occipital bone.

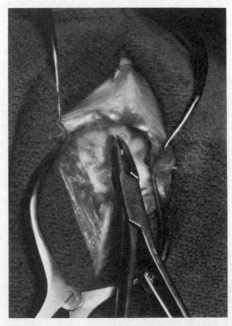

Figure 99–19. Rongeurs are used to remove the occipital bone.

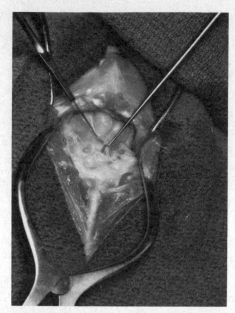

Figure 99–20. The dura mater over the cerebellum is carefully incised.

integrity of the confluens sinuum, the transverse sinuses, and the ventral occipital sinuses, the craniectomy is not extended beyond the external occipital protuberance dorsally, the nuchal crests laterally, and the foramen magnum ventrally.

If the dura mater is intact, a dural hook is used to elevate it from the cerebellum. A No. 11 scalpel blade is used to nick the dura mater (Fig. 99–20), and dural scissors are used to incise it. Sutures placed through the cut edges of the dura mater permit lateral retraction, and the weight of the hemostats used to clamp the sutures prevents retraction. Frequent irrigation is essential.

The cerebellum can be retracted to further assess the ventral and lateral recesses of the caudal fossa. The cerebellar vermis can be elevated to inspect the obex and caudal aspect of the fourth ventricle. A thin membrane, the caudal medullary velum, is interrupted if this is done. A midline incision can be made through the vermis to explore the depths of the cerebellum if a tumor is present. At the termination of caudal fossa exploration, the dura mater is sutured (if possible) and the wound is closed in routine fashion. If the dura mater is not closed, and because no occipital bone flap is used, a fascial graft can be sutured into place over the craniectomy site to reduce or prevent CSF leakage and formation of a cerebellar cicatrix. Routine closure without a graft has apparently not produced complications, and may not be necessary.[20, 43]

This procedure provides excellent exposure to the caudal aspect of the cerebellum, the dorsal aspect of the caudal medulla, and the rostral aspect of the spinal cord. The rostral and rostrolateral cerebellum is not accessible by this approach, which must be combined with caudolateral craniotomy and tentorial cerebellectomy for maximal exposure.[43]

Postoperative Management

Postoperatively, the animal is carefully monitored. Signs of recovery followed by a deterioration in neurological status may signal progressive swelling and edema of the brain, or compression and displacement due to the accumulation of blood and clots. Corticosteroids and antibiotics are indicated, as previously mentioned, and intravenous fluids can be given at maintenance levels. If pharmacological decompression is unsatisfactory, surgery may be necessary to remove the bone flap and permit cerebral decompression or to evacuate a clot and stop hemorrhage. A week or two later, when the animal is stable, a prosthesis may be implanted to protect the brain.

Recovery from brain surgery can be stormy. It is important to be patient and not to expect marked improvement in neurological function too soon. There are no guidelines to predict how quickly or to what extent the animal will recover function. If the surgeon has been careful and a large amount of brain has not been removed or compromised, functional recovery may proceed to a point beyond that expected. The key notes are good nursing care (i.e., assisting with normal evacuations), prevention of infection, maintenance of fluid and electrolyte balance, prevention of decubital ulcers and pneumonia, attention to nutritional and caloric needs, and maintenance of proper sanitation, along with extreme patience and persistence.

PREFRONTAL LOBOTOMY

Prefrontal lobotomy has been described as a surgical means of correcting unacceptable aggressive, destructive, and other socially malfeasant behavior in dogs.[2, 49] Although some animals appear to have derived benefit from this procedure,[2] others are made substantially worse. The consensus of opinion is that prefrontal lobotomy is of limited usefulness and is warranted or justified only as a last resort before euthanasia. The surgical procedure is described in detail elsewhere.[20, 50]

CRANIAL TRAUMA

Head injuries are common in small animal practice. Fortunately, most head injuries result in superficial, ocular, or paracranial injury and sometimes involve brain or cranial injury. When cranial injury occurs, the clinical signs can be variable, confusing, and frustrating. An understanding of the underlying pathophysiology of cranial trauma and neuroanatomy can help to alleviate some of the difficulty with such cases.

Cranial trauma or brain injury consists of three basic types: concussion, contusion, and laceration.[52] A *concussion* is the transient loss of some neurological function as a result of head trauma without persistent evidence of actual parenchymal damage. Associated with concussion is edema. There is no doubt that some animals sustain parenchymal damage, yet reveal no clinical evidence of that damage and are classified as concussive. The term then describes a clinical, not a pathophysiological, distinction.

In a *contusion*, in addition to concussive damage, there is hemorrhage within the parenchyma. Although other extraparenchymal hemorrhage does not constitute a contusion, generally the forces required for epidural or subdural hemorrhage are so great that they create parenchymal contusions. Edema is also associated with contusions. Two types of contusions are distinguished—cerebral and brainstem. *Cerebral contusions* are usually in areas of the cerebral cortex beneath the impact site (*coup*) and appear as petechial and ecchymotic hemorrhages (Fig. 99–21). This type of hemorrhage may appear on the opposite side of the brain from the impact (*contracoup*). Cerebral contusions in general are not severe, but the tremendous amount of cerebral edema associated with this severe an impact frequently causes critical rises in intracranial pressure and shifts or herniation of brain contents (See Chapter 90).

Brainstem contusion is an acute, severe, and life-threatening event. Energy applied to the cranium is distributed more diffusely and concentrated in the base of the skull and brain. The concentration of this energy causes severe disruption of the microvasculature of the brainstem, resulting in a central core of hemorrhage within the brain (Fig. 99–22). The pons and midbrain receive most of the damage.

Clinical signs of brainstem contusion include immediate mental changes (coma or stupor), pupillary changes (dilated, nonresponsive pupils or constricted pupils), and gait changes (nonambulatory, spastic tetraparesis or even decerebrate rigidity). Clinical signs of cerebral contusion or edema include slow insidious onset several hours following trauma, early anisocoria, increasing gait difficulty, and decreasing sensorium.

Laceration of the brain can occur in three ways: as

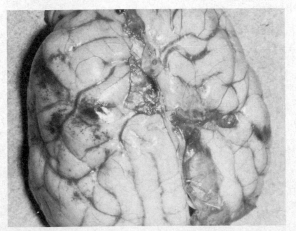

Figure 99–21. The brain of this dog clearly demonstrates a cerebral contusion with ecchymotic and petechial hemorrhages in the left frontoparietal cortex.

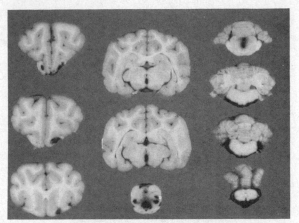

Figure 99–22. Transverse sections of this dog's brain reveal a central core of hemorrhage in the midbrain and rostral pons (brainstem contusion). There is also subdural hemorrhage around the medulla and pons.

a severe acceleration or deceleration injury, on intracranial penetrating injury, or a skull fracture. Acceleration injuries lacerate brain by causing relative movement of the brain over roughened or rigid intracranial surfaces. Contusion injuries are frequently present with this form of brain injury. Missile injuries and stab wounds lacerate brain merely by passing through the tissue. The nature of the penetrating item is important. A high-energy bullet hits the head and creates a concussion or energy wave that damages vast amounts of brain in addition to that damaged by the bullet itself, whereas a slow penetration of a skull usually lacerates brain only and does not produce as much concussive damage.

Skull fractures frequently lacerate brain tissue. The cause of the fracture must be taken into account. A skull fracture produced by impact with a fast-moving automobile involves fracture, laceration, and concussive damage that must be considered. A skull fracture that is caused by a crushing injury lacerates brain tissue, but there is no concussive energy to damage other brain tissue.

The pathophysiological response of brain tissue to injury is discussed in Chapter 90. Emergency complications of brain injury include various types of hematomas and herniations. Three basic types of hematomas exist: epidural, subdural, and intraparenchymal. The epidural hematoma should be suspected if a fracture line crosses the course of the middle meningeal artery. This type of hematoma produces a slowly progressive, compressive brain syndrome that may result in death. The patient may appear normal upon initial examination. Subdural hematomas are more common than epidural hematomas and are usually caused by rupture of the large diploic veins of the subarachnoid space with subsequent hemorrhage. Subdural hematomas are usually rapidly expanding and diffuse, and may easily cover an entire cerebral hemisphere (Fig. 99–23). Progression to severe clinical signs is due to an increase in intracranial pressure. Intraparenchymal hematomas are usually caused by brain laceration most commonly

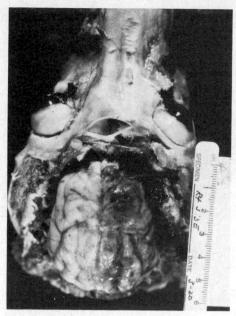

Figure 99–23. This subdural hematoma is extensive, covering nearly the entire hemisphere.

associated with depressed cranial fractures. Decompression of the fracture and removal of the hematoma are critical to prevent additional brain damage.

Brain herniation is a shift of brain contents as a result of increased pressure gradients usually caused by cerebral edema or hemorrhage. The four types of brain herniation are described in Chapter 90. The destructive results of herniation should encourage aggressive action to prevent herniation rather than to wait for and treat it.

Patient Evaluation

In a mild, concussive head injury with no neurological deficits, it is advisable to observe the patient for 24 to 48 hours for signs of deteriorating neurological function. Most cases never need additional care, but in rare instances, a hematoma or edema develops, requiring medical or surgical attention.

In head injury with neurological deficits, the patient is hospitalized and monitored closely if possible, and medical treatment is instituted. Serial evaluations are made and recorded, including (1) state of consciousness, (2) patterns of breathing, (3) size and reactivity of pupils, (4) ocular movements, and (5) motor responses.[12, 52]

In patients that have received a concussion, these five parameters are monitored periodically for 24 to 48 hours. Patients with a contusion are hospitalized and closely monitored. Mental status declines from apathetic through stuporous to coma and death unless adequate medical or surgical intervention is performed. Respiratory patterns are monitored for change, and all changes are recorded. Abnormal patterns include Cheyne-Stokes respiration, CNS hy-

perventilation, and severe ataxic respiratory patterns.[52] A progression from one pattern to another may indicate continuing progression and decline in neurological status.

Pupil size is an important sign. Pupils can be normal, uneven (anisocoria), constricted (miosis), or dilated (mydriasis). The pupillary light reflex should also be determined. Miotic pupils can indicate cerebral concussion or lower brainstem disease. Anisocoria can suggest brainstem disease, ocular disease, or peripheral nerve disease. Dilated, nonresponsive pupils indicate a poor prognosis if coupled with other midbrain signs. A change in pupils toward dilated and nonresponsive is considered a decline in neurological status, and more aggressive therapy should be sought.

Ocular movements are used to test the integrity of extraocular muscle innervation and the vestibular system, providing a general assessment of brainstem function from the midbrain through the pontine medullary junction.

Motor responses are especially important to assess in patients with an early decline of neurological function. The intention of this assessment is to detect mild hemiparesis, lateralization, and early evidence of complications of head injury.

Treatment

Mild concussions causing only transient neurological dysfunction usually do not require therapy. If neurological deterioration occurs (usually as a result of cerebral edema or intracranial hemorrhage), the patient should be treated as one that has just been injured and has neurological signs.

Head trauma alone rarely causes shock. If shock is present following trauma, the clinician should suspect other injury as the cause. Routine emergency management always takes precedence. A patent airway and control of major hemorrhage should be the first concerns. After initial stabilization, the neurological evaluation can be undertaken and appropriate therapy can be begun.

Patients that are delirious, stuporous, or worse are treated initially with corticosteroids. Various regimens have been applied, but the most common consist of high doses of intravenous dexamethasone (2 to 10 mg/Kg) three to four times per day for two to three days. A preliminary dose of a water-soluble steroid, such as methyl prednisolone succinate, and antibiotic therapy are also advisable. The use of osmotic diuretics to treat head injury is controversial. In the face of edema only, 20 per cent mannitol at 2 gm/kg every four to six hours may have benefit; however, the clinician can seldom be sure that no hemorrhage is present. In the presence of hemorrhage, mannitol may have deleterious effects for two reasons: (1) reduction of brain size allows more space for hemorrhage and (2) movement of mannitol-laden blood into extravascular spaces within the cranium may act as a wick and soak up more fluid, thus aggravating the effect of the hemorrhage.[52] Mannitol may be used when intracranial surgery is performed. Moreover, extra care must be undertaken to control hemorrhage. Dimethyl sulfoxide has been reported to be beneficial in treatment of controlled intracranial injury.[5]

If the patient's condition continues to deteriorate following the use of steroids and osmotic diuretics, surgical decompression is advisable. Serial neurological evaluations should indicate which side of the brain is most affected. Radiography may support the localization.

Epidural and often subdural hemorrhage can usually be detected by placing burr holes in the calvarium at locations described for the lateral craniotomy. If a linear fracture that crosses the middle meningeal artery is detected, the burr holes may need to be closer to that junction to facilitate clearance of the hemorrhage.

If subdural or intraparenchymal hematoma is not detected by burr hole placement, a craniotomy may be required. The craniotomy can be performed by connecting the same burr holes in the manner described for the lateral craniotomy. After the durotomy is performed, the surgeon may find that no hemorrhage but significant cerebral edema is present. The craniotomy has been useful to decompress the brain and to rule out life-threatening hemorrhage.

Not all skull fractures require surgical intervention. Fractures that occur deep in the petrous-temporal bone or in the basisphenoid bone are usually not accessible to surgery. Fractures in the frontoparietal region are readily accessible to the surgeon. These fractures may be linear, comminuted, depressed, or compound. Linear fractures of this area produce laceration of branches of the middle meningeal artery and result in epidural hematoma. Dural and brain lacerations may also occur. Linear fractures in this region may or may not require surgery. The decision should rest on the patient's serially evaluated neurological status. Deteriorating patients should be operated on.

Fractures in the frontoparietal region are often comminuted or depressed, causing dural and brain lacerations and extensive hemorrhage within the brain parenchyma. Depressed fractures must be carefully elevated. The bone fragments may be removed by direct grasp, but access to them through appropriately placed burr holes may lessen meningeal or brain damage. Once bone fragments are cleared from the area, malacic brain and hemorrhage may be removed by suction (Fig. 99–24) When hemorrhage is controlled, the dural laceration is repaired or the defect is patched with a fascial graft. Frequently, the bone defect cannot be repaired. In small dogs, this situation may be undesirable because of exposure of brain to future injury. In larger dogs the temporalis muscle usually affords adequate protection. If necessary, a prosthesis can be inserted at a later data.

Complications

Immediate complications include seizures, infection, brain herniation secondary to edema, and death. Seizures can occur from trauma or surgery. If they occur within two weeks of the injury, they are usually the result of hemorrhage or malacia. Hemorrhage due to trauma frequently causes seizures within the first few hours after injury. Seizures following trauma most often have an onset of about one year after trauma and should be treated like idiopathic epilepsy. We recommend the use of prophylactic anticonvulsants for at least six months following brain trauma or surgery, especially if seizures occur within two weeks after the injury.

Infection can occur rapidly, violently, and with devastating results. It is more common in patients with more devitalized tissue and those with reasons for developing sepsis, such as prolonged placement of venous catheters. Patients with fractures through sinuses, blood in the ears, epistaxis, or cerebrospinal fluid rhinorrhea are also more at risk of developing post-traumatic infection. Central nervous system infection can follow cranial fractures by several years.

In general, small animals with head injuries should be monitored carefully. If brainstem signs occur from the initial impact and little improvement is seen in 48 hours, the prognosis is poor. If signs develop slowly, aggressive medical and surgical treatment is often rewarding.

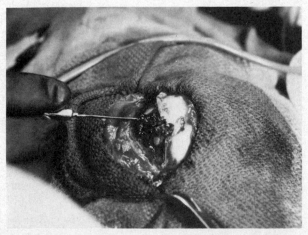

Figure 99–24. A large intraparenchymal hematoma caused by a depressed skull fracture. The skull fracture has been removed and the hematoma and malacic brain are being aspirated from the site. This dog recovered and was walking within 72 hours of surgery.

1. Alford, R. H.: Prevention of bacterial disease by oral and parenteral antimicrobial agents. So. Med. J. 66:32, 1973.
2. Allen, D. B., Cummings, J. F., and deLahunta, A.: Effects of lobotomy on aggressive behavior. Cornell Vet. 64:201, 1974.
3. Bakay, L., and Glasauer, F. E.: *Head Injury.* Little, Brown, Boston, 1980.
4. Bartels, J. E., Hoerlein, B. F., and Boring, J. G.: Neuroradiography. *In* Hoerlein, B. F. (ed.): *Canine Neurology:*

Diagnosis and Treatment. 3d ed. W. B. Saunders, Philadelphia, 1978.

5. Brown, F. D., Johns, L. M., and Mullan, S.: Dimethyl sulfoxide in experimental brain injury with comparison to mannitol. J. Neurosurg. *53*:58, 1980.

6. Chrisman, C. L.: *Problems in Small Animal Neurology.* Lea & Febiger, Philadelphia, 1982.

7. Coxe, W. S.: Intracranial tumors. *In* Eliasson, S. G., Prensky, A. L., and Hardin, W. B., Jr. (eds.): *Neurologic Pathophysiology.* 2d ed. Oxford University Press, New York, 1978.

8. deLahunta, A.: *Veterinary Neuroanatomy and Clinical Neurology.* W. B. Saunders, Philadelphia, 1977.

9. De la Torre, E., Netsky, M. G., and Meschan, I.: Intracranial and extracranial circulation in the dog: anatomic and angiographic studies. Am. J. Anat. *105*:343, 1959.

10. Dorn, A. S.: A standard technique for cerebral angiography. J. Am. Vet. Med. Assoc. *161*:1669, 1972.

11. Fankhauser, R., Luginbuhl, H., and McGrath, J. T.: Tumors of the nervous system. Bull. WHO *50*:53, 1974.

12. Fenner, W. R.: Seizures and head trauma. Vet. Clin. North Am. *11*:31, 1981.

13. Fike, J. R., LeCouteur, R. A., Cann, C. E., and Pflugfelder, C. M.: Computerized tomography of brain tumors of the rostral and middle fossa in the dog. Am. J. Vet. Res. *42*:275, 1981.

14. Fishman, R. A.: *Cerebrospinal Fluid in Diseases of the Nervous System.* W. B. Saunders, Philadelphia, 1980.

15. Galicich, J. A., French, L. A., and Melby, J. C.: Use of dexamethasone in treatment of cerebral edema associated with brain tumors. Lancet *81*:46, 1961.

16. Goodman, S. J., and Stern, W. E.: Cranial and intracranial bacterial infections. *In* Youmans, J. R. (ed.): *Neurological Surgery.* Vol. 6. W. B. Saunders, Philadelphia, 1982.

17. Gordon, E.: The management of acute head injuries. *In Monographs in Anesthesiology.* Vol. 2: *A Basis and Practice of Neuroanesthesia.* 2d Ed. Excerpta Medica, Amsterdam, 1981.

18. Hoerlein, B. F., and Petty, M. F.: Contrast encephalography and ventriculogaphy in the dog—preliminary studies. Am. J. Vet. Res. *22*:1941, 1961.

19. Hoerlein, B. F., Few, A. B., and Petty, M. F.: Brain surgery in the dog—preliminary studies. J. Am. Vet. Med. Assoc. *143*:21, 1963.

20. Hoerlein, B. F., and Oliver, J. E.: Brain surgery. *In* Hoerlein, B. F. (ed.): *Canine Neurology: Diagnosis and Treatment.* 3rd ed. W. B. Saunders, Philadelphia, 1978.

21. Hoerlein, B. F.: Acute trauma to the central nervous system. *In Canine Neurology: Diagnosis and Treatment.* 3rd ed. W. B. Saunders, Philadelphia, 1978.

22. Horsley, V.: Brain surgery. Brit. Med. J. *2*:723, 1886.

23. Ihrke, P. J., Halliwell, R. E. W., and Deubler, M. J.: Canine pyoderma. *In* Kirk, R. W. (ed.): *Current Veterinary Therapy VI: Small Animal Practice.* W. B. Saunders, Philadelphia, 1977.

24. Indrieri, R. J., Holliday, T. A., and Keen, C. L.: Critical evaluation of creatine phosphokinase in cerebrospinal fluid of dogs with neurologic disease. Am. J. Vet. Res. *41*:1299, 1980.

25. Indrieri, R. J., Holliday, T. A., Selcer, R. R., et al.: Choroid plexus papilloma associated with prolonged signs of vestibular dysfunction in a young dog. J. Am. Anim. Hosp. Assoc. *16*:263, 1980.

26. James, C. W., and Hoerlein, B. F.: Cerebral angiography in the dog. Vet. Med. *55*:45, 1960.

27. Jenkins, L. C.: *General Anesthesia and the Central Nervous System.* Williams & Wilkins, Baltimore, 1969.

28. Jennett, B., and Teasdale, G.: *Management of Head Injuries.* F. A. Davis, Philadelphia, 1981.

29. Kallfelz, F. A., deLahunta, A. and Allhands, R. V.: Scintigraphic diagnosis of brain lesions in the dog and cat. J. Am. Vet. Med. Assoc. *172*:589, 1978.

30. Klemm, W. R.: *Animal Electroencephalography.* Academic Press, New York, 1969.

31. Kramer, P. W., Griffith, R. S., and Campbell, R. L.: Antibiotic penetration of the brain: a comparative study. J. Neurosurg. *31*:295, 1969.

32. Langfitt, T. W.: Increased intracranial pressure and the cerebral circulation. *In* Youmans, J. R. (ed.): *Neurological Surgery.* Vol. 2. W. B. Saunders, Philadelphia, 1982.

33. LeCouteur, R. A., Fike, J. R., Cann, C. E., and Pedroia, V. G.: Computed tomography of brain tumors in the caudal fossa of the dog. Vet. Rad. *22*:244, 1981.

34. LeCouteur, R. A., Scagliotti, R. H., Beck, K. A., and Holliday, T. A.: Indirect imaging of the canine optic nerve, using metrizamide (optic thecography). Am. J. Vet. Res. *43*:1424, 1982.

35. Lindberg, A. A.: The influence of longitudinal transection of the corpus callosum upon locomotion in the dog. Biol. Abstr. *13*:4020, 1939.

36. Lowbury, E. J. L., Blowers, R., Cunliffe, A. C., et al.: Aseptic methods in the operating suite. A report to the Medical Research Council by the Sub-committee on Aseptic Methods in Operating Theaters, Committee on Hospital Infection. Lancet *1*:705, 1968.

37. Luginbuhl, H.: Comparative aspects of tumors of the nervous system. Ann. N. Y. Acad. Sci. *108*:702, 1963.

38. Luginbuhl, H.: A comparative study of neoplasms of the central nervous system in animals. Acta Neurochir. Suppl. *10*:30, 1964.

39. Luginbuhl, H., Fankhauser, R., and McGrath, J. T.: Spontaneous neoplasms of the nervous system of animals. *In* Krayenbuhl, H., Maspes, P. E., and Sweet, W. H. (eds.): *Progress in Neurological Surgery.* Vol. 2. S. Karger, Basel, and Year Book Medical Publishers, Chicago, 1968.

40. McGrath, J. T.: *Neurologic Examination of the Dog with Clinicopathologic Observations.* 2nd ed. Lea & Febiger, Philadelphia, 1960.

41. McLean, A. J.: Transbuccal approach to the encephalon in experimental operations upon carnivoral pituitary, pons, and ventral medulla. Ann. Surg. *88*:985, 1928.

42. Oliver, J. E.: Principles of canine brain surgery. Anim. Hosp. *2*:73–88, 1966.

43. Oliver, J. E.: Surgical approaches to the canine brain. Am. J. Vet. Res. *29*:353, 1968.

44. Oliver, J. E., Jr.: Cranial sinus venography in the dog. J. Am. Vet. Rad. Soc. *10*:66, 1969.

45. Parker, A. J., and Cunningham, J. G.: Transfrontal craniotomy in the dog. Vet. Rec. *90*:622, 1972.

46. Parker, A. J.: Some clinical dangers of mannitol therapy. J. Am. Anim. Hosp. Assoc. *10*:175, 1974.

47. Parker, A. J., Devous, M. D., Twardock, A. R., and O'Brien, D. P.: Scintigraphic imaging of acute unilateral lesions in the brain parenchyma of three dogs. J. Am. Anim. Hosp. Assoc. *18*:926, 1982.

48. Petersdorf, R. G., Browder, A. A., and Feinstein, A. R.: Symposium on the chemoprophylaxis of infection. IV: Protection against infection in susceptible individuals. J. Pediat. *58*:174, 1961.

49. Redding, R. W.: Prefrontal lobotomy of the dog. *In: Scientific Proceedings, Annual Meeting, American Animal Hospital Association,* 1972.

50. Redding, R. W.: Prefrontal lobotomy. *In* Bojrab, M. J. (ed.): *Current Techniques in Small Animal Surgery I.* Lea & Febiger, Philadelphia, 1975.

51. Redding, R. W.: Canine electroencephalography. *In* Hoerlein, B. F. (ed.): *Canine Neurology: Diagnosis and Treatment.* 3rd ed. W. B. Saunders, Philadelphia, 1978.

52. Selcer, R. R.: Trauma to the central nervous system. Vet. Clin. North Am. *10*:619, 1980.

53. Sims, M. H., and Redding, R. W.: The use of dexamethasone in the prevention of cerebral edema in dogs. J. Am. Anim. Hosp. Assoc. *11*:439, 1975.

54. Spano, J. S., and Hoerlein, B. F.: Laboratory examinations. *In* Hoerlein, B. F. (ed.): *Canine Neurology: Diagnosis and Treatment.* 3rd ed. W. B. Saunders, Philadelphia, 1978.

55. Stern, W. E.: Preoperative evaluation: complications, their prevention and treatment. *In* Youmans, J. R. (ed.): *Neuro-*

logical Surgery. 2nd ed. Vol. 2. W. B. Saunders, Philadelphia, 1051–1116, 1982.

56. Thornton, G. W.: Antimicrobial therapy in the dog and cat. Vet. Clin. North Am. 5:133, 1975.

57. Verdura, J., White, R. J., and Albin, M.: A new technique for aseptic hypophysectomy in the dog. J. Surg. Res. 3:174, 1963.

58. White, S. D., Ihrke, P. J., Stannard, A. A., et al.: Occurrence of Staphylococcus aureus on the clinically normal canine haircoat. Am. J. Vet. Res. 44:332, 1983.

59. Williams, J. B., and Dart, R. M.: Chloramphenicol (Chloromycetin) concentration in cerebrospinal, ascitic and placental fluids. Boston Med. Q. 1:7, 1950.

60. Zaki, F. A., and Hurvitz, A. I.: Spontaneous neoplasms of the central nervous system of the cat. J. Small Anim. Pract. 17:773, 1976.

Index

Index

Note: Page numbers in *italic* type indicate illustrations; page numbers followed by *t* refer to tables.
To avoid qualifying almost every item in the index with the terms *canine* and *feline*, these adjectives are included only where the distinction is required, that is, in discussions pertaining specifically to the dog or the cat.

Antibiotic eye drops, fortified, preparation of, 1591t
Antibody(ies), as proteins, 183–184
  effector functions of, 184–185
  in defense against tumors, 2401
  in immune response, role of, 182
Antibody-mediated disease, diagnosis of, criteria for, 1471t
Anticholinergic drugs, effect on reproductive function of, 2650
  effect on respiration of, 2625
  placental transfer of, 2654
  preanesthetic, 2596
Anticoagulants, 1105–1106
  in blood transfusions, 76
  in burn injuries, 526
  in treatment of disseminated intravascular coagulation, 1193
Antidiuretic hormone (ADH), 1725
  in regulation of renal fluid, 91
  secretion of, and extracellular volume, 1726
    effect of anesthesia on, 2668
  surgical trauma and, 83, 83
Antigen(s), histocompatibility, 200
  in immune response, role of, 182
  transplantation, 200
  tumor-specific, 2400
  unknown, immune complexes and, 195
Antigen receptors, on B cells and T cells, 184
Antigen-antibody reaction, 185
Antigenic determinants, 181
Antigenicity, 180
  requirements for, 181
Anti-inflammatory drugs, in wound healing, 35–36
  nonsteroidal, in degenerative joint disease, 2300
Antimetabolites, in cancer chemotherapy, 2411t, 2413–2414
Antimicrobial drugs, 52–70. See also *Antibiotics* and names of specific drugs.
  adverse effects of, 52–56, 54–55t
  bacterial sensitivity tests for, errors in interpretation of, 66t
  bacteriostatic vs. bactericidal, 65t
  biological alterations due to, 52–56, 54–55t
  choice of administrative routes for, 65
  combinations of, antagonistic, 65t
  elimination rates of, 60, 61t
  fixed-dose combinations of, 69
  for urinary tract infections, 1761–1762, 1761t
  hypersensitivity reactions to, 52, 54–55t
  in contaminated surgery, 63
  in hepatic disease, 68
  in neonate, 68–69
  in parenteral mixtures, compatibility of, 98t
  in pregnancy, 68
  in renal insufficiency, 67–68, 68t
  in shock, 143
  in surgery, 63–69
    chemoprophylaxis with, 56–63
    indications for, 63
  in uncontaminated surgery, 63
  minimal inhibitory concentration (MIC) of, 58

Antimicrobial drugs (*Continued*)
  new, 69
  pharmacokinetics of, 57, 58, 59t, 61t
  prophylactic use of, for wounds, 438
  regimens for, in dogs and cats, 62t
  time needed for peak concentration of, 57t, 58
  time/dose relationships of, 57, 58, 61t
  tissue distribution of, 59t
  topical, for open wounds, 433–434
  toxic effects of, 52, 54–55t
  treatment failure with, causes of, 67t
Antipyretics, for hyperthermia, 406
Antireflux surgery, 686–689, 687, 688. See also *Gastroesophageal reflux disease.*
Antisepsis, introduction of, 37
Antiseptic(s), definition of, 250
  in wound healing, 36
Anus, and anal sphincter, excision of, 782, 783
  and rectum, 768–794
    anatomy of, 768–770, 768, 788–791
    congenital abnormalities of, 773–774
    prolapse of, 770–773, 771, 772
    surgical diseases of, 770–792
    tumors of, 786–792
  imperforate, 773
  muscles of, anatomy of, 791
Aorta, coarctation of, 1089, 1089, 1090
Aortic arch, anomalies of, surgical correction of, 1112–1114
  double, surgical correction of, 1114
  persistent right, 1089–1090, 1090, 1113
    breed predisposition for, 1070t
    diagnosis of, 1090
    radiograph of, 1090
    surgical correction of, 1112–1113, 1113
Aortic bodies, location of, 930
Aortic embolism, canine, angiogram of, 1154
  feline, surgical management of, 1126
  … … cardiomyopathy, 1154
  surgical treatment of, 1154, 1155
Aortic hiatus, 572
Aortic regurgitation, acquired, 1095
  congenital, 1086
Aortic stenosis, 1084–1086
  angiogram of, 1085
  breed predisposition for, 1070t
  electrocardiogram in, 1060, 1085
  heart failure in, 1049
  pressure changes in, 1085
  radiograph of, 1061, 1084
  stress-volume loop in, 1049
  subvalvular, surgical correction of, 1128–1129, 1128, 1129
    pressure criteria for, 1128t
  types of, 1084
  venous angiogram in, 1062
Aortic-pulmonary window, 1087, 1087
  angiogram in, 1087
  heart chamber pressures in, 1087t
  oxygen saturations in, 1087t
Apicoectomy, 614
Apnea, in operating room emergencies, 394
Apocrine sweat glands, 423
Aponeurosis, abdominal, 567
Appendage tourniquets, hypertension due to, 398

Aqueous drainage, 1568, 1568
Aqueous flare, in glaucoma, 1572
Aqueous production, in glaucoma, procedures for decreasing, 1579–1581
  procedures for increasing, 1576–1579
Arrhenius relationship, in hyperthermia, 2427–2429, 2428
Arrhythmias, in shock, treatment of, 142
  postoperative, 375
Arterial pressure, 356
  evaluation of, 1068
  monitoring of, 356
    equipment for, 356, 2708
    in critical care patient, 2707
    in shock, 140
    normal, 352t
Arterial pulse, 352t, 355
  monitoring of, 355
Arterialization, 102
Arteriography, cerebral, 1318, 1319
Arteriotomy, longitudinal, technique of, 1148, 1150
  technique of, 1148, 1148, 1149
  transverse, technique of, 1148, 1149
Arteriovenous fistula(e), 1051, 1052
  abnormal circulatory pathway in, 1051, 1052
  clinical findings in, 1051
  congenital vs. acquired, 1051
  hepatic, 1169
  local effects of, 1051–1053
  pathophysiology of, 1051–1054
    therapeutic considerations in, 1054
  peripheral, angiogram of, 1153
  radiograph of, 1152
  surgical repair of, 1153
  systemic effects in, 1053–1054, 1053
Artery(ies). See also names of specific arteries.
  bovine, as heterograft, 1105
  cutaneous, 427, 428, 428
    anatomical landmarks for, 473
  esophageal, anatomy of, 653–654
  great, transposition of, 1086, 1086
  hepatic, anatomy of, 795
  intercostal, 537
  intestinal, anatomy of, 719
  of left thorax, anatomy of, 1032, 1032, 1033
  of stomach, 682, 682
  pelvic, anatomy of, 789
  perineal, anatomy of, 790
  pulmonary. See *Pulmonary artery(ies).*
  superficial, of canine trunk, 429
Arthritis. See also *Articular disease* and *Degenerative joint disease.*
  erosive immune-mediated, 2306–2310
  rheumatoid, 2306–2310
    clinical features of, 2307
    diagnostic criteria for, 2308, 2308t
    differential diagnosis of, 2308t
    immune complexes and, 195
    laboratory findings in, 2307
    pathology of, 2309, 2309
    radiography in, 2307–2308, 2308
    treatment of, 2309–2310
  septic, 2030–2034. See also *Septic arthritis.*
  synovial fluid changes in, 2032t
Arthrodesis, 2263–2276

Arthrodesis *(Continued)*
  bone grafting in, 2042–2043
  complications in, 2264
  external skeletal fixation for, 1982, *1983*
  general procedure for, 2263–2264
  in rheumatoid arthritis, 2310
  indications for, 2263
Arthroscopes, sources of, 350
Arthroscopy, 349
Arthus reactions, and related maladies, 195
  characteristics of, 188t
Articular disease. See also *Arthritis; Lupus erythematosus,* systemic; and other specific diseases.
  degenerative. See *Degenerative joint disease.*
  immune-mediated, 2302–2311
    erosive, 2306–2310
    nonerosive, 2302–2306
Arytenoid cartilage, lateralization of, in laryngeal paralysis, 974, *975*
  position of, in laryngeal collapse, *973*
  in laryngeal paralysis, *973*
Ascites, hepatic cirrhosis and, 798–802, *799*
    LeVeen shunt in, 801, *801, 802*
    management of, 800–801
  surgery in, anesthetic aspects of, 2619
Asepsis, definition of, 250
  earliest uses of, 3
  surgical, basic techniques for, 295–297
    historical aspects of, 3, 250–251
    principles of, 250–261
L-Asparaginase, in cancer chemotherapy, 2412t, 2415
Aspiration, of gastric contents, as operating room emergency, 396–397
  postoperative considerations in, 397
  preoperative considerations in, 397
  postoperative problems of, 379
  transtracheal, 2371
Aspiration biopsy, fine needle, 2370
Aspiration pneumonia, postoperative, 167
Aspirin, as anticoagulant, 1106
  for degenerative joint disease, 2300
  for rheumatoid arthritis, 2309
  in wound healing, 35
Asthenia, cutaneous, 428–430, *429*
Astrocytoma(s), breed predilection for, 1275t
  canine, 2500
  features of, 1275t
  of brain, *1274*
  spinal, 2519
Asystole, ventricular, cardiac arrest due to, 159
    electrocardiograph in, *159*
    subsequent management of, 160–161
Ataxia, hereditary, features of, 1280t
Atelectasis, in anesthesia, 2622
  inadequate postoperative ventilation due to, 1028
  respiratory problems due to, 393
Atlantoaxial joint, anatomy of, 1373–1374, *1374*
  developmental, 1374t
  fractures of, complications in, 1379
    postoperative care in, 1378
    surgical treatment of, 1378
  instability of, 1373–1379
    diagnosis of, 1375–1376

Atlantoaxial joint *(Continued)*
  instability of, pathology of, 1374–1375, *1374, 1375*
    prognosis in, 1376
    with dens fracture, 1375, *1375*
  ligaments of, *1374*
    rupture of, *1374, 1375*
  luxations of, complications in, 1379
    diagnosis of, 1375, *1376*
    postoperative care in, 1378
    surgical repair of, 1376–1378, *1376–1378*
      dorsal approach to, 1376–1377, *1376–1377*
      ventral approach to, 1377–1378, *1378*
Atracurium, potency and duration of, in cats, 2681t
  in dogs, 2680t
Atresia ani, 773
  treatment of, 774
  with rectal fistula, 773, *773*
Atrial depolarization, premature, electrocardiography in, 1060
Atrial fibrillation, electrocardiogram of, *1093*
  in mitral regurgitation, 1093
Atrial septal defect, angiogram of, *1074*
  breed predisposition for, 1070t
  heart chamber pressures in, 1074t
  heart failure due to, pathophysiology of, 1046
  oxygen saturations in, 1074t
  physiology of, 1072
  prognosis in, 1074
  radiographs of, *1072, 1073*
  surgical correction of, 1129, *1129*
Atrioventricular node, conduction disorders at, electrocardiography in, 1059
Atrioventricular valves, anatomy of, *1037, 1038*
Atrium(a), anatomy of, *1035,* 1036–1037, *1036*
Auditory evoked responses, 1312, *1312*
Aural hematoma, 1890–1891, *1890*
  treatment of, 1891, *1891*
Auricle. See *Pinna.*
Auricular hematoma, 1890–1891, *1890*
  treatment of, 1891, *1891*
Auscultation, in cardiac disease, 1056–1057
Autoantigens, diseases and, 195
Autoclave, for ethylene oxide sterilization, 267
  loading of, 264
  operation of, 264–265
  preparation of surgical packs for, 264, *265*
  steam pulsing systems for, 263
  types of, 262
Autoimmune diseases, 194
  self-recognition and, 204
Autoimmunity, 194
Autotransfusion, of blood, 79
  in hemothorax, 563, *563*
Axillary nerve, signs of dysfunction of, 1257t
Axon(s), 1244
Axonal migration, in nerve regeneration, 26

Axonopathy, progressive, features of, 1280t
Axonotmesis, 25
Azotemia, postoperative, 168
  postrenal, 169
  prerenal, 169

B lymphocytes, immune responses of, T-cell–independent, 182
  vs. T lymphocytes, distinguishing characteristics of, 180t
Bacillus Calmette Gúerin (BCG), in tumor therapy, 2403
Bacteria, in wound infections, measurement of, 39
  role of, 38
  sources of, 38–39
  resistant, due to antimicrobial therapy, 53
Bacterial diseases, immunological defense mechanisms and, 191, 191t
Balanoposthitis, 1632
  etiologic agents in, 64t
Bandage(s), carpal flexion, *1990,* 1991
  dry, 370
  for closed skin wounds, 456–457
  for fractures, 1988–1991
    Robert-Jones, 1989–1990, *1990*
    soft padded, 1988–1989
    tape stirrups for, 1988, *1989*
  rigid, 371
  tie-over, for skin graft, 499, *499*
  wound dressings and, techniques of, 434–435
Barbiturates, anesthetic, 2607
  complications of, 2607
  effect on cardiovascular system of, 2636
  effect on reproductive function of, 2650
  neuromuscular effects of, 2676
  placental transfer of, 2653
Barium enema, colonic perforation in, *760*
Basal cell carcinoma, of eyelid, 2523
Basal cell epithelioma, of eyelid, 2523
Basal cell tumor(s), 2443–2444
  granular, 2443
  of eyelid, 2523
  of pinna, 1898
Basalioma, 2443
Base excess, in acid-base balance, 115
  measurement of, 118
Basophils, development of, 1178
Basset hound, cancer types in, 2361t
  high-risk cancer sites in, 2361t
Bence Jones proteins, 195
Benzalkonium chloride, sterilization with, 269
Benzodiazepine derivatives, neuromuscular effects of, 2675
Beta cell carcinomas, pancreatic, 1882–1886
Betapropiolactone, sterilization with, 268
Bicarbonate, blood levels of, evaluation of, 126
  in acid-base regulation, 111–112
  reabsorption of, in acid-base regulation, 117
Biceps brachii tendon, origin of, avulsion of, 2354, *2356*
  displacement of, 2357
  translocation of, in shoulder luxation, 2059, *2059*

Bronchoconstriction, respiratory
dysfunction due to, 934
Bronchofiberoscope, 347
Bronchography, in stabilized respiratory
disorders, 944–945
Bronchoscopy, 346t, 347, 948
Bronchoscope(s), 346, 346
sources of, 350
Bronchus(i), anatomy of, 990–991
congenital disease of, 991–992
diagnosis of, 991–992
history in, 991
physical examination in, 991
radiography in, 991–992
external injury to, 998–1000
foreign bodies in, 997–998
diagnosis of, 997
nonretrievable, therapy for, 998
retrieval by bronchotomy, 998, 998
intrathoracic, external injury to, 999
neoplasia of, 1001
resection and anastomosis of, 1006, 1006
Bruton's agammaglobulinemia, 196
Buffer(s), in acid-base regulation,
distribution of, 112
Buffer function, 112–115
evaluation of, 113–115
base measurements in, 115
use of nomograms in, 113–115
Buffer titration curve, 113
Buffering, by bone, 113
by ionic shifts, 113
in extracellular fluids, function of,
112–113
Bullae, of lung, 1011–1012
radiograph of, 1012
Bulldog, cancer types in, 2361t
high-risk cancer sites in, 2361t
Bundle of His, conduction disorders at,
electrocardiography in, 1059
Buphthalmos, in glaucoma, 1571–1572
Burn(s), 516–526
causes of, 517
chemical. See Chemical burns.
control of infection in, 525
disseminated intravascular coagulation
in, 519
electrical. See Electrical injury(ies).
excision of eschars in, 523
first aid for, 521–522
first- and second-degree, in dog, 522
from heat lamp, 216
from heating pad, 216
gastric and duodenal ulceration in,
525–526
immunosuppression in, 517
infections in, etiologic agents of, 64t
initial evaluation of, 521
kerosene, 215
liver damage in, 519
local wound therapy for, 523–525
management of, 521–526
metabolic changes due to, 222–223t
nutritional needs after, 521
pathophysiology of, 517
physiological changes due to, 222–223t
red blood cell loss in, 519
renal failure in, 519
third-degree, from heating pad, 517
Burn hazards, in operating room, 408

Burn shock, 518–519
electrolyte changes in, 518
fluid and electrolyte therapy for, 522
fluid losses and shifts in, 518
myocardial-depressant factor in, 518
treatment of, 522–523
Burn toxins, 519
Burn wound(s), 519–521
dressings for, 525
metabolic response to, 86
third degree, in dog, 520
treatment of, 523–525
Busulfan, in cancer chemotherapy, 2410t
Butyrophenones, neuromuscular effects of,
2675

Calcaneal quartal joint, arthrodesis of,
2260
Calcanean tendon, rupture of, 2350–2352,
2351
repair of, 2351, 2351
Calcaneus, epiphysis of, avulsion of, 2351,
2352
fractures of, 2251–2252, 2251, 2252
Calcitonin, 1875–1876
Calcium, in body fluid, abnormalities of,
93
in cardiopulmonary arrest, 150
renal regulation of, 1728
supplementation with, in
hypoparathyroidism, 1880
Calcium oxalate uroliths, 1814
Calcium phosphate uroliths, 1815
Calcium-phosphorus homeostasis,
physiology of, 1874–1878
Calculolytic diets, in struvite urolith
dissolution, 1818, 1820
Calories, maintenance requirements of,
379
Cancer. See also Tumors, Carcinoma and
other specific names of tumors.
canine breed predilection for, 2361t
chemotherapy for, 2405–2417. See also
Cancer chemotherapy.
distribution of, by anatomical site, 2361t
immunotherapy for, 2400–2405
radiation therapy for, 2386–2400. See
alsos36Radiotherapy.
surgical management of, guidelines for,
2383–2385
Cancer chemotherapy, 2405–2417
alkylating agents in, 2409, 2410t
antibiotics in, 2411–2412t, 2414
antimetabolites in, 2411t, 2413–2414
biological basis of, 2406–2407
combined drugs in, 2408
drug absorption in, 2407
drug distribution in, 2407
drug excretion in, 2408
drug interaction in, 2407
drugs used in, 2409–2415, 2410–2412t
dosages of, 2410–2412t
toxicity of, 2410–2412t
guidelines for, 2409
hormones in, 2412t, 2414–2415
immunodeficiency in, 197
pharmacological factors in, 2407–2409
plant alkaloids in, 2411t, 2414
predictors of response in, 2415–2416

Cancer chemotherapy (Continued)
route of administration in, 2407
toxic effects in, 2407, 2410–2412t
with radiotherapy, for tumors, 2393
with radiotherapy, for tumors, toxic
effects of, 2393t
Canine erythrocyte antigen (CEA), 1195
Canine secretory alloantigen (CSA)
system, 204
Canthoplasty, lateral, lengthening
palpebral fissure by, 1450
Canthotomy, lateral, 1441, 1442
Canthus, lateral, of eye, relocation with Z-
plasty of, 455, 455
Capillaries, pulmonary, perfusion of, 924,
924, 924t
Capillary refill time (CRT), 359
monitoring of, 359
normal values for, 352t
Capitulum (humeral condyle), fractures of,
2077–2092
repair of, 2082, 2083, 2085, 2087
Caprolactum, polymerized, as suture
material, 339, 339
Carbenicillin, adverse effects of, 54t
pharmacokinetic data for, 61t
regimen for, in dog and cat, 62t
time needed for peak concentrations of,
57t
Carbohydrate(s), digestion of, enzymes in,
738t
sources of, in parenteral nutrition, 230
Carbohydrate-in-water solution, for fluid
therapy, 96
Carbohydrate metabolism, in surgical
patient, 85
Carbon, in soft tissue implants, 174
Carbon dioxide, excessive, hypercapnia
due to, 395
total, in acid-base balance, measurement
of, 118
in acid-base evaluation, 115
ventilatory response to, 929, 929, 930
Carbon dioxide pressure, clinical
evaluation of, 110
Carbon dioxide system, 108–115
Carbon dioxide tension, arterial, 116
measurement of, 353
normal values for, 352t
Carbon dioxide transport, hemoglobin-
related, 109–110
in plasma, 109
in respiration, mechanisms of, 928, 929
Carbonic anhydrase, in carbon dioxide
transport, 109
Carcinogens, in etiology of tumors, 2364
Carcinoids, hepatic, 2463
Carcinoma(s). See also Tumor(s) and
names and sites of specific tumors.
basal cell, 2443
of lip, 630, 631
bile duct, 2462–2463
cholangiocellular, 2462–2463
conjunctival, 2528
hepatocellular, 2461–2462, 2462
of prostate, 1643–1645, 1644
of rectum, 787–792
of tongue, 629
peritoneal, secondary, 592
sebaceous, of pinna, 1898
squamous cell, 2446

Lung(s) *(Continued)*
abscess of, treatment of, 1012
acquired diseases of, 1012–1016
and thoracic wall, compliance curves of, *538*
as defense mechanism, in anesthesia, 2624
biopsy of, percutaneous, 2380
bullae of, 1011–1012
radiograph of, *1012*
congenital diseases of, 1011–1012
cryosurgery of, 1016
cysts of, 1011
defense mechanisms of, 931
disorders of, respiratory dysfunction due to, 934
expansion of, in postoperative care, 1027
foreign body in, 1014
functional anatomy of, *913, 916*
laceration of, 1014–1015
repair of, 1014–1015, *1015*
lobectomy of, 1016–1018
needle biopsy of, 1016
normal, physiology of, 919–931
physiological changes in, in cardiac bypass, 1140
radiography of, in stabilized respiratory disorders, 944, *944*
reimplantation of, 1019
surgical procedure for, 1019–1020
smoke injury to, 517
Lung lobe torsion, 1015
diagnosis of, 1015
inadequate postoperative ventilation due to, 1028
treatment of, 1015
Lung tumors, 1016, 2588–2590
diagnosis of, 2589–2590
hypertrophic osteopathy of hindlimb in, *2589*
incidence of, 2588–2589
primary, 2588–2590
prognosis for, 2590
pulmonary nodule in, *2589*
treatment of, 2590
Lupus erythematosus, systemic (SLE), 2302–2306
clinical features of, 2303, *2303*
diagnosis of, 2305, 2305t
hematological involvement in, 2304
incidence of, 2303
mucocutaneous lesions in, 2304
musculoskeletal involvement in, 2303–2304
pathology of, 2303, *2303, 2304*
renal involvement in, 2304
skin lesions in, 2304
treatment of, 2306
Luteinizing hormone (LH), 1842–1843
Lymph nodes, 179, 1224–1235
anatomy of, 1224–1225
disorders of, 1229–1234
diagnostic evaluation of, 1231–1234
enlargement of, classification of, 1229t
Lymph node biopsy, 2375–2376
comparison of impression smears and scrapings in, 1232
complications of, 1234
contraindications to, 1234
cytological examination in, 1233–1234, *1233, 1234*

Lymph node biopsy *(Continued)*
excisional, 1232
fine-needle aspiration, 1231, 2376
incisional, 1232
guillotine method of, 1232, *1232*
wedge technique of, 1232, *1232*
with Tru-cut needle, 1232, *1232, 2376, 2376*
Lymphadenitis, types of, 1229t
Lymphadenopathy, diagnostic approach to, 1230–1234
types of, 1229
Lymphangiectasia, intestinal, 1228–1229
treatment of, 1229
Lymphangiography, 1231
technique of, 1231
Lymphangioma, 1229
Lymphangiosarcoma, 1229
Lymphangitis, 1225
treatment of, 1225
Lymphatic system, 1224–1235
embryology of, 1224
neoplasia of, 1229
peripheral, anatomy of, 1224
disorders of, 1225–1229
physiology of, 1225
Lymphatic vessels, chylous effusions of, 1229
esophageal, anatomy of, 654
neoplasia of, 1229
Lymphedema, primary, 1226
secondary, 1226–1228
causes of, 1227
treatment of, 1228
Lymphedema congenita, 1226
Lymphoblastic leukemia, canine, 2483
Lymphocytes, B and T, identification of, 180, 180t
development of, 1179
differentiation of, 179
in wound healing, 30
Lymphocytic leukemia, canine, 2483
chronic, 2483
feline, 2483, 2485
Lymphoid hyperplasia, benign, biopsy of, *1233*
Lymphoid organs, central, lymphocyte differentiation in, 179
secondary, 179–180
Lymphoid system, 178–180
Lymphoid tumors, 195. See also *Lymphoma* and *Lymphosarcoma*.
Lymphokines, 189
activities of, 190t
Lymphoma, malignant, lymph node biopsy in, *1223, 1234*
renal, in cats, age and sex in, 2564t
in dogs, age and sex in, 2565t
surgical considerations in, 1182
Lymphoproliferative disorders, 2478–2489
Lymphosarcoma, canine, 2478–2482
alimentary, 2479
clinical staging for, 2480, 2481t
chemotherapy for, 2481
adverse effects of, 2481t
combination, results of, 2482t
dosage schedules in, 2481t
classification of, 2479
clinical findings in, 2479
cutaneous, 2479
cytology of, 2480

Lymphosarcoma *(Continued)*
canine, diagnosis of, 2480
frequency of types of, 2479t
hematological findings in, 2480
histopathology of, 2480
hypercalcemia in, 2479–2480
immunotherapy for, 2481–2482
mediastinal, 2479
multicentric, 2479
prognosis in, 2482
radiography in, 2480
radiotherapy for, 2482
thymic, 2479
treatment of, 2480–2482
cardiac, 2474–2475, *2475*
cutaneous, 2449, *2449*
clinical stages of, 2443t
feline, 2483
alimentary, 2485
chemotherapy for, 2486
results of, 2487t
classification of, 2484–2486, 2485t
clinical findings in, 2484–2486
diagnosis of, 2486
intracranial, 2503, *2504*
mediastinal, 2484
multicentric, 2485
prognosis in, 2487
treatment of, 2486–2487
unclassified, 2485
FeLV and, 2484, 2485t
intraocular, 2530–2531, *2531*
Lysosomal enzymes, in shock, 136
Lyssa, resection of, as cure for rabies, 2

Macroglobulinemia, bleeding disorders in, 1188
Macrolides, adverse effects of, 54t
Macropalpebral fissure, surgical correction of, 1451, *1451*
Macrophages, in defense against tumors, 2401
in wound healing, 29
Major histocompatibility complex (MHC), 192–194
association of disease with, 193–194
biological role of, 193
I (immune response) region of, 193
K and D regions of, 192
of dogs, 201–204
biological significance of, 204
structure of, 192, 192t, *193*
Malacia, of brain, 1269–1271
in trauma, 1271, *1271, 1272*
spinal cord, 1278–1279, *1278, 1279*
"Malicious prosecution," malpractice countersuits against, 10
Malleolus, tibial, avulsion fractures of, 2236–2237, *2236, 2237*
Malpractice, causes of actions for, 8–9
definition of, 7
involvement of assistants in, 12
punitive damages in, 17–18
statute of limitations for, 9
veterinarian countersuits in, 9–10
Malpractice insurance, legal aspects of, 19–20
Mammary glands, anatomy of, 505
lymphatic drainage of, *505*

Metronidazole *(Continued)*
  pharmacokinetic data for, 61t
  regimen for, in dog and cat, 62t
Michele trephine, 2375
Microhematocrit, estimation of water loss
    with, 94
Micropalpebral fissure, surgical correction
    of, 1449–1451, *1450*
Microphakia, 1537
Microscope, operating, *288*
  for ophthalmic surgery, 1435, *1435,*
    1436
Microwaves, hyperthermia with, 2432,
    2432
Micturition, disorders of. See also *Urinary*
    incontinence.
  drug therapy for, 1744–1745t
  neurology of, 1730–1731
Midbrain (mesencephalon), anatomy and
    function of, 1248
Midbrain syndrome, 1264
  signs of, 1264t
Middle ear, 1915–1923
  anatomy of, 1915
  congenital abnormalities of, 1917
  diseases of, 1917–1923
    auditory tube insufflation in, 1918
    bulla osteotomy in, 1919–1920
      lateral, 1920
      ventral, 1919, *1919*
    curettage in, 1919
    head tilt in, 1917, *1917*
    in cats, 1921–1922
    treatment of, 1918–1920
      complications of, 1920–1921
      results of, 1920–1921
  drain in, 368
  examination of, 1915–1917
  feline, diseases of, radiography in, 1915,
    1916
  inflammatory polyps of, 1921–1922,
    1922
  infection of, 1917
    clinical signs of, 1917–1918
    osteomyelitis of skull in, 1917, *1917*
    irrigation of, 1918
      equipment for, *1918*
    trauma of, 1917
    tumors of, 1921, *1921*
Minerals, in parenteral nutrition,
    problems of, 238–239
  nutritional needs for, in dog and cat,
    226t, 227–228
  sources of, in parenteral nutrition, 230
Miosis, evaluation of, 1289
Mitosis, cellular, 2386, *2387*
  in tissue regeneration, 22
Mitral atresia-hypoplastic left heart
    syndrome, 1083, *1083*
Mitral regurgitation, 1092–1994
  diagnosis of, 1092
  heart failure due to, pathophysiology of,
    1047–1049
  radiograph of, *1092*
  stress-volume loop in, *1048*
Mitral valve, anatomy of, *1037*, 1038
  congenital disorders of, 1083–1084
  replacement of, 1129–1130, *1130*
Mixed bacterial vaccine (MBV), 2403
Molar gland, anatomy of, *644*, 645

Moll, glands of (ciliary glands), anatomy
    of, 1483
Möller-Barlow's disease, 2313–2314, *2313,*
    2314
Monitoring of surgical patient, 351–365
  general condition in, 351–352
  high risk regimen for, 363, 363t
  indications for, 362
  low risk regimen for, 362, 363t
  moderate risk regimen for, 363, 363t
  pathophysiological basis for, 361–363
  postoperative, 381–385
Monocytes, development of, 1179
  in wound healing, 29
Monorchism, 1620
Monteggia fracture, of ulna, 2100–2102,
    2101, 2102
  repair of, 2101, *2101, 2102, 2103*
Motility, gastric, 683
  effect of anesthetics on, 2612
  in small intestine, 740
Motor nerve conduction, 1310–1311
  in segmental demyelination, *1311*
  technique and waveforms for recording,
    1310, *1310*
Motor vehicle accidents, injuries due to,
    224
Mouth. See also *Oral cavity* and specific
    parts.
  anatomy of, 606–609
  tumors of, 2453–2455
Mucocele, salivary, 647
  clinical signs of, 647
  diagnosis of, 647
  prognosis in, 649
  recurrence of, 649
  treatment of, 647
  zygomatic, 1557–1558
Mucometra, 1665
Mucosa, esophageal, anatomy of, 652, *654*
Multiple exostosis, hereditary, 2314–2315,
    2315
Murmurs, cardiac, 1057
Muscle(s). See also names of specific
    muscles.
  anal, anatomy of, *791*
  and tendons, injuries to, 2331–2358
  contractile process of, 1938
  cutaneous, in cat, *424*
  extraocular, innervation of, 1554t
  of eye, *1551*
  pelvic, anatomy of, *790*
  perineal, anatomy of, *790*
  skeletal, anastomosis of, suture
    techniques for, *2332*
    anatomy of, 2331
    atrophy of, 2339
    canine, fiber types in, 1300, *1302,*
      1303t
      serial sections of, *1302*
    contractures of, 2339
    contusions of, 2331
    fibrosis of, 2339
    healing of, 2331
    human, fiber types in, *1301*
      serial sections of, *1301*
    injuries to, 2331–2342
      classification of, 2331–2332
    lacerations of, 2332
    regeneration of, 23–24

Muscle(s) *(Continued)*
  skeletal, regeneration of,
    cellular events in, *24*
    rupture of, 2332–2335
      in racing greyhound, 2333
      surgical repair of, 2334–2335, *2334*
    sprains of, 2331
    tumors of, 2581–2582
  smooth, regeneration of, 24
  structure of, 1937–1938, *1937*
  superficial, of head and face, in cat, *425*
    in dog, *426*
  thoracic, 537
  types of, 1937
Muscle biopsy, 1299–1302, 2342
  histochemistry in, 1300–1301, 1301t
  morphometry in, 1301–1302
  processing of, 1300
  technique of, 1300
Muscle diseases, anesthetic responses in,
    2683
Muscle surgery, anesthesia in, 2684–2685
Muscularis, esophageal, anatomy of, 653
Musculocutaneous nerve, signs of
    dysfunction of, 1257t
Musculoskeletal system, 1925–2358
  anesthesia and, 2675–2691
  preoperative evaluation of, 248
  tumors of, 2575–2583
Myasthenia gravis, anesthetic response in,
    2684
  thymus and, 1237–1239
Myelin, loss of, 1279
Myeloma, 195
  bleeding disorders in, 1188
  multiple, 2487–2489
    clinical findings in, 2488
    diagnosis of, 2488
    differential diagnosis of, 2489
    hematological findings in, 2488
    prognosis in, 2489
    serum protein abnormalities in, 2488
    spinal, 2512, *2513*
    treatment of, 2489
    urinalysis in, 2488
  surgical considerations in, 1182
Myelomalacia, 1278–1279
Myelopathy, demyelinating, features of,
    1280t
  hereditary, features of, 1280t
Myeloproliferative diseases, 2489–2494
  bone marrow findings in, 2490
  classification of, 2491, 2491t
  diagnosis of, 2490
  etiopathogenesis of, 2489
  hematological findings in, 2490
  necropsy findings in, 2490
  preleukemia syndromes in, 2490
Myeloschisis, 1344, *1344*
Myelosis, erythremic, 2493
Myoblasts, in tissue regeneration, 23, *24*
Myocardial damage, electrocardiography
    in, 1059
Myocardial depressant factor (MDF), in
    shock, 135, 518
Myocardial disease, anesthetic
    management in, 2639
Myocardial heart failure, 1044–1046
  stenotic lesions in, 1049
Myocardial tumors, clinical signs of, 2471
Myocardium, biopsy of, technique of,
    1132, *1132*